Tropical and Geographical Medicine

SECOND EDITION

Associate Editors

Clinical Considerations in the Approach to Tropical Medicine

David A. Warrell, M.A., D.M., F.R.C.P.
Professor of Tropical Medicine and Infectious Diseases, University of Oxford, Oxford, England

Protozoan Diseases

Louis H. Miller, M.D.
Head, Malaria Section, Laboratory of Parasitic Diseases, National Institute of Allergy and Infectious Diseases, National Institutes of Health, Bethesda, Maryland

Metazoan Diseases

Adel A. F. Mahmoud, M.D., Ph.D.
John H. Hord Professor of Medicine, Chairman, Department of Medicine, Case Western Reserve University, Physician-in-Chief, University Hospitals of Cleveland, Cleveland, Ohio

Viral and Chlamydial Diseases

Scott B. Halstead, M.D.
Acting Director, Health Sciences Division, The Rockefeller Foundation, New York, New York

Bacterial, Spirochetal, and Rickettsial Diseases

Charles C. J. Carpenter, M.D.
Professor of Medicine, Brown University; Physician-in-Chief, The Miriam Hospital, Providence, Rhode Island

Fungal Diseases

John E. Bennett, M.D.
Head, Clinical Mycology Section, Laboratory of Clinical Investigation, National Institute of Allergy and Infectious Diseases, National Institutes of Health, Bethesda, Maryland

Nutritional Diseases

Gerald T. Keusch, M.D.
Professor of Medicine, Chief, Division of Geographic Medicine and Infectious Diseases, Department of Medicine, New England Medical Center Hospitals, Tufts University School of Medicine, Boston, Massachusetts

Tropical and Geographical Medicine

SECOND EDITION

Kenneth S. Warren, M.D.

Director for Science, Maxwell Communication Corporation
Professor of Medicine, New York University
Adjunct Professor of Medicine, The Rockefeller University

Adel A. F. Mahmoud, M.D., Ph.D.

John H. Hord Professor of Medicine and Chairman
Department of Medicine, Case Western Reserve University
Physician-in-Chief, University Hospitals of Cleveland

McGRAW-HILL INFORMATION SERVICES COMPANY

New York   St. Louis   San Francisco   Colorado Springs   Auckland   Bogotá
Caracas   Hamburg   Lisbon   London   Madrid   Mexico   Milan   Montreal
New Delhi   Paris   San Juan   São Paulo   Singapore   Sydney   Tokyo   Toronto

TROPICAL AND GEOGRAPHICAL MEDICINE

1234567890 HALHAL 943210

ISBN 0-07-068328-X

This book was set in Times Roman by Waldman Graphics, Inc.: the editors were Dereck Jeffers and Stuart D. Boynton, the production supervisor was Robert Laffler; the designer was Jose Fonfrias Arcata Graphics/Halliday was printer and binder. Cover: map courtesy of Hammond, Maplewood, New Jersey

Library of Congress Cataloging in Publication Data

Tropical and geographical medicine / [edited by] Kenneth S. Warren,
   Adel A. F. Mahmoud.—2nd ed.
      p.   cm.
   Includes bibliographical references.
   ISBN 0-07-068328-X
   1. Tropical medicine.   2. Medical geography.   I. Warren, Kenneth S.
II. Mahmoud, Adel A. F.
   [DNLM: 1. Epidemiology.   2. Tropical medicine.   WC 680 T855]
RC961.T73 1989
616.9′883—dc20
DNLM/DLC
for Library of Congress   89-12967
                                                            CIP

Contents

PART ONE

CLINICAL, BIOLOGICAL, AND EPIDEMIOLOGICAL CONSIDERATIONS IN THE APPROACH TO TROPICAL MEDICINE

PART TWO

PROTOZOAN DISEASES

PART THREE

METAZOAN DISEASES

PART SIX

FUNGAL DISEASES

PART SEVEN

NUTRITIONAL DISEASES

APPENDIXES

List of Contributors

Selwyn J. Baker, M.D., F.R.C.P.(C), F.R.A.C.P.
Professor of Medicine, Chief, Gastroenterology, St. Boniface Hospital, Winnipeg, Manitoba, Canada

John G. Banwell, M.D.
Professor of Medicine, Chief, Division of Gastroenterology, Department of Medicine, Case Western Reserve University and University Hospitals of Cleveland, Cleveland, Ohio

John E. Bennett, M.D.
Head, Clinical Mycology Section, Laboratory of Clinical Investigation, National Institute of Allergy and Infectious Diseases, National Institutes of Health, Bethesda, Maryland

Kathryn Bennett, M.Sc.
Lecturer, Department of Clinical Epidemiology and Biostatistics; Associate Director, McMaster International Clinical Epidemiology Program, McMaster University, Hamilton, Ontario, Canada

Michael Bennish, M.D.
Assistant Pediatrician, New England Medical Center Hospital, Boston, Massachusetts

David R. Bickers, M.D.
Professor and Chairman, Department of Dermatology, Case Western Reserve University and University Hospitals of Cleveland, Cleveland, Ohio

Martin J. Blaser, M.D.
Chief, Infectious Disease Section, Veterans Administration Medical Center; Associate Professor of Medicine, University of Colorado School of Medicine, Denver, Colorado

Philip S. Brachman, M.D.
Professor, Division of Public Health, Emory University, Atlanta, Georgia

Robert W. Bradsher, Jr., M.D.
Associate Professor of Medicine, Director, Division of Infectious Diseases, University of Arkansas College of Medicine, Little Rock, Arkansas

Joel G. Breman, M.D., D.T.P.H.
Chief, Malaria Control Activity, Malaria Branch, Division of Parasitic Diseases, Center for Infectious Diseases, Centers for Disease Control, Atlanta, Georgia

Thomas Buchanan, M.D.
Professor of Medicine, University of Washington; Chief, Immunology Research Lab, Pacific Medical Center, Seattle, Washington

Donald A. P. Bundy, Ph.D.
Director of Field Operations, Parasite Epidemiology Research Group, Department of Pure and Applied Biology, Imperial College of Science, Technology and Medicine, University of London, London, England

Danai Bunnag, M.R.C.P., D.T.M.&H. (Lond.)
Professor of Tropical Medicine, Head, Department of Clinical Tropical Medicine, Director, Bangkok Hospital for Tropical Diseases; Faculty of Tropical Medicine, Mahidol University, Bangkok, Thailand

Thomas Butler, M.D.
Chief of Infectious Diseases, Professor of Internal Medicine, Texas Tech University Health Sciences Center, Lubbock, Texas

Doris Howes Calloway, Ph.D.
Professor of Nutrition, Department of Nutritional Sciences, University of California, Berkeley, California

Charles C. J. Carpenter, M.D.
Professor of Medicine, Associate Director, Brown University International Health Center, Brown University; Physician-in-Chief, The Miriam Hospital, Providence, Rhode Island

Anthony Cerami, Ph.D.
Professor and Head, Laboratory of Medical Biochemistry, The Rockefeller University, New York, New York

A. Barnett Christie, M.D., F.R.C.P.
Honorary Physician in Infectious Diseases, Fayakerly Hospital, Liverpool; Honorary Fellow, Liverpool School of Tropical Medicine, Liverpool, England

Robert Colebunders, M.D.
Senior Investigator, Institute of Tropical Medicine, Antwerp, Belgium

Edward S. Cooper, M.B., M.R.C.P.
Visiting Lecturer, Parasite Epidemiology Research Group, Imperial College of Science, Technology and Medicine, University of London, London, England; Tropical Metabolism Research Unit, University of the West Indies, Kingston, Jamaica

Jose Rodrigues Coura, M.D.
Professor of Tropical Medicine, Federal University of Rio de Janeiro; Director, Oswaldo Cruz Institute, Rio de Janeiro, Brazil

John H. Cross, Ph.D.
Professor of Preventive Medicine, Division of Tropical

Public Health, Department of Preventive Medicine and Biometrics, Uniformed Services University of the Health Sciences, Bethesda, Maryland

Christina Wood-Dahlström, Ph.D.
Clinical Research Scientist, F. Hoffman-La Roche, Basel, Switzerland

Thomas M. Daniel, M.D.
Professor of Medicine, Department of Medicine, Case Western Reserve University and University Hospitals of Cleveland, Cleveland, Ohio

John R. David, M.D.
John LaPorte Given Professor and Chairman, Department of Tropical Public Health, Harvard School of Public Health, Boston, Massachusetts

Roger M. DesPrez, M.D.
Chief, Medical Service, Veterans Administration Medical Center; Professor of Medicine, Vanderbilt University Medical School, Nashville, Tennessee

Robert M. Douglas, M.D., F.R.A.C.P., F.R.A.C.G.P.
Director and Professor, National Centre for Epidemiology and Population Health, Australian National University, Canberra, Australia

Richard J. Duma, M.D., Ph.D.
Professor of Medicine, Microbiology, and Pathology, Chairman, Division of Infectious Diseases, Virginia Commonwealth University, Medical College of Virginia, Richmond, Virginia

Jerrold J. Ellner, M.D.
Professor of Medicine and Pathology, Chief, Division of Infectious Diseases, Department of Medicine, Case Western Reserve University and University Hospitals of Cleveland, Cleveland, Ohio

Paul T. Englund, Ph.D.
Professor of Biological Chemistry, Department of Biological Chemistry, The John Hopkins University School of Medicine, Baltimore, Maryland

Fred M. Feinsod, M.D., D.Sc., M.P.H.
Assistant Professor, Departments of Medicine and of Social and Preventive Medicine, State University of New York–Buffalo School of Medicine, Buffalo, New York

Susan Fisher-Hoch, M.D.
Special Pathogens Branch, Centers for Disease Control, Atlanta, Georgia

Coy D. Fitch, M.D.
Drefs Professor and Chairman, Department of Internal Medicine, St. Louis University Medical Center, St. Louis, Missouri

Jorges Flores, M.D.
Visiting Scientist, Laboratory of Infectious Diseases, National Institute of Allergy and Infectious Diseases, National Institutes of Health, Bethesda, Maryland

Samuel B. Formal, Sc.M., Ph.D.
Chief, Department of Bacterial Diseases, Walter Reed Army Institute of Research, Washington, D.C.; Profes-

sional Lecturer in Microbiology, Georgetown University School of Medicine, Washington, D.C.

John N. Galgiani, M.D.
Associate Professor of Medicine, Chief, Section of Infectious Diseases, Veterans Administration Medical Center, Tucson, Arizona

Herbert M. Gilles, M.D. (Malta), M.Sc. (Oxon.), D.Sc. D.Med.Sc. (Stockholm), F.R.C.P., F.F.M.C.
Emeritus Professor of Tropical Medicine, Senior Research Fellow, Department of Pharmacology and Therapeutics University of Liverpool, Liverpool, England

Frances D. Gillin, Ph.D.
Adjunct Professor of Pathology, Department of Pathology, University of California, San Diego, Medical Center, San Diego, California

Lawrence T. Glickman, V.M.D., Dr.PH.
Head, Veterinary Pathobiology, Department of Pathobiology, Purdue University, West Lafayette, Indiana

Robert A. Goodwin, Jr., M.D.
Professor of Medicine Emeritus, Vanderbilt University Medical School, Nashville, Tennessee

Sherwood L. Gorbach, M.D.
Professor of Community Health and Medicine, Tufts University School of Medicine, Boston, Massachusetts

John R. Graybill, M.D.
Assistant Chief, Medical Service, Audie L. Murphy Memorial VA Hospital; Professor of Medicine, University of Texas Health Science Center at San Antonio, San Antonio, Texas

J. Thomas Grayston, M.D.
Professor of Epidemiology, Department of Epidemiology, School of Public Health and Community Medicine, University of Washington, Seattle, Washington

Bruce M. Greene, M.D.
Professor of Medicine and Microbiology, Director, Division of Geographic Medicine, Department of Medicine, University of Alabama at Birmingham School of Medicine, Birmingham, Alabama

Donald L. Greer, Ph.D.
Associate Professor, Louisiana State University Medical Center, New Orleans, Louisiana

David I. Grove, M.D., F.R.A.C.P., F.R.C.P.A., D.T.M.&H.
Director, Department of Postgraduate Medical Education, Sir Charles Gairdner Hospital, Nedlands, Western Australia

Richard L. Guerrant, M.D.
Professor of Medicine, Head, Division of Geographic Medicine, University of Virginia School of Medicine, Charlottesville, Virginia

Ian D. Gust, M.B.B.S., B.Sc., DipBact (Lond.), F.R.C.P.A., F.R.A.C.P., F.A.T.S.
Professor, Director, Macfarlane Burnet Centre for Medical Research, Fairfield Hospital, Fairfield, Victoria, Australia

Stephen L. Hajduk, Ph.D.
Associate Professor of Biochemistry, Department of Biochemistry, University of Alabama at Birmingham School of Medicine, Birmingham, Alabama

Neal A. Halsey, M.D.
Associate Professor and Director, Division of Disease Control, Department of International Health, The Johns Hopkins University School of Hygiene and Public Health; Associate Professor, Department of Pediatrics, The Johns Hopkins University School of Medicine, Baltimore, Maryland

Scott B. Halstead, M.D.
Acting Director, Health Sciences Division, The Rockefeller Foundation, New York, New York

Khunying Tranakchit Harinasuta, M.D., D.T.M.&H., F.R.C.P.
Professor of Tropical Medicine, Consultant, Hospital for Tropical Diseases, Faculty of Tropical Medicine, Mahidol University, Bangkok, Thailand

R. Brian Haynes, M.D., Ph.D.
Professor of Clinical Epidemiology and Medicine, Chief, Health Information Research Unit, Faculty of Health Sciences, McMaster University, Hamilton, Ontario, Canada

Graeme B. Henderson, Ph.D.
Assistant Professor, Laboratory of Medical Biochemistry, The Rockefeller University, New York, New York

Erik L. Hewlett, M.D.
Professor of Medicine and of Pharmacology, Head, Division of Clinical Pharmacology, University of Virginia School of Medicine, Charlottesville, Virginia

King K. Holmes, M.D., Ph.D.
Professor and Vice-Chairman, Department of Medicine, University of Washington; Physician-in-Chief, Harborview Medical Center, Seattle, Washington

Donald R. Hopkins, M.D., M.P.H., D.Sc.
Senior Consultant, Global 2000, Inc., Atlanta, Georgia

Elizabeth Jacob, M.R.C.(Path), F.R.C.P.(C)
Associate Professor of Medicine, University of Manitoba, St. Boniface Hospital, Winnipeg, Manitoba, Canada

Anthony A. James, Ph.D.
Assistant Professor of Tropical Public Health, Department of Tropical Public Health, Harvard School of Public Health, Boston, Massachusetts

J. S. Job, M.D., M.P.H.
Department of International Health, The Johns Hopkins University School of Hygiene and Public Health, Baltimore, Maryland

Richard Johnson, M.D.
Professor and Director, Department of Neurology, Professor of Microbiology and Neuroscience, The Johns Hopkins University School of Medicine, Baltimore, Maryland

Russell C. Johnson, Ph.D.
Professor, Department of Microbiology, University of Minnesota Medical School, Minneapolis, Minnesota

Jeffrey M. Jones, M.D., Ph.D.
Professor of Medicine, University of Wisconsin Medical School; Assistant Chief of the Medical Service, William S. Middleton VA Medical Center, Madison, Wisconsin

Albert Z. Kapikian, M.D.
Head, Epidemiology Section, Laboratory of Infectious Diseases, National Institute of Allergy and Infectious Diseases, National Institutes of Health, Bethesda, Maryland

Edward Kaplan, M.D.
Professor of Pediatrics, University of Minnesota Medical School; Adjunct Professor, Division of Epidemiology, University of Minnesota School of Public Health; Head, WHO Collaborating Centre for Reference and Research on Streptococci, University of Minnesota, Minneapolis, Minnesota

Ben Z. Katz, M.D.
Assistant Professor, Departments of Pediatrics, and Epidemiology and Public Health, Yale University School of Medicine, New Haven, Connecticut

James W. Kazura, M.D.
Professor of Medicine, Chief, Division of Geographic Medicine, Department of Medicine, Case Western Reserve University and University Hospitals of Cleveland, Cleveland, Ohio

Gerald T. Keusch, M.D.
Professor of Medicine, Chief, Division of Geographic Medicine and Infectious Diseases, Department of Medicine, New England Medical Center Hospitals, Tufts University School of Medicine, Boston, Massachusetts

John N. Krieger, M.D.
Associate Professor, Department of Urology, University of Washington School of Medicine, Seattle, Washington

Cho-chou Kuo, M.D.
Professor, Department of Pathology, School of Public Health and Community Medicine, University of Washington, Seattle, Washington

James E. Loyd, M.D.
Assistant Professor of Medicine, Vanderbilt University Medical School, Nashville, Tennessee

Lucio Luzzatto, M.D.
Professor of Haematology, Royal Postgraduate Medical School; Consultant Haematologist, Hammersmith Hospital, London, England

John T. Macfarlane, M.A., D.M., F.R.C.P.
Consultant Physician in General and Respiratory Medicine, City Hospital, Nottingham, England

Adel A. F. Mahmoud, M.D., Ph.D.
John H. Hord Professor of Medicine, Chairman, Department of Medicine, Case Western Reserve University; Physician-in-Chief, University Hospitals of Cleveland, Cleveland, Ohio

Adolfo Martínez-Palomo, M.D., D.Sc.
Professor and Head, Section of Experimental Pathology,

Center for Research and Advanced Studies, National Polytechnical Institute, Mexico City, Mexico

Joel B. Mason, M.D.

USDA Human Nutrition Research Center on Aging at Tufts University; Assistant Professor, Division of Gastroenterology, Tufts-New England Medical Center, Boston, Massachusetts

Leonardo Mata, M.S., D.Sc.

Professor and Head of Microbiology, Institute for Health Research (INISA), University of Costa Rica, Guadalupe, Costa Rica

V. I. Mathan, M.D., Ph.D., F.R.C.P., F.A.M.S.

Professor of Medicine and Gastroenterology, Head, Wellcome Research Unit and Department of Gastroenterology, Christian Medical College Hospital, Vellore, Tamil Nadu, India

Josip Matovinovic, M.D.

Professor Emeritus, University of Michigan Medical School, Ann Arbor, Michigan

Robert M. May, M.D., F.R.S.

Royal Society Research Professor, Zoology Department, Oxford University, Oxford; Imperial College of Science, Technology and Medicine, London, England

Robert E. McCabe, M.D.

Chief, Section of Infectious Diseases, Veterans Administration Medical Center, Martinez, California; Assistant Professor of Medicine, University of California Medical Center, Davis, California

Joseph B. McCormick, M.D.

Special Pathogens Branch, Centers for Disease Control, Atlanta, Georgia

Michael R. McGinnis, Ph.D.

Professor and Vice Chairman, Department of Pathology, University of Texas Medical Branch, Galveston, Texas

Joseph L. Melnick, Ph.D., D.Sc.

Distinguished Service Professor and Chairman, Virology and Epidemiology; Dean of Graduate Studies, Department of Virology and Epidemiology, Baylor College of Medicine, Houston, Texas

Richard D. Meyer, M.D.

Professor and Director, Division of Infectious Diseases, Cedars-Sinai Medical Center, University of California, Los Angeles, California

Edward H. Michelson, Ph.D.

Professor of Preventive Medicine and Biometrics, Uniformed Services University of the Health Sciences, Bethesda, Maryland

George Miller, M.D.

The John F. Enders Professor of Pediatric Infectious Diseases; Professor of Epidemiology, Department of Pediatrics, Yale University School of Medicine, New Haven, Connecticut

Louis H. Miller, M.D.

Head, Malaria Section, Laboratory of Parasitic Diseases, National Institute of Allergy and Infectious Diseases, National Institute of Health, Bethesda, Maryland

Richard A. Miller, M.D.

Chief, Infectious Disease Division, Seattle Veterans Administration Medical Center; Assistant Professor of Medicine, University of Washington, Seattle, Washington

Malcolm E. Molyneux, M.D., F.R.C.P.

Senior Lecturer in Tropical Medicine, Liverpool School of Tropical Medicine, Honorary Consultant Physician, Merseyside, England

L. N. Mohapatra, M.D. (Patna), Dip.Bact.(Lond.), F.A.M.S.

Director, Regional Medical Research Centre, Bhubaneswar, India

Thomas P. Monath, M.D.

Director, Division of Vector-Borne Viral Diseases, Center for Infectious Diseases, Centers for Disease Control; Public Health Service, Department of Health and Human Services, Fort Collins, Colorado

Anne B. Morrisey, M.S.

Assistant Director, Clinical Microbiology Laboratory, University Hospitals of Cleveland, Cleveland, Ohio

J. W. Mugerwa, M.D.(Ea.)

Professor of Pathology, Makerere Medical School, Kampala, Uganda

Hamish N. Munro, M.B., D.Sc.

Professor of Nutrition, M.I.T.; Senior Scientist and Professor Nutrition, USDA HNRC, Tufts University, Boston

Franklin A. Neva, M.D., M.S.

Chief, Laboratory of Parasitic Diseases, National Institute of Allergy and Infectious Diseases; Member, Laboratory of Clinical Investigation, National Institutes of Health, Bethesda, Maryland

Nadia Nogueira, M.D., Ph.D.

Associate Medical Director, Sandoz Research Institute, East Hanover, New Jersey; Adjunct Professor, Department of Molecular Parasitology, The Rockefeller University, New York, New York

Gideon B. A. Okelo, M.D., F.R.C.P., M.R.C.P., M.B.B.S., D.T.M.&H., C. Biol., MiBiol.(Lond), F.A.M.S.

Chairman and Associate Professor of Medicine, Department of Medicine, University of Nairobi, Nairobi, Kenya

Edward C. Oldfield III, M.D., F.A.C.P., CDR, MSC, USN

Head, Infectious Disease Division, Naval Hospital, San Diego, California

G. Richard Olds, M.D.

Associate Professor of Medicine and Molecular Cell and Developmental Biology; Director, International Health Institute and the Program in Geographic Medicine, Brown University and The Miriam Hospital, Providence, Rhode Island

Charles L. M. Olweny, M.B.Ch.B., M.Med., M.D., F.R.A.C.P.

Director, Medical Oncology, Royal Adelaide Hospital;

Clinical Professor, University of Adelaide, Adelaide, South Australia

John Orley, D.M., M.A., B.Litt, M.R.C.Psych(U.K.)
Senior Medical Officer, Division of Mental Health, World Health Organization, Geneva, Switzerland

Joseph V. Osterman, Ph.D.
Chief Scientist, U.S. Army Medical Research and Development Command, Fort Detrick, Frederick, Maryland

Eric A. Ottesen, M.D.
Head, Clinical Parasitology Section, Laboratory of Clinical Investigation; Senior Investigator, Laboratory of Parasitic Diseases, National Institute of Allergy and Infectious Diseases, National Institutes of Health, Bethesda, Maryland

Zbigniew S. Pawlowski, M.D.
Professor and Head, Clinic of Parasitic and Tropical Diseases, Academy of Medicine, Poznan, Poland

Peter L. Perine, M.D., M.P.H.
Professor and Director of Tropical Public Health; Professor of Medicine, Uniformed Services University of the Health Sciences, Bethesda, Maryland

Elizabeth A. Phelan, A.B.
Research Associate, U.S.D.A. Human Nutrition Research Center on Aging, Tufts University, Boston, Massachusetts

Prida Phuapradit, M.D., M.R.C.P.(U.K.)
Assistant Professor of Medicine, Ramathibodi Hospital, Mahidol University, Bangkok, Thailand

Peter Piot, M.D.
Professor and Head, Department of Microbiology, Institute of Tropical Medicine, Antwerp, Belgium

Thomas C. Quinn, M.D.
Associate Professor of Medicine, Division of Infectious Diseases, The Johns Hopkins University School of Medicine; Associate Professor, Department of Immunology and Infectious Diseases, The Johns Hopkins University School of Hygiene and Public Health; Senior Investigator, Laboratory of Immunoregulation, National Institute of Allergy and Infectious Diseases, National Institutes of Health, Bethesda, Maryland

Jack S. Remington, M.D.
Professor of Medicine, Division of Infectious Diseases, Stanford University School of Medicine; Chairman, Department of Immunology and Infectious Diseases, Marcus A. Krupp Research Chair, Palo Alto Medical Foundation, Palo Alto, California

Mario Rigatto, M.D., Docent
Professor of Internal Medicine, Federal University of Rio Grande do Sul (UFRGS), Brazil; Senior Researcher, National Research Council (CNPq), Porto Alegre, Brazil

Irwin H. Rosenberg, M.D.
Professor of Medicine and Nutrition, Director, Human Nutrition Research Center on Aging, Tufts University, Boston, Massachusetts

Patricia L. Rosenfield, Ph.D.
Program Officer, Carnegie Corporation of New York, New York, New York

Philippe Rossignol, Ph.D.
Assistant Professor, Department of Entomology, Oregon State University, Corvallis, Oregon

Trenton I. Ruebush, II, M.D.
Medical Epidemiologist, Malaria Branch, Division of Parasitic Diseases, Center of Infectious Diseases, Centers for Disease Control, Atlanta, Georgia

Guillermo Ruíz-Palacios, M.D.
Professor and Head, Department of Infectious Diseases, Instituto Nacional de la Nutrition ''Salvador Zubiran,'' Mexico City, Mexico

Robert M. Russell, M.D.
Associate Director U.S.D.A. Human Nutrition Research Center on Aging, Tufts University, Boston, Massachusetts

Manuel Ruz, M.Sc.
Graduate Associate, Applied Human Nutrition Program, Department of Family Studies, University of Guelph, Guelph, Ontario, Canada

David Sack, M.D.
Associate Professor of International Health, Department of International Health, The Johns Hopkins University School of Hygiene and Public Health, Baltimore, Maryland

David L. Sackett, M.D., M.Sc., F.R.C.P.
Professor of Medicine, Professor of Clinical Epidemiology and Biostatistics, McMaster University, Hamilton, Ontario, Canada

David Sacks, Ph.D.
Senior Investigator, Laboratory of Parasitic Diseases, National Institute of Allergy and Infectious Diseases, National Institutes of Health, Bethesda, Maryland

Robert A. Salata, M.D.
Assistant Professor of Medicine, Division of Geographic Medicine, and Director, Traveler's Health Care Center, Department of Medicine, Case Western Reserve University and University Hospitals of Cleveland, Cleveland, Ohio

Gerhard A. Schad, Ph.D.
Professor of Parasitology, Department of Pathobiology, University of Pennsylvania, Philadelphia, Pennsylvania

Peter M. Schantz, V.M.D., Ph.D.
Division of Parasitic Diseases, Center for Infectious Diseases, Centers for Disease Control, Atlanta, Georgia

W. Michael Scheld, M.D.
Professor of Internal Medicine and Neurosurgery, University of Virginia School of Medicine, Charlottesville, Virginia

Richard D. Semba, M.D.
Instructor, The Wilmer Institute, The Johns Hopkins Hospital, Baltimore, Maryland

Robert E. Shope, M.D.
Professor of Epidemiology, Yale Arbovirus Research Unit,

Yale University School of Medicine, New Haven,
Connecticut

Michael Sitrin, M.D.

Assistant Professor of Medicine, Section of Gastroenterology, Department of Medicine, University of Chicago, Chicago, Illinois

David H. Smith, M.B.B.S., F.R.C.P., D.T.M.&H.

Senior Lecturer in Tropical Medicine, Honorary Consultant Physician, Department of Tropical Medicine and Infectious Diseases, Liverpool School of Tropical Medicine, Liverpool, England

Margaret H. D. Smith, M.D.

Professor Emeritus of Pediatrics, New Orleans, Louisiana

Rosemary Soave, M.D.

Assistant Professor of Medicine and Public Health, Division of Infectious Diseases, Department of Medicine, The New York Hospital–Cornell Medical Center, New York, New York

Noel W. Solomons, M.D.

Senior Scientist and Scientific Coordinator, Center for Studies of Sensory Impairment, Aging and Metabolism, Research Branch of the National Committee for the Blind and Deaf of Guatemala, Guatemala City, Guatemala

Andrew Spielman, Sc.D.

Professor of Tropical Public Health, Department of Tropical Public Health, Harvard School of Public Health, Boston, Massachusetts

John B. Stanbury, M.D.

Professor Emeritus of Experimental Medicine and Honorary Physician, Massachusetts General Hospital; Lecturer, Harvard Medical School; Chairman, International Council for Control of Iodine Deficiency Disorders, Boston, Massachusetts

David P. Stevens, M.D.

Professor of Medicine, Chief, Division of General Internal Medicine, Department of Medicine, Case Western Reserve University and University Hospitals of Cleveland, Cleveland, Ohio

David N. Taylor, M.D.

Center for Vaccine Development, Baltimore, Maryland

Hugh R. Taylor, M.D., F.R.A.C.S.

Associate Professor, The Wilmer Institute, The Johns Hopkins Hospital, Baltimore, Maryland

Robert B. Tesh, M.D.

Associate Professor of Epidemiology, Department of Epidemiology and Public Health, Yale University School of Medicine, New Haven, Connecticut

Benjamin Torún, M.D., Ph.D.

Head, Program of Metabolism and Clinical Nutrition, Institute of Nutrition of Central American and Panama (INCAP); Professor of Basic and Human Nutrition, University of San Carlos, Guatemala City, Guatemala

Sriram P. Tripathy, M.B.B.S., M.D., F.A.M.S.

Additional Director General, Indian Council of Medical Research, Ansari Nagar, New Delhi, India

Peter Tugwell, M.D.(Lond.), M.Sc., F.C.A.P.

Professor of Medicine and Chairman, Department of Clinical Epidemiology and Biostatistics, McMaster University; Chief of Medicine, Rheumatic Disease Centre, Chedoke-McMaster Hospital, Hamilton, Ontario, Canada

Aree Valyasevi, M.D., D.Sc.

Professor and Director, Institute of Nutrition, Mahidol University, Nakorn Pathom, Thailand

Athasit Vejjajiva, M.B.(Lond.), F.R.C.P., F.R.A.C.P., F.R.C.P.(T)

Professor of Medicine and Senior Neurologist, Faculty of Medicine, Ramathibodi Hospital, Mahidol University, Bangkok, Thailand

Fernando E. Viteri, M.D.

Division of Disease Prevention and Control, Pan American Health Organization, Washington, D.C.

M. Farid Abdel Wahab, M.D., D.T.M.&H.

Chairman, Tropical Medicine Department, University of Cairo, Cairo, Egypt

Julia A. Walsh, M.D., D.T.P.H.

Assistant Professor, Department of Medicine, Harvard Medical School, Boston, Massachusetts

Peter D. Walzer, M.D.

Chief, Infectious Disease Section, Cincinnati Veterans Administration Medical Center; Professor of Medicine, University of Cincinnati College of Medicine, Cincinnati, Ohio

David A. Warrell, M.A., D.M., F.R.C.P.

Professor of Tropical Medicine and Infectious Diseases, University of Oxford, Oxford, England

Kenneth S. Warren, M.D.

Director for Science, Maxwell Communication Corporation, The Maxwell Foundation; Professor of Medicine, New York University; Adjunct Professor of Medicine, The Rockefeller University, New York, New York

Prawase Wasi, M.D., Ph.D.

Professor of Medicine, Division of Heamatology, Department of Medicine, Faculty of Medicine, Siriraj Hospital, Bangkok, Thailand

Sir David J. Weatherall, M.D., F.R.C.P., F.R.S.

Nuffield Professor of Clinical Medicine, University of Oxford; Honorary Director, MRC Molecular Haematology Unit, Nuffield Department of Clinical Medicine, John Radcliffe Hospital, Oxford, England

Theodore E. Woodward, M.D., M.A.C.P., D.Sc.,

Professor of Medicine Emeritus, University of Maryland School of Medicine, Baltimore, Maryland

Lowell S. Young, M.D.

Director, Kuzell Institute for Arthritis and Infectious Diseases, Medical Research Institute of San Francisco at Pacific Presbyterian Medical Center; Clinical Professor of Medicine, University of California, San Francisco, San Francisco, California

Preface to the Second Edition

The production of a major new textbook is an overwhelming task. One looks forward, from the beginning, to the second edition in which an experienced core of editors, associate editors, and authors is available, inevitable errors can be corrected, and constructive criticism of both readers and, particularly, reviewers can be taken into consideration. Our favorite review dubbed *Tropical and Geographical Medicine* ''a potential classic.'' On the basis of that reviewer's suggestions and those of others, we have striven to ensure that this work achieves its potential. The principal concern was with the clinical or ''patient'' sections of each chapter, and we asked all authors to focus on that area and to include many more illustrations. We also have introduced a series of appendices intended to help with defining clinical syndromes, the geographic distribution of major infectious diseases, and therapeutic approaches.

Clinical Considerations, the opening section of the book, is now written largely from the viewpoint of the tropics. There has been an emphasis throughout the book on authors from the tropics or those with major field experience. We've gone even further in making this not an American or British textbook but an international effort. The authors come not only from the U.S.A. and the U.K. but from 15 other countries, including (in order of frequency) Canada, Thailand, Australia, India, Switzerland, Mexico, Belgium, Guatemala, Brazil, Poland, Uganda, Kenya, Costa Rica, Jamaica, and Egypt. In spite of burgeoning interest in every area of tropical medicine, and the continuing information explosion, the revised and updated book is now 11 pages shorter than the previous edition. Finally, we are pleased to say that our remarkable publishers will be providing a significant number of copies of *Tropical and Geographical Medicine* for distribution in the tropics at an affordable cost.

It is hoped that *Tropical and Geographical Medicine* will provide students, clinicians, researchers, and educators with a broad knowledge of diseases and conditions that affect billions of people worldwide. Credit must be given to those who made possible the production of this text. We are particularly indebted to a group of dedicated contributors for their expertise and scholarship. McGraw-Hill has provided the logistical and technical support particularly of Dereck Jeffers and Stuart D. Boynton. Ms. Linda Ryan of the Department of Medicine at Case Western Reserve University provided most capable editorial and secretarial support.

Kenneth S. Warren
Adel A. F. Mahmoud

Preface to the First Edition

The developing areas of the world have a burden of illness that differs drastically from that of the rest of this globe. The major health problems of the developing countries are generally related to warm climates, overcrowding, rural areas, poverty, and childhood. This markedly different spectrum of diseases requires a textbook devoted specifically to the major infectious and nutritional problems of one-half of the globe's land area and three-quarters of the globe's population. Many of the health problems of the developing world were prevalent in temperate climates just a relatively short time ago, but were largely ameliorated by industrial development and medical technology. While it was expected that similar changes would take place throughout the world, development has not occurred as rapidly as had been hoped.

There has been, however, a remarkable rise in the potential of modern science to provide new means of treatment and prevention of the great tropical and geographical diseases. An augury of the future lies in the development of several excellent new drugs for schistosomiasis, a vaccine for hepatitis B, and a new oral vaccine for typhoid. Many more therapeutic and preventive modalities are in the offing, including a spate of vaccines for malaria. While the scientific capacity in the developing world is increasing, the scientists and physicians of the developed world still have a major role to play. They can and should bring the full scientific power of the developed world, its infrastructure and technology, to bear on these great neglected diseases.

In the last several decades the practice of tropical and geographical medicine has undergone a drastic change. The field essentially arose in Europe. Since World War II, however, there has been a remarkable burgeoning of medical schools throughout the tropical areas of Latin America, Africa, the Middle East, and Asia. These schools, which have recognized the necessity of training their students to deal with their indigenous diseases, have increased the need for a general reference book. Even in temperate areas, however, specialists in tropical and geographical medicine are essential. Some of the parasitic infections such as toxoplasmosis, trichinosis, and enterobiasis are cosmopolitan in distribution. Immunodeficiency states related to age, advanced disease, new therapeutic modalities, and even new diseases such as acquired immunodeficiency syndrome (AIDS) have resulted in the activation of latent protozoan and helminth infections.

Both the growth of biomedical research and the broadening of clinical training have been taken into consideration in the development and organization of *Tropical and Geographical Medicine*. This text is multiauthored with a global representation of 153 contributors from 21 different nations. We have attempted to merge the most up-to-date information on the etiological agents of disease, and the host responses to them, with clinical and field experience. The basic structure of the book reflects an understanding of all infectious agents as parasites in the broad sense of the term. It presents the three crucial facets of the relationship between the infectious agent and host: the parasite, the patient, and the population. We must be aware of each of these elements in order to deal with tropical and geographical diseases not only in the individual patient but, equally important, in populations of infected or diseased individuals. The text has the virtues of drawing on the expertise of many clinicians and researchers.

Furthermore, we have availed ourselves of the lessons of the great modern textbooks of medicine and the invaluable aid of a distinguished group of associate editors. Using the example of *Principles of Internal Medicine*, we have provided general material on clinical areas, genetics, parasitism, and nutrition. This information is followed by sections on protozoan disease; metazoan disease; viral and chlamydial disease; bacterial, spirochetal, and rickettsial disease; fungal disease; nutritional disease; and epidemiology and health care. The book is intended for all those who are studying, researching, or practicing tropical and geographical medicine. It has been planned to provide an adequate and balanced guide for the student, the scientist, and the clinician.

Although we cannot acknowledge all those who have helped in the production of *Tropical and Geographical Medicine*, we would like to thank the contributors, associate editors, and the publisher for the remarkable degree of cooperation which has resulted in the rapid production and publication of this new text. A special acknowledgment is due to Linda Ryan who coordinated the entire project out of the Division of Geographic Medicine at Case Western Reserve University School of Medicine in Cleveland, Ohio.

Kenneth S. Warren
Adel A. F. Mahmoud

Tropical
and
Geographical
Medicine

SECOND EDITION

NOTICE

PART I

Clinical, Biological, and Epidemiological Considerations in the Approach to Tropical Medicine

SECTION A / Clinical Considerations

CHAPTER 1 / Introduction · David A. Warrell

This section is intended mainly for the physician working in a busy clinic or hospital ward in a tropical country. In that situation, facilities for laboratory and other investigations are likely to be limited or even nonexistent so that clinical skills are of paramount importance. A second group of readers is envisaged—physicians working in western industrialized countries who are seeing both their compatriots returned home from tourism or work in the tropics and immigrants from tropical countries. Some returning travelers will be treated at designated tropical units or travelers' clinics, where a high level of expectation of the diagnosis of a tropical disease and special skills and experience necessary for confirming the diagnosis will exist. Increasingly, however, patients with imported tropical diseases are presenting themselves to general practitioners and to nonspecialized general medical clinics. No doctor can now afford to ignore the increasing problem of imported tropical disease created by the boom in travel to tropical areas.

HISTORY TAKING

Language difficulties may prevent the physician from taking a full and precise history. Whenever possible, physicians should try to become fluent in the major languages in the area where they work. Interpreters will be essential in many cases, but what they say should not be accepted uncritically. It is very useful for physicians to know enough of the language to assess whether the interpreter has asked a question precisely. The same rules apply as with all good clinical history taking. The main complaint must be established at the outset, followed by the sequence of events from the initial symptom up until the present time. Leading questions should be avoided and a "veterinary" approach (relying totally on physical examination) should be employed only as a last resort if the language barrier is absolute, sign language fails, or the patient is unconscious and unaccompanied by anyone who can give a history. It must be accepted that, quite apart from language difficulties, the expatriate doctor may lack the understanding of local psychology, religion, and customs that may be necessary for the proper interpretation of the patient's history and behavior. Because of these problems in communication, it is essential that the patient should be given the benefit of the doubt and should not too readily be diagnosed as hysterical or having a "low pain threshold."

The precise timing of events and geographical details is equally important in the endemic area and in the travelers' clinic. Many tropical conditions, infectious and nutritional, have a seasonal peak of incidence, knowledge of which can assist present and retrospective diagnosis. The physician should be aware of major epidemics through reading the World Health Organization's *Weekly Epidemiological Bulletin* and the *Morbidity and Mortality Weekly Review* produced by the Centers for Disease Control in Atlanta. However, awareness of a current epidemic should not close the physician's mind to other diagnoses. For example, during the 1970 cholera epidemic in northern Nigeria, a number of patients with other diseases, such as lobar pneumonia and malaria, were wrongly admitted to rehydration units. Knowledge of the patient's tribe and religion may be important for the diagnosis of some conditions. For example, in Nigeria, peripartum cardiac failure is common only among women living in a restricted area of the north who have observed traditional Hausa practices during pregnancy and the puerperium (these practices include eating Lake Chad salts and lying on a heated bed). There is a high prevalence of hydatid disease among the Turkana of northern Kenya because of the way they live with their animals, and so this condition would be the most likely cause of abdominal swelling in a member of this ethnic group. There are dry season diseases, notably malnutrition and epidemic meningococcal meningitis in the Sahel, and wet season diseases such as malaria and snakebite in many parts of the world, and melioidosis in northeastern Thailand.

TRAVEL HISTORY

When taking a travel history it is inadequate to discover only which countries were visited. It is important to establish if there were any incidental stopovers in the journey where an infection could have been acquired before the final destination was reached. It is very useful to have an atlas in the travel clinic so that the itinerary can be understood. Exact conditions of travel, eating, working, and sleeping in the tropical endemic area are important. For example, tourists who spend their time in air-conditioned hotels in capital cities such as Nairobi and Bangkok run a negligible risk of malaria, whereas those who visit game parks and rural areas may be exposed to bites by infected mosquitoes, especially if they are out of doors after dusk and sleep in the open. In the case of tropical infections, knowledge of the precise dates during which the patient was in the endemic area can be useful to support or exclude diagnosis of the particular infection on grounds of known incubation periods. For example, a patient who develops a fever less than 7 days after entering the endemic area is unlikely to have malaria, and someone who first falls ill more than 3 weeks after leaving west Africa is unlikely, on those grounds alone, to be suffering from Lassa fever.

Patients should be asked about unusual or special events such as the discovery of an attached tick, insect bites, mammal bites, illness among other members of the group, sexual contacts, blood transfusions, injections, or a raw or exotic meal.

Some patients are clearly at greater risk from particular conditions because of their occupation or hobbies: industrial diseases such as silicosis, byssinosis and bagassosis are described in the tropics; zoologists and hunters are at special risk from some zoonoses; and cave explorers may be exposed to cryptococcosis and bat rabies.

Patients may be vulnerable to certain infections because they have not been vaccinated, they have not taken appropriate chemoprophylaxis, or they are immunocompromised or immunodeficient because of pregnancy, splenectomy, a chronic disease such as hepatic cirrhosis, or immunosuppressant drugs.

Finally, it must be remembered that in many parts of the tropical world, traditional forms of treatment remain more popular than western medicines, at least as a first resort. These remedies can produce a vast array of misleading signs and symptoms such as the well-known hypoglycemia after cow's urine treatment in Nigeria, severe vomiting and other gastrointestinal symptoms produced by many herbal medicines, severe toxicity produced by bush teas in the Caribbean, and the bizarre syndrome of severe chemical conjunctivitis, ruptured ear drums, and aspiration pneumonia resulting from ayurvedic treatment of snakebite in Sri Lanka. Always remember to ask patients what treatment they received before seeing you!

PHYSICAL EXAMINATION

The chapters in this section provide detailed advice about examination of the various systems. However, in a busy outpatient clinic in the tropics there may be time for no more than rapid screening or triage. Patients with gross physical signs can quickly be identified. Among those appearing reasonably well, a rapid respiratory rate with flaring of the nostrils is a useful sign of significant respiratory infection or high fever. Thorough examination may be hindered by lack of time, poor facilities, and lack of privacy, and in some cultures, by the patient's extreme embarrassment. For example, in some Muslim countries female patients will not agree to be examined by male doctors. Many important physical signs can be found only by scrupulous examination of the skin and mucous membranes. Hairy areas such as the scalp, axillae, and perineum may conceal a distinctive lesion such as a rash, chancre or eschar, or

an ectoparasite. Ophthalmoscopy (see Chap. 7) and auriscopy should not be omitted. The discovery of lymphadenopathy may provide a valuable clue to local or systemic disease and a site for diagnostic aspiration or biopsy. The site of lymphadenopathy may have diagnostic significance, for example, the bilateral posterior cervical lymphadenopathy of African trypanosomiasis (Winterbottom's sign) and the gross inguinal lymphadenopathy of lymphogranuloma venereum. In tropical countries, patients suffering from sexually transmitted diseases are more likely to present themselves to general rather than specialist clinics. The genitalia must be adequately examined in both sexes: in females this involves vaginal examination and use of the speculum. In patients with acute abdominal symptoms, genitourinary symptoms, and unexplained fever, the rectal examination should never be omitted. This should usually be followed by proctoscopy, which allows examination of the rectal mucosa, biopsy of ulcerated areas, and examination for ova of *Schistosoma mansoni* if this enters into the differential diagnosis (see below).

LABORATORY INVESTIGATIONS

Immediate, simple investigations performed by the physician at the bedside or in the sideroom laboratory provide the best means of confirming the diagnosis of many tropical infections. Blood smears provide the only means for rapid and conclusive diagnosis of malaria and filariasis. Parasites (e.g., plasmodia, trypanosomes, microfilariae) may be seen in standard hematological thin films, but specific stains, concentration methods such as the thick malarial film and microfiltration, and examination of a buffy coat smear may be needed. Other tropical infections can be diagnosed by rapid examination of sputum (e.g., paragonimiasis), urine (e.g., *Schistosoma haematobium*), stool (e.g., protozoa and helminths), lymph node aspirates (e.g., plague and African trypanosomiasis), "sneeze plate" (leprosy), skin scrapings and skin slits (superficial mycoses, onchocerciasis, leishmaniasis, leprosy), and cerebrospinal fluid (pyogenic meningitides, tuberculous meningitis, eosinophilic meningitides, etc.). With several of these investigations, the chances of diagnosis are enhanced by immediate examination of fresh samples or specimens (for example, the hot stool for amebic dysentery and the malarial film).

The timing of samples may be crucial: for example, the examination of urine at about midday for *S. haematobium* ova and blood at midnight for *Wuchereria bancrofti* and midday for *Loa loa* microfilariae.

In conclusion, the physician dealing with patients suffering from tropical and geographical diseases must apply the principles of good general medicine but with special emphasis on precise location of the geographical area where the disease was contracted, precise timing of events to allow interpretation in relation to the incubation periods of specific diseases, epidemiological and public health background, and the use of rapid confirmatory methods often carried out close to the patient rather than in distant laboratories. In some tropical settings, the physician may have to develop clinical screening methods to make the best use of a very limited allocation of time for each patient and may have to rely heavily on clinical techniques where there is a lack of laboratory facilities. Special skills include not only a wide background knowledge of the diseases themselves but awareness of their current geographical distribution and an ability to overcome language difficulties in history taking and in the interpretation of the patient's history and behavior. Finally, the tropical physician may be dependent on a range of simple laboratory skills.

| CHAPTER 2 | *Fevers* · Herbert M. Gilles · David A. Warrell |

Among patients suffering from tropical and geographical diseases, fever is the commonest symptom. In this chapter the approach is pragmatic and intended for three groups of physicians: those working in a health center or rural hospital in the tropics with limited laboratory facilities; those working in a well-staffed district, regional, or teaching hospital in the tropics with adequate laboratory facilities; and those in nonendemic areas essentially concerned with international travelers—a rapidly growing group in the developed world.

GENERAL CONSIDERATIONS

The ability of a healthy individual to maintain the body temperature within a narrow range (1 to 1.5°C) despite extremes in environmental and physical conditions depends on the production of heat within the body and very accurate control of heat loss.

Fever results from disturbances of thermoregulation or from the action on hypothalamic thermoregulatory centers of endogenous pyrogens (such as interleukin-1) released from macrophages under the influence of a variety of stimuli including bacterial endotoxin, other microbial constituents, and immune complexes [1–4].

High temperatures may be recorded in healthy people as a result of individual variations, site of measurement, time of day, phase of the menstrual cycle, pregnancy, age, exercise, anxiety, and stress [4,5]. Diurnal variation may be as much as 2°C, the maximum being between 1700 and 1900 h. Temperature may rise to 38°C in the second half of the menstrual cycle and in pregnancy. Fifty percent of healthy 18-month-old infants were found to have rectal temperatures above 37.8°C. In marathon runners the temperature may exceed 40°C.

For practical purposes, however, the oral temperature can be said to be raised when it is above 37.2°C in a person at bed rest.

The pulse rate usually increases by about 15 beats per minute for every 1°C rise in temperature, but this relationship may be lost in some diseases. Thus, in many cases of typhoid fever during the second week the pulse rate falls short of the expected rate by 20 or more beats per minute; a similar dissociation may occur in brucellosis, leptospirosis, dengue, sandfly fever, Q fever, meningitis, and yellow fever (Faget's sign) and may imply myocarditis. On the other hand, in acute Chagas' disease, rheumatic fever, Rhodesian trypanosomiasis, plague, and tuberculosis, the pulse may be unusually rapid in proportion to the temperature. Injection of large numbers of gram-negative organisms (for example, immunization with the early typhoid vaccines) or the phagocytosis of massive intravascular spirochetemia (for example, the Jarisch-Herxheimer reaction of louse-borne relapsing fever) causes a dramatic sequence of physiological changes known as the *endotoxin reaction* [6,7]. First, the patient feels cold and has a cold, vasoconstricted, goose-pimpled skin. Core temperature, blood pressure, pulse, and respiratory rates increase rapidly; the patient develops a chill or rigor and piles blankets on the bed. Second, core temperature reaches a peak, and there is vasodilatation, a flushed warm skin, increase in pulse pressure, fall in mean arterial pressure, and a tendency to postural syncope. The patient feels insufferably hot, has a throbbing headache, and throws off all the bedclothes. Third, sweating breaks out, and the temperature and other variables return slowly toward normal. These changes can occur in any acute or exacerbated infection when there is a rapid, massive or concerted release of endogenous pyrogens, but is particularly typical of lobar pneumonia, ascending cholangitis, pyelitis, viral hepatitis, and malaria. Noninfective causes include transfusion reactions, massive intravascular hemolysis, and pyrogen reactions.

Fever is associated with an array of metabolic changes, immunological responses, and inflammatory reactions involving humoral mediator systems. Of practical clinical importance is the increased hepatic synthesis of a variety of proteins including fibrinogen (largely responsible for the increase in erythrocyte sedimentation rate) and C-reactive protein.

TYPES OF FEVER

The patterns of fever have diminished in diagnostic importance in the light of improved laboratory facilities, the introduction of modern chemotherapeutic agents, and the increasing use of often irrational self-medication especially in the tropics. Nonetheless, fever patterns are still of some importance to the physician deprived of adequate laboratory facilities, especially in the diagnosis of chronic fevers. It is therefore important to record the temperature every 4 to 6 h to produce a temperature chart.

CONTINUOUS FEVER

With continuous fever, persistent or unremittent diurnal variations are small in the case of typhoid, and greater in sepsis "swinging"—but the temperature rarely falls to normal. Sometimes a double diurnal rise to high peaks occurs, e.g., in miliary tuberculosis, gonococcal endocarditis, and kala azar. Often in kala azar there is also a dissociation between the height of the fever and the subjective symptoms, which are frequently mild, allowing the patients to remain ambulatory and able to carry out normal activities.

REMITTENT FEVERS

Remittent fever is not sustained for more than hours or days but falls to normal or below, daily or periodically (every third or fourth day), as in vivax or quartan malaria, especially when relapses occur.

Undulant fever

Undulant fever is a remittent fever with a gradual rise and a gradual fall to normal or just above normal levels; then, after an afebrile or relatively afebrile period, the pattern reappears, e.g., as in brucellosis. Occasionally this type of fever is seen in deep-seated lymphomas.

Relapsing fever

Exemplified by louse-borne and tick-borne relapsing fevers, this is a remittent fever in which acute febrile episodes persist for several days followed by rapid fall (during an endotoxin-like reaction) and a variable apyrexial interval of weeks before a repetition of the same pattern. There may be several relapses; the spirochetes of the *Borrelia* genus are seen during the pyrexial phases only.

Saddleback fever

A diphasic remittent fever is sometimes seen in patients suffering from alphavirus infections, e.g., dengue. A continuous fever for a few days is followed by a remission and a second bout of continuous fever associated with appearance of a rash and terminating by lysis.

HYPERPYREXIA

Hyperpyrexia is usually defined as a temperature exceeding 41.1°C, irrespective of the etiology. Common contributing fac-

tors associated with hyperpyrexia are *Plasmodium falciparum* and heatstroke. The muscular spasms associated with severe tetanus and status epilepticus sometimes give rise to hyperpyrexia in the hot season in the tropics, and body temperature should be monitored frequently in these cases.

CLASSIFICATION AND DIAGNOSIS OF FEVER

The subject of fever of obscure origin has been well-reviewed [10–12]. Here we describe a practical approach to the diagnosis of acute and chronic fever in tropical countries and in the travelers' clinic. Fever can be conveniently subdivided into acute fevers (less than 2 weeks' duration) and chronic fevers (more than 2 weeks' duration).

ACUTE FEVER

This is a common problem throughout the tropics, and in most instances it can be assumed that the illness is infectious in origin.

Diagnosis at the health center or rural hospital

The history and examination often give the best clues to the particular organ or system involved, especially as there is often delay in seeking medical aid in the tropics, which increases the chances of identifying a localizing sign or symptom. Unfortunately, history and examination in a rural environment are often curtailed because of the sheer numbers of patients. Certain useful clinical signs may be immediately obvious, such as a rapid respiratory rate in patients with lower respiratory tract infections or high fever. One must not overlook examination of the throat and ears in the young and pelvic examination in women.

If there is a polymorphonuclear leukocytosis and parasitemia is scanty, it is likely that the fever is nonmalarial in origin. If in doubt, in areas where malaria is endemic, *always* treat for malaria and monitor the patient's progress. It must be emphasized that *the presence of malaria parasites in nonimmunes dictates immediate treatment irrespective of any other consideration.* A total and differential blood count should be done in *all* cases, complemented by a thick blood film for malaria and other blood parasites.

In countries where malaria is holoendemic, the presence of parasites *in the indigenous population* does not necessarily mean it is the cause of the fever, since a high percentage of persons have asymptomatic parasitemia. The density of parasitemia together with the results of the white blood and platelet counts are often helpful here. If the WBC is normal or reduced, there is thrombocytopenia, and the parasitemia is moderate to high, then malaria is likely to be the cause of the fever. However, leukocytosis is common in severe falciparum malaria.

The following characteristics often indicate the site of infection [11]:

1. Sore throat: streptococcal tonsillitis; diphtheria; Lassa fever
2. Cough, pleuritic pain, rusty sputum: pneumonia
3. Severe pain and swelling in a joint: pyogenic arthritis
4. Severe pain in the head and back of the neck with neck stiffness, headache, and photophobia: meningitis
5. Severe pain in a bone: osteomyelitis with or without SS disease; lymphomas
6. Severe lower abdominal pain: pelvic sepsis
7. Bloody diarrhea: bacillary dysentery; *Campylobacter* infection; *Schistosoma mansoni*
8. Marked localized lymphadenopathy: local sepsis; plague; bancroftian filariasis; tuberculosis; African trypanosomiasis
9. Sharply defined cutaneous inflammation: erysipelas
10. Ill-defined subcutaneous inflammation: cellulitis; pyomyositis; Calabar swelling
11. Tender liver: amebic liver abscess; viral hepatitis

If there are no localizing signs and a polymorphonuclear leukocytosis is present, the likely diagnoses are as follows: septicemias of all kinds, especially meningococcemia; leptospirosis (jaundice and proteinuria may be present); relapsing fever (*Borrelia* spp. will be seen in the blood film during the pyrexial waves); or acute nontyphoid *Salmonella* septicemia (rose spots and splenomegaly occasionally develop).

Of the acute fevers without a raised white cell count, the most common are malaria, togavirus, and rickettsial infections.

Acute Fever with a Rash. A number of diseases in which fever is usually of short duration and somewhat irregular in type are associated with a rash, e.g., togavirus infections, measles, rubella, varicella, scarlet fever, and typhus. If the rash is hemorrhagic, conditions such as Marburg and Ebola virus diseases, dengue, hemorrhagic fever, Congo-Crimean hemorrhagic fevers, Hantaan virus disease, chikungunya, Rift Valley fever, and meningococcemia are possibilities.

Acute Fever with Adenopathy. Human immunodeficiency virus infections, Bancroftian or Malayan filariasis, plague, trypanosomiasis, infectious mononucleosis, lymphogranuloma venereum, or local sepsis may present in this way. Localization of enlarged lymph nodes may be helpful (e.g., cervical—Winterbottom's sign—in African trypanosomiasis).

Acute Fever with Hepatomegaly. Amebic liver abscess or viral hepatitis are common conditions in the tropics. Jaundice can occur in viral hepatitis as well as in falciparum malaria but is uncommon with amebic liver abscess.

Acute Fever with Anemia. Causes include erythrocytic infections such as malaria and bartonellosis; infections associated with a bleeding diathesis such as yellow fever and other viral hemorrhagic fevers and meningococcemia; and any infection in an individual with a preexisting congenital anemia, e.g.,

sickle cell disease, thalassemia, or glucose-6-phosphate dehydrogenase deficiency or preexisting acquired anemia, such as hookworm anemia.

Acute Fever with Eosinophilia. This syndrome suggests acute massive infection with a helminth (e.g., trichinosis if there are acute gastrointestinal symptoms and myositis) or migration of larval helminths (e.g., nematodes such as hookworm, toxocara, and strongyloides if there are pulmonary or cutaneous symptoms). Eosinophilia is associated with katayama fever, infection with schistosomes after 1 to 2 months, and also occurs with fever in early clonorchiasis, paragonimiasis, and in reactions to treatment in onchocerciasis. Eosinophilic meningitis suggests angiostrongyliasis or gnathostomiasis in Asia.

Diagnosis in district, regional, or teaching hospital

This environment often allows a more thorough history to be taken and a more exhaustive physical examination to be carried out. Whenever practicable, the presumptive diagnoses made in the previous section should be confirmed by appropriate investigations, such as culture of a throat swab, blood, urine, or feces; radiology; serology and so on (see also ''Chronic Fever'').

In addition to the WBC the platelet count is often low in malaria infection; this is helpful in differentiating a causative from an incidental parasitemia (but see above). For virological studies culture as well as paired serological tests should be done.

CHRONIC FEVER

In the tropics, chronic fever, defined as fever of more than 2 weeks' duration, is most often caused by infection and malignancy, rarely by connective tissue diseases.

In circumstances where laboratory facilities are rudimentary or very limited, a careful history and thorough physical examination will have to be relied upon to elucidate the problem. Certain essential laboratory examinations to confirm the diagnosis may have to be sent to a more sophisticated laboratory, since in many instances it is impracticable to move the patient. In some circumstances physicians may have to resort to therapeutic trials on the basis of their own findings until the necessary results are received, which in some tropical countries may take a long time.

There is no substitute for a good history. In this respect the following points need to be emphasized: (1) the distribution of the various diseases varies within the same country and their transmission is often seasonal; (2) the ecology of potential vectors is important; (3) the patient's occupation may result in special exposure to infections such as scrub typhus, anthrax, Rift Valley fever, or Kyasanur forest disease; and (4) pets may be the cause of toxocariasis or hydatid disease, while the intake of some foods may be responsible for fascioliasis or trichiniasis. In addition, the patient's immunization record and past history and exposure to venereal disease should be determined. The symptoms of the patient's illness are, of course, of prime importance, as is the presence of spots or sores. Repeated and thorough physical examination, including a rectal examination, is essential. Some patients develop skin lesions, funduscopic changes, enlargement of organs, and masses in the course of their disease. Some areas require daily examination, e.g., skin, eyes, nail beds, lymph glands, abdomen, and heart.

In circumstances where laboratory facilities are good, they should be used intelligently, with the simplest test ordered first and the more complex ones later, as follows: (1) microscopy of blood, (2) examination of urine, (3) hemogram, (4) roentgenogram, (5) sputum, (6) stool, (7) cerebrospinal fluid, (8) repeated cultures, (9) acute and convalescent serum samples for antibody titers, (10) inoculation of blood into laboratory animals, (11) xenodiagnosis, (12) serological tests, (13) virological investigations, and (14) marrow aspiration.

Later such noninvasive procedures as radioactive scans, computed tomography, ultrasound, and lymphoangiography may be required.

Invasive procedures such as biopsy from liver, lymph node, bone marrow, peritoneum, pleura, synovium, or skin for histology and culture may be required for a definitive diagnosis.

It is important to remember that the commonest cause of chronic fever in the tropics is tuberculosis. There is an increasingly obvious association of recrudescent tuberculosis with HIV infections. When the infection is disseminated, the Mantoux test is often negative—an unusual finding in the tropics, where most adults have a positive test unless they are undernourished or otherwise debilitated.

FEVER IN THE INTERNATIONAL TRAVELER

The exponential increase and speed of travel in recent years has resulted in communicable and tropical diseases being encountered in increasing numbers in nonendemic areas. The nature of the infection will depend on the areas of the world that the patient has visited. Thus, travelers to southern Europe may contract enteric fever, legionnaires' disease, kala azar, or brucellosis; those to tropical countries, malaria, trypanosomiasis, filariasis, schistosomiasis, viral hepatitis, dengue, or rare viral infections such as Lassa fever.

The most important single duty of the physician for all patients who have a fever is to take *routinely* a geographical history [*12*] including the following *pertinent* questions: (1) Where exactly have you been and where did you stop on the way? (2) Which prophylactic immunizations did you have before traveling? (3) What precautions, if any, did you take against contracting a communicable disease (e.g., did you eat fresh vegetables or fruit, etc.)? (4) Did you regularly take antimalaria prophylactics and, if so, what? (5) When did you stop taking the tablets? (6) Have other members of your party been ill?

After a thorough physical examination, a blood film for malaria parasites as well as a white blood and platelet count and differential count should be obtained. At this stage, the following courses of action are possible: (1) the physician may have made a confident diagnosis of an infection that can be treated at home; (2) the patient may be referred to a communicable or tropical disease unit for further investigation; or (3) one of the "exotic" viral hemorrhagic fevers, e.g., Lassa fever, may be suspected, in which case the physician must follow the agreed local procedures for dealing with such patients.

Falciparum malaria is a "medical emergency" since early diagnosis and treatment are mandatory. If in doubt, the patient should be treated to avoid a fatal outcome. Safari holidaymakers run the risk of contracting African trypanosomiasis and schistosomiasis.

The most important aspect of "imported fevers" is for physicians to recognize the possibility of their increasing incidence in nonendemic environments.

REFERENCES

1 Dinarello CA, Cannon JG, Wolff SM: New concepts on the pathogenesis of fever. Rev Infect Dis 10:168–189, 1988

2 Dinarello CA, Wolff SM: Molecular basis of fevers in humans. Am J Med 72:799–819, 1982

3 Cooper KE: The neurobiology of fever: Thoughts on recent developments. Ann Rev Neurosci 10:297–324, 1987

4 Murphy PA: Temperature regulation and the pathogenesis of fever, in Mandell GL, Douglas RG Jr, Bennett JE (eds): *Principles and Practice of Infectious Diseases,* 2d ed. New York, Wiley, 1985, pp 334–339

5 Feigin RD: Fever of unknown origin, in Feigin RD, Cherry JD (eds): *Textbook of Pediatric Infectious Diseases.* Philadelphia, Saunders, 1981, pp 787–795

6 Altschule MD, Freedberg AS: Circulation and respiration in fever. Medicine (Baltimore) 24:403, 1945

7 Warrell DA, Pope HM, Parry EHO, et al: Cardiorespiratory disturbances associated with infective fever in man: Studies of Ethiopian louse-borne relapsing fever. Clin Sci 39:123–145, 1970

8 Petersdorf RG, Beeson PB: Fever of unexplained origin: Report of 100 cases. Medicine 40:1, 1961

9 Larson EB, Featherstone HJ, Petersdorf RG: Fever of undetermined origin: Diagnosis and follow-up of 105 cases, 1970–1980. Medicine (Baltimore) 61:269–292, 1982

10 Dinarello CA, Wolff SM: Fever of unknown origin, in Mandell GL, Douglas RG Jr, Bennett JE (eds): *Principles and Practice of Infectious Diseases,* 2d ed. New York, Wiley, 1985, pp 339–347

11 Dinarello CA, Wolff SM: Approach to the patient with fever of unknown origin, in Mandell GL, Douglas RG Jr, Bennett JE (eds): *Principles and Practice of Infectious Diseases,* 2d ed. New York, Wiley, 1985, pp 347–351

12 Bell DR (ed): Fevers in general, in *Lecture Notes on Tropical Medicine,* 2d ed. Oxford, Blackwell, 1985

Gastrointestinal Manifestations

· *V. I. Mathan*

The majority of patients who present to clinicians in tropical countries are likely to complain of some gastrointestinal symptoms. There are no specific ''tropical'' gastrointestinal complaints, but the interpretation of symptoms has to be in the context of local disease patterns. A careful history and physical examination can help to distinguish the symptoms due to problems primarily of the gastrointestinal tract and liver from the gastrointestinal manifestations that may be associated with disease in other organ systems.

Alteration in bowel habits, loss of appetite, abdominal pain, gastrointestinal bleeding, and a feeling of abdominal fullness are the major symptoms of which patients may complain. Among these, the most widely prevalent is diarrhea, an increase in the frequency of stools with increased fecal water content and, sometimes, mucus or blood. For clinical management it is convenient to consider gastrointestinal symptoms in two major groups: diarrhea and other, nondiarrheal symptoms.

DIARRHEA

Diarrhea is only a symptom, the result of failure of adequate absorption of water from the intestinal contents, usually associated with inflammation of the mucosa and motility disorders, with a variety of underlying etiologies. A precise definition of diarrhea is difficult, and most of the accepted definitions are complicated and meant for research purposes, to study etiology, pathogenesis, or therapy. For clinical purposes it is essential to keep in mind that diarrhea is a *symptom* complained of by a patient and that the clinician's responsibility is to manage the patient, detect the underlying pathology, and resolve the symptom. It is useful to divide patients with diarrhea into three groups named for the duration of the symptom: acute diarrhea, persistent diarrhea, or chronic diarrhea.

ACUTE DIARRHEA

Diarrhea of less than 2 weeks' duration is considered acute diarrhea. In a longitudinal morbidity survey in a southern Indian rural community, the median duration of episodes of acute noncholera diarrhea was 2 days and the mean duration 3 days. Only a small proportion of these patients require the attention of a medical practitioner. Acute diarrhea, in addition to being endemic, can also occur in epidemics. The mortality associated with diarrhea is high in most developing countries, and it is estimated that about 15 million deaths due to diarrhea occur worldwide, mostly in tropical countries, mainly in children [1]. Acute diarrhea is not only a problem of children; adults in

tropical developing countries are estimated to suffer from at least one episode of acute diarrhea every 3 to 4 years. In the economy of many developing countries, where the family is dependent on the daily earnings of the adult members, episodes of acute diarrhea in adults can have serious consequences for the welfare of the family. The mortality of acute diarrhea in children and adults can be significantly reduced by oral maintenance of hydration with appropriate liquids containing glucose and electrolytes. This unfortunately does not reduce the morbidity or the economic consequences of diarrhea.

Acute diarrhea is the response of the gastrointestinal tract to a variety of specific infections. As recently as the late 1960s enteric pathogenic microbes could be detected in only about one-quarter of the patients, but the emergence of a variety of new techniques has changed this situation. Current microbiological techniques (culture, stool microscopy, electron microscopy, etc.) can identify enteropathogenic microbes in nearly 80 percent of patients with acute diarrhea. When stool samples from healthy controls in several tropical developing countries were examined using the same microbiological techniques as used for patients with diarrhea, a high prevalence of pathogens was detected (Table 3-1). It is clear that in the unhygienic environment of much of the tropical developing world, there is a large circulation of enteric pathogens in the community [1–3]. At birth children acquire antibodies (predominantly IgA) from the mother transplacentally and through breast milk. The prior experience of the mother could therefore determine the susceptibility of the young infant to a certain extent. It has been shown that exposure to pathogens, even in young chil-

Table 3-1. Rate of isolation of enteric pathogens in a consecutive series of 916 children with acute diarrhea and 587 matched asymptomatic case controls in southern India

Pathogen	Rate of isolation, %*	
	Patients	**Controls**
Salmonella sp.	3.7	6.0
Shigella sp.	19.7	2.7
Enteropathogenic *E. coli*	9.1	6.6
Enterotoxigenic *E. coli*	14.4	7.2
Campylobacter	15.2	13.5
Other bacteria	2.3	2.1
Parasites	19.2	16.4
Rotavirus	17.7	1.2
Other viruses	13.7	9.4

*One-third of the patients with diarrhea and 12% of the controls had more than one pathogen at the same time.

dren, is not necessarily associated with episodes of diarrhea. The factors that determine the emergence of this symptom in each host-pathogen encounter are not yet understood. However, the lower incidence of acute diarrhea in adults in tropical countries, as compared to the children, indicates the development of protective immunity acquired by living in a contaminated environment. Adults from temperate countries who visit tropical developing countries develop episodes of acute diarrhea (travelers' diarrhea, tourista, Delhi belly, Montezuma's revenge, etc.), and a spectrum of agents similar to those isolated from children in that country can be isolated from these adult patients.

Several microbial virulence factors that can initiate pathogenic mechanisms leading to diarrhea have been identified [4]. The production of an exotoxin, enterotoxin, was classically demonstrated in *Vibrio cholerae*, the causative agent of Asiatic cholera. Cholera toxin is a protein with two subunits, the B subunit binding to a specific receptor on the enterocyte surface membrane, following which the A subunit initiates water secretion by the small-intestinal mucosa, with adenylcyclase and cyclic adenosine monophosphate (AMP) acting as mediators. The ability of enterocytes to absorb water along with glucose is intact in such patients and is used in the strategy of oral glucose-electrolyte therapy. A variety of other enteric pathogens also elaborate toxins that can stimulate water secretion. Some microbes (e.g., *Shigellae*, enteroinvasive *Escherichia coli, Entamoeba histolytica*, etc.) can penetrate the epithelial lining of the gastrointestinal tract, damage enterocytes and colonocytes, and lead to diarrhea, usually with blood or mucus in the stool. The majority of such invasive pathogens damage the colon, but viruses such as the rotavirus invade and damage the upper small intestine and usually result in watery diarrhea. Several organisms (e.g., *Shigella, Campylobacter*) are both enteroinvasive and toxin-producing. The relative importance of these two virulence factors is not yet fully elucidated. Another group of organisms are enteroadhesive and produce changes in the enterocyte and colonocyte surface membrane that result in acute diarrhea. Not even one of these three mechanisms of pathogenesis of diarrhea can be demonstrated in all organisms isolated from patients, and in about 20 to 25 percent of patients there are no pathogens recognizable by current methods [1]. Recently it has been suggested on the basis of animal experiments that a neurohumoral-vascular response by the host to as yet unknown trigger signals initiated by microbes may be important in pathogenesis [5–7]. In southern India a vascular lesion was found to be present in the rectal mucosal lamina propria in adults with acute infectious diarrhea. The prevalence of this vascular lesion correlated not with the type of enteric pathogen that was isolated, but with the clinical severity of diarrhea [8]. Ultrastructural studies suggested that this lesion was the result of damage to the endothelial lining of the lamina propria microvasculature by gram-negative bacterial endotoxin [9]. An animal model in which acute diarrhea can be induced by bacterial lipopolysaccharide after appropri-

ate sensitization has been described, and this may be another mechanism of pathogenesis [10]. It is now clear that the response of the host to the microbial pathogen is at least as important as microbial virulence factors.

While a variety of microbial virulence factors and host responses may be operative in the pathogenesis of acute diarrhea, the ultimate result is a reduction in the net absorption of water (due to reduced absorption, increased secretion, or both). The early mortality associated with acute diarrhea is due to dehydration. The strategy of oral rehydration has been devised taking advantage of the fact that glucose-mediated water and sodium absorption is intact even in cholera. The oral rehydration solution recommended by the World Health Organization (Table 3-2) effectively replaces lost body fluids and electrolytes but does not reduce the severity of the diarrhea or provide adequate nutrient energy. There are also problems of availability of the salt-sugar mixture in rural areas and poor acceptability by the mothers of this nontraditional method of management. A variety of studies are being carried out to further modify the composition of the oral rehydration fluids to overcome these drawbacks. Cereal-based fluids or home-available fluids appear to be a promising alternative. They may also overcome the lack of acceptance of the glucose-electrolyte solution in several rural communities by utilizing locally available cereals that may already be used by mothers for children with diarrhea.

Antimicrobials (antibiotics and chemotherapeutic drugs) have a limited role in the management of uncomplicated acute diarrhea [11]. It has been shown that the total fluid loss from the body is significantly reduced in patients with cholera if appropriate antibiotics are given. While antibiotics are thus indicated in patients with cholera, their utility in diarrhea associated with other toxigenic enteropathogens is not established. *Shigella* dysentery requires antibiotic therapy, but multi-drug-resistant *Shigellae* are widely prevalent, and the antibiotic sensitivity pattern in each locality has to be taken into account in planning appropriate therapeutic measures. In certain localities the protozoan parasite. *E. histolytica* may be a more frequent cause of dysentery than *Shigella,* and therapy with metronidazole is essential. Stool microscopy has to be painstaking to identify this pathogen. Except for these specific indications, antimicrobials do not contribute to the successful management of acute diarrhea, while the maintenance of hy-

Table 3-2. Composition of glucose-electrolyte solution useful for oral maintenance of hydration in diarrhea*

Component	g/L
Sodium chloride	3.5
Sodium bicarbonate	2.5
Potassium chloride	1.5
Glucose (sucrose)	20.0 (40.0)

*Each liter contains sodium, 90 meq; potassium, 20 meq; chloride, 80 meq; bicarbonate, 30 meq; glucose, 111 meq.

dration and nutrition is essential in all patients. The use of antibiotics as a prophylactic against travelers' diarrhea has been advocated, but sound hygienic practices are a more acceptable alternative.

Acute diarrhea is generally thought of as an endemic problem, and the magnitude of epidemics of acute diarrhea is seldom recognized. The exceptions were the pandemics due to *S. dysenteriae* 1 in Latin America and south Asia in the late 1960s and 1970s. They were associated with multi-drug-resistant organisms and led to considerable morbidity and mortality. In a 20-year watch for epidemics of acute diarrhea in 200 villages with a continued population of about 200,000 in southern India, nearly 40 epidemics of acute diarrhea were detected. Microbial pathogens that could be causally implicated were found in less than half of these epidemics. They were common source outbreaks, outbreaks due to contaminated water supply, and several in which the mode of spread could not be determined. In most of the common source outbreaks, in that crowded habitat, there was secondary person to person spread. The risk of such outbreaks is high where large groups of people gather or following natural calamities like floods, earthquakes, etc., and it is necessary to ensure adequate hygienic measures under such circumstances and to develop appropriate strategies for control of the epidemic.

PERSISTENT DIARRHEA

Only a very small proportion of all episodes of acute diarrhea in the community persist for longer than 2 weeks. However, in hospitals a significant number of such patients are seen [12,13]. One well-recognized mechanism of persistence is secondary lactose intolerance following infective diarrhea in small children. Exclusion of lactose (milk) from the diet is necessary in the management of such children. The pathogenic mechanisms cannot be clearly defined in many children with persistent diarrhea, although enteroadhesive *E. coli, Giardia lamblia,* and *Cryptosporidium* have been implicated in some studies. In adults with shigellosis, persistence has been attributed to cell-mediated colonocyte damage, mucosal ischemia secondary to vascular lesion, and crypt colonocyte damage due to bacterial endotoxin [14]. Whatever the pathogenesis, the maintenance of nutrition is a challenging problem in the management of such patients. With nutritional support the majority of such patients recover in about 4 weeks.

CHRONIC DIARRHEA

Diarrhea persisting for longer than a month is chronic diarrhea. A large number of clinical conditions can give rise to chronic diarrhea. Many are associated with malabsorption of nutrients, and some are more prevalent in tropical countries. While detailed investigations are necessary to identify the underlying pathology, a clinical classification is useful in dealing with the patients. Patients presenting with chronic diarrhea can be conveniently divided into those with and those without accom-

panying signs of malnutrition. A further clinical division in each category is possible based on the presence or absence of blood in the stool (Table 3-3). The majority of patients who give a history of chronic diarrhea but have no signs of malnutrition and no blood in the stool are likely to be patients with the irritable bowel syndrome, which is as widely prevalent in the tropics as in industrialized countries. They can be distinguished from patients with genuine chronic diarrhea by showing that fecal weight and fecal water are within normal limits. Blood streaking of the stool due to hemorrhoids may be present in such patients. In patients with chronic diarrhea without significant malnutrition but with a history of blood in the stools, the possibility of early neoplastic lesions of the colon or parasite-associated conditions like amebomas, whipworm colitis, or schistosomiasis should be entertained. A large number of conditions can give rise to chronic diarrhea with signs of malnutrition, the majority associated with malabsorption syndromes. Inflammatory bowel disease, especially ulcerative colitis, is being recognized with increasing frequency in tropical countries and should be considered in patients with chronic diarrhea with persistent blood in the stool. Crohn's disease is still recognized less frequently, and in the individual patient tuberculous infection has to be excluded before the diagnosis can be considered. Colonic and rectal neoplasms are also important in patients with persistent blood in the stool. In patients with chronic diarrhea without blood but with signs of nutritional deficiency, an underlying malabsorption syndrome is the likely possibility.

The differential diagnosis of the malabsorption syndromes is particularly difficult in many tropical developing countries, since the many detailed investigations that are necessary are not yet widely available. The aim of investigating such patients is threefold (1) to establish that the patient has malabsorption of nutrients, (2) to evaluate the nutritional sequelae of malabsorption so that adequate supplementation can be given, and (3) to determine the pathogenesis of the malabsorption.

Table 3-3. Clinical classification of chronic diarrhea

No clinical signs of malnutrition:
  No blood in stool
    Irritable bowel syndrome
  Blood present in stool
    Early neoplastic disease
    Ameboma
    Uncomplicated ulcerative colitis
Clinical signs of malnutrition:
  Blood present in stool
    Inflammatory bowel disease (ulcerative colitis)
    Advanced colorectal neoplasia
  No blood in stool
    Malabsorption syndromes
      Primary malabsorption—tropical sprue
      Secondary malabsorption
      Human immunodeficiency virus infection

The widespread prevalence of minor intestinal mucosal morphological abnormalities in the upper small bowel with mild impairment of absorption of nutrients in most apparently healthy indigenous populations of tropical countries has to be kept in mind when patients are evaluated [*15*]. These alterations, termed *tropical enteropathy,* are likely to be an adaptation to life in the contaminated environment of the tropics with its frequent enteric infections and the diet consumed by these populations. Similar morphological lesions have now also been demonstrated in the colons of healthy residents of southern India [*16*]. Expatriates from temperate climates to the tropics develop these changes; they revert to the temperate zone pattern on their return [*17*].

A variety of tests are available to document malabsorption. A simple microscopic examination of a stool smear, stained with a fat stain such as Sudan III, can reveal fat droplets and fatty acid crystals. A more quantitative estimation of fat absorption is possible with fecal fat estimations or a variety of breath estimations after oral intake of labeled fats. There are no specific tests of absorption of nutrient carbohydrates. The xylose absorption test is unlikely to be a measure of nutrient carbohydrate absorption and is more likely to reflect the total intestinal absorptive area [*18*]. Quantitation of fecal calorie excretion is a good measure of total energy absorption [*19*]. Nitrogen balance studies are tedious and have little role to play in the clinical evaluation of patients. The absorption of a variety of other nutrients can also be measured; of particular value is measurement of vitamin B_{12} absorption, which can indicate ileal function. The tests that are usually used in the clinical situation are fecal fat, xylose absorption, and vitamin B_{12} absorption.

The nutritional background of the population has also to be taken into consideration when the nutritional sequelae of malabsorption are being evaluated. Several clinical signs of nutritional deficiency—pallor, edema, glossitis, stomatitis, and skin changes—can provide valuable clues. Objective measurements of hemoglobin concentration and serum concentrations of iron, folate, vitamin B_{12}, vitamin A, albumin, and other nutrients are useful in planning therapeutic supplements. Many of the patients may have megaloblastic anemia. Trace element deficiency may also be a problem.

Malabsorption and the consequent malnutrition is the result of a variety of factors that either damage the enterocyte or interfere in the process of digestion and absorption [*13*]. While nutritional supplementation, correction of dehydration, and symptomatic treatment of diarrhea will help to improve the condition of the patients, it is critical to identify any underlying condition and take appropriate corrective action. The pathogenic mechanisms of a large number of conditions that manifest with malabsorption are well understood, and these can be generally classified as the secondary malabsorption syndromes (Table 3-4). They include inadequate digestion due to luminal factors or deficiencies of exocrine digestive secretions, mucosal damage by a variety of agents, and interference with

Table 3-4. Working classification of malabsorption syndromes

1. Secondary malabsorption
   1.1. Inadequate digestion
   1.1.1. Luminal factors:
       Reduced intestinal bile salt concentration
       Bacterial overgrowth (especially strictures)
       Intestinal pseudoobstruction, Chagas' disease
       Postsurgical alterations
       Gastrojejunocolic fistulas
       Gastrinoma with hyperacidity
       Drug-induced: neomycin, cholestyramine
   1.1.2. Deficiency of digestive secretion:
       Chronic pancreatitis
       Liver disease
       Obstructive jaundice
   1.2. Inadequate mucosal surface area
   1.2.1. Postsurgical, short-bowel syndrome, gastrojejunocolic fistulas
   1.3. Metabolic and endocrine causes:
       Hyperthyroidism, carcinoid syndrome, VIPoma, etc.
       Hypo- or agammaglobulinemia
   1.4. Interference with lymphatic transport:
       Filariasis
       Tabes mesenterica
       Constrictive pericarditis
       Lymphangiectasia
   1.5. Mucosal absorptive defects
   1.5.1. Parasites:
       Giardia lamblia
       Strongyloides stercoralis
       Capillaria philippinensis
       Cryptosporidium
       Coccidia
   1.5.2. Biochemical or genetic disorders:
       Gluten-sensitive enteropathy (celiac sprue)
       Dermatitis herpetiformis
       Abetalipoproteinemia
       Disaccharidase deficiency (especially lactase)
   1.5.3. Other infections:
       Whipple's disease
       Human immunodeficiency virus infection
   1.5.4. Miscellaneous:
       Amyloidosis
       Lymphoma
       Systemic sclerosis
       Mastocytosis
       Eosinophilic enteritis
2. Primary malabsorption syndrome: tropical sprue

transport of nutrients after absorption. Detailed investigation of the patient may include barium meal examination with follow-through studies of the small intestine, small-bowel enemas, barium enema with double-contrast studies, jejunal and colonic mucosal biopsies, examination of the small-intestinal luminal fluid for bacteria, parasites, and bile salts, and evaluation of pancreatic and liver functions. The conditions that

Table 3-5. Tests useful in the differential diagnosis of the malabsorption syndromes and chronic diarrhea

Tests	Useful to diagnose
Barium meal follow-through and small-bowel enema	Strictures, blind loops, diverticula, bypass
Barium enema	Ileocecal tuberculosis, inflammatory bowel diseases
Jejunal biopsies	Celiac sprue, Whipple's disease, lymphoma
	Useful in tropical sprue, eosinophilic enteritis, agammaglobulinemia, parasitic disease
Intestinal luminal fluid	Bacterial overgrowth, bile salt deficiency, parasites

can be diagnosed by these tests are listed in Table 3-5. In a significant proportion of patients with the malabsorption syndrome no specific underlying pathology can be detected, and they must be diagnosed as patients with a primary malabsorption syndrome, or tropical sprue [20,21]. This disease, or, more correctly, syndrome, is one among several conditions that will have to be particularly considered in the differential diagnosis of malabsorption syndromes in the tropics.

Tropical sprue

Tropical sprue is defined as a primary malabsorption syndrome in residents of or visitors to several tropical regions [20]. The syndrome is endemic in most of the tropics, but has not been reported from sub-Saharan Africa or Jamaica, although it is widely prevalent in the other Caribbean Islands. Epidemics of tropical sprue have been reported from the Indian subcontinent, and the available epidemiological evidence suggests an infectious etiology, although no agent has been isolated [20]. Patients present with chronic diarrhea, malabsorption of a variety of nutrients, and signs of extensive nutritional deficiencies. It has been suggested that nutritional deficiencies may be important in the etiology, but the evidence for this is not conclusive, and analysis of data on large number of patients clearly shows that the deficiency states are the consequence and not the cause of malabsorption.

Three major geographically defined groups of patients have been studied extensively: expatriates from the temperate zone resident in south and southeast Asia [22], patients with Caribbean tropical sprue, and native patients with tropical sprue in southern India. There appear to be differences between these three groups of patients, which suggests that tropical sprue is a syndrome with possibly a multiplicity of causes. In both expatriate sprue and Caribbean sprue folate deficiency is a major presenting feature; almost all patients have vitamin B_{12} malabsorption, and the patients respond well to therapy with folic acid and antibiotics [23]. In the Caribbean area chronic colonization of the small intestine with toxin-producing coli-

forms has been shown to be causal and their eradication curative [24]. In contrast, in southern India only two-thirds of patients have folate deficiency or vitamin B_{12} malabsorption, and the response of the patients to folate and antibiotic therapy is variable, with about 50 percent of the patients going into apparently spontaneous cure if nutritional support is maintained. There is no evidence that small-bowel bacterial colonization plays a role in southern Indian tropical sprue [25].

Ultrastructural studies and in vitro organ culture of jejunal mucosal biopsies from patients with tropical sprue in southern India have shown that the primary lesion occurs in enterocytes in the stem cell compartment in the crypts [26]. This lesion can be demonstrated early during the course of illness in epidemic tropical sprue, with persistence in some patients who develop chronic malabsorption and rapid recovery in others. The factors that predispose to recovery or persistence and the agent(s) damaging the stem cell are not yet known. It is also not known whether a similar enterocyte stem cell lesion is present in patients with tropical sprue in other geographical areas.

The colon also is apparently damaged in patients with tropical sprue in southern India, who show defective water and electrolyte absorption. This appears to be the major defect leading to diarrhea [27].

Small-intestinal parasites

Malabsorption syndromes can result from colonization of the small intestine by several parasites, *G. lamblia* [28], *Strongyloides stercoralis* [29], *Cryptosporidium* [30], *Isospora* [31], and *Capillaria philippinensis* [32]. While chronic diarrhea due to these parasites is more common in immunocompromised individuals, they do cause illness in the immunocompetent also. It may be necessary to examine small-intestinal luminal fluid and biopsies repeatedly to make the diagnosis. Appropriate therapy can eradicate the infestation and give relief to the patient.

Abdominal tuberculosis

Tuberculous infection is still widespread in many tropical areas, and abdominal tuberculosis can present in four forms: glandular, tuberculous peritonitis, ileocecal tuberculosis, and tuberculous enteritis [33]. Peritonitis and ileocecal tuberculosis seldom present with chronic diarrhea and malabsorption. Retroperitoneal tuberculous lymphadenitis (tabes mesenterica) can produce malabsorption by lymphatic obstruction but is rare. Tuberculous enteritis can give rise to intestinal strictures and secondary bacterial overgrowth and a malabsorption syndrome. Diagnosis is difficult since visualization of the strictures, usually in the distal small bowel, is difficult even with small-bowel enema examination. A history of persistent pyrexia with evening rise of temperature and episodes of colicky abdominal pain should suggest the possibility. Laparotomy is usually necessary to obtain histopathological proof of the infection. Resections should be limited to the minimum extent possible, since adequate chemotherapy can resolve the lesions.

Lymphoma of the intestine

Focal or diffuse primary intestinal lymphoma is relatively rare. The diffuse form usually involves the proximal small intestine and can give rise to severe malabsorption [34]. This form is more frequent in the Mediterranean littoral but has been reported in other tropical countries. All stages—from diffuse proliferation of the immunocytes to fully developed lymphomas—can be seen in such patients. A fast-moving paraprotein which does not conform to IgA and which contains an α heavy chain can be identified in a high proportion of such patients. This immunoproliferative small-intestinal disorder can be treated in the early stages with long-term tetracyclines, but once a lymphoma is established, antimitotic drugs are necessary.

Tropical pancreatitis

The syndrome of chronic calcific pancreatitis, without prior history of alcohol ingestion, viral infections, or acute pancreatitis is prevalent in certain tropical regions, Central and South Africa, Indonesia, and southern India [35]. This does not also seem to be secondary to a definable chronic nutritional deficiency, although pancreatic atrophy is found in kwashiorkor and severe malnutrition. Severe and unrelenting upper abdominal pain is complained of by a proportion of the patients, although in others the first clue may be the detection of pancreatic calculi on a plain skiagram of the abdomen. The patients have malabsorption with steatorrhea, the fecal fat consisting mainly of unsplit fats, and they can develop diabetes mellitus. The pancreatic lithiasis can extend to total destruction of the organ. Pancreatic enzyme supplementation with food is necessary in the management of these patients.

Human immunodeficiency virus (HIV) infection

Chronic diarrhea, malabsorption, and wasting in patients with HIV infection has led to its local name, ''slim disease,'' in parts of the African continent [36]. The diarrhea and malabsorption have been attributed to secondary opportunistic infection, but have been documented in patients with no demonstrable enteric pathogen. Recent reports that there are morphological alterations in the small-intestinal mucosa unassociated with opportunistic infection raise the question of whether the intestinal manifestations may be the result of HIV infection per se damaging the mucosa [37].

OTHER GASTROINTESTINAL SYMPTOMS

LOSS OF APPETITE

Anorexia, especially of recent onset, should alert the clinician to attempt early diagnosis of neoplastic diseases. Carcinoma of the stomach, especially in the younger age group, is frequent in some tropical countries (in southern India 16 of 100 consecutive patients with carcinoma of the stomach were under 30 years of age). Since atrophic gastritis is also widely prevalent in many such areas, the symptom may be lightly dismissed. All patients with recent onset of anorexia, irrespective of their age, should have upper-gastrointestinal endoscopy, if facilities are available. Anorexia may also be the presentation of a variety of diseases in other organ systems (e.g., congestive cardiac failure or liver disease), as well as of some of the malabsorption syndromes.

ABDOMINAL PAIN

Abdominal pain is a frequent complaint, and, particularly with uneducated patients, it is difficult to characterize the nature and location of the pain accurately. Three major profiles of abdominal pain should be distinguished.

Epigastric pain and heartburn

Peptic ulcer and esophagitis are frequently encountered in many areas of the tropics. The characteristic relationship to food (hunger pains in duodenal ulcer and food-induced pain in gastric ulcer) and posture and the occurrence of nocturnal pain which wakes the patient in the early hours of the morning are helpful in diagnosing organic lesions. All such patients should have upper-gastrointestinal endoscopy, since the syndrome of nonulcer dyspepsia is being recognized with increasing frequency as part of functional bowel disorders. Epigastric pain, usually severe and persistent, may be a manifestation of tropical pancreatitis syndrome.

Colicky abdominal pain

Many patients, particularly young children, are unable to describe the classical episodic crampy abdominal pain of colic. Parasitic infestation, especially with roundworms, tuberculous intestinal strictures, and lead poisoning are particularly important as underlying causes. A ball-rolling movement in the abdomen noted by the patient is often associated with roundworms or intestinal strictures.

Left lower quadrant pain

Crampy or persistent pain localized to the left lower quadrant, often associated with constipation or small, frequent stools, may be dismissed by the clinician as due to an irritable bowel. The sigmoid colon is often palpable, and sigmoidoscopy, preferably with a flexible sigmoidoscope, is essential in all such patients. Inflammatory lesions, especially associated with infection by *E. histolytica*, schistosomes, or other parasites, and with neoplastic lesions have to be excluded.

CONSTIPATION

Since many of the population groups in tropical countries consume a high-residue diet, it might be assumed that constipation as a presenting symptom is rare. This is not so, and while neoplastic and other obstructive lesions of the colon should be considered, primary constipation that might respond to appropriate modifications of the diet is not infrequently encountered in consultant gastrointestinal practice.

GASTROINTESTINAL BLEEDING

Hematemesis and melena are important symptoms with immediate life-threatening sequelae. There are likely to be regional differences in the underlying diseases. In southern India, about 80 percent of such patients have portal hypertension–associated bleeding, while in northern India, the proportion is less.

ABDOMINAL MASSES

Abdominal masses other than hepatosplenomegaly are less frequently encountered. The commonest in many countries are due to tuberculous infections, but patients with gastrointestinal malignancy unfortunately often present when the disease is advanced and large masses are present. Amebic abscesses may also present as abdominal masses unrelated to the liver.

FUNCTIONAL BOWEL DISORDERS

The irritable bowel syndrome and nonulcer dyspepsia are considered by many to be the result of the divorce from nature in industrialized societies. The reality to clinicians in tropical countries is very different, with up to 50 percent of patients in gastroenterology clinics complaining of gaseousness, abdominal distension, dyspepsia, ill-defined abdominal pain, and frequent stools. With the variety of parasitic infection that is widely prevalent in such populations, it is quite feasible to diagnose chronic amebiasis or giardiasis in such patients. However, it must be emphasized that the same spectrum of functional bowel disorders that are prevalent in industrialized countries can be found in tropical developing countries. Before ascribing diagnostic significance to parasitic cysts found in such patients, it is essential to know the prevalence of the parasite in the population and to ensure that therapeutic eradication of the parasite leads to relief of symptoms.

REFERENCES

1 Tzipori S (ed): *Infectious Diarrhoea in the Young*. Amsterdam, Excerpta Medica, 1985
2 Rajan DP, Mathan VI: Prevalence of *Campylobacter fetus,* subsp. *jejuni* in healthy populations in southern India. J Clin Microbiol 15:749–751, 1982
3 Mathan VI, Rajan DP: The prevalence of bacterial enteric pathogens in a healthy population in southern India. J Med Microbiol 22:93–99, 1986
4 CIBA Foundation Symposium 42: *Acute Diarrhoea in Childhood*. Amsterdam, Elsevier, 1976
5 Eklund S, Jondal M, Lundgren O: The enteric nervous system participates in the secretory response to the heat stable enterotoxins of *Escherichia coli* in rats and cats. Neurosciences 14:673–681, 1985
6 Osborne MP, Haddon SJ, Spencer AJ, et al: An electron microscopic investigation of time-related changes in the intestine of neonatal mice infected with murine rotavirus. J Pediatr Gastroenterol Nutr 7:236–248, 1988
7 Collins J, Starkey WG, Wallis TS, et al: Intestinal enzyme profiles in normal and rotavirus-infected mice. J Pediatr Gastroenterol Nutr 7:264–272, 1988
8 Chaudari CP, Mathan M, Rajan DP, et al: A correlative study of etiology, clinical features and rectal mucosal pathology in adults with acute infectious diarrhea in southern India. Pathology 17: 443–450, 1985
9 Mathan M, Mathan VI: Local Shwartzman reaction in the rectal mucosa in acute diarrhoea. J Pathol 146:179–187, 1985
10 Mathan VI, Penny GR, Mathan M, et al: Bacterial lipopolysaccharide induced intestinal microvascular lesions leading to acute diarrhoea. J Clin Invest 82:1714–1721, 1988
11 Holmgren J, Lindberg A, Mollby R (eds): *Development of Vaccine and Drugs Against Diarrhea*. Chartwell-Bratt Ltd, 1986
12 Walker-Smith JA, McNeish AS (eds): *Diarrhoea and Malnutrition in Childhood*. London, Butterworth, 1986
13 Lebenthal E (ed): *Chronic Diarrhea in Children*. New York, Raven, 1984
14 Mathan MM, Mathan VI: Ultrastructural pathology of the rectal mucosa in *Shigella* dysentery. Am J Pathol 123:25–38, 1986
15 Baker SJ, Mathan VI: Tropical enteropathy and tropical sprue. Am J Clin Nutr 25:1047–1055, 1972
16 Mathan M, Mathan VI: Rectal mucosal morphologic abnormalities in normal subjects in southern India. A tropical colonopathy. Gut 26:710–717, 1985
17 Lindenbaum J: Tropical enteropathy. Gastroenterology 64: 637–652, 1973
18 Rolston DDK, Mathan VI: Xylose transport in the human jejunum. Digest Dis Sci, in press
19 Chacko A, Begum A, Mathan VI: Absorption of nutrient energy in southern Indian control subjects and patients with tropical sprue. Am J Clin Nutr 40:771–775, 1984
20 The Wellcome Trust, London: *Tropical Sprue and Megaloblastic Anaemia*. London, Churchill Livingston, 1971
21 Mathan VI: Tropical sprue in southern India. Trans R Soc Trop Med Hyg 82:10–14, 1988
22 Klipstein FA: Tropical sprue in travellers and expatriates living abroad. Gastroenterology 80:590–600, 1981
23 Klipstein FA, Samloff MI, Schenk EA: Tropical sprue in Haiti. Ann Intern Med 64:575–594, 1966
24 Klipstein FA, Holdeman LV, Corcino JJ, et al: Enterotoxigenic intestinal bacteria in tropical sprue. Ann Intern Med 79:632–641, 1973
25 Bhat P, Shanthakumari S, Rajan D, et al: Bacterial flora of the gastrointestinal tract in southern Indian control subjects and patients with tropical sprue. Gastroenterology 62:11–21, 1972
26 Mathan M, Ponniah J, Mathan VI: Epithelial cell renewal and turnover and its relationship to the morphological abnormalities in the jejunal mucosa in tropical sprue. Digest Dis Sci 31:586–593, 1986

27 Ramakrishna BS, Mathan VI: The role of bacterial toxins, bile acids and free fatty acids in colonic water malabsorption and tropical sprue. Digest Dis Sci 32:500–505, 1987

28 Wright SG, Tomkins AM, Ridley DS: Giardiasis: Clinical and therapeutic aspects. Gut 18:343–350, 1977

29 Milder JE, Walzer PD, Kilgore G, et al: Clinical features of *Strongyloides stercoralis* infection in an endemic area of the United States. Gastroenterology 80:1481–1488, 1981

30 Mathan MM, Venkatesan S, George R, et al: Cryptosporidium and diarrhoea in southern Indian children. Lancet ii:1172–1175, 1985

31 Trier JS, Moxey PL, Schimmel PC, et al: Chronic intestinal coccidiosis in man: Intestinal morphology and response to treatment. Gastroenterology 66:923–935, 1974

32 Whalen GG, Strickland GT, Cross JH, et al: Intestinal capillariasis. A new disease in man. Lancet i:13–17, 1969

33 Chuttani HK: Intestinal tuberculosis, in Card WI, Creamer B (eds): *Modern Trends in Gastroenterology*. Butterworth, London, 1970, p 373

34 Ramot B: Malabsorption due to lymphomatous disease. Annu Rev Med 22:19–24, 1971

35 Pitchumoni CS: Pancreas in primary malnutrition diseases. Am J Clin Nutr 26:375–379, 1973

36 Serwadda D, Mugerwa RD, Sewankambo NK, et al: Slim disease: A new disease in Uganda and its association with HTLV-III infection. Lancet ii:849–852, 1985

37 Griffin GE, Miller A, Batman P, et al: Damage to jejunal intrinsic autonomic nerves in human immunodeficiency virus infection. AIDS, in press

CHAPTER 4 / *Hepatic Disorders* · Malcolm E. Molyneux

HEPATIC SYMPTOMS

Some diseases of the liver, e.g., hepatic schistosomiasis, have a restricted "tropical" distribution; others occur throughout the world but are more common in developing than in industrialized countries, e.g., hepatocellular carcinoma. Some hepatic conditions are encountered less often in the tropics then elsewhere, e.g., gallstones. The liver may be the organ primarily involved in a disease, as in hepatitis or liver abscess, or it may be affected by a disorder in another organ, as in congestive cardiac failure. Sometimes hepatic damage is part of a generalized systemic disease such as typhoid fever. A carefully directed history and examination can help toward the diagnosis of common clinical syndromes, and it is usually possible to use simple and inexpensive tests to confirm a diagnosis and guide therapy.

ILLNESS OF RECENT ONSET WITH MALAISE AND JAUNDICE

A characteristic history of symptoms may suggest viral hepatitis. In developing countries most adults are already immune to hepatitis A; more likely possibilities are B, non-A non-B, or δ hepatitis. A preceding history of severe joint pains and swelling, with or without urticarial rash, suggests the preicteric serum sickness–like syndrome of hepatitis B. Enquire about blood transfusion, needle stick injuries, and sexual exposure. In a patient known to be a hepatitis B carrier, the current illness may be due to δ hepatitis (hepatitis D), which is more often fulminant than the other types of hepatitis. Some kinds of hepatitis are reported to be more severe in pregnancy, particularly epidemic non-A non-B hepatitis. If the patient is in the third trimester of pregnancy, consider a diagnosis of "acute fatty liver of pregnancy," a severe form of liver necrosis of unknown cause. Ask about alcohol consumption, and especially about home-distilled spirits, which may be potently hepatotoxic. If several members of the family or community have become ill simultaneously, a food contaminant, e.g., aflatoxin, may be suspected. In areas where yellow fever occurs, this diagnosis must be considered, especially if there have been several recent deaths from acute icteric disease. Enquire about drugs and traditional herbal remedies, although taking these may have been the result rather than the cause of symptoms. A history of severe limb pains is usual in a crisis of sickle cell anemia. Malaria may mimic hepatitis: moderate jaundice is common in falciparum malaria, especially in the nonimmune.

The most important assessment to make on examination is of cerebral function: if there is altered consciousness, immediately look for and correct hypoglycemia, which may complicate hepatitis, malaria, or toxic hepatic necrosis, especially in children. Look for signs of hemorrhage in skin, mucosae, and optic fundi. These may suggest a viral hemorrhagic fever, leptospirosis, relapsing fever, or fulminant hepatic necrosis. Conjunctivitis and meningism are common in leptospirosis. Measure the size of the liver by firm percussion from above and by soft percussion from below. The liver may be enlarged and tender in hepatitis, but if pain and tenderness are severe, consider ascending cholangitis, which in southeast Asia may occur in the fluke infestations opisthorchiasis and clonorchiasis. Reduced hepatic dullness should warn you of possible impending hepatic necrosis. Examine the chest carefully; jaundice commonly complicates lobar pneumonia in some communities, particularly in central Africa.

The most useful investigations are inexpensive. Blood glucose can be measured immediately by glucose-oxidase strip in the patient with altered consciousness. Shake a sample of urine in a test tube; yellow coloration of the froth indicates conjugated bilirubin and hepatocellular or obstructive jaundice. A hematocrit and thin blood film may reveal anemia, sickling of red cells, and other features of hemolysis, or may show the spirochetes of relapsing fever or malaria parasites. Neutropenia and thrombocytopenia may be seen in hepatitis, yellow fever, relapsing fever, and malaria; a leukocytosis suggests leptospirosis, septicemia, or cholangitis. Stool microscopy may reveal the ova of *Opisthorchis* or *Clonorchis*. Conventional "liver function tests" are expensive and too often performed as a routine; they seldom give an unequivocal diagnosis and should, if available, be used selectively, not invariably. Specific serological tests are available for many infections. For hepatitis A, B, and δ, and for infections by other viral agents such as cytomegalovirus or Epstein-Barr virus, a single acute plasma sample is sufficient; for other viruses paired samples give a retrospective diagnosis, which may be important epidemiologically or in research studies but cannot influence immediate management. Non-A non-B hepatitis remains (in 1989) a diagnosis of exclusion.

HEPATOMEGALY

The patient may have been aware of a mass in the upper abdomen. A history of pain is unlikely to distinguish between the causes of liver enlargement; it may be local or referred to the shoulder. Both abscess and tumor may be painless or extremely painful. Severe pain in a rapidly enlarging liver may be the presenting symptom of cardiac tamponade and may be prominent in congestive cardiac failure or right-sided heart failure of any cause. The geographical and occupational history may alert you to the possibility of hydatid disease; hepatic cysts are commonly painless, but may cause increasing discomfort. Recent hemoptysis may be a clue to amebic liver abscess which has ruptured into the lung; but pulmonary tuberculosis is an alternative possibility—occasionally the liver contains multiple or massive tuberculomas. Hepatic vein thrombosis, which may result from the ingestion of bush teas ("venoocclusive disease") or may complicate primary carcinoma, causes painful hepatomegaly of rapid onset, usually with ascites. Alcohol may cause massive fatty enlargement of the liver and eventually cirrhosis, although more cirrhosis in the tropics is related to hepatitis B virus than to alcohol. Diffuse hepatomegaly in a young child in India, or less commonly elsewhere, may be due to Indian childhood cirrhosis.

The commonest error on examination is to neglect cardiac signs, particularly the elusive ones of constrictive pericarditis (usually tuberculous) or endomyocardial fibrosis. Look carefully for pulsus paradoxus and raised venous pressure, and for precordial signs of pericardial effusion or constriction. Ascites is usual in these conditions and may be gross. Jaundice is more common with hepatocellular carcinoma than with amebic liver abscess. Look for stigmata of chronic liver disease; hepatocellular carcinoma usually arises in a cirrhotic liver. Signs of liver failure—fetor, flapping tremor, and encephalopathy—also indicate a background of chronic liver disease. Fever may occur with malignancy or abscess; a hectic spiking fever suggests abscess, but in some patients with chronic amebic abscess the temperature is normal. Make a deliberate point of testing for intercostal tenderness over the right lower chest, a sign that is highly suggestive of amebic liver abscess. A pathological fracture or spinal deposit with myelopathy may be the presenting feature of hepatocellular carcinoma. Diffuse liver enlargement does not exclude carcinoma, which may be multilocular, or abscess, which may be deep and pushing normal liver downward. Careful inspection and gentle palpation may reveal expansile pulsation in cardiac failure. Auscultation over a mass may yield a nonspecific friction rub or the systolic bruit common in primary carcinoma.

Precise diagnosis is important; failure to treat an abscess misdiagnosed as tumor is disastrous, and extensive investigation of the liver for what is primarily a cardiac problem is wasteful. Anemia and neutrophil leukocytosis are usual in amebic liver abscess, but neither is invariable, and both may occur in association with hepatocellular carcinoma. Marked eosinophilia, in conjunction with fever and tender hepatomegaly, may occur in the migratory phase of fascioliasis. Viable *Fasciola* or schistosome ova may be identified by stool microscopy or, if this is negative, by rectal biopsy; in endemic areas the presence of eggs in the bowel does not prove that the hepatic problem is schistosomal. In the investigation of hepatomegaly, plain x-ray of the chest yields more than abdominal x-rays, which, although expensive, are rarely helpful. The chest radiograph may show the raised diaphragm and basal effusion of amebic liver abscess, or metastases in ribs, lung, or spine from a primary tumor in the liver or elsewhere. Pericardial effusion or calcification should be identified or suspected from the physical examination, but can be confirmed radiologically. Where hydatid disease is a possibility, plain abdominal x-ray may show circular calcifications. Ultrasonography, when available, is a particularly useful form of investigation and is entirely noninvasive. It can usually distinguish tumor from abscess or cyst, and can identify deeper lesions not detectable by physical examination. Ultrasonography may also detect or confirm a pericardial or pleural effusion. Liver biopsy may help in the investigation of hepatomegaly; it must only be done if bleeding tendencies have been excluded and the patient can be observed for several hours after the procedure. Biopsy provides a histological diagnosis, although sampling error sometimes reduces its accuracy. Liver biopsy must not be done if hydatid cyst or amebic abscess are possibilities; for each of these a therapeutic trial of specific drug treatment is often the best and safest means of diagnosis. Transaminases and alkaline phosphatase do not differentiate between various causes of liver enlargement. The plasma α-fetoprotein level is raised in most, but not all, patients with hepatocellular carcinoma. A fluorescent antibody test for amebiasis contributes to the diagnosis, but you should know the range of titers prevailing in the healthy local population before drawing conclusions from a raised level in an individual.

PORTAL HYPERTENSION

Portal hypertension is commonly encountered in tropical countries because both cirrhosis and hepatic schistosomiasis may lead to it. The presence of portal hypertension should be suspected in any person with gastrointestinal bleeding and splenomegaly, or with massive splenomegaly for which no cause is evident. Enlarged and tortuous veins on the abdominal wall are found in a minority of patients, but are diagnostic. They seldom take the form of the classical "caput medusae," but can usually be seen to emerge from the region of the umbilicus (Fig. 4-1*A* and 4-1*B*). A loud venous hum, obliterated by moderate pressure, can be heard over the vessels. Esophageal varices may be demonstrated by barium swallow, which must be performed with small quantities of barium and correct posturing to be of any value. Endoscopy is less expensive and more accurate.

Evidence of liver cell failure, which may be exacerbated by gastrointestinal hemorrhage, suggests that the underlying cause of portal hypertension is cirrhosis rather than schistosomiasis. This is because the periportal fibrosis of schistosomiasis does not damage hepatocytes until the disease is advanced. Testicular atrophy, gynecomastia, fetor, encephalopathy, and ascites all suggest cirrhosis, but may develop in advanced schistosomiasis. The liver may be enlarged and nodular in both diseases, but it may become shrunken and impalpable in cirrhosis. In hepatic schistosomiasis (usually due to *S. mansoni* or *S. ja-*

ponicum), the left lobe may extend nearly to the umbilicus in the midline, while the liver edge is not palpable in the anterior axillary line. A systolic bruit may be heard over the spleen or medial to it in portal hypertension of any cause.

A history of umbilical sepsis, sometimes complicating umbilical vein catheterization for exchange transfusion, in a child with portal hypertension suggests that pyogenic thrombophlebitis spread to involve the portal vein in the neonatal period. Hepatic venoocclusive disease most commonly affects young children, and may lead eventually to portal hypertension in later childhood.

Examination of stool may reveal schistosome ova, which may or may not be related to the etiology of the condition. Rectal biopsy is dangerous if there are rectal collaterals or if hemostasis is impaired. Proof of the hepatic histology is not possible without liver biopsy; this procedure is dangerous if the prothrombin time is prolonged or there is excessive ascites, when a presumptive diagnosis may be the best that can be made.

ASCITES

Knowing that ascites is present may contribute to the diagnosis, and also affords a fluid for analysis. It must be looked for carefully where its presence is not immediately obvious and also distinguished from other causes of abdominal distension. Percussion for shifting dullness is the most useful method of examination. General examination will help to distinguish some causes of ascites. Signs of chronic liver disease suggest cirrhosis; signs of cardiac failure or tamponade must be looked for—rapidly accumulating ascites may be a presenting feature of these conditions. Hepatic vein thrombosis presents with painful hepatomegaly and rapidly accumulating ascites. A

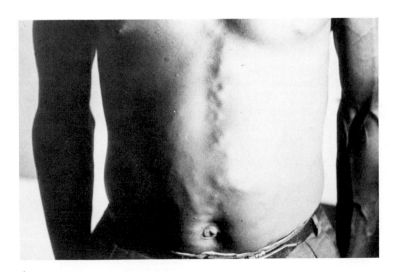

A

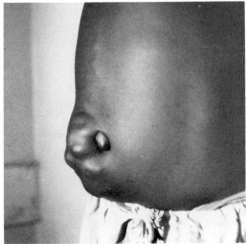

B

Figure 4-1. Caput medusae in two east African patients. One man (*A*) had hepatic schistosomiasis mansoni; the other (*B*) had HBV-related cirrhosis of the liver.

needle sample of peritoneal fluid, taken from the flank with full sterile precautions, serves to distinguish exudate from transudate. This distinction can often be made at the bedside by letting the fluid stand for half an hour, after which a coagulum or web can be seen in an exudate fluid (see Fig. 4-2). Laboratory measurement of proteins and a cell count should be done if possible. In many patients with ascites—particularly in cardiac failure—the fluid concentration is in the intermediate range (1.5 to 3 g/dL) and you cannot confidently identify it as exudate or transudate. Hemorrhagic fluid suggests malignancy, and chylous ascites occurs in lymphoma and occasionally in filariasis. Cirrhosis is the commonest cause of transudative ascites. An exudate with lymphocytes suggests tuberculous peritonitis: peritoneal biopsy with an Abrams needle is more likely to confirm the diagnosis than attempts to stain or culture the mycobacteria. Cytological examination of aspirated peritoneal fluid may identify malignant cells; the accuracy of the procedure depends on the competence of the cytologist. A diagnostic approach to ascites is suggested in Fig. 4-3.

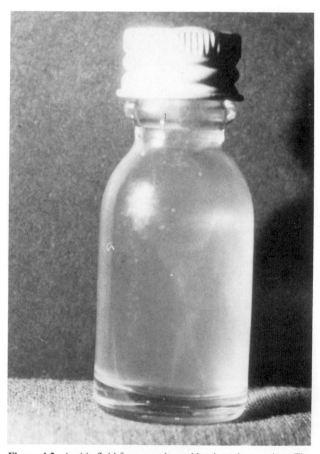

Figure 4-2. Ascitic fluid from a patient with tuberculous ascites. The fluid is faintly opalescent and a ''web'' can be seen after the sample has stood for 15 to 30 min.

CONDITIONS IN WHICH THE HEPATIC CAUSE IS EASILY MISSED

PREICTERIC HEPATITIS

Symptoms that precede jaundice may be severe but nonspecific. Fever may last for several days and be treated in vain with a variety of drugs. Diarrhea is common in hepatitis A, especially in the young. Upper abdominal pain, which may have a sudden onset, may be mistaken for peptic ulcer or myocardial ischemia. The preicteric serum sickness–like immune complex syndrome of hepatitis B may be labeled arthritis or urticaria. Pruritus, especially of the palms of the hands, may be attributed to skin disease.

FULMINANT HEPATIC NECROSIS

When there is rapid liver cell destruction due to a toxin or virus, alterations of consciousness, coma, or convulsions may develop without a clinically obvious hepatic cause. Hypoglycemia may be the mechanism of cerebral changes and should be looked for immediately; if due to hepatic necrosis, it will require continuous monitoring and correction. Signs of chronic liver disease are not present unless there was a preexisting cirrhosis. It is not possible to look for a flapping tremor in the deeply unconscious patient. Jaundice may not develop for hours or days. A reduced area of dullness on careful percussion of the liver is often a helpful sign suggesting the diagnosis.

NONHEPATIC COMPLICATIONS OF PRIMARY HEPATOCELLULAR CARCINOMA

Although seldom listed in standard textbooks, hepatocellular carcinoma (HCC) is a common source of malignant secondary deposits in bone (Fig. 4-4). A pathological fracture or myelopathy due to a vertebral deposit may be the presenting sign. Plain x-ray shows a lytic lesion; in the spine it is distinguished from tuberculosis by the classical site of the metastasis in a pedicle. Occasionally HCC may present with functional abnormalities such as hypercalcemia or hypoglycemia.

UNRECOGNIZED AMEBIC LIVER ABSCESS

A deep or posteriorly situated amebic liver abscess (ALA) may not be obvious clinically and may be the cause of unexplained fever. With a chronic ALA there may be little or no leukocytosis. Hemoptysis due to extension into the lung may continue for many weeks and be misdiagnosed as tuberculosis. Rupture of an ALA into the pericardium is a cause of pericardial effusion that is sometimes difficult to identify. Rupture into the peritoneal cavity causing acute peritonitis may also present a diagnostic dilemma.

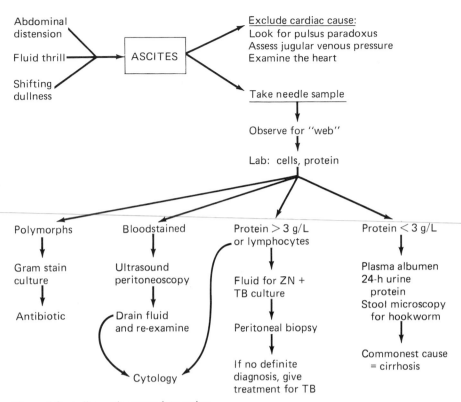

Figure 4-3. A diagnostic approach to ascites.

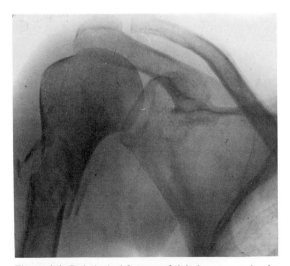

Figure 4-4. Pathological fracture of right humerus at the site of a metastasis from hepatocellular carcinoma in a 41-year-old African man.

NONHEPATIC CONDITIONS THAT MAY BE MISTAKEN FOR LIVER DISEASE

JAUNDICE DUE TO HEMOLYSIS

Suspect hemolysis particularly if there is anemia or a falling hemoglobin level. The dark urine is due to urobilinogen, not bilirubin: the froth on a shaken urine sample does not take on the yellow color that it does with conjugated bilirubin. A thin blood film may reveal features of sickle cell disease, thalassemia, or a nonspecific hemolytic pattern. In malaria jaundice may be due to both hepatic involvement and hemolysis.

HEPATIC CONGESTION SECONDARY TO HEART FAILURE

Ascites, hepatomegaly, and jaundice may be the most obvious features, especially in constrictive pericarditis, endomyocardial fibrosis, and pericardial effusion. Severe pain may result from rapid enlargement of the liver. Ascitic fluid commonly has a protein concentration in the intermediate range between transudate and exudate.

APPARENT HEPATOMEGALY DUE TO LOW DIAPHRAGM

Asthma and chronic airways obstruction may occur in all parts of the world. The physician must check by firm percussion for the upper edge of hepatic dullness to complete the assessment of liver size.

YELLOW SKIN NOT DUE TO JAUNDICE

Carotenemia causes yellowing of skin, identifiable on palms and soles in black races. The sclerae of the eye remain white. Mepacrine, a now obsolete antimalarial drug, is still available and used in some areas, and may have a similar effect on skin color. Again the eyes are unaffected.

REFERENCES

1 Zuckerman AJ (ed): Viral hepatitis. Clin Trop Med Commun Dis 1(2): 1986
2 Sherlock S: The liver in infections, in *Diseases of the Liver and Biliary System,* 7th ed. Oxford, Blackwell, 1985
3 Blumberg BS (consulting reviewer): Oncology Overview: Selected Abstracts on Hepatitis B Virus. U.S. Department of Health and Human Services and National Institutes of Health, 1982
4 Cook GC: *Tropical Gastroenterology.* Oxford University Press, 1980

CHAPTER 5 / # Respiratory and Cardiovascular Symptoms · *John Macfarlane* · *Mario Rigatto*

Respiratory diseases are the commonest cause of hospital admission and attendance, and also of death in many parts of the third world [1]. They accounted for a quarter of both adult and pediatric admissions reported from hospitals in Uganda, Zambia, and Papua New Guinea. Respiratory infections, in particular acute pneumonia and tuberculosis [2,3], are the most common conditions, but asthma and various noninfectious lung diseases are also prevalent in some areas [1,5]. After pulmonary tuberculosis, asthma was the most common chronic chest disease in children seen in Ibadan, Nigeria. About half of the patients seen with a chest complaint at a medical center in the Southern Maldives were diagnosed as having asthma. In countries where tobacco smoking is prevalent, lung cancer is also not uncommon. AIDS is an increasing problem in many areas and the chest is often the site of opportunistic infections caused for example by pneumocystis and atypical mycobacteria, although in Zimbabwe it is reported that *Mycobacterium tuberculosis* infection is the more usual in HIV-positive patients. Therefore the main respiratory syndromes that a physician will encounter commonly include pneumonia and its complications such as lung abscess and empyema, pulmonary tuberculosis, asthma, chronic obstructive lung disease, and also lung cancer. Most of these conditions can be readily diagnosed from careful history and physical examination of the patient and very simple investigations (Table 5-1).

RESPIRATORY SYMPTOMS

The important respiratory symptoms are cough, sputum production, breathlessness, wheeze, and chest pain.

COUGH

Most bronchial conditions, and some lung conditions, are associated with cough. Its timing is important in diagnosis. Cough waking a patient during the night is an important symptom of asthma, even if not associated with wheeze and dyspnea. Cough on rising in the morning is seen with asthma and with chronic bronchitis when the patient clears his or her chest of sputum. Cough after food, on bending or lying down may suggest silent aspiration. Cough always worse when lying on one side may point to pooling of secretions in one lung (Fig. 5-1) (e.g., bronchiectasis or lung abscess).

The duration of cough should be noted. Cough for a few hours or days is seen in someone with acute asthma or infection. In contrast it will have been present for weeks or months in someone with tuberculosis, chronic obstructive airways disease, or lung cancer.

A productive cough is particularly a feature of disease of the airways; a dry cough is seen with conditions of the lung parenchyma.

SPUTUM

Expectoration of mucus from the lower respiratory tract is abnormal. Of the 100 mL of mucus produced by the lower respiratory tract each day, most is swallowed unnoticed. Production of clear sputum largely rules out a respiratory infection whereas mucopurulent sputum is seen in acute bronchitis and pneumonia (Table 5-2) and large quantities of purulent sputum suggest a condition such as bronchiectasis or lung abscess. A fetid smell points to anaerobic infection. Blood in sputum is

Table 5-1. Symptoms, signs, and simple investigation of common respiratory syndromes

	Pneumonia	Lung abscess	Tuberculosis	Pulmonary fibrosis	Lung cancer	Asthma	Chronic obstructive airways disease
Symptom duration	Hours, days	Days, weeks	Weeks, months	Months, years	Weeks, months	Intermittent (hours/days if acute)	Months, years
Cough	++*	++	++	+	+	+	+
Sputum	0*/+	++	+	0	+	0/+	+
	MP*/B*	p	MP/B	0	M*	M/MP	M
Dyspnea	++	0	0	++	+	+++	++
Wheeze	0	0	0	0	+	+++	++
General features	Toxic, unwell, febrile, herpes labialis	Toxic, unwell, febrile, weight loss, finger clubbing	Weight loss, unwell	Well, finger clubbing	Smoker, weight loss, finger clubbing	Well, anxious	Well, smoker
Usual chest signs	Focal creps*	Variable; focal creps	Variable, apical signs	Diffuse basal creps	Variable; focal wheeze	Diffuse wheeze	Diffuse wheeze and creps
Simple tests	CXR*, sputum exam	CXR, sputum exam	CXR, sputum exam (ZN)	CXR	CXR	Peak flow before and after bronchodilators	Peak flow before and after bronchodilators

*Key: + = symptom present; 0 = symptom not present; M = mucoid sputum; MP = mucopurulent; p = purulent; B = blood stained; creps = crepitations; CXR = chest radiograph.

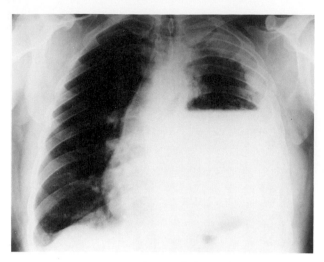

Figure 5-1. Chest radiograph of a man with a left chronic empyema complicated by a bronchopleural fistula. The patient coughed large amounts of purulent sputum when lying on his right side.

usually commented on by the patient. Blood-tinged mucopurulent sputum is not unusual with acute bronchial and lung infections (Table 5-2) for a few days, but intermittent streaks for longer periods may suggest bronchial carcinoma, and blood clots can also be seen with tuberculosis. Sudden hemoptysis with clear or absent sputum can point to pulmonary infarction.

BREATHLESSNESS

Breathlessness can be caused by noncardiorespiratory syndromes, such as metabolic acidosis and psychogenic hyperventilation, but associated respiratory symptoms are usually absent. Determining the timing of the breathlessness is most important. Breathlessness coming on dramatically over minutes points to a diagnosis such as pneumothorax, pulmonary edema, or pulmonary embolus. In contrast the same symptom developing progressively over months or years points more to chronic obstructive airways disease or a fibrosing lung condition such as fibrosing alveolitis. Dyspnea coming on acutely over hours is seen with pneumonia, allergic alveolitis, asthma, and acute heart failure. Subacute symptoms over days and

Table 5-2. Symptoms and signs for 283 adults presenting with acute pneumonia

Sign or symptom	Patients presenting with symptom, %
Productive cough	62
Pleural pain	50
Hemoptysis	17
High fever	62
Bronchial breathing	28
Focal crepitations in chest	73

weeks may suggest a pleural effusion, bronchial carcinoma, or lung infiltration with metastatic tumor or sarcoidosis. Intermittent attacks are a feature of asthma and left ventricular failure. Work-related symptoms will point to occupational asthma or alveolitis.

WHEEZE

This symptom suggests airways disease. Sometimes the wheeze is more noticeable to friends and relatives than to the patient. Stridor produced by large-airways obstruction produces a loud, easily identifiable fixed wheeze and identifies the patient in need of urgent treatment.

CHEST PAIN

Most of the lower airways and lung parenchyma are insensitive to pain, and quite advanced disease can develop before pain is noticed. In contrast the parietal pleura is very sensitive and the characteristic pleural pain, worse on inspiration, coughing, and moving, is noted when inflammation is present. The acute sharp pleural pain is normally felt directly over the site of the inflammation but may be localized to the shoulder tip or neck if the diaphragm is involved. Acute pleural pain developing over minutes or hours is normally seen with pleuropulmonary infection (Table 5-2) or pulmonary infarction, but chest wall pain can mimic it. In this latter situation, local tenderness will be elicited and such conditions as a rib fracture, epidemic intercostal myalgia, or the preeruptive phase of thoracic herpes zoster should be considered. In contrast, pain arising from the mediastinum in conditions such as early lung cancer or glandular enlargement from lymphoma or sarcoidosis usually results in a dull central chest pain. Pain from the upper airways (for example, in acute tracheobronchitis) is characteristically described as a rough, raw, sandpaperlike retrosternal sensation.

GENERAL FACTORS

A past or family history of asthma or atopic disease may be helpful in considering asthma and a childhood history of a severe respiratory infection may be associated with subsequent bronchiectasis. Regular cigarette smoking can be a factor in chronic obstructive airways disease and lung cancer. Occupation may be relevant in asthma, lung shadowing (e.g., from pneumoconiosis), and lung infections (e.g., Q fever in farm workers; psittacosis in bird handlers).

RESPIRATORY SIGNS

The general condition of the patient is of major importance in diagnosis. The febrile, sweating, toxic patient with a rapid respiratory rate, cough, shallow breathing, and obvious pain on inspiration is likely to have acute pneumonia. The less toxic but cachectic-looking individual perhaps with clubbing of the fingers is more likely to have a condition like a lung tumor, suppurative lung disease, or tuberculosis. The age of scars on

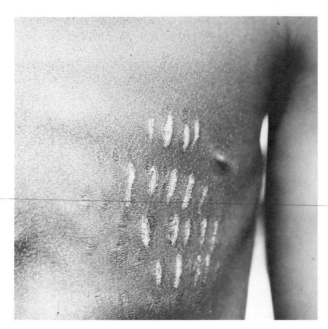

Figure 5-2. The age of the scars from a native doctor's cuts can be helpful in assessing the duration of an illness. This young man with pleurisy has fresh cuts only a few days old, but older, healed scars suggest a similar illness in the past. (*From [1] with permission of the editor.*)

the chest from the native doctor may be useful in timing the duration of an illness (Fig. 5-2).

Even a brief examination of the chest can be very informative. Poor expansion of one side denotes pathology on that side. Polyphonic wheezes or ronchi generally denote diffuse small airways obstruction whereas a monophonic wheeze suggests a large airway narrowing caused, for example, by a tumor or an inhaled foreign body. Crepitations or crackles are heard in alveolar conditions such as pulmonary edema and alveolitis and also in pneumonia where they are far commoner than the "classic" bronchial breathing.

SIMPLE INVESTIGATIONS OF RESPIRATORY SYMPTOMS

A guide to simple investigation of the respiratory symptoms is shown in Table 5-1. Gram staining of mucopurulent sputum may show a predominant organism such as *Streptococcus pneumoniae* or *Staphylococcus aureus* and is a specific but not very sensitive indicator of the cause of the pneumonia. Where laboratory facilities are limited, sputum smear and culture is probably indicated only in those patients with pneumonia who do not respond to initial antibiotic therapy. Sputum smears are essential for the investigation of possible pulmonary tuberculosis. The tuberculin skin test is rarely of practical help except in young children. A chest radiograph is useful in someone

with focal chest signs. For those with symptoms suggestive of airflow obstruction the peak flow rate can be measured simply and quickly using a Wright peak flow meter. A reduced measurement makes the diagnosis, and reversibility can be assessed using treatment such as a bronchodilator aerosol.

INFLUENCE OF SOCIOECONOMIC AND GEOGRAPHICAL FACTORS ON CARDIOVASCULAR DISEASE

The prevalence and types of cardiovascular diseases in a community are directly affected by both its socioeconomic profile and its geographical location. Perhaps no other system in the body has such a direct relationship with affluence and lifestyle. As a rule, the rise of cardiovascular mortality is a good indicator of growing affluence in the population considered [6].

Cardiovascular diseases are, by far, the number one cause of death in the developed countries but not so in the developing ones. There is a positive correlation between income per capita and the percentage of deaths due to cardiovascular diseases. The factors pertinent to this correlation have to do, at least in part, with the greater prevalence in a more developed society of a hypercaloric diet, a more sedentary way of life, better standards of public health care, a longer lifespan, a heavier alcohol and tobacco exposure, and a more widespread use of hormonal contraception. Most of these factors interact—e.g., diet, vaccines, and better housing prolong lifespan. In its turn, a longer lifespan offers a better chance for long-term aggressions—such as tobacco, alcohol, diabetes, hypertension—to unveil their destructive effects.

Socioeconomic status is also a predictor of the types of cardiovascular disease likely to predominate. Areas of poverty, illiteracy, overcrowding, poor sanitary habits, and poor diet favor infections and nutritional diseases. Children are particularly vulnerable. These factors account for the prevalence in such areas of streptococcal diseases (rheumatic fever, nephritis), syphilis (aneurysms), tuberculosis (constrictive pericarditis, kyphoscoliosis, cor pulmonale), trypanosomiasis, diphtheria, scarlet fever (myocarditis), beriberi, and hookworm disease (high-output failure).

Latitude has its role in the determination of regional patterns of cardiovascular health and disease. In great part it adds up to socioeconomic influences. It is well known that the performance of the human being—and consequently the degree of wealth—reaches its peak in the temperate bands of the globe. No developed country has most of its territory either in the tropical or in the arctic bands. However, latitude has an influence of its own on some infectious agents of cardiovascular disease. Tropical bands make the best habitat for the agents of endemic diseases such as *Trypanosoma cruzi* (Chagas' disease) and *Schistosoma mansoni* or *S. haematobium* (bilharziasis).

Altitude (above 3000 m) is also a factor influencing cardiovascular health. Very low ambient oxygen pressure above this altitude challenges respiration and overloads the heart by thickening the blood with erythrocytes, raising cardiac output, and increasing pulmonary vascular resistance. Exhaustion of these mechanisms of adaptation may lead to Monge's disease.

Ethnic composition of some communities may determine a particular profile for cardiovascular diseases. Atherosclerosis, diabetes, hypertension, and rheumatic heart disease are much more prevalent in Trinidad and Tobago than in its neighboring countries.

Brazil, with latitudes ranging from 5° to 34°S, and with three-fourths of its territory in the tropics and one-fourth in temperate South America, provides a vivid illustration of the relationship between the epidemiology of cardiovascular disease and geography. A comparison of Brazil's tropical Northeast Region, close to the Equator (39 million inhabitants), with its temperate South Region (21 million inhabitants) leads to the following contrasts: life expectancy at birth—51.57 years in the Northeast, 66.98 in the South; infant mortality—121.36 per 1000 live births in the Northeast, 61.8 in the South; fecundity rate—6.13 percent in the Northeast, 3.63 percent in the South; vegetative growth of the population—2.16 percent in the Northeast, 1.44 percent in the South; illiteracy rate—46.9 percent in the Northeast, 17.3 percent in the South; gross internal product per capita—3 times higher in the South; cardiovascular mortality as a percentage of the total number of deaths—13 percent in the Northeast, 32.5 percent in the South; myocardial infarction as a percentage of total cardiovascular deaths—33.8 percent in the Northeast, 54 percent in the South; trypanosomiasis and schistosomiasis deaths as a percentage of total cardiovascular deaths—3.7 percent in the Northeast, 1.2 percent in the South (Fig. 5-3).

DIFFERENCES IN FREQUENCY OF CARDIOVASCULAR SYMPTOMS IN VARIOUS GEOGRAPHICAL AREAS

Symptoms of practically all cardiovascular diseases are everywhere, but their frequency may vary significantly.

In a tropical office in Latin America, central Africa, or south Asia, palpitations, dyspnea and fatigue should be the prominent symptoms: palpitations from the dysrhythmias character-istic of Chagas' disease or from atrial fibrillation of rheumatic heart disease; dyspnea from the failing rheumatic or chagasic heart; fatigue from the high-output insufficiency of advanced iron anemia, from cor pulmonale of schistosomiasis, or from thromboembolic disease of young females with many pregnancies.

In a temperate-world medical office, pain, dyspnea, and cerebral symptoms should predominate. The clinician in this setting will see pain of angina or infarction from coronary heart disease or from dissecting aneurysms, pain of intermittent claudication from partially occluded lower-limbs arteries of diabetics or smokers, and pain from arterial thromboembolic episodes stemming from blood and vessel alterations induced by smoke or hormonal contraception; orthopnea from a failing left ventricle of hypertension or ischemic heart disease; dyspnea from hypoxic chronic cor pulmonale due to smoking; effort dyspnea from a failing myocardium handicapped in its vigor by a sedentary life, smoking, and/or alcohol.

In a high-altitude medical office of South America, fatigue, growing cyanosis, lower-limb edema, and difficulty in intellectual concentration are common symptoms of chronic mountain sickness (chronic *soroche*). All of them are reversible with the removal of the patient to sea level.

Some diseases are apparently not influenced, at least discernibly, by socioeconomic and geographical factors. Congenital cardiovascular malformations are among them. Cardiac murmurs and/or cyanosis are leading signs to be looked for in children of any age around the world.

CARDIOVASCULAR SYMPTOMS

Taking the word *symptom* in its broader sense, i.e., subjective and objective (sign), it is appropriate to say that dyspnea, palpitation, chest pain, edema, and cyanosis are the most revealing symptoms of cardiovascular disease [7]. Each will now be discussed.

DYSPNEA

Dyspnea is the leading symptom of a compromised respiration. When of cardiovascular origin, it is most frequently due to pulmonary congestion from left heart failure in the presence

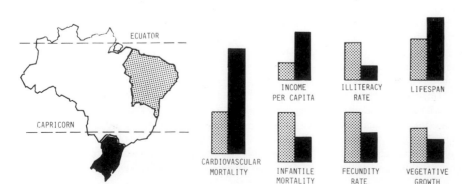

Figure 5-3. Cardiovascular mortality and socioeconomic characteristics of a tropical (Northeast; dotted area) and a temperate (South; black area) region of Brazil. Relative values (for specific values and units see text).

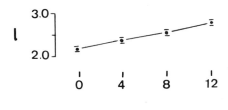

Figure 5-4. Improvement of vital capacity (VC) over 12 days of successful treatment of 27 patients with congestive heart failure. The vertical bars correspond to 2 standard errors of the mean.

of a still competent right heart. Arterial hypertension and ischemic heart disease are the most frequent causes for it in mature and old people. A faulty mitral valve from rheumatic heart disease is the leading cause in children and young adults. Progressive intensity of the pulmonary congestion may lead to cardiac asthma and to frank pulmonary alveolar edema. Pleural effusion, more frequently at the right lung, may intensify the difficulty in moving the chest bellows. Interstitial edema stimulates respiratory frequency. The diminished compliance configurates a restrictive ventilatory insufficiency with a drop in vital capacity, a good indicator to use in following the evolution of the picture (Fig. 5-4). Interstitial edema, following a postural distribution, fosters $\dot{V}/Q$ imbalance and compromises diffusion, leading to an alveolar-capillary pulmonary insufficiency. The alveolar-arterial oxygen difference ($PA_{O_2} - Pa_{O_2}$) is a sensitive indicator of the degree of pulmonary congestion (Fig. 5-5). Situations demanding a higher left ventricular performance, as lying down (orthopnea) or exercising (effort dyspnea) are useful to differentiate dyspnea of cardiovascular origin from that of pulmonary origin. Nevertheless, important overlapping does occur. Orthopnea may be seen in asthmatic patients who may better mobilize their accessory muscles of ventilation in a sitting position. And effort dyspnea may be dramatic in pulmonary emphysema.

The anemic patient, because of poor oxygen carriage to the

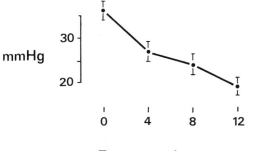

Figure 5-5. Reduction of alveolar-arterial oxygen difference ($PA_{O_2}-Pa_{O_2}$) over 12 days of successful treatment of 27 patients with congestive heart failure. The vertical bars correspond to 2 standard errors of the mean.

respiratory muscles, has the potential for dyspnea. Nevertheless, most anemic patients complain of fatigue instead of breathlessness. Dyspnea may be seen in severe anemia (less than 7 g of hemoglobin per dL of blood) with high-output failure.

PALPITATION

Irregularities of the heartbeat may be noticed by the patient at a rather early moment of a cardiac disease. They are the most notorious symptom of Chagas' disease. Atrial fibrillation, in young people, stems dominantly from rheumatic valve disease or hyperthyroidism. In old people, ischemic heart disease has the lead.

CHEST PAIN

Compressive retrosternal pain, with or without irradiation to the back, the arms, or the neck, more frequently does herald myocardial suffering from ischemia consequent to coronary obstruction. However, it may derive from aortic dissection, from pericarditis, or from sudden and important pulmonary hypertension, as in thromboembolic disease. Other mediastinal sufferings such as tracheobronchitis and esophagitis may present a similar picture. Pleural disease, in its early phase, adds another possible cause to the list. Sometimes high abdominal diseases, as cholecystitis or pancreatitis, may make the differential diagnosis difficult.

Precipitation or intensification of the pain by physical effort and relief by rest favor a cardiovascular origin. Relation to food intake favors digestive problems. A relationship to ventilatory movements points to pleural processes. Nevertheless, in many cases, only electrocardiographic, radiological, ergometric, cine-angiographic, echographic, isotopic, endoscopic, or laboratory tests may ascertain the origin of the pain.

A brief, transitory oppression in the chest may announce to an experienced clinician an episode of pulmonary embolism, particularly if accompanied by an otherwise unexplained tachypnea, more rarely by bronchial wheezing.

EDEMA

Cardiovascular disease is a common cause of pulmonary or peripheral edema. Pulmonary edema, from pulmonary congestion, was considered in the discussion of dyspnea. Peripheral edema is taken as cardiac if accompanied by a raised central venous pressure, detected by jugular congestion in the sitting position or measured through a venous catheter. Right ventricular failure is the commonest cause of peripheral edema of cardiac origin. In the presence of clear lung fields and of normal or small cardiac size, constrictive pericarditis should be considered. Acute pericarditis with pericardial effusion and, eventually, tamponade must be considered in the presence of an enlarged cardiac silhouette. The presence of paradoxical pulse favors pericardial involvement. Echocardiographic studies or cardiac catheterization with an analysis of the morphology of the pressure curves from the right side of the heart facilitate the diagnosis. Patients with hypoxic chronic cor pulmonale frequently have a slight degree of peripheral edema not seldom interpreted as a manifestation of right heart failure. This is not necessarily so. If not accompanied by raised central venous pressure, this edema is usually related to the hypercapnia present in most of these patients.

CYANOSIS

This is a rather difficult symptom to handle. Artificial illumination and variations in the melanin content of the skin make its recognition erratic. Nevertheless, when ascertained, its contribution to the diagnosis is significant. Cyanosis indicates either a poor central oxygenation of the blood, as in pulmonary failure or in intracardiac or pulmonary arteriovenous shunts, or a poor peripheral perfusion with a more than usual removal of oxygen from the blood by the tissues, as in heart failure. In central cyanosis, the extremities are usually warm; in peripheral cyanosis, they are usually cold. Central cyanosis of pulmonary insufficiency is usually corrected by oxygen therapy. Central cyanosis of circulatory origin is uninfluenced by oxygen therapy. Some abnormal hemoglobins, such as meta- and sulfahemoglobin, must be disregarded in the absence of other evidence of cardiac or pulmonary disease. In patients with pulmonary circulation involvement due to schistosomiasis the presence of cyanosis practically rules out pulmonary hypertension. Hypertensive patients do not have cyanosis. Venoarterial shunts are apparently responsible for the phenomenon. If they cause blood to be detoured from the pulmonary arteriolar circulation, the shunts would account for both the cyanosis and the protection against hypertension.

Other symptoms may announce a cardiovascular abnormality. Syncope is by no means rare. It may be either *cardiac* (cardiac standstill by vagal inhibition, ventricular asystole as in Stokes-Adams fit, ventricular fibrillation, ball-valve thrombus or pedunculated myxoma, aortic stenosis, paroxysmal rhythm changes with very rapid ventricular rates, massive pulmonary embolism, hemopericardium with cardiac tamponade) or *vasomotor* (hemorrhage, loss of plasma into wounds, burns, crush injuries, orthostatic hypotension). Hemoptysis, while much more frequently associated with pulmonary diseases, may be an important feature of mitral stenosis, for instance. Hemoptoic sputum is a classic symptom of pulmonary infarction.

Cough, recurrent bronchitis, insomnia, clubbing, anorexia, dementia, systemic embolism, nausea, vomiting, oligemia, and nocturia, are other symptoms of cardiovascular disease, with or without heart failure.

REFERENCES

1 Macfarlane JT: The respiratory physician in a third world district hospital: Appropriate technology. London, British Medical Association, 1985, pp 46–49
2 Allen SC: Lobar pneumonia in Northern Zambia: Clinical study of 502 adult patients. Thorax 39:612–616, 1984
3 Harrico AD, Speare R, Wirima JJ: A profile of respiratory disease in an African medical ward: J R Coll Physicians Lond 22:109–113, 1988
4 Warrell DA, Fawcett IW, Harrison RDW, et al: Bronchial asthma in the Nigerian Savanna Region. Q J Med 44:325–347, 1975
5 Wolstenholme, RJ: Bronchial asthma in the southern Maldives. Clin Allergy 9:325–332, 1979
6 Parry EHO, Rigatto M, Hathirat S: Geographical variation in cardiac disease, in Weatherall DJ, Ledigham JGG, Warrell DA (eds): *Oxford Textbook of Medicine,* 2d ed. Oxford, Oxford University Press, 1987, pp 13-397 to 13-403
7 Wood P: *Diseases of the Heart and Circulation,* 2d ed. Philadelphia, Lippincott, 1956, pp 12–25

CHAPTER 6 / *Skin Disorders* · David R. Bickers

The skin is a major interface between the human body and its environment. As such, cutaneous tissue is subject to a wide spectrum of potentially toxic chemical and physical agents that can cause pathological changes. These can be appreciated by the physician by direct inspection and palpation of the skin without the need for invasive techniques.

The outermost layer of the epidermis, the stratum corneum, is in direct contact with the environment. Essentially a multilayered membrane containing the fibrous protein keratin embedded in an amorphous matrix with numerous, lipid-rich interstices, this compact yet complex structure constitutes the major barrier between the body and the outside world and is the critical impediment to movement of chemicals in and out of the body. The skin is quite sensitive to changes in the water content of the atmosphere. When the relative humidity falls, water evaporates from the stratum corneum, forming air-water interfaces that give the visible appearance of scaling and the texture of dryness. Thus, substantial changes in ambient conditions can influence the expression of disease in cutaneous tissue.

The term *tropical dermatoses* is somewhat misleading. "Tropical" diseases are not influenced simply by climatic conditions but also by social factors; leprosy and endemic syphilis, for example, occur in temperate as well as in tropical climates, and the infectious pyodermas and mycoses that frequently occur in the tropics are also common in temperate regions and are therefore not exclusively tropical diseases. However, diseases of the skin in tropical regions may differ in their incidence, prevalence, and appearance from the identical disorders occurring in more temperate climates as a consequence of different climatic conditions.

The major determinants of any human disease can be broadly divided into factors relating to the host and factors related to the host's environment. The host factors are largely dependent upon the genetic endowment of the individual, and alterations in the gene pool may greatly influence the phenotypic expression of certain disorders. A good example of the influence of genetics on expression of a dermatological disorder is provided by the San Blas Indians of the Cuna tribe, who inhabit islands off the coast of Panama [1]. These Indians are normally dark-complected with ample melanin pigment in their skin. However, a sizable number of individuals in this inbred population are afflicted with oculocutaneous albinism, an autosomal recessive disorder characterized by decreased or absent activity of the enzyme tyrosinase. This results in diminished melanin synthesis, and these hypopigmented individuals, unlike their normally pigmented kin, are at high risk for the development of actinic damage, solar elastosis, and skin cancer as a result of chronic intense sun exposure in this tropical region.

Extrinsic environmental factors that are among the important determinants of tropical dermatoses include climate (temperature, relative humidity, degree of intensity of sun exposure), altitude, exposure to flora and fauna, particularly insects that may function as intermediate hosts, and diet. Furthermore, "tropical dermatoses" also may occur more frequently in these geographical areas because of often poor hygienic techniques.

It is important to emphasize that the etiological agents responsible for most of the tropical diseases are infectious in nature and include viruses, bacteria, fungi, protozoa, spirochetes, and helminths.

Malnutrition is another major cause of disease in these areas.

In many of the tropical dermatoses, the skin is a major site of involvement either primarily or secondarily, but it is often not the only organ involved. Furthermore, primary involvement of internal organs may be accompanied by cutaneous manifestations.

Skin diseases are a major health hazard in the tropics. Although few patients die of tropical skin disease, considerable morbidity accompanies many of these disorders. This chapter will briefly discuss skin diseases commonly encountered in tropical and subtropical regions. Special attention is paid to the factors that influence the clinical appearance of the more common skin diseases in different geographical regions.

There is meager epidemiological information available concerning diseases that occur in tropical areas, and, as a result, our knowledge of the incidence of dermatological disorders is mainly limited to statistics derived from patients attending skin clinics. These data are not based on total populations and are therefore inadequate; however, they do provide a general picture of the prevalence of skin diseases in a given locality.

FACTORS AFFECTING THE INCIDENCE OF SKIN DISORDERS IN TROPICAL REGIONS

RACIAL AND GENETIC FACTORS

Racial characteristics of ethnic groups that may influence the occurrence of skin diseases are difficult to determine, as they are closely interrelated with environmental and socioeconomic factors. In general, it may be said that Congoids have a greater tendency to develop keloids, pseudofolliculitis barbae, and folliculitis keloidalis, while Mongoloids are more prone to lichenification. In comparison to Caucasians, both Congoids and Mongoloids are resistant to actinic damage, solar keratoses, and skin cancer, and, in general it can be stated that the incidence of these diseases decrease in direct proportion to increased pigmentation of the skin.

GEOGRAPHICAL AND CLIMATIC FACTORS

Geographical and climatic factors play an important role in the development of skin diseases. This is particularly evident at different altitudes [2]. In the lowlands, from sea level to 3000 feet, extreme heat and humidity enhance the growth of exuberant vegetation. These climatic conditions favor the development of miliaria (prickly heat), due to sweat duct occlusion, and pityriasis versicolor, a superficial dermatophyte infection due to *Pityrosporum ovale* (Fig. 6-1). Pyoderma, particularly impetigo, is more likely to occur under these conditions, and epidemics of impetigo have occurred repeatedly in tropical regions (Fig. 6-2) [3]. Superficial dermatophyte infections, candidiasis, and pyodermas are exceedingly common and are often more indolent, responding very slowly to appropriate antimicrobial therapy that is quickly effective in a more temperate climate.

At higher altitudes, about 3000 to 6000 feet, the cooler temperatures affect the pattern of disease: Bacterial pyoderma and superficial fungal infections are less common and more easily controlled, while the soil and flora appear to favor deep fungal infections such as sporotrichosis, chromomycosis, and mycetoma.

At the colder, very high altitudes such as the altiplano at the top of the Andes, with a totally different fauna and flora, the pattern of disease again changes. There, with low humidity, one encounters skin diseases common in temperate climates, such as xerosis, or dryness, "winter itch," and even frostbite. Also, because the atmosphere is thinner at high altitude, the intensity of solar radiation is enhanced. This may be even further exaggerated by reflection from snow at higher altitudes,

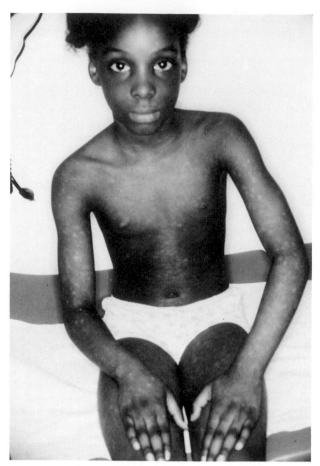

Figure 6-1. Extensive pityriasis versicolor in a young black female. There is considerable depigmentation in the affected areas.

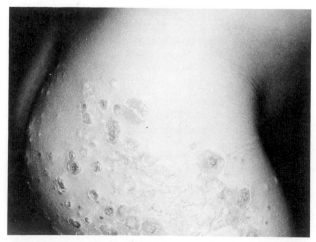

Figure 6-2. Pyoderma is much more common in the tropics. In this patient with bullous impetigo there is extensive involvement of the buttock area.

resulting in increased risk of severe sunburn and of actinic keratoses and nonmelanoma skin cancer in chronically exposed individuals.

Another interesting example of the influence of geographic factors is a form of dermatomycosis and onychomycosis clinically indistinguishable from dermatophyte infections and caused by the mold fungi *Hendersonula toruloidea* and *Scytilidium hyalinum;* it occurs in patients originating from the tropics or subtropics but living in temperate climates [4,5]. Thus, susceptibility to certain infections may be "imported" into temperate areas from tropical ones.

The role of climatic factors is evident in the seasonal variability of various dermatoses. During the rainy season, there is an abundance of pyoderma, especially impetigo and furuncles, as well as insect bites which may be followed by papular urticaria in many individuals.

SOCIOECONOMIC FACTORS

The occupation of an individual may create a predisposition to certain skin diseases. Agricultural workers in rural areas may be directly exposed to saprophytes in the soil or on plants. Inoculation into the skin may result in the development of sporotrichosis or mycetoma. These individuals are also exposed to insects that are vectors of diseases such as leishmaniasis and onchocerciasis. Industrial workers may develop contact dermatitis as a result of occupational exposure to various chemicals. These may cause allergic sensitization or primary irritation.

Dietary deficiency may predispose to certain nutritional disorders. Overcrowded housing and deficient hygienic facilities often enhance the likelihood of infectious diseases ranging from pyoderma to leprosy. Local customs and the use of traditional medicines may lead to unusual cutaneous disorders such as skin eruptions resulting from coin-rubbing, a practice of some Mongoloid ethnic groups. The widespread use of natural substances, particularly herbs, may at times cause skin irritation.

PATTERNS OF SKIN DISORDERS

There is considerable difference in the distribution pattern of skin diseases encountered in tropical, as opposed to nontropical, countries. In the latter, as a result of better health care and preventive medicine, there is a preponderance of noninfective, inflammatory disorders, many of which cause only minor discomfort. In general, deep fungal infections and parasitic disorders are uncommon.

In tropical countries, especially in the poorer, underdeveloped, rural areas, this pattern is reversed. Infectious and parasitic disorders predominate, whereas noninfectious diseases are less frequently seen. Premalignant actinic damage and malignant tumors, especially those precipitated by solar radiation, are decidedly rare in the highly pigmented races inhabiting the tropics.

The ratio of infectious-parasitic to noninfectious-nonparasitic disorders can be considered a crude index of underdevelopment and poor socioeconomic conditions. In urban areas in the tropics, statistics from skin clinics begin to show a reversal of this ratio with predominance of noninfective disorders, especially contact dermatitis. This inverted ratio may be interpreted as one sign of increasing use of more modern techniques of disease control [6].

Statistics obtained from skin clinics in rural areas throughout the tropics show striking similarities in terms of the types of diseases that are encountered. Van Heck and Bugingo in Rwanda showed that parasitosis, especially scabies and mycoses, affected almost 30 percent of their patients [7]. In several rural dispensaries in Central America, Failmezger showed that parasitosis constituted 37 percent, mycoses 15 percent, and pyoderma about 6 percent of all skin disorders [8]. In most Asiatic rural areas a high prevalence of infective parasitic disorders is also evident. This has been shown in India and in Malaysia [9]. In fact, Pettit reported that almost half the patients in Malaysia presented with primary or secondary bacterial infections [10].

Statistics from large urban areas in the tropics demonstrate a clear-cut shift in this historical pattern. In a report from the Institute of Dermatology in Bangkok, Thailand, Kotrajaras showed that parasitosis occurred in 18 percent, pyoderma in 2 percent, and mycoses in 13 percent of the patients, while eczematous dermatitis was observed in 37 percent [11]. This illustrates the concept that urbanization greatly influences the nature of dermatological disease in the tropics.

The age of the patient is another important determinant of the type and incidence of skin diseases. It is well known that the great majority of the population of the tropics is considerably younger and that life expectancy is shorter than that in nontropical western countries. The incidence of skin diseases observed in children also varies with age. Ruiz-Maldonado at the National Institute of Pediatrics in Mexico City reported that in infants from 1 to 12 months the most common disorders were scabies (16.1 percent), prurigo caused by insect bites (14.7 percent), atopic dermatitis (Fig. 6-3) (13.2 percent), and diaper rash (10 percent) [12]. Tamayo, at the same institute, showed that in children from 2 to 6 years of age, the most common skin disorders were prurigo caused by insects (25.3 percent) and atopic dermatitis (15.4 percent), while in schoolchildren 6 to 12 years of age, the most frequent diseases were warts (13 percent) and atopic dermatitis (11.7 percent) [13]. Both pityriasis alba and scabies were seen in 10.3 percent of adolescent children [14].

TROPICAL AND GEOGRAPHICAL VARIATIONS OF THE COMMONEST SKIN DISORDERS AND SOME TROPICAL DERMATOSES

The clinical picture of some of the more common skin disorders encountered in the tropics varies considerably with the geographical location. One important factor in these variations

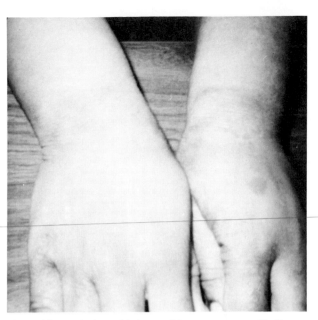

Figure 6-3. Atopic dermatitis is one of the most common skin diseases seen in children.

is the degree of skin pigmentation. In black skin, erythema is difficult to detect because melanin absorbs radiant energy throughout the visible spectrum. Lesions that would appear red in Caucasoid skin are dark gray or copper-colored, and yellow lesions (like xanthoma) appear light brown. In brown skin, the variations are similar but rather less pronounced. Another characteristic of tropical dermatoses is the advanced stage of the eruptions or lesions when first seen by the physician. This is common in patients from rural areas who have little or no access to appropriate medical care.

The following is a brief outline of the major tropical and geographical variations in clinical presentation of the more common skin disorders. In addition, some tropical dermatoses will be briefly discussed. For more comprehensive discussion of these diseases, the reader should consult textbooks dealing with tropical dermatology [15,16].

ECZEMATOUS DERMATITIS GROUP

Atopic dermatitis

Atopic dermatitis is a chronic, pruritic dermatosis observed in genetically predisposed individuals with a familial tendency to allergic diseases such as asthma, urticaria, and hay fever. Atopic dermatitis is common and often severe in Mongoloids and relatively rare in African Congoids. Climate has a definite effect on atopic dermatitis. Hot, dry climates are generally beneficial, while cold or hot, humid weather exacerbates the disease.

The morphology and topography of the eruption varies with the age of the patient. There is an infantile phase manifested by erythematovesicular patches located on the cheeks and ex-

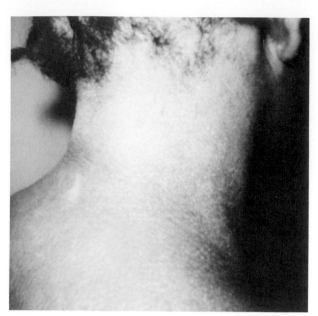

Figure 6-4. Atopic dermatitis involving the neck.

tremities. This is followed by a childhood phase characterized by red, lichenified, and highly pruritic patches in the antecubital and popliteal fossae, neck (Fig. 6-4), groin, and axillae. The adult phase shows persistence of flexural involvement. The skin is dry, irritable, and highly pruritic. A common complication of atopic dermatitis is secondary pyoderma, particularly impetigo or furunculosis. Less common but more worrisome is the secondary dissemination of herpes virus over the eczematous eruption to produce eczema herpeticum.

The course of atopic eczema is generally self-limited, and most cases clear prior to adolescence, but persistence into adulthood seems to be more common in the tropics.

Treatment. Acute stages should be treated with wet compresses, topical fluorinated corticosteroids, and systemic antihistamines to relieve pruritus. Lichenified areas benefit from combinations of corticosteroids and coal tar preparations. Short courses of systemic corticosteroids may help to control acute exacerbations. Secondary pyodermas should be managed with appropriate systemic antibiotics, and antiviral therapy with parenterally administered acyclovir may be lifesaving in eczema herpeticum [*17*].

Contact dermatitis

Contact dermatitis is a common skin reaction caused by cutaneous exposure to environmental agents that may cause irritation or allergic sensitization. Its incidence is rapidly increasing in tropical countries, especially in larger cities. This is due to wider availability of agents capable of causing skin injury such as cosmetics, dyes, chemicals, etc. Also, many emerging industries use special chemicals that are capable of causing contact dermatitis. All races and ages are affected, but for unknown reasons Congoids generally seem to be less susceptible to contact dermatitis.

Contact dermatitis may be caused by two different mechanisms, irritation and allergic sensitization of the skin.

Irritant contact dermatitis is caused by direct damage or toxic effects of chemicals. Absolute irritants damage the skin at first contact, whereas relative irritants act slowly, causing a cumulative type of injury.

Allergic contact dermatitis is a manifestation of delayed hypersensitivity and develops as a result of exposure to topical allergens after a variable period of incubation.

In most tropical countries, many highly advertised "cureall" skin preparations are sold over the counter. These often are a cause of contact dermatitis, since the ingredients of some of these products are notorious sensitizers such as ammoniated mercury, benzocaine, and sulfonamide derivatives.

Clinically, the eruption is an acute, pruritic, eczematous dermatitis manifested by redness, edema, vesiculation, and crusting localized to the areas on contact. Cumulative and chronic eruptions are dry, lichenified and fissured. The hands and face are often affected. Detailed discussion of contact dermatitis can be found in at least two excellent textbooks of medicine [*18,19*].

Treatment. The acute eczematous phase requires moist compresses and topical corticosteroid preparations. Short, tapered courses of oral prednisone (60 mg over 10 days) may be indicated on occasion. Chronic cases benefit from topical corticosteroids, coal tar preparations, and emollients. Systemic antihistamines may relieve pruritus. Patch testing should be done in an effort to identify the etiologic agent since avoidance of exposure is probably the most effective form of management.

Occupational dermatitis

In rapidly developing cities of the tropics, chronic, disabling "cement" dermatitis as a result of chromate sensitivity commonly occurs in those working in the building trade. Rural workers often suffer from contact with woods, plants, insecticides, and fertilizers, etc. Other workers in various industries may develop dermatitis when exposed to different substances. Lists of agents causing dermatitis used in various occupations can be found elsewhere [*20*].

The management of occupational dermatitis must be individualized. Those with extreme sensitivity must avoid further exposure; in others, a process of "hardening" may develop in which repeated exposure results in diminished sensitivity. The mechanism of this phenomenon is unknown. Education of workers regarding the use of protective measures and hygiene can greatly reduce the incidence of occupational dermatitis.

Other eczematous eruptions

Seborrheic dermatitis is often seen in all tropical races, but for unknown reasons, stasis dermatitis caused by insufficient venous drainage, while common in Caucasoids, is unusual in African Congoids and Mongoloids. Infective eczema caused or perpetuated by bacterial infection of the skin is a common occurrence in the tropics. Pityriasis alba, a postinflammatory hypopigmentation, is exceedingly common in children living in tropical areas. Asteatotic, or "winter," eczema is common on the high-altitude plateaus. Lichen simplex chronicus, manifested by lichenification resulting from excoriation, is very common in Asiatic ethnic groups.

There is a nonclassified eczematous eruption which does not fit into the accepted pattern and which may be called "tropical eczema." This is a recalcitrant, extensive, pruritic, weeping eruption that may become secondarily infected with bacteria. Treatment centers on the use of appropriate antibiotics and topical corticosteroids.

BACTERIAL INFECTIONS

Pyoderma

There are many bacterial diseases affecting the skin that occur in people in the tropics. Undoubtedly, one of the most serious and widespread disorders is leprosy (see Chap. 88); however, the commonest, by far, is pyoderma. This term defines an invasion of the skin by pyogenic organisms, specifically *Staphylococcus aureus* and/or group A streptococci (Fig. 6-5). Pyoderma may be primary or secondary. Secondary pyoderma is superimposed on preexisting dermatoses, usually of the eczematous type. This process is often called "impetiginization," since the infection is superficial and impetigo-like. Tropical conditions such as warm climate, high humidity, lack

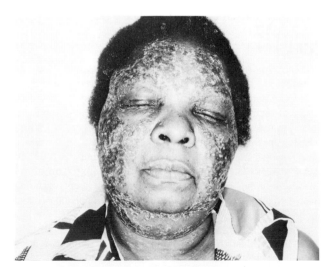

Figure 6-5. Pyoderma (resolving bullous impetigo) involving the face.

of medical care, and deficient hygiene are predisposing factors to impetiginization. This secondary bacterial invasion modifies the dermatological features of primary conditions and may make accurate diagnosis difficult.

Impetigo

Impetigo, caused by *S. aureus* or group A streptococci, or both, is the commonest of all pyodermas [17]. It is a superficial infection affecting mostly the face of children and is manifested by thin-walled vesicles that soon break and form characteristic "stuck-on," honeylike, yellow crusts. A common variety in the tropics is a bullous type with large blisters as a result of infection with particular phage groups of *S. aureus* that elaborate an exotoxin capable of cleaving the epidermis. *Ecthyma* refers to deeper, punched-out, ulcerative lesions covered with brown crusts, mainly involving the legs. Erysipelas and cellulitis often follow skin injury and are common in rural areas. These disorders are characterized by red, hot, tender plaques which may be associated with fever and chills. Other pyogenic disorders that occur commonly in the tropics include streptococcal ulcers, gangrene, and paronychia, an infection of the soft tissue around the nails.

Folliculitis is common in rural workers and often affects the lower extremities. Furuncles and carbuncles are common in the summer and tend to involve the scalp and posterior neck of children and hairy areas of the extremities of adults. Interestingly, sycosis barbae, mainly an infection of facial hair, is rare in most tropical races.

Treatment. General measures include cleansing of the skin and the use of topical antibiotics. Specific systemic antibiotic therapy is also indicated. Drug selection should be guided by culture and sensitivity studies whenever possible.

Erythrasma

Erythrasma is a mild cutaneous disorder caused by the grampositive diphtheroid *Corynebacterium minutissimum* and is common in the tropics. The eruption is manifest by faintly scaly, well-defined patches usually involving the genitocrural areas, the toe webs, and the antecubital and popliteal fossae (Fig. 6-6); pruritus is minimal. The disease may occur together with other superficial corynebacterial infections such as pitted keratolysis and trichomycosis axillaris [21]. It should be differentiated from tinea cruris and candidiasis. Diagnosis is confirmed by demonstrating the typical coral-red fluorescence of the infected skin using a Wood's lamp. Treatment with orally administered tetracycline (1 g/day for 7 days) or erythromycin (1 g/day for 5 days) is usually effective, but the condition frequently recurs.

Tropical ulcer

This is an acute localized necrosis of the skin and subcutaneous tissue affecting predominantly the lower extremities that is en-

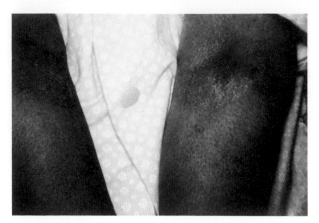

Figure 6-6. Erythrasma involving the antecubital fossae.

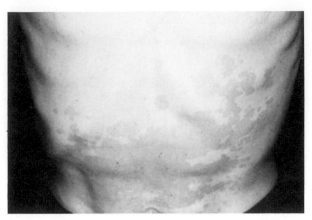

Figure 6-7. Pityriasis versicolor involving the lower abdomen.

demic in, but not confined to, the tropics. The disorder begins as a small papule overlying an area of necrotic dermis and primarily affects male children between the ages of 5 and 15. Recent studies suggest that anaerobes can be isolated from these lesions, particularly fusobacteria and *Bacteroides* [22,23].

FUNGAL INFECTIONS

Tinea imbricata

This is a rare, superficial fungal infection caused by *Trichophyton concentricum* and occurs irregularly in tropical regions. Clinically, there is involvement of large areas of skin with concentric rings of triangular scales, some of which may be loosely adherent. Coalescence of lesions forms a delicate, lace-like pattern that may evolve into a generalized scaling that can mimic exfoliative dermatitis. The disease tends to be chronic, and there may be deficient T-cell responsiveness in these patients [24,25]. Orally administered griseofulvin is effective, but relapses occur. Ketoconazole may also be effective.

Tinea nigra

Tinea nigra is a common, mild, asymptomatic fungal infection caused by varieties of *Cladosporium*. It occurs mainly in coastal regions. The lesions are sharply marginated, brown to black macules, usually found on the palmar surface of the hands and, rarely, on the feet. Confusion with nevi or melanoma may lead to unnecessary surgical removal. Treatment with keratolytic preparations containing salicylic acid such as Whitfield's ointment is effective.

Pityriasis versicolor

Pityriasis versicolor is the most common of the superficial fungal disorders that occur in the tropics. It is usually asymptomatic and in most instances is discovered when the patient seeks medical care for other conditions. It is caused by *Pity-*

rosporum ovale. Clinically, there are numerous, round or oval, scaly macules varying in color from pink to light brown (Fig. 6-7). In dark-skinned patients, a depigmented variety resembling vitiligo or indeterminate leprosy may occur. It is of interest that the organism may elaborate increased amounts of azelaic acid, a dicarboxylic acid that can inhibit tyrosinase activity [26]. The fungus is easily identified microscopically in scrapings examined in KOH wet mounts. Vigorous scrubbing and application of keratolytic preparations such as sodium thiosulfate constitute effective treatment. Application of selenium sulfide preparations and the imidazole antifungals also seems to be effective. Orally administered ketoconazole is said to be curative, but relapses can occur with all forms of therapy.

DEEP FUNGAL INFECTIONS

Ecologic conditions in the tropics favor the growth of numerous fungi capable of causing deep fungal infections. These are discussed in detail in other chapters of this book, but one of them, chromomycosis, will be briefly presented here.

Chromomycosis (chromoblastomycosis)

Chromomycosis is a chronic, progressive, granulomatous disease caused by various fungi such as *Fonsecaea pedrosoi, Cladosporium carrionii,* and others characterized by the dark color of their colonies when grown in vitro. These fungi are found in nature primarily in hot and humid climates, and Caucasians appear to be most susceptible.

Accidental inoculation through puncture injury is followed several weeks later by the onset of a nodule [27]. This grows slowly, becomes verrucous, and years later, a large vegetating plaque may cover most of the extremity. Elephantiasis and bone involvement may cause severe disability.

The diagnosis is made by finding brown "fumagoid" cells in KOH examination and by culture. The differential diagnosis should include verrucous tuberculosis, mycetoma, leishmaniasis, and other verrucous disorders found in the tropics.

Treatment. Early lesions may be destroyed or excised surgically. Large lesions may benefit from teatment with calci-
ferol, 5-fluorocytosine, and amphotericin B. Ketoconazole and
5-fluorocytosine in combination may be more effective than
either alone [*28*]. Relapses are common.

PARASITIC DISEASE

The parasitic diseases are described in their respective chapters. In this section only papular urticaria, a common skin
eruption secondary to insect bites, is discussed.

Papular urticaria

This condition, also known as lichen urticatus, is one of the
most common dermatoses seen in children in the tropics. Papular urticaria is particularly common in populations of low
socioeconomic status. The eruption seems to result from an
allergic reaction to insects. The causative insects are usually
fleas, particularly fleas from dogs (*Ctenocephalides canis*), cats
(*C. felis*), and humans (*Pulex irritans*). Bedbugs (*Cimex lectularius*) may also cause this disorder [*29*]. Initially an urticarial wheal forms, followed by a papule surmounted by a
vesicle. The disease is rare after the age of 7, apparently as a
result of spontaneous desensitization.

The clinical picture includes wheals, often with a central
hemorrhagic punctum, papules, papulovesicles, and residual
hyperpigmented spots. Pruritus is severe, and, as a result, most
lesions are excoriated.

Treatment. Avoidance of insects and the use of insecticides,
particularly DDT, and insect repellents are al¹ helpful. Topical
antipruritics and corticosteroids are beneficial. Systemic antihistamines may reduce itching and thereby diminish excoriations.

DRUG ERUPTIONS

Drug eruptions commonly occur in the tropics. Several factors
contribute to their high incidence. One is the wide range of
medications used, which include those generally employed in
western countries and those administered in the treatment of
tropical diseases. Another factor is that in many tropical areas
drugs can be obtained over the counter without a prescription.
This leads to indiscriminate use of medications and self-treat-
ment without medical supervision.

Drug eruptions may result from immunological and nonimmunological mechanisms. Immunological pathways may be
mediated by IgE or immune complexes, or they may be cell-
mediated. Nonimmunological pathways include side-effects,
overdosage, and drug interactions. General characteristics of
drug eruptions are their sudden onset and generalized distribution and the disappearance of the eruption when the drug is
discontinued. The eruption may reappear when the drug is
readministered.

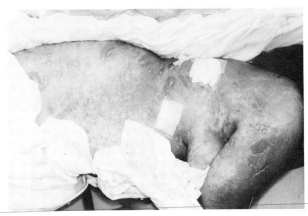

Figure 6-8. Blisters occurring in a patient with barbiturate-induced
toxic epidermal necrolysis.

Clinically, drug eruptions are polymorphous, and all types
of skin lesions may develop. As a rule, most drugs elicit a few
related types of cutaneous reactions. Urticarial and exanthe-
matic rashes (roseoliform, morbilliform, or scarlatiniform) are
the most common ones. They may be elicited by penicillin,
barbiturates, aspirin, and sulfonamides, among other medications.

Some drugs may elicit reactions that resemble specific diseases; thus, thiazide diuretics can produce a lichen planus–like
disease, and procainamide and hydralazine may evoke a lupus
erythematosus–like syndrome. Two other types of drug reaction should be mentioned.

Toxic epidermal necrolysis

This disease closely resembles staphylococcal scalded skin
syndrome, which occurs primarily in children [*30*]. In adults,
the same clinical picture with bullae that break and peel in
large sheets is frequently related to drugs such as dapsone,
long-acting sulfonamides, or barbiturates (Fig. 6-8).

Fixed drug eruptions

This is a common type of reaction that occurs more frequently
in highly pigmented tropical races The lesions are localized,
single or multiple, reddish-purple macules, 2 to 6 cm in diameter, often with a central blister. They heal with increased,
slate-gray pigmentation which may persist for months or years.
Readministration of the drug usually causes exacerbation of
the lesions in the same anatomical area. Common causes of
fixed drug eruptions are phenolphthalein (in laxatives), barbiturates, sulfones, and phenacetin.

TUMORS

It is generally true that the incidence of benign tumors of the
skin found in the tropics is similar to that in western countries,

except for a predisposition to keloids in Congoids. Conversely, the number of nonmelanoma skin cancers is smaller in tropical areas than in nontropical countries. This is mainly due to the protective action of melanin on the skin, which decreases the damaging effect of sunlight in the more pigmented tropical races. As a result, precancerous actinic keratoses or basal cell carcinomas are quite uncommon in these individuals. This contrasts with the high incidence of these diseases in fair-skinned populations, especially when excessively exposed to sunlight in the tropics. Local tumors are important factors in the geographic variations of carcinoma. In southeast Asia, oral cancer is almost 10 times more frequent than in the United States and Europe because of the common habit of chewing tobacco and betel nuts. In Kashmir, so-called Kangri cancer is common in those who use earthenware pots containing hot coals under their clothing to warm their skin [*31*].

Basal cell carcinoma

Basal cell carcinoma is a slowly growing, noninvasive tumor which usually does not metastasize. It begins as a round, dome-shaped, translucent papule which slowly enlarges and becomes ulcerated. In tropical races, the predominant variety is the pigmented type, which shows specks or diffuse, brown-to-black pigmentation. Differentiation from melanoma may be difficult. Favorite sites are sun-exposed areas of the face and trunk. Treatment with destructive methods such as electrodesiccation and curettage or liquid nitrogen cryotherapy is effective. Surgical excision and x-ray therapy are curative.

Squamous cell carcinoma

This occurs much less often in darker races and tends to develop equally in sun-exposed and sun-protected areas. In fair-skinned individuals, squamous cell carcinoma usually occurs on sun-exposed skin. In tropical races, it often originates in areas of chronic ulceration such as phagedenic ulcer, in areas of chronic granulomatous change secondary to deep fungal infections, or in scars. It also occurs on the lips in areas of chronic actinic cheilitis. Onset is gradual, although the course is faster than that of basal cell carcinoma. Early lesions show an indurated base and a warty surface; when fully developed, the lesions present a characteristic cauliflowerlike appearance. Metastases to regional lymph nodes can occur and may disseminate, leading to a fatal outcome. The legs are often affected in tropical races. Surgical excision of the carcinoma and draining lymph nodes is essential.

Kaposi's sarcoma

Kaposi's sarcoma is endemic in equatorial Africa and is an indolent disease in which the initial manifestation is usually edema of the feet and legs followed by the development of bluish-purple plaques and nodules in the same regions (Fig. 6-9) [*32*]. Over a period of years, these lesions gradually en-

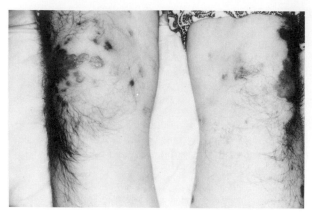

Figure 6-9. Nodular lesions of Kaposi's sarcoma occurring on the knees.

large and coalesce to form tumors. In the past decade, atypical Kaposi's sarcoma has been recognized in Africa; in this form the disease begins at a younger age, there may be no skin lesions at the outset, and those that occur are located atypically. In 8 of 13 African patients so described, there were no initial skin lesions, and the diagnosis was made by biopsy of enlarged lymph nodes [*33*]. This form of the disease behaves aggressively in most patients, and many have died within months of its onset due to widespread metastasis and/or opportunistic infections.

This atypical form of Kaposi's sarcoma occurs as one of the manifestations of the acquired immunodeficiency syndrome (AIDS) [*34*]. The major pathological consequence of AIDS is opportunistic infection, and this is related to specific immune deficits in patients infected with the human immunodeficiency virus (HIV). Histologically, Kaposi's sarcoma is a tumor of endothelial or endothelial-like cells. There is no evidence that these cells are infected with HIV nor do they express CD4 antigens. [*35*].

Melanoma

Melanoma is a less common type of skin cancer which, unlike basal cell and squamous cell carcinomas, may be a highly invasive, malignant tumor. This is a neoplasm of melanocytes. In tropical races, the acral areas (palmoplantar or subungual) are most commonly affected. Treatment is dependent upon depth of invasion, but requires wide excision and regional lymph node dissection.

MISCELLANEOUS

Acne

Acne is a chronic, inflammatory disorder of the pilosebaceous unit manifested by comedones, papules, pustules, nodules, and

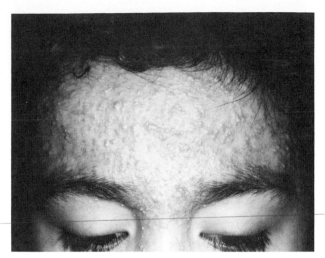

Figure 6-10. ''Mallorca acne'' occurring after extensive sun exposure while on vacation in the tropics.

cysts. The cause is unknown. Genetic, endocrine, and environmental factors may play a role. Acne begins at puberty and disappears spontaneously, usually after the teenage years. Areas rich in sebaceous glands, including the face, neck, and trunk, are most frequently affected. There are geographical and climatic variations. Acne is mild and has a low incidence in races with sparse body and facial hair. It is also rare and mild in the African Congoid. Keloidal scars may occur particularly in highly pigmented ethnic groups. Climatic factors affect the course of acne. Cautious exposure to sunlight usually improves acne, but tropical heat and humidity may exacerbate the disease. Indeed, the name *tropical acne* has been given to a severe nodulocystic form which has occurred in military personnel assigned to tropical climates [*36*]. This differs from typical acne vulgaris in that it involves the upper and lower back, the neck, and buttocks, and it often begins suddenly in older individuals. This disorder has also occurred in warm and humid occupational settings outside of the tropics.

Caucasoids suddenly exposed to a tropical climate may develop a severe form of acne known as *acne aestivalis* or *mallorca acne* (Fig. 6-10) [*37*]. This was first described by Hjörth et al. in Danish females who traveled to Mallorca for a holiday in the sunshine. This is a good example of the exacerbating effect of tropical climate on a common disease.

Treatment. Topical therapy with preparations containing sulfur, resorcin, benzoyl peroxide, or vitamin A acid are helpful. Systemically, the oral administration of broad-spectrum antibiotics such as tetracycline and erythromycin is effective. The photosensitizing properties of the tetracyclines should be kept in mind when prescribing these drugs.

Lichen planus

Lichen planus is an inflammatory dermatosis characterized by a localized or widespread eruption of flat, polygonal, often highly pruritic papules which may coalesce to lichenified plaques. The cause is unknown. Preferential sites of involvement are the flexor aspect of the wrists and forearms, inner thighs, shins, waistline, lumbar region, and penis.

Lichen planus is very common in certain parts of Africa, where some patients may present with large lesions and florid eruption. The individual papules on black skin are gray or black, lacking the characteristic violaceous color seen in fair-complected individuals. A stubborn hypertrophic variant found mainly on the legs occurs frequently in some tropical regions (Fig. 6-11). Residual pigmentation of healed lesions is persistent in most of the highly pigmented tropical races (Fig. 6-12). Lichen planus actinicus is a peculiar variant of the disease, thought to be precipitated by sunlight. It is limited primarily to the light-exposed areas, and the lesions are often annular. Some believe this to be the most common type of lichen planus in tropical regions [*38*].

The differential diagnosis of lichen planus includes secondary syphilis, tuberculoid leprosy, and drug eruptions. The hypertrophic type should be differentiated from verrucous tuberculosis, chromomycosis, lichen amyloidosis, and Kaposi's sarcoma.

Treatment. Topical medications are of little benefit. Severe cases improve with the simultaneous administration of paren-

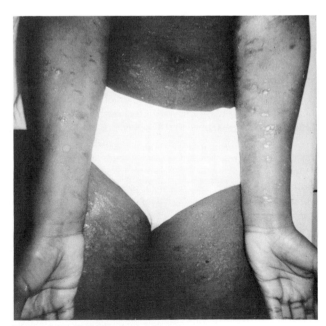

Figure 6-11. Extensive lichen planus.

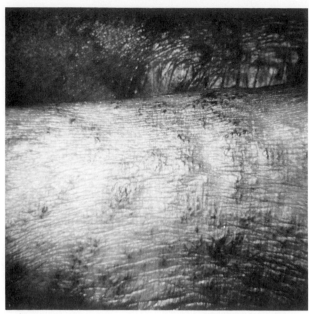

Figure 6-12. Pigmentary changes in the skin following lichen planus.

teral corticosteroids and a tranquilizer. Intralesional injections of a corticosteroid suspension may be of help in selected patients.

Psoriasis

Psoriasis is a chronic, inflammatory, cutaneous disorder manifested by erythematous papules and plaques covered with silvery scales. Pruritus is usually minimal but is occasionally severe. The cause is unknown, but aberrant regulation of epidermal proliferation is probably crucial. The disease has a predilection for aspects of the extremities, especially the knees and elbows, as well as the scalp, lumbosacral region, and genitals. Pitting and onycholysis affect the nails. Seronegative arthritis may occur in 5 to 10 percent of patients. In west Africans and their descendents in the Americas, psoriasis is rare, while in east African Congoids the disease is rather common but tends to run a mild course. In black skin, the scaly lesions appear gray, and when the scales are removed, they show a copperlike color due to retained melanin pigment. In some South American Indians psoriasis is rare, and in Mongoloids the disease is often milder and occurs less often than in Caucasoids. The differential diagnosis includes secondary syphilis, drug eruptions, and, in endemic areas, pinta.

Treatment. Keratolytic preparations containing salicylic acid, coal tar products, and chrysarobin derivatives such as anthralin are helpful. Topical corticosteroid preparations are effective, but their high cost often limits their use in the tropics. Systemic corticosteroids should never be used in psoriasis because of

the risk of a rebound pustular flare during tapering. Ultraviolet phototherapy and PUVA photochemotherapy are effective in more severely affected individuals [*39*].

SUMMARY

Tropical dermatology includes the study of diseases of the skin that may occur anywhere in the world but whose clinical appearance may be influenced or altered by their development in the ethnic groups which inhabit tropical regions. In addition, there are a large number of tropical diseases that occur almost exclusively in these geographical regions. The clinical expression of tropical diseases is dependent upon genetic, socioeconomic, and environmental factors, many of which remain poorly understood.

REFERENCES

1 Mosher DB, Fitzpatrick TB, Ortonne J-P, et al: Disorders of pigmentation, in Fitzpatrick TB et al (eds): *Dermatology of General Medicine,* 3d ed. New York, McGraw-Hill, 1987, pp 794–876

2 Canizares O: Los efectos de la altitud en dermatologica, in *Trans V Ibero Latino Americano Congress of Dermatology,* Buenos Aires, 1963, pp 861–866

3 Potter EV, Ortiz JS, Sharrett AR, et al: Changing types of nephritogenic streptococci in Trinidad. J Clin Invest 50:1197–1204, 1971

4 Hay RJ, Moore MK: Clinical features of superficial fungus infections caused by *Hendersonula toruloidea* and *Scylatidium hyalinum.* Br J Dermatol 110:677–683, 1984

5 Greer DL, Gutierrez MM: Tinea pedis caused by *Hendersonula toruloidea.* J Amer Acad Dermatol 16:1111–1115, 1987

6 Caniazares O: Essays on tropical dermatology. Excerpta Med 12:426–431, 1972

7 Van Heck E, Bugingo G: Prevalence of skin diseases in Rwanda. Int J Dermatol 19:526–531, 1980

8 Failmezger TC: A clinical survey of skin diseases in selected Latin American countries. Int J Dermatol 17:583–587, 1978

9 Canizares O: Dermatology in India. Arch Dermatol 112:93–97, 1976

10 Pettit JHS: Perspectives in dermatology: Malaysia. Int J Dermatol 15:505–510, 1976

11 Kotrajaras R: *Annual Report of the Institute of Dermatology.* Bangkok, Thailand, 1978

12 Ruiz-Maldonado R: Dermatosis mas frecuentes en al lactante y preescolar, in Ruiz-Maldonado R, Saul A, Ibarra G, et al (eds): *Temas de Dermatologic Pediatrica.* Mexico City, F. Mendez Cervantes, 1980, pp 211–214

13 Tamayo L: Dermatosis mas frecuentes en el excolar, in Ruiz-Maldonado R, Saul A, Ibarra G, et al (eds): *Temas de Dermatologica Pediatrica.* Mexico City, F. Mendez Cervantes, 1980, pp 215–217

14 Saul A: Dermatosis mas frecuentes en el adolescente, in Ruiz-Maldonado R, Saul A, Ibarra G, et al (eds): *Temas de Dermatolica Pediatrica.* Mexico City, F. Mendez Cervantes, 1980, pp 219–221

15 Canizares, O (ed): *Clinical Tropical Dermatology.* Oxford, Blackwell, 1975

16 Simons, RDGP: *Handbook of Tropical Dermatology and Medical Mycology,* vols 1 and 2. Amsterdam, Elsevier, 1952

17 Swartz MN, Weinberg AN: Infections due to gram-positive bacteria, in Fitzpatrick TB, et al (eds): *Dermatology in General Medicine,* 3d ed. New York, McGraw-Hill, 1987, pp 2100–2121

18 Fisher AA: *Contact Dermatitis.* Philadelphia, Lea & Febiger, 1986

19 Cronin E: *Contact Dermatitis.* London, Churchill-Livingstone, 1980

20 Adams RM: *Occupational Contact Dermatitis.* Philadelphia, Lippincott, 1983, pp 379–445

21 Sinchuphak W, MacDonald E, Smith EB: Erythrasma: Overlooked or misdiagnosed. Int J Dermatol 24:95–96, 1985

22 Adriaans B, Hay R, Drasar B, et al: The infectious etiology of tropical ulcer—A study of the role of anaerobic bacteria. Br J Dermatol 116:31–37, 1987

23 Robinson DC, Adriaans B, Hay RJ, et al: Clinical and epidemiologic features of tropical ulcer (tropical phagedenic ulcer). Int J Dermatol 27:49–53, 1987

24 Hay RJ: Tinea imbricata: The factors affecting persistent dermatophytosis. Int J Dermatol 24:562–564, 1985

25 Hay RJ, Reid S, Talwat E, et al: Immune responses of patients with tinea imbricata. Br J Dermatol 108:581–586, 1983

26 Nazzaro-Porro M, Passi S: Identification of tyrosinase inhibitors in cultures of pityrosporum. J Invest Dermatol 71:205–208, 1978

27 McGinnis MR: Chromoblastomycosis and phaeohyphomycosis: New concepts, diagnosis and mycology. J Am Acad Dermatol 8:1–16, 1983

28 Silber JG, Gombert ME, Green KM, et al: Treatment of chromomycosis with ketoconazole and 5-fluorocytosine. J Am Acad Dermatol 8:236–238, 1983

29 Rees R, King LE Jr: Arthropod bites and stings, in Fitzpatrick TB, et al (eds): *Dermatology in General Medicine,* 3d ed. New York, McGraw-Hill, 1987, pp 2495–2506

30 Lyell A: Toxic epidermal necrolysis: An eruption resembling scalding of the skin. Br J Dermatol 68:355–363, 1956

31 Mulay DM: Skin cancer in India. Nat Cancer Inst Mono 10:215–219, 1963

32 Taylor JF, Smith PG, Bull D, et al: Kaposi's sarcoma in Uganda: Geographic and ethnic distribution. Br J Cancer 26:483–497, 1972

33 Bayley AC: Aggressive Kaposi's sarcoma in Zambia, 1983. Lancet i:1318–1320, 1984

34 Bayley AC, Cheingsong-Porov R, Dalgleish AG, et al: HTLV-III serology distinguishes atypical and endemic Kaposi's sarcoma in Africa. Lancet i:359–361, 1985

35 Weissman I: Approaches to an understanding of pathogenetic mechanisms in AIDS. Rev Inf Dis 10:385–398, 1988

36 Tucker SB: Occupational tropical acne. Cutis 31:79–81, 1983

37 Hjörth N, Sjölin KE, Sylvest B, et al: Acne aestivalis: Mallorca acne. Acta Dermatol Venereol 52:61–63, 1972

38 Katzenellenbogen I: Lichen planus actinicus (lichen planus in subtropical countries). Dermatologica 124:10–20, 1962

39 Melski JW, Tanenbaum L, Parrish J, et al: Oral methoxsalen photochemotherapy for the treatment of psoriasis: A cooperative clinical trial. J Invest Dermatol 68:328–335, 1977

CHAPTER 7 / *Eye Manifestations* · Hugh R. Taylor · Richard D. Semba

EYE DISEASES IN TROPICAL AREAS

The spectrum of eye diseases in tropical areas differs in many ways from that seen in more temperate areas. There are a number of reasons for this. Common eye diseases, especially infections and trauma, are often seen at a more severe or advanced stage because of delays in patient presentation and the difficulty of obtaining medical attention. Some systemic tropical diseases have secondary ocular involvement. Also, there are a number of specific eye diseases that do not occur (or are no longer seen) in the more ''developed'' areas. The latter include diseases such as trachoma and onchocerciasis.

This chapter will give a general outline of the management of some common tropical ocular problems and will describe the ophthalmic features of trachoma and xerophthalmia (for a more complete description of these conditions see Chaps. 70 and 121). Many of the incidental ocular manifestations of other diseases will be found under the relevant disease sections in various chapters. A detailed description of the ocular manifestations of a comprehensive range of diseases is also available [1].

In the developed countries, blindness is seen with increasing frequency in the elderly. Age-related changes and degenerative diseases are the most important causes of blindness. For the most part, these diseases are poorly understood, and, therefore, they are difficult to prevent. The amount of blindness in developed countries can be taken as an approximate baseline of blindness that is, with some exceptions, unavoidable with the present forms of treatment. If blindness is defined as vision of less than 3/60 (20/400), the rates in most developed countries range from 1.5 to 2.0 per 1000 [2].

In developing areas, however, there is a tremendous ''overburden of unnecessary blindness'' superimposed on this baseline of ''unavoidable blindness'' [3]. In Africa, for example, the rates of blindness may range from 53 to 68 per 1000 [2]. There are probably over 30 million people in developing areas who are blinded by diseases that are either preventable or treatable. Usually, these are common diseases such as infections that respond well to standard treatment. Thus, it is important that all health workers realize that they can play an important role in the prevention of blindness and that the treatment of eye disease is not the responsibility of ophthalmologists alone.

In general, the eye responds to inflammation, whether from infection, trauma, or other causes, in much the same way as other tissues of the body. However, the eye is especially susceptible to loss of function after relatively trivial inflammation. Normal ocular function is dependent on the transparency of the ocular media, and thus a small strategically placed scar can render the eye functionally useless.

THE OPHTHALMIC EXAMINATION

An appropriate history and a careful examination are the foundations of management of all ocular problems [4]. The history should include details of the onset, duration, and characteristics of the presenting complaint and a review of the patient's general health and individual and family history. Specific questions should be asked concerning changes in vision, blurring, flashes or floaters, double vision, visual field loss, night blindness, ocular discharge, pain, and discomfort. It is important to assess visual acuity in any patient complaining of change of vision. Visual acuity is usually measured with a letter chart placed 6 m from the patient [5]. In small children, visual acuity is assumed to be normal if they can fixate and follow a small target with each eye while the other is covered.

A simple examination of the eye with a hand light will reveal gross corneal or conjunctival disease, blood or pus in the eye, cataract, or acute glaucoma. Whenever possible, the front of the eye should be examined with magnification such as with a 2X loupe or a direct ophthalmoscope using the + 10 diopter lens. The pupils should be examined for reflex movement, size, and shape. An ophthalmoscope is needed to examine the back of the eye for retinal and optic nerve disease.

THE PAINFUL RED EYE

Although conjunctivitis is the most common cause of a painful red eye, all patients need to be carefully examined to exclude more serious eye conditions that have a similar presentation.

A simple history and ocular examination will reveal the correct diagnosis in most cases (Table 7-1).

CONJUNCTIVITIS

Conjunctivitis is the most common cause of bilateral red eyes. Conjunctivitis is usually infective, although it can be caused by allergy and trauma. Infectious conjunctivitis typically has an acute onset, and discharge is usually present. With bacterial infection, the discharge is mucopurulent or purulent, whereas the discharge is more watery with viral and chlamydial infections. A frankly purulent discharge is characteristic of gonococcal infection. There is often an accumulation of discharge around the lid margins, which may at times cause the lids to stick together.

Conjunctival "injection" (vascular dilatation and redness) is the hallmark of conjunctivitis. The injection is most prominent on the conjunctiva underneath the eyelids (tarsal conjunctiva) and in the fornices. It is less severe near the cornea. The dilated conjunctival vessels give a bright red injection which, with severe inflammation, may be associated with red blotches of subconjunctival hemorrhage. Pseudomembranes are seen as dirty, gray sloughs on the tarsal conjunctiva, and they occur with severe inflammation. Follicles or germinal centers are common in viral and chlamydial conjunctivitis and are seen as white dots in the tarsal conjunctiva and in the fornix. Giant papillae are characteristic of allergic conjunctivitis. In uncomplicated conjunctivitis, the cornea is clear and bright, the pupil and anterior chamber are normal, and visual acuity is not affected.

Treatment

Bacterial conjunctivitis responds quickly to specific antibiotic treatment. Topical antibiotics such as 0.5% chloramphenicol or gentamicin are given every 1 to 2 h during the day with 1% ointment at night. Antibiotic ointments such as 1% tetracycline

Table 7-1. Differential diagnosis of the painful red eye

	Acute conjunctivitis	Keratitis, corneal ulcer	Anterior uveitis	Acute angle-closure glaucoma
Pain	Itching, irritation	Moderate to severe	Moderate	Severe, nausea, sudden onset
Vision	Normal	Blurred	Blurred	Marked reduction, with halos
Injection	Conjunctiva, bright red	Ciliary or diffuse	Ciliary	Ciliary, purple
Discharge	Moderate to marked, watery to purulent	Variable, mild to marked	None	None
Cornea	Clean and bright	Abrasion, opacity, foreign body	Clear, keratic precipitates	Steamy?
Pupil	Normal	Variable	Small, irregular, sluggish	Large, oval(?), unresponsive
Other features	Very common, all ages	Photophobia	Exclude systemic disease	Usually in elderly; intraocular pressure raised

or gentamicin (3 mg/g) may be used as an alternative and are given four times a day. Ocular ointments are especially useful for children. Antibiotic treatment should be continued for about 1 week. It is important that the eye be kept free of accumulating discharge. To avoid spreading the infection, patients should wash their hands carefully and not share towels or clothes with others.

Gonococcal ophthalmia neonatorum usually develops within the first 2 or 3 days of life [6]. It is a very serious infection and requires prompt treatment with intravenous crystalline penicillin [100,000 units/(kg·day)] in four divided doses [7]. The eyes should be irrigated with saline at least hourly to eliminate discharge. Chlamydial inclusion conjunctivitis characteristically develops between 4 and 12 days after birth [8]. It is best treated with oral erythromycin [50 mg/(kg·day)] given in four divided doses for 2 weeks.

Symptomatic relief can be obtained in viral conjunctivitis with the use of cold compresses and topical vasoconstricting drops such as 0.1% naphazoline or 0.12% phenylephrine given three or four times a day. Vasoconstricting drops also can be used in patients with allergic conjunctivitis. Topical antibiotics are unnecessary in uncomplicated viral conjunctivitis. Topical steroids should never be used in conjunctivitis except under the direct supervision of an ophthalmologist because steroids can have disastrous effects in bacterial and herpetic infections.

KERATITIS, CORNEAL ULCERATION, AND NECROSIS

Keratitis and corneal ulceration are frequent causes of a unilateral painful red eye. Vision is usually reduced, and severe photophobia is often present. Secondary uveitis is common, leading to ciliary injection (a ring of redness around the cornea). Superficial keratitis is common in viral infections. Deep corneal ulceration is more often the result of bacterial infection, and the signs of conjunctivitis are usually present. Herpes simplex is the most important cause of viral corneal ulceration. Fungal corneal ulcers may follow rather minor trauma, and they are not uncommon.

The presence of a corneal defect is the most important diagnostic sign. The cornea may be cloudy or hazy in keratitis, whereas an ulcer will show as a surface defect that distorts the corneal reflex. Ulcers, especially small ulcers such as dendritic ulcers caused by herpes infection, are best seen after the instillation of fluorescein. Large ulcers are often filled with white, sloughed material and debris. Dark tissue may sometimes be seen in the base of an ulcer. This tissue is usually a bit of iris, and this indicates that the ulcer has perforated the cornea and that iris is plugging the hole. Pus may accumulate in the anterior chamber and form a fluid level (hypopyon).

Treatment

Bacterial Keratitis. Intensive local antibiotic therapy is used to treat bacterial corneal ulcers. Microbiological cultures and Gram stains will often assist in the proper management. Intensive local antibiotics are usually given by topical routes [9]. Fortified eye drops are used, in which the antibiotic is diluted in artificial tears. Cephazolin (50 mg/mL) and gentamicin (12.5 mg/mL) are commonly used. Initially, they should be given a few minutes apart every hour. A mydriatic (1% atropine sulfate drops four times a day) is usually prescribed. Subconjunctival antibiotics such as carbenicillin (100 mg) and gentamicin (20 mg) can be used in addition in corneal ulceration due to gram-negative bacteria, especially *Pseudomonas* sp. Topical antibiotics should be continued until the corneal ulcer is completely healed.

Herpetic Keratitis. This commonly presents with the characteristic dendritic ulcer, and there is usually a decrease in corneal sensation. Single dendritic ulcers are best treated with simple debridement with the removal of all the infected epithelium around the edge of the ulcer, followed by the instillation of an antiviral (0.5% idoxuridine ointment) and then patching of the eye for 1 or 2 days [10]. Alternatively, a topical antiviral agent such as 1% trifluorothyoxidine drops or 0.5% idoxuridine ointment may be used every 4 h for at least 1 week. Usually, topical antiviral therapy should not be continued for longer than 2 to 3 weeks because it may cause severe toxic reactions that can mimic herpetic keratitis. In most cases, it is advisable to use a mydriatic (1% atropine sulfate drops four times a day) until the ulcer has healed. Steroids should never be used by nonophthalmologists to treat corneal ulcers and keratitis.

Total necrosis of the cornea is most often caused by xerophthalmia and keratomalacia, and this is the most common cause of blindness in children in Asia [11]. In Africa, many children are blinded by corneal necrosis which follows an attack of measles. Although superficial keratitis is common in measles, well-nourished children do not usually develop severe corneal necrosis after this infection. Blinding corneal necrosis after measles usually results from the precipitation of severe vitamin A deficiency [12]. Other possible contributing factors may include herpetic keratitis or a chemical or bacterial keratitis following the use of traditional herbal remedies on the eye.

OCULAR TRAUMA

A history of trauma can usually be elicited. The signs and symptoms are usually unilateral and are of sudden onset. The sensation of "something in the eye" or pain is often caused by conjunctival foreign bodies. They usually are associated with some degree of conjunctival injection and watering of the eye. Although foreign bodies may be easily seen with simple examination, they sometimes lodge underneath the upper eyelid where they are not seen until the eyelid is everted.

Corneal foreign bodies usually produce more pain and photophobia and frequently cause ciliary injection. Most corneal foreign bodies can be simply removed with a cotton-tipped applicator. Antibiotic ointment or drops should be put into the eye and the eye patched for 24 h. If it is not possible to remove the corneal foreign body easily, the patient should be referred to an ophthalmologist.

Immediate and copious irrigation is the best treatment for chemical burns to the eyes. Although normal sterile saline is the best irrigating solution, it is preferable to use clean tap water than to delay irrigation. Alkali, unlike acid, continues to penetrate the eye for some time. For this reason, the severity of alkaline burns is not always immediately apparent and is often more severe. Although minor burns can be treated with antibiotics, cycloplegia, and patching, all cases of severe burn should be referred to an ophthalmologist.

Conjunctival hemorrhages are common, especially in the elderly. They may be either spontaneous or traumatic. They require no treatment, and they resolve spontaneously with 1 to 2 weeks. Minor conjunctival lacerations heal spontaneously, and they usually do not require suturing, although topical antibiotics may be given for a few days. Penetrating injuries to the eye, including intraocular foreign bodies, are medical emergencies and should be treated by an ophthalmologist. Severe eye injuries can masquerade as minor conjunctival and lid lacerations unless the globe and visual acuity are carefully examined. In case of doubt, refer the patient to an ophthalmologist.

ANTERIOR UVEITIS

Inflammation of the anterior uvea (the iris and the ciliary body) is called anterior uveitis. Compared to conjunctivitis and keratitis, uveitis is a less common cause of a sore red eye. Included in this term are iritis and iridocyclitis. Mild anterior uveitis is frequently seen in association with other ocular conditions, especially corneal trauma and ulceration. Uveitis may occur in association with systemic diseases, although uveitis often occurs as an isolated event with no recognizable cause.

Patients with primary anterior uveitis present with moderate to severe pain and some blurring of vision in one or both eyes. These symptoms are usually of gradual onset. Ciliary injection is the most characteristic sign of anterior uveitis, with the redness being most marked at the corneal limbus. The pupil is usually small and reacts poorly to light. The irregularity of the pupil may be due to adhesions (posterior synechiae) between the pupillary margin and the lens. Inflammatory cells and exudate can be seen in the anterior chamber if the eye is examined with a slit lamp. If the inflammation is more severe, pus may form a fluid level (hypopyon). Inflammatory cells (keratic precipitates) may be seen as clumps on the back of the cornea. Although uveitis may occur as an isolated ocular condition, patients should be examined to exclude the possibility of underlying conditions such as systemic infections, arthropathies, collagen diseases, or other systemic illnesses.

Treatment

Anterior uveitis is best treated with topical steroids (such as 1% prednisolone acetate drops given initially four times a day) and with cycloplegics (for example, atropine sulfate 1% drops four times a day). If patients have severe pain and photophobia, some relief may be obtained with systemic analgesics (aspirin 600 mg every 4 h). Secondary glaucoma and secondary cataracts may develop in patients with severe or chronic uveitis, and these conditions require specific treatment.

ACUTE ANGLE-CLOSURE GLAUCOMA

Acute angle-closure glaucoma is characterized by a sudden increase in intraocular pressure caused by obstruction of the drainage pathways for outflow of the intraocular fluid (aqueous humor). The elevated pressure can cause permanent and total loss of vision within 1 to 2 days; and for this reason, prompt diagnosis and treatment are highly important. Angle-closure glaucoma usually occurs in elderly people, and it is a relatively uncommon cause of a painful red eye. The onset of pain is usually sudden, and the pain may be severe enough to cause nausea and vomiting. Vision is moderately reduced, and the patient may complain of seeing halos or colored rings around lights.

On examination, the most striking features are the hazy or steamy cornea (corneal edema) and the elevated intraocular pressure. Intraocular pressure is best measured by tonometry, but it can be assessed by palpating the eye through closed lids and comparing its degree of resilience with a normal eye. Ciliary injection may be present. On closer examination, the anterior chamber appears very shallow and the iris may seem to touch the cornea. The pupil is irregular, semidilated, and unreactive.

Treatment

Every effort should be made to reduce the intraocular pressure as quickly as possible. Hyperosmotic agents such as oral glycerine (3 mg per kilogram of body weight) should be followed by frequent miotic drops (2 to 4% pilocarpine, 1 drop every 15 min for four doses, then every half-hour for 1 h, and then once every 2 h). Oral carbonic anhydrase inhibitors (acetazolamide, 500 mg orally or intramuscularly) can also be used. Patients frequently require strong analgesia to control the severe pain. Patients with acute angle-closure glaucoma should be referred to an ophthalmologist so that definitive laser treatment or surgery (peripheral iridectomy) can be performed.

CATARACT

A cataract is an opacity in the lens of the eye. In a normal eye with a clear lens, the pupil appears black. When a cataract is present, the pupil will appear white or brown (Fig. 7-1). Although a number of congenital and metabolic disorders are

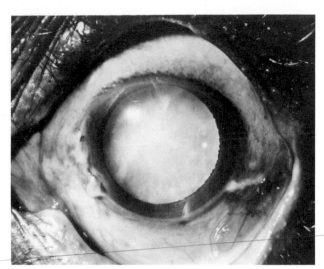

Figure 7-1. Mature cataract obstructing the pupil which now appears milky white.

associated with cataracts, these are relatively uncommon. Most cataracts occur in elderly patients and are termed *senescent* or *senile cataracts*. Although sunlight, especially ultraviolet radiation, and nutritional factors have been proposed as causes of senile cataracts, the etiology of cataract is almost certainly multifactorial [*13,14*]. Secondary cataracts may occur after trauma and intraocular inflammation. Although the causes of senile cataract are unknown, the basic treatment is straightforward: surgical extraction followed by the appropriate "aphakic" refractive correction. Aphakia is the condition existing after the natural lens is removed.

Previously, thick aphakic spectacles were prescribed to patients after cataract surgery; but now for most patients in the United States, a plastic intraocular lens is implanted in the eye at the time of cataract surgery (Fig. 7-2). This gives a significant improvement in postoperative visual function, but because of issues of surgical instrumentation, cost, and safety, implants are not yet in widespread use in developing countries.

Cataracts remain the leading cause of blindness in many parts of the world because of the lack of the appropriate surgical facilities. Measures to overcome this problem can include the training of paramedical staff to perform cataract surgery and the use of mobile cataract camps [*14*]. Although cataract extraction is relatively simple, there is a real risk of operative complications and infection if meticulous care is not paid to all aspects of the surgery. In the absence of other underlying ocular pathology, about 90 percent of patients can be expected to regain good vision with the appropriate refractive correction. Because of the lack of surgical facilities, it has been estimated that worldwide only 20 percent of those people blinded from cataract will ever receive surgical treatment [*15*].

CHRONIC SIMPLE GLAUCOMA

Chronic simple glaucoma or chronic open-angle glaucoma is a common and important cause of blindness. Unlike acute angle-closure glaucoma, which has an acute presentation, the elevation of intraocular pressure in chronic simple glaucoma is very gradual and insidious. Over many years the elevated intraocular pressure slowly destroys the fibers of the optic nerve, thus causing visual field loss [*16*]. This usually goes unnoticed until all the peripheral vision is lost and the central vision begins to be affected. Often at this late stage there is little that can be done to save the remaining "island" of central vision. The signs of chronic simple glaucoma are elevated intraocular pressure, progressive visual field loss, and abnormal cupping and atrophy of the optic nerve head (as a result of nerve fiber destruction).

Diagnosis

Methods for the early detection and diagnosis of glaucoma are at present unsatisfactory. The simplest and most widely used technique is the measurement of intraocular pressure (tonometry). In general, intraocular pressures above 21 mmHg are regarded as abnormal; and the higher the pressure, the more likely the patient is to have glaucoma [*17*]. However, only 1 in 20 of the patients with a pressure greater than 21 mmHg will develop glaucoma, and about half of the patients with glaucoma will have a normal pressure on a single screening examination. The finding of abnormal cupping of the optic nerve head is suggestive of glaucoma as are the classical visual field defects. Glaucoma is usually diagnosed on the basis of

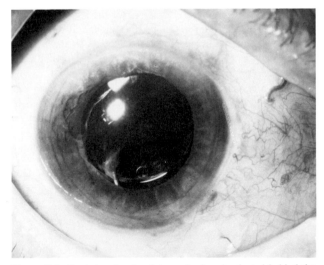

Figure 7-2. Posterior chamber intraocular lens implanted behind the iris at the time of cataract surgery. As the implant is displaced slightly upward, the edge of the lens can be seen as well as a small hole used to position it during surgery.

the presence of two of the triad of signs, elevated pressure, abnormal cupping, and visual field loss.

Treatment

The reduction of intraocular pressure to a safe level is the aim of glaucoma treatment. Although a pressure of 21 mmHg is usually regarded as a safe level, some patients may continue to lose visual field at this pressure and may require even further reduction. Intraocular pressure can be reduced by various topical medications. These include parasympathomimetics (such as pilocarpine, 1 to 4% four times a day), sympathomimetics (such as epinephrine, 1 to 2% two times a day), β-adrenergic blockers (such as timolol maleate 0.25 to 0.5% two times a day). Oral carbonic anhydrase inhibitors (such as acetazolamide 250 mg, four times a day) can also be used. As in the treatment of systemic hypertension, these various medications can be used in combination, and commonly they must be used more or less indefinitely.

In some instances, there is continuing visual field loss despite maximum medical therapy. In these cases, the patients require glaucoma surgery, which may entail the argon laser treatment of the trabecular meshwork or the surgical creation of a small filtering fistula to reduce the intraocular pressure. In many of the developing areas where medication is difficult to obtain, surgery is used as the initial treatment of choice. Filtering surgery is not always successful, however, and it may need to be repeated or the patient continued on antiglaucoma medication.

SENILE MACULAR DEGENERATION

Senile macular degeneration is an important cause of blindness, and it occurs in the elderly. It is one of the major causes of blindness in the developed countries, although in developing areas its importance is usually overshadowed by the tremendous amount of blindness caused by corneal scarring and cataract. Its etiology is unclear, although in some cases it may be familial or associated with hypertension [18]. The disease is slowly progressive, with a gradual reduction of central vision. If the disease is more advanced in one eye, all vision may be lost in that eye without the patient realizing it. Patients may then complain of a sudden loss of vision when their remaining good eye is covered for some reason.

Senile macular degeneration shows a series of progressive changes that can be seen with the ophthalmoscope [19]. Initially, there are small, white retinal dots (drusen) mainly in the macular area and often associated with areas of alteration in the retinal pigment epithelium. With time these changes become more marked and involve a larger area. In some cases, a net of new blood vessels grows from the choroid underneath the retina. Small hemorrhages are then likely to occur and to leave areas of scarring as they resolve (Figs. 7-3, 7-4). Initially, leakage from these vessels often causes minor aberrations in central vision. The vessels are best seen during fluo-

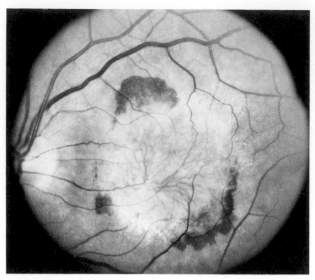

Figure 7-3. Senile macular degeneration showing hemorrhage and scar tissue at the macular region of the retina. The optic nerve is visible to the left.

rescein angiography. If these vessels can be detected at an early stage, they can be sealed in many cases with laser photocoagulation. This will often reduce the likelihood of progressive loss of vision and blindness [20]. Laser photocoagulation represents a major advance in the treatment of this disease. Although senile macular degeneration may destroy the macula and therefore central vision, the peripheral visual field is not affected.

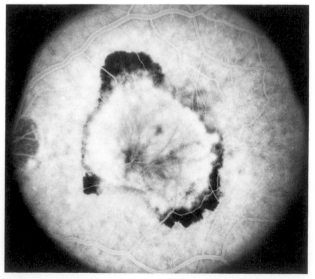

Figure 7-4. Fluorescein angiogram of same eye as in Fig. 8-3. Dye can be seen in the retinal veins and leaking from new vessels in the disciform scar in the macula. (*Courtesy of R. P. Murphy.*)

XEROPHTHALMIA

Xerophthalmia is the major clinical result of vitamin A deficiency, and it can result in blindness. The causes, physiology, and geographical distribution of vitamin A deficiency are presented in detail in Chap. 121. Xerophthalmia is a disease of major importance; each year it affects about 5 million children under the age of 6 [*11*]. It occurs especially in the Indian subcontinent, Indonesia, and the Philippines. It also occurs in widespread areas of the Sahel, in east Africa, in some areas of southeast Asia, and in Central and South America. Recent data have shown that even mild vitamin A deficiency is associated with a significant increase in childhood mortality and that periodic supplementation with vitamin A can dramatically reduce mortality rates [*21*].

OCULAR CHANGES

Chronic progressive vitamin A deficiency initially causes night blindness followed by xerosis of the conjunctiva, then xerosis of the cornea, and finally corneal ulceration and necrosis (keratomalacia) in severe cases. Night blindness is the earliest symptom of vitamin A deficiency and is due to inadequate vitamin A levels in the retina. Mothers will frequently notice that their children lose their way at night or stumble into objects. Local terms denoting night blindness often exist [*17*].

In conjunctival xerosis, thickening and keratinization of the conjunctiva occur. This process is seen first temporally, then nasally, and progresses until the whole conjunctiva becomes xerotic. Clinically, the conjunctiva is no longer smooth and glistening but becomes dry, unwettable, thickened, and skinlike. Frequently, collections of keratin and debris occur and form Bitot's spots which look foamy or cheesy (Fig. 7-5).

The xerotic cornea is dry and irregular, with loss of the clear corneal reflex. The cornea may be mildly opaque. The xerotic

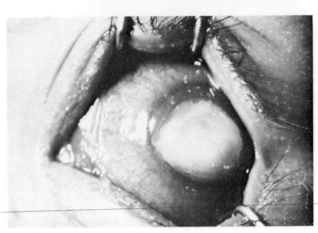

Figure 7-6. Total necrosis of the cornea (keratomalacia). (*Courtesy of A. Sommer.*)

cornea is particularly susceptible to ulceration. Xerophthalmic ulcers are classically round and sharply demarcated. Although small ulcers tend to be peripheral, large ulcers can involve the entire cornea (Fig. 7-6). Corneal ulceration often leads to perforation, which, if small, may become plugged with iris tissue. Larger perforations lead to loss of the eye. Scars are left when the ulcer heals. Small peripheral scars usually do not affect vision, although blindness results when there are large central scars and from atrophy (phthisis) of the perforated eye.

During an acute infection such as measles or gastroenteritis, severe vitamin A deficiency may be precipitated rapidly in children who have borderline vitamin A stores if these stores are rapidly mobilized and then depleted. These children may present with corneal ulceration or keratomalacia without first developing the signs of mild vitamin A deficiency. Frequently, these children are severely malnourished and severely ill.

Small white dots in the retina may be seen in cases of longstanding vitamin A deficiency.

TREATMENT

High doses of vitamin A (200,000 IU) are given orally at the time of diagnosis of xerophthalmia. An additional oral dose should be given the next day and again 1 week later [*22*]. In children with corneal ulceration, topical antibiotics should be used and the eye protected with a firm shield. These children are frequently severely ill and in danger of dying, and they require the appropriate treatment for their malnutrition or systemic infections.

With the exception of corneal ulceration, the signs of xerophthalmia disappear within a few days of receiving high-dose vitamin A. Corneal ulceration will commence to heal within a few days but may take several weeks to heal completely, leaving a permanent scar.

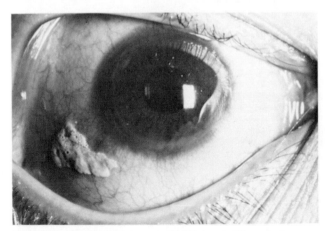

Figure 7-5. Classical foamy temporal Bitot spot. (*From A. Sommer: Field Guide to Detection and Control of Xerophthalmia, Geneva, WHO, 1978.*)

TRACHOMA

Trachoma is a chlamydial infection that occurs epidemically in many developing areas. Although initially acquired in early childhood, blindness from trachoma does not occur until adult life. Blindness is usually caused by corneal scarring which results from progressive scarring and distortion of the upper eyelid [23]. The progressive accumulation of scars can be halted with appropriate intervention, but changes that have already occurred cannot be reversed. Chlamydial infections are dealt with more fully in Chap. 70.

Repeated episodes or reexposure to *Chlamydia trachomatis* appear to be necessary for the development of chronic endemic trachoma. Inclusion conjunctivitis, a self-limited chlamydial infection, develops after a single exposure [24]. In areas of endemic trachoma, the chlamydial infection is not limited to the eyes but also involves other mucous membrane surfaces such as the nasopharynx and gastrointestinal tract [25].

It now appears that in trachomatous areas the majority of the transmission of chlamydia occurs within the family [26]. The presence and severity of trachoma has been correlated with face cleaning behavior [27]. In families in these areas, personal hygiene is usually poor, often because of limited access to water, high fly density, crowding, and so forth. Because of poor hygiene, there is an increased frequency of transmission of chlamydia-infected secretions, and family members are subjected to high rates of reinfection. The presence of infection and ocular discharge feeds into this cycle and facilitates transmission.

Secondary bacterial conjunctivitis may have a synergistic effect with chlamydial infection. The combination can intensify the inflammation, thus leading to increased conjunctival scarring or to corneal ulceration and later corneal scarring. Seasonal epidemics of bacterial conjunctivitis with *Haemophilus, Streptococcus,* and *Neisseria* organisms are common in some areas of north Africa.

OCULAR CHANGES

The clinical signs of trachoma fall into two groups: the signs of active (or reactive) inflammation and the signs of cicatricial changes. The inflammatory signs include follicles in the superior tarsus, limbal follicles, and papillae. These signs indicate the presence of an active inflammatory response to current chlamydial infection. The signs of cicatricial trachoma include scarring of the superior tarsal conjunctiva, trichiasis, corneal pannus, and Herbert's pits. These signs indicate that the patient has had active chlamydial infection in the past, but the signs themselves do not indicate current infection.

Tarsal follicles are seen as large, pale yellow or white spots on the superior tarsus (Fig. 7-7). They may be slightly elevated and are 0.5 to 2 mm in diameter. They are lymphoid germinal centers. Follicles may also form at the limbus, where they appear as a gelatinous gray string of dots. Papillae are small, red pinpoint dots in the superior tarsal conjunctiva. They are

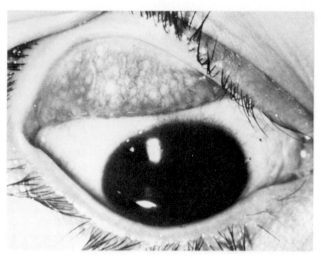

Figure 7-7. Trachoma follicles showing as pale dots in the upper tarsal conjunctiva.

not specific for trachoma and can be seen with almost any conjunctival irritation. A marked inflammatory thickening of the lid indicates more severe disease (Fig. 7-8). This response increases dramatically with secondary bacterial infection. The intensity of the papillary response with inflammatory thickening and the presence of follicles provide a good index of the severity of inflammation and the need for urgent treatment on an individual basis [23].

Conjunctival scars first appear as small, starlike figures, which gradually accumulate to form a basketweave network.

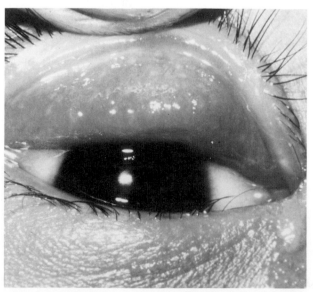

Figure 7-8. Trachomatous inflammation showing both inflammatory thickening and follicles.

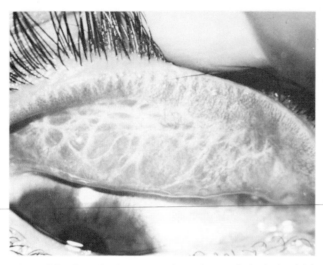

Figure 7-9. Consolidating bands of scarring, typical of cicatricial trachoma.

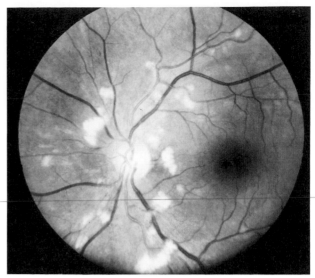

Figure 7-11. Multiple cotton-wool spots in patient with AIDS in Rwanda. (*Courtesy of P. Kestelyn.*)

With time, the scars consolidate to form strong bands that distort the eyelid (Fig. 7-9). This causes the lid margin to roll inward, causing the eyelashes to rub on the eye (trichiasis) (Fig. 7-10). The continuous rubbing of the lashes on the cornea leads to corneal ulceration and opacification (Fig. 7-11). A simplified grading scheme of trachoma has been developed recently by the World Health Organization [28].

The eye is examined with a ×2.5 loupe. The features of trachoma are classified as follows: TF—the presence on the central upper tarsal conjunctiva of at least five follicles 0.5 mm in diameter; TI—inflammatory thickening that obscures more than half the normal tarsal vessels; TS—the presence of easily visible scarring on the upper tarsal conjunctiva; TT—the presence of at least one lash rubbing the eye; and CO—the presence of an easily visible central corneal opacity that blurs the pupil margin.

Inflammatory infiltrates and new vessels may also appear in the superior cornea and produce a characteristic superior corneal "pannus." Pannus may extend several millimeters onto the cornea. Small, clear depressions are left at the sites of limbal follicles. These are known as *Herbert's pits*.

TREATMENT

Chlamydia are susceptible to a number of common antibiotics including sulfonamides, tetracycline, and erythromycin. However, trachoma is basically a disease that occurs in the presence of poor personal and community hygiene. A nonspecific improvement of hygiene is often associated with the disappearance of blinding trachoma. Programs are now underway to develop specific health education programs aimed at improving personal hygiene behavior [29]. It is also theoretically possible to eliminate blinding trachoma in the short term by the appropriate use of antibiotics. Antibiotic treatment aimed at eliminating trachoma must reach all "components" of the community pool of infection. Mass treatment has been used, because all members of the community are potentially part of the infectious pool. The existence of extraocular chlamydial infection also suggests that systemic antibiotics should be used. However, because of the inherent practical difficulties, mass systemic antibiotic treatment for trachoma is not generally recommended at this time.

The presently recommended approach to the treatment of trachoma is the intermittent use of topical ocular antibiotics

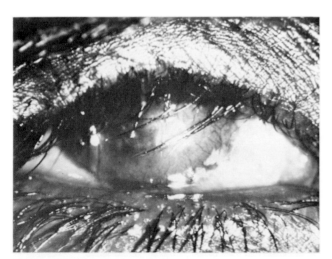

Figure 7-10. Early trichiasis, with the lashes already causing corneal opacification.

[23]. The preferred preparation is 1% tetracycline ointment given twice a day for 6 weeks for an individual. When treating larger groups, the same ointment is given daily for 5 consecutive days once a month for 6 months. This regime is repeated on an annual basis as needed. Intermittent topical therapy will temporarily reduce the ocular chlamydial infection and lessen the ease of transmission. Topical antibiotic therapy will also significantly reduce bacterial secondary infection.

When trichiasis occurs, it should be treated. Epilation is satisfactory treatment for single lashes, although they regrow quickly. It is usually necessary to perform surgery to rotate the lid margin and lashes away from the eye.

ACQUIRED IMMUNODEFICIENCY SYNDROME

The acquired immunodeficiency syndrome (AIDS), a disease caused by the human immunodeficiency virus (HIV), has emerged as a global health problem. AIDS is of particular importance in ophthalmology because approximately 75 percent of patients with AIDS have ocular manifestations.

OCULAR CHANGES

The ocular manifestations of AIDS are protean and are related to either opportunistic infection or neoplasm. The pattern of eye disease seems to vary in different populations [30]. The most common ocular manifestations appear to be cotton-wool spots, Roth spots and intraretinal hemorrhages, perivascular sheathing, cytomegalovirus retinitis, and conjunctival Kaposi's sarcoma [31,32].

Cotton-wool spots are gray, semiopaque lesions with feathery borders that lie in the inner retina (Fig. 7-11); they represent microinfarcts of the retina from arteriolar occlusion. Cotton-wool spots are the most common ocular lesion in AIDS and may represent an underlying vascular disorder. The lesions usually resolve in 4 to 12 weeks, leaving no clinical trace. The cotton-wool spots in AIDS appear to be morphologically identical to the cotton-wool spots commonly seen in diabetic retinopathy.

Roth spots are white-centered intraretinal hemorrhages, and they represent septic emboli which have lodged in the retinal microcirculation. Roth spots are generally seen in patients who have an underlying source for septic emboli, such as subacute bacterial endocarditis, although there may be no obvious source of septic emboli. Perivascular sheathing has been noted and occurs mostly in the peripheral retina of patients with AIDS as an isolated finding or associated with cytomegalovirus infection [31].

Cytomegalovirus (CMV) is a common opportunistic infection among some populations with AIDS, although it appears to be much less common in central Africa than in the United States and Europe [30]. In CMV retinitis, the retinal lesions are white, granular areas in the posterior pole, often associated with hemorrhage and perivasculitis (Fig. 7-12). CMV retinitis generally follows a vascular distribution and is associated with

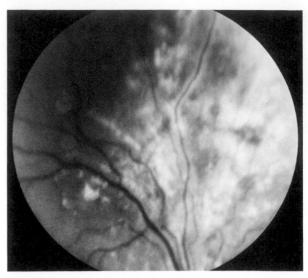

Figure 7-12. Cytomegalovirus retinopathy in a pediatric AIDS patient in Rwanda. (*Courtesy of P. Kestelyn.*)

retinal vascular occlusions that lead to retinal nonperfusion and necrosis. Other opportunistic infections that cause retinal changes include herpes zoster, herpes simplex, *Toxoplasma gondii*, *Candida* sp., and cryptococcus.

Kaposi's sarcoma is the most common malignancy associated with AIDS, and it may first appear on tarsal or bulbar conjunctiva as a bright-red mass which could easily be mistaken for a subconjunctival hemorrhage. When the lesion appears on the eyelids or other skin, it appears as a flat or elevated purplish nodule.

At the present time, treatment for the ocular complications of AIDS is limited to specific treatment for the underlying opportunistic infections. Ganciclovir, an antiviral derivative of acyclovir, has shown some promise in initial clinical trials for treatment of CMV infection, although active CMV lesions have been found in the eyes of patients receiving treatment [33].

REFERENCES

1 Fraunfelder FT, Roy FH: *Current Ocular Therapy*. Philadelphia, Saunders, 1984

2 World Health Organization: Available Data on Blindness (update 1987). WHO Publication 87.14, 1987

3 Jones BR: Eliminating the overburden of avoidable blindness, in Wilson J (ed): *World Blindness and Its Prevention*. Oxford University Press, 1980, pp 36–43

4 Vaughan D, Asbury T: General ophthalmology. Los Altos, Calif, Lange, 1980, pp 14–34

5 World Health Organization: Guidelines for Programmes for the Prevention of Blindness. Geneva, WHO, 1979

6 Chandler JW, Rotkis WM: Ophthalmia neonatorum, in Duane TD (ed): *Clinical Ophthalmology*. Hagerstown, Md, Harper & Row, 1980, vol 4, chap 6

7 Sexually Transmitted Diseases. Treatment Guidelines, 1982. MMWR 31S:41, 1982

8 Rapoza PA, Quinn TC, Kiessling LA, et al: Assessment of neonatal conjunctivitis with a direct immunofluorescent monoclonal antibody stain for Chlamydia. JAMA 255:3369–3373, 1986

9 Abbott RL, Abrams MA: Bacterial corneal ulcers, in Duane TD (ed): *Clinical Ophthalmology,* vol 4. Hagerstown, Md, Harper & Row, 1986

10 Coster DJ, Jones BR, Falcon MG: Role of debridement in the treatment of herpetic keratitis. Trans Ophthalmol Soc UK 97:314–317, 1977

11 Sommer A: *Nutritional Blindness: Xerophthalmia and Keratomalacia.* Oxford University Press, 1982

12 Foster A, Sommer A: Corneal ulceration, measles, and childhood blindness in Tanzania. Br J Ophthalmol 71:331–343, 1987

13 Leske MC, Sperduto RD: The epidemiology of senile cataracts: A review. Am J Epidemiol 118:152–165, 1982

14 Schwab L, Taylor HR: Cataract and delivery of surgical services, in Duane TD (ed): *Clinical Ophthalmology,* vol 5. Hagerstown, Md, Harper & Row, 1984

15 Wilson J: *World Blindness and its Prevention.* Oxford University Press, 1980, pp 1–13

16 Kolker AE, Hetherington J: *Becker-Shaffer's Diagnosis and Therapy of the Glaucomas,* 4th ed. St. Louis, Mosby, 1976

17 Sommer A: *Epidemiology and Statistics for the Ophthalmologist.* Oxford University Press, 1980, pp 11–14

18 Ferris FL: Senile macular degeneration: Review of epidemiological features. Am J Epidemiol 118:132–141, 1983

19 Patz Z, Fine SL, Orth DH: *Diseases of the Macula.* St. Louis, Mosby, 1976

20 Macular Photocoagulation Study Group: Argon laser photocoagulation for neovascular maculopathy: Three year results from randomized clinical trials. Arch Ophthalmol 104:694–701, 1986

21 Sommer A, Tarwotjo I, Djunaedi E, et al: Impact of vitamin A supplementation on childhood mortality: A randomized community trial. Lancet i:1169–1173, 1986

22 World Health Organization: Control of vitamin A deficiency and xerophthalmia. Geneva, WHO, 1982

23 Dawson CR, Jones BR, Tanzzo ML: Guide to Trachoma Control. Geneva, WHO, 1981

24 Taylor HR, Johnson SL, Prendergast RA, et al: An animal model of trachoma: II. The importance of repeated reinfection. Invest Ophthalmol Vis Sci 23:507–519, 1982

25 Schachter J, Dawson CR: Chlamydial infections, a worldwide problem: Epidemiology and implications for trachoma therapy. Sex Trans Dis 8:167–174, 1981

26 Grayston JT, Wang S-P, Yeh LJ, et al: Importance of reinfection in the pathogenesis of trachoma. Rev Infect Dis 7:717–725, 1985

27 Taylor HR, Millan-Velasco F, Sommer A: The ecology of trachoma: An epidemiological study of trachoma in Southern Mexico. Bull WHO 63:559–567, 1985

28 Thylefors B, Dawson CR, Jones BR, et al: A simple system for the assessment of trachoma and its complications. Bull WHO 65:477–483, 1987

29 Taylor HR: Strategies for the control of trachoma. Aust NZ J Ophthalmol 15:139–143, 1987

30 Kestelyn P, Van de Perre P, Rouvroy D, et al: A prospective study of the ophthalmologic findings in the Acquired Immunodeficiency Syndrome in Africa. Am J Ophthalmol 100:230–238, 1985

31 Newsome DA, Green WR, Miller ED, et al: Microvascular aspects of acquired immune deficiency syndrome retinopathy. Am J Opthalmol 98:590–601, 1984

32 Schuman JS, Orellana J, Friedman AH: Acquired Immunodeficiency Syndrome (AIDS). Surv Ophthalmol 31:384–410, 1987

33 Pepose JS, Newman C, Bach MC, et al: Pathologic features of cytomegalovirus retinopathy after treatment with the antiviral agent ganciclovir. Ophthalmology 94:414–424, 1987

CHAPTER 8 / *Neoplasms and Malignancies*
· *Charles L. M. Olweny*

INTRODUCTION

DEFINITIONS

A *neoplasm* is an autonomous purposeless new growth of tissue which is no longer under the control of normal growth-controlling mechanisms. Neoplasms are at times described as "tumors" because more often than not they present as swellings. The abnormal cells of a neoplasm differ from normal cells in their growth and cell surface characteristics as well as in their biochemical and physiological interactions with the host. Neoplasms may be benign ("simple" or "innocent") or malignant. Malignant neoplasms composed of epithelial cells are called *carcinomas*, while those composed of connective tissue are referred to as *sarcomas*.

MALIGNANT NEOPLASMS IN DEVELOPING COUNTRIES

The pattern of diseases in the developing countries is influenced by the predominantly young age of the population and the high prevalence of infectious and communicable diseases. However, according to the World Health Organization (WHO), after the first 5 years of life the causes of death are similar the world over; the three commonest causes are cardiovascular diseases, accidents, and cancer. The types of tumors observed in developing countries are different from those of the developed nations. Lung and colorectal cancers, which are leading causes of death in industrialized countries, are relatively uncommon in most third world countries. On the other hand

Table 8-1. Cancers etiologically associated with infectious agents

Types of cancer	Infective agent
Hepatocellular carcinoma	Hepatitis B virus
Cancer of uterine cervix	Human papilloma virus
Burkitt's lymphoma	Epstein-Barr virus
Nasopharyngeal carcinoma	Epstein-Barr virus
Kaposi's sarcoma	Human immunodeficiency virus
Squamous cell carcinoma of the urinary bladder	*Schistosoma haematobium*

cancers of the liver and uterine cervix are very common in most third world countries. Of interest is the fact that some of the tumors commonly seen in the developing countries are etiologically associated with infective agents (Table 8-1).

GENERAL FACTS ABOUT CANCER

Of the estimated 5.9 million new cases of cancer annually, 2.9 million occur in the developed world and 3 million in the developing countries. The commonest cancers worldwide are shown in Table 8-2. Lung cancer will soon overtake stomach cancer mainly because of increasing smoking in the developing countries. Developing nations accounted for 50 percent of the world's tobacco production in 1961–1963, 58 percent in 1972–1974, and now account for 63 percent of the total. While tobacco consumption is decreasing by 1.1 percent each year in industrialized countries, it continues to increase by 2.2 percent each year in the third world. Cigarettes marketed in these third world countries have a higher tar and nicotine content than those sold in industrialized countries. In China and India, two of the most populous nations on earth, one-quarter to one-third of all males are addicted to tobacco smoking by the time they are 18 to 20 years of age. For some developing countries, such as Malawi and Zimbabwe, tobacco is the major source of foreign exchange earnings, and in other countries, like Malaysia,

Table 8-2. Rank order of twelve commonest cancers in the world, 1980*

Rank	Males	Females	Both sexes
1	Lung	Breast	Stomach
2	Stomach	Cervix	Lung
3	Colorectal	Colorectal	Breast
4	Mouth/pharynx	Stomach	Colorectal
5	Prostate	Corpus uteri	Cervix
6	Esophagus	Lung	Mouth/pharynx
7	Liver	Ovary	Esophagus
8	Bladder	Mouth/pharynx	Liver
9	Lymphatic	Esophagus	Lymphatic
10	Leukemia	Lymphatic	Prostate
11	— — —	— — —	Bladder
12	— — —	— — —	Leukemia

*From [1].

tobacco companies spend exorbitant sums on advertising. WHO has warned that there will be an epidemic of lung cancer in developing countries in the coming decade unless national programs of public information and education are initiated and legislation prohibiting tobacco advertising and sales promotion is enacted forthwith.

CANCER DEATHS

Of the estimated 4.3 million yearly deaths from cancer, 2.3 million occur in developing countries. The highest number of cancer deaths is in Asia (Table 8-3). In 1979, for instance, there were more cancer deaths in India (423,000) than in the United States (409,000). In Shanghai province in China, cancer rose from the sixth to the leading cause of death within two decades from 1960 to 1980. The same can be expected in most other developing countries. Unfortunately, the public and most health administrators are not aware of the magnitude of the problem. In addition, the figures available represent only the tip of the iceberg, as most developing countries only have hospital-based cancer registers or none at all.

In the developing countries the commonest cancers are primary liver, mouth and pharynx, uterine cervix, and esophagus. Burkitt's lymphoma, though numerically unimportant, is of great interest as a ''human tumor model.'' Kaposi's sarcoma has recently gained international prominence because of its association with acquired immunodeficiency syndrome (AIDS).

HEPATOCELLULAR CARCINOMA

DEFINITIONS

Hepatocellular carcinoma (HCC) accounts for over 90 percent of primary liver cancers. The cholangiocellular form and hepatoblastomas occurring in childhood are less common.

EPIDEMIOLOGY

HCC is found mainly in sub-Saharan Africa, southeast Asia, and western Pacific countries. It is the commonest form of cancer in tropical Africa, reaching its highest recorded incidence in Mozambique. However, of the 260,000 new cases estimated yearly, some 40 percent occur in China.

Table 8-3. Estimated yearly cancer deaths by continent

Continent	Estimated deaths
Asia	1,858,000
Europe	1,398,000
North America	449,000
Latin America	291,000
Africa	268,000
Oceania	32,000
Total	4,296,000

ETIOLOGY OF HCC

About 80 percent of HCC cases result from hepatitis B virus (HBV) infection. Epidemiological studies indicate a 200-fold increased risk of developing HCC in individuals infected with HBV [2]. However, in tropical areas other factors, notably aflatoxin contamination, may also play a role. In Swaziland, HBV infection is widespread and the proportion of HBV-exposed individuals is very high (86 percent of men), but the distribution of HCC correlates more closely with levels of aflatoxin contamination and consumption that with HBV infection [3]. It would appear that in most tropical countries HBV infection may be the *initiating* factor and other factors, of which aflatoxin is but one important one, may be the *promoting* factors.

CLINICAL FEATURES

In tropical areas HCC is an aggressive disease, with 90 percent of patients being dead within 3 months of diagnosis. Patients present with right upper quadrant pain and mass, weight loss, ascites, and jaundice. There is almost invariably underlying macronodular cirrhosis and portal hypertension such that hematemesis and melena from ruptured esophageal varices is a common complication. The male-female ratio is 4:1. Most patients present in the third and fourth decades, two to three decades younger than in developed countries. Poor prognostic factors include cachexia, ascites, jaundice, and venous collaterals.

Since colon and rectal cancers are relatively uncommon in the tropics and subtropics, HCC should be suspected in any young adult male with right upper quadrant pain and mass. Detection of α-fetoprotein in serum (positive in 70 percent of cases) increases the suspicion further. The diagnosis is usually made clinically. Liver biopsy is avoided because there is no effective treatment and the associated coagulation abnormalities may make the procedure hazardous. A common differential diagnosis in the tropics is amebic liver abscess.

MANAGEMENT OF HCC

Treatment is palliative. Surgery offers an advantage in survival and possible "cure" in "early" cases diagnosed when there is minimal tumor of less than 3-cm diameter. Hepatic resection is possible even in the presence of cirrhosis in cases of minimal HCC, and radical resection leads to prolonged survival [4]. Radiotherapy is inappropriate except for palliative pain relief, as the liver is very sensitive even to low-dose radiation. Chemotherapy offers limited promise. The only drug that has provided reproducible results is the anthracycline doxorubicin. The overall response rate is about 40 percent. Combination chemotherapy has not improved response rates. A recent anecdotal report has suggested dramatic response in a patient treated with a doxorubicin and cisplatin combination. [5].

PREVENTION OF HCC

Because HCC is almost uniformly fatal, the only hope for this tumor rests with prevention. HCC is invariably associated with HBV infection. Vaccination against HBV is safe and effective. However, in Africa, southeast Asia, and the western Pacific, vertical HBV transmission or very early exposure occurs such that early immunization is necessary. A WHO-sponsored immunization program has started in Gambia in West Africa, but the effect will not be evident for two to three decades. The major constraint with HBV vaccination is the cost of the vaccine, currently $80 to $100 for the three-dose course. This is clearly well beyond the means of most developing nations, whose average annual budget for health services is $2.6 per capita, which is about 1 percent of the gross national product. It is hoped that genetic engineering will provide cheaper vaccines for most third world countries.

CANCER OF UTERINE CERVIX

EPIDEMIOLOGY AND ETIOLOGY

Cervical cancer is particularly common in Latin America, the Caribbean, and most of tropical Africa, where it is estimated that 1 in 1000 women between the ages of 30 and 55 years will develop and probably die from it. The highest recorded incidence rate is in Colombia, with the age-adjusted rate of 53 per 100,000 population. The women at high risk are those from low socioeconomic class. Cancer of the cervix occurs in those with early and frequent sexual experience, multiple sexual partners, exposure to uncircumsized males, and lack of personal hygiene. Recent findings tend to suggest that the sexual behavior of the male is just as important [6]. Even if she has no other sexual partners, the wife may "contract" the disease from a promiscuous husband who has had pre- or extra-marital relationships. Case control studies in western countries show that circumcision status of the husband per se does not protect against cervical cancer in the female partner, and there are areas in Africa where cervical cancer is common despite male circumcision. The Lugbara of Uganda, who are renowned for their meticulous cleanliness, do not circumcise their males and have a low incidence of cervical cancer. These observations suggest that cleanliness is more effective than circumcision. These and other factors suggest, too, that cervical cancer is due to a venereally transmissible agent or agents. Human papilloma viruses types 16 and 18 are now incriminated [7].

CLINICAL FEATURES

The observed peculiar features of cervical cancer in the tropics include advanced stage at presentation and the very young age of the population affected. At the Kenyatta National Hospital (KNH) in Nairobi, Kenya, only 10 percent of patients present with stage I disease, while over 60 percent have disease stages III and IV (Table 8-4). Most women in developing countries at the time of first presentation already have fungating, foul-

Table 8-4. Staging classification of carcinoma of uterine cervix

TNM classification	Figo classification	Descriptive criteria
Tis	O	Carcinoma in situ
T_1	I	Confined to uterus (extension to corpus to be disregarded)
T_2	II	Invades beyond uterus but not to pelvic wall or to lower third of vagina
T_3	III	Extends to pelvic wall and/or involves lower third of vagina and/or causes hydronephrosis or nonfunctioning kidney
T_4	IV	Invades mucosa of bladder or uterus and/or extends beyond true pelvis and/or distant metastases

smelling cauliflowerlike growths and some already have fistulas resulting from direct invasion of surrounding viscera. Unlike Europe and North America, the peak age at presentation is between the third and fourth decades. At KNH over 40 percent of cervical cancer patients are under 40 and over 70 percent are under 50 years of age. Pretreatment investigations should include examination under anesthesia, chest roentgenogram, intravenous pyelography, barium enema, sigmoidoscopy, and cystocopy.

MANAGEMENT OF CERVICAL CANCER

If cytology reveals severe dysplasia or carcinomatous changes, then directed biopsies utilizing Lugol's iodine to highlight glycogen-deficient malignant cells (Scheller test) or colposcopy with 3% acetic acid must be performed. If there is disparity between the cytological and pathological specimens or if microinvasive carcinoma is discovered, the entire squamocolumnar junction is removed (conization). Cancer in situ or intraepithelial cancer (stage 0) is usually treated surgically with total abdominal hysterectomy with or without a small vaginal cuff. If the patient wishes to retain fertility, as is often the case in developing countries, then conization may be adequate. However, this calls for close surveillance. The treatment outcome with either form of treatment is excellent with less than 2 percent developing recurrent in situ disease or invasive carcinoma [8]. Surgery and radiotherapy are recommended for invasive stages I and II. Surgery is usually chosen for younger women who wish to preserve ovarian function and avoid vaginal irradiation. Radiation is preferred for patients in whom surgery is contraindicated and in older patients. Survival at 5 years is 60 to 90 percent with both types of treatment [9]. For patients with advanced disease chemotherapy may be tried.

The best single agent is cisplatin, with response rates approaching 40 percent. Combination of bleomycin, vincristine, or mitomycin C with cisplatin has been reported to give higher response rates, with 10 to 15 percent complete responses [10].

PREVENTION OF CERVICAL CANCER

Although the risk factors for cancer of the cervix are well known, control remains difficult because those at greatest risk are the hardest to reach. Cancer of the cervix is frequently associated with a long history of cervicitis, severe cervical dysplasia, and carcinoma in situ. Longitudinal studies indicate that if left untreated carcinoma in situ can develop into frankly invasive cancer over a period of 3 to 20 years in 70 percent of patients. If detected early, cervical cancer is curable in almost 100 percent of cases. Early detection (secondary prevention) is possible by Pap smear.

In developing countries it will be necessary to train primary health care workers (nurses and midwives) in the techniques of taking Pap smears, as these people see the majority of patients.

CANCER OF THE ORAL CAVITY AND PHARYNX
EPIDEMIOLOGY AND ETIOLOGY

Oral cancer is the commonest form of cancer in southeast Asia, home of one-sixth of the world's population. In Sri Lanka and India approximately 35 to 40 percent of all cancers occur in the oral cavity [11], compared with only 2 to 3 percent in the United Kingdom and the United States. India has the highest recorded incidences, 30 per 100,000 males and 14 per 100,000 females per year. The incidence is also high in Bangladesh, Burma, Kampuchea, Malaysia, and Pakistan. There are more than 100,000 new cases each year. In India there is a high prevalence of oral premalignant lesions such as leukoplakia and oral submucous fibrosis. The high frequency of oral cancer is related in 90 percent of cases to tobacco consumption, especially to betel quid chewing with tobacco as the main ingredient.

PREVENTION AND EARLY DETECTION

It takes up to 15 years for an oral lesion to become cancerous, making this cancer very amenable to early detection and cure by radiotherapy and surgery. Unfortunately most victims seek help only when pain develops, usually at an advanced stage of the disease.

An innovative approach using primary health care workers proved cost-effective in Sri Lanka [12]. In this study 34 primary health care workers who were mostly midwives examined 28,295 subjects over a period of 52 weeks. Of those screened, 1220 subjects (4.2 percent) were found to have lesions needing further examination. Although only 50 percent showed up for reexamination, 90 percent of these were found to need medical care. Poor compliance may have been due to lack of awareness by the community of the serious nature of oral cancer and the value of screening.

BURKITT'S LYMPHOMA

DEFINITION

Burkitt's lymphoma (BL) is a malignant lymphoma of B-cell origin. It is classified as a high-grade malignancy and described as malignant lymphoma of small noncleaved cells of undifferentiated Burkitt type. It is composed of uniformly undifferentiated lymphoid cells with interspersed macrophages giving the so-called starry sky appearance (Fig. 8-1A). The cells have rounded nuclei with two to five prominent nucleoli. The cytoplasm stains deep blue and is often vacuolated (Fig. 8-1B).

EPIDEMIOLOGY AND ETIOLOGY

BL is endemic in most of tropical Africa and parts of Papua New Guinea. In these areas it is the commonest childhood malignancy and often accounts for more than 50 percent of childhood tumors. In Uganda, the annual incidence varies between 0 and 6 cases per 100,000 population and in Papua, New Guinea, between 0.07 and 1.8 per 100,000 population. Outside endemic areas, sporadic cases of BL have been reported from the United States, Europe, and the Middle East. In endemic areas BL occurs in areas with specific climatic conditions [13]: latitudes 10 to 15° north and south, altitudes below 1500 meters, diurnal temperature below 16°C, and annual rainfalls of about 50 cm. Time-space clustering has been observed in Uganda and Tanzania, which suggests an infective origin.

A persuasive etiologic theory has emerged linking endemic BL with Epstein-Barr virus (EBV). EBV transforms B lymphocytes both in vitro and in vivo. In the West Nile district of Uganda 42,000 children were recruited into a WHO-sponsored prospective seroepidemiological study. Serological evidence of EBV infection proved to be a high risk factor for BL. In addition, EBV DNA and EBV-associated nuclear antigen (EBNA) are consistently present in more than 90 percent of BL cases. It is suggested that latently infected B cells are driven by EBV to undergo replications such that one of three specific chromosomal translocations occurs. These are t(8;14)

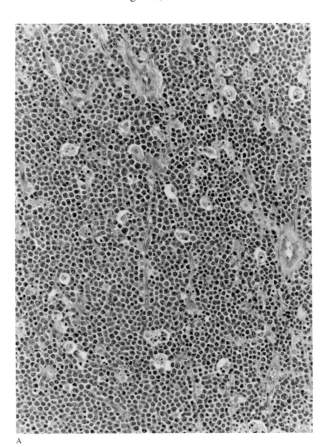

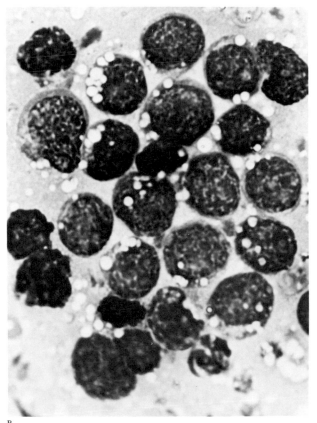

A   B

Figure 8-1. *A.* Uniform immature lymphoid cells with interspersed macrophages giving the "starry sky" appearance. *(Courtesy of Dr. A.S.-Y. Leong.)* *B.* Giemsa-stained imprint of Burkitt's lymphoma. Note uniformly basophilic undifferentiated cells, cytoplasmic vacuoles, and prominent nucleoli. × 1000.

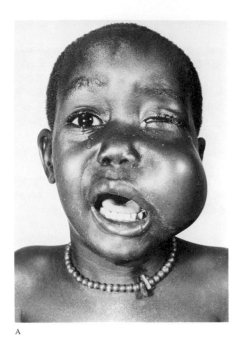

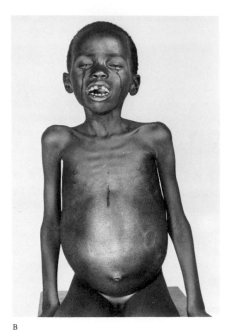

A   B

Figure 8-2. *A.* Jaw tumor in an 8-year-old Ugandan girl with Burkitt's lymphoma. *B.* Abdominal tumor in a 6-year-old Ugandan girl.

seen in more than 80 percent of cases, t(8;22), and t(2;8); they have in common 8q24 band involvement. The chromosomal translocations cause *c-myc* oncogene activation. The role of malaria may be to facilitate the development of lymphoma through polyclonal B-cell activation and/or T-cell immunosuppression.

FEATURES OF BL

BL is a rapidly growing tumor. In endemic areas 75 percent of cases present with jaw swelling (Fig. 8-2*A*), 50 percent with abdominal masses (Fig. 8-2*B*), and 30 percent with central nervous system involvement such as paraplegia or multiple cranial nerve palsies. Nonendemic BL, though morphologically similar to the endemic form, exhibits differences outlined in Table 8-5. Staging criteria are shown in Table 8-6.

Table 8-5. Similarities and differences between endemic and nonendemic BL

Feature	Endemic	Nonendemic
Climatic distribution	Related	Not related
EBV association	Nearly always	Uncommon
Chromosomal translocation	Always	Always
Role of hyperendemic malaria	Possible	Unlikely
Jaw involvement	Common (75%)	Rare (< 5%)
Peripheral adenopathy	Rare	Common (20%)
Marrow involvement	Rare	Common
Survival after single-agent cyclophosphamide therapy	Expected	Unusual

MANAGEMENT OF BL

The goal of management is cure. Patients suspected of having BL must be referred to a central hospital with the necessary skills and facilities. The role of surgery is for diagnosis, surgical debulking, decompression in case of spinal cord compression, and insertion of Ommaya reservoir for intraventricular therapy. BL is radiosensitive, but conventional once-daily therapy is ineffective because of the peculiar cell kinetics of this tumor. Hyperfractionation (three to four fractions per day) is recommended. The role of craniospinal irradiation to prevent CNS relapse is questionable. The treatment of choice for BL is chemotherapy. Cyclophosphamide 40 mg/kg intravenously every 2 to 3 weeks is as effective in inducing remissions as a combination of cyclophosphamide, vincristine, and methotrexate [14]. About 90 percent will achieve complete response with one or two cycles of chemotherapy. However, about 50 percent will relapse, usually with CNS disease. Because BL is extremely chemosensitive, there is a grave danger of patients

Table 8-6. Staging for Burkitt's lymphoma

Stage	Site of involvement	10-year survival rate, %
A	Solitary extraabdominal site	90
AR	Resected extraabdominal tumor	90
B	Multiple extraabdominal sites	50
C	Intraabdominal tumor with or without facial tumors	50
D	Intraabdominal tumor (stage C) with sites of tumor other than facial	30

developing tumor lysis syndrome [15]. Intracellular elements, notably potassium, phosphates, and urates, are released causing hyperkalemia, hyperphosphatemia, hyperuricemia, and secondary hypocalcemia. Patients with bulky tumors, usually in stages C and D, are at high risk of developing this complication within 24 to 72 h of starting treatment. Adequate hydration (100 to 150 mL/h) during that period together with alkalinization of urine is advisable to prevent this dreaded complication, which may cause sudden death in an apparently "well" patient responding rapidly to treatment. In addition allopurinol 300 mg/day is recommended to prevent uric acid nephropathy.

PREVENTION OF BL

There is now a prospect of preventing BL by vaccination. A vaccine has been developed by Professor M. A. Epstein and his group at Oxford England using the high-molecular-weight glycoprotein component of EBV membrane antigen [16]. This vaccine confers 100 percent protection against lymphomagenic EBV dose in cottontop tamarins, the animal of choice for experimental EBV infection. After preliminary trials to establish safety and efficacy in preventing infectious mononucleosis, it will be appropriate to test this vaccine in BL endemic countries.

KAPOSI'S SARCOMA

DEFINITION

Kaposi's sarcoma (pronounced Kawposhi) is characterized by the growth of multiple vascular nodules on the skin of one or more extremities with occasional involvement of internal organs.

EPIDEMIOLOGY

In1961 at an international conference held at Makerere Medical School in Kampala, Uganda, the high incidence of Kaposi's sarcoma (KS) in the black male population of sub-Saharan Africa was noted. At a second conference in Kampala in 1980 particularly high rates were reported from central African countries, especially Zaire, Rwanda, Burundi, Uganda, Malawi, Tanzania, Zambia, Zimbabwe, and Kenya. Incidences decreased toward west and south Africa [17]. Time-space clustering had been observed in the West Nile district of Uganda. The observation that 25 to 30 percent of individuals with AIDS have KS has given considerable prominence to KS. Thus, KS occurs in *sporadic* form (as originally described by Kaposi in southern Europeans), in *endemic* form (as was seen in central African countries prior to the AIDS epidemic), and more recently in *epidemic* form in association with AIDS. The clinicoepidemiological correlation is shown in Table 8-7. In Africa all three epidemiological varieties occur. Recent observations

Table 8-7. Clinicoepidemiological correlation of Kaposi's sarcoma

Epidemiological variety	Clinical variety	Clinical behavior
Sporadic	Cutaneous nodular	Indolent
Endemic	Cutaneous nodular	Indolent
	Locally aggressive (florid/infiltrative)	
	Generalized aggressive (lymphadenopathic)	Aggressive
Epidemic	Generalized aggressive (lymphadenopathic/generalized nodular HIV + ve)	Aggressive

indicate that the epidemic form is on the increase in countries like Uganda [18] and Zambia [19].

CLINICAL FEATURES

The cutaneous nodular variety is the commonest form and often involves one or more extremities. It is indolent in behavior and may even undergo spontaneous regression. The locally aggressive forms are either florid or infiltrative in nature and will cause death within 1 year if not treated. The generalized aggressive form may be lymphadenopathic or nodular. Prior to the AIDS epidemic the lymphadenopathic form was confined to children (Fig. 8-3A) and young females. KS associated with AIDS in Africa is also either generalized nodular or lymphadenopathic. Endoscopy in these individuals reveals disease throughout the gastrointestinal tract (tongue, esophagus, stomach, and ileum). Pleural effusion is common. Oral candidiasis, diarrhea, and wasting are prominent features. Wasting is so prominent that AIDS is referred to as "slim disease" in Uganda. The epidemic form ends in death within 4 to 6 months with or without treatment. Patients with the epidemic form of KS are invariably HIV-positive and are much younger (mean age 30 years) than individuals with sporadic or endemic forms.

TREATMENT

The classical cutaneous nodular form of KS is indolent in behavior and may not need treatment unless a vital structure is involved. Chemotherapy with single oral drugs like Trenimon or Razoxane controls the tumor.

The locally aggressive forms (both florid and infiltrative varieties) and childhood lymphadenopathic form respond best to combination chemotherapy such as actinomycin D plus vincristine plus dacarbazine (Fig. 8-3B) [20]. The generalized aggressive forms associated with AIDS respond very poorly to all forms of therapy [18]. Since treatment of KS in AIDS patients is only palliative, the best-tolerated form of therapy is to be recommended.

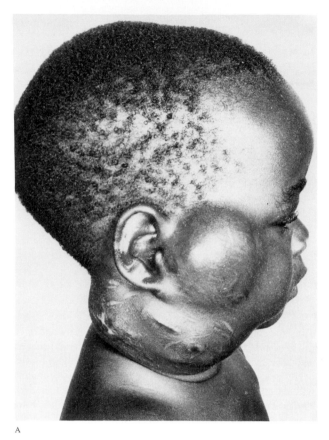
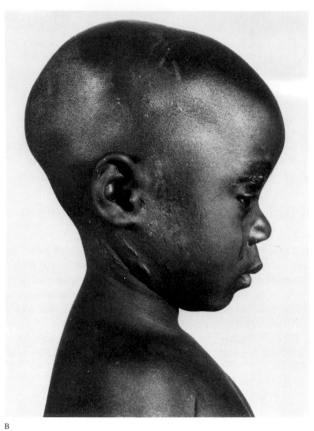

A   B

Figure 8-3. *A.* Aggressive lymphadenopathic Kaposi's sarcoma in a Ugandan 4-year-old girl. Note scarifications prior to hospitalization. *B.* The same child after a course of chemotherapy combining actinomycin D, vincristine, and dacarbazine. Alopecia is a complication of therapy.

REFERENCES

1 Parkin DM, Laara E, Muir CS: Estimates of the worldwide frequency of sixteen major cancers in 1980. Int J Cancer 41:184–197, 1988

2 Beasley RP, Hwang LY, Lin CC, et. al: Hepatocellular carcinoma and hepatitis B virus. Lancet ii:1121–1132, 1981

3 Peers F, Bosch X, Kaldor J, et al: Aflatoxin exposure, hepatitis B virus infection, and liver cancer in Swaziland. Int J Cancer 39:545–553, 1987

4 Nagasue N, Yukaya H, Chang YC, et al: Appraisal of hepatic resection in the treatment of minute hepatocellular carcinoma associated with liver cirrhosis. Br J Surg 74:836–838, 1987

5 Olweny CLM, Johnson R: Rapid response to cisplatin and doxorubicin in hepatocellular carcinoma complicated by hepatitis B reactivation. J Gastroenterol Hepatol 2:533–537, 1987

6 Buckley JD, Harris RWC, Doll R, et al: Case-control study of the husbands of women with dysplasia or carcinoma of the cervix uteri. Lancet ii: 1010–1015, 1981

7 Crum CP, Kenberg I, Richart H, et al: Human papilloma virus type 16 and early cervical neoplasia. N Engl J Med 310:880–883, 1984

8 Baggish MS: A comparison between laser excisional conization and laser vaporization for the treatment of cervical intraepithelial neoplasia. Am J Obstet Gynecol 155:39–44, 1986

9 Perez CA, Camel HM, Kuske RR, et al: Radiation therapy in the treatment of the uterine cervix: A 20-year experience. Gynecol Oncol 23:127–140, 1986

10 Picozzi VJ, Sikia BI, Carlson RW, et al: Bleomycin, mitomycin, and cisplatin therapy for advanced squamous carcinoma of the uterine cervix: A phase II study of the Northern California Oncology Group. Cancer Treat Rep 69:903–905, 1985

11 Pindburg, JJ: Epidemiologic studies of oral cancer. Int Dental J 27:172–178, 1977

12 Warnakulasurinya K, Kanayake E, Sivayoham A, et al: Utilization of primary health care workers for early detection of oral cancers and precancer cases in Sri Lanka. Bull WHO 62:243–250, 1984

13 Burkitt DP: Determining the climatic limitations of children's cancer common in Africa. Br J Med ii:1019–1023, 1962

14 Olweny CLM, Katongole-Mbidde E, Kaddu-Mukasa A, et al: Treatment of Burkitt's lymphoma: Randomized clinical trial of single versus combination chemotherapy. Int J Cancer 17:436–440, 1976

15 Arseneau JC, Bagley CM, Anderson T, et al: Hyperkalaemia, a sequel to chemotherapy of Burkitt's lymphoma. Lancet i:10–12, 1973

16 Epstein MA: Recent studies on a vaccine to prevent EB virus–associated cancers. Br J Cancer 54:1–5, 1986

17 Hutt MSR: The epidemiology of Kaposi's sarcoma, Olweny CLM, Hutt MSR, Owor R (eds): *Kaposi's Sarcoma*. Basel, Karger, 1981, pp. 3–8

18 Serwadda D, Carswell W, Ayuko WO, et al: Further experience with Kaposi's sarcoma in Uganda. Br J Cancer 53:497–500, 1986

19 Bayley AC: Aggressive Kaposi's sarcoma in Zambia. Lancet i: 1318, 1984

20 Olweny CLM, Toya T, Katongole-Mbidde E, et al: Treatment of Kaposi's sarcoma by combination of actinomycin D, vincristine, and imidazole carboxamide (DTIC): Results of randomised trial. Int J Cancer 14:649, 1974

CHAPTER 9 / *Anemia* · *David J. Weatherall* · *Prawase Wasi*

Anemia is one of the commonest causes of ill health in many tropical countries. Although its pathophysiology is similar in tropical and temperate climates, the spectrum of causes is different; the anemias of malnutrition, infection, malabsorption, and the genetic disorders of the red cell predominate in the tropics. Furthermore, severe anemia in the tropics frequently has a complicated, multifactorial basis and results from the interaction of several different mechanisms including deficiency of one or more factors required for hemopoiesis, infection, and a hemoglobinopathy or red cell enzyme defect.

In this chapter we shall describe briefly the prevalence, pathophysiology, and general approach to the investigation and management of anemia, particularly as it relates to tropical practice. The reader is referred to standard textbooks and reviews on the pathophysiology and investigation of anemia for a more extensive account of anemia in general [1–3].

DEFINITION

A functional definition of anemia is the state in which the circulating red cell mass is insufficient to meet the oxygen requirements of the tissues. However, because of the numerous compensatory mechanisms which can be brought into play to increase the efficiency of tissue oxygenation, it is not possible to use this definition in clinical practice. Thus, anemia is usually defined by the hemoglobin level, hematocrit, or red cell count. This approach is complicated by the fact that the "normal" hemoglobin level varies with age, sex, race, and altitude. For a particular age or sex the frequency distribution of normal hemoglobin concentrations approaches a Gaussian curve; if there is an increased prevalence of anemia in a population, it is skewed to the left. Thus it is customary to take an arbitrary cutoff point; a hemoglobin value below this point indicates that there is a high probability that the individual is anemic. The hemoglobin concentrations below which anemia is likely to be present in populations living at sea level, as proposed by the World Health Organization (WHO) [4], are shown in Table 9-1. It should be emphasized that these figures are entirely arbitrary and they are simply the best that can be achieved given our current lack of information about the ethnic differences in normal hemoglobin levels.

EPIDEMIOLOGY

Numerous surveys for the prevalence of anemia have been carried out in tropical populations. Because of differences in methodology and problems of demographic design, it is very difficult to interpret the results and to compare one with another. Data for different populations are given in a WHO publication and in several recent reviews [4–7]. Some indication of the magnitude of the problem was provided recently by Baker [6], who analyzed several large series of studies of hemoglobin levels in pregnant women in different regions of tropical Asia. The prevalence, as judged by WHO criteria, ranged from 6 percent in the urban Chinese populations of

Table 9-1. Hemoglobin concentrations below which anemia is likely to be present in populations at sea level, as proposed by the World Health Organization [4]

	Hemoglobin concentration, g/dL
Children, 6 months to 6 years old	11
Children, 6 to 14 years old	12
Adult males	13
Adult females (nonpregnant)	12
Adult females (pregnant)	11

Singapore to 88 percent in mixed urban and rural populations of India. From other published data it seems likely that in many tropical countries anemia affects a high proportion of the population.

It is extremely difficult to obtain overall prevalence figures for any particular population because most surveys have included only one region or a particular group of people, who may not be representative of the entire population or even of the same poulation during another season of the year. For example, anemia is more prevalent in low-lying regions of the tropics than in drier, highland areas. Furthermore, studies in the Gambia have shown that the mean hemoglobin levels in children vary significantly at different times of the year; anemia is much more common in the wet season when malaria transmission is at its highest [8]. The incidence may vary widely in the same population depending on the level of poverty. In Thailand it is rare among medical students from well-to-do families, while in the poorest northeasterners it reaches a prevalence of over 90 percent [9].

Similar problems exist in trying to determine the relative importance of different causes of anemia in the tropics. Most surveys have concentrated only on one mechanism such as iron or folate deficiency; as already mentioned, tropical anemias are very complex and have to be analyzed against a background of dietary insufficiency, a variety of chronic infections, and genetic disorders of the red cell.

CLASSIFICATION AND PATHOPHYSIOLOGY [1–3]

Anemia can result from either defective production or an increased rate of loss of red cells (Table 9-2). Decreased production follows from a reduced rate of proliferation of red cell precursors or from failure of their maturation leading to intramedullary destruction and ineffective erythropoiesis. Loss of blood may be due to bleeding or hemolysis. In many forms of anemia several of these mechanisms may be operating simultaneously.

DEFECTIVE RED CELL PRODUCTION

Defective proliferation of red cell precursors

The main causes of this group of anemias are an inadequate supply of iron, primary disease of the bone marrow which involves stem cells or later erythroid precursors, or a reduction in the amount of erythropoietin reaching the red cell precursors. In tropical populations a reduced supply of iron is by far the commonest basis for defective erythroid proliferation. It is

Table 9-2. The main groups of anemias

Impaired red cell production:
Decreased or inappropriately increased total erythropoiesis
Greatly increased ineffective erythropoiesis
Increased rate of red cell destruction (hemolysis)
Loss of red cells from the circulation (bleeding)

caused either by dietary deficiency, malabsorption, or infection. In the latter case iron becomes trapped in the storage compartments of the marrow and hence is unavailable to the erythroid precursors, which require a critical level of iron for proliferation as well as for hemoglobin synthesis, which is, in turn, necessary for normal cytoplasmic maturation.

Defective red cell maturation

This may involve the nucleus or the cytoplasm. The important disorders of nuclear maturation in the tropics result from deficiency of either folate or vitamin B_{12}. The main causes of defective cytoplasmic maturation are the inherited disorders of globin synthesis, the thalassemias. In all these conditions the marrow is hyperplastic, but many of the red cell precursors are destroyed before they reach the peripheral blood, i.e., there is ineffective erythropoiesis. This is characterized by erythroid hyperplasia with a relatively low reticulocyte count in the peripheral blood. The disorders of nuclear maturation are usually characterized by megaloblastic erythropoiesis and a macrocytic anemia; those involving cytoplasmic maturation show normoblastic proliferation and a hypochromic, microcytic anemia.

EXCESSIVE LOSS OF BLOOD

Bleeding

Chronic blood loss from the gastrointestinal tract in excess of 15 to 20 mL/day produces a state of negative iron balance. Although iron absorption may be increased, there is a steady drain on the body iron stores, which, in adults, are normally in the region of 1 g. Once the stores are depleted, the hemoglobin level starts to fall, although at this stage the red cell morphology may be relatively normal. It is only when iron deficiency is well established that the typical hypochromic, microcytic red cells appear. In tropical populations hookworm infection is by far the commonest cause of chronic gastrointestinal blood loss.

Hemolysis

A modest shortening of red cell survival may not cause anemia because of compensatory erythroid hyperplasia and an increased rate of red cell production. If the red cell survival is short enough, even a healthy marrow cannot compensate, and anemia results. The accelerated erythropoietic activity in hemolytic anemia is reflected by a raised reticulocyte count and macrocytosis due to the presence of ''young'' cells in the circulation. The increased rate of red cell destruction results in an elevated bilirubin level and increased amounts of urobilinogen in the urine and stool. If it is primarily intravascular, haptoglobins and hemopexin disappear from the plasma, free hemoglobin and methemoglobin appear in the plasma, and there may be hemoglobinuria and hemosiderinuria (Fig. 9-1).

Red cells are destroyed prematurely if their membrane is abnormal in structure or function, if they are exposed to ex-

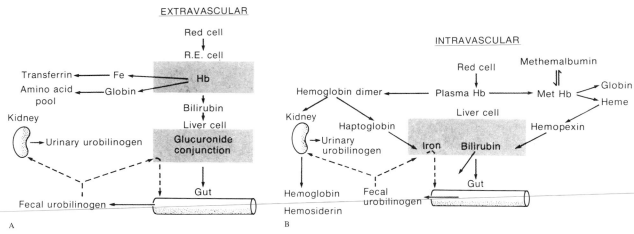

Figure 9-1. The pathophysiology of hemolysis. **A.** Extravascular. **B.** Intravascular. (*From Weatherall DJ, and Bunch C, in Pathophysiology, The Biological Basis of Disease, 2d ed. Smith, L.H., and Thier, S.O., eds. Philadelphia, Saunders, 1985.*)

cessive trauma in the circulation, or if they are unusually rigid due to the precipitation or abnormal molecular configuration of hemoglobin. The cell must be able to undergo considerable deformation as it passes through the microcirculation; this depends on the plasticity of the cell, which in turn is related to its surface-volume ratio. Normal red cell survival relies on the production of energy for transport of sodium and potassium across the membrane and for the renewal of membrane lipids. Abnormalities of any of these functions tend to produce a spherical cell which is not easily deformed and hence is prematurely destroyed. This process occurs in any condition in which the membrane is structurally abnormal and may also result from the interaction of antibodies on the cell surface with macrophages, and by the direct effects of trauma, chemicals, bacteria, or parasites. The pathophysiology of premature red cell damage due to abnormal aggregation or precipitation of hemoglobin molecules is considered in Chap. 14.

COMPENSATION AND CLINICAL FEATURES

COMPENSATION

A variety of compensatory mechanisms are initiated in response to anemia. In young people with a healthy myocardium these are remarkably effective, and such patients may remain free of symptoms at very low hemoglobin levels, provided that the anemia has developed gradually. The main compensatory changes are the modulation of the oxygen affinity of hemoglobin, increased cardiac output, and redistribution of flow between different organs. In addition there may be some ill-defined adaptive changes in tissue enzymes.

An early response to anemia is an increase in the level of red cell 2,3-diphosphoglycerate (2,3-DPG). This shifts the oxygen dissociation curve to the right; with increasing severity of anemia there is a progressive increase in 2,3-DPG which may facilitate oxygen delivery by as much as 40 percent for the same hemoglobin concentration [10]. This is the main adaptive mechanism at hemoglobin values in excess of 7 to 8 g/dL. Below this level there is an increase in cardiac output [11], and a hyperkinetic circulation develops, characterized by tachycardia, arterial and capillary pulsation, a wide pulse pressure, and hemic murmurs. The circulation time is shortened, left ventricular stroke work is increased, and coronary flow increases in proportion to the increased cardiac output. In very severe anemia there may be progression to high-output cardiac failure with cardiomegaly, pulmonary edema, ascites, and peripheral edema.

CLINICAL FEATURES

As mentioned above, there may be no symptoms in patients with mild to moderate anemia of slow onset. As the anemia becomes more severe, there is pallor, dyspnea, tachycardia, palpitations, a variety of cardiac bruits, and, if cardiac failure occurs, basal crepitations, peripheral edema, and ascites. There are associated neuromuscular symptoms including headache, vertigo, faintness, tinnitus, roaring in the ears, and retinal hemorrhages. Gastrointestinal symptoms include weight loss, loss of appetite, nausea, and diarrhea. There are often genitourinary manifestations including menstrual irregularity, urinary frequency, and loss of libido. There may be a low-grade fever.

Several studies in Africa and elsewhere have shown that in pregnancy there is an increased risk of fetal and maternal morbidity and mortality associated with anemia [12,13]. In west Africa it has been found that pregnant women with hemoglobin values below 4 g/dL frequently develop high-output cardiac failure [13].

Studies in Asia [14,15] have suggested that moderate anemia may reduce work capacity, have a deleterious effect on growth rates in young children, and cause an increased proneness to infection. However, much of this data is difficult to evaluate, and further work on these important aspects of tropical anemia is required.

THE MAJOR GROUPS OF ANEMIA IN THE TROPICS

IRON DEFICIENCY (See also Chap 124)

Normal iron balance and requirements

A normal adult male requires about 1 mg of iron per day to meet basal losses. The nonpregnant adult female requires about twice this amount to make up additional loss by menstruation. Iron requirements are increased above these levels during periods of rapid growth or in pregnancy; daily requirements for different ages and sex as recommended by the WHO [16] are summarized in Table 9-3. The average daily intake of iron varies widely; it is usually in the 10- to 40-mg range. Iron-replete individuals absorb approximately 10 percent of ingested iron and hence iron balance is maintained. The relative amount of iron absorbed increases in iron-deficient subjects.

The cause of nutritional iron deficiency anemia is complex. It may, of course, arise simply from a diet deficient in iron. However, the form of iron in the food is also extremely important. For example, it has been estimated that in Venezuela, where 80 to 90 percent of iron intake is of vegetable origin in the form of corn, black beans, and similar vegetables, only 0.6 to 1.0 mg of iron is absorbed per day by normal subjects and from 1 to 2 mg in iron-deficient subjects [17]. Iron derived solely from meat is absorbed less well than when a mixed meal with corn is taken. Studies in India point to an inhibitory effect of cereal-based diets on iron absorption; this may be mediated by their high fiber, polyphenol, phytate, and phosphate content [18]. Work in Thailand has shown that subtle differences in the diet, substitution of grain rice for rice flour, for example, may have profound effects on the level of iron absorption [19].

Table 9-3. Daily requirements for iron (amounts to be absorbed) for different ages and sex as recommended by WHO scientific groups [16]

Group	Iron to be absorbed, mg
Infants, 5 to 12 months	0.7
Children, 1 to 12 years	1.0
Boys, 13 to 16 years	1.8
Girls, 13 to 16 years	2.4
Menstruating women	2.8
Adult males (65 kg)	0.9
Pregnancy, first half	0.8
Pregnancy, second half	3.0
Lactation	2.4

Although these analyses are bedeviled by difficulties of interpretation because of inadequacies of radioactive iron labeling techniques, it is apparent that differences in the diet may have profound effects on iron absorption. It is also clear that the diets in the developing countries are, in many cases, at borderline levels for iron requirements and that, if iron losses are increased, iron deficiency is inevitable [20].

Decreased absorption

Iron absorption is reduced in some patients with tropical sprue and in other tropical malabsorption syndromes [6].

Excessive loss

Hookworm infection is the commonest cause of iron loss in the tropics [21]. Approximately 0.3 mL of blood per worm per day may be lost in *Necator americanus* infection and about 0.2 mL of blood per worm per day in *Ancylostoma duodenale* infection; total blood losses vary from 2 or 3 mL to 100 mL/day with particularly heavy infections. There may be a mild blood loss in association with *Trichuris trichiura* infection; each worm causes blood loss of about 0.005 mL/day. There may be sufficient blood loss from the urinary tract in patients with schistosomiasis to cause chronic iron deficiency anemia.

There is no evidence that there is increased loss of iron through the skin by excess sweating, or through the intestinal tract, in tropical countries.

Clinical effects

Iron deficiency anemia is characterized by a hypochromic, microcytic anemia (Fig. 9-2). There is some evidence [14,15], though not substantiated, that reduced iron stores are associated with diminished work capacity and that severe iron deficiency may be associated with growth retardation. The relationship between iron deficiency and infection is extremely complicated. Some studies have shown that the incidence of bacterial infection is lower in iron-deficient subjects [22]; it has also been suggested that *Plasmodium falciparum* malaria is less severe in the presence of iron deficiency. On the other hand, severe iron deficiency has been shown to have a deleterious effect on cell-mediated immunity. The whole subject of iron metabolism and infection is under active investigation [22] and remains controversial.

Prophylaxis

The prophylaxis of iron deficiency requires a multipronged approach including supplementation of demographic groups at most risk, fortification of one or more stable foods, the control of hookworm and other parasites, and major education programs with the use of iron supplementation during pregnancy. Fortification programs are currently under study in Thailand and elsewhere. Preliminary data suggest that fortifying fish

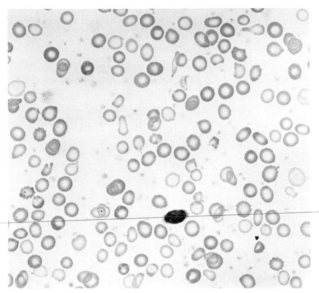

Figure 9-2. A hypochromic, microcytic blood picture (Leishman stain ×600).

sauce with iron may reduce the incidence of nutritional iron deficiency in parts of Thailand [7]. Investigations into salt fortification are currently underway in India [6]; preliminary studies indicate that this approach can result in a significant rise in hemoglobin concentration in children in rural populations.

Principles of management

It is important to attempt to distinguish between dietary iron deficiency and blood loss as the cause of iron deficiency anemia. This is achieved by taking a full history and carrying out a careful clinical examination followed by an analysis of the stools for occult blood and a careful search for hookworm. If there is evidence of gastrointestinal blood loss and hookworm is not the cause, the site of bleeding must be sought by endoscopic and radiological analysis of the gastrointestinal tract. The anemia should be treated with the administration of iron by mouth, either in the form of ferrous sulphate or ferrous gluconate. The hemoglobin level should rise by about 1 g/week. In order to restore the iron stores to normal, therapy

should be continued for 3 to 6 months after a normal hemoglobin level has been achieved.

MEGALOBLASTIC ANEMIA (See also Chap. 119)

While less common than iron deficiency anemia, megaloblastic anemias due to vitamin B_{12} or folate deficiency occur commonly in some tropical countries. The main causes of tropical megaloblastic anemia are summarized in Table 9-4.

Vitamin B_{12} deficiency

The major dietary sources of vitamin B_{12} are liver, meat, and other animal products; fish sauce, which is widely consumed in Thailand and other parts of Asia, is also a rich source [6]. Theoretically, subjects who eat virtually no animal-derived food or fish sauce should have a high prevalence of nutritional vitamin B_{12} deficiency. However, overt vitamin B_{12} deficiency is relatively uncommon. This may be because vitamin B_{12} can be derived from bacterial contamination of food and water; this mechanism has been demonstrated in parts of southern India [6]. It is also possible that some vitamin B_{12} is derived from bacteria in the small bowel.

Vitamin B_{12} combines with intrinsic factor and is absorbed in the ileum. The daily requirements are not known for certain; it has been estimated that they range from 0.3 µg in infancy and childhood to approximately 3 µg/day during pregnancy; the adult requirement is somewhere in the region of 2 µg/day [23].

Probably the commonest form of dietary vitamin B_{12} deficiency occurs in infants born to and suckled by vitamin B_{12}-deficient mothers; this disorder is seen predominantly in Indian populations [6]. Dietary deficiency of vitamin B_{12} is less common in the adult populations of Asia and Africa, although, interestingly, it seems to be increasingly recognized in Indian immigrants to the United Kingdom [6,23]; perhaps this is because there is less bacterial contamination of water and food.

By far the commonest cause of malabsorption of vitamin B_{12} in the tropics is sprue [5,6,24]. The mechanism is not understood, although the fact that it can be corrected by broad-spectrum antibiotics in a high proportion of cases suggests that excessive utilization by an abnormal intestinal bacterial population may be partly responsible. However, intubation studies in which intrinsic factor–vitamin B_{12} complexes have been fed

Table 9-4. Mechanisms of megaloblastic anemia in the tropics

Deficiency	Intake	Absorption	Requirement
Vitamin B_{12}	Inadequate diet in vegetarians; bacterial deviation in gut in sprue	Defective in sprue	Increased in pregnancy and lactation
Folate	Destruction of dietary folate by excessive boiling; possible inhibitors of intestinal conjugase in food; inadequate diet	Defective in sprue	Increased in pregnancy and lactation, malaria, hemoglobinopathy, and iron deficiency.

to patients with sprue suggest that the complex reaches the ileum in normal amounts [25]; hence it is more likely that the bacteria interfere with absorption by producing abnormal intra-luminal conditions which are unfavorable for the binding of the complex or that they produce direct damage to the intrinsic factor–vitamin B_{12} receptors or the ileal entrance sites [6].

Vitamin B_{12} deficiency due to lack of intrinsic factor (true pernicious anemia) seems to be relatively uncommon in Africa, India, and southeast Asia [6,7].

Folic acid deficiency (See also Chap. 119)

There are relatively few data on the prevalence of folate deficiency in tropical countries. Most studies have been confined to pregnant women or hospital populations. The condition seems to be particularly common in parts of India [5,6], where up to 70 percent of women in the last trimester of pregnancy have been found to be folate-depleted. The condition is less common in Asia and Africa, although precise figures are not available. These differences probably reflect both diet and methods of cooking.

The minimal daily requirement for folate estimated as pter-oylglutamic acid is about 50 μg [23]. Folate is present in most foods, especially in liver, vegetables, and yeast; it occurs both as free monoglutamate and in polyglutamate forms. The latter have to be broken down to monoglutamate in intestinal cells before absorption, since free pteroylmonoglutamic acid is more readily absorbed than polyglutamate. Absorption occurs mainly in the upper jejunum. All the folates are heat-labile and readily destroyed by prolonged cooking. Folate requirements are markedly increased during pregnancy and also in any form of chronic hemolytic anemia; increased folate is required by the hyperplastic bone marrow.

Dietary folate deficiency occurs most commonly in pregnancy and during lactation. It is particularly common in parts of India [5,6] where the diet is borderline in folate, but it also occurs in Africa, particularly in communities which practice prolonged cooking of food [7]. Malabsorption of folate is very common in patients with tropical sprue; the exact mechanism is still not understood. Interestingly, the absorption of mono-glutamate may be normal in patients with sprue, even in the presence of severe folate deficiency. On the other hand poly-glutamate malabsorption is common [26]. This may be the result of defective transport of polyglutamate into the entero-cytes or defective intracellular breakdown to monoglutamate; the enzyme responsible for the metabolism of polyglutamate, γ-glutamyl transpeptidase, is present in normal levels in the enterocytes in this disorder, however.

Clinical and hematological changes

Vitamin B_{12} or folate deficiency is characterized by progressive anemia, pallor, hyperpigmentation of the skin and mucous membranes, splenomegaly, low-grade fever, and, in the case of vitamin B_{12} deficiency, a neurological syndrome comprised

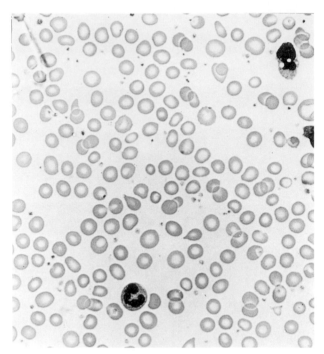

Figure 9-3. A macrocytic blood picture from a patient with folic acid deficiency (Leishman stain ×600).

of peripheral neuropathy and of subacute combined degeneration of the cord. The hematological picture is characterized by a macrocytic anemia (Fig. 9-3) with a megaloblastic bone marrow and there may be marked neutropenia and thrombo-cytopenia. The diagnosis is confirmed by specific assays for serum or red cell folate and serum vitamin B_{12}. The diagnosis of sprue depends on the appropriate clinical findings in association with typical histological appearances on jejunal biopsy.

The syndrome of neonatal vitamin B_{12} deficiency in India is characterized by failure of normal development, involuntary movements, alterations in muscle tone, and hyperpigmentation of the skin and mucous membranes [6]. Unrecognized, this disorder progresses to coma and death.

Principles of management

Megaloblastic anemia always requires full investigation. Some indication of the cause may be ascertained by a full clinical history and physical examination. The levels of serum vitamin B_{12} and serum or red cell folate should be determined. If the cause is not obvious from the clinical history, it is essential to carry out further investigation to determine the reason for the deficiency of either vitamin B_{12} or folic acid. This may require radioactive vitamin B_{12} absorption studies, analysis of small-bowel function and absorptive capacity, or, if the facilities are not available, observation of the hematological responses to pharmacological doses of either vitamin B_{12} or folate. The latter are characterized by a reticulocytosis which occurs 5 to 8 days after the initial dose. Since many patients with megaloblastic anemia are also iron-depleted, it is important to administer oral iron as well as vitamin B_{12} or folate if a full reticulocyte response is to be obtained.

OTHER DEFICIENCY STATES

Although deficiencies of other trace elements or vitamins such as B_6, pantothenic acid, and riboflavin may play a role in the production of anemia in experimental animals, none of these factors has been shown to be a cause of anemia in human beings. Anemia is a major problem in children with the syndrome of protein-calorie malnutrition (kwashiorkor) [7]. This has an extremely complex pathogenesis which is not yet fully understood. These children sometimes have erythroid hypoplasia which may be in part due to protein deficiency, infection, and, possibly, riboflavin deficiency. However, many of them are vitamin B_{12} and folate-deficient and are also iron-depleted. Although there is a hemolytic component, this too may have a complex basis including chronic malaria or vitamin E deficiency. This incidence of megaloblastic erythropoiesis in kwashiorkor is low in tropical Africa [7], but it is quite common in South Africa, Colombia, and Jordan [27]. It is also relatively common in parts of India. Probably the pathophysiology of this syndrome varies between races. The marked erythroid hypoplasia may reflect gross protein deficiency; similar changes have been produced in experimental animals.

THE ANEMIAS OF INFECTION

Most infectious disorders are accompanied by a varying degree of anemia. This has a complex pathophysiology which has, in general, been a neglected area of hematology. The response of the hemopoietic system to infection varies depending on the particular oganism involved. There is a fairly well defined series of changes in iron metabolism, superimposed on which there may be alterations in red cell survival and the effects of hypersplenism; the latter vary considerably depending on the organism involved.

BACTERIAL AND VIRUS INFECTIONS

Information about the changes in the hemopoietic system secondary to acute or chronic infections has been derived from both human and animal studies. Soon after infection there is a fall in the serum iron level and iron binding capacity (TIBC) [28] with a rise in the plasma ferritin level [29]. As the infection becomes established, the changes of what is called "the anemia of chronic disorders" develop [28]. These include a moderate degree of anemia, normochromic or slightly hypochromic red cells, a paucity of iron in the red cell precursors, and an accumulation of iron in the storage elements of the bone marrow. There is sequestration of iron in the iron stores; this is reflected by a poorly proliferating marrow and a slightly

reduced mean cell hemoglobin level. It is possible that the increased ferritin synthesis and the sequestration of iron represents an adaptive mechanism leading to a fall in the serum iron level, hence affording protection against proliferation of bacteria or other organisms. If the infection becomes chronic, a moderate degree of anemia persists together with the accumulation of iron in the storage compartments of the marrow. There may be an associated reduction in red cell survival; this is rarely marked [28]. There is some evidence for an inappropriate erythropoietin response in this form of anemia, although the published data are inconsistent.

Superimposed on the changes outlined above, some infections produce more specific hematological pictures. For example, some bacterial septicemias are associated with disseminated intravascular coagulation and a microangiopathic hemolytic process, i.e., the presence of severe hemolysis with marked morphological changes of the red cells due to damage by fibrin strands in the microcirculation [30]. Some organisms, particularly of the *Clostridium* group, produce specific lecithinases which disrupt the red cell membrane and cause intravascular hemolysis. Viral infections may be complicated by transient red cell aplasia. For example, it has been established that parvovirus infections cause red cell aplasia in patients with sickle cell anemia [31]. A syndrome of acute erythrophagocytosis in association with virus infections has been described [32]; although this seems to occur most commonly in immune-suppressed individuals, there is some evidence that it may occur more widely than has hitherto been realized. This syndrome is characterized by progressive anemia with marked erythrophagocytosis of red cell precursors in the bone marrow. The mechanism for these interactions between viruses and red cell precursors is not understood.

PARASITIC INFECTIONS

Many parasitic infections are associated with some degree of anemia, the pathophysiology of which, in most cases, is complex and ill-defined. The anemia of *P. falciparum* malaria is a good example of our current state of uncertainty about this important problem [33]. In acute infections in nonimmune individuals there is a rapid fall in hemoglobin level which corresponds approximately with the degree of parasitemia, and probably results from disruption of red cells by the parasites and from the entrapment of parasitized cells in the microcirculation. However, after treatment the hemoglobin level may continue to fall for 7 to 21 days, and there is an inappropriate reticulocyte response indicating ineffective erythropoiesis or defective proliferation of red cell precursors. During this stage there is a shortened red cell survival; although some patients at this phase of the illness have a positive direct antiglobulin (Coombs) test, there is no definite evidence for an immune basis for this hemolytic component; its mechanism is not understood. After about 2 weeks there is a reticulocytosis and the hemoglobin level gradually returns to normal. In endemic areas repeated reinfections may produce profound anemia, particularly in childhood. Recent studies indicate that this has a dyserythropoietic basis with minimal hemolysis, probably complicated by hypersplenism in some cases [*34*]. Acute episodes of hemolysis with hemoglobinuria, blackwater fever, are now rarely seen except in patients with fulminating *P. falciparum* infections. Some cases undoubtedly result from glucose-6-phosphate dehydrogenase (G-6-PD) deficiency with a hemolytic response to drugs used in the treatment of malaria. However, the pathophysiology of this condition remains uncertain (see Chap. 14).

Even less is known about the pathophysiology of anemias of other common parasitic disorders. Leishmaniasis is associated with a hemolytic component together with dyserythropoiesis and, in chronic cases, the effects of hypersplenism (see below) [*35*]. There is a major hemolytic component in bartonellosis because of the disruption of the red cells [*30*] by the organism. Schistosomiasis may be associated with severe anemia which results from a combination of the anemia of infection, the pathophysiology of which was discussed earlier, chronic blood loss, and hypersplenism [*35*]. All the chronic anemias of parasitic infection may be complicated by nutritional iron or folate deficiency and, in the case of hookworm and other gut parasites (see above), by the effect of chronic iron loss.

HYPERSPLENISM IN TROPICAL DISORDERS

Although splenomegaly is a feature of many tropical disorders, there is increasing evidence, particularly from work in east and west Africa and New Guinea, that there is a specific entity, the tropical splenomegaly syndrome (TSS), which occurs widely throughout Africa, India, and southeast Asia. This condition is characterized by gross splenomegaly, a high level of immunity to malaria, serum IgM levels at least two standard deviations above the local mean, and a variable response to antimalarial therapy [*7,36,37*].

Etiology and pathophysiology

There is considerable evidence that malaria plays an important role in TSS. Epidemiological studies indicate that differences in the pattern of malarial transmission may be important in determining the incidence of this syndrome and that, in addition, genetic factors may play a part. Patients with the TSS syndrome have higher malarial antibody titers than those who live in the same environment and are unaffected; this seems to involve IgM rather than IgG titers. These observations, together with the partial response to antimalarials and the fact that individuals with the sickle cell trait seem to be partially protected from the TSS syndrome, indicate that the condition probably results from an unusual form of immune response to chronic malarial antigenemia; the mechanism is not clear.

Progressive splenomegaly results in pooling of the formed elements of the blood; in patients with very large spleens one-third to one-half of the total circulating red cell mass may be sequestered. This produces a dilutional anemia which is made worse by an absolute increase in plasma volume which is often associated with massive splenomegaly; the mechanism is unknown. In addition there may be pooling of the neutrophils and platelets resulting in neutropenia and thrombocytopenia.

Clinical and hematological features

There is massive splenomegaly, weight loss, and a variable degree of anemia, neutropenia, and thrombocytopenia. The red cell volume is only moderately decreased, but the plasma volume is elevated in most cases. Isotope dilution studies indicate that there is pooling of red cells in the large spleen, and, as in other forms of hypersplenism, there may be some shortening of red cell survival. There may be an increased proneness to infection due to neutropenia, and bleeding due to thrombocytopenia. The bone marrow shows active erythropoiesis, and there is infiltration with mature lymphocytes, and some lymphocytic infiltration of liver. IgM levels are high, and there is a relative increase of T lymphocytes in the peripheral blood. The serum may show increased cold agglutinin titers and an increase in rheumatoid factor, antibodies to thyroglobulin, antinuclear factor, and circulating immune complexes.

Prognosis and relationship to malignant disease

This condition has remarkably poor prognosis in parts of Africa, with up to a 50 percent mortality rate in some populations. It has been suggested that this disorder may be related to a lymphoma, but so far there is no evidence that this is the case.

Principles of management

This condition is best managed by the use of antimalarial drugs together with long-term antimalarial prophylaxis. There have been many reports of successful reduction of spleen size by the use of agents such as proguanil, although, as mentioned above, the results are variable. There seems to be no place for splenectomy in this condition.

HEMOLYTIC ANEMIA IN THE TROPICS

Hemolytic anemias are common in the tropics (Table 9-5). Many of the disorders outlined in the previous sections may be complicated by the hemoglobinopathies, thalassemia, or G-6-PD deficiency. These conditions are described elsewhere in this book (Chap. 14). The hemolytic complications of bacterial and parasitic infections were considered earlier. There is a hemolytic component to the TSS syndrome and in all patients with splenic enlargement; however, this is minor compared with the effect of pooling of a significant proportion of the circulating red cell mass in these large spleens. While it should be remembered that any form of hemolytic anemia can be encountered in the tropics, the vast majority of cases result from infections and the hemoglobinopathies.

Table 9-5. Main groups of hemolytic anemias

Genetic disorders of the red cell	Acquired disorders of the red cell
Membrane:	Immune:
Hereditary spherocytosis	Isoimmune—Rh or ABO
Hereditary ovalocytosis	Autoimmune—warm or cold
Stomatocytosis	antibody
Other "leaky" membrane	Nonimmune:
disorders	Trauma: microangiopathy,
Acanthocytosis	valve prosthesis, body
Hemoglobin:	suface contact
Sickling disorders	Membrane defects: PNH,*
Hemoglobins C, D, and E	liver disease
Unstable hemoglobins	Parasitic infections
Thalassemia syndromes	Bacterial infections
Energy pathways:	Physical agents, drugs, and
Hexose monophosphate shunt	chemicals
Embden-Meyerhof pathway	Hypersplenism
	Due to defective red cell
	maturation

*PNH = paroxysmal hemoglobinuria

ANEMIA OF PREGNANCY IN THE TROPICS

Anemia in pregnancy is a major public health problem in many parts of the world [3]. Representative data are summarized in Table 9-6.

The major causes of anemia in pregnancy are iron and folate deficiency, malaria, and the hemoglobinopathies. The relative importance of these factors varies in different parts of the world; iron deficiency predominates in India whereas malaria complicated by folate deficiency is the major cause of profound anemia in west Africa (Table 9-6). Malaria is particularly important, as both the frequency and density of parasitemia increase progressively to reach a peak about midpregnancy, especially in first pregnancies.

Severe anemia in pregnancy has serious implications for both mother and fetus. With maternal hemoglobin levels of 3 g/dL or less cardiac failure often occurs and, without treatment, mortality is approximately 50 percent [3]. Fetal hypoxia is reflected by compensatory placental hypertrophy and retarded intrauterine growth. Fetal distress is common, birth

Table 9-6. Prevalence (percent) of anemia (Hb <11.0 g/dL) and iron deficiency (saturation of transferrin <15 percent) during pregnancy

Geographical area	Anemia	Iron deficiency
Latin America	27	49
Nigeria	47	31
Northern India	80	52
Southern India	57	99
Philippines	63	35

Source: From [3].

weights are low, and there is a high perinatal mortality; in Nigerian mothers with hematocrits of 0.23 or less at the time of delivery 50 percent of infants weighed less than 2.0 kg and the perinatal mortality was more than 30 percent.

PRACTICAL APPROACH TO THE ANEMIC PATIENT IN THE TROPICS

By taking a full history, carrying out a competent clinical examination, and performing a few simple hematological investigations it is possible to sort out most causes of anemia and to manage them appropriately. The key features in the history, obtained either directly from an adult or from the parents of affected children, include diet, gastrointestinal symptoms with particular attention to diarrhea, episodic fevers suggesting infection, ingestion of drugs that might cause marrow failure, and any symptoms of bruising or bleeding which might indicate a hemorrhagic diathesis. The clinical examination should include an attempt at an assessment of the degree of anemia from inspection of the mucous membranes, nail beds, and skin creases, a careful and systematic palpation of the lymph node groups, an examination of the oral cavity and tongue for signs of bleeding or glossitis, a full abdominal examination with particular respect to hepatosplenomegaly, a rectal examination with an immediate study of feces for parasites or ova and cysts, a simple occult blood examination of the stool sample, and a full examination of all the systems in the standard way.

Hematological studies will depend on the sophistication of equipment that is available. The most valuable measurement is a hemoglobin or packed cell volume (hematocrit) level. If this is combined with a careful examination of a well-stained blood film, which must include a careful search for malarial parasites, it should be possible to sort out most cases of anemia. If an electronic cell counter is available, considerable help will be obtained from the MCH and MCV because these measurements will make it possible to classify the anemia as microcytic, normocytic, or macrocytic. By and large, microcytic anemias indicate iron deficiency or thalassemia, while normochromic anemias are the rule where infection is the underlying cause. A macrocytic anemia should always be investigated further by a bone marrow examination and estimation of the serum B_{12} and folate levels, where possible. Normochromic or slightly macrocytic anemias should be studied further with a reticulocyte count because if this is elevated it suggests regeneration and the possibility of hemolysis. As mentioned earlier, the most important causes of hemolysis in the tropics are the hemoglobinopathies and infection.

In general, anemia should be managed by treating the underlying cause. However, in cases of profound anemia it may be necessary to transfuse the patient. Particularly if there is splenomegaly, which may be associated with an increased blood volume, great care is required in transfusing profoundly anemic patients. The general rule should be to transfuse no more than 1 U of blood over a 4-h period and to administer a powerful diuretic such as furosemide at the same time that each unit of blood is given. This approach will suffice except in cases of profound anemia with severe heart failure, where it may be necessary to carry out a partial exchange transfusion to raise the hematocrit into a safer range. Again, this should be combined with diuretic therapy.

SUMMARY: ANEMIA AS A PUBLIC HEALTH PROBLEM IN THE TROPICS

Anemia is a major public health problem in most tropical countries. The WHO is promoting control of nutritional anemia, but this is a difficult problem because of lack of adequate health care infrastructures. In many of these countries there are established hematology units staffed by western-trained hematologists. However, the practice and teaching of modern hematology by these units in the last 20 to 30 years has hardly had any impact on the control of anemia in the communities. Their clinical approach is largely doctor- and disease-oriented and a one-to-one form of care and teaching, as practiced in the developed countries. In the developing tropical countries it will be important to revise current approaches to the management of anemia. Like most public health problems, intervention for anemia must be integrated into the primary health care with full support at other levels of health care, including the more sophisticated hematology units [38].

REFERENCES

1 Hardisty RM, Weatherall DJ (eds): *Blood and Its Disorders,* 2d ed. Oxford, Blackwell, 1982

2 Williams WJ, Beutler E, Erslev A, et al: *Hematology,* 4th ed. New York, McGraw-Hill, 1989, in press

3 Fleming AF: Anaemia as a world health problem, in Weatherall DJ, Ledingham JGG, Warrell DA (eds): *The Oxford Textbook of Medicine,* 2d ed. Oxford, Blackwell, 1987, pp 19, 72–79

4 World Health Organization: Nutritional anaemias. Tech Rep Ser 503. Geneva, WHO, 1972

5 Baker SJ: Nutritional anaemia—a major controllable public health problem. Bull WHO, 56:659–675, 1978

6 Baker SJ: Nutritional anaemias: Tropical Asia. Clin Haematol 10:843–871, 1981

7 Masawe AEJ: Nutritional anaemias: Tropical Africa. Clin Haematol 10:815–842, 1981

8 McGregor IA, Williams K, Billewicz WZ, et al: Haemoglobin concentration and anaemia in young West African (Gambian) children. Trans R Soc Trop Med Hyg 60:650–667, 1966

9 Wasi P, Na-Nakorn S, Piankijagum A, et al: The haematocrit values and the incidence of anaemia in the population of Thailand. Siriraj Hosp Gaz 25:584–598, 1973

10 Adamson JW, Finch CA: Hemoglobin function, oxygen affinity and erythropoietin. Annu Rev Physiol 37:351–369, 1975

11 Varat MA, Adolph RJ, Fowler NO: Cardiovascular effects of anemia. Am Heart J 83:415–426, 1972

12 Lawson J: Severe anaemia in pregnancy; a tropical obstetric emergency. Trop Doct 1:77–79, 1971

13 Harrison KA: Blood volume changes in severe anaemia of pregnancy. Lancet i:20–25, 1967

14 Basta SS, Soekirman MS, Karyadi D, et al: Iron deficiency anemia and the productivity of adult males in Indonesia. Am J Clin Nutr 32:916–925, 1979

15 Garby L, Areekul S: Iron supplementation in Thai fish sauce. Ann Trop Med Parasitol 68:467–476, 1974

16 World Health Organization. Control of nutritional anaemia with special reference to iron deficiency. Tech Rep Ser 580. Geneva, WHO, 1975

17 Layrisse M: The aetiology and geographic incidence of iron deficiency, in Plenary Sessions, XIth Cong Internat Soc Haemat. Sydney, Blight, p 95, 1966

18 Venkatachalam PS: Iron metabolism and iron deficiency in India. Am J Clin Nutr 21:1156–1161, 1968

19 Hallberg L, Bjorn-Rasmussen E, Rossander L, et al: Iron absorption from Southeast Asian diets. II, Role of various factors that might explain low absorption. Am J Clin Nutr 30:539–548, 1977

20 Suwanik R, Punyaprateep B, Pleehachinda R, et al: Iron status of Thai population in Bangkok and villagers of Northeastern Thailand. J Med Assoc Thailand 64:283–287, 1981

21 Roche M, Layrisse M: The nature and causes of "hookworm anemia." Am J Trop Med Hyg 15:1031–1102, 1966

22 Bullen JJ: The significance of iron in infection, in *Reviews of Infectious Diseases.* University of Chicago, 1981, vol 3, pp 1127–1138

23 Hoffbrand AV: Vitamin B_{12} and folate metabolism. The megaloblastic anaemias and other nutritional anaemias, in Hardisty RM, Weatherall DJ (eds): *Blood and Its Disorders,* 2d ed. Oxford, Blackwell, 1982, pp 119–263

24 Klipstein FA: Tropical sprue in travelers and expatriates living abroad. Gastroenterology 80:590–600, 1981

25 Kapadia CR, Bhat P, Jacob E, et al: Vitamin B_{12} absorption—a study of intraluminal events in control subjects and patients with tropical sprue. Gut 16:988–993, 1975

26 Bernstein LH, Gutstein S, Weiner S, et al: The absorption and malabsorption of folic acid and its polyglutamates. Am J Med 48:570–579, 1970

27 Pitney WR: Anaemia in the tropics, in Goldberg A, Brain MC (eds): *Recent Advances in Haematology,* 1st ed. Edinburgh, Churchill Livingstone, 1971, pp 337–356

28 Reizenstein P: Annotation, The haematological stress syndrome. Br J Haematol 43:329–334, 1979

29 Halliday JW, Powell LW: Serum ferritin and isoferritins in clinical medicine, in Brown EB (ed): *Progress in Hematology XI.* New York, Grune & Stratton, 1979, pp 229–266

30 Gordon-Smith EC: The non-immune acquired haemolytic anaemias, in Hardisty RM, Weatherall DJ (eds): *Blood and Its Disorders,* 2d ed. Oxford, Blackwell, 1982, pp 515–544

31 Serjeant GR, Topley JM, Mason K, et al: Outbreak of aplastic crises in sickle cell anaemia associated with parvovirus-like agent. Lancet ii:595–597, 1981

32 McKenna RW, Risdall RJ, Brunning RD: Virus associated hemophagocytic syndrome. Hum Pathol 12:395–398, 1981

33 Pasvol G: The anaemia of malaria. Q J Med 58:217–219, 1986

34 Phillips RE, Looareesuwan S, Warrell DA, et al: The importance of anaemia in cerebral and uncomplicated falciparum malaria: Role of complications, dyserythropoiesis, and iron sequestration. Q J Med 58:305–323, 1986

35 Pippard MJ, Moir D, Weatherall DJ, et al: Mechanism of anaemia in resistant visceral leishmaniasis. Ann Trop Med Parasitol 80:317–323, 1986

36 Fakunle YM: Tropical splenomegaly. Part I: Tropical Africa. Clin Haematol 10:963–975, 1981

37 Crane GG: Tropical splenomegaly. Part 2: Oceania. Clin Haematol 10:976–982, 1981

38 Wasi P, Na-Nakorn S: Problems of haematology training in developing countries. Br Med J 283:292–293, 1981

CHAPTER 10 / *Eosinophilia* · *Adel A. F. Mahmoud*

Eosinophilia is one of the most common hematological laboratory findings in patients seen in the developing countries. Although controlled epidemiological data are lacking, an analysis of the presenting features of several major global parasitic infections showed that anemia is the most common hematological finding and that eosinophilia is next in frequency [1]. In spite of the long-known association of eosinophilia with tissue-dwelling worm infections, considerable confusion is involved in defining the clinical conditions associated with increased cell counts. Furthermore, the clinical significance of these cells and the usefulness of detecting changes in their numbers in achieving an etiological diagnosis need to be elucidated. This chapter will discuss eosinophilia as a clinical laboratory feature associated with several disease complexes that are either particularly prevalent in developing countries or of worldwide importance.

Eosinophils are morphologically distinct granulocytes because of their characteristic acid-staining granules. In normal individuals, eosinophils constitute a small portion of leukocytes detected in bone marrow or peripheral blood. Eosinophil precursors constitute approximately 0.5 to 3.0 percent of bone marrow myelocytes and 0.5 to 4.0 percent of metamyelocytes [2]. In the peripheral blood of normal individuals direct counts of eosinophils show a range of 0 to 350 cells per cubic millimeter; rarely it exceeds 500. It must be emphasized, however, that eosinophils appearing in peripheral blood represent only a small fraction of the total eosinophil pool, as has been demonstrated by kinetic studies in experimental animals [3]. Most mature eosinophils are found in storage compartments either in bone marrow or in tissues, particularly those tissues exposed to the environment, such as the gastrointestinal tract, skin, lungs, and uterus. Furthermore, peripheral blood eosinophil counts in normal humans undergo diurnal variation; highest levels are observed at midnight, and lowest at midday. Eosinophil counts also may vary with age of the individual, with administration of drugs (e.g., steroids) or during infections of a wide variety of etiologies [4].

DEFINITIONS

Peripheral blood eosinophilia occurs in association with several well-delineated clinical conditions such as allergies and worm infections [4]. Furthermore, eosinophilia is often noted in many other less well-defined clinical settings such as malignancies or connective tissue disorders. Far less common are the poorly defined hypereosinophilic syndromes in which no etiological mechanisms or associations have yet been identified. As the number of eosinophils seen in peripheral blood represents a fraction of the mature cell pool, clinical evaluation of eosinophil counts in peripheral blood must, therefore, be based on several observations at well-defined time periods and on thorough assessment of other factors which may lead to changes in cell counts. Eosinophil counts based on peripheral blood smears, though suggestive of changes in cell numbers, may be grossly inaccurate; the importance of direct enumeration of eosinophils, using any of several simple counting techniques, cannot, therefore, be overemphasized [5].

Clinically significant eosinophilia that merits further investigations is indicated by an absolute eosinophil count in the peripheral blood exceeding 500 cells per cubic millimeter. This is simply a working definition, and several factors such as drug therapy, known allergies, etc., have to be taken into consideration before embarking on a diagnostic workup. The observation that peripheral blood eosinophil count in an individual is elevated should be confirmed on at least two separate occasions to justify proceeding with further investigations. Eosinophils may also be seen in peritoneal, pleural, or cerebrospinal fluid (CSF); in urine; or in sputum; their presence in these sites is almost always associated with an underlying pathological process.

CLINICAL SIGNIFICANCE OF EOSINOPHILIA

That the peripheral blood eosinophil count of a particular individual is elevated may be a useful feature allowing an etiological diagnosis for the underlying disease process to be made.

Nevertheless, in a small but significant proportion of these cases a definitive diagnosis may not be possible. Because of the lack of adequately controlled clinical observations, most statements are based on reports of eosinophil counts in patient populations. This has resulted in considerable confusion in the literature by including almost all parasitic and other bacterial and mycobacterial infections as conditions associated with eosinophilia [6]. An attempt will be made, therefore, to point to situations in which confirmatory evidence was obtained from either clinical or experimental studies.

Peripheral blood and bone marrow eosinophilia, as well as tissue eosinophilia, are prominent features of those infections caused by worms which migrate through extraintestinal structures of the host. Repeated clinical observations have documented an association between eosinophilia and infection with tissue nematodes, trematodes, or cestodes. In contrast, there are no controlled studies which convincingly demonstrate that worms which do not invade host tissues (e.g., *Enterobius vermicularis*) or any particular protozoal infections are associated with elevated eosinophil counts. Table 10-1 summarizes the location and species of worm infection with clinical or exper-

imentally proven association with significant eosinophilia; the clinical features and diagnosis of each are included in the listed chapter. Because of the specific geographical distribution of these helminths, an important initial step in formulating the workup plans is to obtain appropriate and detailed geographical and travel history.

How and why are tissue-invading worm infections associated with prominent eosinophilia while all other infectious agents including protozoa and helminths that do not migrate in the host are not? Recent evidence suggests that migratory helminths such as *Trichinella spiralis* or *Schistosoma mansoni* are capable of sensitizing the host immune response in such a way as to result in increased production and migration of eosinophils [7,8]. In studies of worm infections in cell-mediated-deficient or nude mice, no peripheral blood or tissue eosinophilia was observed, in contrast to their immunologically intact control littermates. The failure of nude mice to mount an eosinophilic response may be due to their inability to produce detectable or effective eosinophilopoietin or other soluble mediators that stimulate bone marrow precursor cells to produce mature eosinophils [9]. Furthermore, products from host sensitized T cells or mononuclear phagocytes may influence eosinophils either at the level of production or by stimulating them to migrate to sites of parasite invasion [10] or by activating them to kill extracellular targets or generate leukotriene [11,12]. Finally, it has recently been demonstated that eosinophils detected in the peripheral blood of individuals with eosinophilia are different from normal cells in regard to percentage of cells bearing specific surface receptors [12] and in their biochemical activity [13,14]. The significance and biological relevance of these observations and their relation to eosinophil function in vivo is still unclear.

Other clinical conditions which are frequently associated with eosinophilia are listed in Table 10-2. There is no particular predilection for these conditions to occur in the developing countries, the exception being eosinophilic endomyocarditis that has been described in African patients.

Table 10-1. Tissue-invading worm infections that are frequently associated with eosinophilia

Worms	Localization in host	Parasite species
Tissue nematodes	Blood and lymphatics	*Wuchereria bancrofti*
		Brugia malayi
	Subcutaneous tissues	*Loa loa*
		Onchocerca volvulus
		Dracunculus medinensis
		Ancylostoma braziliense
	Gut	*Strongyloides stercoralis*
	Lungs	Migrating larvae of:
		Ascaris lumbricoides
		Necator americanus
		Ancylostoma duodenale
		S. stercoralis
		Toxocara canis
		Toxocara catis
		Tropical pulmonary eosinophilia
	Liver	*T. canis*
		T. catis
	Muscle	*Trichinella spiralis*
	Brain	*Angiostrongylus cantonensis*
Tissue trematodes	Liver	*Schistosoma mansoni*
		Schistosoma japonicum
		Fasciola hepatica
	Lung	*Paragonimus westermani*
	Urinary tract	*Schistosoma haematobium*
Tissue cestodes	Liver, lung, brain	*Echinococcus granulosus*

Table 10-2. Conditions other than worm infections that are frequently associated with eosinophilia

Common:
  Allergies: Hay fever, urticaria, asthma, dermatitis herpetiformis
  Drug reactions: Iodides, erythromycin, sulfonamide, nitrofurantoin, others
  Collagen vascular: Allergic angiitis, fasciitis, polyarteritis nodosa
  Gastrointestinal: Eosinophilic gastroenteritis
  Hypereosinophilic syndromes
  Miscellaneous: Pulmonary infiltrate with eosinophilia
Occasional:
  Fungal infections: Aspergillosis, coccidioidomycosis
  Malignancies: Lymphomas, solid tumors of lungs, stomach, postirradiation
  Miscellaneous: Chronic peritoneal dialysis, hereditary eosinophilia

The role of eosinophils in allergic reactions is related to their response to mediators derived from mast cells; degradation of the latter cells results in the release of many powerful chemotactic and chemokinetic factors that influence eosinophil mobility. There also is a preferential concentration of several enzymes in human eosinophils which are capable of degrading or inhibiting mast cell–derived factors [14,15]. Eosinophil chemotaxis and chemokinesis may be stimulated in vitro by a variety of factors such as complement products, T-cell-related lymphokines, mast cell peptides, and more importantly by products of lipooxygenation of arachidonic acid. Determination of the molecular level at which these stimuli affect eosinophil function is being actively pursued. It seems that the peptide and lipid stimuli act on several classes of eosinophil cell surface receptors, leading to cell activation. Furthermore, it has been demonstrated that some products of the lipooxygenase pathway are released into the extracellular fluid; they selectively increase expression of C3b receptors on eosinophil membrane and enhance the rate of oxidative metabolism and release of lysosomal enzymes [16].

The hypereosinophilic syndromes are a group of heterogeneous clinical conditions characterized by persistent eosinophilia of 1500 cells per cubic millimeter for 6 months or more, lack of etiological diagnosis despite careful workup, and organ system involvement, particularly of the heart, lungs, and nervous system [15]. While the mechanism of eosinophilia in these syndromes is unknown, the possible causal relationship of eosinophils to tissue damage has recently been appreciated. Besides the space-occupying nature of eosinophil infiltrates in several organs, these cells are capable of inducing tissue damage directly, by release of toxic products or via the initiation of thromboembolic sequelae.

A few eosinophils may be seen occasionally in sputum smears. Marked eosinophilia in sputum is, however, seen in pulmonary allergic conditions or during the migratory phase of *Ascaris lumbricoides* and other tissue nematodes (Table 10-1). Eosinophils are not normally seen in other body fluids; their presence in CSF usually indicates a helminthic infection (*Angiostrongylus cantonensis, Taenia solium,* visceral larva migrans) or is associated with malignancy. Similarly, eosinophilia in pleural or peritoneal fluids may be seen in association with migratory worm infections; malignancy; and following repeated peritoneal dialysis; in some instances no etiological diagnosis can be made. Eosinophilia in urinary sediments has recently been described in association with interstitial nephritis of several etiologies [16].

BIOLOGY OF EOSINOPHILS

Eosinophils are distinguished from other granulocytes (neutrophils and basophils) by their crystalloid granules, which take acid aniline stains such as eosin. Production and maturation of eosinophils occur in the bone marrow, although there is suggestive evidence that extramedullary eosinophilopoiesis

may occur in certain tissues. The cells acquire their early distinct eosinophil granules (homogeneous and round) at the promyelocyte stage; prior to this stage, eosinophil precursors cannot be identified by morphological criteria. During cell maturation, the eosinophil granules acquire the characteristic crystalline form with a central dense core and an electron-radiolucent matrix. Eosinophil granules contain several enzymes such as peroxidase, acid phosphatase, and aryl sulfatase, but they lack lysozyme. Some of the eosinophil enzymes differ from those of neutrophils in several ways, including substrate specificity, effect of inhibitors, and antigenicity. Furthermore, eosinophil granules contain other newly characterized proteins such as major basic protein, cationic protein, and neurotoxin [17,18].

The cell surface membrane of human eosinophils has not been well characterized except for receptors for the Fc portion of IgG and for the C3b fragment of complement [13]. Enhancement of the function of these receptors or an increase in the proportion of cells carrying them has been shown following exposure to synthetic chemotactic peptides, and in patients with eosinophilic endomyocarditis. Perturbation of eosinophil membrane leads to a respiratory burst with increased oxygen consumption, generation of hydrogen peroxide and superoxide anion, and degranulation. Complement or antibody-dependent eosinophil degranulation on the surface of nonphagocytosable objects such as worms is associated with increased oxygen consumption and evacuation of granule contents to the outside to be deposited on the parasite surface. This phenomenon of extracellular degranulation is of significance in regard to the functional adaptation of eosinophils to play a role in host protection.

Recently, several factors have been shown to play a role in regulating eosinophil production, maturation, and function. Enough evidence now exists that interleukin 5 is a specific stimulator of eosinophil colony formation [18] in contrast to the less specific action of granulocyte-macrophage colony stimulating factor or interleukin 3 [19]. Furthermore, some of these factors have a profound effect on eosinophils in vitro. For example, recombinant human granulocyte-macrophage colony stimulating factor converts cocultured normodense eosinophils into hypodense cells with marked increase in production of leukotriene C_4 and antibody-dependent killing of *S. mansoni* larvae [20]. The oxidative metabolism of arachidonic acid in human eosinophils differs from that of neutrophils and results in the production of leukotriene C_4, which is vasoactive, resulting in contraction of vascular and nonvascular smooth muscles [21].

FUNCTIONAL SIGNIFICANCE OF EOSINOPHILS

Allergy and helminth infections are the two most consistent pathological conditions associated with eosinophilia. Investigations of both disease states in vitro and in vivo, using humans and experimental animals, have provided the basis for our cur-

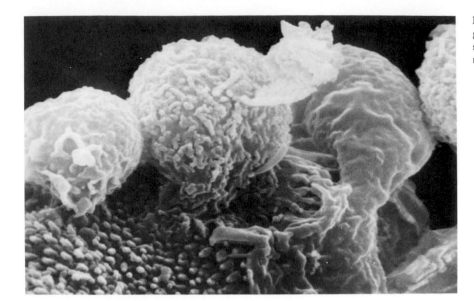

Figure 10-1. Scanning electron micrograph of mouse eosinophils attaching and spreading on the surface of schistosomula of *S. mansoni*.

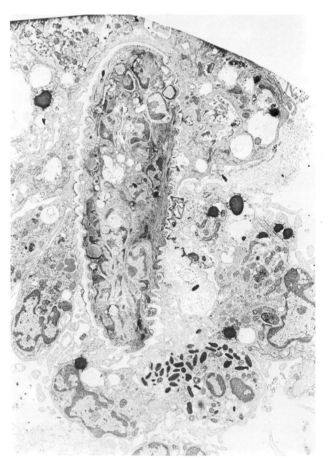

Figure 10-2. Transmission electron micrograph showing the attachment of mouse eosinophils and macrophages to *Trichinella spiralis* larva.

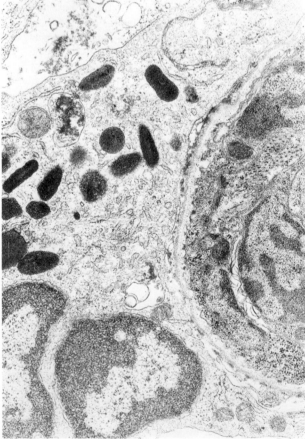

Figure 10-3. Transmission electron micrograph of the tight attachment of mouse eosinophils to the surface of *T. spiralis* larva. Electron-dense material can be seen deposited on the parasite surface.

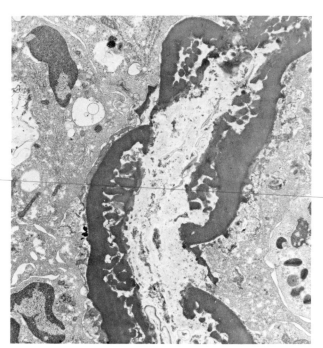

Figure 10-4. Transmission electron micrograph of *T. spiralis* larva showing evidence of worm destruction following incubation with eosinophils and antibodies.

rent understanding of eosinophil function. Eosinophils have been shown to modulate the expression of immediate hypersensitivity reactions. This function is particularly suited to the mature eosinophils, which reside mainly in tissues. Under these conditions, eosinophils are exposed to diverse stimuli arising from the sequence of events involved in the expression of immediate hypersensitivity; these include factors which recruit eosinophils, enhance their receptors and biochemical activity, and may alter their function. The response of eosinophils attracted to sites of mast cell activation and degranulation consists of the release and accumulation of specific factors capable of inhibiting or degrading mediators produced by mast cells. In this capacity, eosinophils seem to play a central homeostatic function in modulating acute allergic inflammation. Recent evidence suggests, however, that eosinophil degranulation results in the release of enzymes and proteins that injure a variety of tissues in vitro including pneumocytes and tracheal epithelium [22]. These eosinophil products include the cell-specific peroxidase [23], major basic protein [24], and eosinophil-derived neurotoxin [25]. What determines whether eosinophil invasion of tissues results in the limiting of the extent of an inflammatory process or the mediation of tissue damage is not, however, clear.

A role for eosinophils in host protection against invasive helminths has recently been demonstrated. Human eosinophils incubated with the larval forms of several helminths such as *S. mansoni* [26], *T. spiralis* [27], and *O. volvulus* [28], in the presence of specific antibodies or complement led to destruction of these organisms. The biological relevance of these in vitro observations was confirmed in mice depleted of their eosinophils by antieosinophil serum; these animals lost their resistance to *T. spiralis* and *S. mansoni* [29]. Eosinophil-mediated killing of these multicellular organisms is initiated by tight attachment of the cells to the parasite surface (Figs. 10-1 and 10-2), followed by extracellular degranulation and deposition of electron-dense material on the parasite surface (Fig. 10-3). Parasite mortality is morphologically demonstrable before significant phagocytosis can be detected (Fig. 10-4). Among the products of eosinophil degranulation, several have been shown to kill multicellular organisms in cell-free systems, such as hydrogen peroxide alone or in the presence of peroxidase and halides, and both major basic and cationic granule proteins.

REFERENCES

1 Warren KS, Mahmoud AAF: *Geographic Medicine for the Practitioner: Algorithms in the Diagnosis and Management of Exotic Diseases,* 2d ed. University of Chicago Press, 1978, pp ix–xi

2 Williams JW, Beutler E, Erslev AJ, et al: *Hematology,* 2d ed. New York, McGraw-Hill, 1977, pp 659–769

3 Foot EE; Eosinophil turnover in the normal rat. Br J Haematol 11:439–445, 1965

4 Beeson PB, Bass DA: The eosinophil, in Smith, LH, Jr (ed): *Major Problems of Internal Medicine.* Philadelphia, Saunders, 1977, vol 14, p 269

5 Dacil JV, Lewis SM: *Practical Hematology,* 6th ed. Edinburgh, Churchill Livingstone, 1984

6 Conrad ME: Hematologic manifestations of parasitic infections. Semin Hematol 8:267–303, 1971

7 Basten A, Beeson PB: Mechanism of eosinophilia. II. Role of the lymphocyte. J Exp Med 131:1288–1305, 1970

8 Mahmoud AAF, Warren KS, Graham RC, Jr: Antieosinophil serum and the kinetics of eosinophilia in schistosomiasis mansoni. J Exp Med 142:560–574, 1975

9 Mahmoud AAF: Eosinophilopoiesis, in Mahmoud AAF, Austen KF (eds): *The Eosinophil in Health and Disease.* New York, Grune & Stratton, 1980, pp 61–75

10 Greene BM, Colley DG: Eosinophils and immune mechanisms. III. Production of the lymphokine eosinophil stimulation promoter by mouse T lymphocytes. J Immunol 116:1078–1083, 1976

11 Veith MC, Butterworth AE: Enhancement of human eosinophil mediated killing of *Schistosoma mansoni* larvae by mononuclear cell products in vitro. J Exp Med 157:1828–1843, 1983

12 Dessein AJ, Lee TH, Elsas P, et al: Enhancement by monokines of leukotriene generation by human eosinophils and neutrophils stimulated with calcium ionophore A23187. J Immunol 136:3829–3838, 1986

13 Kay AB, Anwar ARE: Eosinophil surface receptors, in Mahmoud AAF, Austen KF (eds): *The Eosinophil in Health and Disease.* New York, Grune & Stratton, 1980, pp 207–228

14 Bass DA, Grover WH, Lewis JC, et al: Comparison of human eosinophils from normals and patients with eosinophilia. J Clin Invest 66:1265–1273, 1980

15 Fauci AS: The idiopathic hypereosinophilic syndrome: Clinical, pathophysiologic, and therapeutic considerations. Ann Intern Med 97:78–92, 1982

16 Sutton JM: Urinary eosinophils. Arch Intern Med 146:2243–2244, 1986

17 Gleich GJ, Adolphson CR: The eosinophilic leukocyte structure and function. Adv Immunol 39:177–253, 1986

18 Mahmoud AAF, Austen KF: *The Eosinophil in Health and Disease*. New York, Grune & Stratton, 1980, pp 149–165

19 Metcalf D, Begley CG, Johnson GR, et al: Biologic properties in vitro of a recombinant human granulocyte-macrophage colony stimulating factor. Blood 67:37–45, 1986

20 Owen WF, Rothenberg ME, Silberstein DS, et al: Regulation of human eosinophil viability, density, and function by granulocyte/macrophage colony stimulating factor in the presence of 3T3 fibroblasts. J Exp Med 166:129–141, 1987

21 Owen WF, Soberman RJ, Yoshimoto T, et al: Synthesis and release of leukotriene C_4 by human eosinophil. J Immunol 138:532–538, 1987

22 Davis WB, Fells GA, Sun XH, et al: Eosinophil mediated injury to lung parenchymal cells and interstitial matrix. J Clin Invest 74:269–278, 1984

23 Agosti JM, Altman LC, Ayars GH, et al: The injurious effect of eosinophil peroxidase, hydrogen peroxide, and halides on pneumocytes in vitro. J Allergy Clin Immunol 79:496–504, 1987

24 Caleich GJ, Frigas E, Loegering DA: Cytotoxic properties of the eosinophil major basic protein. J Immunol 123:2925–2927, 1979

25 Durack DT, Ackerman SJ, Loegering DA, et al: Purification of human eosinophil-derived monotoxin. Proc Natl Acad Sci USA 78:5165–5169, 1981

26 Butterworth AE, David JR, Franks D, et al: Antibody dependent eosinophil-mediated damage to ^{51}Cr-labeled schistosomula of *Schistosoma mansoni:* Damage by purified eosinophils. J Exp Med 145:136–150, 1977

27 Kazura JW: Host defense mechanism against nematode parasites: Destruction of *Trichinella spiralis* newborn larvae by parasite stage-specific human antibody and granulocytes. J Infect Dis 143:712–718, 1981

28 Greene BM, Taylor HR, Aikawa M: Cellular killing of microfilariae of *Onchocerca volvulus:* Eosinophil and neutrophil-mediated immune serum-dependent destruction. J Immunol 127:1611–1618, 1981

29 Mahmoud AAF: The ecology of eosinophils in schistosomiasis. J Infect Dis 145:613–622, 1982

CHAPTER 11 / *Neurological Symptoms* · *Prida Phuapradit*

INTRODUCTION

In general neurological symptoms are similar everywhere, but their causes vary to a certain extent in different parts of the world. In tropical countries infectious diseases of the nervous system—meningitis, encephalitis, cerebral abscess, rabies, leprosy—and neurological disorders associated with vitamin deficiencies are common. Cerebrovascular diseases, neoplasms, and degenerative diseases of the nervous system are probably equally common in tropical and temperate countries. Certain diseases, notably pernicious anemia and its neurological complications and multiple sclerosis, are rare in the tropics [1]. Subacute myelooptic neuropathy (SMON) associated with clioquinol intoxication, once a major neurological problem in Japan, is rare in other countries. Thiamine deficiency and beriberi are endemic in certain parts of Asia, but the neurological counterpart, Wernicke's encephalopathy, which is common in the west is virtually never seen in beriberi occurring in Asian people. In southeast Asia Wernicke's encephalopathy was described only in European prisoners of war [2]. A genetic predisposition probably accounts for the racial differences in susceptibility to developing Wernicke's encephalopathy. A similar observation can be made about the rarity of parenchymal forms of neurosyphilis, notably tabes dorsalis, in Asia, although syphilis is a major venereal disease in this part of the world [1]. This chapter deals with some of the common neurological problems encountered in the tropics.

HEADACHE

Tension headache and migraine are universal, and they are also the commonest causes of headache in the tropics. The former is characterized by undulating headache of long duration, usually with an onset in adolescence or adulthood. The hallmark of migraine is paroxysmal headache, which can be either unilateral or bilateral, with onset in adolescence and frequently a family history. The attacks usually last from a few hours to a day and are often accompanied by vomiting and visual disturbances. Common precipitating factors are physical exhaustion and mental stress.

Other causes of headache, although more serious, are much less common than the tension-vascular headache. For example, excruciating generalized headache of sudden onset suggests subarachnoid hemorrhage due to rupture of an intracranial aneurysm or an angioma. Mycotic aneurysms are common in patients with infective endocarditis, and rupture invariably results in fatal subarachnoid hemorrhage. In endemic areas

(Thailand, Laos, Kampuchea) cerebral gnathostomiasis may present with subarachnoid or intracerebral hemorrhages and paralysis of the cranial nerves (Fig. 11-1). The cerebrospinal fluid (CSF) is bloody or xanthochromic and contains many eosinophils [3].

Rapidly progressive headache, developing over hours or days, in association with fever, photophobia, and neck stiffness, is characteristic of meningitis. Bacterial and viral meningitides usually present acutely. As elsewhere *Neisseria meningitides* and *Streptococcus pneumoniae* are the commonest causes of pyogenic meningitis in adolescents and adults. Petechiae, or ecchymoses, a useful sign of meningococcemia, should be sought in the conjunctiva and skin. In pyogenic meningitis papilledema and signs of focal cerebral damage are unusual, and their presence suggests the possibility of brain abscess, space-occupying lesions, or tuberculous meningitis. In developing countries tuberculous meningitis is still common and can present in different ways. The history is usually prolonged, and signs of increased intracranial pressure, communicating hydrocephalus, and arteritis, as results of basal arachnoiditis, are common [4]. The clinical manifestations of cryptococcal meningitis are similar to those of tuberculous meningitis. In endemic areas eosinophilic meningitis may be caused by *Angiostrongylus cantonensis, Gnathostoma spinigerum,* and cysticercosis. Careful examination of the CSF is essential for the diagnosis. The profiles of the CSF findings in various types of meningitis are summarized in Table 11-1. Abrupt onset of fever and headache are also presenting symptoms of viral encephalitis, but symptoms and signs of cerebral dysfunction—such as confusion, hallucination, seizures, disturbances of consciousness, and signs of focal or diffuse cerebral damage—are usually present.

Arthropodborne viruses are important causes of epidemic encephalitis in Asia, America, and central Europe. The most common cause of sporadic encephalitis is herpes simplex. The virus has a predilection for the temporal lobes, causing hemorrhagic necrosis and producing focal neurological signs. In tropical countries encephalitis must be differentiated from cerebral malaria, a severe complication of *Plasmodium falciparum* infection. As there are no diagnostic clinical features of cerebral malaria, constant clinical index of suspicion and

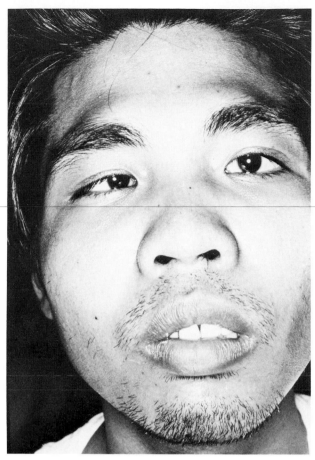

Figure 11-1. Left sixth nerve palsy in a patient with subarachnoid hemorrhage caused by gnathostomiasis.

careful examination of the peripheral blood for the parasite are essential.

Progressive headache of subacute onset, developing over a period of weeks or months suggests increased intracranial pressure or space-occupying lesions. Papilledema and focal neurological signs may be present. These patients deserve full neurological investigations.

Table 11-1. CSF findings in common types of meningitides

	Meningitis				
	Pyogenic	**Viral**	**Tuberculous**	**Cryptococcal**	**Angiostrongylus**
Pressure	↑	N	↑	↑	↑
No. of cells	>1000	<1000	<1000	<1000	<1000
Types of cells	P	L	L + P	L + P	L + E
Glucose	↓	N	↓	↓	N
Protein	↑	↑ or N	↑	↑	↑

Note: ↑ = usually increased; N = usually normal; P = polymorphonuclear cell; L = lymphocyte; E = eosinophil; > = usually more than; < = usually less than.

EPILEPSY

Epilepsy is common worldwide. The diagnosis is based mainly on careful history obtained from the patient and witnesses. An epileptic seizure is usually so dramatic that most descriptions are unmistakable. Practically it is useful to distinguish two groups of epilepsy; the generalized (idiopathic) and the partial (symptomatic) seizures. In the former the seizures are symmetrical without focal features. The age of onset is during the first or second decades of life, and there is commonly a positive family history. Partial seizures are caused by discharges of a group of neurons in a part of the cerebral hemisphere, producing focal epilepsy. However, the focal discharges may spread very rapidly and manifest as generalized convulsions without premonitory symptoms. Partial seizures are acquired and occur in all age groups. Common causes of symptomatic seizures are head injury, cerebral anoxia at birth, sequelae to meningitis, encephalitis, brain abscess, arteriovenous malformation, and cerebral tumors. In the tropics and other endemic areas cerebral cysticercosis is an important cause of epilepsy [5]. Most patients have no abnormal neurological signs, but those with heavy infestation of the cysticerci in the brain parenchyma may present with signs of severe intracranial hypertension [6]. Subcutaneous nodules of cysticerci are present in some patients. The diagnosis is made from the appearance of the cystic lesions in the CT scan and a specific serological test of the CSF.

STROKES

Cerebrovascular disease is a major neurological problem in the tropics, as elsewhere. The usual presentation of stroke is a sudden onset of focal neurological deficit, such as hemiparesis. Common causes of strokes are cerebral infarction from atherosclerosis, cerebral embolism, hypertensive intracerebral hemorrhage, and subarachnoid hemorrhage. In general patients with spontaneous intracerebral hemorrhage are severely ill with headache and dense hemiplegia. Progressive impairment of the level of consciousness may follow. It is invariably the result of hypertension. Fatal intracranial bleeding can also result from severe thrombocytopenia in aplastic anemia and dengue hemorrhagic fever. In endemic areas intracerebral hemorrhage is a manifestation of gnathostomiasis [3].

It is useful to differentiate infarction of the cerebral hemisphere from lacunar infarct. The former produces severe hemiplegia in association with aphasia, hemianopia, and cortical sensory loss and is caused by occlusion of middle cerebral or internal carotid arteries. In these patients evidence of atherothromboembolism from great vessels in the neck and cardiac sources of embolism should be looked for. Lacunar infarct, which is relatively less severe and carries a better prognosis, produces isolated hemiparesis or unilateral sensory loss with no disturbance of higher cerebral function. It is associated with hypertension and diabetes mellitus and is caused by thrombosis of the small perforating branches of the middle cerebral artery.

Cerebral infarction in the young is a common problem in the tropics. By and large it is frequently a complication of the endemic rheumatic valvular heart disease and less commonly Takayasu's disease (pulseless disease). Takayasu's disease is mainly a disease of young women and is more common in the orient than in the west. It is a form of arteritis that involves the aorta and its branches. Pulses of large vessels in the limbs and neck are often diminished or absent, and bruits may be heard over these vessels. A majority of patients with Takayasu's disease have hypertension, which is secondary to unilateral narrowing or occlusion of the renal artery. In the active stage of the arteritis the erythrocyte sedimentation rate (ESR) is often raised. Cerebral infarct is also a well-recognized complication of tuberculous meningitis [8]. It is the result of the intracranial arteritis and usually develops early during the course of the meningitis. Either small perforating branches or large intracranial arteries are involved. Preceding history of fever, headache, and the presence of neck stiffness and examination of the CSF will give the diagnosis. Characteristic appearances of the arteritis can be demonstrated by carotid angiography (Fig. 11-2).

PAINFUL OPHTHALMOPLEGIA

Damage to the third nerve causes ptosis, a fixedly dilated pupil and inability by the eye to perform any movement except abduction. Pain in the eye and forehead is common and can be severe in acute compressive or intrinsic lesions of the nerve. In this situation it is important to examine the pupils carefully. Generally third nerve palsy with a dilated pupil is caused by compressive lesions of the nerve such as aneurysms or infiltrating tumors. By contrast, an intrinsic lesion of the nerve,

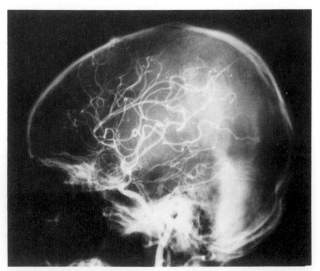

Figure 11-2. Tuberculous arteritis revealed by carotid angiography. Note the narrowing and irregularity of the intracranial portion of the internal carotid artery and its branches.

such as infarction of the nerve in diabetes mellitus, characteristically spares the pupil. Causes of unilateral third nerve palsy are diverse, but as elsewhere, aneurysm of the posterior communicating artery and diabetes mellitus are the most common.

Other, less common causes of painful unilateral third nerve palsy are tumors infiltrating from the base of skull such as carcinoma of the nasopharynx, painful ophthalmoplegia (Tolosa-Hunt syndrome), sphenoidal sinusitis, and neurosyphilis. Painful ophthalmoplegia is a self-limited condition which is common in the tropics [1]. The usual presentation is acute or subacute painful unilateral paralysis of the third nerve (Fig. 11-3). The pupil can be either affected or spared. Adjacent cranial nerves such as the fourth, sixth, and the first division of the fifth cranial nerve may be involved. Painful ophthalmoplegia is caused by a nonspecific granulomatous lesion of unknown etiology in the superior orbital fissure and anterior part of the cavernous sinus [9]. The diagnosis is made by recognition of this condition and exclusion of compressive lesions of the nerve. Treatment with large doses of corticosteroid promptly relieves the pain and leads to rapid improvement of the ophthalmoplegia.

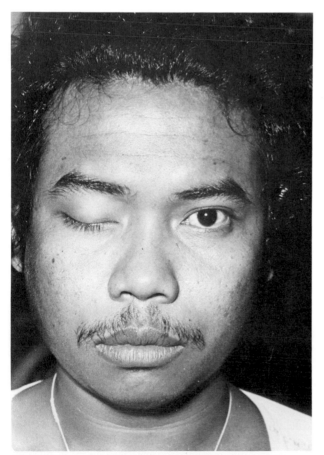

Figure 11-3. Acute, painful ophthalmoplegia in a Thai patient.

WEAKNESS

Approach to patients with muscular weakness requires accurate history to assess the onset and rate of progression of the symptoms. The site of the lesion can be determined by appropriate neurological examination with emphasis on the pattern of weakness, the presence of the upper or lower motor neuron signs, and the presence or absence of sensory loss.

In general myopathies and disorders of the neuromuscular junction produce weakness of the proximal muscles of the limbs and trunk. Wasting of the muscles and loss of reflexes are unusual and occur only in an advanced stage. Ptosis and weakness of the facial, extraocular, bulbar, and limb muscles are common in myasthenia gravis. Bites by cobras and kraits produce similar symptoms, which develop rapidly after the bites. In the tropics polymyositis, muscular dystrophy, and metabolic myopathies are similar to cases seen elsewhere, but some rare muscle disorders, caused by parasites, are encountered in endemic areas. Subacute painful weakness of the muscles with periorbital swelling, splinter hemorrhages, fever, and hypereosinophilia suggest trichinosis. A preceding history of gastrointestinal disturbances may be obtained. The diagnosis is based on history of ingestion of contaminated pork, demonstration of the larvae of *Trichinella spiralis* in the muscle biopsy, and serological tests. Cysticercosis commonly involves the muscles, but usually produces no symptoms. Rarely, cysticercosis presents as bilateral symmetrical enlargement of muscles, notably the thighs, calves, glutei, and shoulder girdles, known as *pseudohypertrophic myopathy* [10]. Proximal weakness of the limbs may be present. The involved muscles are packed with numerous cysts. Hydatid cysts and sparganosis may present as a mass in the muscle, but this mass is painless and does not cause weakness. Rarely acute toxoplasmosis may present with generalized painful muscle weakness resembling polymyositis [11]. Associated features are fever, sore throat, lymphadenopathy, and high and rising titers of toxoplasma antibody.

Bacterial infections of the muscles, which are rare elsewhere, still occur in the tropics. *Staphylococcus aureus* produces pyomyositis, which presents with pain, tenderness, swelling in one or more muscle groups, and fever. The muscles commonly affected are the glutei and quadriceps. In most cases no antecedent or underlying cause is found. Treatment consists of an appropriate antibiotic, incision, and drainage.

Recurrent attacks of episodic weakness of the limbs, lasting several hours in association with hypokalemia are features of hypokalemic periodic paralysis. The severity varies from slight weakness to almost complete paralysis of the limbs and trunk, with sparing of the bulbar, ocular, and respiratory muscles. Familial hypokalemic periodic paralysis, a well-known rare autosomal dominant disorder, occurs worldwide. In Asia, particularly in patients with Chinese and Japanese ancestry, hypokalemic periodic paralysis is most commonly associated with thyrotoxicosis [12]. Several attacks may recur, until the hyperthyroidism is under control. Although thyrotoxicosis is much more frequent in women than in men, patients who develop the paralysis are invariably male. Hypokalemic periodic paralysis is also a manifestation of renal tubular acidosis and hyperaldosteronism. It is of interest to note that the incidence of periodic paralysis in primary hyperaldosteronism is higher in Chinese patients than in Caucasians [13].

Predominantly distal and symmetrical weakness with early loss of reflexes and distal sensory loss are features of peripheral neuropathy. The commonest cause of acute peripheral neuropathy worldwide is Guillain-Barré syndrome. A preceding history of upper respiratory tract infection may be obtained. The weakness may be distal, proximal, or generalized. Bilateral facial weakness, pain in the back and limbs, and limitation on straight-leg–raising test are common. Although in severe cases the weakness progresses rapidly to complete paralysis and respiratory failure, requiring assisted ventilation, the illness is self-limited, and most patients recover fully with supportive treatment. Corticosteroids are not helpful, but plasmapheresis may speed up the recovery. Acute peripheral neuropathy with features similar to Guillain-Barré syndrome can occur in acute beriberi, intermittent porphyria, AIDS, Semple-type rabies vaccination, rabies, infections by cytomegalovirus, Epstein-Barr virus, and hepatitis B virus. In endemic areas paralytic rabies is an important cause of acute peripheral neuropathy and myelitis, which is often misdiagnosed [14]. A history of animal bite, itching or paresthesias at the site of the bite at the onset of the illness, widespread fasciculation in the muscles, myoedema, mental confusion, and spasms of respiratory muscles during inspiration are features of paralytic rabies. Hydrophobia is usually absent. The diagnosis of paralytic rabies during life is difficult. In experienced hands demonstration of rabies antigen in the skin biopsy by immunofluorescent method is the best method and does not give false-positive results [15].

An important cause of acute peripheral neuropathy in the orient is beriberi. Even in Japan, beriberi, which virtually disappeared many years ago, has recently reappeared in adolescents who consume an unbalanced diet containing high carbohydrate and low thiamine, such as instant noodles and milled rice. In acute beriberi the weakness is generalized and severe. Characteristically the calves are tense and tender. In addition to the signs of the neuropathy the patients are often dyspneic with signs of congestive heart failure and hyperdynamic circulation [16]. Beriberi can also be chronic, the so-called dry beriberi. It occurs in the inactive patients who are deficient in both thiamine and calories.

The commonest cause of chronic peripheral neuropathy in the tropics is leprosy. Tuberculoid leprosy produces mononeuritis and mononeuritis multiplex. The most commonly involved nerves are ulnar, median, peroneal, and facial, and the affected nerves are usually enlarged. Depigmented anesthetic skin lesions and anhidrosis are commonly present. Progressive symmetrical sensory peripheral neuropathy occurs in lepromatous leprosy. Early sensory loss appears in the ear lobes and cheeks. Bilateral facial paralysis and weakness of the limbs with

trophic changes in the toes and fingers develop in an advanced stage. A form of neuropathy known as *tropical ataxic neuropathy* has been endemic in Nigeria, Senegal, Uganda, and other parts of Africa. It is a slowly progressive sensorimotor neuropathy with proprioceptive loss and ataxia in the lower limbs. Optic neuropathy, sensorineural hearing loss, and, less commonly, myelopathy are associated features. The neuropathy is related to heavy consumption of cassava, a plant known to contain cyanogenic glycosides. There are several other causes of peripheral neuropathy in the tropics, and the profile is similar to that in other parts of the world.

In contrast to the symmetrical weakness in peripheral neuropathy, acute lesions of the anterior horn cell, typically caused by poliovirus and enterovirus 70, produce patchy and asymmetrical weakness. Fever and back pain are common at the onset. Reflexes in the affected segments are absent. Wasting of the muscles appears early and is usually severe. Enterovirus 70 has produced epidemics and pandemics of acute hemorrhagic conjunctivitis during the last two decades [17]. In Asia following the conjunctivitis a number of adult patients developed an acute paralytic illness with clinical features similar to those of poliomyelitis [18]. The weakness and wasting of the affected muscles are usually severe and permanent (Fig. 11-4). Motor neuron disease, a slowly progressive disorder of the anterior horn cells, is similarly seen in the tropics as elsewhere.

Spinal cord disorders produce weakness of the muscles below the site of the lesion. The pattern of the weakness of myelopathy is characteristic. In the upper limbs the weakness is more in the extensor groups and vice versa in the lower limbs. The limbs are spastic, and reflexes below the lesion are brisk with extensor plantar responses. Sensation is impaired below the site of the lesion, and in the late stage disturbances of the function of the bladder and bowel will occur.

In the tropics acute myelopathy is a common neurological emergency. It is often caused by compressive lesions in the epidural space of the spinal cord. Pain and rapidly progressive paraparesis with sensory level and disturbances of bladder function are the usual presentation. Common causes of the spinal cord compression are metastatic carcinoma, lymphoma, myeloma, epidural abscess, and tuberculosis. X-ray of the spine may show associated bone lesions. Myelogram and surgical treatment should be performed without delay. In endemic areas of southeast Asia acute ascending myelitis is often caused by *Gnathostoma spinigerum* [3] (Fig. 11-5). Severe radicular pain in the limbs often precedes the weakness. A history of painless migratory swellings of the skin may be obtained. The paraplegia is usually severe and permanent (Fig. 11-5). There is hypereosinophilia, and the CSF, which is often bloody or xanthochromic, also contains eosinophils. Other parasitic infections that may produce myelopathies are cysticercosis, hydatid disease, schistosomiasis, and paragonimiasis. In developing countries, where Semple-type rabies vaccine is still used for postexposure prophylaxis, acute myelitis is an important

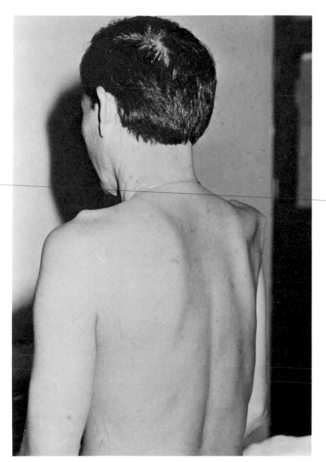

Figure 11-4. A Thai patient with neurological complications of acute hemorrhagic conjunctivitis caused by enterovirus 70. Note the severe and asymmetrical wasting of the muscles.

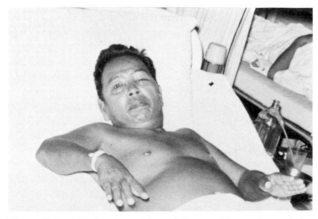

Figure 11-5. A Thai patient with myelitis caused by gnathostomiasis. He was severely paraplegic. Note the swelling around the left eye, caused by migration of the worm.

and serious complication of the vaccine [19]. It usually appears within 7 weeks after the first injection of the vaccine. Other neurological complications are meningoencephalitis and acute peripheral neuropathy.

Subacute combined degeneration of the spinal cord, pernicious anemia, and tabes dorsalis are rare in the tropics [1]. Multiple sclerosis is uncommon, but it does occur. In the Asian patients painful tonic seizure of the limbs is a common presentation, and involvement of the optic nerve is more frequent and severe at the onset when compared with patients in the west [20]. In India progressive cervical myelopathy, caused by congenital atlantoaxial dislocation, is found with unusually high frequency [21]. The dislocation results from the maldevelopment of the transverse ligament and the odontoid process. Transient attacks of quadriparesis, precipitated by neck flexion or extension, are a common presentation. Lathyrism, a form of myelopathy caused by heavy consumption of the neurotoxic pea *Lathyrus sativus,* is now mainly seen in India. It is characterized by a relatively acute onset of pain and weakness of the lower limbs, which progresses to permanent spastic paraparesis. The upper limbs are usually unaffected.

Clusters of chronic myelopathy, known as tropical spastic paraparesis, have been endemic in tropical islands, Japan, India, and Africa [22]. The onset of the paraparesis is gradual, and the progression in most patients is slow; severe neurological deficits develop over a period of several years. Signs of involvement of the posterior column and sensory loss are minimal. Recently the retrovirus human lymphotropic virus type I infection has been shown to be associated with the myelopathy.

REFERENCES

1 Spillane JD: Introduction, in Spillane JD (ed): *Tropical Neurology.* London, Oxford University Press, 1973, pp 1–21

2 De Wardener HE, Lennox B: Cerebral beriberi (Wernicke's encephalopathy): Review of 52 cases in a Singapore prisoner-of-war hospital. Lancet i:11–17, 1947

3 Boongird P, Phuapradit P, Siridej N, et al: Neurological manifestations of gnathostomiasis. J Neurol Sci 31:279–291, 1977

4 Juel-Jensen BE, Phuapradit P, Warrell DA: Bacterial meningitis, in Weatherall DJ, Ledingham JGG, Warrell DA (eds): *Oxford Textbook of Medicine,* 2d ed. London, Oxford University Press, 1987, pp 21.129–21.141

5 Thomson AJ, de Villiers JC, Moosa A, et al: Cerebral cysticercosis in children in South Africa. Ann Trop Paediatr 4:67–77, 1984

6 Rangel R, Torres B, Del Bruto O, et al: Cysticercotic encephalitis: A severe form in young females. Am J Trop Med Hyg 36:387–392, 1987

7 Dalal PM: The aortic arch syndrome—an idiopathic form of noninflammatory occlusive vascular disease, in Spillane JD (ed): *Tropical Neurology.* London, Oxford University Press, 1973, pp 92–98

8 Dalal PM: Observations on the involvement of cerebral vessels in tuberculous meningitis in adults, in Goldstein M et al (eds): *Advances in Neurology.* New York, Raven, 1979, vol 25, pp 149–159

9 Tolosa E: Periarteritic lesions of the carotid siphon with the clinical features of a carotid infraclinoidal aneurysm. J Neurol Neurosurg Psychiatry 17:300–302, 1954

10 Jacob JC, Mathew NT: Pseudohypertrophic myopathy in cysticercosis. Neurology 18:767–771, 1968

11 Rowland LP, Greer M: Toxoplasmic polymyositis. Neurology 11:367–370, 1961

12 McFadzean AJS, Yeung RTT: Periodic paralysis complicating thyrotoxicosis in Chinese. Br Med J 1:451–455, 1967

13 Ma JTC, Wang C, Lam KSL, et al: Fifty cases of primary hyperaldosteronism in Hong Kong Chinese with a high frequency of periodic paralysis: Evaluation of techniques for tumour localisation. Q J Med 61:1021–1037, 1986

14 Phuapradit P, Manatsathit S, Warrell MJ, et al: Paralytic rabies: Some unusual presentations. J Med Assoc Thai 68:106–110, 1985

15 Warrell MJ, Looareesuwan S, Manatsathit S, et al: Rapid diagnosis of rabies and post-vaccinal encephalitides. Clin Exp Immunol 71:229–234, 1988

16 Tanphaichitr V, Vimokesant S, Dhamamitta S, et al: Clinical and biochemical studies of adult beriberi. Am J Clin Nutr 23:1017–1026, 1970

17 Editorial: Lancet i:373–374, 1982

18 Phuapradit P, Roongwithu N, Limsukon P, et al: Radiculomyelitis complicating acute hemorrhagic conjunctivitis: A clinical study. J Neurol Sci 27;117–122, 1976

19 Hemachudha T, Phanuphak P, Johnson RT: Neurologic complications of Semple-type rabies vaccine: Clinical and immunologic studies. Neurology 37:550–556, 1987

20 Kuroiwa Y, Hung TP, Landsborough D, et al: Multiple sclerosis in Asia. Neurology 27:188–192, 1977

21 Wadia NH: Congenital atlanto-axial dislocation and its manifestations due to spinal cord compression, in Spillane JD (ed): *Tropical Neurology*. London, Oxford University Press, 1973, pp 99–107

22 Roman G: The neuroepidemiology of tropical spastic paraparesis. Ann Neurol 23(suppl):S113–S120, 1988

CHAPTER 12 / *Psychiatric Disorders and Mental Health in the Tropics* · J. H. Orley

Epidemiological evidence indicates that mental disorders are no less common in the tropics than elsewhere in the world. They are sometimes caused by tropical diseases; at other times they occur independently. Frequently the symptoms of mental disorder are similar to those of physical disorders and can confuse the unwary physician.

Before dealing with clinical issues of diagnosis and medical treatment, some more general issues relating to the organization of mental health services will be dealt with.

The impression has existed that disturbed behavior, as compared with quiet behavior, during mental illness is more common in the tropics than elsewhere and that mania is more frequent than depression. There were, indeed, early reports that depression did not occur in Africans. A variety of factors probably accounted for this observation. One was that milder depressive symptoms were often presented more as somatic complaints and were missed as depression. An equally important factor is that it is more the need for social control than for treatment that brings those with severe mental disorders to health facilities. An excited, violent patient, for instance, in a manic phase of a manic-depressive illness, may be brought to a hospital within a few days of onset. The same patient in a depressive phase of the illness, just sitting, doing little or nothing, may be kept at home for months or years.

Psychiatrists and other mental health professionals may be rare in the tropics, in which case the general health services have to deal with most psychiatric complaints or they remain unattended to. The general physician therefore should be prepared to give attention to severely disturbed psychiatric patients, who require control. They may be brought to a health facility, either privately or through the police, on an emergency basis, and it is as well for the physician or nurse to have a system of management ready. It is advisable that in a sizable health facility such as a district hospital or larger, there be at least one nurse able to deal with such crises. Such a nurse could have received formal psychiatric nurse training after basic training or might take a special course which lays out a simple system for the identification and management of mental health problems by nonphysicians [1]. This latter kind of preparation has been tested in one setting in which general nurses were given only 13 hours extra training to achieve reasonable knowledge and skills for dealing with the initial presentation [3]. Continued support from and supervision by a trained mental health professional would still be necessary. This might be provided by occasional visits of a professional from some other health facility.

A further reason for physicians to give attention to mental disorders is that they will encounter many that are less obvious but more frequent. It is estimated that between 10 and 20 percent of all patients attending general health clinics have predominantly psychiatric illnesses. In addition is a group of patients sometimes called "functional complainers," who may not have psychiatric illness but may be expressing social and emotional problems through somatic symptoms. If health staff are unaware that both these groups often present with somatic symptoms without physical illness, such patients can unnecessarily use up considerable resources for investigation and treatment of their complaints. It is not that such patients should be rejected by the system, but that they should be given appropriate attention. Otherwise both they and their medical attendants become frustrated by the lack of results and the obvious waste of resources. This chapter will therefore deal with both the severe disorders that often demand emergency treatment and the more frequent but less severe disorders that can place a heavy burden on already busy outpatient clinics.

The physician in the tropics has roles other than purely clinical ones. Even the general physician has a broader public health role and is often in a position to advise governments (local or national) about activities that can be undertaken to promote health, including mental health. Thus, if a new housing scheme is proposed, the physician may be one of the few local people who can help planners to consider health matters. This means attention to matters that affect physical health, such as clean water, drainage, and waste disposal, and also consideration of facilities that may affect mental health, such as adequate day care facilities for children (possibly through cooperatives of mothers), facilities for educating girls as well as boys (the mental life of girls being no less important), and facilities for promoting social contact.

Physical and mental health problems in the tropics are sometimes aggravated by severe social problems, an outstanding example of which are those of being a refugee. Fortunately, acute nutritional and other physical health problems among refugees are often dealt with in the first weeks and months of resettlement. The social and psychological problems may be more persistent and difficult to deal with and may soon present as health problems. This aspect of work among refugee groups needs as much attention as physical needs. The rest of this chapter will, however, deal with the clinical problems presented by the mentally ill.

There is an unfortunate tendency in medical teaching and practice to separate the psychological from the physical. There is growing evidence to suggest, however, that much physical disease can be precipitated by psychological stress. One mechanism that has been demonstrated is depression of the immune system by psychological stress.

There is no doubt that much psychiatric disorder can be precipitated by a physical illness which in one way or another affects the brain, and hence experience and behavior. There is a danger of regarding behavioral disturbances as manifestations only of psychological processes. While this is often so, disturbed behavior may be due to a physical disease. Unfortunately, the nature of the behavior does not usually indicate the nature of the physical disease, or even that physical disease is present. It is, however, frequently the case that where there is a disturbance of brain function due to acute or chronic organic disease involving the brain or other organs, there is impairment of consciousness distinct from the change in mental state occurring in the more purely functional illnesses such as schizo-

phrenia, manic-depressive illness, anxiety states, and other conditions usually referred to as *neuroses*.

The clinical descriptions which follow are therefore divided into:

1. The clearly organic conditions as they appear in the tropics, such as those associated with parasitic or bacterial infections, vitamin and mineral deficiencies, and the problems of drug and alcohol misuse.
2. The functional psychoses, with particular reference to their manifestation and management in tropical settings.
3. The less severe but very widespread psychiatric disorders that present in clinics alongside the physical illnesses but which need to be distinguished from them.

THE CLEARLY ORGANIC DISTURBANCES LEADING TO PSYCHIATRIC DISORDER

Organic disturbances of all kinds tend to produce a similar clinical picture of impaired consciousness. This seems to be because they affect brain function in a fairly nonspecific way. In some cases, however, organic changes can affect structures in the brain, leading to a more specific syndrome, e.g., amnesia (see below). Specific damage to the brain may also produce localizing neurological lesions. Abuse of psychotropic substances also has a fairly general effect on brain function, but amphetamine abuse (see below) produces a schizophrenic picture. In a minority of cases of psychiatric disorder brought on by physical disease, the picture is identical to a purely functional presentation. In the majority, however, there is impaired consciousness, which must be defined.

Impaired consciousness, also called clouding of consciousness, has been described as a state of reduced wakefulness and can vary from a mild reduction in function to a state of delirium. Taken further it becomes a total loss of consciousness, as in coma. In its mildest form there may only be a slowness in responding and a lack of ability to concentrate. Disordered thinking and the presence of delusions and hallucinations are not in themselves signs of impaired consciousness and indeed can easily occur in clear consciousness. (The inexperienced health worker may refer to these as "confusion," but this latter term should be reserved for impaired consciousness.) Drowsiness often occurs in organic states, but patients with acute organic changes may also be excited. The most easily elicited signs are those of disorientation in time, place, and person. Disorientation in these circumstances refers to the patients' lack of awareness of their own identity and failure to recognize the health attendant. It should not be confused with a delusional state, in which the patient may be fully aware but convinced that the hospital is really some special palace and the nurses are really all servants parading as nurses. A patient with impaired consciousness may not understand clearly what is said, may respond vaguely and inappropriately, and may speak in a rambling, incoherent, or even delirious manner. In such states, hallucinations are more commonly visual than auditory. Both misinterpretation of environmental stimuli and hallucinations may make the patient extremely frightened.

Associated with impaired consciousness is loss of recent memory, and inability to remember much from minute to minute. This should be tested by asking the patient to remember something and then to recall it a short while later. This picture of impaired consciousness is seen typically in the disturbed states that accompany systemic infections, such as a pneumonia and typhoid, or infections of the central nervous system such as bacterial or parasitic meningitis and encephalitis. Disturbance of mental function, sometimes with excited behavior can develop with an acute bacterial or parasitic (e.g., malaria) infection. More chronic states of impairment of consciousness can occur with parasitic infections such as trypanosomiasis, paragonimiasis, cysticercosis, schistosomiasis japonicum, and other infections that can directly involve the brain. Although not common nowadays, it should always be borne in mind that a dementia and disinhibited behavior can occur in syphilitic general paralysis of the insane. Whenever impaired consciousness is associated with disturbed behavior and thinking, it is wise to explore the possibility of organic causes. Seizures or other neurological signs always indicate organic disease affecting the central nervous system (CNS), but these features are by no means invariable in organic states.

VITAMIN DEFICIENCY

Some vitamin deficiencies also produce organic brain disease, and some of these are more frequently found in the tropics. Thiamine deficiency (see below) produces a mental state, as part of Korsakoff's syndrome, now better described as the amnesic syndrome, characterized by loss of recent memory and time sense with a relative sparing of general intellect (see Chap. 11).

In its more acute and severe form, thiamine deficiency can produce Wernicke's encephalopathy: ataxia, ophthalmoplegia, and impaired consciousness, even coma. This may be precipitated by infection, diarrhea, or vomiting superimposed on preexisting mild deficiency. Experimental deprivation of thiamine in humans quickly brings on mental symptoms of fatigue, insomnia, irritability, and some impairment of thinking, long before the appearance of classical symptoms of beriberi. In the full-blown form of the encephalopathy, pathological cerebral changes are found in the mammillary bodies, the region of the third ventricle, periaqueductal gray matter, and parts of certain thalamic nuclei. The chronic picture of Korsakoff's syndrome is caused by lesions in the same sites. The syndrome can be caused by factors other than thiamine deficiency. It is typical of chronic alcohol abuse (see below), in which case it is probably attributable to an associated thiamine deficiency.

Pellagra (see below) is another vitamin deficiency disease exhibiting marked mental symptoms which is seen frequently in the tropics. The brain seems particularly susceptible to nicotinamide deficiency, probably because of its very active respiration of glycolysis. This requires the coenzymes I and II derived from niacin. Early symptoms of deficiency may be lassitude, irritability, insomnia, and depression, followed by an acute organic mental disturbance that may appear before the typical three D's: dermatitis, diarrhea, and the more marked dementia which is classically described as a sequel.

Other vitamin deficiencies seldom, if ever, lead to psychiatric disorders.

MINERAL DISORDERS

Iodine and zinc deficiencies are particularly associated with the tropics and have important psychiatric sequelae.

Iodine

Cretinism is caused by iodine deficiency affecting the fetal brain in its early development. This is largely irreversible, and so it is important that no woman of childbearing age be iodine-deficient. It is now becoming apparent that iodine deficiency in childhood and adolescence associated with only mild degrees of goiter is probably associated with a depression of mental function. Crude measurement of IQ is difficult and probably does not provide a good indication of the psychological deficits resulting from iodine deficiency and hypothyroidism. Nevertheless, even studies using these crude measures point to defects which can be reduced by iodine supplementation.

Zinc

The role of zinc in mental functioning has yet to be properly established. Zinc deficiency (see below) is now well described, and it seems likely that, like iodine deficiency, it can produce irreversible change in the fetus if present in early pregnancy. Deficiency leads to dwarfism and an impairment of mental development which may be reversed by zinc supplementation. Animal studies indicate that zinc deficiency may cause violent and aggressive behavior, but this has not been studied in humans.

ALCOHOL AND DRUG ABUSE

Alcohol and drug problems are dealt with here because in many tropical countries these are important causes of morbidity. In their defense it is said that alcohol and drugs have important social functions and that their dangers are minimal when they are used in socially regulated ways. Evidence for this is not convincing, and in any case traditional social controls and values break down so frequently that problems related to alcohol and drug abuse are important. Although traditional ''opaque'' beers may have more nutritive value than commercially brewed ones, the damage caused far outweighs any potential benefits derived from these brews.

Apart from the direct adverse effects of alcohol and drugs on human metabolism and the effects of associated vitamin deficiencies, health is also damaged by accidents at work, while driving, and at other times. Such damage occurs both to the subject and to others in the environment. In particular, a person who spends much of the family income on alcohol or drugs has little left for food or other things that enhance health. Children become neglected, and the general level of development of the home, the family, and the community suffers.

Alcohol

Alcohol has acute and chronic effects on the brain. The immediate effects are well known and may be socially useful. However, the impaired judgment resulting even from relatively low levels of blood alcohol can lead to accidents and deaths. Severe alcohol intoxication leads to coma and associated complications. A syndrome of hypoglycemic coma following acute alcohol intoxication has been described, especially in Africa. This should be recognized by emergency medical services, as it can, of course, be cured with intravenous glucose. Thiamine supplements may be needed by patients already deficient since the extra glucose may further deplete the body of this vitamin.

Chronic use of alcohol has adverse effects on the brain and other organs. Dementia is well recognized. Auditory hallucinations may develop in fully conscious patients. They do not always remit once drinking stops and associated vitamin deficiencies are corrected. Classically, an amnesic syndrome develops with chronic alcohol abuse, and this is associated with thiamine deficiency as described above. This may be associated with cerebral damage irreversible by thiamine.

A further clinical presentation associated with alcohol abuse is delirium tremens. This is usually attributed to a withdrawal state; however, there do seem to be other contributory factors such as infection, head injury, or poor nutrition. The picture is often complicated by the presence of the amnesic syndrome. The typical features of delirium tremens are the presence of illusions or hallucinations (typically but not always visual) which are very frightening for the patient. Although at times the patient may see a comical side to these hallucinations, the overriding emotion is one of terror. Associated with this may be a marked tremor and, later, considerable overactivity. In the early stages the patient will control the tremor (i.e., the morning shakes) by taking more alcohol. Convulsions are not uncommon either in the early phase or during the acute delirium, when impairment of consciousness is also found. Delirium tremens usually ends within 3 to 7 days but is a dangerous condition carrying a risk of death from infections, cardiac failure, or injury. Dehydration and vitamin deficiencies should be corrected; infection should be treated or prevented with antibiotics. The patient should be sedated as necessary using diazepam. Once recovered, patients need to be told firmly that their condition was caused by drink and that they should give it up. Where it is culturally appropriate and sufficient numbers exist, mutual support groups of recovered patients can be formed in the style of Alcoholics Anonymous.

In medical practice there is a danger, however, of assuming that the problems of alcohol consumption are restricted to those "alcoholics" who are obviously heavily addicted. In any population, this relatively small group represents only the tip of the iceberg. For each such person there are many more people in the general population whose health is being adversely affected by alcohol, either directly or indirectly. What is more, preventive measures aimed at the wider group will probably lead to better results than dealing with the crises presented by the identified alcoholic who, sadly, does not respond well to treatment in the long term. Health education in schools, and for social and professional groups, and the control of availability of alcohol are important issues. A paramedical staff member could be assigned the task of working on such health education programs. In particular, the police should be made aware of the problem, since they will enforce control policies more effectively if they understand their importance.

Because alcohol contributes to so many presentations at health clinics in many areas of the world, it is wise for health workers to have a simple set of screening questions which can be asked of most, if not all, adult patients. Fifty years ago syphilitic lesions could mimic most medical presentations and had to be excluded. Nowadays alcohol should occupy this place as a possible cause for most medical presentations, at least in areas where alcohol consumption is widespread.

Drug abuse

There are three categories of drugs which can be abused: those which have been used traditionally in a society and which are to a greater or lesser extent socially sanctioned, like alcohol and tobacco; more recently introduced illicit drugs such as heroin or refined cocaine, which at least in towns are being taken up by the younger generations; and licit drugs which are normally available from chemists on prescription but because of the lack of adequate controls in many tropical areas are fairly freely available; for example, amphetamines and other such stimulants and sedatives, such as short-acting barbiturates and methaqualone.

The Traditional Drugs. It is difficult to make any generalizations about the health damage from traditional drugs, and the damage has to be weighed against some possible social benefits. There is little doubt, however, that opium smoking, in, for instance, some parts of Thailand, is deleterious to the families of those with severely dependent members. The dangers of coca and khat chewing are more contentious. Cannabis taken in one form or another is recognized in many tropical countries as bad for health. Most psychiatrists working in the tropics are convinced of its adverse short- and long-term effects on mental functioning. An acute confusional psychosis can develop. This tends to resolve when the cannabis is stopped.

The Newer Illicit Drugs. Patients affected by these drugs may be brought for treatment because of some criminal behavior or by worried relatives. At the moment use of these drugs is probably not such a major public health problem in the tropics, but it is a growing one to both health and police authorities. In the case of the injected drugs the problem has taken on a new dimension with transmission of AIDS by shared unsterilized needles.

The Licit Drugs. The amphetamines are particularly important. These may be taken by students or long distance drivers. Chronic use can lead to a psychosis identical to schizophrenia with little effect on consciousness. In the poorest countries most people cannot afford seriously to abuse these drugs, and so their adverse effects have not yet reached public health proportions. In other tropical countries, however, their use is widespread.

Before dealing with the functional psychoses in which the level of consciousness is seldom impaired, it should be pointed out that physical diseases do sometimes lead to a picture of a mental disorder without impairment of consciousness. This can be true of any physical disease, and so when a patient presents with mental disturbance in relatively clear consciousness, the physician must remain vigilant and carry out routine examinations for physical diseases and watch for changes in the patient's state which indicate that a physical disease such as typhoid is developing.

THE FUNCTIONAL MENTAL DISORDERS

Functional mental disorders include schizophrenia, manic-depressive psychosis, other psychoses, depressive anxiety, hysterical disorders, and somatization of psychological disorders. Those aspects of presentation or management that are of particular relevance to the tropics will be dealt with here.

CHRONIC SCHIZOPHRENIA

Patients with schizophrenia may be brought for treatment either by relatives or by the police because their behavior has become disturbed, violent, or destructive. Relatives may come to a hospital having exhausted their patience and money on traditional healers; others may go directly to a psychiatric clinic or hospital if it becomes known that such cases are being treated there. An approach to these patients is as follows:

1. Treat any concurrent physical illness. Physical debility and illness can affect mental functioning in chronic schizophrenics more than in normal people.
2. Establish that the patient has chronic schizophrenia. There should be a history of months or years of mental disturbance with thinking disorder occurring without impaired consciousness. If the symptoms are disabling, the patient should be started on a small dose of an antipsychotic medication and the dose increased within the normal therapeutic range over several weeks until the symptoms have diminished sufficiently to allow the patient to function socially. A medication often available is chlorpromazine, which may be effective at a dose of 100 mg daily in relatively quiet patients, although it can be increased to 600 mg daily. Total suppression of symptoms may not be possible. Patients themselves and those who know them may have to decide on an adequate dose. The medication should be stopped if a high dose fails to make any significant difference within, say, 1 month.
3. Patients may need help in reintegrating into their family or community. Although some patients may need residential care of some kind, this very rarely needs to be hospital care. Some form of sheltered accommodation might be adequate, but this provision has to be socially possible and appropriate and has to be developed by local communities wherever possible. Various kinds of sheltered village accommodation have been developed in Africa. However, families should be encouraged and supported to accept their own sick members back.

ACUTE PSYCHOSES

People who become acutely mentally disturbed pose a particular problem to health services, which are expected to provide social control under these circumstances. Initially, such patients may be put in police custody, and it is sensible for a local health worker to establish working relations with the police on procedures for handling the situation. With disturbed patients, some physical restraint may be necessary while assessment is carried out and treatment initiated. This may even be done while the patient is in police custody. Wherever possible, every attempt must be made to exclude a physical cause for the condition. Whatever the cause, the patient's physical needs should not be ignored. In particular the patient may need rehydration and feeding. In severely disturbed patients it may be impossible to carry out an adequate examination of physical and mental status. Some mild clouding of consciousness may be observed even when no physical illness is found. Under these circumstances it may be possible to carry out some symptomatic treatment to settle the patient in the hope of carrying out a more detailed examination when the patient is calmer. Nonorganic causes for acute psychoses include mania (or hypomania), schizophrenia, and psychogenic or reactive psychoses. An acute psychotic syndrome (NOS) without organic cause is particularly common in less developed countries. It tends to have a good prognosis. If the patient needs more than simple physical restraint once physical needs have been tended to, major tranquilizers such as chlorpromazine may be used either orally or intramuscularly. Doses may have to be higher initially than those used in treating chronic schizophrenia. Side effects such as hypotension and parkinsonism will have to be looked for carefully and dealt with. In experienced hands, electroconvulsive therapy (ECT) often with a major tranquilizer may be effective in cutting short an acute psychotic episode.

DEPRESSIVE DISORDER

Epidemiological evidence indicates that serious psychiatric depression is as common throughout the tropics as it is elsewhere in the world. Patients may have a tendency to present somatic symptoms, so physicians must be aware of the syndrome in order to pick out those with depression from the stream of those presenting at general medical clinics. For this purpose a simple screening device such as the Self-Reporting Questionnaire (SRQ) [2] administered by a relatively low level worker can help to pick out such cases. Key symptoms that can alert the health worker to the presence of depression are sleep disturbance, poor appetite with weight loss, fatigue, especially if it is worse in the morning and improves later, and excessive worry. The treatment of depression must take into account possible psychological and social causes. When the depression is severe and causing functional impairment, the use of an antidepressant medication such as amitriptyline or imipramine may be indicated. However patients need warning of possible side effects and on the delay in feeling benefit from treatment.

In particular, depressed patients should be assessed for suicidal risk. Although suicide rates vary throughout the world, a tropical environment has certainly not been identified as a preventive factor. Rates of 5 to 10 per 100,000 per annum have been reported from Africa. Those who are depressed can be sensitively assessed for suicide risk by asking whether they feel life is not worth living or whether they think they would be better off dead. Only if a positive response is obtained to these questions should they be asked if they had actually thought of killing themselves, followed by an enquiry as to concrete plans or even attempts. At other times, relatives may bring a patient to hospital because of a suicide attempt. Where suicidal risk is identified the patient needs constant surveillance by a relative and where it occurs as part of a depressive illness, rapid treatment with antidepressants or ECT. In many cultures, suicide brings great shame to the family and requires special rituals subsequently. All this may require very sensitive handling by health workers should they be involved. A further particular risk period for depression is postpartum. Some women become temporarily emotionally upset at this time, but as many as 10 percent may develop a full-blown depression which in some cases may linger on for many months or even years. This has important implications for the woman's own health as well as for that of her baby. In situations where infants are vulnerable because of malnutrition and infection, a mother's impairment at this time may be yet a further factor contributing to infant mortality.

CONVERSION HYSTERIA

Although not common, the dramatic nature of this condition means that it may require attention. It is a condition which appears to affect girls and young women more frequently than males, and is considered to be the result of a reaction to some life event or difficult social situation, the symptoms enabling the patient to escape from or avoid it. Motor paralysis, aphonia, as well as blindness and other sensory losses may occur. Exploration of possible causes, counseling, and rehabilitation techniques may all help. Quick and dramatic cures are not always possible, but simple tests like getting the patient with aphonia to cough and then to go on to more elaborate phonation can at times produce quick changes.

SOMATIZATION

Although it has already been stated that depression may present with many somatic complaints, it is also true that many patients present with physical complaints (often multiple) which are inexplicable physically and are presumed to be psychological or social in origin. While some of these patients have full-blown depressive or anxiety disorders and others have milder tension, worry, and sleep problems, yet others have little more than the unexplained somatic symptoms. The symptoms commonly encountered as part of this somatization include fatigue, feeling slowed up, weakness, dizziness, insomnia, poor appetite, fainting, nausea, gastrointestinal upset, squeezing of the heart, tension in the neck, shoulders, back, or chest, headache and pressure on the head, heat in the head, burning eyes, peppery sensations, and palpitations.

One particular syndrome, often described, has been called the "brain fag" or "study stress" syndrome. This has been described mostly from tropical Africa and occurs predominantly in secondary school children. The symptoms usually include headache or other symptoms related to the head (pressure, tension), troubles with vision and concentration, and sleeping difficulties, as well as other symptoms of tension. Since the numbers of people affected in a school may be large, it is often better to organize supportive tension-reducing groups within schools than to try and tackle this on an individual basis in clinics. Improving study methods is a more sensible approach than giving tranquilizing or antidepressant medication. Those complaining of symptoms, however, do also need screening for near and distance vision problems and for a history suggestive of sinusitis. As has already been discussed, some of those cases with a psychological cause and requiring a psychological intervention can be picked out using a simple screening device such as the SRQ.

It should always be remembered, however, that psychophysiological symptoms may after all result from physical diseases, especially in parts of the world with high rates of endemic infections. Where physical symptoms do result from psychological causes, however, they may have a use, like hysteria, both as an appeal by a person for help from a doctor, but probably more importantly to deflect attention from an interpersonal conflict within families, to express personal distress, and to solicit comfort and support from others.

As western medicine has become more scientific, its models of explanation have moved away from folk models. This is so in Europe where doctors now seldom explain symptoms to patients in terms of changes in the weather, the winds, dampness, "acidity," or low blood pressure. Patients, however, still use and expect communication in these terms. How much more difficult is it therefore for poorly educated patients, unfamiliar with "science," to communicate easily with scientifically trained doctors. Under these circumstances, patients are "accused" of using the wrong models to express themselves and the doctors complain about the "complainers." Patients with psychophysiological symptoms need a sensitive approach which takes account of their own health belief models.

REFERENCES

1 Essex B, Gosling H: *Programme for Identification and Management of Mental Health Problems*. Edinburgh, Churchill Livingstone, 1982
2 Harding TW, De Arango MV, Baltazar J, et al: Mental disorders in primary health care: A study of their frequency and diagnosis in four developing countries. Psy Med 10:231–241, 1980
3 Meursing K, Wankiiri V: Use of flow-charts by nurses dealing with mental patients: An evaluation in Lesotho. Bull WHO 66(4): 507–514, 1988

CHAPTER 13 / Genetic Factors Modifying Tropical Disorders · Lucio Luzzatto

Every living organism is the product of a set of genes and of a set of interactions with the environment. In considering an individual, it is natural to think of the genome as the fixed component of the organism and of the environment as a variable to which the genome responds. However, the most distinctive feature of living, as opposed to nonliving things, is that the genome has been itself shaped by selective processes in the course of evolution.

The geographical distribution of human diseases clearly reflects the existence of these two components and their interactions, and prominently so in tropical areas. There the prevalence of a number of infectious and parasitic diseases is high because the environment is favorable to the transmission of, say, hepatitis or schistosomiasis; and the prevalence of sickle cell anemia is high because the gene responsible for this condition, $Hb\beta^s$, is common. We now know that the high frequency of $Hb\beta^s$ is in turn the result of selection by malaria, an exogenous factor. Thus, genetics, environment, and their interactions are all equally important in determining the epidemiology of tropical diseases. In addition, because different individuals, depending on their genome, respond differently to environmental pathogenic situations, genetics is also important in considering the clinical features of tropical diseases.

FEATURES OF THE HUMAN GENOME

FORMAL GENETICS

In all organisms except certain viruses, DNA is the genetic material, and in eukaryotic organisms it is arranged in chromosomes. Some numerical data on the human genome are summarized in Table 13-1. It is now clear that only a fraction of DNA consists of genes in the classical sense of the word, i.e., coding for a specific product. While the significance of the rest of the DNA is being keenly debated [1], it cannot be simply assumed that it does not play a role—be it structural or regulatory. However, the reason why genetics has been mainly concerned with DNA expressed in specific products, i.e., genes in the strict sense, is that mutations of individual genes are inherited according to simple, easily recognizable patterns which we call mendelian. While Mendel's laws were derived by observing and quantitating the results of appropriate

crosses (see Fig. 13-1), they can now be seen to be entirely predictable merely from our knowledge of the behavior of chromosomes at meiosis. Thus, we can easily see why a cross between two homozygotes can only yield heterozygotes (Mendel's first law); why a gene is inherited independently from another (Mendel's second law; independent assortment). However, we can also see that if the two genes being examined are in close proximity along the same chromosome, they will tend to be inherited together, or in linkage (an exception to independent assortment).

X-linked inheritance

Whereas any gene located on any of the 22 pairs of autosomes is transmitted as illustrated in Fig. 13-1, genes on the X chromosome exhibit a distinctly different pattern of inheritance. More precisely, since there are two X chromosomes in females, there is no difference from the behavior of autosomes here. By contrast, males are surprisingly haploid with respect to X-linked genes, and these are transmitted only to children who receive the paternal X chromosomes, i.e., to daughters. In male children the father is immaterial as far as X-linked genes are concerned, since they only receive the Y chromosome. The Y chromosome has only very limited homology to a portion of the X, and it contains very few expressed genes. This peculiar state of affairs causes, only with respect to

Table 13-1. Numerology of the human genome

	Approximate* values
Amount of DNA per haploid chromosome set	3.5×10^9 bp
Estimated number of expressed individual genes	5×10^4
Fraction of repetitive DNA	0.5
Average number of genes per chromosome	5×10^3
Number of bp per centimorgan†	10^6

*The emphasis is on the word approximate: only an order of magnitude is claimed as correct.

†bp = base pairs; centimorgan is the unit of genetic linkage, and it is defined as the distance between two genes that gives a recombination frequency of 1 percent. Thus, the last line gives a conversion factor for the size of the genome from genetic to molecular measurements.

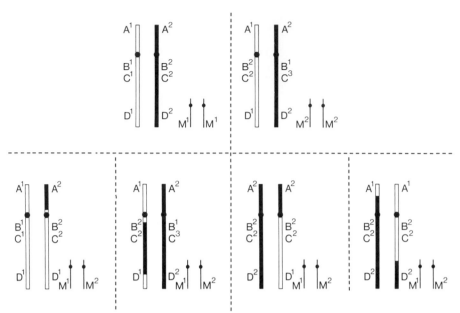

Figure 13-1. Diagram of inheritance of single genes (Mendel's laws). *Top:* parental genotypes. *Bottom:* genotypes of four among many possible offspring. For simplicity, only 2 of the 23 human chromosomes are drawn. Four genetic loci (A, B, C, D) are marked on one pair of chromosomes and one genetic locus (M) is marked on the other. Two alleles are seen at loci A, B, D, M; and three alleles at locus C. The two chromosomes of the longer pair are distinguished in each parent by the empty or full bar. The black dot in each chromosome represents the centromere. The diagram illustrates several points: (1) If both parents are homozygotes at a certain locus (in this case, $M^1M^1 \times M^2M^2$), all offspring will be heterozygotes at that locus (in this case, M^1M^2). If both parents are heterozygous, for instance, at loci A and D, the expected genotype ratios in the offspring will be 1:2:1 for homozygotes (A^1A^1,D^1D^1), heterozygotes (A^1A^2,D^1D^2), and homozygotes (A^2A^2,D^2D^2), respectively. These are all examples of Mendel's first law. (2) If two loci are on different chromosomes, they are inherited independently from each other (this is seen to be true if we consider the M locus *versus* the other four loci). If two loci are on the same chromosome but far apart (e.g., A and B), they still have an equal chance of being transmitted together (4 out of 8 cases), or of being separated by meiotic crossover (4 out of 8 cases). These are examples of Mendel's second law (independent assortment). (3) If two loci are on the same chromosome but relatively near to each other (e.g., C and D), there is a greater chance that they are transmitted together (6 out of 8 cases), rather than segregating as a result of crossover (2 out of 8 cases). If two loci are very near to each other (closely linked; see B and C) they are very unlikely to be separated by crossover (0 out of 8 chances in this illustration). This type of behavior, called genetic linkage, constitutes an important and regular exception to Mendel's second law. Note that the various allelic genes in this illustration (distinguished by superscripts) are assumed to be all codominant. The concepts of "dominant" and "recessive" are not essential in considering their inheritance.

X-linked genes, a unique asymmetry in the two parents' contribution to the male offspring's genetic make-up.

X chromosome inactivation

In principle, one would expect that females having two X chromosomes would express each X-linked gene at twice the level found in males, who only have one X chromosome; in fact, no difference is found in most cases. This very important phenomenon, called *dosage compensation,* is explained by the fact that in each female somatic cell only one of the two X chromosomes is active. The cytological manifestation of the inactive X is the heterochromatic Barr body. Since there may be approximately 5000 genetic loci on the X chromosome (see Table 13-1), it is practically certain that every female will be heterozygous at least at some of them. Cells with the paternal active X will express different alleles from those with the maternal active X. As a result, there will be a physiological somatic cell mosaicism in every woman (a privilege denied to men).

MOLECULAR BASIS OF INHERITANCE

The unique double-stranded structure of DNA is the physical basis of heredity. Its functional features can be defined under three headings.

Replication

Each cell division, including the production of gametes, is preceded by a round of DNA synthesis, whereby a copy of the parent DNA molecule is manufactured. Since each strand dictates the synthesis of its complement, each newly synthesized strand can be "proofread" by comparing it to its preexisting partner, and the cell has mechanisms to correct occasional copying errors. As a result, the outcome of the replication process is astonishingly accurate.

Mutation

The DNA replication machinery is extremely accurate, but being a physical object, it cannot be perfect. Something of the order of one base pair (bp) in 10^8 will be changed at each round of DNA replication; in germ cells, this will be an inheritable *point-mutation*. (If we take the average size of a gene to be 1000 bp, the mutation rate per gene per generation works out to approximately 10^{-5}.) In other, probably even less common, cases, a mutation may consist in loss (*deletion*) or addition (*insertion*) of DNA, or in *duplication* of a segment. We can detect only a fraction of the mutations that take place. Some of them are lethal and will be lost—by definition—as soon as they occur. Others may never be expressed (see below). A number, however, will manifest themselves by causing, for instance, a disease. Because this is the group that is important for medicine, the word *mutation* tends to carry a negative connotation. However, the majority of mutations giving visible effects are not pathological; they simply cause the variability that makes humankind pleasantly diversified, as seen in variations of skin and eye color, or in blood groups and HLA types. In addition, let us never forget that mutations are the raw material on which selection can operate, and the basis for the whole of biological evolution.

Expression

The base-pairing principle which underlies replication of DNA is also the main physical basis for its transcription into RNA. Some of this is incorporated into ribosomes or serves to recognize amino acids as transfer RNA; but the most numerous species consist of messenger RNA molecules, which are subsequently translated, according to the rules of the so-called genetic code, into protein molecules. Thus, most of what we know about gene expression consists in visible characters depending on enzymes or other proteins, such as hemoglobin, or collagen, or components of the cell membrane. If the gene is mutated, the protein product will be structurally changed. On the other hand, important regulatory regions of DNA can be expressed not in the structure, but in the amount of protein made, as in some of the thalassemia syndromes.

GENOTYPE AND PHENOTYPE

While the former term of this heading is unambiguously defined by the genetic makeup of an individual, the latter designates the way it is manifested. As such, phenotype is a relative concept, because what we see depends on how we look. If we consider a single locus A, the genotype of a person is

defined completely by the pair of allelic genes present at that locus. However, the expression of each gene will depend on the particular pair involved, and may be affected by the rest of the genome as well. For instance, the expression of an allele A^1 may be different in genotype A^1A^2 and in genotype A^1A^3; in addition, the expression of any or all the alleles at locus A may be affected by what genes are present in the same person at locus B.

"Dominant" and "recessive" genes

When, in a heterozygote, only one of the two genes at locus A is manifested, we say it is dominant, and we call its allelic opposite number recessive. Dominance is rarely complete; for instance, although red cells with either genotype *A/A* or genotype *A/O* are classified as group A, the number of A substance molecules is less in the latter than in the former. Also, because dominance is defined in terms of gene expression, it is as relative as the concept of phenotype; for instance, the gene for blood group A_2 is dominant with respect to O, but recessive with respect to the blood group A_1 gene. The designation of a gene as dominant is relative in yet another sense, because it depends on which aspect of the phenotype we examine (see Table 13-2). However, from the clinical point of view, it is extremely important to consider whether a particular gene gives a disease only in homozygotes (*recessive* disease) or also in heterozygotes (*dominant* disease). Among the many practical implications, let us note the following: (1) Only dominant diseases will, in general, exhibit vertical transmission; therefore, a negative family history cannot be taken as evidence against the genetic basis of a (recessive) pathological state. (2) Parental consanguinity and inbreeding in general increase the risk only of recessive, and not of dominant, diseases. (3) The risk of recurrence of a genetic disease in the offspring of a particular couple is very different in the two cases.

Table 13-2. Genotype and phenotype in a monogenic disease

Genotype	Clinical disease	Hemoglobins in red cell	Sickling phenomenon
$Hb\beta^A/Hb\beta^A$	0	A	−
$Hb\beta^A/Hb\beta^S$	0[a]	A + S	+
$Hb\beta^S/Hb\beta^S$	+ + +	S	+

Note: It is clear that in terms of the clinical phenotype, *S* is recessive; in terms of the biochemical phenotype, hemoglobins *A* and *S* are co-dominant; in terms of sickling, a commonly used laboratory test, *S* is dominant. This illustrates that the concepts of dominant and recessive are only relative to the particular level of phenotypic expression being considered. It does not mean that these concepts have outlived their usefulness, since obviously clinical disease is the most important from the practical point of view, and to this extent it is appropriate to continue to designate sickle cell anemia as an autosomal recessive condition.

Source: From [2].

Table 13-3. Gene interactions and "polygenic" diseases

Examples	Genes involved A	B	Clinical condition or interaction	Reference
(1)	Hb S	α Thalassemia	B mitigates expression of A	[4]
(2)	HLA-B27		Predisposition to ankylosing spondylitis	[5]
(3)	HLA	Gm	Combination of certain haplotypes of A and B strongly predisposes to thyrotoxicosis	[6]
(4)	HLA-B8-DR3	Gm	Combination of A with certain haplotypes of B predisposes to chronic active hepatitis	[7]

SINGLE GENES VERSUS MULTIGENE CHARACTERS

A genetic disease has been traditionally defined in terms of mendelian inheritance, implying that the disease is essentially determined by a single gene. This is a reasonable simplification in many cases (see Ref. 3) in which a particular genotype is invariably associated with a certain disease; a classical example pertinent to tropical medicine is sickle cell anemia. However, in each individual the entire genome is expressed as a whole, and even in relatively straightforward cases we cannot assume that other genes do not play a role. On the contrary, we know of at least one other gene, that for α thalassemia, which affects the clinical severity of sickle cell anemia (see Table 13-3), and we can conceive of yet others (Chap. 14). In spite of their important clinical effects, these genes do not disturb the biochemical expression of the S gene to the point of making it unrecognizable; therefore, we can still easily follow its inheritance. However, it is not difficult to visualize that if a gene A could only be identified through a clinical syndrome, and this were modified to the point of being fully manifested or fully suppressed by the action of another gene B, and if A and

B assort independently, the syndrome would appear so erratically in families that we might not even realize that it is genetic at all. The situation would become even more complicated—practically beyond recognition by current methodologies—if more than two genes were involved. Thus, we can infer that many conditions which fail to show mendelian inheritance may nevertheless be genetically determined, even to a large extent; they simply depend on a constellation of genes, rather than on a single gene. There are reasons to suspect that this may be true, for instance, in various kinds of cardiovascular, neurological, and other degenerative disorders (see Table 13-3).

GENES AND ENVIRONMENT

The dichotomy between endogenous and exogenous causes is urged upon authors of textbooks by the almost inescapable need to set up some kind of classification of the etiology of diseases. The dichotomy is valid, as long as we realize fully that it is only a first approximation of a more complex state of affairs. A good historical example, within tropical diseases, is the case of leprosy. At some time and in some cultures the

Table 13-4. Examples of genetic modifiers of acquired tropical diseases

Species	Genetic system	Chromosome localization	Cells where expressed	Increased resistance, dominant/ recessive	Tropical disease(s) involved	Reference
Humans	Duffy	1	Erythrocytes	R	Malaria (*P. vivax*)	[9]
	Hemoglobin:*		Erythrocytes	D†	Malaria (*P. falciparum*)	[10]
	α locus	16p13				
	β locus	11p15				
	Glucose-6-phosphate dehydrogenase	Xq28	Erythrocytes	D†	Malaria (*P. falciparum*)	[10]
	HLA	6p21.3	Most cells	R	Leprosy; probably many others	[12]
Mouse	*Lsh*	1	Macrophages	R	Leishmaniasis	[13]
	MHC	17	Most cells	R	Trypanosomiasis? intestinal worms; probably many others	[14]
	Ity	1	Macrophages	D	Salmonellosis	[14]

*Hemoglobin S is certainly involved, and almost certainly β and α thalassemia. Hemoglobin E is also probably involved inasmuch as it gives a mold thalassemia phenotype (Chap. 14). Scanty evidence for other hemoglobin variants.
†Heterozygote advantage. Because heterozygotes are relatively resistant to malaria, in this respect the gene concerns is dominant. However, SS homozygotes do not share the benefit of increased resistance [10].

HARDY-WEINBERG EQUILIBRIUM

Consider, in a certain breeding group, an autosomal locus with two *alleles*, A^1 and A^2. The corresponding possible *genotypes* are obviously

$$A^1A^1 \qquad A^1A^2 \qquad A^2A^2$$

As a result of segregation at meiosis only two types of *gametes* (with respect to that locus) will be produced

$$A^1 \qquad A^2$$

Let us call their frequencies (*gene frequencies*)

$$p_A{}^1 \qquad q_A{}^2$$

or p and q for brevity. If we regard the output of one generation as one pool of gametes, we need two of them to make a zygote, i.e., one individual of the next generation. To obtain a particular combination of two gametes will then be analogous to picking at random two beads out of a bag, where red and green beads are present in large numbers, and the frequency of any particular genotype will depend on the relative abundancies of the two types of gametes: specifically, the probability of picking an A^1 gamete is p, and the probability of picking an A^2 gamete is q. Since compound probabilities are obtained by multiplication, the expected frequencies of the possible genotypes are:

$$
\begin{aligned}
A^1A^1: &\quad p \times p &&= p^2 \\
A^1A^2: &\quad p \times q + q \times p &&= 2\,pq \\
A^2A^2: &\quad q \times q &&= q^2
\end{aligned}
$$

With only two alleles, this formulation can be further simplified by considering that $p = 1 - q$. If we introduce a third allele A^3 with frequency r, the frequencies of the additional genotypes will obviously be

$$
\begin{aligned}
A^3A^3: &\quad r^2 \\
A^1A^3: &\quad 2\,pr \\
A^2A^3: &\quad 2\,qr
\end{aligned}
$$

Thus, the Hardy-Weinberg rule defines fully the relationship between gene frequencies and genotype frequencies. In a two-allele system, if we determine experimentally the frequency of one single genotype, we can, in principle, calculate all other values. For instance, in a particular community it is found that 64 percent of people are A^2A^2, i.e.,

$$A^2A^2: \qquad q^2 = 0.64$$

Then the gene frequencies are

$$q = \sqrt{0.64} = 0.8; \qquad p = 1 - 0.8 = 0.2$$

and the remaining two genotype frequencies are

$$
\begin{aligned}
A^1A^2: &\quad 2\,pq = 2 \times 0.2 \times 0.8 = 0.32 \\
A^1A^1: &\quad p^2 = 0.2^2 = 0.04
\end{aligned}
$$

In practice, it is advisable to determine experimentally all genotype frequencies, if at all possible, because this will permit obtaining a statistically more accurate estimate of gene frequencies. At the same time, it will be a check of whether the particular system under investigation conforms to the Hardy-Weinberg rule.

cause was regarded as exogenous, i.e., punishment for sins committed. Subsequently, as empirical observations began to supersede metaphysical explanations, multiple cases within families suggested that leprosy was inherited [8]. When *Mycobacterium leprae* was discovered by K. Hansen in 1873, it seemed obvious that it, an exogenous microorganism, was the cause of the disease and that clustering of patients in families could be attributed to infectious rather than genetic transmission. However, as epidemiological and clinical studies of leprosy progressed, one wondered why not all people coming into contact with *M. leprae* became infected, and why, among those who did, some developed the lepromatous and others, the tuberculoid form of the disease. Now, it has become clear that while certainly without *M. leprae* there can be no leprosy, the development and the clinical type of the disease are significantly conditioned by genetic factors. At least one of the gene loci involved has been pinpointed to within the HLA complex (see below). Thus, the exogenous and endogenous theories are reconciled.

What we know about this and other examples (see Table 13-4) is hardly a complete explanation of the general question of why different people react differently to infectious agents from the environment. However, it is probably safe to assume that as in leprosy, also in most other cases the host-pathogen interaction can be affected by genetic factors in at least two ways: (1) the growth of the pathogenic organism and (2) the reaction of the host organism (including immune response, tissue reaction, macrophage activity, etc.). Although few model systems are worked out in any detail, they are very useful pointers to how other situations can be investigated.

POPULATION GENETICS

Like the behavior of genes in families (formal genetics), which can be analyzed in a simple way by means of Mendel's laws, the behavior of genes in a breeding community can also be described in terms of a single rule, which goes under the names of W. Hardy and O. Weinberg, and on which the whole of population genetics is based. While the complexities of this subject entail quite awesome algebra, its basic formulation is extremely simple (see "Hardy-Weinberg Equilibrium").

When the rule here derived is satisfied, the population is said to be in Hardy-Weinberg equilibrium with respect to the genes involved. There are four assumptions implicit in the derivation: (1) Mating occurs at random. (2) No mutations take place in the generation(s) analyzed. (3) The breeding group is self-contained. (4) All genotypes and all gametes have the same reproductive fitness. If any of these conditions is not fulfilled, the population is not in Hardy-Weinberg equilibrium. In any case from real life, deviations from expected frequency values will nearly always occur, even though they will be mostly small and therefore difficult to detect. The most common causes of such deviations are the following: (1) Consanguinity will produce matings with identical parental genes more often than would be expected by chance. This phenomenon, often related to sociocultural factors, is called *inbreeding*. It produces an excess of homozygous offspring, and therefore an excess of individuals affected by recessive genetic disease. (2) Mutations produce new alleles, or more rarely the reversion of a previous mutation. Unless the population is very small, the effect will be negligible in one generation, but may become amplified over a number of generations. (3) A population is rarely completely isolated. If people migrate away from it, the effect on genetic structure will not be significant, barring the unlikely event that certain genotypes emigrate more than others. However, if people migrating *into* the population have different genotype frequencies, it is clear that this gene flow will change the genetic structure of the resident population. (4) Most important from the point of view of natural selection, and therefore of tropical medicine, is the possibility that not all genotypes have the same reproductive fitness. In this case it is no longer justified to assume that each gamete has an equal chance of contributing to the following generations' genetic makeup. In other words, if a particular genotype is either subject to a higher mortality rate before reproductive age or is less fit to reproduce, there will be a relative shortage in the next generation of the respective alleles.

It is important to note that while inbreeding will only modify genotype frequencies, mutation, gene flow, and selection will change gene frequencies as well. All of these processes do, by definition, infringe on the Hardy-Weinberg rule. However, its very convenient mathematical form can be retained by introducing, for each of them, appropriate quantitative correction parameters, such as the inbreeding coefficient, the mutation rate, and different fitness values for different genotypes [*15*].

POLYMORPHISM, DRIFT, AND SELECTION

While in the long run mutations are, as mentioned earlier, the main basis of evolution, the gene frequencies in contemporary human populations result mainly from flow and drift of existing genes, on which environmental selection acts differently in different places. When in a particular population two or more allelic genes are present at frequencies higher than can be accounted for by recurrent mutations, we say that the population is polymorphic with respect to that genetic locus.[1] In practice, because mutation rates are difficult to measure, it is safe to assume that a gene is polymorphic when it is found in at least 1 percent of individuals. Although polymorphisms are very common, there are basically only two ways whereby a polymorphism can persist indefinitely in a population (see Table 13-5). If the various genotypes involved have approximately the same fitness, gene frequencies will be stable. Most populations are polymorphic with respect to most blood groups,

[1]In current jargon, the more common allelic gene is often regarded as "normal," and the less common gene is itself called polymorphic. This is not strictly correct, since, by definition, only a population can be polymorphic, not a gene.

Table 13-5. Various kinds of genetic polymorphism

Genotypes	Fitness* values		
	I	**II**	**III**
A^1A^1	1.0	1.0	1.0
A^1A^2	1.1	1.0	1.1
A^2A^2	1.2	1.0	0.5
Fate of polymorphism			
Transient	Stable (neutral)	Stable (balanced)	

*Fitness is defined in terms of reproductive performance, i.e., average number of offspring produced. Each column gives one set of fitness values for the three genotypes concerned, taking as unity, in each case, the fitness of the A^1A^1 homozygote.

probably for this reason. On the other hand, if there are differences in reproductive fitness, the polymorphism will persist only if the heterozygote is the most fit, because he or she will pass on to the next generation either gene with equal probability. This situation has been well characterized for hemoglobin S, and it is referred to as *balanced* polymorphism, because the heterozygote advantage balances the low fitness of the SS homozygote. If one homozygote has a lower fitness than the other and the heterozygote is intermediate in fitness, then selection will tend to eliminate the polymorphic situation. However, since this will take time, and in the meantime other phenomena, such as gene flow, may interfere, it is quite possible that we are presently seeing polymorphisms in many real populations in this nonequilibrium situation (see Table 13-5).

LINKAGE DISEQUILIBRIUM

We have noted that linked genes tend to be inherited as one set (Fig. 13-1), in defiance of Mendel's second law. However, no matter how close two genes lie, over the generations they will eventually be separated by crossover. Thus, while in families we see linkage, in a population we do not expect, a priori, any preferential association of a particular allele at one locus with a particular allele at another, even closely linked locus. In some cases, however, preferential association is found. This finding is called linkage disequilibrium (see box) because the assortment of the two (nonallelic) genes appears not to have been totally randomized, or equilibrated, by recombination. Barring the as yet unproven possibility that this is caused by a relative rarity of crossover in the respective chromosomal region, the only current explanation for this state of affairs is that the particular combination of linked genes, also called a *haplotype,* is favored by selection. The extent of the selective force involved is measured by the value D of linkage disequilibrium.

When investigating the possible association of a disease, or disease susceptibility, with a known gene, which we can call a *marker,* two approaches can be considered: (1) In families, we can look for cosegregation of the disease in question with the marker gene. (2) In populations, we can look for an increased frequency of the marker gene among affected individuals compared to controls. If both associations are complete, the marker gene might itself be the gene responsible for the disease; this would be a rare finding! If only (1) is successful, it means that the disease gene and the marker gene are within measurable genetic distance. If (2) is also successful, even though the association is incomplete, it means that not only the two genes are linked, but they are also in linkage disequilibrium. This type of analysis has been notably successful with respect to the human major histocompatibility complex, HLA.

LINKAGE DISEQUILIBRIUM

The major histocompatibility complex (MHC) is located within a relatively small region of chromosome 6. It comprises several loci coding for cell surface proteins called *histocompatibility loci antigens* (HLA), at least three loci coding for complement components, and other loci. The HLA loci are characterized by the highest variability and the highest rate of polymorphic alleles thus far known in the human species. For instance, there are at least 12 polymorphic alleles known at HLA locus A and even more at HLA locus B.

In a Congolese population the following gene frequencies were measured [17]:

$$\text{HLA-A10:} \quad 0.09$$
$$\text{HLA-B12:} \quad 0.16$$

The probability of finding these two nonallelic genes lined up on the same chromosome is

$$\text{HLA-A10} - \text{B12:} \quad 0.09 \times 0.16 = 0.0144$$

i.e., 1.44 percent of the population would be expected to have these two alleles in linkage. Instead, it is found in 3.8 percent. The difference

$$D = 0.0380 - 0.0144 = 0.0236 = 2.36 \text{ percent}$$

is a measure of *linkage disequilibrium*. The combination of the two genes on the same chromosomes (e.g., A10 − B12) is called a *haplotype* (quite a different concept from genotype, which means a combination of two allelic genes on opposite chromosomes, e.g., A9/A10).

GENETIC FACTORS MODIFYING TROPICAL DISEASES

We have already mentioned that host genetics determines to a significant extent susceptibility or resistance to acquired disease. In principle, we could either consider, for each disease in turn, which genetic systems may be involved, or, for each known genetic system in turn, what disease may be affected. A detailed analysis by either approach is precluded by restrictions of space. Since individual tropical diseases are already discussed systematically throughout this volume, we give here an outline of those genetic factors about which more is known in relation to conditions highly prevalent in tropical areas.

THE IMMUNE SYSTEM

Traditionally immune response has been regarded as the territory of acquired, as opposed to innate resistance to, infectious agents. However, we now know that not only both cellular and humoral immunity are under genetic control (this is a truism, since every component of the body is determined by genes), but most important, these phenomena display extensive genetic variability, and it is with this aspect alone that we are concerned here. Moreover, we must concentrate on factors that are relatively common (polymorphic) and that have some degree of specificity. For instance, it is clear that children with severe combined immune deficiency will respond poorly to most infections; this is fortunately a rare, obviously extreme, and nonspecific situation. By contrast, why some people with a "normal" immune system should respond more or less actively than average to, for instance, a *Leishmania* infection, is far less obvious; but from a practical point of view, this may equally make a difference between life and death, and it may be an important factor in determining the whole pattern of that disease in a particular population in an endemic area. Because of the complexity of the immune system, our knowledge in this area is very limited, but the few glimpses we have suggest that wide vistas are yet to be opened.

HLA

The case of leprosy has already been mentioned, and this is the one on which most information is available. De Vries et al. reported in 1976 [18] nonrandom segregation of HLA types in sibs with the same type (lepromatous or tuberculoid) of the disease. Deviation from randomness was less conspicuous when sibs were discordant for the type of leprosy. Subsequently, preferential inheritance of HLA-DR2 was observed in tuberculoid leprosy [19], and an excess in the inheritance of the same HLA haplotypes was found when several sibs were affected. As a sort of control, the segregation of 31 other genetic markers was found to be random. It is likely that a wealth of older data on the "heredity" of leprosy and of the specific form of the disease [20–22] can be interpreted, in retrospect, as related to HLA. It is still somewhat controversial whether specific HLA alleles affect susceptibility to leprosy per se [21], or rather the development of a particular form of leprosy [22]. The next step in these studies must be to find the mechanism of such genetic determinants of the immune response, and it is very promising that antigen presentation to T-cell clones from leprosy patients has now been analyzed by transfection experiments [23], an approach by which it will be possible to test the role of individual HLA class II molecules encoded by allelic genes.

The message from this work is that genetic variation affects the immune response not only in a general way, but also specifically with respect to individual organisms or antigens. Indeed, there is now evidence that this may be true for viruses, such as hepatitis [7]; for a number of bacteria [23a]; for protozoa, such as trypanosomes (this has been shown thus far only in a mouse model system [13]) and malaria [24]; for metazoa, such as *Schistosoma* [25] and *Trichinella* (again in the mouse [26]).

Macrophage function

The complex role of these cells in the control of infection is discussed elsewhere in this volume (Chap. 17). Certainly it must be at least dual, since macrophages have been shown to be involved in antigen presentation, and they are, by definition, effectors of phagocytosis. Genetic variation of macrophage function is not yet well characterized in humans. However, in mice the number of macrophages that can form in vitro colonies is controlled by a single dominant gene. Also in this species a gene has been identified, and mapped on chromosome 1, that affects dramatically *Leishmania* infection (Table 13-4). The gene is expressed in Kupffer cells and in spleen macrophages, but not in macrophages collected from peritoneal exudates. The sensitivity allele *Lsh^s* is dominant over the resistance allele *Lsh^r* [13], perhaps by an immunosuppressive mechanism [27]. Obviously *Lsh^r* confers to mice a selective advantage in areas of *Leishmania* endemicity, but, interestingly, wild mice that have been tested were uniformly found to have this gene even in parts of the world where the sandfly vector is absent. This suggests that either the *Lsh^s* gene is detrimental in other ways as well, or that *Lsh* is closely linked to some other gene that has selective value. The *Ity* gene, which affects resistance to *Salmonella typhimurium* and which is closely linked to *Lsh,* gives a hint in this direction.

Other immunogenetic determinants

Given the complexity of the immune system, it is likely that there are many other ways in which this can behave differently in different individuals, as a result of genetic variation. For instance, it has been reported that mice with reduced "natural killer" cell activity have greater susceptibility to *P. chabaudi* infection [28]. By contrast, very little is known about biologically significant variation in humoral immunity. Studies of correlations between immunoglobulin allotypes and parasitic infection have often been unrewarding [29]. It is possible that because the immunoglobulin repertoire is vast in all people, appropriate antibodies can always be produced. However, it would be surprising if genetic variation in the number and structure of V genes did not occur, and therefore subtle qualitative and quantitative differences in specific antibody production are likely to be genetically determined and could be important in susceptibility to tropical diseases and the pattern of their clinical expression.

RED CELLS AND MALARIA

The balanced polymorphism of Hb S has become a prototype of our understanding of natural selection in the human species.

Already in 1949 J. B. S. Haldane had clearly identified *P. falciparum* malaria as a good candidate for shaping human evolution, because this disease (1) has been hyperendemic in large parts of the world for centuries or millennia; (2) it causes a high mortality rate; (3) much of this mortality takes place in the prereproductive age. It has been since fully established that AS heterozygotes suffer less high parasitemias, less cerebral malaria, and less mortality than AA homozygotes (reviewed in Ref. 10).

Subsequently, it was suggested that also G-6-PD deficiency might exert a protective effect [30,31], and this has also been confirmed. In this case the genetic situation is made unique by the fact that the G-6-PD gene is X-linked, and therefore female heterozygotes exhibit red cell mosaicism. It turns out that in a mosaic, when both G-6-PD–normal and G-6-PD–deficient red cells are available in the circulation, *P. falciparum* prefers the normal cells [32]. The mechanism for this is not yet clarified [33].

In the case of thalassemia, direct evidence of protection against malaria has been slow to come by. However, there is a very strong argument in favor of this idea, namely the extraordinary genetic heterogeneity of the thalassemia syndromes. This indicates that many mutational events have occurred, all giving rise to a thalassemia phenotype, but all independent from each other. Since these genes are detrimental in homozygotes, it is difficult to conceive how they could possibly have become polymorphic unless they were selected for. The fact that plasmodia are intraerythrocytic parasites, plus geography, suggests that malaria may be the selective force.

While these genetic features of red cells are important against *P. falciparum,* there is no evidence that they affect other plasmodial species. Unexpectedly, in 1975 Miller and his associates [9] discovered that Duffy-negative human red cells would not support the penetration of *P. knowlesi,* a simian malaria parasite regarded as closely related to human *P. vivax.* This finding was of interest, in terms of how plasmodia invade red cells, and also because it might explain the absence of this plasmodium in west Africa, where the entire population is Duffy-negative.

While several genes expressed in red cells seem to have been selected by one and the same environmental agent, malaria, it does not mean that the mechanism of resistance is always the same. On the contrary, there is evidence (Fig. 13-2) that different genes may act on invasion, on intracellular development of the parasite, or on the ultimate fate of parasitized cells.

THE "NEW GENETICS" AND TROPICAL DISEASES

It is likely that we have only skimmed the surface of genetic susceptibility to acquired diseases. Apart from many gaps in our knowledge, there is an important general consideration with respect to infectious and parasitic agents; namely, because they are themselves living organisms, they have their own genetic variation and their own evolution. Indeed, there is am-

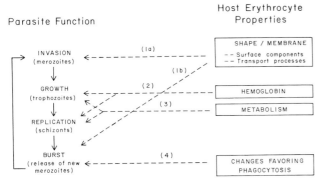

Parasite Function

Host Erythrocyte Properties

Figure 13-2. Interactions between human red cells and plasmodia. On the left is a scheme of the asexual schizogonic cycle of the malaria parasite. On the right are boxed the main features that may be subject to genetic change in the erythrocytes which host the asexual cycle. Broken-line arrows indicate some of the most likely ways in which a genetically determined change in the red cell may interfere with parasite development. 1a is best exemplified by the blockage of penetration of *P. knowlesi* in Fy(−) red cells (see the Duffy antigen). 1b is hypothetical. 2 may apply in various forms of abnormal hemoglobins and thalassemia. 3 may be pertinent to relative resistance of G-6-PD–deficient red cells, as observed in heterozygotes. 4 is likely to take place in *HbAS* heterozygotes, where parasitization produces sickling with consequent removal of parasitized red cells (see section on HbS). This scheme is obviously a gross oversimplification. For instance, shape factors, as in thalassemia (see section on abnormal hemoglobins and thalassemia) or in ovalocytosis may be important at any stage of parasite development, and so may be transport processes, since these are altered in malaria infection. (*From [10]*)

ple evidence that this is true for parasites [*34*] as well as their vectors [*35*].

In addition, there are probably many sorts of interactions that have not even been considered yet. We will quote just two examples here. (1) J. German [*36*] has attempted to connect two apparently totally unrelated epidemiological data: the relatively high prevalence of a genetic disorder, xeroderma pigmentosum (XP), in Egypt and Japan, where schistosomiasis is also endemic. The hypothesis was made that during penetration of the skin by cercariae, these are exposed to ultraviolet sunlight, which might cause DNA damage. If the parasite relies on host enzymes for DNA repair, this might be inadequate in XP heterozygotes, who would thus not allow development of the adult worms. At the moment, this is merely a hypothesis (if it is correct, XP would be another example of balanced polymorphism), but it can be tested experimentally. (2) A monoclonal antibody raised against rat neurone membranes has been found to recognize also a component of *Trypanosoma cruzi* [*37*]. Clearly, this finding could explain major features of the pathogenesis and pathology of Chagas' disease.

Parasitism is unique because two organisms are forced, in a way, to evolve together [*38*]. As they share an ecological niche, they may also share portions of their genome. The mon-

oclonal recombinant DNA revolution has given us the technology to test such possibilities. Indeed, it is not unlikely that various parasites may have in their genomes surprises still in store for the molecular biologist, partly because they belong to a variety of taxonomic groups within protozoa and metazoa, and partly because of their unique feature of coevolving with the host. The most spectacular example of this is in the apparently unique mechanism of antigenic variation in *Trypanosomatidae* [*39*], a novel system ideally suited for the analysis of gene expression. One might say that *Trypanosoma* has already become, in this respect, the *E. coli* of parasitology. In the same family of organisms, parasitic kinetoplast DNA probes are already in use for diagnostic purposes [*40*].

REFERENCES

*1 Lewin B: *Gene III*. New York, Wiley-Interscience, 1987

*2 Luzzatto L: Sickle cell anaemia in tropical Africa. Clin Haematol 10:757–784, 1981

3 McKusick VA: *Mendelian Inheritance in Man*, 8th ed. Baltimore, Johns Hopkins, 1987

4 Embury SH, Dozy AM, Miller J, et al: Concurrent sickle cell anemia and α-thalassemia: Effect on severity of anemia. N Engl J Med 306:270–274, 1982

*5 Sadis JA, Brewerton DA: HLA, ankylosing spondylitis and rheumatoid arthritis. Br Med Bull 34:275–278, 1978

6 Uno H, Sasazuki T, Taura H, et al: Two major genes, linked to HLA and Gm, control susceptibility to Graves' disease. Nature 292:768–770, 1981

7 Whittingham S, Mathews JD, Schanfield MS, et al: Interaction of HLA and Gm in autoimmune chronic hepatitis. Clin Exp Immunol 43:80–86, 1981

8 Daniellssen DC, Boeck W: *Traite de la Spedalskhed*. Paris, Bailliere, 1848

9 Miller LH: Hypothesis on the mechanism of erythrocyte invasion by malaria mesozoites. Bull WHO 55:157–162, 1971

*10 Luzzatto L: Genetics of red cells and susceptibility to malaria. Blood 54:961–976, 1979

11 de Vries RRP, van Rood JJ: HLA and infectious diseases. Arch Dermatol Res 264:89–95, 1979

12 Cooper DN, Clayton JF: DNA polymorphism and the study of disease associations. Hum Genet 78:299–312, 1988

*13 Bradley DJ, Blackwell JM: Genetics of susceptibility to infection, in Michal F (ed): *Modern Genetic Concepts and Techniques in the Study of Parasites*. Basel, Schwabe, 1981

*14 Skamene E, Kongshavn PAL, Landy M (eds): *Genetic Control of Natural Resistance to Infection and Malignancy*. London, Academic, 1980

*15 Cavalli-Sforza LL, Bodmer WF: *The Genetics of Human Populations*. San Francisco, Freeman, 1971

16 Piazza A, Menozzi P, Cavalli-Sforza LL: Synthetic gene frequency maps of man and selective effects of climate. Proc Natl Acad Sci USA 78:2638–2642, 1981

17 Roychoudhury AK, Nei M: *Human Polymorphic Genes—World Distribution*. Oxford, Oxford University Press, 1988

*This article is a review of the literature.

18 de Vries RRP, Lai A, Fat RFM, et al: HLA-linked genetic control of host response to *Mycobacterium leprae*. Lancet ii:1328–1330, 1976

19 Van Elden MJ, de Vries RRP, Mehra NK, et al: HLA segregation of tuberculoid leprosy: Confirmation of the DR2 marker. J Infect Dis 141:693–701, 1980

20 Serjeantson S, Wilson SR, Keats BJB: The genetics of leprosy. Ann Hum Biol 6:375–393, 1979

21 Jazwinska EO, Serjeantson SW: HLA-DR, -DQ DNA genotyping and T-cell receptor RFLPs in leprosy. Dis Markers 6:173–183, 1988

22 van-Eden W, Gonzales NM, de Vries RR, et al: HLA-linked control of predisposition to lepromatous leprosy. J Infect Dis 151:9–14, 1985

*23 Skamene E: Genetic control of resistance of bacterial infections, in Skamene E, Kongshavn PAL, Landy M (eds): *Genetic Control of Natural Resistance to Infection and Malignancy*. London, Academic, 1980

23a Wilkinson D, de Vries RR, Madrigal JA, et al: Analysis of HLA-DR glycoproteins by DNA-mediated gene transfer. Definition of DR2 beta gene products and antigen presentation to T cell clones from leprosy patients. J Exp Med 167:1442–1458, 1988

24 Piazza A, Mayr WR, Contu L, et al: Genetic and population structure of four Sardinian villages. Ann Hum Genet 49:47–63, 1985

*25 Mahmoud AAF: Genetics of schistosomiasis, in Michal F (ed): *Modern Genetic Concepts and Techniques in the Study of Parasites*. Basel, Schwabe, 1981, pp 303–322

26 Wassom DL, David CS, Gleich GJ: MHC-linked genetic control of the immune response to parasites: *Trichinella spiralis* in the mouse, in Skamene E, Kongshavn PAL, Landy M (eds): *Genetic Control of Natural Resistance to Infection and Malignancy*. London, Academic, 1980, pp 75–82

27 Nickol AD, Bonventre PF: Visceral leishmaniasis in congenic mice of susceptible and resistant phenotypes: T-lymphocyte-mediated immunosuppression. Infect Immun 50:169–174, 1985

28 Eugui EM, Allison AC: Malaria infections in different strains of mice and their correlation with natural killer activity. Bull WHO 57(suppl 1):231–238, 1979

29 Yogore MG, Schanfield MS: Immunoglobulin allotypes in Filipinos. I. Lack of association between *Schistosoma japonicum* infection and immunoglobulin allotypes. Immunogenetics 8:419–423, 1981

*30 Motulsky AG: Metabolic polymorphisms and the role of infectious diseases in human evolution. Hum Biol 32:28–44, 1960

31 Allison AC: Glucose 6-phosphate dehydrogenase deficiency in red blood cells of East Africans. Nature 186:531–533, 1960

32 Luzzatto L, Usanga EA, Reddy S: Glucose 6-phosphate dehydrogenase deficient red cells: Resistance to infection by malarial parasites. Science 164:939–941, 1969

*33 Charmot G: Facteurs congenitaux et facteurs genetiques dans la resistance au paludisme a *P. falciparum* en Afrique tropicale. Med Trop (Madrid) 40:657–665, 1980

*34 Walliker D: Genetics of parasites, in Michal F (ed): *Modern Genetic Concepts and Techniques in the Study of Parasites*. Basel, Schwabe, 1981

35 Richards CS: Genetic studies on variation in infectivity of *Schistosoma mansoni*. J Parasitol 61:233–236, 1975

36 German J: *Xeroderma pigmentosum*, defective DNA repair—and schistosomiasis? Ann Genet (Paris) 23:69–72, 1980

37 Wood JN, Hudson L, Jessel TM, et al: A monoclonal antibody defining antigenic determinants of subpopulations of mammalian nemones and *Trypanosoma cruzi* parasites. Nature 296:34–38, 1982

*38 Clark B: The ecological genetics of host-parasite relationships, in Taylor AE, Muller R (ed): *Genetic Aspects of Host-Parasite Relationships*. Oxford, Blackwell, 1976, pp 87–103

39 Wirth DF, Pratt DM: Rapid identification of *Leishmania* species by specific hybridization of kinetoplast DNA in cutaneous lesions. Proc Natl Acad Sci USA 79:6999–7003, 1982

*40 Borst P, Cross GAM: Molecular basis for Trypanosome antigenic variation. Cell 29:291–303, 1982

Common Genetic Disorders in the Tropics · David J. Weatherall

Many genetic diseases occur at about the same frequency in tropical countries as elsewhere. There are some unexplained differences, the relative rarity of cystic fibrosis and phenylketonuria in Africans and Orientals, for example. As in temperate zones, there is some unevenness of distribution of genetic variants in populations due to founder effects and gene drift. However, one group of genetic disorders, the inherited anemias, is extremely common in some tropical countries, probably because heterozygous carriers are or have been protected against *Plasmodium falciparum* malaria.

The two most important types of inherited anemias are the hemoglobinopathies and glucose-6-phosphate dehydrogenase (G-6-PD) deficiency. The hemoglobinopathies occur at very high frequencies in some populations and produce a major public health problem. G-6-PD deficiency, while less of a world health problem, is of considerable importance because it causes hemolytic reactions to drugs used commonly in tropical medicine; it is also responsible for favism, neonatal jaundice, and hemolysis associated with a variety of intercurrent illnesses.

THE HEMOGLOBINOPATHIES

The hemoglobinopathies are genetic disorders of the structure or synthesis of hemoglobin. Before describing them it is necessary to review briefly the structure and genetic control of normal human hemoglobin. Readers who wish to pursue this subject more fully should consult one of the many reviews or monographs that deal with the human hemoglobin field [1–3].

THE STRUCTURE AND GENETIC CONTROL OF NORMAL HUMAN HEMOGLOBIN

Human hemoglobin is heterogeneous at all stages of development. Several embryonic hemoglobins are produced which are replaced by fetal hemoglobin (Hb F) at about 8 weeks' gestation. Just before birth Hb F synthesis declines and by the

age of 1 year the adult hemoglobins, Hb A and Hb A_2, are fully established. In normal adults Hb A_2 makes up about 2.5 percent of the total hemoglobin and only trace amounts of Hb F are produced. The mechanisms which regulate this series of adaptive changes are not understood.

All the human hemoglobins have a similar basic structure; they consist of two pairs of peptide chains, each associated with a heme molecule. Both Hb A and Hb F have a pair of α chains. In adult life these are paired with β chains to form Hb A ($\alpha_2\beta_2$) and with δ chains to form Hb A_2 ($\alpha_2\delta_2$). In fetal life α chains combine with γ chains to form Hb F ($\alpha_2\gamma_2$), which is heterogeneous; there are two varieties of γ chains which differ in their amino acid composition only at position 136, which may contain either glycine or alanine; γ chains which contain glycine at position 136 are called $^G\gamma$ chains and those which contain alanine are called $^A\gamma$ chains. There is an embryonic α-like chain (ζ chain) which combines with ϵ (embryonic β-like) chains and γ chains to form the embryonic hemoglobins Gower 1 ($\zeta_2\epsilon_2$) and Portland ($\zeta_2\gamma_2$). Some α chains are also synthesized early in embryonic life; these combine with ϵ chains to form the other embryonic hemoglobin, Gower 2 ($\alpha_2\epsilon_2$).

The structure and organization of the genetic control of the human hemoglobins is summarized in Fig. 14-1. The genes which encode the α-like and β-like globin chains have been isolated from bacteriophage lambda libraries of human DNA, and their structures have been determined [4]. All the globin genes have one or more noncoding inserts [intervening sequences (IVS) or introns] at a similar position along their length. For example, all the non-α globin genes contain two inserts of 122 to 130 and 850 to 900 bp between codons 30 and 31 and 104 and 105, respectively. These genes are transcribed into a large-molecular-weight precursor messenger RNA (mRNA), and the introns are excised, and the remaining pieces of the mRNA (exons) are spliced together before the definitive mRNA molecule is delivered to the cell cytoplasm

Figure 14-1. The genetic control of human hemoglobin synthesis.

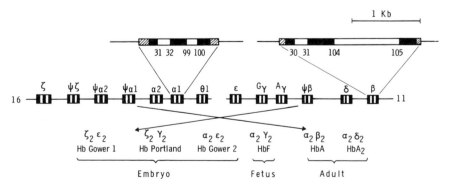

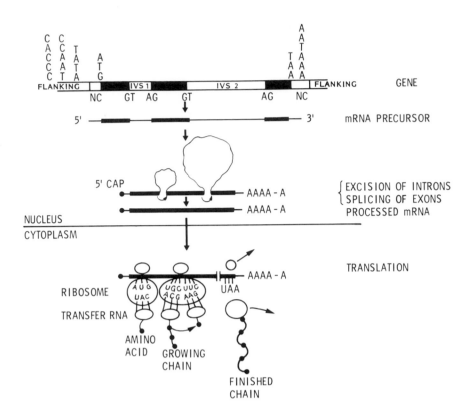

Figure 14-2. The transcription and translation of a human globin gene.

(Fig. 14-2). Very little is known about the regulation of these gene loci; it appears to be mediated mainly at the transcriptional level.

GENETIC DISORDERS OF HEMOGLOBIN

There are three main groups of genetic disorders of hemoglobin. First, there are the structural hemoglobin variants, most of which result from single amino acid substitutions in the α or β globin chains. Second, there are the thalassemias, disorders which are characterized by a reduced rate of synthesis of one or more of the globin chains. Finally, there are conditions in which the switch from Hb F to Hb A synthesis is defective; they are given the descriptive title "hereditary persistence of fetal hemoglobin (HPFH)." They are of no clinical significance except that they can modify the clinical course of some of the more important hemoglobinopathies.

THE STRUCTURAL HEMOGLOBIN VARIANTS

More than 400 structural hemoglobin variants have been detected during the last 25 years, the majority of which have single amino acid substitutions in the α or β chains [1]. A few result from deletions of one or more amino acids, insertions of additional amino acids, chain termination or frame shift mutations, or from other novel molecular lesions. Originally these variants were named by letters of the alphabet, but these have long been used up, and "new" hemoglobin variants are now named after the place of their discovery. Most of them are not associated with disease. Therefore their detection has depended on electrophoretic screening techniques. It has been estimated that 1 in 800 individuals carries an electrophoretic hemoglobin variant; perhaps 1 in 300 has a variant of any sort [5].

Some hemoglobin variants, because they alter the functional properties or stability of the molecule, cause a clinical disorder. For instance, several different amino acid substitutions interfere with heme-heme interaction and hence produce a high-oxygen-affinity hemoglobin which is associated with a familial polycythemia [6]. Others cause permanent methemoglobinemia and hence are responsible for one form of genetically determined cyanosis [1]. Yet another group, in which the amino acid substitutions cause instability of the molecule, is characterized by a chronic hemolytic anemia due to hemoglobin precipitation and Heinz body formation; in some cases the instability is so mild that hemolysis occurs only after the administration of oxidant drugs [7]. Because they have not been selected for, all these variants are rare. They have been described in detail in several recent reviews [1,2,6,7]. Here, we shall concentrate on the structural variants which occur frequently enough to produce a major public health problem—hemoglobins S, C, and E.

Table 14-1. The commoner sickling disorders

Sickle cell anemia
Hemoglobin SC disease
Hemoglobin SD disease
Hemoglobin S–O Arab disease
Hemoglobin S–β thalassemia
Hemoglobin S–α thalassemia
Hemoglobin S–hereditary persistence of fetal hemoglobin

THE SICKLING DISORDERS

The sickling disorders include the homozygous state for the sickle cell gene, sickle cell anemia, and the heterozygous state for the sickle cell gene in combination with genes for either structural hemoglobin variants or different types of thalassemia. These conditions are summarized in Table 14-1.

Etiology and pathophysiology

Hemoglobin S differs from Hb A by the substitution of valine for glutamic acid at the sixth position in the β chain. Although the clinical features of sickle cell anemia should be explainable by this substitution, it is still not absolutely certain why it causes red cells to sickle. In 1950 Harris showed that if a concentrated solution of Hb S is deoxygenated, liquid crystals, or tactoids, are formed [8]. He concluded that sickling of red cells is due to polymerization of abnormal hemoglobin molecules into elongated fibers. Electron micrographs of sickled cells show bundles of long, straight fibers whose axis is parallel to the long axis of the sickle cell. These fibers have a diameter of approximately 17 nm with spacing between them ranging from 18 to 24 nm. Fibers of deoxygenated Hb S transform into needlelike crystals under appropriate conditions. X-ray diffraction analysis shows that the fibers and crystals have a similar structure. In the crystal form, peripheral strands are packed around central strands, either parallel or antiparallel and either half staggered or in register. The contact regions between the strands involve the mutation site β6 Val on one molecule and the hydrophobic residues between the E and F helices of a neighboring molecule in the other strand of the pair. These studies suggest that the pairing of strands and their aggregation may be the molecular basis for sickling [1,2].

When the oxygen tension of Hb S–containing red cells is lowered to a critical point, intracellular polymerization of hemoglobin occurs which leads to the formation of sickled red cells. In Hb S homozygotes sickling occurs first at oxygen saturations below 85 percent and is nearly complete at 38 percent. Red cells containing Hb S go through cycles of sickling and unsickling until, finally, an irreversibly sickled cell (ISC) is formed; variable numbers of ISC can be seen in the peripheral blood of patients with sickle cell anemia. It is believed that sickled cells lose their flexibility after they have given up their oxygen in the tissues and that the resulting increase in mechanical fragility leads to their premature destruction in the microcirculation. It is now apparent that the pathophysiology

of the anemia and vascular occlusion of the sickling disorders has a more complex basis than that outlined above. For example, sickle cells tend to adhere to vascular endothelial cells [9], where they are apparently recognised by monocytes and macrophages, suggesting that one component of the anemia of the sickling disorders is accelerated erythrophagocytosis [10]. Furthermore, because sickle cell membranes have increased amounts of membrane-associated hemichrome, there may also be autooxidative damage to sickle red cells [11,12].

The vascular occlusion that occurs in the sickling disorders may be exacerbated by adherence of sickle cells to the vascular endothelium. Presumably once vascular occlusion has occurred in small vessels, it is amplified by a vicious circle of stasis, sickling, and further occlusion. If this process continues, the end result is infarction of tissue in the region supplied by the blocked vessel.

Thus, sickle cell anemia is characterized by chronic anemia and tissue damage due to recurrent blockage of the microcirculation. Many factors influence the rate of sickling; these include the level of Hb F, the mean cell hemoglobin concentration (MCHC), and the mean cell hemoglobin (MCH), which may be modified by the coexistence of one or more forms of thalassemia [1–3,13].

The distribution of the sickle cell gene

The distribution of the sickle cell gene is summarized in Fig. 14-3. It is found in a broad belt across tropical Africa, sporadically in some Mediterranean populations, in parts of the Middle East, and in large regions of India. The carrier rate in these populations ranges from 5 to 30 percent of the population. Recently, it has been possible to trace the history of the sickle cell gene by analyzing its association with different patterns of restriction endonuclease polymorphisms in the β globin gene cluster [14]. These studies suggest that the mutation has arisen independently in west Africa and somewhere in India or the Middle East (Fig. 14-3).

The sickle cell trait

Individuals with the sickle cell trait have approximately 30 to 35 percent Hb S (Fig. 14-4). The condition is rarely associated with any clinical abnormality. Spontaneous hematuria or splenic infarction has been reported in persons who have flown in unpressurized aircraft at high altitudes or who have become unusually hypoxic during anesthesia.

Sickle cell anemia

Sickle cell anemia is a common and sometimes incapacitating disorder [15–17]. It has been the subject of a monograph [15] and many reviews [1,2,16,17] and will only be described in outline here. The major clinical features include chronic hemolytic anemia, susceptibility to infection, tissue damage, and, most importantly, the occurrence of acute exacerbations or crises which may be life-threatening.

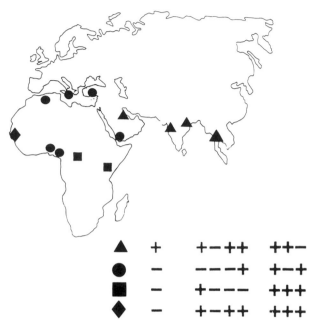

Figure 14-3. The distribution of the sickle cell gene. The different patterns of + and − reflect the presence or absence of particular restriction fragment length polymorphism sites along the β globin gene cluster (β globin gene haplotype). It is clear that the haplotypes in the Middle East and India are different from those in Africa, indicating an independent origin of the sickle cell gene in Africa and the Middle East. (*Based on [14].*)

Presentation and Course. Patients with severe sickle cell anemia usually present in the first year of life, either with anemia following an intercurrent infection, or with attacks of painful swelling of the hands and feet, the ''hand and foot syndrome.'' These episodes, which are due to dactylitis, usually last for several weeks. X-rays of the hands or feet may be normal, although there may be cortical thickening and bone destruction with healing. These episodes usually subside without sequelae, but infarction and destruction of the carpal and metacarpal bones may occur and lead to shortening of the fingers.

The course through childhood is characterized by chronic anemia with mild jaundice; affected children are remarkably active despite their low hemoglobin levels. Apart from pallor and icterus the only characteristic physical finding early in life is splenomegaly. However, because of repeated infarction the spleen gradually regresses and is not usually palpable in children over the age of 12 years.

Anemia. Steady-state hemoglobin values range from 6 to 10 g/dL with an associated reticulocytosis, usually in the 10 to 20 percent range. The peripheral blood film shows anisochromia and a variable number of sickled red cells. There is marked erythroid hyperplasia of the bone marrow.

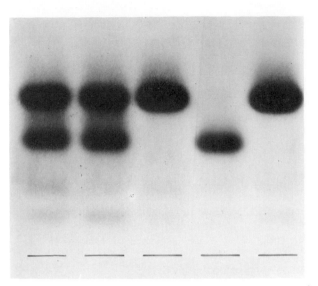

Figure 14-4. The hemoglobin electrophoretic pattern in sickle cell anemia and sickle cell trait. Left to right: 1 and 2, sickle cell trait; 3, normal adult hemoglobin; 4, sickle cell anemia; 5, normal adult. Starch gel electrophoresis, pH 8.5, protein-stained.

Infection. Children with sickle cell anemia are unusually prone to infection, mainly pneumococcal, although other organisms including *Haemophilus influenzae* and members of the typhoid group may play a role [16,17]. The reason for the susceptibility to infection is still not understood. In part it may result from abnormal reticuloendothelial function, particularly hyposplenism [18]. It is not clear, however, why children with hyposplenism are particularly prone to pneumococcal infection. The spleen may be necessary for antibody formation or for antigen processing. Other possible mechanisms include a deficiency of pneumococcal serum-opsonizing activity or a related abnormality in the properdin pathway with impaired fixation of the first component of complement to pneumococci [19].

Sickle Cell Crises. A classification of clinical forms of sickling crises is shown in Table 14-2. Their designation as painful,

Table 14-2. Sickling crises

Vasoocclusive:
  Bone
  Abdominal
  Lung
  Neurological
Hemolytic
Aplastic
Sequestration:
  Spleen
  Liver
Mixed

hemolytic, aplastic, and so on is rather artificial because in many cases more than one pathological mechanism may be occurring simultaneously.

The commonest form is the "painful" crisis. Although these episodes may be triggered by infection and dehydration, often it is impossible to find a precipitating cause. However, it seems likely that the basic defect is intravascular sickling with infarction of tissue. These episodes are characterized by severe pain in the back and limbs; local bone pain may simulate osteomyelitis. Other organs may be involved. The "chest syndrome" is the name given to an acute pulmonary disorder characterized by fever, pleuritic pain, and infiltrates on the chest x-ray. These episodes are probably due to pulmonary vascular occlusion [20]. "Abdominal crises" are characterized by pain associated with generalized tenderness and, sometimes, distension of the abdomen with reduced bowel sounds, which may simulate a perforated viscus. Vasoocclusive episodes may involve the central nervous system, with fits and focal neurological signs. All these different types of vasoocclusive episodes tend to last for a few days, after which they gradually subside. They may leave in their wake a series of complications due to permanent tissue damage.

Hemolytic crises are characterized by rapidly progressive anemia associated with an increase in the reticulocyte count. In aplastic crises there is a "shutdown" of erythropoiesis, and because of the shortened red cell survival, profound anemia may develop over a period of a few hours. Recent work suggests that these episodes are associated with parvovirus infections [21].

Sequestration crises are the commonest cause of infant death in sickle cell anemia [22]. An already enlarged spleen rapidly becomes engorged with blood; most of the circulating red cells may be trapped over a few hours. There is a sudden onset of shock associated with a rapidly enlarging spleen. An infant who has had an episode of this type is likely to have a second one. A similar picture can occur in adults; in this case sequestration of red cells occurs in the liver.

Chronic Tissue Damage. Repeated blockage of small vessels can lead to widespread tissue damage, resulting in a variety of complications. The bones are particularly vulnerable. X-rays of the spine may reveal sclerosis, and repeated infarction of the heads of the humerus or femur may lead to aseptic necrosis [15–17]. Occasionally, bone infarcts become infected; staphylococci or organisms of the *Salmonella* group are usually involved. Recurrent ulceration of the skin over the inner and lower aspects of the tibia is common. There is progressive impairment of renal concentrating capacity with increasing age. In early childhood this is reversible by blood transfusion; this is not the case later in life, and renal failure is a common cause of death in adults [15]. Hematuria due to papillary necrosis is common. Occasionally, a nephrotic syndrome develops. Recurrent priapism may lead to permanent fibrosis and

deformity of the penis. Although commoner in hemoglobin SC disease, ocular abnormalities occur in sickle cell anemia [23]. They are characterized by pallor of the peripheral retina, tortuosity of the vessels, and peripheral arteriovenous anomalies. Cardiovascular abnormalities are less common; there is often cardiomegaly with a variety of flow murmurs due to anemia. There may be chronic impairment of pulmonary function due to repeated pulmonary infarction. Rarely, widespread infarction of the liver leads to fibrosis and permanent impairment of liver function. Gallstones are common, as are cholecystitis and ascending cholangitis. Infarction of the central nervous system may result in chronic epilepsy or in a variety of chronic focal neurological lesions.

Pregnancy is sometimes associated with more frequent vasoocclusive episodes, and there is an increased maternal and fetal morbidity and mortality [24].

Diagnosis. Sickle cell anemia is diagnosed by the characteristic hematological changes together with a positive sickling test, the most reliable of which is to observe sickling in a drop of blood mixed with freshly prepared 2% sodium metabisulfite under a sealed microscope slide [3]. The diagnosis is confirmed by hemoglobin electrophoresis which shows Hb S and Hb A_2 with a variable increase in Hb F; Hb A is absent [3] (Fig. 14-4). Each parent shows the sickle cell trait. The differentiation of sickle cell anemia from the various interactions of the sickle cell and thalassemia genes is considered later.

Prognosis and Racial Variation in Severity. Remarkably little is known about the natural history of sickle cell anemia, although it is becoming apparent that the disease has a very variable course and prognosis, even within members of the same racial group. While survival to adult life is now commonplace in the United States, parts of Europe, and the Caribbean, this is not the case in rural Africa [25]. In a survey in Kenya, although there were approximately 25 percent sickle cell carriers at birth, no adults with sickle cell disease could be found. It seems likely that in these rural populations lack of adequate medical care and health education results in a high mortality early in infancy, due mainly to bacterial infection and malaria [15]. The mortality early in life in Jamaica is approximately 10 percent; death is usually due to sequestration crises [22]. In the United States and Great Britain the early mortality is approximately 5 percent. Again, infection is the main cause, as it is at all ages, although in Jamaica progressive renal failure is an increasingly important cause of death in adults [15].

In parts of Saudi Arabia [26,27] and India [28] the disease is very mild. This may be due to the production of unusually high levels of Hb F. There is also a high incidence of α thalassemia in these populations; studies in the United States and the Caribbean indicate that α thalassemia can ameliorate the clinical course of sickle cell anemia [29]. Whether these two mechanisms are entirely responsible for the mildness of the disorder in these populations or whether climatic, economic, or other genetic factors are also involved remains to be seen.

Other sickling disorders

Hemoglobin SC Disease [1,2,15,30]. This condition runs a milder course than sickle cell anemia; there are fewer crises, and the anemia is less severe. However, it is important because of the occurrence of serious vasooclusive complications. These include ocular lesions characterized by vitreous hemorrhages and retinitis proliferans, sometimes leading to retinal detachment and blindness. Other complications include recurrent hematuria, avascular necrosis of the heads of the femora, and a variety of acute respiratory syndromes. The latter tend to occur late in pregnancy or in the puerperium and are frequently misdiagnosed as pneumonia. Hemoglobin SC disease is diagnosed by the finding of a mild anemia with a blood film which shows many target cells, sickled forms, and cells with crystals; hemoglobin electrophoresis shows Hb S and Hb C; one parent has the Hb S trait and the other the Hb C trait.

With the exception of the different interactions of the sickling disorders with thalassemia, other sickling combinations are rare (Table 14-1). Hemoglobin SD disease may be associated with a clinical picture identical to sickle cell anemia, while Hb SE disease is a much milder condition.

The treatment of the sickling disorders

Prevention. Since the heterozygous state for the sickle cell gene is easily identified, the condition could be prevented by population screening and prospective genetic counseling. However, where this has been tried, it has not been successful, and the only practical approach is to identify carrier females early in pregnancy, and if their husbands are also carriers, to offer the couple the option of prenatal diagnosis and therapeutic abortion. This can be done by fetal blood sampling or by direct analysis of the globin genes in DNA obtained from amniotic fluid or by chorionic villus sampling [31]. The techniques are similar to those which are applied to the prenatal diagnosis of thalassemia. However, because of uncertainty about the prognosis of any individual patient, wide-scale application of this approach is not yet recommended, and it should be reserved for women who have already had one severely affected child and who are particularly keen not to have another child with the disorder.

Management of Established Cases. Between crises, except for good general pediatric care, no special treatment is required. Parents should be warned about the dangers of infection and told to report early if any unusual symptoms develop. Antimalarial drugs and folic acid supplements should be administered regularly. Great care should be taken if an anesthetic is required, and dehydration and hypoxia avoided. Major surgery may require transfusion or exchange transfusion (see

below). It is now common practice to give prophylactic penicillin and/or pneumococcal vaccine to affected children; although the results of extensive trials are not yet available, one study [31a] suggests that daily penicillin will reduce the incidence of life-threatening infection in the early years of life. Similar data obtained in Jamaica are less encouraging [15].

A painful crisis is best treated in hospital with careful clinical and hematological surveillance, hydration with intravenous fluids, oxygen therapy, and adequate analgesia. Although there is the risk of addiction, powerful analgesics should not be withheld. The pain of sickling crisis can be excruciating; usually it lasts for only a few days and the strength of the analgesics can be reduced rapidly. Infection should be treated with appropriate antibiotics. The hematocrit and reticulocyte count should be monitored at regular intervals. During an uncomplicated painful crisis there is no place for blood transfusion. However, if there is hyperhemolysis with a rapidly falling hemoglobin level and climbing reticulocyte count, or if the reticulocyte count falls suggesting an impending aplastic crisis, the patient should receive a blood transfusion. In young infants it is important to examine the abdomen several times a day so that splenic sequestration can be diagnosed early; the cardinal sign is a rapidly enlarging spleen. This complication is also managed by blood transfusion.

In patients with recurrent crises and those who need major surgery or have had neurological or lung crises, it is advisable to reduce the number of sickleable cells below 40 percent. If the initial hematocrit is low, this can be achieved by hypertransfusion; if not, an exchange transfusion is required. The rationale for this approach is that if high hematocrits are obtained without significantly reducing the number of sickleable cells, increased blood viscosity and sluggish flow may lead to further intravascular sickling. Once the level of sickleable cells is reduced below 40 percent, it can be maintained by regular "top-up" transfusions which "shut down" red cell production. The use of hypertransfusion during pregnancy is controversial. If pregnant women are having repeated crises or other complications, it is probably safer to maintain the number of sickleable cells below 40 percent by transfusion until after delivery. On the other hand, many women have a relatively uneventful pregnancy, and routine transfusion is not recommended [24,32]; recent trials have shown it to be of no value.

Occasionally, in early childhood the spleen may enlarge to such a degree that secondary hypersplenism occurs; this complication is usually seen in malarious areas [15–17]. In such cases splenectomy may be indicated. Similarly, because sequestration crises seem to recur in the same infant, one episode may be an indication for splenectomy [22].

Current research is directed toward trying to prevent sickling by the development of agents which inhibit polymerization of Hb S by disrupting intramolecular bonds, decrease the intracellular concentration of deoxy Hb S, or stabilize the red cell membrane [33]. Several promising agents have been produced, but none are yet developed for clinical use. Cyanate, by reacting with free amino groups (carbamylation), maintains Hb S in the oxy configuration and thus inhibits sickling [15]. It is too toxic to give systematically; extracorporeal carbamylation may be a useful form of treatment for severely affected patients if facilities are available.

HEMOGLOBIN C AND E DISORDERS [1,2]

Hemoglobin C occurs mainly in west Africa and sporadically in north Africa and in some of the Mediterranean populations. The homozygous state for Hb C is characterized by a mild hemolytic anemia with splenomegaly. The blood picture is remarkable for the presence of almost 100 percent target cells; there is a mild anemia and a low-grade reticulocytosis. No treatment is required.

Hemoglobin E is the commonest hemoglobin variant in the world population. It occurs in high frequency throughout southeast Asia, Burma, India, and as far west as some scattered pockets in the Middle East. There have been a few reports of the variant in Turkey, but it is not seen in the Mediterranean region. In parts of Thailand and Vietnam the carrier rate approaches 50 percent of the population.

The homozygous state for Hb E is an extremely mild condition characterized by a symptomless anemia and usually the spleen is not palpable. The peripheral blood shows a very similar picture to that of heterozygous β thalassemia. There is hypochromia with a reduced mean cell volume (MCV) and MCH, but no evidence of significant hemolysis. The clinical importance of Hb E is its interaction with β thalassemia. In Thailand several syndromes caused by the interaction of hemoglobin E with α thalassemia have been described [3]. The clinical manifestations of these conditions are due to the effects of α thalassemia.

THE THALASSEMIAS

The thalassemias are genetic disorders of hemoglobin synthesis characterized by a reduced rate of production of one or more of the globin chains [3]. They are classified, according to which chain is affected, into the α, β, δ, $\delta\beta$, and $\gamma\delta\beta$ thalassemias. Clinically, the α and β thalassemias are the most important.

The α thalassemias

Because α chains are shared by both fetal and adult hemoglobin, the α thalassemias affect hemoglobin synthesis in both fetal and adult life. At the phenotypic level several well-defined forms of α thalassemia can be recognized. These are the Hb Bart's hydrops syndrome, Hb H disease, and two carrier states; a more severe and easily recognizable form called α thalassemia 1, or α^0 thalassemia, and a milder or "silent" form, α thalassemia 2, or α^+ thalassemia. The homozygous state for α^0 thalassemia produces the Hb Bart's hydrops syndrome, and the compound heterozygous state for α^+ and α^0 thalassemia results in Hb H disease. In many oriental populations there is a common α chain variant called Hb Constant Spring. Because it is synthesized at a reduced rate, it produces the phenotype of α^+ thalassemia. Hence, Hb H disease can also result from the compound heterozygous state for α^0 thalassemia and Hb Constant Spring.

Distribution [2,3]. The α^+ thalassemias are common in parts of west Africa and in countries with a large west African immigrant population. α^0 Thalassemia is extremely rare in these populations, and hence the Hb Bart's hydrops syndrome and Hb H disease are not seen. Both α^0 and α^+ thalassemia occur frequently in some of the Mediterranean island populations, in parts of Greece, throughout the Middle East, and at a particularly high frequency in a line starting in southern China, passing through Laos, Thailand, and the Malay Peninsula, and ending in some of the island populations of Indonesia and New Guinea. These disorders reach their highest frequency in parts of Melanesia and Polynesia, where up to 80 percent of the population is heterozygous for one or another forms of α thalassemia. Thus Hb H disease and the Hb Bart's hydrops syndrome are frequently seen in southeast Asia, but are less common in the Mediterranean region and the Middle East.

Molecular Genetics and Pathophysiology [1–3,34]. In fetal life defective α chain production results in an excess of γ chains which form γ_4 tetramers or Hb Bart's. Similarly, in adult life excess β chains produced in the presence of defective α chain synthesis form homotetramers with the structure β_4 or Hb H. Hb H and Hb Bart's have an extremely high oxygen affinity and are physiologically useless. Thus, the α thalassemias are characterized by defective hemoglobin synthesis with hypochromic red cells, and the presence in the cells of varying amounts of homotetramers which are of no value for oxygen transport. Furthermore, Hb H is unstable and forms inclusion bodies as red cells age; these rigid structures cause damage to the red cells in their passage through the spleen and hence result in hemolysis.

The α^0 thalassemias, in which there is loss of both linked α globin genes on chromosome 16, all result from deletions. To date, nine such deletions have been described. In all but one variety both α globin genes are removed; in one case the deletion ends approximately 17 kb* upstream from the α globin genes but appears to completely inactivate them.

The α^+ thalassemias, in which one α globin gene is inactivated, can be classified into deletion and nondeletion types. There are a variety of deletions involving one of the α globin genes, the commonest being those that remove either 3.7 or 4.2 kb. It seems likely that these have resulted from misalignment and unequal crossing over; the triplicated α globin gene arrangements, $\alpha\alpha\alpha^{anti-3.7}$ and $\alpha\alpha\alpha^{anti-4.2}$, have been observed in many populations.

*kb = 1000 nucleotide bases.

A variety of molecular forms of α^+ thalassemia in which the genes are not deleted have been observed. These result from a number of different molecular lesions. In some cases there is defective RNA processing. For example, one common form of nondeletion α^+ thalassemia results from the loss of 5 bp at the 5' splice junction of IVS 1 of the α2 globin gene. Another mutation, which is common in the Middle East, involves a base substitution in the polyadenylation signal (see Fig. 14-2) which is reflected by the change AATAAA→AATAAG in the α2 genes. Another class of mutations involves messenger RNA translation. Two of these mutations involve single-base substitutions in the initiator codon. At least four mutations have been described that affect the termination of translation; single-base changes in the α chain termination codon allow the insertion of an amino acid with subsequent read-through of messenger RNA which is not normally translated; hence the synthesis of an elongated α chain. This is the molecular basis for Hb Constant Spring and a family of similar chain termination mutants. Finally, several α^+ thalassemias have been described that result from amino acid substitutions in the α globin genes that cause gross instability in their products. In effect they cause a complete absence of α chain production from the affected locus.

It is becoming apparent that lesions that affect the α2 rather than the α1 gene cause a more severe phenotype. Indeed, recent work suggests that nondeletion mutations of the α2 gene can give rise, in the homozygous state, to Hb H disease [34].

The Hemoglobin Bart's Hydrops Syndrome [3,35]. Affected infants are usually stillborn between 30 and 40 weeks' gestation; if liveborn they take a few gasping respirations and then die. The fetuses are pale with widespread edema, massive hepatosplenomegaly, extramedullary erythropoiesis, and ascites and pleural effusions. There is severe anemia with hypochromic red cells, and many nucleated red cells are seen in the peripheral blood. The hemoglobin consists of Hb Bart's and Hb Portland; Hb A and Hb F are absent. Both parents are heterozygous for α^0 thalassemia.

Hemoglobin H Disease [1–3,35]. This disorder is characterized by moderate anemia, icterus, and splenomegaly. The hemoglobin level is in the 5 to 10 g/dL range, and the red cells are hypochromic with marked variation in shape and size. There is an elevated reticulocyte count. The red cells contain multiple inclusion bodies after incubation of the blood with redox agents such as brilliant cresyl blue; they result from precipitation of Hb H by the redox action of the dye. After splenectomy large, single inclusions are found in some of the red cells. These consist of Hb H which has precipitated in older cells; they are normally removed by the spleen.

The condition runs a variable course with exacerbations of anemia in response to intercurrent infection or the use of oxidant drugs. In some cases there is progressive splenomegaly with hypersplenism and worsening of the anemia. The diagnosis depends on the demonstration of Hb H by electrophoresis and the finding of characteristic inclusion bodies in the red cells. One parent has α^0 thalassemia trait and the other α^+ thalassemia trait. In cases which result from the interaction of α^0 thalassemia with Hb Constant Spring there is 1 to 2 percent Hb Constant Spring in addition to Hb A and Hb H; one parent has α^0 thalassemia trait and the other Hb Constant Spring trait. Recent studies in the Middle East indicate that some patients with Hb H disease are homozygous for nondeletion forms of α^+ thalassemia; in this case both parents show mild α thalassemic changes with reduced MCH and MCV values [2].

Homozygous State for α^+ Thalassemia [36]. This condition, which occurs in 2 to 3 percent of west Africans, is characterized by a mild hypochromic, microcytic anemia with reduced MCH and MCV values and about 5 to 10 percent Hb Bart's at birth; this is not replaced by Hb H in adult life. Globin chain synthesis studies show a deficit of α chain production. The α^+ thalassemia trait is found both in parents and in all offspring.

The Heterozygous Carrier States for α^+ or α^0 Thalassemia [3,35,36]. Heterozygotes for α^+ thalassemia may have normal blood counts or there may be very mild hypochromia with a slightly reduced MCH and MCV; at birth some but not all cases have 1 to 2 percent Hb Bart's.

α^0 Thalassemia heterozygotes are symptomless. They have a mild anemia, reduced MCH and MCV values, hypochromic red cells, and 5 to 10 percent Hb Bart's at birth. This is not replaced by a similar amount of Hb H, although a few cells containing Hb H bodies are found in adults. There is a significant reduction of α chain synthesis, but the only certain way to make the diagnosis is by globin gene analysis.

The α thalassemia carrier states have been found in association with a variety of rare α chain hemoglobin variants such as hemoglobins Q, J Tongariki, and Hasharon [3].

The β thalassemias

The β thalassemias are heterogeneous at both clinical and molecular levels [1–3]. They are classified into β^0 thalassemias, in which no β chains are produced, and β^+ thalassemias, in which some β chains are produced but at a reduced rate. The severe transfusion-dependent forms result from the homozygous states for β^+ or β^0 thalassemia, or from the compound heterozygous state for β^+ and β^0 thalassemia. Furthermore, individuals who are apparently homozygous for β^0 or β^+ thalassemia may in fact be compound heterozygotes for two different molecular forms.

Molecular Basis and Pathophysiology [1–3,34,37,38]. In recent years the β globin genes from children with β thalassemia have been sequenced. These studies have shown that β thalassemia is an extremely heterogeneous condition at the molecular level, and over 50 different mutations have been described. Unlike the α thalassemias deletions are an uncommon cause of β thalassemia. In certain populations from north India a 619-bp deletion has been found that removes the 3′ end of the β globin gene but leaves the 5′ end intact. At least four other deletions have been reported which remove the 5′ end of the β globin gene, although these appear to be rare. But the vast majority of cases of β thalassemia result from point mutations that interfere with transcription, processing of the transcripts, or translation of the products of the β globin genes (see Fig. 14-2).

There are several classes of β thalassemia mutations. First, there are those that involve the upstream promotor sequences (see Fig. 14-2). In most cases they cause a mild reduction of β chain synthesis and the phenotype of β+ thalassemia. Second, there are mutations that involve the processing of messenger RNA. For example, mutations at the intron-exon junctions involving the invariant dinucleotides, GT at the 5′ and AG at the 3′ end, completely inactivate splicing and cause the phenotype of β0 thalassemia. Another group of β thalassemias involves single-base substitutions within the consensus sequence of the IVS 1 donor site. These are remarkably subtle, because a single-base substitution at position 5 of IVS 1 results in severe β0 thalassemia, whereas a T→C change at position 6 causes an extremely mild form of β+ thalassemia. RNA processing can also be affected by mutations that cause new splice sites, within either introns or exons. Finally, just like the mutation that was described as a cause of nondeletion α+ thalassemia, a single-base change in the polyadenylation signal sequence has been found as the basis for one form of β thalassemia.

Another common group of β thalassemias results from mutations that affect RNA translation. These include nonsense mutations which produce premature chain termination codons within coding sequences, and a variety of frame-shift mutations. The latter arise from the insertion or deletion of one or more nucleotides, any number but 3, which throws the reading frame out of phase and leads to the scrambling of the messenger RNA.

These molecular studies have provided a clear basis for understanding some of the phenotypic variability in β thalassemia; the processing mutations in particular provide a wide spectrum of defects in β chain production ranging from almost no gene product to a very mild reduction in the output of β chains. Similarly the transcriptional mutations usually cause a very modest reduction in β chain synthesis.

If β chain production is defective, excess α chains are synthesized. α Chains without partner β chains precipitate in red cell precursors and cause their defective maturation. For this reason all the β thalassemias are characterized by ineffective erythropoiesis, i.e., intramedullary destruction of a large proportion of red cell precursors. Those that reach the peripheral blood contain rigid inclusions and are destroyed in the microcirculation. Hence the anemia of β thalassemia results from a combination of ineffective erythropoiesis and shortened red cell survival. Some red cell precursors retain the ability to synthesize γ chains after birth. These cells are relatively protected in the marrow and blood because some of the excess α chains combine with the γ chains to produce Hb F instead of precipitating. Thus β thalassemia is characterized by a variable increase in the level of Hb F in the peripheral blood. However, cells containing Hb F have a high oxygen affinity, and this, together with the severe anemia, produces severe hypoxia, a marked increase in erythropoietin production, and stimulation of the ineffective erythroid marrow leading to the expansion of the bones and severe skeletal deformities. Constant exposure of the spleen to abnormal red cells causes splenomegaly, and secondary hypersplenism may develop. Finally, there is increased iron absorption from the gastrointestinal tract. This, together with repeated blood transfusions, leads to progressive iron loading with death due to generalized siderosis, particularly of the liver, endocrine glands, and myocardium.

***Distribution* [*3*].** The β thalassemias occur in a broad belt ranging from the Mediterranean and parts of north and west Africa through the Middle East and Indian subcontinent to southeast Asia. The high incidence zone stretches north through Yugoslavia and Rumania and the southern parts of the U.S.S.R., and includes the southern regions of the People's Republic of China.

The Severe Homozygous or Compound Heterozygous Forms of β Thalassemia. These conditions usually present in the first year of life with failure to thrive, poor feeding, intermittent fever, or failure to improve after an intercurrent infection. At this stage affected infants are pale and have splenomegaly. The subsequent course through childhood and adolescence depends on whether the infant is started on an effective transfusion regime [*3*].

In adequately transfused thalassemic children early growth and development are normal and splenomegaly is minimal. However, because of a gradual accumulation of iron, symptoms develop on entering adolescence. There is no adolescent growth spurt, and hepatic, endocrine, and cardiac complications of iron loading produce a variety of complications including diabetes, hypoparathyroidism, adrenal insufficiency, and progressive liver failure. The commonest cause of death, which usually occurs toward the end of the second decade, is progressive cardiac damage; it may be sudden due to an arrhythmia or may follow a period of protracted cardiac failure.

Children who are inadequately transfused have a distressing series of complications throughout childhood. Growth and development are retarded, there is progressive splenomegaly with hypersplenism, hideous deformities of the skull with bossing and overgrowth of the zygomata giving rise to the typical mongoloid appearance (Fig. 14-5), and an increased proneness to infection. Because of massive expansion of the marrow (Fig. 14-6) these children are hypermetabolic, with intermittent fever, loss of weight, and increased requirements for folic acid.

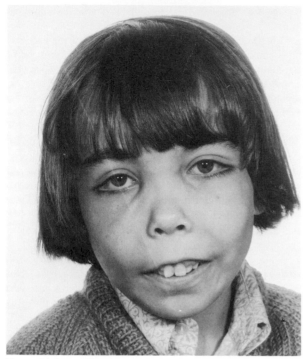

Figure 14-5. A child with homozygous β thalassemia.

There is a bleeding tendency which, although partly due to thrombocytopenia secondary to hypersplenism, may be exacerbated by liver damage associated with iron loading. If these children do not die in childhood from infection and anemia, they develop the same complications of iron loading as well-transfused patients.

At presentation there is a severe anemia with hemoglobin values ranging from 2 to 8 g/dL. The red cells are hypochromic with marked variation in shape and size and many misshapen forms; nucleated red cells are always found in the peripheral blood (Fig. 14-7). After splenectomy many of the nucleated cells and mature erythrocytes contain ragged inclusions. There is a slight elevation of the reticulocyte count. The bone marrow shows marked erythroid hyperplasia, and many of the red cell precursors contain α chain inclusions. The serum iron level rises progressively, and most transfusion-dependent children have totally saturated iron binding capacities; this is mirrored by a high plasma ferritin level, and liver biopsy shows an increase of iron both in the reticuloendothelial and parenchymal cells (Fig. 14-8).

The Hb F level is always elevated. In β^0 thalassemia there is no Hb A and the hemoglobin consists of Hb F and Hb A$_2$ only. In β^+ thalassemia the level of Hb F ranges from 30 to 90 percent; the Hb A$_2$ level may be low, normal, or elevated and is of no diagnostic value.

Heterozygous β Thalassemia. Heterozygous carriers are usually symptom-free, although they may become severely anemic in pregnancy. There is a mild degree of anemia with hemoglobin values in the 9 to 11 g/dL range. The red cells are hypochromic and microcytic with low MCH and MCV values.

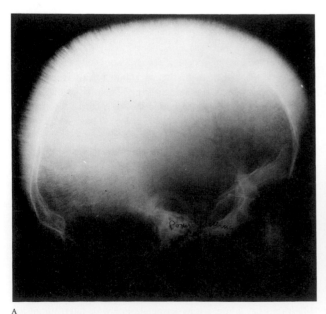

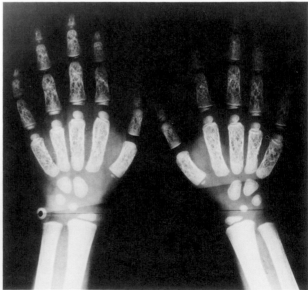

A

B

Figure 14-6. The radiological appearances in homozygous β thalassemia. *A.* Skull. *B.* Hands.

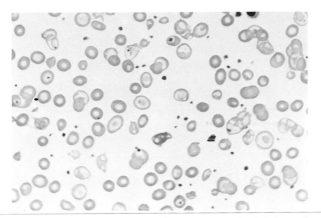

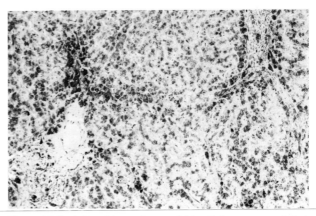

Figure 14-7. Blood film from a child homozygous for β thalassemia. Leishman stain, × 750.

Figure 14-8. A liver biopsy from a child with homozygous β thalassemia showing increased iron deposition. Perl's stain, × 600.

The Hb A_2 level is elevated in the 4 to 6 percent range; there is a slight elevation of Hb F in about 50 percent of cases [3].

Sickle Cell β Thalassemia [3,15,39]. The clinical manifestations which result from the interaction of the β thalassemia and sickle cell genes vary considerably. In Africans there is an extremely mild form of β^+ thalassemia which, when it interacts with the sickle cell gene, results in a condition characterized by mild anemia and few sickling crises. On the other hand, in Mediterranean populations it is quite common for an individual to inherit β^0 thalassemia from one parent and a sickle cell gene from the other. Sickle cell β^0 thalassemia is characterized by a clinical course which is indistinguishable from sickle cell anemia. The diagnosis rests on finding a sickling disorder in association with thalassemic red cell changes, i.e., a low MCH and MCV. In sickle cell β^0 thalassemia there may be an elevated reticulocyte count and sickled red cells on the peripheral blood film. The diagnosis is confirmed by hemoglobin electrophoresis, which in sickle cell β^+ thalassemia shows Hb S together with 10 to 30 percent Hb A and an elevated Hb A_2 value. In sickle cell β^0 thalassemia the hemoglobin consists mainly of Hb S with an elevated level of Hb F and Hb A_2. One parent has the sickle cell trait and the other the β thalassemia trait.

Hemoglobin C Thalassemia [3]. This disorder is restricted to west Africans and some north African and southern Mediterranean populations. It is characterized by a mild hemolytic anemia and splenomegaly. There are numerous target cells and thalassemic red cell indexes with a moderately elevated reticulocyte count. The hemoglobin consists of hemoglobins C and F, or C, A, and F. The diagnosis is confirmed by finding the Hb C trait in one parent and the β thalassemia trait in the other.

Hemoglobin E β Thalassemia [1–3,40]. This is the commonest severe form of thalassemia in southeast Asia and throughout the Indian subcontinent. Hemoglobin E is inefficiently synthesized; hence when a Hb E gene is inherited together with a β^0 thalassemia determinant, which is the commonest type of thalassemia in southeast Asia, there is a marked deficiency of β chain production. The clinical and hemotological changes are variable. There is usually severe anemia and splenomegaly with typical thalassemic bone changes. Although patients with this disorder are not always transfusion-dependent, their hemoglobin values are usually in the 4 to 9 g/dL range. The blood film shows typical thalassemic red cell changes, and there is erythroid hyperplasia of marrow with α chain inclusions in the red cell precursors. The diagnosis is made by finding only Hb E and Hb F on hemoglobin electrophoresis and by demonstrating the Hb E trait in one parent and the β thalassemia trait in the other.

Although very little is known about the natural history of this disorder, in many parts of southeast Asia and India it probably causes a very high mortality in the early years of life [40]. Complications include a proneness to infection, secondary hypersplenism, progressive iron loading leading to liver rather than cardiac damage, a variety of neurological lesions due to tumors caused by extramedullary erythropoiesis extending in from the inner tables of the skull, folate deficiency, and recurrent fractures. However, some patients with Hb E thalassemia grow and develop normally with few complications, and there are many recorded cases of pregnancy in women with this disorder.

The δβ and Hb Lepore Thalassemias [1–3,41]. Disorders due to reduced β *and* δ chain synthesis are much less common than those due to defective β chain production. In some cases they are caused by deletions of the δ and β globin genes, while others result from mispaired synapsis and unequal crossing over between the δ and β globin gene loci with the production of δβ fusion genes. The latter produce δβ fusion chains which combine with α chains to form hemoglobin variants called the Lepore hemoglobins. These conditions are classified into the δβ and Hb Lepore thalassemias. They are found sporadically in many populations; there are no high incidence areas.

δβ Thalassemia homozygotes have a moderate anemia and splenomegaly, but they are usually symptomless except during periods of stress such as infection or pregnancy. Hemoglobin analysis shows 100 percent Hb F. Heterozygous carriers have thalassemic blood pictures, elevated levels of Hb F in the 5 to 20 percent range, and normal levels of Hb A_2. Depending on the structure of the Hb F, these disorders are classified into $^G\gamma$ and $^G\gamma^A\gamma$ forms; they are similar clinically. They all result from deletions of the β globin gene complex. For this reason they are now classified according to the genes that are lost into $(\delta\beta)^0$ and $(^A\gamma\delta\beta)^0$ types.

The homozygous state for Hb Lepore is usually similar to homozygous β thalassemia, although occasionally it is milder and non-transfusion-dependent [41]. The hemoglobin consists of F and Lepore only. Heterozygous carriers have thalassemic blood pictures associated with about 5 to 15 percent Hb Lepore.

There is a group of genetic disorders of hemoglobin production encountered most commonly in black populations which are called collectively hereditary persistence of fetal hemoglobin (HPFH) [3]. Homozygotes have a mild thalassemia-like blood picture but are not anemic; they have 100 percent Hb F. Heterozygotes show no hematological abnormalities and have 20 to 30 percent Hb F. These conditions are due to gene deletions involving the δ and β globin genes and, in effect, are extremely mild forms of δβ thalassemia [1–3].

Thalassemia intermedia [3,42]

Definition and Pathogenesis. The term *thalassemia intermedia* is used to describe patients with thalassemia which, although not transfusion-dependent, is more severe than the disease in α or β thalassemia heterozygotes. Many of the conditions which were described earlier in this section fulfill these criteria, e.g., Hb C or Hb E thalassemia, the various δβ and Hb Lepore thalassemias, and disorders which result from the interactions of the β and δβ thalassemias. However, some individuals with thalassemia intermedia have parents with typical heterozygous β thalassemia; hence they appear to be homozygous for β thalassemia yet have an unusually mild disease. In some patients this is due to the additional inheritance of an α thalassemia determinant [42–44]. This reduces the amount of globin chain imbalance and consequently the severity of the dyserythropoiesis which characterizes homozygous β thalassemia. In other patients, particularly blacks, mild forms of homozygous β thalassemia seem to be due to unusually mild β thalassemia determinants [3,44]. In Asians with β^0 thalassemia intermedia there appears to be an additional genetic determinant causing high levels of fetal hemoglobin production [42].

Clinical and Hematological Changes. The clinical course is extremely variable. Some patients are almost symptom-free

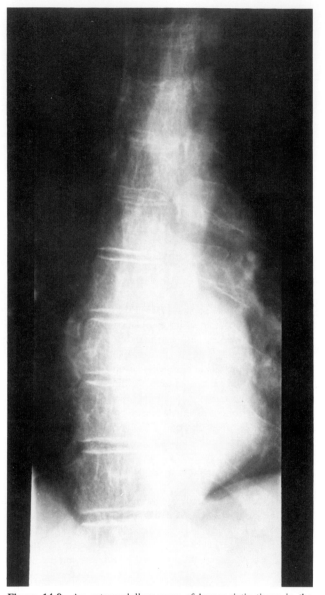

Figure 14-9. An extramedullary mass of hemopoietic tissue in the chest of a child with β thalassemia intermedia.

and have a mild anemia. Others have hemoglobin values in the 5 to 7 g/dL range with marked splenomegaly, skeletal deformities due to expansion of bone marrow, and severe iron loading due to increased intestinal iron absorption. Recurrent leg ulceration, folate deficiency, symptoms due to extramedullary hemopoietic tumor masses in the chest (Fig. 14-9) and skull, gallstones and proneness to infection are particularly characteristic of this group of thalassemias. Because of the extreme heterogeneity of this disorder it is only possible to determine the course that is likely to evolve in any individual patient by careful surveillance from early childhood.

Prevention and treatment

Since there is no definitive treatment and the management of the transfusion-dependent homozygous β thalassemias is such a drain on health resources, prevention of these disorders is becoming a major challenge in countries in which they are common.

Prevention. Since the heterozygous carrier states for the important thalassemias can be identified, it is possible to screen populations and to provide genetic counseling and advice about the choice of marriage partners. However, where this approach has been used, it has not been very effective, and in most high-incidence countries the secondary prevention of the important thalassemias is being carried out by screening in the antenatal clinics and by prenatal diagnosis for those parents who wish it.

Until recently the main approach to prenatal diagnosis of the thalassemias, and sickle cell anemia, involved fetal blood sampling followed by globin chain synthesis studies. Carried out at about 18 weeks' gestation, this has been very successful and has reduced the incidence of new births of homozygous β thalassemics in many populations [45].

More recently prenatal diagnosis of thalassemia has been carried out successfully by fetal DNA analysis, following either amniocentesis or chorionic villus sampling. The latter approach seems likely to be the most attractive because it can be carried out late in the first trimester [46]. Fetal DNA analysis for β thalassemia can be approached in several ways. Sometimes the mutation alters a restriction enzyme site and hence can be seen directly by Southern blotting. Where the mutation is known, oligonucleotide probes can be constructed to detect it directly. In those cases in which the mutation is not known, it is often possible to define which parental chromosome carries the mutation by using restriction fragment length polymorphisms and then by determining whether the fetus has inherited both of the affected parental chromosomes. Several extensive series of prenatal diagnoses have been reported using these approaches [46–48]. The error rate is approximately 1 percent, and the fetal loss rate about 2 percent. Programs of this type are now being set up in many countries round the world.

Treatment. The symptomatic management of severe β thalassemia consists of regular blood transfusion, splenectomy if hypersplenism develops, and the administration of chelating agents to reduce iron overload [3]. When the diagnosis of severe β thalassemia is suspected, the infant should be observed for several weeks to ensure that transfusion is necessary. If so, the hemoglobin level should be maintained between 9 and 14 g/dL by transfusion every 6 to 8 weeks. Either washed or frozen red cells should be used; whole blood should be avoided because of the danger of sensitization to serum or white cell components. The pre- and posttransfusion hemoglobin level should be monitored and transfusion requirements

carefully plotted. If there is a marked increase, hypersplenism should be suspected. Splenectomy should be carried out as late as possible and not in the first 5 years of life because of the high incidence of postsplenectomy infection [3]. Splenectomized children should be maintained on prophylactic penicillin, and the parents warned about the dangers of infection.

The most useful chelating agent for the prevention or treatment of iron overload is deferoxamine (Desferal). It has to be administered systemically, and the best results are obtained by slow subcutaneous infusion using a mechanical pump [49,50]. Deferoxamine therapy should be started as early as possible, usually between the second or third year; the child should be admitted to a hospital and a 12-h, overnight, deferoxamine infusion set up using a "butterfly" needle placed subcutaneously in the anterior abdominal wall. The urinary iron excretion in the 24-h postinfusion period is measured, after which, using the same technique, a dose-response curve is drawn starting with 0.5 g of deferoxamine and increasing until a plateau of iron excretion is reached. This determines the maintenance dose, which the child should then receive on five nights a week with a rest at weekends. Iron excretion is improved by giving 100 to 200 mg of ascorbic acid daily. A careful ophthalmological surveillance for cataract formation should be maintained. Children or parents who cannot manage this treatment should receive daily bolus injections of deferoxamine [3]. Whatever the route that is used, the urinary iron should be monitored regularly to make sure the drug is still effective.

Hemoglobin H disease requires no treatment unless hypersplenism develops; patients should be warned against the use of oxidant drugs which worsen the anemia. Children with β thalassemia intermedia should be watched carefully in early childhood, and if there are signs of growth retardation or increasing bone deformity, they should be placed on a regular transfusion regime.

Future developments in the management of the thalassemias include the synthesis of oral chelating agents and the development of gene therapy. Although bone marrow transplantation has been used in a few centers its widespread application does not seem to be indicated; the problems of graft-versus-host disease and the high mortality following the procedure make it unsuitable for general application [2].

GLUCOSE-6-PHOSPHATE DEHYDROGENASE DEFICIENCY

Glucose-6-phosphate dehydrogenase (G-6-PD) deficiency is by far the commonest red cell enzyme deficiency in the world population. It has been estimated that it affects over 100 million individuals. Although most affected persons show no clinical disability unless exposed to oxidant drugs, the condition is associated with some well-defined clinical disorders including favism, neonatal jaundice, and hemolysis associated with a variety of intercurrent illnesses.

DISTRIBUTION

G-6-PD deficiency is widespread in the populations of Africa, the Mediterranean, the Middle East, and southeast Asia. Figures for the world distribution of G-6-PD deficiency have been summarized by the World Health Organization and in several recent reviews [51–54]. The high gene frequencies are due to protection of carriers against *P. falciparum* malaria.

NORMAL RED CELL METABOLISM

During normal red cell development the mitochondria are lost at about the same time as the nucleus is extruded; mature red cells have little capacity for oxidative energy production. Glucose is metabolized mainly through the anaerobic Embden-Meyerhof pathway with the production of lactate. There is a net production of 2 mol of ATP and the reduction of 2 mol of NAD^+ to NADH per mole of glucose. About half of the ATP produced in this way is used for the red cell to maintain its volume and the integrity of its membrane by pumping sodium and water out of, and potassium into, the cell. The reduction of NAD^+ plays an important role in preventing the oxidation of heme iron. The other major energy pathway is the hexose monophosphate (HMP) shunt in which there is a reduction of $NADP^+$ to NADH. This pathway is stimulated by certain redox compounds and oxidants. One of its major functions is to maintain adequate levels of reduced glutathione which is essential for protection against oxidant damage. G-6-PD is the first, and rate-limiting, enzyme in this pathway.

PATHOGENESIS

G-6-PD deficiency is an inherited condition in which the activity of red cell G-6-PD is diminished. The gene determining the structure of G-6-PD is on the long arm of the X chromosome and therefore the defect is inherited in a sex-linked fashion. Hence it is fully expressed in affected males. Because one X chromosome is inactivated during early development (lyonisation), female heterozygotes have two populations of red cells, deficient and normal. Because the inactivation process is random, the enzyme activity in the blood of female carriers varies markedly, ranging from normal to almost as low as that found in hemizygous males.

G-6-PD deficiency results from the inheritance of any one of a large number of G-6-PD variants which have been defined either by their electrophoretic mobility, thermal stability, pH optima, substrate affinity, or by other techniques of enzyme chemistry [51–53,55]. Normal G-6-PD is called type B. In Africa there is a common variant called A, and G-6-PD deficiency in this population results from the production of a mutant form of this enzyme, called the A^- type. Although this is synthesized in normal quantities, it is unstable, and its level rapidly declines as red cells age. The Mediterranean variant, which is also extremely common, appears to be a structural mutant with reduced enzyme activity. In the form of the G-6-PD deficiency associated with this variant, there are extremely low enzyme values, whereas in the A^- variety of G-6-PD deficiency, there may be easily detectable enzyme levels in affected males. The disorder is extremely heterogeneous in southeast Asia [53]. Among the many variants described, the Mahidol and Canton types are particularly common. Over 100 G-6-PD variants have now been discovered and are named after their place of origin. Although many are harmless, some are associated with drug-induced hemolysis or chronic hemolytic anemia. Recently the amino acid substitutions in seven different G-6-PD variants have been determined [55a].

MECHANISM OF HEMOLYSIS [51,56,57]

The hemolysis of G-6-PD deficiency is characterized by the formation of intracellular inclusions called *Heinz bodies,* which consist of denatured hemoglobin and stromal protein. The mechanism whereby hemoglobin damage and precipitation occurs is still uncertain. Some drugs and chemicals have a direct oxidant action on hemoglobin and also form free radicals which oxidize reduced glutathione to the disulfide form (GSSG) or complex glutathione with hemoglobin to form a mixed disulfide. When oxidation damage of this kind occurs, hemoglobin is irreversibly denatured and precipitates to form Heinz bodies. Normal red cells are protected from this process by reducing GSSG to GSH via the HMP shunt; this is not possible in G-6-PD-deficient cells. This description of the pathophysiology of G-6-PD deficiency may be oversimplified. Oxidative damage to red cells results in the production of irreversible and unstable hemoglobin derivatives called hemichromes and the generation of superoxides and other "excited" intermediates capable of damaging red cell lipids, all of which are related to methemoglobin production which can be caused by many oxidants [56]. Furthermore, none of these mechanisms explains why neonatal hemolysis or sensitivity to fava beans occurs in G-6-PD-deficient individuals.

CLINICAL FEATURES

The clinical consequences of G-6-PD deficiency are summarized in Table 14-3. Hemolysis can occur after exposure to a variety of drugs and other oxidants, without the action of any identified toxic agent in the neonatal period, and after exposure to the bean *Vicia faba*. It has also been reported during intercurrent illnesses. Its relationship to blackwater fever and malaria is uncertain.

Table 14-3. Clinical associations of G-6-PD deficiency

Drug-induced hemolysis
Favism
Neonatal jaundice
Hemolysis due to intercurrent illness
Chronic hemolytic anemia

Table 14-4. Drugs thought to be associated with hemolysis in G-6-PD-deficient individuals*

Aminoquinolines:	Analgesics:
Primaquine	Aspirin
Pamaquine (Plasmoquine)	Acetophenetidin (phenacetin)
Chloroquine	Acetanilide
Sulfones:	Miscellaneous:
Dapsone (Avlosulfon)	Vitamin K (water-soluble
Thiazosulfone (Promizole)	analogues)
Sulfonamides:	Naphthalene (moth balls)
Sulfanilamide	Probenecid (Benemid)
Sulfacetamide (Albucid,	Dimercaprol (BAL)
Sulamyd)	Methylene blue
Sulfafurazole (Gantrisin)	Acetylphenylhydrazine
Sulfamethoxypyridazine	Phenylhydrazine
(Lederkyn, Midicel, Kynex)	p-Aminosalicylic acid
Nitrofurans:	Quinine
Nitrofurantoin (Furandantin)	Quinidine
Furazolidone (Furoxone)	Chloramphenicol
Nitrofurazone (Furacin)	

*This is a partial list; it is impossible to list all the agents suspected of producing hemolysis.
Source: From [52,53].

Drug-induced hemolysis

A list of some of the more important drugs which can produce hemolysis in G-6-PD-deficient individuals is shown in Table 14-4. Sensitivity to individual agents varies depending on the type of enzyme deficiency and the size of the dose. For example, drugs such as chloramphenicol may induce hemolysis in individuals with Mediterranean G-6-PD deficiency but not in blacks with the milder A⁻ variant. Furthermore, hemolytic episodes tend to be self-limiting in individuals with the A⁻ variant, whereas if the drug is continued in those with the Mediterranean form, there may be gross and sometimes fatal intravascular hemolysis.

There is conflicting evidence about the relative degree of hemolysis in response to different antimalarial drugs [53]. Among Africans, Chinese, and Thais primaquine causes mild to moderate hemolysis. Chloroquine has not been reported to cause hemolysis in Africans or in most Orientals, although severe hemolysis was observed in Cambodian soldiers who took a single dose of 600-mg chloroquine; some of these individuals developed renal failure. Quinine does not seem to cause hemolysis in G-6-PD–deficient Africans, although a case has been reported in the newborn period. A single dose of 1 g sulfamethopyrazine, 0.5 g trimethoprim, or 1 g sulfadoxine plus 50 mg pyrimethamine did not cause hemolysis in enzyme-deficient Thais. A single dose of 400 to 1600 mg diformyl-dapsone caused mild to severe hemolysis in G-6-PD–deficient red cells transfused into normal recipients; the same drug given to 12 G-6-PD–deficient Thais caused only a slight shortening of the red cell survival. Weekly administration of diformyl-

dapsone for malaria prophylaxis has been used in G-6-PD–deficient Thai subjects; no hemolysis was observed [53].

An episode of drug-induced hemolysis begins 1 to 3 days after exposure to the drug. There is a sudden onset of anemia and jaundice, and the peripheral blood picture shows the characteristics of hemolysis with Heinz bodies in the red cells. In severe cases there is shivering, backache, abdominal pain, and the passage of dark urine. As mentioned above, in the A⁻ type of G-6-PD deficiency the hemolytic reaction is self-limiting. This is because reticulocytes have relatively normal enzyme activity.

Favism

Severe and sometimes fatal hemolytic reactions due to the action of the bean *Vicia faba* are seen commonly in the Mediterranean region, the Middle East, and indeed anywhere where G-6-PD patients are exposed to the bean or, possibly, even to the pollen of the blossom. The pathogenesis of favism is not understood. It has a seasonal incidence and a peak occurrence in childhood, although some individuals are exposed to the bean for years before the first attack. It spares some G-6-PD families completely. The toxic factor in the bean has not been defined. Extensive studies have implicated the aglycones convicine and vicine [57]. Other genetic factors may be involved in addition to G-6-PD deficiency.

Neonatal jaundice

Jaundice and evidence of mild hemolysis may occur during the first week of life of G-6-PD–deficient infants and may occasionally lead to kernicterus [58]. Despite much work it is not clear why newborn infants who are G-6-PD–deficient develop hyperbilirubinemia. The hemolytic component is relatively mild, and studies in Greece have suggested that this syndrome may require the interaction of a second genetic factor, so far unidentified.

Intercurrent illness

There have been numerous reports of the occurrence of severe hemolytic reactions in G-6-PD–deficient individuals during the course of intercurrent illness such as bacterial and virus infection including hepatitis and diabetic ketoacidosis. Again the mechanism is not clear. G-6-PD deficiency may have contributed to the pathogenesis of "blackwater fever" in patients with malaria, although the association is not well-defined.

Chronic hemolysis

Some of the rare types of G-6-PD deficiency are associated with a continuous hemolytic process, one form of the hereditary nonspherocytic hemolytic anemia [51]. These patients usually present early in life, sometimes with neonatal jaundice, and hemolysis is exacerbated by infection or the administration of drugs. They have splenomegaly and the hematological changes of a chronic hemolytic anemia.

LABORATORY DIAGNOSIS

In the absence of hemolysis most G-6-PD–deficient individuals have a normal blood picture, and the condition can only be identified by an enzyme assay. During hemolytic episodes the hematological changes are as described above with the presence of Heinz bodies in the red cells. It may be difficult to make the diagnosis during an acute hemolytic crisis in an individual with G-6-PD deficiency of the A$^-$ variety. The high reticulocyte count may produce a normal enzyme assay, and hence the test has to be repeated when the hemolytic episode is over. Although this is less of a problem with other varieties of G-6-PD deficiency, the Mediterranean type, for example, red cell enzyme activity may still increase significantly during a hemolytic crisis.

The further characterization of G-6-PD deficiency (e.g., A$^-$, Mediterranean, Canton, etc.) requires a battery of studies including electrophoretic analysis, estimation of Km for NADP and glucose-6-phosphate, pH optima, and the utilization of substrate analogues.

TREATMENT AND PREVENTION

G-6-PD–deficient individuals should avoid drugs which can provoke hemolysis and should be given a list of these agents (Table 14-4). In very severe episodes, blood transfusion may be necessary. Splenectomy has been reported to be of value in the rare cases of chronic hemolysis.

REFERENCES

1 Bunn HF, Forget BG: *Hemoglobin: Molecular, Genetic and Clinical Aspects*. Philadelphia, Saunders, 1986

2 Weatherall DJ, Clegg JB, Higgs DR, et al: The hemoglobinopathies, in Scriver CR, Beaudet AL, Sly WS, et al (eds): *Metabolic Basis of Inherited Disease,* 6th ed. New York, McGraw-Hill, 1989

3 Weatherall DJ, Clegg JB: *The Thalassaemia Syndromes,* 3d ed. Oxford, Blackwell, 1981

4 Maniatis T, Fritsch EF, Lauer J, et al: The structure and chromosomal arrangement of human globin genes, in Stamatoyannopoulos G, Neinhuis AW (eds): *Organization and Expression of Globin Genes.* New York, Alan R Liss, 1981, pp 15–31

5 Harris H: Genetic heterogeneity in inherited disease. J Clin Pathol 27:32–37, 1974

6 Bellingham AJ: Haemoglobins with altered oxygen affinity. Br Med Bull 32:234–238, 1976

7 White JM: The unstable haemoglobin disorders. Clin Haematol 3:333–356, 1974

8 Harris JW: Studies on the destruction of red blood cells. VIII. Molecular orientation in sickle-cell hemoglobin solutions. Proc Soc Exp Biol Med 75:197, 1950

9 Mohandas N, Evans E: Sickle cell adherence to vascular endothelium: Morphologic correlates and the requirement for divalent cations and collagen binding plasma proteins. J Clin Invest 76:1605–1612, 1985

10 Hebbel RP, Miller JW: Phagocytosis of sickle erythrocytes: Immunologic and oxidative determinants of hemolytic anemia. Blood 64:733–741, 1984

11 Hebbel RP, Schwartz RS, Mohandas N: The adhesive sickle erythrocyte: Cause and consequence of abnormal interactions with endothelium, monocytes/macrophages, and model membranes. Clin Haematol 14:141–161, 1985

12 Hebbel RP: Auto-oxidation and a membrane-associated "Fenton reagent": A possible explanation for development of membrane lesions in sickle erythrocytes. Clin Haematol 14:129–140, 1985

13 Evans E, Mohandas N, Leung A: Static and dynamic rigidities of normal and sickle erythrocytes: Major influence of cell hemoglobin concentration. J Clin Invest 73:116–123, 1984

14 Kulozik AE, Wainscoat JS, Serjeant GR, et al: Geographical survey of β^S-globin gene haplotype: Evidence for an independent Asian origin of the sickle-cell mutation. Am J Hum Genet 39:239–244, 1986

15 Serjeant GR: *Sickle Cell Disease.* Oxford University Press, 1985

16 Milner PF: The sickling disorders. Clin Haematol 3:289–331, 1974

17 Luzzatto L: Sickle cell anaemia in tropical Africa. Clin Haematol 10:757–784, 1981

18 Pearson HA, Cornelius EA, Schwartz AD, et al: Transfusion-reversible functional asplenia in young children with sickle cell anemia. N Engl J Med 283:334–341, 1970

19 Johnston RB, Newman SL, Struth AG: An abnormality of the alternate pathway of complement activation in sickle-cell disease. N Engl J Med 288:803–808, 1973

20 Davies SC, Luce PJ, Win AA, et al: Acute chest syndrome in sickle-cell disease. Lancet i:36–38, 1984

21 Serjeant GR, Topely JM, Mason K, et al: Outbreak of aplastic crises in sickle cell anaemia associated with parvovirus-like agents. Lancet ii:595–597, 1981

22 Rogers DW, Clarke JM, Cupidore L, et al: Early deaths in Jamaican children with sickle cell disease. Br Med J 1:1515–1516, 1978

23 Condon PI, Gray R, Serjeant GR: Ocular findings on children with sickle cell haemoglobin C disease in Jamaica. Br J Ophthalmol 58:644–649, 1974

24 Koshy M, Ashenhurst J: Management of pregnancy in sickle cell anemia. Tex Rep Biol Med 40:273–282, 1981

25 WHO Working Group: Hereditary anaemias: Genetic basis, clinical features, diagnosis, and treatment. Bull WHO 60:643–659, 1982

26 Perrine RP, Brown MJ, Clegg JB, et al: Benign sickle cell anaemia. Lancet ii:1163–1167, 1972

27 Perrine RP, Pembrey ME, John P, et al: Natural history of sickle cell anemia in Saudi Arabia. Ann Intern Med 88:1–6, 1978

28 Kar BC, Satapathy RK, Kulozik AE, et al: Sickle cell disease in Orissa State, India. Lancet ii:1198–1201, 1986

29 Higgs DR, Aldridge BE, Lamb J, et al: The interaction of alpha thalassemia and homozygous sickle cell disease. N Engl J Med 306:1441–1446, 1982

30 Serjeant GR, Serjeant BE: A comparison of erythrocyte characteristics in sickle cell syndromes in Jamaica. Br J Haematol 23:205–213, 1972

31 Goossens M, Dumez Y, Kalan L, et al: Prenatal diagnosis of sickle-cell anemia in the first trimester of pregnancy. N Engl J Med 309:831–833, 1983

31a Gaston MH, Verter JI, Woods G, et al: Prophylaxis with oral penicillin in children with sickle-cell anemia: A randomized trial. N Engl J Med 314:1593–1599, 1986

32 Charache S, Scott J, Niebyl J, et al: Management of sickle cell disease in pregnant patients. Obstet Gynecol 55:407–410, 1980

33 Luskey KL, Schechter AN, Hercules JI: New approaches to the therapy of sickle cell disease. Tex Rep Biol Med 40:305–312, 1981

34 Thein SL, Weatherall DJ: The thalassaemias, in Hoffbrand AV (ed): *Recent Advances in Haematology, 5*. London, Churchill, 1988, in press

35 Wasi P, Na-Nakorn S, Pootrakul S: The α thalassaemias. Clin Haematol 3:383–411, 1974

36 Higgs DR, Pressley L, Clegg JB, et al: α Thalassemia in Black populations. Johns Hopkins Med J 146:300–301, 1980

37 Orkin SH, Kazazian HH: The mutation and polymorphism of the human β-globin gene and its surrounding DNA. Ann Rev Genet 18:131–171, 1984

38 Nienhuis AW, Anagnou NP, Ley TJ: Advances in thalassemia research. Blood 63:738–758, 1984

39 Serjeant GR, Ashcroft MT, Sergeant BE, et al: The clinical features of sickle cell β thalassaemia in Jamaica. Br J Haematol 24:19–30, 1973

40 Wasi P, Na-Nakorn S, Pootrakul S, et al: Alpha- and beta-thalassemia in Thailand. Ann NY Acad Sci 165:60–82, 1969

41 Efremov GC: Hemoglobins Lepore and anti-Lepore. Hemoglobin 2:197–233, 1978

42 Wainscoat JS, Thein SL, Weatherall DJ: Thalassaemia intermedia. Blood Rev 1:273–279, 1987

43 Wainscoat JS, Old JM, Weatherall DJ, et al: The molecular basis for the clinical diversity of β thalassaemia in Cypriots. Lancet i:1235–1238, 1983

44 Weatherall DJ, Pressley L, Wood WG, et al: Molecular basis for mild forms of homozygous beta-thalassaemia. Lancet i:527–529, 1981

45 Alter BP: Prenatal diagnosis of hemoglobinopathies and other hematologic diseases. J Pediatr 95:501–513, 1979

46 Old JM, Ward RHT, Petrou M, et al: First trimester diagnosis for haemoglobinopathies: A report of 3 cases. Lancet ii:1413–1416, 1982

47 Old JM, Fitches A, Heath C, et al: First trimester fetal diagnosis for haemoglobinopathies: Report on 200 cases. Lancet ii:763–767, 1986

48 Weatherall DJ: Prenatal diagnosis of inherited blood diseases. Clin Haematol 14:747–774, 1985

49 Pippard MJ, Callender ST, Weatherall DJ: Intensive iron-chelation therapy with desferioxamine in iron-loading anaemias. Clin Sci Mol Med 54:99–106, 1978

50 Graziano J, Piomelli S: Clinical management of β-thalassemia. Tex Rep Biol Med 40:355–364, 1981

51 Beutler E: G-6-PD: Historical perspective and current status, in Weatherall DJ, Fiorelli G, Gorini S (eds): *Advances in Red Blood Cell Biology*. New York, Raven, 1982, pp 297–308

52 Bienzle U: Glucose-6-phosphate dehydrogenase deficiency. Part I: Tropical Africa. Clin Haematol 10:785–799, 1981

53 Panich V: Glucose-6-phosphate dehydrogenase deficiency. Part 2: Tropical Asia. Clin Haematol 10:800–814, 1981

54 Luzzatto L: Malaria and the red cell, in Hoffbrand AV (ed): *Recent Advances in Haematology, 4*. Edinburgh, Churchill, 1985, pp 109–126

55 Persico M, Battistuzzi G, Mareni C, et al: Genetic variants of human glucose-6-phosphate dehydrogenase (G6PD): Studies of turnover and of G6PD-specific mRNA, in Weatherall DJ, Fiorelli G, Gorini S (eds): *Advances in Red Blood Cell Biology*. New York, Raven, 1982, pp 309–318

55a Vulliamy PJ, D'Urso M, Battistuzzi G, et al: Diverse point mutations in the human glucose-6-phosphate dehydrogenase gene cause enzyme deficiency and mild or severe hemolytic anemia. Proc Natl Acad Sci USA 85:5171–5175, 1988

56 Bashan N, Potashnik R, Frazer D, et al: The effect of oxidative agents on normal and G6PD-deficient red blood cell membranes, in Weatherall DJ, Fiorelli G, Gironi S (eds): *Advances in Red Blood Cell Biology*. New York, Raven, 1982, pp 365–374

57 Chevion M, Navok T, Glaser G: Favism inducing agents: Biochemical and mechanistic considerations, in Weatherall DJ, Fiorelli G, Gorini S (eds): *Advances in Red Blood Cell Biology*. New York, Raven, 1982, pp 381–390

58 Chan MCK: Neonatal jaundice, in Hendrickse RG (ed): *Paediatrics in the Tropics*. Oxford, Oxford Medical, 1981, pp 13–26

CHAPTER 15

Parasitism and the Host-Parasite Interface · Kenneth S. Warren

How does parasitism relate to tropical medicine, and if it does bear a relationship, what is its importance relative to other aspects of tropical medicine? A parasite, as defined in the unabridged *Oxford English Dictionary,* literally means one who eats at the table at another's expense and repays him with flattery. Its biological definition is an animal or plant which lives in or upon another organism (technically called its host) and draws its nutriment directly from it. By this definition all infectious agents, viruses, bacteria, fungi, protozoa, and helminths are parasites. Nevertheless, textbooks of parasitology today deal only with protozoa and helminths. Viruses, bacteria, and fungi are presented in textbooks of microbiology. How did this happen? Historically, the answer was not clear because neither scientists nor historians had even posed the question. Michael Worboys' paper "The Emergence of Tropical Medicine" points to the importance of the development of the germ theory of disease in the 1860s, but he notes [1] that until the 1870s "almost all known parasites were flukes or worms." In his *A History of Parasitology* Foster notes that protozoa were first observed in 1681 by Leeuwenhoek examining his own feces [2]. It was not until the early 1800s, however, that parasitic protozoa were first described, and these largely in insects. "The first human protozoan parasite of major importance to be described was the ameba of dysentery by Losch in 1875, but as late as 1886 no parasitic protozoan was generally accepted as the cause of any important human disease" [2]. Bacterial diseases were discovered in that era, but viruses were not described until the early twentieth century. One of the first attempts to categorize these infectious agents occurred around the turn of the century when helminths and protozoa were called "animal parasites," not because they infected animals, but because they themselves were conceived of as animals. At that time bacteria were called "vegetable parasites." Recently, viruses have been characterized as "molecular parasites."

The reasons for this separation of infectious diseases into two completely separate disciplines are not completely clear, but Worboys, in a more recent paper entitled "The Emergence and Early Development of Parasitology," observed that the main impetus was the appearance of tropical medicine, for which parasitology provided the "zoological underpinning" [3]. At his inaugural lecture at the London School of Tropical Medicine in 1899, Sir Patrick Manson stated, "Today the protozoan and the helminth, as regards tropical pathology, are in the ascendent. In this school, although the bacterium will not be neglected, necessarily a large share of your time will be occupied with animal parasites, a subject which I fear has not been sufficiently studied hitherto in our medical schools" [4]. As Edward Kass has shown, bacteriology began to appear in American medical schools in 1885 and became widespread well before 1900 [5]. Thus, different venues for teaching and research in parasitology and in bacteriology-microbiology had occurred early in the development of the fields. Further definition of these disciplines occurred with the development of scientific societies. While the Society of American Bacteriologists (later changed to Microbiologists) was inagurated in 1899, the first parasitological organization, appropriately the Helminthological Society of Washington, was founded in 1911. The American Society of Parasitologists did not appear until 1927, and the British Society did not begin until 1962.

It should now be apparent that the disciplines of parasitology and microbiology, as presently defined both in textbooks and practice, became separated in time and in place in a relatively unplanned manner which bears little relationship to the meaning of the term *parasite.*

As noted above, the *Oxford English Dictionary* defines parasites as animals or plants, but all infectious agents essentially fulfill this definition. Thus, the arbitrary definition of parasitology as a field dealing only with animal parasites and microbiology as concerned with plants cannot be accepted. Since infectious agents run such an enormous gamut in size, this might seem to be a reasonable means of distinction. Yet, the enormous leaps in size from viruses to bacteria, from prokaryotes (bacteria) to eukaryotes (fungi, protozoa), and from unicellular to multicellular (helminths) organisms blur the arbitrary boundaries of microbiology and parasitology. Nevertheless, helminths can be distinguished from all other infectious agents by their multicellularity and associated size. Thus, all species of adult worms are visible to the naked eye; in contrast, all of the other parasites, from protozoa to viruses, require light or electron microscopes to be seen. Furthermore, helminths share a major biological characteristic that differentiates them from all other infectious agents: with rare exceptions, they do not replicate directly within the human definitive host. That this characteristic is not trivial is obvious because of its profound implications for transmission, host immunological responses, treatment, and control [6].

Thus, a subdivision of parasites such as that suggested by the population biologists Anderson and May [7] might be considered:

> Microparasites (viruses, bacteria, protozoa) are characterized by small size, short generation times, extremely high rates of direct reproduction within the host, and a tendency to induce immunity to reinfection in those hosts that survive the initial onslaught. The duration of infection is typically short in relation to the expected life span of the host, and therefore is of a transient nature. . . . Macroparasites which include parasitic helminths and arthropods tend to have much longer generation times than the microparasites, and direct multiplication within the host is either absent or occurs at a low rate. The immune responses elicited by these metazoans generally depend on the number of parasites present in a given host, and tend to be of relatively short duration. Macroparasitic infections, therefore, tend to be of a persistent nature, with hosts being continually reinfected.

Within these broad categories, however, parasite transmission systems are exceedingly heterogeneous. Thus, they are an endless source of fascination for the biologist, but an endless source of frustration for the physician attempting to control them. At a Dahlem workshop on the *Population Biology of Infectious Disease Agents* [8] at least nine major transmission systems were described from direct human-to-human transmission to highly complex systems involving vectors, intermediate hosts, reservoir hosts, and stages in the external environment. In general the simpler systems are most prevalent among the microparasites with the most complex occurring among the macroparasites, i.e., liver flukes which involve human beings, external environment, intermediate host (snail), external environment, paratenic host (fish), and human beings.

Another aspect of heterogeneity and complexity is the localization and migration of parasitic organisms within the human host. Parasites may localize in the dermal, respiratory, intestinal, urinary, hematological, and central nervous systems, and specific areas thereof. They may migrate from one organ to another, e.g., poliovirus from the intestines to the central nervous system, malaria from the liver to the bloodstream, and schistosomes from the skin to the lungs to the liver and then to either the intestinal or vesical venules. Host genetic or environmental factors may determine or facilitate the infective and localization processes.

A crucial aspect of heterogeneity as far as the host is concerned lies in the distinction between infection and disease. These outcomes are affected by a variety of factors determining the virulence of parasite species and strains and the host's capacity, both innate and acquired, to resist infection. Infection is defined as the presence of the living parasite within the host, and disease by overt manifestations of such infection, including symptoms and signs. For the multiplying microparasites, a relatively rare example of a constant association between infection and disease has been smallpox. Examples of variable associations between infection and disease are numerous, including inapparent or subclinical infections with mumps and hepatitis viruses, eclipse phases of herpes and varicella viruses,

dormant infections in tuberculosis, carrier states in typhoid and amebiasis, inapparent infections in toxoplasmosis, and subclinical infections in partially immune individuals with falciparum malaria. For the nonmultiplying helminth infections, the density of the parasites within the host plays an essential role in the occurrence of symptoms and signs of disease. Furthermore, population studies have revealed a negative binomial distribution of infection in human beings with only a small proportion of infected individuals bearing moderate- to high-density infections. Hookworm disease, as manifested by anemia, is never seen in minimal infections, since these are associated with negligible blood loss. In schistosomiasis mansoni, morbidity as manifested by impaired work ability and hepatosplenomegaly is seen only in heavily infected individuals.

Thus, the heterogeneity of infectious diseases is related to parasite transmission systems, the localization and migration of parasites within the human host, and the occurrence of signs and symptoms of disease related to the virulence of the parasite and the resistance of the host.

The basic factors underlying the host-parasite interaction are described in this section, "Parasitism." It deals with all parasitic organisms, both micro and macro. The host-parasite interface begins at the membrane, involving not only permeability but surface antigens, receptors, and genetic markers. It involves biochemistry in terms of substances which are absorbed, secreted, and excreted; the immune response of the host, and its effect not only on the parasite but on itself in the form of immunopathology; the means by which parasites evade (protect themselves from) the host response; and the development of parasites in hosts with compromised or altered responses. Finally, understanding the relationship of populations of parasites with populations of hosts and transmission of the former via vectors and intermediate hosts is essential for coping with the broad and heterogeneous range of infectious disease, and will be discussed in detail.

REFERENCES

1 Worboys M: The emergence of tropical medicine: A study in the establishment of a scientific specialty, in Lemain G, MacLeod M, et al (eds): *Perspectives on the Emergence of Scientific Disciplines.* The Hague, Mouton, 1980

2 Foster WD: *A History of Parasitology.* London, Livingston, 1965

3 Worboys M: The emergence and early development of parasitology, in Warren KS, Bowers JZ: *Parasitology: A Global Perspective.* New York, Springer-Verlag, 1983

4 Manson P: The need for special training in tropical disease. J Trop Med 2:57–62, 1899

5 Kass EH: History of the specialty of infectious disease in the United States. Ann Intern Med 106:745–56, 1987

6 Warren KS: The guerrilla worm. N Engl J Med 282:810–811, 1970

7 Anderson RM, May RM: Population biology of infectious diseases: Part I. Nature 280:361–367, 1979

8 Anderson RM, May RM (eds): *Population Biology of Infectious Disease Agents.* Dahlem Konferenzen. Berlin, Springer-Verlag, 1982

Host-Parasite Interface: Biochemistry and Rational Drug Design

· Graeme B. Henderson · Anthony Cerami

The metabolism of parasitic organisms has inevitably evolved and been refined in response to life within the environment of the mammalian host. The net result of this process of adaptation is an organism that has more or less mastered its particular ecological niche. The cost of this mastery to human health is incalculable. The individual diseases caused by parasitic organisms will be discussed elsewhere in this volume. These diseases represent the foremost human health problem in the world today, and yet available chemotherapy for many of these diseases is either inadequate or nonexistent. In addition, the usefulness of drugs which are available is constantly being undermined by the rapid spread of drug-resistant phenotypes. Lack of progress in the development of antiparasitic drugs is in part a reflection of the economic basis on which pharmacological agents have traditionally been developed; as the populations at risk are also the most economically disadvantaged, expensive drug screening and development programs have rarely been applied to these diseases. However, this is not the only difficulty. Where screening has been applied, as in the malaria drug screening programs, this approach has not met with great success. Problems in developing suitable culture systems for many of the parasitic organisms under study have perhaps been the most important factors impeding progress. The ability to obtain organisms in sufficient quantity in order to study their metabolism outside the mammalian host is a relatively recent advance. This remains a major limiting factor with several parasites. However, in spite of the inherent difficulties which accompany research in this area, our knowledge of parasite biochemistry has reached a point where it is now possible to apply rational approaches to the design of new antiparasitic drugs.

The two basic requirements for the success of the rational approach to drug design as applied to parasitic diseases were first stated in 1902 by Paul Ehrlich: (1) a biochemical process of importance to the parasite must be identified and then inhibited by chemotherapy and (2) such chemotherapy must be tolerated by the mammalian host (i.e., must be selectively toxic to the parasite). Then, as now, it was recognized that the best chemotherapeutic targets are metabolic processes that are distinctly different in the parasite from analogous processes in the mammalian host. Our purpose in this chapter is to describe how the rational approach to drug design is being applied to parasite disease and to illustrate areas to which it might be extended. We begin with a discussion of aspects of parasite nutrition and energy metabolism that are significantly different from analogous host cell processes and then describe some biochemical processes that are unique to the parasite. In a short review of this type, we make no attempt to comprehensively describe any particular area. For supporting data the reader is directed to the references in the text and to some recent monographs on parasite biochemistry and chemotherapy [1–3].

METABOLIC STREAMLINING

One of the most striking metabolic adaptations to parasitism is a phenomenon known as *streamlining*. Life within the nutritionally rich mammalian environment has enabled many parasitic organisms to streamline their metabolic activities, as they are able to obtain essential cellular components from their host [4]. For example, although many parasites synthesize pyrimidines de novo, they invariably import purine bases and transform these into nucleotides via salvage pathways. Similarly, although lipids and sterols are essential components of parasite membranes, these components are also primarily derived from the host. While several parasites have been shown to synthesize or interconvert amino acids, many of the essential amino acids can be obtained from the host by simple diffusion and/or by mediated uptake processes. This streamlining process must have involved the development and refinement of highly sophisticated mechanisms for the import of these and other essential nutrients.

Economically, de novo synthesis makes good sense; the parasites are simply utilizing the raw materials of their environment. This aspect of parasite metabolism offers several interesting opportunities for chemotherapy. For example, the metabolic dependence upon the host for the synthesis of purine bases has been intensively studied [5]. Many pathogenic protozoa of the genera *Leishmania* and *Trypanosoma* import various analogues of purine bases, including the pyrazolopyrimidine derivative *allopurinol*. Allopurinol and analogous structures possess antiparasitic activity by virtue of their metabolism and incorporation into parasite RNA. The conversion of allopurinol by the responsible parasite enzymes, hypoxanthine-guanine phosphoribosyltransferase, succino-AMP synthetase, and succino-AMP lyase, has been studied, and the efficacy of the compound seems to depend on the selectivity of the parasite succino-AMP lyase. This enzyme is somewhat less discriminating than the counterpart mammalian enzyme, which does not accept allopurinol as substrate. Although turnover of the drug is relatively inefficient (V_{max} values being <1 percent of the corresponding values for IMP), nevertheless sufficient conversion takes place to the detriment of the organism. Allopurinol and some derivatives may prove to be therapeutically useful antileishmanial agents. Clinical studies on antimony-resistant leishmaniasis in humans using allopurinol gave apparent cures in some cases [5].

The promising results achieved with allopurinol have encouraged research into the use of purine analogues in treatment of other parasite diseases, notably malaria. Unlike the host cell, erythrocytic stages of the malaria parasite require a continuous source of purine nucleotides in order to proliferate. The source of these bases is erythrocyte adenine nucleotides which are first deaminated to IMP by adenosine deaminase. Adenosine deaminase activity is increased in *Plasmodium falciparum*–infected erythrocytes and appears to be of parasite origin. This enzyme, therefore, seems to be a worthwhile therapeutic target, particularly as treatment of *Plasmodium knowlesi*–infected monkeys with known adenosine deaminase inhibitors has been shown to produce a dramatic reduction in parasitemia [5]. These and other results point to the importance of purine metabolism as a target for the development of antiparasite drugs. More generally, this work illustrates the inherent vulnerability of the streamlined parasite metabolism toward exploitation by chemotherapy.

There is probably no single mammalian cell type which contains in sufficient quantity all of the nutrients that a growing parasite requires; yet many parasites spend a part of their life cycle within intact cells. Leishmania, for example, live inside phagolysosomes within macrophages; *Trypanosoma cruzi* lives in the cytoplasm of muscle cells and in macrophages; and *Plasmodium* lives within erythrocytes and hepatocytes. For these and other parasitic protozoa the maintenance of such a streamlined metabolism must pose special problems. One way around this involves the import of nutrients from the surrounding medium by insertion of appropriate receptor molecules into the host cell membrane. Analysis of the membranes of parasitized host cells reveals a number of parasite-derived pro-

teins, and it is likely that many of these are involved in the process of nutrient import. The study of the mechanisms of uptake of nutrients by both extra- and intracellular parasites is in its infancy. Much more research in this area is warranted.

ENERGY METABOLISM

If the de novo synthetic activities of parasites may be said to be streamlined, such economy does not extend to parasite energy metabolism, which, when compared to that of the mammalian host, appears almost profligate. The oxidation of 1 molecule of glucose by normal aerobic metabolism yields a total of 36 molecules of ATP. While all protozoan and helminth parasites metabolize glucose, many do it extremely inefficiently. Few, if any, parasites possess an active tricarboxylic acid cycle, and many lack cytochromes or a classical electron transport system. In addition, most parasitic organisms do not oxidize lipid, a process which provides valuable energy to mammalian systems. To a certain extent, this particular metabolic adaptation to parasitism also reflects the nutritionally rich nature of the mammalian host; raw energy in the form of carbohydrate is generally not limited. However, energy metabolism in parasite systems is not simply a pared down or underdeveloped version of the mammalian process. There are several features of energy metabolism in parasites that are novel and potentially vulnerable to chemotherapeutic attack.

With the discovery that the classical enzymes of glycolysis are compartmentalized within a subcellular organelle, the *glycosome,* energy production in bloodstream African trypanosomes has been the subject of much recent investigation [6]. The glycosome (Fig. 16-1) is a membrane-bound organelle that has been identified in all trypanosomatids examined to date. The glycosome contains the first seven enzymes of glycolysis,

Figure 16-1. Intermediary metabolism of bloodstream forms of African trypanosomes showing the site of action of salicylhydroxamic acid (SHAM).

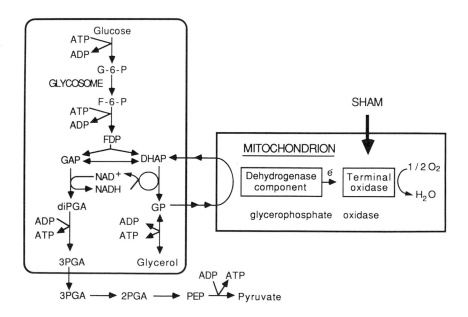

two enzymes of de novo pyrimidine biosynthesis, glycerol phosphate dehydrogenase, glycerol kinase, adenylate kinase, as well as enzymes of CO_2 fixation. As these enzymes are usually located in the cytoplasm of other organisms, the functional significance of the glycosome is a mystery. It has been suggested that such packing of the glycolytic enzymes might promote enzyme-enzyme interactions that somehow facilitate rapid "tunneling" of the glycolytic intermediates through the organelle, but there is, as yet, little evidence for this. It is certainly true that some trypanosomes possess an extraordinarily high rate of glycolysis; for example, bloodstream forms of *Trypanosoma brucei* consume the equivalent of their own dry weight of glucose every hour. The reason for this is evident on examination of Fig. 16-1. These organisms possess a highly unusual respiratory mechanism in which NADH generated during glycolysis is reoxidized by means of a glycerophosphate shuttle, which involves glycosomal glycerol phosphate dehydrogenase and a glycerol phosphate oxidase located in the mitochondrion. Thus, under aerobic conditions, trypanosomes obtain just two molecules of ATP per glucose molecule oxidized.

The glycerophosphate oxidase of bloodform African trypanosomes represents a particularly attractive target for drug development. This complex catalyzes four-electron reduction of O_2 to H_2O, does not contain cytochromes, and can be blocked by a variety of metal chelating agents, notably salicylhydroxamic acid (SHAM). When bloodstream *T. brucei* organisms are exposed to SHAM, the aerobic component of their energy metabolism is blocked. However, this does not alter the rate of glucose metabolism. Although inhibition of glycerophosphate oxidase should reduce net ATP production to zero, in fact, ATP production continues by means of the glycosomal

glycerol kinase, which transfers phosphate to ADP from accumulating glycerol phosphate. Based on this analysis, it was predicted that a combination of SHAM and glycerol would have a lethal effect on the organism. This has been shown to be correct in vitro and in vivo. While this drug combination has not proved clinically useful (because of problems of glycerol administration and distribution), this strategy deserves further study. The synergism observed between SHAM and glycerol relies on a simple mass-action effect on glycerol kinase; a more systematic analysis and characterization of this enzyme would seem worthwhile.

The glycerophosphate shuttle is an elegant expedient that compensates for the lack of a functioning citric acid cycle. Other parasites that also lack a functioning citric acid cycle employ other devious (but metabolically similar) tricks. For example, parasitic helminths metabolize glucose incompletely to phosphoenol pyruvate (PEP). In mammalian systems this compound is processed to acetate, which enters the citric acid cycle, but in most helminths, PEP is further processed as outlined in Fig. 16-2. This pathway was first described in *Ascaris lumbricoides* and appears to operate in other helminths [7,8]. PEP is first converted to oxaloacetate, which is subsequently reduced to malate and transported into the intramembranous space of the mitochondrion. Here malate is converted to either pyruvate or fumarate, which enters the mitochondrion; pyruvate is then oxidized to acetate and CO_2, and fumarate is reduced to succinate. The oxidation of pyruvate produces NADH, which must be reoxidized. Many helminths have a rudimentary respiratory chain that can couple NADH oxidation to O_2 reduction, H_2O_2 being the apparent product. However, this does not appear to be the preferred route. Most parasitic helminths do not require O_2; NADH oxidation is more usually

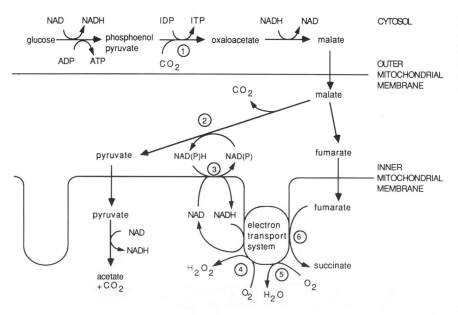

Figure 16-2. Intermediary metabolism of *Ascaris*. 1, phosphoenolpyruvate carboxykinase; 2, malic enzyme; 3, transhydrogenase; 4, cytochrome o terminal oxidase; 5, cytochrome aa terminal oxidase; 6, fumarate reductase.

coupled to fumarate reduction to succinate, which is then secreted, or in some cases, metabolized to propionate. The fumarate reductase activity is accompanied by the phosphorylation of ADP to ATP via an electron transport chain which involves flavoproteins, rhodoquinone, and cytochrome proteins. A similar pathway from PEP to succinate possibly occurs in *Trypanosoma cruzi,* the agent of South American Chagas' disease.

A number of parasitic organisms live in anaerobic or partially anaerobic environments; examples include the intestinal pathogens *Entamoeba histolytica* and *Giardia lamblia* and the venereal pathogen *Trichomonas vaginalis.* Because of the low O_2 tension in these environments, none of these organisms possess mitochondria, citric acid cycle, or classical electron transport systems and all depend heavily on glycolysis for ATP production. There are a number of unusual features associated with energy production in these organisms. *E. histolytica* and *G. lamblia,* for example, convert pyruvate anaerobically to acetaldehyde and CO_2. Under anaerobic conditions, the acetaldehyde is reduced, thereby regenerating NAD. *T. vaginalis* utilizes lactate dehydrogenase for the same purpose. This organism also possesses a novel organelle, the hydrogenosome. Within the hydrogenosome, pyruvate oxidation is coupled to proton reduction with concomitant production of hydrogen gas. This system is similar to oxidation-reduction systems found in anaerobic bacteria such as *Clostridia* spp.

UNUSUAL METABOLIC PROCESSES ELUCIDATED BY STUDIES ON THE MODE OF ACTION OF EXISTING DRUGS

To a certain extent the biochemical processes described in the previous sections can be rationalized in terms of the parasite habit. There are, however, aspects of the metabolism of parasites which seem to be unique and which, at present, defy explanation. These areas of parasite biochemistry are naturally of great interest from a pharmacological standpoint, as they represent opportunities to develop drugs which inhibit processes that differ significantly in the host or are perhaps absent altogether. Three examples from the biochemistry of parasitic protozoa illustrate this point.

The tripeptide *glutathione* (GSH) is found in high concentration in both prokaryotic and eukaryotic cells, where it is thought to have a number of important functions, which include thiol-disulfide redox control and isomerization, free radical scavenging, and hydrogen peroxide reduction. Interest in glutathione metabolism in trypanosomatids has recently been stimulated by the finding that these organisms conjugate this compound to the polyamine spermidine and that the bis-glutathionylspermidine adduct, which has been given the trivial name *trypanothione,* serves as a redox carrier for reducing equivalents between NADPH and peroxides [9]. Trypanothione is maintained in the reduced (dithiol) form within the cell by an NADPH-dependent flavoprotein disulfide reductase

(trypanothione reductase) and appears to be a specific cofactor for a trypanosome peroxidase activity. In this capacity trypanothione therefore appears to be a parasite equivalent of glutathione. As these organisms lack classical glutathione reductase and peroxidase activities, the inhibition of the enzymes responsible for trypanothione biosynthesis or the enzymes responsible for its metabolism represent important new targets for chemotherapy. The GSH-based antioxidant system seems to suffice for almost all other aerobic organisms; it is therefore not obvious why the kinetoplastida carry out this more elaborate process. One is inclined to believe that trypanothione (or the process of conjugation of GSH to spermidine) must have some other function within trypanosomatids. The enzyme trypanothione reductase has now been purified and characterized from representative trypanosomatids, and specific inhibitors of this enzyme have been shown to be trypanocidal in an in vitro *T. cruzi* test system [10]. Trypanothione may also mediate the selective toxic effects of aromatic arsenicals in African trypanosomes. It has been shown that trypanothione can form a relatively stable adduct with trivalent arsenicals such as melarsan oxide [9]. More recently, the two enzymes which are responsible for the biosynthesis of trypanothione, N^1-glutathionyl-spermidine synthetase and trypanothione synthetase, have been purified from the insect trypanosomatid *Crithidia fasciculata* (Henderson et al. unpublished).

GSH conjugation to spermidine links thiol and polyamine metabolism in trypanosomatids. In the last few years, polyamine metabolism in parasitic protozoa has become the subject of much research [11]. Difluoromethylornithine (DFMO) is an irreversible inhibitor of ornithine decarboxylase (ODC), a key enzyme in the biosynthesis of polyamines. Administration of DFMO to African trypanosomes blocks ODC (which leads to a depletion of intracellular putrescine and spermidine) in the parasite as it does in mammalian cells. African trypanosomes are susceptible to DFMO treatment in vitro and in vivo. DFMO is currently undergoing clinical trials in the Sudan and has proved useful in treating late-stage arsenical refractory cases of *T.b. gambiense* sleeping sickness. Given the high doses required for efficacy [200 to 500 mg (kg/day) for 6 to 8 weeks], DFMO appears to be generally well tolerated. This has encouraged research into its use in the treatment of other protozoan diseases including leishmania and malaria [11].

Folates serve as cofactors for various one-carbon transfer reactions in most cells. In the synthesis of thymidylate, the enzyme thymidylate synthetase catalyzes transfer of a methyl group equivalent from $N^{5,10}$-methylene tetrahydrofolate to dUMP; in this process, tetrahydrofolate becomes oxidized to dihydrofolate. To complete the cycle dihydrofolate is reduced by the enzyme dihydrofolate reductase. Folate metabolism is central to pyrimidine biosynthesis; as protozoa synthesize pyrimidines de novo and do not possess salvage pathways for these nucleotides, it has long been a target for the development of antiparasitic agents. Several antimalarial drugs, for example, proguanil and pyrimethamine, work by inhibiting folate metabolism in *Plasmodium*. On characterization of the thymidylate synthase–dihydrofolate reductase of parasitic protozoa, both activities have been shown to be associated with a bifunctional dihydrofolate reductase (H_2-folate)–thymidylate synthase (TS) enzyme [*12,13*]. This enzyme complex is overexpressed in antifolate-resistant protozoa. Drug resistance is a major problem in the chemotherapy of parasite diseases (as in all microbial diseases), and resistance to the antimalarial dihydrofolate reductase inhibitors is now widespread. It is hoped that study of the protozoan H_2-folate–TS complex will lead to a new generation of antimalaria folate inhibitors and better understanding of the mechanisms of drug resistance in these organisms.

On close examination, the biochemistry of glutathione, polyamine, and folate metabolism in parasitic protozoa has been shown to be significantly different from the analogous mammalian processes. In each case the initial stimulus for research was to understand the mechanism and specificity of existing antiparasitic drugs. It is likely that further study in these areas will lead to a new generation of antiparasitic agents.

NOVEL ASPECTS OF BIOCHEMISTRY ASSOCIATED WITH A PARASITIC LIFESTYLE

In order to enjoy the nutritionally rich environment of the mammalian host, parasitic organisms have had to develop highly sophisticated methods of evading or tricking the host immune response. Investigation of this aspect of parasite biochemistry is providing many new targets for future rational drug design. One evasive tactic is to "hide" within host cells. The mechanisms by which parasites first identify and then gain entry into particular host cells are for the most part obscure. This is particularly true of many groups of intracellular protozoa which infect nonphagocytic cells. Such organisms appear to gain entry to susceptible host cells by a process of "induced endocytosis." Most is known about the entry of malarial merozoites into host erythrocytes, at least at the morphological level. The apical end of the merozoite first makes contact with the surface of an erythrocyte and there forms a small depression in the erythrocyte membrane. The red cell then invaginates around the merozoite, and entry is complete in 20 to 30 s when the red cell plasma membrane seals behind the internalized parasite. The biochemistry of this process is now being investigated. Recent studies point to the importance of parasite proteolytic enzymes [*14*] and host cell ATP [*15*]. Once inside the erythrocyte, the maturing malaria parasite is relatively safe from direct contact with antibodies and other humoral and cellular factors. However, as discussed above, intracellular maturation necessitates the insertion of parasite proteins into the red cell. As these perturbed host cells are recognized by the phagocytic cells of the reticuloendothelial system (RES), some species of malaria, notably *P. falciparum,* have developed an additional method of avoiding the RES. This organism induces the formation of "knobs" on the erythrocyte membrane which cause the parasitized red cells to adhere to the endothelial lining of capillaries. In this way the parasitized erythrocytes evade filtration by the RES. Recent studies have identified the receptor for the parasite knob proteins as thrombospondin, a common surface protein of endothelial cells [*16*].

Perhaps the most remarkable method of evading the host immune response has been devised by African trypanosomes. These organisms are surrounded by a glycoprotein coat which is about 7-nm thick. In each parasite, the coat is composed of a single glycoprotein. After 5 to 7 days in the bloodstream the host mounts a powerful immune response against this parasite surface antigen. This response eliminates most of the parasite population, but a small percentage of the parasites now possess a different surface glycoprotein which is antigenically distinct. It has been estimated that the number of variable-surface glycoprotein (VSG) genes which can be potentially expressed by a clonal African trypanosome population may range from 300 to 1000; thus, host immune response can never totally eliminate a circulating population. This phenomenon is responsible for the waves of chronic disease observed in human beings and in domestic animals, which continue until the hapless mammal lapses into the chronic stages of the disease. The elucidation of the molecular mechanisms which control the expression of a single gene from the vast VSG gene repertoire has been the subject of much elegant work [*17,18*]. Expression appears to be controlled at the level of transcriptional activation and may involve genomic rearrangements similar to those which occur in B cells on expression of the V_H gene repertoire. The biosynthesis of the VSG protein and its interaction with the trypanosome membrane has also been investigated. The parasite VSG mRNA encodes a protein containing a short carboxy-terminal hydrophobic domain. On completion of protein synthesis, this terminal sequence is rapidly (within 1 min) removed and replaced by a glycosyl-phosphatidylinositol (G-PI) moiety. The complete structure of the *T. brucei* G-PI has now been determined [*19*]. The carboxy terminal of the processed VSG is linked to an ethanolamine residue, which bridges the VSG protein to a mannose-galactose–containing glycan that terminates with a glucosamine residue directly linked to dimyristylphosphatidylinositol. In the trypanosome, the G-PI lipid serves to anchor the VSG to the cell surface. Recently, similar glycosylated phosphoinositides have been described in other biological systems. Examples include the mannosylphosphatidylinositols of mycobacteria and the complex acidic lipophosphoglycans of *Leishmania donovani*. In addition, phosphatidylinositolglycans have recently been reported to mediate the action of insulin in mammalian cells [*19*]; these also contain a $GlcNH_2$-inositol linkage which may be structurally related to the trypanosome G-PI anchor.

CONCLUDING REMARKS

The need to develop new treatments for the diseases caused by protozoan and helminthic parasites is unanimously acknowledged by all of the major national and international organizations concerned with human health. It has traditionally been the case that antiparasitic drugs were found by screening procedures rather than on a basis of the biochemistry of the parasites. As we have tried to show in this chapter, this approach need not be relied upon in the future. The foregoing illustrations are just a few of innumerable areas in which the biochemistry of parasitic organisms differs from that of the host. Future investigation of these processes at the molecular level is the most sensible approach to the development of the urgently needed new antiparasite drugs.

REFERENCES

1 Trager W: *Living Together, The Biology of Animal Parasitism.* New York, Plenum, 1986

2 Campbell WC, Rew RS: *Chemotherapy of Parasitic Diseases.* New York, Plenum, 1986

3 Peters W: *Chemotherapy and Drug Resistance in Malaria,* 2nd ed. New York, Academic, 1987, vols 1&2

4 Cox FEG: *Modern Parasitology.* London, Blackwell, 1982

5 Hope DJ: Nucleotide metabolism in parasitic protozoa. Bailey DM (ed), Ann Rev Med Chem 21: 247–255, 1986

6 Fairlamb AH, Opperdoes FR: Carbohydrate metabolism in African trypanosomes, with special reference to the glycosome, in Morgan MJ (ed): *Carbohydrate Metabolism in Cultured Cells.* New York, Plenum, 1986, pp 183–224

7 Barrett J: *Biochemistry of Parasitic Helminths.* Baltimore, University Park Press, 1981

8 Saz H: Energy metabolism of parasitic helminths: Adaptations to parasitism. Ann Rev Physiol 43:323–341, 1981

9 Henderson GB, Fairlamb AH: Trypanothione metabolism, a chemotherapeutic target in trypanosomatids. Parasitol Today 3:312–315, 1987

10 Henderson GB, Ulrich P, Fairlamb AH, et al: "Subversive" substrates for the enzyme trypanothione disulfide reductase: Alternative approach to chemotherapy of Chagas' disease. Proc Natl Acad Sci USA, 85:5374–5378, 1988

11 Bacchi CJ, M'Cann PP: Parasitic protozoa and polyamines, in M'Cann PP, Pegg AE, Sjoerdsma A (eds): *Inhibition of Polyamine Metabolism.* New York, Academic, 1987, pp 317–344

12 Ferone R, Roland S: Dihydrofolate reductase/thymidylate synthase, a bifunctional polypeptide from *Crithidia fasciculata.* Proc Natl Acad Sci USA 77:5802–5806, 1980

13 Coderre JA, Beverley SM, Schimke RT, et al: Overproduction of a bifunctional thymidylate synthetase–dihydrofolate reductase and DNA amplification in methotrexate-resistant *Leishmania tropica.* Proc Natl Acad Sci USA 80:2132–2136, 1983

14 Bernard F, Schrevel J: Purification of a *Plasmodium berghei* neutral endopeptidase and its location in merozoites. Mol Biochem Parasitol 26:167–174, 1987

15 Olson JA, Kilejian A: Involvement of spectrin and ATP in infection of resealed erythrocyte ghosts by the human malarial parasite, *Plasmodium falciparum.* J Cell Biol 95:757–762, 1982

16 Roberts DD, Sherwood JA, Spitalnik SL, et al: Thrombospondin binds falciparum malaria-parasitized erythrocytes and may mediate cytoadherence. Nature 318:64–66, 1985

17 Boothroyd JC: Antigenic variation in African trypanosomes. Ann Rev Microbiol 39:475–502, 1985

18 Parsons M, Nelson RG, Agabian N: Antigenic variation in African trypanosomes: DNA rearrangements program immune evasion. Immunol Today 5:43–50, 1984

19 Ferguson MAJ, Homans SW, Dwek RA, et al: Glycosyl-phosphatidylinositol moiety that anchors trypanosoma brucei variant surface glycoprotein to the membrane. Science 239:753–759, 1988

CHAPTER
17

Host-Parasite Interface: Immune Evasion · John R. David

The biology of parasitism has many fascinating aspects. High on the list is the diversity with which parasites have evolved to evade the natural and acquired defenses of the host. At the same time, the host has developed mechanisms for keeping parasites in check and, in some cases, eliminating them. This parasite-host interaction is an excellent window into the evolution of adaptation of both host and parasite for survival. This chapter will briefly review the mechanisms parasites use to escape host defenses (see Table 17-1). Effective immune mechanisms against particular parasites are described in other chapters.

ANTIGENIC VARIATION BY TRYPANOSOMES AND OTHER PROTOZOA

The African trypanosome responsible for sleeping sickness has evolved a most sophisticated form of immune evasion: antigenic variation [1]. Infection by these trypanosomes in humans or animals causes waves of parasitemia, peaking every 7 to 10 days. Trypanosomes isolated from each of these waves are covered on their surfaces by different glycoproteins of around 55 kD, which are called *variable surface glycoproteins,* or VSGs. Each of these has a different amino acid sequence, and,

Table 17-1. Mechanisms of immune evasion

Mechanisms	Parasite examples
Antigenic variation	Trypanosomes
	Malaria, giardia
Evasion from macrophages	
Prevention of phagolysosomal fusion	*T. gondii*
Escape from lysosomal toxic molecules	Leishmania
Escape into cytoplasm	*T. cruzi*
Modulation of macrophage function	Leishmania
Uptake of host antigen	Schistosomes, *T. vivax*
Antigen mimicry	Schistosomes
Shedding of antigen	Schistosomes, trichinella
Intrinsic membrane changes	Schistosomes
Cleaving of antibody	Schistosomes, *T. cruzi,* filaria
Immune suppression	Leishmania, filaria
Resistance to complement lysis	Schistosomes, *T. cruzi*
Production of anti-inflammatory molecules	*T. taeniaeformis,* amoeba
Armor-plated surface immune to attack	Guinea worm
Enhancement by insect vector saliva	Leishmania

as a group, they are coded for by several hundred distinct VSG genes. The organisms switch from one VSG to another, thus evading elimination by antibodies reproduced to previously exhibited VSGs. However, the switching from one VSG gene to another is not dependent on antibody. The molecular mechanism involving the duplication of a particular VSG gene and its expression is one of the most interesting problems in the molecular biology of parasites.

Antigenic variation in malaria was first described in *Plasmodium knowlesi* in rhesus monkeys [2]. For example, the serum of an infected animal would agglutinate schizont-infected erythrocytes from all infected erythrocyte samples obtained from an animal before the serum sample but not from subsequently isolated infected red cells. The antigen was called SICA for schizont-infected cell agglutination. Each wave of parasitemia has a distinct SICA antigen. Cloned parasites exhibit the same variation, and the SICA antigens have been shown to be a family of proteins of approximately 200 kDa [3]. Antigenic variation was subsequently identified for *P. falciparum* by surface immunofluorescence of infected erythrocytes [4]. With infection, successive waves of parasite-infected erythrocytes exhibited different surface antigens that were also strain-specific. Antigenic variation also has been shown in *P. fragili* [5].

Recently, antigenic variation was reported in *Giardia lamblia* and appears to be associated with a family of cysteine-rich proteins of 170 kDa [6]. More details as to the mechanism of antigenic variation in trypanosomes and the other parasites can be found in the chapters covering these organisms.

EVASION OF KILLING BY MACROPHAGES

It is remarkable that various microorganisms evade the cytocidal armamentarium of one of the host's major defenses, the macrophage. And yet many do. A number of mechanisms underlie this evasion. These include prevention of fusion of the phagosome containing the organism with lysosomes carrying toxic molecules and hydrolases, neutralization of macrophage toxic substances, and escape by the organism into the cytoplasm, which presumably is free of such lethal molecules.

INHIBITION OF PHAGOSOME-LYSOSOME FUSION

Mycobacterium tuberculosis, Toxoplasma gondii, and *Legionella pneumophila* are examples of organisms that prevent the fusion of phagosomes with primary lysosomes [7,8]. Living intact organisms are required for this to occur. Indeed, damaged organisms, or even organisms coated with antibody which itself is not harmful, will not prevent the fusion of phagosomes with lysosomes. Until recently, the mechanism was poorly understood. Fusion could be prevented by some polyanionic substances such as acidic sulfatides from the cell wall of mycobacteria. Of interest, the excretory factor of leishmania, which is also polyanionic, does not do this. Recently, it has been shown that the prevention of fusion appears to be due to the inhibition of saltatory movement of the periphagosomal lysosomes [9]. The saltatory movement of these lysosomes slowed or stopped after ingestion of live but not dead *Mycobacterium microti,* an organism that prevents the fusion of phagosomes with lysosomes. Furthermore, the normal fusion of phagosomes containing *Saccharomyces cereviseae* with lysosomes was inhibited in macrophages that had previously been fed live but not dead *M. microti.*

ESCAPE FROM MACROPHAGE-KILLING MOLECULES

Organisms such as leishmania [10] and *M. leprae* live and multiply well inside phagolysosomes, somehow evading the many toxic molecules in these organelles. The leishmania promastigote is much more susceptible to killing by macrophages than the transformed amastigote. The mechanisms for this resistance are not well understood. Some experiments suggest that leishmania do not significantly inhibit the lysosomal digestive enzymes, whereas others suggest that they may alter these processes by the release of substances such as excretory factors that have antilysosomal activity. The search for molecules that are present in greater quantity on amastigotes than promastigotes should help in further understanding this mechanism of escape. It should be stressed that under certain circumstances macrophages can be activated, for instance, by interferon γ [11] or granulocyte-macrophage colony-stimulating factor (GM-CSF) [12], and can overcome the evasion mechanisms of the parasites.

ESCAPE FROM THE PHAGOLYSOSOMES

Mycobacteria leprae and *Trypanosoma cruzi* [13] can escape from the phagolysosomes and then multiply in the cytoplasm. Studies using electron microscopy showed the parasite was first surrounded by two sets of membranes, its own and that of the phagolysosome, and subsequently only by its own. Again, as in leishmania, the insect form of the parasite was killed by the macrophage whereas the transformed trypomastigote was not. Macrophages that were activated overcame this escape mechanism and killed the parasites.

ESCAPE FROM OR NEUTRALIZATION OF TOXIC OXYGEN METABOLITES

Phagocytosis of microorganisms is usually accompanied by a respiratory burst resulting in the production of toxic oxygen metabolites including superoxide, hydrogen peroxide, singlet oxygen, and hydroxyl anions. Activation of macrophages can lead to an increase in this respiratory burst and increased production of hydrogen peroxide. Some organisms appear to inhibit this burst. For instance, live but not dead *T. gondii* are ingested by resident mouse macrophages without stimulating a respiratory burst [14]. Similarly, amastigotes of *Leishmania donovani* failed to elicit a respiratory burst, whereas promastigotes did [15]. Killing or coating amastigotes with antibody did not change their behavior in this respect, suggesting that the decrease or lack of stimulation of a respiratory burst was due to a property of the amastigote surface. Again, search for substances found on amastigotes but not promastigotes should be of special interest. Leishmania have a superoxide dismutase [16] but lack scavengers of oxygen peroxide such as catalase or glutathione peroxidase. In contrast, *T. gondii* have both catalase and glutathione peroxidase, which may play a part in their survival [17]. *Plasmodium berghei* decrease the production of reactive oxygen by macrophages, and *Schistosoma mansoni* also diminish the respiratory burst of murine peritoneal macrophages.

PARASITE MODIFICATION OF MACROPHAGE FUNCTION

The activation of macrophages by a number of stimulants including interferon-γ, GM-CSF, or muramyl dipeptide (MDP) is accompanied by modulation of the expression of macrophage genes for Ia, IL-1, and TNF [18]. It has been shown that *L. donovani* suppresses the normal IL-1 response [19] and expression of class I and II major histocompatibility gene products. *L. major* also fails to induce the elaboration of IL-1 by human monocytes [20]. How different protozoa affect macrophage lymphokine and surface receptor activities will be of special interest. Recent findings indicate that both *Listeria monocytogenes* and the phenolic glycolipid of *M. leprae* diminish the normal processing of antigen by mouse macrophages [21]. Further, *Trypanosoma brucei* appears to be able to mediate immune dysfunction through macrophages by IL-1 secretion. The production of this cytokine may be responsible for some of the polyclonal activation and prostaglandin E_2 production that may mediate immune suppression [22].

IMMUNE ESCAPE BY SCHISTOSOMES: A CONCERT OF EVASION MECHANISMS

Some organisms have evolved many different mechanisms to evade the host's immune defenses. The schistosomes are an excellent example. Rather than describe each of these under the separate general headings, it seems appropriate to describe all of them together, especially as multiple mechanisms may function in concert. Some of these mechanisms may explain the phenomenon of *concomitant immunity,* a descriptive term for the survival of the invading parasite despite the protective immune response it has stimulated in the host against subsequent invaders.

MASQUERADE BY THE UPTAKE OF HOST ANTIGENS

One mechanism of special interest is the ability of schistosomes to disguise themselves by taking host antigens onto their surfaces. It was found that when adult worms were transferred from the blood vessels of a mouse to a monkey, they lived perfectly well, whereas worms transferred from the blood vessels of a mouse to a monkey that previously had been immunized with murine red blood cells were killed. Analysis of this form of masquerade has shown that various host molecules are taken up by the schistosomes; these include blood group glycolipids [23], major histocompatibility complex (MHC) glycoproteins [24], fibronectin [25], and nonspecific host immunoglobulins (bound by their Fc portion) [26]. It has been more difficult to show unequivocally that the uptake of host antigen by the parasite is the actual mechanism for their protection. Support for the view that uptake of host antigen is important in immune evasion by adult schistosomes comes from experiments which show that such worms can be killed by antibody-dependent cell-mediated cytotoxicity in vitro using antibodies directed to the host MHC antigens that have been taken up [27]. On the other hand, lung worms, also covered by MHC molecules of the host, were resistant to antibodies directed against these molecules, findings consistent with previous studies that had suggested other mechanisms described below.

The protozoan *Trypanosoma vivax* also appears to take up sialoglycoproteins of host origin. Further, it has been proposed that pathogenic *Trypanosomatidae* have Fc receptors to take up host immunoglobulins for protection.

HOST MOLECULE MIMICRY

One of the early suggestions for immune evasion was that schistosomes were capable of synthesizing antigens that cross-reacted with host molecules. Although this may be so for the antigens on the schistosome's surface which cross-react with α_2-macroglobulin [28], present evidence suggests that other antigens, such as MHC molecules, are of host and not of parasite origin. First, schistosome DNA fails to hybridize with murine MHC recombinant probes [29]. Further, MHC glycoprotein recovered from the surface of schistosomes has molecular weight and serological characteristics indistinguishable from those of the host MHC [29].

SHEDDING OF SCHISTOSOME SURFACE ANTIGENS

One-day-old schistosomula fail to bind antibodies. Although this could be due to the uptake of host antigens, an alternate possibility is that the antigenic sites are shed. Studies with schistosomula cultured in vitro in the absence of host molecules have shown that they lose their ability to bind rat antibodies [30], human antibodies [31], and C3 and concanavalin A [32] after 18 h of transformation. However, some antigens detected by mouse monoclonal antibodies can be detected for 48 or 96 h. Recent studies have shown that when schistosomula cultured for 6 days were injected intravenously into the lungs of mice, they had lost their parasite antigens when recovered 30 min later at a time when no host antigen was detected [33]. Shedding of antigens has also been described for *Trichinella spiralis*, *Fasciola hepatica*, *Entamoeba histolytica*, *T. cruzi*, and *T. gondii*.

RESISTANCE DUE TO INTRINSIC MEMBRANE CHANGES

Studies on schistosomula suggest that resistance to immune attack at the lung stage may be due to intrinsic membrane changes and not the lack of surface antigen secondary to shedding or host antigen acquisition. The surfaces of skin and lung stage schistosomula were made to contain equal amounts of a hapten antigen, trinitrophenyl (TNP), and the susceptibility to attack by anti-TNP antibodies and complement or eosinophils in vitro or by immune mechanisms of mice immunized with TNP on bovine γ-globulin in vivo was examined. Whereas the skin stage schistosomula were killed by these in vitro and in vivo effector mechanisms, the lung stage hapten-covered schistosomula were resistant. These experiments indicated that lung stage schistosomula were resistant for reasons other than their low surface antigenicity [34].

Schistosomula cultured in vitro with serum become resistant to complement and antibody-dependent cell-mediated cytotoxicity [35,36]. Resistance is correlated with the uptake of cholesterol and triglycerides from the serum [37]. Further, the escape induced by concanavalin A or sera from the damage caused by antibody and complement may be due in part to the methylation of phospholipids by methyltransferases produced by the schistosomula [38]; inhibition of the methyltransferases enhances the killing. The methylation of phospholipids is associated with increased fluidity of the membrane. The schistosomular surface also elaborates lysophosphatidylcholine,

which can act as a detergent; a number of interactions of schistosomula with cells, including the fusion of neutrophil cell membrane with the schistosomular surface, the lysing of red blood cells, and the inhibition of mast cell degranulation can all be attributed to the elaborated lysophosphatidylcholine [39].

Recent studies also indicate that resistant schistosomula, but not susceptible early skin schistosomula, possess a membrane pump/carrier which may reverse the damage that would follow from ion imbalance caused by the immune attack; this is discussed in a review [40].

RESISTANCE TO COMPLEMENT

The cercariae are covered by a carbohydrate-rich glycocalyx which triggers the alternate complement pathway, and they are sensitive to complement lysis [41]. Although freshly transformed skin schistosomula are also susceptible, they rapidly lose this sensitivity. After 24 to 48 h, whether cultured in vitro or recovered in vivo, they are resistant, as are lung stage schistosomula. Whereas some resistance to complement may be due to surface changes that no longer allow the activation of the alternate complement pathway, other studies have shown that schistosomula develop resistance to complement lysis through surface changes despite the binding of all complement components onto the surface [42].

OTHER MECHANISMS FOR ESCAPING IMMUNE ATTACK

In addition to the above, there are a number of further evasion mechanisms that have been proposed for schistosomes. They have been shown to release a soluble factor called SDIF which inhibits mast cell degranulation and T-lymphocyte proliferation and could enhance survival of the parasite [43]. They possess proteolytic enzymes which can cleave antibody at the Fc region, thus disarming the antibodies that must bind effector cells through their Fc. However, the in vitro studies demonstrating the effectiveness of antibody-dependent cell-mediated cytotoxicity suggest that this enzyme may not play an important role. Further, immune complexes formed by the combination of antibody and shed schistosome antigen could block cells mediating antibody-dependent cell-mediated cytotoxicity. Indeed, immune complexes following infections by leishmania and malaria might also enhance immune evasion by those organisms.

PARASITE EVASION OF ANTIPARASITE ANTIBODY

Many of the mechanisms described above such as shedding of antigen, masquerading with host antigens, formation of complexes, and intrinsic membrane changes are ways that parasites evade the effects of antiparasite antibodies. Other mechanisms may involve the destruction of the antibodies themselves. For example, *T. cruzi* produces a protease that will split the Fc domains from the antibody leaving the Fab fragments bound to the surface. Without the Fc portion, the antibody is unable to bind either complement or the Fc receptor of effector cells [44]. This has been called *fabulation*. Proteases that cleave antibodies have also been described for *Fasciola hepatica, S. mansoni* schistosomula, and *Brugia malayi*.

EVASION BY IMMUNE SUPPRESSION

A number of parasites induce specific immune suppression in the host. For example, *Leishmania donovani* induces a specific suppression of T-cell responses. Despite the large amounts of specific antibody produced, these patients do not exhibit delayed-type hypersensitivity to leishmania antigen, and their T cells do not respond in vitro to this antigen. The parasite suppresses the production of IL-2 and interferon-γ [45]. Marked T-cell suppression is also seen in cases of diffuse cutaneous leishmaniasis [46]. Extensive studies by a number of investigators using BALB/c mice have shown that spread of *L. major* is due in part to T cells that function as suppressor cells but are of the L3T4 phenotype, not the Lyt 2, the usual suppressor phenotype [47,48]. Further studies indicate that BALB/c appear to have a higher proportion of these L3T4 cells than do resistant C57 black mice. When the number of L3T4 cells is decreased in vivo by means of a monoclonal antibody, the BALB/c mice become resistant to *L. major*. However, if all L3T4 cells are removed, the mice are susceptible, indicating the probable existence of suppressor and helper L3T4 cell subsets [49].

Studies with the filaria *B. malayi* indicate that microfilariae also induce a state of specific antigen immunosuppression. Delayed skin reactivity and T-cell proliferation to microfilarial antigen is diminished, and the number of CD8 cytotoxic/suppressor cells is increased [50]. Further, extracts of *B. malayi* contain factors that are immunosuppressive [51]. The transplacental transfer of rodent microfilariae induced antigen-specific tolerance in rats which could also blunt the host's defenses [52].

PARASITE EVASION OF CYTOTOXICITY BY COMPLEMENT

Whereas epimastigotes of *T. cruzi* (the stage in the insect vector) are highly sensitive to lysis by the alternative complement pathway, the metacyclic trypomastigotes (the infective stage) are resistant [53]. Treatment of blood trypomastigotes with trypsin and to a lesser extent with neuraminidase converts these protozoa into activators of the alternative pathway and thus sensitive again. Further studies showed that the protection of the trypomastigotes by a trypsin-neuraminidase-sensitive molecule required protein synthesis [54]. Treatment of metacyclic trypomastigotes with pronase almost completely reversed their resistance to serum lysis, and partial reverse was seen with *N*-glycanase and neuraminidase [55]. With enzyme treatment, there was an increase in the deposition of C3 and C9 on these organisms. Further, it was shown that the hemolytic inactive fragment, iC3b, was the main form of the molecule on the

resistant trypomastigotes, whereas the hemolytic active C3b was the main form on the enzyme-treated and sensitive trypomastigotes. This appears to be due to a developmentally regulated glycoprotein doublet of 90 to 115 kDa on the surface which is pronase-sensitive [55]. Further, the C3 binds by a covalent ester linkage to surface molecules of different molecular weight on the sensitive epimastigote and resistant trypomastigote. Evasion of the complement system by schistosomes is discussed above.

For a long time it has been known that various leishmania are lysed by complement. Of interest is the finding that different species of leishmania show differing susceptibility to complement lysis. Amastigotes of *L. tropica*, which causes cutaneous lesions, were shown to be very susceptible to lysis by fresh human serum, but not heated serum [56]. Further studies showed that the membrane attack was a consequence of the alternative complement pathway. In contrast, *L. donovani*, which causes visceral leishmaniasis, was 10 times less susceptible to killing by normal serum. The marked difference between the susceptibility of these organisms to lysis by serum may explain, in part, the ability of *L. donovani* to escape the site of inoculation and disseminate.

PARASITE ENZYMES, PROTEINASE INHIBITORS, AND OTHER MOLECULES CAN COUNTER HOST DEFENSES

It can be seen from the various sections that some parasites produce enzymes and other molecules that can counter the host's defenses. These have been recently reviewed [57] and are listed in Table 17-2. A number of investigators have proposed that proteinase inhibitors could be important in the parasite's ability to evade host defense. A proteinase inhibitor from the metacestode *Taenia taeniaeformis*, called taeniastatin, has been described that inhibits complement activation and inhibits lymphocyte proliferation, neutrophil chemotaxis, and aggregation [57].

SURVIVAL OF PARASITES IN HOSTS WITH GENETICALLY DETERMINED LOW IMMUNE RESPONSE

Studies with inbred animals indicate that susceptibility to some parasites is genetically determined. Examples include *L. don-*

Table 17-2. Molecules produced by parasites can counter the host's defenses

Cleave antibodies
Inactivate complement components
Consume complement
Inactivate leukotrienes, prostaglandins
Inactivate platelet activating factor (PAF)
Inactivate chemotactic factors
Inhibit lymphocyte proliferation

ovani [58], *L. tropica* [59], and *T. spiralis* in mice [60]. This has been reviewed, and the possibility that the continued transmission of parasites in human beings is partly affected by genetic susceptibility is discussed in the review [61].

The possibility that the survival of parasites despite an immune attack is due to the selection of resistant subsets of parasites has been addressed. In the case of *S. mansoni* surviving the protective mechanisms of mice immunized with irradiated cercariae, it was shown that five generations of survivors were no more resistant than the original organisms. Similarly, the exoerythrocyte form (EEF) of *P. berghei* that resists the inhibitory effects of interferon-γ does not appear to be a resistant subset of parasite. However, over a much longer period of time, parasites probably have evolved ways of resisting the host's defenses through the process of selection.

IMMUNE MODULATION THROUGH MATERNAL-FETUS INTERACTION

There is some evidence that offspring of parasite-infected mothers have an altered immune response to the parasite. For instance, *B. malayi* infection in the mother predisposed the offspring of gerbils to patent infection after inoculation with infective larvae [62]. The prenatal induction of tolerance from mother to newborn has been described. Mice born of *S. mansoni*-infected mothers have less acute granuloma than normal controls. Some studies suggest that this may be due to the passage of antigen from the mother to the fetus or newborn through the placenta or colostrum. Other experiments suggest that an idiotypic–anti-idiotypic network may affect the offspring's immune response to schistosomes. Indeed, the presence of anti-idiotypic T cells in cord blood was recently demonstrated [63]. This is an exciting area of research which may lead to a better understanding of the host response to parasites in endemic areas.

INSECT VECTOR SALIVA CAN ENHANCE TRANSMISSION OF PARASITES

Saliva of arthropod vectors such as mosquitoes, ticks, reduviid bugs, and sand flies contain molecules that prevent blood coagulation of the host or are anti-inflammatory [64]. Recently, it was shown that the injection into mice of saliva from sand flies *Lutzomyia longipalpus* with *Leishmania major* promastigotes markedly increased the size of the lesions and the number of parasites found in the lesions [65]. As little as 10 percent of a salivary gland was effective. The saliva did not act directly on the leishmania, but on the host. Salivary gland extracts from mosquitoes, ticks, and reduviid bugs had no effect on the transmission of leishmania. The extracts of sand fly salivary gland were found to contain a molecule with potent vasodilatory activity. Of interest, the sand fly saliva extract when preincubated with human monocyte-derived macrophages prevented their activation by interferon-γ. These studies indicate that the saliva from an insect vector may enhance the transmission of the parasites, helping them to evade the host's defenses.

REFERENCES

1 Cross GAM: Identification, purification and properties of clone-specific glycoprotein antigens constituting the surface coat of *Trypanosoma brucei*. Parasitology 71:393–417, 1975

2 Brown IN, Brown KN, Hills LA: Immunity to malaria: The antibody response to antigenic variation in *Plasmodium knowlesi*. Immunology 14:127–138, 1968

3 Howard RJ, Barnwell JW, Kao V: Antigenic variation in *Plasmodium knowlesi* malaria: Identification of the variant antigen on infected erythrocytes. Proc Natl Acad Sci USA 80:4129–4133, 1983

4 Hommel M, David PH, Oligino LD: Surface alterations of erythrocytes in *Plasmodium falciparum* malaria. J Exp Med 157:1137–1148, 1983

5 Handunnetti SM, Mendis KN, David PH: Antigenic variation of cloned *Plasmodium fragile* in its natural host *Maca sinica*. J Exp Med 165:1269–1283, 1987

6 Adam RD, Aggarwal A, Altataf AL, et al: Antigenic variation of cysteine-rich protein in *Giardia lamblia*. J Exp Med 169:109–117, 1988

7 Armstrong JA, D'Arcy Hart P: Response of cultured macrophages to *Mycobacterium tuberculosis*, with observations of fusion of lysosomes with phagosomes. J Exp Med 134:713, 1972

8 Jones TC, Hirsch JG: The interaction between *Toxoplasma gondii* and mammalian cells. II. The absence of lysosome fusion with phagocytic vacuoles containing living parasites. J Exp Med 136:1173–1194, 1972

9 D'Arcy Hart P, Young MR, Gordon AH, et al: Inhibition of phagosome-lysosome fusion in macrophages by certain mycobacteria can be explained by inhibition of lysosomal movement observed after phagocytosis. J Exp Med 166:933–946, 1987

10 Alexander J, Vickerman K: Fusion of host cell secondary lysosomes with parasitophorous vacuoles of *Leishmania mexicana*-infected macrophages. J Protozool 22:502–508, 1975

11 Murray HW, Rubin BY, Rothermel CD: Killing of intracellular *Leishmania donovani* by lymphokine-stimulated human mononuclear phagocytes: Evidence that interferon-gamma is the activating lympokine. J Clin Invest 72:1506–1510, 1983

12 Weiser WY, Van Neil A, Clark SC, et al: Recombinant human granulocyte/macrophage colony stimulating factor activates intracellular killing of *Leishmania donovani* by human monocyte-derived macrophages. J Exp Med 166:1436–1446, 1987

13 Kress Y, Bloom BR, Wittner M, et al: Resistance of *Trypanosoma cruzi* to killing by macrophages. Nature 257:394–396, 1975

14 Wilson CB, Tsai V, Remington JS: Failure to trigger the oxidative burst by normal macrophages: Possible mechanisms for survival of intracellular pathogens. J Exp Med 151:328–346, 1980

15 Murray HW: Susceptibility of *Leishmania* to oxygen intermediates and killing by normal macrophages. J Exp Med 153:1302–1315, 1981

16 Meshnick SR, Eaton JW: Leishmanial superoxide dismutase: A possible target for chemotherapy. Biochem Biophys Res Commun 102:970–976, 1981

17 Murray HW, Nathan CA, Cohn ZA: Macrophage oxygen-dependent antimicrobial activity. IV. Role of endogenous scavengers of oxygen intermediates. J Exp Med 152:1610–1624, 1980

18 Vermeulen MW, David JR, Remold HG: Differential mRNA responses in human macrophages activated by interferon-γ and muramyl dipeptide. J Immunol 139:7–9, 1987

19 Reiner NE: Parasite accessory cell interactions in murine leishmaniasis: I. Evasion and stimulus-dependent suppression of the macrophages interleukin 1 response by *Leishmania donovani*. J Immunol 138:1919–1925, 1987

20 Crawford GD, Wyler DJ, Dinarello GA: Parasite-monocyte interactions in human leishmaniasis: Production of interleukin-1 in vitro. J Infect Dis 152:315–322, 1985

21 Leyva-Coban F, Unanue E: Intracellular interference with antigen presentation. J Immunol (in press)

22 Askonas BA, Bancroft GJ: Interaction of African trypanosomes with the immune system. Phil Trans Soc Lond (B) 307:41–50, 1984

23 Goldring OL, Kusel JR, Smithers SR: *Schistosoma mansoni:* Origin in vitro of host-like surface antigens. Exp Parasitol 43:82–93, 1977

24 Sher A, Hall BF, Vadas MA: Acquisition of murine major histocompatibility complex gene products by schistosomula of *Schistosoma mansoni*. J Exp Med 148:46–57, 1978

25 Ouaissi MA, Cornette J, Capron A: Occurrence of fibronectin antigenic determinants on *Schistosoma mansoni* lung schistosomula and adult worms. Parasitology 88:85–96, 1984

26 Kemp WM, Merritt SC, Bogucki MS, Rosier JG, Seed JR: Evidence for adsorption of heterospecific host immunoglobulin on the tegument of *Schistosoma mansoni*. J Immunol 119:1849–1854, 1977

27 McLaren DJ, Terry RJ: The protective role of acquired host antigens during schistosome maturation. Parasit Immunol 4:129–148, 1982

28 Damian RT, Greene ND, Hubbard WJ: Occurrence of mouse α$_2$-macroglobulin antigenic determinants on *Schistosoma mansoni* adults, with evidence on their nature. J Parasitol 59:64–73, 1973

29 Simpson AJG, Singer D, McCutchan TF, et al: Evidence that schistosome MHC antigens are not synthesized by the parasite but acquired from the host as intact glycoproteins. J Immunol 131:962–965, 1983

30 Samuelson JC, Sher A, Caulfield JA: Newly transformed schistosomula spontaneously lose surface antigens and C3 acceptor sites during culture. J Immunol 124:2055–2057, 1980

31 Dessein A, Samuelson JC, Butterworth AE, et al: Immune evasion by *Schistosoma mansoni:* Loss of susceptibility to antibody- or complement-dependent eosinophil attack by schistosomula cultured in medium free of macromolecules. Parasitology 82:357–374, 1981

32 Samuelson JC, Caulfield JP, David JR: Schistosomula of *Schistosoma mansoni* clear concanavalin A from their surface by sloughing. J Cell Biol 94:355–362, 1982

33 Pearce EJ, Basch PF, Sher A: Evidence that reduced surface antigenicity of developing *Schistosoma mansoni* schistosomula is due to antigen shedding rather than host molecule acquisition. Parasite Immunol 8:79–94, 1986

34 Moser G, Wassom DL, Sher A: Studies of the antibody dependent killing of schistosomula of *Schistosoma mansoni* employing haptenic target antigens. I. Evidence that the loss in susceptibility to immune damage undergone by developing schistosomula involves a change unrelated to the masking of parasite antigens by host molecules. J Exp Med 152:41–53, 1980

35 Tavares CAP, Soares RC, Coelho PMZ, et al: *Schistosoma mansoni:* Evidence for a role of serum factors in protecting artificially transformed schistosomula against antibody-mediated killing in vitro. Parasitology 77:225–233, 1978

36 McLaren DJ, Incani RN: *Schistosoma mansoni:* Acquired resistance of developing schistosomula to immune attack in vitro. Exp Parasitol 53:285–298, 1982

37 Rumjanek FD, McLaren DJ: *Schistosoma mansoni:* Modulation of schistosomular lipid composition by serum. Mol Biochem Parasitol 3:239–252, 1981

38 Parra JFC, França RCS, Kusel JR, et al: *Schistosoma mansoni:* Phospholipid methylation and escape of schistosomula from in vitro cytotoxic reaction. Mol Biochem Parasitol 21:151–159, 1986

39 Golan DE, Brown CS, Cianci CML, et al: Schistosomula of *Schistosoma mansoni* use lysophatidylcholine to lyse adherent human red blood cells and immobilize red cell membrane components. J Cell Biol 103:819–828, 1986

40 Pearce EJ, Sher A: Mechanisms of immune evasion in schistosomiasis. Contr Microbiol Immunol 8:219–232, 1987

41 Samuelson JC, Caulfield JP: Cercarial glycocalyx of *Schistosomula mansoni* activates human complement. Infect Immun 51:181–186, 1986

42 Ruppel A, McLaren DJ, Diesfield HJ, et al: *Schistosoma mansoni:* Escape from complement-mediated parasiticidal mechanisms following percutaneous primary infection. Eur J Immunol 14:702–708, 1984

43 Capron A, Dessaint JP: Schistosome as a potential source of pharmacological agents, in Capron (ed): *Clinics in Immunology and Allergy*. Philadelphia, Saunders, 1982, vol 2, p 613

44 Krettli AU, Eisen H: Escape mechanisms of *Trypanosoma cruzi* from the host immune system. Semaine Inserm Seillac, France, 1980

45 Carvalho EM, Badaro R, Reed SG, et al: Absence of gamma interferon and interleukin 2 production during active visceral leishmaniasis. J Clin Invest 76:2066–2069, 1985

46 Petersen EA, Neva FA, Oster N, et al: Specific inhibition of lymphocyte-proliferation responses by adherent suppressor cells in diffuse cutaneous leishmaniasis. N Engl J Med 306:387–392, 1982

47 Howard JG, Hale C, Liew FY: Immunological regulation of experimental cutaneous leishmaniasis. IV. Prophylactic effect of sublethal irradiation as a result of abrogation of suppressor T cell generation in mice genetically susceptible to *Leishmania tropica*. J Exp Med 153:557–568, 1981

48 Titus RG, Lima GC, Engers HD, et al: Exacerbation of murine cutaneous leishmaniasis by adoptive transfer of parasite-specific helper T cell populations capable of mediating *Leishmania major*-specific delayed type hypersensitivity. J Immunol 133:1594–1600, 1984

49 Titus RG, Ceredig R, Cerottini JC, et al: Therapeutic effects of anti-L3T4 monoclonal antibody GK 1.5 on cutaneous leishmaniasis in genetically-susceptible BALB/c mice. J Immunol 135:2108–2114, 1985

50 Piessens WF, Partono F, Hoffmann SL, et al: Antigen-specific suppressor T lymphocytes in human lymphatic filariasis. N Engl J Med 307:144–148, 1982

51 Wadee AA, Vickery AC, Piessens WF: Characterization of immunosuppressive proteins of *Brugia malayi* microfilariae. Acta Tropica 44:343–352, 1987

52 Haque A, Capron A: Transplacental transfer of rodent microfilariae induces antigen-specific tolerance in rats. Nature 299:361–363, 1982

53 Joiner K, Sher A, Gaither T, et al: Evasion of alternative complement pathway of *Trypanosoma cruzi* results from inefficient binding of factor B. Proc Natl Acad Sci USA 83:6593–6597, 1986

54 Kipnis T, David JR, Alper C, et al: Enzymatic treatment transforms trypomastigotes of *Trypanosoma cruzi* into activators of alternative complement pathway and potentiates their uptake by macrophages. Proc Natl Acad Sci USA 78:602–605, 1981

55 Sher A, Hieny S, Joiner K: Evasion of the alternative complement pathway by metacyclic trypomastigotes of *Trypanosoma cruzi:* Dependence on the developmentally regulated synthesis of surface protein and *N*-linked carbohydrate. J Immunol 137:2961–2967, 1986

56 Hoover DL, Berger M, Nacy CA, et al: Killing of *Leishmania tropica* amastigotes by factors in normal human serum. J Immunol 132:893–897, 1984

57 Leid RW, Suquet CM, Tanigoshi L: Parasite defence mechanisms for evasion of host attack: a review. Vet Parasitol 25:147–162, 1987

58 Blackwell J, Freeman J, Bradley DJ: Influence of H-2 complex on acquired resistance to *Leishmania donovani* infections in mice. Nature 283:72–74, 1980

59 Howard JG, Hale C, Liew FY: Genetically-determined susceptibility to *Leishmania tropica* infection is expressed by haematopoietic donor cells in mouse radiation chimaeras. Nature 288:161–162, 1980

60 Wassom DL, Wakelin D, Brooks BO, et al: Genetic control of immunity to *Trichinella spiralis* infections of mice: Hypothesis to explain the role of H-2 genes in primary challenge infections. Immunology 51:625–631, 1984

61 Wakelin D: Evasion of the immune response: Survival within low responder individuals of the host population. Parasitology 88:639–657, 1984

62 Schrater AF, Spielman A, Piessens WF: Predisposition to *Brugia malayi* microfilaremia in progeny of infected gerbils. Am J Trop Med Hyg 32:1306–1308, 1983

63 Colley D: Personal communication

64 Ribeiro JMC: Role of saliva in blood-feeding by arthropods. Ann Rev Entomol 32:463–478, 1987

65 Titus RG, Ribeiro JMC: Salivary gland lysates from the sand fly *Lutzomyia longipalpus* enhance leishmania infectivity. Science 239:1306–1308, 1988

CHAPTER
18

Immunocompromised Host
· Jerrold J. Ellner

The pandemic of acquired immunodeficiency syndrome (AIDS) changes traditional notions about the immunocompromised host. Formerly, immunocompromise was a rare condition, particularly in developing countries. Congenital immunodeficiencies are infrequent and generally produce rapidly lethal infections. Severe forms of acquired immunodeficiency usually result from the treatment of malignancy, particularly leukemias or management of patients following organ transplantations. This deliberate immunocompromise is a by-product of medical progress and represents a well-recognized and studied situation often approached in a stereotypical fashion; for example, the neutropenic patient with fever is treated with antibiotics.

AIDS changes all this. In March 1988, the World Health Organization estimated that 5 to 10 million persons had been infected with the human immunodeficiency virus (HIV), and only 2 to 3 million of them were residents of the United States and Europe. Neither the ultimate spread of HIV infection nor its natural history in developing countries is clear. In the United States the question of whether a patient is at high risk for AIDS (male homosexual, intravenous drug abuser, hemophiliac, recipient of blood transfusion before 1985) has become essential for assessing the possibility of opportunistic infection in many clinical settings. In much of the world, heterosexual spread of HIV predominates, so that any sexually active person, particularly one with multiple sexual contacts and sexually transmitted diseases, must be considered potentially immunocompromised.

The interactions of infectious agents with humans are modified sometimes drastically, when the usual immune response is subverted [1–7]. The result is increased frequency of severe infections caused by organisms ordinarily of low virulence comprising mucosal and skin flora or agents normally maintained in a latent stage.

Most commonly, immunity is compromised by a preexisting and serious underlying disease. The immunocompromised state is not, however, an all-or-none phenomenon. The nature and extent of immunosuppression vary with the predisposing disease and are in turn predictive of the spectrum of infectious agents with increased pathogenicity for the host (Table 18-1). Although neoplasm and its treatment, and infection with HIV constitute the most significant forms of immunocompromise, common diseases such as diabetes mellitus and uremia also alter host immunity. Demonstrated defects in the immune response often are subtle, however, and of uncertain significance. Infectious diseases themselves may depress immunity,

Table 18-1. The relationship between immune deficit
and infectious complications

Immune deficit	Infectious organism
Antibody	Encapsulated aerobic bacteria
Cell-mediated immunity	Latent microbes, facultative intracellular pathogens
Neutropenia/severe neutrophil dysfunction	Organisms constituting normal flora or ubiquitous in the environment

too, either directly through immunosuppressive bacterial products and activation of suppressor mechanisms, or indirectly through associated fever, anemia, and malnutrition. The influence of one infectious disease on the predilection for other infections has not been evaluated in most instances and is a major issue in areas of high prevalence of HIV infection.

This chapter explores the relationship between diseases associated with specific and profound disorders of the immune response and related susceptibility to infection. Clinical observation of this relationship has provided vital insights into mechanisms of host resistance and microbial pathogenicity and affords a logical approach to diagnosis and management of such patients.

DISEASES PRODUCING IMMUNOSUPPRESSION

DISORDERS OF CELL-MEDIATED IMMUNITY

Cell-mediated immunity is the major host defense mechanism operative against a restricted group of pathogens. Most of these organisms are facultative intracellular pathogens; that is, they have the capacity to survive within mononuclear phagocytes. Such agents usually elicit granulomatous tissue responses.

The interaction of specifically sensitized T lymphocytes with mononuclear phagocytes is critical to an effective cell-mediated immune response [8,9]. The first step in this interaction is ingestion of the parasite by mononuclear phagocytes in host tissues. These resident macrophages are not capable of destroying the organism but may limit its proliferation. The macrophages present antigen derived from the causative agent to specifically sensitized T lymphocytes. The T lymphocytes are thereby activated to release glycoprotein products termed *lymphokines.* Chemotactic lymphokines attract mononuclear phagocytes to the site of infection and initiate granuloma formation. At the local site, macrophages are activated by lymphokines and in some instances directly by bacterial products to become more efficient in the phagocytosis and killing of organisms. The activated macrophage develops the capacity to overcome the defenses of the intracellular organism and destroy it.

The primary defect in most diseases associated with impaired cell-mediated immunity occurs at the level of the T lymphocyte. Clinical assessment of T-cell function usually consists of determining delayed skin test reactivity. The list of diseases, as well as the situations associated with impaired

Table 18-2. Conditions associated with suppression
of delayed hypersensitivity

Infections:
   Viral: Human immunodeficiency virus infection, measles, cytomegalovirus, infectious mononucleosis, varicella-zoster
   Bacterial: Typhoid fever, pneumonia, tuberculosis, leprosy
   Fungal: Coccidioidomycosis, histoplasmosis, blastomycosis
   Other: Onchocerciasis, trypanosomiasis
Vaccinations:
   Measles, mumps, varicella
Tumors:
   Hodgkin's disease, lymphomas, advanced solid tumors
Drugs:
   Corticosteroids, cytotoxic drugs, niridazole
Miscellaneous diseases:
   Sarcoidosis, uremia, diabetes mellitus, malnutrition
Other conditions:
   Surgery, anesthesia, old age, leukocytosis, anemia, fever, burns

delayed hypersensitivity, is long and is constantly growing (Table 18-2) [10]. Not all of these conditions are associated with increased susceptibility to infection with intracellular organisms. In most, defects in T-cell function presumably are too subtle or too transitory to produce a clinically significant diathesis to infection.

Frequent infection with unusual organisms sometimes provides the first clue that a patient or group of patients has an acquired immunodeficiency. In fact, the opportunistic infection represents the AIDS-defining condition. The AIDS epidemic also highlights the importance of adequate microbiology and pathology in establishing that a patient has an opportunistic infection. Lacking such laboratory support, the clinical case definition proposed by the WHO can be used to establish the diagnosis of AIDS, but is of no help in identifying the specific opportunistic infection.

Clinical observation permits a trimmed-down list of diseases associated with defective cell-mediated immunity and increased risk of infection. Foremost among these are AIDS, Hodgkin's disease and other lymphomas [13], hairy-cell leukemia [14], and advanced solid tumors; patients with severe malnutrition or those receiving treatment with high-dose corticosteroids, cytotoxic drugs, or radiotherapy [3] show a similar predilection for infections. Congenital immunodeficiencies are associated with severe infections early in childhood and will not be considered here.

Patients with these acquired immunodeficiencies are susceptible to the group of organisms shown in Table 18-3. This list, again, is based on clinical observation and includes some but not all intracellular parasites. The spectrum of opportunistic agents in AIDS is somewhat different and has unexplained geographic variation [11,12,51]. AIDS is associated with most of the infections shown in Table 18-3, although some, such as *Listeria,* are curiously infrequent. Additional organisms, particularly *Mycobacterium avium* and JC virus, the cause of pro-

Table 18-3. Infectious agents with increased pathogenicity in patients with defective cell-mediated immunity

Viruses:
  Varicella-zoster, herpes simplex, cytomegalovirus
Fungi:
  Pathological: *Histoplasma, Coccidioides*
  Saprophytic: *Cryptococcus, Candida, Nocardia*
Bacteria:
  *Listeria, Nocardia, Mycobacterium tuberculosis, Legionella
    pneumophila*
Other:
  Pneumocystis carinii, Toxoplasma gondii, Cryptosporidium sp.,
    Strongyloides stercoralis

gressive multifocal leukoencephalopathy, are more common in AIDS patients, as are diarrheal pathogens such as *Cryptosporidium* species. The unique susceptibility to *M. avium* that is found in up to 50 percent of AIDS patients at autopsy is not understood but probably relates to exposure to the organism in the environment rather than reactivation of latent infection. As regards geographical differences, *Pneumocystis carinii* is the most common opportunistic infection in the United States. It is one-third as frequent in Haiti [11], and bilaterial pulmonary infiltrates presumed to be *Pneumocystis* are similarly infrequent in Zaire. Recent studies from Uganda in which material obtained by brochoalveolar lavage was stained for *Pneumocystis* failed to reveal this organism in 45 consecutive patients with AIDS and pulmonary infiltrates (Serwadda, D, et al., personal communication). *M. avium* also is rare, if it occurs at all, outside of the developed countries, whereas tuberculosis is not only common but the main communicable infection found in AIDS patients. Besides infection with facultative intracellular organisms, patients (particularly children) with AIDS develop severe bacterial infections and certain tumors, most frequently Kaposi's sarcoma and lymphomas. The interaction of HIV with the other viral agents or exposures leading to endemic Kaposi's sarcoma or Burkitt's lymphoma in regions such as Uganda is not well understood. Based on limited observations, HIV infection does not seem to exacerbate other endemic diseases such as malaria. Exposure is clearly a major factor in the selection of intracellular parasites actually causing infection in a deficient host. For example, *Mycobacterium leprae,* although an intracellular parasite, is limited in geographical distribution. Relevant observations as to its pathogenicity in the defective host need to be made in endemic areas. The mechanisms of intracellular persistence associated with particular infectious agents have been reviewed [15].

Clinical observation of the natural history of infectious diseases in the immunocompromised host has provided circumstantial evidence for the overriding importance of cell-mediated immunity in resistance to certain etiological agents. For example, the frequent exacerbation of latent viral infections in patients with defective cell-mediated immunity suggests a

dominant role for this effector mechanism in immunological surveillance and maintenance of the latent state [16]. The recognition of the increased occurrence of *Legionella pneumophila* in immunosuppressed patients provoked studies demonstrating that it too is a facultative, intracellular organism [17]. Documentation of the hyperinfection syndrome associated with *Strongyloides stercoralis* (abdominal pain, distension, shock, gram-negative sepsis, meningitis) similarly must reflect the importance of cell-mediated immunity in preventing such progression in the normal host [18]. Scientific confirmation of the role of cell-mediated immunity in resistance to this multicellular helminth lags behind clinical observation.

Thus, depression of cell-mediated immunity alters the outcome of exposure to certain infectious agents. Latent infections with viruses, fungi, protozoa, or mycobacteria reactivate or progress to cause disease [19]. Nonetheless, certain biases restrict our understanding of the totality of the relationship between defects in cell-mediated immunity and infectious disease. Occurrence and recognition of the immunocompromised state are greatest in areas in which modern diagnostic technology and antitumor and immunosuppressive therapy are available and used; the occurrence of certain parasitic diseases is rare in such settings. So, little is known of the effect of immunocompromise on the natural history of many diseases endemic in developing countries. For example, the activated macrophage appears to be an important effector cell in the host response to *Schistosoma mansoni* [20]. Clinical evidence regarding the effect of immunocompromise on the natural history of human schistosomiasis is limited. Autopsy studies are available on one patient with chronic schistosomiasis who underwent renal transplantation and was treated with prednisone and azathioprine [21]. The patient died from septicemia. At postmortem examination, *S. mansoni* eggs were found in the liver and colon. However, no granulomas or macrophages were present around the eggs. Thus, in humans, as in experimental animals, depression of delayed hypersensitivity is associated with diminished granulomatous hypersensitivity. Theoretically, decreased granuloma size in such individuals might result, paradoxically, in amelioration of disease manifestations. The pandemic of AIDS may clarify the role of cell-mediated immunity in the clinical expression of schistosomes.

Although the association between defective cell-mediated immunity and the infections discussed is clear-cut, treatment of the underlying disease and its progression are complicating factors because they tend to produce a more severe and generalized immunocompromised state which predisposes to other infectious agents. For example, during intensive chemotherapy for lymphoma, bacterial infections predominate [22]. Progression of the underlying disease results in local factors also favoring bacterial infections: mucosal breakdown, masses obstructing bronchi, ureters, or the biliary tract. The result is an increase in severe bacterial infection and septicemia late in the course of most diseases associated with impaired cell-mediated immunity. In fact, even in the disease considered the prototype of abnormal T-lymphocyte function, Hodgkin's disease, the most common infectious complications are bacterial [13,52].

DISORDERS OF HUMORAL IMMUNITY

Phagocytosis of encapsulated organisms by neutrophils initially is limited to the inefficient process of surface phagocytosis. Bacteria are trapped between the neutrophil and tissues (alveolar wall, fibrin meshwork, other neutrophils). Opsonization is essential for effective ingestion of the organisms by phagocytic cells. Deposit of C3b on the microbe, via the alternate or classical complement pathway, leads to facilitated attachment to neutrophils through C3b receptors and a burst of phagocyte metabolic activity [23]. Opsonization by specific antibodies increases attachment of bacterium to phagocyte, internalization, and degranulation as well as the oxidative burst. The action of heat-labile (complement) and heat-stable (antibody) opsonins is synergistic and promotes killing as well as internalization of organisms.

Although a number of mechanisms of containment of parasites may be adversely affected in hypogammaglobulinemic states, the opsonic defect appears to be most critical. Depressed levels of antibody may be due to decreased production or loss. The acquired diseases in the former category associated with increased frequency of infection are common variable immunodeficiency, chronic lymphocytic leukemia, multiple myeloma, B-cell lymphoma, and AIDS. The paraproteinemic states belong in this category because of secondary hypogammaglobulinemia. Therapy with cytotoxic drugs may produce a similar abnormality. Infections due to the pneumococcus, *Haemophilus influenzae,* streptococci, and *Neisseria* predominate early in the course of the immunodeficiency associated with these diseases. Giardiasis and progressive enteroviral infection also occur. As the underlying disease progresses, infections due to enteric gram-negative bacilli become more frequent [24]. Treatment of the malignancy with corticosteroids and cytotoxic drugs also causes additional defects in cell-mediated immunity predisposing to infections with the group of pathogens already discussed. Antibody deficiency states are of particular importance because of the relative simplicity of replacement therapy with intravenous γ-globulin, which is effective in protecting the patient against lethal systemic infection. Intravenous immunoglobulin also is of use in preventing infection in patients with chronic lymphocytic leukemia [53]. Limited access to such treatment modalities, however, may prevent appropriate management.

In sickle cell anemia, a different kind of opsonic activity is abnormal. Depletion of alternative complement pathway components activated by erythrocyte stroma causes impairment of opsonization of pneumococci, *H. influenzae,* and *Salmonella* species and is associated with frequent infections with these organisms. Impaired reticuloendothelial system function due to erythrophagocytosis and functional asplenia also may predispose to serious bacterial infections in patients with sickle

cell disease. Also of note, terminal complement deficiencies, for example, of C5, 6, and 7, are associated with a predilection for neisserial infection [47], as is dysfunctional properdin [54]. This reflects the importance of bactericidal activity of serum in preventing systemic infection with these organisms.

IMPAIRED NEUTROPHIL FUNCTION

Neutrophil function is impaired in a large array of inherited and acquired diseases. However, the clinical importance of specific abnormalities often is uncertain. Impaired chemotaxis is a significant fact   in patients with inherited C3 and C5 deficiencies, who are subject to frequent bacterial infections [25]. Corticosteroid therapy also produces impaired chemotaxis. Whereas circulating neutrophil counts may be normal or increased in the patient treated with corticosteroids, the related dysfunction in localization of these cells to the site of infection is profound. Defective cell-mediated immunity also contributes to the spectrum of infections promoted by corticosteroids. Circulating inhibitors of chemotaxis have been demonstrated in Hodgkin's disease, sarcoidosis, leprosy, and cirrhosis, but are of uncertain relevance.

Intrinsic defects in neutrophils are rare but vital to an understanding of the microbicidal mechanisms of this cell line. For example, neutrophils from patients with chronic granulomatous disease (CGD), inherited as an X-linked recessive trait, cannot develop an oxidative burst [26]. They are predisposed to serious, deep-seated infections with catalase-producing organisms such as staphylococci, *Serratia, Nocardia,* and *Aspergillus* [27,48]. These organisms produce hydrogen peroxide; however, concurrent production of catalase prevents intracellular destruction by neutrophils from patients with CGD. Catalase-negative organisms produce sufficient net hydrogen peroxide to permit their own killing by CGD neutrophils through the myeloperoxidase pathway.

Patients with inherited myeloperoxidase deficiency have relatively few bacterial infections. The absence of myeloperoxidase-dependent feedback control mechanisms allows exaggerated production of directly microbicidal oxidative products [28]. The result is slight delay in bacterial killing in vitro, without an attendant predisposition to bacterial infection.

The most severe intrinsic neutrophil defects occur in the Chédiak-Higashi syndrome [29]. Patients with this autosomal recessive trait have giant granules in their leukocytes and defective microtubule assembly. The result is impaired chemotaxis, abnormal phagolysosomal fusion, delayed bacterial killing, and recurrent infections. Diagnosis of this syndrome is aided by phenotypic abnormalities: partial albinism, depigmentation of the iris, peripheral neuropathies, and nystagmus.

Neutropenia

As the neutrophil count drops below 500 per microliter, a dramatic increase occurs in the frequency and severity of infections [30,31]. While most reliable data originate from pa-

Table 18-4. Infections in neutropenic patients

Bacteria:
  Pseudomonas, Klebsiella, Serratia, Escherichia coli,
  Staphylococcus aureus, Staphylococcus epidermidis,
  Corynebacterium J-K
Fungi:
  Candida, Aspergillus, Zygomycetes, *Cryptococcus*
Viruses:
  Cytomegalovirus
Protozoa:
  P. carinii

tients with acute leukemia, granulocytopenia of other etiologies is associated with comparable risk of infection [*32*]. In inherited and acquired neutropenias, mononuclear phagocytes compensate, at least partly, for the antibacterial function of the missing neutrophils. Thus, in patients with chronic and cyclical neutropenias the susceptibility to infection varies inversely with the monocyte count. This is not the case in acute leukemia. Following chemotherapy of acute leukemia, neutropenia usually is sustained and associated with damage to mucosal barriers to infection. Patients become susceptible to ''opportunistic'' agents which are ubiquitous in the environment and ordinarily comprise the normal flora (Table 18-4). This list necessarily is incomplete; other unusual opportunistic agents have been reported to cause disease in patients with leukemia and may become particular problems at individual centers [*33,34*]. About one-fifth of febrile episodes in neutropenic patients represent bacteremia or fungemia. [*49*]. Because infections may be fulminant, standard practice is to institute therapy with nafcillin or vancomycin plus an anti-*Pseudomonas* penicillin, or Ceftazidime or Imipenem plus an aminoglycoside [*50,58*]. If there is a clinical response, antibiotics are continued until the neutrophil count exceeds 1000 per microliter. If there is no response despite 5 to 7 days of antibiotics, amphotericin B is added empirically [*57*].

SPLENECTOMIZED PATIENTS

Splenectomy imposes a great risk of fulminant, often lethal infections, particularly in children with hemolytic and other anemias [*35*] or Hodgkin's disease [*36*], and in adults within the first 3 years following the procedure [*37*]. Impairment of antibody response to capsular polysaccharide antigens and removal of a site of clearance of opsonized intravascular organisms are important factors in the compromised status of splenectomized patients [*38*]. These individuals also lack alternate complement pathway components and ''tuftsin,'' an immunoglobulin-like tetrapeptide [*39*].

Splenectomized patients are at particular risk of developing severe infections with encapsulated bacteria such as *Streptococcus pneumoniae*, other streptococci, *H. influenzae*, and *Neisseria meningitidis*. Less virulent bacteria also may cause septicemia in splenectomized patients; an example is the organism classified as DF-2 which often is introduced by dog bites [*40*]. Loss of the spleen also is associated with a more virulent course in patients with typhoid fever, malaria, and babesiosis [*41*], diseases in which reticuloendothelial clearance of the parasite is an essential feature of the host response.

It must be emphasized that splenectomy should be avoided, when possible, in the interest of preventing immunocompromise. For example, although a large number of splenectomies are performed to treat schistosomiasis, the therapeutic benefit of this procedure has not been validated in most instances. In view of the long-term serious infectious morbidity, avoidance of unnecessary splenectomies is crucial. In fact, awareness of the problems ensuing from splenectomy has popularized spleen-sparing surgical procedures, such as limited resections in trauma victims. The frequent occurrence of life-threatening bacterial infections in splenectomized individuals also indicates the importance of administration of pneumococcal and meningococcal polysaccharide vaccines to them. When possible, vaccination should be undertaken prior to splenectomy and institution of cytotoxic drugs [*42,43*].

IMMUNOSUPPRESSION BY INFECTIOUS DISEASES

Specific and generalized immunosuppression develops during many chronic infectious diseases. Suppression and suppressor mechanisms restricted to antigens derived from the causative organism have been observed in leishmaniasis, schistosomiasis, filariasis (*Brugia malayi*), leprosy, and tuberculosis [*44,45*]. Specific immunosuppression may well affect the expression and natural history of the primary infection. However, specific immunosuppression often is superimposed on nonspecific immunosuppression, which theoretically could influence the course of unrelated infectious diseases. In this regard, it is of interest that in two populations in Upper Volta having similar overall prevalence of leprosy, the prevalence of lepromatous leprosy is twice as high in the area hyperendemic for onchocerciasis [*46*].

ASSESSMENT OF IMMUNE FUNCTION

Optimal assessment of immune function requires both quantification of leukocyte number and determination of functional activity [*56*]. Cellular immunity is assessed by delayed hypersensitivity skin testing, quantitation of lymphocytes and, as available, total T cells and T-cell subpopulations (CD4 = helper-effector, CD8 = suppressor-cytotoxic). Humoral immunity is assessed by serum protein electrophoresis and quantitation of immunoglobulins; antibody activity is assessed by measuring isoagglutinins or antibody to a vaccine the patient has received (polio, diphtheria, tetanus). Complement is assessed as CH50 or by measurement of C3 and C4. Additional testing usually requires access to research laboratory facilities.

CONCLUSIONS

Observations of infectious complications in immunocompromised hosts have clarified the importance of particular host defense mechanisms in the containment of specific infectious agents. The degree of immunocompromise and its nature need to be considered in determining likely etiologies of infection. No substitute yet exists, however, for early biopsy and culture of involved tissue. Paradoxically, the least common and most severe forms of immunocompromise are best understood. While the relative efficacy of sophisticated and expensive new modalities of treatment of acute leukemia is being debated, more attention needs to be placed on understanding immunological and other defects associated with and predisposing to parasitic infections of humans and the impact of infection with human immunodeficiency virus on the course of infectious agents endemic to developing countries.

REFERENCES

1 Twomey JJ: Infections complicating multiple myeloma and chronic lymphocytic leukemia. Cancer 13:1240–1253, 1960

2 Levine AS, Graw RG, Jr, Young RC: Management of infections in patients with leukemia and lymphoma. Semin Hematol 9:141–179, 1972

3 Winston DJ, Gale RP, Meyer DV, et al: Infectious complications of human bone marrow transplantation. Medicine 58:1–31, 1979

4 Young LS: Nosocomial infections in the immunocompromised adult. Am J Med 70:398, 1981

5 Rubin RH, Wolfson JS, Cosimi AB, et al: Infection in the renal transplant recipient. Am J Med 70:405–411, 1981

6 Abraham, J: Management of the immunocompromised host. Med Clin N Am 68:617, 1984

7 Pizzo PA, Young LS: Limitations of current antimicrobial therapy in the immunosuppressed host. Am J Med 76:78–82, 1984

8 Mackaness GB: The influence of immunologically committed lymphoid cells on macrophage activity in vivo. J Exp Med 129:973–992, 1969

9 Johnston RB, Jr. Monocytes and macrophages. N Engl J Med 318:747–752, 1988

10 Kantor FS: Infection, anergy and cell-mediated immunity. N Engl J Med 292:629–634, 1975

11 Pope JW, Liautant BM, Thomas F, et al: The acquired immunodeficiency syndrome in Haiti. Ann Intern Med 103:674–678, 1985

12 Selek RM, Starcher ET, Curran JW: Opportunistic diseases reported in AIDS patients: Frequencies, associations and trends. AIDS 1:175–182, 1987

13 Casazza AR, Duvale CP, Carbone PP: Summary of infectious complications occurring in patients with Hodgkin's disease. Cancer Res 26:1290–1296, 1966

14 Mackowiak PA, Demian SE, Sutker WL, et al: Infections in hairy-cell leukemia. Clinical evidence of a pronounced defect in cell-mediated immunity. Am J Med 68:718–724, 1980

15 Edelson PJ: Intracellular parasites and phagocytic cells: Cell biology and pathophysiology. Rev Infect Dis 4:124–135, 1982

16 Merigan TC: Host defenses against viral disease. N Engl J Med 290:323–329, 1974

17 Horwitz MA, Silverstein SC: Legionnaire's disease bacterium (*Legionella pneumophila*) multiplies intracellularly in human monocytes. J Clin Invest 66:441–450, 1980

18 Igra-Siegman Y, Kapila R, Sen P, et al: Syndrome of hyperinfection with *Strongyloides stercoralis*. Rev Infect Dis 3:397–407, 1981

19 Kaplan MH, Armstrong D, Rosen P: Tuberculosis complicating neoplastic disease. Cancer 33:840–858, 1974

20 James SL, Sher A, Lazdins JK, et al: Macrophages as effector cells of protective immunity in murine schistosomiasis. II. Killing of newly transformed schistosomula in vitro by macrophages activated as a consequence of *Schistosoma mansoni* infection. J Immunol 128:1535–1540, 1982

21 Hillyer GV, Cangiano JL: *Schistosoma mansoni* granuloma in immunosuppressed man: Report of a case. Trans R Soc Trop Med Hyg 73:331–333, 1979

22 Bishop JF, Schimpff SC, Diggs CH, et al: Infections during intensive chemotherapy for non-Hodgkin's lymphoma. Ann Intern Med 95:549–555, 1981

23 Goldstein IM, Kaplan HB, Radin A , et al: Independent effects of IgG and complement upon human polymorphonuclear leukocyte function. J Immunol 117:1282–1287, 1976

24 Meyers BR: Current patterns of infection in multiple myeloma. Am J Med 52:87–92, 1972

25 Gallin JI, Wolff SM: Leukocyte chemotaxis: Physiological considerations and abnormalities. Clin Haematol 4:567–607, 1975

26 Hohn DC, Lehrer RI: NADPH oxidase deficiency in X-linked chronic granulomatous disease. J Clin Invest 55:707–713, 1975

27 Lazarus GM, Neu HM: Agents responsible for infection in chronic granulomatous disease of childhood. J Pediatr 86:415–417, 1975

28 Klebanoff S, Pincus S: Hydrogen peroxide utilization in myeloperoxidase-deficient leukocytes: A possible microbicidal control mechanism. J Clin Invest 50:2226–2229, 1971

29 Bheme RS, Wolff SM: The Chédiak-Higashi syndrome: Studies in four patients and review of the literature. Medicine 51:247–280, 1972

30 Bodey GP, Buckley M, Sathe YS, et al: Quantitative relationships between circulating leukocytes and infection in patients with acute leukemia. Ann Intern Med 64:328–329, 1966

31 Singer C, Kaplan MM, Armstrong D: Bacteremia and fungemia complicating neoplastic disease. Am J Med 62:731–742, 1977

32 Guwith MJ, Brunton JL, Lank BA, et al: Granulocytopenia in hospitalized patients. I. Prognostic factors and etiology of fever. Am J Med 64:121–132, 1978

33 Pearson TA, Braine HG, Rathbun HK: *Corynebacterium* sepsis in oncology patients: Predisposing factors, diagnosis and treatment. JAMA 238:1737–1740, 1977

34 Winston DJ, Jordan MC, Rhodes J: *Allescheria boydii* infections in the immunosuppressed host. Am J Med 63:830–835, 1977

35 Smith CH, Erlandson ME, Stern G, et al: Post-splenectomy infection in Cooley's anemia: An appraisal of the problem in this and other blood disorders with consideration of prophylaxis. N Engl J Med 266:737–743, 1962

36 Chelcote RR, Baehner RL, Hammond D, et al: Septicemia and meningitis in children splenectomized for Hodgkin's disease. N Engl J Med 295:798–800, 1976

37 Bisno AL, Gopal V: Fulminant pneumococcal infections in "normal" asplenic hosts. Arch Intern Med 137:1526–1531, 1977

38 Ellis EF, Smith RT: The role of the spleen in immunity: With

special reference to the post-splenectomy problem in infants. Pediatrics 37:111–119, 1966

39 Likhite VV: Immunologic impairment and susceptibility to infection after splenectomy. JAMA 236:1376–1377, 1976

40 Butler T, Weaver RE, Ramani TKV, et al: Unidentified gram-negative rod infection: A new disease of man. Ann Intern Med 86:1–5, 1977

41 Fitzpatrick JEP, Kennedy CC, McGeown MG, et al: Human case of piroplasmosis (babesiosis). Nature 217:861–862, 1968

42 Siber GR, Weitzman SA, Aisenberg CA, et al: Impaired antibody response to pneumococcal vaccine after treatment for Hodgkin's disease. N Engl J Med 299:442–448, 1978

43 Ammar AJ, Addiego J, Wara DW, et al: Polyvalent pneumococcal polysaccharide immunizations of patients with sickle cell anemia and patients with splenectomy. N Engl J Med 297:897–900, 1977

44 Ellner JJ: Suppressor cells of man. Clin Immunol Rev 1:119–214, 1981

45 Petersen EA, Neva FA, Oster CN, et al: Specific inhibition of lymphocyte proliferation responses by adherent suppressor cells in diffuse cutaneous leishmaniasis. N Engl J Med 306:387–392, 1982

46 Proust A, Nebout M, Rougemont A: Lepromatous leprosy and onchocerciasis. Br Med J: 589–590, 1979

47 Ross SC, Denson P: Complement deficiency states and infection: Epidemiology, pathogenesis and consequences of neisserial and other infections in an immune deficiency. Medicine 63:243, 1984

48 Tauber AI, Borregard N, Simons E, et al: Chronic granulomatous disease: A syndrome of phagocyte oxidation deficiencies. Medicine 62:286, 1983

49 Pizzo PA, Commers J, Cotton D, et al: Approaching the contro-

versies in antibacterial management of cancer patients. Am J Med 76:436–449, 1984

50 Pizzo PA, Robichand KJ, Gill FA: Empiric antibiotic and antifungal therapy for patients with prolonged fever and granulocytopenia. Am J Med 72:101–111, 1982

51 Mann JM, Snider DE, Frances H, et al: Association between HTLV-III/LAV infection and tuberculosis in Zaire. JAMA 3:346, 1986

52 Notter DT, et al: Infections in patients with Hodgkin's disease: A clinical study of 300 consecutive adult patients. Rev Infect Dis 2:761, 1980

53 Cooperative Group for the Study of Immunoglobulin in Chronic Lymphocytic Leukemia: Intravenous immunoglobulins for the prevention of infection in chronic lymphocytic leukemia. N Engl J Med 319:902–907, 1988

54 Sjoholm AG, Kuijper EJ, Tijssen CC: Dysfunctional properdin in a Dutch family with meningococcal diseases. N Engl J Med 319:33–37, 1988

55 Malech HL, Gallin JI: Neutrophils in human diseases. N Engl J Med 317:687–694, 1987

56 Hony R: Evaluation of immunity. Immunol Invest 16:453–499, 1987

57 Diamond RD: Fungal infections in the compromised host—an overview. Adv Exp Med Biol 202:119–126, 1986

58 Pizzo PA, Hathorn JW, Hiemenz J, et al: A randomized trial comparing ceftazidime alone with combination antibotic therapy in cancer patients with fever and neutropenia. N Engl J Med 315:552–558, 1986

CHAPTER 19 / *Ecology and Population Biology* · Robert M. May

There is fascination in the recondite details that make each association between host and parasite unique. The present textbook makes this plain, as chapter after chapter chronicles the individual complexities of specific infections. This is of course necessary, because effective intervention must be based on full understanding of such detailed complications.

This chapter, however, focuses on the overall population biology of associations between hosts and parasites, emphasizing broad themes that are common to most systems. In pursuit of such generality, this chapter defines *parasite* in a wide sense to include viruses, bacteria, protozoans, and fungi, along with the more conventionally defined helminth and arthropod parasites. One advantage of this approach is that it provides a framework within which a vast array of information about parasitic infections may be organized in an orderly way, giving emphasis to the similarities and differences among the various parasites, and identifying the ecologically based patterns of

relationship among epidemiological parameters (such as transmission rates, virulence, life span of the parasite within a host).

Another advantage of the approach is that it directs attention to the processes of infection and immunity within the population as a whole, as opposed to within individuals. Public health programs in general, and programs of vaccination and chemotherapy in particular, require such appreciation of the effects of herd immunity, along with the more immediately apparent effects of individual immunity that are discussed in other chapters in this book.

In what follows, I first outline some basic concepts. These include the definition of microparasite and macroparasite (a rough dichotomy that cuts across conventional taxonomic lines), the basic reproductive rate of a parasite, and some broad patterns to be found in transmission (thresholds and breakpoints) and in the prevalence of parasitic infections. The concepts are then applied in a discussion of strategies for vaccination or chemotherapy against specific microparasitic and macroparasitic infections. This discussion highlights some instances (including malaria and rubella) where considerations of herd immunity and of individual immunity can intersect in complicated ways. Next, some aspects of the coevolution of hosts and parasites are briefly indicated. The chapter concludes with mention of wider aspects of the way parasitic infections may influence the population size of their animal hosts, including human beings in the past, the present, and the future.

BASIC CONCEPTS

MICROPARASITES AND MACROPARASITES

Microparasites may be defined as those parasites having direct reproduction—usually at very high rates—within the host [1]. They tend to be characterized by small size and short generation times; hosts that recover from infection usually acquire immunity against reinfection for some time, and often for life. Although there are many exceptions, the duration of infection is typically short in relation to the expected life span of the host, and therefore is of a transient nature. Most viral and bacterial parasites fall broadly into the microparasite category.

For microparasites, thus defined, it usually makes sense to divide the host population into relatively few classes of individuals: susceptible, infected, and recovered-immune. Such a compartmental model for the dynamic interaction between parasite and host populations is depicted schematically in Fig. 19-1 [1–4]. Greater detail and realism can be attained by adding more compartments to the model (for example, a class of latent, but not yet infectious, individuals). The essential feature of these compartmental models, however, is that little or no account is taken of the degree of severity of the infection; the reality of infected individuals with differing nutritional, environmental, or genetic status is replaced by the simplified abstraction of some average "infected" individual. Most of the biological and epidemiological parameters (host birth and death rates, disease-induced death rates, recovery rates, rates of loss of immunity) represented in Fig. 19-1 can be measured by appropriate studies. The transmission rate, however, combines many biological, social, and environmental factors, and (as discussed further below) is rarely amenable to direct measurement.

Macroparasites may be defined as those having no direct reproduction within the host [1]. This category embraces essentially all parasitic helminths and arthropods. Macroparasites are typically larger and have much longer generation times than microparasites, with the generation time often being an appreciable fraction of the host life span. When an immune response is elicited, it usually depends on the number of parasites present in the host and tends to be of relatively short duration. Thus macroparasitic infections are typically of a persistent nature, with hosts being continually reinfected.

For macroparasites, the various factors characterizing the interaction—egg output per parasite, pathogenic effects upon

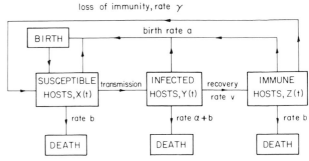

Figure 19-1. Schematic representation of the population dynamics of a microparasitic infection, described by a compartmental model. The flow rates between the compartments are as indicated. Transmission processes can be complicated; in the simplest case, the overall transmission rate is taken to be βXY. For a fuller discussion, see Ref. 1.

the host, evocation of an immune response in the host, parasite death rates, and so on—all generally depend on the number of parasites present in a given host. Mathematically, this means that the relatively simple compartmental models must be replaced by more complicated models that take full account of the distribution of parasites among the hosts [2,5–7]. Typically, the parasites are not distributed in an independently random way but show an aggregated or "clumped" distribution, with often a minority of the host population harboring the majority of the parasite population; for many macroparasites, it is common to find 70 percent or more of the parasites contained in 20 percent or fewer of their human hosts.

More significant from a public health point of view, for many macroparasites an important distinction can be made [8,9] between infection (harboring one or more parasites) and disease (harboring a parasite burden large enough to produce pathogenic symptoms, or even host death). For a canonical microparasitic infection, such as smallpox, it is reasonable to assume that a given host either does, or does not, "have smallpox"; for a macroparasite, such as hookworm or *Ascaris* or schistosomiasis, there is a real distinction between being infected with one or two worms, and carrying a worm load large enough to cause illness.

The division into microparasites and macroparasites is necessarily a rough one, essentially corresponding to two ends of a continuum [1]. Many parasites do not fit easily into this dichotomy. A lot of protozoan parasites, for instance, may to a good approximation have their epidemiology described by the compartmental models that are characteristic of microparasites, while on the other hand their patterns of persistence within the host population, with hosts being continually reinfected, are characteristic of macroparasites. Thus, as discussed in the examples below, an account of the degree of immunity that can naturally be elicited against malaria requires a model intermediate between the two extremes. Explicit acknowledgement of the effects of age structure within the host population is a further necessary complication in the realistic evaluation of control programs.

In short, the paradigmatic notions of microparasite and macroparasite are deliberate oversimplifications, aimed at elucidating some basic ideas. Realistic refinements can then be grafted on, layer by layer, as we proceed from basic understanding to detailed application.

BASIC REPRODUCTIVE RATE OF A PARASITE

The basic reproductive rate, R_0, is essentially the number of successful offspring that a parasite is intrinsically capable of producing [10–15]. It is, in effect, Fisher's "net reproductive value" for the parasite. Clearly a parasitic species must have $R_0 > 1$ if it is to be capable of establishing itself within a host population.

For a microparasite (represented mathematically by a compartmental model), R_0 is more precisely defined as the average number of secondary infections produced when one infected individual is introduced into a host population where everyone is susceptible [10–15]. For example, for transmission of HIV-AIDS within a particular risk group, we have $R_0 = \beta c D$, where β is the average probability that an infected individual will infect a susceptible partner, c is the appropriately averaged rate at which new partners are acquired (i.e., the average number of new partners per unit time), and D is the average duration of infectiousness.

As such a microparasitic infection becomes established in a host population, the fraction that remains susceptible decreases. Eventually an equilibrium may be attained, with the rate at which susceptible individuals are lost to infection being balanced against the rate at which newly susceptible hosts appear (usually by birth, but possibly also by immigration or by loss of immunity). At equilibrium, each infection will on average produce exactly one secondary infection [2,15], that is, at equilibrium the parasite reproductive rate is $R = 1$. If we assume that there is homogeneous mixing within the host population [2–4], so that the number of secondary infections produced by an infected individual is linearly proportional to the probability that a random contact is with a susceptible, we have in general that $R = R_0 x$, where x is the fraction of the host population that is susceptible. Thus, under the plausible assumption of homogeneous mixing, the equilibrium condition $R = 1$ leads to an important relation between the basic reproductive rate R_0 for a microparasite and the fraction x^* of the host population that is susceptible at equilibrium [12,13]:

$$R_0 x^* = 1 \qquad (19\text{-}1)$$

For a macroparasite (represented mathematically by a distributional model), R_0 is the average number of female offspring produced throughout the lifetime of a mature female parasite, which themselves achieve reproductive maturity in the absence of density-dependent constraints [7,14,17,18].

The factors governing equilibrium in a host-macroparasite system are more complex than those in host-microparasite systems. In the absence of any density-dependent constraints, a macroparasite with $R_0 > 1$ could attain arbitrarily high population levels, as hosts with high parasite burdens continued to put out large numbers of eggs, leading to yet higher parasite burdens per host. In reality, various kinds of density-dependent processes intervene to halt such exponential growth: egg output per parasite declines as the number of parasites in a host increases; hosts with high burdens may be less likely to acquire further infections, for a variety of possible reasons; parasite death rates may increase as the number of parasites in a host increases; the overall transmission rate may saturate to some upper limit when the parasite population is large; and a high burden may simply kill the host [5–7]. Precisely which of these density-dependent factors, individually or in combination, will be primarily responsible for establishing equilibrium is likely to vary from one host-parasite association to the next. Some examples will be discussed below.

TRANSMISSION: THRESHOLDS AND BREAKPOINTS

These general ideas about the essential character of the parasite and about its overall reproductive rate are valid, independent of the details of the transmission process. We now turn to consider some implications of the various kinds of direct and indirect transmission of parasites [2,14] which are illustrated schematically in Fig. 19-2.

For *direct* transmission, depicted in Fig. 19-2A, the transmission stages of the parasite pass directly from one host to the next. Some parasites, including many viruses and bacteria, pass by direct contact between hosts or in vapor droplets. Others, such as hookworm and other helminths, have free-living transmission stages of the parasite. These transmission stages may be capable of surviving for a long time in the external environment, as is the case, for example, for anthrax and for many fungal infections. As indicated schematically in Fig. 19-2A, for direct transmission one concatenates the various factors into an overall transmission factor T_1, which gives R_0.

As a specific formal example, consider a directly transmitted microparasitic infection whose engagement with its host pop-

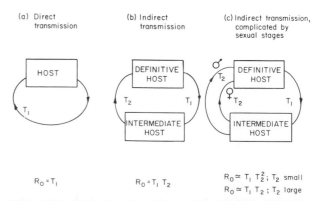

Figure 19-2. Schematic representation of the main kinds of transmission processes for parasites. For a discussion, see the text.

ulation is described by Fig. 19-1. Assume further that the rate at which new infections appear is βXY; that is, the number of new infections to appear per unit time is proportional to the number of binary encounters between susceptible individuals X, and infected individuals, Y, with the proportionality constant or "transmission rate" being β [1–4,11,12]. Then, if one infectious individual is introduced into an infection-free population of N susceptible individuals, the number of secondary infections produced per unit time is βN. The average duration of infectiousness, on the other hand, is $1/(\alpha + b + v)$, where v is the recovery rate, b the natural mortality rate, and α the disease-induced mortality rate (see Fig. 19-1). It follows that the basic reproductive rate for this infection is

$$R_0 = \frac{\beta N}{\alpha + b + v} \qquad (19\text{-}2)$$

This result could be arrived at via a much more mathematical route [1], but the qualitative derivation given here contains the essentials. From Eq. 19-2 R_0 could, in principle, be calculated in terms of the basic biological and epidemiological parameters. Although N, α, b, and v can usually be estimated, in practice it is effectively impossible to measure the transmission parameter β directly.

Thresholds

Equation 19-2 could alternatively be rewritten as

$$R_0 = \frac{N}{N_T} \qquad (19\text{-}3)$$

where the threshold population density is defined here as $N_T = (\alpha + b + v)/\beta$. The criterion $R_0 > 1$ for establishment of the parasite is thus equivalent to the requirement that the population exceed some threshold magnitude, $N > N_T$ [1–4,12,19]. If the population is below N_T, then $R_0 < 1$ and the infection cannot persist within the host population. For most directly transmitted microparasitic infections of humans, such as measles or smallpox, rough estimates put the threshold population size around 300,000 or more [2,15,20,21]. Such infections, which are of short duration and usually leave recovered individuals immune, need these large populations in order to maintain, by births, a sufficient stream of new susceptible hosts. It is clear, however, that infectious diseases (in combination with malnutrition) kill many people—particularly children—in developing countries today. Some recent assessments of the likely effects of campaigns of immunization against, for example, measles, pay explicit attention to this fact. See McLean and Anderson [37] for a discussion of the epidemiological data required in order to design an effective, community-based immunization program aimed at the eradication of measles; these authors also discuss the likely demographic consequences of such a campaign. By the same token, the current epidemic of HIV-AIDS in large cities in central Africa is likely to have significant demographic implications;

one effect will be eventual reduction in rates of population growth, possibly even leading to population decline in some regions; another effect will be significant changes in the age structure within the severely affected populations [16].

More generally, R_0 is likely to increase as the population of hosts increases, but not necessarily according to the simple linear relation of Eqs. 19-2 and 19-3. Data for measles and for pertussis in Britain, for example, can be seen to obey a more general power-law relation, $R_0 = (N/N_T)^v$, with $v < 1$ [13,22]. Likewise for macroparasites various effects can lead to R_0 increasing less fast than linearly with increasing host density [7,23]. The essential idea of a threshold host density for maintenance of the parasite, however, retains its validity.

There remains an exceptional class of parasitic infections, which includes most sexually transmitted diseases, where the probability for a given susceptible individual becoming infected is likely to be wholly independent of the total population size [2,24]. In this event, R_0 does not depend on N at all (although R_0 will change in response to social changes which, for example, affect the average rate of acquisition of new sexual partners).

Other complications arise when the "homogeneous mixing" assumption breaks down because there are two or more qualitatively distinct categories of hosts [25–28]. For example, while typhoid usually runs a relatively short course of infection from which the host either recovers or dies, a few hosts ("typhoid Marys") will be asymptomatic yet will carry and can transmit the infection for a relatively long time, possibly even lifelong; it is not obvious which is more important in transmission, the much larger number of much shorter infections, or the small number of long and asymptomatic infections. Such complexities can be encompassed within the definitions of R_0 and N_T, but they complicate matters [25,28,29].

When transmission is *indirect*, as illustrated in Fig. 19-2B and C, the parasite (micro or macro) passes through one or more species of intermediate hosts in completing its life cycle [1,2]. In simple cases, as indicated in Fig. 19-2B, the basic reproductive rate will be a product of the factors involved in transmission from the definitive to the intermediate host, T_1, and those from the intermediate back to the definitie host, T_2: $R_0 = T_1 T_2$. Thus, for malaria and a wide class of similarly transmitted parasites, we have [2,10,30,31]

$$R_0 = \frac{ma^2 bce^{-\mu T}}{\mu r} \qquad (19\text{-}4)$$

Here m is the average number of mosquitoes per human host, a is their biting rate, b the probability that an infected human will infect a biting mosquito, c the probability that an infectious mosquito will infect a bitten human, μ the mosquito death rate, T the latent period in the mosquito, and r is the recovery rate of malarious humans. This well-known formula is compounded from $T_1 = mab/r$ and $T_2 = (ac/\mu)e^{-\mu T}$. Some applications and shortcomings of this result are discussed below; the purpose of the present discussion is mainly to emphasize that the concept of R_0 embraces both direct and indirect transmission.

For Eq. 19-4, the criterion $R_0 > 1$ translates into the threshold condition $m > m_T$. That is, the number of mosquitoes per human host must exceed some threshold value. At first sight, this is an odd result: increasing human numbers will dilute the efficacy of mosquito transmission and reduce R_0. This is because anopheline mosquitoes take a fixed number of blood meals; if the intermediate vectors simply bit any human host they chanced upon (as is the case for many other parasitic infections), R_0 would be proportional to the product of the magnitudes of definitive and intermediate host populations [11,25]. Whatever the details, it is clear that the maintenance of indirectly transmitted infections does not typically require the very large host populations that are needed for directly transmitted microparasitic infections.

Figure 19-2C illustrates an additional complication that arises for the many macroparasites with a sexual stage in the definitive host. In this case, as first emphasized by Macdonald for schistosomiasis [17], it is necessary to have a mated pair of adult macroparasites in the definitive host. If the average level of transmission from intermediate to definitive host, T_2, is low, then the probability of having one mated pair scales approximately as T_2^2, and $R_0 \simeq T_1 T_2^2$. Conversely, at high transmission levels, a host is likely to acquire several parasites, whence these complications are not important and $R_0 \simeq T_1 T_2$. Macdonald's numerical studies of his models for schistosomiasis [32] were inadvertently carried out mainly for low values of T_2, which led him to conclude that "safe water supplies [low T_2] are more important than latrines [low T_1]." This is indeed true (although it neglects supervening sociological and economical factors) in the limit he studied when $R_0 \simeq T_1 T_2^2$, but both factors are equally important in the more common event that T_2 is somewhat large and $R_0 \simeq T_1 T_2$; for a more rigorous discussion, see [33].

Breakpoints

Macdonald's [17] concept of a "breakpoint" has potential importance for the control of macroparasites with sexual stages in the definitive host. For most parasites with high R_0, unremitting vigilance is necessary even after the infection has been eradicated from a region, because the basic biology is such that the infection will tend to reestablish itself if a few infected individuals are introduced. But for schistosomes and other macroparasites with transmission cycles of the kind depicted in Fig. 19-2C, there can be two alternative stable states for the host-parasite association at high R_0: when parasites are reintroduced at low densities, the chances of a given host acquiring a mated pair are low; once parasites are reintroduced at densities above the "breakpoint," such pairing does occur, and the infection then "takes off" to realize its high reproductive potential, R_0.

This notion of a breakpoint is obviously attractive. It offers the seductive hope that macroparasites could be eradicated by

a one-time reduction below breakpoint densities, without the environmental or social changes that are needed if R_0 itself is to be reduced below unity. Unfortunately, recent work [33,34] suggests that the patterns of parasite aggregation or clumping found for most host-macroparasite systems have the implication that such breakpoint densities are too low to be of practical significance. Specific estimates for *Ascaris* and for hookworm infections find breakpoint densities to be of the order of 0.3 to 0.5 worms per host [18]. Although still open to debate, one recent consensus was that the breakpoint is, for all practical purposes, a beguiling chimera [35].

PREVALENCE

Before we proceed to examples, which ultimately give way to the particularities of specific parasites, one more generality deserves attention. Figure 19-3 applies to essentially all parasitic infections and shows the prevalence of infection P at equilibrium as a function of the parasites' basic reproductive rate R_0 [35]. (For both macroparasites and microparasites, the prevalence is defined as the fraction of the host population harboring one or more parasites; the prevalence may attain almost 100 percent for infections like malaria, hookworm, schistosomiasis, or *Ascaris* in regions of high endemicity, or it may average very low values for infections like measles or mumps.)

Although the detailed shape of the curve, and the scaling of the y axis, may vary from parasite to parasite, all share the common property that the equilibrium prevalence is zero if R_0 is below unity. Above this threshold value of R_0, prevalence will rise, saturating to some limiting value for $R_0 \gg 1$.

Figure 19-4 illustrates the breakpoint phenomenon. For $R_0 > 1$ there are now two alternative equilibrium values for prevalence, one finite and the other zero. If the prevalence can

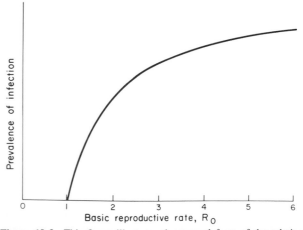

Figure 19-3. This figure illustrates the general form of the relation between the prevalence (or "amount") P of infection in the host population at equilibrium and the basic reproductive rate R_0 of the micro- or macroparasite. Note the threshold at $R_0 = 1$. For discussion (and explanation of the arbitrary scale on the P axis) see the text.

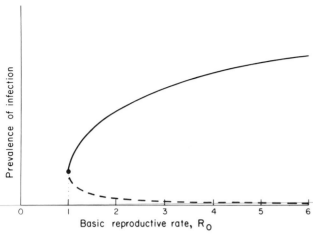

Figure 19-4. This figure is analogous to Fig. 19-3 but shows the prevalence P of infection as a function of the basic reproductive rate R_0 in the case where there are two alternative stable states—one at finite prevalence, and one at zero prevalence—above the transmission threshold at $R_0 = 1$. The dashed line corresponds to the "breakpoint" level of prevalence discussed in the text.

be depressed below the (dashed) breakpoint value, then the system will move spontaneously toward the disease-free state, $P = 0$, even if R_0 is large. The discouraging remarks made earlier about the breakpoint amounts to the suggestion that, in practice, the dashed breakpoint curve in Fig. 19-4 is indistinguishable from the x axis, so that Figs. 19-3 and 19-4 are indistinguishable.

EXAMPLES, APPLICATIONS, AND COMPLICATIONS

ESTIMATING R_0 FOR MICROPARASITES

We have seen that, assuming homogeneous mixing in the host population, R_0 and x^* for microparasites are related according to Eq. 19-1, which can be rewritten as

$$R_0 = \frac{1}{x^*} \qquad (19\text{-}5)$$

If accurate and complete serological studies are available, the fraction x^* of the population that is susceptible can be calculated, and R_0 thus determined. Unfortunately, such paragons of studies are not common. And we have already explained, following Eq. 19-2, that direct assessment of R_0 in terms of basic biological and epidemiological parameters is infeasible due to the impossibility of measuring the transmission parameter β.

For microparasites that induce lifelong immunity, a rough estimate of R_0 can be made if the age A at which hosts acquire infection is known. By assuming hosts are susceptible up to age A, and infected or immune thereafter, we arrive at the approximation $x^* \simeq A/L$; here L is the life expectancy of the average host. We thus have

$$R_0 \simeq \frac{L}{A} \qquad (19\text{-}6)$$

More exact expressions for R_0 in terms of A and L begin by assuming that individual hosts experience a "force of infection" λ that is independent of age and measures the probability of becoming infected in some unit time interval. In a homogeneous population at equilibrium, the fraction of hosts of age a that remains susceptible may be shown to be [2,11,12]

$$x(a) = e^{-\lambda a} \qquad (19\text{-}7)$$

It follows that the average age at infection is related to λ by $A = 1/\lambda$. To calculate the proportion of the total population that is susceptible, x^*, we need to know the probability of survival to age a; x^* is then the appropriate average over $x(a)$. One simple assumption (which is not very realistic for humans) is that hosts have a constant, age-independent death rate b; b and L are related by $b = 1/L$. Under this assumption about survivorship, it can be shown [11,12] that $x^* = A/(A + L)$; thus

$$R_0 = 1 + \frac{L}{A} \qquad (19\text{-}8)$$

Another simple assumption (which is closer to reality for many human populations) is that all hosts live to exactly age L, whereupon they die. This leads to the result

$$R_0 = \frac{(L/A)}{1 - \exp(-L/A)} \qquad (19\text{-}9)$$

Actual survivorship curves, such as that shown in Fig. 19-5C, are intermediate between these two extremes, though generally closer to the second. Many recent discussions of R_0 in human populations, however, have used Eq. 19-8. I mention all this so that the reader who wishes to pursue these matters further will be able to place particular analyses in context.

Table 19-1 lists estimates of R_0 for a variety of microparasitic infections, mainly in developed countries. These estimates are drawn from several sources. The figure for smallpox in the third world before the global eradication campaign is a crude guess, essentially based on Eq. 19-6. Similarly, the figures for *Plasmodium falciparum* and *P. malariae* are based on a rough assessment of the average age at first infection; Macdonald's earlier estimates [30], based directly on the formula Eq. 19-4, give values of R_0 for malaria in India and Africa ranging from around 10 to several hundreds. The other values of R_0 given in Table 19-1 are for directly transmitted microparasitic infections in developed countries and are more accurately based on Eq. 19-1 in conjunction with data on the age-specific incidence (rate of appearance of new infections).

CONTROL OF MICROPARASITIC INFECTIONS BY VACCINATION

A first step toward the control of a communicable infection is the development of a safe, effective, and relatively inexpensive vaccine that gives lasting (ideally, lifelong) protection. Once this problem of providing individual immunity has been solved, there arise questions about immunity within the population as a whole ("herd immunity").

Criterion for eradication

Under the conventional assumption of homogeneous mixing, the criterion for eradication of an infection can be stated in simple and general terms. Suppose a proportion p of the total population are protected by some specific vaccination program. Then, in the absence of infection, the fraction of the population remaining susceptible is $x^* = 1 - p$, and the reproductive rate of the microparasite is $R_0 (1 - p)$ (see Eq. 19-1). The microparasitic infection cannot persist if its reproductive rate is less than unity, which leads to the eradication criterion [12,40]

$$p > 1 - \frac{1}{R_0} \tag{19-10}$$

The larger R_0, the greater the proportion of the host population that must be protected by vaccination in order to eradicate the infection.

The final column in Table 19-1 is based on Eq. 19-10, and it shows this critical value of p for the various infections. Some tentative, but interesting, conclusions emerge.

Smallpox appears to have one of the smallest values of R_0 of these tabulated diseases, suggesting that a vaccination coverage of around 70 to 80 percent in the neighborhood of known cases may be sufficient for eventual eradication. This fact, in conjunction with the apparency of the disease and the availability of an effective vaccine, may help explain the success of the global eradication campaign [36]. Although the etiology of measles is similar to smallpox, with the infection always being apparent and running a relatively short course, the tentative estimate that R_0 is probably around 10 to 15 (corresponding to p around 90 percent or higher) for measles in developing countries may make its global eradication much more difficult than was the case for smallpox.

The very high values of R_0 for malaria suggest that its eradication is likely to be very difficult, whatever the control method. In particular, a campaign against *P. falciparum* in Nigeria based wholly on use of an effective vaccine would appear to require that 99 percent of the population be protected for eradication to be achieved [38].

Evaluation of the prospects for a particular vaccination program requires much more detailed analysis, taking full account of the available data for age-specific rates of acquisition of infection and age-specific vaccination rates, along with birth and death rates. Such age-specific information is then used to compute the overall proportions of the total population that are susceptible, infected, and immune. An example of the kind of information that is needed is given in Fig. 19-5, which pertains to measles and to pertussis in England and Wales. It can be

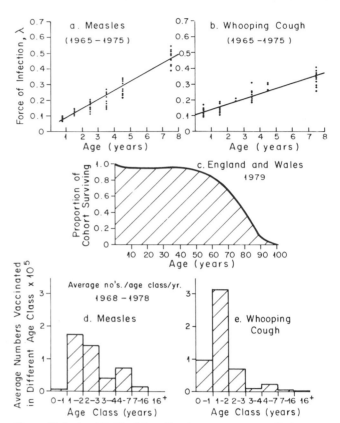

Figure 19-5. *A* and *B*. The "force," or instantaneous rate, of infection λ as a function of age for measles and pertussis, respectively, in England and Wales. *C*. The corresponding survivorship curve. *D* and *E*. The number of individuals vaccinated against measles and pertussis, respectively, in various age classes. For sources of data and further discussion, see Ref. 13.

estimated that, with the age-specific vaccination schedules shown in Fig. 19-5, and making the dubious assumption that vaccines are 100 percent effective, the coverage needed to eradicate measles in England and Wales is around 96 percent, and for pertussis is also around 96 percent [13]. These percentages could be slightly diminished by concentrating vaccination toward 1-year-olds [13]. Coverage of this magnitude has not been achieved in Britain, although in the United States it has for measles, which appears to be essentially eradicated.

The assumption of homogeneous mixing

As emphasized at the outset, most of the above analysis assumes homogeneous mixing within the host population. In reality, transmission rates will tend to vary both among different social groupings (family, school, etc.) and in response to environmental factors (transmission may exhibit seasonality, or some groups may frequent locations such as riverbanks where vectors are more likely to be found). Such inhomogeneities almost invariably exist, and the question is to what extent their effects may average out to make the assumption of homogeneous mixing a reasonable approximation [2,25–27,41]. The answer will vary from infection to infection, depending on the specific circumstances.

An interesting empirical test of the assumption of homogeneous mixing has recently been made for measles in Britain by Fine and Clarkson [41]. This test begins by noting an important corollary of Eq. 19-1, that was derived from the homogeneous mixing assumption: under *any* vaccination program that falls short of eradicating the infection, the fraction of the population remaining susceptible at the new equilibrium is identical with that in the original, prevaccination population, being simply $x^* = 1/R_0$. It is clear that this result follows from Eq. 19-1, independent of the details of the vaccination schedule; the only way to alter x^* (short of vaccinating so high a proportion that the upper limit to x^*, $1 - p$, is driven below $1/R_0$) is to make environmental or social changes that alter R_0 itself. Fine and Clarkson then analyze the data that are available for age-specific incidence and immunity levels for measles in England and Wales since 1950. They find that although [41] "there has been a dramatic and complicated shift in the age pattern of measles immunity in the population," the "total number of individuals susceptible to measles has remained relatively constant" (at around 4 to 4.5 million, corresponding to $x^* \simeq 0.09$ and R_0 around 11 to 12, in accord with the independent estimate in Table 19-1). As Fine and Clarkson emphasize, there are biases and deficiencies in the available data (having to do mainly with the notification of cases), and methods of correcting for such biases depend to a degree on the assumption of homogeneous mixing. Thus the test of this assumption is not altogether free of some circularity. I think, however, that Fine and Clarkson's analysis is important and elegant, showing that homogeneous mixing represents a useful working approximation for measles in England and Wales, and therefore possibly for broadly similar infections elsewhere.

Herd immunity versus individual immunity

Although the total number of susceptible individuals may remain constant under a vaccination program that stops short of eradication, the number of individuals experiencing infection will decrease. That is, the number of individuals moving from the susceptible to the immune class as a result of vaccination will be counterbalanced by a decrease in the number of individuals making this passage as a result of natural infection and recovery. Consequently the "force of infection" λ will decrease, and the average age at which infection is acquired will increase [42,43].

If the reaction of the host to the infection is the same at all ages, any reduction of the overall prevalence as a result of a vaccination program is simply a good thing. But many infections elicit significantly more severe responses when experienced in later years rather than in infancy. Poliomyelitis, mumps, and possibly measles are in this class. Rubella is not particularly worrisome if experienced when young, but can cause the damaging congenital rubella syndrome (CRS) in the offspring of women who contract the infection in the first trimester of pregnancy. For such infections, the result of a vaccination program that falls short of eradication is to decrease the total number of infections, but to increase the fraction of these cases that are found in older age groups. The net outcome of these countervailing effects will depend on the details of the infection and of the vaccination schedule, but it can be that the total number of infections in older age classes actually increases under vaccination.

Knox [42] and Dietz [43] have used epidemiological data

Table 19-1. Estimates of the basic reproductive rate R_0 for various infections

Infection	Geographical location (time period)	R_0	p, %	References
Smallpox	Developing countries (before global campaign)	3–5	70–80	[36]
Measles	England and Wales (1956–1968)	13	92	[38]
	Various places in U.S. (1910–1930)	12–13	92	[13]
Pertussis	England and Wales (1942–1950)	17	94	[38]
	Maryland, U.S. (1908–1917)	12	92	[13]
Rubella	England and Wales (1979)	6	83	[13]
	West Germany (1972)	7	86	[13]
Chickenpox	Various places in U.S. (1913–1921; 1943)	9–10	90	[13,38]
Diphtheria	Various places in U.S. (1910–1947)	4–6	~80	[13,38]
Scarlet fever	Various places in U.S. (1910–1920)	5–7	~80	[13]
Mumps	Various places in U.S. (1912–1916; 1943)	4–7	~80	[13]
Poliomyelitis	Netherlands (1960); United States (1955)	6	83	[13]
P. falciparum	Northern Nigeria (1970s)	~80	99	[38,39]
P. malariae	Northern Nigeria (1970s)	~16	94	[38,39]

Note: The estimate of p, the proportion that must be protected by vaccination in order to achieve eradication, assumes "homogeneous mixing" as discussed in the text.

Source: Unless otherwise noted, these estimates are from [13] where references are given to the primary sources from which the basic data came.

from rubella vaccination programs in Britain to show that the incidence of CRS can indeed increase under some vaccination programs. Such a perverse outcome is more likely if a proportion of all boys and girls are vaccinated at an early age than if a similar proportion of only girls are vaccinated around 12 to 13 years of age; this is because the latter strategy affords more scope for the early acquisition of immunity by natural infection in addition to that provided to those who are vaccinated.

Figure 19-6 illustrates the basic principles. We assume a constant force of infection λ in the host population before vaccination begins, so that the fraction susceptible at age a, $x(a)$, is given by Eq. 19-7. The survivorship curve is taken to be rectangular, with all hosts dying at exactly age L. Recalling that $\lambda = 1/A$, we see that λ may be related to the microparasites' basic reproductive rate R_0 by Eq. 19-9: $R_0 = \lambda L/[1 - \exp(-\lambda L)]$. Now let us establish a vaccination program whereby a fraction p of all individuals are vaccinated, within a year or so of birth (with a correction, if necessary, to account for the protection afforded by maternal antibodies), using a vaccine that confers lifelong immunity. The fraction of individuals of age a that are now susceptible is

$$x(a) = (1 - p)e^{-\lambda'a} \qquad (19\text{-}11)$$

Here λ' is the (diminished) force of infection in this postvaccination population, which can be calculated from the relation $R_0 (1 - p) = \lambda'L/[1 - \exp(-\lambda'L)]$. Given the values of R_0 and L, we can now calculate the number of individuals who

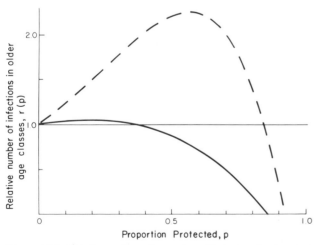

Figure 19-6. This figure shows the number of infections in older age groups (specifically, between 18 and 35 years, in a population where the average life expectancy is 70 years) when a proportion p of the population are protected by vaccination soon after birth; the number of infections is calculated as a ratio $r(p)$ to the corresponding number before vaccination (that is, with $p = 0$). The solid and dashed curves depict $r(p)$ for infections with $R_0 = 7$ and 13, respectively. The derivation and implications of these results are discussed more fully in the text and elsewhere [44].

are infected between age a_1 and age a_2 when a proportion p are vaccinated at birth, as a ratio to the number of individuals acquiring infections in this age range before vaccination was introduced [44]. The solid curve in Fig. 19-6 shows this ratio, $r(p)$, as a function of p for $R_0 = 7$, $L = 70$, $a_1 = 18$, and $a_2 = 35$ (which roughly corresponds to infection with rubella among women in the main childbearing years in a western country). In this simple caricature, the incidence of CRS can increase slightly under such a vaccination program when p is less than 0.3 or so. Using the same parameter values but with $R_0 = 13$ (roughly corresponding to measles), we obtain the dashed curve in Fig. 19-6, which exhibits a very marked increase in the incidence of infection among adults when the vaccination coverage is in the range 0.2 to 0.7.

I have deliberately dwelled on this topic, because it offers a clear example where individual immunity can be at odds with herd immunity; for some infections, individuals who are vaccinated are indeed better off, but the total number of serious cases within the population can actually increase under certain programs of vaccination.

POPULATION DYNAMICS OF MACROPARASITES

Models for the population dynamics of macroparasites usually need to take account of the way the parasites are distributed among the host population [5,6,23]. In practice, this distribution can almost invariably be described by a negative binomial distribution, in which a "clumping parameter" k describes the degree to which the parasites tend to aggregate: small values of k correspond to high aggregation or "overdispersion," with relatively few hosts harboring most of the parasites; the limit $k \to \infty$ corresponds to a Poisson distribution, in which the parasites are distributed independently randomly. The k values characterizing the negative binomial distribution of specific macroparasites in human host populations are listed in Table 19-2. These distributions typically have $k < 1$, which is also characteristic of most macroparasites in nonhuman animal hosts [6].

The dynamics of the association between hosts and macroparasites tends to be further complicated by the variety of different time scales for different processes. Characteristic time scales for particular components of these associations are dis-

Table 19-2. Degree of aggregation of adult macroparasites within human host populations*

Parasite	Geographical location	k
Ascaris lumbricoides	Iran	0.2–3
Necator americanus	India	0.03–0.6
N. americanus and		
Ancylostoma duodenale	Taiwan	0.05–0.4
Schistosoma mansoni	Brazil	0.03–0.5

*Measured by the clumping parameter k of the negative binomial distribution; the smaller k, the more clumped the distribution.
Source: From [18], where references to primary sources are given.

Table 19-3. Characteristic time scales for different components in the overall association between human hosts and some specific macroparasites

Parasite	Typical life expectancies		
	Humans, years	Adult parasite in humans, years	Transmission stage of parasite (infective stage or intermediate host)
Ascaris lumbricoides	40–60	1–2	1–3 months (egg)
Trichuris trichiura	40–60	2–3	1–2 months (egg)
Necator americanus	40–60	2–4	3–10 days (L_3 larvae)
Schistosoma mansoni	40–60	3–4	3–6 weeks (infected snail)
Onchocerca volvulus	40–60	8–14	1–3 weeks (dipteran vector)
Wuchereria bancrofti	40–60	12–16	1–2 weeks (dipteran vector)

Source: From [18], where references to the primary sources are given.

played in Table 19-3, where some patterns can be seen to emerge. The life span of adult parasites in their human hosts tends to range from around 1 to around 10 years, which is roughly one to two orders of magnitude smaller than the life span of the average host. The life spans of the transmission stages of the parasite (which often involve intermediate vector hosts) range from weeks to months and are significantly less than those of the adults. Notice one practical implication of this latter fact: a control program that interrupts a transmission cycle by removing intermediate hosts will need to be maintained at least as long as the life span of a typical adult parasite (unless combined with chemotherapy to kill adult parasites), or else the system is liable to bounce back as soon as the insecticide, molluscicide, or whatever is withdrawn—the comparatively long life of the adult parasite provides buffering against fluctuations in transmission levels.

For many purposes, we can take advantage of the systematically different time scales apparent in Table 19-3 to focus on the population dynamics of the adult parasites [14,18], regarding the host population as constant (because it changes relatively slowly) and regarding the population of transmission stages as always having the appropriate equilibrium value (because it changes relatively fast). In this event, the interesting variable is the mean number of adult parasites per host at time t, $M(t)$. If these parasites are distributed in negative binomial fashion, the prevalence of infection is [18,34]

$$P = 1 - \left(1 + \frac{M}{k}\right)^{-k} \tag{19-12}$$

Here k is the clumping parameter mentioned above.

The mean parasite burden M obeys a differential equation of the form [18]

$$\frac{dM}{dt} = \mu M[R_0 f(M, k, z) - 1] \tag{19-13}$$

Here the negative term on the right-hand side describes the loss of adult parasites, which have a death rate μ (or an average life span $B = 1/\mu$). The basic reproductive rate R_0 gives the number of successful offspring produced over the life span of

the adult parasite, so that the effective per capita birth rate is R_0/B or μR_0. The factor $f(M, k, z)$ describes density-dependent effects that will act to depress the effective value of the per capita parasite reproductive rate as parasite burden increases; these density-dependent effects will depend on the mean load M, on the distribution pattern (characterized by k), and on the precise nature of the density-dependent effects (abstractly characterized here by the parameter z); these density-dependent effects may be influenced by immune responses in host individuals [59,63,64]. In the low-density limit, $M \to 0$, density-dependent effects will be negligible and $f \to 1$; in this limit, the gain term in Eq. 19-13 becomes simply $\mu R_0 M$.

From Eq. 19-13, R_0 can be estimated in two ways. First, if average worm burdens have been driven to low values (for example, by a chemotherapy program), the initial rise back toward high levels will be exponential at the rate $\mu(R_0 - 1)$; in such circumstances, careful monitoring can lead to an assessment of R_0. Second, if the system has settled to an endemic, equilibrium state, we have $R_0 f(M^*, k, z) = 1$. R_0 can now be estimated if we know the equilibrium mean parasite load M^*, the aggregation parameter k, and the character of the density-dependent processes that determine the functional form of f [along with the parameter(s) z]. Anderson and May [18] have used data from hookworm, *Ascaris,* and schistosome infections to argue that density-dependent reduction in per capita egg output may be a predominant regulatory effect for many macroparasites. These authors show that a reduction in per capita egg production of the general form $\exp(-ci)$, where i is the number of parasites in a given host, fits the various data sets. In conjunction with the assumption that the parasite distribution is negative binomial, this leads to an explicit formula for the density dependence factor f:

$$f(M, k, z) = \left[1 + (1 - z)\left(\frac{M}{k}\right)\right]^{-(k+1)} \tag{19-14}$$

with $z = \exp(-c)$. An estimate of R_0 thus follows if M^*, k, and c are known. For a more explicit discussion, see Ref. 18.

Estimates of R_0 are presented in Table 19-4 for four macroparasitic infections of humans. All but one of these R_0 values

Table 19-4. The basic reproductive rate R_0 for some macroparasites

Parasite	Geographical location	Rough estimate of R_0
Onchocerca volvulus (filariasis, river blindness)	Sudan	5–35
Ascaris lumbricoides (roundworm)	Iran	4–5
Necator americanus (hookworm)	India	2–3
Schistosoma mansoni (schistosomiasis)	Brazil	1–2

Source: These estimates are from [*18*]; the data on which the estimates are based are from references given in [*18*].

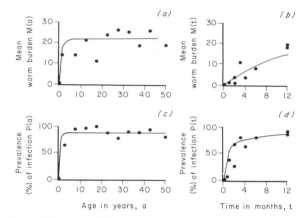

Figure 19-7. *A* and *C.* Data from a horizontal epidemiological survey [*46*] and theoretical curves [*18*] for the rise in the average worm burden and in the prevalence of infection, respectively, with host age, for *Ascaris* infections in Iran. *B* and *D.* Data [*46*] and theoretical curves [*18*] for the rise in the average worm burden and in the prevalence, respectively, over time in a sample of people who were cleared of worms by antihelminthic treatment at time $t = 0$.

are relatively low. It would be a mistake, however, to assume that such macroparasites may be relatively easy to eradicate because they have low values of R_0. As emphasized by Bradley [*45*] and others, the density-dependent mechanisms possessed by most macroparasites endow their populations with a considerable degree of resilience.

Equations 19-13 and 19-12 can be used to predict how the average parasite burden and the prevalence change in response to control measures or other perturbations. In particular, Figs. 19-7*B* and *D* show the increase over time in intensity and prevalence of *Ascaris* infection in a population of hosts who were cleared of worms by chemotherapy at time $t = 0$. The data are from a study in Iran [*46*], and the theoretical curves are from Eqs. 19-13 and 19-12 with Eq. 19-14 for f and $k = 0.57$, $z = 0.96$, $\mu = 1$ year^{-1}, $M^* = 22$ (and consequently $R_0 = 4.3$). The rapidity with which the mean worm burden, and especially the prevalence, return to their pristine levels is typical of many such macroparasitic infections in regions of high endemicity.

More generally, we may wish to describe changes in the mean parasite burden both over time t and as a function of the age a of the host. The result is a partial differential equation for $M(t, a)$ which I will not discuss in detail here, but whose basic structure is an appropriate generalization of Eq. 19-13 [*18*]. In the steady state, the age-specific parasite burden does not vary with time, and we get an ordinary differential equation for $M(a)$ and thence for the age-specific prevalence $P(a)$. Figures 19-7*A* and *C* show data pertaining to the rise in the average intensity and prevalence, respectively, of *Ascaris* infections; the data come from a horizontal epidemiological survey of the Iranian population mentioned above. The steady-state theoretical curves describing the rise in average intensity and prevalence with age are calculated using the same values for the epidemiological parameters k, z, μ, and R_0 as were employed above for Figs. 19-7*B* and *D* [*18*]. It is encouraging that this relatively simple model gives a reasonable fit to a range of different kinds of data.

MACROPARASITES AND CHEMOTHERAPY

Figure 19-8 aims to show how macroparasitic infections change, as a simultaneous function of time and host age, under specific regimes of chemotherapeutic intervention. The mathematical model is as outlined above, with the parameters chosen to have the values corresponding to *Ascaris* in Iran [*18*]. In Fig. 19-8 the infection is at its endemic equilibrium value for the first 20 years; during this time the age-specific intensity and prevalence, $M(a)$ and $P(a)$, remain steady (corresponding to Figs. 19-7*A*, *C*). For the next 10 years, 20 percent of the population (selected at random) is treated each month with a drug of 95 percent efficacy. After 10 years of such chemotherapy, the treatment is stopped and the host-parasite system allowed to return to its precontrol equilibrium. Figure 19-8*A* shows that the mean parasite burden falls relatively quickly to low levels under this program, but that the original high level is rapidly recovered once chemotherapy stops (as shown for the host population as a whole in Fig. 19-7*B*). Figure 19-8*B* shows that the prevalence falls much more slowly, remaining at about 30 percent in older age groups even after 10 years of treatment in this empirically based example; the prevalence also returns rapidly to its saturation level once chemotherapy is withdrawn (as seen also in Fig. 19-7*D*).

There are several messages to be read from Fig. 19-8. It was emphasized earlier that for macroparasites there is an important distinction between infection (harboring one or more parasites) and disease (harboring a parasite burden large enough to produce pathogenic effects). The amount of infection is measured by the prevalence P, while the amount of disease depends on the mean parasite burden M. In this sense, Fig. 19-8 shows that a control program might be successful in

clumped or aggregated way; often relatively few hosts carry the relatively high burdens that cause disease. In this circumstance, it could make sense to target chemotherapy selectively against the heavily infected hosts, thus aiming to reduce or eliminate disease without necessarily eradicating infection from the population [8,9]. A disadvantage of such a selective program could lie in the difficulty or cost of identifying the heavily infected hosts. An offsetting advantage is that fewer people need to be treated than in a "scattershot" program, thus reducing the cost, slowing down the evolution of parasite resistance to the drug, and avoiding any risk of toxic side-effects in administering the drug to individuals who are only lightly infected. These benefits will be enhanced if, as has been suggested, the hosts who are identified as most heavily infected are predisposed to this state, not by chance, but as a consequence of genetic, behavioral, or social traits.

The same mathematical models that have been sketched above, and whose dynamic workings are depicted in Figs. 19-7 and 19-8, can be used to get a rough idea of the consequences of targeting chemotherapy selectively against more heavily infected individuals. This question is explored in detail elsewhere [18]. Table 19-5 summarizes some typical findings (for a system where the original mean parasite burden is M^* = 40, where the drug is assumed 95 percent effective, and

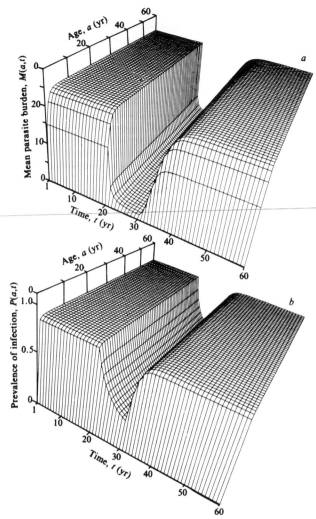

Figure 19-8. These "three-dimensional" figures show how (A) mean parasite burden and (B) prevalence vary as functions of host age and of time. The infection is assumed to be at equilibrium for the first 20 years; for next 10 years a chemotherapy program is maintained, under which 20 percent of the population are treated each month; and beginning in year 30 the program is withdrawn and the infection allowed to regain its endemic level. The implications and underlying assumptions are discussed in the text; for a fuller account, see Ref. 18.

significantly reducing, or even effectively eliminating, disease (reducing M to low levels; Fig. 19-8A), without coming anywhere close to eradicating infection (leaving P at a relatively high level; Fig. 19-8B). Notice also that even though M is held at low levels for almost 10 years, both M and P bounce quickly back if control is withdrawn.

Figure 19-8 corresponds to a situation in which the chemotherapy was administered at random. But for the *Ascaris* infection on which Fig. 19-8 is based, and for macroparasites in general, the parasites are distributed among their hosts in a

Table 19-5. The potential advantages of a program of selective chemotherapy that focuses on heavily infected hosts*

Comparison of random versus "selective" treatment, assuming the parasite clumping parameter is $k = 0.5$

	Fraction of host population to be treated		
	0.40	0.20	0.10
Percentage reduction of mean parasite burden if treatment is at random	40	20	10
Percentage reduction of mean parasite burden under "selective" treatment" defined above	75	38	19

Proportion of host population that must be treated to achieve 50% reduction of mean parasite burden, as a function of the "clumping parameter" k for the parasite distribution

	$k = 0.05$ (high aggregation)	$k = 0.5$ (significant aggregation)	$k \to \infty$ (Poisson: random distribution)
Random treatment	53	53	53
Selective treatment, as defined above	8	28	53

*Specifically, the program of "selective treatment" is assumed to concentrate (albeit with an element of uncertainty) on hosts with parasite burdens above or around the pristine average value. For a much more detailed and explicit account, see Ref. 18.

where the parasite distribution among hosts is negative binomial with clumping parameter k).

It is clear from Table 19-5 that significant efficiencies can accrue to a program of selective chemotherapy, especially if the goal is to reduce the incidence of disease (i.e., reduce the average parasite burden), rather than the more heroic goal of eradicating infection (i.e., reducing prevalence to zero).

MALARIA: TRANSMISSION AND IMMUNITY

The formula Eq. 19-4 for the basic reproductive rate of malaria has been used in many discussions of control programs by Macdonald [10,30] and others. It indicates, for instance, that increasing the death rate μ of adult mosquitoes is likely to be more effective in reducing R_0 than is reduction of mosquito density m by decreasing survivorship of larval stages [because R_0 depends on μ exponentially through the factor $\exp(-\mu T)$, but only linearly on m]. In other words, insecticides are likely to be more effective than larvicides [32].

In practice, some of the oversimplifications in Eq. 19-4 have serious consequences. Thus the "average mosquito density" fails to account for inhomogeneities in mosquito distribution. Mosquitoes that rest outdoors (exophilic) can have very different survival under a spraying program than those resting indoors (endophilic), which can undercut simple estimates of the impact of insecticides [47]. The effects of superinfection, and of age structure and other inhomogeneities in the character of host populations, can lead to further departures from an idealized compartmental model [32,39,47,48].

In regions where malaria is endemic, older age groups appear to exhibit some degree of acquired immunity, so that the clinical pathology is more common among younger people. Moreover, there is evidence (for a review, see Ref. 31) to suggest that maintenance of such immunity depends on continued exposure to infection; the immunity may be boosted, as it were, by bites from infected mosquitoes. Under these circumstances, mathematical models need to take account both of an immune class and of a rate of loss of immunity that depends on the intensity of transmission. Figure 19-9 is the outcome of one such model, showing the prevalence of malaria

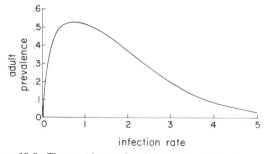

among adults as a function of the infection rate [31]. The figure shows that, at relatively high transmission levels, reduction of the infection rate (by a program of chemotherapy or by mosquito control) can lead to increased prevalence among adults; the prevalence falls when transmission is reduced to very low levels. A certain amount of field data (summarized in Ref. 31) seems to support the pattern indicated in Fig. 19-9.

In short, theoretical studies of the population biology of malarial infections illustrate that simple models can be a useful guide to basic principles, but that in practice the details matter. In particular, Fig. 19-9 provides another striking example where control programs can have perverse and counterintuitive effects on herd immunity: in some situations, reduction of transmission by programs of chemotherapy, vaccination, or vector control may actually make things worse for the adult population as a whole by diminishing the average level of naturally acquired immunity.

COEVOLUTION OF HOSTS AND PARASITES

The foregoing discussion pays no attention to the coevolution of hosts and parasites. In many control programs, however, the evolution of resistance by parasites to drugs, or by vectors to insecticides or molluscicides, cannot be ignored.

Many (though not all) naturally occurring host-parasite associations, on the other hand, appear to have settled into an evolutionary equilibrium. In this event, the received wisdom set forth in most medical texts, and elsewhere, is that "successful" or "well-adapted" parasites are relatively harmless to their hosts. This idea is reasonable, at first sight: all else being equal, it is to the advantage of both host and parasite for the parasite to inflict little damage. Moreover, a certain amount of anecdotal information supports the view [49]. Thus, for instance, in regions of Africa where trypanosomiasis is endemic, indigenous ruminants suffer mild infections with insignificant morbidity, while domestic ruminants that have been bred for a long time in the region suffer more severely, and recently imported exotic ruminants suffer virulent infections which are usually fatal if untreated.

On theoretical grounds, it would indeed appear that parasites evolve to be avirulent, provided that transmissibility and duration of infectiousness are entirely independent of virulence. This assumption, however, is not generally valid; the damage inflicted on their hosts by viral, bacterial, protozoan, and helminth parasites is often directly associated with the production of transmission stages. Once these complications are introduced into the theoretical models, it appears that many coevolutionary paths are possible, depending on the details of the interplay between the virulence and the transmissibility of the parasite [7,14,50–53].

The introduction of the myxoma virus into wild populations of rabbits in Australia and England in the early 1950s provides an unusually well-documented and interesting example [54]. At first the disease was highly virulent, but throughout the

Figure 19-9. The prevalence of malaria among adults (people over 20 years of age) is shown as a function of the infection rate. The curve derives from a model in which immunity is maintained by reinfection; for details, see Ref. 31.

subsequent decade successively less virulent strains of the virus began to appear. Since the mid-1960s, the virus appears to have come to an equilibrium with its rabbit host (in both Australia and England), with the predominant strain of the virus being one of intermediate virulence. The data can be analyzed to get a rough estimate of the relationship between the virulence α and the transmissibility of the various strains of the myxoma virus, as measured by $\beta(\alpha)$ and $v(\alpha)$ [50]. Substituting these empirical relations for $\beta(\alpha)$ and $v(\alpha)$ in Eq. 19-2 for the basic reproductive rate R_0 of the myxoma virus, we obtain an estimate of the overall dependence of R_0 on α. In this particular instance, it turns out that strains with intermediate virulence α have the largest R_0 and may thus be expected to predominate [50].

There are other circumstances where the evolutionary pressures on the parasite are likely to promote virulence. The various baculoviruses, which kill their insect hosts and effectively turn them into masses of viral transmission stages, are likely examples.

In brief, although parasite "harmlessness" may characterize many old-established associations, neither a priori theoretical arguments nor empirical evidence points to its being a general rule [50,53].

REGULATION OF HOST POPULATIONS BY PARASITES

Throughout this chapter, we have focused on endemic infections which are present in populations at steady levels (give or take periodic fluctuations around some long-term average [13–15], as is the case for measles, chickenpox, and the like), rather than on epidemic infections which occasionally sweep through populations but are otherwise absent [2–4].

The human host populations have, furthermore, been treated as constant or at least changing on a time scale that is slow in comparison with those relevant to the dynamics of parasitic infection. It is likely, however, that many nonhuman animals have their population densities regulated, wholly or in part, by parasites (defined broadly, as above, to include viruses, bacteria, protozoans, and helminths).

To explore this possibility [1], we need an analytic framework departing from conventional epidemiology in that the host population is itself a dynamic variable, interacting with the parasite population. The basic such model shows that the criterion for a microparasite to be able to regulate the host population density is [1]:

$$\alpha > r \left(1 + \frac{v}{b + \gamma} \right) \qquad (19\text{-}15)$$

Here α is the host death rate associated with the infection (the virulence), r is the intrinsic population growth rate per capita (birth rate less death rate, b) in the disease-free population, v is the recovery rate, and γ is the rate of loss of acquired immunity. Additional criteria may need to be satisfied for a par-

ticular microparasite to be capable of regulating its host population, but Eq. 19-15 is the basic condition. The criterion may be generalized in various ways to encompass depression of the reproductive rate of infected hosts, dependence of virulence on stress or on the nutritional state of the host, and so on [1,55]. An expression broadly similar to Eq. 19-15 applies to the possibility that a macroparasite may regulate a host population [6,7].

In general, the condition Eq. 19-15 suggests that it will be easier for a host population to be regulated by a parasite if the hosts have a relatively small r value, or if there is no acquired immunity (corresponding to $\gamma \to \infty$, whence the criterion for regulation is simply $\alpha > r$). This latter observation implies that, other things being equal, invertebrate populations may be regulated by parasites more commonly than vertebrates, which typically do possess acquired immunity against many infections. Holmes [56] has independently advanced this suggestion, on purely empirical grounds.

As emphasized by Holmes [56], although anecdotes abound concerning the havoc that diseases can wreak in natural populations of plants and animals, it is very difficult to assess the extent to which such diseases are important as regulatory agents. For example, in some species of wildfowl in North America some 80 to 90 percent of the individuals not shot by hunters die of diseases each year, yet it is arguable that availability of breeding sites remains the primary factor regulating population density. The various causes of death in natural populations are hard to disentangle, and, particularly for vertebrate populations, it may be that regulatory mechanisms often depend on the interplay of several factors [57].

Theoretical studies show that when a parasitic infection does regulate its host population, the outcome may be a steady, constant value or it may be a stable cycle in which host density and disease prevalence rise and fall in periodic fashion [14,55]. Such dynamic host-parasite models have been shown to give good fits to laboratory data for experiments in which animal populations are regulated by infection; in particular, the Greenwood et al. experiments on laboratory mice populations infected with ectromelia or with *Pasteurella muris* can be analyzed in detail in this way [1]. In the field, such models have been applied to suggest that the 5–12 year cycles observed in many univoltine forest insects, and the 9–10 year cycle of the larch budmoth in Switzerland in particular, may possibly derive from specific viral or microsporidian protozoan infections [55]. The models have also been used tentatively to explain the population dynamics of foxes in those parts of Europe where rabies is now endemic, and where fox densities appear to cycle around average levels that are significantly lower than the disease-free ones (set primarily by territoriality) [58].

In short, the possibility that many nonhuman animal populations are regulated by parasites is important both for ecological theory and for practical applications [57]. But systematic collections of data are scarce.

In any assessment of the impact of disease on natural populations, humans must be considered as a special case, if only because the patterns of accelerating growth of human populations over the past century and more are without parallel elsewhere in the animal kingdom. Changing life expectancies in human populations, particularly over the past two centuries in the developed world and since World War II in the developing world, are almost wholly due to reduced mortality from infectious diseases [60–62]. Although these diminished mortality rates—and their demographic consequences—are clear, the relative importance of the contributions made to them by better nutrition, improved hygiene, medical advances, and other factors remains the subject of sharp and unresolved debate [57–60]. For sexually transmitted diseases (STDs) such as HIV-AIDS, R_0 is likely to depend on behavioral habits within the population (such as the average rate of acquiring new sexual partners, c) rather than upon population density as such.

As other chapters in this book make plain, both microparasitic and macroparasitic infections continue to exact a toll of mortality and morbidity in human populations, especially in developing countries [62]. As better understanding of the processes of individual immunity and of herd immunity are combined with more effective delivery of primary health care, this toll could diminish. But supervening social and economic considerations will determine the ultimate outcome of such shifts in the dynamic association between human hosts and their parasites. The topics covered in this chapter are no more than a tiny piece in a large and complex mosaic.

REFERENCES

1 Anderson RM, May RM: Population biology of infectious diseases: Part I. Nature 280:361–367, 1979

2 Bailey NJT: *The Mathematical Theory of Infectious Diseases,* 2d ed. New York, Macmillan, 1975

3 Hoppensteadt FC: *Mathematical Theories of Populations: Demographics, Genetics and Epidemics.* Regional Conference Series in Applied Mathematics, 20. Philadelphia, Society for Industrial and Applied Mathematics, 1976

4 May RM, Anderson RM: Transmission dynamics of HIV infection. Nature 326:137–142, 1987

5 Crofton HD: A quantitative approach to parasitism. Parasitology 63:179–193, 1971

6 Anderson RM, May RM: Regulation and stability of host-parasite population interactions. I. Regulatory processes. J Anim Ecol 47:219–247, 1978

7 May RM, Anderson RM: Regulation and stability of host-parasite population interactions: II. Destabilizing processes. J Anim Ecol 47:249–267, 1978

8 Warren KS: The control of helminths: Non-replicating infectious agents of man. Annu Rev Public Health 2:101–115, 1981

9 Smillie WG: Control of hookworm disease in South Alabama. South Med J 17:494–499, 1924

10 Macdonald G: The analysis of equilibrium in malaria. Trop Dis Bull 49:813–829, 1952

11 Dietz K: Transmission and control of arbovirus diseases, in Ludwig D, Cooke KL (eds): *Epidemiology.* Philadelphia, Society for Industrial and Applied Mathematics, 1975, pp 104–121

12 Dietz K: The incidence of infectious diseases under the influence of seasonal fluctuations, in Berger J, Buhlen W, Repges R, Tautu P (eds): *Mathematical Models in Medicine; Lecture Notes in Biomathematics, II.* Berlin, Springer-Verlag, 1976, pp 1–15

13 Anderson RM, May RM: Directly transmitted infectious diseases: Control by vaccination. Science 215:1053–1060, 1982

14 May RM, Anderson RM: Population biology of infectious diseases: II. Nature 280:455–461, 1979

15 Yorke JA, Nathanson N, Pianigiani G, et al: Seasonality and the requirements for perpetuation and eradication of viruses in populations. Am J Epidemiol 109:103–123, 1979

16 Anderson RM, May RM, McLean AR: Possible demographic consequences of AIDS in developing countries. Nature 332:228–233, 1988

17 Macdonald G: The dynamics of helminth infections, with special reference to schistosomes. Trans R Soc Trop Med Hyg 59:489–506, 1965

18 Anderson RM, May RM: The population dynamics and control of human helminth infections. Nature 297:557–563, 1982

19 Kermack WO, McKendrick AG: A contribution to the mathematical theory of epidemics. Proc R Soc A 115:700–721, 1927

20 Bartlett MS: Measles periodicity and community size. J R Stat Soc Ser A 120:48–70, 1957

21 Black FL: Measles endemicity in insular populations. Critical community size and its evolutionary implication. J Theor Biol 11:207–211, 1966

22 Anderson RM, May RM: Vaccination against rubella and measles: Quantitative investigations of different policies. J Hyg 90:1–67, 1983

23 May RM: Dynamical aspects of host-parasite associations. Crofton's model revisited. Parasitology 75:259–276, 1977

24 Hethcote HW, Yorke JA: *Gonorrhea Transmission Dynamics and Control,* Springer Lecture Notes in Biomathematics, no 56. New York, Springer-Verlag, 1984

25 Dietz K: Models for vector-borne parasitic diseases, in Barigozzi C (ed): *Vito Volterra Symposium on Mathematical Models in Biology; Lecture Notes in Biomathematics, 39.* Berlin, Springer-Verlag, 1980, 264–277

26 May RM, Anderson RM: Spatial heterogeneity and the design of immunization programs. Math Biosci 72:83–111, 1984

27 Kemper JT: On the identification of superspreaders for infectious disease. Math Biosci 48:111–128, 1980

28 Dietz K, Molineaux L, Thomas A: A malaria model tested in the African savannah. Bull WHO 50:347–357, 1974

29 Cooke KL: Models for endemic infections with asymptomatic cases: I. One group. Math Modelling 3:1–15, 1982

30 Macdonald G: Theory of the eradication of malaria. Bull WHO 15:369–387, 1956

31 Aron JL, May RM: The population dynamics of malaria, in Anderson, RM (ed): *Population Dynamics of Infectious Diseases.* London, Chapman Hall, 1982, pp 139–179

32 Macdonald G: Collected papers, in Bruce-Chwatt LJ, Glanville VJ (eds): *Dynamics of Tropical Disease.* Oxford, Oxford University Press, 1973

33 May RM: Togetherness among schistosomes: Its effects on the dynamics of the infection. Math Biosci 35:301–343, 1977

34 Bradley DJ, May RM: Consequences of helminth aggregation for

the dynamics of schistosomiasis. Trans R Soc Trop Med Hyg 72:262–273, 1978

35 Fine PEM: Control of infectious diseases (group report), in Anderson RM, May RM (eds): *Population Biology of Infectious Diseases*. New York, Springer-Verlag, 1982, pp 121–147

36 Anderson RM: The control of infectious disease agents: Strategic models, in Conway GR (ed): *Pest and Pathogen Control: Strategy, Tactics and Policy Models*. New York, Wiley, 1983

37 McLean AR, Anderson RM: Measles in developing countries. Part I: Epidemiological parameters and patterns. Epidemiol Inf 100:111–133, 1988

38 Anderson RM: Transmission dynamics and control of infectious disease agents, in Anderson RM, May RM (eds): *Population Biology of Infectious Diseases*. New York, Springer-Verlag, 1982, pp 149–177

39 Molineaux L, Gramiccia G: The Garki Project: Research on the Epidemiology and Control of Malaria in the Sudan Savanna of West Africa. Geneva, WHO, 1980

40 Smith CEG: Prospects for the control of infectious disease. Proc R Soc Med 63:1181–1190, 1970

41 Fine PEM, Clarkson JA: Measles in England and Wales: II. The impact of the measles vaccination programme on the distribution of immunity in the population. Int J Epidemiol 11:15–25, 1982

42 Knox EG: Strategy for rubella vaccination. Int J Epidemiol 9:13–23, 1980

43 Anderson RM, May RM: Age-related changes in rate of disease transmission: Implications for the design of vaccination programs. J Hyg 94:365–436, 1985

44 May RM: Vaccination programs and herd immunity. Nature 300:481–483, 1982

45 Bradley DJ: Regulation of parasite populations: A general theory of the epidemiology and control of parasitic infections. Trans R Soc Trop Med Hyg 66:697–708, 1972

46 Croll NA, Anderson RM, Gyorkos TW, et al: The population biology and control of *Ascaris lumbricoides* in a rural community in Iran. Trans R Soc Trop Med Hyg 76:187–197, 1982

47 Molineaux L, Shidrawi GR, Clarke JL, et al: Assessment of insecticidal impact on the malaria mosquito's vectorial capacity, from data on the man-biting rate and age-composition. Bull WHO 57:265–274, 1979

48 Molineaux L, Dietz K, Thomas A: Further epidemiological evaluation of a malaria model. Bull WHO 56:565–571, 1978

49 Allison AC: Coevolution between hosts and infectious disease agents, and its effects on virulence, in Anderson RM, May RM (eds): *Population Biology of Infectious Diseases*. New York, Springer-Verlag, 1982, pp 245–267

50 May RM, Anderson RM: Coevolution of parasites and hosts, in Futuyma D, Slatkin M, Levin B, Roughgarden J (eds): *Coevolution*. Sunderland, Mass, Sinauer, 1983, pp 186–206

51 Levin SA, Pimentel D: Selection of intermediate rates of increase in parasite-host systems. Am Natur 117:308–315, 1981

52 Bremermann HJ: Sex and polymorphism as strategies in host-pathogen interactions. J Theor Biol 87:671–702, 1980

53 Levin BR: Evolution of parasites and hosts (group report), in Anderson RM, May RM (eds): *Population Biology of Infectious Diseases*. New York, Springer-Verlag, 1982, pp 213–243

54 Fenner F, Ratcliffe FN: *Myxomatosis*. Cambridge, Cambridge University Press, 1966

55 Anderson RM, May RM: The population dynamics of microparasites and their invertebrate hosts, Phil Trans R Soc B 291:451–524, 1981

56 Holmes JC: Impact of infectious disease agents on the population growth and geographical distribution of animals, in Anderson RM, May RM (eds): *Population Biology of Infectious Diseases*. New York, Springer-Verlag, 1982, pp 37–51

57 Hassell MP: Impact of infectious diseases on host populations, in Anderson RM, May RM (eds): *Population Biology of Infectious Diseases*. New York, Springer-Verlag, 1982, pp 15–35

58 Anderson RM, Jackson H, May RM, et al: The population dynamics of fox rabies in Europe. Nature 289:765–771, 1981

59 Anderson RM, Crombie J: Experimental studies of age-prevalence curves for *Schistosoma mansoni* infections in populations of *Biomphalaria glabrata*. Parasitology 89:79–105, 1984

60 McKeown T: *The Modern Rise of Population*. London, Edward Arnold, 1976

61 Wrigley EA, Schofield RS: *The Population History of England, 1541–1871*. Cambridge, Mass, Harvard University Press, 1981

62 Pereira MS: The impact of infectious disease on human demography today, in Anderson RM, May RM (eds): *Population Biology of Infectious Diseases*. New York, Springer-Verlag, 1982, pp 53–64

63 Crombie JA, Anderson RM: Population dynamics of *Schistosoma mansoni* in mice repeatedly exposed to infection. Nature 315:491–493, 1985

64 Anderson RM, May RM: Herd immunity to helminth infection and implications for parasite control. Nature 315:493–496, 1985

Transmission of Vector-Borne Disease · Andrew Spielman · Anthony A. James

In public health, the entomological objective is to protect non-immune human populations from exposure to vector-borne agents of disease. This discipline synthesizes ecological, genetic, and physiological methodologies to analyze the complex relationships that link vectors to their hosts, the pathogens that are transmitted, and the influence of the environment. We seek a permanent improvement in health rather than a rapidly reduced prevalence of infection. In this review, we examine these relationships in order to explain how component variables affect transmission of pathogens. We seek to provide a conceptual basis for programs aiming to regulate transmission.

VECTOR-ENVIRONMENT RELATIONSHIPS

Vectors of the pathogens that cause human disease generally exploit disturbed environments. These insects, ticks, and mites prefer newly created sites, where they rapidly become abundant. In temperate zones, seasonal weather changes and predators can interfere with the growth of newly established vector populations. However, environmental disturbances in tropical sites are particularly conducive to vector-borne disease because these regions are climatically stable and may permit year-round proliferation of an opportunistic vector. Increased economic productivity in tropical regions often creates disturbances that produce an increased burden of disease. This dilemma constitutes the main focus for agencies concerned with the health of the residents of developing countries.

Efforts to limit the transmission of tropical disease are facilitated when the crucial environmental features exploited by the vector can be identified. Vector-parasite and vector-host relationships modify these environmentally dependent patterns of transmission. The following discussion describes the major features of these relationships for certain of the major vectors. Details of the life history, taxonomy, and importance to health of insect and acarine vectors can be obtained from standard medical entomology texts [1–3]. The more important vectors and some infections that they transmit are listed in Table 20-1.

Each of the various vectors exploits its environment in a characteristic manner. Common themes can be identified and will be described for the major groups. Of the vector arthropods, flies depend more upon external environmental factors than do lice, while other vectors occupy intermediate positions on this scale of environmental constraint. Those hematophagous arthropods most dependent upon breeding conditions created by human activity similarly tend to depend upon human hosts for food. Such narrowness of host range promotes the efficiency of these organisms as vectors of pathogens specific to the human host. This relationship would provide a first clue to the identity of particular vectors.

MOSQUITOES

Mosquitoes transmit many of the infections usually thought of as "tropical." In general, these vectors are opportunistic. They rapidly exploit newly created bodies of water and lead the chain of succession. Natural seasonal change provides abundant opportunity for mosquitoes in temperate regions, but in the tropics human activity creates the disturbed conditions most commonly exploited by mosquitoes. Monsoons and other periodic climatic events also create transient bodies of water that may be fertile sources of mosquitoes.

In general, mosquitoes of the genus *Aëdes* adapt most readily to the extremes of transient environmental conditions. The egg is deposited on moist substrates at margins of receding bodies of water. The embryo develops and after a few days becomes resistant to desiccation. Depending upon the species, such embryos can survive for months or even years until water levels rise once again to submerge the egg. Consequent reduction in

Table 20-1. Principal insect, mite, and tick vectors and the main infections that they transmit

Common name	Genus	Infections
Mosquitoes	*Aëdes*	Dengue
		Yellow fever
		Viral encephalitis
	Anopheles	Malaria
	Culex	Lymphatic filariasis
Blackflies	*Simulium*	Onchocerciasis
Sand flies	*Phlebotomus,*	Leishmaniasis
	Lutzomyia	Papatasi fever
		Bartonellosis
Biting midges	*Culicoides*	Visceral filariasis
Deerflies	*Chrysops*	Eyeworm
Tsetse	*Glossina*	African sleeping sickness
Kissing bugs	*Triatoma, Rhodnius,*	Chagas' disease
	Panstrongylus	
Fleas	*Xenopsylla*, etc.	Plague
		Murine typhus
Lice	*Pediculus*	Epidemic typhus
		Relapsing fever
		Trench fever
Chigger mites	*Trombicula*, etc.	Tsutsugamushi
Mouse mites	*Lyponyssoides*	Rickettsialpox
Hard ticks	*Dermacentor*	Spotted fever
	Ixodes	Babesiosis
		Lyme disease
	Hyalomma	Crimean-Congo hemorrhagic fever
Soft ticks	*Ornithodorus*	Relapsing fever

oxygen tension stimulates hatching, often within minutes. This rapid response to flooding obviates the several days of delay in hatching otherwise required if eggs (always nonembryonated) were laid directly upon the water. Larval *Aëdes* browse upon organic matter that has accumulated on the bottom of the body of water; their mouthparts are adapted for chewing or scraping. They can derive nutrients from organic material already present in the breeding site at the time of flooding or carried into the site from nearby vegetation. No infusion need develop. Certain *Aëdes* can develop in water that stands for a week or less, and pupae can develop even when stranded. *A. aegypti* and similar mosquitoes in the subgenera *Stegomyia* and *Finlaya* exemplify this pattern of adaptation to transient habitats. Automobile tires provide ideal breeding sites, particularly when placed beneath overhanging vegetation. Water can remain in them for a least 1 week, even under conditions of extreme drying. Proliferation of the automobile coupled with the durable nature of this by-product of transportation has resulted in an impressive accumulation worldwide of potential *Aëdes* breeding sites. Increased risk of dengue, yellow fever, and California encephalitis accompanies this particular aspect of economic development.

Anopheline mosquitoes, in general, are adapted to more permanent conditions than *Aëdes* mosquitoes. The boatlike egg is deposited directly upon the water, often while the female hovers some distance above the surface. Lateral air chambers, or, occasionally, a hydrophobic fringe, keep the dorsal surface in contact with air. Submersion during the first 3 to 4 days drowns the developing embryo. Hatching follows embryonic maturation. Some species appear capable of surviving for a week or so if the egg becomes stranded, but the natural role of such estivation has not been demonstrated. Absence of an air tube permits the larva to lie against the surface, often in the line of intersection formed by air, water, and emergent vegetation, and this sequestration appears to protect against predators. The larva feeds mainly upon material contained in the surface film. Pollen may be an important nutrient. Taken together, these features demonstrate that anophelines have adapted to a more permanent aquatic habitat than *Aëdes*. The water must remain for several weeks or more; the surface must be free of mold; and particular vegetation may be required. Generally, predators reduce anopheline larval density with the passage of time. Particular species exploit different variations on this theme.

In Africa, *Anopheles gambiae* exploits open sunlit pools such as the brick pits used for making mud-brick for home construction. Because mud-brick buildings require constant repair, the brick pits are located close to homes, and villages tend to develop where the water table is high enough to flood the pits. Maximum breeding densities are reached soon after the onset of seasonal rains. A companion African vector, *An. funestus,* becomes most abundant with onset of the dry season. Sunlit pools containing emergent marginal vegetation provide the main breeding sites. Thus, clearing of forests near developing villages renders human populations vulnerable to risk of

perennial malaria, even where rainfall is seasonal. Combined transmission by *An. gambiae* and *An. funestus* results in seasonally constant transmission patterns. Similarly constant transmission patterns due to a combination of vectors characterize the Indian subcontinent. In that region, *An. culicifacies* exploits irrigated fields and the ditches that drain them. The rainy season is the period of maximum productivity of that vector, while drying conditions promote maximum abundance of *An. stephensi,* a mosquito that breeds in water puddled in the beds of streams. Similar perennial transmission can occur where multiple vectors are present.

Such ecological generalities, however, cannot automatically be applied across broad regions. For example, Sri Lankan *An. culicifacies* breeds in water-filled hollows left in the sandy beds of receding rivers. Therefore, in contrast to the situation in nearby India, *An. culicifacies*–transmitted malaria in Sri Lanka follows drought. The abundance of this vector increases reciprocally with intensity of irrigation, due to increased puddling as the river level is lowered when water is diverted to irrigate crops. Neither the fields themselves nor the ditches that drain them support *An. culicifacies* in Sri Lanka.

Agricultural practices pose a special problem when the vector breeds directly in irrigated fields and drainage ditches. Such mosquitoes, in particular, are likely to develop insecticide resistance in response to agricultural spray [4]. The absence of winter makes tropical agriculture dependent upon pesticides; cotton, tobacco, and rice receive frequent treatment to protect against numerous arthropod pests.

Economic development can promote multiplication of different *Anopheles*. Fish ponds in Indonesia support *An. sundaicus* and *An. subpictus*. In the Philippines, construction of villages in upland regions results in increased human exposure to *An. minimus,* a vector that exploits eddies along the margins of mountain streams. Wherever human activity creates environmental change, collections of water may be exploited by particular vector *Anopheles.*

Culex mosquitoes are adapted to conditions intermediate in stability between those exploited by *Aëdes* and by *Anopheles* species. Eggs are deposited directly on the water, cemented together in geometric clusters. Each stands on a cuticular pedicel that holds the body of the egg vertically well above the water. Larvae hatch after 3 or 4 days; the eggs cannot withstand drying. Larval *Culex* are filter feeders that hang from the surface by means of a long, slender air tube. The more important vector species breed in highly contaminated ground pools including cesspools, ditches, sewage waste lagoons, etc. Such water stands long enough to develop an infusion but not so long as to permit the water to clarify. The erect position of the egg and the long air tube appear to adapt *Culex* mosquitoes to the scum often present on such water, while filter feeding exploits rich supplies of suspended nutrient.

Culex pipiens mosquitoes become abundant in proportion to the amount of waste water accumulated near human dwellings. These insects are absent or scarce where houses are constructed without altering the natural contours of the land and where feces are deposited upon the ground rather than in pits. They become abundant where drainage ditches must be constructed and where fecal deposits are flushed by water. In temperate regions, indigenous *C. pipiens pipiens* generally do not bite human hosts, but tropical *C. p. quinquefasciatus* are highly anthropophagic. Thus, urbanization in the tropics carries particular risk of filariasis.

Both male and female mosquitoes require frequent intake of nectar, honeydew, or similar carbohydrate nutrients. Blood is ingested solely by females in preparation for oogenesis or perhaps for hibernation. Depending on feeding and reproductive habits, a vector mosquito may be exposed to potential hosts every 3 or 4 days. Longevity, and hence total number of host contracts, depends upon availability of carbohydrates, permissive nature of the climate, and predators of the adult stage. These generalities apply to the adult stage of blackflies, sand flies, midges, and horseflies.

BLACKFLIES

In constrast to the still water adaptation of mosquitoes, blackflies (*Simulium*) develop in rapidly flowing water. Eggs are cemented to vegetation or other substates close to the breeding site or, in certain species, laid directly on the water. Embryos survive until inundation and consequent hatching. The larvae of most species attach to submerged rocks or vegetation by means of specialized suckers and prolegs. They tend to be sessile, concentrating at points where the current is greatest. Anchored strands of silk aid downstream movement. Feeding is a passive process, depending upon the current for particulate matter to collect in a basketlike filter. Rapid flow of water maximizes feeding efficiency, and consequent aeration facilitates the cutaneous respiration upon which these larvae depend. Pupae form in a silken cocoon spun where the larvae feed. Large, leathery wings enable the emerging adult to take flight immediately after contact with air; other insects must rest while their wings harden. This combination of characteristics enables blackflies to exploit rapidly flowing water such as spillways of dams, narrow points in rivers, and mountain streams. The *S. neavei* group of species (largely in eastern Africa) attaches to freshwater crabs and prawns, which permits them to exploit mud-bottomed, slow-moving rivers.

Attempts to harness water power and to manage streams frequently increase the velocity of water flow near points of concentrated human activity. Construction of dams provides an obvious case in point, but other activities produce similarly pernicious effects. Ferry crossings generally are placed at narrow points of rivers, and the river may further be narrowed by abutments constructed as landing points on opposite banks. Ferry operators would be exposed to blackflies at points of maximum vector density and might serve as potent sources for blackfly-transmitted parasites. In other locations, stream straightening due to erosion would increase water velocity where agricultural practices are faulty or where forests are denuded. Taken together, these environmental trends increasingly maximize transmission of onchocerciasis, particularly in western Africa.

SAND FLIES

Sand flies (such as *Phlebotomus* and *Lutzomyia*) exploit moist recesses of forest litter, loose soils, termite nests, cracks in dried mud, animal burrows, or tree holes, where they feed on decaying organic matter. The caterpillarlike larvae are terrestrial but require humid conditions. Adults are poor fliers, tending to fly only short distances. Even at rest, their wings are held upright, making them vulnerable to wind. Adults rest near the breeding sites and emerge to feed at night when wind and humidity are most favorable.

Different flies exploit diverse features of the environment. Around houses, accumulation of organic matter due to domestic animals, poor sanitation, or use of dung for fuel promotes their abundance. In contrast, close contact with rodent burrows, termitaria, forest litter, or similar natural breeding sites exposes human hosts to the zoonotic cycle of sand fly–borne pathogens. Expanding human communities dependent on animal husbandry or forest clearing may be vulnerable to one or both of these threats. However, as economic development proceeds toward urbanization, human populations experience reduced contact with wild or domestic animals, and sites favoring fly breeding tend to be destroyed by trampling or by pavement.

Because of their short flight pattern, sand flies are readily destroyed by residual insecticides; consequently, antimalaria programs commonly have caused leishmaniasis to disappear. However, cessation of spray programs has rendered certain human communities vulnerable to resumed transmission of leishmaniasis.

BITING MIDGES

Biting midges (*Culicoides, Leptoconops*), vectors of *Mansonella ozzardi* and of Oropouche virus, exploit bodies of water containing soggy, decaying vegetation. Larvae are aquatic and move in an undulatory manner. The adults are minute, remaining near larval breeding sites. Disturbed drainage due to human intervention promotes breeding of these flies, particularly when decaying vegetation accumulates in water. Locations such as beaches, rivers, and marshes are sensitive to human intervention and to the enhanced fly breeding that results.

DEERFLIES

Deerflies (such as *Chrysops*) are vectors of loiasis in Africa as well as pests of people and animals worldwide. Deerflies breed in soggy soil in marshes and other moist habitats. The larvae feed on various invertebrates, developing over a year or more.

The adults are strong-flying daytime or crepuscular feeders, attracted to their prey mainly by sight and carbon dixoide. Because breeding sites and habits are poorly known, human impact on breeding is not clear and control is difficult.

TSETSE FLIES

Tsetse flies (*Glossina*) reproduce in a fashion unique among human-biting flies; a female develops a single larva at a time within her body and takes several blood meals while each larva matures. After a week or so, the mature larva is deposited on soil, burrows in, and pupates without feeding. Adults are strong daytime fliers and locate their hosts mainly by sight. Both sexes blood-feed, and most species are specific in their habitat and host preference. An exception is the riverine species of the *Glossina palpalis* group, which feed opportunistically. Such flies were responsible for the spread of sleeping sickness along the major rivers and lakes of Africa following the explorations at the beginning of the century. Other tsetse exploit forests or savannahs, feeding mainly on suids or bovids.

Risk of tsetse-borne trypanosomiasis may be increased by human intervention depending on the type of fly as well as the parasite. For example, settlement near and exploration of rivers bring human hosts into close contact with species of the *palpalis* group, vectors of Gambian sleeping sickness. Absence of other vertebrate hosts intensifies transmission. In contrast, risk of acquiring Rhodesian sleeping sickness, a zoonosis, is greater where human hosts are associated with wild or domestic animals in the savannah breeding grounds of species of the *morsitans* group. Overall, tsetse flies have been difficult to eliminate, resulting in a constant disease burden in many parts of Africa and preventing human settlement of vast regions in that continent.

FLEAS

Fleas (*Xenopsylla, Pulex*) generally parasitize mammals that form nests or that return each night to a particular resting place. Eggs are laid individually and hatch after a few days. The caterpillarlike larvae crawl over the nest material, feeding on particles of organic matter, particularly dried granules of undigested host blood expelled from the anus of the adult. This requirement for host blood focuses the activities of all stages of the flea around the nest. Larvae are sensitive to drying. In the absence of hosts, adult fleas may delay emergence from the pupal cocoon. The adult feeds solely on blood, but feeding may be delayed for weeks.

Plague and typhus are maintained in zoonotic foci by particular fleas associated with their characteristic rodent hosts. Transmission to human hosts generally follows contact with nests of infected reservoir hosts. Risk of being bitten by a host-specific, zoophilic flea is increased following death of the normal host as well as by direct effects of the plague bacillus on the flea. Typhus rickettsiae seem to be relatively nonpathogenic in the vector.

Chigoe fleas (*Tunga penetrans*) may be anthroponotic in sites where people congregate. Larvae develop in soil from which the adults emerge and attach to human or animal hosts. The engorging bodies of the female become pea-sized tumors that cause great discomfort.

LICE

The body louse (*Pediculus humanus*) is the only one of the three louse parasites of human hosts that perpetuates zoonoses (typhus and relapsing fever). Maturation proceeds through a series of similar developmental stages. Human blood provides the sole nutrient for all stages, and a meal is required at least daily. Body lice remain in direct contact with the host only a few minutes, long enough to imbibe blood. Between meals, these insects remain in the outer layer of clothing, apparently seeking an optimal temperature somewhat cooler than the skin of the human host. The body louse is really a "clothes louse," and its abundance depends upon the host continuously wearing an outer layer of clothing. Indigent, older persons are particularly vulnerable to infestation. Periods of warfare or other disasters promote conditions in which large human populations remain fully clothed for extended periods of time, producing epidemics of louse-borne disease.

Head lice (*P. capitis*) and the venereally transmitted crab lice (*Phthirus pubis*) are transmitted by direct contact between people. These pediculoses may be highly prevalent, even in affluent societies.

KISSING BUGS

The bloodsucking kissing bugs (*Triatoma, Rhodnius, Panstrongylus*) become abundant in the site in which their diurnal hosts sleep. In the sylvan environment, they generally parasitize rodents, marsupials, or armadillos. These are burrow-inhabiting mammals, and the bugs remain in the burrows. Anthropophilic species have become adapted to human residences, where they inhabit crevices in walls or furniture or thatch. All stages feed solely on blood. Adult kissing bugs differ from nymphs in that they are winged and those of some species can fly. But in general, bugs are restricted to the immediate vicinity of resting hosts. Bugs can feed every week or so, but survive 8 or 10 weeks without feeding.

House construction is the main determinant of abundance of the species that transmit Chagas' disease. Mud and wattle construction or thatched roofs generally provide the necessary cover in Latin America for these crevice-dwelling insects.

MITES

Chiggers (trombiculids) and mouse mites (dermanyssids) are the only mites known to serve as vectors of human disease, and of these, chiggers are more important. They proliferate in grassy bottomland, where small rodents and other animal life are abundant. Larval chiggers are parasitic, attaching to a host for a week or more and imbibing lymph through a tunnellike structure (the stylostome) that develops as an intradermal extension of the larval mouthparts (human hosts generally abrade the externally attached larva, leaving the stylostome to provide continued antigenic stimulus). The nymphal and adult stages that follow the single larval stage are insectivorous and feed on small soil-dwelling arthropods. Chiggers depend upon relatively natural conditions; scrub typhus (tsutsugamushi) affects human hosts mainly when people intrude into these zoonotic foci. Military activities as well as farming in new developments provide this rodent-chigger-human contact.

In contrast, the mites that transmit rickettsial pox are domestic. They develop through a series of similar nymphal stages, each entirely hematophagous. Feeding is completed in 5 or 10 min and takes place in the nests of the rodent hosts, generally the common house mouse. Classically, human exposure to these mites follows removal of garbage or trash that has accumulated in a human residence. Mouse populations increase as trash accumulates but are displaced following trash removal. Thus, local outbreaks of rickettsial pox have followed the clean-up process associated with repair of domestic incinerators.

Scabies mites (*Sarcoptes scabiei*) produce an anthroponotic infection acquired by direct contact between people. The dermatitis induced in sensitized hosts can be highly debilitating.

TICKS

Soft ticks (argasids) develop through a series of similar and entirely hematophagous nymphal and adult stages. Soft ticks generally withstand drying conditions and survive for years in the absence of hosts. They seek hosts within the nest, feeding for 15 or 20 min. Relapsing fever is zoonotic in many parts of the world; transmission to human hosts follows prolonged contact with *Ornithodoros*-infested rodent burrows. However, in Africa *O. moubata* infests human residences, and sleeping people serve as reservoirs of the spirochete and also sustain the vector. Residence in dirt-floored traditional housing promotes transmission.

Hard ticks (ixodids) differ markedly from soft ticks. Development proceeds through three stages: larval, nymphal, and adult. Prolonged attachment, as long as a week or more, permits each stage of the tick to imbibe and concentrate enormous quantities of blood, thereby permitting unusually large increments of growth between stages. Ixodid vectors of human pathogens drop from their hosts following each of the three periods of engorgement (three-host ticks). Others remain through one molt (two-host ticks) or continuously through both molts (one-host ticks). Engorged ticks then enter the soil and later molt or oviposit. Adults die following egg laying. When questing for hosts, these ticks mount vegetation to a height that optimizes contact with certain hosts. Many populations are highly

specific in host range. For example, the brown dog tick (*Rhipicephalus sanguineus*) in North America rarely attaches to human hosts. This tick may be abundant in households that harbor domestic dogs, but will parasitize dogs exclusively. However, in north Africa, this tick bites humans and is an important vector of a human rickettsial infection.

Certain vector ticks appear to be increasing in abundance and distribution. The dog tick (*Dermacentor variabilis*), vector of Rocky Mountain spotted fever in North America, is favored by the current popularity of dogs as pets. Similarly, landscape changes and the consequent multiplication of deer in many temperate regions of the world appear to favor the *Ixodes* deer ticks that transmit Lyme disease and babesiosis. Thus, practices that encourage increased abundance of domestic or peridomestic animals may incur certain risks to human health. In this manner, affluence may promote vector-borne zoonoses.

NONHEMATOPHAGOUS ARTHROPODS

The guinea worm (*Dracunculus medinensis*) is the agent of the most important anthroponosis transmitted by nonhematophagous arthropods. Dracontiasis results when infected cyclopoid copepods contaminate drinking water. Adult worms develop subcutaneously and release larvae via a blister in the skin when stimulated by water contact. Larvae, in turn, are eaten by copepods, in which they develop to the infective stage. Arid conditions or periodic drought maximizes transmission by concentrating human activities around open wells or other small bodies of water.

The lung fluke (*Paragonimus westermani*) is zoonotic in wild carnivores, notably felids, and is transmitted by freshwater crabs or crayfish. Human infection arises when poorly cooked or pickled meat of these crustaceans is ingested.

The rat tapeworm (*Hymenolepis diminuta*) is endemic where grain is prepared in a manner that fails to ensure thorough heating. Scarcity of fuel, as in the African Sahel, would promote this practice. Stored grain is contaminated by rodents harboring the adult tapeworms. Various grain-contaminating beetles then eat feces containing excreted eggs and are eaten, in turn, by human hosts when grain is prepared by inadequate baking in the sun.

POPULATION STRUCTURE

Many morphologically distinct vector arthropods now have been divided into arrays of reproductively isolated populations that vary in their ability to transmit agents of human disease. Specific names applied to vectors, therefore, may be misleading if they include groups of diverse populations. The term *species complex* has been applied to such problem designations. Indeed, many of the more widely distributed vectors are locally heterogeneous, and the number of described species complexes continues to multiply.

The blackfly vectors of onchocerciasis present an extraordinary example of such complexity. The *Simulium damnosum* complex in Africa has been divided into dozens of "cytospecies," based on chromosomal banding patterns [5]. As many as six of these species are abundant and presumably important as vectors. Recently discovered morphological criteria now permit recognition of various of these formerly obscure taxa. Application of isozyme technology [6] has been used to identify these insects.

The *An. gambiae* complex of African malaria vectors contains six members. These include two brackish water species present on opposite coasts, three freshwater species, and a species that breeds in mineral-rich water in a restricted location in Uganda. Two of the freshwater forms, *An. gambiae* and *An. arabiensis,* are strongly anthropophilic and are effective vectors of malaria. But these species cannot be distinguished by conventional means. However, hybrids resulting from intermating are nonfertile, and this provided the original clue pointing toward a species complex. Later the component populations were distinguished by banding patterns of polytene chromosomes [7] or by isozyme characteristics [8]. More recently, chromatographic analysis of cuticular waxes [9] and specific molecular probes [10,11] proved useful in distinguishing members of this and other species complexes. Such cryptic species, which represent genetically discrete intrabreeding units, seem to be the rule among mosquito populations. The number of examples grows as knowledge of vector biology increases and with improvement in the techniques used to resolve differences.

Further epidemiological complication derives from growing evidence that certain local vector populations may not comprise genetically distinct entities. *A. aegypti* populations, for example, are structured in a complex manner; in east Africa, house-entering populations differ genetically from nearby forest populations. However, hybrid larvae are abundant in peridomestic sites, particularly when rainfall is abundant. This partial and seasonally varying genetic isolation illustrates the difficulty of defining vector populations both for epidemiological studies and as targets for intervention.

Populations of the common house mosquito (*C. pipiens*) are structured in another manner and seem still more difficult to define. Genetically hematophagous populations (anautogenous) may coexist with others (autogenous) that need not feed on blood. Autogenous *C. pipiens* seem to provide a homogeneous, exclusive target for control or study.

These limitations of taxonomy become acute when environmental change selects some genetic component of a vector population. For example, use of insecticide may select for resistant organisms in local populations of a species. Later, local populations would come to differ in vulnerability to insecticidal interventions. Public health workers seek to designate particular vector characteristics as a basis for study or intervention, but conventional species designations are chosen by evolutionists seeking to describe genetic discontinuity. Exclusionary definitions, based on description of genetic boundaries, can fail to meet the epidemiological need for inclusionary descriptions of vectors.

VECTOR-PATHOGEN RELATIONSHIPS

The term *vector competence* designates those properties of an arthropod that affect its suitability as a host for a pathogen. Factors that affect pathogen uptake, development, and output determine this epidemiological parameter. This three-part concept, originally devised to quantify observations that flea species differ in their ability to transmit plague, was expressed as the product of the proportion of fleas ingesting the plague bacillus, the proportion of infected fleas that sustained sufficient bacterial growth to block their guts, and the proportion of blocked fleas transmitting bacilli to a host. Similar uptake, development, and output relationships characterize other vector-pathogen combinations. *Vector competence* has come to replace the original, narrowly defined term, *vector efficiency*. Any genetically determined behavioral or structural property of a vector affecting uptake or delivery of pathogens is included within the concept of vector competence.

Uptake of pathogens potentially is affected by a variety of diverse physiological characteristics of the vector. Placement of a hematophagous arthropod's mouthparts determines its access to pathogens. For example, only vectors that feed from subcutaneous pools of blood, such as blackflies, and not those that cannulate blood vessels, such as mosquitoes, can ingest the skin-dwelling microfilariae of *Onchocerca volvulus*. Probability of ingestion would be further increased if microfilariae were to concentrate over certain regions of the host's body on which particular locally abundant blackflies most frequently fed.

The correspondence between the night biting behavior of particular vectors and the nocturnal periodicity of microfilariae of certain populations of *Wuchereria bancrofti* presents another obvious and well-established component of uptake efficiency. Although such filarial worms develop in laboratory-infected *A. aegypti*, their crepuscular feeding habits prevent these insects from ingesting these pathogens, thereby precluding any vector role for these mosquitoes.

Certain pathogens may accumulate at the vector's mouthparts in response to a stimulus secreted by the biting vector. It may be that microfilariae are attracted to the mouthparts of feeding mosquitoes [12], an adaptation that would enhance uptake by concentrating the pathogen. The bite-stimulated shower of bluetongue virus particles into the peripheral blood [13] provides another example of concentration. On the other hand, ingested microfilariae may be destroyed by the pharyngeal teeth of certain mosquitoes [14].

Various factors affect the *development* of pathogens once ingested by the vector. Significant interactions exist between pathogens and the vector's midgut, hemolymph, and salivary glands as well as certain other tissues. Although the digestive enzymes of the midgut constitute a medium that is potentially hostile to the survival of ingested pathogens, enhancing factors may also be present. The midgut milieu includes properties that affect exflagellation of the gametocytes of malarial parasites. Viral penetration of the midgut wall appears to be affected by binding properties between arboviral particles and the midgut wall [15]. The peritrophic membrane may limit passage of microfilariae [16], African trypanosomes [17], and *Babesia* kinetes [18]. In addition, viral particles [19] or microfilariae [20] may not traverse the midgut wall. Bluetongue virus can penetrate a fly's midgut only in association with microfilariae [21], and similar coingestion of virus and filarial worms greatly enhances viral infection of the salivary glands of mosquitoes [22].

Melanization [23] or the action of such antimicrobial factors as attacins and cecropins [24] may limit development within the hemolymph. Associations of pathogens with other tissues, as in the case of filarial worms with flight muscles and malpighian tubules, are poorly understood but essential to development.

Many pathogens must penetrate into the lumen of the salivary glands in order ultimately to be transmitted to the vertebrate host, and recognition of the gland's surface may be prerequisite to penetration. Malaria sporozoites, for example, invade only salivary tissues and only those of particular vector species [25]. These organs present yet another level of complexity because their apical surfaces are cuticular. Malaria sporozoites must cross a basement lamina, a cell layer, and a cuticular surface before entering the lumen from which they will be released. The dynamics of these tissue tropisms and membrane relationships affect the number of pathogens that lie within the lumen of the salivary glands and limit the infectious inoculum.

The size of the infectious inoculum, which constitutes the *output* component of vector competence, may also be determined by behavioral traits of the vector as well as developmental interactions between pathogens and vectors. The defecation patterns of Chagas' disease–infected bugs illustrate behavioral influences on vector competence. The timing and placement of the vector's feces determine effective output. Additional effects on the output component of vector-competence are exemplified by features of the transmission of plague. The massive overgrowth of bacilli in the proventriculus of infective fleas obstructs the digestive tract, thereby depriving the vector of food. Such starving fleas feed frequently and indiscriminately. Another case in which pathogen-vector interaction maximizes vector competence is provided by the tsetse-trypanosome interaction. The trypanosomes form rosettes around sensory structures in the food canal of infected flies, thereby physically obstructing the flow of the ingested blood. Such obstructed flies feed more slowly than do noninfected flies and presumably deliver correspondingly more pathogens. Similarly, the number of sporozoites inoculated by *Plasmodium gallinaceum*–infected *A. aegypti* is increased because of the salivary pathology caused by the infection [26].

Inherited infections present special problems in evaluating vector competence. Transovarial transmission of pathogens occurs in two discrete patterns: (1) *nonstable infection*, in which the pathogen survives in the vector across only one generation, and (2) more or less *stable infection*, in which the pathogen resides within the vector for two or more generations. Transmission of cattle babesiosis by one-host ticks exemplifies nonstable transmission. Adults transmit acquired infection to their progeny via the egg; resulting subadult ticks transmit the infection to their vertebrate hosts and lose the infection before maturing to the adult stage. Another cycle of transmission requires that these adults reacquire the infection. Pathogen uptake, development, and output each retain their importance as components of vector competence in nonstable transmission. In contrast, when inherited infection is stable, as in bunyavirus-infected mosquitoes, pathogen uptake becomes less important. Once infection becomes established, a transovarial line of infected vectors will exist. Recent work [27,28] suggests that California encephalitis virus may be maintained by inherited infection alone. This vertical mode of transmission can be amplified by supplementary infections acquired directly from vertebrate hosts. When pathogens are inherited in a stable manner, extrinsic incubation periods (duration of development in the vector) as well as multiple feedings are eliminated as absolute requirements for transmission. Interepidemic perpetuation of an arboviral agent is facilitated when it is inherited by the vector population [29,30]. Of course, an agent cannot be perpetuated by inherited infection alone unless all of the progeny of an infected vector inherit the agent.

The saliva that hematophagous arthropods inject into their host's skin alters the feeding site in a manner that may enhance the site's receptivity to the delivery of pathogens [31]. This dimension of vector competence was recognized during the 1980s with the discovery that saliva contains antihemostatic and immunosuppressive components. Apyrase activity, which appears to be universal in hematophagous arthropods, prevents platelet aggregation. Such components as prostaglandin E_2 and others having anticomplement and antianaphylatoxin activities convey particular properties that may facilitate transmission. Indeed, the salivary product of a vector sand fly enhances leishmanial infection under experimental conditions [32]. These anti-inflammatory properties of saliva illustrate the extraordinary example of adaptation of vector and host.

VECTOR-HOST RELATIONSHIPS

The term *vector* applies to hematophagous arthropods that actively carry pathogens to reservoir hosts. The host-seeking behavior of these organisms provides ''direction'' to transmission. In contrast, nonhematophagous carriers of infection lack direction because they must be ingested in the course of the reservoir host's own feeding activities. As in mathematics, *scalar* seems appropriate to describe the passive counterpart of *vector*. Scalar arthropods, without direction, carry a quantity of infection that vertebrate hosts accidentally ingest. Hematophagous directionality greatly enhances communicability; the *basic reproduction rate* of a vector-borne pathogen generally exceeds that of other pathogens. Each primary vector-borne infection may be communicated to hundreds of secondary infections.

Vectorial capacity represents an entomological restatement of the basic reproduction rate of a vector-borne pathogen, synthesizing all variables that affect communicability. Pathogens must mature rapidly and abundantly in the vector, and must be delivered to a suitable host. The relevant variables generally are considered to include effective density relative to the reservoir host, frequency of feeding, and longevity of the vector.

In the 1950s, Macdonald [33] developed a predictive model for malaria incidence. This work stimulated field studies that eventually proved the concept's usefulness and practicality. Macdonald's model constitutes an important basis for epidemiological entomology. The model calculates the number of secondary cases that a certain vector population will generate from a single case originally introduced into a region. This convention represents the basic reproduction rate. If the equation is simplified to consider the number of potentially infective bites, only entomological parameters need be considered, greatly simplifying field work. This simplified equation is now termed *vectorial capacity*. Although basic reproduction rate has proved difficult to evaluate because of human variables [34], vectorial capacity is somewhat more amenable to study.

Vectorial capacity may be expressed as follows: an infective human host entering an endemic focus will be exposed to some measurable number of vectors m per day, an anthropophagic proportion that will deliver a number a of bites per day. (The product ma represents the human-biting rate.) A proportion p of these blood-fed vectors survives each day. Because none is infective before the parasite reaches the ducts of the salivary glands (in the case of malaria), they must survive this period of time (the extrinsic incubation period), which lasts n days. Thus, a proportion p^n remains alive after this period. These surviving and infected vectors then have a life expectancy of $-1/(\ln P)$, during which time a proportion a will bite human hosts each day. The product represents vectorial capacity (VC):

$$\text{VC} = \frac{ma^2p^n}{-\ln p}$$

Vectorial capacity would express basic reproduction rates if vector competence were perfect. Every vector biting an infective human host would become infected, and every infective bite would infect the host. Of course, this assumption is oversimplified.

Entomological inoculation rates measure potential incidence as the product of effective vector density ma and infection rate s (or sporozoite rate in the case of malaria). Such rates always exceed the *parasitological inoculation rates,* an estimate of actual incidence corresponding to prevalence of infection in infants that are 1 year old. Local discrepancies between these

rates (generally expressed as b) have been estimated [44], but their causes remain unexplained.

These considerations permit ranking of the various components of vectorial capacity in a hierarchy important to epidemiological studies and interventions. Most powerful in non-inherited anthroponoses are the vector's life expectancy p, which contributes exponentially; narrowness of host range a and frequency of feeding, which contribute as the square; and vector abundance m and vector competence, which provide linear contributions. When transmission is stably inherited, narrowness of host range and abundance both contribute linearly.

An important paradox is inherent in transmission of zoonotic disease. Narrowness of host range is essential for maintaining the enzootic cycle; transmission of zoonotic pathogens to human hosts is extraneous to that cycle, thereby resulting in some reduced vectorial capacity. An epidemic "bridge" must permit transmission to human hosts; but it must be narrow enough to maintain the basic reproduction rate of the pathogen. The challenge of zoonosis research is thus to explain how the bridge is directed toward human hosts.

Two principal zoonotic patterns characterize the epidemic bridge: (1) one derives from "overflow" due to episodic events; (2) the other from paucity of alternative hosts. As an example of the first, eastern equine encephalitis (EEE) perpetuation depends upon *Culiseta melanura*, a mosquito specifically adapted to wetland birds. Mammals rarely are bitten [35]. Episodes of human disease occur when other mosquitos, of lesser vectorial capacity, enter the cycle in large numbers. Their presence seems irrelevant to the enzootic cycle in nature. An example of the second is Lyme disease and human babesiosis in island situations, where the vector tick (*Ixodes dammini*) tends to be non-host-specific [36]. The scarcity of alternative, noncompetent hosts focuses vector activity on the rodent reservoir, preserving vectorial capacity. Human infection follows intrusion into such zoologically restricted regions. This condition characterizes islands, deserts, or environments disturbed by human activity.

Because programs intended to limit outbreaks of disease are "reactive," they must respond to the results of epidemiological surveillance. Two kinds of *transmission indexes* have been used for this purpose: (1) purely entomological estimates that reflect vector abundance and (2) estimates based on microbiological factors. These useful measures are derived empirically on the basis of local experience and are intended to predict outbreaks of human disease.

Entomological transmission indexes employ insect-trapping devices, human-biting rates, spray knockdown catches, collections of larvae, etc., in the case of malaria. In one location in Kenya, for example, the resting density critical to malaria transmission lay between 0.14 and 1.2 anophelines per house. Various indexes have been derived for *A. aegypti*–borne disease, based variously on egg-collection traps, on proportion of houses infested, or on proportion of infested containers per house. One *Xenopsylla cheopis* per rat is said to represent a critical transmission index for plague.

Recently, immunological [37] and molecular biological techniques have been applied to determine entomological inoculation rates. Pathogen-specific DNA diagnostic probes have been used to assay the frequency of *Leishmania* parasites in sand flies [38]. At present, these techniques fail to distinguish between infective and noninfective parasites.

Microbiological transmission indexes are used for evaluating onchocerciasis and filariasis suppression programs. An "annual transmission potential" is calculated. This represents the number of infective-stage filarial larvae per person per year, and is calculated from an estimate of the number of vectors biting each person per year multiplied by wormload per fly. Between 1200 and 2000 larval *O. volvulus* per person per year seems to represent the threshold for 70 percent prevalence of infection in human hosts [39]. Lacking is a threshold estimate that might serve as a baseline indicator of human disease. Similar estimates are available for lymphatic filariasis; a transmission potential of 10,000 larvae per person per year may serve as the threshold-sustaining transmission rate in Rangoon [40]. Informal indexes to predict outbreaks of encephalitis have been based on discovery of virus in pooled mosquitoes or of virus or antibody in birds.

HOST-PATHOGEN RELATIONSHIPS

Antivector interventions distinguish between infection and disease. The concept that parasitic infection need not result in disease grew from the early studies of hookworm infection. A balanced diet compensates for the loss of blood resulting from the presence of a few worms, and immunity reduces both worm burden and loss of blood due to each worm. Indeed, chronically infected hosts adapt to their condition by enhanced erythropoiesis. This nonequivalence of infection and disease characterizes parasites in general, particularly those vector-borne agents possessing a repertoire of adaptive strategies for evading the host's immune response [41].

Vector-transmitted filarial infection commonly is asymptomatic, even when microfilaremia is patent [42]. Presumably, immune status of the host determines severity of disease, but the mechanisms remain elusive. The "paradox of the heavy exposure to infective mosquito bites coupled with a lack of severe (filarial) disease" [42] occurs locally.

Death attributed to malaria is associated with epidemics rather than with situations in which transmission is constant. The Ceylon experience of the 1930s, the World War II experience in Italy, and the events following introduction of *An. gambiae* into Brazil and Egypt exemplify the catastrophic conditions that accompany such epidemics. In contrast, malaria-related mortality under highly endemic conditions mainly occurs in a narrow age cohort of the human population. In Kisumu in Kenya, this "window of mortality" spanned the fourth to eighth months of life (Fig. 20-1) [43]. Maternal antibody

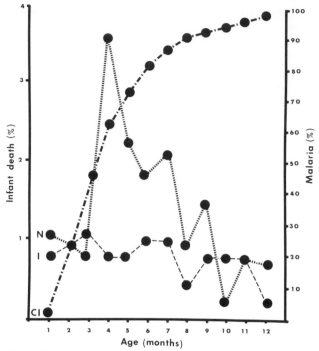

Figure 20-1. Cumulative incidence (CI) of malaria in a region in Kenya sprayed with fenitrothion. Age-specific infant mortality rates in this intervention region (I) are compared with those in a nearby nonintervention region (N). *(Compiled from Tables 2 and 6 in D. Payne, B. Grab, and R.E. Fontaine, Bull WHO 54:369–377, 1976.)*

protects during the first 3 months of life, and infection becomes universal by the ninth month. About half of the infants initially became infected while protected by maternal antibody. After indoor residual spraying of fenitrothion, transmission was reduced to the extent that only 14 percent of children became infected within the first year of life. The "severe complications of malaria may become more common among older African children in the future, as they acquire infection at older ages and with little or no prior exposure" [44]. By reducing malaria incidence, the Kisumu spray interventions may have "widened the window of mortality," but the availability of antimalarial drugs would have masked this potential enhancement of disease. Perhaps the presently increasing drug resistance in Africa renders this protection temporary. In regions in which prevalence of malaria is less (i.e., about 50 percent in a village in El Salvador), infants seem to lack maternal protection, and insecticidal intervention may be less destabilizing. "Interrupted transmission and low endemicity lead to the production of an unstable immunity that in turn inclines to the precipitation of periodic epidemics. Steady transmission, not materially changing from year to year, leads on the other hand to the production of a firm immunity that protects the community against outbreaks of disease" [45].

MANAGEMENT OF ARTHROPOD-BORNE DISEASE

Ultimately, disease control programs seek to reduce the burden of ill health borne by defined human populations. Prompt, total, and permanent elimination of certain pathogens represents the highest ideal of the goal, and smallpox eradication represents the one great success of this kind. Five features of smallpox rendered it uniquely vulnerable to eradication: easily recognized cases, absence of nonhuman reservoir hosts, a long incubation period, absence of subclinical cases in nonvaccinated persons, and availability of a vaccine effectively preventing disease even after initial infection. Case finding was facilitated because infection was always patent, producing characteristic skin lesions. Epidemiological intelligence based upon such clinical diagnosis guided vaccination of all possible contacts and eventual eradication worldwide. None of the vector-borne pathogens express these vulnerabilities. In particular, malaria frequently produces subclinical infection and may be difficult to treat. Fortunately, the importance of vector longevity and the effectiveness of DDT provided another kind of vulnerability that was exploited in the recently attempted massive campaigns in the Americas and in Asia. Certain of these time-limited campaigns have attained their goals, particularly on such islands as Jamaica, Taiwan, Mauritius, and Sardinia. But, on larger landmasses, malaria eradication failed. Efforts to limit transmission continue, but a philosophy of "control" has replaced that of eradication, at least for the immediate future. Focusing on a longer period of time, "the member governments of the Pan American Health Organization (PAHO) have reaffirmed that malaria eradication is the ultimate goal of the malaria program in the Americas and that any control activities represent an intermediate stage toward that goal" [46]. In addition, the organization retains the goal of "eradication of the vector of urban yellow fever" (*Aëdes aegypti*).

The history of antimalaria activities in Sri Lanka illustrates the recent evolution of "intensified" programs designed to reduce the burden of vector-borne disease. Numerous malaria outbreaks have been recorded since 1858 when systematic records were first maintained, but the first large-scale control effort responded to the disastrous episode of 1934 to 1935. As a consequence, larvicidal oils were applied to riverbeds, and about 13 million treatment days of quinine were administered to fever patients. DDT was first applied in residential residual treatments in 1945 and continued until 1954 when malaria appeared to have disappeared as a public health problem. But the disease subsequently returned, and spraying was resumed in 1957. Eradication was adopted as a formal goal in 1958 and was attained for a few months in 1963, but DDT spraying was resumed because local outbreaks continued. The endemic region remained in a prolonged "modified attack" phase of eradication. This continued until 1967, when a major outbreak of *P. vivax* infection began. DDT resistance had emerged in *An. culicifacies,* the presumed vector. In 1968, a WHO-sponsored

evaluation recommended that the region revert to an "intensified attack phase of eradication," and the consumption of DDT increased threefold. In spite of this effort, prevalence of *P. vivax* continued to increase through 1970 and that of *P. falciparum* began to rise. Another review, conducted in 1972, recognized the presence of DDT resistance but concluded that failure of eradication was due to incomplete spray coverage. Accordingly, DDT spraying was reintensified, including experimental use of malathion in certain limited foci. Another *P. vivax* outbreak ensued (1973–1976), and *P. falciparum* continued its gradual emergence. Evidence of operational ineffectiveness of DDT had become incontrovertible, causing the program to shift to malathion. By this time, the goal of eradication was abandoned, and an "intensive malaria control program" was implemented in May 1977. This formal control program aimed to eradicate *P. falciparum* and reduce the prevalence of *P. vivax* to a low, sustainable level in 1981 (1 case per 10,000 population). All houses in endemic regions would be sprayed with malathion four times each year. A schedule of spraying was anticipated. Each year thereafter, the 12 million residents of the endemic region were protected by about 4.2 million pounds of malathion and 20 million antimalaria tablets. Unfortunately, this profligate drug distribution appears to have destroyed surveillance. The number of patients reporting to "passive case detection indicator institutions" declined. In 1978, the antimalaria budget required about $14 million per year, consuming 21 percent of the Sri Lankan budget for health care. Health care expenses consumed about 5 percent of the national budget, with about 30 percent of the budget for malaria deriving from national funds. By the mid-1980s, malathion had lost much of its effectiveness against the vector [47], and chloroquine resistance had become common in *P. falciparum*. Prevalence of infection abruptly rose once again, and the direction of this antimalaria effort became uncertain. Although temporary successes were registered, this intensified effort could not successfully be deintensified.

The philosophy of encephalitis control in the state of Massachusetts represents a different approach toward disease control. Only 57 cases of human eastern equine encephalitis (EEE) have been recorded, but the disease is so severe that local residents demand protection from outbreaks. Human infections occur sporadically: 34 in 1938, 4 in 1955, 12 in 1956, 1 in 1970, 2 in 1973, 3 in 1974, and 1 in 1975. Sporadic cases have continued to occur during the decade of the 1980s. The region experienced extended silent periods in which no virus was isolated even from birds or mosquitoes. Following the 1956 episode, a surveillance station was staffed in the most affected part of the region and an action doctrine was proposed as follows: When a human infection is detected, surveillance for EEE activity is to be intensified and antimosquito measures prepared. Efforts to reduce abundance of vector mosquitoes are to follow confirmation of a second human case. This doctrine remained untested until 1973, when the surveillance network detected an intense, developing epizootic [48]. EEE virus was isolated repeatedly from mosquitoes, birds, and horses. Aerial ultra-low-volume (ULV) spraying recently had become available and provided a highly effective means for destroying adult mosquitoes. The authorities decided to preempt any impending human outbreak and ordered ULV spraying for the eastern third of the state. Only two human cases were recorded, and these patients were infected just before the region around their homes was treated. From this experience, new action guidelines were established based mainly on entomological surveillance. Aerial ULV spraying would be applied to regions 8 km in diameter. However, this program was thrown into disarray the following summer when three fatal human infections were confirmed. The entomological indicators had failed to register warning. The state then returned to its original pre-1973 doctrine and ordered local ULV spraying about 2 weeks after the third patient died, more than a month after the first death. In 1975, one human fatality occurred early in the transmission season (mid-July), prompting the authorities to prepare for a spray campaign. No further human infections were recognized that year, but entomological indicators began to rise during August. Regional ULV applications then were ordered to prevent the outbreak of human infection that seemed imminent. This reactive effort aiming to contain outbreaks can be sustained indefinitely.

Intensified antimalaria control campaigns, as practiced in Sri Lanka, seek to reduce prevalence of infection. Such preemptive efforts to suppress transmission are seen as a step toward eradication. Spray operations are conducted according to prearranged plan. Some prescribed number of nearly complete (at least 80 percent of houses) spray rounds is scheduled, and the work is carried out until the end of the planned campaign. The numer of spray rounds may be adjusted, within limits. That is, "problem" villages generally receive more frequent insecticide coverage than do others, a procedure that tends to increase development of insecticide resistance. *Intensified* is a well-defined term, implying a need for external resources. A national intensified-control program requires sponsorship by another country or external agency.

Eradication doctrine demands operational perfection because success depends upon elimination of the last indigenous infection. In the case of malaria, the strategy requires that all local residences be treated with insecticide. Failure to reduce malaria prevalence implies incomplete coverage, a lapse that must be corrected promptly in order to forestall insecticide resistance in the vector. In contrast, *intensified-control doctrine* permits *slippage* because a certain specified level of transmission is tolerable (by definition). In the Sri Lankan intensified-control program, 80 percent spray coverage and 80 percent effectiveness of the spray against the target vector is considered satisfactory.

In place of perfection, intensified-control programs may seek to apply combinations of techniques. The Sri Lankan campaign distributes antimalaria tablets, attempts to flush puddled streambeds, and experiments with biological control in addition to household spraying. Instead, "integration" of diverse techniques replaced "perfection" of application.

The agricultural concept of *integrated pest management* (IPM) has been borrowed by public health entomologists. The damage produced by agricultural pests generally is proportional to the abundance of the pest, so control efforts mainly attempt to reduce pest populations. Similarly, mosquito abatement operations seek to reduce pest numbers. Source reduction, generally directed against larvae, is most cost-effective. An IPM program directed against pest mosquitoes might employ larvivorous fish, improved drainage, and larvicidal applications as well as aerosol applications of adulticide. The results are additive, each incrementally reducing the risk of mosquito bite, a goal consistent with pest reduction but questionable if the goal is to prevent human disease.

In contrast to pest control, the objective of vector control is to reduce vectorial capacity, a model in which vector abundance is a linear function only. Narrowness of host range contributes as the square, and longevity contributes exponentially. In the case of malaria, residential residual spraying may affect all these functions. Adult mosquitoes face increased daily mortality, and those that feed on human hosts are more at risk than are those that feed on other animals. Reduced abundance depends upon the feeding and resting habits of the particular mosquito in question and on its ability to increase. Conceivably, transmission could be broken, but without apparent effect upon vector abundance if the vector population were highly reproductive and short-lived. Other scenarios could be constructed. Aerial ULV spraying destroys those mosquitoes (or other vectors) that are adult at the time of treatment. The effect upon abundance can be transitory when the environment produces great numbers of mosquitoes. However, for a week or more, mosquitoes that are old enough to transmit infection would be scarce or absent.

Source reduction, as by larvicide, effectively reduces the abundance of biting mosquitoes, but the effect upon disease transmission can be complex. For example, local residents might seek protection from a vector when biting mosquitoes are abundant. Thus, mosquito control might paradoxically promote transmission if larvicides were directed against nonvector species. Furthermore, measures that reduce vector abundance might actually increase vectorial capacity. Crowded larvae give rise to small adults with impaired hormonal function; frequency of blood-feeding and longevity may be affected. At least in the case of container-breeding species, availability of food seems to limit this aspect of adult quality. As a result, incomplete or short-lived larvicidal operations as well as introduction of predators or parasites might increase vectorial capacity of the target population. It follows that biological control efforts directed against larvae, under certain circumstances, might serve to increase transmission. Conversely, residual insecticides applied to the resting places of adult vector insects might destroy natural predators or parasites of the adult stage, and this too would increase transmission. Attempts to reduce transmission by destroying vectors require well-defined objectives.

Zooprophylaxis [49], which implies diversion of zoophilic vectors to nonhuman hosts, affects the "host-range" component of vectorial capacity. The resurgence of malaria in Guyana following displacement of draft animals by motor vehicles demonstrated the power of this subtle environmental factor [50]. The ratio of competent to noncompetent hosts seems to be a critical determinant of transmission. Specific vectors are diverted by specific noncompetent or nonhuman hosts [49]. However, host abundance can affect transmission in a complex manner, particularly in the case of zoonoses. For example, intensity of transmission of *Babesia microti* seems to vary inversely with the abundance of the main reservoir host. This would result if vector abundance were independent of that of the main reservoir for the parasite. Thus, host contact would increase as host abundance decreased. Efforts to reduce transmission by destroying the reservoir host would be counterproductive. Repellents, use of bednets, etc., affect host contact, but those techniques seem applicable mainly for protecting individuals or groups of travellers. In fact, such measures for personal protection of an indigenous population can increase vectorial capacity by concentrating the vector population on a smaller set of people. Nonprotected people might suffer an increased number of infectious inocula.

Environmental management aims to alter particular conditions that promote the abundance of vectors. These measures include water-level fluctuation to strand larval *Anopheles* [51], installation of tide gates to reduce brackish-water breeding [52], or drainage to eliminate standing water altogether [53]. The objective is to neutralize the basic conditions that originally promoted transmission. Generally, these measures seek to stabilize aquatic conditions.

Ill-planned attempts to destroy aquatic larvae may actually destabilize bodies of water. For example, oiling of a pond effectively destroys larval mosquitoes as well as many of the insects that feed on mosquitoes. Eventually, the oil disappears, leaving transient conditions that may encourage extraordinary abundance of the target population. Chemical larvicides rarely are used in vector control because of (1) this destabilizing effect, (2) increased risk of insecticide resistance, and (3) minimal impact on vectorial capacity. Because human disturbance of the environment often is the root cause of unacceptable patterns of tropical disease, measures directed at these specific conditions would provide long-term corrections and control.

The pressing challenge is to devise rational reactive progams that stabilize transmission yet preserve the usefulness of insecticide. For example, two epidemiological indicators seem promising as signals for application of indoor residual insecticide for malaria control. Locally increased consumption of antimalaria drugs would provide one such signal. In this conservative program, baseline drug consumption for villages would be reported periodically, perhaps weekly, and spray rounds would be ordered if cerain experiential baselines were exceeded. Insecticide use would result in reduced drug use. The other indicator might exploit "malaria-contributed mortality." The total number of deaths would be recorded as a denominator, and the presence of blood-borne parasites would be determined. Spray rounds would be signaled by a rise in the incidence of local residents dying while parasitemic, whatever the attributed cause of death. By inference, these measures might serve to indicate malaria's contribution to morbidity and mortality rates. Evaluation of such a program would be facilitated because denominators might readily be derived and because "active" and "passive" case detection would not be confused. Thus, future efforts could be justified and chemical assets conserved.

In public health, entomological intervention seeks to manage transmission of infection in order to reduce the burden of disease borne by indigenous human populations. Suppression efforts may raise epidemic conditions where infection might otherwise be nonpathogenic. In contrast, containment efforts that aim to prevent or terminate episodes of increased infection would reduce disease.

CONCLUSIONS

Certain principles derive from this discussion of the role of vectors in transmitting tropical diseases:

1. Tropical diseases generally are vector-borne, and most are transmitted by arthropods that exploit disturbed environments, particularly disturbances caused by human activity. In this manner, economic development in the tropics creates special potential for ill health.
2. The burden of tropical disease is greatest during episodes of increasing prevalence of a pathogen, and such "epidemics" result from increased abundance either of vectors or of nonimmune hosts.
3. Each kind of vector exploits its own characteristic environmental niche. Broadly distributed species tend to be complexes of reproductively isolated populations that may differ in vectorial capacity.
4. The competence of arthropods as vectors for pathogens may be influenced by factors affecting uptake, development, and quantity of infectious pathogens delivered to the reservoir host, as well as receptivity of their site of placement. In the case of stably inherited infection, uptake is eliminated as a component of vector competence. Output is eliminated in the event that the pathogen-infected arthropod (scalar) is ingested passively by the vertebrate host. Intensity of disease in the human host relates, in part, to pathogen output from the vector.
5. The capacity of an arthropod to transmit an anthroponosis depends upon its vector competence (a linear function), abundance (contributing linearly), narrowness of host range

(contributing as the square), frequency of feeding (contributing as the square), and longevity (an exponential function). In the event that the pathogen is inherited in a stable fashion by the vector, transmission depends upon vector competence, abundance, and narrowness of host range, each contributing linearly. Sustained transmission of zoonotic disease requires that vectorial capacity (operating between the vector and natural reservoir hosts) is disturbed minimally by loss of pathogens to human or other nonreservoir hosts. Such a bridge to human hosts is possible if paucity of alternative hosts maximizes contact with human hosts or when episodic abundance of vectors causes overflow of the pathogen into an epidemic cycle.

6. Efforts seeking to limit transmission aim to reduce particular components of vectorial capacity. Abundance may be reduced by habitat destruction, by host removal, or by insecticide or biological agents applied against immature stages of the target population. Host range is affected by increasing abundance of particular diversionary hosts. Longevity is reduced by attacks on the adult stage, using insecticide either in a residual formulation or as a space spray. Transmission may be enhanced if efforts directed against larvae reduce competition. Reducing abundance of reservoir hosts or using repellants may increase vector abundance relative to the remaining hosts and increase transmission.

7. Insecticide resistance in a vector population intensifies due to destruction of the vector by a chemical. Agricultural use of the chemical enhances resistance only if the vector's breeding or resting habits expose it to lethal amounts of chemical.

8. Disease prevention programs seek either to contain or to suppress transmission. Containment programs aim to prevent or terminate epidemics, responding to epidemiological indicators (transmission indexes or manifestations of disease) and operate without limit of time. Suppression programs generally operate according to some predetermined schedule of action, seeking an irreversible goal within a finite period of time. Suppression programs are more costly and are more conducive to innsecticide resistance. In the event of failure, suppression programs promote epidemics because nonimmune human hosts may have become more abundant than they were prior to the program and chemical assets may have been lost.

9. A program aiming to prevent vector-borne disease should seek first to prevent or reduce epidemics. Within that constraint, the goals must be worthwhile and attainable, producing results that are subject to evaluation.

REFERENCES

1 Busvine JR: *Insects and Hygiene,* 3d ed. London, New York, Chapman and Hall, 1980

2 Harwood RF, James MT: *Entomology in Human and Animal Health,* 7th ed. New York, Macmillan, 1979

3 Smith KGV (ed): *Insects and Other Arthropods of Medical Importance.* London, British Museum (Natural History), 1973

4 Georghiou GP: Studies on resistance to carbamate and organophosphorus insecticides in *Anopheles albimanus.* Am J Trop Med Hyg 21:797–806, 1972

5 Vajime CG, Dunbar RW: Chromosomal identification of eight species of the subgenus *Edwardsellum* near and including *Simulium (Edwardsellum) damnosum* Theobold (Diptera: Simuliidae). Tropenmed Parasitol 26:111–138, 1975

6 Meredith SEO, Townson H: Enzymes for species identification in the *Simulium damnosum* complex from West Africa. Tropenmed Parasitol 32:123–129, 1981

7 Coluzzi M, Sabatini A: Cytogenetic observations in species A and B of the *Anopheles gambiae* complex. Parassitologia 9:73–88, 1967

8 Mahon RJ, Green CA, Hunt RH: Diagnostic allozymes for routine identification of adults of the *Anopheles gambiae* complex (Diptera, Culicidae). Bull Ent Res 66:25–31, 1976

9 Carlson DA, Service MW: Identification of mosquitoes of *Anopheles gambiae* species complex A and B by analysis of cuticular components. Science 207:1089–1090, 1980

10 Gale KR, Crampton JM: Use of a male specific DNA probe to distinguish female mosquitoes of the *Anopheles gambiae* species complex. Med Vet Entomol 2:77–79, 1988

11 Panyim S, Yasothornsrikul S, Tungpradubkul S, et al: Identification of isomorphic malaria vectors using a DNA probe. Am J Trop Med Hyg 38:47–49, 1988

12 Obiamiwe BA: Relationship between microfilarial density, the number of microfilariae ingested by mosquitoes, and the proportion of mosquitoes with larvae. Ann Trop Med Parasitol 71:491–500, 1977

13 Luedke AJ, Jones RH, Walton TE: Overwintering mechanisms for bluetongue virus: Biological recovery of latent virus from a bovine by bites of *Culicoides variipennis.* Am J Trop Med Hyg 26:313–325, 1977

14 McGreevy PB, Bryan JH, Oothuman P, et al: The lethal effects of the labial and pharyngeal armature of mosquitoes on microfilariae. Trans R Soc Trop Med Hyg 72:361–368, 1978

15 Sundin DR, Beaty BJ, Nathanson N, et al: A G1 glycoprotein epitope of La Crosse virus: A determinant of infection of *Aëdes triseriatus.* Science 235:591–593, 1987

16 Duke BOL, Lewis DJ: Studies on factors influencing the transmission of onchocerciasis. III. Observations on the effect of the peritrophic membrane in limiting the development of *Onchocerca volvulus* microfilariae in *Simulium damnosum.* Am Trop Med Parasitol 58:83–88, 1964

17 Yorke W, Murgatroyd F, Hawking F: The relation of polymorphic trypanosomes, developing in the gut of *Glossina,* to the peritrophic membrane. Ann Trop Med Parasitol 27:347–354, 1933

18 Rudzinska MA, Spielman A, Lewengrub S, et al: Penetration of the peritrophic membrane of the tick by *Babesia microti.* Cell Tissue Res 221:471–481, 1982

19 Kramer LD, Hardy JL, Presser SB, et al: Dissemination barriers for western equine encephalomyelitis virus in *Culex tarsalis* infected after ingestion of low viral doses. Am J Trop Med Hyg 30:190–197, 1981

20 Schrater AF, Rossignol PA, Hamill B, et al: *Brugia malayi* microfilariae from the peritoneal cavity of birds vary in their ability to penetrate the mosquito midgut. Am J Trop Med Hyg 31:292–296, 1982

21 Mellor PS, Boorman J: Multiplication of bluetongue virus in *Culicoides nubeculosus* (Meigen) simultaneously infected with the virus and the microfilariae of *Onchocerca cervicalis* (Railliet and Henry). Ann Trop Med Parasitol 75:463–469, 1980

22 Turell MJ, Mather TN, Spielman A, et al: Increased dissemination of dengue 2 virus in *Aëdes aegypti* associated with concurrent ingestion of microfilariae of *Brugia mayali*. Am J Trop Med Hyg 37:197–201, 1987

23 Christensen BM, Sutherland DR: Defense reactions of mosquitoes to filarial worms: Comparative studies on the response of three different mosquitoes to inoculated *Brugia pahangi* and *Dirofilaria immitis* microfilariae. J Invert Pathol 44:267–274, 1984

24 Boman HG, Hultmark D: Cell-free immunity in insects. Ann Rev Microbiol 41:103–126, 1987

25 Rosenberg R: Inability of *Plosmadium knowlesi* sporozoites to invade *Anopheles freeborni* salivary glands. Am J Trop Med Hyg 34:687–691, 1985

26 Rossignol PA, Ribeiro JMC, Spielman A: Increased biting rate and reduced fertility in sporozoite-infected mosquitoes. Am J Trop Med Hyg 33:17–20, 1986

27 Tesh RB, Shroyer DA: The mechanism of arbovirus transovarial transmission in mosquitoes: San Angelo virus in *Aëdes albopictus*. Am J Trop Med Hyg 29:1394–1404, 1980

28 Turrell MJ, Hardy JL, Reeves WC: Stabilization of California encephalitis virus in *Aëdes dorsalis* and its implications for viral maintenance in nature. Am J Trop Med Hyg 31:1252–1259, 1982

29 Bailey CL, Eldridge BF, Hayes DE, et al: Isolation of St. Louis encephalitis virus from overwintering *Culex pipiens* mosquitoes. Science 199:1346–1349, 1978

30 Rosen L, Tesh RB, Lien JC, et al: Transovarial transmission of Japanese encephalitis virus by mosquitoes. Science 199:909–911, 1978

31 Ribeiro JMC: Role of saliva in blood-feeding by arthropods. Ann Rev Entomol 32:463–478, 1987

32 Titus RG, Ribeiro JMC: Salivary gland lysates from the sandfly *Lutzomyia longipalpes* enhance *Leishmania* infectivity. Science 239:1306–1308, 1988

33 Macdonald G: The analysis of equilibrium in malaria. Trop Dis Bull 49:813–828, 1952

34 Garrett-Jones C: The human blood index of malaria vectors in relation to epidemiological assessment. Bull WHO 30:241–261, 1964

35 Magnarelli L: Host feeding patterns of Connecticut mosquitoes (Diptera: Culicidae). Am J Trop Med Hyg 26:547–552, 1977

36 Spielman A, Etkind P, Piesman J, et al: Reservoir hosts of human babesiosis on Nantucket Island. Am J Trop Med Hyg 30:560–565, 1981

37 Collins FH, Procell PM, Campbell GH, et al: Monoclonal antibody-based enzyme-linked immunosorbent assay (ELISA) for detection of *Plasmodium malariae* sporozoites in mosquitoes. Am J Trop Med Hyg 38:283–288, 1988

38 Rogers WO, Burnheim PF, Wirth D: Detection of Leishmania within sandflies by kinetoplast DNA hybridization. Am J Trop Med Hyg, in press

39 Thylefors B, Philippon B, Prost A: Transmission potentials of *Onchocerca volvulus* and the associated intensity of onchocerciasis in a Sudan-Savanna area. Tropenmed Parasitol 29:346–354, 1978

40 Hairston NG, De Meillon B: On the inefficiency of transmission of *Wuchereria bancrofti* from mosquito to human host. Bull WHO 38:935–941, 1968

41 Bloom BR: Games parasites play: How parasites evade immune surveillance. Nature 279:21–26, 1979

42 Piessens WF, McGreevy PB, Ratiwayanto S, et al: Immune responses in human infections with *Brugia malayi*: Correlation of cellular and humoral reactions to microfilarial antigens with clinical status. Am J Trop Med Hyg 29:563–570, 1980

43 Payne D, Grab B, Fontaine RE, et al: Impact of control measures of malaria transmission and general mortality. Bull WHO 54:369–377, 1976

44 Molineaux L, Gramiccia G: *The Garki Project*. Geneva, WHO, 1980

45 Macdonald G: *The Epidemiology and Control of Malaria*. London, New York, Oxford University Press, 1957

46 Health for All by the Year 2000: Plan of Action for the Implementation of Regional Strategies. Washington, DC, Pan American Health Organization, official document no 179, 1982

47 Herath PRJ, Hemingway J, Weerasinghe IS, et al: The detection and characterization of malathion resistance in field populations of *Anopheles culcifiacies* B in Sri Lanka. Pestic Biochem Physiol 29:157–162, 1987

48 Grady GF, Maxfield HK, Hildreth SW, et al: Eastern equine encephalitis in Massachusetts, 1957–1976: A prospective study centered upon analysis of mosquitoes. Am J Epidemiol 107:170–178, 1978

49 Hess AD, Hayes RO: Relative potentials of domestic animals for zooprophylaxis against mosquito vectors of encephalitis. Am J Trop Med Hyg 19:327–333, 1970

50 Giglioli G: Ecological change as a factor in renewed malaria transmission in an eradicated area. Bull WHO 29:131–145, 1963

51 Darrow EM: Factors in the elimination of the immature stages of *Anopheles quadrimaculatus* Say in a water level fluctuation cycle. Am J Hyg 50:207–235, 1949

52 Hackett LW: *Malaria in Europe*. London, Oxford University Press, 1937

53 Carmichael GJ: Anopheline control through water management. Am J Trop Med Hyg 21:281–286, 1972

Snail Intermediate Hosts

· Edward H. Michelson

The Mollusca constitute one of the major divisions of the animal kingdom and are of unusual interest in regard to both diversity of organization and the multitude of species. Although the basic organization of the Mollusca is relatively simple, diversification and adaptive radiation of the basic theme make an all-inclusive definition difficult. The Mollusca may be considered, however, as tripoblastic, coelomic, (generally) nonsegmented invertebrates which possess a shell or rudiments of a shell during some period of their life. They occur in the marine, aquatic, and terrestrial biotopes—ranging from the poles to the tropics and from the depths of the oceans to altitudes exceeding 14,000 feet. In size, they range from minute snails (< 1 mm) to gigantic squids (> 15 m). Conservatively, there are approximately 50,000 described species, of which 75 percent are gastropods (snails and slugs). There are six classes of mollusks: Monoplacophora, Amphineura, Scaphopoda, Gastropoda, Bivalvia, and Cephalopoda. The Gastropoda and Bivalvia are of primary medical importance, the Cephalopoda of rare concern, and the remainder are entirely marine and of little medical significance. Two of the several subclasses of the Gastropoda, the Prosobranchia and the Pulmonata, contain the majority of the medically important species. The Prosobranchia have gills, an operculum which closes the shell, a single pair of tentacles, and are dioecious. They are principally marine in habit; however, it is the aquatic forms that are of medical interest. The Pulmonata respire by means of a "lung" or respiratory sac, have either one or two pairs of tentacles, are monoecious, and are primarily terrestrial (order Stylommatophora) or aquatic (order Basommatophora). Most of the medically important species belong to the Basommatophora and, in particular, to the families Planorbidae and Lymnaeidae.

ASSOCIATION OF HUMANS AND MOLLUSKS

Shell middens and archaeological sites attest that humans and mollusks have been intimately associated since prehistoric time. Over the centuries, the mollusk has not only provided humans with a source of food but has also served as a model and inspiration for architecture, literature, and personal ornamentation. In addition, mollusks have served as religious objects, currency, and as curative agents for a variety of afflictions. Pliny the Elder prescribed the use of slugs and snails for the relief of stomach and headaches and as cures for "ague, corns, web in the eye, scorbutic affections, hectic fevers, pleurisy, asthma, obstruction, dropsy, swelling joints" and other conditions. Likewise, the ingestion of raw slugs and snails was practiced in parts of England until the late 1800s as a cure for consumption, and the practice continues today in some parts of the world for a variety of conditions.

MOLLUSKS AND DISEASE TRANSMISSION

It is difficult to ascertain when mollusks were first associated with the transmission of disease. The biblical admonition against the use of shellfish as food provides no specific evidence that the prohibition was for reasons of health. However, as early as 1793, there were published accounts associating the ingestion of shellfish with the syndrome of mussel toxemia. Although several earlier investigators had suggested that fascioliasis and schistosomiasis were snailborne diseases, it remained for Thomas and Leuckart, in 1881, to demonstrate independently the essential role of the snail *Lymnaea truncatula* in the life cycle of *Fasciola hepatica*. Another 32 years elapsed before Miyari and Suzuki demonstrated the transmission of *Schistosoma japonicum* by the snail *Oncomelania nosophora,* a feat which enabled Leiper to identify species of *Biomphalaria* and *Bulinus* as the respective hosts of *S. mansoni* and *S. haematobium.*

Mollusks of medical importance may be categorized as follows: (1) Those which act as passive agents for the dispersal of microbial pathogens and toxins. This category consists mainly of bivalves (clams and oysters), which when eaten may transmit species of *Salmonella, Shigella,* various viruses, and toxins. (2) Those which may actively inject a neurotoxin, as, for example, species of *Conus.* (3) Those which serve as intermediate hosts for helminthic parasites. This latter category is of prime importance since it is now recognized that *all trematode parasites of humans and their domestic animals are required to spend a portion of their life cycle in a suitable molluscan host.* Frequently, this host is a snail and, in the case of most of the trematodes infecting humans, it is aquatic or amphibious. Table 21-1 lists the major parasitic diseases of humans in which a snail host is required.

Table 21-1. Some of the more important snailborne diseases of man and domestic animals

Trematode etiology:	
Schistosomiasis	Fasciolopsiasis
Fascioliasis	Heterophyiasis
Paragonimiasis	Metagonimiasis
Clonorchiasis	Paramphistomiasis
Ophisthorciasis	Dicroceliasis
Nematode etiology:	
Angiostrongyliasis	
Cestode etiology:	
Davainiasis	

SPECIES OF MEDICAL IMPORTANCE

HOSTS OF HUMAN SCHISTOSOMES

The snail species which serve as hosts for *Schistosoma mansoni*, both in Africa and in the western hemisphere, are members of the genus *Biomphalaria* of the family Planorbidae. These species are generally aquatic, have a discoidal shell which in the adult stage measures 7 to 30 mm in diameter, and a hemolymph (blood) characterized by the presence of free hemoglobin.

In the western hemisphere, 20 to 22 species of *Biomphalaria* occur but only three of the species, *B. glabrata*, *B. straminea*, and *B. tenagophila*, have populations which have been found infected in nature. *B. glabrata* has the highest host competency, a wide distribution, and is the most important of the three species with respect to disease transmission. In the Caribbean area, it is found in Haiti, Dominican Republic, Puerto Rico, Vieques, St. Martin, St. Kitts, Antigua, Guadeloupe, Martinique, and St. Lucia. In South America, the species occupies the coastal regions of Venezuela, Surinam, and French Guiana, then extends itself throughout northeastern and southeastern Brazil. *B. straminea* has a wider distribution than *B. glabrata* but is less competent as a host, and natural infections rarely exceed 0.2 percent. Its range extends from the islands of Martinique, Grenada, and Trinidad to Costa Rica and Panama in Central America, and then to Venezuela, Surinam, Guiana, French Guiana, throughout Brazil, and into Paraguay, northern Argentina, and portions of Bolivia and Peru. Except for Brazil, where it is an important host in the northern and northeastern regions, it has not been found infected in any other portion of its range. *B. tenagophila* appears to be restricted to Bolivia and to the southern part of South America and serves as a host only in a limited region of southern Brazil.

Approximately a dozen nominal species of *Biomphalaria*, several with multiple subspecies, have been recognized in Africa. In accordance with the scheme proposed by Mandahl-Barth [1], these species are organized into four species complexes: the *pfeifferi* group, the *alexandrina* group, the *sudanica* group, and the *choanomphala* group. Although most species of African *Biomphalaria* are considered to be susceptible to at least some strains of *S. mansoni*, host competency of the various species and their populations differs. At least one species, *B. arabica*, occurs in the Arabian peninsula and is responsible for oasis transmission.

The snail hosts of *S. haematobium* in Africa and the Middle East are members of the genus *Bulinus* of the family Planorbidae [2]. Approximately 36 species of *Bulinus* are presently recognized in this area, but all are not schistosome hosts. The taxonomy of the genus is complex and the delimitation of species is still in a state of flux. At present, the genus is divided into two subgenera (*Bulinus* and *Physopsis*) which comprise four species complexes—the *forskalii* group, the *truncatus* group, the *tropicus* group, and the *africanus* group. In addition to serving as hosts for *S. haematobium*, several species of *Bulinus* serve as hosts for *S. intercalatum*, *S. bovis*, *S. mattheei*, and several other trematodes.

Species of two additional genera, *Planorbarius* and *Ferrissia*, have also been incriminated as hosts of *S. haematobium* but are of limited importance. *Planorbarius metidjensis* serves as a host in Portugal, but although it occurs in north Africa, it is incapable of transmitting African strains of the parasite. *Ferrissia tenuis*, a member of the family Ancylidae, appears to be the host of a *haematobium*-like parasite in Bombay State, India.

The Asiatic species of schistosomes, *S. japonicum* and *S. mekongi*, utilize species of *Oncomelania* and *Tricula*, respectively, as their intermediate hosts. The genus *Oncomelania*, as presently conceived, consists of two species, one of which is polytypic (*O. hupensis*) and whose subspecies serve as hosts for the various geographical strains of the parasite: *Oncomelania hupensis hupensis* (China), *O. h. nosophora* (Japan), *O. h. formosana* (Taiwan), *O. h. lindoensis* (Indonesia), and *O. h. quadrasi* (Philippines) [3]. The snail hosts responsible for the transmission of the schistosome species found in the Malaysian peninsula have been identified as *Roberstiella kaporensis* and *R. gismanni* [4].

Tricula aperta is the only known snail host of *S. mekongi* [5]. The species appears to be restricted to the Mekong and Mum rivers in Laos and Thailand and has been divided into three "races" based on slight differences in morphology. Although all three "races" can be infected in the laboratory, only the gamma race has been found naturally infected [6].

Species belonging to several freshwater and marine genera serve as host for nonhuman schistosomes which cause the syndrome of schistosomal dermatitis, or "swimmer's itch." Members of the freshwater genera *Lymnaea*, *Physa*, *Bulinus*, *Indoplanorbis*, *Amerianna*, and *Segmentina* serve as hosts for various species of *Trichobilharzia*, *Schistosomatium*, and several dermatitis-inciting cercariae whose adult stages are unknown. The marine genera *Littorina*, *Nassarius*, *Haminoea*, and *Pyrazus* serve as hosts for *Microbilharzia*, *Austrobilharzia*, and numerous dermatitis-producing cercariae.

HOSTS OF FASCIOLA

The snail hosts for the several species of *Fasciola* belong to the molluscan family Lymnaeidae. There is some disagreement as to the taxonomy of the family, since some authorities recognize but a single genus, *Lymnaea*, while others recognize additional genera. Members of the family are aquatic or amphibious in habit, have conical or oblong shells, are distributed worldwide with the greatest concentration of species in the temperate regions. Some of the major hosts are as follows: *Lymnaea truncatula*, in Europe; *L. natalensis*, in Africa; *L. tomentosa*, in Australia; *L. auricularia*, in the Indian subcontinent; *L. cubensis*, in the West Indies and southern United States; *L. bulimoides*, *L. columella*, and *L. modicella*, in North America. Many of these species exhibit strain specificity with respect to their susceptibility and can only be infected with particular geographical strains of the parasite [7].

HOSTS OF PARAGONIMUS

The snail hosts of *Paragonimus westermani*, the principal species which infects humans, belong to genera comprising the prosobranch families Thiaridae (*Thiara, Brotia*) and Pleuroceridae (*Semisulcospira*). The taxonomy of these families and of their genera and species is controversial, and records of species incriminated as hosts are in need of further study. The more important of the host species are *Semisulcospira libertina* in Japan and China and *Brotia asperta* from the Philippines. The identities of the snails responsible for the transmission of the African species *P. africanus* and *P. uterobilateralis* are not know with certainty, although species of *Potadoma* are suspected. In Latin America, *Araopyrus columbiensis* is the host of *P. caliensis* in Colombia, and *A. costaricensis* has been incriminated as the host of *P. mexicanus* in Costa Rica. Peruvian species of *Paragonimus* are thought to use *A. columbiensis* and *Littoridina cumingii* as hosts. The North American species, *P. kellicoti,* has *Pomatiopsis lapidaria* as its host [8].

HOSTS OF *CLONORCHIS* AND *OPISTHORCHIS*

The two main snail species which serve as hosts for *Clonorchis* are *Parafossarulus manchouricus* and *Bithynia fuchsiana*. *Alocinma longicornis* is also considered to be a host but appears to be of less importance. Hosts of the related species *Opisthorchis viverrini* are also members of the genus *Bithynia* (*B. laevis, B. funiculata, B. goniomphalus*). *Opisthorchis felineus,* which occurs in central and eastern Europe and occasionally infects humans, has *Bithynia leachii* as its host.

HOSTS OF MISCELLANEOUS HELMINTHS

Although it is not possible in a brief presentation to list all the parasites and their snail hosts that on occasion infect humans, some mention appears warranted for those which have some impact in the limited areas in which they occur even though they are still not generally considered to be of worldwide importance. These include *Heterophyes heterophyes* and its hosts *Cerithidea cingulata* and *Pirenella conica; Metagonimus yokogawai,* in which *Semisulcospira* and *Thiara granifera* serve as hosts; and a number of species of Echinostosomes which use a wide variety of freshwater pulmonates as hosts. As noted previously, the nematode parasite *Angiostrongylus cantonensis,* the etiological agent of eosinophilic meningoencephalitis, shows little host specificity, and a wide variety of terrestrial slugs and snails as well as freshwater species serve as its host. Some of the major host species are the slugs *Veronicella alte* and *V. siamensis,* the terrestrial snails *Achatina fulica* and *Bradybaena similaris,* and the freshwater prosobranchs *Pila scutata, P. ampullacea,* and *Viviparus javanica.* In Central America, *Angiostrongylus costaricensis* appears to be transmitted by the slug *Vaginulus plebius* and possibly by several species of terrestrial snails.

TAXONOMY OF HOST SPECIES

The taxonomy of the molluscan intermediate hosts is exceedingly complex and beyond the purview of the present chapter. Those who desire to delve further into the subject or find the need to identify specimens for themselves are encouraged to consult the following sources: the monograph by Malek [8] and the keys prepared by Paraense [9] for the identification of neotropical Planorbidae and other Latin American hosts; the recent text by Brown [2] for the identification of African freshwater mollusks; papers by Davis for an insight into the hosts of oriental schistosomes; the update, prepared by SEAMEO-TROPMED [10], on the snail hosts occurring in southeast Asia; and for a general overview, the monograph by Malek [11].

HOST CAPACITY AND COMPETENCE

The snail host-parasite relationship is not haphazard and, in most instances, exhibits some degree of specificity. Some parasites, to be sure, show little or no specificity in their choice of a molluscan host, but this appears to be the exception among species infecting humans. In some relationships, species of several snail genera may serve as hosts for a particular parasite (*S. haematobium* and the genera *Bulinus, Planorbarius,* and *Ferrissia*) or species of only one genus may serve as hosts (*S. mansoni* and *Biomphalaria*). The relationship may be even more restrictive in that only certain strains or populations of a species may serve as a suitable host [12]. This phenomenon is common among the mammalian schistosomes and their respective hosts as well as among the snail hosts of *Fasciola*. It may, in fact, be more common than presently recognized.

The capacity of a snail to serve as a host and acquire an infection with a particular parasite depends on a variety of environmental factors, both physiochemical and biotic. These include water temperature, salinity, and habitat parameters such as depth, surface area, etc., as well as the presence or absence of decoy organisms, miracidial predators, and hyperparasites. The competence of a snail species to serve as a host and its role in the transmission of disease depends, in addition, on factors innate to both snail and parasite. Thus, the genetic makeup of the host snail, its age and size, nutritional status, ability to produce miracidial attractants, and its defense mechanisms tend to influence competency. The parasite strain, the quantum of infectious stages, and their viability likewise serve as determinants of host competency and its importance in disease transmission. The role of these various factors is poorly understood and warrants further study.

CONTROL METHODOLOGY

The objectives of snail control programs may be broadly characterized as either (1) the eradication of the snail hosts in a given area, or (2) the reduction of the snail population to a level at which disease transmission ceases or is significantly reduced. The first objective is seldom practical or possible and the advisability of its implementation requires precise knowledge of the role of the snails on the balance of the biotic community. This type of information is difficult to acquire and is often not available. Successful attainment of the second objective has been hampered largely by insufficient data relevant to the biology, ecology, and sampling of the snail hosts. To answer the question, At what level must we reduce a snail population to affect transmission significantly, is not presently possible and undoubtedly will vary from habitat to habitat. Surveys in many endemic areas of schistosomiasis indicate that the prevalence rates of human infection may be on the order of 20 to 60 percent when snail infection rates are 1 percent or less. However, in schistosomiasis and many other snailborne diseases, snails are not truly "vectors," and infection may be more dependent on the frequency of water utilization and human-water contact than on the frequency of infected snails. It must also be remembered that, in the case of trematode infections, the intramolluscan stage is a multiplicative process, and from one miracidium hundreds or thousands of cercariae develop. Moreover, field and laboratory observations suggest that once a snail becomes infected, it remains so for many months and possibly for the remainder of its life.

Methods used to control snail populations include (1) the application of molluscicides—chemical toxicants which are applied either focally or areawide; (2) environmental management—application of engineering or hydrological techniques to destroy or modify existing habitats; and (3) biological control—the use of natural or introduced predators, competitors, and parasites.

MOLLUSCICIDES

The concept of controlling snail hosts with molluscicides was first proposed in 1915 by Narabayashi and has been used on an ever-expanding scale during the subsequent six decades. A recent WHO report stated that as of 1976, 31 of 55 countries endemic for schistosomiasis were employing molluscicides as a means of snail control [13].

The molluscicide of choice and the WHO standard by which all available and potential compounds are compared is niclosamide. It is of interest to note that no new compounds have been approved for use by the WHO since they published their list of acceptable compounds in 1973, and that several molluscicides available at that time (yurimin, trifenmorph) are no longer being produced or are of limited availability [14]. The probability of newer molluscicides being developed is not promising in view of the following factors: (1) high develop-

ment and testing costs; (2) uncertainty of world markets and the affordability of these products by developing countries; and (3) increasing demands that such products be proved environmentally safe. It would appear, therefore, that the effective use of molluscicides in the future will depend on the development of newer formulations of existing compounds, newer methods of application, and the possible use of natural products that exhibit toxicity to the snail hosts. Recent initiatives in the development of sustained-release matrices and investigations of potential plant molluscicides, such as Endod, appear promising.

As noted, two strategies are presently employed in applying molluscicides, focal and areawide applications. The former depends upon a precise knowledge of snail foci, seasonal variation in transmission, and water use and contact by the population at risk. Although this strategy appears to be the most cost-effective, it may not be applicable in situations in which the human population is dense, has intimate and continual contact with water, and in which water-contact sites are multiple and ill-defined, e.g., extensive irrigation schemes. In this type of habitat, one must resort to areawide methods in consort with water management.

ENVIRONMENTAL MANAGEMENT

Environmental alterations of existing snail habitats have the advantage of permanence and avoid the necessity for repeated treatments. They are, however, costly, although in the long term the initial costs may be vitiated by savings in labor, chemicals, and by economic benefits derived from land reclamation. Methods which have been employed in the destruction or alteration of snail habitats include the lining of irrigation canals with cement, fluctuation of water levels in storage ponds, increase in water flow rates, elimination of aquatic vegetation, improvement of irrigation drainage systems, and land fill. Frequently, snail habitats may be altered or destroyed not by intent, but as a consequence of social or economic pressure. For example, in the San Juan area of Puerto Rico, many former habitats have been replaced by small factories, shopping centers, and asphalt parking lots. Similarly, in Japan, former areas of wet rice cultivation have been drained and replanted with more economically valuable crops.

BIOLOGICAL CONTROL

As a consequence of both a heightening awareness of environmental safety and the need for more economical methods of control, increasing efforts have been directed toward the possible use of biological methods as an alternative to chemicals. The concept is not new with respect to snail control, and attempts to control the hosts of *Clonorchis* biologically were made by Nagano more than 50 years ago. Subsequently, a large variety of biological agents (including fish, birds, insects, helminths, and microbial pathogens) have been suggested, but few appear to be of practical value or have been investigated other than in the laboratory. The only agent which has been extensively studied and has had a degree of field evaluation is the predatory snail *Marisa cornuarietis*. Experience with this snail, particularly in Puerto Rico, has demonstrated its effectiveness in controlling and eliminating the schistosome host *Biomphalaria glabrata* [*15*]. Recent attempts to use the freshwater pulmonate *Helisoma duryi* as a competitor of schistosome snail hosts appear promising both in the laboratory and in limited field trials [*16*].

COST-EFFECTIVENESS

Information relevant to the cost of snail control usually refers to the cost of chemical treatment. The need for recurrent treatments and long-term commitments increases costs and may place an inordinate demand on the limited resources of developing countries. Jobin [*17*] developed an analysis which allowed him to compare the costs of control projects from different geographical areas and found that costs per 100 m³ of snail habitat treated ranged from $1.40 to $40 (in 1972 U.S. dollars). Costs were cheaper in projects in which the habitats were clustered and rainfall limited. One study in which *Marisa* was used as the sole control agent suggested that in this particular situation, biological control was more than 60 times cheaper than if conventional molluscicides were used.

Increasing demands for cheap hydroelectric power and the need to increase agricultural productivity by extensive irrigation in many of the developing countries will increase the number of habitats suitable for snail colonization and consequently increase the potential for disease transmission. Technology for the control of snail populations is both adequate and available; however, past experience dictates that transmission cannot be substantially reduced if attacking the snail hosts is the sole means of control. Control of disease depends, therefore, on the intelligent and imaginative use of these techniques in consort with a total control strategy that incorporates chemotherapy, water management, and improved environmental sanitation. A total strategy implies not only the integration of health disciplines and professionals, but also integrated input of economic planners, engineering professionals, and agriculture specialists.

REFERENCES

1 Mandahl-Barth G: Intermediate Hosts of Schistomiasis. Geneva, WHO, 1958, pp 5–132

2 Brown DS: *Freshwater Snails of Africa and Their Medical Importance*. London, Taylor & Francis Ltd, 1980, p 487

3 Davis GM: Snail hosts of Asian *Schistosoma* infecting man: Evolution and coevolution, in Bruce JT et al (eds): *The Mekong Schistostome*. Malacol Rev suppl 2, 1980, pp 195–238

4 Graer GJ, Ow-Yang CK, Yong H-S: *Schistosoma malayensis* N.SP.: A *Schistosoma japonicum*–complex schistosome from peninsular Malaysia. J Parasitol 74:471–480, 1988

5 Kitikoon V: Studies on *Tricula aperta* and related taxa, the snail intermediate hosts of *Schistosoma mekongi:* III. Susceptibility studies. Malacol Rev 14:37–42, 1981

6 Kitikoon V, Schneider CR, Sommani S, et al: Mekong schistosomiasis: II. Evidence of the natural transmission of *Schistosoma japonicum* Mekong strain at Khong Island, Laos. Southeast Asian J Trop Med Public Health 4:350–358, 1973

7 Boray JC: Experimental fascioliasis in Australia, in Dawes B (ed): *Advances in Parasitology*. Academic, New York, London, 1969, 7:95–210

8 Malek EA: Snail hosts of schistosomiasis and other snail-transmitted diseases in tropical America: A manual. Pan Am Health Org Sci publication 478, 1985

9 Paraense WL: Estado atual da sistemática dos planorbideos brasileiros. Arq Mus Nac RJ 55:105–128, 1975

10 SEAMEO-TROPMED: Snails of medical importance in Southeast Asia. Southeastern Asia J Trop Med Public Health 17:282–322, 1986.

11 Malek EA: *Snail-Transmitted Parasitic Diseases*. Boca Raton, CRC Press, 1980, vols 1 and 2

12 Michelson EH, DuBois L: Susceptibility of Bahian populations of *Biomphalaria glabrata* to an allopatric strain of *Schistosoma mansoni*. Am J Trop Med Hyg 27:782–786, 1978

13 Iatrotski LS, Davis A: The schistosomiasis problem in the world: Results of a WHO questionnaire survey. Bull WHO 59:115–127, 1981

14 Epidemiology and control of schistosomiasis. WHO Expt Comm Rep 643, Geneva, WHO, 1980

15 Jobin WR, Ferguson FF, Berrios-Duran LA: *Effect of Marisa cornuarietis* on populations of *Biomphalaria glabrata* in farm ponds of Puerto Rico. Am J Trop Med Hyg 22:278–284, 1973

16 Frandsen F, Christensen NØ: Effect of *Helisoma duryi* on the survival, growth, and cercarial production of *Schistosoma mansoni*–infected *Biomphalaria glabrata*. Bull WHO 55:577–580, 1977

17 Jobin WR: Cost of snail control. Am J Trop Med Hyg 28:142–154, 1979

SECTION D / Nutrition

CHAPTER 22 / Nutritional Needs and Evaluation
· Christina Wood-Dahlström · Doris Howes Calloway

The existence of national and international nutrient intake standards (usually called *recommended allowances*) should not imply that these are immutable statistics or that an individual's requirements can be estimated with precision by consulting such tables. There is considerable variability among individuals in their requirements for energy and for each of the approximately 45 essential nutrients; therefore, a particular person's requirements can only be determined by direct measurement. In practice, this is never done. Nutrient allowances are generally based on requirement studies conducted on a few individuals of a population. The results are averaged and adjusted for interindividual variability and efficiency of absorption to derive an allowance figure intended to cover the requirements of most individuals of that population (Fig. 22-1).

Determination of nutritional status involves (1) physical examination and measurement of the most appropriate biochemical and anthropometric indexes, (2) characterization and quantification of the dietary intake, and (3) correlation of the intake data with the biochemical and anthropometric findings. The third point must be considered with the understanding that dietary data can indicate that nutrients may be deficient in the diet at the time of study, while anthropometric and biochemical data can reflect remote past as well as present nutrient deficiencies. Occasionally, isolated nutrient deficiencies (vitamin A, iodine, etc.) are observed in a population; however, most often a syndrome of mixed nutrient deficiencies occurs as a result of too little food being consumed and that often of poor quality.

Expression of dietary allowances as specific nutrients does not imply that nutrients are to be provided as separate entities. Allowances for many nutrients are not as yet established due to lack of definitive studies in human beings. If a diet provides adequate levels of the specified nutrients *from foods,* the need for the less-studied nutrients is likely to be met as well. Nutritional supplements and food fortification (as, e.g., addition of iodine to salt) have a place but cannot be relied upon to satisfy wider nutritional requirements. The ability of the diet to fulfill an individual's requirements depends on the composition and digestibility of each food consumed and the efficiency of absorption of the nutrients.

NUTRIENTS

Food is composed of nutrients, water, and nonnutrients, including nonabsorbable material and pharmacoactive, and occasionally toxic, components such as caffeine and cyanogenic glycosides. Carbohydrates, fats, proteins, and alcohol can provide energy; carbohydrates and proteins yield about 17 kJ (4 kcal)/g, fat about 38 kJ (9 kcal)/g, and alcohol 29 kJ (7 kcal)/g. Enough carbohydrate and fat should be present in

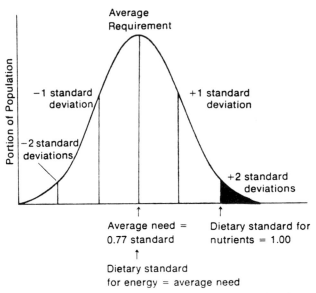

Figure 22-1. Dietary standards for protein, vitamins, and minerals are intended to cover the needs of almost all healthy people in a population; they are set at two standard deviations above the mean requirement, where that is known. Thus, only 2.5 percent of a normally distributed pouplation of requirers (the darker colored area) will fail to meet their needs if their diets meet the standard. The standard deviation is about 0.15 of the mean requirement in the few instances where valid information exists. Thus the average need is about 77 percent of the standard, and the requirement of half the individuals will be met by intakes at this level. However, the standard for energy is set at the mean requirement, so the needs of half a population are not met by intakes that equal the standard. *(From [1] with permission.)*

the diet to spare proteins for their specific role in muscle, organ, enzyme, and hormone structure and function. A healthy adult needs about 180 g of glucose per day, derived from carbohydrates or some amino acids, to supply the energy needs of brain and blood. There is no specific requirement for dietary carbohydrate, but about 75 to 100 g/day is enough to prevent excessive protein breakdown for gluconeogenesis and ketosis from incomplete fat oxidation [2]. In addition to energy supply, dietary fat is also a source of the essential polyunsaturated fatty acids: linoleic, linolenic, and arachidonic. Infants require and adults should consume at least 3 percent of energy in the form of essential fatty acids, 4.5 percent during pregnancy, and 5 to 7 percent during lactation. In tropical countries, especially among the poor, the portion of energy derived from fat is often as low as 10 percent, but to meet essential fatty acid requirements a level of 15 to 20 percent is recommended [3].

Protein is required to provide the constituent amino acids, nine of which are essential, i.e., they cannot be made from precursors in the human body. These are histidine, isoleucine, leucine, lysine, methionine, phenylalanine, threonine, tryptophan, and valine. Cystine can substitute, in part, for methionine, and tyrosine for phenylalanine. The other 10 amino acids present in all common proteins may be used as such or as precursors, and thus reduce the need for the essential amino acids. With rare exceptions, ordinary mixed diets that meet total protein allowances also meet the need of adults and older children for specific amino acids, but amino acid supply may sometimes be an issue for preschool children [4].

The water-soluble vitamins (B complex-thiamine, riboflavin, niacin, folacin, vitamin B_6, vitamin B_{12}, pantothenic acid, biotin, and choline and vitamin C) and the fat-soluble vitamins (A,D,E, and K) have diverse functions in metabolism of other nutrients as well as specific roles (vitamin A in vision, vitamin K in blood clotting, etc.). The needs for biotin and vitamin K usually are met by a combination of diet and synthesis by enteric microflora; vitamin D is made by activation of a precursor in the skin on exposure to sunlight and is also present in a few animal foods. The need for all other vitamins must be met by diet alone. The macrominerals (sodium, potassium, chlorine, calcium, phosphorus, and magnesium) and the trace elements (iron, iodine, copper, manganese, zinc, fluorine, selenium, chromium, molybdenum, nickel, vanadium, silicon, and possibly some others) have a wide variety of structural and metabolic functions. Relatively little is known about the role of trace elements recently established as being essential, nor about their distribution in foods. It is characteristic of trace elements that the range between minimum requirement and toxicity is fairly narrow.

NUTRIENT REQUIREMENTS

Recommended dietary or nutrient allowances have been developed for many countries and population groups [5]. The figures presented here are the standards developed by inter-national agencies [4,6–10] and should be valid for conditions in most tropical countries.

ENERGY

It is currently believed that inadequate intake of food, and thus, amount of energy, often together with the catabolic effects of infection (see Chap. 23), is the primary cause of most malnutrition in the world. This view differs from the consensus of the 1960s, when protein deficiency was considered to be the most serious condition. Components of the total energy requirement include basal metabolic rate (BMR) and energy expenditure for physical activity, plus the costs of tissue deposition in growing children and pregnant women and of milk secretion in lactation (Table 22-1). Standards for children below age 10 years are based on observed energy intakes of healthy children in developed countries. Energy requirements of other groups are based on BMR (which is, in turn, related to body size and composition) and the energy cost of occupational and desirable nonoccupational activity. People eating less than the specified amounts tend to compensate by reducing discretionary activities, with perceived detrimental physical and social consequences. No adjustment for climate is necessary unless clothing and shelter are insufficient for protection against low nighttime and seasonal temperatures; exposure to cold would then increase energy demand. Recommendations for any specific adult group should be adjusted for their observed height, appropriate weight, and activity patterns (see Table 22-1). Underfed children are undersized, and their allowances should be based on body size appropriate to their age rather than observed body size. This proportionately increased allowance will permit catch-up growth. Standards assume that the diet is as digestible as the diet consumed by reference populations; if the diet is coarse and high in fiber, digestibility may be 95 to 97 percent of reference, and allowances should be increased accordingly.

PROTEIN

In contrast to energy, for which the figures are the average requirement, the FAO/WHO/UNU Safe Level of Protein Intake is calculated to meet the needs of the average plus two standard deviations (Table 22-1). For young infants the recommendation is based on the intake of healthy breast-fed babies. Adult levels are amounts of protein (nitrogen × 6.25) required to maintain nitrogen balance in metabolic experiments. Safe levels for children provide for maintenance and growth and take account of the marked variation in growth rate within and between children. Extra allowances for pregnancy are based on the composition of tissue gained and for lactation, on the amount of milk protein secreted, adjusted in both cases for the efficiency with which dietary protein is converted to tissue protein by young infants. Where body weight and, in the case of children, height are low, allowances for specific groups should be based on standard rather than observed body size.

Table 22-1. Recommended energy and protein allowances[a]

Age yr	Body weight,[b] kg	Basal metabolic rate/kg[c] In kcal	Basal metabolic rate/kg[c] In kJ	Recommended allowances reference diet[d] (kg/day) Average energy requirement,[e] ×BMR	Recommended allowances reference diet[d] (kg/day) Average energy requirement,[e] In kcal	Recommended allowances reference diet[d] (kg/day) Average energy requirement,[e] In kJ	Safe protein intake, g	Example application tropical low-cost diet[f] (kg/day) Energy In kcal	Example application tropical low-cost diet[f] (kg/day) Energy In kJ	Example application tropical low-cost diet[f] (kg/day) Protein, g
0.25–0.50	7				100	418	1.85	Not suitable		
0.5–0.75	8.5			– – –	95	397	1.65	Not suitable		
0.75–1.0	9.5	54	225	– – –	100	418	1.50	105	440	2.75
1–2	11			– – –	105	439	1.20	110	460	1.95
2–3	13.5			– – –	100	418	1.15	105	440	1.90
3–5	16.5			– – –	95	397	1.10	100	415	1.80
5–7	20.5	47	195	– – –	88	366	1.00	92	385	1.65
7–10	27			– – –	72	303	1.00	76	320	1.25
Males:										
10–12	34.5	36	155	1.75	64	267	1.00	67	280	1.25
12–14	44	32	135	1.68	55	228	1.00	57	240	1.20
14–16	55.5	30	125	1.64	48	202	0.95	51	210	1.10
16–18	64	28	115	1.60	44	184	0.90	46	190	1.05
18–30	65	26	110	1.78	46	193	0.75	49	200	0.90
30–60	65	25	105	1.78	44	186	0.75	47	195	0.90
60+	65	22	90	1.55	34	140	0.75	36	145	0.90
Females:										
10–12	36	33	140	1.64	54	226	1.00	57	240	1.25
12–14	46.5	28	120	1.59	45	190	0.95	48	200	1.10
14–16	52	26	110	1.55	41	172	0.90	43	180	1.05
16–18	54	26	105	1.53	39	163	0.80	41	170	0.95
18–30	55	24	100	1.64	39	164	0.75	41	170	0.90
30–60	55	24	100	1.64	39	164	0.75	41	170	0.90
60+	55	22	90	1.56	34	140	0.75	36	145	0.90
Add *per day:*										
Pregnant					200[g]	850[g]	6	210[g]	900[g]	11[i]
Lactating					500[h]	2100[h]	15	525[h]	2205[h]	28[i]

[a]Adapted from [4]. Energy figures are average requirements: the "safe level of protein intake" is the average requirement + 2 standard deviations. See text.

[b]Through age 18 years, NCHS median figures at mid-point age range; adult figures are representative but arbitrary.

[c]Calculated from formulas given in Ref. 4, Table 5 or Tables 42–48. Figures have been rounded.

[d]"Reference diet" assumes energy digestibility typical of diet pattern of industrialized countries and protein quality and digestibility of eggs, milk, meat, fish, and poultry.

[e]Energy requirement of older children and adults is stipulated as multiples of BMR to allow adjustment for body weight and for varying times and intensity of physical activity. For adults whose occupational work is classified as light, moderate, and heavy, BMR factors are, respectively: men 1.55, 1.78, and 2.10; women, 1.56, 1.64, and 1.82. Herein adult figures assume moderate activity through age 60 and light activity after age 60. Requirements figures for children below age 10 are derived from observed intake of healthy children in Canada, Sweden, the United Kingdom, and the United States.

[f]This example calculation is based on Nigerian cassava-based diet, Ref. 4, Table 40: Corrected requirement = energy standard requirement × 1/0.95 for reduced digestibility (95% of ref.); protein standard safe level × 1/0.85 for reduced digestibility (85% of ref.) The × factor for reduced quality is as follows: 1/0.64 to age 1 yr; 1/0.72 ages 1–6 yr; 1/0.95 ages 6–12 yr. The limiting amino acid in this diet is lysine; enough lysine is provided per g of protein to meet adult requirements, so no quality correction is required for adults.

[g]Assumes some reduction in physical activity; if not, increase allowances shown by 40%.

[h]Assumes some fat deposited in pregnancy available to support lactation during the first 6 months; if not, increase allowances shown by 40% during that period. Breast milk is not sufficient to meet infant energy needs beyond the first 3 months.

[i]Specific amino acid requirements for pregnancy and lactation are unknown. Calculation assumes *additional* need is same as infant pattern.

Food proteins are grouped according to biological quality. High-quality proteins are those having patterns of amino acids closest to the human requirements pattern, a high proportion of the essential amino acids, and near-perfect digestibility; included in this group are eggs, milk, meat, fish, poultry, and some soybean foods (tofu, tempeh, soy "milk"). The amino acid most likely to be limiting in dietary proteins is lysine; others sometimes in short supply are tryptophan, and, very rarely, threonine and methionine-cystine. When one or more amino acids are low, it is necessary to increase the total protein intake to meet the requirement for the amino acid(s) or to add a complementary protein to the diet (e.g., beans with rice). Most ordinary mixed dietary proteins provide enough essential amino acids, and protein allowances need only be corrected for digestibility. Diets low in animal foods and legumes may be marginal for young children; an example of how allowances are to be adjusted in that case is given in Table 22-1. Amino acid composition warrants special consideration in the case of infant formulas and weaning foods. In practice, a diet in which 10 percent of energy derives from protein will meet or exceed the requirements of almost all healthy people beyond infancy, provided that the energy need is met.

Protein utilization is influenced by energy intake in that if the amount of energy consumed is insufficient, some protein will be used for energy, thereby increasing the effective protein requirement. Physical activity is anabolic, leading to improved utilization of protein even when there is no apparent increase in muscle mass. Loss of nitrogen due to heavy sweating is compensated by reduced urinary nitrogen, an adjustment possible at recommended protein intake levels. Stressors have a catabolic effect on protein metabolism, and there is a need for increased protein during recovery from illness and other trauma.

VITAMINS AND MINERALS

Allowances for vitamins and minerals usually are set by determining the amount required to correct or prevent deficiency symptoms (physical, physiological, and biochemical) with an adjustment to cover the requirements of most people (Table 22-2). Because information is lacking, no allowances have been set for some of the micronutrients, but a range of probably safe intakes has been published for some of these [10,11].

Single micronutrient deficiencies, as differentiated from a generally poor intake, are rare. Iodine deficiency is found where the soil and water and hence the total food supply are low in this element; this situation may exist for some other trace elements (e.g., selenium), but no other clinical syndromes have been identified to date. Vitamin A deficiency, leading to blindness, is prevalent in Asia and parts of Africa and South America; in this instance, deficiency is due to failure to consume foods containing a nutrient that is not widely distributed. Classical scurvy, caused by vitamin C deficiency,

reflects the same type of nutrient distributional problem, but it is rarely seen today. Iron deficiency is common but usually is associated with blood loss, as with menstruation and hookworm infection, with increased need, as in pregnancy, or, often, with a marginal diet. Deficits of niacin and zinc also occur fairly commonly, but always in conjunction with an inadequate diet overall. Rickets due to vitamin D deficiency in the tropics is found where exposure to sunlight is reduced by clothing (bundling infants, purdah) or by staying indoors. Deficiencies of the intestinally synthesized vitamin K and biotin sometimes occur as a result of administration of antibiotics that suppress intestinal microflora. Nutritional deficiency diseases are discussed in more detail in Chaps. 114 to 122.

Where an isolated nutrient deficiency is identified, fortification of a widely used, cheap food is a reasonable societal solution. Salt, soy sauce, and sugar are currently studied vehicles for this purpose. Individual supplements can also be given if individuals can be reached effectively, but this may be costly. Most problems yield to improved diets and associated health measures.

The only natural micronutrient toxicity commonly found is dental mottling and, in the extreme, skeletal deformity due to excess fluorine. Hemosiderosis has been ascribed to habitual consumption of beverages brewed in iron pots and hence very high in iron. Other micronutrient excesses sometimes result from overenthusiastic dosage with pills or nostrums containing high levels of vitamin A or D.

WATER

The need for adequate water intake is more critical in the short term than the need for food. Serious consequences of acute dehydration result from a loss of 6 to 10 percent of body weight as water, and a 20 to 22 percent loss is fatal [1]. Marginal intake of water results in formation of concentrated urine, contributing to the formation of kidney stones, a common problem in the tropics. In mild climates, the requirement for water is estimated to be 1 mL per 4 kJ (1 kcal) of expended energy, and the requirement is increased by about 1 L/day during lactation. With hard work and intense heat, sweat loss can reach 8 to 10 L/day and requires continuous replacement with lightly salted water (2 g NaCl per liter) or with water and salty food. Water need is increased by high salt and high protein intakes, sometimes a problem in infants; by fever; and by losses due to vomiting and diarrhea. Drinking water is also a source of some essential minerals, notably calcium and fluorine. The provision of adequate amounts of safe drinking water to populations in less developed countries is one of the foremost health problems today.

OTHER CONSIDERATIONS

An individual's nutrient requirements are influenced by factors affecting absorption and by interactions between foods and

Table 22-2. Dietary standards for daily vitamin and mineral intake[a]

Age group	Vitamin A,[b] µg	Vitamin D,[c] µg	Thiamine, mg	Riboflavin, mg	Niacin, mg	Folacin, µg	Vitamin B₁₂, µg	Ascorbic acid, mg	Calcium, g	Iron,[d] mg	Zinc,[e] mg
Children:											
less than 1 yr	350	10.0	0.3	0.5	5.4	26	0.1	20	0.5–0.6	7–21	3–12
1–3	400	10.0	0.5	0.8	9.0	50	0.5	20	0.4–0.5	5–12	4–16
4–6	400	10.0	0.7	1.1	12.1	50	0.7	20	0.4–0.5	5–14	4–16
7–9	500	2.5	0.9	1.3	14.5	102	0.9	20	0.4–0.5	8–23	4–16
Male adolescents:											
10–12	500	2.5	1.0	1.6	17.2	102	1.0	20	0.6–0.7	12–23	7–28
13–15	600	2.5	1.2	1.7	19.1	170	1.0	30	0.6–0.7	12–36	7–28
16–19	600	2.5	1.2	1.8	20.3	200	1.0	30	0.5–0.6	8–36	7–28
Female adolescents:											
10–12	500	2.5	0.9	1.4	15.5	102	1.0	20	0.6–0.7	12–23	7–26
13–15	600	2.5	1.0	1.5	16.4	170	1.0	30	0.6–0.7	13–40	6–22
16–19	500	2.5	0.9	1.4	15.2	170	1.0	30	0.5–0.6	16–48	6–22
Male adults	600	2.5	1.2	1.8	19.8	200	1.0	30	0.4–0.5	8–23	5–22
Female adults	500	2.5	0.9	1.3	14.5	170	1.0	30	0.4–0.5	16–48	6–22
Pregnant women (latter half of term)	600	10.0	+0.1	+0.2	+2.3	370	1.4	30	1.0–1.2	f	8–30
Lactating women (first 6 mos.)	850	10.0	+0.2	+0.4	+3.7	270	1.3	30	1.0–1.2	f	14–54

[a]Values are recommended daily allowances and are intended to meet the requirements of 97.5 percent of the population. Values are from Refs. 6–10.

[b]As retinol. 1 µg retinol = 1 retinol equivalent = 6 µg β-carotene = 12 µg other provitamin A carotenoids based on human studies. International units (IU), based on rat studies, are sometimes used, wherein 1 retinol equivalent = 3.33 IU retinol.

[c]As cholecalciferol.

[d]The lower value applies when a large proportion of the calories in the diet come from animal foods; the higher value applies when the diet contains negligible amounts of animal foods. Amounts required to prevent anemia are less than values shown, which are intended to allow storage.

[e]The lower figure is for diets containing generous amounts of animal foods and refined cereals (zinc absorption, 30 percent)—and the higher figure is for diets based on coarse cereals and legumes (zinc absorption, 10 percent).

[f]For women whose intakes of iron throughout life have been at the level recommended in this table, the daily intake of iron during pregnancy and lactation is the same or less than that recommended for women of childbearing age who are not pregnant or lactating. For women whose status with respect to iron is not satisfactory at the beginning of pregnancy, the requirement is increased, and in the extreme situation of women with no stores of iron, the requirement can probably not be met without supplementation.

nutrients that affect their availability. The effects of tropical enteropathy and sprue, prevalent malabsorption syndromes, on nutritional status and protein requirements have been well reviewed [12]. The absorption of vitamins and minerals can either be hindered or enhanced by dietary factors. For instance, tea, dietary fiber, and phytate (present in cereal bran and legumes) all interfere with iron absorption; ascorbic acid, amino acids, and sugars have enhancing effects on the absorption of nonheme iron that are even stronger than the inhibitory effects just mentioned. Absorption of heme iron is 10 times more efficient than that of nonheme iron and is less subject to the influence of other dietary components.

Efficiency of absorption of some nutrients, particularly iron and calcium, is regulated according to physiological need. Homeostatic regulation is also achieved by storage and selective excretion. This regulatory capability allows maintenance of effective tissue levels of nutrients in the face of low or episodic intakes. More studies are needed on the long-term consequences (or lack thereof) of such adaptation to low and high intakes of nutrients.

With regard to metabolism, deficiency or excess of certain nutrients influences the need for other nutrients. For example, diets high in carbohydrate require an increased intake of thiamine, a B-complex vitamin functioning as a coenzyme in carbohydrate metabolism. Similarly, an increased intake of protein demands a higher vitamin B₆ intake, and diets containing large amounts of vegetable oil (high in polyunsaturated fatty acids) require greater amounts of vitamin E, an antioxidant. A thorough presentation of vitamin and mineral interactions is contained in Ref. 13.

The use and abuse of alcohol is so prevalent throughout the world that its effects on the nutritional condition of a population under study should always be considered. Loss of money for food due to purchase of alcohol and drunkenness may impair the nutritional state of whole families. Excessive alcohol consumption damages the liver, intestinal mucosa, and eventually the nervous system. Chronic alcoholics are reported to have low blood levels of zinc and vitamin A [14] as well as decreased absorption of thiamine, vitamin B_6, and folacin [15]. Alcoholic beverages often displace food energy with an attendant reduction in intake of essential nutrients. However, some local brews (e.g., pulque) which are low in alcohol content and are consumed unfiltered make a useful contribution of vitamins and minerals.

EVALUATION OF NUTRITIONAL STATUS

A determination of nutritional status of an individual involves an understanding of the living conditions, an examination for the physical and physiological symptoms known to be associated with nutritional deficiency, and correlation of the diagnosis with an analysis of the food intake. It is important to distinguish between acute and chronic malnutrition, and this can be accomplished to some degree with appropriate anthropometric indexes. Useful biochemical measurements include hemoglobin and/or hematocrit, serum albumin, and levels of vitamins and minerals and/or metabolic activities dependent upon them (e.g., transketolase activity for thiamine) (Table 22-3) [16]. Measurement of some nutrients in serum may not provide a useful reflection of the nutrient's status. For example, vitamin A is stored in the liver and serum levels are finely regulated, making vitamin A status difficult to determine. However, serum levels of β-carotene, a precursor of vitamin A, directly reflect intake and therefore give a better indication

of vitamin A status. With the realization that malnutrition affects not only an individual's physical and biochemical parameters, but also diverse physiological, psychological, and social functions, new indexes for malnutrition (e.g., immune responsiveness, reproductive ability, cognitive development) are being sought.

The most accepted anthropometric indicators are height for age and weight for height, compared to reference standards [17]. WHO [18] has accepted for this purpose data from a probability sample of the U.S. population, recognizing that privileged children in all countries tend to grow at similar rates. It is recognized that height and other physical measurements reflect growth-inhibitory situations throughout life, including disease episodes as well as malnutrition. Nevertheless, height for age remains the most useful index of chronic food deprivation, whereas weight for height reflects the current nutrition situation and is a reliable index when precise age cannot be determined, as is often the case (Fig. 22-2).

Field experience indicates that the latter is more predictive of morbidity and mortality than is stunting [17]. Other indexes useful for population-based studies include the QUAC stick, which measures arm circumference (AC) in relation to height. The QUAC stick offers the advantages of being independent of age, quick, and simple and requiring minimal equipment. The measuring stick contains two scales, one at the 50th centile of standard AC and the second at 85 percent of that, against which a child's AC is compared. In a study in Bangladesh, the relative risk of mortality among children aged 1 to 9 years was 3.4 for those whose measurements were at or below the lower cutoff scale [20].

Table 22-3. Table of current guidelines for criteria of nutritional status for laboratory evaluation

Nutrient and units	Age of subject, yrs	Criteria of status		
		Deficient	Marginal	Acceptance
Hemoglobin[a] (g/dL)	6–23 mo.	Up to 9.0	9.0–9.9	10.0+
	2–5	Up to 10.0	10.0–10.9	11.0+
	6–12	Up to 10.0	10.0–11.4	11.5+
	13–16M	Up to 12.0	12.0–12.9	13.0+
	13–16F	Up to 10.0	10.0–11.4	11.5+
	16+M	Up to 12.0	12.0–13.9	14.0+
	16+F	Up to 10.0	10.0–11.9	12.0+
	Pregnant (after 6 mo.)	Up to 9.5	9.5–10.9	11.0+
Hematocrit[a] (packed cell volume in percent)	Up to 2	Up to 28	28–30	31+
	2–5	Up to 30	30–33	34+
	6–12	Up to 30	30–35	36+
	13–16M	Up to 37	37–39	40+
	13–16F	Up to 31	31–35	36+
	16+M	Up to 37	37–43	44+
	16+F	Up to 31	31–37	37+
	Pregnant	Up to 30	30–32	33+
Serum albumin[a] (g/dL)	Up to 1	—	Up to 2.5	2.5+
	1–5	—	Up to 3.0	3.0+
	6–16	—	Up to 3.5	3.5+
	16+	Up to 2.8	2.8–3.4	3.5+
	Pregnant	Up to 3.0	3.0–3.4	3.5+

Table 22-3. (*Continued*)

| Nutrient and units | Age of subject, yrs | Criteria of status | | |
		Deficient	Marginal	Acceptance
Serum protein[a] (g/dL)	Up to 1	—	Up to 5.0	5.0+
	1–5	—	Up to 5.5	5.5+
	6–16	—	Up to 6.0	6.0+
	16+	Up to 6.0	6.0–6.4	6.5+
	Pregnant	Up to 5.5	5.5–5.9	6.0+
Serum ascorbic acid[a] (mg/dL)	All ages	Up to 0.1	0.1–0.19	0.2+
Plasma vitamin A[a] (μg/dL)	All ages	Up to 10	10–19	20+
Plasma carotene[a] (μg/dL)	All ages	Up to 20	20–39	40+
	Pregnant	—	40–79	80+
Serum iron[a] (μg/dL)	Up to 2	Up to 30	—	30+
	2–5	Up to 40	—	40+
	6–12	Up to 50	—	50+
	12+M	Up to 60	—	60+
	12+F	Up to 40	—	40+
Transferrin saturation[a] (percent)	Up to 2	Up to 15.0	—	15.0+
	2–12	Up to 20.0	—	20.0+
	12+M	Up to 20.0	—	20.0+
	12+F	Up to 15.0	—	15.0+
Serum folacin[b] (ng/mL)	All ages	Up to 2.0	2.1–5.9	6.0+
Serum vitamin B_{12}[b] (pg/mL)	All ages	Up to 100	—	100+
Thiamine in urine[a] (μg/g creatinine)	1–3	Up to 120	120–175	175+
	4–5	Up to 85	85–120	120+
	6–9	Up to 70	70–180	180+
	10–15	Up to 55	55–150	150+
	16+	Up to 27	27–65	65+
	Pregnant	Up to 21	21–49	50+
Riboflavin in urine[a] (μg/g creatinine)	1–3	Up to 150	150–499	500+
	4–5	Up to 100	100–299	300+
	6–9	Up to 85	85–269	270+
	10–16	Up to 70	70–199	200+
	16+	Up to 27	27–79	80+
	Pregnant	Up to 30	30–89	90+
RBC transketolase-TPP-effect[b] (ratio)	All ages	25+	15–25	Up to 15
RBC glutathione reductase-FAD-effect[b] (ratio)	All ages	1.2+	—	Up to 25
Tryptophan load[b] (mg xanthurenic acid excreted)	Adults (Dose: 100 mg/kg body weight)	25 + (6 h)	—	Up to 25
		75 + (24 h)	—	Up to 75
Urinary pyridoxine[b] (μg/g creatinine)	1–3	Up to 90	—	90+
	4–6	Up to 80	—	80+
	7–9	Up to 60	—	60+
	10–12	Up to 40	—	40+
	13–15	Up to 30	—	30+
	16+	Up to 20	—	20+
Urinary N'-methyl-nicotinamide[a] (mg/g creatinine)	All ages	Up to 0.2	0.2–5.59	0.6+
	Pregnant	Up to 0.8	0.8–2.49	2.5+
Urinary pantothenic acid[b] (μg)	All ages	Up to 200	—	200+
Plasma vitamin E[b] (mg/dL)	All ages	Up to 0.2	0.2–0.6	0.6+
Transaminase index[b]				
EGOT[c]	Adult	2.0+	—	Up to 2.0
EGPT[d]	Adult	1.25+	—	Up to 1.25

[a]Adapted from the Ten State Nutrition Survey.
[b]Criteria may vary with different methodology.
[c]Erythrocyte glutamic oxalacetic transaminase.
[d]Erythrocyte glutamic pyruvic transaminase.

Source: From [22].

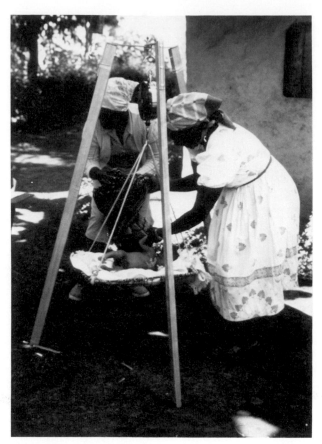

Figure 22-2. Monitoring growth of infants and young children is a key element in their own nutrition assessment and is a good indicator of community nutrition conditions. Simple equipment for field use is shown in use in Kenya. *(Courtesy of C. Neumann, UCLA.)*

EVALUATION OF DIETARY INTAKE

Food intake records provide much useful information beyond nutrient intake per se, for development of economic indicators, identification of commonly used foods as a guide for fortification policy, price supports, agricultural planning, and the like. If such records are to be used as an indicator of nutritional status, however, the record must be valid and representative of usual or habitual intake, and the nutrient content of the foods must be known. With suitable caution, intake may then be compared with recommended allowances.

All of the nutrient allowances except that for energy are intended to cover the actual requirements of 97.5 percent of the population, so it is evident that the nutrient allowances are greater than the actual requirements of most individuals. Because an individual's own requirement is not known, comparison of that individual's intake with the allowance can only indicate the level of risk that the individual's requirement is not being met at a particular intake. Obviously, if the person is consuming a nutrient at the allowance level, the risk of deficiency will be quite low. Dietary intake data should be interpreted in terms of probability of deficiency at a particular intake level, and the variability of requirements is an important factor in determining the probability of deficiency at substandard intake levels. For population data, the variabilities of both requirements and intakes as well as the correlation between the two variabilities must be used [4,21].

Accurate measurement of dietary intake in a field situation is a difficult task. The methods used fall into two broad categories: (1) direct, on-the-spot observation and/or weighing and (2) recording of food intake and recall questionnaire. Weighing methods are time-consuming and intrusive; the mere presence of an investigator is likely to alter the usual eating patterns. Recall questionnaires involve the subject's recounting of the foods eaten within the last few days, or a "diet history" of the foods usually consumed. Validity depends on the subject's ability to remember the foods eaten (a problem for children and old people), the willingness to divulge what was actually eaten rather than what is thought should have been eaten, and the investigator's skill in interviewing. A review of procedures and problems of dietary intake methods has been published by the National Academy of Sciences [21].

Food composition tables have been prepared for many major geographical areas [refer to FAO and U.S. Department of Agriculture (USDA) publications]. The nutrient composition of agricultural products varies among regions and even seasonally due to differences in climate and soil; therefore, it is desirable to use local food composition tables when evaluating food intake data. Food preparation habits within households also may affect nutrient composition and availability. For example, iron content is greatly enhanced by cooking acidic food in an iron pot, and the use of lime in preparing maize tortillas not only enriches the calcium content but also renders niacin more available, an important pellagra-preventive factor.

Staple diets are those in which 60 to 80 percent of energy is provided by one food. In tropical countries the staple food is usually a cereal grain (rice, maize, sorghum, wheat, millet) or other starchy food (cassava, yam, plantain, taro, breadfruit). All of these foods contain a high percentage of carbohydrate and little or no fat. The starchy foods are low in protein; the cereal grains contain more protein, but rice is relatively low in protein, maize and sorghum are intermediate, and whole wheat is relatively high. Protein in this class of foods is low in lysine content; maize is notably low in tryptophan; and rice in threonine. As a generalization, B vitamins and minerals tend to occur along with protein, so the foods higher in protein tend also to be better sources of micronutrients. Milling of cereal grains, which removes the bran and germ, markedly reduces vitamin and mineral content and also dietary fiber, with a resultant increase in digestibility of protein and energy.

Other foods consumed with the staple usually complement

the nutrient composition of the staple and make the diet adequate. Complementary amino acids are provided by beans, peas, nuts, seeds, leaves, and animal foods; these foods also provide B vitamins and minerals. Dark-green leafy vegetables supply vitamins A and C, folacin, riboflavin, magnesium, and also iron, calcium, and other minerals, though at limited bioavailability. Vitamins A and C are derived from other green and deep-yellow vegetables (e.g., peppers, squash), fruits (papaya, mango), and tomatoes.

A minimally adequate, low-cost diet contains at least a staple plus beans or nuts, leafy green vegetables, and a source of vitamin B_{12}. The quality of the basic staple is far less important if the diet contains generous amounts of the protective foods: milk, eggs, meat, beans, nuts, and vegetables.

The energy (caloric) density of foods refers to the amount of energy per weight of food. It is an important consideration in infant and child nutrition as well as in repletion of malnourished children. When the staple food is bulky (i.e., high in fiber and/or water) and low in fat, such as cassava or the lower quality cereals, the child may not be able physically to consume enough to meet energy needs. For example, a 4- to 6-year-old child would have to eat 1.7 kg of maize tortillas per day to fulfill 80 percent of his or her energy requirement.

An extension of this concept concerns the protein, vitamin, and mineral density of food. With many mixed diets, the amount of food necessary to satisfy energy requirements will also contain adequate amounts of essential nutrients. However, diets based heavily on low-protein staples and diets in which a large part of the energy is derived from refined fats and oils and sugar may be lacking in this regard, especially for small children and the aged.

REPLETION OF MALNOURISHED INDIVIDUALS

When severe malnutrition is identified, acute-phase repletion is best handled in a hospital situation. An understanding of the physiological disturbances associated with protein-energy malnutrition is essential. Dehydration, infection, and anemia with cardiac and renal dysfunction must be addressed, and rehydration and restoration of electrolyte balance must be accomplished with frequent monitoring. Ashworth [25] has reported the successful treatment methods used in Jamaica. When oral feeding is reinitiated, small, frequent meals with low initial protein levels are recommended. Catch-up growth after a period of malnutrition or infection is based on reestablishing the proper weight for height. Catch-up growth requires a high-energy and nutritious diet.

The real problem with repletion of malnourished children occurs when they resume the family diet. If their dietary intake and health conditions are not altered, they will more than likely return shortly to the malnourished state. Therefore, proper repletion requires education of the parents in the preparation of the most appropriate, economical combination of locally available foods to fulfill the child's energy and protein requirements regularly.

CONCLUSION

For optimal function, the human body requires water and certain amounts of nutrients that are provided by consumption of foods. While some measure of adaptation to low intakes is possible through regulation of absorption and excretion, inadequate food intakes lead to growth retardation and a wide range of physiological, psychological, and social dysfunctions. The demands of growth in infants, young children, and pregnant and lactating women as well as the social and cultural habits of food allocation put these groups at most risk for development of malnutrition. Nutritional rehabilitation and prevention of deficiency require overall consideration of the social-environmental system in which the malnutrition is created.

REFERENCES

1 Briggs GM, Calloway DH: *Nutrition and Physical Fitness,* 11th ed. New York, Holt, Rinehart and Winston, 1984

2 FAO/WHO: Carbohydrates in Human Nutrition. FAO Food and Nutrition Paper no 15, Rome, 1980

3 FAO/WHO: Dietary Fats and Oils in Human Nutrition. FAO Food and Nutrition Ser no 20, Rome, 1980

4 FAO/WHO/UNU: Energy and Protein Requirements. WHO Tech Rep Ser 724, Geneva, 1985

5 International Union of Nutritional Science: Report of Committee on International Dietary Allowances. Nutr Abstr Rev 45:89–111, 1975

6 FAO/WHO: Requirements of Vitamin A, Thiamine, Riboflavin and Niacin. FAO Nutrition Meetings Rep Ser no 41, Rome, 1967

7 FAO/WHO: Requirements of Ascorbic Acid, Vitamin D, Vitamin B-12, Folate, and Iron. FAO Nutrition Meetings Rep Ser no 47, Rome, 1970

8 FAO/WHO: Calcium Requirements. FAO Nutrition Meetings Rep Ser no 30, Rome 1962

9 FAO/WHO: Requirements of Vitamin A, Iron, Folate and Vitamin B-12, in press

10 WHO: Trace Elements in Human Nutrition. WHO Tech Rep Ser 532, Geneva, WHO, 1973

11 Food and Nutrition Board: *Recommended Dietary Allowances,* 9th ed. Washington, DC, National Research Council, 1979

12 Rosenberg IH, Scrimshaw NS (eds): Proceedings of a workshop on malabsorption and nutrition. Am J Clin Nutr 25:1046–1133; 1226–1289, 1979

13 Levander OA, Cheng L (eds): *Micronutrient Interactions: Vitamins, Minerals and Hazardous Elements.* New York, New York Academy of Science, 1980

14 McClain CJ, Van Theil DH, Parker S, et al: Alterations in zinc, vitamin A, and retinol binding protein in chronic alcoholics: A possible mechanism for night blindness and hypogonadism. Alcoholism Clin Exp Res 3:135–141, 1979

15 Baker H, Frank O, Zetterman RK, et al: Inability of chronic alcoholics with liver disease to use food as a source of folates, thiamin, and vitamin B-6. Am J Clin Nutr 28:1377–1380, 1975

16 Christakis G (ed): Nutritional assessment in health programs. Am J Public Health 63(suppl):34–35, 1973

17 Martorell R, Habicht J-P: Growth in early childhood in developing countries, in Falkner F, Tanner JM (eds): *Human Growth, A Comprehensive Treatise,* 2d ed. New York, Plenum, 1986, pp 241–262

18 WHO: A Growth Chart for International Use in Maternal and Child Health Care: Guidelines for Primary Health Care Personnel. Geneva, WHO, 1978

19 Waterlow JC: Classification and definition of protein-energy malnutrition, in Beaton GH, Bengoa JM (eds): *Nutrition in Preventive Medicine.* Geneva, WHO, 1975

20 Sommer A, Lowenstein MS: Nutritional status and mortality: A prospective validate of the QUAC stick. Am J Clin Nutr 28:287–292, 1975

21 Food and Nutrition Board: Nutrient adequacy: Assessment using food consumption surveys. Washington, DC, National Academy Press, 1986

22 Food and Nutrition Board: Diet and Health: Implications for reducing chronic disease risk. Washington, DC, National Academy Press, 1989

23 Poirier LA, Newborne PM, Pariza MW (eds): Essential nutrients in carcinogenesis, New York, Plenum, 1986

24 Shils ME, Young VR (eds): *Modern Nutrition in Health and Disease,* 7th ed. Philadelphia, Lea & Febiger, 1988

25 Ashworth A: Progress in the treatment of protein-energy malnutrition. Proc Nutr Soc 38:89–97, 1979

CHAPTER 23 / *Nutrition and Infection* · Leonardo Mata

The association of famine and pestilence has been recognized since the beginning of history, but it was not until the late 1950s that it was scientifically documented [1]. The presence of infectious disease was also noted in the early accounts of kwashiorkor, but its role in the genesis of malnutrition was generally overlooked until synergistic and antagonistic interactions between malnutrition and infection were recognized [1]. *Synergism* is when malnutrition exacerbates the outcome of infection and infection aggravates nutritional deficiency: the outcome is assumed to be greater than the summation of both effects. This interaction occurs frequently in populations of developing countries in which infectious diseases are highly prevalent and diets are often deficient. In contrast, *antagonism* results when a deficiency in one or more nutrients impairs the replication of an infectious agent. This can be demonstrated in the laboratory, but it rarely occurs in nature; it may be observed, for instance, under extreme nutritional deprivation [2].

Long-term field studies in deprived rural societies have revealed the importance of the interactions of nutrition and infection in determining morbidity, growth failure, acute malnutrition, and mortality [3–5]. In such societies, growth faltering generally begins at about 3 to 6 months among infants at the breast or even earlier among those prematurely weaned to the bottle [4,6]. It is not yet clear if stunting is primarily related to inadequate food supplementation when mother's milk becomes insufficient or is related to infectious disease or to an association of both. While a decrease in the supply of human milk without proper supplementation is common in developing societies, the striking event during weaning is the repeated occurrence of infectious diseases [4].

CLINICAL AND LABORATORY STUDIES

ANIMAL MODELS

Experimental animals deprived of calories, protein, vitamins, amino acids, or trace elements show increased clinical responses to viruses, rickettsias, bacteria, and protozoa. The course of infection is more severe, more prolonged, and more lethal than in control well-nourished animals [1]. Enhanced clinical responses relate to alterations in host-specific and nonspecific immune competence. On the other hand, infectious organisms are capable of altering the nutritional state of animals inoculated by natural or unnatural routes. Animal studies, fundamental for understanding nutrition-infection interactions, may not be applicable to human situations because (1) artifical nutritional deficiencies that lead to host resistance in experimental animals do not easily occur in human populations; and (2) type, dose, specificity, and route of infection used in animal models are not those observed naturally in humans.

THE HUMAN HOST

Clinical studies in confined volunteers demonstrated that virtually all metabolic pathways are altered during the course of infection. Viral, rickettsial, bacterial, and parasitic infections diminish appetite, increase catabolism after the anabolic phase, and induce metabolic alterations leading to nutrient overutilization, nutrient wastage, nutrient sequestration and nutrient diversion [7]. Abnormalities occur even with mild or asymptomatic infections. There are absolute losses of nitrogen, sodium, potassium, bicarbonate, chloride, and phosphate in systemic infections [7]. There is also increased synthesis of liver enzymes and of acute-phase reactant proteins (nutrient diversion) and a decrease of circulating trace elements (zinc, iron and copper) and concentration in hepatic cells (nutrient sequestration).

EFFECT OF NUTRITION ON RESISTANCE

Intrauterine growth retardation impairs immune competence, and small-for-gestational-age infants exhibit a higher incidence of infection and mortality in the first years of life [4,8]. Breast-feeding is the most important defense barrier against infection in the first months of life [6]. Other defense mechanisms are gastric acidity, intestinal motility, intestinal microflora, and immune response and its amplification [9]. Well-nourished individuals better withstand dehydration, nutrient losses, and other infection-induced alterations.

In postnatal undernutrition, whether of nutritional origin (as in famine) or due to nutrition-infection interactions (the most common form in developing countries) there are alterations in integrity of skin and mucosae, hypochlorhydria, and abnormalities in intestinal microbiota. Severely malnourished children may exhibit decreased lymphoid cells, impaired function of T and B lymphocytes, and diminished synthesis of complement and secretory IgA [8,9]. Undernourished children experience greater severity, chronicity, and mortality due to infections. Duration of disease and the carrier state of certain agents is generally longer in undernourished as compared to well-nourished individuals [1,4].

With severe food deprivation, depletion of host stores may actually suppress infection, and starved individuals can develop acute infectious disease upon nutritional recuperation [2]. While acute infections generally enhance immunity, some agents, e.g., measles, commonly induce secondary immunodeficiency [10]. The important public health implications of infections in the undernourished are enhanced symptoms, duration, the precipitation of acute protein-energy malnutrition, and augmented mortality from the two processes [1,4,11].

EFFECT OF INFECTION ON NUTRITION AND GROWTH

Epidemiological evidence shows that infection is the most important factor inducing malnutrition and growth retardation in less developed societies. In these, high rates of infection are determined by deficient social, cultural, and economic conditions which favor deficient sanitation and poor personal hygiene.

PRENATAL LIFE

Infections with viruses, bacteria, and protozoa in the pregnant woman may reach the placenta and fetus. The risk of maternal infection is enhanced by physiological alterations during gestation. The risk for the fetus is low, and not more than 2 percent of infants are infected; this increases during epidemics, for instance, of rubella, and is particularly worrisome in populations affected by acquired immunodeficiency syndrome (AIDS). Intrauterine or intrapartum infection may not result in clinical manifestation in the mother or fetus; in a few cases, however, there is interruption of pregnancy, preterm delivery, fetal growth retardation, embryopathy, overt disease in the infant, or acute or chronic sequelae [12]. Mechanisms include decreased placental blood flow, permeability to metabolites and antigens, decreased cell multiplication, cell proliferation, inflammation, and necrosis.

Maternal infection is significantly more frequent in traditional than in industrial societies [4]. In poor urban and rural areas, high levels of cord IgM as well as intrauterine infections occur in greater frequency than in populations with better conditions [4,12]. For instance, in Guatemala, Peru, and Colombia, a high proportion of newborns have high levels of serum IgM [13,14], suggesting common fetal antigenic stimulation; this, in turn, might be related to fetal growth retardation. Such greater occurrence, however, does not explain the high incidence of prematurity and fetal growth retardation observed in deprived populations throughout the world, which may reach as much as 40 percent [4]. The finding, however, deserves scrutiny, as an alternative hypothesis to that of inadequate diet in the mother. The effects of food supplements during pregnancy on pregnancy outcome are not striking.

POSTNATAL LIFE

Early neonatal infection

During exclusive breast-feeding, infections with *Giardia, Entamoeba histolytica, Shigella,* and *Salmonella* are rare and usually asymptomatic [4]. With weaning, infection increases to high rates by the end of the first year and particularly during the second and third years of life. Multiple and chronic infections are more often seen at these ages. Virus shedding occurs as early as the first weeks of life, increases in the second semester, and in the second and third years constitutes a virtual "viral flora" [4,15].

The implications of excessive infections are (1) precocious development of serum IgG and IgM to very high levels in the first year of life; and (2) damage to the intestinal mucosa resulting in inflammation and malabsorption. [4].

Infectious disease

High morbidity rates become obvious in individual growth charts of children in the first 3 years of life (Fig. 23-1). Infectious diseases are exceedingly common; in Sta. Maria Cauqué, Guatemala, children averaged seven episodes per year in the first 3 years of life [4,16]. Respiratory and diarrheal disease were most common in infancy. The latter increases with age to reach the highest incidence in the second year of life. Infections induce anorexia, nutrient losses, metabolic alterations,

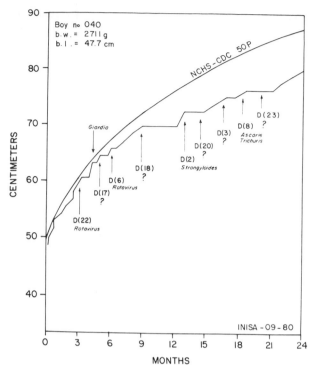

Figure 23-1. Growth curve, diarrheal episodes, and enteric agents of a Cauqué child who exhibited adequate fetal development. Length followed the 50th percentile of the National Center for Health Statistics reference curve up to 6 months of age; thereafter, growth faltering resulted in stunting evident at 1 year of age [*24*]. All diarrheas were associated with periods of stunting which were of short duration during exclusive breast-feeding (the first 5 months of life), and lasted longer during weaning. Growth faltering was observed regardless of etiological agent involved. b.w. = birth weight; b.l. = birth length; D = diarrheal disease; ? = agent not diagnosed.

hormonal imbalances and alterations in immune function (see Chap. 24) and lead to wasting, stunting, acute malnutrition and death.

Reduced food consumption

In enteric disease, anorexia, fever, diarrhea, and vomiting are important causes of reduced food consumption by village children [*4,15*]. Food withdrawal and inappropriate treatment and feeding during convalescence are common responses derived from cultural tradition, taboos, and beliefs and further reduce dietary intake. Energy and protein consumption are reduced by 20 to 60 percent during infectious disease. As much as 16 percent of the overall dietary calories and 18 percent of the protein may not be consumed by weaned children as a result of diarrhea [*15*]. This is more significant in regions where food consumption is already below 80 percent of the recommended level. Profound anorexia is found in acute respiratory disease, whooping cough, and measles, but some reduction in food

consumption is observed even with mild infections like the common cold.

Altered digestive-absorptive processes

Diarrhea accelerates transit through the intestinal tract, potentially interfering with food digestion. The mucosal surface can be physiologically altered by *Giardia* or bacteria, or it may be structurally damaged by invading viruses, bacteria, and parasites. Microscopic jejunal mucosal lesions concurrent with bacterial colonization are seen in persons living in the tropics [*16*]; jejunitis and the accompanying malabsorption of sugar, fats, and vitamins disappear spontaneously in such individuals when they move to a more protected environment with better sanitation [*17*]. Bacterial enterotoxins stimulate formation of cAMP and cGMP, impairing "net absorption" of sodium and water [*18*]. Certain bacteria split bile salts, reducing micelle formation and fat absorption and increasing the bile acid pool, which irritates the mucosa; microbial overgrowth in the small intestine is related to malnutrition in children [*4*]. Dehydration is a serious consequence of diarrhea or other febrile processes, and, if brisk, may lead to obtundation and death within a matter of hours in the already malnourished child. Rehydration results in prompt return to normality and has a profound influence on recuperation from nutritional sequelae.

Altered immune response

Infectious agents may alter one or more cell types and functions of the immune system [*1,2,4,7,10*]. Viral infections depress the immune system, inducing anergy. The most severe effects, however, are those mediated by replication of the human immunodeficiency virus (HIV) within CD4 lymphocytes, macrophages, and Langerhans cells. Progressive depletion of CD4 lymphocytes favors replication of opportunistic agents and tumors, resulting in AIDS [*19*].

Wasting and stunting effect

Repetitive infectious bouts result in progressive deterioration of nutritional status, manifested as weight faltering and impaired linear growth. Such changes are evident in growth curves of breast-fed children of Sta. Maria Cauqué village, who were observed prospectively from birth to school age [*4,15*]. The rate of low-birth-weight babies in this population was around 40 percent.

In general, growth velocity during exclusive breast-feeding (3 to 6 months) in these Mayan Indian children was comparable to that of reference curves of the National Center for Health Statistics (NCHS). Onset of supplementary feeding was associated with growth faltering. In infants maintained at the breast for prolonged periods, there was subtle starvation; however, the striking alterations in growth during weaning more often than not reflected documented infectious diseases, particularly diarrhea. The origin of infection was primarily from weaning foods contaminated with pathogens [*15*] or contaminated hands, water, and utensils.

Figure 23-1 shows body length, enteric infections, and episodes of diarrhea of a typical child who had adequate fetal growth. Diarrheas were associated with stagnation in linear growth, regardless of infectious etiology. Acute weight loss (5 to 10 percent) was common. Wasting (deficit of weight for height greater than 80 percent) persisted for weeks or months, contributing to the genesis of marasmus [*4*] and was complicated in some instances by inadequate feeding during convalescence. Wasting and stunting also occur in conjunction with other diseases, notably measles and pertussis. Growth impairment was greater if infants had fetal growth retardation or had been prematurely weaned.

Severe malnutrition

Undernourished children become critically ill after acute watery diarrhea, dysentery, measles, pertussis, and other infectious diseases, often accompanied by social and psychological stress or neglect [*20*]. Sudden falls in serum albumin after measles, hookworm, and diarrhea may usher in clinical kwashiorkor [*21*]; a protein-losing enteropathy has been recognized in rotavirus and *Shigella* diarrheas [*22*]. Severe malnutrition may develop weeks after bouts of diarrhea, measles, or malaria, often quite independently of food availability.

Infectious disease may be especially virulent in malnourished children who are weak and failing to grow well, who are born premature or with fetal growth retardation, or who suffer from immunological, genetic, or other degenerative disorders. With inadequate or absent family, maternal technology [*23,24*], health services, and oral rehydration therapy (ORT), infectious diseases become the main factors inducing malnutrition and death in children in developing countries.

SUMMARY AND CONCLUSIONS

Attempts to intervene in these complex interacting events must be based on an understanding of pathogenesis. It has been difficult in field studies to demonstrate that malnutrition increases susceptibility to infection. Clearly, infection depends on the frequency of host exposure to infectious agents, and high acquisition rates of infection in tropical regions are largely due to the level of microbial contamination in the environment and inadequate host hygiene.

Infection has negative effects on the pregnant woman, the fetus, infant, and young child; its results are growth retardation, morbidity, malnutrition, and often death. The role of infection as a determinant of malnutrition in developing countries is certain. Even when poor village children consume adequate calories and protein during disease-free episodes, infection reduces food consumption.

The nutritional damage inflicted by infection is enhanced by inappropriate child care, lack of prompt use of ORT for diarrhea or of treatment for other infections, and inadequate feeding during convalescence [*23*]. Recurrent diarrhea, anorexia, and fever—coupled with poor diets and hygiene—lead to marasmus and/or kwashiorkor. The risk of death increases for preterm infants and those small for gestational age [*4*], particularly if they have become wasted and/or stunted [*4,11*]. The well-nourished child, however, is also at risk of death from infectious disease if the environment is hostile. Survivors tend to remain stunted, and women previously undernourished may, in turn, give birth to preterm and growth-retarded neonates, perpetuating the dreadful cycle.

Field studies emphasize the need to improve environmental sanitation, personal hygiene, and child-rearing practices, using a holistic approach, for promotion of children's nutrition and health. However, populations suffering from acute food shortages represent an exception, and food distribution should be the first priority.

A practical way of knowing whether to choose infection or diet as the target of intervention in a given ecosystem is to assess the prevalence of undernutrition and mortality. If an excess occurrence of malnutrition and death is observed for all ages and social classes, then food probably is the limiting factor, as, for instance, during famines. The common constraint in developing countries, however, does not appear to be food intake, because even in very poor villages, children frequently consume more than 90 percent of the recommended calories and protein. In such cases, undernutrition is generally restricted to infants and young children, and occasionally to the very old and feeble. In these instances, the greater importance of infection is apparent.

Epidemiological evidence shows that control and prevention of infectious disease, particularly diarrhea, correlate with improved nutrition, growth, and survival [*24*]. It is expected that widespread application of ORT, improved water supplies, expanded primary health services (immunization, family planning), and health education will improve nutrition worldwide without unjustified emphasis on food distribution programs except for populations affected by a proven shortage in supplies.

REFERENCES

1 Scrimshaw NS, Taylor CE, Gordon JE: Interactions of nutrition and infection. Am J Med Sci 237:367–403, 1959.

2 Murray MJ, Murray AB: Starvation suppression and refeeding activation of infection. Lancet i:123–125, 1977

3 McGregor IA, Rahman AK, Thomson AM, et al: The health of young children in a West African (Gambian) village. Trans R Soc Trop Med Hyg 64:48–77, 1970

4 Mata LJ: *The Children of Santa Maria Cauqué: A Prospective Field Study of Health and Growth.* Cambridge, MIT Press, 1978

5 Whitehead RG, Coward WA, Lunn PG, et al: A comparison of the pathogenesis of protein-energy malnutrition in Uganda and the Gambia. Trans R Soc Trop Med Hyg 71:189–195, 1977

6 Jellife DB, Jellife EFP: *Human Milk in the Modern World: Psychosocial, Nutritional, and Economic Significance.* Oxford University Press, 1978

7 Beisel WR: Magnitude of the host nutritional responses to infection. Am J Clin Nutr 30:1236–1247, 1977

8 Chandra RK, Newberne PM: *Nutrition, Immunity and Infection: Mechanisms of Interactions*. New York, Plenum, 1977

9 DuPont HL, Pickering LK: *Infections of the Gastrointestinal Tract. Microbiology, Pathophysiology and Clinical Features*. New York, Plenum, 1980

10 Targett GAT: Malnutrition and immunity to protozoan parasites, in Isliker H, Schurch B (eds): *The Impact of Malnutrition on Immune Defense in Parasitic Infestation*. Bern, Has Huber, 1980, pp 158–179

11 Chen LC, Alauddin-Chowdhury AKM, Huffman SL: Anthropometric assessment of energy-protein malnutrition and subsequent risk of mortality among preschool-aged children. Am J Clin Nutr 33:1836–1845, 1980

12 Alford CA, Foft JW, Blankenship WJ, et al: Subclinical central nervous system disease of neonates: A prospective study of infants born with increased levels of IgM. J Pediatr 75:1167–1178, 1969

13 Mata L, Urrutia JJ, Serrato G, et al: Viral infections during pregnancy and early life. Am J Clin Nutr 30:1834–1842, 1977

14 McMurray DN, De Aly AC, Rey H: Serum IgM as an indicator of intrauterine infection in Colombian newborns. Bull Pan Am Health Organ 14:376–385, 1980

15 Mata LJ, Kronmal RA, Urrutia JJ, et al: Effect of infection on food intake and the nutritional state: Perspectives as viewed from the village. Am J Clin Nutr 30:1215–1227, 1977

16 Gangarosa EJ, Beisel WR, Benyajati C, et al: The nature of the gastrointestinal lesions in Asiatic cholera and its relation to pathogenesis: A biologic study. Am J Trop Med 9:125–135, 1971

17 Lindebaum J, Gerson CD, Kent TH: Recovery of small-intestinal structure and function after residence in the tropics. I. Studies in Peace Corps volunteers. Ann Intern Med 74:218–222, 1971

18 Field M: Intestinal transport of water and electrolytes, in McClung HJ (ed): *Etiology, Pathophysiology, and Treatment of Acute Gastroenteritis*. Columbus, Ross Laboratories, 1978, pp. 57–61

19 Gotlieb MS: Immunologic aspects of the acquired immunodeficiency syndrome and male homosexuality, in Cooney TG, Ward TT (eds): *AIDS and Other Medical Problems in the Male Homosexual*. Philadelphia, Saunders, pp 651–664

20 Goodall J: Malnutrition and the family: Deprivation in kwashiorkor. Proc Nutr Soc 38:17–28, 1979

21 Whitehead RG: Infection and how it influences the pathogenesis of protein-energy malnutrition, in Isliker H, Schurch B (eds): *The Impact of Malnutrition on Immune Defense in Parasitic Infestation*. Bern, Hans Huber, 1981, pp 15–25

22 Wahed A, Rahaman MM, Gilman RH, et al: Protein-losing enteropathy in diarrhea: Application of alpha one antitrypsin assay. Dhaka, International Centre for Diarrhoeal Disease Research, Bangladesh, 1981

23 Mata L: The malnutrition-infection complex and its environment factors. Proc Nutr Soc 38: 29–40, 1979

24 Mata L: Malnutrition and concurrent infections: Comparison of two populations with different infection rates, in MacKenzie JS (ed): *Viral Diseases in South-East Asia and the Western Pacific*. Sydney, Australia, Academic, 1982, pp 56–76

CHAPTER
24

Nutrition and Immune Function

Gerald T. Keusch

The frequency of infectious diseases among the people in the developing world is astounding. The reasons for this enormous morbidity and mortality are well described in ecological terms in the preceding discussion (Chap. 23) by Leonardo Mata. Faced with constant exposure to pathogenic organisms, each individual must mobilize host defenses to the maximum in order to survive the onslaught. In the process, host metabolism is significantly altered to a catabolic state in which muscle stores of protein and lipid from fat depots are consumed, resulting in a transient malnutrition. Unless these deficits are restored during convalescence, there will be long-lasting nutritional consequences. Unfortunately, it is now quite certain that the various forms of malnutrition prevalent among the same developing world populations adversely affect the functioning of the immune system. Thus, it is almost inevitable that a cyclical interaction develops in which infection results in malnutrition, in turn impairing host defenses and increasing susceptibility to infection. These interactions, described as

synergistic, were first clearly recognized by Scrimshaw, Taylor, and Gordon [1].

Investigations of nutrition–immune function interactions have been conducted in both humans and experimental animals. It must be recognized that human malnutrition is more complex than experimental deficiencies in animal models. For example, malnutrition in humans is rarely of a single nutrient, is usually complicated by other stress such as infection, and generally develops irregularly over time, unlike the steady and controlled process imposed upon an experimental model. All of these features can alter the apparent immunological impact of changes in nutritional state in humans.

ALTERED HOST METABOLISM IN INFECTION

For unclear physiological reasons, the infected host changes his or her pattern of behavior and metabolism, as if guided by the principle that there will be no food available, and, in fact, anorexia (or loss of appetite) is one of the early manifestations of infection [2]. To meet the energy needs, glucose is produced from endogenous stores, while body protein is broken down to provide amino acids for new protein synthesis [3]. A remarkable synchrony in these events permits surprising efficiency in the reutilization of substrates. For example, proteolysis of muscle releases amino acids which are taken up by the liver and used for conversion to glucose (by gluconeogenic pathways) as well as for synthesis of host proteins used in the inflammatory response. These proteins, known collectively as acute phase reactants, include complement components, various enzyme inhibitors, and transport or binding proteins for a few minerals that appear to play a role in host responses to infection, such as iron, zinc, and copper [2,4].

One of the most common signs of infection is fever, which increases energy demands in a predictable fashion, no matter how it is induced, even by enclosing subjects in a heat chamber [3]. In septic patients, resting energy expenditures can increase by as much as 40 percent. Behavioral changes compensate for this in part, and the host becomes sleepy and usually will reduce voluntary activity to conserve energy as much as possible. Metabolically, muscle now relies on in situ oxidation of branched-chain amino acids released by muscle proteolysis, as "functional insulin resistance" reduces glucose uptake in the tissue [3]. To further compensate for new protein synthesis (including proliferation and production of immunologically competent cells and proteins and the other acute phase reactants) the synthesis of less critical proteins, such as albumin or transferrin, is shut off, resulting in hypoalbuminemia and hypotransferrinemia, two clinical hallmarks of infection [2,3].

These events are regulated by small peptides (cytokines) that are released from infected macrophages and other cells (Fig. 24-1) [5]. In addition to their metabolic role, they also function to regulate the immune response [6]. The regulator proteins include interleukin 1 (IL-1), IL-6, and cachectin/tumor necrosis factor (C/TNF). IL-1 is the principal endogenous pyrogen causing fever [7], as well as a critical regulator of T lymphocytes because it can induce the T-cell IL-2 (T-cell growth factor) receptor and stimulate synthesis of IL-2 [5]. Human IL-1, a 17,000-MW peptide, has been cloned as well as expressed. It has many metabolic properties (Table 24-1), at least some of which are due to its ability to increase production of prostaglandin E2.

Some events triggered by production and release of IL-1 are secondary to IL-1 induction of the synthesis of other cytokines, for example, IL-1 induction of IL-2 in the activation of T-cell responses [6]. IL-1 also activates B cells for antibody production, a property now known to be due to induction of other cytokines acting on the B cell, including IL-3 and IL-6 [5]. IL-6 has metabolic effects as well. It is a potent activator of the hepatic acute phase protein response [8], and it may be the actual regulator of some events now attributed directly to IL-1.

In addition, lipid metabolism is often altered in infection.

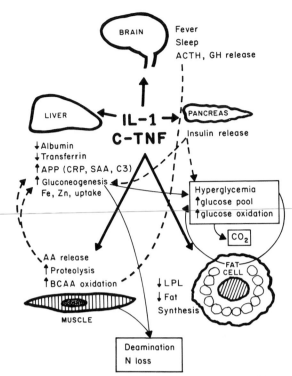

Figure 24-1. Schematic diagram of the tissue targets (bold arrows) for interleukin 1 (IL-1) and cachectin/tumor necrosis factor (C/TNF) in the metabolic response to infection. The tissue responses are listed and interactive pathways are shown by fine arrows. The dashed arrows show the roles of hormonal intermediates in the metabolic responses listed.

Clearance of fatty acids from plasma [9] and fat synthesis by adipocytes and utilization of ketones [10] may be impaired. The hypertriglyceridemia is due to depression of lipoprotein lipase activity, whereas impaired fat synthesis is due to a reduction in the anabolic enzymes. A powerful cytokine regulatory mechanism for these events has been uncovered in the past few years [11]. This molecule, first named *cachectin* be-

Table 24-1. Metabolic effects of interleukin 1 or IL-1 fragments

Results in fever (endogenous pyrogen)
Induces slow wave sleep
Alters appetite (anorexia)
Increases central ACTH and growth hormone release
Increases insulin release from pancreatic islets
Leads to muscle proteolysis and amino acid release
Enhances hepatic amino acid uptake, upregulates acute phase protein synthesis, and downregulates albumin and transferrin synthesis
Decreases plasma Fe/Zn
Accelerates hepatic gluconeogenesis
Inhibits lipoprotein lipase production and adipocyte fat synthesis

cause of its ability to deplete lipid stores and cause weight loss, is a macrophage product similar in molecular weight to IL-1. With purification and sequencing of its primary structure, its identity with a previously described factor, tumor necrosis factor (TNF), was demonstrated. C/TNF acts to inhibit activation of the genes for lipoprotein lipase and the lipid anabolic enzymes without affecting transcription of genes for other proteins [12]. As a consequence, mRNA for these enzymes is not made and the enzymes cannot be produced.

Another example of metabolic shifts in infection is the rapid uptake of plasma iron and zinc by liver and mononuclear cells and the release of copper-ceruloplasmin [3]. These changes are due to (1) the release of lactoferrin from granulocytes under the control of IL-1, which leads to uptake of iron-lactoferrin complexes by the liver, (2) IL-1-enhanced synthesis of metallothionine, the intracellular zinc-binding protein, and (3) the cytokine-mediated upregulation of synthesis of the acute phase protein ceruloplasmin, which carries copper into circulation [2]. The resulting hypoferremia may protect the host from the infection by depriving invading microorganisms of iron needed for growth and production of virulence factors; the uptake of zinc may prime the proliferative response of lymphocytes, since the key DNA synthetic enzymes are all zinc metalloenzymes; while the circulating copper ceruloplasmin may mitigate the adverse effects of hypoferremia on erythropoiesis by means of its ferrioxidase enzyme activity, which increases the efficiency of iron uptake for hemoglobin synthesis by red cell precursors.

THE T LYMPHOCYTE AND CELL-MEDIATED IMMUNITY

PROTEIN-ENERGY MALNUTRITION (PEM)

The most common nutritional problem in the world is deficiency in dietary intake of protein, energy, or both. PEM occurs in two related forms, kwashiorkor, a greater relative deprivation in protein, and marasmus, a more balanced deficit in both protein and energy (see Chap. 118). Immune deficits are more frequent, diverse, and severe in kwashiorkor [2].

The first link between PEM and altered cell-mediated immunity came from studies demonstrating diminished tuberculin responsiveness in malnourished individuals with active tuberculosis following bacillus Calmette-Guérin (BCG) immunization or living in a highly endemic area for *Mycobacterium tuberculosis* [4]. Numerous studies in the past decade have demonstrated that the absolute number and percentage of mature peripheral E (erythrocyte)-rosetting T lymphocytes in circulation is diminished in kwashiorkor patients and to a variable extent in marasmic individuals [4]. In contrast the proportion of B lymphocytes, assessed by the presence of surface immunoglobulin or C3b receptors on B cells, is normal [4,13]. As a result there is an increase in a population of non-T, non-B cells possessing neither the E rosette nor surface Ig markers (null cells). Some evidence suggests that these are immature cells of the T lineage. For example, there is a 10-fold increase in the activity of terminal deoxynucleotidyl transferase (Tdt) in peripheral blood lymphocytes from PEM children compared to well-nourished age- and sex-matched controls [13]. Tdt activity is a marker for pre- or intrathymic T cells and correlates significantly with the proportion of null cells in individual subjects. Second, these null cells express natural cytotoxic (NC) activity to cultured mouse (DBA/2) fibroblasts [14]. Third, thymic hormones increase the expression of mature T-cell markers in vitro in PEM peripheral blood lymphocytes [15].

These alterations in circulating T-lymphocyte populations are associated with thymic abnormalities consisting of a marked depletion of thymocytes, especially from the cortex, with relative prominence of epithelial and reticular tissues, loss of differentiation between cortex and medulla, and a decrease in Hassall's corpuscles [4]. Spleen, tonsil, and lymph node also demonstrate changes in regions populated by T cells, including paracortical and periarteriolar collections, with preservation of B-lymphocyte-rich germinal centers and primary follicles. Thymic hormones incubated in vitro with peripheral blood lymphocytes from malnourished children result in a significant induction of the E-rosette marker in PEM patients with decreased numbers of circulating mature T cells [15].

As a consequence, functional tests of peripheral blood lymphocytes are abnormal in PEM [4]. The most commonly reported defect is a depression in the proliferative response to mitogenic lectins such as phytohemagglutinin (PHA). The PHA response is uniformly blunted in kwashiorkor, whether assessed as the morphological transformation of unstimulated small lymphocytes to large, blastic proliferating cells, or as the incorporation of [³H] thymidine into DNA. In contrast, studies in marasmic individuals are often, but not always, normal, indicating a difference in the ability of the protein-deprived individual to support a proliferative response of activated lymphocytes in contrast to the less severe limitations in the marasmic patient. However, cellular proliferation is of fundamental importance to immune responses since clonal expansion of specifically responsive cells is the heart of the system.

PEM also reduces delayed type skin test responsivity to recall antigens and diminishes the incidence of positive reactions to sensitization with BCG or dinitrochlorobenzene (DNCB). PPD or DNCB reactivity correlates with plasma albumin levels, indicating that the most severe defect is likely to be in the kwashiorkor patient. The afferent (sensitization) limb appears to be functional, however, since repeat challenge when the nutritional deficits are corrected is often positive, even without repeat sensitization doses [16]. The failure of the delayed type hypersensitivity (DTH) response is therefore explainable by several possible mechanisms: limited proliferative responses, reduced mediator production, or defective inflammatory reactions in response to lymphokines. Reduced proliferative capacity to respond to PHA has already been noted, and lymphokine production in PEM is reduced in response to appropriate stimuli. The inflammatory response in skin per se may also be depressed due to cellular or humoral chemotactic defects or both.

MINERAL AND VITAMIN DEFICIENCIES

Figure 24-2 indicates the presumed locus of action of several specific nutrients on T lymphocytes. Studies primarily in animal models suggest that zinc deficiency may mimic the central effects of PEM on the thymus [4,17]. This may be because many of the enzymes needed for proliferative responses (including thymidine kinase, DNA polymerase, and DNA-dependent RNA polymerase), as well as thymic hormone factors and terminal deoxynucleotidyl transferase, are zinc-containing metallopeptides. Limited human studies are consistent with this mechanism [4]. Iron deficiency in humans appears to affect peripheral blood T lymphocytes, reducing both E-rosette formation and PHA responsiveness, as well as DTH responses [4,17]. In vitro responses to PHA are restored by addition of iron salts to the medium. Modulation of E-rosetting and mixed lymphocyte responses by addition of iron in vitro has also been shown. These effects may relate to receptors on the lymphocyte surface for iron, ferritin, or transferrin. Copper deficiency may impair the generation by T helper cells of the lymphokine interleukin 2 (IL-2), necessary for the induction of cytotoxic effector cells and B-cell response to T-dependent antigens [4,18].

Vitamin A in supplemental doses seems to function as an immunoadjuvant in the generation of cytotoxic T-cell responses in animals [4]. States of vitamin A deficiency have not been well studied, but in animals appear to affect both T- and B-cell maturation. B vitamin deficiencies, particularly of pyridoxine, reduce the antibody response to T-dependent antigens [4] and suppress DTH response to PPD as well as the granulomatous response to *Schistosoma mansoni* eggs. These defects may in part be localized to the thymus, as evidenced by the failure of thymic epithelium from pyridoxine-deficient mice to induce functional differentiation of T-cell precursors in vitro [19]. In contrast, normal thymic epithelium induces precursors from normal or pyridoxine-deficient animals equally well. Vitamin C has been studied in both deficiency and supplementation states [4,17]. Deficiency induces a T-cell lesion affecting the generation of cytotoxic effectors in vivo and in vitro, and impairs the DTH response to PPD, but not antibody production to T-dependent antigens.

THE B LYMPHOCYTE AND ANTIBODY RESPONSES

PROTEIN-ENERGY MALNUTRITION

Serum antibody responses to vaccines used as probes for antibody production in human PEM have been variously reported to be normal or depressed [4,20]. Some antigens, such as tetanus toxoid, reliably induce a protective antibody response, even in severe PEM. The response to other protein antigens, for example, flagellin, may be suboptimal unless a dietary protein supplement is fed at the time of immunization. Antibody to either the protein H antigen or polysaccharide O antigen of *Salmonella typhi* is often depressed in PEM and may also be enhanced by protein supplements [20]. The frequent impairment of the antibody response to the T-independent polysaccharide O antigen suggests a defect at the level of the antigen presenting cell.

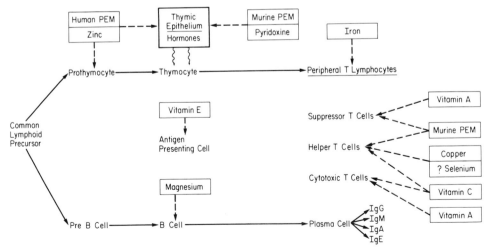

Figure 24-2. Localization of the effects of nutrients on the immunological network. This diagram is based on human and experimental animal studies, extensively reviewed in [2]. *(Reproduced with permission from G.T. Keusch, C.S. Wilson, S.D. Waksal: Nutrition, host defenses and the lymphoid system, in J.J. Gallin, A.S. Fauci (eds.): Advances in Host Defense Mechanisms, vol. 2, New York, Plenum, 1982.)*

Nevertheless, B-cell numbers in circulation and in B-cell regions of peripheral lymphoid organs are only minimally altered, and plasma immunoglobulin levels are normal to increased in human PEM, presumably due to frequent antigenic stimulation. Vaccines such as measles and smallpox are clinically effective even in severe PEM, and serum antibody responses to polio vaccine are also intact [21,22]. In contrast, levels of secretory IgA and antibody in secretions are often depressed, although many fewer studies have been reported thus far [4,22,23]. Defective mucosal immune responses, however, could explain the frequency and severity of diarrheal and respiratory diseases in PEM subjects.

PHAGOCYTIC CELLS AND COMPLEMENT

PROTEIN-ENERGY MALNUTRITION

The frequency of bacterial infections in malnourished subjects could be the result of acquired phagocytic cell dysfunction and/or defects in complement. A modest impairment in microbicidal activity against *Staphylococcus aureus, Escherichia coli,* or *Candida albicans* has been shown in some studies [24]. In

a few instances this defect has been correlated with decreased iodination of bacteria via the myeloperoxidase–hydrogen peroxide–halide system. Since myeloperoxidase (MPO) is an iron-requiring enzyme and similar defects in bactericidal function and iodination have been shown in "pure" iron deficiency, it has been suggested that concomitant iron deficiency may complicate human PEM and contribute to leukocyte functional lesions [25].

IRON AND ZINC

Iron deficiency is reported to depress bactericidal activity of polymorphonuclear leukocytes, presumably via diminished MPO activity [17,25]. Similarly, oral or intramuscular administration of excessive iron in the PEM subject with severely depressed serum transferrin may increase the virulence of certain microorganisms. As the unbound iron in serum is increased, it becomes freely available for microbial utilization [26]. Zinc deficiency results in impaired chemotactic activity of PMLs, which is corrected by repletion of the mineral. At the same time, excess zinc in vitro reversibly inhibits phagocytosis, the oxidative burst, and microbicidal activity of both

Table 24-2. Summary of effects of human protein-energy malnutrition on components of the immune system

T Lymphocytes		B Lymphocytes	
Parameter	**Observation**	**Parameter**	**Observation**
Thymus gland	Atrophy and lymphocyte depletion; decreased thymic hormone in serum	Peripheral lymphoid organs	Relative preservation of cellularity of B-lymphocyte regions
Peripheral lymphoid organs	Depletion of cells from T-dependent areas	Circulating lymphocytes	Normal number
Circulating lymphocytes	Relatively normal numbers but decreased proportion of identifiable mature T lymphocytes	Serum immunoglobulins	Normal-elevated levels
Mitogen responses in vitro	Depressed	Secretory immunoglobulins	Decreased levels
Mediator production	Inadequate data but appears to be decreased	Serum antibody responses	Variable—especially poor to polysaccharide antigens
Delayed type skin hypersensitivity	Impaired, particularly efferent limb	Secretory antibody responses	Impaired

Phagocytic cells		Complement	
Parameter	**Observation**	**Parameter**	**Observation**
Chemotaxis	Delayed	Classical pathway activation	Impaired
Mobilization of marrow reserves	Depressed	Alternative pathway activation	Impaired
Particle ingestion	Normal	Component levels	Decreased, except for C4 and ? factor P
Lysosomal fusion	Normal	Regulatory proteins (C1 inhibitor, β1H)	Relatively normal
Degranulation	Normal	Opsonic function	Diminished
Oxidative burst	Blunted	C3 conversion products	Present in vivo
Iodination	Impaired	Immunoconglutinin	Increased
Bactericidal activity	Decreased to a variable extent		

PMLs and macrophages [27]. The importance of this effect in humans is unclear.

THE COMPLEMENT SYSTEM

Measures of hemolytic complement activity by either classical or alternative pathways are abnormal in many patients with PEM, more so in those infected at the same time [28]. This is certainly due, in part, to consumption of complement since C3 activation products may be detected in serum [29]. In otherwise normal individuals, C3 generally behaves as an acute phase reactant, rising in concentration as it is being consumed. The failure of this rise to occur in PEM suggests that biosynthesis may be limiting as well; the result is a deficiency in complement bioactivity necessary for normal phagocyte function, including chemotactic and opsonic functions [28,30]. These defects may, in fact, be quantitatively more important than intrinsic abnormalities of the phagocyte itself and would also amplify any cellular defect present.

SUMMARY AND CONCLUSIONS

Infection exerts a profound influence on host nutritional status and, together with dietary inadequacies, is the major cause of malnutrition in children in developing countries [31]. The metabolic alterations in infection are due to the action of several small peptides, known as cytokines, that also function to regulate the immune response. These metabolic and immunological responses are thus intricately linked in the host response to infection.

Nutritional alterations can, in turn, affect the functional activity of host defenses at several different levels (Table 24-2). Profound impairment in maturation and function of the T lymphocyte due to malnutrition leads to significant defects in cell-mediated immunity, and via the regulatory role of T cells, to alterations in B-cell function and antibody production. The complement system is also severely affected in PEM, presumably due to both increased consumption and decreased synthesis. Complement abnormalities act synergistically with modest impairment of phagocytic cells to produce important deficits in phagocytosis and microbicidal activity in vivo. The consequence is to increase severity and duration of infections. It seems clear that rapid nutritional rehabilitation is required for optimal host survival in acute infections and to reduce risk from subsequent infections. Any program to reduce malnutrition must address the problem of frequent infection or be doomed to partial or total failure.

REFERENCES

1 Scrimshaw NS, Taylor CE, Gordon JE: Interactions of nutrition and infection. WHO Monogr Ser 57, Geneva, WHO, 1968

2 Farthing MJG, Keusch GT: Nutrition and Infection. Ann Rev Nutr 6:131–154, 1986

3 Beisel WR: Magnitude of the host nutritional response to infection. Am J Clin Nutr 30:1236–1247, 1977

4 Keusch GT, Wilson CS, Waksal SD: Nutrition, host defenses and the lymphoid system, in Gallin JI, Fauci AS (eds): *Advances in Host Defense Mechanisms.* New York, Raven, 1983, vol 2, pp 275–359

5 Dinarello CA, Mier JW: Lymphokines. N Engl J Med 317:940–945, 1987

6 Dinarello CA: The multiple biological properties of interleukin-1 influencing immunocompetent cells, in Gupta S, Paul WE, Fauci AS (eds): *Mechanisms of Lymphocyte Activation and Immune Regulation.* New York, Plenum, 1987, pp 103–114

7 Dinarello CA, Cannon JG, Wolff SM: News concepts on the pathogenesis of fever. Rev Infect Dis 10:168–189, 1988

8 Gauldie J, Richards C, Harnish D, et al: Interferon B2/B-cell stimulatory factor type 2 shares identity with monocyte-derived hepatocyte-stimulating factor and regulates the major acute phase protein response in liver cells. Proc Natl Acad Sci USA 84:7251–7255, 1987

9 Kaufmann RL, Matson CF, Beisel WR: Hypertriglyceridemia produced by endotoxin: Role of impaired triglyceride disposal mechanisms. J Infect Dis 133:548–555, 1976

10 Beisel WR, Wannemacher RW: Gluconeogenesis, ureagenesis, and ketogenesis during sepsis. J Parent Enteral Nutr 4:277–285, 1980

11 Beutler B, Cerami A: Cachectin and tumor necrosis factor as two sides of the same coin. Nature 320:584–588, 1986

12 Torti FM, Dieckmann B, Beutler B, et al: A macrophage factor inhibits adipocyte gene expression: An *in vitro* model of cachexia. Science 229:867–869, 1985

13 Chandra RK: T and B lymphocyte subpopulations and leukocyte terminal deoxynucleotidyl transferase in energy-protein undernutrition. Acta Paediatr Scand 68:841–845, 1979

14 Chandra RK: Lymphocyte subpopulation in human malnutrition: Cytotoxic and suppressor cells. Pediatrics 59:423–427, 1977

15 Keusch GT, Cruz JR, Torun B, et al: Immature circulating lymphocytes in severely malnourished Guatemalan children. J Pediatr Gastroenterol Nutr 6:265–270, 1987

16 Koster F, Gaffar A, Jackson TM: Recovery of cellular immune competence during treatment of protein-calorie malnutrition. Am J Clin Nutr 34:887–891, 1981

17 Beisel WR: Single nutrients and immunity. Am J Clin Nutr 35(suppl):417–468, 1982

18 Flynn A, Yen BR: Mineral deficiency effects on the generation of cytotoxic T-cells and T helper cell factors in vitro. J Nutr 111:907–913, 1981

19 Willis-Carr JI, St. Pierre RL: Effects of vitamin B6 deficiency on thymic epithelium cells and T lymphocyte differentiation. J Immunol 120:1153–1159, 1978

20 Chandra RK: Immunoglobulins and antibody response in protein-calorie malnutrition—a review, in Suskind RM (ed): *Malnutrition and the Immune Response.* New York, Raven, 1977, pp 155–168

21 Ifekwunigwe AE, Grasset N, Glass R, et al: Immune response to measles and smallpox vaccinations in malnourished children. Am J Clin Nutr 33:621–624, 1980

22 Chandra RK: Reduced secretory antibody response to live attenuated measles and poliovirus vaccines in malnourished children. Br Med J 2:583–585, 1975

23 McMurray DN, Rey H, Casazza LJ, et al: Effect of moderate malnutrition on concentrations of immunoglobulins and enzymes in tears and saliva of young Colombian children. Am J Clin Nutr 30:1944–1948, 1978

24 Keusch GT: Nutrition and infection, in Remington JS, Swartz MN (eds): *Current Clinical Topics in Infectious Diseases*. New York, McGraw-Hill, 1984, pp 106–123

25 Prasad JS: Leukocyte function in iron-deficiency anemia. Am J Clin Nutr 32:550–552, 1979

26 Murray MJ, Murray AB, Murray MB, et al: The adverse effect of iron repletion on the course of certain infections. Br Med J 2:1113–1115, 1978

27 Chvapil M, Stankova L, Weldy P: The role of zinc in the function of some inflammatory cells, in Brewer GJ, Prasad AS (eds): *Zinc Metabolism: Current Aspects in Health and Disease,* New York, Alan R. Liss, 1977, pp 103 122

28 Keusch GT, Torun B, Johnston RB, et al: Impairment of hemolytic complement activation by both classical and alternative pathways in sera from patients with kwashiorkor. J Pediatr 105:434–436, 1984

29 Chandra RK: Serum complement and immunoconglutinin in malnutrition. Arch Dis Child 50:225–229, 1975

30 Keusch GT, Urrutia JJ, Guerrero O, et al: Serum opsonic activity in acute protein calorie malnutrition. Bull WHO 59:923–929, 1981

31 Keusch GT, Scrimshaw NS: Selective primary health care. XXIII. Control of infection to reduce the prevalence of infantile and childhood malnutrition. Rev Infect Dis 8:273–287, 1986

CHAPTER 25 / *Estimating the Burden of Illness in the Tropics* · Julia A. Walsh

The burden of illness is a major concern for all societies. It includes not only the suffering, pain, and discomfort of each sick person and the grief and anguish of relatives and friends, but also the burden on the family in caring for and accommodating a sick member in the household. In addition, the losses to the economy from deaths, disability, and disease can be substantial. Finally, the burden includes the costs to the family and society for services for prevention of disease and care for the sick.

Measurement of this burden takes on special significance in the face of scarce resources. Such limitations should challenge our skill in setting priorities for the allocation of the few available resources and in evaluating health service programs and biomedical and behavioral research. Health services should be planned to alleviate the maximum amount of morbidity and mortality. When health services planners and providers recognize the contribution that each disease makes to the burden of illness in the community, they can direct their efforts and resources toward those health problems causing excessive death and disablement. Similarly, biomedical and behavioral research can be concentrated on those important diseases for which methods of prevention or treatment are inadequate.

Each of the multitude of health problems facing both westernized and developing nations varies greatly in the amount and kind of medical care required for alleviation of the disease. Each differs in the effects on the community in terms of pain and suffering and losses in productivity due to illness, disability, and death. For example, the poliomyelitis viruses infect essentially everyone in developing countries during early childhood. Very few of those infected become paralyzed, and an even smaller number die, but those permanently disabled represent a long-term encumbrance or drain on the resources of the family and the community. In contrast, measles infects all small children. Three percent or more die, but the rest recover from the 10- to 14-day illness and remain immune for life. Another example is Chagas' disease, which infects fewer people than either polio or measles. Only a small proportion of these will suffer from clinical disease, but adults in the economically productive years are most seriously affected by this long-term progressive disability.

Within a population, some age and socioeconomic groups have a much greater likelihood of experiencing illness and dying. Infants and children less than 5 years of age constitute between 5 and 15 percent of the population in most developing countries but represent 25 to 40 percent of the deaths [1,2]. In addition to the "usual childhood diseases," polio, whooping cough, diphtheria, and measles, these young children suffer more frequently than adults from diarrhea, respiratory infections, malnutrition, tetanus, and malaria. A health care facility attempting to minimize morbidity and mortality in a community should direct its efforts at treating this particularly high risk group. Nonetheless adults, particularly those over 55 years of age, constitute the majority of patients contacting the health services. Elders may have more time to visit health facilities than mothers with children. The mothers are involved with their many responsibilities: child care, household chores, water drawing, farming, wood gathering, or other occupational efforts.

The poorest and the most destitute are another group with excessive risk for sickness and early demise and again are frequently inadequately served by the health care system. How can a health care system most effectively improve public health and decrease the burden of illness unless it serves the most afflicted groups?

METHODS FOR MEASUREMENT

UNITED STATES

The indicators of burden of illness that can be most easily measured are the distribution of deaths, the cost of services provided, and the losses in output. The dimensions of the burden for the family and for the suffering individual are not so easily quantified.

In the United States, the economic costs of many specific illnesses have been estimated, including studies of peptic ulcers, heart and circulatory diseases, alcoholism, syphilis, cancer, stroke, mental illness, digestive diseases, and influenza. The National Academy of Sciences' Institute of Medicine recently studied the economic and social burden of infectious diseases in order to determine priorities for vaccine research and development [3]. A parallel study estimated disease burden of potentially vaccine-preventable infections in developing countries [4].

In developing countries, only meager health and disease statistics are available, and studies on the economic consequences of illness are rare. If more useful information were available, choices for the allocation of the scarce resources designed to reduce the overall burden of illness could be made more rationally. For the United States, the National Center for Health Statistics has developed an array of indexes of burden, including potential years of life lost by disease, distribution of causes of death and years of life lost per death, distribution of inpatient days by disease, causes for physician contacts, distribution of work-loss days, and health expenditures. Most of the data are taken from their national data systems. Diagnostic data, of varying degrees of precision, are available from the Vital Statistics System, Hospital Discharge Survey, Health Interview Survey, Ambulatory Medical Care Survey, Nursing Home Survey, and the Health Examination and Nutrition Survey. These indexes are presented in the major diagnostic groups, categorized according to the International Classification of Diseases, Adapted (ICDA).

Table 25-1 shows the distribution of the potential years of

Table 25-1. Estimated years of potential life lost (YPLL) before age 65 and cause-specific mortality by cause of death—United States, 1986

Cause of mortality (ICD, 9th revision, codes)	YPLL for persons dying in 1986	Cause-specific mortality, 1986,* rate/100,000
All causes (Total)	12,054,242	870.8
Unintentional injuries† (E800–E949)	2,371,024	39.7
Malignant neoplasms (140–208)	1,821,682	193.3
Diseases of the heart (390-398,402,404–429)	1,534,607	318.7
Suicide/homicide (E950–E978)	1,342,693	22.0
Congenital anomalies (740–759)	651,523	5.1
Prematurity‡ (765–769)	438,351	2.8
Sudden infant death syndrome (798)	313,555	2.0
Acquired immunodeficiency syndrome§	246,823	3.6
Cerebrovascular disease (430–438)	232,583	61.3
Chronic liver diseases and cirrhosis (571)	225,028	10.9
Pneumonia and influenza (480–487)	166,389	29.2
Chronic obstructive pulmonary diseases (490–496)	127,889	31.3
Diabetes mellitus (250)	126,652	15.1

*Cause-specific mortality rates as reported in the National Center for Health Statistics' Monthly Vital Statistics Report are compiled from a 10% sample of all deaths.
†Equivalent to accidents and adverse effects.
‡Category derived from disorders relating to short gestation and respiratory distress syndrome.
§Reflects Centers for Disease Control surveillance data.

Table 25-2. Estimated years of potential life lost before age 65 according to disease category of underlying cause of death—United States, 1986

Cause of mortality (ICD category)	Years
All causes	6
Unintentional injuries	25
Malignant neoplasms	4
Diseases of the heart	2
Suicide/homicide	25
Congenital anomalies	54
Prematurity	65
Sudden infant death syndrome	65
Acquired immunodeficiency syndrome	29
Cerebrovascular disease	1.6
Chronic liver diseases and cirrhosis	8.6
Pneumonia and influenza	2.4
Chronic obstructive pulmonary diseases	1.7
Diabetes mellitus	3.5

life lost by disease. This is based on the age-specific death rates from various disease categories and the expectation of life in each age group. For example, a child born in the United States in 1984 could expect to live 74.7 years. In contrast, an individual 65 years of age in 1984 could expect to live 16.8 years more [5]. Table 25-2 lists the estimated years of potential life lost (YPLL) before age 65 per death according to disease category of underlying cause of death in the United States in 1986.

Diseases of the heart account for the greatest number of deaths and injuries for the largest total number of potential years of life lost before age 65. Since the early 1970s, the number of deaths and potential years of life lost from heart diseases has declined in this country for reasons that are not fully understood, while the percentage resulting from chronic obstructive pulmonary disease and diabetes has increased. All infectious diseases, including parasites, pneumonia, influenza, and acquired immunodeficiency syndrome (AIDS) account for about 3 to 5 percent of the deaths and of the potential years of life lost. In contrast, as demonstrated below, in developing countries infectious diseases account for the largest percentage of deaths and potential years of life lost.

Since the last edition of this book AIDS has steadily risen in importance. Each year the number of deaths and the potential years of life lost from this condition have risen. However, other infectious diseases that can be easily prevented and/or treated, such as respiratory disease, diarrhea, and measles still cause more deaths in the developing world. Some demographers predict that AIDS may eventually result in population reductions in Africa early in the next century unless transmission stops.

The years of life lost from a particular cause is a function of the age distribution of the population and the age-disease-specific mortality rate and life expectancies at various ages.

For example, among Americans, suicide, homicide, and unintentional injuries account for more than 30 percent of the potential years of life lost, even though they cause only 7 percent of the deaths. Each death results in an average of 25 years of life lost because young people (men three times more than women) are primarily affected. In the United States, more potential years of life and a greater proportion of lives are lost from these causes than in European and most developing countries.

The economic costs to the United States of various illnesses are better delineated by the analysis of causes of hospitalization, physician visits, days lost from work, and health expenditures. Table 25-3 lists the distribution of inpatient days by disease category of diagnosis in acute care hospitals. The total number of inpatient days in nursing homes is almost twice the number of acute care hospital days. Table 25-4 lists the distribution of physician office visits. These two tables indicate the relative burden of various diseases in terms of demands on medical care resources. Hospital and nursing home care together account for more than half of the total personal health care expenditures in the United States. In developing countries fewer inpatient and outpatient facilities are available, and many people who might benefit from medical attention never receive this care. Particularly in these countries, but also in the United States, the use of health resources is a function of a complex set of circumstances. Incidence, prevalence, severity, and du-

Table 25-3. Number of patients and days of care for patients discharged from short-stay hospitals and average length of stay, by selected first-listed diagnostic categories—United States, 1985*

Diagnostic category*	Discharged patients, number in thousands	Days of care, number in thousands	Average length of stay, days
All conditions[†]	35,056	226,217	6.5
Females with deliveries (V27)	3,854	12,640	3.3
Normal deliveries	1,386	3,470	2.5
Complicated deliveries	2,468	9,170	3.7
Heart disease (391–392.0, 393–398, 402, 404, 410–416, 420–429)	3,584	26,082	7.3
Acute myocardial infarction (410)	755	7,152	9.5
Atherosclerotic heart disease (414.0)	304	2,016	6.6
Other ischemic heart disease (411–413, 414.1–414.9)	992	5,379	5.4
Cardiac dysrhythmias (427)	511	3,148	6.2
Congestive heart failure (428.0)	557	4,459	8.0
Malignant neoplasms (140–208, 230–234)	1,911	17,001	8.9
Malignant neoplasms trachea, bronchus, and lung (162, 197.0, 197.3)	315	2,884	9.2
Malignant neoplasm of breast (174, 175, 198.81)	208	1,489	7.2
Fractures, all sites (800–829)	1,129	9,864	8.7
Cerebrovascular disease (430–438)	916	9,600	10.5
Pneumonia, all forms (480–486)	854	6,788	7.9
Psychoses (290–299)	701	10,435	14.9
Intervertebral disc disorders (722)	508	3,693	7.3
Benign neoplasms and neoplasms of uncertain behavior and unspecified nature (210–229, 235–239)	500	2,740	5.5
Diabetes mellitus (250)	480	3,901	8.1
Cholelithiasis (574)	474	3,558	7.5
Arthropathies and related disorders (710–719)	465	3,584	7.7
Asthma (493)	462	2,275	4.9
Noninfectious enteritis and colitis (555–556, 558)	457	2,241	4.9
Diseases of the central nervous system (320–336, 340–349)	425	4,092	9.6
Alcohol dependence syndrome (303)	388	4,169	10.7
Inguinal hernia (550)	384	1,231	3.2
All abortions, including ectopic and molar pregnancies (630–639)	382	821	2.1
Calculus of kidney and ureter (592)	325	1,217	3.7
Chronic disease of tonsils and adenoids (474)	288	437	1.5
All newborn infants	3,794	144	3.8

*National Center for Health Statistics.
[†]Includes data for diagnostic conditions not shown in table.
Discharges are from nonfederal short-stay hospitals. Diagnostic groupings and code number inclusions are based on the International Classification of Diseases, 9th revision, clinical modification code.

Table 25-4. Distribution of physician office visits by whether the condition was chronic or acute and the type of acute condition—United States, 1982–83

	Physician office visits, in 100s	Percent distribution
All conditions	660,967	100.0
Chronic conditions	421,499	63.8
Acute conditions	239,467	36.2
Types of acute conditions		
Respiratory conditions	65,605	9.9
Injuries	55,612	9.8
Infective and parasitic diseases	23,382	3.5
Digestive system conditions	7,552	1.1
All other acute conditions:	87,316	13.2
Acute ear conditions	15,425	2.3
Skin conditions	8,476	1.2
Acute back, spine, and neck pain	1,162	0.2
Other musculoskeletal conditions	10,223	1.5
Selected chronic conditions		
Circulatory	84,410	12.7
Skin and musculoskeletal	58,738	8.9
Visual impairments	49,634	7.5
Diabetes	17,805	2.7
Digestive	15,485	2.2
Respiratory	50,352	7.5
All other chronic conditions	145,075	22.0

Source: National Center for Health Statistics.

ration of a specific disease may play even less of a role than the availability of scientific and technological advances and societal, cultural, economic, and legal factors. Especially in developing countries, the use of existing health resources may poorly measure the costs of illness because of the uneven availability of facilities.

The cost of disease in terms of loss of economic output is another method for measuring the burden of illness. Table 25-5 lists the causes of absence from work in the United States by chronic disease category. The table reflects only short-term or temporary illness causing loss of days of work among those currently employed. Respiratory disorders (chronic bronchitis plus emphysema) and accidents (disc, back, or spine disorders) are the main causes of absences from work, accounting for almost half of the total.

Health expenditures are another burden of illness. In the United States in 1980, the mean amount paid out-of-pocket by all "multiple-person families" was $575 per family.[1] This does not include long-term care and health insurance premiums. The major components include: dental care, $159; physician care, $126; inpatient hospital care, $79; and prescription medications, $69. The total health care expenditure was $2111 [6].

DEVELOPING COUNTRIES

The systems available for measuring burden of illness in developing countries are much less sophisticated than those of

[1]The term *multiple-person families* refers to families with an average size of 1.5 persons or more during the survey year.

Table 25-5. Days lost from work associated with selected reported chronic conditions per currently employed person 18–64 years of age with condition per year and prevalence of these conditions among currently employed persons, by age and condition—United States, 1983

Chronic condition	Work-loss days per currently employed person with condition per year			Prevalence of condition, in thousands		
	18–64 years	18–44 years	45–64 years	18–64 years	18–44 years	45–64 years
Heart conditions, excluding rheumatic and hypertensive	3.6	*	6.4	4989	2200	2780
Hypertension	0.5	0.7*	0.4*	9934	4040	5894
Chronic bronchitis	2.1	2.5	1.1*	3505	2446	1058
Emphysema	*	*	*	413	71*	342
Ulcer of stomach and duodenum	1.6	2.6	*	2145	1335	810
Hernia of abdominal cavity	5.1	0.9*	8.4	1677	728	949
Arthritis	0.5	*	0.8	9443	3354	6089
Intervertebral disc disorders	8.4	6.4	10.5	1622	823	799
Diabetes mellitus	1.0*	3.5*	*	1633	479	1153
Impairments (except paralysis) of back or spine	2.9	2.0	4.9	6742	4560	2182

*Very small numbers.

Source: National Center for Health Statistics.

Table 25-6. Death rates per 100,000 population for all age groups according to causes in Matlab, Bangledesh—1981

Case	Rate per 100,000
Tetanus	202
Respiratory	166
Dropsy	104
Dysentery	101
Acute	33
Chronic	68
Fever	78
Rheumatism	56
Measles	50
Diarrhea	42
Acute	24
Chronic	17
Old age	42
Drowning	39
Gastrointestinal	37
Liver	23
Jaundice	16
Heart	11
Childbirth	10
Other	333
All causes	1311

Source: From [7].

the United States National Center for Health Statistics and are based on much less data. Only a few studies following relatively small groups of people in diverse geographical areas provide some indication of the causes and the social cost of disability and death. These usually do not follow ICDA classification so that comparability with U.S. data is limited. For example, Table 25-6 lists the causes of death in Matlab, Bangladesh [7]. Infectious diseases cause at least 40 percent of the deaths in these least industrialized countries, compared with about 1 percent in the United States. Heart disease probably causes 7 to 10 percent, and congenital anomalies and diseases of early infancy, 15 to 20 percent [8]. Of all these categories, infectious diseases are the most easily prevented and cured with available technology. Control of these has resulted in the enormous increases in life expectancy that have occurred in the United States and other developed countries in the last century. For example, in England in 1881, when life expectancy at birth was only 47 years, the probability of eventually dying from an infectious disease was more than 40 percent, while in 1964, when life expectancy at birth was 70+ years, there was only a 13 percent probability of eventually dying from infections [8].

In the last 30 years, mortality rates around the world have declined enormously. Infant mortality rates have declined between 2 and 5 percent per year in practically every developing country. In the middle income countries, chronic diseases and injuries have supplanted the infectious disease as the major killers. Table 25-7 presents the major causes of death in Thailand, which in 1985 had a per capita gross national product of $800 and an infant mortality rate of 45 per thousand live births [9].

Table 25-7. Leading causes of death in Thailand by rate (per 100,000 population) according to ICD, 9th revision, 1979 and 1983

Cause of death	ICD(9)	1979 Order	1979 Rate	1983 Order	1983 Rate
Accidents, injuries, homicide, & suicide	800–848 900–929 950–969	1	67.2	1	49.9
Heart disease	410–429	3	28.6	2	33.2
Respiratory system	460–466 470–478 480–519	2	44.6	5	20.5
Digestive system	530–579	4	24.2	3	22.4
Neoplasms	150–165 190–199	5	17.3	4	21.3
Cerebrovascular system	430–438	9	10.3	6	11.8
Tuberculosis	010–018	6	15.1	7	11.2
Nervous system	320–359	8	12.1	8	10.7
Intestinal infections	001–009	7	12.5	9	7.3
Urinary system	580–599	10	5.6	10	6.9
Hypertensive diseases	401–405	11	3.7	11	3.6
Endocrine and metabolic diseases, immunity disorders	240–259 270–279	12	2.8	12	3.8
Nutritional deficiencies	260–269	13	2.6	13	1.4

Source: Modified from Division of Health Statistics, Office of the Permanent Secretary, Ministry of Public Health, Thailand, Public Health Statistics, 1980–1983.

Table 25-8. Causes of death for individuals of all ages in the developing world

Conditions	Infections[1]	Deaths[1]	Disease episodes[1]
Respiratory disease (upper & lower)	—	10,000[2]	15,000,000[3]
Circulatory system[4]	—	8,000	*
(Low birth weight[5])	—	(5,000)	(19,000)
Diarrhea	—	4,300	28,000,000
Measles[6]	67,000	2,000	67,000
Injuries	—	2,000	*
(Malnutrition[8])	—	(2,000)	(5-8,000)
Neoplasms[9]	—	2,000	*
Malaria	2,600,000[10]	1,500	150,000
P. falciparum	—	1,350	120,000
Tetanus	—	1,200	1,800
Tuberculosis	1,000,000	900	7,000
Hepatitis B[11]	300,000	800	3,700
Whooping cough	55,000	600	51,000
Typhoid	70,000	600	35,000
Maternal mortality	—	500	—
Meningitis	—	350	1,000,000
Schistosomiasis	200,000	250-500	10,000
Syphilis[12]	15,000	200	250
Amebiasis	500,000	70	40,000

[1]Thousands per year. Episodes means yearly incidence and prevalence of disease.

[2]4 million of these deaths occur in children under 5 years old.

[3]25 million episodes of acute lower respiratory tract infectious disease and 15 billion episodes of acute upper respiratory tract infectious disease.

[4]This category includes cardiovascular diseases and certain degenerative diseases (nephritis, cirrhosis of the liver, ulcers of stomach and duodenum, and diabetes).

[5]Low birth weight is the underlying cause of death, although the immediate cause may be respiratory, diarrheal, or other disease; therefore, these deaths have also been counted in the other categories.

[6]A small proportion of these deaths may also be counted in the diarrheal disease category.

[7]Occurrences of injury are probably 100 times more frequent than deaths, but extremely few reliable data are available on incidence.

[8]Severe malnutrition is the underlying cause of death, although the immediate cause may be respiratory, diarrheal, or other disease; therefore, these deaths have also been counted in other categories.

[9]Includes neoplasms of all types except hepatitis B–related hepatocellular carcinoma, which is listed separately.

[10]This is the population at risk inhabiting infected areas; 365,000,000 live in highly endemic areas.

[11]The infections are the asymptomatic carriers of hepatitis B surface antigen present in the world. Episodes include acute hepatitis, cirrhosis, and primary hepatocellular carcinoma.

[12]The deaths are primarily excess perinatal deaths among the 10% of seroreactive women giving birth in sub-Saharan Africa. No good information is available on adult deaths from tertiary syphilis or extent of disease in other parts of the world.

Causes of death

Table 25-8 lists the number of infections and the deaths caused by the major diseases in developing countries during 1986 [*10*]. Those suffering most are infants and children and those living in the poorest, most destitute areas. In those extremely deprived areas where life expectancy is the shortest, infectious diseases cause more than half of the deaths.

Occurrence of infection and episodes of infectious disease differ for many of these conditions. The infecting agent may coexist in or on an individual without producing any recog-nizable symptoms. This phenomenon is most recognizable among populations infected with the helminthic and protozoan parasites. For example, in many parts of the developing world the majority of individuals carry a small number of ascarides or hookworms in their intestines, but extremely few, fewer than 1 percent of those infected, have any symptoms. Only those continually exposed to infection and carrying a huge number of worms develop any disease. The disease episode column lists estimates of the numbers of people who suffer some type of illness and are at risk of dying. The infections column and the column of disease episodes combine preva-

Table 25-8. Causes of death for individuals of all ages in the developing world (*Continued*)

Conditions	Infections[1]	Deaths[1]	Disease episodes[1]
Human immunodeficiency virus (HIV)	4,000	50-70	140
South American trypanosomiasis	24,000	60	1,200
Rheumatic fever and heart disease	—	52	2,200
Hookworm	800,000	50	1,500
Rabies	35	35	35
Diphtheria	60,000	30	600
Dengue	*	15	48
Hepatitis A	*	14	5,000
Yellow fever	*	9	82
Japanese B encephalitis	*	7	28
Ascariasis	700,000	10	700
Giardiasis	250,000	10	500
Poliomyelitis	150,000	2	220[13]
Leprosy	1,000	1	1,000
Leishmaniasis	1,000	1	1,000
Trichuriasis	500,000	1	100
Filariasis	90,000	1	1,000
Dracunculiasis	1,000	1	1,000
Onchocerciasis[14]	1-5,000	1	*
African trypanosomiasis	*	1	*
Other[15]		1-2,000	

[13]Cases of paralysis.

[14]No systematic survey of prevalence and incidence has occurred since the beginning of the onchocerciasis control program in West Africa, which has markedly diminished the occurrence of infection and disease.

[15]Deaths of unclear etiology or disease with relatively small numbers of cases.

Note: —not applicable; *no data.

Source: From [*10*].

lence and incidence data. Prevalence refers to the number of cases that are present at a specified period of time. Incidence refers to the number of new cases of a disease occurring in the population during a specified period of time (in this case during 1 year). In general, for chronic diseases and infections prevalence is given, while for those producing short-term illness, such as measles and whooping cough, incidence estimates are listed.

The data in Table 25-8 have been culled primarily from World Health Organization publications and are not usually based on disease notifications, since case reporting is rarely complete even in highly developed countries and becomes sporadic and irregular in the developing countries. Instead, these figures have usually been calculated from disease and mortality surveys performed in a variety of specific populations. These surveys represent small groups of people, and the generalizability of these results may be questioned. But from most parts of the developing world, very little information on disease surveillance and cause of death is available. These estimates are presented with acknowledged reservations in order to attempt to set priorities for disease control.

Respiratory diseases together with diarrheal disease cause one-half to two-thirds of the morbidity and mortality from communicable diseases in developing countries. Like diarrhea, respiratory infections produce severe morbidity and mortality, particularly in infants and young children. Many different microbes cause this group of diseases—viruses such as influenza, parainfluenza, and adenoviruses, and bacteria such as the pneumococcus and *Hemophilus influenza B*—but the etiology in the majority of cases remains unknown. Surveys of the incidence of respiratory infection are difficult to find, particularly since case definitions can vary from the common cold to severe acute lower respiratory infection, bronchiolitis, or pneumonia. The common cold occurs in most adults throughout the world at least one to two times a year and in preschoolers three to five times a year. But the incidence of lower respiratory tract and chronic respiratory disease is much less available. Because of this difficulty in defining terms and finding incidence data, the columns for estimates of infection and disease incidence have been left blank. Data on deaths are somewhat easier to obtain, and these diseases seem to cause one-third or more of the deaths in children aged 5 and under and 15 percent or more of the deaths in all age groups [*11,12*].

Diseases of the circulatory system affect primarily adults and the elderly, and few simple, efficacious preventive or treatment measures are available to control them. Hypertension treatment, diet, smoking prevention, and exercise may have some influence on mortality rates. These require long-term changes in behavior. Deaths in this category will certainly increase in the future as people live longer, their diet and exercise patterns change, and smoking increases.

Low birth weight means a weight at birth of 2500 g or less. In some parts of the developing world almost 50 percent of babies begin life with this disadvantage. In contrast, in industrialized countries, this occurs in as few as 4 percent of all births. The consequences of low birth weight include: enormously greater risk of dying in infancy and childhood, developmental disabilities, and retardation in mental and motor skills. Small improvements in the incidence of low birth weight will markedly decrease the infant and child mortality rate. For example, a fall from 30 to 15 percent could result in 25 percent more infants surviving (a fall in infant mortality rate from 160 to 120 per thousand) [13]. The risk factors associated with low birth weight are myriad. More research is needed into the causes and possible preventive measures, particularly regarding gestational infections precipitating early delivery and affecting intrauterine growth rates [14].

Many different organisms can cause diarrhea, for example, *Escherichia coli, Vibrio cholera, Salmonella, Shigella,* and rotavirus. Amebiasis, giardiasis, and intestinal helminths are considered separately. Because of the numerous etiologies for diarrhea plus the tendency of many of these microbes to infect humans asymptomatically, the infection column in Table 25-8 has been left blank. In developing countries, adults usually suffer from at least one episode of mild diarrhea yearly. In contrast, children under 5 have an incidence of 2 to 10 episodes of diarrhea annually, averaging about 4 in most poor communities, and this dehydrating illness lasts several days to a week. Assuming that 450 million children under age 5 reside in developing countries and suffer from an average of three episodes of diarrhea yearly and 3 billion adults have one episode yearly, there would be 1.4 billion cases among the children and 3 billion adult cases. The case fatality rate from diarrhea varies from 1 in 100 cases among the poorest, malnourished, and youngest children to less than 1 in 1000 among adults. Diarrhea and malnutrition interact closely. The anorexia and malabsorption caused by diarrhea results in weight loss and can precipitate malnutrition. Malnourished individuals have an increased risk of prolonged illness and death when stricken with diarrhea [15]. The use of oral rehydration therapy seems to avert some of this risk of malnutrition.

Measles appears to be the next most common cause of death in developing countries. Essentially, everyone who is not immunized and who survives beyond the first 6 months of life becomes infected and suffers from the illness. Particularly in infants and malnourished children, the disease is severe and prolonged with multiple complications including diarrhea, pneumonia, otitis media, and weight loss that can lead to malnutrition. Case fatality rates in community studies range from 1 to 10 percent; therefore, this preventable infection may cause 5 percent or more of all the deaths in all age groups (see Table 25-5). This deadly disease can be entirely prevented by immunization of infants [16].

Young adults and children have the greatest risk of injuries, usually as a result of exposure to hazards in the home, community, and at work. Injuries result most often from motor vehicle accidents, burns, and falls [17]. The loss of these healthy, productive individuals incurs an inordinately great societal cost. Little is presently known about risk factors or the appropriate interventions to prevent these episodes.

Malnutrition is not an infectious disease, but nutrition and infection interact closely with each other. Infections, particularly diarrhea, exert a negative impact on nutritional status, while malnutrition predisposes the individual to an increased risk of morbidity and mortality from various infections. Malnutrition was the underlying cause in more than 50 percent of the child deaths in Latin America [18]. In Bangladesh, the mortality rate of the children in the lowest decile according to weight for age or height for age was about four times the rate of those in the top decile. Epidemiological studies in Guatemala, the Gambia, and Bangladesh have demonstrated a marked negative relationship between infections and a child's physical growth and development [19]. Diarrhea, measles, and malaria appear to have the greatest impact on nutrition. These probably exert their effect through the mechanisms of decreased food intake, malabsorption, and loss of nutrients in the gastrointestinal tract during certain diarrheal diseases. Control of these infections should greatly lessen the burden of malnutrition in society.

Only a few of the less common types of neoplasms can occasionally be cured, such as childhood leukemia and Hodgkin's disease. However, one of the most common types in the developing world, hepatitis B–related hepatocellular carcinoma (listed separately in Table 25-8) can now be prevented through immunization. Adults and the elderly are the age groups most commonly affected by cancers. Lung cancer is the most rapidly increasing, following the epidemic increase in the use of tobacco.

Particularly in sub-Saharan Africa, malaria causes an enormous number of deaths. In the equatorial areas, because of both the particularly vigorous, difficult to control vector mosquito, *Anopheles gambiae,* and the high degree of endemicity of virulent *Plasmodium falciparum,* malaria remains the primary or contributing cause in one-third or more of the deaths. In areas where malaria has been controlled, usually through intensive insecticide campaigns, the crude death rate has declined by one-third or more and the infant mortality rate by the same or greater degree [20]. In other parts of the developing world, malaria continues as an endemic or epidemic seasonal disease of lower intensity but is still a cause of substantial morbidity and mortality. Official surveillance reports markedly underrepresent the number of deaths. They embrace a range of case definitions from patients suffering febrile episodes in association with positive blood smears (malaria may not be the primary cause) to smear-positive individuals who may be asymptomatic but are discovered in community surveys. None of the usual surveillance methods can estimate the disability caused by chronic infection or by the occasional febrile episode that is self-limited or self-treated. The data on declines in mortality associated with malaria control give the best indication of its devastating effect on holo- or hyperendemically infected populations. The greatest burden certainly is on infants and small children, but even adults who have supposedly developed immunity suffer an excess mortality [21].

Probably at least 150 million clinical cases of malaria occur yearly. Most of these occur in young children in equatorial Africa, but some also occur among those residing in unprotected areas of Asia and America: 1800 million live in areas where they are at risk for acquiring the infection. Eight hundred million people is a conservative estimate of the number of individuals who may become infected with the malaria parasite during the year (most asymptomatically infected). Conservatively, this protozoan causes at least 1.5 million deaths annually; again, most of these occur in Africa, the epicenter of malaria.

From numerous studies, it is known that tetanus is a disease of great importance in most developing countries. It accounts for between 5 and 61 percent of all neonatal deaths, and surveys from Bangladesh, India, Indonesia, and other countries demonstrate an incidence of 15 per 1000 live births or more. The incidence appears higher in rural than in urban areas. Approximately 1 billion people live under circumstances associated with this high incidence. Nonneonatal tetanus occurs as a result of dirty wounds. Underlying these cases are injuries; adding these to the injury category increases the evidence for the enormity of the societal burden from injuries. Infant deaths are preventable by immunization of pregnant women every 3 to 5 years, and the nonneonatal cases are preventable by vaccination of young children and providing boosters every 5 years.

Tuberculosis remains a major health problem throughout Asia, South America, and Africa. Despite BCG (bacillus Calmette-Guérin) immunization and chemotherapy, the incidence of new cases and deaths from tuberculosis remains high, even though these have declined to some extent in the past 30 years. In parts of Asia, annual incidence rates exceed 300 to 500 per 100,000 population per year. The estimates listed in Table 25-8 extrapolate from reported cases and deaths and from surveys. The tubercle bacillus infects 1.5 billion people throughout the developing world as judged by positive skin tests, and the annual risk of infection in some areas exceeds 2 percent. The prevalence of active cases of tuberculosis is approximately 6 to 8 million and approximately 900,000 die yearly. Adult

men over age 25 in the economically productive years of life sustain the highest incidence rates for active disease and death, heavily burdening families dependent upon them for support and countries attempting to advance.

Infection with the hepatitis B virus (HBV) causing hepatitis and eventual hepatocellular carcinoma and cirrhosis has only recently been recognized as a major cause of death and disability. Like TB, its most devastating effects are primarily in men over age 25 to 30. HBV infection peaks during childhood, and in high incidence areas, such as east Asia and west Africa, 10 to 15 percent of the population eventually become chronic carriers. Only 10 percent of children infected ever develop clinical hepatitis, but for the chronic carriers, the eventual results of these benign childhood infections are premature death from primary hepatocellular carcinoma (PHC) and cirrhosis. Three hundred million people chronically carry HBV; 800,000 die yearly from PHC and cirrhosis. PHC is uniformly fatal within a year. Those afflicted with cirrhosis live slightly longer, but this end-stage liver disease is also incurable [22].

Whooping cough, like measles, is highly contagious and infects almost all who are not immunized. Some 80 percent of all children are infected with *Bordetella pertussis* before they reach the age of 5 years. Half suffer a clinically recognizable illness with a spasmodic cough and retching lasting several weeks. The other infections may be asymptomatic or only mildly symptomatic. Infants have the most severe disease, and in older children and adults the disease becomes less symptomatic. Case fatality rates usually vary from 1 to 3 percent in community studies, but this does not take account of late deaths from malnutrition resulting from pertussis [23].

The categories of disease listed above appear to be the leading causes of ill health and death globally. More detailed descriptions of these and of the others listed in Table 25-8 can be found in other chapters in this text. The relative importance within an individual country, region, district, or neighborhood can vary. Efficacious, feasible interventions that can allay disease and disability from many of these are available within the developing world. However, research can still help to find easier, less expensive methods of prevention and treatment.

In general, the major scourges of a century ago in industrialized countries continue to be the primary problems in developing countries. These illnesses have been controlled in the west, but the populations in warm climate countries still suffer their consequences. Certainly for health care systems to be most effective in alleviating the burden of illness, their resources should be directed toward the control of these diseases, since many can be easily treated or prevented with existing technology.

Morbidity

The causes of illness in developing countries are quite different from the causes of death. Most illnesses disable without kill-

Table 25-9. Prevalence of illnesses in a cohort of 197 rural Bangladeshi children aged 2–60 months studied in 1978–1979

Illness	Days	Prevalence per 100 child-days
Upper respiratory illness	37,111	60.3
Diarrhea	7,904	12.8
Impetigo	5,119	8.3
Scabies	4,206	6.8
Other skin infection	2,969	4.8
Chronic otitis	2,457	4.0
Stomatitis	2,449	4.0
Conjunctivitis	1,363	2.2
Asthma	269	0.4
Pneumonia	175	0.3
Measles	138	0.2
Hepatitis	69	0.1
Eczema	55	0.1
Varicella	41	0.1
Tonsillitis	35	0.1
Typhoid fever	20	0.03
Other recorded illnesses	15	0.02
Mumps	14	0.02
Pertussis	7	0.01

Source: From [2].

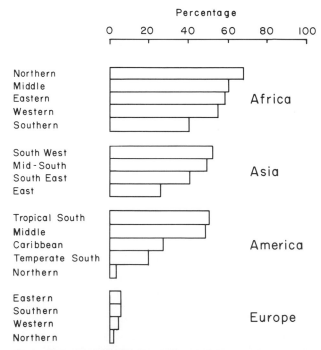

Figure 25-1. Contribution of mortality of children under 5 years to deaths of all ages. (*From* [2].)

ing. Table 25-9 lists the prevalence of illness in rural Bangladeshi children younger than 5 years of age. The days of illness from respiratory, diarrheal, and skin diseases totals more than 90 percent of a child's life [24]. Even less is known about the causes of disability in adults.

Age distribution of deaths

Children under 5 years bear the brunt of disability and deaths from infectious diseases. Children comprise approximately 15 percent of the population in Africa, Asia, and South America, but their mortality rate is so high that their deaths contribute to between 40 and 60 percent of deaths at all ages (Fig. 25-1) [2]. Table 25-10 compares the child and maternal mortality rates found in less developed countries with those in industrialized countries [2]. The highest levels characterize the rates found in Africa or Asia, while the lowest levels are those found in western Europe or the United States. The mortality rate and life expectancy for those over age 5 approaches that of westernized countries. For example, in Matlab, Bangladesh, the life expectancy for a 5-year-old is 63 years and the crude death rate for this group is 7.6 per 1000. In contrast, in the United States the crude death rate in 1984 was 8.5 per 1000 population. The age structure of the American and Matlab populations is strikingly different. The U.S. population has many more individuals over 60, whose risk of death is quite high from heart and circulatory disease, neoplasms, etc. The mortality rate for those over 60 is probably quite similar in developed and less developed countries. In contrast, the mortality rate for those between 5 and 45 years in Matlab and other tropical areas exceeds that of westernized populations, but does not reach the ratios demonstrated in Table 25-10.

Fifteen million infant and child deaths occur annually. From 90 to 97 percent occur in the less developed regions. The risk factors for death include poverty, low level of maternal education, birth interval less than 24 months, birth weight less than 2500 g, neonatal tetanus, breast-feeding less than 6

Table 25-10. Comparison of extreme levels of national maternal and child mortality rates

	Highest levels (1)	Lowest levels (2)	Ratio of (1)/(2)
Perinatal mortality*	120	12–15	8–10
Infant mortality*	200	8–10	20–25
Childhood mortality†	45	0.4–1	45–75
Maternal mortality‡	1000	5–10	100–200

*Per 1000 live births.
†Per 1000 population.
‡Per 100,000 live births.

Source: World Health Organization. Reprinted with permission.

months, pertussis, respiratory infections, inadequate water supply, diarrhea, malaria, poor nutritional status, and measles. To prevent these deaths, these detrimental factors must be allayed.

Potential years of life lost

Another method for assessing burden of illness for developing regions is the calculation of the impact of the disease on a community by measuring the healthy days of life lost through illness, disability, and death as a consequence of the disease. Table 25-11 present such an estimation for Ghana [25]. This measure is derived by combining information for each illness on the incidence rate, the case fatality rate, and the extent and duration of disability produced by the disease. Table 25-11 is not exactly comparable to Table 25-1 for the United States because different disease classifications are used, and because Table 25-11 includes both days of life lost because of disability and days of life lost by deaths. If the Ghana data are recalculated to include only days of life lost by mortality (as measured in Table 25-1), the ranking of the first 10 diseases

Table 25-11. Disease problems of Ghana—ranked order of healthy days of life lost

Rank order	Disease	Days of healthy life lost	Percent of total
1	Malaria	32,600	10.2
2	Measles	23,400	7.3
3	Pneumonia (child)	18,600	5.8
4	Sickle cell disease	17,500	5.5
5	Malnutrition	17,500	5.5
6	Prematurity	16,800	5.2
7	Birth injury	16,400	5.2
8	Accidents	14,900	4.7
9	Gastroenteritis	14,500	4.5
10	Tuberculosis	11,000	3.5
11	Cerebrovascular disease	10,400	3.3
12	Pneumonia (adult)	9100	2.9
13	Tetanus (neonatal)	6900	2.2
14	Cirrhosis	6600	2.1
15	Congenital malformations	6000	1.9
16	Complications of pregnancy	5900	1.8
17	Hypertension	5100	1.6
18	Intestinal obstruction	4900	1.6
19	Typhoid	4800	1.5
20	Meningitis	4600	1.5
21	Hepatitis	4600	1.5
22	Pertussis	4600	1.5
23	Other birth diseases	4600	1.5
24	Tetanus (adult)	4500	1.4
25	Schistosomiasis	4400	1.4
	Total of first 25 diseases	270,200	84.9

Source: From [25].

changes slightly. The new ranking becomes measles, pneumonia (child), malaria, malnutrition, prematurity, sickle cell disease, birth injury, gastroenteritis, accidents, and tuberculosis. Again, the importance of infections as causes of illness burden and deaths becomes evident.

This type of ranking inherently places a greater value on the death of a newborn than on the death of an older person since the life expectancy at birth is greater. If a society values its newborns more than its health care, resources should be used to control these top-ranked disease problems. If a society decides that other groups should receive priority, for example, young adults in the economically productive years of life, then its resources would most effectively be directed at controlling other disease problems. Also, this type of ranking tends to undervalue diseases causing chronic disability rather than death, such as poliomyelitis and leprosy. A severely maimed individual may represent both the loss of an economically and socially productive person and a chronic drain on the community resources.

If we carefully analyze the causes of death and disability in the economically productive age groups, again infectious diseases cause the majority of the illness. Schistosomiasis, hepatitis virus–associated cirrhosis and hepatoma, Chagas' disease, tuberculosis, filariasis, guinea worm, and amebiasis affect older age groups more than children, but diarrhea, malaria, and respiratory infections also contribute to disability. In setting priorities for health services, value judgments concerning age groups and diseases of importance for the community should be recognized.

Health expenditures

A final method for measuring the burden of illness is comparison of health care expenditures. Public and private spending on health care in developing countries averages about $9 per capita in low-income countries and $31 in middle-income countries. These figures are low compared with an average of $670 in industrialized countries and the average U.S. health expenditures mentioned above. Despite this remarkable difference, the proportion of total national income devoted to health ranges from 2 to 12 percent in almost all countries [26]. Private household expenditures amount to about half of this.

CONCLUSION

This chapter has attempted to delineate the major diseases causing illness in developing countries. These are frequently not the exotic parasitic diseases usually associated with tropical medicine, but are primarily bacterial and viral infectious diseases that once were endemic in industrialized countries but now are controlled through improvements in immunization, hygiene, nutrition, housing, water supply, and socioeconomic status. In order to improve health in tropical countries, these should be the priorities for allocation of health resources [27].

REFERENCES

1 Chen LC, Rahman M, Sardar AM: Epidemiology and causes of death among children in a rural area of Bangladesh. Int J Epidemiol 9(1):1, 1980

2 Anonymous: Towards a Better Future—Maternal and Child Health. Geneva, World Health Organization, 1980

3 Institute of Medicine: *New Vaccine Development: Establishing Priorities,* vol 1, Diseases of Importance in the United States. Washington, DC, National Academy Press, 1984

4 Institute of Medicine: *New Vaccine Development: Establishing Priorities,* vol 2, Diseases of Importance in Developing Countries. Washington, DC, National Academy Press, 1986

5 Trends in years of potential life lost due to infant mortality and perinatal conditions, 1980–1983 and 1984–1985. Morbid Mortal Week Rep 37(16):249–256, 1988

6 Sunshine JH, Dicker M: Family Out-of-Pocket Expenditures for Health Care: United States, 1980. National Center for Health Statistics, 1985

7 Zimicki S, Nahar L, Sarder AM, D'Souza S. Demographic Surveillance System—Matlab, vol 13, Cause of Death Reporting in Matlab. Source Book of Cause-specific Mortality Rate. Dhaka, International Centre for Diarrhoeal Disease Research, scientific report no 63, Bangladesh, October, 1985

8 Preston S, Keyfitz N, Schoen R: *Life Tables for National Populations.* New York and London, Seminar Press, 1972

9 The Fact Finding Commission, National Epidemiology Board of Thailand: Review of the Health Situation in Thailand: Priority Ranking of Diseases. Bangkok, National Epidemiology Board of Thailand, 1987

10 Walsh JA: Establishing Health Priorities in the Developing World. New York, United Nations Development Programme, 1988

11 Berman S, McIntosh K: Respiratory infections. Rev Infect Dis, in press

12 Bulla A, Hitze KL: Acute respiratory infections: A review. Bull WHO 56:481, 1978

13 Ashworth A, Feachem RG: Interventions for the control of diarrhoeal diseases among young children: Prevention of low birth weight. Bull WHO 63(1):165–184, 1985

14 Walsh JA, Hutchins S: Group B streptococcal disease: Its importance in the developing world and prospects for prevention with vaccines. Ped Infect Dis, in press

15 Rohde JE: Acute diarrhea, in Walsh JA, Warren KS (eds): *Strate-gies for Primary Health Care: Technologies Appropriate for the Control of Diseases in the Developing World.* University of Chicago Press, 1986, pp 14–29

16 Walsh JA: Selective primary health care: Strategies for control of disease in the developing world. IV. Measles. Rev Infect Dis 5(2):330–340, 1983

17 Manciaux M, Romer CJ: Accidents in children, adolescents and young adults: A major public health problem. World Health Stat Q 39(3):227–31, 1986

18 Puffer RR, Serrano CV: Patterns of mortality in childhood. Washington, DC, PAHO, scientific publication no 262, 1973

19 Keusch GT, Scrimshaw NS: Control of infection to reduce the prevalence of infantile and childhood malnutrition, in Walsh JA, Warren KS (eds): *Strategies for Primary Health Care: Technologies Appropriate for the Control of Disease in the Developing World.* University of Chicago Press, 1986, pp 298–313

20 Kuznetsov RL: Malaria control by application of indoor spraying of residual insecticides in tropical Africa and its impact on community health. Trop Doct 7:81–91, 1977

21 Reubush TL III, Breman JG, Kaiser RL, et al: Malaria, in Walsh JA, Warren KS (eds): *Strategies for Primary Health Care: Technologies Appropriate for the Control of Disease in the Developing World.* University of Chicago Press, 1986, pp 47–60

22 Francis DP: Hepatitis B virus and its related diseases, in Walsh JA, Warren KS (eds): *Strategies for Primary Health Care: Technologies Appropriate for the Control of Disease in the Developing World.* University of Chicago Press, 1986, pp 289–298

23 Hewlett EL: Pertussis and diphtheria, in Walsh JA, Warren KS (eds): *Strategies for Primary Health Care: Technologies Appropriate for the Control of Disease in the Developing World.* University of Chicago Press 1986, pp 85–93

24 Black RE, Brown KH, Becker S, et al: Longitudinal studies of infectious diseases and physical growth of children in rural Bangladesh. I. Patterns of morbidity. Am J Epidemiol 115(4):305–314, 1982

25 Ghana Health Assessment Project Team: A quantitative method of assessing the health impact of different diseases in less developed countries. Int J Epidemiol 10(1):73–80, 1981

26 World Bank: Financing Health Services in Developing Countries: An Agenda for Reform. Washington, DC, World, 1987

27 Walsh JA, Warren KS: Selective primary health care: An interim strategy for disease control in developing countries. Soc Sci Med 14C:145–163, 1980

Social Determinants of Tropical Disease · Patricia L. Rosenfield

Systematic scientific investigations focused on understanding the etiology and ecology of tropical diseases were initiated more than 100 years ago [1]. Hypotheses and propositions about disease transmission were closely related to factors in the human environment, but stopped short of seriously examining the interaction of human behavior and disease transmission. With the rapidly increasing sophistication of biomedical research throughout the twentieth century, the more traditional concern about environmental causation of disease rapidly gave way to laboratory investigations starting with the macroscopic and culminating in the genetic-level investigations of the 1970s and 1980s. These investigations were originally directed toward illuminating the transmission and life cycles, and then toward pinpointing vulnerable sites for drugs and vaccines to kill the parasite, and pesticides to kill the vectors of vectorborne tropical diseases. Only the entomologists sustained concern about the environmental factors, including vector-human contact [2].

The increasing environmental consciousness of the late 1960s and early 1970s brought those concerned with the spectrum of problems in human ecology into contact with diseases such as malaria and schistosomiasis because of the close association of the life cycle of those diseases with environmental changes from construction of dams and irrigation systems [3]. This linking of human ecology with tropical disease research also provided the impetus for the expanded development of the field of medical anthropology. Together, the different discipline lines began to converge in the study of disease transmission and control, as exemplified by the pioneering works of Benjamin Paul, George Foster, and Frederick Dunn [4]. These scholars and others gave prominence to the interdisciplinary diagnosis of the social determinants of tropical diseases; the center of attention became the role of individuals, and occasionally communities, in influencing patterns of disease transmission. From anthropological-ecological studies, recommendations generally focused on improving people's attitudes toward health and hygienic practices and on changing their behavior. The health educators, borrowing heavily from this research, argued that by developing better education programs, people would know why they should change their attitudes and their behaviors; their receptiveness to health and disease control programs would increase.

Unfortunately the tropical diseases did not decline in prevalence or incidence as a result of these well-intentioned education programs [5]. Social science and medical researchers have recently realized that changing attitudes and behavior is not sufficient to reduce disease transmission and improve ac-

ceptability of control programs. The scope of "social determinants" has now been broadened to take into account contributing factors other than individual (or community) behavior and attitudes. This recognition has resulted from studies exploring the reasons for the lack of success of programs which did incorporate human behavior and attitudes through health education measures, and yet were not achieving the anticipated goals. The experiences of education programs conducted under the auspices of the national and international malaria eradication programs began to raise these concerns, which were further emphasized by studies supported by the global United Nations Development Program/World Bank/WHO Special Program for Research and Training in Tropical Diseases (TDR) and by other WHO programs [6]. The emphasis has now shifted from that of "blaming" the individuals at risk for their attitudes and behavior to examining more systematically the social and economic conditions which influence transmission and control of tropical diseases, and, as importantly, the design, organization, management, and implementation of disease control programs.

This expanded definition of the social determinants of tropical diseases parallels the findings in agriculture and family planning research concentrating on the acceptance and use of agricultural technologies and contraceptives, respectively [7]. Results from research in those fields have increased understanding of the broader range of factors that influence decision making on the part of individual farmers and women and have led to more socially sound research and operations.

In this review of social determinants of tropical diseases, the extended range of factors influencing or affecting disease transmission and the effectiveness of disease control is described. The factors are drawn from individual, household, community, and broader societal conditions. When taken together they form the basis of a more suitable scientific diagnostic approach for analyzing the particular conditions influencing the transmission and control of tropical diseases than what has been customarily used. Because research on social determinants is not an end in itself—that is, because the aim of such research is to contribute to the improvement of disease control programs and reduction in incidence and prevalence of disease—attention is also given to social factors that influence the effectiveness of disease control programs.

As part of the presentation and discussion of an analytical framework for social diagnoses of tropical diseases, results of studies are reviewed to illustrate with field examples the different components of the framework. A brief discussion of methods for interdisciplinary studies indicates further the feasibility of applying the basic concepts. The next steps to take in achieving use of this broader diagnostic algorithm are suggested in the concluding section.

A FRAMEWORK FOR ANALYSIS OF SOCIAL DETERMINANTS

The framework proposed for use in analyzing the social determinants of tropical disease is drawn from the experiences of the TDR Social and Economic Research (SER) program and is given in Fig. 26-1 [8]. This framework has been modified from the one used to guide strategic decisions in the TDR/SER program as to which research to emphasize under which conditions. Briefly, the factors incorporated sequentially in the framework include the baseline historical influences shaping individual, community, and societal interactions, linked to those factors relating to disease transmission and control. The framework can be used to guide analysis of these interacting relationships with the aim of improving the effectiveness of disease control strategies within a particular societal context.

The following review emphasizes how the different components of the framework can be analyzed from the perspective of the individual, household, community, and society, and in relationship to parasite and vector conditions. Such analyses, as discussed below, necessitate an interdisciplinary team approach, the team including a parasitologist, vector biologist, epidemiologist, and control program staff along with social scientists (anthropologist, sociologist, economist, etc.) as appropriate to the problem being investigated. The examples presented below are intended to demonstrate that these issues are not merely theoretical concerns, but rather are issues which

can be studied in the field to contribute to understanding the broadly defined social determinants of tropical diseases.

INDIVIDUAL CHARACTERISTICS

To evaluate the individual characteristics influencing transmission and control of tropical diseases, it is crucial to understand people's beliefs and levels of knowledge about diseases, disease vectors, and control measures. However, the beliefs and attitudes concerning particular health conditions do not emanate solely from experience with a disease, but often from a general perception of disease impact. As indicated in a study from the Philippines, it has been the perceived impact of a disease (in this instance, schistosomiasis) which has influenced decisions as to where to locate, what kinds of agricultural activities to engage in, and expectations of future earnings as well as of employment and marriage possibilities. Those people who have not had exposure to the disease and who may not know much about the disease were those who often took the most severe measures to avoid the disease in response to their perceived fear of the disease [9].

Such perception also may lead the individual to decide that the disease is not serious enough to warrant changing behavior, and, therefore, even though the person at risk may be fully aware of the etiology of the disease and its impact, he or she will continue to engage in disease-transmitting behavior, as do, for example, migrants moving to new colonization projects where they may be exposed to new diseases. Research in the Amazon region of Brazil has demonstrated that economic necessity often overwhelms the risk of disease in relation to individual behavior. In the state of Rondonia, a team of social

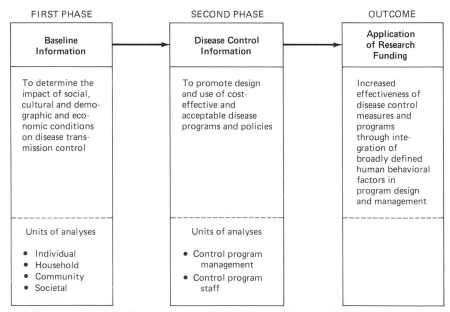

Figure 26-1. A conceptual framework for the analysis of social determinants of tropical diseases. (*Modified from the Strategic Plan for Research presented in* [8].)

and medical scientists, including disease control program staff, has shown that settlers fully know the risk of contracting malaria but continue to clear the jungle in the hope of improving their economic conditions. In 1985, "there were nearly 12,000 officially reported cases of malaria for a total population averaging 5000 people—more than two cases per person per year" [10]. The settlers know about the availability of chemotherapy and therefore choose to run the risk of becoming infected (and possibly dying since for many this is their first exposure to the disease), and then seeking treatment. Unfortunately, access to preventive measures (e.g., improved housing or protective clothing) has been limited due to economic constraints, and thus the cycle of infection-debility-treatment— infection-debility-treatment is maintained at potentially damaging cost to the long-term well-being of the individual. Because people have moved to these new colonization projects out of economic necessity, they are willing to run the risk of malaria in order to achieve short-term economic success.

Much of the baseline work on understanding people's knowledge about disease and disease vectors, and their attitudes toward control measures, has focused on traditional beliefs as well as the lack of knowledge about the etiology of the disease. Studies from countries in Africa, Asia, and Latin America have demonstrated that traditional beliefs often influence people's behavior with regard to transmission of disease [11]. While people may recognize the symptoms, they often do not understand the causes or else have developed an explanatory system for the causes that leads to use of ineffective preventive measures and/or influences the acceptability of more effective curative measures. The assumption behind many of the studies on understanding attitudes and beliefs is that lack of knowledge and awareness concerning disease-transmitting behavior or limited acceptance of control programs could be improved by incorporating the relevant social, cultural, economic, and ecological information into health education programs. For example, in peninsular Malaysia, in a rural setting, some villagers were unaware of the relationship between mosquitoes and filariasis. Their traditional explanation for the symptoms of elephantiasis was that the swollen legs were due to the anger of the elephant gods in a swampy area near their villages, who sent the disease to afflict them [12]. Others associated the disease with particular foods and drinks. Only 9.2 percent were aware of the epidemiology of the disease [13]. The researchers proposed an education program based on their findings but recognized that even with such knowledge, the resulting actions may not be implemented unless people feel that avoiding the disease is worth the extra effort required to practice preventive measures, such as eliminating or clearing mosquito breeding places.

Leprosy is one of the diseases still prevalent in the tropics for which there is a wide variety of traditional and modern explanations. An extensive study in Sarawak, Malaysia, of the traditional beliefs about leprosy led to design of health education material for villagers based on different cultural back-

grounds and different living conditions. This study involved individuals at risk and infected as well as control program staff to develop different educational materials such as cartoons, articles, posters, and tape-slide shows and consequently may lead to improved use of control services [14]. The results of these newly designed health education efforts are now being evaluated by the control program and Ministry of Health staff.

However, as indicated by the results of agriculture and family planning studies referred to earlier, it is likely that revisions and improvements in health education materials, albeit desirable, are necessary but not sufficient actions to convince people to change their behavior. This is demonstrated by a review of studies on water contact behavior influencing schistosomiasis transmission that was conducted in 1979 and resulted in a wide range of topics for study and recommendations about factors influencing how to change water-related behavior [15]. Studies on this topic indicate that even when knowledge is increased, if the appropriate water supplies are not available, it is obviously impossible for people to change their behavior. A recent study in Egypt examined the relationship between the use of domestic water supplies and prevalence of schistosomiasis [16]. Women continued to use schistosome-infected canal water because hand pumps were not repaired; even when the pumps worked, they were not popular because water quality from those pumps was not acceptable and the pumps were not conveniently located. These results complement the findings of other researchers over the past 10 years and illustrate the need to adopt a broader approach to changing or facilitating change in individual behavior.

Health education based on broad knowledge of social determinants can contribute to enabling "people and communities to make their own decisions on matters of health" [17]. The diagnosis of individual decision making and behavior with regard to disease-transmitting activities, as indicated in Table 26-1, includes careful examination of both traditional beliefs and attitudes towards the disease and more modern perceptions of the impact of the disease, and of how those perceptions are influenced, modified, or discounted because of the basic necessity to earn money, grow food, provide shelter, or provide water for the individual and the family. Other factors are indicated in Table 26-1 and could be expanded or elaborated on in relation to the particular problem or set of problems being analyzed.

HOUSEHOLD AND COMMUNITY CHARACTERISTICS

Many of the vectorborne, water-related tropical diseases are related to community hygiene; even the broader understanding of individual behavior described above would not provide enough information for improving health conditions. For example, with diseases such as guinea worm and schistosomiasis, individuals play a crucial role in contaminating the water supply with the parasite that can ultimately become infective to others who then use that water source. With diseases such as

Table 26-1. Illustrative characteristics influencing individual attitudes and behavior toward tropical disease transmission and control

Perception of disease and its impact
Attitudes toward disease, control measures, and control program

Knowledge of disease transmission and control processes
Economic conditions (including agricultural practices)
Living conditions (including availability of protected water supplies and sanitation facilities, and housing conditions)

Educational levels
Access to alternative traditional providers of health care
Use of modern governmental or private health care providers

malaria and filariasis which are mosquito-borne, the individual often has limited control over the conditions of the mosquito habitats; it requires a community effort to ensure protected water supplies and sustain elimination of breeding places. With a disease such as Chagas' disease, the situation is slightly more complicated. If an individual improves his or her housing, but others in the community do not, it is likely that the one family may be protected but the vectors of Chagas' disease, namely the triatomine bugs, will infest unprotected housing and vegetation in the vicinity.

Community action is needed in all these cases to reduce the risk of disease to the community as a whole and to individuals. However, as is well known from work in environmental economics on similar kinds of community problems, it is often most difficult to achieve community action to reduce disease-transmitting habitats or to modify disease-transmitting behavior if an individual recognizes that he or she does not have to act if their neighbors act to improve the situation [18]. The combination of the "free-rider" and "externality" effects is an important concern to take into account as actions are proposed to modify human behavioral influences on transmission of diseases. Studies on the role of community participation in disease control, particularly those focusing on vector control, have demonstrated that it is difficult to promote and sustain community participation for the good of the community.

In Kenya and Tanzania, studies have shown that both vector control and distribution of chemotherapeutic agents, respectively, are difficult to sustain. In the first instance, in a project focusing on community-based malaria control in Kenya, because of people's limited available time, they preferred to focus on income-generating activities and not work collectively and continually to control mosquito population. The population did participate in the distribution of chloroquine, after appropriate training and incentives were put in place [19]. In Tanzania, the official government political structure was used as the basis of community participation for chloroquine distribution; this did not succeed for a number of reasons including the unavailability of the local distributor when the mothers came to pick up the drugs [20].

In Sri Lanka, community participation was successfully promoted for anopheles control but only in the context of a larger voluntary effort, the Sarvodaya program, which incorporated malaria as part of overall community development efforts. Disease vector control was placed in the context of socially acceptable effort to improve everyone's social and economic conditions without making anyone worse off [21]: those who donated time and effort for vector control shared responsibilities with others who worked on community hygiene, education, and nutrition improvements.

Particularly with regard to the vectorborne tropical diseases, analyzing and diagnosing individual behavior and then aggregating the findings to obtain an understanding of community behavior is not sufficient. The aggregation process tends to smooth out the complexities; different sets of questions should be asked focusing on interactions between households and within the community. The community is more complicated than the sum of its parts; data are required on a wide range of factors to increase understanding about how to achieve disease control. Questioning individuals specifically about their personal disease-related behavior should be complemented by examining communitywide housing, water, and economic-related conditions. A thorough review of these issues was undertaken in 1983 and indicated that it is crucial to define for each instance the relevant community and the most effective, acceptable control measures so that the appropriate people are involved in activities that will have some lasting impact. The question of time availability or competing demands on the time of individuals participating on behalf of the community emerged as a key element for assessing the sustainability of community activities for disease control [22]. Using the conceptual framework presented in Fig. 26-1, a strategic plan for research was developed to guide researchers in identifying specific community characteristics influencing disease transmission and control (see Fig. 26-2).

CONTROL PROGRAM CHARACTERISTICS

As indicated at the beginning of the chapter, understanding of individual and community behavior should be enhanced by examining the role of control programs and their staff as another key to achieving an understanding of the broad-based factors influencing both disease transmission and the acceptability and use of control measures. If the control program is not implemented in an acceptable manner in a community, it is not going to have an impact on the control of the disease. People will not utilize the services, and the disease will continue to be prevalent in that area despite expenditures of time and money on control activities. Thus, any analysis of the social determinants of tropical diseases should include information on the control program as well as the community being served.

The most dramatic demonstration of the need for such information is the continual problem with acceptability of house

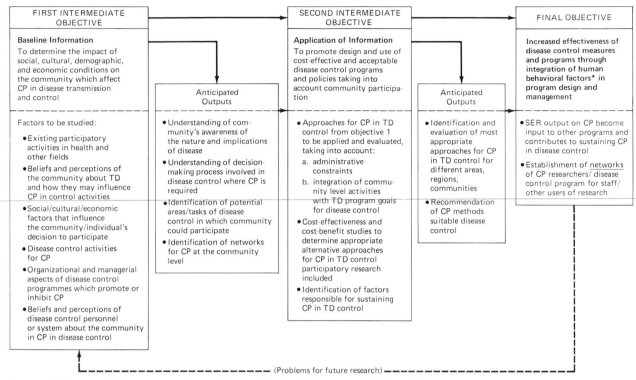

FIRST INTERMEDIATE OBJECTIVE		SECOND INTERMEDIATE OBJECTIVE		FINAL OBJECTIVE
Baseline Information To determine the impact of social, cultural, demographic, and economic conditions on the community which affect CP in disease transmission and control		**Application of Information** To promote design and use of cost-effective and acceptable disease control programs and policies taking into account community participation		**Increased effectiveness of disease control measures and programs through integration of human behavioral factors* in program design and management**

Factors to be studied:	Anticipated Outputs		Anticipated Outputs	

• Existing participatory activities in health and other fields
• Beliefs and perceptions of the community about TD and how they may influence CP in control activities
• Social/cultural/economic factors that influence the community/individual's decision to participate
• Disease control activities for CP
• Organizational and managerial aspects of disease control programmes which promote or inhibit CP
• Beliefs and perceptions of disease control personnel or system about the community in CP in disease control
	• Understanding of community's awareness of the nature and implications of disease
	• Understanding of decision-making process involved in disease control where CP is required
	• Identification of potential areas/tasks of disease control in which community could participate
	• Identification of networks for CP at the community level
		• Approaches for CP in TD control from objective 1 to be applied and evaluated, taking into account:
		  a. administrative constraints
		  b. integration of community level activities with TD program goals for disease control
		• Cost-effectiveness and cost-benefit studies to determine appropriate alternative approaches for CP in TD control participatory research included
		• Identification of factors responsible for sustaining CP in TD control
			• Identification and evaluation of most appropriate approaches for CP in TD control for different areas, regions, communities
			• Recommendation of CP methods suitable disease control
				• SER output on CP become input to other programs and contributes to sustaining CP in disease control
				• Establishment of <u>networks</u> of CP researchers/disease control program for staff/other users of research

(Problems for future research)

Figure 26-2. Research plan on community participation in tropical disease control. (*From* [22].)

spraying for malaria and filariasis control, and of case finding and case holding for leprosy control. Control of these diseases has tended to be organized vertically. That is, disease control efforts are not incorporated into any other health activity. Thus the staff in those programs have specialized in controlling the specific disease and often have worked for many years on that particular disease problem. Years of effort have led to, in many cases, a sense of frustration because the disease is still widely prevalent and work has become unsatisfactorily repetitive [23]. Those many years of frustrated effort often lead to negative attitudes toward those individuals who are at risk or infected, and may generate the population's resistance to house spraying or case-finding and case-holding activities.

For example, careful analyses of people's health-seeking behavior with regard to malaria control have been carried out in Thailand [24]. The major determinants of treatment-seeking behavior were related in part at least to confidence in the effectiveness of the control activities as well as to the usual factors of costs of disease and costs of treatment. In a thorough analysis of the acceptance of household spraying against anopheles mosquitos, it was the attitude toward the householders of the people doing the spraying that influenced whether or not the spraying would be accepted. The project team also analyzed health-seeking behavior, demonstrating that the population would first utilize locally and socially acceptable

treatment providers, starting with self-medication, lay doctors, drugstores, with malaria clinics being the last resort. A separate economic analysis of the costs of a malaria control program in Thailand has resulted in fuller understanding of the need to have programs that are perceived to provide effective service for the time and money that the patient spends to obtain that service [25].

SOCIETAL CONTEXT CHARACTERISTICS

Further complicating the diagnosis of social determinants of tropical diseases is the increasingly recognized fact that understanding the following:

> Human behavior and attitudes concerning tropical diseases
> Intracommunity relations influencing disease transmission
> Control program–community interactions (for community control programs)

is not sufficient for complete analysis of the social determinants of tropical diseases and the identification of the most appropriate kinds of control actions. The tropical diseases of concern here are diseases closely linked to poverty; indeed, ''poverty has become the underlying cause of ill health . . . [and] in such situations there is little the individual *per se* can do to improve his/her health'' [26]. Thus an analysis of the underlying social and economic context is essential for contributing to understanding why there is continued transmission of the tropical diseases despite the generally well-established knowledge of their etiology and the availability of at least some effective control measures. While the clinician might be dismayed by the increased complexity of the social diagnosis, those concerned about continued morbidity and mortality resulting from tropical diseases must understand that individual, community, and control program actions, even when well integrated, will not be sufficient for successful, sustainable control unless political, economic, and social support is provided on a continuing basis.

Such commitment and support could lead to a reorientation of the resource allocation process, as discussed fully in analyses of the situations in China; Kerala State, India; Sri Lanka; and Costa Rica at a conference analyzing good health at low cost (as summarized in Fig. 26-3), and as demonstrated by programs of intersectoral actions for health sponsored by WHO [27]. While these elements may appear to be beyond the immediate control of individuals, communities, and control programs, experiences from the countries referred to above indicate that when there is sufficient citizen participation in the

decision-making process, along with an educated population, and when the government has recognized the relationship between disease and development, sufficient resources are regularly made available to sustain control program activities. In Sri Lanka and Costa Rica, in particular, malaria control has been a very high priority of the governments; in Sri Lanka, the relationship to new settlement projects has recently been under study, and in Costa Rica for decades there has been explicit recognition of the economic impact of malaria and the need for well-organized, sustained control programs.

Knowledge of the political, economic, and social systems can complement the interpretation of findings from studies on the individual, community, and control program. For example, the project in the Amazon region of Brazil referred to earlier had to include analysis of the political and economic decisions that led to the decision to invest in colonizing the jungle—e.g., the decision to build houses and roads, and to obtain loans from the World Bank. This in turn had to be related to (1) where settlers were attracted from, (2) their previous exposure to and knowledge of malaria, (3) the location of housing and roads in relation to mosquito-breeding sites, and (4) the availability of funds for providing preventive and control

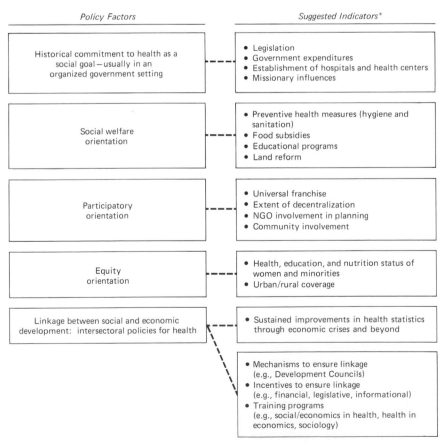

Figure 26-3. Social and political policy factors contributing to improved health status in China, Costa Rica, Kerala State (India), and Sri Lanka. (*From* [27].) *Indicators are suggested for assessing the relative strengths of the different policy factors in the examples.

Policy Factors

Historical commitment to health as a social goal—usually in an organized government setting

Social welfare orientation

Participatory orientation

Equity orientation

Linkage between social and economic development: intersectoral policies for health

Suggested Indicators*

- Legislation
- Government expenditures
- Establishment of hospitals and health centers
- Missionary influences

- Preventive health measures (hygiene and sanitation)
- Food subsidies
- Educational programs
- Land reform

- Universal franchise
- Extent of decentralization
- NGO involvement in planning
- Community involvement

- Health, education, and nutrition status of women and minorities
- Urban/rural coverage

- Sustained improvements in health statistics through economic crises and beyond

- Mechanisms to ensure linkage (e.g., Development Councils)
- Incentives to ensure linkage (e.g., financial, legislative, informational)
- Training programs (e.g., social/economics in health, health in economics, sociology)

measures. Recommendations from the research are already leading to increased attention to these issues in new loans to Brazil under consideration by the World Bank.

Understanding the broad range of determinants affecting the transmission and control of tropical diseases can improve the design of disease control strategies by (1) incorporating social and economic factors into new types of health education programs, into the training of control program staff, and into the design or reorientation of control programs; (2) changing the level of resources allocated to the control of tropical diseases on a continuing basis in order to increase the effectiveness and sustainability of control efforts; and, (3) in parallel with the governmental changes, changing the risk-taking behavior of individuals, households, and communities with respect to the tropical diseases.

FEASIBILITY OF BROAD-BASED DIAGNOSIS OF THE SOCIAL DETERMINANTS OF TROPICAL DISEASES

To the non-social scientist, the components of this broader-based approach to the diagnosis of social determinants of tropical diseases may seem related but difficult to analyze coherently. The conceptual framework given in Fig. 26-1 provides a simple algorithm for assessing the social determinants of tropical disease. Use of this algorithm demands an interdisciplinary approach, linking several different disciplines in the social sciences with epidemiologists who can relate these findings to levels of disease, and control program staff who, by their involvement throughout this process, can contribute their knowledge and can increase their own sensitivity to and understanding of the determining factors. This kind of team was organized for most of the projects mentioned here. While each individual contributes his or her special knowledge to the study, having a commonly agreed to problem or set of problems to analyze has facilitated the research process. Ideally, research teams move from the initial research on social determinants to assessing the feasibility of implementing recommendations from the study, thus contributing to the improvement of disease control programs.

An example of this is a project on leprosy in the Philippines where the first stage of the research provided thorough analysis of the individual and community factors influencing people's attitudes toward the disease and their use of control services [28]. The initial study combined social, linguistic, psychological, and epidemiological research techniques to determine the subtle sources of prejudice against leprosy patients as indicated by language and the range of beliefs that led to limited use of control services—many were based on religious and cultural traditions not met by taking a drug requiring long-term use for effectiveness.

For the second stage of the research, the team joined forces with the control program to analyze both staff attitudes toward patients and the organization of the control program, including

the shift from a vertical to an integrated program. Using a combination of social science and management research methods, the team uncovered several possibilities for reducing staff biases, improving program management, and increasing service utilization by the population. Special training programs were recommended by the team as well as improved management measures to ensure easy and discreet access to services for the patients. Starting from a concern about understanding social determinants, the research team developed the capacity to analyze and recommend changes in program design and management.

Another approach for combining baseline social analyses with concern about community participation is that of participatory research, an approach which brings together, in the research activity itself, the population in the study area, the researchers, and the control program staff. This approach has been used effectively in the study of several tropical diseases, notably Chagas' disease, malaria, and schistosomiasis. These studies have led to a series of recommendations from researchers as to the best way of organizing participation in the baseline research in order to develop acceptable and effective interventions to facilitate changing behavior to reduce disease transmission and increase the effectiveness of disease control activities [8,29].

An example from a study in Brazil on Chagas' disease shows how such an approach may be used to improve understanding of the disease and develop control programs acceptable to the community and to individuals [30]. The researchers and community members worked together to study the transmission of the disease so as to identify the most effective control measure (housing improvements), to determine the constraints against implementing those improvements (money), and to decide how to meet those constraints (initiate income-generating activities). The control program staff were also included in the discussions and actions, which led to measurable reduction in disease incidence in the 0- to 4-year-old age range. A program of community-determined housing improvements and income-generating activities has initiated effective Chagas' disease control. A participatory approach also has the extra benefit of increasing contact between the control program staff and the population, enabling staff to achieve increased acceptance of the program, resulting in increased program effectiveness.

NEXT STEPS

While individual research projects have demonstrated the feasibility of analyzing social determinants from a broad, interdisciplinary, and applied perspective, more work is needed to demonstrate the applicability of the diagnostic results to improving control program activities. Greater attention must be given to the policy implications of research, including how to present the findings to those responsible for resource allocation. This means employing disciplines different from those usual in our work, namely political science and economics.

Moreover, since the process of achieving policy change is often sensitive to local nuances, the interest of national researchers in examining these problems should be strengthened to increase the likelihood that research results will be listened to by their compatriots. The projects described here have indicated that when national investigators work in partnership with control programs and communities, change can result. In addition to obtaining important academic results, projects so organized can yield practical results to improve the control of tropical disease by recommending approaches which integrate changes in human behavior with changes in control program implementation and overall development policies [31]. Only when the diverse social and medical science disciplines work together with control program staff to obtain the broad understanding of social determinants of tropical diseases can sustainable disease control be achieved.

Note: Work reported here is drawn from the author's tenure as Secretary of the Scientific Working Group and Steering Committee on Social and Economic Research of the UNDP/World Bank/World Health Organization Special Programme for Research and Training in Tropical Disease.

REFERENCES

1 Bruce-Chwat LJ: *Essential Malariology,* 2d ed. London, William Heinemann Medical, 1985, pp 1–11; Jordan P: *Schistosomiasis: The St. Lucia Project.* Cambridge, Cambridge University Press, 1985, pp 1–2; Jordan AM: *Trypansomiasis Control and African Rural Development.* Essex, Longman, 1986, pp 30–43

2 Youdeowei A and Service MW: *Pest and Vector Management in the Tropics.* Essex, Longman, 1983, pp 1–44

3 Rosenfield PL: The Management of Schistosomiasis: Research Paper R-16. Washington, DC, Resources for the Future, 1979

4 Dunn F: Social determinants in tropical disease, in Warren KS, Mahmoud ADF (eds): *Tropical and Geographical Medicine,* 1st ed. New York, Mcgraw-Hill, 1985, pp 125-1 to 125-21

5 Gramiccia G: Health education in malaria control—why has it failed? World Health Forum 2:385–393, 1981

6 World Health Organization: WHO Expert Committee on Malaria 18th Report. Geneva, World Health Organization, 1986

7 Freedman R: The contribution of social science research to population policy and family planning program effectiveness. Studies in Family Planning 18:57–82, 1987; Matlon P, Cantrell R, King David Benoit-Catlin M: Coming Full Circle: Farmers' Participation in the Development of Technology. Ottawa, International Development Research Centre, 1984

8 UNDP/World Bank/WHO Special Programme for Research and Training in Tropical Diseases: chap 12, Social and economic research, in Seventh Programme Report, January 1983–31 December 1984. Geneva, World Health Organization, pp. 12/1–12/12

9 Herrin AN: Perception of disease impacts: what can they tell us? Paper prepared for meeting on the economics of tropical diseases, School of Economics, University of the Philippines, Manila, September 2–5, 1986

10 Sawyer DR: Malaria on the Amazon frontier: economic and social aspects of transmission and control. Southeast Asian J Trop Med Public Health 17:342–345, 1986

11 Rosenfield PL: Social and economic research, in Maurice J, Pearce AM (eds): Tropical Disease Research: A Global Partnership, Eighth Programme Report of UNDP/World Bank/WHO Special Programme for Research and Training in Tropical Diseases. Geneva, World Health Organization, 1987, pp 149–159

12 Mohd Riji H: Cultural factors in the epidemiology of filariasis due to *Brugia malayi* in an endemic community. Final Report Project 810065, available from UNDP/World Bank/WHO Special Programme for Research and Training in Tropical Diseases, Geneva, 1983, pp 137–149

13 Mohd Riji H: Comparison of knowledge on filariasis and epidemiologic factors between infected and uninfected respondents in a Malay community. Southeast Asian J Trop Med Public Health 17:457–463, 1986

14 Chen PCY: Longhouse dwelling, social contact and the prevalence of leprosy and tuberculosis among native tribes of Sarawah. Soc Sci Med 26:1073–1077, 1988; Chen PCY, Sim HC: The development of culture-specific health education packages to increase care-finding of leprosy in Sarawak. Southeast Asian J Trop Med Public Health 17:427–432, 1986

15 UNDP/World Bank/WHO Special Programme for Research and Training in Tropical Diseases (TDR): Workshop on the Role of Human/Water Contact in Schistosomiasis Transmission, TDR/SER-HWE/79.3. Geneva, 1979

16 Khairy AEM: Domestic water supplies and community self-help in Sidi Ghazzi area–Nile Delta, a strategy for schistosomiasis control: Part I. Water supplies and the prevalence of schistosomiasis. Bull High Institute Public Health 16:9–19, 1986

17 Brieger WR, Ramakrishna J: Health education: social marketing does not have all the answers. World Health Forum 8:385, 1987

18 Fisher AC, Peterson FM: The environment in economics: A survey. J Econ Lit 14:1–33, 1976

19 Kaseje DCO, Sempebwe EKN, Spencer HC: Community leadership and participation in the Saradidi, Kenya, Rural Health Development Programme. Ann Trop Med Parasitol 81suppl:46–55, 1987

20 MacCormack CP, Lwihula G: Failure to participate in a malaria Chemosuppression programme: North Mara, Tanzania. J Trop Med Hyg 86:99–107, 1983

21 Silva KT: A popular approach towards malaria control. Project ID 810420 available from UNDP/World Bank/WHO Special Programme for Research and Training in Tropical Diseases, Geneva, 1987

22 UNDP/World Bank/WHO Special Programme for Research and Training in Tropical Diseases (TDR): Community Participation in Tropical Disease Control: Social and Economic Research Issues—Report of the Scientific Working Group on Social and Economic Research. TDR/SER-SCO G(4)/CP/83.3, Geneva, TDR, 1983

23 World Health Organization Study Group: Malaria control as part of primary health care. WHO Tech Rep Ser 712, Geneva, World Health Organization, 1984

24 Hongvivatana T, Leerapan P, Chaiteeranuwatsiri M: Knowledge Perception and Behavior of Malaria. Bangkok, Monograph Series Centre for Health Policy Studies, Mahidol University, 1985

25 Kaewsonthi S, Harding AG: Cost and performance of malaria surveillance: the patients' perspectives. Southeast Asian J Trop Med Public Health 17:406–412, 1986

26 World Health Organization/Rockefeller Foundation: Intersectoral Action for Health: The Way Ahead. New York/Geneva, Rockefeller Foundation/World Health Organization, 1986, p 18

27 Halstead SB, Walsh JA, Warren KS: Good Health at Low Cost. New York, The Rockefeller Foundation, 1985; World Health Organization: Intersectoral Actions for Health for All: Promoting Health Through Public Policy. WHO/SHS/ISC/88.1. Geneva, World Health Organization, 1988

28 Valencia LB, Ventura ER, Paz CJ, et al: Society and Leprosy: A Study of Knowledge, Attitudes and Practices of Philippine Ilocanos—Social and Economic Research Project Reports No. 2; Managing Triadic Interaction: A Guide to Hansen's Disease Control—Social and Economic Research Project Reports No. 3. Geneva, UNDP/World Bank/WHO Special Programme for Research and Training in Tropical Diseases, 1988

29 Elder M: Sharing the research work: participative research and its role demands, in Reason P, Rowan J (eds): *Human Inquiry: A Sourcebook of New Paradigm Research*. Chichester, England, Wiley, 1981, pp 253–266

30 Dias RB, Pinto Dias JC: A migracao vista por Chagasics. Rev Soc Bras Med Trop 17(supp):56, 1984; Dias RB: Chagas' Disease, Popular Knowledge and New Strategies of Control, Final Report 810351. Geneva, UNDP/World Bank/WHO Special Programme for Research and Training in Tropical Diseases, 1986

31 Rosenfield PL: Linking theory with action: the use of social and economic research to improve the control of tropical parasitic diseases. Southeast Asian J Trop Med Public Health 17:323–332, 1986

CHAPTER
27

Relative Risks, Benefits, and Costs of Intervention · Kathryn Bennett · Peter Tugwell · David Sackett · Brian Haynes

Those who provide, plan, or pay for health care must decide which health services should be provided to whom in order to effectively and efficiently reduce the burden of disease, disability, and untimely death. Such decisions demand a critical appraisal of existing evidence about the relative risks, benefits, and costs of intervention and, if required, a call for new evidence.

The approach described in this chapter, an outgrowth of work by Cochrane [1], Sackett [2], and Evans [3], provides a framework for assembling the specific subset of information that is most likely to help in reducing the burden of both morbidity (symptoms; physical, emotional, social and functional impairment) and mortality for a disease. This is accomplished by subdividing the spectrum of health information inquiries into steps that constitute a logical progression—from quantifying the burden of illness, to identifying its likely causes, to validating interventions that prevent or ameliorate it and evaluating their efficiency, to monitoring the application of these interventions, and, coming full circle, to determining whether the burden of illness is reduced. Each of the six steps in the "measurement loop" (Fig. 27-1; Table 27-1) poses a different type of research or evaluation question and calls for a specific set of methodological standards applicable to either the critical appraisal of existing information or, if required, the generation of new evidence. The loop format emphasizes the importance of monitoring after implementing a health intervention to determine whether the planned reduction in the burden of illness is achieved. This process is *iterative,* since in almost all health care situations, the burden of illness is reduced by only a small proportion and repeated cycles of the "loop" are needed to

eradicate even that portion for which effective interventions exist.

In the discussion that follows we show how an evaluation of relative risk, benefits, and costs can contribute to health decisions in less developed countries (LDCs). The measurement loop provides a practical guide to research methods of use to both (1) the "consumers" of research—health professionals and policymakers who wish to decide whether to apply the results of research investigations to health care decisions; and (2) the "doers" of research—those individuals involved in the planning and implementation of health research. Immunization for the prevention of measles and the use of oral rehydration salts (ORS) for the treatment of acute diarrhea of childhood are examples used to illustrate how the approach can be used to summarize the available evidence and make recommendations for action.

As will be discussed, application of the measurement loop approach can contribute to areas of concern to LDCs in at least four ways. First, the loop provides a framework for assembling and critically evaluating the evidence necessary to rank alternative health interventions in terms of both burden of illness and cost-effectiveness and to thereby determine priorities among interventions under consideration for implementation. Ranking of interventions within the context of health planning is of high relevance in situations of competing priorities and scarce resources. When the cost of a package of interventions outstrips the available resources, those actions with the greatest potential to reduce disease burden in terms of costs and effects given the available budget can be identified.

Second, the loop can contribute to the transfer of appropriate

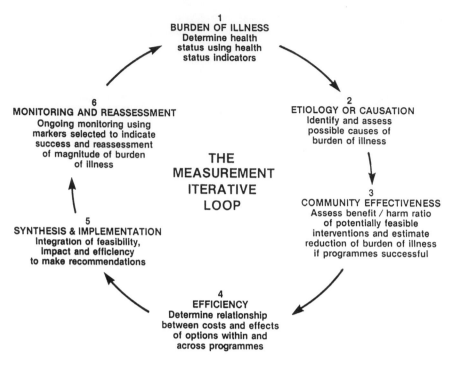

Figure 27-1. The measurement iterative loop.

technology to LDCs by assisting with the critical assessment and appropriate evaluation of medical innovations developed by industrialized nations, as the assumptions upon which the effectiveness of procedures developed in the west are based may not be valid in specific LDC settings.

Third, the loop emphasizes the importance of monitoring health programs after implementation. This is crucial to ensure that expected benefits are achieved and to reassess the health status of the population served. This is particularly relevant to large-scale community-based programs such as the provision of basic child and maternal health care. For example, monitoring of the quality of care provided by village and clinic health workers and of the availability of essential drugs is fundamental to the effectiveness of basic primary health care initiatives. If the cold chain is not monitored, the effectiveness of measles vaccination programs can be as low as zero [4,5]. If oral rehydration therapy is not used appropriately by mothers, the massive campaigns to promote it will not result in the levels of reduction in mortality that are possible by this simple intervention. In all these cases huge amounts of scarce resources could be wasted.

Fourth, the loop approach can assist in identifying gaps in the empirical data base, as will be illustrated with our two examples. Recent critical analyses to estimate the impact of a number of interventions relevant to LDC health problems have underlined this problem, with the authors needing to make a number of assumptions due to the lack of necessary data [6–9]. As is recognized by these authors, although evidence is available to support the efficacy (performance under ideal conditions) of many of the individual components of what is being recommended, (community) effectiveness under field conditions in actually reducing death and disability is untested in most instances. Further research under field conditions to validate recommendations is needed to ensure that the minimum magnitude of impact on health acceptable for a given intervention is achieved. This ''essential national health research'' [97,98] is the responsibility of researchers at the local or regional level and is a fruitful area for collaboration between individuals from industrialized and LDC countries.

MEASUREMENT LOOP STEP 1: BURDEN OF ILLNESS

The first step determines the current levels of morbidity (in terms of physical, emotional, and social function; symptoms) and mortality (death rates, healthy years of life lost). Good examples of studies carried out to assess the magnitude of health needs are: (1) a survey of health in seven countries directed by an international group of collaborators under the aegis of the World Health Organization [10]; and (2) a study of the major causes of illness and death in Ghana reported by the Ghana Health Assessment Project Team [11]. Both of these studies quantitatively assess functional health deficits as well as mortality; in fact, the latter study describes an interesting approach which quantifies the burden of illness by combining functional health deficits and mortality into units designated as ''healthy days of healthy life lost.''

The magnitude of burden due to measles and acute diarrhea

Table 27-1. Measurement iterative loop: Classification of health research and evaluation

1. *Burden of illness:* Quantification of current levels of morbidity (functional impairment; physical, emotional, and social symptoms) and mortality (death rates; healthy days of life lost).
   a. *Avoidable burden of illness:* Those components of disability, symptoms, and mortality for which feasible, effective prevention or cure exists.
   b. *Unavoidable burden of illness:* Those components of disability, symptoms, and mortality for which no effective, feasible prevention or cure currently exists.
2. *Etiology:* Studies aimed at establishing the contribution of potential causal factors to the burden of illness.
3. *Community effectiveness:* How well an intervention known to be efficacious works when applied in the less than optimal conditions of clinical or field settings; community effectiveness is the product of five factors:

$$\frac{\text{Community}}{\text{effectiveness}} = \text{efficacy} \times \frac{\text{diagnostic}}{\text{accuracy}} \times \frac{\text{provider}}{\text{compliance}} \times \frac{\text{patient}}{\text{compliance}} \times \text{coverage}$$

   Efficacy is the assessment of whether the maneuver, procedure, or service does more good than harm under conditions of optimal patient and provider compliance; *diagnostic accuracy* is the extent to which patients with the condition of interest are correctly discriminated from those without the condition; *provider compliance* is the extent to which the appropriate diagnostic and management (preventive, therapeutic, and/or rehabilitative) actions are complied with by the health provider; *patient compliance* is the extent to which patients comply with the health provider's recommendations and treatment; and *coverage* is the assessment of whether a specific health intervention, known to be effective, is being appropriately utilized by all patients who could benefit from it, calculated by determining the proportion of people in need of the specific intervention who are offered it.
4. *Efficiency:* The assessment of the extent to which the maneuver, procedure, or service is being delivered to those who would benefit from it, with an optimal use of resources, in terms of the impact obtained for a specific cost.
5. *Synthesis and implementation.* The integration of burden of illness, clinical-community effectiveness, efficiency, and feasibility to make recommendations for implementation.
6. *Monitoring and reassessment:* Ongoing monitoring of the progress of the program using "markers" (short-term, intermediate, or long-term) to indicate progress selected according to the individual project; assessment of the success of the specific therapy or health intervention in achieving the predicted reduction in the burden of illness; and, if this is not achieved, identification of the specific factors responsible so they can be corrected.

of childhood is well documented, with both consistently ranked among the top five killers of the under-5 population in LDCs. The incidence of acute diarrhea in children under 5 is in the range of 2.2 to 3 episodes per year with an associated case fatality rate in the range of 0.5 to 1 percent, or approximately 4.6 million deaths per year worldwide [12]. The impact of multiple episodes of diarrhea on nutritional status and the ability to withstand infection further increases the associated burden in terms of increased risk of disease.

The risk of measles in the absence of immunization is essentially 100 percent. Although a relatively benign disease in industrialized nations, the case fatality rate in LDCs ranges between 1 to 5 percent due to the frequent and severe complications that include marked weight loss due to diarrhea, poor appetite, and general malaise [13,14]. Severity of complications and risk of death are significantly increased in malnourished children. Maternal antibodies, which protect against measles, begin to wane around 6 months of age in LDC pop-

ulations; the optimal age for immunization now recommended is 9 months.

To make judgments about the quality of information concerning burden, three guidelines are applied. First, Is the attribute selected for the measurement relevant to the question being asked? The most appropriate and efficient method or indicator will vary according to the aspects of morbidity or mortality under consideration and the existing setup for collection of routine health statistics. For example, mortality rates indicate nothing about the magnitude of pain, mental suffering, or disability. These aspects of the burden of illness are equally as important as, or more important than, mortality rates for illnesses such as polio, malaria, schistosomiasis, leprosy, or trachoma, in which mortality contributes a relatively small proportion of the overall burden.

Second, Are the measurement methods accurate? This includes two components: (1) the ability of the indicator to reflect meaningful differences in the magnitude of the burden of illness and (2) the precision of the method. For example, mortality rates are assessed accurately in many (although by no means all) parts of the world where there is a legal requirement to report births and deaths, and these can be checked against other sources of existing information such as a census. Cause of death is rarely documented accurately (even in industrialized countries), and most components of morbidity will require specially designed surveys.

Cause-specific mortality rates for measles and acute diarrhea are particularly susceptible to problems of inaccuracy due to the need to rely on the report of family members or lay persons. Inaccuracy is also introduced by the likelihood that other diseases and chronic disorders such as malnutrition and infection may be present simultaneously. As a result, it is often impossible (and inappropriate) to attribute death to a specific cause. In fact, in Bangladesh, malnutrition is thought to be the cause of death in over 50 percent of all deaths, with concurrent diseases increasing the level of malnutrition and eventually precipitating the death [15].

Caution should be exercised when surrogate measures such as utilization or supply are used as indicators of burden, because they have been shown to be at variance with good survey data in some situations [10]. It is important to distinguish the burden of illness or need as assessed by health status information from three other types of measures often inappropriately substituted for need: want, utilization, or supply. *Want* refers to the public's perceptions of wants, expectations, and rights; it can be estimated by population surveys of self-perceived health status and expectations but more often is expressed by acts of individuals or groups (e.g., citizen groups formed to encourage the opening or discourage the closing of local health facilities). The "seven countries" survey carefully assessed several such aspects of health in 12 study populations

Table 27-2. Comparison of data on the wants and needs for health services in seven countries

Country	Want		Need			
	Proportion of adults reporting any chest pain		Proportion of adults with definite angina pectoris		Mortality per 1000 from arteriosclerotic and degenerative heart disease	
	%	Rank	%	Rank	%	Rank
Finland	45	1	2.5	1	3.4	2
Poland	41	2	1.7	3	1.4	6.5
Canada	36	3	0.8	7	2.7	4
Yugoslavia	30	4	0.8	6	1.4	6.5
United States	28	5	1.0	5	4.3	1
United Kingdom	25	6	1.4	4	2.9	3
Argentina	16	7	1.7	2	1.9	5

Source: Adapted from [10].

[10]. From Table 27-2 it is clear that self-perceived complaints (wants) may differ sharply from place to place irrespective of the prevalence of the disease of interest; for example, over twice as many Poles as Argentineans reported chest pain, while the prevalence of true angina pectoris in adults was the same.

Utilization data are abundant, as they are gathered in the course of providing most health services and are collated and reported by many governments. The data in Table 27-3 demonstrate the contrast between utilization data and the data for want and need shown in Table 27-2. Because of the abundance and low cost of routinely collected utilization data and under the assumption that use equals need, utilization data tend to be substituted for other measures in the evaluation of need. The shortcomings of substituting either want or use are important to emphasize since such information is frequently used as the basis for major health policy decisions (including targeting of research). Careful assessment of health status information should be insisted upon unless substitution of "want" or "use" data is judged acceptable.

The results of data collection must be easy to interpret and apply. Summary statistics for indicators, such as diarrhea-specific mortality rates, the proportion suffering lameness from polio, or the incidence rate for measles, are usually sufficient without any sophisticated mathematical transformation. Health indexes that combine several attributes or indicators of a disease into one number are often used to express disease burden. However, the assumptions and relative weights assigned to factors that make up the indexes need to be explicitly stated so that users can interpret the index and decide whether they can apply it in their setting.

The use of indexes that combine morbidity and mortality have the potential to be exceedingly helpful in quantifying the burden of illness and assessing the relative impact of different diseases. Such indexes quantify and then combine the healthy days of life lost due to both the disability and death associated with a specific disease. The result is a single measure of the overall impact of a disease providing a common unit of measure for comparison between different diseases. Weighting of the disability component according to severity can be used to increase the sensitivity of the index to the actual impact of an illness on an individual.

As mentioned above, the Ghana Health Assessment Project (Table 27-4) combined morbidity and mortality into a single index, "healthy days of life lost" (HDLLs) [11]. Details of the relative contribution of each are provided so that the results are meaningful to those utilizing them. Using this approach, the HDLLs due to 48 diseases or disorders were determined and ranked. Measles was the second-ranked disease, responsible for the loss of 23,400 HDLLs (96.6 percent due to premature death); acute diarrhea was ranked ninth, responsible for 14,500 HDLLs (93.3 percent due to premature death).

However, the design, application, and use of such indexes is often not straightforward. Adequate data on disability days and years of life lost may not be easily obtainable, and deter-

Table 27-3. Utilization of health services in seven countries, %

Country	Immunized within past 12 months	Taking prescribed medicine past 2 days	Consulted a physician within past 2 weeks	Consulted a dentist within past month	Admitted to hospital within past 12 months
Finland	17	28	12	12	11
Poland	59	19	16	12	10
Canada	23	30	15	11	12
Yugoslavia	26	18	14	9.9	9.5
United States	36	34	16	12	14
United Kingdom	14	24	18	8.5	7.9
Argentina	38	30	20	11	6.5

Source: Adapted from R.J.C. Pearson, B. Smedby, R. Berfenstam, et al: Hospital caseloads in Liverpool, New England, and Uppsala, Lancet ii:559, 1968

mining weights for the disability component is a complex and controversial task requiring a number of assumptions to be made. The Ghana team used expert opinion to estimate disability weights and recognized that special studies are needed to validate such assumptions. Application of this approach is also subject to value judgments regarding time preferences (a healthy day of life in the present has a greater value to an individual than one in the future) and the relative economic productivity of an individual at different ages. Prost and Prescott [16] and Barnum [17] have evaluated the effect of incorporating weighting for these factors into rankings using the HDLL approach. Their work has demonstrated that taking into account these factors can change the favored program(s) from those aimed at children to those aimed at "productive" adults.

BURDEN OF ILLNESS AND THE NATURAL HISTORY OF DISEASE

An important component to consider in determining the burden of illness is the natural history of a disease. The information gathered in natural history studies provides accurate information about the probability and magnitude of a change in health status over time in patients with specified conditions or in citizens with specified risk factors and predicts the burden of illness on a society. The study of tuberculosis reported by Doege [18] is an example of this type of study. In addition, the placebo group in randomized controlled trials can sometimes provide useful information on prognosis. Studies providing information on risk factors and the identification of

Table 27-4. Use of healthy days of life lost by Ghana Health Assessment Project: Specification of morbidity and mortality components

Disease	Average age at onset	CFR %	Average age at death	Disablement to death, %	Permanently disabled, %	Disablement, %	Days of temporary disablement	Incidence	Days of life lost	Due to premature death, %
1. Cholera	15	7.6	15	....	0	....	14	0.05	65	99.0
2. Typhoid	20	7.3	20	....	0	....	60	4.00	4,755	95.3
3. Gastroenteritis	2	1.0	2	....	0	....	14	70.00	14,470	93.3
4. Tuberculosis	20	35.0	25	25	0	....	200	2.00	11,005	94.6
5. Diphtheria	3	7.0	3	....	0	....	30	0.01	14	98.0
6. Pertussis	1	1.0	1	....	0	....	30	21.00	4,643	86.6
7. Meningitis	10	20.0	10	....	0	....	30	1.25	4,650	99.3
8. Polio	3	5.0	3	....	95	25	....	0.22	1,227	17.4
9. Measles	2	3.0	2	....	0	....	21	39.00	23,358	96.6
10. Malaria	1	2.3	1	....	97.7	2	....	40.00	32,567	54.1

Details of how days of healthy life lost have been determined

# of days of healthy life lost by the community attributable to the disease

Source: Adapted from [*11*], Table 1, "Disease problems of Ghana measured in terms of the days of healthy life which each costs the community (per 1000 persons per year)."

high-risk groups (for example, prediction of birth complications in pregnant women) are also included in this group.

Trend analysis is receiving increasing attention in the assessment of future health needs. The expanding elderly population and the AIDS crisis are two good subjects for trend analysis. A study has been done in China showing the social and economic consequences of the aging of the Chinese population in the twenty-first century and, accordingly, policy implications for old age support and health care needs [19].

AVOIDABLE AND UNAVOIDABLE BURDEN OF ILLNESS

The burden of illness can be usefully divided into "avoidable" and "unavoidable" to reflect whether efficacious methods of reducing the burden of illness are known. Unavoidable burden of illness includes those aspects of disability, symptoms, and mortality for which no feasible, efficacious prevention or cure currently exists. Clearly, allocation of resources to research into potentially reversible or curable etiological factors and the identification and testing of the efficacy of interventions are needed to reduce this component of the burden of illness.

Avoidable burden of illness includes those aspects of disability, symptoms, and mortality for which feasible, efficacious prevention or therapy exists. Demonstrated efficacy should be a requirement for the allocation of resources to study community effectiveness and efficiency and should guide the subsequent decisions by clinical or community health services.

To distinguish avoidable and unavoidable burden requires knowledge about possible causes of the burden and whether efficacious preventive, therapeutic, or rehabilitative strategies are available. The next two steps of the loop address these issues.

MEASUREMENT LOOP STEP 2: ETIOLOGY

The second step focuses on determining the causes of the health problems contributing to the burden of illness identified in step 1. Elucidation of causal factors requires a careful review of all the biological and behavioral attributes that might contribute to the specific health problem of interest; the "hypothesis space" (Fig. 27-2) is explored, and the most likely potential causes assessed. This involves a wide array of techniques ranging from the laboratory to the clinic and the community. For multiple causal factors, the relative contribution of each to a health problem is difficult to estimate but is crucial given the consequent commitment of time and money to developing interventions to reverse their effects. This is particularly relevant to the care of the under-5 population of LDCs, in whom malnutrition and infection interact to increase the morbidity and mortality associated with other diseases of childhood [15].

Guidelines for assessing evidence for causation relationships originated with the work of Robert Koch in the late 1900s, looking at infections [20]. Virologists subsequently modified Koch's guidelines, introducing the concept of using an exper-

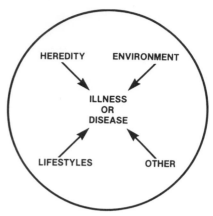

Figure 27-2. The hypothesis space.

imental approach wherein the investigator controls exposure to the putative cause. These guidelines have been modified for use in noninfectious disease by Bradford Hill [21] and further developed [22] by the Department of Clinical Epidemiology and Biostatistics at McMaster University (Table 27-5).

The cause of measles is well-established, an RNA paramyxovirus that affects only humans [13,14]. Acute diarrhea of childhood, on the other hand, is known to be caused by numerous infectious and parasitic organisms. In only 50 to 70 percent of cases can an underlying cause be identified [23,24].

The application of these commonsense principles involves two stages. First, the reader should scan the report to see whether the research methods used were strong or weak. Second, the reader should apply the set of "diagnostic tests" for causation to the methods and to the results. These two steps are elaborated upon below.

STEP 1: THE RESEARCH METHODS

Suppose, for example, an investigator wanted to find out whether vitamin A deficiency is a cause of acute diarrhea in the under-5 population in LDCs. What would be the most powerful sort of study to be found in the literature? Most investigators, it is hoped, would select a true experiment in humans: a study method in which children under 5 years of age with vitamin A deficiency would be randomly allocated (by a system analogous to tossing a coin) to receive or not to receive vitamin A supplements and then followed to see if the incidence of diarrhea was reduced in the children who received supplements. Evidence from such a randomized trial (class 1 evidence) is the soundest that can be obtained, whether it concerns etiology, therapeutics, or any other causal issue. The basic architecture of the randomized trial is shown in Fig. 27-3.

A randomized controlled trial of vitamin A supplementation has been implemented in Sumatra and shows a reduction in overall mortality rates among children aged 12 to 71 months

Table 27-5. Development of a set of guidelines for assessing evidence for causation

A. Koch's postulates—1882
  1. Causative agent must be demonstrated in every case of disease
  2. Causative agent should not be in any other disease
  3. Causative agent should be capable of producing disease in experimental animals
  4. Causative agent must be recovered from the experimental disease produced
B. Diagnostic tests for causation for noninfectious agents
  STEP 1: Strength of basic methods of studies
  1. Is the research design appropriate? In decreasing order of validity:
       Class 1 evidence: Randomized controlled trial
       Class 2 evidence: Cohort analytic study; before-after study
       Class 3 evidence: Case-control study
       Class 4 evidence: Descriptive study
  2. (a) Were the major sources of bias avoided or, if present, measured?
     (b) Were the sampling, assessment of exposure, and analysis at an acceptable level?
  STEP 2: The nine diagnostic tests for causation
  1. Is there *evidence* from appropriately designed studies in humans?
  2. Is the association strong? Is the association stronger than for alternative explanations?
  3. Do other investigators *consistently* find this same result?
  4. Is the *temporal* relation in the proper direction?
  5. Is there a *gradient* or dose-response relationship?
  6. Does the association make *epidemiological sense*?
  7. Is the association *biologically sensible*?
  8. Is the association *specific*?
  9. Is the relationship *analogous* to another, well-accepted relationship?

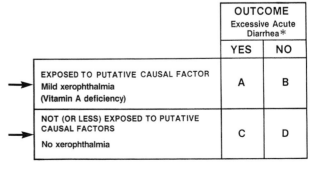

Figure 27-3. A randomized trial.

[25]. Unfortunately, diarrhea-specific morbidity and mortality was not assessed. Some controversy exists in the literature regarding the results of this trial, with questions raised regarding potential confounding associated with the uncertain baseline comparability of the control and supplemented villages and the lack of placebos and blind outcome assessments [26–32]. Further demonstrations of this relationship are needed.

Although the true experiment (randomized trial) would give the most accurate or valid answer to a question of causation, it cannot always be used for reasons of ethics and feasibility. For example, no researcher would ever consider conducting an experiment that would deliberately cause urinary tract schistosomiasis in a random half of a group of people to see whether they were more prone to developing bladder cancer. Thus, nonexperimental studies into issues of causation are much more likely to be encountered.

The next most powerful study method would identify two groups (or cohorts) of children, one mildly xerophthalmic (as an indicator of vitamin A deficiency) and the other not. These

two cohorts would then be followed forward in time to determine the diarrhea-related morbidity and mortality that occurred in each (see Fig. 27-4). If the rates were higher in the xerophthalmic cohort, this would constitute reasonably strong evidence that vitamin A deficiency led to increased diarrhea-specific morbidity and mortality.

However, such a cohort analytic study (class 2 evidence) is not as strong as a randomized trial: the reason becomes apparent if we consider the potential for lack of comparability of the study groups. The cohort study could provide a distorted answer to the causal question if children at high risk of diarrhea for extraneous reasons were not equally distributed between the cohorts of those who were and those who were not xerophthalmic. Are xerophthalmic children less likely to utilize the local health care facilities as often as nonxerophthalmic children? Are xerophthalmic children more likely to have mothers who are less well educated? Are xerophthalmic children generally less well and living under conditions more conducive to vitamin A deficiency? Yes. Therefore, a nonexperimental study such as the cohort study should be viewed with some caution. Documentation of the similarity of the two cohorts on potentially confounding factors can help in dealing

		OUTCOME Excessive Acute Diarrhea*	
		YES	NO
EXPOSED TO PUTATIVE CAUSAL FACTOR Mild xerophthalmia (Vitamin A deficiency)		A	B
NOT (OR LESS) EXPOSED TO PUTATIVE CAUSAL FACTORS No xerophthalmia		C	D

——— Direction of Inquiry ——→

＊i.e. > 2.2 episodes per year

Figure 27-4. Cohort and prospective analytic surveys.

with this problem, but usually even with this information uncertainty will still exist. A prospective cohort study of the relation between mild xerophthalmia and the incidence of diarrhea has been done, showing a threefold increase in the incidence of diarrhea in mildly xerophthalmic children when compared to children with normal eyes [33]. This association was independent of both age and anthropometric status (weight for length).

Before-after studies have similar problems with comparability. For example, if diarrhea-related morbidity and mortality rates are compared before and after the implementation of a vitamin A supplementation program, it is difficult to control contemporaneous changes in other relevant factors that might also influence diarrhea incidence, such as a measles epidemic.

Finally, the case-control study (class 3 evidence) also deserves caution in interpretation (Fig. 27-5). In a case-control study, the investigator identifies two groups of children, one with and one without the outcome of interest: ''cases'' (children with more than the expected number of bouts of diarrhea per year) and ''controls'' (children with equal to or less than the expected number of bouts of diarrhea per year). In this case, the direction of inquiry is backward in time. Both groups of infants are then assessed for vitamin A deficiency; if children with excessive bouts of diarrhea are found more often to have vitamin A deficiency, this would constitute evidence, although not very strong evidence, that vitamin A deficiency might contribute to the risk of diarrhea.

Why is the case-control study low on the scale of strength of evidence? It is because it is so liable to bias. In addition to the biases noted with the cohort study, it is also susceptible to several other biases [34]. For example, given that diarrhea is associated with an increased risk of death, some children will not survive long enough to be included in a case-control study, much less to be assessed for vitamin A deficiency. As a result, an increased risk from vitamin A deficiency could appear to be absent when, in fact, deficiency was lethal for some children. Furthermore, if the diarrhea altered a child's eating habits or ability to absorb vitamin A, then vitamin A deficiency would follow the diarrhea, not cause it. In fact, this issue is still the source of some debate [26]. Accordingly, the results of case-control studies are not as compelling as the more rigorous designs.

One final type of study deserves mention. This is the case-series or descriptive study (class 4 evidence), in which it is noted that a substantial proportion of children with repeated cases of acute diarrhea are vitamin A–deficient. No comparison group of any sort is provided, although there will often be reference to other studies by other investigators using different eligibility criteria (often called *historical controls*). About all that can be concluded is that higher diarrhea-related morbidity and mortality rates might (but will not necessarily) follow vitamin A deficiency in children. In terms of strength, such studies are best used to stimulate other, more powerful investigations.

In summary, then, readers of reports purporting to show etiology or causation should decide whether the research design used was strong or weak. Class 1 evidence from randomized trials provides the best basis for making decisions about causation, providing the trial is implemented reasonably well. A cohort study, although weaker than a randomized trial, is always to be preferred over a case-control study and can sometimes be trusted. For example, useful knowledge about the effectiveness of oral rehydration therapy comes from a large cohort study conducted in two communities in Bangladesh [35]. A cohort study conducted in Taiwan has provided us with the best evidence currently available on the risk of liver cancer due to hepatitis B virus [36]. The case-control study is a weak design, and has led to erroneous conclusions in the developed world, such as the now discarded link between reserpine and breast cancer [37]. However, for some extremely rare disorders (especially rare adverse drug reactions) case-control studies may be the only ones available. Finally, case reports should clearly be passed over when stronger evidence is available.

STEP 2: APPLYING THE NINE DIAGNOSTIC TESTS FOR CAUSATION

As noted above, in making a causal decision information should be sought relative to some commonsense rules of evidence, herein called diagnostic tests and listed in Table 27-5. These are discussed below in order of decreasing importance, and Table 27-6 indicates the impact of each upon causal decisions.

Appropriateness and strength of study design

As discussed above, any consideration of causation should begin with a search for the best evidence. The appropriateness of the design for answering the question posed and, accordingly, the strengths and weaknesses in terms of the potential for bias should be identified.

	OUTCOME	
	CASES	CONTROLS
	Children With Excessive Diarrhea*	Matched Children Without Excessive Diarrhea*
EXPOSED TO PUTATIVE CAUSAL FACTOR (Vitamin A deficiency)	A	B
NOT (OR LESS) EXPOSED TO PUTATIVE CAUSAL FACTORS (No Vitamin A deficiency)	C	D

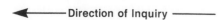
◄——— Direction of Inquiry ———

* i.e. > 2.2 episodes per year

Figure 27-5. Case-control studies.

Table 27-6. Importance of individual diagnostic tests in making the causal decision

Diagnostic test	Effect of test result on causal decision*		
	Test result positive	**Test result neutral**	**Test result reverse of hypothesis**
Design:			
Human experiments	+ + + +	– – – –	– – – –
Cohorts	+ + +		
Case comparison	+		
Strength:			
From experiment	+ + + +		
From cohort study	+ + +	– – –	– – –
From case-comparison study	+	0	–
Consistency	+ + +	– – –	– – –
Temporality	+ +	– –	– –
Gradient	+ +	– –	– –
Epidemiological sense	+ +	– –	– –
Biological sense	+	0	–
Specificity	+	0	–
Analogy	+	0	0

*Symbols: + = Causation supported; – = causation not supported; 0 = causal decision not affected. The number of +'s or –'s indicates the relative contribution of the diagnostic test to the causal decision.

Strength of association

Strength here means the odds favoring the outcome of interest with, as opposed to without, exposure to the putative cause. The higher the odds, the greater the strength. There are two strategies for estimating the strength of the association. Both randomized trials and cohort analytical studies permit direct calculations of relative risk (strength) by comparing outcome rates in exposed and unexposed persons (Table 27-7). In case-control studies, however, relative risk can only be indirectly estimated by calculation of relative odds (Table 27-7).

Etiological fraction (EF) (Table 27-7) can be used to quantify the magnitude of the contribution of the putative cause to the outcome. It tells us the portion of outcomes observed in a

community or population that are related (or "due") to exposure to the putative cause, which would not have occurred in its absence (if it were, indeed, the cause). The important advantage of etiological fraction is that it quantifies the maximum reduction in the burden of illness that can be achieved in a specific population by interventions designed to modify the factor being assessed. For example, suppose a cohort analytic study of 200 children was conducted (of whom 100 had received vitamin A supplements and 100 had not) to investigate the relation between vitamin A deficiency and acute diarrhea. The results obtained are displayed in Table 27-8; the relative

Table 27-7. Strategies for estimating strength of association

		Outcome of interest	
		Yes	No
Exposure to putative cause	Yes	a	b
	No	c	d

For class 1 & 2 studies:
Relative risk (RR) = $a/(a + b) - c/(c + d)$

Etiological fraction (EF) = $\dfrac{\theta(RR - 1)}{\theta(RR - 1) + 1}$

For class 3 studies:
Relative odds (RO) = ad/bc

Etiological fraction (EF) = $\dfrac{\theta(RO - 1)}{\theta(RO - 1) + 1}$

θ = prevalence of exposure in the population being considered.

Table 27-8. Relation between vitamin A supplements and excessive acute diarrhea*

		Excessive diarrhea		
		Yes	No	
Vitamin A supplements	No	20	80	100
	Yes	10	90	100
		30	170	200

$RR = \dfrac{20/100}{10/100} = \dfrac{0.2}{0.1} = 2$

$EF = \dfrac{\theta(2 - 1)}{\theta(2 - 1) + 1} = \dfrac{\theta}{\theta + 1}$

In this population θ is 50% since half of the children were not "exposed" to vitamin A supplements (100/200)

$\therefore EF = \dfrac{.5}{.5 + 1} = .33$

*For example, > 2.2 episodes per year.

risk is 2.0, and the etiological fraction 33 percent (0.33 × 100). From this it can be concluded that children receiving no vitamin A supplementation are more than twice as likely to experience excessive bouts of diarrhea as children receiving them, and that 33 percent of the excessive diarrhea found in this study was "due to" vitamin A deficiency and therefore possibly avoidable.

Consistency

Consistency refers to the repetitive demonstration of an association between exposure to the putative cause and the outcome of interest, using different strategies and different settings. For example, the link between hepatitis B and liver cancer has been reported consistently in studies carried out in Africa and Asia [36,38]. The consistency of these findings in a Caucasian population [38] lends strength to the causal relationship, greatly reducing the likelihood that other factors, whether toxic, genetic, racial, or nutritional in nature, may be responsible.

Temporality

Temporality refers to a consistent sequence of events—exposure to the putative cause followed by the occurrence of the outcome of interest. For example, as outlined above, if one were studying the relationship between vitamin A deficiency and diarrhea in children in a case-control study, it would not be possible to sort out whether the vitamin A deficiency predisposed to acute diarrhea or vice versa. Although this diagnostic test looks easy to apply, it is not. What if a predisposing factor is responsible both for low vitamin A levels and for diarrhea?

Gradient

Gradient refers to demonstrable increasing risk or severity of the outcome of interest in association with an increased "dose" or duration of exposure to the putative cause. Increasing rates of acute diarrhea associated with progressively increasing severity of xerophthalmia would satisfy this guideline. Studies of schistosomiasis investigating the relationship between the magnitude of worm burden and clinical disease show that light infections produce little impact on the individual while heavy worm loads are associated with significant clinical consequences [40]. Reverse gradients are useful, too; for example, if rates of diarrhea progressively decreased with increasing amounts of vitamin A supplementation, this would be a *reverse gradient*.

Epidemiological sense

This criterion refers to agreement with our current understanding of the distribution of causes and outcomes. The reason for this criterion being low on the list is that it does not require evidence that the exposure and outcomes affected the same individual. Vitamin A deficiency is not found in areas with a ready, natural supply of vitamin A. Indeed, initiation of investigations of the link between hepatitis B and liver cancer began based on observations that the incidence of liver cancer seemed to be associated with high levels of hepatitis B infection [41].

Biological sense

Biological sense refers to agreement with our current understanding of the responses of cells, tissues, organs, and organisms to stimuli. It is by this yardstick that nonhuman experimental data should be measured. Laboratory or animal studies have been responsible for many of the major advances in medicine, and such basic research plays a vital role in our understanding of the cellular basis for disease. For example, specific defects in cellular immune response have been documented in malnourished persons, suggesting a link between infection and nutrition [42].

Some biological observations are compelling [20,43]. However, biological sense is relatively low among the criteria because, while it frequently provides essential explanatory information, virtually any set of observations can be made biologically plausible (given the ingenuity of the human mind and the vastness of the supply of contradictory biological facts).

Specificity

Specificity refers to the limitation of the association to a single putative cause and a single effect. One of the minor diagnostic tests, this is only moderately useful, and then only when it is present. The weakness of this test is underscored when considering teratogens, which commonly produce multiple effects in several organ systems.

Analogy

Analogy refers to the similarity of the association to another previously demonstrated causal relationship. The last and least of the diagnostic tests, an appropriate example in relation to diet and disease would be the possible relationship between the diarrhea found in pellagra due to deficiency of another vitamin, niacin [44].

Summary

When confronted by a question of causation, these nine diagnostic tests can be used to distill one's prior knowledge and, with the assistance of judgments such as those shown in Table 27-6, reach a causal conclusion. The diagnosis of causation is not simply arithmetic, and the strategies and tactics for making this judgment are still primitive. The diagnostic tests presented here are a start. It is suggested that their use, particularly when clearly specified before a review of relevant data, will lead to more rational—albeit less colorful—discussions of causation in human biology and health care.

This model can also be applied when assessing the effectiveness of interventions as well as causal agents in general. The emphasis in assessing effectiveness will be upon the first few criteria, since it is usually possible to find information from more rigorously designed studies concerning an intervention than concerning causal agents.

Although knowledge of causes is very important for identifying possibly efficacious interventions, it is not always necessary to insist upon a complete understanding of the etiology of disease prior to intervention (John Snow took off the pump handle 50 years before the etiological agent for cholera was discovered).

MEASUREMENT LOOP STEP 3: COMMUNITY EFFECTIVENESS

Step 3 looks at information on how well an intervention with potential for reducing burden will work when applied in the community. Disability and disease for which effective, feasible interventions exist can then be identified as avoidable.

Community effectiveness is determined by five factors: efficacy, screening and diagnostic accuracy, health provider compliance, patient compliance, and coverage. Evidence of efficacy may be transportable from country to country, but patient compliance, health provider compliance, and coverage are more likely to differ both between and within countries. Definitions and methodological guidelines for evaluating the quality of evidence relating to each of these five components are discussed below.

EFFICACY

Efficacy asks the question, Can it work? It is defined as the extent to which a specific health intervention does more good than harm to patients (citizens) who are diagnosed correctly and appropriately cared for and who fully comply with recommendations or treatment. That is, the evaluation of efficacy assumes optimal diagnostic accuracy, health provider compliance, and patient compliance. Careful attention to these factors is required when deciding whether a study is truly assessing efficacy. Efficacy is the "anchor point" when estimating the benefit of interventions applied in a community setting and quantifying the upper bound or maximum benefit that can be achieved; it is regarded to be more stable and less liable to fluctuation in different circumstances than the four other components of community effectiveness.

Methodological standards for the assessment of efficacy are summarized in Table 27-9. It is unusual for a single study to fully comply with all seven standards for reasons such as the nature of the disorder in question, the limitations introduced by the experimental setting, or the cost of the assessments required. However, each of these standards should be considered when assessing or designing studies in order to determine whether the failure to satisfy a given standard invalidates the trial.

Table 27-9. Methodological standards for studies of the efficacy of therapeutic or preventive health interventions

1. Is the research design appropriate?
   a. Were the major sources of bias avoided or, if present, measured?
   b. Were the methods used for sampling, assessment of exposure, and analysis acceptable?
2. Were all relevant outcomes reported?
3. Were the study patients or population recognizably similar to your own?
4. Were both clinical-community and statistical significance considered?
5. Is the therapeutic maneuver feasible in your setting?
6. Were all patients who entered the study accounted for at its conclusion?
7. Are the study results consistent with those of others?

Do we have evidence for the efficacy of measles immunization and ORS? We believe that the efficacy of both are well established [45,47]. The major evidence for the efficacy of measles vaccine comes from a randomized trial conducted in Great Britain by the British Medical Research Council, which showed an 85 percent reduction in the incidence of measles due to measles vaccine [46]. Other trials are also available focusing on seroconversion and reporting rates of up to 95 percent.

Although the comparative efficacy and safety of ORS for rehydration relative to intravenous fluid (IV) replacement has been clearly established in randomized trials [47,48], ethical considerations rule out randomized trials of ORS efficacy against no treatment, as such a design would necessitate withholding treatment from a dehydrated child. However, the efficacy of ORS compared to no treatment can be derived from descriptive studies, particularly those of severely ill cholera patients, many of whom would be expected to die in the absence of treatment. Accordingly, as will be discussed below, ORS represents an unusual case wherein sufficiently dramatic results have been observed in descriptive studies to draw conclusions about the efficacy of ORS. Based on the available evidence, when applied to patients with mild to moderately severe dehyration, ORS is considered to be 95 to 100 percent efficacious [47,49]. In cases of severe dehydration, IV treatment is recommended for initial rehydration with ORS administered subsequently for maintenance.

Is the research design appropriate?

Random Allocation. As was the case for determining causation, the well-executed randomized trial provides the strongest evidence for efficacy. In any disease that is not uniformly fatal, improvement unrelated to the intervention can best be taken into account by identifying and following a control group of patients who are similar in as many ways as possible to those receiving the intervention.

The comparability of the control subjects is absolutely crucial if the results are to be valid. The best way of achieving comparability is to ensure that every patient who enters the study has the same, known probability (typically 50 percent) of receiving one or the other of the treatments being compared; thus, assignment to one treatment or another should have been carried out by a system analogous to flipping a coin. It is usually easy to decide whether this was done, for key terms such as *randomized trial* or *random allocation* should appear in the abstract, the methods section, or even the title of such articles. A formal explanation for this strict rule is lengthy, but its conclusion is straightforward. As discussed above in measurement loop step 2 (causation), random allocation eliminates many of the biases that lead to false results in nonrandomized trials. Instances are numerous in which the developed world has been misled by accepting evidence from nonrandomized trials. For example, clofibrate was growing in popularity in the developed world before publication of a randomized clinical trial showed that it actually increased mortality rates; the drug was subsequently banned in several countries [50]. Furthermore, it has been estimated that 2500 gastric freezing machines had been purchased to treat tens of thousands of peptic ulcer patients by the time that a randomized clinical trial demonstrated the lack of efficacy of this procedure [51]. Similarly, a randomized trial was required in which angina patients were randomly allocated to undergo or not undergo internal mammary ligation only after the arteries had been surgically exposed to demonstrate how often symptomatic improvement can follow placebo medications and procedures [52]. Finally, the risk of relying on poorly designed trials is underlined by the work of Sacks, Chalmers, and Smith [53]. Their review of 50 articles evaluating six different therapies revealed that poorly designed, uncontrolled studies claimed important benefit 79 percent of the time, while well-designed, controlled trials claimed important benefit only 20 percent of the time.

The review of Bacillus Calmette-Guérin (BCG) vaccination by Clemens provides an excellent example relevant to LDC health problems. It is particularly interesting in that it addresses this same issue from the other direction—namely, poor methodology leading to rejection of a potentially useful intervention [54]. Their review concludes that the best available evidence (keeping in mind that these studies were conducted in industrialized settings) for the efficacy of BCG vaccination suggests a high efficacy for the vaccine for clinical tuberculosis. Undoubtedly, additional instances relevant to the major health problems in the developing world will arise as more information from controlled trials becomes available.

The efficacy of polio immunization [55] is accepted by virtually all providers and consumers of health care, as is the efficacy of antimicrobial prophylaxis in the secondary prevention of acute rheumatic fever [56]. On the other hand, the long-term efficacy of health education programs remains hotly con-

tested [57]. The major reason for consensus in the first two cases and its absence in the third concerns the nature of the available evidence on the efficacy of these preventive maneuvers. The claims of the efficacy of polio immunization and rheumatic fever prophylaxis arise from placebo-controlled, randomized trials. Neither the subjects nor their clinicians knew who had received the active agent and who had received the placebo (thereby making the trial double-blind). In each case, the intervention was judged efficacious when it found that the target disorder was far less likely to befall individuals who received the intervention than those who did not.

It is widely acknowledged that nonexperimental evidence (the cohort, before-after, case-control, and case-series designs described previously) can provide important information about etiology and the adverse effects of therapy. However, those most familiar with these nonexperimental approaches agree that frequently they are not suited to the demonstration of efficacy, and this conclusion is substantiated in the requirements for experimental validation of new drugs and, increasingly, new surgical procedures. This conclusion is also true for the validation of health care services; the realization of the pitfalls of research designs has led to the recognition that nonexperimental evidence is often insufficient in judging the efficacy of these services as well.

Skeptics insist upon evidence from true experiments in which, for example, individuals at risk for a given health problem are randomly allocated either to undergo or not to undergo early diagnostic and subsequent treatment procedures. Such experiments are now commonplace and have documented both the clear-cut advantages of early detection and treatment of moderate and severe hypertension [58], and the failure of the hospital admission laboratory screening for this problem to benefit either patients or those who care for them [59].

There are three exceptions to this requirement for experimental evidence. First, when a disorder is associated with a uniformly fatal outcome, any maneuver that saves lives is efficacious, and no randomized trial is necessary. Thus, experimental evidence was not required to validate the efficacy of treatment of tuberculosis meningitis with streptomycin [60]. Similarly, as noted above, initial experience with ORS in severely ill cholera patients showed a dramatic reduction in the case-fatality rate that could only be attributed to this simple intervention [49,61]. Secondly, when a disorder producing substantial mortality rates is uniformly cured, a controlled trial is also unnecessary—as, for example, with the use of penicillin for treatment of pneumonia in patients without other morbidity [62].

The third exception to the requirement for experimental evidence on the benefit of a health service occurs when random allocation to receive or not receive the maneuver is judged unethical or would be politically unacceptable. However, this latter exception is closely tied to geography and local practice. For example, in the developed world randomized trials to evaluate coronary care units were considered unethical in the United States at the same time that such trials were in progress in the United Kingdom.

In summary, then, although the randomized trial can sometimes produce an incorrect conclusion about efficacy (especially when it is a small trial), it is by far the best tool currently available for identifying the clinical maneuvers or health services that do more good than harm.

Comparability of Study Groups and Prognostic Stratification. Although random allocation is the method most likely to produce comparable study groups, this method does not guarantee similarity of groups with respect to all important variables. The use of prognostic stratification prior to randomization is one way to ensure that study groups are comparable with respect to known important prognostic factors.

For example, the underlying risk of developing and dying from the target condition should be identified for members of the study population. If subgroups in the study population vary widely in risk, consideration should be given to stratification. For example, if periodic screening tests for bladder cancer were being performed upon individuals with schistosomiasis, it would be important to stratify these subjects in terms of their tobacco use, a previously identified risk factor for bladder cancer. The investigator should also look for stratification in primary prevention trials of a new vaccine if members of the study population vary widely in their risk of developing the target infection; in fact this particular problem may have influenced the results of the major randomized trial of BCG vaccine conducted in India [63]. In the presentation of the results of such trials, the effect of this stratification upon the subsequent outcomes should be described in detail.

Were all relevant outcomes reported?

Mortality and Morbidity. The outcomes assessed should include (or predict) all those components of health status relevant to the intervention being assessed, including quality of life and patient preference. The World Health Organization's definition of health (optimal physical, emotional, and social well-being) can be broken down to cover the spectrum of health in measurable terms utilizing the 10 D's: death, disease, distress, discomfort, disability, dysfunction, disharmony (family impact), dissatisfaction, disposition (risk factors), and debt [64]. For example, when looking at measles immunization it is important (although more difficult) to determine the incidence of measles rather than simply seroconversion rates. This was done in the Medical Research Council trials conducted in Great Britain, which is a major strength of that data. Increasing attention is being directed toward the importance of including an assessment of the impact of the intervention on the patient's quality of life. Such assessments address health status, changes in functional abilities, and patient preferences for alternative treatments or health states [65–67].

Explicit, Objective Outcome Criteria. Outcome criteria should be reproducibly defined, and for each outcome the following issues should be considered when deciding whether the results are likely to be meaningful:

1. Credibility of the assessment method used: For outcomes other than death that require a set of criteria for definition or an index or other instrument for measurement, credibility refers to the extent to which the method appears to measure what it is intended to measure and is therefore acceptable to those health professionals who might want to use the results of the study.
2. Reproducibility: This concerns the extent to which the measurement instrument produces the same result on repeated applications.
3. Whether the results are assessed by blind observers: Assessments performed by individual(s) unaware of specific characteristics of the patient that might influence the assessment (e.g., the study group to which the patient belongs, previous diagnosis, and/or aspects of the patient's history) are necessary to minimize the likelihood of bias.
4. Responsiveness to change: This refers to evidence that the instrument or measurement approach used can detect a change in outcome when it is known to exist by other accepted assessment methods.

Were the study patients (population) recognizably similar to your own?

This criterion has two elements. First, the study patients must be recognizable: that is, how they were selected, what diagnostic criteria were used, and the patients' clinical and sociodemographic status must be described in sufficient detail for you to be able to recognize the similarity between the study patients and your own patients. Second, the study patients must be similar to patients in your practice or community. To put it another way, you should ask yourself, Are the patients in the study so different from those I am concerned with that I could not apply the study results? When both recognizability and similarity are satisfied, you will be able to predict, with confidence, the outcomes to be expected from the application of the specific therapy or program to specific patients or populations.

The reports of the community-based studies of measles immunization and ORS [35,68] could each have benefited from inclusion of further details about the populations studied. Information on the age, sex, and socioeconomic status of the population is needed to allow readers to recognize the populations studied and judge the applicability of the results to the settings in which they work.

In summary, answers to the following three questions are needed to fulfill this criterion:

1. Were study subjects drawn from a random population sample or from a population of patients at some health facility?

2. Exactly how were they diagnosed or detected, including diagnostic criteria?
3. What were the patients' sociodemographic status and clinical status (e.g., severity and duration of condition)?

Were clinical-community and statistical significances considered?

Clinical-Community Significance. Clinical-community significance here refers to the importance of a difference in health outcomes between treated and control patients. Differences observed between treatment and control patients are considered significant clinically or in regard to the community when they lead to changes in health provider or planner clinical or community-related behavior (i.e., decision making).

Clinically significant changes are usually reported in terms of relative risk reduction. For example, in the measles immunization trial carried out in the Kasongo [68], the relative risk reduction was 55 percent [(36 − 16)/36]; that is, the risk of measles for a vaccinated individual would be less than half that of an unvaccinated individual. On the other hand, changes significant to the community are usually reported in terms of absolute risk reduction. For example, in the Kasongo report, the absolute risk of measles was 36 percent in the unvaccinated group and 16 percent in the vaccinated group, reflecting an absolute risk reduction for a vaccinated child of 20 percent.

It is important to note that although these assessments are often made from the perspective of the clinician or those making decisions about specific communities of individuals, clinical and community significance could also be defined from the patient's perspective in terms of "important differences in the quality of life." Utility measurement techniques, which quantify the strength of an individual's preference for alternative health outcomes or interventions is an approach that has been used to address this issue in a number of diseases [66,67] but has not yet been widely applied in developing country settings.

A new perspective on clinical significance, the number needed to be treated (NNT), has recently been developed [69]. NNT is determined as the reciprocal of the absolute risk reduction (the difference in event rates between treated and untreated groups of patients). The advantage of this approach is that it combines the baseline risk of the patient for a target event with the consequences of treatment, which is not the case with either the relative risk reduction or the odds ratio. It is useful to the health provider in that it provides a yardstick for determining the number of patients who must be treated in order to prevent one adverse event. For example, using the measles data from the Kasango project summarized above, the absolute risk reduction was 20 percent, or 0.2. Taking the reciprocal (1/0.2) yields an NNT of 5; that is, five children must be immunized to prevent one case of measles.

Statistical Significance. By contrast, statistical significance merely tells us whether a difference is likely to be real, not whether it is important or large. More precisely, the statistical significance of a difference is nothing more than a statement about the likelihood that this difference is due to chance alone.

The determinants of clinical and community significance are therefore the determinants of change in clinical or community action. If the results of a study lead you to manage your patients differently or to abandon an established program for a new one, the difference in the effects of these programs is thereby of clinical or community significance. The determinants of the statistical significance of any given result rises (that is, the *p* value falls) when the number of subjects in the study is increased, when the health outcomes show less fluctuation from day to day or from patient to patient, and when the measurement of this health outcome is both accurate and reproducible.

Adequacy of the Sample Size or β Error. On the basis of the foregoing, the busy reader can develop quick yardsticks to use when reading therapeutic articles. First, is the reported difference of clinical or community significance? Readers must scrutinize the difference in clinical outcomes in the studies to see whether they are of potential significance. If so, is the difference statistically significant—if yes, then the results are both real and worthy of implementing.

Second, if the difference is not statistically significant, is the number of patients large enough to show a significant difference clinically or in the community if it should occur? As discussed in the previous paragraph, the number of patients in a study is one of the determinants of statistical significance. Thus, if a study is huge, the difference in health outcomes can be statistically significant ("real") even when its magnitude is not clinically significant. Conversely, however, if a study is too small, even large differences of enormous potential clinical or community significance may not be statistically significant. For example, in the recent report on measles vaccination effectiveness by the Kasongo project team [68], no difference in overall mortality was found. However, examination of the death rates in the two groups suggests that an important difference may exist which was not found to be statistically significant due to insufficient sample size. The observed death rates were 4.5 percent in vaccinated group 1 and 7 percent in unvaccinated group 2, a risk reduction of 35 percent. Consideration of such a difference in the planning stages of this study would have revealed that to be 80 percent confident that a risk reduction of this size or greater would not be missed would require about 460 children per group (*p* = .05, one-tailed) rather than the approximately 250 children per group studied [68].

Is the maneuver or health intervention feasible in your setting?

Replicable Description of Maneuver or Health Intervention. The health care maneuver or intervention has to be described in sufficient detail for readers to replicate it with precision.

How were the patients diagnosed? Who did what to whom, with what formulation and dose, administered under what circumstances, with what dose adjustments and titrations, with which searches for and responses to side effects and toxicity, for how long and with what clinical criteria for deciding that therapy should be given, increased, tapered, or terminated? This issue presents special problems in trials evaluating the impact of a "package" of interventions. Such is the case in a community-based trial of ORS where the intervention consisted not only of ORS packets but also of a training program for volunteer depot holders and promotional activities related to the availability of ORS and how to use it [35].

Contamination and Cointervention. When reading the description of the maneuver in a published report, readers should note whether the authors avoided two specific biases in its application: contamination (in which control patients accidentally receive the experimental treatment—this results in a spurious reduction in the difference in outcomes between the experimental and control groups) and cointervention (the differential application of additional diagnostic or therapeutic acts to either experimental or control patients that could influence clinical outcomes and thereby bias the magnitude of difference observed between experimental and control groups). It should be apparent that cointervention is prevented by "blinding" both study patients and their clinicians as to who is receiving which treatment.

Cointervention due to unequal access of the two treatment areas to health care was a possibility in the Rahaman study of community-based distribution of ORS [35]; the fact that BCG vaccination leaves a scar may have alerted health workers to look more or less intensively for the occurrence of tuberculosis [63].

Were all patients who entered the study accounted for at its conclusion?

The astute reader will note how many patients entered the study (usually the numbers of experimental and control patients will be almost identical) and will tally them again at its conclusion to make certain that they correspond.

Again, the major trial of BCG in India provides an example [63]. Although the authors tell us exactly how many individuals received each of the three vaccination schedules being tested, it is not clear how many of these individuals were followed up and included in the results. Clearly, in a study such as this there are many practical difficulties in meeting this criterion, but it is crucial to the results. Perhaps representative samples (of adequate number statistically) could be identified after the maneuver is administered and carefully followed, thereby ensuring the validity of the results and reducing the number of intensive, expensive follow-ups required.

What can the reader do when outcomes are not reported for missing subjects? One approach (admittedly conservative and therefore liable to lead to the β error) is to arbitrarily assign a bad outcome to all missing members of the group with the most favorable outcomes. If this maneuver fails to shift the statistical or clinical significance of the results across a decision point, the reader can accept the study's conclusions.

Are the study results consistent with those of others?

This guideline concerns whether or not the study results agree with those of others. As is illustrated by Clemens' review of the trials of BCG conducted to date, different results can often be explained by the strength of the research methods used [54].

With the foregoing seven guidelines, both planners and providers of health care should be able to critically assess and judge the validity, applicability, and gaps in our knowledge about the efficacy of a specific health intervention.

SCREENING AND DIAGNOSTIC ACCURACY

Information on diagnostic accuracy can be obtained from studies of the extent to which patients with the condition of interest are correctly discriminated from those without the condition. This is not confined to technological or laboratory tests and includes the assessment of the accuracy of clinical signs (history, physical examination) or other paraclinical investigations (laboratory, x-ray, etc.). Detection or screening of patients with remedial health needs is necessary to establish the denominator of the population at risk. Screening of children under 1 year of age for measles susceptibility might be carried out in settings where it is judged that the cost of such screening is outweighed by the reduction in the number of children subsequently vaccinated and, accordingly, cost.

Unavoidable health needs (i.e., those for which no therapy is currently available) should not be the focus of screening, not only because of expense but also because of the negative consequences to health of the "labeling" that results. Hypertension, a health problem receiving increasing attention in developing countries, provides an excellent example of the potential impact of labeling. A study involving careful follow-up of steelworkers screened for hypertension revealed that absenteeism rose among previously unaware hypertensives labeled as a result of the screening process [70]. This led the authors and three Canadian task forces on hypertension to recommend that detection of hypertension only be carried out in settings where adequate therapy and long-term follow-up was ensured. In this way the disadvantages associated with being labeled hypertensive could be countered by the long-term benefits of blood pressure control.

Diagnostic accuracy with regard to measles is usually not an issue given that intervention in LDC settings is most often in the form of mass immunization programs with all children in a specified age range vaccinated. In the case of diarrhea among the under-5s, in some settings it may be necessary to discriminate acute from dysenteric and chronic diarrhea since the efficacy of ORS in these indications is not established [9].

EVALUATION OF HEALTH PROVIDER COMPLIANCE

Health provider compliance is assessed by whether the appropriate diagnostic and management actions (prevention, therapy, and rehabilitation) are performed by the health provider. The literature on quality of care calls these actions "clinical process" to differentiate them from "structure" (the supply of facilities and qualified personnel) and "outcome" (patient's health status). Studies of health provider compliance should be restricted to situations in which the causal relationship between the process of care and patient outcome is established, i.e., for a demonstration of efficacy.

Information from evaluations of the ability of different health professionals to apply efficacious interventions is included in this category. A study carried out in Thailand to compare the health care and outcomes of women receiving postpartum tubal ligations by either specially trained nurse midwives or doctors provides an example of this type of evaluation [71].

For both measles immunization and acute diarrhea, provider compliance can drastically alter the impact of treatment. Crucial to measles immunization is maintenance of the cold chain. As previously noted, studies have shown that vaccine effectiveness can be as low as zero due to lack of care by providers in ensuring that the vaccine is maintained at the appropriate temperature [4,5].

Turning to ORS, provider compliance concerns not only appropriate management of diarrhea by the provider (i.e., the decision to treat and the vigor of treatment applied) but also the ability to effectively train others responsible for administering the ORS to the sick child, particularly mothers and other members of the child's household. Studies are available that suggest that adequate levels of ORS preparation skills can be achieved in special training programs [47].

The appropriate use of antibiotics is a major concern in the treatment of acute diarrhea with their use considered to be appropriate in less than 10 percent of cases [24,72]. Inappropriate use of antibiotics for undifferentiated acute watery diarrheas can lead to harmful overgrowth of organisms such as *Clostridium difficile* and may actually prolong duration in some cases [24].

EVALUATION OF PATIENT COMPLIANCE

Patient compliance is determined by whether patients follow the health provider's recommendations and treatment. Immunization programs that involve more than one painful injection in children can fail for this reason alone. Oral rehydration salts for acute diarrhea of childhood provides another good example. Effective treatment requires compliance by both the mother and infant. The effectiveness of most community-based programs depends upon the mother accepting ORS as a treatment and learning to correctly prepare and administer the ORS liquid. The extent to which mothers accept that ORS fluids will stop diarrhea, as opposed to causing it, may influence whether mothers comply with recommendations for its use. Studies of mothers' knowledge and behavior related to ORS preparation and administration have reported varying levels of compliance ranging from 80 to 5 percent [45]. An unannounced assessment of fluid composition revealed that solutions prepared by village workers were on the average satisfactory, while those prepared by mothers tended to be diluted [73].

EVALUATION OF COVERAGE

Coverage refers to the proportion of the target population, i.e., all patients (citizens) in need of a specific, efficacious intervention who are offered it. Coverage should be differentiated from patient compliance: *coverage* describes whether or not an individual in need of a specific health intervention makes contact with the health professional, while *patient compliance* encompasses the adherence by the patient to the subsequent advice. Moreover, as coverage estimates do not take into account the other components of community effectiveness, such estimates do not reflect the proportion of all patients in need who are effectively treated [74].

For example, coverage for ORS will depend upon whether the delivery system is health center or home-based. Clearly, home-based distribution systems should result in close to 100 percent coverage. Rahaman's study of health center–based distribution found that between 60 to 70 percent of children with diarrhea attended a clinic for care of an episode [35]. He also showed that coverage declined with distance from the health facility; 90 percent of diarrheal cases within 1 mile attended the clinic, while less than 70 percent within 2 miles did.

Coverage evaluation requires that the use of health services be related to the need for them in a defined population during a specified time period. Utilization of services in the form of activity-to-population ratios, although very popular, is rarely accurate as a measure of availability since it fails to incorporate information about need. For example, mass measles immunization campaigns in LDCs usually target the specific age group of infants (usually 7 to 9 months of age) considered most at risk (i.e., most likely to be susceptible to measles). Since the proportion of susceptibles is expected to be very close to 100 percent, no actual assessment of susceptibility is usually obtained. It is worth noting that coverage estimates for measles immunization usually reflect how many children were actually immunized rather than how many children were offered an injection, and therefore incorporate patient compliance. The report by McBean on a measles immunization campaign for children 6 to 36 months of age in the Cameroons illustrates the impact that need can have on measles immunization coverage of susceptible children [75]. Overall 78 percent of children in the target age group were taken to the measles immunization sessions. However, this study found that only 40 percent of children in this age range were susceptible to measles, and, of these, only 51 percent were given vaccination during the campaign. In fact, children not susceptible were more likely to present for vaccination than those who were (53 percent of those who remained at home were susceptible versus 36 percent of those who attended). Thus, although 78 percent of children attended, coverage of those in need was only 51 percent.

Availability and acceptability of effective health services

Utilization of effective health services by those in need depends upon availability and acceptability. *Availability* concerns whether efficacious health services are accessible to those in need and they are aware of their being available. This can be measured by estimating the supply of services (the resource-population ratio), taking into account the distribution. Awareness of the availability of these services by those in need is also relevant here. This component is important in screening studies to ensure that there is appropriate linkage of identified patients with the condition of interest to the health provider, so that they get treated rather than just "labeled," as in the hypertension example above [70]. For both measles immunization and ORS, promotional campaigns are required to enhance levels of coverage.

Quantification of acceptability can best be obtained from surveys and should not be confined to users of health services, since the latter statistic does not tell us how many individuals in need of an intervention fail to receive it. Measurement of the acceptability of health services can usefully be divided into patients' perceptions of (1) the resources or facilities, (2) the behavior of health professionals and their staff, and (3) the benefits expected from the health service. The acceptability to mothers of ORS as described above provides a useful example.

PREDICTION OF THE MAGNITUDE OF COMMUNITY EFFECTIVENESS

It is important to be able to estimate the impact of specific treatment interventions when assessing whether a program is achieving its full potential, or when assessing the economic efficiency of the whole program or looking at alternatives for improving the program. All of the economic approaches described in the next step of the loop except for cost-minimization require an estimate of community effectiveness. It is important to point out that the lack of rigorous and valid evidence on clinical-community effectiveness limits the validity of economic evaluations [76]. Given that assumptions must be made in conducting cost-effectiveness, cost-benefit, and cost-utility analyses, it is important to minimize sources of inaccuracy in estimates of impact.

The relationship between the five factors that determine community effectiveness is most accurately estimated by using a multiplicative conditional probabilities model (see boxed text). Unfortunately, the necessary information on conditional probabilities is rarely available. However, an acceptable alternative [77] is to use a simple multiplication formula. This assumes that all the factors are independent. It is unlikely that the factors are highly correlated, (e.g., many patients given optimal care do not comply), but research is needed to confirm the robustness of the simple multiplicative formula. When community effectiveness is expressed in terms of the burden of illness (for example, healthy days of life lost), the percent reduction in the total overall burden of illness in a community (identified in step 1) that might be achieved by a specific health intervention can be estimated.

Conditional Probabilities

The multiplicative law of combining conditional probabilities [77] states that the chance of two events, x and y, both happening is $P(x \text{ and } y) = P(x)P(y)$, assuming both events are independent. When one event is dependent upon the other, such as y is dependent upon x, this is expressed as $P(x \text{ and } y) = P(y/x) P(x)$. Community effectiveness can therefore be stated as follows:

Community effectiveness* (or probability of benefit)
$= P(\text{coverage})$
$\times P(\text{diagnostic accuracy/coverage})$
$\times P(\text{health provider compliance/coverage and diagnostic accuracy})$
$\times P(\text{efficacy of treatment/coverage and diagnostic accuracy and health provider compliance})$
$\times P(\text{patient compliance/coverage and diagnostic accuracy and health provider compliance and efficacy of treatment})$

Under the assumption of independence this can be simplified to:

Community effectiveness $=$ Efficacy $\times$ diagnostic accuracy $\times$ health provider compliance $\times$ patient compliance $\times$ coverage

*Determinants of community effectiveness are organized according to the sequence in which they occur in the process of delivering and receiving health care.

Table 27-10. Sample calculations for community effectiveness: Measles immunization

Type of estimate	Efficacy	Diagnostic accuracy	Provider compliance	Patient compliance	Coverage	Community effectiveness (measles incidence)	Percent of efficacy achieved in the community
"Best evidence" estimate	69% reduction in measles incidence					35% ↓	$\frac{35}{85} = 41\%$
Range of evidence estimate							
From studies combining all components	49.5–69% reduction in measles incidence				51–54%	25–35% ↓	$\frac{25}{85}-\frac{35}{85} = 29\text{–}41\%$
From studies of individual components	**85% reduction in measles incidence**	100%	0–95%	100%*		0–44% ↓	$\frac{0}{85}-\frac{44}{85} = 0\text{–}52\%$
Under improved conditions of provider compliance and coverage	85%	100%	90%	100%*	90%	69%	$\frac{69}{85} = 82\%$

*Assuming coverage incorporates compliance (see text).

Table 27-10 shows some sample calculations for our two examples using the simple multiplication formula. The purpose of these sample calculations is to illustrate the effect on efficacy estimates (obtained under ideal circumstances) of the other factors that influence community effectiveness. These calculations are "best estimates" based on currently available evidence, and we fully appreciate that they may be subject to error. However, we feel that they serve the purpose of illustrating the relative magnitude of the difference between efficacy estimates for an intervention and its impact when implemented under community conditions. In addition, by examining each of the individual components of community effectiveness we can identify the ones that, if improved, would have the greatest impact on increasing community effectiveness.

There are several approaches for deriving best estimates based on the results of multiple studies. These include voting (based on a tabulation of study results and assessment of study quality), delphi and nominal group techniques, consensus, and statistical approaches (meta-analysis, overview analysis) for combining results from two or more studies [78]. For our purposes, meta-analysis constitutes the approach of choice, as this quantitative technique would provide us with the best estimate based on the currently available evidence in the literature [79]. However, we were not able to employ this technique because for both of our examples the current data base did not meet the requirements and assumptions necessary to do so [45,47]. Instead, as will be discussed in detail below, we have used a systematic approach to reviewing the literature using the methodological criteria discussed above. We have defined as our best estimate the results of the study considered to be the strongest according to the methodological standards applied. We have also summarized the range of results, including all of the studies reviewed.

For measles immunization, our estimate of efficacy comes from randomized trials conducted in developed country settings. From these data, we estimate the efficacy of measles immunization in reducing the incidence of measles to be 85 percent. Community-based studies of measles immunization conducted in LDC settings are available, reflecting the collective impact of the other factors that determine effectiveness at the community level with the exception of coverage. None of the studies available include an assessment of coverage—that is, the proportion of children susceptible to measles who received a vaccination. Therefore, in using these studies to estimate community effectiveness, an adjustment must be made to take into account the effect of less than 100 percent coverage on the overall impact in the community. For others interested in deriving estimates for use in their own setting, it will often be worthwhile to carry out local checks on compliance and coverage to ensure accuracy (given that the cost of the expansion of health services warranted the expense of conducting the check). Efficacy should be reasonably stable and therefore suitable for generalization to most populations [76].

The Kasongo study provides the best estimate of community effectiveness, according to the methodological guidelines discussed above, reporting a 69 percent reduction in the incidence of measles in children 7 to 35 months of age. Adjusting this for coverage, estimated to be in the range of 50 percent [75,80], suggests the reduction in measles incidence due to an immunization program is approximately 35 percent. It is important to point out that a comprehensive review of the literature reveals a wide range of results, suggesting that the community impact of measles immunization programs may vary significantly [45]. As is evident from the literature, provider compliance and coverage can have a major impact, causing suboptimal levels of community effectiveness. For example, cold chain problems have been shown to have resulted in the administration of a completely ineffective vaccine [*4,5*]. Regarding coverage, there is clearly room for improvement, and successful programs will need to include strategies to maximize coverage in their overall activity plan.

As is shown in Table 27-10, the potential for a major loss of measles immunization efficacy is great. The Kasango results reflect a 59 percent loss, and taking into account other available data suggests the loss could be as great as 100 percent. If provider compliance and coverage could be raised to a more optimal level (90 percent for each), and it seems reasonable that this could be achieved given the appropriate motivation and commitment of those involved, community effectiveness could be improved to 69 or 82 percent of the maximum possible impact based on efficacy estimates.

For oral rehydration salts (Table 27-11), our estimate of efficacy comes from several initial studies; in particular, the report of the experience under extraordinarily adverse conditions in a Bangladesh refugee camp where the dramatic reduction of the cholera case fatality rate to 3.6 percent was observed [*61*]. It is hence reasonable, as has previously been discussed, to conclude that efficacy under ideal conditions is at least as great as 95 percent. Estimates for community effectiveness and the other components of the equation are based on community-based field trials of ORS and studies targeting the specific individual components [*47*]. Again, for others interested in deriving estimates for use in their own setting it will often be worthwhile to carry out local checks on compliance and coverage to ensure accuracy. Also, as has been pointed out in the literature, the overall impact of ORS on a community may depend upon the proportion of acute watery diarrhea compared to dysentric or chronic diarrhea for which the effectiveness of ORS is not yet established [*9*].

The impact of ORS has been evaluated in several community-based studies. Accordingly, the results of these trials reflect the collective impact of all five factors. The best evidence,

according to the guidelines outlined above, comes from the trial conducted by Rahaman in Bangladesh [*35*]. The results of this community-based trial suggest that we can expect a 79 percent reduction in diarrhea case fatality rates with the implementation of health center–based distribution programs. The magnitude of the impact observed should be interpreted with some caution and taking into account that this study represents an extremely intensive community-based effort that may not be easily replicated in other settings because of resource limitations. As well, total mortality was not reported, leaving some uncertainty as to the accuracy of the cause-specific rates reported by unblinded observers. Once again it is important to point out that a comprehensive review of the literature reveals an extremely wide range of results suggesting that the impact of ORS programs can vary significantly [*47*]. As is evident, patient compliance and coverage can have a major impact, causing suboptimal levels of community effectiveness. For example, it is estimated that home-based distribution programs may actually be less effective than health center–based programs in terms of reduction in case fatality rates [*47*]. Patient compliance, in particular, the attitudes and behavior of the mother, is the most likely source of this loss of efficacy. Accordingly, as is shown in Table 27-10, although there is evidence that up to 83 percent of the maximum efficacy of ORS may be achieved at the community level, reflecting a loss of less than 20 percent of efficacy, impact could be as low as 3 percent of efficacy, reflecting a virtual loss of efficacy. If patient compliance and coverage could be raised to a more optimal level (again, 90 percent for each seems reasonable) community effectiveness could be improved to 66 or 70 percent of the maximum possible impact based on efficacy estimates. (Given the results of Rahaman, where 83 percent of efficacy was maintained, this estimate of 70 percent should be viewed as the minimum target under improved conditions of health service delivery.)

Table 27-11. Sample calculations for community effectiveness: Oral rehydration salts

Type of estimate	Efficacy	Diagnostic accuracy	Provider compliance	Patient compliance	Coverage	Community effectiveness (case fatality rate)	Percent of efficacy achieved in the community
"Best evidence" estimate		79% reduction in case fatality rate				79% ↓	$\frac{79}{95} = 83\%$
Range of evidence estimate							
From studies combining all components		56–79% reduction in case fatality rate				56–79%	$\frac{56}{95} - \frac{79}{95} = 59\text{–}83\%$
From studies of individual components	**95–100%** ↓ in case fatality rate	95–100%	87–100%	59.5–80%	60–70%	28–56%	$\frac{28}{95} - \frac{56}{95} = 30\text{–}59\%$
Under improved conditions of provider compliance and coverage	95	95	90	90	90	66	$\frac{66}{95} = 70\%$

It should be noted that for simplicity we have ignored the iatrogenic complications of therapy in these examples. For example, measles vaccination can include complications of both morbidity and mortality, although the risk is considered to be very small. ORS, when inappropriately administered, can result in severe electrolyte imbalances, particularly hyper- and hyponatremia.

These estimates also do not tell us to what extent the community as a whole would be better off if an intervention were implemented. The reduction in the overall burden of illness experienced by the community will depend upon two factors. First, the proportion of the total burden accounted for by a specific disorder will determine the overall community impact of interventions targeted at this disorder. Second, the effect of competing risks will determine the overall influence on the health of the community. For example, it is well known in LDC settings that children who avoid measles may simply succumb to some other disease.

MEASUREMENT LOOP STEP 4: EFFICIENCY

Step 4 provides information on whether the intervention is being delivered to those who would benefit from it with an optimal use of resources, and involves the relationship between the costs and effects.

$$\text{Efficiency} = \text{patient benefit (outcome)/cost}$$
$$\text{or}$$
$$= \text{net costs (\$)} - \text{net benefits (\$)}$$

Efficiency is expressed as effects (the number of lives saved, number of disability days avoided) obtained for a specific cost (expressed in dollars). Again, the assessment of efficiency should not be conducted in the absence of evidence of efficacy and community effectiveness, although in research, the study of efficiency may be combined with that of efficacy and community effectiveness. Other issues that should be considered in the assessment of efficiency have been discussed by Stoddart [81,82]. The most widely used approaches to evaluating efficiency are as follows: (1) Cost-effectiveness: effectiveness is measured in a common unit of health impact such as lives saved, levels of function restored, or proportion of patients in whom symptoms are controlled. This may be derived from efficacy studies in tightly controlled situations or from studies incorporating variable numbers of the other components that make up community effectiveness. (2) Cost-benefit:effectiveness (benefit) is measured in the appropriate unit (lives saved, functional improvement, symptom control) and then converted into monetary units (i.e., dollars and cents). (3) Cost-utility: effectiveness (utility) is measured in the appropriate unit (lives saved, functional improvement, symptom control) and then converted into "utility units" that are measures of the relative social value (importance) of these outcomes.

The cost-effectiveness of measles vaccination has been investigated in a number of developing country settings [83–87]. This work has considered the relative costs and consequences

of measles immunization alone as well as with other immunizations within the context of the WHO expanded program of immunization (EPI). Overall, these studies suggest measles immunization is cost-effective. As these studies show, cost-effectiveness is influenced by the number of children vaccinated and whether measles vaccine is given alone or is incorporated into other vaccination schedules. In contrast, although some information is available on the cost of ORS [72] and two studies examining the relationship between costs and estimates of deaths averted have appeared in the literature [88,89], a formal evaluation incorporating the methodological issues relevant to conducting an economic evaluation alluded to above has not yet been carried out.

MEASUREMENT LOOP STEP 5: SYNTHESIS AND IMPLEMENTATION

The fifth step integrates feasibility with the estimates of community effectiveness and efficiency obtained in the previous steps to make recommendations for action. This step identifies: (1) the possible limiting constraints on the effectiveness and efficiency estimates in the setting where the intervention will be implemented; and (2) whether and to what extent these constraints can be removed or reduced. Conclusions can then be drawn as to the likely impact of the intervention or program on the burden of illness. Constraints include social, cultural, and political barriers as well as adequacy and availability of facilities and manpower and budgetary considerations.

Inherent in this step is the setting of goals, important both for defining realistic objectives and for assessing success. Estimates of community effectiveness and efficiency can be used to evaluate the success of the intervention over time.

MEASUREMENT LOOP STEP 6: MONITORING

The sixth step is ongoing monitoring of the impact of a health program. Monitoring needs to be tailored to the individual program and may consist of short, intermediate, and long-term criteria of success selected to profile progress. Monitoring methods usually focus on one or more of the following categories: (1) structure: buildings built and equipped and qualifications of health workers; (2) health care and administrative process; the appropriateness of case finding and care of patients with the target disorder; and (3) patient or citizen health outcomes: changes in symptoms, disability, and mortality. The selection of markers needs to take into account the representativeness of the spectrum of disease and age groups, accuracy, and feasibility [90].

The use of "sentinel sites" and community diagnosis systems as monitoring strategies has received attention recently [91]. Sentinel sites are chosen according to the extent to which they are judged as representative of the surveillance targets of interest. Hence, problems identified at these selected sites can be used as indicators of problems in the overall setting where a program is being implemented. At these sites, a small amount of additional manpower may be provided to ensure careful reporting of the data of interest.

Community diagnosis techniques consist of population-based monitoring of the health events of interest rather than the selection of specific sites and can include indicators relevant to monitoring specific programs. This approach involves an annual census plus regular reporting of events by community health workers or appropriate others generated through regular surveillance of all homes in a predefined area.

Finally, case-control and cohort studies have been proposed as cost-effective, time-efficient methods for monitoring the impact of vaccination programs [92–94]. The impact of BCG mass immunization programs in Sri Lanka has been assessed using the case-control approach with the results suggesting an unacceptable level of impact [94].

As is evident from the review of community effectiveness presented above, monitoring is crucial in the successful implementation of community-based programs of measles immunization and ORS. The selection of indicators relevant to provider and patient compliance and coverage (e.g., potency of measles vaccine, number of children effectively immunized, inappropriate use of antibiotics in the treatment of acute diarrhea, willingness of mothers to administer fluids to their sick child) will provide the information needed to identify problems and institute the changes necessary to keep the program on target with regard to the expected decrease in measles incidence and diarrhea case fatality rates.

CLOSING THE LOOP: REASSESSING THE BURDEN OF ILLNESS

Reassessment of health needs and the burden of illness is essential to assess the overall success of interventions—the loop is ''closed,'' returning again to the residual burden of illness. With regard to our two examples, this entails periodic surveys of the incidence of measles and diarrhea case fatality rates.

CAN THE LOOP BE USEFULLY APPLIED TO CLINICAL AND POLICY DECISIONS?

The usefulness of the loop approach in clinical and policy decisions can be illustrated in two ways. First, the loop can be applied to the available evidence on measles immunization and ORS to make recommendations for needed research. Measles immunization is one example where adequate information exists for each step in the loop to the extent reasonable and possible. Currently available evidence should provide a sound foundation in most settings for clinical and policy conclusions. All children are potentially susceptible to measles without vaccination. Efficacy has been studied in rigorous randomized trials that examined the impact of vaccination on the actual incidence of measles. Even though conducted in an industrialized setting, there is no evidence to suggest that the efficacy estimate of 85 percent is not appropriate for developing country settings. Estimates of the other components of community ef-

fectiveness, however, are certainly subject to variation between different settings, but it should be possible to approximate these or carry out quick surveys to obtain the required information. Improved methods for cost-effective, accurate monitoring of priority health problems continue to be called for in the literature [95]. The standardized cluster sampling technique developed by WHO's EPI has proved to be extremely useful and is applied regularly to assess immunization uptake [91]. Finally, new and potentially better vaccines, such as Edmonston-Zagreb, suggest even higher levels of efficacy may be possible [99].

ORS, on the other hand, is an intervention where, by applying the loop to assemble the available information, we can identify gaps in our knowledge and make recommendations for needed research. Although there is no question about the potential of ORS to reduce deaths due to the dehydration caused by diarrhea, significant gaps remain regarding optimal strategies for its delivery including (1) methods to enhance compliance by the mothers and coverage and (2) the role and appropriate use of home-based fluids; further information on the cost-effectiveness and cost-utility of alternative strategies is also needed.

Second, several examples exist where substantial problems could have been avoided through the use of the loop in formulating clinical and policy decisions. For example, the widespread implementation of nutrition programs in the developing world in the 1960s and 1970s could have benefited from consideration of the issues summarized by the loop. Gwatkin, in his review, highlights the role of the various factors that determine community effectiveness and their relation to the poor performance of the programs undertaken [96].

Finally, through the application of the loop to summarize the evidence on measles immunization and ORS, the wide range in the available evidence becomes evident, as is shown in Tables 27-10 and 27-11. With such wide ranges in the estimates, it is extremely difficult to establish rankings that allow the analyst or health care planner to determine the relative impact and costs of the various alternatives under consideration, for example, the top three interventions in terms of maximum health impact per dollar spent relevant to diseases of the under-5 population of LDCs.

An important, associated point concerns the validity of rankings based on efficacy estimates, as opposed to community effectiveness. The two examples used here illustrate the potential impact that the other factors that influence community effectiveness can have. It seems reasonable to conclude that high levels of efficacy may not necessarily translate into high levels of community effectiveness, and, accordingly, rankings based on efficacy estimates should be viewed with caution.

CONCLUSIONS

These guides will not and should not be expected to provide the answer to the question of which programs should be recommended for funding. It is fully appreciated that only rarely (or never) will ideal information be available. Rather, they are intended to provide a set of commonsense guidelines that can be useful as a framework for identifying some of the important factors and assessing the quality of information used in decision making in health care.

On the other hand, the amount of evidence available to decision-makers can be substantial, as our two examples illustrate. Nevertheless, because there are almost always gaps in the evidence, it is important to systematically organize the available information and explicitly identify the gaps so that an informed decision may be made, whether it be a recommendation for funding or for further study. It is recognized that policymakers at all levels have to make decisions *now* on the basis of the best available information, but it is crucial to recognize a weak information base when it exists. All involved in the planning and provision of health care have a responsibility to identify the strengths and weaknesses of the evidence upon which decisions are made. Researchers have a responsibility to generate evidence that can be used by policymakers. Policymakers need to capitalize on the expertise and insights that health researchers can bring to the decision-making process and setting of priorities. Thus, we can iterate toward a higher standard of information on which decisions are based.

Finally, it cannot be overemphasized that the issues discussed above are not unique to LDC settings. However, given the extreme scarcity of resources for health, the severity of many of the problems of LDCs, and the explosion of expensive new medical technologies, the need to set priorities and to identify strategies that maximize the impact of the health resources that are available is of extreme importance to LDCs. What we have presented raises issues common to all involved in the planning and provision of health care worldwide. As has already begun to evolve, the challenges and opportunities offered by this common need set the stage for international partnership and a worldwide sharing of ideas and strategies for solution.

REFERENCES

1 Cochrane AL: Effectiveness and Efficiency: Random Reflections on Health Services. The Nuffield Provincial Hospitals Trust, 1972
2 Sackett DL: On the evaluation of health services, in Last J (ed): *Preventive Medicine and Public Health,* 11th ed. New York, Appleton Century Crofts, 1980
3 Evans JR: Measurement and Management in Medicine and Health Services. New York, Rockefeller Foundation, 1981
4 Abdurrahman MB, Taqi AM: Measles immunity and immunization in developing countries of Africa: A review. Afr J Med Sci 10:57–62, 1981
5 Hendrickse RG: Problems of future measles vaccination in developing countries. Trans R Soc Trop Med Hyg 69:31–34, 1975
6 UNICEF: Assignment Children: A Child Survival and Development Revolution, 1983
7 Grant JP: The State of the World's Children, 1987. New York, United Nations Children's Fund, 1987

8 Walsh JA, Warren KS: Selective primary health care: An interim strategy for disease control in developing countries. N Engl J Med 301: 967–974, 1979
9 Feachem RG: Preventing diarrhea: What are the policy options: Health Policy and Planning 1:109–117, 1986
10 Kohn R, White KL (eds): *Health Care: An International Study.* Toronto, Oxford University Press, 1978
11 Ghana Health Assessment Project Team: A quantitative method of assessing the health impact of different diseases in less developed countries. Int J Epidemiol 10:73–1048, 1981
12 Synder JD, Merson MH: The magnitude of the global problem of acute diarrhoeal disease: A review of active surveillance data. Bull WHO 60:605–613, 1982
13 Walsh JA: Measles, in Warren KS, Walsh JA (eds): *Strategies for Primary Health Care: Technologies Appropriate for the Control of Disease in the Developing World.* University of Chicago Press, 1986, pp 60–71
14 Black FL: Measles, in Warren KS, Mahmoud AAF (eds): *Tropical and Geographical Medicine.* New York, McGraw-Hill, 1984, pp 586–593
15 Walsh JA: Estimating the burden of illness in the tropics, in Warren KS, Mahmoud AAF (eds): *Tropical and Geographical Medicine.* New York, McGraw-Hill, 1984, pp 1073–1085
16 Prost A, Prescott N: Cost-effectiveness of blindness prevention by the onchocerciasis control programme in Upper Volta. Bull WHO 62:795–802, 1984
17 Barnum H: Evaluating healthy days of life gained from health projects. Soc Sci Med 24:833–841, 1987
18 Doege TC: Tuberculosis mortality in the United States 1900 to 1960. JAMA 192:1045–1048, 1965
19 Liang J, Tu EJC, Chen XM: Population aging in the People's Republic of China. Soc Sci Med, in press, 1986
20 Koch R: Die etiologic de tuberculose. Berlin Klin Wochenschlir 19:221–230, (1882 English translation, de Rouville W: Medical Classic 2:853–880, 1973)
21 Hill AB: *Principles of Medical Statistics,* 9th ed. London, Lancet, 1971
22 Department of Clinical Epidemiology and Biostatistics: How to read clinical journals. V. To distinguish useful from useless or even harmful therapy. Can Med Assoc J 124:985–990, 1981
23 Guerrant RL: Unresolved problems and future considerations in diarrheal research. Pediatr Infect Dis 5:S155–S161, 1986
24 Rohde JE: Acute diarrhea, in Warren KS, Walsh JA (eds): *Strategies for Primary Health Care: Technologies Appropriate for the Control of Disease in the Developing World.* University of Chicago Press, 1986, pp 14–28
25 Sommer A, Tarwotjo I, Djunaedi E, et al: Impact of vitamin A supplementation on childhood mortality: A randomized controlled community trial. Lancet i:1169–1173, 1986
26 Feachem RG: Vitamin A deficiency and diarrhea: A review of interrelationships and their implications for the control of xerophthalmia and diarrhea. Trop Dis Bull 84:1–16, 1987
27 Costello AM de L: Vitamin A supplementation and childhood mortality. Lancet ii:161, 1986
28 Gray RH: Vitamin A supplementation and childhood mortality. Lancet ii:161–162, 1986
29 Martinez H, Shekar M, Latham M: Vitamin A supplementation and child mortality. Lancet ii:451, 1986
30 Sommer A, West KP: Vitamin A supplementation and child mortality. Lancet ii:451–452, 1986

31 Gopalan C: Vitamin A deficiency and child mortality. Bull Nutr Found India 7:3–7, 1986

32 Cohen N: Vitamin A supplementation and child mortality. Xerophthalmia Club Bull. 34:1–2, 1986

33 Sommer A, Katz J, Tarwotjo I: Increased risk of respiratory disease and diarrhea in children with pre-existing mild vitamin A deficiency. Am J Clin Nutr 40:1090–1095, 1984

34 Sackett DL: Bias in analytic research. J Chron Dis 32:51–63, 1979

35 Rahaman MM, Aziz KMS, Patwan Y, et al: Diarrhoeal mortality in two Bangladesh villages with and without community-based oral rehydration therapy. Lancet ii:809–813, 1979

36 Beasley RP, Hwang LY, Lin CC, et al: Hepato-cellular carcinoma and hepatitis B virus. Lancet ii:1129–1133, 1981

37 Labarthe DR: Methodologic variation in case-control studies on reserpine and breast cancer. J Chron Dis 32:95–104, 1979

38 Trichopoulus D et al: Hepatitis B and primary hepatocellular carcinoma in a European population. Lancet (ii):1217–1219, 1978

39 Gwatkin DR, Wilcox JR, Wray JD: Can Health and Nutrition Interventions Make a Difference? Overseas Development Council, monograph no 13, February, 1980

40 Warren, KS: The control of Helminths: Non-replicating infectious agents of man. Annu Rev Public Health 2:101–115, 1981

41 Zuckerman AJ et al: Prevention of primary liver cancer. Lancet (i):463–465, 1983

42 Law DK, Dudrick SJ, Abdon NI: Immunization competence of patients with protein-calorie malnutrition. Ann Intern Med 79:545, 1973

43 Minot GR, Murphy WP: Treatment of pernicious anemia by a special diet. JAMA 87:470, 1926

44 Goldsmith GA: Experimental niacin deficiency. J Am Dietetic Assoc 32:312, 1956

45 Bennett KJ, Tugwell P: Measles immunization—A critical review of the evidence for community effectiveness. Submitted for publication

46 Medical Research Council Measles Vaccine Committee: Vaccination against measles: A clinical trial of live measles vaccine given alone and live vaccine preceded by killed vaccine. Br Med J i:441–446, 1966

47 Bennett KJ, Tugwell P: Oral rehydration—A critical review of the evidence for community effectiveness. Submitted for publication

48 Santosham M, et al: Oral rehydration therapy in infantile diarrhea: A controlled study of well-nourished children hospitalized in the United States and Panama. N Engl J Med 306:1070–1076, 1982

49 Levine M: Case study A—Oral rehydration therapy for diarrheal diseases, in Status of Biomedical Research and Related Technology for Tropical Diseases. US Congress, Office of Technology Assessment, OTA-H-258, September, 1985

50 Oliver MF, Heady JA, Morris JN, et al: A co-operative trial in the primary prevention of ischemic heart disease using clofibrate. Report from the committee of principal investigators. Br Heart J 40: 1069–1118, 1978

51 Mias LL: Gastric freezing: An example of the evaluation of medical therapy by randomized clinical trials, in Bunker JP, Barnes BA, Mosteller F (eds): *Costs, Risks and Benefits of Surgery*. New York, Oxford University Press, 1977

52 Glover RP, Davila JC, Kyle RH, et al: Ligation of the internal arteries as a means of increasing blood supply to the myocardium. J Thorac Cardiovasc Surg 34:661–678, 1957

53 Sacks HS, Chalmers RC, Smith H: Sensitivity and specificity of clinical trials. Arch Intern Med 143:753–755, 1983

54 Clemens JD, Chuong JJH, Feinstein A: The BCG controversy—A methodological and statistical reappraisal. JAMA 249:2362–2369, 1983

55 Francis T Jr, Korns RF, Voight RB, et al: An evaluation of the 1954 poliomyelitis vaccine field trials. Am J Public Health 45 (pt 11):1, 1955

56 Evans JAP: Oral penicillin in the prophylaxis of streptococcal infection and rheumatic relapse. Proc R Soc Med 43:206, 1950

57 Robertson L, Kelley A, O'Neil B, et al: A controlled study of the effect of television messages on safety belt use. Am J Public Health 64:1071–1080, 1974

58 Veterans Administration Co-operative Study Group on Antihypertensive Agents: Effects of treatment on morbidity in hypertension II—results in patients with diastolic blood pressure averaging 90 through 114 mmHg. JAMA 213:1143–1152, 1970

59 Durbridge TC, Edwards F, Edwards RG, et al: An evaluation of multiphasic screening on admission to hospital. Med J Aust 1:703–705, 1976

60 Hinshaw HC, Feldman WH, Pfuetze KH: Treatment of tuberculosis with streptomycin: Summary of observations on 100 cases. JAMA 132:778–782, 1946

61 Mahalanabis D, Choudhuri AB, Bagchi NG, et al: Oral fluid therapy of cholera among Bangladesh refugees. Johns Hopkins Med J 132:197–205, 1973

62 Louria DB, Brayton RG: The efficacy of penicillin regimens: With observations on the frequency of superinfection. JAMA 186:987–990, 1963

63 Tuberculosis prevention trial. Trial of BCG vaccines in South India for tuberculosis prevention: First report. Bull WHO 57:819–827, 1979

64 White KL: Improved medical care: Statistics and the health services system. Public Health Rep 82:847–854, 1967

65 Guyatt GH, Bombardier C, Tugwell P: Measuring disease specific quality of life in clinical trials. CMAJ 134:889–895, 1986

66 Torrance GW: Measurement of health state utilities for economic appraisal. J Health Econ 5:1–30, 1986

67 Torrance GW: Utility approach to measuring health related quality of life. J Chron Dis 40:593–600, 1987

68 The Kasongo Project Team: Influence of measles vaccination on survival pattern of 7–35 children in Kasongo, Zaire. Lancet i:704–761, 1981

69 Laupacis A, Sackett DL, Roberts RS: An assessment of clinically useful measures of the consequences of treatment. N Engl J Med 318:1728–1733, 1988

70 Haynes RB, et al: Absenteeism from work after the detection and labelling of hypertension. N Engl J Med 299:741–744, 1978

71 Dusitsin N, Varakamin S, Ningsanon P, et al: Post-partum tubal ligation by nurse-midwives and doctors in Thailand. Lancet i(8169):638–639, 1980

72 Lerman SJ, Shepard DS, Cash RA: Treatment of diarrhea in Indonesian children: What it costs and who pays for it. Lancet ii:651–654, 1985

73 Chen LC, Black RE, Sarder AM, et al: Village-based distribution of oral rehydration therapy packets in Bangladesh. Am J Trop Med Hyg 29:285–290, 1980

74 Tanahashi T: Health service coverage and its evaluation. Bull WHO 56:295–303, 1978

75 McBean AM, Foster SO, Hermann KI, et al: Evaluation of a mass measles immunization campaign in Yaounde, Cameroun. Trans R Soc Trop Med Hyg 70:206–212, 1976

76 Mills A: Economic evaluation of health programmes: Application of the principles in developing countries. World Health Statist Q 38:368–382, 1985

77 Colton T: *Statistics in Medicine*. Boston, Little, Brown, 1974

78 Fink A, Kosecoff J, Shassin M, et al: Consensus methods: Characteristics and guidelines for use. Am J Public Health 74:979–983, 1984

79 Oxman A, Guyatt GH: Guidelines for reading literature reviews. Can Med Assoc J 138:687–705, 1988

80 Breman YG, Coffi E, Raphael Bomba-ire K, et al: Evaluation of a measles-smallpox vaccination campaign by sero-epidemiologic method. Am J Epidemiol 102:564–571, 1975

81 Stoddart GL, Drummond MF: Clinical epidemiology rounds: How to read clinical journals. VII. To understand an economic evaluation (part A). Can Med Assoc J 130:1428–1434, 1984

82 Stoddart GL, Drummond MF: Clinical epidemiology rounds. How to read clinical journals. VII. To understand an economic evaluation (part B). Can Med Assoc J 130:1542–1549, 1984

83 Shepard DS, Sanoh L, Coffi E: Cost-effectiveness of the expanded program on immunization in the Ivory Coast: A preliminary assessment. Soc Sci Med 22:369–377, 1986

84 Barnum H, Tarantola D, Setiady IF: Cost-effectiveness of an immunization program in Indonesia. Bull WHO 58:499–503, 1980

85 Robertson RL, Davis JH, Jobe K: Service volume and other factors affecting the costs of immunizations in the Gambia. Bull WHO 62:729–736, 1984

86 Robertson RL, Foster SO, Hull HF, et al: Cost-effectiveness of immunization in the Gambia. J Trop Med Hyg 88:343–351, 1985

87 Ponninghaus JM: The cost/benefit of measles immunization: A study from Southern Zambia. J Trop Med Hyg 83:141–149, 1980

88 Oberle MW, Merson MH, Shafiqul Islam M, et al: Diarrhoeal disease in Bangladesh: Epidemiology, mortality averted and costs at a rural treatment centre. Int J Epidemiol 9:341–348, 1980

89 Horton S, Claquin P: Cost-effectiveness and user characteristics of clinic-based services for the treatment of diarrhea: A case study in Bangladesh. Soc Sci Med 17:721–729, 1983

90 Tugwell P: A methodologic perspective on process measures of the quality of medical care. Clin Invest Med 2:113–119, 1979

91 Walsh JA: Prioritizing for primary health care: Methods for data collection and analysis, in Warren KS, Walsh JA (eds): *Strategies for Primary Health Care: Technologies Appropriate for the Control of Disease in the Developing World*. University of Chicago Press, 1986, pp 1–13

92 Smith PG, Rodrigues LC, Fine PEM: Assessment of the protective efficacy of vaccines against common diseases using case control and cohort studies. Int J Epidemiol 13:87–93, 1984

93 Smith PG: Evaluating interventions against tropical diseases. Int J Epidemiol 16(2):159–166, 1987

94 Smith PG: Retrospective assessment of the effectiveness of BCG vaccination against tuberculosis using the case-control approach. Tubercle 62:23–25, 1982

95 White KL: A new look at health information. World Health Forum 4:368–373, 1983

96 Gwatkin DR, Wilcox JR, Wray JD: The policy implications of field experiments in primary health and nutrition care. Soc Sci Med 14C:121–128, 1980

97 Independent International Commission on Health Research for Development (editorial). Lancet ii:1076–1077, 1987

98 Chen LC, Cash R: A decade after Alma Ata. Can primary health care lead to health for all? N Engl J Med 319:946–947, 1988

99 Aaby P, Hansen HL, Tharup J et al: Trial of high-dose Edmonston-Zagreb measles vaccine in Guinea-Bissau: Protective efficacy. Lancet ii:809–814, 1988

CHAPTER 28 / # *Infectious Diseases in Travelers and Immigrants* · Robert A. Salata · G. Richard Olds

International travel for business or pleasure has increased dramatically over the past decade. Ten percent of the United States population will travel abroad and return each year. Annually, more than 8 million Americans will travel to developing countries, and 1 million will visit malaria-endemic areas [1–3]. At the same time, the number of immigrants to our country has markedly increased. In 1982 alone, 182 million foreign visitors entered the United States, with 69 percent originating from countries that are ecologically different from our own [3]. Since 1973, more than 1 million refugees have come into this country from southeast Asia, Cuba, South and Central America, the Caribbean, Iran, and Africa [3].

These major increases in international travel and immigration, accompanied by the importation of malaria and other "exotic" diseases, have brought the issues of prevention and management of health problems in travelers and immigrants into every physician's office. Provision of health care to these groups has become so expansive and complex that it has been viewed by some as a new area of medical care. The term *emporiatrics,* from the Greek words *emporus,* "to go on board ship," and *iatrike,* "medicine," has been coined to focus attention on this new discipline [4].

Few physicians educated in the developed world are familiar with the health hazards related to travel or illnesses seen in immigrant populations. Because of this information gap, illnesses in these groups have frequently been misdiagnosed and mistreated [5]. In this chapter, the important aspects of pretravel health advice and immunizations will be discussed first. In the second part of the chapter, the major disease syndromes encountered in returning travelers and immigrants will be reviewed.

PRETRAVEL HEALTH ADVICE

GENERAL RECOMMENDATIONS

After consideration of the traveler's itinerary, the duration and nature of the trip, and the traveler's age and medical, allergy, and immunization history, an individualized program can be designed to ensure health abroad. General advice to the traveler must first include an extensive discussion of careful eating and drinking habits, since the majority of travel-related health problems occur through the ingestion of contaminated food or water [6,7].

General consultation before departure should include a discussion about the common problems related to international travel including jet lag, altitude sickness, environmental exposures, the hazards of insects as vectors of many infections (malaria, yellow fever, dengue, filariasis, trypanosomiasis, onchocerciasis, etc.), and the means to avoid these vectors. Travelers to remote areas must be warned about venomous animals, rabies (predominantly transmitted by domestic dogs and cats), and exposure to rodents (because of plague), as well as the hazards of fresh water swimming (schistosomiasis, noncholera vibrios, or leptospirosis). In the end, most of the illnesses that develop in travelers are related to behaviors that can be modified with proper advice.

With the acquired immunodeficiency syndrome (AIDS) becoming more prevalent abroad [8,9], the hazards of casual sexual encounters as well as of needle and blood and blood product exposure must be emphasized. Blood sources in developing countries currently must be suspect [9]. Travelers should consider having their blood type determined prior to traveling so that transfusions from family members or travel companions with similar blood types are possible in dire emergencies. Several agencies can provide emergency evacuation to industrialized countries if the situation dictates. There is no documented evidence that human immunodeficiency virus (HIV) is transmitted through casual contacts, sources of food or water, contact with inanimate objects, or mosquitoes or other insect vectors.

Although some countries are now requiring HIV testing for entering travelers, it is the opinion of the World Health Organization that the small benefits of screening travelers would not justify the diversion of resources from educational programs and measures to protect blood supplies [10]. Individuals who are known to be HIV-positive and who wish to travel abroad will be subject to increasing restrictions, depending on the severity of their condition and entrance requirements of specific countries.

Patients with other preexisting medical problems are traveling more extensively and are in greatest need of consultation prior to departure. Conditions which have the greatest impact on travel include chronic cardiopulmonary disease, diabetes, allergies, and gastrointestinal problems, especially diarrhea (malabsorption or inflammatory bowel disease) [11]. Special arrangements must be made for patients with bleeding disorders, those on anticoagulation therapy, and those who require hemodialysis.

Patients with chronic medical conditions should take along a brief medical summary and a recent copy of an electrocardiogram or chest x-ray, if pertinent. For those individuals requiring care by specialists, an international directory for that specialty can be consulted. In addition, a directory of physicians worldwide who speak English and who have met certain qualifications is available from the International Association for Medical Assistance to Travelers [736 Center St., Lewiston, N.Y. 14092; telephone: (716) 754-4883]. If medical care is needed urgently when abroad, sources of information include the American embassy or consulate, hotel managers, travel agents catering to foreign tourists, and missionary hospitals. Patients should be counseled, however, to take with them a sufficient supply of prescription medications and to make sure that bottles are clearly marked. A travel health kit consisting of prescription medications and nonprescription items is also often useful. Travelers also need to ascertain whether their hospital insurance will cover medical care abroad.

Pregnancy presents several unique problems for international travel. These include difficulties in the administration of pretravel vaccinations (see section on immunizations) and prescribing of antibiotics (see "Travelers' Diarrhea" below). Malaria is a major consideration in pregnancy and can make international travel to some areas unadvisable. There is an additional concern that air travel late in pregnancy could precipitate premature labor. For traveling small children, particularly infants, additional concerns relate to inadequate primary immunizations, lack of demonstrated efficacy and safety of many vaccines in infants, excretion of prophylactic drugs in breast milk, and increased morbidity and possible mortality associated with some diseases acquired abroad [12]. Careful counseling of pregnant women and parents must, therefore, be accomplished prior to departure.

IMMUNIZATIONS FOR TRAVEL

It is important to recognize that vaccination is only one feature of a comprehensive disease prevention program for travelers. No vaccine is completely safe or effective; benefits and risks should, therefore, be considered for use of all immunizations. Only immune globulin administered as passive protection against hepatitis A has been shown to be highly cost-effective in all susceptible travelers [13]. The most common mistake

Table 28-1. Immunizations for international travel

Vaccine	Indications	Efficacy	Duration of protection	Comments
Required				
Yellow fever	For travel to tropical and subtropical Africa and South America	Very high	10 years	Immune globulin has been administered simultaneously without change in antibody response.
Cholera	Only when necessary for entry	Low	5–6 months	Only 1 dose required by law. New oral vaccine in near future.
Recommended				
Typhoid	For travel to most third world countries, especially as care with food and water decreases or with longer duration of travel	High	3 years	Frequent local and systemic side effects. New oral or injectable vaccines in the near future.
Tetanus	Update every 10 years for travel, especially in older adults	Very high	10 years	Especially important in the tropics. Most frequently given with diphtheria toxoid in adults.
Polio	For travel to tropics, especially in older adults	Very high	Lifelong	If previous vaccine status in adult uncertain, give IPV as primary or booster. Immune globulin given with OPV has not resulted in decreased antibody responses.
Measles	Consider for those born in U.S. after 1956	Very high	Lifelong	Not in pregnancy. Consider giving as MMR if indicated. Should not administer immune globulin simultaneously.
Immune globulin	For travel to most third world countries, especially in younger adults	Very high	1–3 mo for low dose and 4–5 mo for high dose	No risk for HIV transmission. Antibody testing for hepatitis A may be cost-effective in frequent travelers.
Special				
Hepatitis B	For high risk of needle or blood exposure or sexual exposure in endemic areas of far east, sub-Saharan Africa, Amazon Basin, Haiti, or Dominican Republic	High	Lifelong	Not to be given in gluteal area. Equivalent efficacy from both available vaccines (plasma-derived versus recombinant). Optimal immunization should begin 6 mo before departure.
Rabies	For those residing in areas where risk is constant and veterinarians, animal handlers, spelunkers, and certain laboratory workers	High	Every 2 yr or when antibody levels fall below acceptable levels	Chloroquine phosphate may interfere with immune response with low-dose ID vaccination. Preexposure vaccination *does not* eliminate the need for additional therapy after rabies exposure.
Meningococcal A,C,Y,W-135	For travelers to areas of sub-Saharan Africa, India, Nepal, and Saudi Arabia	High	Lifelong	Safety not established in pregnancy.
Plague	For those at high risk of exposure because of research or field activities	High	6 mo–1 yr	Epidemic plague in Vietnam.
Japanese encephalitis	For those residing for prolonged periods in endemic areas of China, Korea, Burma, Bangladesh, Nepal, Thailand, Laos, Vietnam	Very high	Lifelong	Currently unavailable in United States. Travelers may be advised to obtain in endemic area.
Pneumovax	Elderly individuals or those in risk category for pneumococcal infection	Moderate	Lifelong	Reimmunization of persons previously vaccinated with 14-valent vaccine not recommended.
Influenza	Elderly individuals and those in high-risk categories during season	High	Seasonal	Need to know activity in country entered.

made with immunizations is to confuse what is required by law with what is recommended. Currently, only two vaccines, yellow fever and cholera, are required by law for international travel to certain countries (Table 28-1) [12,14]. Foreign governments have no interest in the traveler's health; requirements are established only to block importation of disease. Many vaccines may be far more essential for health and should be strongly recommended (Table 28-1) (typhoid, tetanus, polio, measles, immune globulin). Still, others, such as rabies, plague, hepatitis B, or meningococcal vaccines, should only be administered in special circumstances. The most authoritative sources of health information and requirements for international travel are the publications of the Centers for Disease Control [12], the World Health Organization [14], and the American College of Physicians [15].

In general, a person should allow 4 to 6 weeks before departure for the optimal administration of vaccines, since some vaccines require more than one dose for full protection and some vaccines are incompatible with others. In general, inactivated vaccines can be administered simultaneously although both local and systemic adverse reactions may be cumulative. Field observations have indicated that the simultaneous administration of live virus vaccines does not impair antibody responses [16]. Theoretically, one live virus vaccine may, however, impair the immune response to a second live virus immunization administered within 1 month after the first. Passively acquired antibody from immune globulin administration may also interfere with the antibody responses to live, attenuated vaccines. Therefore, live virus vaccines are generally given together as the first vaccines administered to a traveler, while γ-globulin is given last. Recent prospective studies, however, have indicated that immune globulin does not interfere with antibody responses to oral polio vaccine or yellow fever [17], and thus simultaneous administration can be performed if time does not permit separation of these biologicals.

Vaccine products produced in eggs may contain allergenic substances and cause hypersensitivity responses including anaphylaxis in persons with known egg sensitivity. Screening individuals by history of inability to eat eggs without adverse effects is a reasonable way to identify those at risk from receiving yellow fever, measles, mumps, or influenza vaccines. Bacterial vaccines such as cholera, plague, DTP, and typhoid are frequently associated with local or systemic adverse effects that do not appear to be allergic in nature [15].

Because of a theoretical risk to the developing fetus, live, attenuated virus vaccines are generally not given to pregnant women or those likely to become pregnant within 3 months of immunization [18]. Administration of some vaccines, such as rubella, mumps, and measles, is contraindicated during pregnancy. Yellow fever and oral polio vaccine can be given to pregnant women at substantial risk of exposure to infection [12]. If vaccination of pregnant women is undertaken, waiting until the second or third trimester appears prudent.

Rapid viral replication after administration of live, attenuated virus vaccines has been observed in patients with immunodeficiency disorders [12,15]. These include patients with lymphoreticular malignancies, generalized malignancies, acquired immunodeficiency syndrome (AIDS), or who are undergoing therapy with corticosteroids, alkylating agents, antimetabolites, or radiation. These conditions may also reduce the immune response to inactivated vaccines and toxoids.

The Immunization Practices Advisory Committee of the Centers for Disease Control has recommended that asymptomatic HIV-infected children be given the live, attenuated virus vaccines usually administered in childhood [19,20]. Completely asymptomatic HIV-positive adults may also be immunized with live virus vaccines if they are at high risk of exposure, although a case of disseminated vaccinia has been described in an asymptomatic HIV-positive military recruit after smallpox vaccination [21]. Pneumococcal vaccine should be considered for all HIV-infected individuals, given the increased incidence of pneumococcal infection in this group.

SPECIFIC VACCINATIONS

Yellow fever

Yellow fever is a mosquito-borne viral illness sharing many features with other hemorrhagic fevers, but with more severe hepatic involvement [22]. Yellow fever exists only in Africa and South America in two epidemiological forms—urban and jungle [22]. These forms are etiologically and clinically indistinguishable. Yellow fever vaccine is a live, attenuated vaccine developed in chick embryos and is extremely safe and effective [16]. Yellow fever vaccination is required by law by some countries for travelers arriving from a yellow fever–endemic area. Occasionally this includes countries where yellow fever is not currently reported but in which yellow fever has historically occurred (old yellow fever zones). Medically, all persons 6 months of age or older traveling to or living in areas within countries where yellow fever exists should be vaccinated [16]. Infants under 6 months of age and pregnant women should be considered for vaccination if traveling to high-risk areas when travel cannot be postponed and a high level of protection against mosquito exposure is not feasible. Some studies have demonstrated reduced antibody responses when yellow fever and cholera vaccines are administered simultaneously or within 3 weeks of each other [23]. Therefore, when feasible, these vaccines should be administered separately. Simultaneous administration of γ-globulin can be performed if time does not permit separation, as discussed earlier.

Cholera

Cholera is an acute noninflammatory diarrheal illness caused by *Vibrio cholera* O group 1 acquired through the ingestion of contaminated food or water. At present, careful eating and drinking habits remain the most important strategies in preventing cholera. Although there is continued spread of the seventh pandemic of cholera, which began in 1961, the risk to U.S. travelers is thought to be exceedingly low. Only 10 cases of cholera in U.S. travelers have been reported since 1961 [24,25]. It has been estimated that for American tourists the chance of acquiring cholera is less than 1 in 500,000 [33].

The available cholera vaccine is not very effective even for indigenous populations, with a demonstrated efficacy of only 50 percent in reducing clinical illness following vaccination [26]. In addition, both local and systemic adverse reactions are frequent with this killed bacterial vaccine [26]. Most countries do not require cholera vaccination, and there is no country that currently requires proof of vaccination for direct travel from the United States [12]. Vaccination may be a requirement for travel between certain countries, particularly in Africa. A single dose of vaccine is sufficient to satisfy these international health regulations [12,14]. The complete primary series is recommended only for those who live and work in endemic areas under less than adequate sanitary conditions and those with compromised gastric defense mechanisms (antacid or histamine H_2 blocker therapy, achlorhydria, gastrectomy). More effective vaccines are currently under development [27].

Typhoid

Salmonella typhi, the etiological agent of typhoid fever, is transmitted by contaminated food and water and is prevalent in Africa, Asia, and Central and South America. Annually, hundreds of thousands of cases are reported worldwide. In the United States, approximately 500 cases are reported annually, 60 percent of which are imported [28]. The estimated attack rate for American tourists is about 1 in 10,000 to 1 in 50,000. From 70 to 90 percent of vaccine recipients appear protected, depending in part on the degree of subsequent exposure [29], since the protective effect of this vaccine can be overcome by an increased inoculum. Travelers, including vaccine recipients, must therefore still exercise caution in selecting food and water.

Given this less than ideal efficacy, as well as the fairly frequent adverse side effects of the vaccine, immunization recommendations against *S. typhi* must be individualized. In general, vaccination is indicated for extended (>3 weeks) visits to third world countries or when risk of infection is great (achlorhydria, use of broad-spectrum antibiotics, less than sanitary conditions, etc.). Typhoid vaccination can be given to older children, but no data are available on its efficacy and safety in infants. Better vaccines, including a live, attenuated oral vaccine, are currently under development [30,31].

Diphtheria-tetanus

Tetanus is a global health problem particularly prominent in the tropics [32]. The strategy of choice to prevent neonatal and wound-related tetanus is immunization [32]. In developing parts of the world, as well as in the United States, clinical tetanus primarily occurs in unimmunized or incompletely immunized individuals [32]. Although imported cases of tetanus are unusual, frequently travelers have not had a booster shot within the last 10 years. Since no additional immunizations are required after penetrating wounds if a booster has been administered within the last 5 years, timely pretravel (<5 years) immunization will also reduce the necessity of receiving a needle injection of unknown sterility overseas. As diphtheria still remains a worldwide problem, most adults should be immunized with the combined diphtheria-tetanus vaccine. Young children should also receive the pertussis component of the mixed vaccine.

Polio

Poliomyelitis is still encountered in developing countries, particularly in the tropics [33]. Worldwide, over 250,000 cases were reported in 1986 [34]. This is an eightfold increase in the numbers reported to the World Health Organization in recent years.

Travelers to countries where the risk of exposure to wild polio virus is increased should be fully immunized. Trivalent oral polio vaccine (OPV) is the immunization of choice for all infants, children, and adolescents (up to 18 years old) if there are no contraindications. For unvaccinated adult travelers and for those whose immunization status is unknown primary immunization with inactivated polio vaccine (IPV) is recommended [12,15], since there is a slightly increased risk of vaccine-associated poliomyelitis in adults receiving OPV. Adults incompletely vaccinated with OPV or IPV should complete a full primary series with their original vaccine regardless of the interval since the last dose. Adults who have completed a full primary series with OPV or IPV in childhood should be given one supplemental dose of their original vaccine. This is particularly important in older adults as antipoliomyelitis antibody titers are negligible in many Americans 40 years of age or older [33]. The need for additional doses has not been established.

As noted previously, immunocompromised individuals should not receive live, attenuated virus vaccines; thus, IPV should be used. If OPV is inadvertently administered to a household contact of an immunodeficient individual or a nonimmunized adult, close contact between the patient and the recipient of OPV should be avoided for 1 month after vaccination.

Measles

Although the incidence of measles has continued to decline in the United States, a larger percentage of cases are being imported. Imported measles and associated cases together accounted for 20 percent of all reported cases in the United States in 1985 [35,36]. With the decreasing exposure to natural cases of measles in the United States, unvaccinated persons may reach adulthood still susceptible.

Immunity to measles can be established only in individuals with physician-documented measles, positive serology, or proof of adequate immunization at or after 12 months of age. Most persons born before 1956 are likely to have been naturally infected. Some individuals may have received an inactivated measles vaccine during the 1960s and should be reimmunized with the live vaccine. A single dose of live, attenuated virus induces antibody formation in up to 95 percent of recipients. For children, measles immunization is often combined with mumps and rubella. Measles vaccine should be given at least 14 days before, or deferred for 6 weeks to 3 months after, administration of immune globulin.

Immune globulin

Hepatitis A infection occurs worldwide. Hepatitis A is, in fact, the most frequent serious illness observed in travelers (Fig. 28-1) [37]. Studies have suggested that the risk to short-term travelers (<2 weeks) for acquiring hepatitis A in Africa or southeast Asia may be as high as 1 in 150 [37]. After acute hepatitis A, convalescence may be quite prolonged.

In addition, cases of fulminant hepatitis, chronic disease, and systemic complications are being increasingly recognized in the spectrum of hepatitis A infection [38]. Randomized, double-blind controlled studies have substantiated that passive immunization against hepatitis A with immune globulin is highly effective in preventing hepatitis A and may also provide some protection against hepatitis B and non-A non-B hepatitis [39].

The risk of acquiring hepatitis for U.S. travelers varies with living conditions, duration of stay, and incidence of hepatitis A in the area visited. Travelers to most developed countries are at no greater risk of infection than in the United States. Travelers to developing countries, where risk is high, can decrease their exposure to hepatitis A by avoiding contaminated food and water, particularly raw shellfish. Immune globulin prophylaxis is, however, recommended for travelers to all third world countries. Generally, adults are given 2 mL IM for trips less than a month, while 5 mL is given for longer stays. Individuals planning to reside for long periods of time in developing countries should receive immune globulin regularly (5 mL every 4 to 6 months) [12]. For frequent travelers, screening for anti-hepatitis A virus antibody may be cost-effective and eliminate unnecessary injections for immune individuals.

Theoretical concerns have been raised regarding the potential transmission of HIV through the use of immune globulin. HIV antibodies have been measurable transiently for up to 6 months after the infusion of older immune globulin preparations produced prior to HIV screening of donor blood [40]. Epidemiologically, no cases of AIDS or even HIV antibody conversion have ever been associated with immune globulin administration [40]. Present lots of immune globulin are free of detectable HIV by culture or DNA hybridization techniques [40]. Furthermore, the fractionation process involved in manufacturing immune globulin removes all exogenously added virus [40]. Given the demonstrated safety of immune globulin and the serious nature of hepatitis A infection, passive immunization should be encouraged in all travelers to developing countries.

SPECIAL VACCINES

Hepatitis B vaccine

The prevalence of hepatitis B virus carriers is high (5 to 20 percent) in all socioeconomic groups in sub-Saharan Africa, southeast Asia including China, Korea, and Indonesia, South Pacific Islands, the interior Amazon Basin, Haiti, and the Dominican Republic [41]. Carrier rates of 1 to 5 percent are seen in north Africa, south central and southwest Asia, Japan, eastern and southern Europe, the U.S.S.R., and South America. Hepatitis B vaccination is always recommended for travelers who have direct contact with blood [12]. Vaccination should

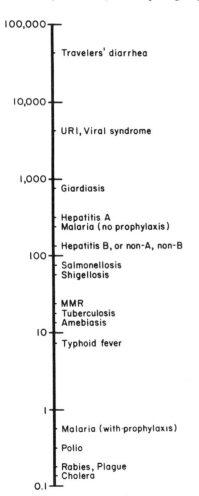

Figure 28-1. Incidence of selected infections per 100,000 short-term travelers to developing countries.

also be considered for travelers residing for long periods (>6 months) in highly endemic areas and for individuals having sexual contact with residents. Two hepatitis B vaccines are currently available in the United States. Recent studies have demonstrated equivalent immunogenicity and efficacy for the plasma-derived and recombinant vaccines.

Vaccination should ideally begin at least 6 months before travel to complete the full series of three doses; some protection is, however, provided by one or two doses. The duration of protection and need for booster doses has not been determined. The optimal site of injection in adults is the deltoid muscle.

Meningococcal meningitis vaccine

Epidemics of meningococcal meningitis have been reported in New Delhi, Nepal, sub-Saharan Africa, and most recently in Mecca and Medina, Saudi Arabia. Cases in American travelers in such areas are infrequent; however, prolonged contact with the local populace could increase the risk of infection and makes vaccination a reasonable precaution. Serogroup A is the most common cause of epidemics outside the United States, but serogroups C and, rarely, B have been associated with epidemics. A quadrivalent A,C,Y,W-135 meningococcal vaccine is currently available in the United States. Clinical efficacy of 85 to 95 percent against serogroup A has been demonstrated for at least 1 year [42]. The need for booster doses has not been established.

Japanese B encephalitis vaccine

Japanese B encephalitis is a mosquito-borne viral encephalitis that occurs in epidemics during rainy summer months in India, Bangladesh, China, Korea, Laos, Nepal, Burma, Vietnam, the eastern part of the U.S.S.R., and northern Thailand [43]. In endemic areas of southeast Asia (including Indonesia, southern Thailand, Sri Lanka, Malaysia, and the Philippines), the risk is lower and there is no seasonal distribution. The risk to short-term travelers who confine their visits to urban centers of epidemic and endemic areas is low, but the prudent use of insect repellent and mosquito netting is probably indicated. Persons at greatest risk are those living for extended periods (>3 months) in endemic or epidemic areas. A highly effective vaccine against Japanese B encephalitis virus is produced by several companies in Japan but is currently not available for distribution in the United States. Until administrative problems in procurement are resolved, high-risk travelers may inquire about the availability of the vaccine at American embassies in countries where Japanese encephalitis is endemic or epidemic [44].

Human diploid rabies vaccine

Travelers to areas where rabies is endemic should be cautioned about the risks of infection related to contact with wild or domestic animals [12]. Although dogs are the main reservoir for infection in developing countries, the epidemiology of infection in animals differs significantly worldwide. Thus, any animal bite or scratch should prompt aggressive local treatment, and consideration should be given to postexposure prophylaxis [12]. Preexposure prophylaxis with human diploid cell rabies vaccine is recommended for persons in high-risk groups such as those living in or visiting countries (>30 days) where rabies is a constant threat [45]. Prophylaxis can be administered intramuscularly or intradermally (half the cost of intramuscular injection); however, concomitant chloroquine administration has recently been shown to interfere with antibody response induced by intradermal administration [46]. Preexposure vaccination does not, however, eliminate the need for additional therapy after a rabies exposure.

Other vaccines

Plague vaccination is rarely indicated for travelers except for those at particularly high risk because of research or field activities in epizootic areas. Activities that may be associated with higher rates of exposure include work with wild rodents or rabbits or laboratory work with *Yersinia pestis* [12]. In most countries of Asia, Africa, and the Americas where plague is reported, the risk of exposure is primarily in rural mountainous or upland areas [12].

Typhus and paratyphoid vaccines are no longer available in the United States and have limited indications for travelers. Bacillus Calmette-Guérin (BCG) vaccine is used extensively overseas but is not available in the United States; it may be indicated for individuals residing in developing countries semipermanently.

Vaccination for influenza or pneumococcal infection may be indicated in selected travelers depending on destination, age, and the underlying medical condition of the traveler. These two vaccines should be considered especially in the elderly.

MALARIA PROPHYLAXIS

This mosquito-borne infection is the leading parasitic cause of death worldwide [47]. Of the four *Plasmodium* species that infect humans, *P. falciparum* causes the greatest morbidity and mortality [47]. In the United States, a growing number of malaria cases are being reported annually in travelers and immigrants. In 1986, 1123 cases of malaria had been reported in the United States [48]. Between 1975 and 1983, *P. falciparum* infections acquired by U.S. citizens traveling to east Africa increased 21-fold [49]. Given this major resurgence of malaria, physicians in developed countries will be increasingly called upon to give advice on the prevention, as well as the diagnosis and treatment, of malaria.

Measures to avoid the insect vector, including the use of appropriate clothing, netting, and insect repellents, are extremely important and must be stressed. Prophylactic medication has also been shown to be extremely effective [47]. Unfortunately, only 28 percent of the 410 U.S. citizens with

P. falciparum malaria acquired in Africa between 1980 and 1984 were using a recommended drug for prophylaxis [*50*]. A recent survey of 4042 returning U.S. travelers to Africa and Haiti demonstrated that 58 percent of these individuals didn't take recommended prophylactic agents regularly [*50*]. Travelers are more likely to take prophylactic antimalarial drugs if appropriate recommendations and education are provided to them by physicians before departure [*50*]. However, in one survey, only 14 percent of persons who sought medical advice obtained correct information regarding malaria prevention and prophylaxis [*51*].

Resistance of *P. falciparum* to the first-line chemoprophylactic agent, chloroquine, is rapidly increasing worldwide (Table 28-2) [*52*]. Because of this growing problem of resistance, second-line agents are being increasingly utilized. In the United States pyrimethamine-sulfadoxine (Fansidar) was given concurrently to travelers visiting areas of chloroquine-resistant *P. falciparum* malaria between 1982 and 1985. During that period, however, numerous cases of severe cutaneous reactions and seven deaths were reported in individuals taking long-term prophylaxis [*53*]. As a result, the current recommendations for malaria prophylaxis have changed several times in the past few years [*52*].

Several factors are important in choosing appropriate chemoprophylactic regimens for malaria. The travel itinerary should be thoroughly reviewed in relation to information on areas of risk within a given country. The risk for acquiring chloroquine-resistant *P. falciparum* malaria should also be determined (Table 28-2). Finally, allergic and/or other known adverse reactions to antimalarials should be considered, as well as the availability of medical care during travel.

Chloroquine is still the mainstay of chemoprophylaxis for travel to most malaria-endemic areas. *P. vivax, P. ovale,* and *P. malariae,* and the other species infecting humans remain chloroquine-sensitive. In areas where *P. falciparum* is developing resistance to chloroquine, sensitive strains coexist. In a study from the Netherlands, decreased parasitemia and milder illness were also found in individuals who took chloroquine but still developed chloroquine-resistant falciparum malaria [*54*]. Malaria chemoprophylaxis should begin 1 to 2 weeks before departure to ensure adequate serum levels and to screen for adverse effects. Chloroquine should be also continued for 6 weeks after leaving an endemic area.

Travelers to areas where chloroquine-resistant malaria exists should be cautioned about the possibility of acquiring resistant malaria and supplied with three tablets of pyrimethamine-sulfadoxine for presumptive treatment if a febrile illness develops [*12,52*]. For travelers to chloroquine-resistant areas of Thailand and Burma, where resistance to pyrimethamine-sulfadoxine is quite common, no clear consensus exists on what is the best chemotherapeutic agent. Alternative prophylactic drugs that can be considered include doxycycline or mefloquine used alone or proguanil used in combination with chloroquine [*14*]. All of these drugs have current problems. Daily doxycycline

Table 28-2. Areas with reported chloroquine-resistant *Plasmodium falciparum*

Africa:	Asia:
Angola	Burma
Benin	China (Hainan Island and
Burundi	southern provinces)
Central African Republic	Indonesia
Comoros	Kampuchea
Gabon	Laos
Kenya	Malaysia
Madagascar	Philippines (Luzon, Basilan,
Malawi	Mindoro, Palawan, and
Mali	Mindanao Islands, Sulu
Mozambique	Archipelago)
Namibia	Thailand
Nigeria	Vietnam
Rwanda	Oceania:
Sudan (northeastern)	Papua New Guinea
Tanzania	Solomon Islands
Uganda	Vanuatu
Zaire (northeastern)	Indian subcontinent:
Zambia (northeastern)	Bangladesh (north and east)
South America:	India
Bolivia	Pakistan (Rawalpindi)
Brazil	
Ecuador	
French Guiana	
Guyana	
Panama (east of the Canal Zone)	
Peru (northern provinces)	
Surinam	
Venezuela	

has been recommended for short-term travelers to rural, forested areas of Burma and Thailand or those who are sulfa-allergic [*52*]. Extensive controlled studies of the tetracyclines as prophylactic agents are lacking and the sun-sensitizing effects of this class of antibiotics has been a concern [*16*]. Weekly mefloquine prophylaxis has been recommended by the WHO [*14*] for travelers to chloroquine-resistant areas and southeast Asia. However, this drug is not currently available in the United States and has very limited availability around the world. Additional concerns include long-term toxicity, cost, and the development of drug resistance. Outside the United States, proguanil and chlorproguanil are frequently prescribed when chloroquine resistance is a consideration. In a recent prospective study by Fogh et al. [*55*], daily proguanil combined with chloroquine was a highly effective and safe chemoprophylactic regimen for short-term travelers to east Africa. Proguanil, however, is unavailable in the United States, and has not been successful in preventing malaria in southeast Asia.

Primaquine therapy, given after travel for the prevention of relapses of *P. vivax* and *P. ovali,* can be considered in returning travelers who have stayed for extended periods in endemic areas. Pretherapy screening for glucose-6-phosphate deficiency may be prudent.

Malaria poses a serious threat to both a pregnant woman and her fetus [47]. Chloroquine has been found to be safe in pregnancy and should be utilized in pregnant women who must travel to malaria-endemic areas. The safety of pyrimethamine-sulfadoxine in pregnancy has not been completely established, although pregnant women have been treated for over 30 years with pyrimethamine combined with sulfamides for toxoplasmosis [56]. Ideally, women who are pregnant should not travel to areas where chloroquine-resistant *P. falciparum* malaria exists. Doxycycline is contraindicated in pregnancy and in children less than 8 years of age. Children of any age can be safely given chloroquine at a dose of 5 mg (base)/(kg·week). Pyrimethamine-sulfadoxine is contraindicated in infants less than 2 months of age.

TRAVELERS' DIARRHEA

Up to 40 percent of all travelers will develop diarrhea overseas [6]. The highest risks occur in Africa, Latin America, southeast Asia, and India [57]. Intermediate risks occur in Mediterranean countries, China, and Israel, while low risks are associated with travel to North America, Europe, Japan, and Australia. The risk for developing travelers' diarrhea correlates with breaks in food and water precautions [7]. Despite the old adage ''Don't drink the water,'' recent studies have implicated food as the source of travelers' diarrhea in 90 percent of cases [6]. Some of the common pitfalls include the use of ice cubes made with contaminated water, the use of tap water for brushing teeth, salads, unpasteurized milk products, street vendor food, and airplane food on the trip home.

Etiologically, enterotoxigenic *E. coli* are responsible for 40 percent of cases of travelers' diarrhea, while *Shigella, Salmonella, Campylobacter,* and rotavirus account for a smaller percentage of cases [6]. Unknown or miscellaneous causes are seen in up to 25 percent of cases. Chronic diarrhea after travel is most frequently associated with *Giardia lamblia* infection [58].

Studies have established the success of antibiotics such as trimethoprim-sulfamethoxazole, trimethoprim alone, or doxycycline in prophylaxis against travelers' diarrhea [59]. Unfortunately, adverse effects have been observed in up to 25 percent of travelers taking these antibiotics for 2 or more weeks [59]. In addition, the etiological agents of travelers' diarrhea are increasingly developing resistance to frequently utilized prophylactic antibiotics [59]. Patients who take prophylactic antibiotics may, therefore, be at higher risk for developing infection with drug-resistant organisms [60]. A recent study has shown that norfloxacin, the new carboxyquinolone, is very effective as prophylaxis for travelers' diarrhea, and no resistant fecal flora emerged during therapy [61]. These drugs, however, are quite expensive. Oral bismuth subsalicylate (Pepto-Bismol)

(two tablets qid) has also been used as a safe and effective prophylactic agent against diarrhea [62], but the amount required often prohibits its use for long trips. Available controlled studies indicate that prophylactic diphenoxylate (Lomotil) actually increases the incidence of travelers' diarrhea in addition to increasing the occurrence of serious side effects [60]. In general, therefore, antibiotic prophylaxis should be reserved for very short trips, and emphasis should be given to the prevention and appropriate treatment of diarrhea when, and if, it appears.

Travelers' diarrhea is usually a mild, self-limited process, with complete recovery even in the absence of therapy. Fluids and appropriate electrolyte replacement are the highest priorities. Fluid and electrolyte balance can be maintained by fruit juices, soft drinks, and salted crackers. Alternatively, oral rehydration formulas may be purchased or prepared [12,60]. Bismuth subsalicylate may be used (two tablets or 1 oz every 30 min for eight doses) and is often sufficient for early and mild cases of travelers' diarrhea. Recent studies have demonstrated that this agent can inhibit the growth of enterotoxic *Escherichia coli* as well as the toxins of *E. coli* and *V. cholera* [63]. In children, mortality and morbidity from infection caused by *Salmonella* and *Shigella* are higher with Lomotil therapy [63]. These dangers in adults are less clear. Most authorities believe that antimotility agents can be used safely if given noncontinuously for mild to moderate diarrhea (< four to five stools per day) [60]. It is often difficult, however, to ensure that these drugs will be utilized in this manner.

Antimicrobial agents such as trimethoprim alone, trimethoprim-sulfamethoxazole, doxycycline, bicozamycin, norfloxacin, and ciprofloxacin have been used quite successfully to dramatically shorten the course (to less than 24 h) or lessen the severity of travelers' diarrhea. These medications are often prescribed prior to travel and carried for presumptive treatment of diarrhea.

A small percentage of travelers will have persistent diarrhea despite empirical antibiotic therapy or will have diarrhea associated with serious fluid loss, fever, and blood or mucus in the stool. These symptoms suggest a more serious illness, and medical attention should be obtained. Chronic diarrhea as a result of travel is unusual, occurring in less than 10 percent of travelers. In this setting, evaluation for parasitic infection, especially giardiasis, chronic campylobacterioses, antibiotic-associated colitis, bacterial overgrowth, or tropical sprue, is in order.

RETURNING TRAVELERS, IMMIGRANTS, AND FOREIGN VISITORS

Many physicians educated in the developed world are unfamiliar with tropical diseases and international health issues. Malaria is the classic example [5]. Appropriate malaria chemoprophylaxis is often not recommended by American physicians prior to overseas travel [50,51]. Cases of malaria in travelers or in immigrants are generally misdiagnosed (>80 percent of the time) on first contact with American physicians resulting in a significant mortality rate (6 to 9 percent) [5]. Almost all of these fatalities should have been preventable with prophylactic medications, as well as early diagnosis and appropriate treatment.

The most frequent complaints observed in returning ill travelers include diarrhea (30 to 35 percent), upper respiratory infection symptoms (12 to 15 percent), fever or rash (10 percent), and abdominal pain or malaise (5 percent) [37,64,65]. The most frequent diagnoses made in returning ill travelers include diarrhea, upper respiratory illnesses, sexually transmitted diseases, giardiasis, hepatitis A, and malaria (Fig. 28-1). In general younger travelers (ages 20 to 29) are twice as likely as older individuals (ages 40 to 69) to contract illness, presumably due to less care in avoiding risky practices [37]. With longer stays abroad, particularly in more primitive settings, diseases such as filariasis, invasive amebic disease, or tuberculosis enter into the differential. Finally, permanent immigrants or foreign visitors can present with illnesses which are totally unfamiliar to physicians in temperate zones such as leishmaniasis, leprosy, or trypanosomiasis. The problem is magnified by the fact that some illnesses acquired abroad may have very long incubation periods or may remain asymptomatic for many years (e.g., schistosomiasis, leprosy, or *Clonorchis sinensis* infection).

Fortunately, the majority of returning ill travelers will have "common" illnesses. However, specific syndromes such as persistent diarrhea, fever, hepatosplenomegaly, skin lesions, or eosinophilia include in their differential many "exotic" diseases that could have been acquired abroad. The first and most important question to ask travelers or immigrants is, "Where have you been?" A careful physical examination is imperative with particular attention to the presence of fever, liver and spleen size, lymphadenopathy, edema, skin lesions, and neuro-logical deficits. High fever, prostration, shock, hemorrhagic manifestations, severe diarrhea, dyspnea, or central nervous system disturbances suggest that the patient has acquired a potentially life-threatening disease abroad [3].

FEVER

Fever in a returning traveler, recent immigrant, or foreign visitor is a relatively common clinical problem, but one which requires prompt attention. The most important consideration is differentiating falciparum malaria from other more familiar etiologies such as influenza or other acute viral illnesses (Table 28-3).

Infection with *P. falciparum* is a major health risk to recent immigrants or refugees and is a growing problem for tourists. Returning travelers from east Africa, for example, have experienced a 21-fold increase in reported cases of malaria from 1975 to 1983 [49], and the majority of U.S. citizens do not take appropriate prophylaxis [51].

Malaria is also a great "mime" of other diseases [5]. Although fever at some point in time is universal, it may not be present at the time a patient seeks medical attention (paroxysms of fever). Approximately 50 percent of imported cases of malaria will have hepatic and/or splenic enlargement [5]. Associated symptoms often include back pain, nausea and vomiting, or diarrhea, which can lead physicians away from the correct diagnosis.

Once suspected, the diagnosis can generally be made by examining thin and thick blood smears for malarial parasites. The thin smear allows identification of the species of *Plasmodium*. Having appropriately diagnosed malaria, it is important to identify the species, since this will determine the clinical management. Other considerations which affect therapy are the frequency and degree of drug resistance found in the country where the infection was acquired (Table 28-2) and the severity

Table 28-3. Classification by incubation period and clinical course of some febrile illnesses in returning travelers

Short incubation		Long incubation	
Acute course	**Prolonged or relapsing course**	**Acute course**	**Prolonged or relapsing course**
Malaria	Typhoid fever	Malaria	Tuberculosis
Influenza	Brucellosis	Hepatitis B	Amebiasis
Childhood viruses	Relapsing fever	Amebiasis	Brucellosis
Hepatitis A	Schistosomiasis (Katayama	Leptospirosis	Filariasis
Bacterial dysentery	syndrome)	Amebiasis	Leishmaniasis
Arbovirus infection	Q fever	Actinomycosis	Trypanosomiasis
Yellow fever		Trypanosomiasis (African)	Melioidosis
Brucellosis		Rabies	Paragonimiasis
Plague			Strongyloidiasis
Tularemia			Schistosomiasis (Katayama
Rickettsiosis			syndrome)
Legionnaire's disease			
Typhus			
Rat-bite fever			

of clinical symptoms (cerebral involvement, renal failure, pulmonary edema, and the degree of parasitemia) [66]. In general, all suspected or confirmed cases of *P. falciparum* should be admitted to the hospital. A negative thin blood film does not exclude the diagnosis of malaria, and thus a thick blood smear should also be obtained to increase the diagnostic yield. Thick blood slides for malaria, however, are often difficult to interpret for the novice and generally require a trained parasitologist. Malaria can also occur even in the face of combination prophylaxis [67]. When in doubt always initiate therapy for *P. falciparum,* since delays in treatment can be associated with increased morbidity and mortality. A complete discussion of the diagnosis, treatment, and management of malaria is contained in Chap. 30.

When malaria has been excluded, several other diagnoses should be considered. The most common serious infectious disease contracted by travelers is hepatitis A [37]; it commonly presents with fever and malaise. Generally the incubation period ranges from 2 to 6 weeks. Although infection with hepatitis A is common, hepatitis B, non-A non-B hepatitis, and δ virus infection can all cause similar clinical pictures. Yellow fever, typhoid fever, amebic liver abscess, and malaria can also be confused with acute hepatitis A.

Clinical suspicion of acute hepatitis can generally be confirmed by laboratory studies. Serum glutamic oxaloacetic transaminase (SGOT), for example, is almost universally elevated even during the preicteric phase of illness. A specific etiological diagnosis, however, requires several serological tests obtained over time. Acute hepatitis is a relatively uncommon cause of fever in immigrants or foreign visitors, since most have been exposed to these viruses during childhood.

Typhoid fever has a much lower attack rate in returning tourists (less than 1 in 10,000) [37] than hepatitis A but is a more common cause of fever in recently arrived immigrants and foreign visitors. In the United States, 60 percent of cases of typhoid fever are imported [68]. Since gastric acidity is a major barrier to infection, individuals taking H_2 blockers or antacids or who have had a partial gastrectomy are at increased risk. Even prior immunization with typhoid vaccine can be overcome with a large inoculum of *Salmonella typhi.*

The illness typically has an incubation period of 1 to 2 weeks, and patients are generally quite ill with a sustained elevated fever. Unfortunately, typhoid can be relatively free of characteristic signs and symptoms [69], but typically patients have high fever, relative bradycardia, headache, and abdominal pain. Diarrhea is uncommon as part of the initial clinical presentation, while constipation is more frequent. The diagnostic skin lesions (rose spots), dry cough, and delirium generally appear during the second week of illness [69]. The diagnosis of suspected cases can easily be made by culturing the stool and blood for *Salmonella typhi.* Bone marrow cultures remain positive for months. Serological tests (such as the Widal test) are of value only if positive in diagnosing an acutely ill patient [70], since false-negatives are common early in infection. Typhoid fever, even with appropriate antibiotic treatment, still carries a significant mortality rate (3 to 10 percent), and drug resistance is now emerging as a serious impediment to successful therapy.

With acute fulminant febrile illnesses, consideration should also be given to various arboviruses including dengue and viral hemorrhagic fevers. These viruses can present with a variety of hemorrhagic manifestations in addition to fever. A petechial rash is common in dengue, while a maculopapular rash is seen in Ebola and Marburg infection. In the Americas, fatal hemorrhagic complications of dengue infection are being increasingly recognized in Brazil and Puerto Rico [71]. The diagnosis of these occasionally fatal viral infections must be suspected on clinical and epidemiological grounds since accurate diagnosis often depends on convalescent serologies. A key observation is that hemorrhagic fever is very unlikely to occur in travelers more than 3 weeks after return. Suspicion is important since Lassa fever can be successfully treated with ribavirin [72]. In addition, fatal nosocomial infections can occur, and suspected cases demand strict isolation procedures.

Despite the fact that tuberculosis is endemic throughout the developing world, mycobacterial infections are rarely contracted by short-term travelers [37,64]. The risk, however, increases with duration of stay. Tuberculosis is prominent in the differential diagnosis of chronic fever in immigrants or foreign visitors. Unfortunately, PPD skin reactivity is often difficult to interpret. Other diseases that often masquerade as tuberculosis include paragonimiasis and melioidosis, both of which can produce a radiographic picture indistinguishable from tuberculosis. Because of the likelihood of isoniazid resistance, all suspected cases should be confirmed by appropriate culture and antibiotic sensitivity tests performed.

African trypanosomiasis, brucellosis, visceral leishmaniasis, and many helminth infections may also cause chronic febrile illnesses presenting weeks, months, and even years after departure from an endemic country.

DIARRHEA

The most common complaint of returning travelers is diarrhea (Table 28-4). Acute travelers' diarrhea is generally caused by enterotoxigenic *E. coli* [57]. Since the average duration of untreated illness is only 5 to 7 days, the likelihood of this diagnosis decreases dramatically in patients with persistent diarrhea or in diarrhea which is unresponsive to empirical antibiotic treatment.

Persistent diarrhea in the returning traveler is most commonly caused by *G. lamblia.* Patients commonly complain of loose, nonbloody, foul-smelling stools, flatulence, and upper intestinal bloating. Fecal leukocytes are not found. Diarrhea may also persist despite antibiotic treatment due to transient lactose intolerance. Food poisoning and infections with *Vibrio* species, including *V. cholerae,* Norwalk agent, rotavirus, and cryptosporidium, also cause a noninflammatory diarrhea, but

Table 28-4. Differential diagnosis of diarrhea in returning travelers

Acute	Bloody	Chronic
Travelers' diarrhea	Campylobacteriosis	Giardiasis
Lactose intolerance	Noncholera vibrios	Cryptosporidiosis
Food poisoning	Shigellosis	Clonorchiasis
Cholera	Salmonellosis	Strongyloidiasis
Malaria	Enteropathogenic *E. coli*	Trichuriasis
Schistosomiasis	*Yersinia* infection	Tropical sprue
	Amebiasis	Posttravelers' diarrhea
	Plesiomoniasis	Antibiotic-associated colitis
	Aeromonas infection	Isosporiasis
	Balantidiasis	Schistosomiasis
	Antibiotic-associated colitis	Chronic campylobacteriosis

stools are usually more liquid in character. In contrast, the finding of blood or fecal leukocytes suggests an invasive pathology. *Shigella* is the most common cause of travelers' dysentery, but other organisms, such as *Campylobacter jejuni*, *Yersinia enterocolitica*, enterohemorrhagic *E. coli* (015 serotype), *E. histolytica*, and *Salmonella*, need to be considered. *Echinostoma* is a parasitic cause of diarrhea in travelers returning from Africa and is associated with eosinophilia. Lastly, empirical antibiotic treatment of travelers' diarrhea may induce antibiotic-associated colitis due to *Clostridium difficile* [73].

In general, it is not cost-effective to initiate a laboratory investigation until bloody diarrhea lasts at least 48 h or loose stools have lasted for at least 5 days. Patients should be instructed to maintain fluid hydration and discontinue dairy products and alcohol. Routine travelers' diarrhea is often shortened by empirical treatment with trimethoprim-sulfamethoxazole, doxycycline, or one of the newer oral quinolones [74]. These latter drugs also treat most other bacterial causes of diarrhea.

With persistent or recurrent diarrhea, fresh liquid stool should be examined at least three times for ova and parasites (*Giardia* and amoeba) and cultured for bacterial pathogens including *Campylobacter*, *Yersinia*, and *Vibrio* species as well as *Salmonella* and *Shigella*. Cultures for enterohemorrhagic *E. coli*, *Aeromonas hydrophilia*, or *Plesiomonas* can be considered if the diagnosis remains unclear. Examination of the stool for occult blood and fecal leukocytes may suggest invasive disease. Gram stain of the stool may reveal the "gull wing" morphology of *Campylobacter*, while *Cryptosporidium* may be visualized by acid-fast staining. If the traveler has had previous antibiotic treatment, a *C. difficile* toxin assay is in order.

If diarrhea persists despite the initial workup, *Giardia* should still be suspected, since up to one-third of cases will have negative stool exams. Duodenal aspiration or a "string test" will help make the diagnosis, or an empirical trial with anti-*Giardia* medications may be indicated. If white or red cells persist in the stool and no etiological agent is identified, sigmoidoscopy or colonoscopy with biopsy and culture should be performed. Positive serology in cases of suspected amebic colitis may also help establish the diagnosis [75].

EOSINOPHILIA

Eosinophilia is an uncommon laboratory abnormality in short-term travelers but can be found in up to 80 percent of refugees, immigrants, or foreign visitors [76,77]. Because the eosinophil is a relatively uncommon cell in the peripheral white cell population, the degree of eosinophilia should always be confirmed by an absolute eosinophil count. The "normal" eosinophil count of immigrants and foreign visitors is often higher than the 300 eosinophils per cubic millimeter upper limit of normal of most laboratories. Most would consider a level of >700 eosinophils per cubic millimeter abnormal even in these populations.

A variety of nontropical etiologies of eosinophilia should always be considered in the differential diagnosis including allergic reactions to medications, malignancy, and collagen vascular diseases. These can generally be excluded by a careful history and physical examination. The vast majority of travelers, immigrants, and foreign visitors have a helminthic etiology to their eosinophilia [77]. The migratory phases of hookworm, strongyloides, and other intestinal nematodes are common causes of eosinophilia in all groups [77]. Other etiologies have a more regional distribution. Filariasis, for example, is the most common cause of eosinophilia in Caucasians returning from Africa [78] but is found in only 2 percent of southeast Asian immigrants [77]. Similarly, clonorchiasis, onchocerciasis, and schistosomiasis all have well-defined geographical distributions.

Initial laboratory evaluation generally includes an absolute eosinophil count, IgE level, stool examinations for ova and parasites, and chest x-ray (tropical pulmonary eosinophilia). If the diagnosis is still unclear, day and night blood tests for microfilariae, skin snips for onchocerciasis, and superficial rectal mucosal biopsies (rectal snips) for schistosome ova may be indicated. If these examinations are negative, the physician should consider serological testing. Serological evaluation is most helpful in travelers with a single short-term exposure to the tropics. Specific serological tests are available for *Strongyloides stercoralis* [79], schistosomiasis, visceral larva migrans, and recently *Onchocerca volvulus*. All forms of human filariasis cross-react with dog heartworm antigens, and thus a positive *D. immitis* titer is helpful in suggesting the correct diagnosis.

Even after clinical investigation, between 30 and 50 percent of immigrants and travelers will have persistent eosinophilia for which a specific diagnosis or etiology is not determined [*77,78*]. Most have a helminth infection that has escaped diagnosis. Patients should, therefore, receive empirical therapy with thiabendazole or mebendazole. Occasionally therapeutic trials with praziquantel or diethylcarbamazine (DEC) are also indicated. A systemic reaction to DEC is almost pathognomonic for a filarial worm infection (loa loa, lymphatic filariasis, or onchocerciasis).

SEXUALLY TRANSMITTED DISEASES

In a recent study of 7886 Swiss travelers, gonorrhea was as common as giardiasis, hepatitis, and amebiasis, particularly among male travelers [*54*]. Prostitution remains a major problem in developing countries and has been responsible for the importation of syphilis, chancroid, and drug-resistant strains of gonorrhea into the United States.

Gonorrhea is often resistant to both penicillin and tetracycline, and patients should, therefore, be treated with ceftriaxone. Chancroid, granuloma inguinale, and lymphogranuloma venereum are rarely seen in the United States, but their global incidences exceed that of syphilis. Each of these venereal diseases requires specific diagnosis tests and different curative chemotherapy. In many areas of southeast Asia and Africa asymptomatic hepatitis B antigenemia is found in 10 to 18 percent of the population. As a result, sexual transmission of hepatitis B infection is a risk for any susceptible individual engaged in sexual activity abroad.

Infection with the human immunodeficiency virus represents a new risk to the traveler, and documented transmission has occurred among men patronizing prostitutes in Africa. As of March 1988, over 28,000 cases of AIDS have been reported in over 135 countries outside the United States [*8*]. In west Africa, an additional concern exists for HIV-2 infection, which causes a similar syndrome as HIV-1 but cannot be differentiated in present assay systems for HIV-1 [*9*]. Several studies have suggested that HIV-1 transmission is more likely if ulcerative lesions (syphilis, chancroid, or lymphogranuloma venereum) are present [*80*]. At the present time there is no reliable laboratory test that can detect incubating HIV infection prior to the development of a specific antibody (3- to 6-month delay). Acute HIV infection should be considered in travelers with a suggestive history (sexual contact with a prostitute in Africa, for example) who present with aseptic meningitis, acute mononucleosis, or an unusual rash or neurological complaint.

TROPICAL SKIN LESIONS

Many tropical diseases present initially with cutaneous manifestations. It is important to differentiate common self-limited skin conditions such as pityriasis, vitiligo, superficial dermatophyte infections, and insect bites from the presentations of more serious systemic diseases. Typical anesthetic hypopigmented lesions of lepromatous leprosy or recurrent Calabar swellings of loa loa are repeatedly misdiagnosed by American physicians, leading to long delays in the initiation of appropriate treatment.

A single nonhealing skin lesion needs to be evaluated for tuberculoid leprosy and leishmaniasis. Less common diagnoses include tuberculosis, *Mycobacterium ulcerans*, blastomycosis, and several other fungal infections. Biopsy of the lesion is often the only way to make the definitive diagnosis. Visualization of *M. leprae* requires modification of the acid-fast stain, so that the pathologist needs to be alerted to this possible diagnosis. Intracellular leishmania can be visualized on hematoxylin and eosin sections but can also be cultured on special media. Blastomycosis and other fungal infections can be visualized with methenamine silver staining or grown in culture.

A pruritic rash may be due to allergies to medications, sun exposure dermatitis during tetracycline treatment, or ectoparasites (fleas, mites, or scabies). Persistence, however, increases the differential and necessitates a punch biopsy. Secondary syphilis and lepromatous leprosy additionally require a specific serology or a nasal scraping, respectively. Intensely pruritic migratory swellings (Calabar swellings) occur over distal joints and are often misdiagnosed as chronic urticaria. These symptoms are pathognomonic for loa loa. Many helminth larvae produce an intense pruritic reaction at the point of penetration e.g., swimmer's itch (schistosomes), ground itch (hookworm or strongyloides), and cutaneous larva migrans.

Boils, impetigo, or cellulitis are major problems in the tropics, particularly in children. These infections are generally caused by staphylococcus or streptococcus and respond to appropriate antibiotics. Other conditions, however, can masquerade as bacterial infections. Some flies in Africa (tumbu flies) lay eggs on moist clothes or the ground. In South and Central America botfly larvae are transmitted to humans by biting insects. In both cases larvae are capable of penetrating into viable tissues, where they mature. These present clinically as boils, but do not resolve with antibiotics. The mature larvae emerge weeks later to the horror of both doctor and patient.

ASYMPTOMATIC TRAVELERS, IMMIGRANTS, AND FOREIGN VISITORS

No screening tests are recommended for short-term tourists. Individuals who have stayed for extended periods of time in primitive conditions (Peace Corps workers or missionaries) should probably have a single stool examination for ova and parasites, an absolute eosinophil count, and a purified protein derivative (PPD) 2 to 3 months upon return. Travelers who are sexually active should have at a minimum a VDRL; HIV testing is also recommended for individuals who have had contact with prostitutes.

Guidelines for evaluation of permanent immigrants to the United States are published and are generally performed prior to arrival in their new host country. Minimal or no screening occurs, however, with individuals arriving on student or visitor visas. A complete history and physical examination is indicated. Special attention should be paid to the cardiac exam (rheumatic heart disease is still quite common overseas), the genitourinary examination, lymphatics, and the skin.

Initial laboratory examinations include a complete blood count with differential, absolute eosinophil count, SGOT, BUN, and serological test for syphilis and hepatitis B surface antigen. Hemoglobin electrophoresis, iron, folate, and B_{12} studies are drawn as indicated for anemia. Skin testing with PPD should be begun with a 1-TU dose, since larger doses may evoke a vigorous delayed hypersensitivity response. A chest x-ray is deemed necessary if the skin test is positive or a past history of BCG vaccination is elicited. Stools for ova and parasites have a high yield for both pathogenic and non-pathogenic parasites (no treatment is required for latter). HIV screening is still controversial but is indicated for individuals from high-risk groups.

It is particularly important to identify young women as hepatitis B antigen carriers since a combination of active and passive immunization with hepatitis B hyperimmune globulin and vaccine will significantly reduce transmission of this virus to newborns [81]. This will also result ultimately in a dramatic reduction in chronic liver disease or hepatocellular carcinoma induced by this virus.

REFERENCES

1 Jones TC: Health advice and immunizations for travelers. Curr Clin Top Infect Dis 6:40–65, 1985

2 Cahill KM, Gorbach SL, Mitler MM, et al: Preparing patients for travel. Patient Care June 14, 1987, pp 217–241

3 Halstead SB, Warren KS: *Disease of Travelers and Immigrants*. Kalamazoo, Mich, Scope, 1987

4 Schultz MG: Emporiatrics—Travellers' health. Br Med J 285:582, 1982

5 Kean BH, Reilly PC: Malaria—The mime: Recent lessons from a group of civilian travelers. Am J Med 61:159–164, 1976

6 MacDonald KL, Cohen ML: Epidemiology of travelers' diarrhea: Current perspectives. Rev Inf Dis 8(suppl 12):S117–S121, 1986

7 Kozicki M, Sheffen R, Schar M: "Boil it, cook it, peel it, or forget it!": Does this rule prevent travelers' diarrhea? Int J Epidemiol 14:169–172, 1985

8 World Health Organization: Acquired immunodeficiency syndrome. WHO Wk Epidemiol Rec 63:69, 1988

9 Quinn TC, Mann JM, Curran JW, et al: AIDS in Africa: An epidemiologic paradigm. Science 234:955–969, 1986

10 World Health Organization: Acquired immunodeficiency syndrome (AIDS): Consultation on international travel and human immunodeficiency virus (HIV). WHO Wk Epidemiol Rec 62:77–78, 1987

11 Steffen R, Van der Linde F: Intercontinental travel and its effects on pre-existing illness. Aviation Space Environ Med 52:57–58, 1981

12 U.S. Department of Health and Human Services, Public Health Services, Centers for Disease Control: *Health Information for International Travel*. Health and Human Services publication (CDC):85-8280, 1987

13 Allard R: Problems in adequately immunizing international travelers. Can Med Assoc J 128:40–41, 1983

14 World Health Organization: *Vaccination Certificate Requirements and Health Advice to Travelers*. WHO Publication Center, 1988

15 Committee on Immunization: *Guide for Adult Immunization*. Philadelphia, American College of Physicians, 1985

16 Centers for Disease Control, Immunization Practices Advisory Committee: Yellow fever vaccine. Ann Intern Med 100:540–542, 1984

17 Kaplan JE, Nelson DB, Schenberger LB, et al: The effect of immune globulin on trivalent oral polio and yellow fever vaccinations. Bull WHO 62:313–315, 1984

18 Immunization during pregnancy. Am Coll Obstet Gynecol Techn Bull 64: 1982

19 Centers for Disease Control: Immunization of children infected with human T-lymphotropic virus type III/lymphadenopathy-associated virus. Morbid Mortal Wk Rep 35:595–598, 603–606, 1986

20 Centers for Disease Control: Immunization of children infected with human immunodeficiency virus: Supplementary ACIP statement. Morbid Mortal Wk Rep 37:181–183, 1988

21 Redfield RR, Wright DC, James WD, et al: Disseminated vaccinia in a military recruit with human immunodeficiency virus (HIV) disease. N Engl J Med 316:673–676, 1987

22 Manath TP: Yellow fever: A medically neglected disease: Report on a seminar. Rev Infect Dis 9:165–175, 1987

23 Felsenfeld O, Woif RH, Gym K, et al: Simultaneous vaccination against cholera and yellow fever. Lancet i:457–458, 1973

24 World Health Organization: Cholera in 1978. WHO Wk Epidemiol Rec 54:129–131, 1979

25 Snyder JD, Blake PA: Is cholera a problem for US travelers? JAMA 274:2268–2269, 1982

26 Centers for Disease Control: Cholera vaccine. Morbid Mortal Wk Rep 27:173–174, 1978

27 Clemens JD, Blake PA: Is cholera a problem for US travelers? JAMA 274:2268–2269, 1982

28 Greenblatt LL, Valdini AF: Imported typhoid fever. J Fam Pract 23:484–486, 1986

29 Warren JW, Hornick RB: Immunization against typhoid fever. Ann Rev Med 30:457–572, 1979

30 Wandan MH, Serie C, Cerisier Y, et al: A controlled field trial of live *Salmonella typhi* strain TY 21a oral vaccine against typhoid: Three year results. J Infect Dis 145:292–295, 1982

31 Acharya IL, Lowe CU, Tharpa R, et al: Prevention of typhoid fever in Nepal with the Vi capsular polysaccharide of *Salmonella typhi*. N Engl J Med 317:1101–1104, 1987

32 Schofield F: Selective primary health care: Strategies for control of disease in the developing world. XXII. Tetanus: A preventable problem. Rev Infect Dis 8:144–156, 1986

33 Horstmann DM, Quinn TC, Robbins FC (guest ed): International symposium on poliomyelitis control. Rev Infect Dis 6(suppl 2):51–56, 1984

34 World Health Organization: Poliomyelitis—The child crippler. Update 6, 1988

35 Amler RW, Bloch AB, Orenstein WA, et al: Imported measles in the United States. JAMA 248:2129–2133, 1982

36 Katz S: Measles—Forgotten but not gone. N Engl J Med 313:577–578, 1985

37 Steffen R, Rickenbach M, Wilhelm V, et al: Health problems after travel to developing countries. J Infect Dis 156:84–91, 1987

38 Gocke DJ: Hepatitis A revisited. Ann Intern Med 105:960–961, 1986

39 Conrad ME, Lemon SM: Prevention of endermic icteric viral hepatitis by administration of immune serum gamma globulin. J Infect Dis 156:56–63, 1987

40 Centers for Disease Control: Safety of therapeutic immune globulin preparations with respect to transmission of human T-lymphotropic virus type III/lymphadenopathy-associated virus infection. Morbid Mortal Wk Rep 35:231–233, 1986

41 Robinson WS, Lutwick LI: The virus of hepatitis, type B. N Engl J Med 295:1168–1174, 1231–1236, 1976

42 Lepon ML, Gold R: Meningococcal A and other polysaccharide vaccines: A five-year progress report. N Engl J Med 308:1158–1160, 1983

43 Umenai T, Krzysko O, Bektimov TA, et al: Japanese encephalitis: Current worldwide status. Bull WHO 63:625–631, 1985

44 Denning DW, Kaneko Y: Should travelers to Asia be vaccinated against Japanese encephalitis? Lancet i:863–854, 1987

45 Fishbein DB, Pacer RE, Holmes DF, et al: Rabies preexposure prophylaxis with human diploid cell rabies vaccine: A dose-response study. J Infect Dis 156:50–55, 1987

46 Pappaloanou M, Fishbein DB, Dreesan DW, et al: Antibody response to preexposure human diploid cell rabies vaccine given concurrently with chloroquine. N Engl J Med 314:280–284, 1986

47 Wyler DJ: Malaria: Resurgence, resistance, and research. N Engl J Med 308:875–878, 934–940, 1983

48 Centers for Disease Control: Summary of notifiable diseases United States, 1986. Morbid Mortal Wk Rep: 35(suppl) 1–57, 1987

49 Lobel HO, Campbell CC, Chwarz IK, et al: Recent trends in the importation of malaria caused by *Plasmodium falciparum* into the United States from Africa. J Infect Dis 152:613–617, 1985

50 Lobel HO, Campbell COC, Pappaloanou M, et al: Use of prophylaxis for malaria by American travelers to Africa and Haiti. JAMA 257:2626–2627, 1987

51 Catino D, Catino JS: Malaria prophylaxis among travelers. JAMA 248:2111–2112, 1982

52 Centers for Disease Control: Revised recommendations for preventing malaria in travelers to areas with chloroquine-resistant *Plasmodium falciparum* malaria. Morbid Mortal Wk Rep 37:277–284, 1988

53 Miller KD, Lobel HO, Satriable RF, et al: Severe cutaneous reactions among American travelers using pyrimethamine-sulfadoxine (Fansidar) for malaria prophylaxis. Am J Trop Med Hyg 35:451–458, 1986

54 Wefsteyn JCFM, de Geus A: Chloroquine-resistant falciparum malaria imported into the Netherlands. Bull WHO 63:101–108, 1985

55 Fogh S, Schapira A, Bygbjerg IC, et al: Malaria chemoprophylaxis in travelers to East Africa: A comparative prospective study of chloroquine plus proguanil with chloroquine plus sulfadoxine-pyrimethamine. Br Med J 296:820–822, 1988

56 Remington JS, Desmonts G: Toxoplasmosis, in Remington JS, Klein JS (eds): *Infectious Diseases of the Fetus and Newborn*. New York, Saunders, 1983, p 143

57 Steffen R, van der Linde F, Gyr K, et al: Epidemiology of diarrhea in travelers. JAMA 249:1176–1180, 1983

58 Giannella RA: Chronic diarrhea in travelers: Diagnostic and therapeutic decisions. Rev Infect Dis 8(suppl 2):S223–S226, 1986

59 Sack RB: Antimicrobial prophylaxis of travelers' diarrhea: A selected summary. Rev Infect Dis 8(suppl 2):S160–S166, 1986

60 Consensus conference. Travelers' diarrhea. JAMA 253:2700–2704, 1985

61 Johnson PC, Ericsson CD, Morgan DR: Lack of emergence of resistant fecal flora during successful prophylaxis of travelers' diarrhea with norfloxacin. Antimicrob Ag Chemother 30:671–674, 1986

62 Dupont HL, Ericsson CD, Johnson PC, et al: Prevention of travelers' diarrhea by the tablet formulation of bismuth subsalicylate. JAMA 257:1347–1350, 1987

63 Ericsson CD, Dupont HL, Johnson PC: Nonantibiotic therapy for travelers' diarrhea. Rev Infect Dis 8(suppl 2):S202–S206, 1986

64 Cossar JH, Reid D, Grist NR, et al: Illness associated with travel: A ten-year review. Travel Med Int 3:13–18, 1985

65 Gore S, Stutkin G: Infectious diseases of travelers and immigrants. Emerg Med Clin North Am 2:587–622, 1984

66 White NJ: The treatment of falciparum malaria. Parasitol Today 4:1014, 1988

67 Miller KD et al: Failures of combined chloroquine and fansidar prophylaxis in American travelers to East Africa. J Infect Dis 154:689–691, 1986

68 Taylor DN, Pollard RA, Blake PA: Typhoid in the United States and the risk to the international traveler. J Infect Dis 148:599–602, 1983

69 Klotz SA, Jorgensen JH, et al: Typhoid fever; an epidemic with remarkably few clinical signs and symptoms. Arch Intern Med 144:533–537, 1984

70 Buck RL, Escamilaa J, Sangalang RP, et al: Diagnostic value of a single, pre-treatment Widal test in suspected enteric fever cases in the Philippines. Trans R Soc Trop Med Hyg 81:871–873, 1987

71 Centers for Disease Control: Dengue and dengue hemorrhagic fever in the Americas, 1986. Morbid Mortal Wk Rep 37:129–131, 1988

72 McCormick et al: Lassa fever: Effective therapy with ribavirin. N Engl J Med 314:20–26, 1986

73 Lyerly DM, Krivan HC, Wilkins TD: *Clostridium difficile:* Its disease and toxins. Clin Micro Rev 1:1–18, 1988

74 Ericsson CD, Johnson PC, Dupont HL, et al: Ciprofloxacin or trimethoprim-sulfamethoxazole as initial therapy for travelers' diarrhea. Ann Intern Med 106:216–220, 1987

75 Ravdin JI, Guerrant R: Current problems in the diagnosis and treatment of amebic infections. Curr Clin Top Infect Dis 7:82–111, 1986

76 Tittle BS, Harris JA, Chase PA: Health screening of Indochinese refugee children. Am J Dis Child 136:697–700, 1982

77 Nutman TB, Ottesen EH, Ieng S, et al: Eosinophilia in Southeast Asian refugees: Evaluation at a referral center. J Infect Dis 155:309–313, 1987

78 Harries AD, Myers B, Bhattacharrya D: Eosinophilia in Caucasians returning from the tropics. Trans R Soc Trop Med Hyg 80:327–328, 1986

79 Gain AA, Neva FA, Krostoski WA: Comparative sensitivity and specificity of ELISA and IHA for serodiagnosis of strongyloidiasis with larval antigens. Am J Trop Med Hyg 37(1):157–161, 1987

80 Piot P, Plummer FA, Rey MA, et al: Retrospective seroepidemiology of AIDS virus infection in Nairobi populations. J Infect Dis 155:1108–1112, 1987

81 Centers for Disease Control: Update on hepatitis B prevention. Morbid Mortal Wk Rep 36:353–366, 1987

PART II / Protozoan Diseases

CHAPTER 29

Introduction · Louis H. Miller

The protozoan section of this edition will reflect the activity of research at the molecular level, research that will in the long run have an impact on the control of protozoan diseases. It will also reflect the effect of acquired immunodeficiency syndrome (AIDS) on the types and presentations of these diseases. For example, *Cryptosporidium* is now the focus of the chapter on coccidiosis, whereas previously it was only given brief mention. Medical entomology and vector biology remains a neglected field, and, if anything, research interest has declined since the first edition of this book. How can this be, when new and imaginative methods of attacking the vectors offer the best hope for controlling American trypanosomiasis, African trypanosomiasis, and malaria in Africa? Insecticides, although useful today, do not appear to be the long-term solution to these problems. It is only through an overview like the one in these chapters that the neglected disciplines can be identified and from such an understanding the search for solutions can be intensified.

The chapters on Protozoa include parasites of worldwide distribution, parasites largely limited to the tropical world, and parasites limited to regions in the tropics. The clinical setting and epidemiology of worldwide diseases may differ for the tropics. For example, *Pneumocystis carinii* pneumonia, a worldwide disease, primarily affects malnourished, premature infants in underdeveloped countries; it is a disease of immunosuppressed patients in the developed world. Based on ribosomal genes, *P. carinii* has been reclassified as a fungus. Diseases such as malaria, which occurs throughout the tropics, have markedly different epidemiological patterns in each region. These differences have a profound influence on the effectiveness of specific control measures. For example, the malaria eradication programs of the 1950s and 1960s that centered on the use of DDT could not be applied to areas of tropical Africa where highly efficient vectors fed outside the houses, not exposed to insecticide-covered walls.

The scientist, the clinician, and the public health worker need an overview of protozoology. Scientists must continuously reevaluate their work in relation to a disease as it occurs in the tropics and not be limited to a study of the infection in animal models. Clinicians and public health workers in the tropics are the advisers for government policy and can contribute to the understanding of a disease in their part of the world. They must be able to weigh the advances in basic science for their application to health policy and planning. For example, why did the malaria eradication program of the 1950s result in reduced support for malaria research even though these methods were not applicable to areas of Africa? Could informed health planners from that region have changed the course of events? Could a similar situation be arising today where the limited research on vectors has not kept pace with the activity of research on improved chemotherapy and vaccines?

Scientists in the developed world have been attracted to the study of protozoa because of the parasites' unusual lifestyles and mechanisms for evading the host immune system. Parasitic protozoa can multiply to unlimited numbers except where limited by innate resistance or immunity. The molecular basis for parasitism is little understood. It is known, for example, that *Toxoplasma gondii* evades lysosomal fusion and *Leishmania* live and multiply within lysosomes, but it is unknown how these parasites control their distribution within the cell or how *Leishmania* survive within lysosomes. Receptors are known to exist for malaria parasite entry into erythrocytes, and identification of the parasite components involved in invasion is just now being made, and their potential for inducing protective immunity (i.e., antigens for vaccines) is being explored. The molecular basis for antigenic variation in African trypanosomes is becoming understood. The irony may be that despite this knowledge we will be no closer to controlling African trypanosomiasis. It is unquestionable, however, that our rapidly growing knowledge of parasitic protozoa will eventually lead to new methods of therapy and disease control.

The first human trials of malaria vaccines recently completed highlight the promise and the problems ahead. Although the variant surface antigen of African trypanosomes does not look to be a promising target for vaccines, research in this area has identified unique enzymes that may be susceptible to a new class of drugs.

The chapters in this part of the book combine the broad disciplines of the biological sciences, so that a reader, from any perspective, can gain new insights that will contribute to the improvement of health in the tropics. The "magic bullets" of previous decades such as insecticides and antiparasitic drugs have offered only temporary amelioration. The spread of multidrug-resistant *Plasmodium falciparum* is one stark example. Some protozoan diseases will remain the problem in the year 2000 that they were 100 years previously, when the biology of many was first discovered, unless better methods of disease control are developed now.

CLASSIFICATION

The classification has been revised since the first edition and will continue receiving scrutiny because of new data from molecular biology and other areas of biochemistry. The present classification is taken from *An Illustrated Guide to the Protozoa,* edited by J. J. Lee, S. M. Hunter, and E. C. Bovee, and published by the Society of Protozoologists in 1985.

Table 1. Taxonomy of parasitic protozoa

Phylum Sarcomastigophora: Flagella, pseudopodia, or both
  types of locomotor organelles
  Subphylum Mastigophora: One or more flagella typi-
    cally present in trophozoites
    Class Zoomastigophorea
      Order Kinetoplastida
        Suborder Trypanosomatina
          Leishmania, Trypanosoma
      Order Diplomonadida
        Suborder Diplomonadina
          Giardia
      Order Trichomonadida
        Dientamoeba, Trichomonas
  Subphylum Sarcodina: Pseudopodia or locomotive pro-
    toplasmic flow without discrete pseudopodia
    Superclass Rhizopoda
      Class Lobosea
        Subclass Gymnamoebia
          Order Amoebida
            Suborder Tubulina
              Entamoeba
            Suborder Acanthopodina
              Acanthamoeba
          Order Schizopyrenida
            Naegleria

Phylum Apicomplexa: Apical complex, generally consisting
  of polar ring(s), rhoptries, micronemes; conoid and subpellicular microtubules present at some stage
  Class Sporozoasida
    Subclass Coccidiasina
      Order Coccidiasina
        Suborder Eimeriorina
          Isospora, Toxoplasma, Cryptosporidium
        Suborder Haemospororina
          Plasmodium
    Subclass Piroplasmasina
      Babesia
Phylum Ciliophora: Simple cilia or compound ciliary organelles typical in at least one stage of life cycle; two types
  of nuclei; sexuality involving conjugation, autogamy, and
  cytogamy
  Class Litosomatea
    Subclass Trichostomatia
      Order Vestubuliferida
        Balantidium

CHAPTER 30

Malaria · Louis H. Miller · David A. Warrell

Malaria is caused by four species of *Plasmodium*, *P. falciparum*, *P. vivax*, *P. ovale*, and *P. malariae*, each with its own morphology, biology, and clinical characteristics (Table 30-1). *P. falciparum* causes the most morbidity and mortality and presents the therapeutic problem of chloroquine resistance. Control of malaria in endemic areas will require determination on the part of governments and health workers because the available tools are expensive and difficult to apply. Research on vaccines and toward new methods of vector control should facilitate the ultimate goal of eradication.

PARASITE

LIFE CYCLE IN HUMANS (Fig. 30-1)

Female anopheline mosquitoes, during a blood meal, inoculate sporozoites which disappear from the circulation within 1 h. Sporozoites enter liver parenchymal cells, where they prolif-

erate into thousands of individual merozoites. Development in liver cells requires about 1 week for *P. falciparum* and *P. vivax* and 2 weeks for *P. malariae*. In *P. vivax* and *P. ovale*, some sporozoites after entry into liver cells remain dormant (hypnozoites) for months to years before proliferating. Merozoites rupture from a liver cell containing a mature schizont and pour into the bloodstream to invade erythrocytes.

Development of the intraerythrocytic parasite follows one of two pathways: asexual proliferation or differentiation into sexual parasites, the gametocytes. Asexual parasites develop from young ring forms through trophozoites to the dividing form, the schizont. Each mature schizont contains 6 to 24 merozoites, the number varying with the particular species.

Merozoites, on rupture of infected erythrocytes, are released to invade other erythrocytes and thus continue the cycle. Parasites proliferate until death of the host (most commonly in *P. falciparum*) or until they are controlled or terminated by the host's immune response or antimalarial drugs. Some erythro-

Table 30-1. Summary of clinical and diagnostic features

	P. falciparum	P. vivax	P. ovale	P. malariae
Clinical features	High parasitemia, severe anemia, renal failure, cerebral malaria, pulmonary edema, shock, jaundice, death	Splenic rupture, anemia		RBC infection persists for years; nephritis
Chloroquine resistance	Yes	No	No	No
Incubation period*	8–25 days (avg., 12)	8–27 days (avg., 14)	9–17 days (avg., 15)	15–30 days
Asexual cycle	48 h	48 h	48 h	72 h
Relapse†	No	Yes	Yes	No
Characteristic on thin blood film	Rings predominate, multiply infected RBCs, rings with threadlike cytoplasm, double nuclei. Banana-shaped gametocytes	Enlarged RBC with Schüffner's dots, trophozoite cytoplasm amoeboid, 12 to 24 merozoites in mature schizont	Oval RBC with fringed edges, Schüffner's dots, trophozoite cytoplasm compact, 6 to 16 merozoites in mature schizont	Trophozoite cytoplasm compact (band forms), 6 to 12 merozoites in mature schizont; RBC unchanged

*Incubation period: Interval from mosquito bite until clinical symptoms (fever). Chemoprophylaxis may suppress initial attack of *P. falciparum* for months and of *P. vivax* and *P. ovale* for months to years.
†Relapse: Recurrent erythrocytic infection derived from latent parasites in liver parenchymal cells after a mosquito-induced infection.

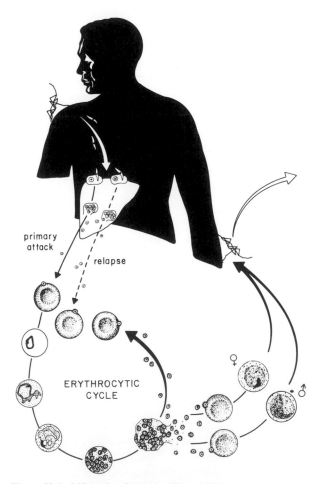

primary attack

relapse

ERYTHROCYTIC CYCLE

♀

♂

Figure 30-1. Life cycle of malaria. *(From [5].)*

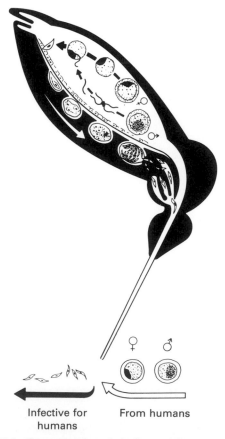

♀   ♂

Infective for humans

From humans

Figure 30-2. The sporogonic cycle in the mosquito.

cytic parasites differentiate into gametocytes that after full maturation await ingestion by the mosquito.

The sporogonic cycle in the mosquito (Fig. 30-2)

When male and female gametocytes are ingested by a mosquito during a blood meal, they lyse the erythrocyte to become extracellular. Gametogenesis proceeds rapidly with the formation by the male gametocytes into eight motile, spermlike male gametes. Fertilization of female gametes occurs rapidly. Within 24 h, zygotes transform into ookinetes which penetrate the mosquito midgut wall to form oocysts. Nine to fourteen days later, the oocysts rupture, releasing sporozoites which invade the salivary glands. Infectious sporozoites are injected into humans during the next blood meal.

PARASITE BIOLOGY, INTRACELLULAR PHYSIOLOGY, AND BIOCHEMISTRY

Sporozoites

Studies on rodent malaria (*P. berghei*) sporozoites have demonstrated that an internal 53,000-MW protein is converted to a 44,000-MW protein that covers the surface of the sporozoite, the *circumsporozoite* (CS) *protein* [1]. Similar sporozoite proteins are seen in all malarias. This protein probably determines molecular specificity in the interaction between sporozoites and liver cells. The conservation of two regions of this protein among malarial species separated in evolution suggested that they were involved in reception [2]. The peptide derived from one of these regions binds to liver cells [3]; the other region has a high degree of homology to thrombospondin, a crosslinking host protein.

Relapses in* P. vivax *and* P. ovale *(Hypnozoites). Some sporozoites develop immediately after entering the hepatic parenchymal cells and, on entering the bloodstream a week or more later, lead to the primary attack. Other parasites remain in liver cells as small, dormant parasites with a single nucleus; these are called *hypnozoites* [4]. Relapses occur when the hypnozoites begin to divide within liver cells months to years after the original bite of the infected mosquito. Different strains of *P. vivax* have their own characteristic patterns of relapse [5]. Some strains (e.g., from New Guinea) relapse monthly after the primary attack. Others relapse 6 months or longer after the primary attack or may not have a primary attack.

Asexual erythrocytic parasites

Merozoite Invasion of Erythrocytes (Fig. 30-3). Merozoites attach to erythrocytes by specific receptors [6], form a junction between the anterior end of the merozoite and the erythrocyte membrane, create a vacuolar membrane continuous with the erythrocyte membranes, and enter within the vacuole by a moving junction around the merozoite. Erythrocytic determi-

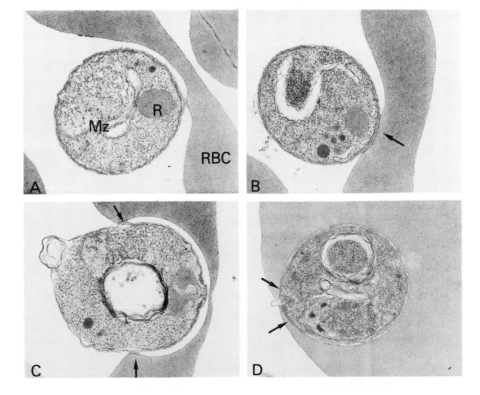

Figure 30-3. Merozoite (MZ) invasion of an erythrocyte (RBC). *A.* Attachment; *B.* junction formation (arrow); *C* and *D.* movement of junction around the merozoite, bringing the merozoite into a vacuole within the erythrocyte [7].

nants required for *P. vivax* and *P. falciparum* invasion are the Duffy blood group system and glycophorin, respectively. Blacks who are Duffy blood group-negative (*FyFy*) are refractory to erythrocytic infection by *P. vivax*. Because *P. vivax* could not be cultured, the molecular mechanism of resistance was determined for *P. knowlesi*, a monkey malaria that is also unable to invade these human erythrocytes. Initial attachment to erythrocytes appears normal, but the merozoites are unable to form a junction with Duffy-negative erythrocytes.

P. falciparum clones demonstrate receptor heterogeneity. Some require sialic acid on glycophorin; others invade by an unknown sialic acid– and glycophorin-independent pathway of unknown specificity [7,8]. Parasites also appear to have alternative pathways for invasion which can be used in the absence of a particular erythrocyte ligand or possibly when they are under immune attack.

Three human malarias, *P. vivax*, *P. ovale*, and *P. falciparum*, invade reticulocytes preferentially. *P. falciparum*, however, can infect erythrocytes of all ages and produces high parasitemias with the resultant morbidity and mortality. *P. malariae* infects mature erythrocytes.

Some of the parasite receptors for invasion by falciparum and knowlesi merozoites have been identified [9,10]. The *P. knowlesi* receptor binds specifically to the Duffy blood group glycoprotein; presumably a similar receptor exists for *P. vivax*.

The Membranes of Infected Erythrocytes. Each malaria induces characteristic morphological changes on the infected erythrocyte membrane: knobs by asexual parasites of *P. falciparum*; knobs by sexual and asexual parasites of *P. malariae*; and Schüffner's dots, caveolar-vesicle junctions, by sexual and asexual parasites of *P. vivax* and *P. ovale*. Knobs on the membrane of *P. falciparum*–infected erythrocytes mediate attachment to venular endothelium [11]. This sequestration explains the predominance of young parasites, ring forms, in the peripheral blood. Knobs may be a factor in obstruction of cerebral vessels leading to cerebral malaria. A submembrane histidine-rich parasite protein forms part of the knoblike protrusion in the erythrocyte membrane [12]. The molecules mediating cytoadherence are probably high-molecular-weight parasite proteins of variant antigenicity [13] and the host proteins, CD36 [14] or thrombospondin [15]. It is unclear whether sequestration in venules of many organs throughout the body during uncomplicated malaria and the binding of parasitized erythrocytes to cerebral endothelium in cerebral malaria or to placental vessels during pregnancy are mediated by the same host molecules.

Parasite Metabolism (see [16].) Malaria parasites derive energy from anerobic glycolysis of glucose to lactic acid. The primate malarias, *P. falciparum* and *P. knowlesi*, lack a functional citric acid cycle. The fact that pantothenate analogues inhibit in vitro growth of *P. falciparum* and *P. coatneyi* suggests that the parasite cannot synthesize CoA and requires intact CoA acetylation reactions. Enzymes of the pentose phosphate shunt exist in malaria parasites, including the first enzyme, glucose-6-phosphate dehydrogenase. Despite the presence of a shunt, reduction of NADP may occur via glutamine dehydrogenase. Limited data exist on electron transport and cytochromes in malaria. Cytochrome oxidase has been identified.

Ingestion of hemoglobin occurs via a specialized organelle, the cytostome, which buds off food vacuoles from its base. Digestion of hemoglobin occurs within the food vacuole with formation of malarial pigment, hemozoin, which consists of monomers and dimers of ferriprotoporphyrin IX, methemoglobin, and plasmodial proteins.

Pyrimidines are synthesized de novo. Para-aminobenzoic acid (PABA) is converted to folate; the folate enzymes associated with pyrimidine biosynthesis have been identified. Parasites obtain their purines from the erythrocyte or the plasma. DNA synthesis is thought to occur prior to schizogony, the period of nuclear division.

The membrane of schizont-infected erythrocytes is more permeable to molecules such as sorbitol than that of normal erythrocytes. During parasite development, the intraerythrocyte Na^+ increases and K^+ decreases. Excessive K^+ leak, such as in *P. falciparum*–infected hemoglobin SA erythrocytes grown at low oxygen tension, is detrimental to the parasite [17]. The parasite's requirement for a high-K^+ environment may explain the absence of malaria in animals with high-Na^+ erythrocytes (e.g., cats, dogs, and cattle).

In Vitro Culture. The continuous culture of the asexual erythrocytic parasites by Trager and Jensen [18] has been a major stimulus for research on malaria parasite physiology, biochemistry, and chemotherapy.

Gametocytes

The rate at which asexual parasites differentiate into gametocytes varies considerably during successive rounds of schizogony. Gametocyte production is modulated by environmental conditions [19], although the trigger for gametocyte formation and where in the asexual cycle commitment to differentiation occurs are unknown.

P. falciparum gametocytes take 10 days to mature from rings to fully mature gametocytes. Young falciparum gametocytes sequester in spleen and bone marrow to appear again in the peripheral blood as mature crescent-shaped parasites within the erythrocyte membrane. The mature gametocytes may survive in the circulation for up to 2 to 3 weeks. In contrast, *P. vivax* gametocytes probably mature in 36 h and remain in the circulation for only about 1 day.

The triggers for gametogenesis (gametocytes to extracellular gametes) in the mosquito midgut include a drop in temperature below 30°C, a rise in pH as a result of the drop in PCO_2, and an unidentified mosquito midgut factor.

The proteins in the membranes of male and female gametes,

zygotes, and ookinetes have been identified [20]. However, the proteins involved in recognition and fusion of male and female gametes have not been identified.

PARASITE GENETICS

The asexual erythrocytic parasite has a haploid genome [21]. The asexual parasites differentiate into male and female gametocytes under environmental influences. Fertilization leads to a diploid zygote. Meiosis has been observed in the ookinete, the stage in the mosquito midgut. Sporozoites are again haploid. The *P. falciparum* genome consists of 14 chromosomes. Variation in chromosome length among parasite clones is caused by deletions in the subtelomeric regions. Genetic markers for asexual erythrocytic parasites include isoenzymes, drug resistance, virulence in rodent malaria, and restriction fragment length polymorphism (RFLP). It should be possible to follow populations of parasites within a community using polymerase chain reaction (PCR) and DNA sequence of highly variant genes such as the 195-kDa glycoprotein on the surface of falciparum merozoites.

PARASITE EVOLUTION

Malaria is classified into saurian, rodent, avian, and primate malaria according to the host in which it is found. This makes the inherent assumption that the malaria parasites evolved with their hosts. By analysis of deoxyguanosine · deoxycytidine (dG · dC) content, cross-hybridization of genes, and ribosomal sequence, *P. falciparum*, the most important human malaria, was found to have derived from avian malaria and to be distant from all other primate malarias [22]. Regions of homology between falciparum and other primate malarias are likely to be conserved as a result of functional constraints.

PATIENT

INNATE RESISTANCE

Genetically determined host factors influence susceptibility to malaria. Certain polymorphisms have been associated with the distribution of *P. falciparum* in the world [e.g., hemoglobin S, thalassemia, and glucose-6-phosphate dehydrogenase (G-6-PD) deficiency]. The evidence for a selective advantage of polymorphisms in malarious areas is most convincing for sickle trait (HbA/S) [23]. Children who die from malaria in west Africa rarely have sickle trait, although the frequency of this phenotype is high in this region. Thus, sickle trait (HbS/A) provides a selective advantage over the homozygous HbA/A or HbS/S. Where the heterozygote has an advantage over either homozygote, a balanced polymorphism results, with the frequency of each gene determined by the relative survival of each homozygote. The mechanism of protection at the cellular level appears to be inhibition of growth in HbS/S or HbS/A erythrocytes at low oxygen tension [24]. The intracellular K^+ decreases in HbS/A erythrocytes under low O_2 tension and causes the death of the parasite [17]. It is presumed that suppression of parasite multiplication in vivo is a consequence of the sequestration of parasitized erythrocytes along venular endothelium where the O_2 tension is low.

Black Africans who have the Duffy blood group–negative genotype (*FyFy*) are resistant to infection by *P. vivax* [25]. This is probably because the erythrocytes lack a receptor for merozoite invasion.

Ovalocytosis occurs throughout lowland tropical areas of southeast Asia and Melanesia, which are endemic for malaria. Invasion of ovalocytic erythrocytes by *P. falciparum* in culture is greatly reduced [26].

IMMUNITY TO ASEXUAL ERYTHROCYTIC PARASITES

Immunity only develops after prolonged or repeated infection. Immunity is usually not sterile, but the infection causes no symptoms or is of much reduced severity. The symptomatic person, however, can infect mosquitoes and can transmit the infection directly to others through blood transfusion. Immunity wanes in a few years when the person is unexposed to reinfection. Recurrence of disease may occur in an immune person immediately after surgery, after splenectomy, or during pregnancy.

Immunity is species-specific (e.g., immunity to *P. falciparum* does not protect against *P. vivax*). Further, the immunity against *P. falciparum* is strain-specific, indicating variant antigens among strains [27]. One such variant antigen is the soluble, heat-stable antigen (S antigen) which shows great heterogeneity within the Gambia [28]. Monoclonal antibodies against surface antigens on *P. falciparum* merozoites also demonstrate antigenic heterogeneity within each region.

Passive transfer of antibody from adult west Africans to east or west African children killed malarial parasites [29]. Antibody may block invasion, kill developing intraerythrocytic parasites, or function through antibody-dependent cytotoxic cells (ADCC). Alternatively, antibody, through formation of immune complexes, may present antigen to the immune cells to boost immunity more efficiently. Sera obtained after a *P. falciparum* infection were most active in suppressing reinvasion in vitro of the homologous, infective strain. The mechanism by which *P. knowlesi* immune serum blocks invasion of rhesus erythrocytes appears to be by merozoite agglutination, since F(ab)' fragments are inactive [30].

The spleen is of primary importance in host survival against malaria. One mechanism may involve antibody and cells within the spleen (ADCC). Alternatively, parasites may be killed by macrophages through antibody-independent mechanisms.

Immune response to malaria may be under the influence of Ir genes. The association between certain HLA-A and -B haplotypes and malaria may result from linkage to specific Ir genes.

Mechanisms of immune induction and immunoregulation in malaria have been studied primarily in the mouse system (see review by Jayawardena [*31*]), but are now being studied in humans in relation to specific antigens. Helper T cells are required for immune induction. T- and B-cell function as measured by antibody production and cell-mediated immune responses is suppressed during infection.

Immunity to sporozoites and gametes

Antibody to the CS protein on the sporozoite surface occurs in naturally infected populations in Africa but probably plays little role in immunity, as humans with antibodies are reinfected [*32*]. Monoclonal antibodies to the CS protein of *P. berghei* or their Fab fragments block infection [*33*]. After immunization of mice with irradiated sporozoites, however, immunity to high-sporozoite challenge is dependent on CD8 + T cells (probably cytotoxic T cells) and not antibody [*34*].

Gamete immunity does not appear to occur in naturally infected populations. Antibodies induced by immunization in animals block fertilization, induce complement-dependent lysis, and block ookinete invasion of the midgut.

PATHOGENESIS AND PATHOLOGY

The asexual erythrocytic cycle is responsible for the symptoms and pathology. Fever and the associated symptoms of headache, nausea, and muscular pain occur at the time schizont-infected erythrocytes rupture and new ring forms appear (Fig. 30-4). Endogenous pyrogen (interleukin 1) has been identified in the blood of patients during a malarial crisis. Endotoxemia has been reported, and mediators such as kinins and cachectin (tumor necrosis factor) have also been found but not yet convincingly related to pathogenesis. The parasitemia (the concentration of asexual parasites in the blood) at which symptoms occur differs from patient to patient. Nonimmune patients gen-

erally develop symptoms at lower parasitemia than semi-immune patients.

P. falciparum malaria causes a diffuse encephalopathy. Erythrocytes containing schizonts and other mature forms with malarial pigment obstruct cerebral capillaries and venules [*35*], and ring hemorrhages develop around some obstructed vessels (Fig. 30-5). The cerebrospinal fluid opening pressure at lumbar puncture is usually normal, and there is no evidence of increased permeability of the blood–cerebrospinal fluid barrier [*36*]. In a few patients cerebral edema may develop as a result of agonal hypoxia. Sequestration of parasitized erythrocytes in the brain and other tissues (retina, bone marrow, hepatic sinusoids, intestine, kidney, and placenta) results from cytoadherence of knoblike protuberances on the erythrocyte surface to endothelium (see ''Membranes of Infected Erythrocytes''). Decreased deformability of infected erythrocytes may contribute to sluggish microvascular flow. Cerebral anaerobic gly-

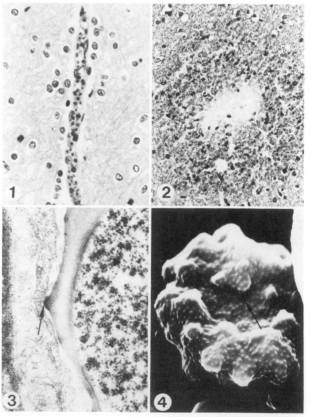

Figure 30-5. *1.* A cerebral capillary from a cerebral malaria patient showing blockage with infected erythrocytes. *2.* Ring hemorrhage around a blocked vessel. *3.* Scanning electron micrograph showing knobs (arrow) over the *P. falciparum*–infected erythrocyte surface. *4.* Electron micrograph showing adhesions (arrow) between electron-dense knobs on infected erythrocytes and capillary endothelial cells. *(From M. Aikawa, Am. J. Trop. Med. Hyg. 39:3, 1988.)*

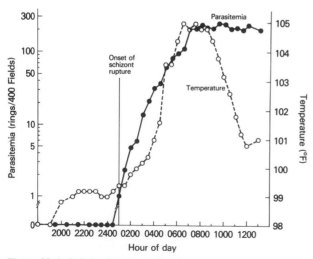

Figure 30-4. Relation between schizont rupture (appearance of rings in erythrocytes) and fever. *(From [5].)*

colysis and reduced cerebral oxygen transport have been demonstrated in patients with cerebral malaria [37].

Anemia is caused by hemolysis of infected erythrocytes, abnormally rapid splenic removal of nonparasitized erythrocytes, and dyserythropoiesis. Immune hemolysis has rarely been demonstrated. Reticulocytosis may be delayed, especially if there are complicating infections. Oxidant drugs can cause severe hemolysis in G-6-PD–deficient patients. Thrombocytopenia is most likely to be caused by sequestration in the spleen. There is no evidence of decreased platelet production or immune lysis.

Acute renal failure is associated with histological appearances of acute tubular necrosis. Possible mechanisms include ischemia resulting from hypovolemia, renal vasoconstriction, or microvascular obstruction by parasitized erythrocytes; and pigment nephropathy secondary to hemolysis. Histopathological features of glomerulonephritis may be found in convalescence. In the liver, Küpffer cells contain malaria pigment, and there is evidence of mild hepatocyte damage (microvesiculation) and, unusually, centrilobular necrosis. The spleen is large, engorged, and heavily pigmented, containing many phagocytic cells which have ingested erythrocytes and malaria pigment.

Most patients who die of malaria have edematous lungs. Pulmonary capillaries and venules are packed with inflammatory cells including neutrophils and monocytes, and there is endothelial and interstitial edema. Bronchopneumonia is a common finding. Large numbers of parasitized erythrocytes are found in the myocardial blood vessels, occasionally associated with subendocardial and epicardial hemorrhages. There is no myocarditis. The intestinal mucosa may be congested and ulcerated, and capillaries of the lamina propria of the jejunum and elsewhere may be packed with parasitized erythrocytes. These appearances may explain the occurrence of endotoxemia, secondary gram-negative septicemias, and impaired intestinal absorption in severe malaria.

Especially in African children, *P. malariae* produces chronic progressive immune complex glomerulonephritis leading to nephrotic syndrome (Fig. 30-6). In the glomeruli there are subendothelial deposits of immunoglobulins, C3, and *P. malariae* antigen. It remains uncertain as to whether only *P. malariae* initiates this condition and why relatively few infected children develop it.

CLINICAL MANIFESTATIONS

The acute attack

No sign or symptom is pathognomonic of malaria, and since delay in treatment of *P. falciparum* increases mortality, the diagnosis should be considered in all febrile patients who have traveled in endemic areas or received blood transfusions. The incubation period (Table 30-1) ranges from 7 to 18 days and is longest (up to 40 days) for *P. malariae*. Immunity, chemoprophylaxis, or partial chemotherapy may prolong incubation

for months to years in the relapsing malarias (*P. vivax* and *P. ovale*), but 65 to 95 percent of patients with imported *P. falciparum* infection present within a month of returning from the malarious area. A typical malarial paroxysm lasts about 8 to 12 h and consists of a cold stage (rigor, chill), a hot stage (high fever, febrile convulsion), and a defervescent stage (sweating). The paroxysm begins with a sudden chilly feeling, followed by teeth-rattling, bed-shaking rigors, and rapid rise in temperature (cold stage). There is intense peripheral vasoconstriction so that the skin appears pale and goose-pimpled, with cyanosis of the lips and nail beds. The patient experiences headache and nausea and may vomit. Within the next 1 to 2 h the temperature rises to between 39 and 41°C and the patient feels hot with a flushed, dry skin, throbbing headache, and palpitations (hot stage). As the temperature falls, a drenching sweat breaks out, and the exhausted patient often sleeps.

The classical periodicity of fever and paroxysms develops only if the patient is untreated until the infection becomes synchronized so that the majority of infected erythrocytes contain mature schizonts and rupture at the same time. The interval is determined by the length of the asexual erythrocytic cycle: 48 h in *P. vivax* and *P. ovale*, producing paroxysms on alternate days (or days 1 and 3, hence tertian); 72 h for *P. malariae*, causing paroxysms on days 1 and 4 (hence quartan). Classical tertian or subtertian fever is rarely seen in falciparum malaria: persistent spiking fever or a daily paroxysm is more usual. Other common symptoms include unproductive cough, backache, myalgias, postural hypotension, diarrhea, and persistent weakness. Common physical signs include anemia, mild jaundice, and moderate tender enlargement of the spleen and liver. Rashes (apart from labial herpes) and lymphadenopathy suggest a diagnosis other than malaria.

Abnormalities in routine laboratory investigations in uncomplicated malaria include evidence of hemolytic anemia, leukopenia resulting from decreased granulocytes and lympho-

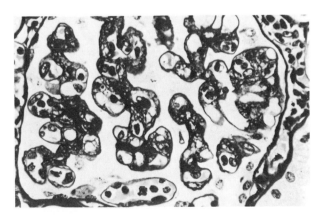

Figure 30-6. Membranoproliferative glomerulonephritis in *P. malariae* infection. *(Courtesy of M. Aikawa.)*

cytes, thrombocytopenia which recovers rapidly after treatment, and minimal albuminuria.

Severe and complicated malaria

The acute mortality of *P. vivax* malaria may result from anemia in severely debilitated patients and from splenic rupture, which is more common than in falciparum malaria. Fatal acute *P. malariae* infection has been described in immunocompromised patients infected by blood transfusion [*38*], but, especially in Africa, *P. malariae* may cause chronic nephrotic syndrome in children which is often fatal.

P. falciparum is responsible for most malarial deaths. Impairment of consciousness (cerebral malaria) is the principal clinical manifestation. A few days after the start of the illness, the level of consciousness may decline gradually, or the patient may remain deeply comatose after a generalized convulsion. High fever alone can cause irritability, confusion, and delirium and, in children, febrile convulsions. For research purposes, the term *cerebral malaria,* implying encephalopathy specifically related to *P. falciparum* infection, should be restricted to patients in unrousable coma (no purposive motor response to noxious stimuli) who have evidence of acute *P. falciparum* infection and in whom other causes of unconsciousness, such as bacterial and viral encephalitides and a recent convulsion, have been excluded [*38*]. However, from the clinical point of view, any alteration in the level of consciousness indicates severe disease requiring urgent treatment. Other signs of cerebral malaria include meningism, retinal hemorrhages, bruxism, and dysconjugate gaze with intact pupillary, corneal, oculocephalic, and oculovestibular reflexes. There are signs of symmetrical upper motor neuron dysfunction: hypertonia, increased tendon reflexes with ankle clonus, extensor plantar responses, and absent abdominal reflexes (useful in distinguishing hysteria). Extensor posturing occurs with and without demonstrable hypoglycemia but is associated with hypoglycemia in other clinical conditions. It consists of decerebrate or decorticate rigidity or even opisthotonos, associated with pouting, and stertorous breathing. Generalized convulsions are common, but focal seizures and localizing neurological signs are uncommon. Less than 10 percent of adults have persisting neurological sequelae, but the incidence may be as high as 40 percent in children with cerebral malaria complicated by hypoglycemia [*39*]. Acute transient and reversible cerebellar ataxia with hypotonia and nystagmus has been described, especially in India and Sri Lanka, in patients with otherwise uncomplicated *P. falciparum* infections.

Anemia is an inevitable consequence of severe falciparum malaria. It is most marked in African children, many of whom may have preexisting chronic anemia, and in patients with high parasitemias and other complications such as renal impairment and secondary bacterial infections. Massive intravascular hemolysis with hemoglobinuria can result from high parasitemia or destruction of G-6-PD–deficient erythrocytes by oxidant an-

timalarial drugs. Classical blackwater fever was characterized by scanty or absent parasitemia, renal failure, and a high mortality among northern Europeans working in Africa. Intermittent quinine treatment or prophylaxis was thought to have induced immune hemolysis in these people.

Hyperpyrexia, which may develop in otherwise uncomplicated attacks of malaria, can damage the central nervous system, cause febrile convulsions, and, in women nearing the end of pregnancy, cause fetal distress.

Spontaneous systemic hemorrhage (e.g., from the nose, gums, or gastrointestinal tract) is a manifestation of disseminated intravascular coagulation found in less than 10 percent of patients with cerebral malaria.

Renal failure resulting from acute tubular necrosis develops in about 30 percent of adult patients with cerebral malaria but is much less common in children. In tropical countries, patients are commonly dehydrated and relatively hypovolemic when they present with severe falciparum malaria. Electrolyte abnormalities include hyponatremia, hypocalcemia (caused by hypoalbuminemia), and hypophosphatemia. Acute pulmonary edema may be caused by excessive fluid replacement or, in patients with normal pulmonary artery wedge pressures, may resemble adult respiratory distress syndrome. This complication is usually fatal.

Algid malaria (hypotension and shock) resembles gram-negative septicemia and may be attributable to secondary gram-negative infections. Metabolic acidosis is found in association with hyperparasitemia, hypoglycemia, shock, and renal failure and is usually caused by accumulated lactate. Gastrointestinal symptoms such as vomiting and diarrhea, which may be profuse and watery, are prominent and misleading symptoms in some falciparum infections. Jaundice is common in adults. It results from hemolysis and hepatocyte dysfunction, which is rarely severe. Hepatic failure is extremely rare.

Hypoglycemia is emerging as a major complication of falciparum malaria in patients with severe disease, pregnant women, and young children [*39,40*]. In pregnant women, hypoglycemia may be asymptomatic, but most patients convulse or have impaired consciousness and extensor posturing.

Severe falciparum malaria may be complicated by a variety of secondary infections including aspiration bronchopneumonia, gram-negative septicemias, nontyphoid *Salmonella* septicemia, and parvovirus infections. Malaria is particularly dangerous in pregnancy, causing maternal death, abortion, stillbirth, premature delivery, and low birth weight in tropical countries. Primiparae are particularly vulnerable.

Laboratory investigations show evidence of severe hemolysis, neutrophil leukocytosis, thrombocytopenia, prolonged prothrombin and partial thromboplastin times, and other evidence of disseminated intravascular coagulation (DIC) including reduced antithrombin III concentrations. Lumbar puncture is important in patients with cerebral malaria to exclude other treatable encephalopathies. The cerebrospinal fluid (CSF) opening pressure is normal in 80 percent of adult cases. The

CSF may contain a few lymphocytes and increased protein concentration. High CSF lactate and low glucose concentrations indicate a bad prognosis. Blood glucose must be checked frequently, especially in children, pregnant women, and severe cases. Urine commonly contains protein, erythrocytes, hemoglobin, and red cell casts.

Asymptomatic infection, recrudescence, and relapse

Partial therapy or immunity reduces parasitemia, and symptoms may disappear. Despite persistent erythrocytic infection during these asymptomatic periods, parasites are difficult to locate on blood films. Periodic rises in parasitemia cause recurrent clinical attacks *(recrudescence)*. The total duration of erythrocytic infection varies for each malaria. Most falciparum infections are eliminated in 1 year; a few persist for up to 3 years. *P. malariae* may persist as an asymptomatic infection for the life of the patient. How *P. malariae* evades the immune response for years while infecting new erythrocytes every 72 h remains a mystery. The asymptomatic erythrocytic infection poses two potential risks to others. First, donated blood induces malaria in the recipient. Second, the asymptomatic patient can infect vector mosquitoes. *Relapse* differs from recrudescence in that the infection that induces the relapse persists in a latent form in hepatic parenchymal cells [*4*]. Relapses occur only in *P. vivax* and *P. ovale*. Drugs that cure the latent infection in the liver differ from those that destroy asexual erythrocytic parasites (see ''Treatment''). Relapses never occur from a blood-induced infection (e.g., transfusion malaria) because the asexual erythrocytic parasite cannot infect liver parenchymal cells.

Bloodborne malaria infections

Congenital malaria is extremely rare except in infants born to nonimmune mothers. It is diagnosed by detecting parasitemia in the neonate within 7 days of birth or later if there is no possibility of postpartum mosquito-borne infection. Transfusion of infected whole blood, packed cells, leukocyte or platelet concentrates, bone marrow aspirate, and fresh plasma have been responsible for transfusion malaria. Malaria may also be transmitted by organ transplants and between intravenous drug abusers.

Diseases associated with falciparum malaria

Tropical Splenomegaly Syndrome (Hyperreactive Malaria Splenomegaly) [*41,42*]. Some residents of malarious areas develop progressive massive splenomegaly with associated hepatomegaly. Other features of tropical splenomegaly syndrome include elevated serum IgM and malarial antibody levels, hepatic sinusoidal lymphocytosis, hypersplenism with profound anemia and neutropenia, and clinical and immunological responses to antimalarial prophylaxis, with death from overwhelming bacterial infections in untreated patients (see Chap. 9).

Endemic Burkitt's Lymphoma. This common childhood tumor of the jaw or abdomen occurs in areas of holoendemic falciparum malaria. Immune surveillance of B lymphocytes chronically infected with Epstein-Barr virus may be reduced by *P. falciparum* infection, allowing chromosomal translocations which activate the oncogene responsible for malignant transformation [*43*] (see Chap. 8).

Diagnosis

Malaria should be suspected in any febrile patient who has been in the tropics, who has received a blood transfusion, or who has been punctured by a contaminated needle. Outside the endemic area, people living near international airports may be bitten by imported infected mosquitoes. The diagnosis is confirmed by identifying malaria parasites in Giemsa-stained thick and thin blood films. Blood examination should be repeated at 12-h intervals, as the parasitemia may fluctuate. Parasites may be undetectable during the first few days of the initial attack, in asymptomatic semi-immune people, and in those who have taken antimalarial drugs. Early treatment is very important. Examination of blood films should not be delayed until there is a paroxysm, and if malaria is strongly suspected on clinical grounds, a therapeutic trial should be instituted despite repeatedly negative blood films. In nonimmunes, a retrospective serological diagnosis may be made. using the indirect fluorescent antibody test.

Well-prepared and properly stained thick and thin blood films simplify diagnosis. Slides should be thoroughly cleaned with alcohol, dried, polished, and labeled with the patient's name, the date, and the time. For the thick film, one drop of blood at one end of the slide should be evenly spread in a circular motion to a diameter of 2 cm using the edge of another slide. For the thin film part of a second drop of blood should be spread on the slide as for routine hematological examinations. After the blood films are completely dry, the thick film should be lysed with water and the thin film fixed with absolute methanol. Both should be stained with Giemsa at pH 7.0 to 7.2.

Once malaria parasites are identified in the blood film, the most important distinction is between *P. falciparum* and other species, as this will influence treatment. Mixed infections may occur, and so the finding of *P. vivax,* for example, does not exclude *P. falciparum*. *P. falciparum* may be multi-drug-resistant, and response to treatment must be closely monitored. All other species are sensitive to chloroquine. Crescent-shaped gametocytes are diagnostic of *P. falciparum*. Other features suggestive of this species include high parasitemias (>5 percent), the predominance of small ring forms, multiple infected erythrocytes, rings with double nuclei, and appliqué forms. Except at high parasitemias, trophozoites and schizonts are rarely seen, because infected erythrocytes adhere to venular endothelium. Immature large erythrocytes are not infected. Pink stippling (Schüffner's dots) of the cytoplasm of infected erythrocytes is typical of *P. vivax* and *P. ovale*. (See Table 30-1 for diagnostic characteristics of *P. vivax, P. ovale,* and *P. malariae*.) Common artifacts resembling malaria parasites are superimposed platelets, particles of stain, pits in the slide, and erythrocyte inclusions (e.g., Howell-Jolly bodies and siderocytes). Other erythrocyte infections such as bartonellosis and babesiosis may be confused with malaria.

Serological tests have no place in the diagnosis of the acutely ill patient; however, recently developed DNA probes [44] and the indirect fluorescent antibody test may prove useful in screening potential blood donors and for epidemiological studies.

Differential diagnosis

Malaria enters into the differential diagnosis of any acute severe fever, especially those commonly associated with rigors, impaired consciousness, jaundice, spontaneous bleeding, diarrhea, shock, renal failure, and respiratory distress. In western countries, imported malaria is commonly misdiagnosed as influenza, viral hepatitis, travelers' diarrhea, and viral encephalitis. Important differential diagnoses include yellow fever and other viral hemorrhagic fevers, leptospirosis, relapsing fevers, heatstroke, and enteric fevers. Cerebral malaria must be distinguished from other infective meningoencephalitides, metabolic comas, intoxications, and psychoses.

TREATMENT

P. falciparum

Chemotherapy must be started as soon as possible, especially in patients with severe falciparum malaria in whom there is a highly significant relationship between delayed chemotherapy and mortality. Outside the endemic area patients are likely to be nonimmune, and falciparum malaria should be regarded as a medical emergency requiring admission to the hospital. Patients who appear stable on admission may deteriorate rapidly. The choice of antimalarial drug will depend on the origin of the infection, for chloroquine resistance is now prevalent in most parts of the endemic area with the exception of parts of west Africa, the Middle East, Central America, and the Caribbean (Table 30-2). Even in areas of predominant drug sensitivity, such as west Africa, drug-resistant parasites occur. Drug resistance is divided into three types: RI, defined by disappearance of parasites on blood films and clinical recovery followed by recrudescence weeks later; RII, reduction in parasitemia and clinical symptoms followed by a rise in parasitemia; and RIII, no response to therapy. Since treatment failure may occur with any drug regimen and with parasites from any part of the world, the course of parasitemia must be followed

at 12-h intervals. Failure to reduce parasitemia in the first 24 to 48 h of treatment should raise the possibility of parasite resistance to that treatment. No asexual parasites should be detectable in smears 4 to 5 days after completing a course of chloroquine; persistence after the fifth day indicates drug failure. A simple method of estimating parasitemia from the thin blood film is as follows: at low parasite densities, the number of infected erythrocytes in 25 oil immersion fields is counted; at high parasite densities, the number of infected erythrocytes per 500 erythrocytes is counted.

Gametocytes may persist in the blood for weeks after asexual forms have been successfully eliminated. Gametocytes do not cause disease, and their presence does not indicate treatment failure.

RI-resistant parasites recrudesce up to 2 months after treatment in a nonimmune. The patient should be warned that any febrile episode weeks to months after treatment may indicate drug failure and requires evaluation for malaria.

Chloroquine resistance is widespread (Table 30-2). Chloroquine is still recommended for the treatment of *P. falciparum* infections acquired in west Africa, the Middle East, Central America, and the Caribbean. Infections acquired elsewhere, or those of high parasitemia, are assumed to be chloroquine-resistant and are treated with quinine. Sulfonamide-pyrimethamine combinations (Fansidar) are still effective for chloroquine-resistant *P. falciparum* infections in Africa, but carry the risk of severe hypersensitivity reactions to sulfonamide such as erythema multiforme, Stevens-Johnson syndrome, and toxic epidermal necrolysis. In the United States, the risk of fatal reactions to Fansidar prophylaxis has been calculated as 1 in 11,000 to 25,000. Quinine resistance, usually at the RI level, is emerging in southeast Asia and parts of Africa. In these areas, quinine is combined with tetracycline (except in young children and pregnant women).

Table 30-2. Worldwide distribution of chloroquine-sensitive *P. falciparum*

Latin America:
Central America north of Panama
Dominican Republic
Haiti
Asia:
The Middle East
West Africa:*
Chad
Equatorial Guinea
Guinea
Guinea-Bissau
Liberia
Senegal
Sierra Leone

*Chloroquine resistance of *P. falciparum* is rapidly spreading throughout Africa.

Symptomatic and supportive measures

High fever contributes to headaches, muscular pain, and other symptoms of malaria and causes febrile convulsions in children and fetal distress in pregnant women. Temperature should be kept below 38.5°C by fanning the patient after sponging the skin with tepid water, by the use of a cooling blanket, or by antipyretic drugs such as acetaminophen (15 mg/kg in tablets by mouth, as a powder washed down a nasogastric tube, or as a suppository). Patients should be nursed in bed because of their postural hypotension.

Chemotherapy of chloroquine-sensitive *P. falciparum*

Chloroquine-sensitive strains occur in west Africa, the Middle East, Central America, and the Caribbean (Table 30-2). Adults should be given 300 mg of chloroquine *base* three times on the first day and 300 mg once on the second and third days. This regimen is well-tolerated, but Africans may experience severe itching of the palms of the hands and soles of the feet without any obvious skin abnormalities and without serious sequelae. Because of the possibility of chloroquine resistance, parasitemia should be followed closely during treatment and alternative drugs instituted if indicated. Fever occurring weeks after therapy may indicate a recrudescence.

Treatment of chloroquine-resistant *P. falciparum*

Patients who have acquired *P. falciparum* malaria in an area of known chloroquine resistance (Asia, east and central Africa, South America), who have a life-threatening infection, in whom the infection has broken through chloroquine prophylaxis, or in whom the origin of the infection is uncertain should not be treated with chloroquine. Adults should be treated with quinine sulfate 600 mg three times a day for 7 days; children should receive 10 mg of the salt per kilogram three times per day for 7 days. In areas of emerging quinine resistance, such as southeast Asia, adults and children over the age of 8 years, but not pregnant women, should be given tetracycline in a dose of 250 mg every 6 h for 7 days. In some parts of the world, such as Africa, addition of a single dose of the pyrimethamine-sulfonamide combination (for example three tablets of Fansidar) at the beginning or end of the course of quinine is effective. Mefloquine (Lariam) has recently been marketed in France and Switzerland and has been widely used as a first-line treatment of confirmed *P. falciparum* infection in Thailand. The adult dose is 20 mg/kg given as two doses 8 h apart.

Treatment of severe and complicated malaria

In patients with *P. falciparum* asexual parasitemia, the following features indicate severe disease and the need for urgent intravenous chemotherapy: impaired consciousness (cerebral malaria), renal failure, pulmonary edema, hypoglycemia, circulatory collapse, spontaneous systemic bleeding, repeated generalized convulsions, acidemia, hyperparasitemia (for example, more than 100,000 parasitized erythrocytes per microliter), jaundice, hyperpyrexia, severe normocytic anemia, and inability to swallow tablets. Chloroquine is less toxic than quinine and may be more rapidly effective against chloroquine-sensitive strains of *P. falciparum*; however, physicians may prefer to use quinine in all cases of severe falciparum malaria because of the risk of chloroquine resistance even when the infection has been acquired in a predominantly chloroquine-sensitive area of the world. Treatment should be initiated with a loading dose of 16.7 mg quinine *base* per kilogram in a suitable volume of isotonic fluid given by intravenous infusion over 4 h. Subsequent maintenance doses of 8.3 mg *base* per kilogram are infused over 4 h every 8 h until the patient can swallow tablets and complete a full 7 days of quinine treatment. If quinine or mefloquine have been taken within the previous 12 h, the initial dose of intravenous quinine should be 8.3 mg *base* per kilogram. In patients who require more than 72 h of intravenous treatment, the dose should be reduced to 5.6 mg *base* per kg given every 8 h. If parenteral quinine is not available, quinidine gluconate may be used. The regimen recommended in the United States is a loading dose of 10 mg quinidine gluconate per kilogram infused over 1 h followed by a continuous infusion of 0.02 mg/(kg·min) by infusion pump for up to 72 h or until the patient can swallow quinine tablets. Quinidine is more cardiotoxic than quinine, so ECG and blood pressure should be monitored throughout the infusion period [45].

Patients with severe malaria should, whenever possible, be treated in an intensive care unit. Convulsions can be prevented by a single intramuscular injection of phenobarbital, 3.5 mg/kg [46]. Dexamethasone in a dose of 2 or 11 mg/kg in 48 h has been found to increase morbidity and not to reduce mortality [47,48]. Other suggested ancillary treatments include osmotic or diuretic agents such as mannitol, dextrans, epinephrine, and heparin, but there is no convincing evidence of benefit to outweigh their potentially deleterious effects.

Excessive or rapid parenteral fluid replacement and blood transfusion carry the risk of precipitating acute pulmonary edema. Fluid therapy must be strictly controlled by measurement of urine output, daily weighing, fluid balance charts, and monitoring of central venous pressure. Cautious transfusion of fresh compatible whole blood will be required if the hematocrit falls below 20 percent. The majority of patients with a falling urine output and elevated blood urea nitrogen and serum creatinine concentrations can be treated conservatively by cautious correction of hypovolemia. Isotonic saline is infused, but the central venous pressure must not be allowed to rise above +5 cmH$_2$O. Diuretics and renal vasodilators such as dopamine, 2.5 to 5 μg/(kg·min), are effective in some cases. Peritoneal dialysis, hemodialysis, or hemofiltration is indicated once renal failure is established. Metabolic (lactic) acidosis must be treated by improving pulmonary gas exchange, correcting hypovolemia, and treating associated septicemias. The value of bicarbonate and dichloroacetate, which stimulates pyruvate dehydrogenase, is uncertain. Pulmonary edema associated with elevated central venous or pulmonary artery wedge pressures should be treated by acute reduction of cardiac filling pressure by posturing, venesection, and vasodilator drugs. When acute pulmonary edema is associated with normal or reduced right heart pressures, it should be treated like adult respiratory distress syndrome (ARDS). In patients with hypotension and shock, circulatory disturbances should be corrected (for example, with plasma expanders and selective vasoconstrictors such as dopamine). Hemocultures should be taken, and broad-spectrum antimicrobial treatment started immediately because of the risk of septicemia. Blood glucose should be measured frequently, especially in patients at high risk of developing hypoglycemia (see above). In any patient with proven or suspected hypoglycemia 50% glucose should be injected intravenously. Continuous intravenous infusion of 5% dextrose, 80 mL/(kg·24 h), prevented hypoglycemia in African children with cerebral malaria who were normoglycemic before the start of quinine treatment [39]; however, in Thai adults, hypoglycemia sometimes arose despite continuous intravenous infusion of 5 or 10% dextrose. Quinine- or quinidine-induced hyperinsulinemia can be prevented by the somatostatin analogue SMS201-995. A single dose of 50 μg by subcutaneous injection followed by 1 mg glucagon was effective.

When more than 10 percent of erythrocytes are infected, the prognosis is very poor. In these cases, exchange transfusion may reduce parasite burden more rapidly than chemotherapy alone and has other possible benefits such as removal of harmful circulating factors and replacement of platelets and clotting factors. More than 30 patients have been treated with encouraging results.

Malaria in pregnancy

In pregnancy, the high risk of maternal and fetal mortality demands early diagnosis and rapid treatment of malaria. Chloroquine and quinine can be used safely but sulfonamide-pyrimethamine, tetracycline, primaquine, and aspirin are contraindicated in late pregnancy. In late pregnancy it is important to start fetal monitoring before the first dose of quinine so that effects of the disease are not confused with drug toxicity. Hypoglycemia is particularly common in women with malaria, both before treatment and as a result of quinine- or quinidine-induced hyperinsulinemia. Fetal distress is usually the result of placental insufficiency but may be associated with high maternal temperature and hypoglycemia. Early obstetrical intervention should be considered for the benefit of mother and fetus. Fluid balance is particularly critical in pregnancy. It is dangerous for a woman to go into labor while fluid-overloaded, as the sudden increase in peripheral vascular resistance post partum may precipitate pulmonary edema. Exchange transfu-

sion has proved an effective way of managing severe anemia with high-output cardiac failure.

Malaria in children

In hyperendemic areas children under the age of 6 years may suffer from severe infections while they are acquiring immunity. Febrile convulsions are common under the age of 4 years even in association with uncomplicated falciparum malaria or benign malarias. However, if the patient remains unconscious for more than about 30 min after the febrile convulsion, cerebral malaria should be suspected. There is a suggestion, as yet unproven, that protein-calorie malnutrition and iron deficiency may protect children from severe falciparum malaria. The clinical pattern of severe malaria differs in children and adults. Children have a shorter history of fever before becoming comatose (average about 2 days) and may remain unconscious for only 24 h. Cough, vomiting, diarrhea and convulsions are particularly common; corneal and vestibulo-ocular reflexes may be lost; pupillary responses may be asymmetrical; and there may be a general reduction in muscle tone. Jaundice, pulmonary edema, and renal failure are uncommon, but anemia is common and severe, as is hypoglycemia and its neurological sequelae. Hypoglycemia is usually detected on admission to hospital and before antimalarial treatment has been started. Plasma insulin concentrations are appropriately low; blood levels of lactate, alanine, and counterregulatory hormones are high; and there is no evidence of starvation ketosis [39]. Parasitemias may be very high in partially immune children with severe malaria, who may have surprisingly mild symptoms.

The principles of management are the same as for adults. It is important to reduce fever, correct severe anemia by cautious blood transfusion, avoid fluid overload, and prevent convulsions. Chloroquine tablets can be made more palatable for children if their bitter taste is obscured by grinding them up with honey or jelly. In an emergency, solutions or suspensions of chloroquine, quinine, and mefloquine can be given by nasogastric tube. Loading doses of quinine (see above) have been used safely in children with severe malaria.

Treatment of *P. vivax*, *P. ovale*, and *P. malariae*

Acute attacks by any of these species should be treated with chloroquine (see above). *P. vivax* and *P. ovale* infections acquired through mosquito bites may have persistant hepatic forms (hypnozoites). These must be eliminated with primaquine to prevent relapses. The dose is 7.5 mg twice daily for 14 days [children 0.25 mg/(kg·day) for 14 days] except in areas where the primaquine-resistant Chesson strain of *P. vivax* is prevalent (for example, in New Guinea, and Indonesia) where the dose should be doubled. In patients with mild G-6-PD deficiency, primaquine-induced hemolysis can be reduced by giving 45 mg/week for 8 weeks [for children 0.75 mg/(kg·week) for 8 weeks], but in patients with severe

G-6-PD deficiency, chloroquine prophylaxis or treatment of relapses is preferable to primaquine treatment. Primaquine is not indicated in the treatment of transfusion malaria because erythrocytic parasites of blood-induced infection do not infect the liver.

Sites of action of antimalarial drugs

Pyrimethamine has a greater affinity for parasite than host dihydrofolate reductase and blocks folate metabolism. Pyrimethamine resistance results from point mutations in the active site of the gene encoding dihydrofolate reductase [49]. Sulfonamides block utilization of PABA.

Chloroquine, quinine, and quinidine are concentrated in the parasite's food vacuole, raising its pH and so perhaps interfering with enzymatic digestion. Chloroquine resistance is associated with increased efflux of chloroquine from these vacuoles, an effect that can be prevented in vitro by calcium channel–blocking agents such as verapamil [50,51]. Quinine and chloroquine also bind ferriprotoporphyrin IX, producing a toxic complex which cannot be detoxified by binding to the hemin-binding protein. The antimalarial action of artemisinine (ginghaosu) is dependent on an endoperoxide bridge which may act by altering membrane permeability.

Prevention

While physicians in western countries will seldom see malaria patients, they will frequently be asked for advice by travelers to endemic areas. In the past, recommendation of a single drug, chloroquine, would have sufficed. Today, because of chloroquine-resistant *P. falciparum* and the lack of a completely satisfactory alternative drug, textbooks can only give the broad principles of prophylaxis. Specific chemoprophylactic regimens are constantly changing because of new reports of toxicity and the data from trials of chemoprophylaxis. One drug under study, mefloquine, could become the drug of choice in the near future. Updated recommendations on chemoprophylaxis can be obtained, for example, from publications from the Centers for Disease Control, Atlanta, Georgia. The basic principles are as follows: First, no drug today guarantees absolute protection from malaria; *P. falciparum* resistance has been ascribed to all antimalarial drugs. Therefore, the traveler should be warned that fever during or following travel in endemic areas may be caused by malaria, even though the traveler is on drug suppression. Second, the traveler should actively avoid contact with evening- and night-biting anophelines. Measures include screening of housing, use of bed netting impregnated with permethrin emulsifiable concentrate, use of mosquito repellent such as Off (*N,N*-diethyltoluamide) and insecticide aerosol (a synthetic pyrethroid), and wearing of protective clothing (e.g., trousers, long-sleeved shirt, and boots). Third, the risk of malaria varies with the area visited. As a generalization, the risk of acquiring *P. falciparum* is high in sub-

Saharan Africa and New Guinea, moderate in the Indian subcontinent, and low in southeast Asia and Latin America. In some countries, the area visited will influence the risk. For example, a visitor to Thailand would be at very low risk in Bangkok and at high risk of multi-drug-resistant infections in some rural areas. Fourth, the length of stay in an endemic area will influence the choice of regimen. A cumulative dose of chloroquine exceeding 100 g (more than 5 years' prophylaxis at normal dosage), or even less in the elderly, may cause macular degeneration of the retina. Doxycycline prophylaxis cannot be recommended for periods longer than a few months, because there is a lack of data on its long-term use. Fifth, the intelligence and reliability of the traveler and the traveler's access to medical treatment will influence the choice of regimen. These considerations can be used in deciding whether to give the traveler a curative regimen for self-medication in case of drug failure in isolated regions.

Chloroquine is a safe antimalarial drug effective against chloroquine-sensitive *P. falciparum* and against the other three species of human malaria. Chloroquine phosphate, 500 mg once weekly, should be started 2 weeks before travel and continued until 6 weeks after leaving an endemic area. In chloroquine-resistant areas where the risk of infection is high, other drugs may be combined with chloroquine such as proguanil, 200 mg daily, or doxycycline, 100 mg daily. There is increasing evidence for the efficacy of proguanil, the safest antimalarial drug, against *P. falciparum*, but the optimal regimen has not yet been determined. The side effects of doxycycline include photosensitivity and fungal esophagitis and vaginitis. The drug is contraindicated during pregnancy and in young children. Mefloquine may become the prophylactic of choice when more information becomes available on its toxicity and efficacy. Fansidar, pyrimethamine combined with a long-acting sulfonamide, sulfadoxine, is no longer recommended because of fatal cutaneous reactions in approximately 1 in 20,000 people taking the drug.

Travelers who were heavily exposed to malaria and are not G-6-PD–deficient should receive primaquine on return from an endemic area to eliminate hepatic forms of *P. vivax* and *P. ovale* (dosage as above.)

Chemoprophylaxis during pregnancy and in young children

As discussed above, chemoprophylaxis in areas of high risk for chloroquine-resistant *P. falciparum* is inadequate; therefore, pregnant women and young children should not travel to these areas unless travel is essential and warrants the risk. Chloroquine is safe for use in both groups. The prophylactic dose of chloroquine base in children is 5 mg/(kg·week) up to the maximum adult dose of 300 mg/week. Because of the bitter taste of chloroquine, a liquid suspension of chloroquine sulfate (Nivaquine) is available in the tropics. Doxycycline is not recommended for pregnant women or children under 8 years of age because of damage to bone and teeth.

Because of its risk to mother and child, acute malaria should be treated according to the regimens outlined above (see ''Therapy''). Primaquine should not be used during pregnancy.

POPULATION

EPIDEMIOLOGY

The endemicity is determined by vectorial capacity [52], host factors such as immunity, and the character of the parasite. The most widely used classification of endemicity of *P. falciparum* derives from spleen rates in children 2 to 9 years of age and in adults.

Hypoendemic: Spleen rate less than 10 percent in children.
Mesoendemic: Spleen rate 10 to 49 percent in children.
Hyperendemic: Spleen rate constantly over 50 percent in children and high in adults.
Holoendemic: Spleen rate constantly over 75 percent in children and low in adults.

Malaria transmission from year to year may be subject to various degrees of fluctuation, which determines stability. Transmission in areas of stable malaria is relatively constant over the years, even in the presence of relatively large environmental changes. Endemicity is usually high in areas with a high vectorial capacity. An example of stable malaria would be *P. falciparum* malaria in tropical Africa transmitted by the *A. gambiae* complex and *A. funestus*. The high degree of immunity in the older population and multiple reinfection each year from high vectorial capacity stabilize the parasite rate in the community.

Transmission in regions of unstable malaria is marginal with low vectorial capacity. Marked increase in vectorial capacity as a result of unusual environmental conditions may cause epidemics.

The factors in the epidemiology of malaria can be analyzed from the vector (vectorial capacity), parasite, and human host.

The vector (vectorial capacity)

The central concept in understanding malarial transmission in any part of the world is vectorial capacity [52], which is defined as the expected number of new infections produced per infective case per day. It is determined by the interaction of the vector mosquito and its biology with the environment and the parasite.

$$\text{Vectorial capacity} = (ma)\,(x)\,(a)\left(\frac{p^n}{-\ln p}\right)$$

The definition and implications for each term in the equation are described below.

1. The number of mosquito bites per person per day (ma). This factor will be influenced by the host preference of the vectors (a) and the vector density (m). Vector populations vary according to availability of breeding sites (e.g., rainy season in the tropics) and warm seasons in temperate zones. Great increases in vector population may result from unusual climatic

Table 30-3. Methods for the control of malaria

Target	Method	Example	Limitations
Mosquito larvae	Removal of breeding sites	Drainage of swamps Cover cisterns	Limited to areas of high population density
	Alternating irrigation	Cotton & cereal crops	Not useful for rice
	Larviciding	Abate in wells	Not effective if breeding surfaces extensive
	Biological control	Larvivorous fish	Breeding sites must be stable
Adult mosquitoes	Kills adults	Pyrethroids	Short-lasting
	Residual insecticides	Intradomiciliary spraying with DDT, malathione, propoxur	Expensive, resistance, behavioral avoidance, exophilic mosquitoes, mobile population, outdoors at night
	Ultralow volume spray (ULV)	ULV spraying from air to control epidemics in Haiti	Expensive, insecticide resistance, short-lasting effect
	Block contact with humans	Screens, netting, repellent	Expensive, requires high individual motivation
Asexual erythrocytic parasite	Treatment of cases	Chloroquine and primaquine	Not proven to have major impact on transmission
	Mass drug prophylaxis	Weekly chloroquine	Expensive, difficult to maintain cooperation of population
		Medicated salt	May accelerate onset of drug resistance

conditions such as puddling of streams in Sri Lanka during unusually dry periods. Control measures (Table 30-3) would be directed at reducing mosquito populations and blocking access to human beings (e.g., mosquito netting).

2. Efficiency with which malaria parasites infect mosquitoes and complete the sporogonic cycle (x). For unknown reasons, only anopheline mosquitoes can transmit human malaria. More than one *Anopheles* species may exist within a region, but some may not be susceptible to infection. Some mosquitoes may be excellent vectors of the local malarial parasites but do not transmit the same malarial species from another region. An ideal target for genetic engineering of mosquito populations would be the introduction of a gene for refractoriness to malaria. A single gene for refractoriness to malaria was demonstrated for *P. gallinaceum* in *Aedes aegypti* [53] and a multigene system for encapsulation of malaria parasites in the midgut of *Anopheles gambiae* [54].

3. The host preference of vectors (a). A mosquito must feed twice on a human to transmit malaria, once to become infected and once to transmit the infection. The frequency with which mosquitoes feed on hosts other than humans will influence vector efficiency. One of the mysteries during the early part of this century was why increases in populations of *A. maculipennis* were not associated with epidemics of malaria in one part of Europe, although it was the vector in other parts. Mosquitoes from both regions could be infected with malaria when fed directly on humans. It was later discovered that *A. maculipennis* was not one species but a species complex. The nonvector species had a genetically determined behavior of feeding predominately on animals. It might be possible in the future to introduce a gene into the mosquito population which would change the feeding preference from humans to animals.

4. Expectation of life of infected mosquitoes after completion of sporogonic development ($p^n/-\ln p$). This contains two terms: p, the daily mosquito survival rate, and n, the time required for completion of sporogonic development (time from ingestion of an infected blood meal to infectious sporozoites in salivary glands). Residual insecticides, the most important tool for the control of malaria, shorten mosquito survival, a factor taken to the nth power.

The second term, n, sporogonic development, is greatly influenced by temperature. Sporogony of *P. vivax* ceases below 16°C, that of *P. falciparum* below 20°C. For this reason *P. vivax* is better transmitted in temperate regions than *P. falciparum*. It is evident from Fig. 30-7 that sporogony of *P. vivax* requires 55 days at 16°C and only 7 days at 28°C. Malaria is rarely transmitted above 2500 m because of low temperature.

Parasite

Low temperatures block sporogonic development [see ''The Vector (Vectorial Capacity)'']. In regions of long-standing transmission, the parasite adapts to local anthropophilic mos-

quitoes. A more dramatic example of adaption is the fact that the relapse pattern of *P. vivax* corresponds to vector population densities [5]. Relapses occur soon after the primary attack in tropical regions where transmission is perennial. In contrast, relapses occur 6 months or longer after the primary attack in other regions where winter or the dry season in the tropics causes marked seasonal fluctuations in vector populations. Thus, relapses occur when the vector density is high.

P. falciparum appears to suppress concurrent infections with *P. vivax* or *P. malariae*.

Human host

Humans through their patterns of life influence the intensity of malaria transmission. First, poor water management (e.g., in agriculture) increases breeding sites. Second, practices such as nocturnal outdoor activities and use of mosquito netting will affect exposure to the vector. Third, population migration may cause the spread or the reintroduction of malaria. Fourth, wars, limited resources, and mismanagement may interfere with ongoing malaria control measures. Fifth, large-scale use of insecticides in agriculture may select for insecticide resistance in the malaria vector.

Innate resistance and immunity determine the distribution of infection and disease in a community. For example, Africans who are Duffy blood group–negative are refractory to *P. vivax* [25]. Immunity in holoendemic areas of tropical Africa largely limits severe disease to preschool children. From the viewpoint of transmission, however, the immune older children and adults still have asexual parasitemia and gametocytemia and,

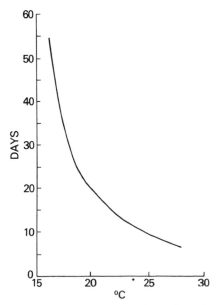

Figure 30-7. Duration of sporogony of *Plasmodium vivax* at various temperatures. *(After [55].)*

although asymptomatic, are important reservoirs for infection of mosquitoes.

Epidemiology of malaria in nonendemic areas

Most malaria patients seen in Europe and in the United States are infected in Africa, Asia, and Latin America (imported cases). Mosquito vectors capable of transmitting malaria still exist in countries where malaria has been eradicated (e.g., *Anopheles freeborni* in the western United States). In these areas, episodes of transmission have occurred following infection of local mosquitoes by individuals infected in the tropics (introduced cases). Congenital infection probably occurs more frequently than estimates from areas with high malaria endemicity would suggest because transplacental immunity suppresses parasite multiplication. Other causes of infection in nonendemic areas include blood transfusion and communal use of syringes by drug addicts. The single most important factor in preventing transfusion malaria is the exclusion of donors who have lived or traveled in endemic areas until their risk of infection is negligible, since chronic infections are often asymptomatic. Most falciparum-infected individuals undergo self-cure in 3 years; a rare case may persist for 4 years. *P. vivax* and *P. ovale* may last for 3 to 5 years. *P. malariae* may persist as an asymptomatic erythrocytic infection for decades. Since *P. falciparum* and *P. vivax* are the most serious problems, donors should be excluded for 4 years after return from the tropics.

Distribution of malaria

Malaria in large measure remains a tropical disease; eradication has eliminated malaria from the United States, Cuba, Jamaica, Puerto Rico, the Antilles, Chile, Israel, Japan, Lebanon, Taiwan, North Korea, Europe, and Australia.

Africa. Sub-Saharan tropical Africa is the major focus of malaria in the world with high morbidity and mortality in preschool children. *P. falciparum* predominates followed in frequency by *P. malariae*. *P. ovale* has replaced *P. vivax* in west Africa and occurs in east Africa in the distribution of the Duffy-negative blood group genotype (*FyFy*). Low-level transmission, predominantly of *P. vivax*, occurs in north Africa. Chloroquine resistance is now relatively widespread in Africa and can be of a high level in east and central Africa, where resistance to Fansidar also occurs.

Asia. The recurrence of malaria, predominantly *P. vivax*, in India, Pakistan, and Sri Lanka occurred in the late 1960s and 1970s. Malaria has again been brought under control in this region at heavy cost to the health budget. Chloroquine-resistant *P. falciparum* occurs commonly in Burma, Thailand, Laos, Kampuchea, Vietnam, Philippines, Malaysia, and southern China with extension south and east into Indonesia, New Guinea, the Solomon Islands and Vanuatu and west to central India. Fansidar resistance is common in Thailand and bordering regions.

Sporadic cases of *P. ovale* have been reported from southeast Asia and New Guinea.

Americas. *P. vivax* predominates in Central America. *P. falciparum* in Haiti, and both *P. falciparum* and *P. vivax* in South America. Multi-insecticide-resistant *A. albimanus* presents control problems in Central America, largely as a result of aerial spraying of cotton crops. Chloroquine-resistant *P. falciparum* occurs in South America and north to the Panama Canal. Fansidar resistance occurs in Brazil.

Pacific Islands. Hyperendemic *P. falciparum* occurs in the coastal regions of Papua New Guinea. Malaria occurs in Vanuatu and the Solomon Islands. Chloroquine-resistant *P. falciparum* extends eastward through New Guinea to the Solomon Islands and Vanuatu.

MALARIA CONTROL AND ERADICATION

The major tools for the control of malaria have been directed against the vector. Antimalarial drugs, especially chloroquine, reduce morbidity and mortality, although in some instances they have been used as primary tools for achieving malaria control, especially where malaria is unstable, where the malarious areas are small and confined by natural boundaries of transmission, and where the people are easily accessible.

The methods for the control of malaria are summarized in Table 30-3. When malaria eradication was first instituted as a program of WHO in the 1950s, the program depended mainly on spraying walls with residual insecticides, malaria case detection, and treatment of patients with antimalarial drugs. With the failure of this program a new approach called integrated control was instituted. This means the intelligent use of all tools available (Table 30-3), taking into consideration mosquito bionomics, population distribution, and feasible control targets within the financial and administrative capabilities of the countries involved. Because of widely distributed breeding areas and the difficulty of defining the best method of attack from district to district within a country, residual insecticides will remain the mainstay of most programs, which highlights the importance of insecticide resistance. Health workers and agricultural planners must cooperate to minimize this problem, since indiscriminate use of insecticides on crops has, in large measure, caused insecticide resistance.

Malaria control has not been considered feasible in much of tropical Africa; the countries depend on the widespread availability of antimalarial drugs for limiting disease. The high vectorial capacity and the outdoor feeding and resting of vectors such as *A. arabiensis* [55] make control impossible at this time. Therefore the goal of the program in this area is improved diagnosis and treatment for early cure of infections and prevention of death.

Problems in antimalarial control operations

The methods for control, even where successful, demand militarylike organization and heavy financial investment. It is not surprising, then, that financial, administrative, political, and operational difficulties would often interfere with these programs. For example, integration of antimalarial programs into other health programs such as mother-child health and population control in part explained the resurgence of malaria in India. Human factors such as population movements and outdoor sleeping habits cause additional problems for malaria control programs.

Since residual insecticides are the mainstay of any program, insecticide resistance, behavioral avoidance of sprayed surfaces, and outdoor feeding have created major problems. In addition, the spread of multi-drug-resistant *P. falciparum* will probably increase morbidity and mortality in regions of resurgent malaria.

There is no question that new tools for malaria control are sorely needed in the decades ahead.

MALARIA RESEARCH

It is peculiar that the use of DDT as a residual insecticide in the 1950s was felt to have eliminated malariology as a viable field for young investigators, since sub-Saharan Africa was largely untouched by this method. This experience would argue that the countries most affected by malaria should develop their own capabilities for research toward its elimination. Research on malaria must be three-pronged. First, there is the immediate need for new drugs and insecticides or insecticidelike agents (e.g., *Bacillus thuringiensis israeliensis*). Second, vaccines which should become available during the next decade or two will reduce morbidity and offer additional tools for malaria control and eradication in some areas. Third, novel approaches to vector control would offer hope to areas such as tropical Africa where the available methods are too expensive and may have only limited success.

Research for new antimalarial drugs

There is an immediate need for new blood schizontocidal drugs to replace chloroquine wherever this rapid-acting, inexpensive, and safe drug has lost its efficacy against *P. falciparum*. Mefloquine, a new antimalarial drug developed by the Walter Reed Army Institute of Research, is highly effective against chloroquine-resistant *P. falciparum* [56]. If resistance develops to mefloquine, a quinoline methanol, cross-resistance may exist for other new antimalarials being developed by Walter Reed such as the phenanthrene methanols. A drug derived from a traditional Chinese herbal remedy for malaria, qinghaosu, appears effective against chloroquine-resistant strains of *P. falciparum* and is undergoing clinical trials. Other drugs under development include halofantrine, enpiroline, arte-ether (a qinghaosu derivative), and synthetic trioxanes.

Drugs for radical cure of *P. vivax* and *P. ovale* (i.e., that kill latent forms in the liver) are needed as replacements for primaquine, an 8-aminoquinoline, which is toxic and requires a long course of treatment. Walter Reed has synthesized other 8-aminoquinolines to reduce toxicity and increase efficacy. No new class of drugs with radical curative activity has been identified.

Clinical research

There is a need to understand pathophysiological mechanisms in humans so that treatment of the disease can be put on a rational basis. Pharmacological studies are necessary in human patients of different ages, races, and severities of disease so that drug regimens can be optimized. The use of ancillary treatments must be critically tested, not merely used on the basis of anecdotal reports.

Vector research

Vector research has immediate needs for new, cheap insecticides, new methods of larviciding, and better use of available tools. In the long term, new methods for vector control are needed, especially in areas of high vectorial capacity where residual insecticides and other presently available techniques are ineffective. Vaccines would probably not, of themselves, eliminate transmission in these areas and may not protect young children, the main victims. Therefore novel approaches to vector control would change the present bleak prospects for malaria control and eradication. For example, introduction of a gene in the mosquito population for refractoriness to malaria could eliminate malaria transmission. Research on the use of bed nets impregnated with pyrethroids is under study, but the effect on disease as well as infection rates must be evaluated. It is theoretically possible that such a method would decrease the attack rate but increase morbidity and mortality.

Vaccine development

There is no question that vaccines will be developed against malaria; vaccines have been successful in every animal model tested. The form that vaccines will take and when they will be available is unpredictable. The ultimate vaccine will probably contain antigens from different species (e.g., *P. falciparum* and *P. vivax*) and against different stages in the parasite's life cycle (sporozoite, asexual, and gamete). Such a vaccine would reduce or eliminate morbidity and mortality and block transmission of the parasite to others.

Sporozoite Vaccines. This is the only vaccine successfully applied to humans [57]. Vaccination, however, required large numbers of x-ray-attentuated sporozoites, clearly impractical for mass vaccination. The mechanism of immunity in humans after immunization with irradiated sporozoites is unknown. In mice, cytotoxic T cells are of primary importance [34]. One epitope for cytotoxic T cells has been defined for the CS protein of *P. falciparum*, but the epitope is variant among clones [58], complicating subunit vaccine development. Vaccine trials in humans to induce antibodies to the repeating epitope of the falciparum CS protein have been largely unsuccessful [34].

Clearly, if effective, a sporozoite-based vaccine would eliminate the disease and transmission as well. However, if one sporozoite escapes the immune system, a fully virulent infection could occur. Since the sporozoites leave the circulation within minutes after being injected and enter the protected environment of the liver, they must be eliminated immediately on entering the body. Thus, there is no opportunity for the infection to boost immunity. Therefore, the immune system must be at a high level at all times. The question remains whether this vaccine will be useful in the developing world where repeated vaccination at short intervals would be impractical.

Vaccines against Liver Stages. Vaccines against this stage have a potential advantage over those against sporozoites in that the parasites are within these cells for at least 7 days, which should allow adequate time for their elimination. As in the case of sporozoites, if any parasites escape immune surveillance, severe infection could result.

Vaccines against Asexual Stages. Protection against the asexual erythrocytic parasite, the cause of the disease, would probably be the centerpiece of any vaccine. In every animal malaria studied to date, it has been possible to immunize against this stage. In most cases, an adjuvant has been necessary to induce protective immunity [20]. The vaccines have usually consisted of whole parasitized erythrocytes, merozoites (the extracellular invasive forms), or partially purified antigens. In these studies, the infection has been modified, allowing survival of the host, but usually the infection has not been prevented.

The major focus of research today is to identify antigens that can be synthesized. The two major points of attack are the antigens on the erythrocyte surface and the merozoite antigens. Malaria induces changes in the erythrocyte membrane such as the protrusion of knobs that are found on erythrocytes infected with *P. falciparum*. These knobs are responsible for the parasite's attachment to endothelium; the determinants for such attachment may be parasitic in origin.

Antibodies to merozoites could block invasion either by agglutinating merozoites or by specifically blocking receptors for attachment to erythrocytes. Monoclonal antibodies that block invasion in vitro are being sought.

Gamete Vaccines. This is an altruistic vaccine because it would bring no protection to the recipient. Such a vaccine could be used in areas where vectorial capacity is relatively low (e.g., Sri Lanka) to help in the eradication of malaria or to control renewed epidemic spread.

Gamete immunity is mediated by antibody that blocks fertilization in the mosquito's stomach [20]. Monoclonal antibodies have been identified that mimic the effect of immune serum. One target antigen on falciparum ookinetes consists of four epidermal growth factor–like domains [59]; this is being developed for vaccine trials.

Problems in Vaccine Development. Even if the immunogens were identified, they may not be effective without the use of adjuvants [20]. The question remains, what adjuvant to use and how to test for it. An adjuvant may be highly effective in one animal system but may be ineffective in another. For example, malarial antigen with Freund's complete adjuvant protects monkeys against lethal *P. knowlesi* but induces no protection in the rodent systems.

Another problem with vaccine development is that immunity to asexual erythrocytic infection with *P. falciparum* tends to be strain-specific [27]. Multiple strains exist within one area, each with unique antigens. In addition, some malarial parasites can change their antigens in response to the host immune response (antigenic variation). Clearly, the immunogen must be common to all parasites or have limited variability to be of use for vaccines. We are just entering the era of defining the antigens so that we can know their potential variability. Subunit vaccines may face the further problem that the malarial proteins that are targets of immunity have evolved to be poor immunogens, that is, they have few T-cell epitopes.

One last consideration will be the effectiveness of vaccines in young children and in semi-immune adults, many of whom may be infected at the time of vaccination.

REFERENCES

1 Yoshida N, Potochjak P, Nussenzweig V, et al: Biosynthesis of Pb44, the protective antigen of sporozoites of *Plasmodium berghei*. J Exp Med 154:1225–1236, 1981

2 Dame JB, Williams JL, McCutchan TF, et al: Structure of the gene encoding the immunodominant surface antigen on the sporozoite of the human malaria parasite *Plasmodium falciparum*. Science 225:593–599, 1984

3 Aley SB, Bates MD, Tam JP, et al: Synthetic peptides from the circumsporozoite proteins of *Plasmodium falciparum* and *Plasmodium knowlesi* recognize the human hepatoma cell line Hep G2-A16 *in vitro*. J Exp Med 164:1915–1922, 1986

4 Krotoski WA, Garnham PCC, Bray RS, et al: Observations on early and late post-sporozoite tissues in primate malaria. I. Discovery of a new latent form (hypnozoite), and failure of the immunofluorescence technique to detect hepatic forms within the first 24 hours after infection. Am J Trop Med Hyg 31:24–35, 1982

5 Miller LH: Transfusion malaria, in Greenwalt, TJ, Jamieson GA (eds): *Transmissible Disease and Blood Transfusion*. New York, Grune & Stratton, 1975, pp 246–249

6 Hadley T, Klotz FW, Miller LH: Invasion of erythrocytes by malaria parasites: Cellular and molecular overview. Ann Rev Microbiol 40:451–477, 1986

7 Mitchell GH, Hadley TJ, McGinniss MH, et al: Invasion of erythrocytes by *Plasmodium falciparum* malaria parasites: Evidence for receptor heterogeneity and two receptors. Blood 67:1519–1521, 1986

8 Hadley TJ, Klotz FW, Pasvol G, et al: Falciparum malaria parasites invade erythrocytes that lack glycophorin A and B (M^kM^k). Strain differences indicate receptor heterogeneity and two pathways for invasion. J Clin Invest 80:1190–1193, 1987

9 Camus D, Hadley TJ: A *Plasmodium falciparum* antigen that binds to host erythrocytes and merozoites. Science 230:553–556, 1985

10 Haynes JD, Dalton JP, Klotz FW, et al: Receptor-like specificity of a *Plasmodium knowlesi* malarial protein binds to Duffy antigen ligands on erythrocytes. J Exp Med 167:1873–1881, 1988

11 Luse S, Miller LH: *Plasmodium falciparum* malaria: Ultrastructure of parasitized erythrocytes in cardiac vessels. Am J Trop Med Hyg 20:650–655, 1971

12 Kilekian A: Characterization of a protein correlated with the production of knob-like protrusions on membranes of erythrocytes infected with *Plasmodium falciparum*. Proc Natl Acad Sci USA 76:4650–4653, 1979

13 Leech JH, Barnwell JW, Miller LH, et al: Identification of a strain-specific malarial antigen exposed on the surface of *Plasmodium falciparum* infected erythrocytes. J Exp Med 159:1567–1575, 1984

14 Barnwell JW, Ockenhouse CF, Knowles DM: Monoclonal antibody OKM5 inhibits the *in vitro* binding of *Plasmodium falciparum* infected erythrocytes to monocytes, endothelial, and C32 melanoma cells. J Immunol 135:3494–3497, 1985

15 Roberts DD, Sherwood JA, Spitalnik SL, et al: Thrombospondin binds falciparum malaria parasitized erythrocytes and may mediate cytoadherence. Nature 318:64–66, 1985

16 Sherman IW: Biochemistry of *Plasmodium* (malarial parasites). Microbiol Rev 43:453–495, 1979

17 Friedman MJ, Roth EF, Nagel RL, et al: *Plasmodium falciparum*: Physiological interactions with the human sickle cell. Exp Parasitol 47:73–80, 1979

18 Trager W, Jensen JB: Human malaria parasites in continuous culture. Science 193:673–675, 1976

19 Carter R, Miller LH: A method for the study of gametocytogenesis by *Plasmodium falciparum* in culture: Evidence for environmental modulation of gametocytogenesis. Bull WHO 57 (suppl 1):38–67, 1979

20 Miller LH, Howard RJ, Carter R, et al: Research toward malaria vaccines. Science 234:1349–1356, 1986

21 Walliker D, Carter R, Sanderson A: Genetic studies on *Plasmodium chabaudi*: Recombination between enzyme markers. Parasitology 70:19–24, 1975

22 McCutchan TF, Dame JB, Miller LH, et al: Evolutionary relatedness of *Plasmodium* as determined by the structure of DNA. Science 225:808–811, 1984

23 Allison AC: Polymorphism and natural selection in human populations. Cold Spring Harbor Symp Quant Biol 29: 137–149, 1964

24 Friedman MJ: Erythrocytic mechanism of sickle-cell resistance to malaria. Proc Natl Acad Sci USA 75:1994–1997, 1978

25 Miller LH, Mason SJ, Clyde DF, et al: The resistance factor to *Plasmodium vivax* in Blacks. N Engl J Med 295:302–304, 1976

26 Kidson C, Lamond G, Saul A, et al: Ovalocytic erythrocytes from Melanesians are resistant to invasion by malaria parasites in culture. Proc Natl Acad Sci USA 78:5829–5832, 1981

27 James SP, Nicol WD, Shute PG: A study of induced malignant tertian malaria. Proc R Soc Med 25:1153–1186, 1932

28 Wilson RJM: Serotyping *Plasmodium falciparum* malaria with S-antigens. Nature 284:451–452, 1980

29 Cohen S, McGregor IA, Carrington SP: Gammoglobulin and acquired immunity to human malaria. Nature 192:733–737, 1961

30 Cohen S, Butcher GA: Properties of protective malarial antibody. Immunology 19:369–383, 1970

31 Jayawardena AN: Immune responses in malaria, in Mansfield JM (ed): *Parasitic Diseases*, vol 1, *The Immunology*. New York, Dekker, 1981, pp. 85–136

32 Hoffman SL, Oster CN, Plowe C, et al: Naturally acquired antibodies to sporozoites do not prevent malaria: Vaccine development implications. Science 237:639–642, 1987

33 Potochjak P, Yoshida N, Nussenzweig RS, et al: Monovalent fragments (Fab) of monoclonal antibodies to a sporozoite surface antigen (Pb44) protect mice against malarial infection. J Exp Med 151:1504–1513, 1980

34 Good MF, Berzofsky JA, Miller LH: The T cell response to the malaria circumsporozoite protein. An immunologic approach to vaccine development. Ann Rev Immunol 6:663–688, 1988

35 MacPherson, GG, Warrell MJ, White NJ, et al: Human cerebral malaria: A quantitative ultrastructural analysis of parasitized erythrocyte sequestration. Am J Pathol 119:385–401, 1985

36 Warrell DA: Pathophysiology of severe falciparum malaria in man. Parasitology 94(suppl):S53–S76, 1987

37 Warrell DA, White NJ, Veall NJ, et al: Cerebral anerobic glycolysis and reduced cerebral oxygen transport in human cerebral malaria. Lancet, ii:534–538, 1988

38 World Health Organization Malaria Action Programme: Severe and complicated malaria. Trans R Soc Trop Med Hyg 80(suppl):1–50, 1986

39 Taylor TE, Molyneux ME, Wirima JJ, et al: Blood glucose levels in Malawian children before and during the administration of intravenous quinine for severe falciparum malaria. N Engl J Med 319:1040–1047, 1988

40 White NJ, Warrell DA, Chantahvanich P, et al: Severe hypoglycemia and hyperinsulinemia in falciparum malaria. N Engl J Med 309:61–66, 1983

41 Crane GG: Tropical splenomegaly. Part II. Oceania. Clin Haematol 10:976–982, 1981

42 Fakunle YM: Tropical splenomegaly. Part I. Tropical Africa. Clin Haematol 10:963–975, 1981

43 Whittle HC, Brown J, Marsh K: T-cell control of Epstein-Barr virus–infected B cells is losing during *P. falciparum* malaria. Nature 312:449–450, 1984

44 Barker RH Jr, Suebsaeng L, Rooney W, et al: Specific DNA probe for the diagnosis of *Plasmodium falciparum* malaria. Science 231: 1434–1436, 1986

45 Rudnitsky G, Miller KD, Padva T, et al: Continuous infusion of quinidine gluconate for treating children with severe *Plasmodium falciparum* malaria. J Infect Dis 155:1040–1043, 1987

46 White NJ, Looareesuwan S, Philips RE, et al: Single dose phenobarbitone prevents convulsions in cerebral malaria. Lancet ii:64–66, 1988

47 Warrell DA, Looareesuwan S, Warrell MJ, et al: Dexamethasone proves deleterious in cerebral malaria. A double-blind trial in 100 comatose patients. N Engl J Med 306:313–319, 1982

48 Hoffman SL, Rustama D, Punjabi NH, et al: High-dose dexa-

methasone in quinine-treated patients with cerebral malaria: a double-blind, placebo-controlled trial. J Infect Dis 158:325–331, 1988.

49 Peterson D, Walliker D, Wellems T: Evidence that a point mutation in dihydrofolate reductase–thymidylate synthase confers resistance to pyrimethamine in falciparum malaria. Proc Natl Acad Sci USA 85:9114–9118, 1988

50 Martin SK, Oduola AMJ, Milhous WK: Reversal of chloroquine resistance in *Plasmodium falciparum* by verapamil. Science 235:899–901, 1987

51 Krogstad DH, Gluzman IY, Kyle DE, et al: Efflux of chloroquine from *Plasmodium falciparum:* Mechanism of chloroquine resistance. Science 238:1283–1285, 1987

52 Garrett-Jones C, Shidrawi GR: Malaria vectorial capacity of a population of *Anopheles gambiae.* An exercise in epidemiological entomology. Bull WHO 40:531–545, 1969

53 Kilama WL, Craig CB: Monofactorial inheritance of susceptibility of *Plasmodium gallinaceum* in *Aedes aegypti.* Ann Trop Med Parasitol 63:419–432, 1969

54 Collins FH, Sakai RK, Vernick KD, et al: Genetic selection of a *Plasmodium* refractory strain of the malaria vector *Anopheles gambiae.* Science 234:607–610, 1986

55 Coluzzi M, Sabatini A, Petrarca V, et al: Behavioral divergences between mosquitoes with different inversion karyotypes in polymorphic populations of the *Anopheles gambiae* complex. Nature 266:832–833, 1977

56 Sweeney TR: The present status of malaria chemotherapy: Mefloquine, a novel antimalarial. Med Res Rev 1:281–301, 1981

57 Clyde DF, Most H, McCarthy V, et al: Immunization of man against sporozoite-induced falciparum malaria. Am J Med Sci 266:166–177, 1973

58 Kumar SJ, Miller LH, Quakyi IA, et al: Cytotoxic T cells specific for the circumsporozoite protein of *Plasmodium falciparum*. Nature 334:258–260

59 Kaslow DC, Quakyi IA, Syin C, et al: A vaccine candidate on sexual stages of human malaria that contains EGF-like domains. Nature, 333:74–76, 1988

60 Boyd MF (ed): *Malariology*. Philadelphia, Saunders, 1949

61 Garnham PCC (ed): *Malaria Parasites and other Haemosporidia*. Oxford, Blackwell, 1966

62 Spitz S: The pathology of acute falciparum malaria. Milit Surg 99:555–572, 1946

63 Pant CP, Rishikesh N, Bank YH, et al: Progress in malaria vector control. Bull WHO 59:325–333, 1981

64 Brown AWA: Insecticide resistance in mosquitoes: A pragmatic review. J Am Mosq Control Assoc 2:123–140, 1986

65 Davidson EW, Sweeney AW: Microbial control of vectors: A decade of progress. J Med Entomol 20:235–247, 1983

CHAPTER 31 / *Babesiosis* · Trenton K. Ruebush II

Babesia is a tick-transmitted protozoan parasite of animals. The disease it causes, babesiosis or piroplasmosis, is characterized by fever, hemolytic anemia, hemoglobinuria, and renal failure. Occasional human *Babesia* infections occur when humans intrude on the natural cycle of transmission of the organism between the tick vector and the vertebrate host.

Babesiosis is of historical importance because *Babesia bigemina,* the cause of Texas cattle fever, was the first organism shown to be transmitted by an arthropod, predating by several years the discovery of the routes of transmission of malaria, filariasis, and yellow fever.

PARASITE

LIFE HISTORY

Babesiosis is transmitted in nature by ixodid, or hard-bodied, ticks, including members of the genera *Dermacentor, Ixodes,* and *Rhipicephalus.* Organisms are ingested by the tick when it feeds, multiply within the epithelial cells of the tick's gut, and then spread throughout its body. In some species of ticks, such as *Ixodes ricinus* infected with *Babesia bovis,* organisms invade the ovaries and are passed through the egg to the developing larval stage (transovarial transmission). Organisms are then transmitted to the vertebrate host in the salivary secretions during the tick's next blood meal. Thus, the tick can serve as both vector and reservoir for the parasite. In other tick species, such as *I. dammini* infected with *B. microti,* infections are acquired during the larval or nymphal stage and are transmitted by the subsequent stage after the tick has molted (transstadial passage) [1].

Within the vertebrate host *Babesia* is an intraerythrocytic parasite; however, unlike malaria, it does not appear to have an exoerythrocytic stage of development. *Babesia* multiplies asexually by budding within red blood cells, usually producing two or four daughter parasites. When the infected red blood cell ruptures, other erythrocytes are invaded and the cycle is repeated.

MORPHOLOGY

Organisms of the genus *Babesia* are intraerythrocytic protozoan parasites. They range in shape from single, round or piriform bodies, to ameboid or ring forms, to dividing forms, usually made up of two or four daughter cells. *Babesia* may resemble malaria parasites morphologically, but they show no evidence of pigment formation in infected red blood cells.

Although more than 70 species of *Babesia* have been described, there is considerable confusion in the taxonomy of this genus; organisms that apparently belong to the same species may carry several different names. An example of this is *B. divergens,* the cause of several cases of human babesiosis, which is probably identical to *B. bovis*. The application of techniques such as isoenzyme analysis and DNA homology studies to strain identification should help to resolve some of these problems.

RESERVOIR HOSTS

Babesia are parasites of various wild and domestic animals including cattle, horses, sheep, wild and domestic cats and dogs, deer, raccoons, and rodents. The only known route of transmission of the parasite among animals is by tick bite. It is unlikely that humans play a role in maintaining the parasite in nature.

PATIENT

PATHOGENESIS

The major clinicopathological features of babesiosis include hemoglobinemia, hemoglobinuria, jaundice, and renal insufficiency or failure. They are the result of the multiplication of organisms within, and the subsquent destruction of, the red blood cells. Erythrocyte destruction is usually far greater than would be expected based on the level of parasitemia. This may be due to an autoimmune reaction against the erythrocyte membrane, since several patients infected with *B. microti* have been reported to have positive direct antiglobulin tests with non-complement-binding IgG antibody coating their red blood cells [2].

In animals, *Babesia* parasitemia may persist for many years after an infected tick bite. During this period the host is usually clinically healthy and immune to reinfection. Parasitemia persisting for up to 4 months has been documented in human *B. microti* infections. These prolonged parasitemias are probably due to the ability of *Babesia* organisms to alter the specificity of their antigens in response to exposure to specific antibody. Both humoral and cell-mediated immune responses have been demonstrated in *Babesia* infections; however, cell-mediated immunity seems to play the most important role in the control of parasitemia and acquisition of immunity to reinfection.

The response of a vertebrate host to *Babesia* infection may be influenced by the species of parasite causing the infection, the host's age, and the presence or absence of a spleen. In cattle and horses, severity of infection is related to the host's age; infections in older animals are usually associated with much more severe manifestations, while younger animals often have mild or even asymptomatic infections. A similar associ-

ation between age and severity of illness has been noted in human beings infected with *B. microti*. Symptomatic infections are more common in persons older than 40 years [3].

A functioning spleen is also important in immunity to *Babesia*. Splenectomized individuals are more susceptible to infection with *B. divergens* than persons with intact spleens. Furthermore, asplenic patients infected with *B. microti* and *B. divergens* tend to have higher levels of parasitemia and more severe illnesses, and the majority of deaths due to babesiosis have occurred in such patients. In nonhuman animals with subclinical *Babesia* infections, splenectomy frequently causes a recurrence of parasitemia and symptoms.

CLINICAL MANIFESTATIONS

Babesia microti infections

Human *B. microti* infections range in severity from asymptomatic to prolonged, severe illnesses [4]. In most patients there is a gradual onset of irregular fever, chills, diaphoresis, generalized myalgia, and fatigue. Although symptoms tend to fluctuate in severity, no true periodicity has been noted. Many patients do not remember a tick bite; in those who do, the incubation period ranges from 1 to 4 weeks.

On physical examination the only findings are fever, pallor, and occasional mild hepatosplenomegaly. Most patients have a mild to moderately severe hemolytic anemia and a normal or slightly depressed white blood cell count. Hemoglobinuria is rare, but reduced serum haptoglobin levels do occur. In about half the cases, there are slight elevations of alkaline phosphatase, serum glutamic-oxaloacetic acid transaminase, and bilirubin. The level of parasitemia is rarely higher than 10 percent.

The acute illness may last from a few weeks to a month or more. Although relapses, such as are seen in malaria, have not been observed with *B. microti* infections, complete recovery is often delayed by prolonged weakness and malaise. Parasitemia may persist at low levels with or without symptoms for up to 4 months after the onset of illness. *Babesia microti* infections and Lyme disease may occur simultaneously [5].

Splenectomized patients infected with *B. microti* tend to have more severe illnesses than persons with functioning spleens. Although self-limited infections have been reported, both the level of parasitemia and the severity of hemolytic anemia are generally greater in asplenic persons [6,7]. In spite of this, all such patients have recovered from their infections, suggesting that *B. microti* is less pathogenic for humans than *Babesia divergens*.

Babesia divergens infections

Most of the reported patients with *B. divergens* infections had undergone splenectomies before becoming infected. The reasons for the splenectomies included trauma, surgical accidents, portal hypertension, and lymphoma.

Human *B. divergens* infections are characterized by a rapid onset of chills, high fever, nausea, vomiting, and severe hemolytic anemia, which progress within a few days to jaundice, hemoglobinemia, hemoglobinuria, and renal insufficiency or failure [8,9]. Fever, hypotension, and jaundice are the major findings on physical examination. Anemia is generally quite severe with elevated reticulocyte counts and nucleated red blood cells on peripheral blood smears. Marked elevations of bilirubin, liver enzymes, blood urea nitrogen, and creatinine are common. Most of the reported human *B. divergens* infections have been fatal.

DIAGNOSIS

The diagnosis of babesiosis should be considered in any patient with a fever and a history of a tick bite or exposure to ticks. If the patient is asplenic or has the cutaneous lesions of Lyme disease, the probability of babesiosis is greater. Anemia is usually present but may not be severe, particularly in *B. microti* infections. Although nearly all reported cases of human babesiosis have been acquired in Europe and North America, the diagnosis should not be ruled out in patients from other parts of the world since *Babesia* infections in lower animals are worldwide in distribution.

The diagnosis of human babesiosis depends on the microscopic identification of characteristic parasites on thin or thick blood smears. Giemsa stain is preferable to Wright's stain for identification of these organisms. In patients with low-level parasitemia, examination of repeated blood smears may be necessary to make the diagnosis. In human blood smears *B. microti* usually appears as a small ring form indistinguishable from the young trophozoites of *Plasmodium falciparum* [10]. Older stages contain more abundant chromatin and cytoplasm. Unlike *Plasmodium* sp., no pigment is produced in erythrocytes infected with *Babesia* parasites, but this distinguishing characteristic is of value only in the more mature stages of the parasite. Dividing forms of *B. microti* (tetrad forms), made up of four daughter cells held together by thin strands of cytoplasm, are rarely seen in human blood films. *Babesia divergens* in human blood smears ranges from round, oval, or piriform shapes to small ring forms. Dividing parasites usually consist of two daughter cells.

An indirect immunofluorescent antibody test has been used to aid diagnosis in suspected cases of *B. microti* infection but should not be considered a substitute for examination of blood smears [11]. Serum antibody titers rise 2 to 4 weeks after the onset of illness and then gradually fall over 6 to 12 months. Serological cross-reactions occur with other species of *Babesia* and with malaria parasites, but antibody titers are generally highest to the infecting organism.

In suspected cases of human *B. microti* infection in which organisms cannot be identified in blood smears, intraperitoneal or intravenous inoculation of blood into hamsters or gerbils may be helpful in diagnosis [4]. Parasitemia usually appears within 2 to 4 weeks after the animals are inoculated. Although *B. divergens* seems to have a narrower host range than *B. microti,* attempts to infect gerbils have been successful, suggesting that inoculation of this animal might also help in the diagnosis of suspected cases.

MANAGEMENT

Evaluation of the various therapeutic regimens used for human babesiosis is complicated by the small number of cases and the fact that *Babesia* is resistant to most antiprotozoal drugs used in human medicine. Furthermore, in many of the reported cases of human babesiosis it is not clear whether the patient responded to antimicrobial therapy or would have recovered spontaneously. Chloroquine, which had initially been reported to be effective in human *B. microti* infections, seems to act primarily as an anti-inflammatory agent rather than as an antibabesial drug [4,6]. Pentamidine isethionate, a drug effective against some species of *Babesia* in animals, has been reported to reduce fever and parasitemia in several cases, but organisms were not eliminated from the blood [6]. A combination of quinine (650 mg orally three times a day) and clindamycin (600 mg orally three times a day or 1.2 g parenterally twice a day) for 5 to 10 days has been effective in several severely ill patients as well as in trials in animals [12]; however, a recent report indicates that this combination may not eliminate parasites from the blood [13].

Human *B. microti* infections in patients with functioning spleens are generally self-limited. Although symptoms and parasitemia may persist for several months, no permanent sequelae have been observed. Since no completely effective drugs have been identified for the treatment of these infections, symptomatic therapy is probably sufficient in most cases. In asplenic patients and patients with functioning spleens who have severe infections, quinine and clindamycin is the treatment of choice. Exchange blood transfusion has been used successfully in several splenectomized patients with severe *B. microti* infection, but this technique should be considered only when all other therapy has failed [7].

The treatment of human *B. divergens* infections presents special problems due to the fulminant course of the infection. The only two patients who have recovered were managed with blood transfusions and renal dialysis [14]. No chemotherapeutic agents have been shown to be effective in such cases; however, pentamidine is a logical choice for treatment since it is known to be effective against several species of *Babesia* in animals.

POPULATION

EPIDEMIOLOGY

Babesia infections in wild and domestic animals are distributed worldwide but are most prevalent in tropical and subtropical areas. In many countries they are responsible for serious economic losses for the livestock industry.

Human babesiosis is a zoonotic disease. Infection is acquired accidentally when humans intrude in the natural cycle of the parasite between the tick vector and its domestic or wild animal hosts. Human beings play no role in transmission of the disease.

Most cases of human *B. microti* infection were acquired along the northeast coast of the United States on Nantucket Island and Martha's Vineyard Island, Massachusetts, Long Island and Shelter Island, New York, and the nearby mainland. Recently a case was reported from Wisconsin. *Babesia microti* is a parasite of rodents that is transmitted by *I. dammini*, the northern deer tick. This tick normally feeds on rodents during its larval and nymphal stages and on deer in its adult stage, but the nymphal stage also feeds readily on human beings [*1*]. The parasite apparently overwinters in the larval stages of the tick vector and is then transmitted by nymphs during the late spring and summer, when most human cases are diagnosed.

Cases of *B. divergens* infection have been sporadic in occurrence and widely distributed geographically. Infections in humans have been reported from Yugoslavia, Ireland, France, Great Britain, the Soviet Union, and Spain. The causative organism is a parasite of cattle. All of the infections occurred in persons who had previously had splenectomies, a factor which is believed to have increased their susceptibility to this organism. The vector in the European cases is probably *I. ricinus*, the tick responsible for transmission of the parasite among cattle.

Cases of human babesiosis in which the species of the infecting organism could not be identified have been reported from the United States (California and Georgia) and from Mexico.

Babesia infections can also be transmitted by transfusion of blood or blood products. The risk of transmission by this route is greatest with *B. microti,* because this parasite tends to cause prolonged asymptomatic parasitemia [*6,7*].

INFECTION AND DISEASE

Babesia infections in animals range from asymptomatic cases to severe, occasionally fatal illnesses. Subclinical infections are most common in younger animals, but asymptomatic parasitemia persists in many older animals following the acute illness.

Evidence from serological surveys in the northeastern United States indicates that asymptomatic babesiosis is also common in human beings. Approximately 4 percent of the human population of endemic areas have antibodies to *B. microti,* suggesting past or current infections [*4*]. Based on these findings and the worldwide prevalence of *Babesia* infections in animals,

it seems likely that human *Babesia* infections occur in other parts of the world but are not diagnosed as such.

PREVENTION

The only effective means of preventing *Babesia* infections is by avoiding exposure to ticks. Insect repellents are of doubtful value. Evidence suggests that ticks do not transmit infective *Babesia* organisms until they have been feeding for several hours. Therefore, persons at risk should search their bodies for ticks as soon as possible after exposure. In view of the low prevalence of human *B. microti* infection, serological screening of prospective blood donors and the exclusion of persons from endemic areas who have a history of fever in the preceding 6 to 12 months to prevent transfusion-induced babesiosis is not practical.

REFERENCES

1 Spielman A, Wilson ML, Levine JF, et al: Ecology of *Ixodes dammini*–borne human babesiosis and Lyme disease. Ann Rev Entomol 30:439–460, 1985

2 Wolf CFW, Resnick G, Marsh WL, et al: Autoimmunity to red blood cells in babesiosis. Transfusion 22:538–539, 1982

3 Ruebush TK II, Juranek DD, Spielman A, et al: Epidemiology of human babesiosis on Nantucket Island. Am J Trop Med Hyg 30:937–941, 1981

4 Ruebush TK II: Human babesiosis in North America. Trans R Soc Trop Med Hyg 74:149–152, 1980.

5 Grunwaldt E, Barbour AG, Benach JL: Simultaneous occurrence of babesiosis and Lyme disese. N Engl J Med 308:1166, 1883.

6 Teusch SM, Etkind P, Burwell EL, et al: Babesiosis in postsplenectomy hosts. Am J Trop Med Hyg 29:738–741, 1980

7 Jacoby GA, Hunt JV, Kosinski KS, et al: Treatment of transfusion-transmitted babesiosis by exchange tranfusion. N Engl J Med 303:1098–1100, 1980

8 Skrabalo Z, Deanovic Z: Piroplasmosis in man: Report on a case. Doc Med Geogr Trop 9:11–16, 1957

9 Fitzpatrick JEP, Kennedy CC, McGeown MG, et al: Human case of piroplasmosis (babesiosis). Nature 217:861–862, 1968

10 Healy GR, Ruebush TK II: Morphology of *Babesia microti* in human blood smears. Am J Clin Pathol 73:107–109, 1980

11 Chisholm ES, Ruebush TK II, Sulzer AJ, et al: *Babesia microti* infection in man: Evaluation of an indirect immunofluorescent antibody test. Am J Trop Med Hyg 27:14–19, 1978

12 Wittner M, Rowin KS, Tanowitz HB, et al: Successful chemotherapy of transfusion babesiosis. Ann Intern Med 96:601–604, 1982

13 Smith RP, Evans AT, Popovsky M, et al: Transfusion-acquired babesiosis and failure of antibiotic treatment. JAMA 256: 2726–2727, 1986

14 Bazin C, Lamy C, Piette M, et al: Un nouveau cas de babesiose humaine. Nouv Presse Med 5:779–800, 1976

African Trypanosomiasis · Stephen L. Hajduk
· Paul T. Englund · David H. Smith

The trypanosomiases of Africa are infections caused by sub-species of the hemoflagellate *Trypanosoma brucei* known as *T. brucei gambiense,* which is the cause of the chronic so-called African sleeping sickness, and *T. brucei rhodesiense,* which results in a more acute syndrome. The closely related parasite *T. brucei brucei,* a scourge of domestic ungulates, has a considerable effect on human nutrition. All of these subspecies are transmitted to humans through the bite of tsetse flies of the genus *Glossina* whose habitat consists of the region of Africa between latitudes 15°N and 15°S. Control is difficult, as treatment is toxic and vaccines have not been effective because of the trypanosomes' ability to vary their suface antigens. Vector management is also difficult because of the presence of animal reservoirs, the wide distribution of the flies, and the underground habitat of their pupal stages.

The lack of success in the development of effective vaccines and trypanocidal drugs has stimulated the investigation of the basic biochemistry and molecular biology of these organisms. The basic premise for these studies is that the ultimate control of the diseases resides in the identification of novel biochemical and molecular properties of the parasite that can be exploited to develop effective chemotherapy or immunotherapy for infected patients.

PARASITE

T. brucei has been the most intensively investigated of the African trypanosomes, and recent studies have focused on its antigenic variation, its kinetoplast (mitochondrial) DNA, its unusual metabolic and genetic processes, and its complex pathways of differentiation. In this section we shall emphasize these properties of *T. brucei.*

LIFE CYCLE OF THE TRYPANOSOMES

T. brucei is transmitted by the tsetse fly *Glossina,* within which it undergoes important developmental changes [1,2] (Fig. 32-1). The tsetse ingests parasites when taking a blood meal from an infected animal. In the insect midgut the trypanosomes then rapidly differentiate into procyclic forms. The procyclic forms differ in three important ways from the bloodstream stages. First, they lack the dense surface coat, composed of the variant surface glycoprotein, which is found on animal bloodstream forms (Fig. 32-2). Second, in contrast to the bloodstream forms, the mitochondrion of these cells is fully active and has abundant cristae. Third, the procyclic forms are noninfectious for the mammalian host.

The procyclic trypanosomes multiply in the midgut of the tsetse, often reaching high cell densities. After 2 to 3 weeks the trypanosomes migrate to the insect's salivary glands where they change morphologically into epimastigotes. Epimastigotes are multiplicative and are usually seen attached to the surface of the salivary gland epithelium. The epimastigotes ultimately differentiate into metacyclic trypanosomes. These are non-multiplicative and arise from the epimastigotes first as forms attached to host cells and later as forms free in the lumen of the salivary glands. The metacyclics morphologically resemble the animal bloodstream form. They are coated by characteristic variant surface glycoproteins and, most importantly, are the only insect developmental stage in insects which is infectious to the mammalian host.

When the fly bites another mammal, the parasites present in the saliva are injected into the blood, where they quickly develop into long slender bloodstream forms. These cells divide rapidly by binary fission and begin to undergo antigenic variation, the process by which they continually change their surface glycoproteins and therefore evade the immune system of the host (see below). As the infection proceeds, the long slender trypanosomes differentiate further into short stumpy bloodstream forms. These forms are nondividing, and it is generally believed that they are preadapted to life in the insect. After another tsetse takes its blood meal from the infected animal, the short stumpy trypanosomes complete the life cycle by transforming into procyclics in the insect midgut.

In the mammalian host the trypanosome is restricted to extracellular spaces: the bloodstream, tissue fluids, and, in later stages of infection, the spinal fluid. Intracellular stages have not been detected. Whereas pleomorphic strains can exist as either long slender forms or short stumpy forms, some laboratory strains of *T. brucei* are monomorphic. These strains, consisting exclusively of long, slender trypanosomes, grow to very high parasitemias and usually kill the host within a few days. They do not generate significant numbers of short, stumpy forms and infect the tsetse with difficulty, if at all. They survive in the laboratory only by syringe passage. Pleomorphic strains become monomorphic after repeated syringe passage.

The developmental stages of *T. brucei* differ dramatically in their metabolism [3–6]. In the procyclic forms, present in the fly midgut, the parasite's single mitochondrion is fully active and has abundant cristae. These cells have Krebs cycle enzymes, and they actively respire using a cyanide-sensitive electron transport system. In contrast, the long slender bloodstream forms have completely suppressed many mitochondrial functions. Their mitochondrial volume is reduced, and they have few cristae. They are completely deficient in cytochromes and several Krebs cycle enzymes, and their ATP-generating mechanism depends exclusively on glycolysis (see ''Biochemical Pharmacology'').

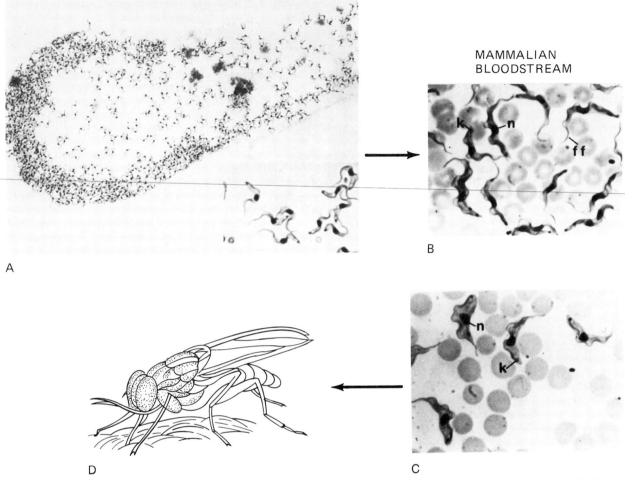

Figure 32-1. The life cycle of *T. brucei*. Infections are transmitted by the injection of saliva containing metacyclic trypanosomes (*A*) during a blood meal. Saliva from a heavily infected tsetse collected on a microscope and stained with Giemsa shows a large number of metacyclics. At higher magnification the kinetoplast and nucleus are clearly visible (inset). Giemsa-stained bloodsmears of long, slender (*B*) and short, stumpy (*C*) developmental stages show the nucleus (n), kinetoplast (k), and free flagellum (ff). *D*. The tsetse fly *Glossina* is the insect vector of African trypanosomiasis.

The life cycle of *T. brucei* is, indeed, complex. However, a deeper understanding of this differentiation process may provide clues that could lead to better therapy of trypanosomiasis. For example, the disease might be treated by blocking the switch from nondividing metacyclics to rapidly dividing long slender bloodstream forms or inducing the differentiation from long slender forms to nondividing short stumpy forms.

MORPHOLOGY OF TRYPANOSOMES

Live preparations of the long slender African trypanosomes observed by phase contrast microscopy in fresh blood preparations are extremely active, undulating rapidly about the microscopic field. These parasites measure approximately 26 by 2.5 μm, and they have a prominent undulating membrane and a long, free flagellum measuring approximately 6 μm. In contrast, the short stumpy developmental stage of African trypanosomes is sluggish in its movements in fresh blood preparations. The short stumpy trypanosomes also differ from the long slender trypanosomes in their size (19 by 3.5 μm) and the complete lack of a free flagellum [1]. Figure 32-1 shows micrographs of long slender and short stumpy forms. In trypanosomes stained with Giemsa a centrally located nucleus is seen along with another intensely stained granule at the base of the flagellum. This granule, known as the *kinetoplast,* is actually a huge network of mitochondrial DNA, a structure unique to the order Kinetoplastida (see "Kinetoplast DNA").

At the ultrastructural level (Fig. 32-2) trypanosomes have several unique features [7]. First, they have a single mitochondrion per cell. Within the mitochondrion, near the basal

A

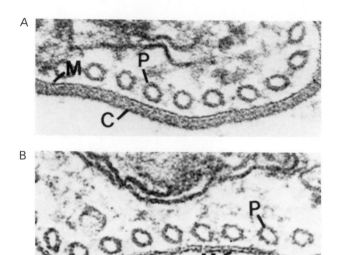

B

C

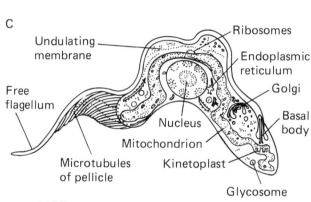

Figure 32-2. Thin-section electron micrographs of bloodstream (*A*) and midgut (*B*) forms of *T. brucei* showing the surface coat (C), plasma membrane (M), and pellicular microtubules (P). A diagram of the *T. b. rhodesiense* bloodstream form (*C*) indicates the typical trypanosome ultrastructural features. [*A and B reprinted from Ref. 62; C from Ref. 61 with permission.*]

body of the flagellum, the kinetoplast DNA (kDNA) is seen as an electron-dense band of regularly aligned fibers. Second, they have small microbody-like vesicles, termed *glycosomes* [*8*], which contain the first nine enzymes of glycolysis. Third, all animal bloodstream forms, as well as the metacyclic forms in the tsetse salivary glands, have a 12- to 15-nm-thick proteinaceous surface coat [*9*] (Fig. 32-2*A*). This coat, composed of the variant surface glycoprotein, covers the entire cell and appears to be an adaptation to life in the immunologically active mammalian host (see "Antigenic Variation of Trypanosomes"). This coat is not present on the procyclic forms in the tsetse midgut (Fig. 32-2*B*). Fourth, beneath the plasma membrane they have a girdle of pellicular microtubules that runs the entire length of the cell (Fig. 32-2*A* and *B*). These microtubules act as a cytoskeleton that gives the cell rigidity

and also may facilitate the morphological changes the trypanosomes undergo during their life cycle.

KINETOPLAST DNA

The kDNA network of trypanosomes is an extraordinary structure composed entirely of topologically interlocked circular DNA molecules [*10–13*] (Fig. 32-3). Each cell contains a single network representing about 10 percent of the total cellular DNA. Why trypanosomes alone in nature have evolved such a complex structure is completely unknown.

The major component of the kDNA network is the minicircle, comprising about 95 percent of the network mass. Each *T. brucei* minicircle is about 1000 base pairs, and there are roughly 5000 per network. Minicircles have unusual properties, which suggest that they have a novel function. First, they evolve extremely rapidly. There is little similarity in nucleotide sequence between minicircles from different species of trypanosomes. In fact, they evolve so rapidly that even within a period of 2 years in continuous culture, the restriction enzyme fragmentation pattern of minicircles from a related insect trypanosomatid, *Crithidia,* changes detectably [*14*]. Minicircles from all species have a conserved GGGGTTGTGAA sequence which is part of the replication origin [*15*]. Third, minicircles have unique physical properties [*16*]. Some minicircle restriction fragments from *T. brucei* and from other trypanosomatid species have a natural curvature. This bending of the DNA helix, most strikingly visualized by electron microscopy [*17*], is probably caused by periodic placement of A runs along the DNA helix. Except for sequences in the replication origin, the bending of the DNA helix in kinetoplast minicircles is the only feature of these molecules known to be conserved in several species of these parasites, and it almost certainly is of major importance to minicircle function. The bending of the helix within these molecules may facilitate the assembly and stabilization of the massive network into its compact and highly organized conformation within the mitochondrion [*18,19*].

Recent studies have shown that the minicircles of *T. brucei* are transcribed [*20*]. The major minicircle transcript is a 240-nucleotide RNA that is present in both the bloodstream and insect developmental stages of the parasite. The 5′ terminus of this transcript has been mapped to a site immediately adjacent to the GGGGTTGTGAA sequence, which is where replication of one of the minicircle strands initiates. Although the function of the 240-nucleotide transcript is unknown, its map position and its presence in all trypanosome developmental stages suggest a relationship to the RNA primer for minicircle replication.

The other component of the kDNA network is the maxicircle [*13*]. Maxicircles have a structure and coding function not unlike that of mitochondrial DNA in other eukaryotic cells. The maxicircle of *T. brucei* is about 20 kb, and the major maxicircle transcripts are 9 and 12 S mitochondrial ribosomal RNAs. Other maxicircle transcripts include messenger RNAs

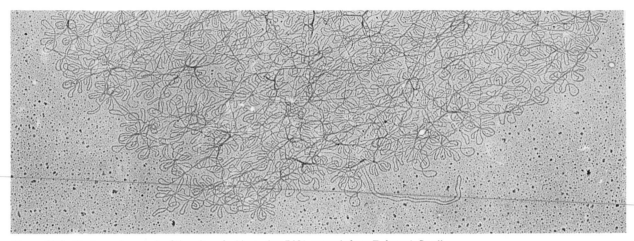

Figure 32-3. Electron micrograph of the edge of a kinetoplast DNA network from *T. brucei*. Small loops are minicircles. (*Electron micrograph from James Ntambi.*)

for cytochrome b, subunits I and II of cytochrome oxidase, and subunits 5 and 6 of the mitochondrial NADH dehydrogenase complex.

Despite the similarity of the maxicircle to other mitochondrial DNAs, there are several unique aspects to the structure and expression of these molecules. First, the maxicircles of trypanosomes are not free in the mitochondrial matrix, but instead are threaded through the network of thousands of minicircles. Each kDNA network contains 25 to 50 maxicircles, all of which appear to have the same sequence with no similarity to that of minicircles. Second, the expression of the maxicircle genes is developmentally regulated during the life cycle of *T. brucei*. In the bloodstream form of the parasite the steady state levels of the maxicircle transcripts are repressed. The level of the maxicircle transcripts increases 60 to 400-fold as the trypanosomes differentiate to the insect developmental stages. The amount of maxicircle transcripts present in the developmental stages of *T. brucei* is not a reflection of differences in the rate of transcription of the maxicircle genes, but of the stability of the maxicircle transcripts. The maxicircle transcripts in the insect developmental stages are more stable than those in the long slender bloodstream forms. The low level of maxicircle transcripts is consistent with absence of functional mitochondria in the bloodstream developmental stages of *T. brucei* [21]. Third, and most remarkably, maxicircle transcripts can be modified, either during or after transcription, by the addition of uridines that are not encoded by the maxicircle genes. These modifications, which are unprecedented in nature, have several consequences. The addition of four uridine residues in the transcript for cytochrome oxidase subunit II corrects a frameshift in the coding sequence for the protein [22]. Furthermore, addition of a uridine to the cytochrome b transcript leads to the creation of an AUG translation initiation codon in this transcript [23]. This novel form of RNA

modification is developmentally regulated in the case of both the cytochrome b and cytochrome oxidase subunit II transcripts. The addition of uridines occurs in the procyclic insect developmental stage and the short stumpy bloodstream forms but not in the long slender stage [24].

Because of its network structure, the replication of kinetoplast DNA presents problems not found with any other DNA [25]. Replication requires doubling the number of minicircles and maxicircles and the distribution of the progeny circles into two daughter networks each indistinguishable from the parent network. These daughter networks then segregate into the two daughter cells during cell division. There is now considerable information at the molecular level about kinetoplast DNA replication. Minicircle synthesis requires release of individual minicircles from the network. The free minicircles undergo replication, and their progeny are then reattached to the network. Release and reattachment of minicircles is probably catalyzed by topoisomerases. Because two minicircles are reattached for every one removed, the network grows until it finally reaches double size. Then the double-size network splits in two. The splitting of the double-size network, which requires unlinking of minicircles from its neighbors, probably also depends on topoisomerase activity. Maxicircles replicate by a mechanism different from that of minicircles; they replicate while still attached to networks.

There are three medically important reasons for studying kinetoplast DNA. First, an increased understanding of its biochemistry may lead to new concepts of chemotherapy to use against these parasites. None of the host organisms of these parasites has DNA that resembles kinetoplast DNA. Therefore, it may be possible to inhibit specifically its replication or expression. This inhibition of expression should result in the selective killing of trypanosomatid pathogens such as *Leishmania donovani* or *Trypanosoma cruzi*, which appear to require kinetoplast gene products in all stages of their life cycle. In contrast, the animal bloodstream forms of *T. brucei* do not have active mitochondria and therefore might not be killed by inhibitors of kinetoplast function. Inhibition of kDNA replication or expression would, however, prevent the transformation to the stages found in the tsetse where mitochondrial activity is required.

Second, characterization of kinetoplast DNA sequences appears to be useful in identification of strains of these parasites for diagnostic or epidemiological purposes. Many of the *Trypanosoma* strains are morphologically and biochemically very similar, and more tools are needed to distinguish strains that may differ in host range or virulence. Substantial progress has already been made in diagnosis and the distinguishing of strains by kinetoplast DNA hybridization or by comparing restriction digests of minicircles [*26*].

Third, several trypanocidal compounds, for example, berenil, ethidium, and pentamidine, may interact preferentially with kDNA [*27*]. An increased understanding of kDNA structure and metabolism may be useful in determining the mode of action of these drugs and in developing new ones.

ANTIGENIC VARIATION OF TRYPANOSOMES

During the course of infection of an animal, the number of trypanosomes in the blood and lymphatic fluids fluctuates in a characteristic fashion (Fig. 32-4). This relapsing parasitemia is due to the host's immune response to the trypanosomes. Each decline in parasite number is the consequence of antibody-mediated destruction of trypanosomes bearing a particular variant surface glycoprotein (VSG). Each new wave of parasitemia represents the growth of a trypanosome population expressing an antigenically distinct VSG. This process of antigenic variation is a feature of all African trypanosomes [*11,28,29–31*]. Since each trypanosome expresses only one VSG at a time and has as many as 1000 different VSG genes, the number of different variable antigen types (VATs) that can be expressed during a trypanosome infection is high. The process of antigenic switching occurs spontaneously in trypanosomes and has frustrated all attempts at immunization against African trypanosomiasis.

The expression of the VSG is developmentally regulated in *T. brucei*. Bloodstream trypanosomes ingested by the insect vector rapidly lose the VSG from their surface. The loss of VSG in the midgut of the tsetse fly corresponds with the loss of infectivity for the mammalian host. In the salivary glands of the tsetse fly the metacyclic trypanosome reacquires the VSG surface coat and infectivity for the mammalian host. The antigenic diversity of the metacyclic trypanosomes is far less extensive than that of the bloodstream trypanosomes. It appears that metacyclic trypanosomes, from a given strain, can express only about 10 to 15 different VSGs [*32–34*]. Why certain VSG genes cannot be expressed by the metacyclics is completely unknown. When a mammal is infected with metacyclic trypanosomes, the first VATs detected in the bloodstream are antigenically the same as the infecting metacyclics. The trypanosomes expressing these VATs rapidly disappear, and the first wave of parasitemia in the animal is extremely heterogeneous, with at least 20 different VATs being expressed during the first 10 days of infection. The realization of the complexity of the tsetse-induced infection has diminished expectation for a vaccine against trypanosomiasis using the metacyclic VSGs as antigens.

Antigenic variation is expressed through the VSG [*31*]. About 10^7 molecules of VSG (about 10 percent of the cellular protein) form a coat on the surface of the bloodstream trypanosome, and their function apparently is to shield all subsurface molecules from attack by host antibodies. VSGs contain roughly 600 amino acid residues, and their sequence differs strikingly in different trypanosome variants. Recently the three-dimensional structures of two different VSGs have been determined by x-ray crystallography [*35*]. VSGs contain roughly 10 percent of their mass as carbohydrates. They have one or more asparagine-linked oligosaccharides, and they also have a glycolipid covalently attached to their carboxy terminus. This glycolipid consists of dimyristoylphosphatidylinositol and several sugars [*36*]. The myristoyl moieties insert into the lipid bilayer of the plasma membrane and thereby anchor the VSG to the cell surface. Trypanosomes contain a phospholipase C, known as VSG lipase, which cleaves this glycolipid anchor [*37*]. Because this enzyme is highly specific for the VSG glycolipid, it probably plays an important role in VSG metabolism; however, its function is not yet known.

The study of the molecular mechanism of antigenic variation in African trypanosomes has led to the discovery of another unique feature of the biology of trypanosomes. Transcription of protein-encoding genes in trypanosomes is discontinuous. All trypanosome mRNAs contain an identical 39-nucleotide sequence at their 5' end that is encoded separately in the trypanosome genome. The 39-nucleotide RNA, termed the *mini-exon*, is transcribed from a 1.4-kb sequence which is present

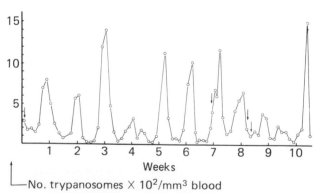

Figure 32-4. Graph showing the fluctuations in parasite number in the blood of a sleeping sickness patient. [*Reprinted from Vickerman (1974) with permission.*]

as a tandem repeat of approximately 200 copies. The initial transcript from the miniexon repeat is the 135-nucleotide miniexon-derived RNA (med RNA). The 5' terminal 39 nucleotides of the med RNA are added in a reaction which is at least superficially similar to splicing of precursor mRNAs from protein-encoding genes of other eukaryotic cells. Functionally the 39-nucleotide miniexon is thought to provide a 5' terminal cap structure for trypanosome mRNAs. This novel mechanism of RNA processing, termed *trans-splicing* since the RNAs joined come from different primary transcripts, might provide a target for drug design. The fact that all trypanosome mRNAs contain the same 5' sequence has led to the proposed use of complementary synthetic oligonucleotides to selectively block trypanosome protein synthesis. Oligonucleotides complementary to the miniexon have been used to successfully block trypanosome mRNA translation using in vitro translation systems [30]. If modified complementary oligonucleotides can be synthesized that are taken up by trypanosomes in the mammalian bloodstream, then this might represent a novel and highly effective chemotherapeutic approach to trypanosomiasis.

DEVELOPMENT OF NEW THERAPEUTICAL APPROACHES

Biochemical pharmacology

To develop novel agents for the treatment of trypanosomiasis a rational approach to drug design is advocated. This requires a thorough understanding of the basic biochemical differences between parasite and host and the design of effective drugs to interfere selectively with the parasites' biochemical pathways. As already outlined in this chapter, trypanosomes have many unique molecular structures and pathways which might be effective targets for new drugs.

The use of a combined treatment of salicylhydroxamic acid (SHAM) and glycerol on bloodstream trypanosome infections is an example of this type of approach [38,39]. This treatment exploits the fact that in the animal bloodstream trypanosomes rely entirely upon high rates of glycolysis for ATP production. They have a novel mitochondria oxidase that indirectly mediates the reoxidation of NADH produced during glycolysis. This enzyme, glycerophosphate oxidase, is inhibited by SHAM, causing the trypanosome to switch to anaerobic glycolysis for ATP production. This switch is inhibited by glycerol in a mass action effect on glycerol kinase. The combination of SHAM and glycerol effectively kills all bloodstream trypanosomes, although the effectiveness on infections involving the central nervous system is less impressive.

Another promising chemotherapeutic agent for African trypanosomiasis, DL-α-difluoromethylornithine (DFMO), has recently been described [40]. DFMO is a potent, irreversible inhibitor of ornithine decarboxylase, which is an essential cellular enzyme required for the de novo biosynthesis of polyamines in all eukaryotic cells. Infections of *T. brucei* in mice and *T. gambiense* in human beings have been cured by treatment

with this drug [41]. DFMO has little or no effect on in vivo polyamine biosynthesis in mammalian cells even though it inhibits the mammalian ornithine decarboxylase in vitro. The molecular basis for the selective action of DFMO on trypanosomes is probably due to the faster turnover rate of the mammalian ornithine decarboxylase relative to the trypanosome enzyme. The trypanosome enzyme lacks the carboxy-terminal 36 amino acids that are responsible for the instability of the mammalian enzyme [42]. Inhibition of polyamine biosynthesis by DFMO might be particularly harmful to trypanosomes. Trypanosomes are unique in that they lack any detectable glutathione reductase activity, and the reduction of glutathione is mediated by a novel glutathione analogue, N^1,N^8-bis (glutathionyl) spermidine (trypanothione), which is capable of rapid nonenzymatic disulfide exchange between enzymatically reduced trypanothione and oxidized glutathione [43]. Since glutathione is the major source of thiol in trypanosomes, alterations in its reduction state might be lethal to the parasite.

Therapeutic natural products

An attractive alternative approach to drug development is to identify naturally occurring substances that would confer resistance to trypanosomes.

T. brucei brucei, a bovine parasite, is noninfectious to human beings. The host range of this parasite is restricted due to its sensitivity to a nonimmune lytic factor in human serum. The human sleeping sickness trypanosomes, *T. b. rhodesiense* and *T. b. gambiense*, are resistant to this natural killing factor. The lytic activity in human serum has been shown to purify with a unique, minor subspecies of high density lipoprotein (HDL) [44,45]. The expression of this human-specific factor in cattle might lead to a new approach to the control of animal trypanosomiasis.

PATIENT

HOST-PARASITE INTERFACE

The major pathological sequelae of African trypanosomiasis occur at three anatomical locations: at the site of inoculation, in the hemolymphatic system, and in the meningoencephalitic tissues. At the site of the tsetse bite, a small nodule forms (trypanosomal chancre) from which organisms may be isolated. It is a self-limited lesion characterized by parasite invasion and multiplication, and by a mononuclear cell infiltrate. Invasion of the bloodstream by the trypanosomes leads to the systemic, or hemolymphatic, phase of the disease. This occurs weeks or months after the onset of the chancre and is characterized by fever, lymphadenopathy, and, occasionally, splenomegaly. Histopathological examination of enlarged lymph nodes shows hypercellularity caused by increased numbers of lymphocytes and the appearance of pale-staining mononuclear cells. The late phase of African trypanosomiasis, so-called sleeping sickness, results from central nervous system (CNS) invasion and the resulting meningoencephalitis. Lesions are predominantly seen in the basal ganglia and manifest as chronic meningitis associated with lymphocyte, plasma cell, and morular cell infiltration. The cellular infiltrates extend into the brain substance, resulting in a characteristic perivascular cuffing. Similar lesions in the myocardium have been described in fatal cases of African trypanosomiasis.

The most striking feature of African trypanosomiasis relates to the oscillation of parasitemia. The trypanosomes appear in the peripheral blood of infected individuals in waves, and if untreated, the phenomenon persists for years (Fig. 32-4). Each parasite wave consists largely of serologically distinct organisms [29]. The host response, in turn, consists of variant-specific antibodies that may account for the destruction of most organisms. Complete elimination of parasites does not, however, occur because of the emergence of a new immunologically distinct parasite population. These specific biological features of the organisms causing African trypanosomiasis and their immunological sequelae in the host may be related to the pathogenesis of disease. For example, patients with African trypanosomiasis show a marked increase in serum immunoglobulins including specific and unrelated antibodies, autoantibodies, and immune complexes [46]. This generalized state of B-cell activation (polyclonal) may be caused either by interference with host T-lymphocyte control of antibody production or by a B-cell mitogen released by the parasites. In addition, several other immunological impairments have been demonstrated in patients with African trypanosomiasis including increased IgM levels in cerebrospinal fluid, which are independent of their elevated level in the blood, reduced antibody response to typhoid vaccination, and decreased skin reactivity to recall antigens.

The etiology of disease manifestations in African trypanosomiasis is unknown [46]. Greenwood outlined a hypothesis suggesting a dominant role of B-lymphocyte proliferation that starts in lymph nodes of infected individuals and results in massive IgM levels in peripheral blood [47]. Central nervous system disease may also be attributable to B-lymphocyte infiltration of the meninges and brain. The relationship between B-lymphocyte proliferation, infiltration, and migration to specific tissues sites and trypanosome infection remains, however, unknown. Furthermore, several extracts of the trypanosomes have been shown to induce an increase in vascular permeability, thrombocytopenia, or hemolytic anemia, but none of these postulated mechanisms of tissue injury has been shown to be biologically important. Other studies in experimental animals have suggested that the trypanosomes induce a metabolic imbalance in the host resulting in accumulation of lactic and pyruvic acids, but the clinical relevance of these observations has not been evaluated. Finally, the multiple immunological sequelae of African trypanosomiasis have led to the postulation of an immunopathological basis for the observed disease syndromes.

CLINICAL MANIFESTATIONS

The course of infection in African trypanosomiasis occurs in three stages [46]. Soon after inoculation of metacyclic trypanosomes by an infected tsetse fly, an inflammatory lesion develops at the site of inoculation, the trypanosomal chancre. Trypanosomes then invade the local lymphatics and later the bloodstream causing hemolymphatic trypanosomiasis. After a variable time parasites invade the choroid plexus and thus enter the brain and cerebrospinal fluid causing meningoencephalitic trypanosomiasis, from which the term *sleeping sickness* arises. There is considerable variation in both the severity and speed of evolution of the clinical picture. In *T. b. rhodesiense,* chancres are common; the hemolymphatic stage is severe and rapidly progresses to a fatal meningoencephalitis, often within months of infection, while in *T. b. gambiense,* chancres are infrequent, the hemolymphatic stage is mild or even inapparent, and the meningoencephalitis progresses slowly, often over several years. However, in either infection, there is a wide spectrum of clinical manifestations.

TRYPANOSOMAL CHANCRE

The lesion occurs within days of an infected bite, starting as a raised disc several centimeters in diameter, surrounded by a zone of erythema and induration. The chancre increases in size and is warm, painful, and tender. Chancres subside spontaneously within 3 weeks, leaving residual scarring and depigmentation. Ulceration occurs in a small proportion, when secondary infection may occur, and residual scarring is more severe. As the chancre evolves, a lymphadenopathy develops in the lymph glands draining the area. These glands are discrete, moderately enlarged, and nontender. Chancres occur in up to 30 percent of *T. b. rhodesiense* infections, although they vary geographically. In suspected clinical cases careful examination of the skin for evidence of a healed chancre is rewarding. The site of the chancre is dependent on the feeding habits of particular vectors and is usually on exposed surfaces (Figs. 32-5 and 32-6).

HEMOLYMPHATIC STAGE

This stage develops during or after the period when the chancre is active. The characteristic features are a periodic fever with episodes of remittent fever, general malaise, joint pains, and headache, lasting for about a week and interspersed with relatively asymptomatic periods. The cyclical pattern is related to fluctuating parasite densities due to changing parasite VSG antigens and partially effective antibody responses.

The hemolymphatic stage is dominated by febrile episodes, which in *T. b. rhodesiense* may be prostrating. In addition, there is a generalized lymphadenopathy often including enlargement of the posterior cervical lymph nodes (Winterbottom's sign), characteristic of *T. b. gambiense.* Lymph nodes

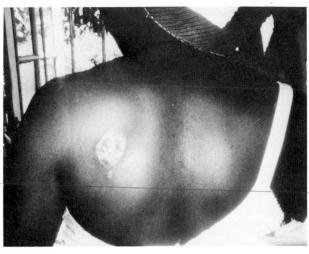

Figure 32-5. Healing chancre on the left shoulder. *T. b. rhodesiense infection.*

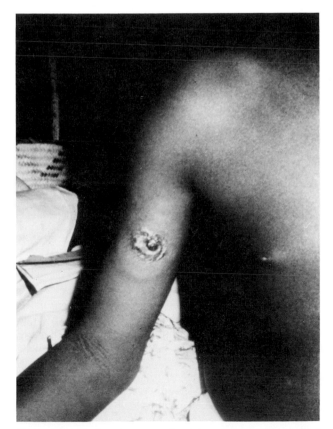

Figure 32-6. Active chancre on the right upper arm. Note central ulceration with surrounding zone of erythema and induration. *T. b. rhodesiense.*

are firm, discrete, and nontender. There is a moderate splenomegaly and hepatomegaly. During febrile episodes a rash may be observed, especially on the trunk. This is a fleeting, circular, nonirritant erythema, often with central unaffected areas, described as circinate erythema, and may be unnoticed by patients. It is not recognizable in pigmented races. Edema occurs in a variety of forms including periorbital edema, facial puffiness, dependent edema, and various serous effusions, including ascites and pleural and pericardial effusions. Evidence of organ damage also occurs. Myocarditis is particularly common and may lead to early mortality in *T. b. rhodesiense.* Jaundice occurs both from hemolysis and hepatic damage when it is accompanied by elevated enzyme levels.

In addition, there may be anemia and hypoalbuminemia. Rarely patients present with a coagulopathy and hemorrhagic manifestations. The total white blood cell count is either normal or modestly elevated, with a relative lymphocytosis. The sedimentation rate is markedly elevated. γ-Globulin levels are elevated. The serum IgM is frequently elevated more than IgG. Circulating immune complexes, heterophil antibodies, and rheumatoid factor are increased.

MENINGOENCEPHALITIC STAGE

The meningoencephalitic stage is characterized by increasing and persistent headache, specific abnormalities in sleep patterns, extrapyramidal and cerebellar signs, progressive alteration in level of consciousness, and abnormal behavior. These occur early in *T. b. rhodesiense* and run an acute course together with the hemolymphatic phase. In contrast, they occur late in *T. b. gambiense,* are usually more slowly progressive, and are not accompanied by a patent peripheral parasitemia.

Headache is severe, bilateral, and often is located in the frontal region. Patients frequently exhibit sleep disorders with diurnal somnolence, inappropriate episodes of sleeping, and nocturnal insomnia. Conscious level declines, and patients become stuporous and lapse into progressive, irreversible coma. The full picture of chronic neurological manifestations is usually seen in individuals infected with *T. b. gambiense.* These include ataxia, tremors, choreic or athetotic movements, hyperreflexia, delayed hyperesthesia (Kerandel's sign), and, less frequently, focal neurological lesions. Pyramidal tract features are unusual. Psychological features progressively accompany these neurological changes: variation in mood, apathy, mania, loss of cognitive function, inappropriate and bizarre or antisocial behavior, and personality change. Gross psychiatric manifestations include hallucinations, delusional states, and overt psychoses.

Other features associated with late stage disease that are probably endocrinologically mediated include impotence, amenorrhea, gynecomastia, and forme bouffie. Iridocyclitis and retinitis have been described. Obesity may occur, rarely, although wasting, emaciation, and nutritional deficiencies are

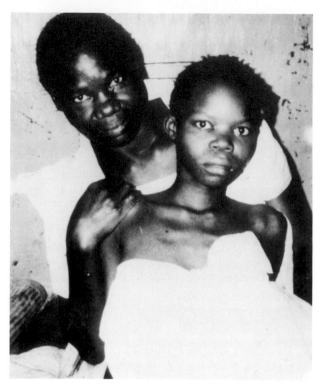

Figure 32-7. Late meningoencephalitis *T. b. rhodesiense* infection. Dull, vacant facies. Stuporous and wasted.

more usual; they are progressive in the later stages of meningoencephalitic trypanosomiasis. The immunosuppression associated with trypanosomiasis leads to a variety of secondary infections (Fig. 32-7).

DIAGNOSIS

Outside endemic areas, diagnosis initially requires a high index of clinical suspicion, especially in view of the wide spectrum of illness ranging from severe febrile disease to slowly progressive meningoencephalitis. Parasitic diagnosis is usually easier in *T. b. rhodesiense* infections and especially in the early stages of infection.

Parasitic diagnosis

Patent parasitemia is more common during febrile episodes and can be detected by examining a wet preparation or thin and thick blood films stained with Giemsa or Field's stain. In *T. b. gambiense,* frequent examination of the blood may be required. More sensitive concentration techniques include microhematocrit centrifugation (MHCT) and examination of the buffy coat [48]. The minianion exchange column (MAEC) [49] is a more sensitive method but may be difficult to use under field conditions. Aspiration of chancres before patent parasitemia may confirm the diagnosis. Lymph gland aspiration is

particularly valuable in *T. b. gambiense*. Trypanosomes can also be detected in the cerebrospinal fluid (CSF), preferably following centrifugation [50]. The CSF should be examined immediately following collection. Trypanosomes may also be detected in the bone marrow and in serous effusions. Animal inoculation using rats or mice is the most sensitive diagnostic method in *T. b. rhodesiense*.

Immunodiagnostic tests

A variety of immunodiagnostic tests have been used in evaluation of trypanosomiasis, notably, indirect immunofluorescence (IIF) and ELISA. Problems with both specificity and sensitivity reduce their value in clinical diagnosis. The card agglutination test (CATT), a latex test utilizing a frequently occurring variant antigen of *T. b. gambiense,* has been found of value as a screening test in *T. b. gambiense* but is of no value in *T. b. rhodesiense*. Newer diagnostic tests are now being pursued, including DNA hybridization and polymerase chain reaction.

Examination of CSF

CSF examination is mandatory both in the investigation of disease and the management of confirmed patients. In confirmed infection, the presence of meningoencephalitis is confirmed by an increase in CSF cells, predominantly lymphocytes, to greater than 5 per centimeter, and by elevation of CSF total protein, raised CSF IgM, or the presence of morular cells (Mott cells) or motile trypanosomes.

CHEMOTHERAPY

Early-stage disease

Before meningoencephalitis has developed, two drugs are effective in clearing infection. Suramin is effective in both *T. b. rhodesiense* and *T. b. gambiense* infection, while pentamidine is effective only in early *T. b. gambiense* infection (Table 32-1).

Suramin. This is administered as an IV solution containing 100 g/L. It is reconstituted prior to use. A test dose of 2 to 5 mg/kg is given initially followed in 48 h by a dose of 10 mg/kg. Thereafter a total dose of 5 g is given in weekly doses of 20 mg/kg. Suramin administration is associated with a rare (1 in 20,000) but potentially fatal hypersensitivity reaction. This risk is increased in the presence of concurrent onchocerciasis. More frequent side effects include various skin reactions and exfoliative dermatitis. The drug is nephrotoxic, and urinary protein and casts should be monitored during treatment.

Pentamidine. Pentamidine isethionate or pentamidine methanesulfonate is administered for 7 to 10 doses daily or alternate-daily by IM injection. The dose is 4 mg/kg (i.e., 2 mL of pentamidine isethionate or 4 mL of pentamidine meth-

Table 32-1. Treatment of early-stage African trypanosomiasis

Drug	Organism	Dose
Suramin	*T. b. rhodesiense* or *T. b. gambiense*	5 mg/kg IV day 1 (2.5 mL),* 10 mg/kg IV day 3 (5.0 mL)* 20 mg/kg IV day 5 (10.0 mL),* then 20 mg/kg IV weekly × 4
Pentamidine methanesulfonate	*T. b. gambiense*	4 mg/kg IM (5.0 mL) daily × 7–10 days
Pentamidine isethionate	*T. b. gambiense*	4 mg/kg IM (2.0 mL)* daily × 7–10 days

*Volume for 50-kg adult.

anesulfonate for a 50-kg adult). The important side effects are syncope, hypotension, and hypoglycemia. Other side effects are vomiting, abdominal pain, and a peripheral neuropathy.

Late-stage disease

The only drug widely used in the treatment of late-stage disease is melarsoprol. Melarsoprol is a 3.6% solution of melarsen oxide and dimercaprol in propylene glycol. The maximum single dose is 3.6 mg/kg (5 mL for a 50-kg adult). It is administered by IV injection. Various regimens have become established in different geographic areas. In general, groups of three daily injections separated by a week's rest period, to a total dose of 35 to 37 mL are used. Most regimes employ low dosages initially, increasing thereafter. A widely used regimen modified from Apted [51] and used in Kenya, Uganda, and Zambia is shown in Table 32-2.

Melarsoprol is an extreme irritant. Thrombophlebitis is common, and severe tissue damage results from extravascular injection. Other side effects include a Jarisch-Herxheimer reac-

Table 32-2. Treatment of late-stage African trypanosomiasis, *T. b. rhodesiense* or *T. b. gambiense*

1. Pretreatment of hemolymphatic infection with suramin on days 1, 3, and 5 (see Table 32-1 for details)
2. Examination of cerebrospinal fluid
   Raised total protein, >5 cells per cubic millimeter; trypanosomes; raised IgM
3. Melarsoprol

Day	7	8	9
mg/kg	0.36	0.72	1.1
Volume*	0.5	1.0	1.5
Day	16	17	18
mg/kg	1.4	1.8	2.2
Volume*	2.0	2.5	3.0
Day	25	26	27
mg/kg	2.2	2.9	3.6
Volume*	3.0	4.0	5.0
Day	34	35	36
mg/kg	3.6	3.6	3.6
Volume*	5.0	5.0	5.0

*Volume in milliliters for 50-kg adult.

tion, hepatic damage, and exfoliative dermatitis. The most important complication is a reactive arsenical encephalopathy, which may occur in up to 5 percent of treated patients. It is fatal in up to 75 percent [52]. It occurs most frequently in the 10 days following the start of treatment, often between the first and second course of injections. Patients present with sudden neurological deterioration, deepening coma, convulsions, or psychotic reactions. Recommended treatment includes withdrawal of melarsoprol, corticosteroids, and diazepam to control convulsions.

A small proportion of infected individuals may become resistant to melarsoprol. Recent trials have suggested that the anticancer drug (α difluoromethylornithine) DFMO and Nifurtimox (a 5-nitrofuran) are effective in *T. b. gambiense* patients refractory to melarsoprol. DFMO, an ornithine decarboxylase inhibitor, is available for oral and parenteral use but is difficult to administer. It has been given in doses of up to 400 mg/kg for 4 to 6 weeks [53]. Nifurtimox has been used in doses of 15 mg/kg for 4 to 6 weeks [54].

GENERAL MANAGEMENT

In parasitologically proven disease, it is usual practice to give IV suramin initially to clear the peripheral parasitemia before carrying out lumbar puncture in view of the risk of introducing trypanosomes. General supportive care is very important in management. The associated immunosuppression leads to a variety of intercurrent infections, especially bronchopneumonia. Such infections require specific chemotherapy. The general condition of severely emaciated patients, especially those with *T. b. gambiense*, should be improved before commencing specific therapy. In *T. b. rhodesiense,* however, the rapid progress of meningoencephalitis demands the early introduction of specific therapy. Under these circumstances, it is prudent to reduce initial doses of melarsoprol and administer it on alternate days. Corticosteroids have been recommended for the treatment of meningoencephalitic trypanosomiasis, but their value has not been confirmed in carefully controlled trials. Following appropriate specific therapy, parasitemias rapidly decline. A Jarisch-Herxheimer reaction may occur, especially when melarsoprol is used in the initial treatment. The clinical features of meningoencephalitis rapidly improve over the early days of treatment. After completion of chemotherapy patients must be followed up for at least 2 years to identify relapse. Follow-up should include CSF examination.

RELAPSE

A proportion of patients relapse after appropriate therapy. Relapse rates are high when initial therapy is inadequate or inappropriate. Relapse often presents with a chronic progressive meningoencephalitis, and parasitic confirmation may be impossible. Under these circumstances increasing CSF pleocytosis and rising total protein level are indications for treatment. Relapse should be treated with further full course of melarsoprol. As infection with African trypanosomiasis does not confer immunity to repeat infection, reinfection may occur. It presents as a new infection, and chancres have been observed in such cases.

Chemoprophylaxis

Pentamidine has been used as a chemoprophylactic in areas of endemic *T. b. gambiense*. Its use, however, may induce parasite resistance and may mask the early features of disease. The use of pentamidine prophylactically can therefore only be justified in very high risk situations.

POPULATION

Epidemiology

T. brucei is widely distributed throughout sub-Saharan Africa. Its occurrence has profoundly influenced human settlement and domestic animal husbandry. In recent years human trypanosomiasis has increased in several regions in Africa. Human conflict, increasing population pressure, migration, and land development programs have led to increased disease transmission. Countries with increasing transmission or epidemics of African trypanosomiasis include Uganda, Zaire, Sudan, Angola, and Mozambique. Official estimates of 10,000 to 20,000 cases annually are doubtless substantial underestimates. Integration of disease-specific control programs into primary health care programs is presently being attempted.

Subdivision into three subspecies, *T. b. brucei, T. b. rhodesiense,* and *T. b. gambiense,* was based on the parasites' differing host responses to infection. *T. b. brucei* does not infect human beings while *T. b. gambiense* and *T. b. rhodesiense* cause differing patterns of human disease. The morphological similarity in *T. brucei* has complicated investigation of the transmission of trypanosomiasis from wild and domestic animals to human beings. Confirmation of the wild game reservoir of *T. b. rhodesiense* was established by human volunteer inoculation of *T. brucei* trypanosomes from a bushbuck *Tragelaphus scriptus* [55]. More recently, the blood incubation inoculation test (BIIT) has also been used to screen potential human pathogenic trypanosomes [56]. Such studies have indicated that bushbuck, wildebeest, and waterbuck are potential

hosts for human infection. More recently analysis of isoenzymes and kDNA as genetic markers has been exploited [57]. Parasites with identical isoenzyme characteristics are termed *zymodemes*. Although no definitive markers of human pathogenicity have been conclusively identified, isoenzyme profiles supplemented by the blood incubation inoculation test have provided evidence that in west Africa both wild and domestic animals harbor the same trypanosome zymodemes, while in *T. b. rhodesiense* substantial differences exist between isolates from southeast and east Africa. In east Africa such studies have confirmed that cattle trypanosomes are identical to isolates obtained from human disease in the same geographical area. In the Lambwe Valley, Kenya, 10 percent of cattle had trypanosomes identical to the dominant zymodemes occurring in a subsequent human outbreak [58]. In eastern Uganda, cattle also harbored trypanosomes identical to those from human beings. Epidemics of *T. b. rhodesiense* are characterized by a wide diversity of zymodeme types [59].

In *T. b. rhodesiense* animal reservoirs play an important and at times an exclusive role in human transmission. Important domestic animal reservoirs include cattle, sheep, and goats; dogs rapidly succumb to infection and are unlikely to be an important reservoir. The bushbuck is perhaps the most important wild animal reservoir, but various other game animals and carnivores harbor *T. brucei* parasites (Table 32-3).

In *T. b. gambiense* a variety of wild and domestic animals have been found to harbor parasites from zymodemes identical to human parasites. Such studies challenge the long-held view that transmission is exclusively person to person. The epidemiological significance of animal infection in relation to human disease transmission is unknown (Table 32-3).

Human trypanosomiasis is transmitted biologically by species of tsetse fly (*Glossina*). The genus *Glossina* comprises three groups: *Austenia* (fusca group), *Nemorhina* (palpalis group), and *Glossina* (morsitans group). Two groups are important in transmission of human disease. The palpalis group of flies include *G. palpalis, G. fuscipes,* and *G. tachynoides*. These species are catholic feeders, inhabiting riverine, lacustrine, and forest habitats; they transmit *T. b. gambiense*. Ep-

Table 32-3. Animal reservoirs of African trypanosomiasis

Organism	Domestic	Wild	
T. b. rhodesiense	Cattle*	Bushbuck*	*Tragelaphus scriptus*
	Sheep	Reedbuck	*Redunca redunca*
	Goat	Waterbuck	*Kobus ellipsiprymnus*
	Dog	Hartebeest*	*Alcelaphus buselaphus*
		Lion*	*Panthera leo*
		Hyena	*Crocuta crocuta*
T. b. gambiense	Pig	Kob	*Kobus kob*
	Cattle	Hartebeest	*Alcelaphus buselaphus*
	Dog*		
	Sheep		

*Human pathogenicity confirmed by volunteer infection.

idemic *T. b. rhodesiense* is also transmitted by the palpalis group of flies in western Kenya and eastern Uganda (*G. f. fuscipes*). The morsitans group of flies include *G. morsitans, G. swynnertoni, G. longipalpis, G. pallidipes,* and *G. austeni.* They inhabit woodland savannah and are generally more host-specific feeders. They transmit *T. b. rhodesiense* infections.

Tsetse flies are hardy and long-lived. They demand shade for resting and produce a single larva at a time. Both sexes take blood meals. Infection rates in flies rarely exceed 0.1 percent. They are attracted to large moving objects (including animals, people, and vehicles) and by dark colors and specific odors.

T. b. gambiense occurs focally through large areas of west and central Africa, west of a line through Sudan, Uganda, and Angola. Human infection can attain high prevalence rates, and transmission is predominantly person to person via the palpalis group of tsetse flies. Human-fly contact is often high at watering points and in association with agricultural activities. The importance of animal reservoirs remains uncertain.

T. b. rhodesiense usually occurs sporadically, especially in east and southeast Africa in open woodland savannah. Infection is often in herders, hunters, honeygatherers, game wardens, and tourists. The infection is transmitted by morsitans group tsetse flies from wild or domestic animals, and human beings play no role as a reservoir of infection.

In contrast, epidemics of *T. b. rhodesiense* have occurred in recent years in Uganda and Kenya in areas close to Lake Victoria, notably in Busoga, Uganda. In this situation, the disease is transmitted by *G. f. fuscipes,* which has become established peridomestically, utilizing for resting and larviposition the introduced bush, *Lantana camara,* which now occupies previously cultivated land. The proximity of the vector to human beings has permitted epidemics involving all age groups and both sexes. The role of person-to-person transmission is uncertain, and both domestic cattle and wild animals may provide a reservoir.

CONTROL

In the past, heroic measures have been employed to control trypanosomiasis, although often predominantly aimed at domestic animal disease. This has included massive clearance of tsetse habitats, destruction of wild game, restriction of human settlement, and enforced relocation of entire populations. With the advent of insecticides, efforts were directed toward more specific control of *Glossina* species using focal spraying, aerial spraying, and most recently traps and screens as vector control methods. The highest public health priority must be the provision of adequate diagnostic and treatment facilities.

SURVEILLANCE AND TREATMENT

Passive surveillance is effective in *T. b. rhodesiense* except in epidemics, where active surveillance and case detection be-

come cost-effective in view of the large numbers of cases. Facilities are required for effective and accurate diagnosis and standardized treatment. In *T. b. gambiense,* active surveillance is of particular importance in view of the prolonged course of infection and the importance of human beings as the reservoir of infection.

VECTOR CONTROL

Vector control techniques depend on the habits of the vector species. Insecticides can be applied focally on the ground or by air, using fixed wing airplanes and helicopters. Extensive use of low-cost traps, such as the pyramidal trap [60], and screens has been shown to reduce tsetse populations to very low levels. Traps and screens can be impregnated with insecticides and in some instances can be improved by the use of attractant odors. Local clearance of vegetation around homesteads, along footpaths, and at watering points will also help to reduce human-fly contact. In the past control programs were disease-specific. Increasingly, attempts are being made to introduce control measures through existing health services, with improved health education and community participation. Long-term control demands community participation in surveillance and the use of appropriate low-cost trapping techniques.

REFERENCES

1 Hoare CA: *The Trypanosomes of Mammals: A Zoological Monograph.* Oxford, Blackwell, 1972
2 Vickerman K: Polymorphism and mitochondrial activity in sleeping sickness trypanosomes. Nature 208:762–766, 1965
3 Bowman IBR, Flyn IW: Oxidative metabolism of trypanosomes, in Lumsden WHR, Evans DA (eds): *Biology of Kinetoplastida.* London, Academic, 1976, pp 435–476
4 Hill GC: Electron transport systems in kinetoplastida. Biochim Biophys Acta 456:149–193, 1976
5 Gutteridge WE, Coombs GH: *Biochemistry of Parasitic Protozoa.* Baltimore, University Park, 1977
6 Fairlamb A: Biochemistry of trypanosomiasis and rational approaches to chemotherapy. Trends Biochem Sci 7:249–253, 1982
7 Vickerman K, Preston TM: Comparative cell biology of the kinetoplastid flagellates, in Lumsden WHR, Evans DA (eds): *Biology of Kinetoplastida.* London, Academic, 1976, pp 35–130
8 Opperdoes FR: Compartmentation of carbohydrate metabolism in trypanosomes. Ann Rev Microbiol 41:127–151, 1987
9 Vickerman K: On surface coat and flagellar adhesion in trypanosomes. J Cell Sci 5:163–193, 1969
10 Simpson L: The kinetoplast of the hemoflagellates. Intern Rev Cytol 32:139–207, 1972
11 Englund PT, Hajduk SL, Marini JC: The molecular biology of trypanosomes. Ann Rev Biochem 51:695–726, 1982
12 Stuart K: Kinetoplast DNA, mitochondrial DNA with a difference. Mol Biochem Parasitol 9:93–104, 1983
13 Simpson L: The mitochondrial genome of kinetoplastid protozoa: genomic organization, transcription, replication, and evolution. Ann Rev Microbiol 41:363–382, 1987

14 Hoeijmakers JHJ, Borst P: Kinetoplast DNA in the insect trypanosomes *Crithidia luciliae* and *Crithidia fasciculata*. II. Sequence evolution of the minicircles. Plasmid 7:210–220, 1982

15 Ntambi JM, Shapiro TA, Ryan KA, et al: Ribonucleotides associated with a gap in newly replicated kinetoplast DNA minicircles from *Trypanosoma equiperdum*. J Biol Chem 261:11890–11895, 1986

16 Marini JC, Levene SD, Crothers DM, et al: A bent helical structure in kinetoplast DNA. Proc Natl Acad Sci USA 79:7664–7668, 1982

17 Griffith J, Bleyman M, Rauch CA, et al: Visualization of the bent helix in kinetoplast DNA by electron microscopy. Cell 46:717–724, 1986

18 Marini JC, Levene SD, Crothers DM, et al: A bent helix in kinetoplast DNA. Cold Spring Harbor Symp Quant Biol 47:279–283, 1983

19 Silver LE, Torri AF, Hajduk SL: Organized packaging of kinetoplast DNA networks. Cell 47:537–543, 1986

20 Rohrer SP, Michelotti EF, Torri AF, et al: Transcription of kinetoplast DNA minicircles. Cell 49:625–632, 1987

21 Michelotti EF, Hajduk SL: Developmental regulation of trypanosome mitochondrial gene expression. J Biol Chem 262:927–932, 1987

22 Benne RJ, Van den Burg J, Bradenhoff JPJ, et al: Major transcript of the frameshifted coxII gene from trypanosome mitochondria contains four nucleotides that are not encoded in the DNA. Cell 46:819–826, 1986

23 Feagin JE, Jasmer DP, Stuart K: Developmentally regulated addition of nucleotides within apocytochrome b transcripts in *Trypanosoma brucei*. Cell 49:337–345, 1987

24 Feagin JE, Stuart K: Developmental aspects of uridine addition within mitochondrial transcripts of *Trypanosoma brucei*. Molec Cell Biol 8:1259–1265, 1988

25 Ryan KA, Shapiro TA, Rauch CA, et al: The replication of kinetoplast DNA in trypanosomes. Ann Rev Microbiol 42:339–358

26 Ole-MoiYoi OK: Trypanosome species-specific DNA probes to detect infection in tsetse flies. Parasitol Today 3:371–374, 1987

27 Hajduk SL: Influence of DNA complexing compounds on the kinetoplast of trypanosomatids, in Hahn FE (ed): *Progress in Molecular and Subcellular Biology*. Berlin, Springer-Verlag, 1978, vol 6, pp 158–200

28 Donelson JE, Rice-Ficht AC: Molecular biology of trypanosome antigenic variation. Microbiol Rev 49:107–125, 1985

29 Boothroyd JC: Antigenic variation in African trypanosomes. Ann Rev Microbiol 39:475–502, 1985

30 Borst P: Discontinuous transcription and antigenic variation in trypanosomes. Ann Rev Biochem 55:701–732, 1986

31 Turner MJ: Biochemistry of the variant surface glycoproteins of salivarian trypanosomes. Adv Parasitol 21:69–153, 1982

32 LeRay D, Barry JD, Vickerman K: Antigenic heterogeneity of metacyclic forms of *Trypanosoma brucei*. Nature 273:300–302, 1978

33 Hajduk SL, Cameron CR, Barry JD, et al: Antigenic variation in cyclically transmitted *Trypanosoma brucei:* Variable antigen type composition of metacyclic trypanosome populations from the salivary glands of *Glossina morsitans*. Parasitology 83:595–607, 1981

34 Esser KM, Schoenbechler MJ, Gingrich JB, et al: Monoclonal antibody analysis of *Trypanosoma rhodesiense* metacyclic variable antigen types. Fed Proc 40:1011, 1981

35 Metcalf P, Blum M, Freymann D, et al: Two variant surface glycoproteins of *Trypanosoma brucei* of different sequence classes have similar 6 Å resolution x-ray structures. Nature 325:84–86, 1987

36 Ferguson MA, Homans SW, Dwek RA, et al: Glycosyl-phosphatidylinositol moiety that anchors *Trypanosoma brucei* variant surface glycoprotein to the membrane. Science 239:753–759, 1988

37 Englund PT, Hereld D, Krakow JL, et al: Glycolipid membrane anchor of the trypanosome variant surface glycoprotein: Its biosynthesis and cleavage, in Englund PT, Sher A (eds): *The Biology of Parasitism*. New York, Alan R Liss, vol 9, 1989, pp. 401–412

38 Clarkson AB, Brohn FH: Trypanosomiasis: An approach to chemotherapy by the inhibition of carbohydrate metabolism. Science 192: 204–206, 1976

39 Fairlamb AH, Opperdoes FR, Borst P: New approach to screening drugs for activity against African trypanosomes. Nature 265:270–271, 1977

40 Bacchi CJ: Content, synthesis and function of polyamines in trypanosomatids: Relationship to chemotherapy. J Protozool 28:20–27, 1981

41 Sjoeidsma A, Schechter PJ: Chemotherapeutic implications of polyamine biosynthesis inhibition. Clin Pharmacol Ther 35:287, 1984

42 Phillips MA, Caffino P, Wang CC: Cloning and sequencing of the ornithine decarboxylase gene from *Trypanosoma brucei*. J Biol Chem 262:8721–8727, 1987

43 Fairlamb AH, Blackburn P, Ulrick P, et al: Trypanothione: A novel bis(glutathionyl)-spermidine cofactor for glutathione reductase in trypanosomatids. Science 227:1485–1487, 1985

44 Rifkin MR: Identification of the trypanocidal factor in normal human serum: High density lipoprotein. Proc Natl Acad Sci USA 75: 3450–3454, 1979

45 Hajduk SL, Moore DR, Vasudevacharya J, Siqueira H, Torri AF, Tytler EM, Esko JD: Lysis of *Trypanosoma brucei* by a toxic subspecies of human high density lipoprotein. J Biol Chem, 264: 5210–5217, 1989

46 Molyneux DH, deRaat R, Seed JR: African human trypanosomiasis, in Gilles HM (ed): *Recent Advances in Tropical Medicine*, Edinburgh, Churchill Livingstone, 1984, pp 39–62

47 Greenwood BM, Whittle HC: The pathogenesis of sleeping sickness. Trans R Soc Trop Med Hyg 74:716–725, 1980

48 Woo PTK: The haematocrit centrifugation technique for the diagnosis of African trypanosomiasis. Acta Tropica 35:384–386, 1970

49 Lumsden WAR, Kimber CD, Evans DA, et al: *Trypanosoma brucei:* Miniature anion exchange and centrifugation technique for detection of low parasitaemias—adaption for field use. Trans R Soc Trop Med Hyg 73:312–317, 1979

50 Epidemiology and Control of African Trypanosomiasis. Tech Rep Ser 739, World Health Organization, Geneva, 1986

51 Apted FIC: Clinical manifestations and diagnosis of sleeping sickness, in Mulligan HW (ed): *The African Trypanosomiases*. London, George Allen & Unwin, 1970, pp 661–683

52 Haller L, Adams H, Merouze F, et al: Clinical and pathological aspects of human African trypanosomiasis (*T. b. gambiense*) with particular reference to reactive arsenical encephalopathy. Am J Trop Med Hyg 35(1):94–99, 1986

53 Van Nieuwenhove S, Schechter PJ, Declercq J, et al: Treatment of Gambian sleeping sickness in the Sudan with oral DFMO (difluoromethylornithine) an inhibitor of ornithine decarboxylase: First field trial. Trans R Soc Trop Med Hyg 79:692–698, 1985

54 Van Nieuwenhove S, Declercq J: Nifurtimox (Lanpit) treatment in late stage of Gambian sleeping sickness. Proceedings of International Scientific Council for Trypanosomiasis Research and Control, 17th Meeting, Arusha, Tanzania. OAU/STRC Publication no 112, 1986, pp 206–208

55 Heisch RB, McMahon JP, Manson-Bahr PEL: The isolation of *Trypanosoma rhodesiense* from a bushbuck. Br Med J ii: 1203–1204, 1958

56 Rickman LR: The blood infectivity test (BIIT) as an epidemiological tool in the study of African trypanosomiasis (sleeping sickness), in *New Approaches to the Identification of Parasites and their Vectors*. Basel, Schwabe & Co, 1984, pp 199–216

57 Godfrey DG: Molecular biochemical characterisation of human parasites, in Gilles HM (ed): *Recent Advances in Tropical Medicine*. Edinburgh, Churchill Livingstone, 1984, pp 289–319

58 Gibson WC, Wellde B: Characterisation of trypanozoon stocks from the South Nyanza sleeping sickness focus in Western Kenya. Trans R Soc Trop Med Hyg 79:671–676, 1985

59 Gibson WC, Gashyumba JK: Isoenzyme characterisation of some trypanozoon stocks from a recent trypanosomiasis epidemic in Uganda. Trans R Soc Trop Med Hyg 77:114–118, 1983

60 Gouteaux JP, Lancien J: Le piège pyramidal a tsé tsé (Diptera: Glossinidae) pour a capture et la lutte essais comparatifs et description de nouveaux systèmes de capture. Trop Med Parasitol 37: 61–66, 1986

61 Vickerman K: Antigenic variation in African trypanosomes, in Porter P and Knight J (eds): *Parasites in the Immunized Host: Mechanisms of Survival*. Ciba Foundation Symposium 25 (new series). Amsterdam, Associated Scientific Publishers, 1974, pp 53–80.

62 Vickerman K: Ultrastructure of Trypanosoma and relation to function, in Mulligan HW (ed): *The African Trypanosomiases*. London, George Allen & Unwin, 1970, pp 60–66

American Trypanosomiasis (Chagas' Disease) · Nadia Nogueira

CHAPTER 33 · *Jose Rodrigues Coura*

American trypanosomiasis is a zoonosis caused by *Trypanosoma cruzi* which can be transmitted to humans by bloodsucking insects of the genera *Triatoma, Rhodnius,* and *Panstrongylus*. The disease was described by Carlos Chagas in 1909, and his accomplishment is a unique instance in medical history. As a single researcher, he was responsible for the description of a new disease, the discovery of its etiology, its vectors, and its reservoirs.

PARASITE

LIFE CYCLE, MORPHOLOGY

In the invertebrate host, *T. cruzi* grows extracellularly in two distinct forms. Epimastigotes multiply in the insect gut and differentiate into metacyclic trypomastigotes, the infectious forms for the mammalian host. These are released with the feces close to the site of the bite and enter the host via the damaged skin or through contamination of mucous membranes. Once in the vertebrate host, metacyclic trypomastigotes readily enter cells, where they replicate as rounded amastigote forms. Amastigotes then differentiate intracellularly into trypomastigotes, which are released in the vasculature, where they circulate as bloodstream-form trypomastigotes. These do not replicate until they enter another cell or are withdrawn by another insect vector (Fig. 33-1).

Blood-form trypomastigotes appear in stained preparations as S-shaped flagellates 15 to 20 μm in length. A central nucleus

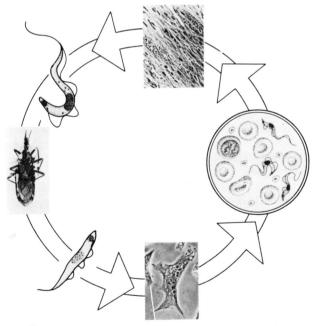

Figure 33-1. Life cycle of *T. cruzi*. Counterclockwise, beginning with the insect vector: Metacyclic trypomastigote left in the feces of the triatomid bug; amastigotes (arrows) within a macrophage; trypomastigotes in peripheral blood; amastigotes (arrow) in heart cells; blood from trypomastigotes ingested by triatomid bug.

and a large terminal kinetoplast can be easily identified. Amastigotes, the vertebrate host's forms, appear as oval aflagellates of approximately 3- to 6-μm diameter. Epimastigotes, the replicative form in the digestive tract of the insect vector, are 20 μm in length, and have a prominent central nucleus and a kinetoplast which is anterior to the nucleus.

T. cruzi can be grown in acellular cultures, where they multiply as epimastigotes and differentiate to a certain degree into metacyclic trypomastigotes, thereby reproducing the growth pattern in the insect vector. The vertebrate stages of the parasite can be obtained either from the blood of infected hosts or from infected cells maintained in vitro.

Surface antigens

Cell surface molecules of *T. cruzi* have spurred considerable interest due to their potential for both specific diagnostic tests and vaccines. Several surface antigens have been identified, and most have been found to be glycosylated. These include a 90,000-dalton glycoprotein [1,2], an 85,000-dalton blood trypomastigote–specific glycoprotein [3] which has been recently cloned, a lipophosphopeptidoglycan (LPPG), a 72,000- to 75,000-dalton glycoprotein specific to the insect stages of the organism [4], and a 70,000- to 84,000-dalton glycoprotein specific to the intracellular amastigote stage [5]. No evidence of antigenic variation has been demonstrated in either these [6] or any other surface antigen of *T. cruzi*. Immunoprecipitation patterns obtained with sera from infected humans and experimental animals (mice, rabbits) reveal a similar pattern in which these moieties appear as major components. This suggests that these surface antigens may be the dominant immunogenic components of *T cruzi*. In conjunction with their ubiquitous presence in all *T. cruzi* strain studies and the absence of antigenic variation in these organisms, it is possible that these glycopeptides will offer possibilities as immunoprophylactic agents. In immunization trials in mice, the 90,000-dalton cell surface glycoprotein has provided protection to challenge with virulent blood forms of the organism. It is therefore possible that these moieties could be of relevance in protective immunization regimens in humans as well. The use of recombinant DNA techniques may prove to be of value in providing large amounts of these antigens for cost-effective vaccines if trial immunizations are successful.

Metabolic pathways of possible therapeutic importance

A number of biochemical differences between the metabolism of trypanosomatids and that of their mammalian hosts may be exploited as targets for chemotherapy. Among these is the high sensitivity of trypanosomes toward agents that promote free radical damage. Trypanosomatids do not possess catalase or glutathione reductase glutathione peroxidase, key enzymes in the antioxidant process. In contrast, all species of trypanosomatids possess instead an unusual NADPH-dependent flavoprotein disulfide reductase (trypanothione reductase). For this reason, drugs that either stimulate H_2O_2 generation or prevent its utilization may prove to be potentially good trypanocidal agents. In this respect, Nifurtimox, a nitrofuran derivative, one of the most effective drugs used for the treatment of acute Chagas' disease, has been shown to be capable of inducing maximal stimulation of superoxide anion and hydrogen peroxide in all the life-stage forms of *T. cruzi* [7]. This fact supports the view that the trypanocidal action of Nifurtimox may be mediated by products of partial reduction of oxygen. Therefore, other drugs that subvert the flow of electrons from the water-producing pathway to the superoxide anion pathway would represent promising chemotherapeutic agents for Chagas' disease. However, the same mechanisms may be responsible for the toxic side effects for the mammalian host observed with this drug at high dosage levels.

Cloning and characterization of parasite strains: Zymodemes and schizodemes

The exact cause of the differences displayed by different strains of *T. cruzi* in both humans and experimental animals is not known, although there is evidence for the involvement of both host and parasite factors. For this reason some effort has been directed toward characterization and identification of different *T. cruzi* stocks. Isozyme analysis has been used to classify strains of *T. cruzi* into several distinct isozyme groups (or zymodemes) [8]. Variation in kinetoplast DNA (kDNA) buoyant density has been reported between different strains of *T. cruzi* isolates [9]. More recently, comparison of restriction endonuclease–generated fragments of kDNA minicircles between several strains and clones of *T. cruzi* has resulted in a classification of subpopulations having similar gel profiles, or schizodemes [10]. This method has revealed heterogeneity in some well-established *T. cruzi* stocks. Schizodemes and zymodemes have not always shown a direct correlation. So far, association between clinical manifestations of the disease and any particular classification has not been demonstrated.

PATIENT

HOST-PARASITE INTERACTIONS

It is generally accepted that soon after their penetration into the mammalian host metacyclic trypomastigotes are engulfed by macrophages, where they multiply as amastigotes. From these cells, trypomastigotes erupt and reach the blood and other tissues. In laboratory animals, *T. cruzi* strains have been shown to display selective parasitism for different tissues under certain specific experimental conditions. Most strains are considered to be myotropic, invading mostly smooth, skeletal, and heart muscle, whereas others have been called *macrophagotropic* owing to what is seen as an interaction predominantly with macrophages. The basis for such differences has not been identified. Whether differences in tissue tropism also exist in humans has not yet been demonstrated.

Despite some controversial findings, most evidence favors the concept that *T. cruzi* enters macrophages by a phagocytic mechanism [*11*]. The organisms are taken up within membrane-bound vacuoles. No evidence has been found at the electron microscopic level of fusion between parasite and host cell membranes or dissolution of the host cell surface membranes to justify a direct penetration mechanism. Trypomastigotes are found in membrane-bound vacuoles at first, but soon lyse the phagosome membrane and escape into the cytoplasm, where they replicate. The mechanism of escape from the phagocytic vacuole is not well understood. Similar electron microscopic findings have been observed with nonprofessional phagocytic cells (HeLa, 3T3, and L cells).

Parasite attachment and interiorization by macrophages is mediated by protease-sensitive receptor-like molecules on the macrophage surface. These might interact with parasite surface components to initiate ingestion. Interestingly, blood-form trypomastigotes are very resistant to interiorization by macrophages, in contrast to the rapid uptake of metacyclic trypomastigotes. This antiphagocytic effect can be overcome either by removal of an antiphagocytic factor from the parasite surface by trypsin treatment or by opsonization with specific IgG-class antibodies [*12*]. Trypsinization of the parasite surface removes the 90,000-dalton glycoprotein, and the antiphagocytic effect is regained as the glycoprotein is inserted back on the surface [*2*]. This reversal can be blocked by preventing protein synthesis with cycloheximide. This suggests a role for the mammalian-stage-specific 90,000-dalton glycoprotein in avoiding the effector function of macrophages, as will be described below.

IMMUNOLOGY

The precise immune mechanisms involved in resistance to *T. cruzi* and control of the parasitism during the chronic phase of infection are not completely understood. Despite the establishment of strong acquired immunity, there is no parasitological cure. This may be because the organisms are sheltered in the cytoplasm of nonimmune cells and therefore not exposed to the host's immune defense system. Other evasion mechanisms may still occur to permit the parasite to overcome the host's immune response.

The importance of antibodies in resistance to *T. cruzi* seems to be primarily associated with the chronic phase of the infection [*13*]. The protective antibodies were found to belong to the IgG class, and their effects may depend primarily on mediation of immunophagocytosis of the organisms by macrophages [*12,14*] rather than on immune lysis in the presence of complement.

Procedures known to interfere with cell-mediated immune mechanisms have been found to increase the severity of infection by *T. cruzi*. More specifically, there is increased evidence both in vivo and in vitro that macrophages play a major role in protection against *T. cruzi* infection, particularly in the acute

phase. In the nonimmune host, macrophages provide a favorable environment for the growth and replication of the organisms. In contrast, in the immune host, macrophages become activated to a microbicidal state in which they are capable of destroying the interiorized organisms [*15*]. This activated microbicidal state of mouse and human macrophages [*14,16*] can be induced under in vitro conditions by soluble products of sensitized T lymphocytes stimulated by the specific antigen (lymphokines). Interferon γ appears to be one of the principal lymphokines that can activate macrophages to kill *T. cruzi*. In vivo administration of interferon γ in mice prevented acute disease, immune suppression, and death in experimental *T. cruzi* infection [*17*].

Under in vitro conditions, opsonization by IgG-class antibodies enhances the uptake of the organisms by both normal mouse and human macrophages without modifying their intracellular fate. In activated macrophages opsonization by IgG results in increased uptake accompanied by increased killing of interiorized organisms [*12,14*], suggesting that in vivo the protective role of antibodies may depend on the presence of concomitant cell-mediated immunity.

Mechanism of intracellular killing in macrophages

On the basis of the observation that variations in virulence of bacteria-parasitizing macrophages appeared to be linked to their resistance to H_2O_2, earlier workers [*18*] had postulated that macrophage production of H_2O_2 might be the biochemical basis for acquired cellular immunity. Similarly, a direct correlation has been found between macrophage production of H_2O_2 and the ability to kill intracellular trypomastigotes of *T. cruzi* [*19*]. The two parameters increased in parallel when macrophages were activated either in vivo by *T. cruzi* infection or in vitro, by exposure to cytokines, such as IFN-γ and GM-CSF. Similarly, both functions decreased following removal of the cytokines. As described earlier, the exquisite sensitivity of trypanosomes to H_2O_2 and the amount of H_2O_2 generated by activated macrophages allow one to calculate that such concentrations of H_2O_2 within phagosomes would amount to several thousand lethal doses for the organisms.

Immunosuppression in Chagas' disease

Depression of the immune response during acute *T. cruzi* infection in both humans and experimental animals has been described, involving depression of both humoral and cell-mediated immune mechanisms. It has been suggested that this immunosuppression is mediated by a subpopulation of thymus-derived lymphocytes. However, the importance of this event in relation to the clinical pleomorphism of Chagas' disease is not well understood.

GENETIC CONTROL OF RESPONSES TO *T. CRUZI*

The factors determining the severity of the acute and chronic phases of *T. cruzi* infections are uncertain. However, factors related to the parasite (strain, size of the inoculum) as well as to the host (state of health, genetic background) are likely to be involved. In experimental animals, sex and age have been found to influence the resistance to infection. In addition, a spectrum of resistance has been found in mice, ranging from highly susceptible to resistant strains. The immune response was found to be necessary for survival in resistant mice, since impairment of the immune system led to fatal parasitemias.

To investigate the role of immune response genes in resistance to acute infection with *T. cruzi*, an attempt was made to correlate resistance or susceptibility with the major histocompatibility complexes of mice (H-2 locus). Results implicate a polygenic regulation or resistance to *T. cruzi* and the presence of an H-2 effect on susceptibility to the parasite [20].

A direct correlation was found between in vitro cell-mediated effector mechanisms and in vivo susceptibility in inbred strains of mice [21]. Spleen cells from resistant mice were able to generate higher levels of lymphokines, at earlier times after infection, than those from susceptible mice. The cellular basis for these differences was not identified, but it could be related to differences in suppressor activity.

The role of genetic factors on the outcome of human infections with *T. cruzi* has not been well investigated. Correlation between severity of infection and HLA haplotypes has not been reported.

PATHOLOGY AND PATHOPHYSIOLOGY

The most important histopathological findings in acute Chagas' myocarditis involve three elements: first, an infiltrate of mononuclear cells into the interstitial space; second, a degenerative process in myocardial fibers; and third, the appearance of the so-called pseudocysts. The intensity of the inflammatory infiltrate is variable, and, depending on its extent, changes in heart morphology may or may not be found.

In chronic Chagas' cardiomyopathy the histological picture is characterized by the presence of fibrosis, degenerating myocardial fibers, and infiltrates of mononuclear cells. The degree of fibrosis is varied. The fibrotic focuses may be small and few, or, in contrast, dense and forming larger fibrotic plates which thin the ventricular wall. The myocardial fibers frequently show degenerative changes in the fibrotic areas. The morphology of the heart in chronic Chagas' cardiomyopathy depends on the extent of the fibrotic process, which leads to both dilation and hypertrophy. These alterations are frequently associated with intramural thrombi, mainly at the apex of the left ventricle (Fig. 33-2). Thinning of the ventricular wall by large fibrotic plates becomes the starting point for the formation of aneurysms. For reasons that are not quite clear, these are often found at the apex of the left ventricle or the posterior area of the mitral valve.

The pathophysiological mechanisms underlying the severe myocarditis which can occur during the chronic phase of Chagas' disease have not been established. The low level of parasites in the tissues as well as in the circulation has prompted investigators to suggest that heart lesions are not produced at this stage by direct destruction of tissue. Immunological causes have been suggested as underlying these chronic lesions. Both humoral and cell-mediated immune phenomena have been implicated [22], but the evidence for both cases is still a matter of controversy.

Sera from both acute and chronic cases of Chagas' disease show reactivity with *T. cruzi*, as well as with normal endocardial tissue, vessels, and interstitium of striated muscle, in what has been called the EVI pattern [23]. These antibodies were not found in other heart diseases examined. More recently, it has been found that these antibodies react with connective tissue structures, namely, laminin, a basement membrane glycoprotein which mediates the attachment of epithelial

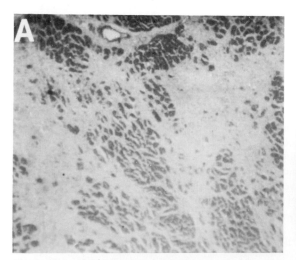
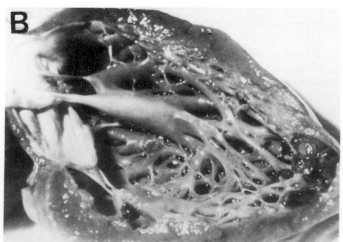

Figure 33-2. Chronic Chagas cardiomyopathy in human being. *A*. Heart fibrosis. *B*. Heart hypertrophy with dilation of the cavity and apical aneurysm of the left ventricle with thrombosis.

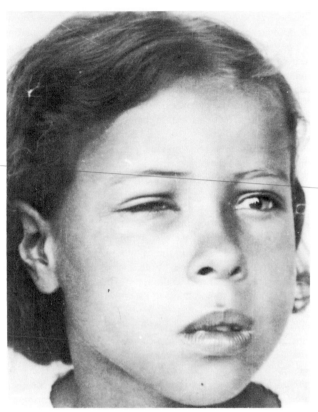

Figure 33-3. Romaña's sign in acute case of Chagas' disease. (*Courtesy of Dr. Joao Carlos Pinto Dias.*)

and endothelial cells to type IV collagen [24]. The reactivity with laminin can explain the EVI pattern, but the significance of these antibodies to the pathology of Chagas' disease is still unclear. These antibodies could damage blood vessels and endocardium, leading to the endocardial fibrosis found in Chagas' disease. The changes would start in the acute phase, when the titers of these antibodies were higher. The nature of the parasite moiety that cross-reacts with laminin is still unclear.

Participation of cell-mediated autoimmune reactions has also been suggested [25], with cytotoxic lymphocytes recognizing cross-reacting moieties in the surface of myocardial cells, resulting in damage to nonparasitized heart cells.

Finally, the lesions could be simply explained by the extent of direct damage produced by the parasites and resulting inflammation during the acute phase. Damage to the conductive tissue could explain the conductive defects that ensue. The resulting fibrosis would be superimposed on other myocardial alterations associated with age, genetic factors, and nutrition, leading to anoxia, further damage, and fibrosis.

The histopathology of the affected esophagus and colon involves the presence of mononuclear cell infiltrates between smooth muscle cells and sometimes granuloma formation. A drastic reduction of neurons in the myoenteric plexus is commonly seen. This destruction of neurons in the ganglia has

been suggested to be the anatomopathological basis for the Chagas' megadisease, since it will result in hyperactivity and hypertrophy of the smooth muscles regulating organ mobility.

CLINICAL MANIFESTATIONS

In humans, the disease begins with a local lesion at the site of inoculation, the primary chagoma, which is followed by acute and chronic manifestations of systemic illness.

The primary chagoma

Following penetration of broken skin or healthy mucous membranes, metacyclic trypomastigotes are phagocytized by macrophages and other local cells. The organisms multiply within the cytoplasm of the host cells, causing them to rupture and generating an inflammatory reaction of variable intensity. In most cases, this reaction is mild and clinically imperceptible.

The initial cutaneous lesion, or "inoculation chagoma," consists of a small nodule 1 to 3 cm wide, raised, reddish, and mildly painful, with an indurated base. It is generally accompanied by satellite swelling of lymph nodes. When the route of inoculation is the ocular mucosa, a characteristic unilateral conjunctivitis and edema of the eyelids may occur, Romaña's sign (Fig. 33-3). Despite its relative rarity, this sign has proved useful in the diagnosis of a large number of cases because of its noticeable location.

The acute phase

In most cases, the clinical symptoms during the acute phase are either mild or absent. As a result, despite the large number of chronic cases in endemic areas, the number of cases with a past clinical history compatible with the acute phase of the disease is rather small. A 16-month follow-up of 554 people with negative serology for Chagas' disease in an endemic area of Brazil revealed the appearance of 14 new cases. Among these, only 5 (35 percent) displayed any clinical manifestations specific for the acute phase of the disease. The acute manifestations of the disease are usually seen in young children [26], where they are serious and often fatal. Initially, this was thought to be due to an increased prevalence of infection in young children. However, cross-sectional serological studies in endemic areas have shown increasing prevalence of infection up until the third or fourth decade of life, indicating that the acute phase is less obvious in older individuals.

The classical manifestations of the symptomatic acute phase are daily fever; cervical, axillary, and iliac adenitis; hepatosplenomegaly; erythematous rash; and acute myocarditis. Several fatal cases of acute meningoencephalitis have been described since the publication of the original papers by Chagas, particularly in infants.

Fever is usually moderate, around 38°C, with peaks occurring in the evenings. Chagas [26] related the cases of high fever to the intensity of the parasitemia and to the severity of the infection. However, they seem more related to the individual response.

Systemic signs usually appear around the second and third weeks of infection. Subcutaneous edema may be present in the face, legs, or feet. This edema is not related to the site of entry or to cardiac failure. It is believed to be of lymphatic origin. The generalized enlargement of lymph nodes, liver, and spleen seems to be related to the response of the mononuclear phagocyte system to the infection. Lymph nodes are usually isolated, nonadherent, and painless. Hepatosplenomegaly is also moderate.

Diffuse acute myocarditis, sometimes accompanied by serious pericarditis and endocarditis, is very frequent during the initial stage of Chagas' disease. This myocarditis can only be differentiated from myocarditis of other etiologies by epidemiological data and isolation of the causative agent. Clinical and radiological manifestations do not always reflect the intensity of the anatomopathological alterations, which are most often indicated by the electrocardiogram. ECG changes in acute disease are noncharacteristic, in contrast to what is seen in the chronic cardiomyopathy of Chagas' disease. Thus, the increased interstitial space produced by edema and cellular infiltration causes a disturbance in oxygen diffusion and the appearance of negative T waves or positive deviations of ST-T segments in the leads oriented toward the lesions. Inflammatory infiltrations of the AV conduction system alter the propagation of the supraventricular impulse, resulting in conduction blocks of all kinds. Sinus tachycardia is the most common finding, and it has been attributed to the destruction of parasympathetic ganglion cells in the heart, leading to a relative predominance of the sympathetic system. Intensity of the second heart sound is often decreased. Functional murmurs occur as a result of valvular incompetence produced by dilatation of the valvular rings.

The majority of all acute cases of Chagas' disease resolve over a period of 2 to 3 months to a subacute stage, and from this to an asymptomatic chronic stage. The first case described by Carlos Chagas, Berenice, exemplifies this progression. A 2-year-old girl at the time of diagnosis, Berenice was still alive and without clinical manifestations of the disease at the age of 72. Twenty years earlier (1961) the "Berenice strain" of *T. cruzi*, which has been used for several experimental studies [27], had been reisolated from her blood.

The chronic phase

For clarity, the chronic phase of Chagas' disease will be divided into an asymptomatic and symptomatic form. The symptomatic form may involve cardiac manifestations, digestive manifestations, or both, as well as other less frequent clinical syndromes.

The chronic asymptomatic form (indeterminate form) appears in patients without apparent symptoms or signs of disease. Over 40 percent of serologically positive cases are classified under this group, when assessed by routine examinations alone. However, when more sophisticated diagnostic methods are employed, or a long-term follow-up is undertaken, large numbers of these patients are in fact found to display clinical signs of disease. This fact is also supported by the finding of focuses of inflammation and fibrosis of the heart in postmortem examination of patients within this group who died suddenly [28].

It should be noted that regional variations in the severity of the disease seem to occur, perhaps accounting for the marked differences in morbidity from one geographical area to another. In a long-term study of 260 chronic cases from different areas of Brazil [29], 40.7 percent were found to have the indeterminate (asymptomatic) form. However, important regional differences were found in the distribution of the clinical forms. This number of patients in the asymptomatic group is greater in the younger age groups. With increasing age, there is a progressive increase in the number of patients presenting electrocardiographic abnormalities (Table 33-1).

Chronic Chagas' Cardiomyopathy. This is the most serious and most frequent of the clinical manifestations of Chagas' disease. Its incidence is greater from the second to fourth decade of life, and no apparent correlation is found between its presence and the sex or race of the patient. The clinical manifestations generally occur from 5 to 15 years after infection.

The signs and symptoms of chronic Chagas' cardiomyopathy are secondary to heart failure, arrhythmia, endomyocardial disorders, as well as embolic complications. In a group of 100 patients with chronic Chagas' cardiomyopathy whose ages ranged from 9 to 70 years (average, 36.8 years), dyspnea and palpitations were found to be the most common complaints [30].

The electrocardiographic irregularities found in chronic Chagas' cardiomyopathy fall into three categories: (1) disturbances in the origin of the stimulus, the most common of which are uni- or multifocal ventricular extrasystoles, and, less frequently, atrial flutter and fibrillation, and atrial and nodal extrasystoles; (2) disturbances in the propagation of the stimulus, which include atrioventricular blocks and right bundle branch blocks—the latter are among the most common electrocardiographic findings in Chagas' disease, particularly when associated with left anterior hemiblock, and no other cardiomyopathy shows such a high prevalence of this disorder (30 to 60 percent); (3) primary alterations of the T wave—these may appear with characteristics of subepicardial ischemia, probably due to inflammatory phenomena (Fig. 33-4).

In some cases of chronic chagasic cardiopathy the standard ECG may appear normal, particularly in those cases presenting rare extrasystoles. On the other hand, it is well known that ECG tracings of chronic Chagas' cardiomyopathy may display changes similar to those seen in coronary heart disease: from elevation of the ST wave, suggestive of acute infarct, to the

Table 33-1. Correlation between age groups and clinical forms in 260 patients infected with *T. cruzi* [29]

| Age group, years | Clinical form (number of patients) | | | | |
	Asymptomatic	Cardiomyopathy	Megaesophagus	Megacolon	Total
0–9	4	0	0	0	4
10–19	13	3	2	0	18
20–29	27	25	10	1	63
30–39	36	41	7	4	88
40–49	12	27	7	1	47
50–59	10	11	5	0	26
60 or more	4	6	1	3	14
Total	106	113	32*	9†	260
	(40.76%)	(43.46%)	(11.53%)	(3.46%)	(100%)

*Sixteen with cardiomyopathy.

†Two with cardiomyopathy, two with megaesophagus, and one with cardiomyopathy and associated megaesophagus.

presence of a deep Q wave, suggestive of an electrically inactive zone. These are thought to be areas of blocked stimulus passage and rarely areas of fibrosis.

In the study described above [30], the distribution of ECG abnormalities was as follows: right bundle branch block (50 percent, 17 percent of which had associated left anterior hemiblock), ventricular extrasystoles (39 percent), AV block (29 percent), and primary disorders of the T wave (23 percent).

X-ray examination of the heart does not usually correlate with ECG patterns. Heart rate disorders and heart block appear long before one can find any radiological manifestations. Enlargement of the cardiac area appears only in more advanced

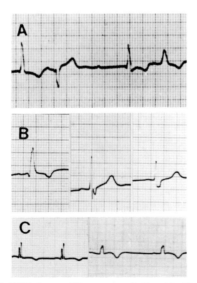

Figure 33-4. ECG abnormalities commonly found in Chagas' disease. *A*. Complete AV block with multifocal ectopic beats (D1). *B*. Right bundle branch block (V$_1$, V$_3$, and V$_5$). *C*. Left anterior hemiblock (V$_6$) and primary T-wave inversion (V$_5$).

and serious cases of the disease, when heart failure develops (Fig. 33-5).

Chronic Digestive Forms. The digestive manifestations of Chagas' disease appear to result from denervation due to destruction of the myoenteric plexus. This results in alterations in the motility of the digestive tract. Although neuronal destruction can occur throughout the entire GI tract, it is in the esophagus and colon that the clinical manifestations are more evident (Fig. 33-6).

The prevalence of the digestive manifestations of Chagas' disease has been reported to vary widely according to the geographical area involved. Thus, in Brazil, the prevalence of functional alterations or dilatation of the esophagus in patients with positive serology for Chagas' disease is around 10 percent, while only 3 percent present colon alterations. In Argentina, the prevalence of digestive manifestations in patients with Chagas' disease is about 3.5 percent, with megacolon being more frequently observed than megaesophagus. In Chile, the digestive forms of Chagas' disease seem to be more important than the cardiac forms. As in Argentina, megacolon is more frequently found than megaesophagus. In Uruguay, Paraguay, and Peru cases of Chagas' megacolon and megaesophagus have also been described. On the other hand, megaesophagus and megacolon are rarely seen in Chagas' disease in Venezuela and Central America. The basis for these regional differences in the clinical manifestations of disease is not yet understood.

Megaesophagus. Although isolated cases of autonomic disorders of the esophagus have been described in the acute phase of Chagas' disease, achalasia, cardiospasm, aperistalsis, and enlargement of the esophagus are more frequently found in the chronic phase. These esophageal disorders tend to precede the appearance of clinical manifestations of cardiomyopathy. In one study of 1592 cases of Chagas' megaesophagus in Goiás, Brazil, the age distribution of the patients was from 2 to 86

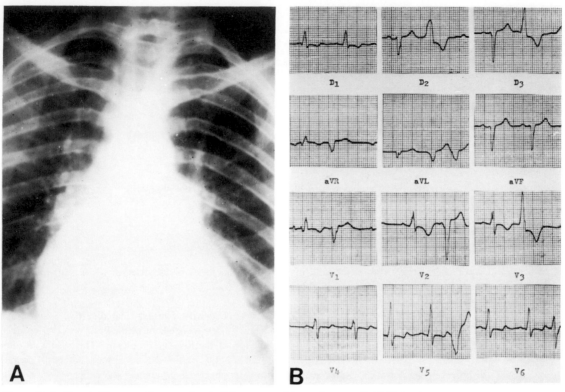

Figure 33-5. Chronic Chagas cardiomyopathy. *A*. Enlargement of the cardiac area. *B*. ECG showing complex arrhythmia and right bundle branch block.

years, the majority (78 percent) occurring between the ages of 20 and 59 [*31*]. The same study reported a predominance of this clinical entity (66 percent) in male patients, a fact reported by other groups as well. No explanation has been found for the sex difference.

The most common signs and symptoms of the Chagas' megaesophagus are dysphagia, odynophagia, and malnutrition. Dysphagia is the most frequent complaint, and it is always related to the contractility of the lower esophagus. It is initially related to ingestion of solid foods and later even to liquids. Odynophagia is related to both the intensity of esophageal contractility as well as with esophagitis caused by food retention or reflux. Heartburn, hiccups, and cough are common findings. Excessive salivation is also a frequent symptom of Chagas' megaesophagus, usually associated with dysphagia and odynophagia. Salivary gland hypertrophy, particularly of the parotids, may occur. Finally, malnutrition with progressive emaciation may result owing to difficulty in swallowing or the regurgitation of foods.

Radiologically, esophageal involvement may be classified into four groups: I—contrast retention in the lower esophagus without dilatation; II—moderate dilatation, lack of motor coordination, with significant contrast retention; III—esophagus dilated and hypotonic, with contrast retention up to its upper third; IV—bulky, elongated, and atonic esophagus generating a right paracardiac shadow in the frontal chest x-ray (dolichomegaesophagus).

Megacolon. The diagnosis of megacolon is rather difficult during the initial stage of the disease since the only evident symptom at first is constipation. In addition, colon x-ray with barium enema, which is recommended for diagnostic confirmation in advanced cases, is expensive, unpleasant for the patient, and of low accuracy in the initial stages. Thus, from a practical standpoint, any patient with positive serology for Chagas' disease who displays frequent constipation lasting more than 1 week should be investigated for Chagas' megacolon. The highest incidence of this clinical form is found in the fifth decade of life, and is also predominant in males [*31*].

The most important clinical manifestations of Chagas' megacolon are constipation, meteorism, difficulty in discharging even soft feces, and abdominal pain. Colon distension by gases results in meteorism, and despite great effort of the abdominal muscles, the patient does not manage to discharge feces, probably due to achalasia of the internal anal sphincter. The abdominal pain results from the distension of the colon by gases and intense contractions. On clinical examination, the abdomen is distended and voluminous, often showing the bulg-

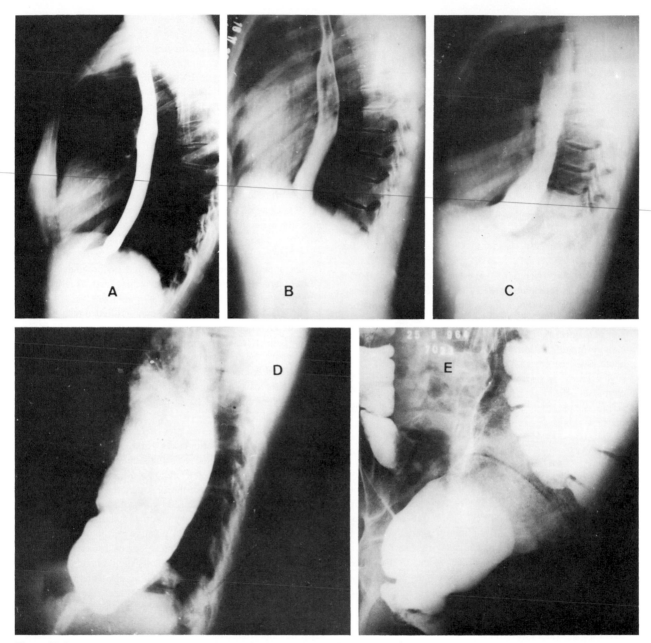

Figure 33-6. Megaesophagus and megacolon in chronic Chagas' disease. *A*. Achalasia of the cardia (contrast retention). *B, C, D*. Progressive enlargements of the esophagus. *E*. Megacolon.

ing of the sigmoid flexure, which may be easily palpable. Fecalomas are common.

Complications. Among the most frequent complications of chronic Chagas' cardiomyopathy are the thromboembolic phenomena [*32*], particularly pulmonary embolism, which is a frequent cause of death. Renal, spleen, and cerebral embolism may also occur.

Esophagitis and cancer of the esophagus represent the most common complications of megaesophagus. The esophagitis is usually the result of mechanical action and food stasis. It could evolve to become ulcerative, with hemorrhage, fibrosis, and stenosis of the esophagus. Cancer seems to occur in 6.6 percent of the cases of Chagas' megaesophagus [*33*].

One of the major complications of megacolon is the presence of fecalomas, with fecal obstruction of the rectum and rectosigmoid. Fecalomas from the upper parts of the colon are less frequent, but can be more serious, often requiring surgery. Volvulus also occurs as a major complication.

Congenital Chagas' disease

Chagas' disease has been found to be transmitted to the fetus possibly by traversing the placental villi. In these, amastigotes are found in Hofbauer cells. Trypomastigotes are released from them and can reach the fetal circulation. In the majority of the reported cases of congenitally transmitted Chagas' disease the mother has been found to be asymptomatic.

The most common findings [34] in congenital cases of Chagas' disease are:

1. Small size for gestational age or prematurity; newborns weigh less than 2500 g.
2. Hepatosplenomegaly, found in the majority of the cases described.
3. Cardiovascular alterations: Acute myocarditis, similar to that found in the acute phase of acquired Chagas' disease.
4. Neurological alterations: Fairly common, with meningoencephalic symptoms such as tremors of the face or limbs, and generalized convulsions.
5. General manifestations: Edema similar to that found in the acute phase of Chagas' disease is frequently found. In the severe cases, hemorrhages may be present (petechiae, ecchymoses, bleeding). Fever is not very frequent as in the acquired cases of Chagas' disease. Most infants die during the first 4 days of life.

PROGNOSIS

The prognosis of Chagas' disease depends on the clinical form and on the complications arising during its evolution. In the acute stage, it depends on the age of the patient and on the intensity and location of the clinical manifestations. As a rule, the acute phase is most serious in children up to 2 years of age and almost always fatal in those displaying heart failure or meningoencephalitis. Prognosis is also serious in the congenital form—in these cases, only a minority survive. Most survivors presented severe neurological sequelae, with mental deficiency or behavioral and learning disabilities.

The prognosis and evolution of chronic Chagas' cardiomyopathy vary considerably from one case to another [35,36]. Patients with minimal lesions (isolated branch block; occasional one-focus extrasystoles) tend to remain stable, and most survive for a long time, usually dying of causes other than Chagas' disease. Patients displaying complex arrhythmia, multifocal ventricular extrasystoles, paroxysmal tachycardia, atrial fibrillation, third-degree AV block, or heart failure with extensive enlargement of the heart have a poor prognosis, usually dying suddenly within a few years. A third group of patients with slight increase in the cardiac area, variability of electrocardiogram, and clinical manifestations have a very uncertain prognosis.

In a study of an endemic area of Minas Gerais, Brazil [37], mortality from Chagas' disease was shown to increase progressively with age, predominating between the ages of 30 and 59. The final estimate of this work for an area with an approximate prevalence of 10 percent of Chagas' infection revealed an overall rate of death from Chagas' disease of 20 out of 100,000 inhabitants. This rate increases two to three times among 30- to 59-year-old people. A study of mortality from Chagas' cardiomyopathy in seven Latin American cities revealed a great variation from one city to another which depended on the prevalence and morbidity of the infection in each area [38].

According to the clinical classification adopted by WHO and PAHO, Chagas' disease may be divided into four grades: I—infection without manifestations of heart lesion; II—infection with moderate cardiac manifestations; III—infection with evident cardiac manifestations; IV—infection with pronounced cardiac manifestations. Cases classified under grades III and IV have a poor prognosis. In these groups, death usually results within 5 years, from cardiac arrest, pulmonary embolism, or irreducible heart failure. The cases classified under grade II have an uncertain prognosis. They may result in sudden death of the patient, or the patient may remain stable and live for many years. For cases classified under grade I, the prognosis is good and compatible with a normal life.

The prognosis of patients with the digestive form is usually good, except for those cases displaying the aforementioned complications.

There are, however, two types of problems with "indeterminate," or asymptomatic, cases. First, cases that are not well studied clinically and are classified under the asymptomatic form may result in sudden death. Second, particularly in countries such as Brazil, where the prevalence of cardiomyopathy is high, social problems, caused by misconceptions about Chagas' disease, may arise for asymptomatic patients. Patients are denied jobs on the basis of a positive serology for *T. cruzi* infection when they have no clinical sign of disease. Therefore, from the social point of view, patients should be classified into three labor-related categories: (1) Those classified under grade I, according to WHO and PAHO, who are bearers of the infection alone, without illness, can live a normal life, and perform regular work; (2) those under grade II, including those with the digestive form, should do work which requires little effort and which does not jeopardize the health of the community; (3) those in grades III and IV should only do very moderate work as occupational therapy.

DIAGNOSIS

The diagnosis of Chagas' disease should be made through the combination of clinical, epidemiological, and laboratory data since the symptoms and clinical signs of the disease are nonspecific. On the other hand, a patient coming from an area where Chagas' disease is endemic may have positive serology for Chagas' disease and even have *T. cruzi* isolated from the blood, but can be an asymptomatic (indeterminate) case of Chagas' disease.

The strongest clinical and epidemiological evidence of a carrier of Chagas' disease is that of a young or middle-aged patient, without hypertension or signs of congenital or rheumatic cardiomyopathy, who has lived in an endemic area and shows signs of cardiomyopathy, megaesophagus, or megacolon. The evidence is particularly strong when associated with electrocardiographic alterations such as right bundle branch block with left anterior hemiblock, AV block, and/or ventricular extrasystoles.

The laboratory diagnosis of American trypanosomiasis can be made by the demonstration of the parasite by direct or indirect methods, by histopathological examinations, and by serological demonstration of anti-*T. cruzi* antibodies.

In the acute stage of the disease, when the parasite is sought directly in the fresh blood or in leukocyte concentrates, the result is almost always positive. The sedimentation of heparinized blood cells with the addition of phytohemagglutinin [39] has been used as a form of parasite concentration. Direct search for the fresh (living) parasite should always be supplemented by its morphological study, after staining on slide by the Giemsa method or other basic dyes, particularly in areas where there is simultaneous human infection by *Trypanosoma rangeli*.

In the acute stage, hemoculture employing NNN, Bonacci, Warren, LIT, and other culture media, as well as inoculation of the patient's blood into laboratory animals, is almost always positive 5 to 15 days after the planting or inoculation. Xenodiagnosis is always positive in the acute stage. However, as it is a long, drawn-out process (30 to 60 days) and disagreeable to the patient, it is not recommended at this stage of the disease, when other simpler methods of parasite isolation exist.

Muscle and lymph node biopsy can be positive for tissue (amastigote) forms of *T. cruzi* in the acute stage of Chagas' disease. However, it is an aggressive examination and not very efficient for diagnosis.

Among the serological tests for diagnosing Chagas' disease in the acute stage, immunofluorescence test for anti-IgM antibodies specific for *T. cruzi* stands out, presenting high, early, and constant titers during this stage [40]. Precipitation and direct agglutination tests of parasite suspension or of its polysaccharide fractions with the serum of the patient in the acute stage of the disease have been used but the cross-reactions and titer variations limit their reliability.

In the chronic stage of the disease, either inapparent or symptomatic, isolation of *T. cruzi* can be done by xenodiagnosis and, less frequently, by hemoculture. Xenodiagnosis has been standardized with 40 third- to fifth-stage *Triatoma infestans* nymphs, divided into four groups of 10 each. The triatomids, which are laboratory-cultivated from the egg state and therefore uninfected, are not fed for 3 to 4 weeks, and then set to suck the suspected individual's blood by applying

boxes containing the bugs to the anterior part of the forearm for 30 min. The triatomids are then kept at 27 or 30°C with an environment of 85 percent relative humidity for 30 days, after which the intestinal contents of the bugs are examined under the microscope. Should the initial examination prove negative, they are reexamined at 60 days. By this method, *T. cruzi* has been isolated in up to 50 percent of chronic cases. Some authors recommend inoculation of the triatomid's intestinal contents into laboratory animals when direct examination is negative.

With hemoculture it has been possible to isolate the parasite in no more than 45 percent of the chronic cases. In the chronic stage of the infection, parasite isolation by inoculation in laboratory animals gives very poor results.

Serological tests to determine anti-*T. cruzi* antibodies are the most important for indirect diagnosis of the chronic infection because of their high positivity and relative specificity. Among them, the most outstanding are the complement-fixation test (Guerreiro-Machado test), immunofluorescence tests [41], indirect hemagglutination [42], and, more recently, the ELISA test [43]. Cross-reactions with leishmaniasis, pemphigus foliaceous, and infectious mononucleosis have been noted with low titers; these cross-reactions can be avoided by selective absorption or by inhibition of heterologous antibodies.

Other serological tests such as direct agglutination, fast hemagglutination, and latex agglutination have produced controversial results because of instability of the antigens or lack of specificity in the chronic stage of Chagas' disease.

MANAGEMENT AND THERAPY

For the treatment of Chagas' disease both specific and symptomatic therapy are indicated, as well as prevention and treatment of complications.

Numerous drugs have been tried in the treatment of *T. cruzi* without results, owing either to low efficacy or to high toxicity. Nitrofurazone has been used with excellent results in mice experimentally infected with *T. cruzi* [44]. However, the drug was found to be too toxic for human use, considering the doses and duration of treatment required [45]. More recently, two drugs have been utilized with promising results in the acute stage of the disease: Nifurtimox (Bayer 2502) and Benzonidazole (RO-7-1051). These, when used on a long-term basis (from 30 to 120 days), daily doses of 8 to 10 mg/kg for Nifurtimox and 5 to 7 mg/kg for Benzonidazole, have been shown to be effective in suppressing parasitemia and clinical manifestations in the acute stage. In a study of 232 patients [46] treated in the acute stage with Nifurtimox for 120 days, 81 percent were considered cured after 2 years' observation. The same study described favorable results in long-term treatment of chronic cases with Nifurtimox, showing suppression of the parasitemia in 96.5 percent of the cases. However, these results have not been confirmed in Brazil [47]. A study of 309 cases treated with Benzonidazole with various therapeutic plans in 10 clinics in Brazil [48] concluded that suppression of the parasitemia was obtained in 78 percent of the cases treated. Both drugs—Nifurtimox and Benzonidazole—can produce individual side effects of moderate to severe intensity such as gastric upset, peripheral polyneuropathy, psychic excitation, dermatitis, and leukopenia. In summary, it can be said that both Nifurtimox and Benzonidazole temporarily suppress parasitemia in the human infection by *T. cruzi* and can cure acute or recent cases of the disease. There is no evidence that chronic disease can be reversed by chemotherapy. However, their side effects limit their use on a larger scale. On the other hand, it has been shown that therapeutic results differ greatly depending on the *T. cruzi* strain and the drug used [49–52].

Treatment of heart failure and arrhythmias, as well as prevention and treatment of thromboembolism, follow the regimens applied to other cardiomyopathies: the use of diuretics, digitalis, anti-arrhythmics, and anticoagulants. Attention should be drawn to the high frequency of digitalis intoxication in patients with Chagas' cardiomyopathy and to the low level of response to rhythm-regulating drugs. In serious cases of heart blocks the use of pacemakers may be necessary. A light, balanced diet should be recommended for cases of megaesophagus, avoiding irritating and excessively hot or cold food. Food should be well chewed and calmly swallowed. Heavy meals and the use of medication at night should be avoided, due to retention, fermentation, and regurgitation during sleep. Gaseous and alkaline drinks before sleeping are recommended to "clean" the esophagus. Atropine has been used with uncertain and contradictory results for relieving spasm and pain. Cardia dilation by probe provides temporary results in incipient cases of achalasia. Pneumatic dilation has been found to be relatively safe and effective, with beneficial effects lasting at least for the 1-year follow-up. Extramucosal cardiotomy (Heller's technique) has provided satisfactory results. Cardioplasty or cardial resection with the use of intestinal loop interposition have been reported to give good results. However, in view of surgical complications, there is a tendency among clinicians to remain more and more conservative nowadays.

Treatment of megacolon is essentially surgical. For incipient cases, or for those with temporary or permanent contraindications, treatment should be conservative, on the basis of diets and laxatives which stimulate intestinal peristalsis.

POPULATION

ECOLOGY

The existence of reservoirs and vectors of *T. cruzi* and, particularly, the socioeconomic and educational level of the population are the most important factors in determining the appearance of Chagas' disease.

Three ecological cycles can be considered in the onset of trypanosomiasis of Latin America: (1) the *wild cycle*, where

T. cruzi circulates among wild animals and triatomids (this is considered the original cycle of the infection); (2) the *paradomestic cycle*, in which wild animals (opossum, guinea pigs in Bolivia and Peru, and rats in Panama and Costa Rica) and triatomids come around human dwellings and occasionally penetrate them, or, in contrast, when domestic animals (dogs and cats) and humans penetrate the wild cycle (this is considered an intermediate cycle); and (3) the *domestic cycle*, when triatomids adapt themselves to human dwellings and transmit the infection to domestic animals, from human to human, and from domestic animals to humans.

Poor and low-income-level populations build their houses in endemic areas, using raw wood obtained from the nearby woods. The walls are made of a mixture of sticks, straw, and clay (mud houses), covered with thatching. These houses offer an excellent habitat for triatomids, which adapt themselves to the human's home and live in the cracks in the walls, the ceiling, and in the cracks of the beds and mattresses themselves. Wild triatomids are brought into the dwelling and to its surroundings on the wood used to build the houses and annexes (e.g., chicken coops and pens) and also with the firewood, stacked near or inside the house, to be used in the kitchen. Occasionally the wild triatomids enter the house, attracted by the light. On the other hand, deforestation by humans around the house pushes away wild animals, leaving the triatomids with no other alternative but to feed on the blood of domestic animals and humans, after adapting to the dwelling, thus setting up the domestic cycle of the disease.

EPIDEMIOLOGY

The most important mechanism of transmission of *T. cruzi* to humans is through contamination by the feces of infected triatomids. This form of transmission is responsible for the existence of the endemic infection in the American continent. Indeed, the world distribution of the disease corresponds exactly to the areas where the vector *Triatoma* species have contacted humans. In this respect, vector control has resulted in dramatic decrease and interruption of the transmission of the infection to humans, as has been the case in some highly endemic areas of Brazil [53].

Since the housing conditions are extremely important in the transmission chain, the prevalence and incidence of infection will vary with the degree of adaptation of the triatomids to the human dwellings, as well as the vector capacity of the species. Thus, the species of higher epidemiological importance will be those with better adaptation to the human homes, such as *Triatoma infestans* in Argentina, Bolivia, Brazil, and Chile; *Panstrongylus megistus* and *Triatoma sordida* in certain areas of Brazil; *Rhodnius prolixus* in Venezuela; and *Triatoma dimidiata* in Central America (Fig. 33-7). The process of adaptation to houses results from alteration in their natural environment, as discussed above. The species complex *Triatoma protacta* has been found to be infected by *T. cruzi* in the United

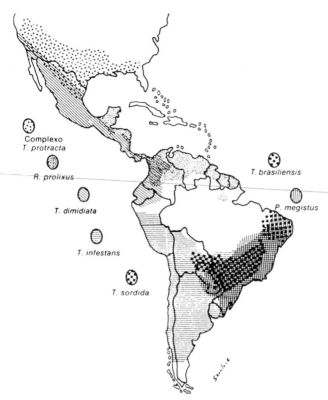

Figure 33-7. Geographical distribution of the most important species of triatomids transmitting *T. cruzi*. (*From* [55].)

States, particularly in California, Arizona, and New Mexico. This species, however, is not a good vector of *T. cruzi* since it does not defecate immediately after the blood meal, and therefore does not leave metacyclics on their human prey. The degree of endemicity of a certain area will depend on the density of the triatomids adapted to the human environment. That is to say, the transmission will depend on the number of infected triatomids in the house and their degree of infection by *T. cruzi*, as well as the characteristics of the species (e.g., frequency of blood meals, agility, host preference).

Transplacental transmission has been estimated at about 2 percent of premature births in 500 cases studied. The incidence was 10.5 percent if only infected mothers were considered. Congenital transmission is thought to occur only in previously deficient or injured placentas.

Transmission of *T. cruzi* by blood transfusion is an important mechanism in the endemic areas or in the large cities nearby, where control of blood donors is not adequately performed. The incidence of donors in blood banks in Latin America with positive Chagas' disease serology can reach 28 percent, although the number of proven cases of transmission by blood transfusion is small. Transmission through breast milk has already been demonstrated, but it seems to be a mechanism of little importance. Speculations have been made about the pos-

sibility of transmission through foods contaminated with feces of triatomids or through undercooked meat of infected animals. Accidental transmission in laboratories is important.

Natural infection by *T. cruzi* in animals, in triatomids, and in humans has been reported from the southern United States to southern Argentina and Chile, in areas where more than 50 million people live. It is estimated that more than 10 million are infected. In the southern United States, two or three sporadic human cases have been reported. In Mexico, the illness becomes endemic, with various cases being reported in that country, in Guatemala, in El Salvador, Honduras, Costa Rica, and Panama. In Belize (former British Honduras), Coura and Petana [54] reported 2.7 percent of the population of a rural area with positive serology for Chagas' infection.

In South America Chagas' disease has been described with a high incidence in practically the whole continent, as shown in inquiries carried out in Columbia, Venezuela, Ecuador, Peru, Bolivia, Paraguay, Uruguay, Chile, Argentina, and Brazil. Venezuela, Argentina, and Brazil have the largest concentration of human cases studied on the continent.

As mentioned above, the prevalence and incidence of the infection correlate with the degree of adaptation of the triatomids to the human dwelling. For example, in Belize, where there has not yet been adaptation of the triatomids to human homes, the prevalence of human infection is very low; the same is true in certain areas of other countries where the disease is considered endemic, as, for example, in the Brazilian Amazon area.

The process of internal migration is a factor of great importance in the spreading of Chagas' disease. This is due not only to the migration of infected humans from one place to another, but also to the domestic animals which accompany them. In addition, house-adapted triatomids may be carried among belongings such as suitcases, clothes, and furniture, thereby creating new focuses of disease. The migration of infected individuals to urban centers also increases the number of blood donors with risk of transmitting the disease.

VECTOR CONTROL

The most important areas to address in terms of the prophylaxis of Chagas' disease are vector control, house improvement, health education, and control of donors at blood banks.

The most efficient measure of vector control has been the use of insecticides. Among those, the most commonly used are the chlorinated compounds, BHC (in Brazil and Argentina), and dieldrin (in Venezuela). Resistance of *R. prolixus* and *T. maculata* to BHC and dieldrin has been described in some areas of Venezuela.

BHC has given good results when the deposition over the surface corresponds to the minimal dose of 0.5 g of the γ isomer per square meter. Its residual action lasts up to 30 days. It is relatively safe when used properly and is inexpensive. Two successive applications a year, 60 to 90 days apart, should be made.

Dieldrin has an initial action of lower efficiency than BHC, but its residual action lasts for several months. Good results have been obtained by the application of 1 g/m². Dieldrin is, however, more expensive than BHC and highly toxic.

Organophosphorous insecticides (malathion and fenthion) and the carbamates (propoxur, or Baygon) have been also used with good results. Their importance may increase with the appearance of resistance to the organochlorous insecticides.

The treatment of the houses with insecticides has to be thorough. The insecticides should be applied not only on the walls (inside and out) but also in the ceilings and roof. Cracks and fissures, including those in furniture, should receive larger amounts of insecticides. Particular attention should be given to the beds and mattresses.

Synthetic insect growth regulators (e.g., juvenile hormone analogues) to block the evolution of the triatomids and attractants such as pheromones have been used experimentally; however, their use in control of the insects has not yet been possible. Biological control through fungi, bacteria, and viruses, although it reduces the triatomid population, has proved incapable of eliminating them completely. Experiments by means of biological competition with sterilized male triatomids have not been promising.

Public health education of the population, as well as improvements in housing, are the permanent measures capable of long-term control of the transmission of the disease. Information should be given about the risk of infection, the habits of the triatomids, and the way to combat them by means of a thorough cleaning of the house, furniture, clothes, and utensils, the use of insecticides, and repair of walls and ceilings so that they do not offer insect shelter. Similar measures should be applied to the annexes to the home. A strict program of improvement and development of dwellings should be oriented by public health services with the support of the government in endemic areas.

Blood donors should be rigorously selected through serological reactions to detect *T. cruzi* infection. Seropositive donors should be turned down. In endemic areas where there is a high number of seropositive donors, the addition of gentian violet to the suspected blood has been used with absolute success. This is accomplished by adding gentian violet at a concentration of 0.25 g per liter of blood, at least 24 h before transfusion.

VACCINES

Attempts to obtain a vaccine against *T. cruzi* have not been very successful [22]. The most important aim of such a vaccine would be to prevent the late complications of the disease. One of the major concerns in the quest for a vaccine against *T. cruzi* is the possibility that a protective moiety or moieties cross-reacting with host tissue would induce or accentuate disease due to autoimmune reactions. In this respect, the use of the 90,000-dalton surface glycoprotein has provided encouraging results in protection experiments in mice. Neither this surface antigen [6], nor the insect-stage-specific 75,000-dalton surface glycoprotein seems to display cross-reactivity with human heart or connective tissue components. Therefore, they may be good candidates for a vaccine. The use of recombinant DNA techniques for antigen production could provide cost-effective preparations for immunization and diagnostic methods.

With the present knowledge of the immune response to this infection, immunization schedules should be oriented toward induction of both cell-mediated and humoral immunity. The target population for immunization purposes in endemic areas should be children from birth to 2 years, who are usually serologically negative. Two aspects must be raised in relation to a vaccination trial against *T. cruzi*. First, it would have to include a very large number of individuals. Second, if the vaccination does not succeed in blocking infection, an assessment of its efficacy in preventing the late complications of the chronic phase would require a follow-up of 15 to 20 years, the time usually required for these clinical forms to appear.

REFERENCES

1 Snary D, Hudson L: *Trypanosoma cruzi* cell surface proteins: Identification of one major glycoprotein. FEBS Lett 100:166–170, 1979

2 Nogueira N, Chaplan S, Tydings J, et al: *Trypanosoma cruzi*: Surface antigens of blood and culture forms. J Exp Med 153:629–639, 1981

3 Peterson DS, Wrightsman RA, Manning JE: Cloning of a major surface antigen gene of *T. cruzi* and identification of a nonapeptide repeat. Nature 322:566–568, 1986

4 Snary D, Ferguson MAJ, Scott MT, et al: All surface antigens of *T. cruzi*: Use of monoclonal antibodies to identify and isolate an epimastigote specific glycoprotein. Mol Biochem Parasitol 3:343–356, 1981

5 Andrews NW, Robbins ES, Ley V, et al: Developmentally regulated, phospholipase C–mediated release of the major surface glycoprotein of amastigotes of *Trypanosoma cruzi*. J Exp Med 167:300–314, 1988.

6 Snary D: *Trypanosoma cruzi*: Studies on the cell surface glycoprotein, no evidence for antigenic variation. Exp Parasitol 49:68–77, 1980

7 DoCampo R, Moreno SNJ, Stoppani AOM, et al: Mechanism of nifurtimox toxicity in different forms of *Trypanosoma cruzi*. Biochem Pharmacol 30:1947–1951, 1981

8 Miles MA, Toye PJ, Oswald SC, et al: The identification of isoenzyme patterns of two distinct strain-groups of *Trypanosoma cruzi* circulating independently in a rural area of Brazil. Trans Soc Trop Med Hyg 71:217–225, 1977

9 Baker J, Miles M, Godfrey D, et al: Biochemical characterization of some species of *Trypanosoma schistotrypanum* from bats. Am J Trop Med Hyg 27:483–491, 1978

10 Morel C, Chiari E, Plessmann Camargo E, et al: Strains and clones of *Trypanosoma cruzi* can be characterized by patterns of restric-

tion endonuclease products of kinetoplast DNA minicircles. Proc Natl Acad Sci USA 77:6810–6814, 1980

11 Nogueira N, Cohn Z: *Trypanosoma cruzi*: Mechanism of entry and intracellular fate in mammalian cells. J Exp Med 143:1402–1420, 1976

12 Nogueira N, Chaplan S, Cohn Z: *Trypanosoma cruzi*: Factors modifying ingestion and fate of blood form trypomastigotes. J Exp Med 152:447–451, 1980

13 Krettli AU, Brener Z: Protective effects of the specific antibodies in *Trypanosoma cruzi* infections. J Immunol 116:755–760, 1976

14 Nogueira N, Chaplan C, Reesink M, et al: *Trypanosoma cruzi*: Induction of microbicidal activity in human mononuclear phagocytes. J Immunol 128:2142–2146, 1982

15 Nogueira N, Gordon S, Cohn Z: *Trypanosoma cruzi*: Modification of macrophage function during infection. J Exp Med 146:157–171, 1977

16 Nogueira N, Cohn Z: *Trypanosoma cruzi*: In vitro induction of macrophage microbicidal activity. J Exp Med 148:288–300, 1978

17 Reed SG: In vivo administration of recombinant IFN-γ induces macrophage activation, and prevents acute disease, immune suppression, and death in experimental *T. cruzi* infections. J Immunol 140:4342–4347, 1988

18 Coleman CM, Middlebrook G: The effects of some sulphhydryl compounds on growth of catalase-positive and catalase-negative tubercule bacilli. Am Rev Tuberc Pulm Dis 74:42–46, 1956

19 Nathan C, Nogueira N, Juangbhanich C, et al: Activation of macrophages in vivo and in vitro. Correlation between H_2O_2 release and killing of *Trypanosoma cruzi*. J Exp Med 149:1056–1068, 1979

20 Wrightsman R, Krassner S, Watson J: Genetic control of responses to *Trypanosoma cruzi* in mice: Multiple genes influencing parasitemia and survival. Infect Immun 36:637–644, 1982

21 Nogueira N, Ellis J, Chaplan S, et al: *Trypanosoma cruzi*: In vivo and in vitro correlation between T-cell activation and susceptibility in inbred strains of mice. Exp Parasitol 51:325–334, 1981

22 Brener Z: Immunity to *Trypanosoma cruzi*. Adv Parasitol 18:247–293, 1980

23 Szarfman A, Cossio PM, Schmunis GA, et al: The EVI antibody in acute Chagas' disease. J Parasitol 63:149–152, 1977

24 Szarfman A, Terranova VP, Rennard SI, et al: Antibodies to Laminin in Chagas' disease. J Exp Med 155:1161–1171, 1982

25 Santos-Busch CA, Teixeira ARL: The immunology of experimental Chagas' disease. III. Rejection of allogeneic heart cells "in vitro." J Exp Med 140:38–53, 1974

26 Chagas C: Nova entidade morbida do homem. Rezumo geral de estudos etiologicos e clinicos. Mem Inst Oswaldo Cruz 3:219–275, 1911

27 Salgado JA: O centenario de Carlos Chagas e a menina Berenice. Mem Inst Oswaldo Cruz 75:193–194, 1980

28 Lopes ER, Chapadeiro E, Almeida HO, et al: Contribuicao ao estudo da anatomia patologica dos coracoes de chagasicos falecidos subitamente. Rev Soc Bras Med Trop 9:269–283, 1975

29 Coura JR: Evolutive pattern in Chagas' disease and the life span of *Trypanosoma cruzi* in human infection. New Approaches in American Trypanosomiasis Research. Scientific Publication 318, Pan American Health Organization, 1976, pp 378–382

30 Coura JR: Contribuicao ao Estudo da Doenca de Chagas no Estado da Guanabara. Thesis, Universidade Federal do Rio de Janeiro, 1965, 143 pp

31 Resende JM: Manifestacoes digestivas, in Grener Z, Andrade Z: *Tripanosoma cruzi e Doenca de Changas*. Rio de Janeiro, Ed. Guanabara Koogan S.A., 1979

32 Andrade ZA: Fenomenos trombo-embolicos na cardiopatia cronica chagasica. Annu Cong Internac Doenca de Chagas, Rio de Janeiro, 1:73–84, 1959

33 Camara-Lopes LH: Carcinoma of the esophagus as a complication of megaesophagus. An analysis of seven cases. Am J Dig Dis 6:742–756, 1961

34 Bittencourt AL: Congenital Chagas' disease, a review. Am J Dis Child 130:99–103, 1976

35 Prata A: Prognostico e complicacoes da doenca de Chagas. Rev Goiana Med 5:87–96, 1959

36 Laranja FS, Dias E, Nobrega G, et al: Chagas' disease. A clinical, epidemiologic and pathologic study. Circulation 14:1015–1060, 1956

37 Abrev LL: Doenca de Chagas. Estudo da mortalidade no municipio de Pains, Minas Gerais. Thesis, Universidade Federal do Rio de Janeiro, 1979

38 Puffer RR, Griffith GW: Patterns of Urban Mortality. Washington, D.C., Scientific Publication 151, Pan American Health Organization, 1967

39 Yaeger RG: A method of isolating trypanosomes from blood. J Parasitol, 46:288, 1960

40 Camargo ME, Amato Neto V: Anti *T. cruzi* antibodies as a serological evidence of recent infection. Rev Inst Med Trop Sao Paulo 16:200–202, 1974

41 Fife EH, Muschel LA: Fluorescent antibody technique for serodiagnosis of *Trypanosoma cruzi* infection. Proc Soc Exp Biol Med 101:540–543, 1959

42 Neal RA, Miles RA: Indirect hemagglutination test for Chagas' disease with a simple method survey work. Rev Inst Med Trop Sao Paulo 12:325–332, 1970

43 Voller A, Draper CC, Bidwell DD, et al: Microplate enzyme-linked immunoabsorbent assay for Chagas' disease. Lancet i:426–429, 1975

44 Brener Z: Ativadade terapêutica do 5-nitro-2-furaldeidosemicarbazona em esquemas de duracão prolongada na infeccao experimental de camundongos pelo *Trypanosoma cruzi*. Rev Inst Med Trop Sao Paulo 3:43–49, 1961

45 Coura JR, Ferreira LF, Morteo RE, et al: Tentativa terapêutica com a nitrofurazona (furacin) na forma crônica da doenca de Chagas. O Hospital 60:425–429, 1961

46 Cerizola JA, Rabinovitch A, Alveres M, et al: Enfermedad de Chagas y la transfusion de sangre. Bol Sanit Panam 73:203–221, 1972

47 Cancado JR, Salgado AA, Marra MD, et al: Ensaio terapêutico clinco na doenca de Chagas cronica com o Nifurtimox em três esquemas de duracâo prolongada. Rev Inst Med Trop Sao Paulo 17:111–121, 1975

48 Coura JR, Brindeiro PJ, Ferreira I: Benzonidazole in the treatment of Chagas' disease. Current Chemotherapy. Intern Cong Chemotheapy 1:161–162, 1978

49 Andrade SG, Figueira RM: Estudo experimental sobre a ação Terapêutica da droga RO-7-1051 na infecção por differentes cepas do *Trypanosoma cruzi*. Rev Inst Med Trop Sao Paulo 19:335–341, 1977

50 Andrade SG, Figueira RM, Carvalho ML, et al: Influência da cepa do *Trypanosoma cruzi* na resposta terapêutica experimental pelo

Bayer 2502 (Resultados do tratamento a longo prazo). Rev Inst Med Trop Sao Paulo 17:380–389, 1975

51 Brener Z, Costa CAG, Chiari C: Differences in the susceptibility of *Trypanosoma cruzi* strains to active chemotherapeutic agents. Rev Inst Med Trop Sao Paulo 18:450–455, 1976

52 Schlemper Jr BR, Loures MAL, Peralta JM, et al: Terapêutica experimental da doenca de Chagas: Susceptibilidade de cepas de *Trypanosoma cruzi* isoladas de duas áreas endêmicas. An. VII. Reunião Anual sobre Pesquisa Básica em Doenca de Chagas. Caxambú, Minas Gerais, 1980

53 Dias JCP: Perspectivas para o controle da doenca de Chagas humana pelo emprego domiciliar de inseticidas de acao residual. Experiencia de Bambui, M.G. Thesis, Fac. Medicine Universidade de Minas Gerais, 1974

54 Coura JR, Petana WB: American trypanosomiasis in British Honduras. I. The prevalence of Chagas' disease in el Cayo District. Ann Trop Med Parasitol 61:244–250, 1967

C H A P T E R 34 / *Leishmaniasis* · Franklin Neva · David Sacks

Leishmaniasis is an infection caused by intracellular protozoan parasites transmitted by various species of sand flies. Depending mainly upon the species of leishmanial parasite, but also upon the immunological status and response of the human host, expression of disease can be quite variable. Human infection may be entirely inapparent or subclinical, or it may display a spectrum of manifestation from cutaneous involvement to late destruction of mucous membranes, to generalized systemic disease with fatal outcome. Parasites are able to evade destructive action of their host cells, macrophages. A normal cell-mediated immune response is critical for ultimate cure of the infection. Diagnosis is established by demonstration of parasites in infected tissues, but serological or delayed-hypersensitivity skin tests may also be useful. Leishmaniasis has a worldwide distribution, with a variety of ecological interactions between vector sand flies, animal reservoirs, and human contacts determining epidemiology of the disease. Treatment still relies mainly on pentavalent antimony but is not uniformly effective. There is no chemoprophylaxis, vaccines are under study but not yet available, and vector control is feasible only in certain epidemiological situations.

PARASITE

TAXONOMY

Since there are few morphological differences between the various members of the genus, a classification has been developed that was initially based on the clinical disease produced, and which was supported subsequently by a variety of biological and epidemiological characteristics. As yet, no universally accepted classification has been produced. However, a generally agreed upon list of the major species and subspecies producing disease in humans is given in Table 34-1. The area that pro-

duces most disagreement concerns the assignment of species or subspecies rank to the recognized entities, since these have rarely been made on the basis of standardized or uniformly accepted taxonomic criteria. Efforts to establish more suitable taxonomic characters have occupied a major focus of research on *Leishmania* for many years. Methods of identification currently in use are listed in Table 34-2. At present, the most commonly used method to identify strains at the species or intraspecies level is isoenzyme characterization. A new methodology based on DNA probes specific for the various *Leishmania* species was developed to provide a direct diagnosis of patients with leishmaniasis and to eliminate the need for culturing parasites before species identification [1]. This methodology allows direct diagnosis from lesion material without requiring isolation of the parasite. The basis for the DNA probes is the *minicircle,* which is a highly repeated small circular DNA molecule found within the mitochondria of the parasite. It has no apparent function but does have a high rate of DNA sequence divergence. Probes based on total kinetoplast DNA can differentiate the major species complexes in the new world. More recently, recombinant kDNA probes have been developed which can differentiate species, subspecies, and even distinct isolates of the parasite. These methods are currently limited to only a few laboratories. They require not only the availability of the probes and the facilities with which to carry out hybridization studies, but also the availability of standard reference material against which the unknown isolate can be compared.

MORPHOLOGY AND ULTRASTRUCTURE

Leishmania are *digenetic* (existing in two forms) protozoa which exist as flagellated extracellular promastigotes in the sandfly vector (or axenic in in vitro culture) and as aflagellar

[handwritten notes at top:] DCL like L. Leprosy. –anergic / c/w L. recidivans. Like tuberculoid. non anergic

[handwritten note upper right:] DCL often anergic to Leish. Ag. Not ulcerative — papule w/ satellite lesions

Table 34-1. Geographical distribution of and clinical disease caused by different species of *Leishmania*

Species	Geographical distribution	Clinical manifestations
L. mexicana complex *L. m. mexicana,* *L. m. amazonensis,* *L. m. venezuelensis,* (? others)	New world—from southern U.S. through Central America, northern and central South America, Dominican Republic	Cutaneous ulcers; small proportion of cases may develop diffuse cutaneous (DCL) or mucocutaneous (MCL) leishmaniasis
L. braziliensis complex *L. b. braziliensis,* *L. b. guyanensis,* *L. b. panamensis,* *L. b. peruviana*	New world—from Central America through parts of South America, including Brazil, Venezuela, Bolivia, Peru, to northern Argentina	Cutaneous ulcers; some cases may later develop MCL (probably more likely if cutaneous lesion not treated adequately)
L. major	Northern Africa, Middle East, central Africa, and southern Asia	Cutaneous ulcers
L. tropica	Middle East and south Asia	Cutaneous ulcers and chronic relapsing cutaneous disease (recidivans form)
L. aethiopica	Ethiopia and contiguous countries	Cutaneous ulcers, rarely DCL
L. donovani	Old world—East Africa and south of Sahara, south Asia, including India and Iran	Visceral leishmaniasis; small proportion may develop post-kala azar dermal leishmaniasis
L. infantum (? separate species)	Old world—North Africa and southern Europe	Visceral leishmaniasis
L. chagasi (? separate species)	New world—foci in several areas of Brazil, Venezuela, and Colombia, and isolated cases in Central and South America	Visceral leishmaniasis

[handwritten annotations:] chiclero ear. (next to L. mexicana); espundia, of "forest yaws" (papillomas) (next to L. braziliensis); rural / moist, multiple. / L. tr. major (next to L. major); urban / dry, single ulcer / L. tr. minor (next to L. tropica); Rx Pentamidine > Sb (next to L. aethiopica)

obligate intracellular amastigotes within mononuclear phagocytes of their vertebrate hosts (Fig. 34-1). The various species are not easily distinguishable morphologically from one another. Romanowsky dyes (e.g., Giemsa) stain chromatin of the nucleus and nucleic-acid-containing kinetoplast a brilliant red or violet, whereas the cytoplasm is stained a pale blue. Amastigotes appear as round or oval bodies ranging from 2 to 3 μm in major diameter. The size of amastigotes from different species is known to vary. The cytoplasm of the amastigotes often stains the same as the host cell cytoplasm, and only the nucleus and kinetoplast can be distinguished. The nucleus of the parasite occupies a central position in the cell and the kinetoplast lies adjacent to it. The kinetoplast, which stains more densely than the nucleus, is variable in shape, being round, oval, rod-shaped, or curved in profile. In all *Leishmania*

Table 34-2. Identification methods for *Leishmania*

Biological characters
   Development in sand flies
   Virulence in rodents
   Thermosensitivity
Immunological characters
   Excreted-factor serotyping
   Monoclonal antibodies
Genetic and biochemical characters
   kDNA hybridization
   Isoenzyme characterization

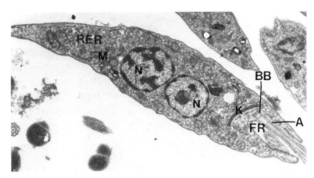
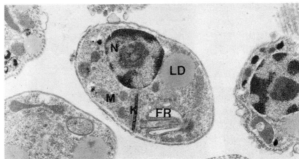

Figure 34-1. Electron micrograph showing *Leishmania* ultrastructure. Promastigote (top) × 13,000; amastigote (bottom) × 15,000. (N = nucleus; K = kinetoplast; M = mitochondria; RER = rough endoplasmic reticulum; A = axoneme; FR = flagellar reservoir; BB = basal body; LD = lipid droplet.) *(Courtesy of Dr. Paulo Pimenta)*

species, as with all trypanosomatids, the primary enzymes of the glycolytic pathway are located inside unique organelles termed *glycosomes*.

The flagellar promastigote forms measure 10 to 20 μm in length, not including the length of the flagellum, which may equal the body length. The pale blue–staining cytoplasm contains a centrally placed nucleus. The kinetoplast lies about 2 μm from the anterior end, and the flagellum emerges anteriorly. The overall shape is that of a spindle with the posterior end gradually tapering to a point.

The plasma membrane of all stages of *Leishmania* is a typical, trilaminar unit membrane 2 to 4 nm in width beneath which lie the subpellicular microtubules which impart shape and flexibility to the parasite. The plasma membrane of the flagellar reservoir is not lined with microtubules. Desmosomes can be seen between the parasite body and flagellum and are usually present at several points where the flagellar and reservoir membranes are closely opposed. The plasma membrane of the reservoir functions as a site of intake and secretion of macromolecules by pinocytosis and exocytosis. The pulsating action of the flagellum is thought to facilitate these processes.

LIFE CYCLE

With the rare exception of the now archaic practice of deliberate vaccination by scarification, human infection is exclusively initiated by the bite of an infected female phlebotomine sand fly (order Diptera; family Psychodidae). The transmission of oriental sore to humans by bite was proven by Adler and Ber (1941) [2] and of kala azar to humans by Swaminath et al. in 1942 [3]. When the sand fly takes a blood meal from an infected host, minute amounts of blood, lymph, and infected macrophages are ingested (Fig. 34-2). Sand flies are considered to be pool feeders and take blood from a small hemorrhage in the skin made by the mouthparts. The number of amastigotes ingested is thought to be extremely low, even when flies engorge directly on cutaneous lesions. Engorgement is quickly followed by the production of a peritrophic membrane which is secreted by the epithelial cells lining the midgut. This membrane retains the developing promastigotes during the first 72 h, and there is evidence that some promastigotes become embedded in it. The parasites lie in the blood meal in nests of actively dividing parasites. As digestion proceeds, the membrane breaks up and free-swimming promastigotes escape to initiate the establishment of infection in the midgut or, in the *braziliensis* group, in the hindgut. An association of the flagella with the microvilli of the midgut or an attachment to the cuticular entema of the hindgut (pylorus and ileum) are characteristic of the replicating forms of *Leishmania* in the sand fly [4]. The initial establishment of infection in both instances is followed by an anterior migration to the thoracic midgut, attachment to the stomodeal (esophageal) valve, and invasion of the mouthparts (esophagus, pharynx, cibarium, and proboscis). Forms in the mouthparts are never seen in division. While for

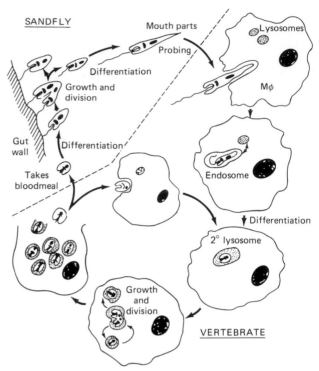

Figure 34-2. Life cycle of *Leishmania*. *(Courtesy of Dr. Paul Bates.)*

some *Leishmania* species several morphologically distinct forms of promastigotes can be found in different parts of the alimentary tract, there is little evidence that these changes reflect development of promastigotes into a form which is uniquely adapted to life in the vertebrate. That there is sequential development of promastigotes from a noninfective to an infective stage is clear from the observation that midgut promastigotes obtained 3 to 7 days after an infective feed demonstrate progressively increased virulence with time for a susceptible vertebrate host [5]. These infective forms are referred to as *metacyclic promastigotes,* by analogy with the term used to denote the infective stages of other hemoflagellates. While metacyclics do not bear any obvious morphological identity, for *L. major* they appear to be small, highly motile promastigotes with a long, free flagellum. They neither divide nor attach to the wall of the alimentary tract. They arise from dividing forms within the midgut 3 or more days after an infecting feed; they are the only parasites seen in the proboscis and are undoubtedly deposited in the skin when the sand fly bites. Although transmission is easily accomplished when metacyclics are in the proboscis, the possibility cannot yet be dismissed that infective promastigotes can be regurgitated from further back in the alimentary tract as a result of changes in the biting behavior of infected flies due presumably to blockage of mouthparts. The saliva of sand flies has several potent pharmacological activities, and these have been recently shown to enhance the survival of inoculated promastigotes [6]. The duration of the existence of promastigotes inoculated by sand flies in the extracellular environment at the site of the bite is dependent on the rate of recruitment of macrophages to the bite, thought to be a matter of hours. After phagocytosis, transformation to dividing amastigotes occurs within 24 h. Reproduction at all stages of the life cycle is believed to occur by binary fission; no sexual stage has been identified, and ploidy has not been determined.

IN VITRO CULTIVATION

Cell biology and biochemistry

Most *Leishmania* species can be readily cultivated axenically as promastigotes in diphasic systems, such as NNN medium composed of a solid agar with rabbit blood and an overlay of salt solution or medium, and monophasic enriched liquid media, either completely defined or containing serum. Amastigotes can be grown in macrophages, macrophagelike tumor lines (e.g., P388D, U937), dog sarcoma lines, and fibroblasts. Extracellular cultivation of aflagellate *Leishmania* of some species *(L. mexicana amazonensis)* has been reported, and their similarity to tissue-derived amastigotes is supported by their reactivity with amastigote-specific monoclonal antibodies. Because of the difficulty in extracting very clean preparations of amastigotes from infected tissue, there is little information on the physiology and biochemistry of these forms relative to axenically derived promastigotes. There is even uncertainty as to whether promastigotes maintained in vitro are reflective of those derived from the sand fly. The importance of medium standardization is reinforced by various reports that virulence and infectivity can be profoundly influenced by culture conditions, and that attenuation almost always accompanies repeated subculture. These differences are now believed to be due, at least in part, to the degree to which different culture conditions support the transformation of promastigotes to the metacyclic stage, which, to emphasize, is not a readily distinguishable event but nonetheless can be expected to occur during the stationary growth phase. The signals which control these developmental events (e.g., nutrient depletion, accumulation of metabolic products) remain undefined.

The focus of much of the recent research on *Leishmania* has been to define those unique aspects of their cell biology and biochemistry which promote their successful parasitism. In order to survive within even nonimmune vertebrate hosts, *Leishmania* must resist killing by two highly evolved antimicrobial defense mechanisms. The first is the potentially lethal effect of normal serum, to which metacyclic promastigotes and tissue amastigotes are presumably exposed prior to uptake by mononuclear phagocytes. Whereas noninfective, dividing promastigotes are extremely sensitive to killing by serum, via activation of the alternative complement pathway, metacyclic promastigotes and amastigotes are relatively resistant. Paradoxically, it does not appear that complement resistance is a consequence of inefficient complement activation, because metacyclic *L. major* promastigotes incubated in serum have been shown to be heavily opsonized with C3b, which as discussed below, has very important implications in terms of attachment to macrophages. Rather, the resistance seems to be due to ineffective deposition of the terminal lytic complement components.

Having survived their brief sojourn in the extracellular milieu, *Leishmania* must then survive a barrage of macrophage microbicidal systems which may include the lethal products of oxygen metabolism, lysosomal hydrolases, low pH, and cationic proteins. Studies involving *Leishmania*-macrophage interactions have focused most intensely in recent years on the receptors and ligands which determine parasite attachment and uptake. A most consistent observation has been the role of C3 deposition on the promastigote surface, which dramatically enhances the attachment and uptake of the parasite by C3 receptors expressed on the macrophage plasma membrane [7]. The parasite surface constituents which appear to be responsible for complement activation and C3 deposition are the two major surface glycoconjugates of *Leishmania*: the surface lipophosphoglycan (LPG) and the promastigote surface protease, g.p. 63. The latter molecule has recently been shown to bind to C3 receptors in an apparently complement-independent manner, presumably via an intrinsic amino acid sequence (RGDS) which provides a common recognition site for cells. The macrophage mannose-fucose receptor (MFR) has also been implicated in the binding of some *Leishmania* species, with the likelihood that it recognizes mannose-containing oligosaccharides in LPG and/or g.p. 63.

Attachment of *Leishmania* amastigotes and metacyclic promastigotes to macrophages leads to extremely rapid phagocytosis of the organisms, particularly when the organisms have been serum-opsonized. Phagocytosis is generally accompanied by a respiratory burst and the consequent production of oxygen metabolites such as superoxide and hydrogen peroxide, which have been shown to be toxic to all stages of the parasite. Amastigotes and metacyclic promastigotes appear to evade oxygen-dependent destruction by triggering a minimal respiratory burst during infection. This may be due to the use of C3 receptors for internalization, since these receptors are known to be uncoupled from cellular activation. It may also be due to the presence of the LPG and a membrane-bound acid phosphatase, both of which have been shown to inhibit the oxygen burst. After phagocytosis the parasite resides in a parasitophorous vacuole which then fuses with secondary lysosomes to form a phagolysosome where the organisms survive and replicate. Thus *Leishmania* challenge successfully the very heart of the cell's defensive machinery containing powerful hydrolytic and oxidative enzymes which kill and digest most living organisms. The phagosome is known to be functional because other material sharing the same vacuole can be seen undergoing digestion. How do *Leishmania* survive? This fundamental aspect of *Leishmania* parasitism has not been explained. Survival may be due to the resistance of the parasite's exposed surface to enzyme attack (perhaps because the presence of LPG makes it so highly negatively charged), or, alternatively, the parasite may excrete inhibitors which prevent this attack (such as the well-described soluble acid phosphatase or the surface protease, g.p. 63). The probability that the phagosomal membrane is modified in some way by the parasite is suggested by the different behavior of the membrane depending upon the species of *Leishmania*. With *L. mexicana*, the phagosome becomes greatly enlarged, and each parasite adheres to the membrane at one end. With *L. donovani*, on the other hand, each parasite is usually surrounded by its own closely opposed, individual membrane.

Since the parasite lies in a functioning phagosome, it must have available to it nutrients ingested by the host cell. Leishmanial acid phosphatases may play a nutritive role by hydrolyzing organic phosphates. The same functions might be served by the unique nucleotidases present on the surface. *Leishmania*, as well as other *trypanosomatids*, cannot synthesize purines de novo and are therefore dependent upon an exogenous supply of preformed purines which can be utilized by leishmanial 3'- and 5'-nucleotidases [8]. Since normal phagolysomal pH falls to between 4.5 and 5.0, the parasite requires a way of maintaining its own intracellular pH. This is accomplished by the action of a membrane-proton-translocating ATPase which is located on the cytoplasmic side of the parasite surface membrane and acts by coupling ATP hydrolysis to proton-pumping activity. This creates a proton electrochemical gradient across the membrane which drives active transport of nutrients, such as glucose and proline, which are vital sources of energy.

PATIENT

PATHOLOGY

Pathology of cutaneous and mucocutaneous disease

The histopathological features of cutaneous leishmaniasis will depend upon a variety of factors, including the species of causative organism, presence or absence of an immune response on the part of the host, and the stage or duration of the disease. Except in a few instances of experimental infections, observations on very early histological changes are not available. However, from studies of infections in experimental animals the earliest lesion consists of a few infected cells and a minimal infiltration of lymphocytes. With an increase of numbers of infected cells the inflammatory reaction in the dermis composed of lymphocytes, plasma cells, and macrophages becomes more prominent, and small foci of necrotic cells and scattered polymorphonuclear leukocytes may be seen. Compromise with the blood supply does not seem to be the cause of necrosis and ulceration of the skin which occurs in cutaneous leishmaniasis; it is more likely the consequence of an intense immunological reaction occurring in the skin, but the exact

mechanism of the process is not known. Later changes occur in the epidermis—such as hyperkeratosis, acanthosis, and pseudoepithelioma formation. Sometimes relatively large numbers of organisms in infected cells are present in lesions, but at other times they are very scanty and may not be seen at all. With the passage of time the acute inflammatory reaction subsides, and the histology is that of a chronic granuloma, with foreign body giant cells frequently present.

The histological picture in mucocutaneous disease is generally similar to that of the cutaneous form except that parasites are much fewer in number and more difficult to find. In addition, the specific histopathology may be greatly altered by the presence of necrosis of affected tissue and superficial bacterial infection. Unfortunately, because of the inaccessibility of tissue specimens in mucocutaneous disease, representative pathological specimens for study have not been available. Therefore, our knowledge of the histopathology of mucocutaneous disease is rather sketchy. The infected macrophages in cutaneous lesions caused by members of the *L. mexicana* complex of organisms tend to have larger vacuoles and often multiple organisms within the vacuoles. This appearance—namely the large vacuolated infected cells—is also typical of diffuse cutaneous leishmaniasis (DCL). Another feature of DCL, in addition to infected macrophages with large vacuoles, is the scarcity of inflammatory cells in the lesion. Also, the overlying epidermis is generally intact.

Large numbers of organisms within swollen phagocytic vacuoles and few infiltrating lymphocytes are also typical of lepromatous leprosy. Similarities in the clinical spectra as well as in the histopathology of leprosy and leishmaniasis have been thoroughly described.

Pathology of visceral leishmaniasis

The organs mainly affected are the liver, spleen, bone marrow, and elements of the reticuloendothelial system at various sites. These organs and tissues hypertrophy,with the increased cells made up of parasitized macrophages but little or no lymphocytic infiltration. Generalized enlargement of lymph nodes is not a consistent finding, but hyperplasia of lymphoid tissue in certain anatomical locations is not unusual. For example, the lamina propria of the small and large intestine and Peyer's patches may be infiltrated with infected macrophages, sometimes leading to ulceration of the mucosa. Endothelial proliferation occurs in certain organs, as within septa of pulmonary alveoli and in renal glomeruli.

The spleen is enlarged, sometimes to tremendous size, but is firm and the capsule is not under pressure. The nature and chronic course of the enlargement make the spleen relatively resistant to tears from an aspirating needle. This makes splenic puncture for diagnosis a less hazardous procedure in this disease than in many other diseases in which splenic enlargement occurs more rapidly. Enlargement of the liver is due to hyperplasia of the Kupffer cells which are packed with the intracellular amastigote forms of the parasite. Only rarely are parenchymal cells of the liver parasitized. There may be focal granulomas and some fibrosis in the liver in chronic untreated cases.

The bone marrow is infiltrated with parasitized macrophages, a process that may impair production of other hematopoietic elements. The enlarged spleen undoubtedly also contributes to the anemia and thrombocytopenia which are characteristic of visceral leishmaniasis. There is a striking polyclonal B-cell activation that results in high IgG and total serum protein values. Some organs, most notably the kidneys, may show pathological changes secondary to deposition of immune complexes.

In the early stages of visceral leishmaniasis, small nodules in the skin containing parasites have been described at or near the site of inoculation. There are a few reports of parasites being demonstrable even in apparently normal skin. A more obvious type of skin involvement, although variable by geographical location, is post-kala azar dermal leishmaniasis (PKDL). This is the development in some patients, after recovery from disease, of a variety of skin lesions which may at times contain large numbers of parasites.

IMMUNOLOGY

Clinical studies

Immunological studies of leishmanial infections in humans have focused primarily on the nature of the immune mechanisms responsible for control and resolution of infection, and resistance to reinfection. Self-cure, which is associated with most forms of cutaneous leishmaniasis, is due to the immune response which the infection evokes, and it was recognized as long as 60 years ago that cell-mediated immunity develops early during cutaneous infection and persists long after healing is complete. Evidence for this cellular reactivity includes ulceration of the lesion, the histopathological evidence, the positive delayed-hypersensitivity (DTH) leishmanin skin test, and the ability of lymphocytes to respond in vitro to leishmanial antigens [9]. Healing is accompanied by low or undetectable levels of specific antibody. It is well established that immunity develops following recovery. The cellular immunity responsible for control and resolution of primary infection, and for resistance to reinfection, is thought to be mediated by sensitized CD4+ T lymphocytes which produce lymphokines capable of activating parasitized macrophages for intracellular killing. Macrophage-activating lymphokines have been shown to enhance both oxygen-dependent and -independent killing mechanisms. One lymphokine clearly implicated in these effects is γ-interferon, which has been shown to be produced by antigen-stimulated lymphocytes from patients with cutaneous leishmaniasis, and to activate human macrophages to kill intracellular organisms.

Cutaneous leishmaniasis is sometimes considered to constitute a polar disease, akin to leprosy, the two rare polar forms being diffuse cutaneous leishmaniasis (DCL) and leishmaniasis recidivans. In DCL, multiple cutaneous granulomata develop which contain abundant parasites but little lymphocyte infiltration. DCL seems to be the result of host unresponsiveness rather than parasite invasiveness. DCL patients demonstrate antigen-specific impairment of DTH reactivity in the presence of a humoral antibody response. Leishmaniasis recidivans is characterized by a predominantly lymphocytic lesion and persistence of low numbers of parasites within macrophages despite the presence of strong DTH reactivity. It is similar in this regard to mucocutaneous leishmaniasis, which is due to metastasis of organisms to mucosal sites from a primary cutaneous lesion. The persistence of leishmanial lesions in the face of strong cellular reactivity remains unexplained for both mucocutaneous disease and leishmaniasis recidivans.

The critical immunological feature of visceral leishmaniasis is the complete absence of cellular reactivity to leishmanial antigens. This results in uncontrolled parasitization of the mononuclear phagocyte system, which is especially prominent in the spleen. The disease is characterized by extremely high titers of antileishmanial antibodies, circulating immune complexes, and raised nonspecific IgM and IgG levels due to extensive polyclonal B-cell activation. The profound impairment of DTH is usually specific, but may extend to other antigens. Nonspecific immunity, if lost, is regained within weeks of recovery after treatment. Specific cellular immunity is regained only slowly after successful treatment, generally within 1 year. Patients who have recovered from infection are normally considered immune to reinfection. In addition, subclinical or asymptomatic infections with *L. donovani* are now thought to be the more usual outcome of exposure since within endemic areas individuals with no history of kala azar display a high frequency of positive leishmanin skin test and/or specific antibody.

Experimental studies

These clinical observations have led to a number of extremely useful lines of immunological research in experimental systems. The first involves the identification of host factors which must play a major role in determining the severity and outcome of disease, since, as is clear from the examples of DCL, recidiva, and subclinical versus acute kala azar, different individuals can respond to the same parasite strain with very different disease profiles. Studies on leishmanial infection in inbred mice have established that the genetic constitution of the host exerts a profound influence on both innate susceptibility and the subsequent outcome of infection. The strain spectrum of acute susceptibility to *L. donovani* follows precisely that of two other obligate intramacrophage pathogens, *Salmonella typhimurium* and *Mycobacterium bovis,* each of which is controlled by a single gene located on chromosome 1 [10]. This gene seems to influence the innate ability of liver macrophages to control the initial intracellular growth of the parasite.

Subsequent immunological control of *L. donovani* infections within acutely susceptible mouse strains has been shown to be influenced, not surprisingly, by major histocompatibility (H-2) linked genes. Genetic analyses of cutaneous disease have relied heavily on the observation that BALB/c mice are uniquely susceptible to infection by *L. major;* the primary cutaneous lesion expands without restraint, leading to metastasis and fatal visceralization. The lack of any immune control in infected BALB/c mice suggests the likelihood that a very high level of innate susceptibility might in some way override the curative potential of any acquired immunity. This acute susceptibility was found to segregate according to a single autosomal non-H-2 linked gene, provisionally mapped to chromosome 8 and hence clearly different from the gene controlling acute susceptibility to *L. donovani*. This explains why the strain susceptibilities to visceral *L. donovani* and cutaneous *L. major* infections are so different, and emphasizes fundamental differences in the pathobiology of these diseases. The relevance of genetic determinants of susceptibility in rodent models to human disease awaits investigation.

The persistence of parasites despite the presence of strong cell-mediated immunity, as in mucocutaneous disease and recidivans, has prompted experimental studies demonstrating two possible immune evasion strategies. The first is that amastigotes of some species or strains of *Leishmania* are resistant to killing by activated macrophages of certain hosts. A spectrum in the susceptibility of leishmanial amastigotes to killing by lymphokine-activated mouse macrophages in vitro has been shown, with some strains *(L. m. amazonensis)* being completely resistant to killing. A second strategy has also been implicated, in which amastigotes which are normally sensitive to intracellular killing mechanisms infect macrophage subpopulations, such as inflammatory macrophages, which are deficient in their ability to be activated by lymphokines. The ability of macrophages to respond to lymphokine activation has also been shown to be influenced by temperature; intracellular killing decreases proportionately at temperatures below 37°C. Since skin temperatures are 5 to 10°C below body core temperature, this effect might contribute to the persistence or slow healing of cutaneous and mucocutaneous lesions.

A final focus of experimental studies has been to define more precisely the cellular and molecular components of cellular immunity, with a particular view to understanding the regulatory events which result in such profound cellular unresponsiveness as that which is characteristic of DCL and kala azar. The most extensively studied laboratory models of cutaneous leishmaniasis have been *L. enrietti* infections in the guinea pig, *L. enrietti* being a natural pathogen of these rodents, and infection with human cutaneous strains in inbred mice. Both models have utilized adoptive transfer of sensitized T lymphocytes to establish immunity, and in both cases have convincingly supported the conclusions drawn from clinical studies that cell-mediated immunity as opposed to humoral response is responsible for acquired resistance to leishmaniasis. The ability of B-cell-depleted antibody-deficient mice to control cutaneous infections is clearly incompatible with an essential protective role for antibody.

The regulation of cell-mediated immunity has been extensively studied in the susceptible BALB/c mouse. The absence of cell-mediated immunity in these mice is known to be due to the activities of parasite-specific CD4+ T lymphocytes which are generated during infection, because removal of these cells prior to infection by a variety of protocols (adult thymectomy, sublethal irradiation, treatment with anti-CD4 antibodies) confers resistance to these animals [11]. It is not clear how these disease-promoting T cells function, either by classically suppressing the activation or expression of other resistance-promoting CD4+ cells, or by elaborating factors which regulate the availability of appropriate macrophage target cells in which the parasite can grow. Apart from antigen-specific T lymphocytes, unresponsiveness in *L. major*–infected BALB/c mice and *L. donovani*–infected hamsters has been shown to be at least partially due to the activities of prostaglandin-producing nonspecific suppressor cells, which are presumably activated macrophages. What role, if any, these regulatory cells have in the evolution of cellular unresponsiveness in humans remains to be established.

CLINICAL MANIFESTATIONS

Human leishmanial infections can result in three main forms of disease, sometimes with dual manifestations in the same patient. The major factor determining the form of disease produced is the infecting species of parasite, but the immune response of the host may also play a role in influencing clinical features and outcome. *Cutaneous* disease is characterized by one or more indolent ulcers, but a wide spectrum of skin involvement can occur. When parasites from skin lesions sometimes metastasize to produce later destructive lesions of the oronasopharynx, the result is *mucocutaneous* leishmaniasis. The *visceral* form (kala azar) is systemic leishmanial disease with parasites in the reticuloendothelial system, and the clinical picture is characterized by hepatosplenomegaly, fever, weight loss, leukopenia, and ultimately death if untreated.

Cutaneous leishmaniasis

Although the different species of *Leishmania* are restricted to certain geographical areas of the world, the basic clinical features of cutaneous leishmaniasis are very much the same. Members of the *L. braziliensis* and *L. mexicana* complexes cause cutaneous leishmaniasis in the western hemisphere, while *L. (tropica) major* and *L. tropica (minor)* cause cutaneous leishmaniasis in Asia, Africa, and southern Europe. Thus, designations of new and old world leishmanial disease are appropriate. *L. aethiopica* is restricted to Ethiopia and contiguous countries, as its name indicates. Cutaneous lesions caused by all of the above species begin as small erythematous papules on exposed areas of the body where infected sandfly vectors have fed. The incubation period may be as short as 1 to 2 weeks up to as long as 1 to 2 months. A tiny vesicle often develops in the center of the papule and oozes some serous fluid; the lesion then gradually enlarges, forming an ulcer with characteristic firm, raised, and reddened edges (Fig. 34-3). The early lesion may be pruritic, but the ulcer, even rather large ones, is not painful. The ulcer can remain relatively dry with a central crust (dry form), or it may exude seropurulent material (wet form). Multiple lesions may be present in the same area of the body, and there may even be multiple lesions over widely distributed sites, depending upon the nature and intensity of exposure to infected sandflies. Subcutaneous nodules sometimes develop in a centripetal direction from the ulcer (sporotrichoid form), presumably along lymphatics, but the nodules are collections of infected macrophages with an accompanying inflammatory reaction, rather than actual lymph nodes. Cutaneous leishmanial lesions will eventually heal spontaneously, but they can persist for up to a year or more without treatment. Lesions caused by some species of *L. major,* especially in the Middle East, may heal within a few months untreated. Secondary bacterial infection of a leishmanial ulcer will make it more difficult to demonstrate organisms for a specific diagnosis and will delay healing. Regional adenopathy with uncomplicated cutaneous leishmaniasis is frequently absent.

The location and appearance of cutaneous leishmaniasis in the affected population may be characteristic for certain geographical regions. For example, involvement of the pinna of the ear by *L. mexicana* in forest workers of Central America who harvest chicle gum from plants is called *chiclero ulcer*.

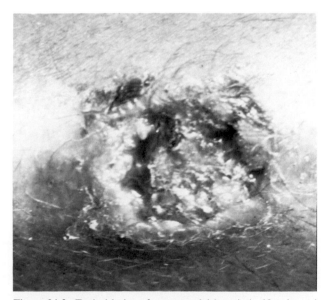

Figure 34-3. Typical lesion of cutaneous leishmaniasis. Note heaped up, indurated edges of the ulcerative lesion.

Pian-bois (''forest yaws'') is the term given to hyperkeratotic or papillomatous lesions seen in northeastern South America and caused by *L. b. guyanensis*. In the Middle East cutaneous leishmaniasis due to *L. tropica* or *L. major* was referred to as *oriental sore* or *Baghdad boil*. The upper face, near the eyes and nose, is a common location of lesions in Ethiopia. The prominent flat, depigmented facial scars seen so often in inhabitants of Iraq, Iran, Afghanistan, and Ethiopia are a telltale badge of previous cutaneous leishmaniasis.

Mucocutaneous leishmaniasis (espundia)

This disease is generally a late complication or sequel to cutaneous leishmaniasis, caused most commonly by members of the *L. braziliensis* complex of organisms. Mucocutaneous leishmaniasis (MCL) is encountered with greatest frequency in Brazil, Bolivia, Ecuador, Peru, and other countries of northern and central South America, with the infecting species believed to be *L. b. braziliensis* in most cases. But the infecting organism is frequently not isolated, and even less often has it been speciated when recovered, so the proportion of MCL due to other species is not clearly established, especially in various regions of Latin America. *L. b. panamensis* in Colombia and Panama can cause MCL, as well as *L. b. guyanensis* in northeastern South America. *L. m. amazonensis* has also been documented as the causative organism in some cases of MCL in Brazil. In addition, a few patients with the unusual anergic form of diffuse cutaneous leishmaniasis (DCL) due to *L. m. mexicana* may have mucous membrane involvement, such as a perforated nasal septum. Therefore, while *L. b. braziliensis* is clearly most frequent, it is not the exclusive cause of MCL, as stated by many textbooks.

Virtually all patients with MCL have a history and/or a typical scar of previous cutaneous disease. Mucosal involvement generally does not become manifest until the initial skin lesion(s) have healed, often many years later. However, in a few instances it may develop while the skin lesion is still active. The likelihood that MCL will later develop in a patient with regular CL cannot be predicted, except that it is encountered with greater frequency in certain geographical regions, it is more commonly associated with *L. b. braziliensis* than other species, and presumably is more likely to occur if there has been no or inadequate treatment of the original cutaneous disease. MCL undoubtedly represents metastatic spread of leishmanial organisms to naso-oropharyngeal tissues from a more peripheral site. It has been suggested that leishmanial organisms causing MCL prefer cooler temperatures of the upper respiratory tract; this is supported by the relative heat sensitivity of western hemisphere species of *Leishmania,* as well as by the lack of evidence for their dissemination to visceral organs. However, the critical factors in the pathogenesis of this disease process that is late to develop and characterized by scanty numbers of organisms but prominent tissue destruction are still largely unknown.

Earliest signs and symptoms of mucosal disease commonly involve the nose. Stuffiness and intermittent nosebleeds may be interpreted as chronic sinusitis. The pathological process may go no further than to destroy a portion of the nasal septum, with or without similar involvement of nasal turbinate tissues. With continued progression, the nose and surrounding tissues become swollen and inflamed, and nasal breathing is further compromised. In order to examine these patients thoroughly it is necessary to debride away crust of necrotic tissue and obtain proper visualization with fiber-optic instruments. Such preparation will often disclose active granulomatous polyps or papillomas along with eroded necrotic areas. The former type of lesions are clearly better sites to biopsy for culture of leishmania. In more advanced cases further tissue destruction results in obvious nasal deformity; it may progress forward to destroy the entire nose, involve the upper lip, or extend down to involve hard and soft palate and even the larynx. Complications of MCL include secondary bacterial infections and aspiration pneumonia. A distinction as to pathogenesis should be made between the mucous membrane involvement that occurs as a result of direct extension from a facial lesion as compared to the metastatic sequel of a cutaneous lesion in western hemisphere MCL.

Visceral leishmaniasis (kala azar)

The generalized form of leishmanial disease in which organisms multiply in the liver, spleen, bone marrow, and lymph nodes is caused by organisms belonging to the *L. donovani* complex. The clinical features of kala azar caused by these species are similar, but they have different epidemiological features. The parent species, *L. donovani,* occurs in Asia (northeastern China, India, and Iran) and Africa (primarily Sudan, Kenya, and Ethiopia), and can affect people of all ages. The parasite which causes kala azar in countries bordering the Mediterranean, in southern Europe as well as north Africa, affects primarily young children and infants. It also differs sufficiently from *L. donovani* to be given species status as *L. d. infantum.* In the western hemisphere also, kala azar is mainly a disease of very young children, with the causative organism, *L. d. chagasi,* being closely related to but slightly different from *L. donovani.* The major geographical foci of visceral leishmaniasis in Latin America are in northern and northeastern Brazil, but small foci are found in northern Argentina, Colombia, and Venezuela. Sporadic cases are also found in some of the Central American countries, including Mexico; these may flare into small but protracted epidemics as occurred in Honduras between 1975 and 1988.

The incubation period of visceral leishmaniasis is usually long, often 1 to 3 months, but it can be as short as a few weeks. There are now well-documented instances in which unsuspected latent infections of unknown duration have been activated under conditions of immunosuppression. The onset of kala azar is generally insidious; fever, sweating, weakness, and weight loss, gradually become noticeable. These symptoms, perhaps including nonproductive cough and abdominal discomfort due to an enlarging spleen and liver, may continue for months with the patient still up and about. In some patients the course of disease is more rapid, with high fever and chills. The most prominent physical findings are fever, hepatosplenomegaly, and cachexia, which is especially evident in the shoulder girdle and thorax (Fig. 34-4). While the fever pattern can be variable, ultimately it often exhibits twice-daily elevations to 38 to 40°C. Moderate generalized adenopathy is seen in patients from some geographical areas, but it is seldom striking in degree. Pigmentary changes in the skin are sometimes present: facial and circumoral hypopigmentation in dark-skinned patients, or hyperpigmentation in those with lighter skin. (The term *kala azar* is Hindi for "black sickness.") The skin may also show petechiae or ecchymoses. Splenic enlargement can be extreme in this disease, often reaching the iliac fossa, and the organ is firm and nontender. Characteristic laboratory findings include anemia, leukopenia (generally <4000 total white blood cells per cubic millimeter) thrombocytopenia, hypoalbuminemia, and a polyclonal hyperglobulinemia which, if the illness is of long duration, results in an elevated total

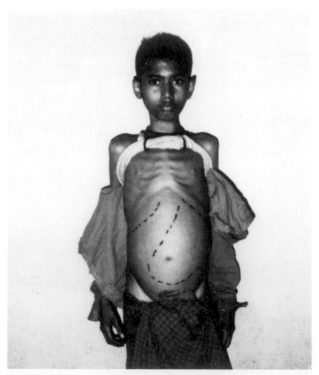

Figure 34-4. Indian kala azar. Hepatosplenomegaly is outlined. Note the emaciation that is especially prominent in thorax and shoulder girdle.

serum protein. In advanced cases edema and ascites can develop, there can be episodes of bleeding from the nose or gums, and deaths are due to secondary bacterial infections such as pneumonia, tuberculosis, or dysentery. Factors contributing to such complications include the granulocytopenia, probable impairment of granulocyte migration, and depressed cell-mediated immune function. Although circulating immune complexes are readily demonstrable in patients with active kala azar, they do not live long enough to develop renal disease or other consequences of this condition.

Rarer forms of leishmaniasis

Chronic Relapsing or Recidiva Form of Cutaneous Disease.
A form of chronic cutaneous leishmaniasis which either persists or reactivates after the original ulcer has healed is known as *chronic relapsing, lupoid,* or the *recidivans* type. The lesions typically are papular and nonulcerating, and they occur beyond the borders of the original scar as satellite lesions, or in the center of a healed area. The histological picture is that of an active granuloma, and while organisms are scanty, they

can generally be cultured from biopsies. *L. tropica* is the species most commonly causing the recidiva-type lesions, and they respond to antileishmanial treatment.

Diffuse Cutaneous Leishmaniasis (DCL).
This striking but uncommon complication of cutaneous disease, associated with anergy to leishmanial antigens, is seen in certain individuals infected with *L. m. mexicana* or *L. aethiopica* (Figs. 34-5, 34-6). It starts as a regular ulcerative cutaneous lesion, but then progresses to involve multiple sites as nonulcerative nodules or plaques on cooler areas of the body as in lepromatous leprosy. However, ulceration does occur in lesions overlying bony prominences and sites of trauma. Histologically the lesions are distinctive in that enormous numbers of amastigotes are present in large phagosomal vacuoles, with scanty lymphocytic infiltrate among the infected macrophages. While lesions may improve and even disappear with aggressive chemotherapy, patients usually relapse. Most cases of DCL have been reported from Ethiopia, Venezuela, Brazil, the Dominican Republic, and Mexico. Although the exact mechanism of failure of immune response in DCL has yet to be defined, the parasite

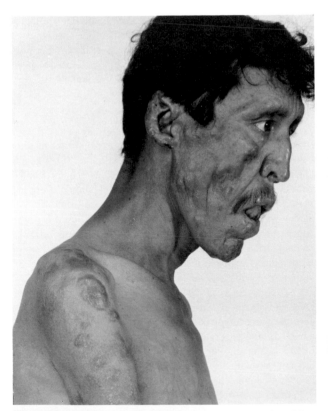

Figure 34-5. Diffuse cutaneous leishmaniasis in a patient from Mexico. Note nodular, nonulcerative lesions involving cheeks, lips, chin, ears, and shoulder. Disease present 15 years.

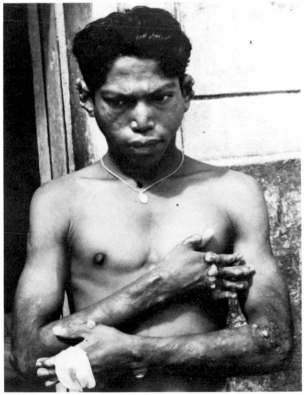

Figure 34-6. Diffuse cutaneous leishmaniasis in a Brazilian from Amazon region. Note nodular nonulcerative lesions of ears, arms, and fingers. Disease present many years.

species must also play a role since DCL does not seem to occur with *L. major* or even members of the *L. braziliensis* complex.

Post-Kala Azar Dermal Leishmaniasis (PKDL). Another cutaneous manifestation of leishmanial disease, PKDL, is seen after treatment and recovery from kala azar. In this situation the patient is otherwise well, without evidence of systemic illness. The lesions can be quite variable, often consisting of small maculopapules around the nose and mouth. They may enlarge to form nodules, or regress and leave hypopigmented areas of the skin. Whether or not there is an immunological basis for this unusual cutaneous sequel to previous visceral leishmaniasis is not clear; presence of apparently normal cell-mediated immunity in some cases has been reported. Parasites can be isolated readily from papular or nodular, but not from hypopigmented, lesions.

DIAGNOSIS

The first element in differential diagnosis is a history of exposure to leishmanial infection. Naturalists studying flora and fauna of the American jungles, archaeologists on Middle Eastern digs, tourists, Peace Corps volunteers, or news correspondents to these areas are potential candidates for cutaneous leishmaniasis. Acquisition of the visceral disease is likely to require more than casual exposure. The differential diagnosis of cutaneous leishmaniasis includes fungal (especially sporotrichosis), mycobacterial (e.g., *M. marinum* or *M. leprae*), or even bacterial infections. Midline granuloma and South American blastomycosis may resemble mucocutaneous leishmaniasis. Tropical splenomegaly syndrome of chronic malaria, hepatosplenic schistosomiasis, chronic brucellosis, leukemia, or lymphoma may resemble kala azar.

Demonstration of *Leishmania* from infected tissue, preferably by culture, is the most reliable method of diagnosis. In the case of CL and MCL, needle aspiration from the edge or scrapings from a slit into the lesion is a convenient way to obtain material for culture or smears, especially under field conditions. However, if tissue is obtained by biopsy, not only is the likelihood of positive culture increased, but cultures for bacteria or fungi can be performed and tissue sections can be made if a wider differential diagnosis is to be considered (Fig. 34-7). Splenic aspirates, bone marrow aspirates or biopsy, or liver biopsy, in that order, are the preferred specimens in suspected kala azar to demonstrate leishmanial organisms by culture or strained smears. With proper precautions as described by Chulay and Bryceson [*12*] the risks of splenic puncture can be minimized to make use of this procedure for diagnosis and monitoring response to therapy in kala azar. Culture of aspirated material from lymph nodes has also been used for diagnosis of visceral leishmaniasis.

For primary isolation of leishmanial organisms a diphasic medium such as NNN or Senekjie, using 15 to 30% defibrinated rabbit blood in the solid phase, is preferable. Several types of liquid media are commercially available, but varia-

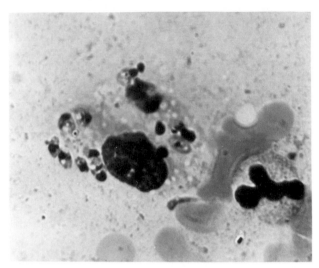

Figure 34-7. Stained impression smear from edge of biopsy specimen of cutaneous leishmaniasis. Note oval intracellular amastigotes in or adjacent to cell; some show characteristic kinetoplast. × 1000.

bility in lots of fetal bovine serum which such media require may compromise their utility. Leishmanial cultures are maintained at 22 to 26°C and should not be discarded as negative before 4 weeks. Inoculation of hamsters, over the nose or base of the tail, may sometimes permit recovery of fastidious *L. b. braziliensis* when cultures fail, but this method is not very practical.

THERAPY

Even though there are promising new developments in drug treatment of leishmaniasis, pentavalent antimony (Sb^5) is still the drug of choice. The preparation available in the United States, Pentostam, is considered an investigational drug and must be obtained from the Centers for Disease Control in Atlanta. Another Sb^5 preparation, Glucantime, is used in Latin America and in French-speaking countries. In recent years the recommended basic course of Sb^5 treatment for all forms of leishmaniasis has been increased to a daily dose of 20 mg per kilogram of body weight for a period of 15 to 20 days. The use of larger doses of Sb^5 has resulted from the finding that about 90 percent of Sb^5 is excreted in the urine within 24 h and that these larger doses are generally tolerable. However, a number of factors may impose variations on this basic course of Sb^5 treatment. For example, some authorities advise that the daily dose of Sb^5 not exceed 850 mg, while others do not hesitate to administer more than 1 g daily in adults.

Patients with MCL and kala azar are likely to require two to three separate 20-day courses of treatment for cure. Although Sb^5 can be given intramuscularly, the larger-sized doses now used virtually require administration of the drug by IV drip over 30 min in 100 to 150 mL of glucose or saline. Patients

allopurinol

treated with Sb[5] should be checked periodically with liver function tests, electrocardiograms, and total white blood counts. Modest elevations in liver enzyme values are common, and mild nonspecific ECG abnormalities may occur. As the cumulative dose of Sb[5] increases, arthralgias commonly develop and general weakness may be noted. Rigorous physical activity should be curtailed until treatment has been completed.

Amphotericin B should be considered for treatment of cutaneous or mucocutaneous disease that has not responded to Sb[5]. It would probably also be effective in kala azar that has not responded to conventional therapy. Of course, amphotericin B is more toxic than Sb[5], but with manipulation of the total time and conditions of intravenous administration in 500 mL of 5% dextrose, either daily or every other day, the drug can be tolerated. One to two grams of amphotericin B are generally sufficient, and further details of its use are discussed elsewhere (see Chap. 116, ''Treatment of the Systemic Mycoses'').

Patients with kala azar in certain regions of the world present the greatest problems in treatment. In Kenya, for example, up to 30 percent of cases relapse within 6 months after receiving a full course of Pentostam. Treatment failures probably represent lack of immunological responsiveness rather than resistance of the parasite to the drug; this latter situation is very difficult to demonstrate, even if attempted experimentally. Another treatment regimen for kala azar is pentamidine, in a dose of 2 to 4 mg per kilogram of body weight every other day for 10 doses. Allopurinol in a dosage of 15 mg/(kg · day) has been found to have some antileishmanial activity, and has been shown to be effective in combination with Pentostam in some cases that failed to respond to Pentostam alone.

Effectiveness of many different drugs has been reported for treatment of cutaneous leishmaniasis. In this regard it should be remembered that infections caused by *L. major,* especially in the Middle East, will often heal spontaneously within 6 months. Therefore, without comparison with untreated controls or with a standard treatment regimen, it may be difficult to evaluate a new drug. Also, there may be considerable differences in response to drugs between species and even strains within a species of parasite. There are several reports that ketoconazole in a daily dose of 400 to 600 mg was as effective as Pentostam, but it had to be given for 4 weeks. Of even greater convenience than oral ketoconazole would be some form of locally applied medication. Encouraging results have been reported with a preparation containing a mixture of 15% paromomycin sulfate with 12% methylbenzethonium chloride in a paraffin ointment that was simply rubbed onto lesions several times a day. If these initial trials can be independently confirmed and extended to cutaneous disease caused by a wider variety of leishmanial species, such a local treatment would be a significant advance. However, without careful evaluation it may not be wise to use local therapy for treatment of cutaneous lesions caused by leishmanial species capable of producing later mucocutaneous disease. The application of local heat (40

to 41°C) for 25 h or more over a period of 4 or 5 days has been shown to eradicate viable leishmania in lesions caused by certain of the *L. mexicana* complex organisms. If some of the technical problems associated with liposomal encapsulation of drugs (such as uniform size and stability of liposomes) can be overcome, the effectiveness of certain proven drugs (Pentostam and amphotericin) could be greatly enhanced.

POPULATION

VECTORS AND RESERVOIRS

The subfamily Phlebotominae contains about 600 species and subspecies, and among these, 70 are proven or suspected vectors of leishmaniasis. In the old world they belong to the genus *Phlebotomus,* and in the new world to the genus *Lutzomyia.* Sand flies generally breed in soil that is rich in humus and which must be damp. The duration of the gonotrophic cycle, which corresponds to the time from one blood meal to the next, has been established for only a few species. *P. ariasi* can undergo at least three gonotrophic cycles, each lasting 7 to 18 days. Some species (e.g., *P. papatasi*) will feed more than once during the development of the eggs. This behavior increases contact between sand flies and vertebrate hosts, including humans. A female sand fly lays 50 to 100 eggs at each oviposition. Depending upon temperature and larval diet, the time from egg laying to the emergence of adults ranges from 35 to 60 days. Freshly emerged adult sand flies disperse from the breeding site to find sugar or a blood meal, or to mate.

Depending on the species, flight ranges of unengorged sand flies vary between 200 m and 2000 m. Preliminary observations on host-finding behavior suggest that female sand flies cannot detect humans at distances greater than 10 m. A sand fly that acts as a vector for humans must be anthropophilic and able to support the full development of the parasite, in particular the anterior migration of infective forms. The timing of blood feeding in relationship to promastigote development in the gut (requiring 4 to 14 days) is of considerable importance in determining the ability of the female sand fly to transmit infection. Other factors which determine vector competency are poorly defined, but recent evidence suggests that the types of sugars and frequency with which they are taken are critical for promastigote survival and development.

Most *Leishmania* species are maintained by wild animals in natural foci of infection. With the important exception of some *L. donovani* subspecies and *L. tropica,* the human is an accidental host who plays little role in maintaining the survival of the parasite. Various rodent species are the primary reservoir of *L. major* in Soviet central Asia, Iran, north Africa, and the Middle East. The main characteristic shared by old world reservoir hosts is a high population density associated with sedentary life in burrows, caves, or houses. The hyrax has been found frequently infected with *L. aethiopica* in Ethiopia and Kenya. In the new world, although a variety of sylvatic species are found infected with *L. braziliensis,* the primary reservoir for *L. b. panamensis* and *L. b. guyanensis* in Central America and Brazil, respectively, is thought to be the sloth. The natural reservoir of *L. b. braziliensis* is not yet known. An extraordinarily long list of mammals has been found naturally infected with *L. mexicana*. Most of these are rodents, but marsupials, primates, and carnivores are also infected. Among domestic animals, the dog is the primary reservoir of *L. donovani* from northeast China to western Africa and South America. Dogs have also been found infected with *L. peruviana* in Peru. In the epidemic areas of India and central Kenya humans are thought to be the only reservoir of visceral leishmaniasis caused by *L. donovani*. Most workers have concluded that *L. tropica* is also maintained by humans, who may be the source of infection for other animals.

Factors determining transmission rates to humans will include occupation, habits, recreational activities, and location and type of housing, all of which can bring humans into close proximity with flies and reservoirs. Human-fly contact is increased by sleeping out of doors and by temporary visits to areas with infected flies during the time of peak biting activity. The possibility of transmission is increased in settlements in neotropical forests, in places infested by infected rodents, and in semiarid foci on the periphery of certain towns. Any type of house construction in which cracks develop will permit sandfly breeding so long as humidity is maintained. Stone walls with crevices, hollow trees, or rodent burrows serve as breeding sites in rural areas.

CONTROL

Most of the leishmanial parasites are transmitted as a zoonosis—i.e., with animal reservoirs and vectors that do not require participation of humans in the cycle. In these circumstances, elimination of sylvatic animal reservoirs and vectors is impractical and unrealistic, particularly in the forest and jungle. If the sandfly vector is peridomestic and enters houses, elimination of breeding sites, such as piles of rubble around houses, and use of residual insecticides may be helpful. If the domestic dog is a reservoir, destruction of infected dogs, especially strays, can be instituted. This has apparently been an effective measure in China. In several parts of the world, especially in the Mediterranean region and in India, the use of residual insecticides for control of malaria resulted in a secondary or fortuitous sharp reduction in cutaneous and visceral leishmaniasis. With malaria control achieved and with cessation of spraying insecticides, visceral leishmaniasis began to appear again in Italy and India. In those circumstances where animal reservoirs and vectors are sylvatic, use of insect repellents and protective clothing may help in reducing the risk of acquiring leishmaniasis.

The fact that resistance to reinfection follows from natural or drug-induced cure of leishmaniasis augurs well for the development of a preventive vaccine. In the past, nomadic populations of the Middle East deliberately induced cutaneous leishmanial infections by scarification from active cases in female children on the extremities or trunk to avoid later scars

of the disease on the face. Immunization by inoculation of living organisms from culture that were believed to be attenuated has been practised on a limited scale in Israel, Iran, and the U.S.S.R. Unfortunately, this type of immunization or "leishmanization" with living organisms, whose virulence cannot always be predicted, can be dangerous. Therefore, the practice has been discontinued in Israel and the U.S.S.R. It is clear that many of the dangers of leishmanization could be eliminated using a killed *Leishmania* preparation. Experimental results using a killed *L. major* vaccine have been encouraging. Susceptible mouse strains have been protected using radioattenuated promastigotes or crude soluble antigen fractions. The vaccine requires adjuvant and IV or ip administration. More recently, successful immunity has been induced using two molecularly defined vaccines: LPG and g.p. 63. Coinciding with the stimulus of animal studies, human trials using a killed *Leishmania* vaccine (a mixture of five merthiolate-treated promastigote strains) began in Brazil in 1979. While these vaccine trials have been severely hampered by field conditions, significant protection was apparent in vaccinees who converted to a positive skin test.

REFERENCES

1 Wirth DF, Pratt DM: Rapid identification of *Leishmania* species by specific hybridization of kinetoplast DNA in cutaneous lesions. Proc Natl Acad Sci USA 70:6099–7003, 1987

2 Adler S, Ber M: The transmission of *Leishmania tropica* by the bite of *Phelbotomus papatasii*. Indian J Med Res 29:803–809, 1941

3 Swaminath CS, Shortt HE, Anderson LAP: Transmission of Indian kala-azar to man by the bites of Phlebotomus argentipes. Indian J Med Res 30:473–477, 1942

4 Killick-Kendrick R: Biology of *Leishmania* in phlebotomine sandflies, in Lumsden WHR, Evans DA (eds): *Biology of Kinetoplastida*. London/New York, Academic, 1979, pp 395–460

5 Sacks DL, Perkins PV: Identification of an infective stage of Leishmania promastigotes. Science 223:1417, 1984

6 Titus, RG, Ribeiro JMC: Salivary gland lysates from the sand fly *Lutzomyia longipalpis* enhance *Leishmania* infectivity. Science 239:1306, 1988

7 Moser DM, Edelson PJ: Activation of the alternative complement pathway by *Leishmania* promastigotes: parasite lysis and attachment to macrophages. J Immunol 132:1501–1506, 1984

8 Dwyer DM, Gottlieb M: The surface membrane chemistry of *Leishmania*: its possible role in parasite sequestration and survival. J Cell Biochem 23:35–45, 1983

9 Pearson RD, Wheeler DA, Harrison LH, Kay DH: The immunobiology of leishmaniasis. Rev Infect Dis 4:907–922, 1983

10 Bradley DJ, Taylor BA, Blackwell J: Regulation of *Leishmania* populations within the host. III. Mapping of the locus controlling susceptibility to visceral leishmaniasis in the mouse. Clin Exp Immunol 37:7–14, 1979

11 Howard JG: Immunological regulation and control of experimental leishmaniasis. Int Rev Exp Pathol 28:79–116, 1986

12 Chulay JD, Bryceson ADM: Quantitation of amastigotes of *Leishmania donovani* in smears of splenic aspirates from patients with visceral leishmaniasis. Am J Trop Med Hyg 32:475–479, 1983

Toxoplasmosis · *Robert E. McCabe*
· *Jack S. Remington*

In recent years *Toxoplasma gondii* has become increasingly recognized as an important pathogen of humans and domestic animals. It is one of the most common causes of latent infection in humans the world over. The acute infection poses greatest hazard to the infant in utero and to the immunocompromised patient, particularly patients with AIDS. As a cause of congenital infection, it may result in serious and debilitating, untoward sequelae. The personal and societal costs of this infection and disease and the relatively simple, inexpensive measures for its prevention are just beginning to be appreciated.

For purposes of definition, *toxoplasmosis* refers to clinical disease caused by the sporozoan, *T. gondii,* whereas *toxoplasma infection* refers to presence of either the trophozoite form or the cyst form in tissues irrespective of clinical disease.

PARASITE

LIFE CYCLE

T. gondii is an obligate intracellular protozoan and is classified as a coccidian [1]. The definitive hosts in nature are members of the cat family. In the cat, the organism has both an enteroepithelial and an extraintestinal cycle, while in incidental hosts such as humans, all orders of mammals, birds, and probably reptiles as well, it exists only in the extraintestinal cycle. There are three forms of the organism, the *trophozoite* (previously known as *tachyzoite*), the *tissue cyst* (which contains intracystic organisms termed *bradyzoites*), and the *oocyst* (in which sporozoites are formed). Oocysts excreted by cats are transmitted to incidental hosts as well as cats. The organisms, released from oocysts by the digestive process, invade intestinal epithelium and then disseminate widely to all host tissues, where the organisms encyst. When this occurs in domestic animals used for meat ingestion, it is a mechanism for transmission of infection. As many as 25 percent of mutton and 25 percent of pork samples surveyed have been shown to contain tissue cysts [1]. Cysts have rarely been demonstrated in samples of beef.

Trophozoites

This form of the organism, depicted in Fig. 35-1*A* and *B*, is 4 to 8 μm in length, motile, and stains well with Wright's and Giemsa stain. In the laboratory trophozoites are propagated in mouse peritoneum and mammalian tissue cell culture. Trophozoites can invade every kind of mammalian cell except nonnucleated erythrocytes and can be found in multiple tissues during the acute stage of infection. Once they are within host cells, trophozoites multiply by endodyogeny, a continuous process in which two daughter cells form within the mother cell. Freezing and thawing, desiccation, and normal gastric secretions that contain pepsin and hydrochloric acid are lethal to trophozoites.

Cysts

A single tissue cyst, as depicted in Fig. 35-1*C*, may measure up to 200 μm in diameter and contain as many as 3000 organisms. The cyst wall is argyrophilic and stains weakly with periodic acid Schiff (PAS) stain. Bradyzoites stain strongly positive with PAS.

Tissue cysts can develop within any organ, are found most often in brain, heart, and skeletal muscle, and remain viable throughout the life of the host. Cysts are a major means by which the organism is transmitted to carnivores, including humans who ingest undercooked meat. Peptic and tryptic digestive juices can disrupt the cyst wall, with liberation of viable organisms that can initiate infection. It has been postulated that tissue cysts latent within immunodeficient patients may disrupt, with dissemination of toxoplasma to other organs and cause clinical disease. Tissue cysts have also been postulated to be a cause of chorioretinitis in immunocompetent older children and adults, although the pathogenesis is controversial. Freezing to −20°C, desiccation, or heating above 66°C is lethal for cysts.

Oocysts

Oocysts, shown in Fig. 35-1*D*, are oval, measure 10 to 12 μm in diameter, and are produced only in the intestines of members of the cat family [1]. After ingestion of cysts or oocysts, oocysts are produced in the small intestine following an asexual cycle (schizogony) and a sexual cycle (gametogony) by the organisms. Up to 10 million oocysts per day are passed in the feces for a period of 7 to 20 days. Passage of oocysts begins 3 to 24 days after ingestion of the organism; the latent period depends on whether tissue cysts, trophozoites, or oocysts are ingested.

The infectious form of toxoplasma develops only after the oocysts are excreted and sporulation occurs. Sporulation requires 2 to 3 days at 24°C, 14 to 21 days at 11°C, and does not occur above 37°C or below 4°C. The oocysts can remain infectious in moist soil for more than 1 year, but dry heat greater than 66°C or nearly boiling water renders them noninfectious. If a cat becomes reinfected with toxoplasma, oocyst excretion rarely recurs.

PATIENT

PATHOGENESIS

Replicating organisms disrupt host cells and then either invade contiguous cells, often with the production of necrotic foci, or

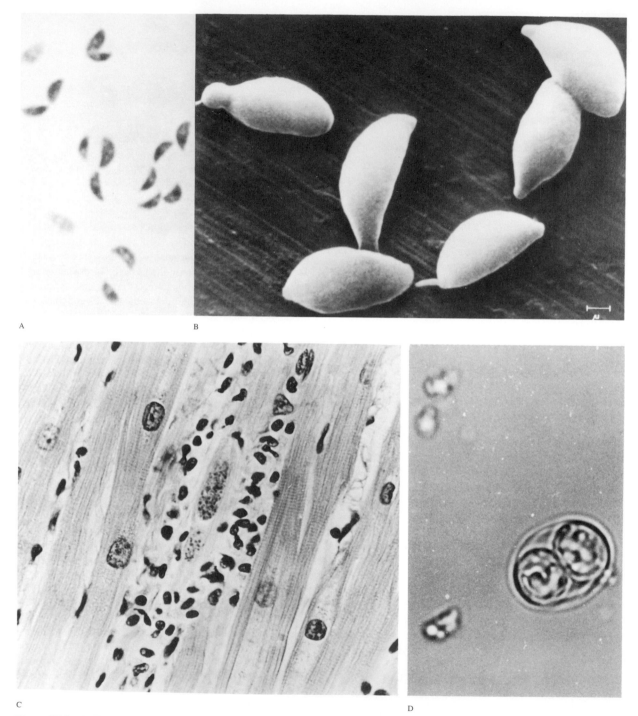

Figure 35-1. *A*. Trophozoites from peritoneal fluid of an infected mouse. *B*. Scanning electron micrograph of toxoplasma trophozoites from the peritoneal fluid of mice. (*From A.S. Klainer, J.L. Krahenbuhl, J.S. Remington: J. Gen. Microbiol. 75: 111–118, 1973.*) *C*. Tissue cysts. *D*. Sporulated oocyst.

disseminate widely throughout the body via the bloodstream or lymphatics. Antibody plus complement can effectively kill extracellular trophozoites. Intracellular trophozoites are protected and can go on either to cause cell destruction or to form cysts. Within macrophages, toxoplasma can block fusion of lysosomes with phagosomes and acidification of phagosomes. Lymphokines such as γ interferon and interleukin 2 appear to play key roles in host defense against toxoplasma by regulation of oxygen-dependent and independent host cell microbicidal activity and function of cytotoxic T cells. Of note is that human neonatal mononuclear phagocytes are deficient in generation of and response to macrophage-activating factors (e.g., γ interferon), which may play a role in pathogenesis of congenital disease. Termination of tissue destruction depends upon emergence of cell-mediated immunity and an antibody response. Cell-mediated immunity may take weeks or months to develop. The barrier to transfer of antibody in the eye and central nervous system may allow organisms to continue to proliferate and destroy tissue at the same time that other organisms are disappearing from extraneural tissue. Cysts form at the same time as tissue destruction occurs, and cysts probably persist for the life of the host. In the immunuocompromised patient, infection often progresses unabated in multiple vital organs, such as brain, lung, and heart, and frequently results in death of the patient. In normal individuals inflammatory reactions are rarely found associated with tissue cysts. Some workers propose that chorioretinitis and its resulting symptoms are a consequence of the immune response to toxoplasma antigen released from cysts. Others contend that cysts rupture and that resultant trophozoite multiplication is responsible for ocular inflammation and symptoms [2]. Cyst rupture has also been postulated as a cause of disseminated toxoplasmosis in immunosuppressed patients.

Reinfection may occur in the normal host, but its frequency and significance are unclear.

PATHOLOGY

Most pathology data are derived from congenitally infected infants and immunocompromised patients with disseminated infection. In infants the degree of organ and tissue involvement varies considerably, but the central nervous system is never spared. In immunocompromised patients, the findings at autopsy are usually dominated by central nervous system involvement, but pneumonitis, myocarditis, and pancreatitis are frequent. Data from immunologically normal adults are limited principally to results obtained from biopsied lymph nodes.

Lymph nodes

The histopathological changes in toxoplasmic lymphadenitis are distinctive and often diagnostic in older children and adults. Reactive follicular hyperplasia, irregular clusters of epithelioid histiocytes that encroach upon and blur the margins of germinal centers, and focal distension of sinuses with monocytoid cells

form a diagnostic triad. Giant cells of the foreign body or Langerhans type, trophozoites, or cysts are rarely demonstrated [3].

Central nervous system

Acute infection produces a focal or diffuse meningoencephalitis characterized by necrosis and microglial nodules [4]. Vascular involvement by trophozoites produces variable but often extensive necrosis of brain parenchyma; areas of coagulation necrosis may range from millimeters to several centimeters in diameter. Trophozoites and cysts are demonstrable in and near inflammatory foci as well as in uninflamed normal tissue. The lesions are usually multiple and are found frequently in gray matter, particularly in the cortex, but may involve almost any location, including cerebellum, spinal cord, brainstem, and basal ganglia. Although the lesions in adults and infants are generally similar, in infants periaqueductal and periventricular vasculitis and necrosis are distinctive of toxoplasmosis. Necrotic tissue may slough into the ventricles, the periventricular necrotic areas may calcify and lead to striking radiographs suggestive but not pathognomonic of toxoplasma infection, or the necrotic areas may become cystic [4]. Impressive hydrocephalus may result from either an obstructive ependymitis or periventricular necrosis or inflammation. Leptomeningeal reactions may be found in both infants and immunocompromised adults but are most marked in infants. In immunocompromised adults, the major pathological finding is necrotizing encephalitis of gray matter with the production of multiple, small, and diffusely distributed lesions; but occasionally single or large abscesses can be detected by computed tomography (CT) scanning or magnetic resonance imaging [5,6]. Such abscesses occasionally calcify in adults or older children.

Eye

Invading trophozoites produce a necrotizing retinitis. Secondarily a mass of budding capillaries can invade the vitreous; granulomatous inflammation of the choroid may appear; and papillitis, iridocyclitis, glaucoma, and cataracts can evolve [1].

Heart

Myocardial fibers may contain cysts or large aggregates of organisms without surrounding inflammation, while separate areas are infiltrated by mononuclear cells without demonstrable organisms. Myocarditis is attributed to rupture of parasitized cells. In immunocompromised patients, areas of necrosis may be widespread.

Other sites

Organisms have been found in almost all organs and may or may not be accompanied by an intense inflammatory response [1]. Several features deserve note. In the kidney, glomerulonephritis with deposition of toxoplasma antigen and antibody in glomeruli has been reported but appears to be rare. Skeletal muscle involvement is similar to that of cardiac muscle, and a widespread myositis or dermatomyositis may be evident. Although hepatomegaly is not uncommon, the entity of toxoplasma hepatitis is controversial and has not been proven to exist. Pulmonary infiltrates on chest radiographs may occur during acute toxoplasma infection, but signs and symptoms are rarely severe in the immunocompetent patient.

CLINICAL MANIFESTATIONS

Acute acquired toxoplasmosis

Only 10 to 20 percent of toxoplasma infections in the adult are symptomatic [7]. In this group of patients, toxoplasmosis most often presents as cervical lymphadenopathy, but pectoral and submental lymph node enlargement is also common, and any or all lymph node groups may be affected. Often only a single lymph node is enlarged, usually to less than 3 cm in diameter. The nodes are usually discrete, vary in firmness, may be tender, but do not suppurate. Fever, malaise, myalgia, fatigue, headache, sore throat, maculopapular rash sparing palms and soles, hepatosplenomegaly, hilar and mediastinal lymphadenopathy, radiographic lung infiltrates, abnormal liver function tests, and atypical lymphocytes may be present. Mesenteric or retroperitoneal lymphadenitis may produce abdominal pain and high fever, and toxoplasmosis may present as fever of unknown origin. The course of acute, acquired toxoplasmosis is self-limited and is most often benign in normal patients, but signs and symptoms may persist or recur for as long as 1 year. Rarely, persons presumed to be immunologically normal develop clinically overt visceral involvement with encephalitis, pneumonitis, or myocarditis which can result in death of the patient. Toxoplasmosis is difficult to diagnose clinically from history, physical examination, and routine laboratory tests since its manifestations mimic many other diseases. Less than 1 percent of syndromes of infectious mononucleosis have been shown to be caused by toxoplasma.

Congenital toxoplasmosis

If primary toxoplasma is acquired during pregnancy, the organism is transmitted to the fetus in up to 61 percent of the cases [1]. The only unequivocal cases of documented transmission of toxoplasma to the fetus from a chronically infected woman occurred in immunocompromised women. Thus, women at risk of delivering an infected infant are those who acquire the infection just prior to or during gestation. The former event is rare.

Both the incidence of toxoplasma infection and the clinical severity of disease in the offspring vary markedly with the trimester of pregnancy during which maternal toxoplasma infection is acquired [1]. For untreated mothers, maternal infection acquired during the third trimester resulted in congenital infection in approximately 65 percent of the infants; the large majority of the infected offspring had no signs of disease.

Infection acquired by the mother in the second trimester produced infection in 54 percent of the offspring, and about 72 percent of these infected offspring had no clinical signs of disease. Infection acquired in the first trimester resulted in congenital infection in 25 percent of the infants, but disease was severe in most of these infants, including a number of stillbirths. Treatment of the mother during gestation reduces the incidence of congenital toxoplasmosis by approximately 60 percent. Congenital disease (as contrasted with infection) is more severe the earlier in gestation that the mother acquires infection.

Toxoplasma infection has been implicated in spontaneous abortions, stillbirths, and premature births. On rare occasions, toxoplasma has been isolated from the abortuses of women with chronic infection. The frequency of toxoplasma infection as a cause of abortion is unknown and controversial.

Clinical manifestations of congenital toxoplasmosis are numerous and include cataracts, glaucoma, microphthalmia, mental and psychomotor retardation, anemia, jaundice, rash, petechiae due to thrombocytopenia, encephalitis, pneumonitis, microcephaly, intracranial calcification, hydrocephalus, strabismus, vomiting, diarrhea, hypothermia, and nonspecific illness. Toxoplasma infection is not known to cause fetal malformation by affecting host DNA. Detailed examination of infants may be needed to detect signs of the infection. In a prospective study, 116 congenitally infected infants without signs of infection were identified. More detailed examination revealed abnormal cerebrospinal fluid in 22 infants; chorioretinitis in 12 infants (usually bilateral); and intracranial calcifications on radiographs in 10 infants [8].

If clinical signs of infection are evident in the neonate, sequelae, as a rule, are severe [1]. Delayed onset disease may be severe or mild. Premature infants often suffer severe central nervous system and ocular disease in the first 3 months of life. Full-term infants frequently develop a milder disease manifested by signs of generalized infection such as hepatosplenomegaly and lymphadenopathy that usually appear in the first 2 months of life. Disease reflecting damage to the central nervous system may occur later, and eye disease may occur months to years after birth.

Recent data suggest that the majority of infants with subclinical infection at birth develop signs or symptoms if the patients are observed into adolescence. In one study [9], clinical evaluation during childhood to a mean age of 8.3 years revealed that 11 of the 13 infected children who were clinically normal in the newborn period suffered sequelae, and in each child the initial manifestation was chorioretinitis that appeared at a mean age of 3.7 years. Three children had unilateral blindness, while the remainder had chorioretinitis without loss of visual function. Five of the 11 children developed neurological sequelae, including one child with delayed psychomotor development, microcephaly, and seizure disorder and two children with minor cerebellar signs. Sensorineural hearing loss occurred in 3 of the 10 children evaluated. Other studies have confirmed the frequent occurrence of disease after infancy due to congenital infection. Treatment of the infant in the first 6 to 12 months of life probably reduces incidence of sequelae.

Ocular toxoplasmosis

Toxoplasma infection is one of the most common causes of chorioretinitis in the United States, Europe, and probably the world. The vast majority of cases of toxoplasma chorioretinitis are a result of congenital infection. Patients are often asymptomatic until later in life. The peak incidence of ocular toxoplasmosis occurs from ages 15 to 20. In these patients, systemic signs and symptoms of infection are uncommon. Signs of congenital ocular toxoplasmosis include microphthalmia, small cornea, posterior cortical cataracts, anisometropia, nystagmus, and optic neuritis, with symptoms of blurred vision, photophobia, scotomas, pain, and epiphora. Strabismus may be an early sign of congenital infection in children. The characteristic focal necrotizing retinitis initally appears in the fundus as yellowish-white, elevated cotton patches with indistinct margins, usually on the posterior pole. These often appear in small clusters in which the individual lesions are of varying ages. With healing, the lesions atrophy, pale, and develop black pigment. Panuveitis may occur, sometimes accompanied by glaucoma and cataracts, but anterior uveitis is never discovered as an isolated finding. Relapses of chorioretinitis are common. The disease may ultimately result in the necessity for enucleation. In the patient with chorioretinitis, additional features on ophthalmoscopic examination that suggest toxoplasmosis include bilateral macular involvement, massive chorioretinal degeneration but with normal-appearing retina surrounding the typical punched out lesions, rapid development of optic nerve atrophy, and frequent clarity of the vitreous and aqueous humor [10].

Immunocompromised patients

Patients who are being treated for Hodgkin's disease, hematological malignancy, or organ graft rejection or who have AIDS are at greater risk for toxoplasmosis. All forms of toxoplasma infection that occur in normal adults can develop in immunocompromised patients. Patients with AIDS who have prior serological evidence of toxoplasma infection are at particularly high risk for development of toxoplasmic encephalitis. Five to 10 percent of AIDS patients in the United States and 25 percent of AIDS patients in much of western Europe are estimated to develop toxoplasmic encephalitis [11–13]. Toxoplasmosis in AIDS patients and in most other immunodeficient patients usually results from reactivation of latent infection. Exceptions include seronegative recipients of a transplant organ from a seropositive donor or recipients of blood products from donors with parasitemia [14]. Persistent parasitemia can be found in normal patients for as long as 1 year after acquisition of infection, but this is a rare occurrence. Patients with chronic myelogenous leukemia with high titers of toxoplasma

antibody, however, seem to have a significant incidence of parasitemia, and use of their blood products for transfusion may pose a special risk for the immunocompromised patient. Organisms may survive in whole citrated blood for up to 50 days at 4°C.

The majority of cases of toxoplasmosis in the immunocompromised patient present with signs referable to the central nervous system due to encephalitis, meningoencephalitis, or mass lesions. Brain involvement frequently leads to death of the patient. None of the clinical signs are pathognomonic, and frequently other diagnoses are entertained such as progressive multifocal leukoencephalopathy, herpes simplex encephalitis, lymphoma or brain abscess(es) due to *Mycobacterium tuberculosis,* fungi, or bacteria. The cerebrospinal fluid usually reveals a mononuclear pleocytosis, elevation of protein concentration, and a normal glucose titer. CT scanning and magnetic resonance imaging [5,6] may help direct diagnostic efforts such as brain biopsy or aspiration. Magnetic resonance imaging (MRI) may be useful either when the CT scan is normal or when attempts to find a lesion accessible to biopsy or aspiration are unsuccessful. Dissemination of the organisms to extraneural tissue is frequent and often results in clinically overt myocarditis and pneumonitis.

DIAGNOSTIC TESTS

Acute infection is diagnosed by isolating toxoplasma from blood or body fluids; demonstration of trophozoites in histological sections of tissue or cytology preparations of body fluids; finding characteristic lymph node histology; demonstration of characteristic serological test results; or demonstration of toxoplasma cysts in placenta, fetus, or neonate. Isolation of toxoplasma from tissues of older children or adults may only reflect the presence of cysts, except, perhaps, for isolation from lymph node tissue in adults, which may reflect presence of trophozoites [1]. Finding numerous cysts in tissue sections suggests, but does not prove, acute infection.

Isolation of the organism

To isolate toxoplasma, suspect material is inoculated subcutaneously and intraperitoneally into laboratory mice or into tissue cell culture [1]. Use of tissue cell culture is a more convenient and rapid method for demonstration of the parasite, but may be less sensitive than mouse inoculation. If storage of specimens prior to attempt at isolation is unavoidable, the material should be refrigerated at 4°C. At this temperature, trophozoites may survive in tissue or blood clots for several days, and cysts may survive as long as 2 months. Formalin treatment kills the organism. When attempting isolation from blood (often successful in neonates with congenital infection), the buffy coat layer (white blood cells) should be separated. If the blood is clotted, the clot may be triturated with mortar and pestle and then homogenized, or broken with a syringe and needle. Biopsy samples of tissues can be treated in the same manner: 0.5 to 2.0 mL of the sample suspended in saline is injected intraperitoneally and subcutaneously into mice. Larger samples of tissue can be minced with scissors and then digested with trypsin (0.25% in buffered saline, pH 7.2). Between 5 and 10 days after intraperitoneal injection of the suspect material, peritoneal exudate is examined for the presence of organisms. If mice die before 6 weeks, peritoneal fluid and impression smears of liver, spleen, and brain are examined in Giemsa-stained preparations. If organisms are not demonstrable, spleen and brain should be inoculated into fresh mice. Mice that survive for 6 weeks should be tested for the presence of specific antibody. For definitive diagnosis, the organisms must be demonstrated in the tissues of the seropositive mouse [1]. A rapid method for diagnosis of toxoplasmic encephalitis is examination of air-dried, Wright-Giemsa–stained sediment of centrifuged specimens of cerebrospinal fluid.

In proven cases of congenital toxoplasma infection, it is usual to recover organisms from placenta [1]. Attempts at isolation of the organism from the placenta should be made whenever there is clinical suspicion of congenital toxoplasma infection.

Histological diagnosis

Although demonstration of trophozoites in tissue establishes the diagnosis as being acute, their often sparse distribution makes such demonstration difficult. They may be seen in histological sections stained with conventional stains, but the immunofluorescent technique and the peroxidase-antiperoxidase

method markedly increase sensitivity of detection [15]. These techniques can be used for unfixed or, following appropriate treatment, for formalin-fixed, paraffin-embedded tissue sections. Other methods that have been used for diagnosis, but with limited experience, include enzyme-linked immunosorbent assay to detect antigen in unfixed tissues, fluorescein-labeled monoclonal antibodies to detect toxoplasma in touch preparations, and electron microscopy.

SEROLOGICAL TESTS (see Table 35-1)

The problem of diagnosis of toxoplasma infection by serology is complicated by the high prevalence of circulating antibody among almost all human populations. In addition, antibody titers may persist at high levels for years in the otherwise normal individual. Serodiagnosis of the acute infection requires demonstration of rising antibody titers (at least two tubes) from a negative or low titer (e.g., 1:16) to a high titer (e.g., ≥ 1:1000) or the combination of a high IgG and a high IgM titer. A single high antibody titer in any test is suggestive, but not diagnostic, of acute infection. The most useful tests are the Sabin-Feldman dye test; agglutination test; indirect fluorescent antibody test, which can be adapted to measure IgG or IgM antibody or both; and double sandwich IgM enzyme-linked immunosorbent assay (ELISA). The recently developed ELISA technique for detection of antigenemia appears promising. Refinements of these tests may occur in the future as specific monoclonal antibodies and specific antigens are isolated.

Table 35-1. Guidelines for interpretation of results of serological tests for antibodies against toxoplasma[a]

Test	Positive titer	Titer in acute infection	Titer in chronic infection	Duration of elevated titer
Sabin-Feldman dye test (DT)[b]	1:4; undiluted[c]	≥1:1000	1:4–1:2000	Years
Indirect fluorescent antibody test (conventional IFA)	1:10	≥1:1000	1:4–1:2000	Years
Indirect hemagglutination test (IHA)[d]	1:16	≥1:1000	1:16–1:256	Years
Complement fixation test	1:4	Varies among laboratories	Negative to 1:8	Years
Agglutination test[e]	1:20	1:20≥1:1000	≤1:12,000–1:64,000	Years
IFA for IgM antibodies (IgM-IFA)[f]	1:2 infants[g]	≥1:2[g]	Negative	Weeks to months
	1:16 adults[g]	≥1:64	1:20	Weeks to months
Double sandwich ELISA for IgM (IgM-ELISA)[h]	1.0 infants	≥1.4	[i]	[i]
	1.7 adults	≥1.7	Negative to 3	Months to years

[a]Exceptions to these generalizations may occur. Also, values obtained in different laboratories may differ significantly.
[b]The World Health Organization has recommended that DT titers be expressed in international units per milliliter.
[c]In toxoplasma chorioretinitis, the DT may be positive in undiluted serum only.
[d]The IHA may give false-negative results early in infection. Therefore, IHA should not be used to detect congenital infection or infection during pregnancy.
[e]The agglutination test titers agree closely with DT titers. See [37].
[f]The IgM-IFA and the conventional IgM-ELISA (but not the double sandwich IgM-ELISA as described by Naot and Remington [19]), may give false-postive results in sera containing rheumatoid factor or antinuclear antibody.
[g]"Naturally occuring" IgM antibodies occur in older children and adults but not in the newborn. This is the reason for difference in titers considered positive between infants and adults.
[h]Titers are expressed as numerical values. See [38].
[i]Unknown at this time.

Sabin-Feldman dye test (dye test)

If living trophozoites are incubated with serum containing toxoplasma antibody and complement, they will lyse and fail to stain with alkaline methylene blue [16]. The titer is that dilution of serum in which half of the organisms are lysed. This titer can be converted into international units by comparison to a reference serum as recommended by the World Health Organization. The antibodies usually appear 1 to 2 weeks after infection, reach high titers ($\geq$ 1:1000) in 6 to 8 weeks, and then slowly decline over months to years. Low titers (1:16 and 1:64) commonly persist for life. The titers of the dye test, as well as those of the other tests, do not correlate with clinical severity of disease.

Indirect fluorescent antibody test (IFA)

Slide preparations of killed trophozoites are incubated with serial dilutions of the patient's serum, and a specific antigen-antibody reaction is detected by a fluorescein-tagged antiserum prepared against serum IgG, IgM, or total immunoglobulin. For IgG, the results agree qualitatively with those obtained in the dye test, but titers are somewhat higher [17]. Although the IFA test is more widely available, the dye test is quantitatively more reliable. This is of special importance in congenital infection and in comparing serial sera from pregnant women.

Antibodies in the IgM-IFA test appear as early as 5 days after infection, rise rapidly to titers of 1:10 to $\geq$ 1:1000, and then fall to low titers and usually disappear within a few weeks or months. In some patients, low titers may be detected for 1 year or more. This test is negative in some immunodeficient patients, most patients with active ocular toxoplasmosis, and approximately 75 percent of infants with congenital toxoplasma infection. In some patients with acute acquired toxoplasma infection, high levels of IgG toxoplasma antibodies interfere with the IgM-IFA test and cause false-negative results. Antinuclear antibodies may cause false-positive reactions in both the IFA and the IgM-IFA tests.

IgM-ELISA

The double sandwich ELISA test for IgM toxoplasma antibody avoids the false-positive results in the IgM-IFA test caused by antinuclear antibodies and rheumatoid factor and has proved to be significantly more sensitive than the IgM-IFA test in detecting cases of acute acquired and congenital toxoplasma infection [18,19]. The double sandwich IgM-ELISA test detects 70 to 80 percent of congenitally infected infants compared to the IgM-IFA test, which detects only approximately 25 percent.

Indirect hemagglutination test (IHA)

Red blood cells that are sensitized with trophozoite antigen agglutinate when incubated with serum containing toxoplasma antibody [20]. Usually the IHA test measures different antibodies than the dye and IFA tests. The appearance of IHA titers may lag several weeks or more behind those measured in dye or IFA tests and can persist at higher levels for even longer periods. Since the rise in IHA titers in acute infection may not occur for months, this test must not be used as a screening test in pregnant women. Furthermore, IHA titers have often been negative in cases of congenital toxoplasma infection and must never be used as the sole serological test in suspect cases of congenital toxoplasma infection. The IHA test may be useful in epidemiology studies and to detect a rise in titer in cases in which dye or IFA titers have already risen to high levels.

Complement fixation test (CF)

As with the IHA test, a rise in CF titer may not occur for months. This test is used to detect a rise in antibody titers when the dye or IFA titers have already reached high levels. Antigens have not been standardized for use in this test or for the IHA test. If "whole" or "heavy" trophozoite antigen is used, CF titers may parallel those of the dye and IFA tests.

Direct agglutination test

This test uses formalin-fixed, intact trophozoites or antigen-coated latex particles and is read similarly to the IHA test by pattern [21]. This method is valuable as an accurate, sensitive, and inexpensive screening test. Naturally occurring IgM antibodies induce nonspecific agglutination. This problem has been overcome by use of 2-mercaptoethanol in the serum diluent. The test should only be used for detection of IgG antibodies.

DIAGNOSIS OF SPECIFIC CLINICAL ENTITIES
(see Table 35-1)

Acute acquired toxoplasmosis

A negative dye or IFA test virtually excludes toxoplasma infection in an immunologically normal individual. Acute acquired infection is confirmed by seroconversion from a negative to a positive titer or a two-tube rise from a low to a high titer in sera run in parallel and drawn at 3-week intervals. A single high titer (e.g., dye or IFA test $\geq$ 1:1000) is only suggestive of acute infection [22]. If, in addition, there is a high IgM antibody titer, diagnosis of acute infection is highly probable. A low titer in the double sandwich IgM-ELISA test makes acute infection quite unlikely. In the immunodeficient patient, the above criteria apply, but serodiagnosis may be difficult due to a depressed antibody response. The ELISA technique for detecting toxoplasma antigens may be useful in such cases. Antibody tests may not be valid if performed on sera from patients who have recently received blood transfusions.

Congenital toxoplasma infection

Serological diagnosis of congenital toxoplasma infection is difficult due to the high prevalence in childbearing populations of IgG toxoplasma antibody, which can be passively transferred across the placenta to the infant in the absence of congenital infection [1]. Thus, IgG antibody titers in newborns may merely reflect recent or remote infection in the mother. These antibodies have a serum half-life of 21 days and may persist in the infant for 6 to 12 months after birth. The duration of persistence depends upon the original antibody titer at birth. In the neonate, serodiagnosis is predicated upon finding persistent or rising titers in the dye or IFA tests or finding IgM antibody that can be produced in utero by the infected fetus. The double sandwich IgM-ELISA test is preferred to the IgM-IFA test, since it avoids the false-positive results caused by rheumatoid factor made by the fetus against maternal IgG and the false-negative results due to maternal IgG antibody [18]. If maternal IgM antibody has been transferred to the infant via a placental leak, the IgM titer of the infant will fall markedly over the first week of life due to the short half-life of IgM antibody.

Infants do not produce toxoplasma IgG antibodies until the second or third month of life, or as late as the sixth to ninth month of life if treated for toxoplasma infection. If the toxoplasma IgM antibody titer is negative, a repeat serology for both IgG and IgM antibody should be performed at least at monthly intervals. Tests for IgG antibody are to differentiate between the transferred maternal and infant IgG antibody, and the specific antibody load can be calculated to determine when the infant begins to synthesize toxoplasma antibody [1].

Cerebrospinal fluid should be tested for the presence of IgM antibody. If the cerebrospinal fluid is positive for IgM antibody and the serum is negative for IgM antibody, central nervous system toxoplasma infection is highly probable. The cerebrospinal fluid should also be assayed for toxoplasma antigen if this test is available. Lymphocyte transformation to toxoplasma antigen is both sensitive (85 percent) and specific (100 percent) in congenital infection, but this has only been established for infants older than 2 months of age.

French investigators have pioneered prenatal diagnosis of congenital toxoplasmosis [23]. They were able to diagnose more than 90 percent of congenitally infected fetuses by inoculating mice with amniotic fluid and fetal blood obtained at 20 to 24 weeks of gestation and by using ultrasound to detect enlargement of cerebral ventricles. Use of tissue culture rather than mice should allow more widespread prenatal diagnosis, which permits targeted, aggressive, specific chemotherapy of the mother during gestation and of the infant at birth, and informed decision regarding abortion.

Toxoplasmosis in the immunodeficient patient

Criteria for diagnosis of acute toxoplasmosis in the immunocompetent adult apply to immunodeficient patients but are fre-

quently not met despite active disease. Diagnosis of toxoplasmosis frequently depends upon demonstration of the organism in smears or tissues. A negative toxoplasma IgG antibody titer may be useful for exclusion of toxoplasma as an etiology for clinical disease, but cases of toxoplasmosis have occurred in patients with negative IgG antibody tests. The large majority of patients with toxoplasmic encephalitis have a CT scan that shows nodular or ring enhancement at the time of presentation; magnetic resonance imaging may be more sensitive [5,6]. Since lesions on CT scans may be caused by many different treatable organisms or neoplasms, a specific diagnosis is highly desirable. Interpretation of needle aspirates of toxoplasmic brain abscesses is complicated by false-negative results [13,24], and open biopsy with use of peroxidase-antiperoxidase histological techniques is preferred. The cerebrospinal fluid may be normal in toxoplasmic encephalitis, but more frequently shows a modest mononuclear pleocytosis, elevated protein, and normal glucose titer. An index greater than 1 (demonstrating local formation of antibody in the CNS) calculated by the following formula has proved useful for diagnosis of 70 percent of cases of toxoplasmic encephalitis in one series: Index = [CSF dye test titer (reciprocal) × total serum IgG]/[total CSF IgG × serum dye test titer (reciprocal)] [25].

Ocular toxoplasmosis

Low dye or IFA test titers are common in this entity. Ocular toxoplasmosis is probably excluded if titers are negative in undiluted sera, while it is likely if titers are positive, and the retinal lesions are typical of those described for toxoplasmosis. Because of the high prevalence of toxoplasma antibody in the general population, it is hazardous to assume that retinal lesions atypical of ocular toxoplasmosis are due to toxoplasma infection. High antibody titers in the aqueous humor suggest ocular toxoplasmosis, and an index can be calculated for secure diagnosis [26].

TREATMENT

With the lack of controlled trials and the variable course of toxoplasmosis, treatment regimens are difficult to evaluate. The following guidelines are derived from clinical experience at different medical centers. Immunologically normal patients with the acquired lymphadenopathic form of disease should not be treated unless the symptoms are unusually severe or persistent or visceral involvement is clinically manifest. Infections acquired by laboratory accident or transfusion of blood products should be treated. Immunocompromised patients should always be treated when the infection is diagnosed as acute. In one experience, treatment of immunocompromised patients resulted in improvement in 80 percent of the patients [27]. In AIDS patients with toxoplasmic encephalitis, clinical improvement is seen in about 90 percent of patients, usually within 1 week of the start of treatment, and CT scan lesions improve within 2 to 4 weeks [5,28,29]. At this time there is no indication for treatment of the immunocompromised patient diagnosed as having the chronic infection. Patients with active chorioretinitis due to toxoplasma should receive specific therapy.

Data indicate that treatment of the acutely infected pregnant woman does not eliminate fetal infection but does decrease its incidence by 60 percent [1]. The goal of treating the acutely infected pregnant woman is to prevent passage of toxoplasma from the mother to the fetus. In the early months of pregnancy, there is significant delay in transmission of the organism from the placenta to the fetus. The infant with congenital toxoplasma infection should be treated to prevent further tissue damage, whether or not there is clinical evidence of the infection.

Optimal duration of therapy is not known. In the immunologically normal person with severe disease, treatment for 2 to 4 weeks is recommended. In immunocompromised patients, treatment should be continued for 4 to 6 weeks beyond complete resolution of all signs and symptoms of active disease. When therapy is stopped in AIDS patients with toxoplasmic encephalitis, usually due to drug toxicity, relapse is frequent and usually occurs within 6 weeks. Thus lifelong treatment may be needed [13,28,29]. For congenitally infected infants, the guidelines of Desmonts and Couvreur are presented in Table 35-2. If spiramycin[1] is not available, treatment for 1 year

[1]This drug has not been approved by the U.S. Food and Drug Administration at the time of publication.

with pyrimethamine and sulfadiazine is recommended. Controlled studies have not been conducted to evaluate the role of corticosteroids, the length of the total treatment course or the individual treatment course, the matching of indications for treatment with the specific regimens, or therapeutic efficacy. For the pregnant woman with acute toxoplasma infection, two different regimens have proved efficacious. Spiramycin, 3 g each day given as three or four divided doses, can be given throughout pregnancy. After the first trimester, pyrimethamine and sulfadiazine can be used. Pyrimethamine should not be used in the first trimester because it is teratogenic in laboratory animals. Variations of these regimens have been used with apparent success [23].

For active ocular toxoplasmosis, pyrimethamine and sulfadiazine are administered for 1 month. Within 10 days, the borders of the retinal lesions should sharpen and the vitreous haze should disappear. A favorable clinical response is seen in 60 to 70 percent of cases. If response is unfavorable, repeated courses of pyrimethamine and sulfadiazine are needed. Systemic corticosteroids are administered if vision is endangered by lesions involving the macula, optic nerve head, or papillomacular bundle. Photocoagulation has been used to treat active lesions and to provide prophylaxis against spread of lesions, since the majority of new lesions appear contiguous to old lesions. Occasionally, vitrectomy and lensectomy may be necessary to restore visual acuity.

Table 35-2. Guidelines for the treatment of congenital toxoplasmosis*

Drugs

1. Pyrimethamine + sulfadiazine: 21-day course.
   a. Pyrimethamine: 1 mg/(kg·day), oral route. (Since the half-life of the drug is 4 to 5 days, the dose can be given every 2 to 3 or even 4 days.)
   b. Sulfadiazine: 50 to 100 mg/(kg·day), oral route in two daily divided doses.
2. Spiramycin†: 30- to 45-day course. 100 mg/(kg·day), oral route in two daily divided doses.
3. Corticosteroids (prednisone or methylprednisolone): 1 to 2 mg/(kg·day), oral route in two divided doses. Continued until the inflammatory process (e.g., high cerebrospinal fluid protein, chorioretinitis) has subsided; dosage then to be tapered progressively to nothing.
4. Folinic acid: 5 mg twice weekly during pyrimethamine treatment.

Indications

1. Overt congenital toxoplasmosis: Pyrimethamine + sulfadiazine: 21 days. Folinic acid to be given as soon as possible. During the first year of life, the child is given 3 to 4 courses of pyrimethamine + sulfadiazine, separated with spiramycin courses of 30 to 45 days. No treatment is usually given after 12 months of age.
2. Overt congenital toxoplasmosis with evidence of inflammatory process (chorioretinitis, high cerebrospinal fluid protein content, generalized infection, jaundice): As in no. 1 above + corticosteroid treatment.
3. Subclinical congenital toxoplasma infection: As in no. 1 above.
4. Healthy newborn in whom serology testing has not provided definitive results but definite maternal infection was acquired during pregnancy: 1 course of pyrimethamine + sulfadiazine for 21 days, followed by spiramycin. Then wait for laboratory evidence for the diagnosis.
5. Healthy newborn born to a mother with high dye-test titer—date of maternal infection undetermined. Spiramycin alone, until laboratory evidence for the diagnosis is definitive. It must be borne in mind that in certain cases the indication for treatment is difficult to define due to the lack of information about the pregnancy and lack of isolation attempts from the corresponding placenta.

*Recommendations of Dr. Jacques Couvreur, Laboratoire de Serologie Neonatale et de Recherche sur la Toxoplasmose, Institut de Puericulture, Paris.
†Not presently available in the United States, but can be obtained in Europe, Canada, and Mexico.

Drugs

Pyrimethamine, sulfadiazine (or trisulfapyrimidine), and spiramycin are the most useful drugs for treating toxoplasma infection [1]. Pyrimethamine is a folic acid antagonist, and folinic acid (6 to 10 mg/day, or up to 50 mg/day for AIDS patients; oral or parenteral) should be added to the regimen, and peripheral blood counts should be checked twice weekly.

Sulfadiazine and trisulfapyrimidines (sulfapyrazine, sulfamethazine, and sulfamerazine) are equally effective. Other commonly used sulfonamides are not as active. The combination of pyrimethamine and sulfadiazine (or trisulfapyrimidine) acts synergistically against toxoplasma. Their combined use is always recommended except in the first trimester, when pyrimethamine is contraindicated due to teratogenic effects demonstrated in laboratory animals. Spiramycin is a macrolide antibiotic which is administered by the oral route. It has been used in the treatment of infected pregnant women and infants with the congenital infection. The activity of the combination of trimethoprim and sulfamethoxazole is significantly less than that of the pyrimethamine and sulfonamide combination, and its efficacy in human cases has not been proven [30]. AIDS patients have developed toxoplasmic encephalitis while receiving spiramycin or trimethoprim-sulfamethoxazole. Thus, neither drug is recommended for treatment of toxoplasmosis in immunodeficient patients.

The loading doses for pyrimethamine differ according to the age of the patient. In adults it is 200 mg given in two divided doses on the first day only; in children it is 2 mg/kg for the first 2 to 3 days; in infants it is 1 mg/kg. For immunocompetent patients, pyrimethamine is usually given at a dosage of 25 to 50 mg/day, although administration at 2- to 4-day intervals has been suggested in view of its 4- to 5-day half-life. Pyrimethamine has been used at 25 mg qod to treat the acute infection acquired during pregnancy. For ocular toxoplasmosis, pyrimethamine at doses up to 50 mg/day is used. For immunodeficient patients, pyrimethamine is given for a minimum of 4 to 6 weeks at 25 to 50 mg/day. For AIDS patients, 75 to 100 mg/day is being used routinely for 3 to 6 weeks and then maintenance therapy is used. Optimal maintenance therapy for AIDS patients has not yet been determined. At present, 50 mg of pyrimethamine daily plus 2 g of sulfa daily, or Fansidar two tablets once weekly are being used. Pyrimethamine and sulfa can be used at the above doses three times weekly if compliance is not a problem.

The loading dose of sulfonamides for older children and adults is 50 to 75 mg/kg (oral or parenteral) followed by 75 to 100 mg/(kg·day) divided into four doses. The maintenance dose of sulfadiazine for AIDS patients is 500 mg by mouth every 6 h. The loading dose for infants is 50 to 100 mg/kg followed by a maintenance dose of 100 to 150 mg/kg divided into two to four doses daily.

Toxicity due to the combination of pyrimethamine and sulfadiazine is common, particularly in AIDS patients, of whom half require discontinuation of treatment due to toxicity [28,29]. Toxicity is usually either bone marrow suppression or skin rash, the latter attributed to the sulfonamide. Desensitization to sulfa has been reported to be successful [31]. Alternatively, clindamycin (1200 to 4800 mg parenterally or intravenously) has been used successfully [32,33]. A macrolide, roxithromycin, and a folic acid antagonist, trimetrexate, are active against toxoplasma in vivo and may be available in the near future. γ Interferon is also active in vivo and is synergistic with roxithromycin against toxoplasma in mice. Spiramycin is given by mouth in a dose of 3 g/day in three to four doses.

PREVENTION

Prevention is most important in seronegative pregnant women and immunodeficient patients. The goal is to avoid ingestion of tissue cysts or sporulated oocysts. Tissue cysts are rendered noninfectious by heating meat to 66°C or by smoking or curing. Freezing is less reliable and requires a −20°C temperature which is not attained by most home freezers. Hands should be washed thoroughly after handling meat, and eggs should not be eaten raw.

Cat feces should be avoided altogether. If this proves impossible, disposable gloves should be worn while disposing of cat litter material, working in the garden, or cleaning a child's sandbox. Oocysts are killed if the cat's litter pan is treated with nearly boiling water for 5 minutes. Vectors such as filth flies and cockroaches should be controlled, and fruits and vegetables should be carefully washed. Serological testing of cats is of no value since it does not detect the acutely infected cat that passes oocysts.

Transmission of toxoplasma by transfusion of leukocyte-rich blood products or by organ transplantation to immunosuppressed patients poses a real danger. It may occur frequently enough to warrant toxoplasma antibody screening for blood product donors and possibly to exclude seropositive people as organ donors to toxoplasma antibody–negative organ recipients.

Serological screening of pregnant women is performed by law in France and Austria. Whether this should be performed in all countries is controversial and would depend upon the epidemiology of the infection in a given country, the cost of such a program, its cost-effectiveness, and its feasibility. We have recommended that a serological test equal in sensitivity, specificity, and reproducibility to the Sabin-Feldman dye test (e.g., IFA or agglutination test) be performed in all pregnant women as early as possible, but at least by 10 to 12 weeks' gestation [34]. Testing of women prior to pregnancy would identify those at risk. Those pregnant women who are seronegative initially should then be tested again within 20 to 22 weeks to allow sufficient time for prenatal diagnosis (see "Diagnosis," above), a decision on possible therapeutic abortion, or initiation of treatment. A third test would be performed near or at term to detect all women who acquire primary infection during pregnancy, so that they and their offspring could be identified and appropriately managed. A woman whose serum is positive upon initial testing would have a test for IgM antibodies performed on the same serum to detect recent infection. If the IgM antibody test were positive or clinical signs suggestive of acute toxoplasmosis were present, a follow-up IgG-IFA or comparable test would be performed to attempt to demonstrate a significant rise in titer. In patients with a positive IgG-IFA test of any titer, a negative IgM antibody test in the first trimester, and no clinical signs of acute toxoplasmosis, no further testing would be performed since the probability of these women being acutely infected is low. Because the risk of transmission of the infection to the fetus is low (approximately 15 percent) in the first trimester and because the incidence of congenital toxoplasmosis can be reduced significantly by antepartum therapy, some authorities recommend treatment rather than therapeutic abortion, reasoning that this would result in a significant number of healthy fetuses. The decision about mode of therapy ultimately must be made with a well-informed pregnant patient who is aware of the risks discussed above. There are no carefully controlled studies to support the contention that a pregnant woman who has toxoplasma antibody and a history of habitual abortion will benefit from treatment.

POPULATION

EPIDEMIOLOGY

Toxoplasma is found in herbivorous, carnivorous, and omnivorous animals, including all mammals throughout the world. The high prevalence of the organism in meat and the fact that oocysts have been found in the feces of approximately 1 percent of cats in diverse parts of the world, including Costa Rica, Japan, and the United States, account for its frequency in nature. Though it is possible that toxoplasma can be perpetuated in nature in the absence of cats (carnivorism, transplacental transmission), felids are primarily responsible for transmission of toxoplasma infection in most parts of the world, particularly in areas where only well-cooked meat is consumed.

A large body of data is available on the prevalence of toxoplasma antibody in many different geographical locations and in different societies within a given location. In general, prevalence is less in cold regions, hot or arid areas, and at high elevations. Many exceptions to these generalizations occur. In France, the prevalence of toxoplasma antibody is very high. Witu, an island in New Guinea without cats, has a prevalence of 7 percent. Human populations on three atolls within 80 miles of each other in Micronesia have markedly different prevalences of antibody. Although there has been much speculation, the causes of these disparities have not been elucidated.

Serological evidence of infection increases with age and reaches 90 percent in some societies by the fourth decade. At present, no consistent correlation has been noted between an-

tibody and sex or occupation, although slaughterhouse workers may be at higher risk of acquiring the infection. Outbreaks within families and other closed groups have been reported frequently [35]. Many of those with the acute infection were asymptomatic in these outbreaks.

Of importance is the prevalence of antibody in pregnant women. Populations with widely different prevalences of positive antibody may have similar incidences of congenital toxoplasmosis. The reason for this is that a population with high prevalence of antibody contains a small group of pregnant women at high risk for acquiring infection during pregnancy, while the group of pregnant women from a population with a low prevalence of antibody is larger but at a lower risk of acquiring infection during pregnancy. Reported incidence figures for congenital toxoplasmosis tend to support this; the rate is 2 per 1000 live births in Mexico City, 1.3 in New York City, 3 in Paris, and 6.5 in the Netherlands [1]. More recent figures are 0.12 cases of congenital toxoplasma infection per 1000 live births in Birmingham, Alabama; 1 in Basel, Switzerland; 2 in Melbourne, Australia; and 2 in Brussels, Belgium. The postulated seroconversion rate among women of childbearing age in the United States is approximately 0.8 percent per year., One would anticipate from this figure that of every 1000 pregnant women in the United States, 6 will acquire primary infection with toxoplasma during a 9-month gestation. In Oregon, where approximately 8 percent of pregnant women have a positive antibody test, it has been estimated that 1 of every 200 pregnancies is associated with a primary infection [36]. In this age of increased travel, a population moving from an area of low infection prevalence to an area with a higher prevalence may be at special risk, such as immigrants to France or missionaries to South America.

REFERENCES

1 Remington JS, Desmonts G: Toxoplasmosis, in Remington JS, Klein JO (eds): *Infectious Disease of the Fetus and Newborn Infant*, 2d ed. Philadelphia, Saunders, 1983, pp 143–263

2 O'Connor GR: The influence of hypersensitivity on the pathogenesis of ocular toxoplasmosis. Trans Am Ophthalmol Soc 68: 501–47, 1970

3 Dorfman RF, Remington JS: Value of lymph-node biopsy in the diagnosis of acute acquired toxoplasmosis. N Engl J Med 289: 878–81, 1973

4 Frenkel JK: Pathology and pathogenesis of congenital toxoplasmosis. Bull NY Acad Med 50:182–91, 1974

5 Post MJ, Kursunoglu SJ, Hensley GT, et al: Cranial CT in acquired immunodeficiency syndrome: Spectrum of diseases and optimal contrast enhancement technique. AJR 145:929–40, 1985

6 Zee CS, Segall HD, Rogers C, et al. MR imaging of cerebral toxoplasmosis: correlation of computed tomography and pathology. J Comput Assist Tomogr 9:797–99, 1985

7 McCabe RE, Brooks RG, Dorfman RF, Remington JS. Clinical spectrum in 107 cases of toxoplasmic lymphadenopathy. Rev Infect Dis 9:754–74, 1987

8 Couvreur J, Desmonts G, Tournier G, et al: Étude d'une série homogène de 210 cas de toxoplasmose congénitale chez des nourissons agés de 0 à 11 mois et dépistés de façon prospective. Ann Pediatr 31:815, 1984

9 Wilson CB, Remington JS, Stagno S, et al: Development of adverse sequelae in children born with subclinical congenital toxoplasma infection. Pediatrics 66:767–74, 1980

10 Koch FLP, Wolf A, Cowen D, et al: Toxoplasmic encephalomyelitis. VII. Significance of ocular lesions in the diagnosis of infantile or congenital toxoplasmosis. Arch Ophthalmol 29:1–25, 1943

11 Luft BJ, Brooks RG, Conley FK, et al: Toxoplasmic encephalitis in patients with acquired immune deficiency syndrome. JAMA 252:913–17, 1984

12 Wong B, Gold JWM, Brown AE, et al: Central-nervous-system toxoplasmosis in homosexual men and parenteral drug abusers. Ann Intern Med 100:36–42, 1984

13 Luft BJ, Remington JS: Toxoplasmic encephalitis. J Infect Dis 157:1–6, 1988

14 Luft BJ, Naot Y, Araujo FG, et al: Primary and reactivated toxoplasma infection in patients with cardiac transplants: Clinical spectrum and problems in diagnosis in a defined population. Ann Intern Med 99:27–31, 1983

15 Conley FK, Jenkins HT, Remington JS: *Toxoplasma gondii* infection of the central nervous system: Use of the peroxidase-antiperoxidase method to demonstrate toxoplasma in formalin-fixed, paraffin-embedded tissue sections. Hum Pathol 12:690–698, 1981

16 Sabin AB, Feldman HA: Dyes as microchemical indicators of a new immunity phenomenon affecting a protozoon parasite (toxoplasma). Science 108:660–663, 1948

17 Walton BC, Benchoff BM, Brooks WH: Comparison of the indirect fluorescent antibody test and methylene blue dye test for detection of antibodies to *Toxoplasma gondii*. Am J Trop Med Hyg 15:149–152, 1966

18 Naot Y, Desmonts G, Remington JS: IgM enzyme-linked immunosorbent assay test for the diagnosis of congenital Toxoplasma infection. J Pediatr 98:32–36, 1981

19 Naot Y, Remington JS: An enzyme-linked immunosorbent assay for detection of IgM antibodies to *Toxoplasma gondii*: Use for diagnosis of acute acquired toxoplasmosis. J Infect Dis 142:757–766, 1980.

20 Welch PC, Masur H, Jones TC, et al: Serologic diagnosis of acute lymphadenopathic toxoplasmosis. J Infect Dis 142:256–64, 1980

21 Desmonts G, Remington JS: Direct agglutination test for diagnosis of toxoplasma infection: Method for increasing sensitivitiy and specificity. J Clin Microbiol 11:562–568, 1980

22 Brooks RG, McCabe RE, Remington JS: Role of serology in the diagnosis of toxoplasmic lymphadenopathy. Rev Infect Dis 9:1055–1062, 1987

23 Daffos F, Forestier F, Capella-Pavlovsky M, et al: Prenatal management of 746 pregnancies at risk of congenital toxoplasmosis. N Engl J Med 318:271–75, 1988

24 Wanke C, Tuazon CU, Kovacs A, et al: Toxoplasma encephalitis in patients with acquired immune deficiency syndrome: Diagnosis and response to therapy. Am J Trop Med Hyg 36:509–16, 1987

25 Potasman I, Resnick L, Luft BJ, et al: Intrathecal production of antibodies against *Toxoplasma gondii* in patients with toxoplasmic encephalitis and the acquired immunodeficiency syndrome (AIDS). Ann Intern Med 108:49–51, 1988

26 Desmonts G: Definitive serological diagnosis of ocular toxoplasmosis. Arch Ophthalmol 76:839–851, 1966

27 Carey RM, Kimball AC, Armstrong D, et al: Toxoplasmosis: Clinical experiences in a cancer hospital. Am J Med 54:30–38, 1973

28 Haverkos HW: Assessment of therapy for toxoplasma encephalitis: The TE study group. Am J Med 82:907–914, 1987

29 LePort C, Raffi F, Matheron S, et al: Treatment of central nervous system toxoplasmosis with pyrimethamine/sulfadiazine combination in 35 patients with acquired immunodeficiency syndrome: Efficacy of long-term continuous therapy. Am J Med 84:94–100, 1988

30 Grossman PL, Remington JS: The effect of trimethoprim and sulfamethoxazole on *Toxoplasma gondii* in vitro and in vivo. Am J Trop Med Hyg 28:445–55, 1979

31 Smith RM, Iwamoto GK, Richerson HB, et al: Trimethoprim-sulfamethoxazole desensitization in the acquired immunodeficiency syndrome. Ann Intern Med 106:335, 1987

32 Rolston KVI, Hoy J: Role of clindamycin in the treatment of central nervous system toxoplasmosis. Am J Med 83:551–554, 1987

33 Danneman BR, Israelski DM, Remington JS: Treatment of toxoplasmic encephalitis with intravenous clindamycin. Arch Intern Med 148:2477–2482, 1988

34 Wilson CB, Remington JS: What can be done to prevent congenital toxoplasmosis? Am J Obstet Gynecol 138:357–363, 1980

35 Luft BJ, Remington JS: Acute toxoplasma infection among family members of patients with acute lymphadenopathic toxoplasmosis. Arch Intern Med 144:53–56, 1984

36 Beach PG: Prevalence of antibodies to *Toxoplasma gondii* in pregnant women in Oregon. J Infect Dis 140:780–783, 1979

37 Desmonts G, Remington JS: Direct agglutination test for diagnosis of Toxoplasma infection: Method for increasing sensitivitiy and specificity. J Clin Microbiol 11:562–568, 1980

38 Siegel JP, Remington JS: A comparison of methods for quantitating antigen-specific IgM antibody using a reverse enzyme-linked immunosorbent assay. J Clin Microbiol 18:63–70, 1983

Primary Amebic Meningoencephalitis

· Richard J. Duma

Primary amebic meningoencephalitis (PAM) is an infection of the central nervous system (CNS) produced by free-living amoebas (FLA) of the genera *Naegleria* and *Acanthamoeba*. It may be *acute, subacute,* or *chronic,* is usually fatal, and is to be distinguished from secondary CNS infections due to *Entamoeba histolytica* [1].

Since the first report by Fowler and Carter in 1965 [2], over 125 cases have occurred worldwide (Fig. 36-1), occasionally in epidemics. However, the true incidence of the disease and whether or not infections may be subclinical are both unknown.

PARASITE

The responsible organisms are *N. fowleri* and species of *Acanthamoeba,* most notably *A. culbertsoni, A. castellanii, A. polyphagia, A. astronyxis,* and *A. rhysodes.* However, several as yet unidentified FLA also produce the disease, but they probably account for only a small percentage of cases.

ECOLOGY, MORPHOLOGY, AND IDENTIFICATION

Pathogenic and nonpathogenic FLA exist widely in nature, particularly in soil and in thermally enriched fresh or brackish waters. They also may be isolated occasionally from the oropharynxes of normal individuals. No animal reservoir is known to exist, though a variety of natural infections of terrestrial and marine animals occur.

FLA are classified according to morphology, motility, mitotic division patterns, and biochemical and immunological characteristics. The classification most useful to the clinician is the one suggested by Page [3].

Naegleria and *Acanthamoeba* vary considerably in size, ranging from 7 to 20 μm. *Naegleria* are generally limax (slug-like) in shape and exist in three forms—trophozoite, cyst, and flagellate; *Acanthamoeba* have characteristic filose pseudopodia and exist in only two forms—trophozoite and cyst (Fig. 36-2). Both amoebas have a single contractile vacuole and may contain ingested red blood cells. Their morphology in the natural state differs from that seen in fixed preparations, as fixation causes rounding up and distortion. The identifying hallmark of FLA is the nucleus, which can be readily seen in the cyst and trophozoite and, with *Naegleria,* even in the flagellate form. It is singular, and consists of a large, dark central karyosome surrounded by a clear halo and a fine nuclear rim.

Cysts of *Naegleria* and *Acanthamoeba* can be readily distinguished from one another, as *Naegleria* are round and double-walled and contain several pores through which excystation occurs; while *Acanthamoeba* are stellate, possess an exocyst as well as an endocyst, and contain opercula for excystation. In diseased tissues or clinical specimens infected by *Acanthamoeba,* cysts may be found; however, they are not found in infections due to *Naegleria.*

Naegleria may be suspected by identifying a flagellate stage,

Figure 36-1. Worldwide distribution of PAM due to all species of free-living amoebas as of January 1982.

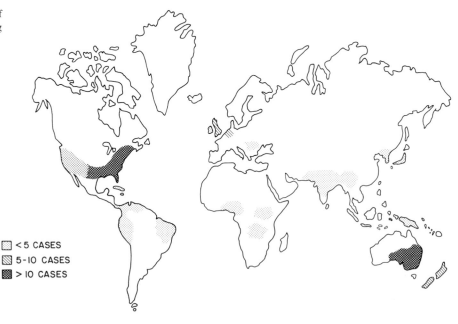

□ <5 CASES
▨ 5-10 CASES
■ >10 CASES

ENTAMOEBA HISTOLYTICA | ACANTHAMOEBA CASTELLANII

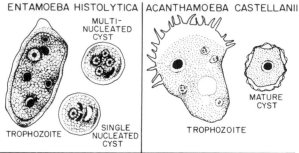

NAEGLERIA FOWLERI

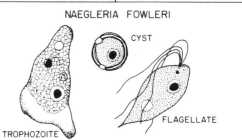

Figure 36-2. Drawings of *Entamoeba histolytica, Acanthamoeba castellanii,* and *Naegleria fowleri.* Note large, centrally located karyosomes and fine nuclear rims of the free-living amoebas compared with the tiny karyosome and chromatin collections about the nuclear rim of *E. histolytica.*

which can be induced by placing the flagellates in distilled water. Flagellates appear as elliptical, uninuclear, highly motile cells, containing a single contractile vacuole and 4 to 6 flagellae on their anterior ends. Flagellates are not found in infected tissues, secretions, or body fluids.

The most effective stain for morphological differentiation of such amoebas is iron hematoxylin, although they are seen readily with hematoxylin and eosin (H&E). Cysts are most easily stained with Gomori's methenamine silver. Electron microscopy may be of aid in distinguishing FLA from *E. histolytica,* as mitochondria are present in the former but not in the latter; however, ultrastructural interspecies differences within genera of free-living amoebas are difficult to discern.

Immunological differences between genera and species exist, so that species-specific antisera may be utilized for identification purposes. However, immunological methods are not reliable in distinguishing pathogenic from nonpathogenic strains.

Fluorescent-labeled antibody stains are often employed in detecting amoebas, especially in tissues suspected of being infected. Similarly, specific indirect immunoenzymatic (peroxidase) staining also is used successfully, even in formalin-fixed paraffin sections. Lysates of amoebas may be studied with immunodiffusion and with isoelectric focusing, in which immunologically distinct bands and isoenzyme patterns, respectively, are identified for each species.

BIOCHEMISTRY AND PHYSIOLOGY

FLA are highly aerobic. *Naegleria* are destroyed by $\leq 0.5\%$ NaCl and grow within narrow pH limits, ideally at pH 6.5. On the other hand, *Acanthamoeba* survive readily in solutions of NaCl, some being isolated from ocean waters containing up to 30 ppt salinity [4].

The optimal growth temperatures for these amoebas vary. Pathogenic *Naegleria* grow best at 37°C but also at 44°C, the latter temperature being used to isolate pathogenic strains. *Acanthamoeba* grow best at 33°C, but some grow at 44°C.

Axenic growth of both pathogenic *Naegleria* and *Acanthamoeba* may be obtained in defined liquid media. For *Naegleria,* hemin and L-methionine appear to be essential nutrients. Chang's medium [5], containing casein yeast and liver extract supplemented with calf serum, is especially useful for pathogenic *Naegleria.* Neff's medium, supplemented with Page's saline, is generally used for culture of *Acanthamoeba.* In such media mean generation times range from 5 to 14 h. With repeated in vitro subculturing, *Naegleria* may lose its pathogenicity, but it may be regained by passage in mice.

Both *Naegleria* and *Acanthamoeba* grow readily on plain 2.5% agar seeded with Enterobacteriaceae (monoxenic cultures). When FLA are inoculated onto such plates, plaques develop, much like those seen in phage typing. FLA may also be cultured on a variety of tissue culture cell lines, i.e., monkey kidney (MK), African green monkey, Vero, and HeLa. Growth rates and cytopathic effects (CPE) may be utilized to identify some amoebas. The value of utilizing CPA for characterizing a strain as pathogenic may be limited, as *N. gruberi,* a nonpathogen, readily infects rat neuroblastoma cell lines [6].

Trophozoites of both *Naegleria* and *Acanthamoeba* are extremely sensitive to drying and freezing. Room temperature (23°C) is recommended for storage or handling of all specimens containing these amoebas.

The membranes of pathogenic amoebas have not been extensively studied, but *Naegleria* contain ergosterol, which probably explains their susceptibility to the polyene antibiotic amphotericin B. On the other hand, membranes of *Acanthamoeba* (Neff) contain 60% 7-dehydrostigmasterol, 40% ergosterol, and a unique lipophosphoroglycan; yet they are highly resistant to amphotericin B.

ANIMAL MODELS AND INTERMEDIATE HOSTS

Naegleria and *Acanthamoeba* appear capable of producing PAM in virtually any animal species. Since mice are exquisitely sensitive to *Naegleria* ($LD_{50} = 10^4$ intranasally instilled trophozoites), this animal is used for studying PAM. However, the LD_{50} will vary with the age, stage of growth, virulence, and inoculum size of the trophozoites, as well as with the age and immune status of the mice.

No intermediate hosts or animal reservoirs appear to exist. However, a variety of terrestrial animals (dogs, beavers, buffalo, and bulls) besides humans and many marine animals (fish, freshwater mollusks, mussels, sea anemones, and crabs) may acquire natural infections.

PATIENT

N. fowleri results exclusively in acute PAM. However, on *rare* occasions the organism may be isolated from the noses of healthy humans. On the other hand, *Acanthamoebae* often produce acute, subacute, or chronic PAM and frequently are cultured from the noses and throats of healthy people and people with upper respiratory tract infections. In immunodeficient patients they can be "opportunistic" (see Table 36-1).

PORTAL OF ENTRY, PATHOLOGY, AND PATHOGENESIS

For *Naegleria* the major portal of entry is the nose, with invasion of the olfactory neuroepithelium. Spread to the CNS is

via the fila olfactoria. *Acanthamoeba* may also invade along this route, but they usually infect other areas of the body first (e.g., eye, lung, skin, uterus), and secondarily invade the CNS via hematogenous spread. Against *Naegleria,* polymorphonuclear leukocytes are the most important cells in host defense, while in subacute and chronic infections due to *Acanthamoeba,* lymphocytes and macrophages are vital. In acute PAM hemorrhagic necrosis of cerebral matter occurs, while in the subacute or chronic form, granuloma formation with giant cells and vasculitis is seen.

Naegleria initially invade the superficial gray and later the deep white matter and cerebellum. The olfactory and frontotemporal regions are prominently involved. A wake of hemorrhage and necrosis follows advancing amoebas. Trophozoites are readily seen in diseased tissues, especially in perivascular spaces, where they invade vessels and avidly consume red blood cells (Fig. 36-3). The spinal cord is rarely involved, but when it is, demyelinization may be present. The subarachnoid

Table 36-1. Differential features of various forms of primary amebic meningoencephalitis

Factors	Acute	Subacute or chronic
Responsible organism	*N. fowleri* (occasionally *Acanthamoeba*)	*Acanthamoeba* spp.
Age	Child or young adult	Any age
Sex	Males 3:2	Males 5:1
Health	Good	Often immunodeficient or chronically debilitated
Incubation period	3–7 days	Unknown
Portal of entry	Nose	Extracerebral (e.g., eye, skin, lung, prostate, etc.)
Route of invasion of CNS	Fila olfactoria	Hematogenous
Clinical picture	Resembles acute bacterial meningitis	Resembles brain abscess
Course	Fatal in 48–72 h if untreated	Fatal in 2–3 weeks
Pathology	Diffuse necrotizing, hemorrhagic necrosis with neutrophilic response	Granulomatous encephalitis and single or multiple abscesses
Location	Typically olfactory, frontal, and cerebellar; involves gray matter	Deep midline and midbrain structures; involves principally white matter
CSF studies	Predominantly PMNs and low sugar	Predominantly round cells and normal or low-normal sugar
Diagnostic studies	Amoebas seen in CSF on direct observation; culture of CSF for amoebas useful; serology not helpful	Amoebas not seen or cultured from CSF; brain biopsy of involved area may be definitive; serology useful
Forms present	Trophozoites	Trophozoites and cysts
Treatment	Amphotericin B; may add rifampin, tetracycline, or minocycline; imidazoles possibly helpful, but also antagonistic to amphotericin B	Surgery; no satisfactory chemotherapy available

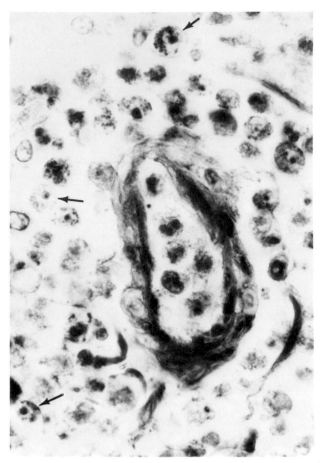

Figure 36-3. *Naegleria* surrounding a small blood vessel within the brain. The extravascular space is filled with amoebas (arrows point to several), some of which are undergoing degeneration (H&E × 1000). Note the single, large centrally located karyosomes surrounded by clear halos (see text).

in central tissues but infrequently in the subarachnoid space. Cysts may also be present.

The pathogenesis of free-living amoebas is poorly understood, but both *N. fowleri* and *Acanthamoeba* possess phospholipases, which may aid in their ability to invade brain substance. Nevertheless, ingestion appears to be the main mechanism through which amoebas destroy other cells. Myocarditis in the absence of amoebas suggests that cellular toxins may be released by some organisms.

CLINICAL MANIFESTATIONS AND DIAGNOSIS

The onset of acute PAM due to either *Naegleria* or *Acanthamoeba* is similar to acute bacterial meningitis. The patient experiences sudden onset of a severe, unrelenting, bifrontal headache associated with fever, nausea, and vomiting. The neck is stiff. Seizures, confusion, and coma may occur. Focal signs, such as paralysis, appear early and persist. Olfactory involvement may be suspected if a history of abnormal patterns of taste or smell is given. The course of acute PAM is one of rapid deterioration and death after 48 to 72 h. Pulmonary congestion, heart failure (probably due to myocarditis), and brainstem herniation are the usual causes of death.

The CSF in acute PAM contains a preponderance of neutrophils (usually 95 percent), low sugar (usually < 10 mg/dL), moderate to high protein, and commonly red blood cells (Table 36-2). If *Naegleria* is the responsible agent, highly motile trophozoites are present. Cultures of the CSF for bacteria, viruses, and fungi are invariably negative.

The onset of *subacute* or *chronic* PAM due to *Acanthamoeba* may be insidious (Table 36-1). Immunodeficient or chronically ill people are often affected, but otherwise healthy people are also reported. The clinical picture is consistent with brain abscess. Headache is prominent, and focal seizures are common. Signs of meningeal irritation occur but are overshadowed by signs of multifocal, deep cortical involvement. Brain scanning

space is invaded early, and a prominent (95 percent) neutrophilic pleocytosis occurs, resembling that seen with bacterial meningitis. Rarely *Naegleria* may disseminate [7]. Also, diffuse myocarditis in the absence of amoebas may occur, often resulting in death.

Acanthamoeba, in addition to producing a clinicopathological picture indistinguishable from that due to *Naegleria,* usually produce a clinical and pathological syndrome of subacute or chronic encephalitis or multiple brain abscesses. Multiple involvement of the midline, deep structures and bilateral frontotemporal areas occurs, suggesting hematogenous spread from a distant focus. In subacute or chronic PAM, unlike that due to *Naegleria,* olfactory areas are spared, and the histopathological picture consists of a preponderance of monocytes, plasma cells, and giant cells. Trophozoites are readily found

Table 36-2. CSF findings in free-living amebic infections of the CNS

	Acute PAM due to *Naegleria*	**Subacute and chronic PAM due to *Acanthamoeba***
Opening pressure	Elevated	Elevated
Protein	Moderately elevated	Moderately elevated
Sugar	Usually low	Normal to low-normal
WBC	Elevated (sometimes up to 10,000)	Low to moderately elevated (usually < 500)
PMN	90–95%	< 70% (round cells often predominate)
Amoebas	Present	Absent

*Occasionally *Acanthamoeba* may produce acute PAM. In such an instance CSF findings may be similar to those produced by *Naegleria* except that amoebas may not be seen.

by computed tomography (CT) may be useful but is not specific. The course of subacute or chronic PAM is one of steady deterioration, with death occurring usually 2 to 3 weeks after onset.

Examination of the CSF is seldom of value diagnostically in subacute or chronic PAM, except to confirm the presence of meningitis (Table 36-2). A preponderance of monocytes occurs. The cellular exudate consists of a preponderance of monocytes. The CSF sugar is normal or slightly low (about 20 to 30 mg/dL), the protein is slightly high, and amoebas are not generally seen in the fluid.

In *Naegleria* infections of the CNS, the diagnosis may be readily made from examination and culture of the CSF (see above). Trophozoites with characteristic limaciform motility are present. Serological tests are of no value because the illness is too brief. In instances in which the diagnosis is sought at autopsy, fluorescent- or immunoperoxidase-tagged antibody stains are useful.

In infections due to *Acanthamoeba,* serological tests are valuable because the course of illness may last several weeks and because *Acanthamoeba* cannot be seen or isolated from the CSF. A variety of serological techniques are employed: motility inhibition, agglutination, precipitation, and indirect fluorescent antibody assays. Diagnosis may also be made by brain biopsy, in which case cultured brain tissue may be positive for organisms.

ADDITIONAL DISEASES

No infection other than PAM is produced by *Naegleria*. However, *Acanthamoeba* may infect the eye and respiratory passages. Many serious ocular infections, usually corneal ulcers, have been reported, mostly from Britain and the United States. Such infections are commonly preceded by local trauma or are associated with soft contact lenses. Corneal ulcers first appear as shaggy, irregular lesions, which may be mistaken for herpes. Subsequently, a characteristic 360° or paracentral stromal ring infiltrate with recurrent epithelial breakdown appears. The diagnosis is usually made from histological studies and cultures of scrapings. Satisfactory therapy is not available, and destruction of the cornea often occurs. Often a penetrating keratoplasty or corneal transplant is necessary. The source of *Acanthamoeba* is believed to be contaminated soil and/or water instilled at the time of trauma or insertion of the contact lens. Amoebas may disseminate from this site to the CNS to produce PAM.

Acanthamoeba infections of the respiratory system may also occur. In England in 1968, a cytopathic agent provisionally called the "Ryan virus" but subsequently identified as *A. castellanii* was isolated with swabs of the upper respiratory tract from patients with fever and influenza-like symptoms [8]. In Czechoslovakia, a statistically significant relationship between the presence of *Acanthamoeba* in people's nasal cavities and upper respiratory tract symptoms was demonstrated [9].

MANAGEMENT

Only three survivors of acute PAM due to *Naegleria* are reported; none is reported for any form of well-documented PAM due to *Acanthamoeba*.

For PAM due to *N. fowleri* the most effective therapeutic agent is amphotericin B, most organisms being killed in vitro in 6 h or less by ≤ 0.75 μg/mL [10]. Imidazoles are also effective, but much less so and unpredictably. Rifampin, tetracycline, or minocycline may also be used, but their value is questionable. Amphotericin B is given intravenously in progressively increasing doses. However, a dose of 1 mg per kilogram of body weight per day should be reached by the second day of therapy. Supplemental intrathecal, intracisternal, and intraventricular injections may be used, but because of brain edema and increased intracranial pressure associated with the disease, such injections may be hazardous. Imidazoles if added may be antagonistic to amphotericin B, since they interfere with sterol synthesis. Nevertheless, in one surviving case of well-established PAM due to *N. fowleri,* combined therapy with miconazole and amphotericin B was effective; and the responsible strain of amoeba was thought to be inhibited in vitro by both agents [11]. Therapy should be continued at least 10 days in uncomplicated cases.

None of the standard agents used to treat amebiasis is effective against FLA. Emetine should especially be avoided because of its myocardial toxicity.

No satisfactory therapy exists for infections due to *Acanthamoeba*. However, since the chronic form frequently presents as a brain abscess or abscesses, surgery may be useful; nevertheless, since multiple abscesses frequently occur, the value of surgery may be limited. Flucytosine (5-fluorocytosine) is suggested as possibly useful, but it does not appear to be effective against all strains of *Acanthamoeba* (particularly pathogenic ones), resistance develops easily, and it must be given orally. Polymyxin B is another potentially useful agent, but it has yet to be employed. In vitro tests suggest it may act synergistically when combined with flucytosine and it is well tolerated intrathecally. Sulfas are also suggested, since they prevent infections in therapeutic mice. However, therapeutic effectiveness of sulfas has not been satisfactorily demonstrated, and their value in PAM is doubtful.

In ocular infections due to *Acanthamoeba,* a variety of agents with limited success have been used: polymyxin B, primacin, paromomycin, hydroxystilbamidine, and pentamidine isethionate.

POPULATION

EPIDEMIOLOGY

PAM due to *Naegleria* and *Acanthamoeba* occurs worldwide, having been reported from at least 18 countries (Fig. 36-1). Approximately 80 percent of the cases are due to *N. fowleri,* the remainder to *Acanthamoeba* or unidentified FLA. In the United States, Europe, and Australia, major epidemics have occurred. In the United States more than 50 cases have been reported from 14 states, most of which are located in the eastern and southwestern parts of the country.

Both in natural and experimental infections, PAM due to *Naegleria* occurs in males twice as frequently as in females. In almost every instance, intimate contact with fresh water occurs. The incubation period is 3 to 7 days. Acquisition of infection depends on several factors, but inoculum size and intranasal instillation appear to be the most important. In Nigeria during the harmattan period, it is believed that PAM due to *Naegleria* may be dust-borne; probably through aerosolized cysts deposited upon the olfactory mucosa [12]. However, people in Nigeria instill water into their noses as a practice in bathing.

The epidemiology of PAM due to *Acanthamoeba* is unknown, but since the natural habitat of these amoebas is soil and water, a relationship to these factors probably exists. *Acanthamoeba* infections occur most often in immunosuppressed individuals; thus, it is also possible that the offending pathogen may reside in certain body cavities (e.g., oropharynx) and at an "opportune" time invade the host. The ratio of PAM due to *Acanthamoeba* in males to females is 5:1.

Naegleria may result in common-source epidemics, usually traced to a single, freshwater warm spring, lake, or heated swimming pool. Both *Naegleria* and *Acanthamoeba* species are also readily found in aquariums and hospital hydrotherapy pools.

In South Australia a unique situation was reported in which the public water supply became contaminated [13]. Organisms were concentrated by the warming of water, which occurred when it was transported via aqueducts over a hot, arid land. Chlorination was difficult to maintain and was ineffective. Nearly a dozen fatal cases resulted from this situation.

PREVENTION, PROPHYLAXIS, VACCINES, AND CONTROL

The only way to prevent PAM due to *Naegleria* is to avoid warm, fresh waters where they reside, and especially to avoid instilling such waters into the nasal cavity. Because mice depleted of complement are highly susceptible to *Naegleria*, humans who are known to be complement-deficient should particularly abstain from contact with such water. Nose clips may be used if swimming is essential. Since the epidemiology of PAM due to *Acanthamoeba* is unknown, no protective measures can be advised. However, ocular infections associated with soft contact lenses may be avoided by storing the lens in sterile water. Although laboratory accidents with *Naegleria* and *Acanthamoeba* are unknown, they are certainly possible. A protective mask should be worn over the nose if organisms are to be aerosolized. In addition, potentially contaminated hands should be kept away from the nose at all times.

Although prophylaxis against FLA is not recommended, it could be considered theoretically useful if a common-source epidemic of *Naegleria* is occurring, to prevent further cases of PAM in a defined population at risk. Amphotericin B, although the most effective therapeutic agent against *Naegleria*, should not be used prophylactically unless *Naegleria* is well established as the cause of the epidemic and unless the epidemic is sizeable. Amphotericin B is highly toxic and has serious side effects.

Vaccines against free-living amoebas are not available, although the possibility of constructing one against *Naegleria* exists. Mice may be protected through immunization with either *N. fowleri* or nonpathogenic *N. gruberi* injected subcutaneously, intraperitoneally, intravenously, or intranasally.

To date no satisfactory method of control for PAM exists. Warm, freshwater lakes commonly used by the public for recreation and bathing can be examined for pathogenic *Naegleria*, and if such organisms are repeatedly isolated from the water or bottom soil, use of the lake should be restricted. Thermal pollution of lakes frequented by the public should be discouraged. Disinfectants such as chlorine and iodine should not be added to natural fresh water since adequate halogen levels cannot be maintained. In addition, such chemicals may adversely affect the competitors and predators of such amoebas, possibly to the selective advantage of pathogenic species.

The waters of indoor swimming pools or baths should be tested frequently for adequate chlorine levels, since concentrations in excess of 1 ppm are lethal to trophozoites. However, superchlorination may be necessary to eradicate cysts.

Filters should be examined and cleaned frequently, as they often serve as concentrating devices, permitting amoebas to continuously reinfect the pool or bath. Chemical or heat sterilization of such filters should be performed on a periodic basis.

REFERENCES

1 Duma RJ: Primary amoebic meningoencephalitis. Crit Rev Clin Lab Sci 3:163–192, 1972

2 Fowler M, Carter RF: Acute pyogenic meningitis probably due to *Acanthamoeba* sp. Br Med J 2:740–742, 1965

3 Page FC: A revised classification of the gymnamoebia (Protozoa: Sarcodina). Zool J Linnean Soc 58:61–77, 1976

4 Sawyer TK, Visvesvara GS, Harke BA: Pathogenic amoebas from brackish and ocean sediments with a description of *Acanthamoeba hatchetti*, n sp. Science 196:1324–1325, 1977

5 Chang SL: Small, free-living amebas: Cultivation, quantitation, identification, classification, pathogenesis and resistance. Curr Top Comp Pathobiol 1:201–254, 1974

6 Marciano-Cabral FM, Bradley SG: Cytopathogenicity of *Naegleria gruberi* for rat neuroblastoma cell cultures. Infect Immunol 35:1139–1141, 1982

7 Duma RJ, Ferrell HW, Nelson CE, et al: Primary amebic meningoencephalitis. N Engl J Med 281:1315–1323, 1969

8 Pereira MS, Marsden HB, Corbitt G, et al: Ryan virus, a possible new human pathogen. Br Med J 1:130–132, 1966

9 Dvořák R, Skočil VS: Relationship of amoebas of the group limax to nasal mucous membrane. Čs Otelaryng 21:279–284, 1972

10 Duma RJ, Finley R: In vitro susceptibility of pathogenic *Naegleria* and *Acanthamoeba* species to a variety of therapeutic agents. Antimicrob Agents Chemother 10:370–376, 1976

11 Seidel JS, Harwatz P, Visesvara GS, et al: Successful treatment

of primary amebic meningoencephalitis. N Engl J Med 306:346–348, 1982

12 Lawande RV, Abraham SN, John I, et al: Recovery of soil amebas from the nasal passages of children during the dusty harmattan period in Zaria. Am J Clin Pathol 71:201–203, 1979

13 Anderson K, Jamieson A, Jadin JB, et al: Primary amoebic meningoencephalitis. Lancet i:672, 1973

CHAPTER 37 / *Amebiasis* · Adolfo Martínez-Palomo
· Guillermo Ruíz-Palacios

Amebiasis is the infection of humans with the protozoan *Entamoeba histolytica*, which has a worldwide distribution. The motile form of the parasite, or trophozoite, usually lives as a commensal in the lumen of the large intestine, where it multiplies and eventually differentiates into the cyst, the resistance form, responsible for the transmission of the infection. As a commensal, *E. histolytica* induces no signs or symptoms; this condition is known as *luminal amebiasis*. As a pathogen, it is the cause of invasive amebiasis, which is prevalent in certain developing countries. Pathogenic strains invade the intestinal mucosa and produce dysentery or ameboma, and through bloodborne spreading give rise to extraintestinal lesions, mainly liver abscesses. The human being is the only reservoir and source of infection [1,2].

PARASITE

The genus *Entamoeba* comprises several species of human parasites; *E. histolytica* Schaudinn, 1903; *E. hartmanni* von Provazek, 1912; *E. coli* (Grassi, 1879) Hickson, 1909; and *E. gingivalis* (Gros, 1849) Smith and Barrett, 1914. Of these, *E. histolytica* is the only species of *Entamoeba* capable of causing disease in human beings. The classification of the species of *Entamoeba* is based on the number of nuclei in the mature cysts; either eight, four, or one. *E. coli* belongs to the eight-nucleated cyst group. Uninucleate cysts of *E. polecki*, a common parasite in pigs, have occasionally been found in humans. In the four-nucleated cyst group, *E. histolytica* can be differentiated from *E. hartmanni* on the basis of the diameter of the cysts, which is less than 10 μm in the latter. With the recognition of *E. hartmanni* as a nonpathogenic species, it should no longer be designated by the term "small race." A fourth group is formed by *E. gingivalis*, for which no cyst form is known.

Another variety of four-nucleated *Entamoeba* are the *E. histolytica*–like Laredo-type isolates. Notwithstanding that the Laredo strains have not been classified as separate species, there are important differences from *E. histolytica*. The Laredo strains are nonpathogenic, have distinct isoenzyme patterns, and their DNA is characteristically different. Simple criteria such as size and the ability to grow at low temperatures can be used to distinguish *E. hartmanni* and Laredo-type amoebas from *E. histolytica*. In addition, another four-nucleated *Entamoeba*, *E. moshkovskii*, present in sewage in various areas of the world, shows many properties in common with the Laredo organisms, except that it is a free-living amoeba.

LIFE HISTORY AND ECOLOGY

The complex life cycle of *E. histolytica* consists of various consecutive stages, namely, trophozoite, cyst, and metacyst. Trophozoites dwell in the colon, where they multiply by binary fission and encyst, producing typical four-nucleated cysts after two successive nuclear divisions. A single four-nucleated metacystic amoeba produces eight uninucleate amoebas after division [3]. Cysts are found in the formed stools of carriers as round or slightly oval hyaline bodies, 8 to 20 μm in diameter, with a rigid wall that protects amoebas outside the human gastrointestinal tract. These cysts never develop in tissues. Trophozoites are of no importance in the transmission of the disease, since they are short-lived outside the body and do not survive exposure to hydrochloric acid and digestive enzymes in the gastrointestinal tract. In contrast, cysts may survive in feces for several days; when ingested in contaminated water or food they survive passage through the stomach and excyst in the terminal ileum, thus completing the life cycle of the parasite (Fig. 37-1).

Pathogenic and nonpathogenic zymodemes

Two of the most puzzling aspects of the biology of *E. histolytica* are the unexplained variability of its pathogenic potential and the restriction of human invasive amebiasis to certain geographical areas despite the worldwide distribution of the para-

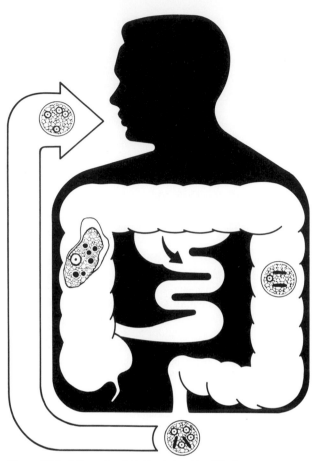

Figure 37-1. Life cycle of *E. histolytica* (simplified).

site. *E. histolytica* comprises an unknown number of pathogenic and nonpathogenic strains, the former with varying degrees of virulence. The most virulent strains appear to be prevalent in regions where invasive amebiasis is common, while those of low virulence may have a cosmopolitan distribution. Under normal conditions, *E. histolytica* acts as a commensal, living in the intestinal lumen without producing ulceration, but under unspecified conditions it can behave as a pathogenic organism whose virulence varies according to the specific strain [4].

Although nonpathogenic strains can be differentiated from invasive strains, there is still insufficient evidence to warrant their designation as separate species. In 1925 the French parasitologist E. Brumpt proposed that invasive amebiasis is produced by a biologically distinct species of amoeba restricted to a few regions, different from nonpathogenic amoebas, which would have a worldwide distribution. For almost 50 years nothing was done to refute or to prove this hypothesis, until differences in surface properties were found between *E. histolytica* isolated from carriers and those obtained from invasive

cases of amebiasis [5]. Sargeaunt et al. [6,7] applied the isoenzyme technique to some 6000 isolates of amoebas obtained from several continents over a 10-year period. The technique is based on the analysis of band patterns obtained after gel electrophoresis with the enzymes hexoquinase and phosphoglucomutase. They found that invasive amebiasis is produced by strains that have characteristic isoenzyme patterns, or *zymodemes,* while most carriers harbor amoebas with nonpathogenic zymodemes. This finding is of great relevance for understanding the epidemiology of amebiasis, both in endemic and nonendemic countries. While the classification of *E. histolytica* into pathogenic and nonpathogenic groups seems firmly established on the bases of zymodeme epidemiological data, a laboratory observation recently has challenged the concept of the stability of pathogenic traits. Under experimental conditions, changes in the bacterial flora associated with cultures of *E. histolytica* may result in the conversion of a nonpathogenic zymodeme into a pathogenic one, and vice versa [8]. So far, there is no indication that these changes take place in the human intestine [7].

MORPHOLOGY AND ULTRASTRUCTURE

The diameter of the amoebas is of practical importance because it can be used to differentiate *E. histolytica* from the small nonpathogenic *E. hartmanni*. Trophozoites obtained from liver or intestinal lesions are generally large, measuring 20 to 40 μm in diameter, while those found in nondysenteric stools measure 10 to 30 μm. The finding of hematophagous trophozoites in feces has traditionally been considered the best evidence of the invasive nature of the amoebas.

The trophozoite, or motile, form of *E. histolytica* is a highly dynamic, pleomorphic cell whose form and motility are extremely sensitive to changes in the physicochemical environment. The pleomorphism of the amoebas is evident under the scanning electron microscope. Amoebas are elongate in form, with protruding lobopodia and a trailing uroid. Less active cells tend to be spherical and have varying amounts of macro- or micropinocytotic vesicles opened to the external surface. Filopodia are filamentous surface projections present on the basal surface of the amoebas which extend several micrometers in length; they apparently are involved in attachment to the epithelial surface (Fig. 37-2) [4].

The plasma membrane of *E. histolytica* is approximately 10 nm thick and is covered on the outer surface by a barely detectable coat composed mainly by glycoproteins. After interaction with lectins or antibodies, there is a surface redistribution of membrane components [4]. As a result, certain surface coat molecules accumulate at the uroid through this "capping" process and are later eliminated into the medium.

The endoplasm of *E. histolytica* contains abundant vacuoles embedded in a cytoplasmic matrix and having the appearance of ground glass. Many vacuoles contain lysosomal enzymes,

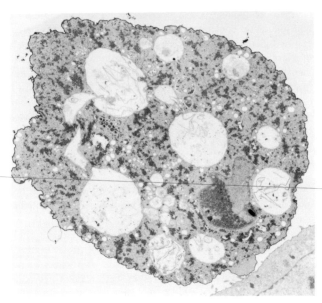

Figure 37-2. Transmission electron micrograph of a trophozoite of *Entamoeba histolytica*. × 2000.

several of which are bound to the vacuolar membrane. The submicroscopic organization of the cytoplasm is characterized by the absence of most of the differentiated organelles found in "typical" eukaryotic cells, i.e., mitochondria, Golgi apparatus, endoplasmic reticulum, centrioles, and microtubules. Ribosomes are usually ordered in helical arrays that aggregate in large crystalline inclusions up to several micrometers in length, constituting the classical "chromatoid bodies" seen with the light microscope, which form under conditions of reduced protein synthesis. Actinlike microfilaments may be identified with immunofluorescence and electron microscopy; however, they differ from other eukaryotic microfilaments both biochemically and morphologically. Microtubules are absent in both the cytoplasm and nuclei of nondividing amoebas, but they are present in the nuclei of dividing *E. histolytica* trophozoites [4]. Several virus and viruslike particles have been identified in *E. histolytica* in cultures, but their relationship with the virulence of the parasite has eluded experimental demonstration.

Cysts can be found in the feces of carriers by the zinc sulfate flotation methods. They appear as round or slightly oval hyaline bodies, 8 to 20 μm in diameter, with a refractive wall, a colorless cytoplasm, and one to four nuclei clearly discernible in specimens stained with iodine. With iron-hematoxylin stain the cytoplasm appears vacuolated and glycogen deposits are visible as clear spaces, while chromatoid bodies are stained blue-black and are rod-shaped with blunt or rounded ends [9]. Electron microscopy has demonstrated the filamentous nature of the cyst wall.

BIOCHEMISTRY, PHYSIOLOGY, AND IN VITRO CULTURE

The large intestine provides an environment with a low oxygen tension, a requirement for the optimal growth of amoebas in culture. Trophozoites of *E. histolytica* are not absolute anaerobes, however, as has traditionally been thought. Amoebas are able to consume oxygen in spite of the lack of mitochondria and can grow in atmospheres containing up to 5% oxygen. Below this concentration, amoebas are able to detoxify the products of oxygen reduction [10].

The metabolism of the parasite is puzzling since *E. histolytica* is a facultative aerobe with peculiar glycolytic enzymes that are also found in certain bacteria. This protean metabolism may be an advantage, enabling the parasite to shift from the environment of the intestinal lumen at low oxygen pressure to the one encountered upon invasion of solid organs with an abundant blood supply.

Carbohydrates are the main source of energy for the parasite. The uptake of glucose involves a specific transport system that provides an amount approximately 100 times that incorporated by endocytosis. Amebic catabolism of glucose differs considerably from that of most eukaryotic cells, owing to the presence of uncommon glycolytic enzymes and the absence of mitochondria, cytochromes, and a citric acid cycle. An unusual adaptation is that inorganic pyrophosphate, generally considered to be an end product of metabolism, is used as an energy source, replacing ATP in several glycolytic reactions. The lipid composition of *E. histolytica* is unusual in that phosphatidylethanolamine predominates over phosphatidylcholine. Furthermore, the presence of the phospholipid ceramide aminoethyl phosphonate in the plasma membrane may confer biological advantages, since this compound is resistant to hydrolysis and many enable the parasite to resist its own phospholipase action. The plasma membrane contains at least 12 different polypeptides, several of which are mannose- or glucose-containing glycoproteins [4,10].

Trophozoites are highly mobile cells; this motility is related to the formation of pseudopodia (lobopodia and microfilopodia). The prominent endocytic functions are carried out through micro- and macropinocytosis, as well as phagocytosis. Exocytosis may play a role in the liberation of toxic substances.

Cultivation of fecal material for the isolation and growth of *E. histolytica* is of diagnostic value, enabling the confirmation of a doubtful microscopic diagnosis. The availability of axenic cultures has had a significant impact on the realization of biochemical and immunological investigations, although the development of a chemically defined medium has yet to be achieved. With Diamond's medium [11] a 100-fold increase in the number of amoebas is obtained in 72 h of incubation at 37°C. So far, nonpathogenic strains have not been cultured in axenic culture media. The differentiation of trophozoites into cysts involves the deposition of a rigid fibrillar wall containing chitin. Encystation in vitro appears to be triggered by local depletion of nutrients and changes in the osmolarity of the medium, but has not yet been obtained under axenic conditions.

Restriction enzyme digestion patterns of total genomic DNA have revealed the presence of highly repeated DNA in *E. histolytica,* which can be differentiated from other amoebas based on digestion patterns [12]. Initial efforts to clone genes of pathogenic amoebas have concentrated on the actin gene [13,14].

ANIMAL MODELS

Although experimental infection with *E. histolytica* has been produced in a variety of mammals, natural susceptibility to an infection that reproduces the main characteristics of invasive amebiasis has only rarely been found in some animals. At one time, experimental intestinal and hepatic lesions were produced in animals by inoculation with trophozoite cultures in association with undefined bacterial flora. At present, hepatic amebiasis can be induced by the direct inoculation of axenic trophozoites into the liver of newborn or young hamsters or by intraportal injection [15,16], and ulcerative lesions of the colonic mucosa can be produced in guinea pigs with axenic amoebas [17]. Those experiments demonstrate the intrinsic pathogenicity of certain *E. histolytica* strains.

PATIENT

Trophozoites usually live as commensals in the lumen of the large intestine; in this phase the infection known as luminal amebiasis produces no signs or symptoms in carriers. No specific host factors have been shown to play a decisive role in the establishment of intestinal or liver lesions in humans. Consideration has been given to a variety of host factors including geographical location, race, sex, age, nutritional and immunological status, diet, local climate, alcoholism, and sexual habits. Pathogenic strains of *E. histolytica* can invade the intestinal mucosa and give rise to amebic dysentery or bloody diarrhea, and less frequently to ameboma, appendicitis, or fulminant colitis. Through bloodborne spreading they may produce extraintestinal lesions, mainly liver abscesses. Less common sites of infection are the brain and lungs. Visceral lesions may reach the skin and genitalia and produce extensive damage.

Whether trophozoites actually are transformed from harmless commensals into aggressive invaders remains hypothetical. The specific designation of the amoeba as *histolytica* by Schaudinn in 1903 clearly indicated the lytic action of trophozoites on human tissues. Less clear, however, is the mechanism through which trophozoites produce cytolysis. Several properties differentiate pathogenic from nonpathogenic strains. Thus, pathogenic strains show (1) characteristic zymodemes distinguished by the presence of a β band and the absence of an α band in the enzyme phosphoglucomutase, and by fast running bands in hexoquinase in most patterns; (2) higher rate

of erythrophagocytosis; (3) a greater propensity to agglutinate with the lectin concanavalin A, reflecting a higher number of exposed glucose- and mannose-containing receptors; (4) a lack of overall surface charge, which may facilitate interaction with the negatively charged mammalian cells; (5) the ability to grow in semisolid media; (6) a more potent cytopathic effect in vitro; (7) the capacity to produce liver and intestinal destructive lesions in rodents; and (8) resistance to complement-mediated lysis [4,6,7,18]. Another surface property, adhesion, is partially mediated by lectins of amebic origin [19,20], but the degree of adhesion is not related to the pathogenicity of the strain.

Toxins with proteinase activity have been identified in homogenates of cultured trophozoites, but they are not cytolethal and their effect is reversible [21,22]. In addition, a collagenase activity [23] and a protein that creates irreversible ion channels in membranes [24,25] have been detected in trophozoites of *E. histolytica.* The role of these and other substances in the lytic activity of the parasite, as well as their mode of liberation from intact amoebas, remain to be studied.

The interaction between trophozoites of *E. histolytica* and cultured mammalian cells that leads to cytopathic effects is as follows: (1) adhesion of the amoebas to target cells; (2) contact-dependent cytolysis, probably through the liberation of enzymes and the pore-forming protein; (3) phagocytosis of lysed cells; and (4) intracellular degradation of the ingested cells [26–28].

Much has been written but little is known about the relationship between amebic virulence and association with pathogenic bacteria. On the one hand, liver lesions are easily produced in susceptible animals with axenically grown amoebas. On the other, these bacteria-free amebic cultures can only induce intestinal ulceration in newborn guinea pigs under conditions which facilitate the close interaction of the amoebas with the mucosal surface; reassociation with bacteria is needed in order to produce colonic lesions in other mammals. The biological basis for this requirement is still unknown. A clue to the understanding of this change may lie in the local conditions at the interface between the mucous lining of the colon and the bacterial flora associated with the amoebas. Anaerobic conditions and bacteria ingested by the trophozoites apparently favor the lowering of the redox potential in the parasite, thus facilitating its electron transport system, the first by virtue of oxygen deprival, with bacteria acting as broad-range scavengers for oxygen molecules [29]. Efforts to demonstrate a virus-induced transformation from harmless commensal to active invader have been fruitless so far.

In summary, the lytic and invasive characteristics of pathogenic strains of *E. histolytica* are related to the striking motility and phagocytic capacity of the trophozoites and to the possible liberation of toxic substances and enzymes following contact with epithelial tissues. The human being appears to be the only mammal genetically susceptible to infection with *E. histolytica.* Much remains to be learned from the study of the factors that determine the genetic resistance of animals to amebic infection.

IMMUNOLOGY

Antigenic activity has been identified in subcellular fractions containing lysosomal, ribosomal, or soluble components of *E. histolytica* trophozoites in culture; up to 32 precipitin peaks have been demonstrated in these fractions by double immunoelectrophoresis. Amebic antigens have been identified in the sera or feces of patients with invasive amebiasis.

In both human and experimental amebiasis the humoral immune response is characterized by the prompt appearance of circulating antibodies. These do not appear to be protective. The detection of circulating antibodies by counterimmunoelectrophoresis, indirect hemagglutination, or ELISA has important practical application in the diagnosis of invasive amebiasis and in seroepidemiological surveys. Antiamebic coproantibodies have been found in feces, but their significance has not been determined.

Immune serum produces rapid lysis of trophozoites in vitro; antiamebic globulin produces a similar although less potent effect, even in the absence of complement. Both effects seem to be antibody-dependent, because they are neutralized by adsorption with antigens from *E. histolytica*. To a lesser extent, complement alone also induces the lysis of certain amebic strains, probably through the activation of the alternative pathway. Possible means of evasion of the humoral immune response utilized by virulent trophozoites of *E. histolytica* include membrane resistance to complement, capping of antigen-antibody complexes, and shedding of surface components.

The cell-mediated immune response is depressed in the initial phase of invasive amebiasis but appears after clinical recovery, as revealed by the presence of a delayed hypersensitivity skin reaction and in vitro tests.

Acquired resistance to reinfection has been demonstrated in experimental animals. In humans the recurrence of liver abscess after successful treatment is extremely rare. In severe forms of amebic colitis, recurrence is also exceptional. On the basis of clinical experience, partial or complete resistance appears to occur in humans after recovery from invasive amebiasis, mostly as a consequence of the stimulation of cellular immune responses. For further details, recent reviews are available [30–32].

PATHOGENESIS AND PATHOLOGY

In biopsy samples of human intestinal tissue infected with *E. histolytica*, inflammatory reactions with edema, hyperemia, and thickening of the colonic mucosa have been described and are probably nonspecific precursor lesions of focal ulcerations. A focal depletion of mucin from the surface of epithelial cells and microulcerations are also found in the preinvasive stage [33]. These early changes are unrelated to the presence of amoebas near the lesions. Both in human and experimental

intestinal amebiasis, invasion of the colonic and cecal mucosa begins in the interglandular epithelium, a site of lowered resistance where the shedding of intestinal cells normally takes place as the final stage in the constant renewal of the epithelium [4,33].

During the early stages of invasion ulceration is superficial; tissue necrosis and cell infiltration at the site of invasion are minimal. Reactive hyperplasia is seen in the areas where lymphoid aggregates are present. Ulcerations may both deepen and progress superficially, forming typical ''flask ulcers'' which extend through the mucosa and muscularis mucosae into the submucosa. Neutrophils and eosinophils are only infrequently seen in these invasive lesions. Amoebas are usually confined to the regions of epithelial lysis and the surface exudate composed of necrotic material, erythrocytes, bacteria, fibrin, and a few inflammatory cells. Only occasionally is there a sizeable infiltration of neutrophils.

Macroscopically, ulcers are initially superficial with hyperemic borders, a necrotic base, and normal mucosa between the sites of invasion. Ulceration may become more extensive and confluent, with progressively smaller areas of intervening edematous mucosa (Fig. 37-3). Further advancement of the lesions produces a loss of the mucosa and submucosa covering

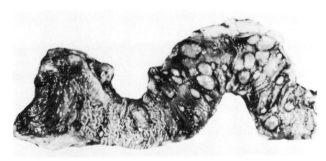

A

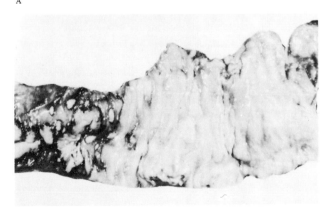

B

Figure 37-3. *A.* Colon with multiple amebic ulcers. *B.* Colon with amebic ulcers (*left*) and a large ameboma (*middle* and *right*). (*Courtesy of Dr. J. Aguirre.*)

the muscle layers, and eventually the rupturing of the serosa [*34*].

The ameboma is an uncommon form of intestinal amebiasis characterized by pseudotumoral lesions with necrosis, inflammation, granulation tissue, ulceration, and slight fibrosis. Those lesions greatly thicken the wall of the intestine, bestowing a gross appearance that can easily be mistaken for that of a malignant tumor (Fig. 37-3*B*).

Complications of intestinal amebiasis include perforation, direct extension to the skin, and dissemination, mainly to the liver. Amoebas probably spread from the intestine to the liver through the portal circulation. The presence and extent of liver involvement bears no relationship to the degree of intestinal amebiasis, and these conditions do not necessarily coincide. The early stages of hepatic amebic invasion have not been studied in humans. In the hamster, an animal particularly susceptible to amebic infection, inoculation of *E. histolytica* trophozoites into the portal vein produces periportal foci of neutrophil accumulations, followed by focal necrosis and granulomatous infiltration. As the lesions extend in size, the granulomas are gradually substituted by necrosis, until the lesions coalesce and necrotic tissue occupies large portions of the liver. The lesions can then develop into areas of liquefied necrotic material surrounded by a thin capsule of fibrous appearance. It is at this stage that liver abscesses have usually been microscopically studied in humans. Whether the initial stages occurring in hamsters are also present in human beings is not yet known. Human liver abscesses consist of areas in which the parenchyma has been completely substituted by material, usually of a semisolid or liquid consistency, composed of necrotic matter and few cells (Fig. 37-4). Neutrophils are generally absent, and amoebas tend to be located at the periphery of the abscess. Liver abscesses may heal, rupture, or disseminate.

Invasive amebic lesions in humans, whether localized in the large intestine, liver, or skin, almost invariably heal without the formation of scar tissue if properly treated. The absence of fibrotic tissue following necrosis is striking, particularly in the liver, since scarring is the usual consequence of severe hepatic infection, irrespective of the etiology. The complete anatomical and functional restitution of liver integrity after treatment of liver abscesses can be assessed by scintillography. Similar recovery can be followed radiologically or endoscopically in cases of severe amebic intestinal infection such as ameboma. To date there is no adequate explanation for the absence of scarring after recovery from invasive amebic lesions. The obvious explanation, i.e., the production of factors that inhibit both fibroblast recruitment and multiplication and the deposition of collagen during infection, awaits experimental demonstration.

In contrast to other infectious processes, no alterations attributable to immunopathological reactions have been described in amebiasis. While circulating antigen-antibody complexes have been found in patients with invasive amebiasis, a

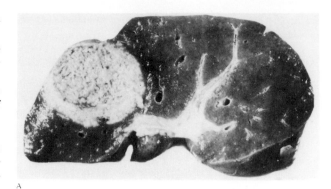

A

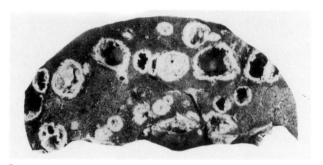

B

Figure 37-4. *A.* Liver with a large amebic abscess. *B.* Liver with multiple amebic abscesses. (*Courtesy of Dr. J. Aguirre.*)

pathogenic role has not been demonstrated for them, except perhaps in a small group of patients with arthritis and amebic colitis [*32*].

CLINICAL MANIFESTATIONS

Intestinal amebiasis

The clinical spectrum of intestinal *E. histolytica* infection ranges from asymptomatic carrier state and acute colitis, to fulminant colitis with perforation. However, a variety of patterns of disease occurs in each category (Table 37-1) depending on the time course of the disease, the susceptibility of the host, including age and, probably, differences in the degree of virulence of amebic strains.

Table 37-1. Clinical presentations of intestinal amebiasis

Asymptomatic cyst carriers
Chronic nondysenteric syndrome
Acute rectocolitis (with or without blood)
Fulminant necrotizing colitis (toxic megacolon)
Postdysenteric colitis
Other manifestations:
    Ameboma
    Amebic appendicitis
    Painless rectal bleeding

Asymptomatic Carriers. The true illness-to-infection ratio of intestinal amebiasis is unknown and variations according to geographical areas and hygiene practices have been noted [35]. In countries where amebiasis is an important health problem, the majority (approximately 80 percent) of individuals with colonic *E. histolytica* infections are carriers, while the remaining 20 percent have invasive intestinal amebiasis. In some studies only 10 percent of cyst passers were reported to have associated mild to severe gastrointestinal symptoms [36]. Excretion of cysts in the stools is intermittent and differs between samples and individuals [37]. In general, asymptomatic carriers excrete small numbers of cysts, although some healthy cyst passers may excrete several millions of cysts daily [38]. The risk for asymptomatic carriers to further develop diarrhea or invasive amebiasis is unknown. In a study in which 15 asymptomatic carriers were followed for up to 18 months, all had spontaneous eradication of the parasite and none developed symptoms of invasive amebiasis [39] suggesting either that these individuals carried nonpathogenic strains or that their immune system was able to clear the cysts. On the other hand, patients with nondysenteric amebic colitis inadequately treated had a greater risk of recurrence or developing amebic abscess, which may suggest that these patients harbored pathogenic strains that were not cleared.

It is then possible that most of the asymptomatic infections are due to nonpathogenic strains, as has been suggested in several studies using isoenzyme profiles (zymodemes) to distinguish pathogenic from nonpathogenic strains [7]. In a study of 303 *E. histolytica* strains isolated from asymptomatic carriers, pathogenic zymodemes were found only in 5 percent [40]. Nevertheless, truly controlled prospective studies are needed to evaluate the outcome of asymptomatic infections with amoebas harboring the so-called pathogenic and nonpathogenic zymodemes or with other virulence markers yet to be defined.

Chronic Nondysenteric Syndrome. There is great controversy on the existence of chronic colitis with *E. histolytica* infection.

Contrary to previous belief, recent data indicates that *E. histolytica* may not be responsible for a syndrome associated with abdominal colic and chronic alterations in bowel habits. In this study there were no differences in symptoms and histological and serological findings between culture-positive and culture-negative subjects, suggesting that the clinical picture may correspond to an irritable bowel syndrome in passers of nonpathogenic amoeba cysts [39]. On the other hand, one must not mistake this irritable bowel syndrome and coincidental isolation of cysts for an early stage of invasive enterocolitis of insidious presentation associated with abdominal colic and intermittent diarrhea lasting several weeks before the initiation of acute rectocolitis [41,42].

Acute Rectocolitis. This is a well-defined syndrome in which the clinical manifestations depend on the location and extension of the lesions in the colon and the time course of the disease. Most patients present a nontoxic dysenteric syndrome, and constitutional symptoms are not as prominent as in *Shigella* dysentery (Table 37-2). Patients with colonic amebiasis have an appearance of well-being, and only one-third of them develop low-grade fever. Children on the other hand, are more likely to have fever exceeding 38°C; and they may also have anorexia, irritability, and vomiting [43]. Abdominal pain occurs virtually in all children, at times so severe that it can be misdiagnosed as acute abdomen or appendicitis. Dehydration occurs frequently in children, although rarely in adults [44].

The onset of acute rectocolitis is gradual, and 85 percent of patients complain of intense abdominal pain. Initially there are loose watery stools that rapidly become blood-stained with mucus. Tenesmus occurs in half of the patients and is always associated with rectosigmoidal involvement. Watery diarrhea or loose stools without blood may be present for few days, particularly when higher regions of the colon are involved, including the cecum. *Typhlitis* is a syndrome characterized by subacute loose or watery diarrhea associated with localized abdominal tenderness on the right lower quadrant and characteristic changes on the barium enema x-rays.

Table 37-2. Comparison between amebic and bacillary dysenteries

	Amebic	Bacillary
Onset	Gradual	Sudden
Clinical appearance	Toxic in infants and children In adults usually nontoxic	Often toxic
Dehydration	Common in children, unusual in adults	Common
Tenesmus	Severe	Moderate
Hepatomegaly	Common	Uncommon
Stool appearance	Blood and mucus; may be semiformed	Blood and mucus; usually liquid
Fecal leukocytes	Uncommon	Common
Colonic ulcerations	Usually segmental	Diffuse

Source: From [43,44].

Rectosigmoidoscopy and colonoscopy of benign cases show small ulcerations with linear or oval contours, 3 to 5 mm in diameter, covered by a yellowish exudate containing many trophozoites. The mucosa between the ulcers may be hyperemic or may have a normal appearance. In more advanced lesions, ulcers are larger and more numerous, with submucosal hemorrhages [41,42,45].

Fulminant Necrotizing Colitis. This is a severe and life-threatening form of intestinal amebiasis that progresses rapidly, although occasionally starts as a nonspecific gastroenteritis and then progresses to the fulminant stage, particularly when diagnosis and treatment are delayed. This severe presentation is more commonly seen in malnourished infants, in the elderly, and in the immunocompromised patient, or after inappropriate use of corticosteroids [46,47]. The disease is characterized by numerous bloody stools with a characteristic foul odor, 20 or more in 24 h, generalized abdominal pain, and rectal tenesmus which tends to be constant and intense. Fever may be high (40°C), nausea and vomiting frequently occur, and the patient appears sick, dehydrated, with low blood pressure and prostration. Profuse rectal bleeding and signs of intestinal perforation and peritonitis occur at the end of this stage. Colonic perforation is a common complication of fulminant colitis and is present in more than 70 percent of the cases; it could be single or multiple. Toxic megacolon occurs rarely and is characterized by marked distension of the abdomen. Necrotizing colitis may be associated with amebic liver abscess, septicemia, and stricture formation [46].

Leukocytosis with a moderate degree of anemia is frequently present in necrotizing colitis. Abdominal films may reveal a paralytic ileus localized in the area of the colon if perforation is associated. Free air in the peritoneal cavity may be found or characteristic findings of toxic megacolon could be seen, such as generalized distension of the colon with intramural gas.

The diagnosis of this entity is based on the abrupt onset of a dysenteric syndrome in a rapidly deteriorating patient with signs of acute abdomen, the presence of amebic trophozoites in the stools, a positive serology, and characteristic changes in the abdominal x-rays. It is not uncommon, particularly in areas where amebiasis is rare, that patients who develop fulminant disease have received corticosteroid therapy for the erroneous diagnosis of chronic idiopathic inflammatory bowel disease.

This severe form of amebiasis has a high mortality rate, up to 60 percent, as a consequence of perforation and septicemia. Early diagnosis and specific therapy are determinant for the outcome. It is still debatable whether surgery has any benefit in the treatment of necrotizing colitis, even if it is complicated with perforation, because of high mortality [48]. There is now a tendency for a more conservative approach with antiamebic and antibacterial drugs, postponing surgery only when there is a residual abdominal abscess. On the other hand, toxic megacolon will require total colectomy and antiamebic and antibacterial therapy.

Postdysenteric Colitis. In a small percent of patients with acute amebic rectocolitis the dysenteric symptoms disappear, but the patient may continue with intermittent watery diarrhea that gradually subsides, leaving loose stools until there is complete resolution without treatment after several months. Repeated stool examinations fail to reveal *E. histolytica*, and repeated antiamebic therapy does not alter the course. Rectosigmoidoscopy shows an edematous, hyperemic, and fragile mucosa. This entity is more frequent among patients who had severe acute rectocolitis and may be a consequence of extensive bowel damage.

Ameboma. Ameboma is found in 0.5 to 1.5 percent of cases of invasive amebiasis of the colon (Fig. 37-5). It is a segmental lesion, single or multiple, that occurs more often in the cecum and ascending colon [34,49], characterized by a thickening of the intestinal wall accompanied by a thin and ulcerated mucosa, producing a rather large (up to 30 cm) mass protruding into the lumen. Seventy percent of the cases are presented as acute dysentery without any signs of an accompanying abdominal mass, and therefore the diagnosis of ameboma is usually made by the radiologist rather than by the clinician. Occasionally the ameboma may present as chronic diarrhea and a palpable abdominal or rectal mass, or, more rarely, as an intestinal occlusion that may be misdiagnosed as carcinoma of the colon. Also, in rare instances, it may present as extensive lesions, resembling advanced Crohn's disease (Fig. 37-5*B*). Differential diagnosis should be made with carcinoma of the colon, chronic idiopathic inflammatory disease, and tuberculosis of the colon. Wet mount preparations taken directly from the lesion and biopsies should be made, even when the diagnosis of amebiasis is highly suspected. Serology is always positive at high titers in this form of amebiasis.

Appendicitis. This is an infrequent presentation described as one of the clinical forms of invasive intestinal amebiasis. Even though ileocecal involvement in this entity is relative high (24 percent), only less than 1 percent of cases of amebic colitis present the characteristic clinical picture of acute appendicitis [48]. In these cases, the symptoms are similar to those of polymicrobial appendicitis, although a few patients can have bloody diarrhea with mucus preceding the symptoms of acute appendicitis, and the diagnosis is made after surgery based on histopathological changes. In a study of 1000 surgical specimens of acute appendicitis, amebic trophozoites were seen in only four; even though amebic appendicitis is rare, in endemic areas histopathology studies are justified in all cases of appendicitis. If the diagnosis is not made and treatment started promptly, the patient with amebic appendicitis develops acute bloody diarrhea and complications such as perforation and fistula. One-third of the patients with amebic appendicitis simultaneously develop liver abscess.

Painless Rectal Bleeding. Hematochezia without diarrhea associated with intestinal amebiasis may be seen, particularly in

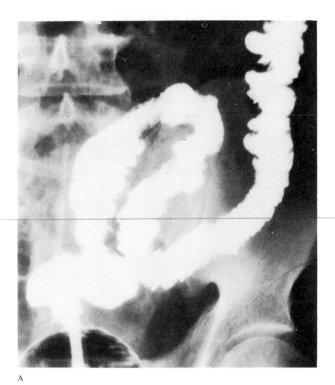 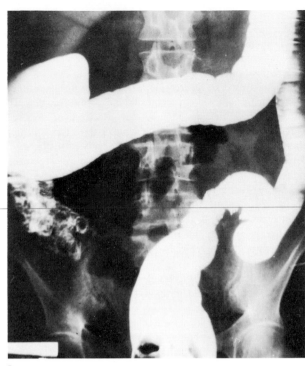

A   B

Figure 37-5. *A.* Amebic colitis. X-ray film showing a rigid intestinal wall of decreased caliber and loss of haustra. *B.* X-ray film of an ameboma of cecum and ascending colon. (*Courtesy of Dr. L. Landa.*)

older children [*50–52*]. The rectal bleeding is intermittent, painless, and frequently chronic, and may last for several weeks; less than 50 percent of the patients have a history of dysentery prior to rectal bleeding. Diagnosis is made by proctoscopy, which reveals an edematous, congestive colitis without ulcers, although rarely there may be a single ulcer with profuse bleeding. Wet mount preparations virtually always show *E. histolytica* trophozoites.

Diagnosis. In the great majority of cases of invasive colonic amebiasis, rectosigmoidoscopy and immediate microscopic examination of rectal smears for the presence of motile, hematophagous trophozoites of *E. histolytica* are the most important diagnostic procedures. Rectosigmoidoscopy and colonoscopy of benign cases show small ulcerations with linear or oval contours (3 to 5 mm), covered by a yellowish exudate containing many trophozoites. The mucosa between the ulcers may either be hyperemic or have a normal appearance. In more advanced lesions, ulcers are larger and more numerous, with submucosal hemorrhages.

The cornerstone in the diagnosis of intestinal amebiasis is still the microscopical observation of cysts and trophozoites of *E. histolytica* in the stools or scraping of affected mucosa. At present, a reliable, easy to perform, sensitive, and rapid assay, such as immunoassay or hybridization using gene probes, is in

the research phase and not available to the clinical laboratory. The direct observation of amoebas has several drawbacks. The examination is tedious and time-consuming, it requires expert eyes, the sensitivity is relatively low, several samples are required in the case of cyst passers, fresh samples are needed for the identification of trophozoites, and the techniques for staining trophozoites maintained in preservative substances, such as polyvinyl alcohol and formalin, are cumbersome. Stool culture of amoebas is in general not applicable as a routine method [*53*].

All these inconveniences make both overdiagnosis and underdiagnosis common problems in clinical laboratories, not only in community health facilities, but also in teaching institutions, where a third or more of the laboratories cannot correctly identify *E. histolytica*. False positives usually result from the misinterpretation of leukocytes, including macrophages or other parasites, mainly *E. hartmanni*, and fecal debris in the stools of patients with inflammatory diarrhea or ulcerative colitis. This is a frequent mistake even in endemic areas, where there is more experience. False negatives, although less frequent, may cost the lives of patients by a delay in the correct diagnosis and treatment.

When trophozoites of *E. histolytica* containing ingested red blood cells are found in stools in association with gastrointestinal symptoms, a diagnosis can be easily made. Problems in diagnosis arise when cysts are identified in stools of healthy or diarrheic individuals, because nonpathogenic strains cannot be distinguished microscopically from pathogenic amoebas, and unfortunately, at present no rapid method is available to differentiate the two types of strains.

Methods used to identify *E. histolytica* in intestinal infections can be direct or by concentration of the samples. The direct method, the wet mount, may use fresh or preserved samples. When made from fresh samples three types of preparations should be included for each specimen: using saline solution (to observe amebic motility in a warm specimen), adding saline plus iodine (to differentiate *E. histolytica* cysts from other amebic species and parasite ova), and saline plus methylene blue (to distinguish cysts from leukocytes, which stain blue). Direct methods should always be used in fresh, diarrheic specimens and with samples taken directly from the lesions through endoscopy. Areas with mucus and blood, when present, are ideal to be tested.

In addition to the wet mount preparation, a portion of the sample should be fixed in 5% polyvinyl alcohol and stained with trichrome or iron-hematoxylin to confirm the morphology of the cysts. This is a useful method when records need to be kept, since cyst morphology remains stable for years [*54*].

Concentrations methods are useful and should be considered complementary to the direct observation, since cyst detection increases several times when the sample is concentrated. Techniques used to concentrate a fixed sample include flotation and sedimentation procedures. The flotation techniques, such as the zinc sulfate method, have been supplanted by the more sensitive and safer sedimentation tests, which are also cleaner and faster. These may use formalin-ether, formalin-ethyl acetate (FEA, a modification that is safer for being less flammable), or Merthiolate-iodine-formalin. Sedimentation procedures detect 30 to 50 percent more *E. histolytica* cysts than the direct-stained or unstained smears, the zinc-sulfate flotation technique, or even the formalin-ether concentration method alone.

The serological detection of antiamebic antibodies is positive in approximately 75 percent of cases of colonic invasive amebiasis. Other laboratory tests are of little use in diagnosis. In children, associated infections with *Salmonella*, *Shigella*, or pathogenic *Escherichia coli* are not uncommon. In severe cases of intestinal amebiasis, leukocytosis with neutrophilia, hyponatremia, and hypokalemia may be found.

Prognosis. Most cases of invasive intestinal amebiasis are completely controlled following the administration of proper chemotherapy. In general, full clinical recovery, the disappearance of mucosal lesions as confirmed by endoscopy, and a negative microscopy examination of feces or rectal smears follow adequate management. True relapses are rare, and in case of new dysenteric attacks, other etiological causes, mainly *Shigella* infection, should be considered. The prognosis may be fatal only in severe clinical forms of the disease, which constitute less than 10 percent of cases of invasive intestinal

amebiasis. In cases of fulminant colitis, 55 percent of patients who can be operated on survive. Amebic appendicitis has a mortality rate of 20 percent due to the frequent perforation of the cecum. Colonic ameboma may have a benign prognosis when a prompt diagnosis is followed by adequate chemotherapy; when surgical resection of the colon due to an incorrect diagnosis is performed or intestinal perforation occurs, mortality increases to 16 percent.

Various authors have stated that invasive amebic colitis frequently has a sequel of chronic lesions of the intestinal wall that are either inactive, appearing as fibrous strictures, or active, such as chronic amebic colitis [*41*]. However, both conditions are only rarely found in areas where invasive amebiasis is most frequent. Furthermore, there is no higher incidence of colonic carcinoma in patients who have suffered from amebic colitis.

Extraintestinal amebiasis: Amebic liver abscess

Amebic liver abscess is the most common extraintestinal form of invasive amebiasis. Amebic abscesses may be found in all age groups, but are ten times more frequent in adults than in children, predominantly in the group of people 20 to 60 years of age. There is a higher frequency in males than in females (3:1 to 6:1). Liver abscesses are more common in the poorest sectors of urban populations; only infrequently are they found

Table 37-3. Clinical and laboratory findings in amebic liver abscess

	Range of percentage
Length of symptoms:	
0–2 weeks	37–66
2–4 weeks	20–40
4–12 weeks	16–42
>12 weeks	5–11
Fever	71–98
Abdominal pain	62–98
Diarrhea	14–66
Cough	10–32
Weight loss	33–53
Tender liver	80–95
Hepatomegaly	43–93
Epigastric tenderness	22
Rales, ronchi	8–47
Jaundice	10–25
WBC >10,000	63–94
Hb <12 g	25–90
Elevated transaminases	26–50
Alkaline phosphatase	38–84
Elevated bilirubin	10–25
Increased ESR	81

Source: Modified from [*57,78*].

in hospitals for the more affluent sectors. In countries in which invasive amebiasis is prevalent, hepatic abscess constitutes a frequent and severe complication. For example, it has been estimated that 1 to 2 percent of all adult patients admitted to general hospitals in Mexico have this condition, and hepatic abscesses have been found in 5.8 percent of 3000 autopsies performed in a large hospital in Mexico City. The reasons for a higher incidence and more severe clinical manifestations in certain age and sex groups, as well as in certain geographical areas, are not well known. Hygiene conditions, overcrowding, disposal of excreta, health education, host immunity, and culinary habits may be contributing factors.

Even though liver abscess is caused by translocation of amoeba from the intestinal lumen, rarely the patients also have amebic rectocolitis (9 percent). *E. histolytica* has been found in the feces in only 22 percent of cases of amebic liver abscess. On the other hand, autopsies of cases with liver abscess showed intestinal involvement in 38 percent [*34,55*].

Amebic liver abscess is usually single; imaging techniques have revealed two or more lesions in only 20 percent of the cases. The same techniques have shown that liver abscesses are found in the right lobe in 83 percent of patients, most frequently in the posterior, external, and superior portions [*55*].

In most patients, mainly young individuals less than 30 years old and children, the clinical presentation and course of the disease are typical. Clinical and laboratory findings in amebic liver abscess reported may vary according to the population studied (Table 37-3) [*55–57*]. The onset is abrupt, with pain in the upper abdomen and high fever. The pain is intense and constant, radiating to the scapular region and right shoulder; it increases with coughing, deep breathing, or when the patient rests on the right side. When the abscess is located in the left lobe, the pain tends to be felt in the epigastrium and may radiate to the left shoulder. Fever is present in 98 percent of the cases; it varies between 38 and 40°C, frequently in spikes, with rigors and profuse sweating in the upper half of the body, especially at night. There is anorexia and rapid weight loss; approximately one-third of the patients have nonproductive cough. Nausea and vomiting may occur, and in some cases diarrhea or dysentery may be present.

Physical examination reveals a pale, wasted patient with an enlarged, tender liver. In most cases digital pressure in the right lower intercostal spaces or fist percussion will produce intense pain. Movement of the right side of the chest and diaphragm is greatly restricted, as well as the intensity of respiratory sounds. In about one-fourth of the cases there is moderate jaundice. There is leukocytosis, >15,000 cells per cubic millimeter, and in 5 percent of the cases a leukemoid reaction is present. Alkaline phosphatase is elevated, this being the most reliable biochemical indicator of amebic liver abscess. Other liver function tests are normal or slightly elevated.

On the other hand, one-third of the patients present with a chronic and milder, nonspecific febrile illness. This generally occurs in older individuals; some of them may in fact be diag-nosed as having fever of unknown origin and weight loss. The fever is continuous and low-grade (<39°C); the patients do not complain of abdominal pain or any other symptom. There are hepatomegaly, anemia, and abnormal liver function tests; alkaline phosphatase is elevated, with levels that are directly proportional to the duration of the illness.

Diagnosis. The diagnosis of amebic liver abscess is sometimes difficult to make. In endemic areas or when there is a history of travel to these countries, amebic abscess should always be suspected in patients who present with spiking fever, weight loss, and abdominal pain in the upper right quadrant or epigastrium with tenderness in the liver area; in addition such patients will have leukocytosis, elevated alkaline phosphatase, and an elevated right diaphragm in the chest films (Fig. 37-6). In this situation the available liver imaging techniques (Fig. 37-7) are indicated, although the sonography or computed tomography (CT) scan (Fig. 37-8) are preferred [*55,58–63*]. These procedures will demonstrate a space-occupying lesion in 75 to 95 percent of the cases, according to the procedure and the course of the illness. Hepatic magnetic resonance imaging gives information comparable to less expensive imaging procedures.

Once the presumptive diagnosis of a space-occupying lesion in the liver is made, the next step to define the etiology is

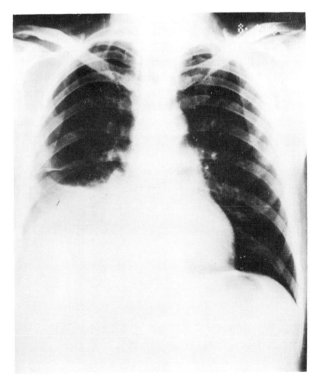

Figure 37-6. Hepatic abscess. X-ray film showing elevation of right hemidiaphragm and pleural effusion. (*Courtesy of Dr. L. Landa.*)

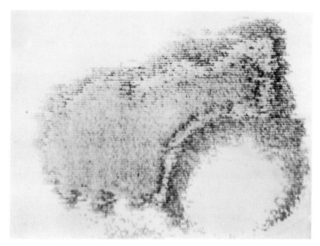

Figure 37-7. Scintillogram showing a large liver abscess produced by *E. histolytica.* (*Courtesy of Dr. L. Landa.*)

serology to detect antiamebic antibodies. This test is accurate in more than 90 percent of cases, although it may be negative, especially in the early stages of the illness or in malnourished patients with chronic abscesses, in which case the test should be repeated 1 or 2 weeks later.

In the past, amebic liver abscess was an important cause of fever of unknown origin (FUO) in developing countries. With the availability of modern imaging techniques and serology it is now a rare cause of FUO, but in places where these techniques are not yet available or where the disease is rare and thus a lack of experience is the rule, it is not uncommon that patients with amebic liver abscess are misdiagnosed in late stages of the disease and develop complications [63].

Differential diagnosis of amebic liver abscess when a space-occupying mass is found in the liver should include pyogenic abscess and neoplasm. The pyogenic abscess is more frequent in older patients with a previous history of hepatobiliary dis-

ease, abdominal sepsis, appendicitis, diverticulitis, or abdominal surgery. These patients are more likely to present with jaundice, pruritus, and septic shock; hepatomegaly and an elevated diaphragm in the chest x-rays are uncommon, and amebic serology is negative. In the presence of a space-occupying lesion with negative serology, aspiration is indicated for microscopy and culture.

Liver neoplasm is a differential diagnosis when the patient is febrile and wasted with vague abdominal discomfort. Neoplasms show distinct images, particularly in the CT scan, and tumor markers such as α-fetoproteins or carcinoembryonic antigen are useful.

Stool microscopy for the identification of trophozoites or cysts is of little value for the diagnosis of amebic liver abscess, since, as was mentioned earlier, only few patients have associated intestinal amebiasis.

Serology. Detection of antibodies to *E. histolytica* is widely used for the diagnosis of liver amebiasis. More than ten different tests have been developed during the last 20 years, although those currently used in most routine laboratories are indirect hemagglutination (IHA), counterimmunoelectrophoresis (CIE), and enzyme immunoassays (EIA). Serological techniques for antibody detection are useful only in amebic liver abscess, invasive intestinal amebiasis, and as a tool for epidemiological studies on amebiasis [32].

Serology is very useful in amebic liver abscess since antibodies are present at high titers in most patients. The antibody response in this entity is directly related to the duration of illness. Serology may be negative during the first week after onset; titers reach a peak by the second or third month, decreasing to lower, still detectable levels by 9 months, although a small portion of the patients may continue with high titers for years [64]. The fact that antibodies, even at high titers, remain present after amebic liver abscess, plus the high prevalence of positive serology in populations of endemic areas,

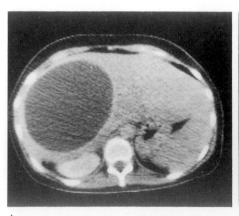
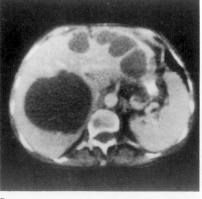

A   B

Figure 37-8. *A.* Single large amebic abscess seen with computed tomography. *B.* Multiple amebic liver abscesses visualized by means of computed tomography. (*Courtesy of Dr. M. Stoopen.*)

Table 37-4. Sensitivity and specificity of indirect hemagglutination for antiamebic antibodies in serum

	Sensitivity			Predictive value*	
Type of amebiasis	No. samples	No. with titer >1:128	%	Positive	Negative
Liver abscess:					
More than 10 days	99	97	97	67.8	98.6
Less than 20 days	10	5	50	9.8	99
Invasive diarrhea	37	32	86	41	98
Chronic diarrhea	21	11	52.3	19.2	99
Control	551	46	8.3	—	—

*The specificity of the test was 91.6%.

render this test less specific. The opposite can be said in countries where amebiasis is not prevalent, in which case serology is specific. In studies using IHA, a greater sensitivity was observed in liver abscess of more than 10 days and in invasive intestinal amebiasis with dysentery (Table 37-4).

Complications. Thoracic complications are common, particularly pleurisy with a nonpurulent pleural effusion, which occurs in more than half of the cases. It is manifested by a nonproductive cough, thoracic pain, and dyspnea related to the extent of the effusion. The rupture of a liver abscess into the bronchi can be accompanied by the sudden development of a cough and the discharge of an abundant anchovy sauce–like exudate in the sputum. Less commonly, the liver abscess may rupture into the pleural cavity accompanied by sudden sharp pain and severe dyspnea with impending shock. The least frequent thoracic complication is amebic pericarditis that may be present when the abscess is in the left lobe of the liver and is characterized by intense precordial pain, anxiety, dyspnea, tachycardia, regurgitation of the jugular veins, and softened cardiac sounds; paradoxical pulse and shock may also occur.

Rupture of an amebic liver abscess into the abdomen occurs in approximately 8 percent of patients. The onset is abrupt, with signs of generalized peritonitis. Only rarely do abscesses rupture into the gallbladder, stomach, duodenum, colon, or inferior vena cava. Occasionally an abscess may erode the abdominal wall and reach the skin.

Secondary bacterial infection of amebic liver abscesses is an uncommon complication which can be suspected when a severe toxi-infectious state is present together with lack of response to antiamebic chemotherapy.

Prognosis. In the past century when treatment of amebic liver abscess was limited to surgery, mortality was approximately 82 percent. The introduction of emetine in 1913 considerably decreased the mortality rate, although a decade ago mortality still approached 10 percent in adults and 20 percent in children, even when treated in hospitals with adequate facilities. A further reduction has been obtained during recent years, lowering the mortality rate to approximately 2 percent [41]. This decrease has been attained only where modern hospital facilities are available; under other conditions mortality probably still exceeds 10 percent.

Other extraintestinal locations

In a few cases invasive hepatic or colonic amebiasis may propagate through the blood to the lungs and brain. *E. histolytica* may invade the skin of the perianal region in cases of rectocolitis, the skin of the abdomen in cases of colostomy or other surgical interventions in patients with amebic colitis, as well as the skin of the chest in cases of spontaneous rupture of an amebic liver abscess. Invasive amebic lesions may affect the vulva, vagina, uterine cervix, and penis. Cutaneous and genital amebic lesions are frequently mistaken for carcinomas; the identification of trophozoites in the lesions facilitates the differential diagnosis. For all these locations, the detection of specific circulating antibodies may be of value in diagnosis. Radiological examination of the thorax is useful in cases of metastatic pulmonary abscesses, as is computed tomography for cerebral abscesses.

TREATMENT

The new amebicides have contributed greatly to decreasing the morbidity and mortality of amebiasis. Antiamebic drugs may be classified in three groups: luminal amebicides; tissue amebicides; and mixed amebicides, effective both in the intestinal lumen and in tissues. The most frequently used amebicides with luminal action are diiodohydroxyquin, diloxanide furoate, and paramomycin. The amebicides effective in tissues are emetine hydrochloride and dehydroemetine, which act in the liver, intestinal wall, and other tissues, and chloroquine, which acts only in the liver. Emetine and dehydroemetine are given intramuscularly and may have a toxic effect on the myocardium. Amebicides effective in both tissues and the intestinal lumen include metronidazole and the nitroimidazole derivatives secnidazole, nimorazole, and tinidazole. In addition to the advantages of being active both in tissues and intestinal lumen, and having an oral route of administration, these drugs are the most therapeutically effective. They are generally well tolerated, and in spite of their reported carcinogenic effect in rodents and their mutagenic potential in bacteria, no such effects have been reported in humans [65]. For these reasons, metronidazole and related compounds are the drugs of choice in the treatment of invasive amebiasis.

Symptomatic and asymptomatic cyst passers

The treatment of choice is luminal agents such as diloxanide furoate or diiodohydroxyquin (Table 37-5). Metronidazole is not recommended in this form of amebiasis; it is not as effective in eliminating the cysts because it is rapidly absorbed and the concentrations reached in stools are not adequate. A 10 percent relapse has been reported. Therefore, metronidazole should be reserved for the invasive forms of the disease.

Diloxanide furoate is as effective as diiodohydroxyquin, and treatments are shorter [66]; unfortunately, this drug is available in only a few countries. In the United States it is only available through the Centers for Disease Control.

Other drugs have been and are still being used, including tetracycline and paromomycin, but these are being replaced by the newer amebicides. A new agent that may be used in the future is quinfamide, a quinolone derivative, which is very active and requires a single-day treatment of three doses of 100 mg by mouth [67].

Great controversy exists in the treatment of asymptomatic cyst passers, particularly those from endemic areas. The reasons for not treating the symptomless carriers include the fact that short-term reinfections due to a constant exposure have been demonstrated. Also, the majority of cyst passers seem to have nonpathogenic strains, as was demonstrated in a study where cyst passers did not develop amebic colitis, at least in 1 year of follow-up [39]. In another series, however, some asymptomatic patients were carriers of amoebas with pathogenic zymodemes, and 10 percent of them developed amebic colitis [68]. Male homosexuals are another group in which symptomless carriage of cysts is frequent, and they have been found to carry amoebas with nonpathogenic zymodemes [69,70]. The controversy as to whether to treat symptomless carriers or not may come to an end when simple methods to define pathogenic strains become available.

The indiscriminate use of amebicides, especially of metronidazole, seems to have had an important effect on the reduction of invasive intestinal amebiasis, and the hospital admis-

Table 37-5. Chemotherapy for amebiasis

Clinical manifestation	Drug	Dose Adult	Children
Cyst passers, symptomatic or asymptomatic	1. Diloxanide furoate	500 mg PO tid for 10 days	20 mg/(kg·day) PO tid for 10 days
	2. Iodoquinol	650 mg PO tid for 20 days	30 mg/(kg·day) PO tid for 20 days
	3. Paromomycin	500 mg PO tid for 5–10 days	30 mg/(kg·day) PO tid for 7 days
Invasive intestinal amebiasis	1. Metronidazole or	500–800 mg PO tid for 5 days	30/50 mg/(kg·day) PO, tid for 5–10 days
	tinidazole plus	2 g PO once a day for 1–3 days	30–35 mg/(kg·day) PO, once a day for 1–3 days
	diloxanide or iodoquinol	See above	
	2. Dehydroemetine	1.5 mg/(kg·day) IM for 5 days (max. 90 mg/day)	1.5 mg/(kg·day) IM in 2 doses for 5 days
Liver abscess	1. Metronidazole or	PO, see above 500 mg IV q 6 h for 5–10 days	See above
	tinidazole or	2 g PO once a day for 3 days	See above
	ornidazole	2 g PO once a day for 3 days	

sions of patients with liver abscess have decreased dramatically in some countries.

Invasive intestinal amebiasis

The nitroimidazoles are the cornerstone in the treatment of these forms of amebiasis (Table 37-5) and should be given for 5 to 10 days, always associated with a luminal agent at the same doses recommended for cyst carriers. Since a shorter treatment is required with tinidazole, this may be the choice when available; it has fewer side effects and equal efficacy compared with other nitroimidazoles, including metronidazole. When amebic colitis is complicated by perforation, surgery is probably not indicated, and a more conservative approach is recommended. Intravenous antibiotics should be used for enteric bacteria plus metronidazole, which also covers anaerobes, at the same doses used in amebic liver abscess (Table 37-5).

Two of the severe forms of invasive intestinal amebiasis require surgery in addition to chemotherapy; toxic megacolon and amebic appendicitis. In fulminant colitis associated with toxic megacolon total colectomy is usually required. Acute amebic appendicitis requires surgery as in the case of bacterial appendicitis; however, the mortality associated with the former is much higher due to the frequent occurrence of lesions of the colon and liver. Colonic ameboma may be cured with metronidazole [48].

Amebic liver abscess

Amebic liver abscess should be treated with chemotherapy; surgery is rarely indicated. The treatment of choice is with nitroimidazoles, orally or, when not tolerated, intravenously (Table 37-5). Although it is a common belief that combined therapy with dehydroemetine is more effective than the nitroimidazole alone, particularly in severe cases, there are no well-controlled comparative studies that demonstrate advantages for the combined therapy.

Failure in the treatment of amebic liver abscess with metronidazole has been reported in up to 10 percent of cases [71]. It is questionable whether a true metronidazole resistance exists in some cases of amebic liver abscess, since treatment was considered a failure when there was lack of response at 72 h; the idea prevails that response should be dramatic and immediate, and it is hard to know whether prolonged treatment of these cases could have resulted in cure. In vitro studies, although limited, have not demonstrated the existence of metronidazole-resistant strains of amoeba.

Indications for percutaneous drainage are: imminent rupture of a large abscess; as a complemental therapy to shorten the course of the disease when response to chemotherapy has been slow; when pyogenic or mixed infection is suspected; and in the case of false-negative serology [48,60,61,72].

Percutaneous drainage should be done with ultrasound or CT scan guidance; catheters should not be left for drainage and should be rapidly removed to avoid contamination.

Indications for surgical drainage include imminent rupture of inaccessible liver abscess, especially of the left lobe, when there is a risk of peritoneal leakage of necrotic fluid after aspiration, and in rupture of a liver abscess.

POPULATION

ECOLOGY

Invasive amebiasis is still a major health and social problem in certain areas of Africa, Asia, and Latin America. In these parts of the world inadequate sanitary conditions may combine with the prevalence of highly virulent strains of *E. histolytica* to sustain a high incidence of intestinal amebiasis, frequent in all age groups, and liver abscesses, mostly in adult males. Conditions in afflicted areas may have deteriorated during recent years as rural populations have tended to migrate to urban areas. Unless prompt diagnosis is followed by adequate treatment, both forms of invasive amebiasis, and particularly liver abscess, may be fatal. In temperate zones where affluent societies prevail, the number of severe cases of amebiasis is much lower. Nevertheless, knowledge of the disease in these regions is also important since the failure to identify an amebic infection may result in a lethal outcome, e.g., intestinal amebiasis may be treated as chronic ulcerative colitis. In addition, high infection rates can exist among certain immigrant groups, and epidemic outbreaks can occur in institutions such as schools or mental hospitals.

The disease characteristically occurs in endemic form in areas of high prevalence, probably due to constant reinfection. Epidemic outbreaks of amebiasis are uncommon, and when present are due to a heavily contaminated water supply. High rates of luminal and invasive amebiasis in mental institutions are probably maintained by person-to-person transmission of the infection.

High levels of seropositivity in the general population correlate with various indexes of poverty: crowding, illiteracy, lack of safe drinking water, and inadequate disposal of human excrement. As in the case with other "tropical" diseases, the prevalence of amebiasis is more related to poverty than to climate.

Luminal amebiasis has a worldwide distribution. There have been estimates that as much as 10 percent of the world's population harbors *E. histolytica*. However, the problems associated with a diagnosis based on stool examination greatly limit the value of this figure. From a general survey of reported cases of amebic liver abscess, Elsdon-Dew [73] concluded that invasive amebiasis is prevalent in west and southeast Africa, the whole of southeast Asia, Mexico, and the western portion of South America. It has been recently estimated that in 1981 there were 500 million people infected with the parasite; of these, 38 million developed disabling colitis or amebic liver abscess and at least 40,000 deaths were attributable to amebiasis [74]. Therefore, on a global scale, amebiasis comes third among parasitic causes of death, behind only malaria and schistosomiasis.

In a national serological survey of nearly 20,000 serum samples from 46 Mexican communities, the average frequency of individuals with serum positive for antiamebic antibodies was 5.95 percent (range, 1 to 20 percent), demonstrating the endemic character of the disease in Mexico. Seropositivity increased after 5 years of age, and maximal levels were obtained in children between 5 and 10 years of age [35].

A major increase in luminal amebic infections has recently been detected in male homosexual populations in several U.S. cities. Point prevalence rates varying from 20 to 31 percent have reached hyperendemic levels. Most reported cases are asymptomatic or present diffuse symptoms, and manifestations of severe invasive amebiasis are generally absent.

INFECTION

Transmission of amebiasis from one individual to another may be accomplished through a variety of mechanisms. Asymptomatic carriers passing large numbers of cysts in their stools are an important source of infection, especially if they are engaged in the preparation and handling of food. The cysts may remain viable and infective for a few days in feces. Since they are killed by desiccation, cyst-laden dust is not infective. They are also killed by temperatures higher than 68°C, so that boiled water is safe. The amount of chlorine needed to purify ordinary water is insufficient to kill cysts; high levels of chlorine are effective, but the water must be subsequently dechlorinated before use. Houseflies and cockroaches ingest cysts present in feces and can pass them from their guts following periods as long as 24 h.

Fecal contamination of water may occur by means of surface runoff into springs, unprotected shallow wells and streams, or by discharge of sewage into rivers. Occasionally, siphonage of sewage into the water supply system has been responsible for outbreaks of infection. Freshening of vegetables and fruits with contaminated water and use of human excreta as fertilizer may produce heavy contamination of vegetables and fruits, which customarily are eaten raw [75,76].

PREVENTION

The basic means of preventing amebic infection is the improvement of living conditions and education in countries where invasive amebiasis is prevalent. Methods of attack by health personnel should be aimed at the following targets: (1) sanitation of the environment, (2) detection and treatment of infections, and (3) health education [76,77].

The most effective preventive measure consists in the adequate disposal of human feces through drainage or the use of septic tanks. Purified water should be distributed through pipelines to avoid contamination. In areas where amebic infection is common, the drinking water should be either filtered or

chlorinated using higher levels of chlorine than those generally used to eliminate bacterial contamination, with subsequent dechlorination. As an alternative, drinking water may be boiled for 10 min.

Freshening of vegetables and skinned fruits with contaminated water and the use of excrement as fertilizer should be avoided. People should be instructed to clean vegetables carefully with uncontaminated running water, because treatment with iodine, chlorine, or silver solutions gives unreliable results. Food handlers should be periodically checked for intestinal infection and treated if found positive. Houseflies and cockroaches should be controlled, and food adequately protected from them.

Cases of invasive amebiasis require prompt chemotherapy and all asymptomatic carriers should be treated. Mass chemotherapy of high-risk populations has been attempted, in mental institutions, for example, with only partially successful results. Individual or collective chemoprophylaxis is not indicated.

Elementary hygienic practices such as the washing of hands always after defecation and before eating, the boiling of drinking water, and avoiding the consumption of raw vegetables and exposed food should be constantly reiterated in schools, health care units, and periodic campaigns using the mass media.

Health personnel should be trained to improve the accuracy of their examinations of stool. Doctors should be constantly reminded of the problem and informed on advances in diagnostic and therapeutic procedures; their active participation in prevention programs should be encouraged.

The introduction of protective immunity is in an experimental stage. It has been shown that rodents can be immunized against intrahepatic challenge with pathogenic strains, using live trophozoites as well as crude or purified *E. histolytica* antigens. It may be possible to obtain safe and effective antigens to be tested in human volunteers, which may lead to the development of an antiamebic vaccine.

REFERENCES

1 Martínez-Palomo A (ed): *Amebiasis*. Amsterdam, Elsevier, 1986
2 Ravdin JI (ed): *Amebiasis. Human Infection by* Entamoeba histolytica. New York, Wiley, 1988
3 Dobell C: Researches on the intestinal protozoa of monkeys and man. I. General introduction. II. Description of the whole life-history of *Entamoeba histolytica* in cultures. Parasitology 20:357–412, 1928
4 Martínez-Palomo A: *The Biology of* Entamoeba histolytica. Chichester, Research Studies Press/Wiley, 1982
5 Martínez-Palomo A, González-Robles A, de la Torre M: Selective agglutination of pathogenic strains of *Entamoeba histolytica* induced by con A. Nature NB 245:186–187, 1973
6 Sargeaunt PG, Jackson TFHG, Simjee AE: Biochemical homogeneity of *Entamoeba histolytica* isolates, especially those from liver abscess. Lancet 1:1386–1388, 1982

7 Sargeaunt PG: The reliability of *Entamoeba histolytica* zymodemes in clinical diagnosis. Parasitol Today 3:40–43, 1987

8 Mirelman D: Effect of culture conditions and bacterial associates on the zymodemes of *Entamoeba histolytica.* Parasitol Today 3:37–40, 1987

9 Spencer FM, Monroe LS: *The Color Atlas of Intestinal Parasites.* Springfield, Charles C Thomas, 1961

10 McLaughlin J, Aley S: The biochemistry and functional morphology of *Entamoeba.* J Protozool 32:221–240, 1985

11 Diamond LS: Lumen dwelling protozoa: *Entamoeba,* trichomonas, and *Giardia,* in Jensen JJ (ed): *In Vitro Cultivation of Protozoan Parasites.* Boca Raton, CRC Press, 1983, pp 65–110

12 Bhattacharya S, Bhattacharya A, Diamond LS: Comparison of repeated DNA from strains of *Entamoeba histolytica* and other *Entamoeba.* Mol Biochem Parasitol 27:257–262, 1988

13 Edman U, Meza I, Agabian N: Genomic and cDNA actin sequences from a virulent strain of *Entamoeba histolytica.* Proc Natl Acad Sci USA 84:3024–3028, 1987

14 Huber M, Garfinkel L, Gitler C, et al: *Entamoeba histolytica:* Cloning and characterization of actin cDNA. Mol Biochem Parasitol 24:227–235, 1987

15 Tanimoto M, Sepúlveda B, Vázquez-Saavedra JA, et al: Lesiones producidas en el hígado del hámster por inoculación de *Entamoeba histolytica* cultivada en medio axénico. Arch Invest Med (Mex) 2(suppl 1):275–284, 1971

16 Mattern CFT, Keister DB: Experimental amebiasis. II. Hepatic amebiasis in the newborn hamster. Am J Trop Med Hyg 26:402–411, 1977

17 Anaya-Velázquez F, Tsutsumi V, González-Robles A, et al: Intestinal invasive amebiasis: An experimental model in rodents using axenic or monoxenic strains of *Entamoeba histolytica.* Am J Trop Med Hyg 34:723–730, 1985

18 Reed SL, Curd JG, Gigli I, et al: Activation of complement by pathogenic and nonpathogenic *Entamoeba histolytica.* J Immunol 136:2265–2270, 1986

19 Orozco E, Rodríguez MA, Murphy ChF, et al: *Entamoeba histolytica:* Cytopathogenicity and lectin activity of avirulent strains. Exp Parasitol 63:157–165, 1987

20 Meza I, Caizares F, Rosales-Encina JL, et al: Use of antibodies to characterize a 220-kilodalton surface protein from *Entamoeba histolytica.* J Infect Dis 156:798–805, 1987

21 Lushbaugh WB, Hofbauer AF, Pittman FE: Proteinase activity of *Entamoeba histolytica* cytotoxin. Gastroenterology 87:17–27, 1984

22 Keene WE, Petitt MG, Allen S, et al: The major neutral proteinase of *Entamoeba histolytica.* J Exp Med 163:536–549, 1986

23 Muñoz ML, Calderón J, Rojkind M: The collagenase of *Entamoeba histolytica.* J Exp Med 155:42–51, 1984

24 Lynch EC, Rosenberg IM, Gitler C: An ion-channel forming protein produced by *Entamoeba histolytica.* EMBO J 1:801–804, 1982

25 Young JDE, Young TM, Lu LP, et al: Characterization of a membrane pore-forming protein from *Entamoeba histolytica.* J Exp Med 156:1677–1690, 1982

26 Ravdin JI: Pathogenesis of disease caused by *Entamoeba histolytica:* Studies of adherence, secreted toxins, and contact-dependent cytolisis. Rev Infect Dis 8:247–260, 1986

27 Gitler C, Mirelman D: Factors contributing to the pathogenic behavior of *Entamoeba histolytica.* Annu Rev Microbiol 40:237–261, 1986

28 Martínez-Palomo A: The pathogenesis of amoebiasis. Parasitol Today 3:111–118, 1987

29 Mirelman D: Ameba bacterium relationships in amebiasis. Microbiol Rev 51:272–284, 1987

30 Trissl D: Immunology of *Entamoeba histolytica* in human and animal hosts. Rev Infect Dis 4:1154–1184, 1982

31 Healy GR: Immunologic tools in the diagnosis of amebiasis: Epidemiology in the United States. Rev Infect Dis 8:239–246, 1986

32 Kretschmer RR: Immunology of amebiasis, in Martínez-Palomo A (ed): *Amebiasis.* Elsevier, Amsterdam, 1986, pp 95–167

33 Prathap K, Gilman R: The histopathology of acute intestinal amebiasis. Am J Pathol 60:229–246, 1970

34 Pérez-Tamayo R: Pathology of amebiasis, in Martínez-Palomo A (ed): *Amebiasis.* Elsevier, Amsterdam, 1986, pp 45–94

35 Gutiérrez G, Ludlow A, Espinosa G, et al: National serologic survey. II. Search for antibodies against *Entamoeba histolytica* in Mexico, in Sepúlveda B, Diamond LS (eds): Proceedings of the International Conference on Amebiasis, Mexico, Instituto Mexicano del Seguro Social, 1976, pp 609–618

36 Knight R: Surveys for amebiasis. Interpretation of data and their implications. Ann Trop Med Parasitol 69:35–48, 1975

37 Bray RS, Harris WG: The epidemiology of infection with *Entamoeba histolytica* in the Gambia, West Africa. Trans R Soc Trop Med Hyg 71:401–407, 1977

38 Feachem RG, Bradley DJ, Garelick H, et al: *Sanitation and Disease: Health Aspects of Excreta and Water Management.* New York, Wiley, 1983

39 Nanda R, Baveja U, Anand BS: *Entamoeba histolytica* cyst passers: Clinical features and outcome in untreated subjects. Lancet ii:301–303, 1984

40 Jackson TFHG, Gathiram V: Seroepidemiological study of antibody responses to the zymodemes of *Entamoeba histolytica.* Lancet i:716–718, 1985

41 Adams EB, MacLeod IN: Invasive amebiasis. I. Amebic dysentery and its complications. Medicine 56:315–323, 1977

42 Juniper K: Acute amebic colitis. Am J Med 33:377–380, 1962

43 Fuchs G, Ruíz-Palacios GM, Pickering LK: Amebiasis in the pediatric population, in Ravdin JI (ed): *Amebiasis, Human Infection by* Entamoeba histolytica. New York, Wiley, 1988, pp 594–613

44 Gutiérrez-Trujillo G; Características principales de la amibiasis invasora en el niño. Arch Invest Med (Mex) 11(suppl 1):281–286, 1980

45 Blumecranz H, Kasen K, Romeu J, et al: The role of endoscopy in suspected amebiasis. Am J Gastroenterol 78:15–20, 1983

46 Cardoso JM, Kimura K, Stoopen M, et al: Radiology of invasive amebiasis of the colon. J Roentgenol 128:935–946, 1977

47 Balikian JP, Bitar JG, Rishani KK, et al: Fulminant necrotizing amebic colitis in children. Am J Proctol 28:69–78, 1977

48 Guarner V: Treatment of amebiasis, in Martínez-Palomo A (ed): *Amebiasis.* Amsterdam, Elsevier, 1986, pp 190–212

49 Radke RA: Ameboma of the intestine: An analysis of the disease as presented in 78 collected and 41 previously unreported cases. Ann Intern Med 43:1048–1066, 1955

50 Kalani BP, Sogani KC: Amoebic rectal bleeding in children. Am J Proctol 26:67–75, 1975

51 Merrit RJ, Coughlin E, Thomas DW, et al: Spectrum of amebiasis in children. Am J Dis Child 136:785–793, 1982

52 Jammal MA, Cox K, Ruebner B: Amebiasis presenting as rectal

bleeding without diarrhea in childhood. J Pediatr Gastroenterol Nutr 4:294–298, 1985

53 Krogstad DJ, Spencer HC, Healy GR: Current concepts in parasitology: Amebiasis. N Engl J Med 298:262–265, 1978

54 Akhtaruzzaman KM, Bienzle U, Rosenkaimer F, et al: Comparison of different methods for the detection of intestinal protozoa and helminths in stool. Trop Med Parasitol 29:427–436, 1978

55 Sepúlveda B, Treviño-García Manzo N: Clinical manifestations and diagnosis of amebiasis, in Martínez-Palomo A (ed): *Amebiasis.* Amsterdam, Elsevier, 1986, pp 170–188

56 Adams EB, MacLeod IN: Invasive amebiasis. II. Amebic liver abscess and its complications. Medicine 56:325–334, 1977

57 Dehesa M, Cairo A, Wolpert E: Estudio retrospectivo de 125 enfermos con absceso hepático amibiano. Rev Invest Clin 27:129–133, 1975

58 Sukov RJ, Cohen LJ, Sample WF: Sonography of hepatic amebic abscess. Am J Radiol 134:911–915, 1980

59 Katzenstein D, Rickerson V, Braude A: New concepts of amebic liver abscess derived from hepatic imaging, serodiagnosis, and hepatic enzymes in 67 consecutive cases in San Diego. Medicine 61:237–246, 1982

60 Conter RL, Pitt HA, Thompkins RK, et al: Differentiation of pyogenic from amebic hepatic abscesses. Surg Gynecol Obstet 162:114–120, 1986

61 Barnes PF, De Cock KM, Reynolds TN, et al: A comparison of amebic and pyogenic abscess of the liver. Medicine 66:472–483, 1987

62 Elizondo G, Wiessleder R, Stark DD, et al: Amebic liver abscess: Diagnosis and treatment evaluation with MR imaging. Radiology 165:795–800, 1987

63 Quinn MJ, Sheedy PF, Stephens DH, et al: Computed tomography of the abdomen in evaluation of patients with fever of unknown origin. Radiology 136:407–410, 1980

64 Knobloch J, Mannweiler E: Development and persistence of antibodies to *Entamoeba histolytica* in patients with amoebic liver abscess: Analysis of 216 cases. Am J Trop Med Hyg 32:727–732, 1983

65 Beard CM, Noller KL, O'Fallon WM, et al: Lack of evidence for cancer due to use of metronidazole. N Engl J Med 301:519–522, 1979

66 Wolfe MS: Nondysenteric intestinal amebiasis: Treatment with diloxanide furoate. JAMA 224:1601–1603, 1973

67 Guevara L, García Tsao G, Uscanga LF: A study with quinfamide in the treatment of chronic amebiasis in adults. Clin Ther 6:43–48, 1983

68 Gathiram V, Jackson TFHG: A longitudinal study of asymptomatic carriers of pathogenic zymodemes of *Entamoeba histolytica.* S Afr Med J 72:669–672, 1987

69 Allason-Jones E, Mindel A, Sargeaunt P, et al: *Entamoeba histolytica* as a commensal intestinal parasite in homosexual men. N Engl J Med 315:353–356, 1986

70 Mathews HM, Moss DM, Healy GR, et al: Isoenzyme analysis of *Entamoeba histolytica* isolated from homosexual men. J Infect Dis 153:793–795, 1987

71 Thompson JE, Forlenza S, Verma R: Amebic liver abscess: A therapeutic approach. Rev Infect Dis 7:171–179, 1985

72 Ralls PW, Barnes PF, Johnson MB, et al: Medical treatment of hepatic amebic abscess: Rare need for percutaneous drainage. Radiology 165:805–807, 1987

73 Elsdon-Dew R: Amebiasis as a world problem. Bull NY Acad Med 47:438–447, 1968

74 Walsh JA: Problems in recognition and diagnosis of amebiasis: Estimation of the global magnitude of morbidity and mortality. Rev Infect Dis 8:228–238, 1986

75 Martínez-Palomo A, Martínez-Báez M: Selective primary health care: Strategies for control of disease in the developing world. X. Amebiasis. Rev Infect Dis 5:1093–1102, 1983

76 Martínez-Palomo A: Amoebiasis. Clin Trop Med Commun Dis 1:587–601, 1986

77 Walsh J, Martínez-Palomo A: Control of amebiasis, in Martínez-Palomo A (ed): *Amebiasis* Amsterdam, Elsevier, 1986, pp 241–260

78 Reed SL, Braude AI: Extraintestinal disease: Clinical syndromes, diagnostic profile and therapy, in Ravdin JI (ed): *Amebiasis. Human Infection with* Entamoeba histolytica. New York, Wiley, 1988

CHAPTER 38 / *Giardiasis* · David P. Stevens · Frances D. Gillin

INTRODUCTION

It is suspected that *Giardia* was the first protozoan seen by van Leeuwenhoek with his primitive microscope in 1681. In an often-quoted description of van Leeuwenhoek's notebooks, Dobell [1] has referred to the motile "animicules" that are thought to have been *Giardia* found in van Leeuwenhoek's own watery stool.

Giardiasis is of worldwide distribution and is both endemic and epidemic. It is the most frequently encountered protozoan disease in the United States and the most common identified cause of waterborne enteric disease. It frequently poses both diagnostic and treatment problems, since therapy may not result in its eradication. The contribution of giardiasis to the malnutrition and mortality caused by diarrheal diseases in developing countries has been incompletely assessed. Its high prevalence in such a setting, however, suggests a significant role for this ubiquitous protozoan. Insights have been gained using animal models of this infection, in vitro cultivation of the trophozoites, and detailed study of its biochemistry and cell biology.

THE PARASITE

MORPHOLOGY AND LIFE CYCLE

Infection with *Giardia lamblia* is initiated by ingestion of cysts in contaminated water or food. Once ingested, cysts are triggered to excyst by exposure to low gastric pH. It is crucial that the trophozoite not emerge until the cyst passes into the duodenum since trophozoites are killed by gastric acid. The newly emerged trophozoite immediately divides into two daughters which can multiply, colonize the upper small intestine, and cause symptoms.

The binucleate trophozoite of *G. lamblia* is shaped like half a pear (Fig. 38-1). It uses four pairs of flagella to swim freely in the intestinal lumen, where it is exposed to bile and changing mixtures of nutrients, digestive enzymes, and their products. Trophozoites also penetrate the mucous layer and use their ventral adhesive disc to attach to the underlying epithelial cells (Fig. 38-2). This attachment is important for maintenance of infection since parasites that do not attach or actively swim upstream would be swept downstream by the flow of intestinal fluid. Prolonged (greater than 2 years) multiplication of trophozoites in the human upper small intestine is well-documented.

If *Giardia* trophozoites move downstream, they must either complete their life cycle by encysting or die, since trophozoites do not naturally survive long outside the host. In contrast, cysts are well-adapted to survival and remain viable for months in cold water. Relatively little is known about the cyst form of *Giardia*, largely because encystation has only recently been induced in vitro. Earlier studies were conducted with cysts isolated from the feces of infected humans or animals.

The cysts of *G. lamblia* are quadrinucleated oval bodies with a long axis of 8 to 12 μm. The most striking difference from the trophozoite is the cyst wall, which contains chitin and stage-specific antigens. It is likely that the wall is responsible for the great resistance of cysts to hypotonic lysis and disinfection by chlorination.

STRAINS AND HOST RANGE

Giardia isolates from many mammals cannot be distinguished from *G. lamblia* morphologically and are referred to as *duo-*

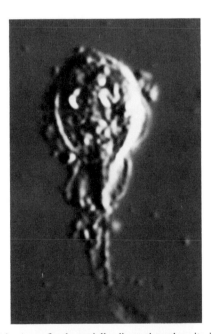

Figure 38-1. An unfixed, partially digested trophozoite in the fluid phase of a duodenal aspirate from a patient with chronic symptomatic giardiasis, photographed with Nomarski differential interference contrast optics. × 4000. This patient exhibited typical symptoms of giardiasis (alternating periods of diarrhea and constipation, abdominal cramping, flatulence, bloating, and extreme fatigue) over a period of several years. Three stools were negative for ova and parasites, and the diagnosis was made by direct microscopic examination of fluid aspirated just below the ligament of Treitz.

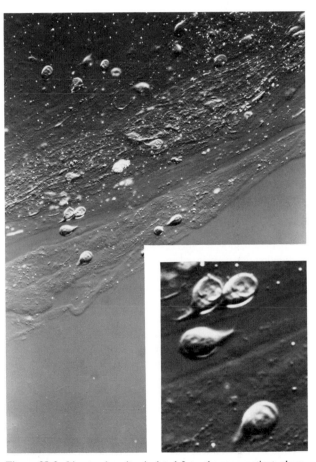

Figure 38-2. Live trophozoites isolated from the same patient, showing association with intestinal mucus. Photographed with Nomarski differential interference contrast optics. Inset: higher magnification, × 2000.

denalis type. Other groups of strains from rodents or amphibians differ in subcellular morphology.

It is not clear, at present, whether a single *Giardia* strain can infect multiple host species, because the results of cross-species transmission studies are conflicting. Confusion in the taxonomy of the genus *Giardia* may soon be resolved by studies of the DNA and protein relationships of isolates from different hosts [2].

ANIMAL MODELS

An animal model of *Giardia muris* infection in mice [3] has facilitated the study of the host's immune reactivity to this infection. Techniques for quantification of trophozoites in small intestine and of cysts in stool provided the means to measure the intensity of infection. In immunologically competent mice, infection reached its peak at about 7 days after inoculation. Thereafter it trailed off and was usually cleared in 6 to 8 weeks. Congenitally thymus-deficient nude mice could be chronically infected [4]. This finding suggested an important role for thymus-dependent immunity in the host's defense against this infection. The biological role for humoral immunity in the murine model was less clear, although specific antibodies developed in serum, intestinal secretions, and milk.

In another model [5], gerbils infected with *G. lamblia* isolates spontaneously cleared the infection and were resistant to challenge with both the same and heterologous strains. They could be infected with both trophozoites and cysts. Cyst excretion by infected animals was intermittent. Trophozoites were found predominantly in the upper small intestine except when infection was heavy, when they were found more widely throughout the intestine.

THE PATIENT

PATHOPHYSIOLOGY

Neither the pathogenic mechanisms nor the extreme variability in duration and severity of giardiasis are currently understood. Untreated infections either may be self-limited or may persist for years. Symptoms may be extremely debilitating and include severe diarrhea, malabsorption, and failure to thrive. Other presentations include weakness, anorexia, vomiting, and abdominal cramps. Alternatively, infection may produce no apparent symptoms, regardless of the duration of infection.

Pathogenesis of this protozoan infection probably results from a complex combination of parasitic factors and host responses. The small-bowel epithelium may be altered morphologically in giardiasis with shortened villi and elongated crypts (Fig. 38-3). Populations of both lymphocytes and polymorphonuclear leukocytes may be increased in the submucosa. Viewed by electron microscopy, epithelial cells are often deformed with blunting of microvilli. Proposed mechanisms for these changes include the physical blockage by *Giardia* covering the epithelium, competition between the parasite and the

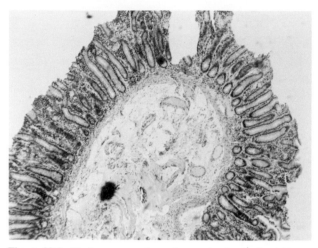

Figure 38-3. Medium-power photomicrograph of a duodenal biopsy obtained from an infected subject with symptoms of diarrhea, steatorrhea, and weight loss. A picture typical of small-intestinal malabsorption is seen with shortened villi and elongated crypts. H&E, × 600.

host for nutrients, direct damage of the intestinal epithelium by overlying and adherent trophozoites, cellular inflammatory reaction in the submucosa, and other mechanisms mediated by the host's immune system. None of these hypothetical mechanisms is exclusive, and there is no direct evidence for any of them.

Three factors that seem important for susceptibility to infection are age, previous exposure to the parasite, and compromised immune status. Children seem to be more frequently infected than adults. Whether this represents cumulative acquired resistance by adults or is more related to hygienic practices is unclear. Previous exposure in humans makes subsequent infection less likely. In a study in Colorado where giardiasis was endemic, the attack rate for visitors was higher than that for long-term residents. On the other hand, in certain less-developed countries, virtually all residents may pass cysts at some time during the course of a year.

The presence of certain immune abnormalities seems to render the human host more susceptible. Symptomatic giardiasis does not appear to be a major problem in patients with AIDS. *Giardia* infection, however, has been associated with nodular lymphoid hyperplasia of the small bowel, dysgammaglobulinemias, and so-called hypogammaglobulinemic sprue. Circulating immunoglobulins do not seem to play a role in protection against *Giardia*, although a role for secretory IgA has been postulated.

A potential role for breast-feeding as a protective measure in giardiasis has been suggested by experimental studies [6]. Female mice that were previously infected with *G. muris* were bred. After delivery of their litters, the mothers shed large numbers of cysts in their stool. When the offspring were weaned, the cyst excretion ceased spontaneously. The litters, on the other hand, were protected against *Giardia* infection by breast-feeding on immune mothers. Breast-fed offspring that were wet-nursed on immune mothers were protected against infection with the same strain, while those born to immune mothers and wet-nursed on nonimmune mothers were susceptible. It is suspected that gut-associated lymphoid tissue that has been primed by antigens of *Giardia* migrates to the breast during lactation. This may render the mother vulnerable to multiplication of the trophozoites in the unprotected small intestine [6].

Studies of human milk have shown that it kills *Giardia* trophozoites in vitro [7]. Fresh human milk from which IgA has been removed similarly kills *Giardia*. Killing appears to be mediated by unsaturated fatty acids that are released from milk triglycerides by bile salt–stimulated lipase of human milk [8]. On the other hand, human intestinal mucus probably protects trophozoites from killing by milk and fatty acids.

CLINICAL PICTURE: STUDIES OF HUMAN VOLUNTEERS AND TRAVELERS

The human volunteer studies of Rendtorff in the mid-1950s [9] showed that the great majority of infected subjects remained asymptomatic. The prepatent period averaged 9 days; cyst excretion tended to be erratic.

Recently, Nash and coworkers infected volunteers by duodenal intubation with axenically cultured trophozoites [10]. Three of five subjects exhibited the typical symptoms of giardiasis. Attempts to reinfect this group led to active infection in two of four rechallenged subjects, but typical symptoms were not observed.

In 324 North Americans who returned from Russia with giardiasis, diarrhea was by far the most common symptom [11]. As seen in Table 38-1, weakness, weight loss, cramping, and nausea were the other common symptoms.

The classical observations of Hoskins and coworkers [12] demonstrated that *Giardia* caused mucosal dysfunction char-

acterized by steatorrhea, D-xylose malabsorption, disaccharidase deficiency, and vitamin B_{12} deficiency. These pathophysiological changes resolved after successful treatment. Clinically, lactase deficiency and milk intolerance often may resolve slowly after successful treatment, presumably due to slow reestablishment of mucosal enzyme activity.

DIAGNOSIS AND TREATMENT

The index of suspicion for giardiasis must be high in any patient with diarrhea, especially in patients with typical epidemiological and clinical histories. Physical findings are nonspecific although abdominal tympany, hyperactive bowel sounds, and diffuse mild tenderness are frequent. Rectal and sigmoidoscopic exams are normal. The hemogram is normal. While barium studies have no place in the evaluation for giardiasis, edema of the small intestine should raise the suspicion of giardiasis when it is seen in gastrointestinal x-rays done for other indications. Examination of up to three stool specimens for cysts may be necessary to establish the diagnosis since the stool exam is frequently negative. If the stool is negative for cysts or trophozoites, duodenal contents may be examined for trophozoites (Fig. 38-4). This may be accomplished by aspiration of duodenal contents, or, more easily, by use of the Enterotest (HEDECO, Mountain View, Calif.). This device employs a string that is contained in a gelatin capsule (Fig. 38-5). The string unfolds out of an opening in one end as the capsule is swallowed. Trophozoites adherent to the string, which is later retrieved, can be scraped onto a slide and identified microscopically (Fig. 38-6). The simplicity and economy of this technique often obviates referral of the patient for specialized consultation.

Patients may be treated with quinacrine hydrochloride, 100 mg for adults or 2 mg/kg for younger children, three times daily for 7 to 10 days. Alternatively, metronidazole, 250 mg

Table 38-1. Symptoms in travelers who returned from Russia with giardiasis

Symptom	Prevalence, %
Diarrhea	96
Weakness	72
Weight loss	62
Abdominal cramps	61
Nausea	60
Greasy stools	57
Abdominal distension	42
Flatulence	39
Vomiting	29
Belching	26
Fever	17

Source: From [*11*].

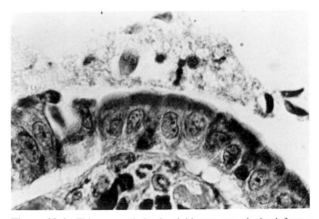

Figure 38-4. This per oral duodenal biopsy was obtained from a subject with giardiasis. *Giardia* trophozoites are seen in the mucous layer overlying the mucosal epithelium. H&E, × 2000.

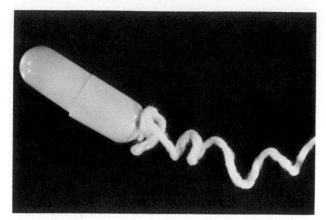

Figure 38-5. The Enterotest is a gelatin capsule containing a nylon string that unfolds out of an opening in one end as the capsule is swallowed. The string is later retrieved, and bile-stained duodenal contents are expressed onto a microscope slide for examination in search of motile *Giardia* trophozoites.

for adults or 5 mg/kg for children, three times daily for 7 days may also be used. The use of the latter drug in giardiasis is not listed in the package insert but is recommended by the Centers for Disease Control. The reports of potential mutagenesis or carcinogenesis with metronidazole in experimental settings require that it be used with caution in children or pregnant women. Treatment failure occurs in 5 to 20 percent of infections, and repeated treatment may be necessary.

In the developing world *Giardia* is a frequent isolate in surveys for stool pathogens but often is not associated with recognizable disease in adults. Inadequate water purification and sewage disposal are incriminated as the dominant cause of its high prevalence. In this setting giardiasis in children has been associated with significant reduction in rate of weight gain and growth, both of which are corrected by treatment [13].

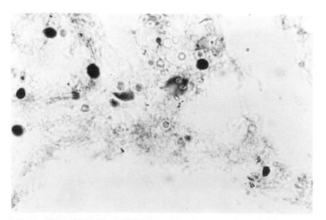

Figure 38-6. *Giardia* trophozoites are seen in a light micrograph of mucus obtained from the duodenum of an infected subject. H&E, × 2000.

POPULATION

EPIDEMIOLOGY

Giardiasis in North America is generally found in four epidemiological settings. First, breakdown in water purification systems has been associated with outbreaks of infection. Second, hikers or travelers returning from highly endemic areas such as the Rocky Mountains, Central America, Russia, and India are at increased risk. Third, several animal reservoirs may be associated with human infections. Finally, person-to-person spread has been documented and poses a particular problem in day-care centers [14]. Foodborne outbreaks have been reported less frequently.

Breakdown of water purification

Craun documented 90 outbreaks of waterborne giardiasis in the United States in the 20-year period between 1967 and 1986, accounting for 23,765 individual cases of giardiasis [15]. Sixty-nine percent of these outbreaks were associated with breakdown in filtration systems. It is of note that the level of chlorination normally found in water purification systems is not adequate to inactivate *Giardia* cysts.

Animal reservoirs

Although *Giardia* has no intermediate host, cysts have been isolated from feces of many animal species. However, most of these same animal hosts are probably not susceptible to human *Giardia*. Two notable exceptions appear to be the beaver and the dog [16]. The beaver has been incriminated by circumstantial evidence in that colonies are frequently found upstream from water supplies that serve as sources of *Giardia* infection in humans. Cross-infectivity of *Giardia* between humans and dogs has been reported.

CONTROL

The strategy for control of *Giardia* infection requires at least three components: (1) treatment of all infected persons; (2) water purification programs; and (3) development of an effective vaccine [17].

Treatment of infected communities results in improvement of growth and development in preschool-age children, even if subsequent reinfection might be anticipated [13]. Such treatment reduces the human reservoir of infection and, consequently, reduces the opportunity for water supply contamination and person-to-person spread.

Repeated treatment of individuals will have little long-term impact if water filtration and sewage disposal systems are not improved. The cost of such programs in developing countries is difficult to justify for anti-*Giardia* programs alone and is most readily supported as part of an effort to control all waterborne enteric infections [17].

Development of an effective vaccine for use in travelers to endemic areas and children residing in endemic areas seems justified. Further research in the mechanism of the host's immune response and refinement of understanding of immunizing antigens of the infecting organism may lead to an effective vaccination strategy for this infection. In the interim, effective pharmacological treatment and efforts to improve water and sewage management in at-risk communities are appropriate intermediate goals.

REFERENCES

1 Dobell C: Discovery of intestinal protozoa in man. Proc R Soc Med 13:1–15, 1920

2 Nash TE, McCutchan T, Keister D, et al: Endonuclease restriction analysis of DNA from 15 *Giardia lamblia* isolates obtained from man and animals. J Infect Dis 152:64–73, 1985

3 Roberts-Thomson IC, Stevens DP, Mahmoud AAF, et al: Acquired resistance to infection in an animal model of giardiasis. J Immunol 117:2037–2037, 1976

4 Stevens DP, Frank DM, Mahmoud AAF: Thymus dependency of host resistance to *Giardiasis muris* infection: Studies in nude mice. J Immunol 120:680–682, 1978

5 Belosevic M, Faubert GM, MacLean JD, et al: *Giardia lamblia* infections in Mongolian gerbils: An animal model. J Infect Dis 147:222–226, 1983

6 Stevens DP, Frank DM: Local immunity in murine giardiasis: Is milk protection at the expense of maternal gut? Trans Assoc Am Phys 91:268–272, 1978

7 Gillin FD, Reiner DS, Wang CS: Human milk kills parasitic intestinal protozoa. Science 221:1290–1292, 1983

8 Gillin FD, Reiner DS, Gault MJ: Cholate-dependent killing of *Giardia lamblia* by human milk. Infect Immunol 47:619–622, 1985

9 Rendtorff RC, Holt CJ: The experimental transmission of human intestinal protozoan parasites. IV. Attempts to transmit *Entamoeba coli* and *Giardia lamblia* cysts by water. Am J Hyg 60:327–338, 1954.

10 Nash TE, Herrington DA, Losonsky GA, et al: Experimental human infections with *Giardia lamblia*. J Infect Dis 156:974–984, 1987

11 Brodsky RE, Spencer HC, Schultz MG: Giardiasis in American travelers to the Soviet Union. J Infect Dis 130:319–323, 1974

12 Hoskins LC, Winawer SJ, Broitman SA, et al: Clinical giardiasis and intestinal malabsorption. Gastroenterology 53:265–279, 1967

13 Gupta MC, Urrutia JJ: Effect of periodic antiascaris and antigiardia treatment on nutritional status of preschool children. Am J Clin Nutrition 36:79–86, 1982

14 Keystone JS, Krajden S, Warren MR: Person-to-person transmission of *Giardia lamblia* in day-care nurseries. CMAJ 119:241–258, 1978

15 Craun GF: Waterborne giardiasis in the United States 1965–84. Lancet 2:513–514, 1986

16 Davies RB, Hibler CP: Animal reservoirs and cross-species transmission of *Giardia,* in Jakubowski W, Hoff JC (eds): Waterborne Transmission of Giardiasis. U.S. Environmental Protection Agency, 104–126, 1979

17 Stevens DP: Selective primary health care: Strategies for control of disease in the developing world. XIX. Giardiasis. Rev Infect Dis 7:530–535, 1985

CHAPTER 39 / # Balantidiasis and Other Intestinal Protozoa · John H. Cross

Balantidiasis is infection with the large ciliated protozoon *Balantidium coli*. Most ciliated protozoa live as commensals in the guts of vertebrates and invertebrates, and *B. coli* is the only member of the group that infects human beings and causes disease. There are free-living ciliates in water, and many are found in the rumen of ruminants and the large intestines of equines where they are involved with the animal's digestive processes.

PARASITE

LIFE CYCLE

B. coli is usually found in the trophozoite stage in the lumen of the large intestine of human beings and animals. It feeds on material in the intestine, including cellular debris, bacteria, starch, and mucus. The trophozoite divides by transverse binary fusion (asexual phase) and sometimes by conjugation in which nuclear material is exchanged between two organisms (sexual phase). Cysts are formed in the lumen of the colon or in freshly evacuated feces by a rounding up of the trophozoite, partial retraction of cilia, and secretion of a cyst wall.

The cyst is the infectious stage and is acquired by the host by ingestion of food and water contaminated with infected feces. Excystation occurs in the small intestine, and the parasite colonizes in the colon and terminal ileum.

MORPHOLOGY [1]

The trophozoites are ovoid organisms covered by a thin pellicle, with projecting longitudinal rows of slightly oblique cilia which can propel the organism rapidly forward or backward. The trophozoites range from 40 to 55 by 30 to 150 μm in size. The anterior end is narrower and contains a funnel-shaped depression, the periostome, which communicates with a cy-

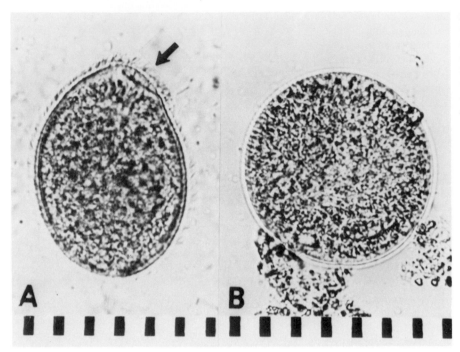

Figure 39-1. *Balantidium coli* in wet unstained preparation. *A.* Trophozoite, arrow pointing to periostome. *B.* Cyst with cilia still visible, Scale in 10-μm units. (*From M. Paulson (ed): Gastroenterologic Medicine, Lea & Febiger, Philadelphia, 1969, p. 501, Fig. 24–27, by permission.*)

tostome and cytopharynx. At the posterior end there is a barely visible tiny opening, the cytopyge, which has an excretory function. The cytoplasm contains a large, kidney-shaped mass of chromatin, the macronucleus, which regulates cytoplasmic activity. A much smaller vesicular micronucleus, concerned with reproduction, lies in the notch of the macronucleus. The cytoplasm contains a large contractile vacuole near the cytopyge, another large vacuole near the center of the body, and numerous small food vacuoles containing starch granules and sometimes red blood cells. (See Fig. 39-1*A*.)

The cyst is round or ovoid, measures 40 to 65 μm in length, and has an opaque, dirty, faintly greenish-yellow tint in fresh preparations. The cilia and cytostome may be visible during encystment but thereafter are not visible. Barlike, colorless cytoplasmic inclusions also are visible in fresh preparations but disappear on staining. The macronucleus is not visible in fresh preparations (see Fig. 39-1*B*).

PATIENT

HOST-PARASITE INTERFACE [1]

Trophozoites of *B. coli* are facultative anaerobes and require a normal intestinal bacterial flora for their growth. They find the colon of the host the most favorable site to colonize. Whether or not mucosal invasion occurs in asymptomatic human infections is not known. When circumstances are favorable, trophozoites invade the mucosa, mechanically by ciliary action and their ability to secrete hyaluronidase and probably other enzymes.

PATHOGENESIS [1–4]

Trophozoites produce mucosal lesions similar to those of amebiasis. The ulcers are shallow, rounded, or occasionally irregular, and vary from pinpoint size to 1 to 2 cm in diameter with little tendency for undermining of the edge. The ulcers are most numerous in the rectosigmoid but involve the entire colon, and occasionally the appendix and terminal ileum. There is little tissue reaction about the ulcers unless secondary bacterial infection occurs. The mucosa between the ulcers is normal except for occasional small hemorrhages. Trophozoites have been found invading all layers and the blood vessels of the wall of the colon, and even in the regional lymph nodes, in unusually severe infections in debilitated patients. Perforation of the colon has been reported and there are scattered reports of the parasite in extraintestinal locations, such as the vagina, liver, and lungs.

CLINICAL MANIFESTATIONS [1–5]

About one in five infections is symptomatic in reported series. Usually the course is chronic with episodes of intermittent diarrhea of varying severity and constipation. Dysentery, similar to that seen in amebiasis, may develop. There may also be abdominal pain, tenderness over the colon, anorexia, nausea, weight loss, and weakness. The course can be fulminating and fatal in debilitated patients. Bowel movements can number from 5 to 24, are mushy or watery, contain mucus and sometimes blood, and have a pigpen odor. The patient's breath also can be fetid, and weight loss can be severe.

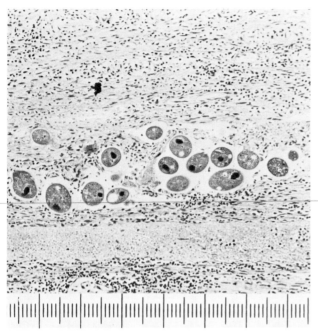

Figure 39-2. *Balantidium coli* trophozoites in tissue of cecal ulcer in a chimpanzee. H&E, scale in 10-μm units. (*Specimen courtesy of Dr. Harold McClure, Yerkes Primate Center, Emory University, Atlanta, Georgia.*)

DIAGNOSIS [1–5]

Diagnosis is made by demonstrating the organism in feces or in scrapings or by endoscopic biopsy of an ulcer (see Fig. 39-2). *B. coli* is shed irregularly, and repeated examinations may be necessary. Usually only the trophozoite stage is found, cysts being found in only 10 percent of cases. The organisms are easily mistaken for plant cells or other debris because of their large size and dirty, opaque appearance. Trophozoites disintegrate rapidly in defecated fecal specimens, so fresh specimens must be examined rapidly or placed in preservative solutions. The macronucleus of *B. coli* is the feature that permits differentiation from free-living ciliates which can occasionally contaminate fecal specimens. The feces typically contain Charcot-Leyden crystals but few polymorphonuclear leukocytes.

MANAGEMENT [6]

In the past, before specific therapy became available, balantidiasis was fatal in up to 30 percent of cases, with malnutrition undoubtedly playing an important role. The infection is cured by administration of 500 mg of tetracycline qid for 10 days [40 mg/(kg·day) up to 2 g daily for children]. Metronidazole (750 mg tid for 5 days) and iodoquinol (600 mg tid for 20 days) are also reported effective.

POPULATION

RESERVOIR [1–3]

B. coli is a zoonosis and has been found in hogs, wild boars, sheep, horses, bovines, guinea pigs, rats, fowl, turtles, cockroaches, and a number of higher primates. Of these animals, the hog is the most commonly and heavily parasitized. Usually the organism is a commensal in pigs, but on occasion it can cause a mild to severe enteritis with ulcerations, hemorrhage, and death. Rat association with domestic pigs may be important in maintaining reservoir infections in both animals.

EPIDEMIOLOGY

The pig is the most important animal reservoir for human infection. About 25 percent of infected persons give a history of contact with pigs. Water contaminated by pigs was believed to be the source of an outbreak of 110 cases of balantidiasis in Truk after a typhoon reported in 1973 [7]. The infection also can be transmitted from human to human, which was the likely source of a 4.9 percent infection rate found in 142 patients examined in a mental hospital in South Carolina and reported in 1939. [8].

Infections have been reported from most parts of the world including Russia, Scandinavia, Germany, Italy, Cuba, North and South America, Africa, Sunda Isles, China, and the Philippines. Most surveys for intestinal parasites which mention *B. coli* were taken prior to 1960. The parasite was known to be endemic in the Seychelles Islands for many years, and in a 1979 report 80 cases were documented. Most were chronic and asymptomatic [9]. In Papua New Guinea the prevalence of infection is high (2 to 29 percent) with women most often infected; pigs sleep in "women's houses" [10]. In stool surveys conducted throughout the Philippine Islands, *B. coli* was found in less than 1 percent of the over 30,000 specimens examined [11]. In Peru, 6 percent of a studied population was found to be infected with the parasite [12]. Sporadic infrequent infections have been reported in the United States and Canada in the past, but balantidiasis now is quite rare in these countries. Probably healthy humans are quite resistant to infection with *Balantidium*. Achlorhydria, an unusually heavy inoculum, and debilitation are likely to predispose to human infection. About one in five cases becomes symptomatic.

PREVENTION

Balantidiasis is a problem only in those countries where sanitation and hygiene are poor and malnutrition is common. Improvements in these areas should eliminate most human contact with the parasite.

CONTROL

Elimination of the infection from animal reservoirs does not appear practical. Reducing human contact with infected pigs and possibly rats and with contaminated food and water and restoring resistance to infection by improving nutrition are the methods for control.

REFERENCES

1 Arean VM, Koppisch E: Balantidiasis: A review and report of cases. Am J Pathol 32:1089–1115, 1956
2 Rivasi F, Giannotti T: *Balantidium coli* in cervico-vaginal cytology: A case report. Pathologica 75:439–442, 1983
3 Auz JL: Absceso hepatico balantidiano. Rev Med Panama 9:51–55, 1984
4 Dauodal P, Wagschal G, Delacour IL, et al: Balantidiose pulmonaire: Un case en Franche-Comté. Presse Med 15:257, 1986
5 Castro J, Vazquez-Iglesias JL, Arnal-Monreal F: Dysentery caused by *Balantidium coli*: Report of two cases. Endoscopy 15:272–274, 1983
6 Drugs for parasitic infections. Med Lett Drugs Ther 30:15–24, 1988
7 Walzer PD, Judson FN, Murphy KB, et al: Balantidiasis outbreak in Truk. Am J Trop Med Hyg 22:33–41, 1973
8 Young MD: Balantidiasis. JAMA 113:580–584, 1939
9 Nuti M, Sanguigni S, DeBac C: Osservazioni su di un Focolaio Endemico di Balantidiasi (Studio di 80 casi). Ann Med Nav 84:641–646, 1979
10 Radford AJ: Balantidiasis in Papua New Guinea. Med J Aust 1:238–241, 1973
11 Cross JH, Basaca-Sevilla V: Biomedical surveys in the Philippines. NAMRU-2 SP47:1–117, 1984
12 Bouree P, David P, Basset D, et al: Enquête epidémiologique sur les parasitoses intestinales en Amazonie peruvienne. Bull Soc Path Exot Filiales 77:690–698, 1984.

CHAPTER 40

Human Coccidial Infections: Cryptosporidiosis and Isosporiasis

• *Rosemary Soave*

CRYPTOSPORIDIOSIS

Cryptosporidiosis is an infection of the gastrointestinal tract that is caused by the coccidian protozoan parasite *Cryptosporidium*. First recognized over three-quarters of a century ago, this parasite was for many years considered a benign commensal; it was subsequently regarded solely as a pathogen of animals. In the early 1980s, detection of *Cryptosporidium* in patients with AIDS and severe enteritis led to increased awareness and knowledge of the parasite's disease-causing potential in the human host [1–3]. Human infection is characterized by watery diarrhea, cramping abdominal pain, malabsorption, and weight loss that is usually self-limited in the immunologically intact host but severe and unremitting in the immunocompromised patient. No effective therapy is yet known for this disease. Although the true prevalence of cryptosporidiosis is unknown, recent studies suggest that it is a common cause of diarrhea worldwide, particularly in young children. Laboratory investigation of *Cryptosporidium* has been exceptionally difficult due to inability to cultivate it in vitro, the absence of a symptomatic small animal model of the disease, its small size, and its defiance of biological rules. *Cryptosporidium*, which means "hidden spore" in Greek, was aptly named, since many years after its discovery it continues to elude practitioners of both human and animal medicine.

PARASITE

Historical aspects

Cryptosporidium was first described in 1907 by Tyzzer, who found it in the gastric glands of asymptomatic mice [4]. Initially thought to be nonpathogenic, it was first recognized as a cause of disease in poultry in 1955 [5]. In subsequent studies, *Cryptosporidium* was found to cause serious disease in several animal species, including calves and lambs; it is now considered to be responsible for major agricultural losses yearly in the United States [1–3,6].

The first seven cases of human cryptosporidiosis were reported between 1976 and 1981 [1–3]. Since most of the patients were immunocompromised, the parasite was thought to be opportunistic, and the disease was believed to occur rarely. By the end of 1982, identification of *Cryptosporidium* in 47 patients with AIDS stimulated the medical community's interest in the parasite. Soon thereafter, reports of outbreaks in animal handlers [7] and travelers [8,9] led to the realization that *Cryptosporidium* is also an important diarrheal pathogen in the immunocompetent host, as well. Popularization of stool examination for detection of the parasite has facilitated diagnosis. As more physicians have looked for the parasite, the number of reported cases has steadily increased, and crypto-

Figure 40-1. Life cycle of *Crypto-sporidium*. *(Modified from J.R. Navin, D.D. Juranek, Rev Infect Dis 6:313-327, 1984.)*

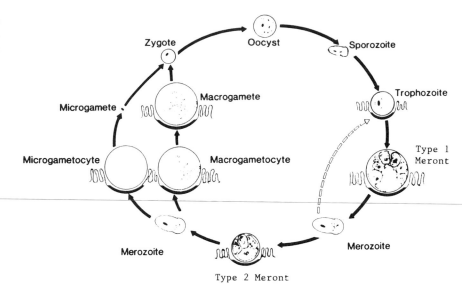

sporidiosis has become recognized as an important public health problem worldwide.

Taxonomy and nomenclature

Based on its having aflagellar but motile sporozoites with an apical complex, *Cryptosporidium* has been assigned to the phylum Apicomplexa, class Sporozoasida [10]. As a member of the order Eucoccidiorida, it is taxonomically related to *Isospora, Eimeria, Toxoplasma, Sarcocystis*, and *Plasmodium* species. *Cryptosporidium* is distinguished from other coccidia by its ability to develop just under the host epithelial cell membrane, an intracellular but extracytoplasmic position. Particularly interesting, however, is the parasite's morphological and biological similarities to the unclassified protozoan *Pneumocystis carinii*. Although 20 species of *Cryptosporidium* have been named for the host in which they were found, recent cross-transmission studies indicate a lack of host specificity and suggest that a much smaller number of species is valid [11]. *Cryptosporidium parvum*, originally described by Tyzzer (1912), and recently validated by Levine [10], as well as Upton and Current [12], is believed to be responsible for cryptosporidial enteritis in humans and cattle.

Life cycle

Unlike other coccidia such as *Toxoplasma* and *Isospora, Cryptosporidium* develops entirely within a single host (monoxenous) (Fig. 40-1). The acid-fast oocyst is 2 to 5 μm in diameter (Fig. 40-2) and when fully mature (sporulated) contains four naked (no sporocyst) sporozoites. Dissolution of a single suture on the oocyst wall allows the flat, thin, (2 to 4 by 6 to 8 μm) sporozoites to exit (excystation) (Fig. 40-3). They move by gliding and implant in the host epithelial cell, where they develop into trophozoites. Asexual multiplication (merogony) re-

sults in the formation of type 1 and type 2 meronts (schizonts). Type 1 meronts release 6 to 8 merozoites that reinvade the host and reinitiate merogony. The four merozoites released from type 2 meronts differentiate into micro (male) and macro (female) gametocytes and initiate sexual multiplication (gamogony). Fertilized macrogametes develop into oocysts that can either reinfect the same host or exit the body in search of a new host. Investigators have reported that variation in oocyst morphology determines outcome, i.e., thin-walled cysts reinfect, whereas the hardy, thick-walled cysts are expelled into the environment [13]. The characteristics of the *Cryptosporidium* life cycle impart to it a tremendous potential for reinfection within a single host, thus providing a mechanism for the sustained infection manifested by the immunocompromised host.

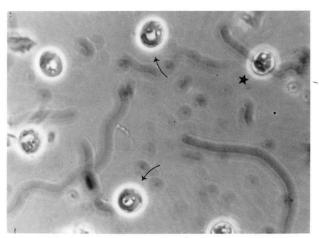

Figure 40-2. Human stool–derived unsporulated (arrows) and sporulated (star) *Cryptosporidium* oocysts. Phase contrast, × 630.

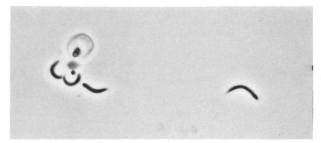

Figure 40-3. Excystation of *Cryptosporidium* oocyst with release of four sporozoites. Phase contrast, × 630.

PATIENT "HOST"

Pathology and pathogenesis

The histopathology of human cryptosporidial infection is based on study of biopsied tissue obtained predominantly from immunocompromised (AIDS) patients [*14,15*]. Although most commonly found attached to epithelial cells of the small intestine (Fig. 40-4), in these patients *Cryptosporidium* has also been detected in the pharynx, esophagus, stomach, duodenum, colon, rectum, gallbladder, bile, and pancreatic ducts. Ultrastructural studies of infected intestine have revealed endogenous stages of the parasite nestled between microvilli and enclosed within a parasitophorous vacuole, i.e., just under the host cell membrane in a unique intracellular yet extracytoplasmic location (Fig. 40-5). Histological changes are nonspecific and variable, ranging from minimal to moderate, and they do not correlate with the degree of infection (Fig. 40-4). Changes include villous atrophy, crypt elongation, and lamina propria infiltration with lymphocytes, polymorphonuclear leukocytes, and plasma cells.

Cryptosporidial infection of the gallbladder and biliary tract has only been described in a small number of AIDS patients who were found to have organisms in bile and adherent to

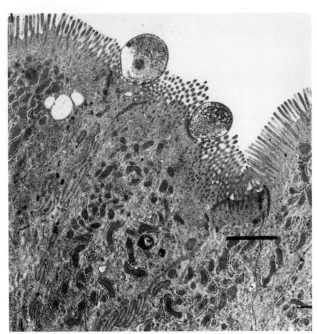

Figure 40-5. Cryptosporidial trophozoites in the brush border of the small intestine. Bar = 5 μm. (*Reproduced from* [*14*].)

gallbladder epithelium with edema, lymphocytic infiltration, and destruction of the underlying mucosa [*16*]. Organisms have also been seen in association with bronchial epithelium and in sputum, but it is not known whether they represent colonization or true infection [*17*]. Neither biliary tract nor pulmonary cryptosporidiosis has been described in immunologically normal individuals.

The intestine is the site most commonly infected in animals with cryptosporidiosis; however, pulmonary, gastric, and biliary tract involvement have been documented as well. In contrast to the pathology described for the human host, histological lesions in animals vary with the degree of infection [*18*]. Blunted, fused villi, flattened enterocytes, focal necrosis, and a greatly reduced microvillous surface have been seen in association with both naturally occurring and experimental infections in calves and pigs [*1–3*].

The pathogenic mechanisms by which *Cryptosporidium* causes disease have not been elucidated. The voluminous, secretory diarrhea reminiscent of cholera suggests an enterotoxin-mediated process, but other mechanisms that interfere with intestinal absorption may be operative.

Clinical manifestations

The incubation period for cryptosporidiosis appears to be between 2 and 14 days. Infected persons characteristically have copious, watery diarrhea, cramping abdominal pain, weight loss, and flatulence. Nausea, vomiting, myalgias, and fever

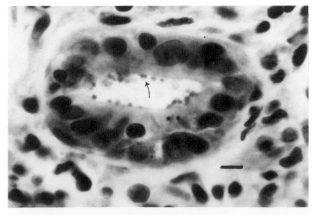

Figure 40-4. Cryptosporidia (arrow) on epithelium of small bowel from an infected patient. Hematoxylin and eosin; bar = 20 μm.

are less common. Symptoms often wax and wane, and some patients describe exacerbation of diarrhea immediately upon ingestion of food. Cryptosporidial oocysts and mucus are present in feces, but blood and leukocytes are uncommon. Peripheral eosinophilia has been reported in some cases. Fat, carbohydrate, and vitamin B_{12} malabsorption as well as reversible lactose intolerance have also been documented in *Cryptosporidium*-infected patients. Radiographic findings are usually nonspecific and include prominent mucosal folds and disordered motility.

The severity and duration of cryptosporidial enteritis are determined by immunocompetence [7,14]. In the immunologically intact individual, symptoms often have an explosive onset and last an average of 10 to 14 days but may be more prolonged [19]. Clearance of the parasite from feces frequently lags behind clinical resolution of illness by 1 to 2 weeks [20]. Although self-limited, illness is often severe enough to warrant therapeutic intervention were it available.

Infection in patients with AIDS or other types of immunocompromise often begins insidiously and escalates in severity as the immune defect becomes more pronounced. Symptoms may persist for months. Frequent voluminous bowel movements often lead to severe dehydration, electrolyte imbalance, profound malnutrition, and weight loss requiring hospitalization.

AIDS patients with biliary cryptosporidiosis have been reported to have signs and symptoms of cholecystitis, including right upper quadrant pain, nausea, and vomiting. The serum alkaline phosphatase level is usually elevated, but the serum transaminases and bilirubin are normal. Radiographic evaluation may reveal a thickened gallbladder wall and bile duct changes reminiscent of sclerosing cholangitis.

Diagnosis

Initially, the diagnosis of cryptosporidiosis was based on microscopic examination of intestinal biopsy specimens. Since 1981, various stains for detecting the parasite in fecal smears have been popularized [1–3]. Most widely used have been several modifications of the acid-fast techniques which differentiate red-staining, acid-fast oocysts from yeasts which, though similar in size and shape, are not acid-fast [21,22]. Although there can be variability in stain uptake, it is generally agreed that experienced observers have little difficulty in detecting oocysts. Since the number of negative specimens required to confirm the absence of cryptosporidial infection is not known and fecal oocyst shedding can be intermittent, at least two smears appear to be required for diagnosis. Recently, a more sensitive and specific direct fluorescent antibody stain which uses a murine monoclonal antibody directed against the oocyst wall has been made commercially available (Meridian Diagnostics, Cincinnati, Ohio) [23,24]. Concentration techniques that optimize detection of oocysts in specimens in which they are rare (e.g., formed stool, environmental samples) are

not necessary for diagnosis during acute illness. Since these techniques pose a risk of exposure by aerosolization, special caution is advised when they are used.

Antibodies to cryptosporidia have been detected in immunocompetent as well as immunocompromised patients by immunofluorescent (IFA) and enzyme-linked immunosorbent (ELISA) assays. Using the IgG and IgM ELISA, 95 percent of *Cryptosporidium*-infected patients (including those with AIDS) were found to have detectable antibody [25]. These methods for serodiagnosis are not commercially available.

Treatment

There is currently no known effective therapy for human cryptosporidiosis. Inability to cultivate the organism in vitro and the absence of a symptomatic small animal model of the disease have hindered the identification of potentially active agents. Fluid and electrolyte replacement is of prime importance in management. Although infection is self-limited in the immunologically normal host, there have been reports of severe enteritis requiring intravenous hydration. Illness will resolve in persons receiving corticosteroids or cytotoxic drugs if the immunosuppressive agents are discontinued. Because of the severity of cryptosporidial infection in AIDS patients, they have been given a vast array of antidiarrheal, antiparasitic, and immunomodulating agents, as well as special diets, with little benefit. Due to lack of toxicity and anecdotal reports of success in palliating diarrhea, the macrolide antibiotic spiramycin has been used extensively in patients with AIDS. This agent, which is given orally at a dose of 2 to 3 g daily, is investigational in the United States and may be obtained from Rhone Poulenc Pharmaceuticals and dispensed with permission from the Food and Drug Administration. Results of a multicenter, placebo-controlled, clinical trial of spiramycin are currently being evaluated. The ornithine decarboxylase inhibitor α-difluoromethylornithine has demonstrated modest efficacy in a small number of cases, but bone marrow and gastrointestinal toxicity have limited further studies. Promising preliminary results have also been obtained with novel agents such as oral bovine transfer factor and hyperimmune bovine colostrum. Failure of therapy for cryptosporidiosis in patients with AIDS may not simply reflect lack of drug efficacy but may also be related to their profound immune dysfunction, multiple concomitant infections and therapies, or poorly understood features of cryptosporidial infection such as a potential biliary tract reservoir.

POPULATION

Epidemiology

Cryptosporidial infection has been described in at least 30 countries spanning six continents [1–3,26]. Large-scale surveys reveal prevalence rates that range from 0.6 to 20 percent in developed countries and 4 to 32 percent in underdeveloped countries. Children are more commonly affected than adults. Although most of these surveys have sampled patients with diarrhea and therefore do not reflect true prevalence, they do indicate that the parasite is ubiquitous. In the United States, 3 to 4 percent of patients with AIDS have cryptosporidial enteritis, undoubtedly an underestimate since it is not looked for in all patients. In contrast, more than 50 percent of the patients with AIDS in Haiti and Africa have cryptosporidiosis.

Although still controversial, some reports suggest that breastfeeding protects against acquisition of *Cryptosporidium*, and a seasonal variation may exist for the disease, manifestations being more common during warm and humid months. Asymptomatic carriage of the parasite has also been described.

Transmission

Animal-to-human transmission of *Cryptosporidium* has been well-documented but may not be as common as spread from either other infected humans or contaminated water. The occurrence of infection in (1) day care center attendees, (2) household contacts of index cases, and (3) health care workers by nosocomial spread suggests that person-to-person transmission is important [1–3,26]. Contaminated water has been implicated as the source of infection in travelers and for various outbreaks in the United States [8,27]. Recently, *Cryptosporidium* oocysts have been detected in Washington State and California rivers [28], as well as in New Mexico and Arizona surface water [29]. Spread of the parasite via sexual activity, aerosolization, fomites, and contaminated food has been suggested but not confirmed.

Control

The cryptosporidial oocyst is quite hardy and resistant to a number of disinfectants, including 3% hypochlorite solution, iodophors, cresylic acid, benzalkonium chloride, and 5% formaldehyde. Heat (65°C for 30 min) and prolonged treatment with bleach or 10% formalin in combination with either bleach or 5% ammonia appear to reduce infectivity. Studies aimed at the identification of more practical and effective ways to destroy cryptosporidial viability are ongoing.

The detection and eradication of *Cryptosporidium* in environmental waters is a particularly troublesome problem. The filtration techniques used to detect *Giardia lamblia* were found to be ineffective for *Cryptosporidium*. Using new methods that employ polypropylene cartridge filters, *Cryptosporidium* oocysts have been found in untreated as well as treated sewage and in surface waters [29,30]. Since chlorination does not kill *Cryptosporidium*, the potential for contamination of drinking water is, in fact, quite real. Improved methods to test and ensure the purity of our water supply are currently being developed.

ISOSPORIASIS

Human isosporiasis is a gastrointestinal tract infection caused by the coccidian protozoan parasite *Isospora belli*. It is a poorly understood infection that is endemic in certain parts of South America and southeast Asia, but it appears to be rare in the United States.

PARASITE

The *I. belli* oocyst is elliptical in shape and approximately 22 to 33 by 10 to 15 μm in size. Within the oocyst, there are two sporocysts, each of which contains four sporozoites. Isosporiasis is acquired through ingestion of sporulated oocysts; the infective dose for humans is not known. The parasite undergoes the asexual (schizogony) and sexual (gametogony) phases of its life cycle in the cytoplasm of intestinal epithelial cells, and unsporulated oocysts are shed in the feces.

PATIENT "HOST"

The pathogenic mechanisms by which *I. belli* causes diarrhea are not known. Histopathological study of biopsies of the small intestine from infected patients revealed atrophic mucosa, shortened villi, hypertrophic crypts, and infiltration of the lamina propria with inflammatory cells, particularly eosinophils [31–33]. Electron-microscopic examination has revealed organisms within cytoplasmic vacuoles in cells with microvillous shortening [34]. Extraintestinal dissemination of the parasite to lymph nodes has been documented in cats [35]. There is only one report of extraintestinal involvement (lymph node) with *Isospora* in a person with AIDS [36].

The spectrum of clinical illness in humans with isosporiasis ranges from self-limited enteritis to chronic diarrhea which may persist for months. Chronic, severe infection has been described in patients with AIDS [36–38] as well as in non-AIDS infants and children [39]. The clinical manifestations of isosporiasis include watery, nonbloody diarrhea, cramping abdominal pain, and weight loss. Fat malabsorption and eosinophilia are common in patients with isosporiasis.

Diagnosis is established by the identification of *Isospora* oocysts in fecal specimens. The latter are acid-fast and can be easily distinguished from cryptosporidia on the basis of shape and size (Fig. 40-6). *Isospora* can also be detected with the fluorescent auramine stain, but the numerous other techniques described for cryptosporidia have not been evaluated for isosporiasis. *Isospora* oocysts may be shed intermittently and in smaller numbers; thus, concentration methods may be useful in diagnosis.

In marked contrast to cryptosporidiosis, isosporiasis responds promptly to therapy. A clinical and parasitological cure may be achieved with oral trimethoprim-sulfamethoxazole (TMP-SMX) usually within a week of initiating treatment [36,37]. Patients with AIDS have a high frequency of recur-

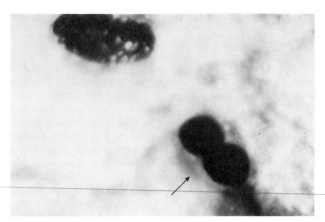

Figure 40-6. Acid-fast sporulated (arrow) and unsporulated *Isospora belli* oocysts in the feces of an infected patient × 630. (*Courtesy of Madeleine Boncy, Port au Prince, Haiti.*)

rence, which responds to retreatment [*37*]. Because of the high rate of recurrence, AIDS patients are often maintained indefinitely on suppressive therapy with TMP-SMX at a lower dose or weekly pyrimethamine-sulfadoxine (Fansidar). Controlled studies to compare different regimens and determine optimal dose and duration of therapy for isosporiasis have not been done. Both success and failure have been reported, anecdotally, with the use of agents such as metronidazole, quinacrine, and nitrofurantoin for isosporiasis.

POPULATION

Although *I. belli* is distributed ubiquitously in the animal kingdom, its prevalence in humans is not known. It is more prevalent in tropical and subtropical climates, and, in fact, is endemic in parts of South America (Santiago, Chile), Africa, and southeast Asia [*31,40*]. It has been implicated in various institutional outbreaks in the United States [*31,40*]. *Isospora* infections have been documented in less than 0.2 percent of patients with AIDS in the United States and 15 percent of AIDS patients in Haiti. Undoubtedly both figures are underestimated since not all patients are examined for the parasite. Transmission of *Isospora* to humans from infected animals and via contaminated water is suspected but not documented.

REFERENCES

1 Fayer R, Ungar BLP: *Cryptosporidium* spp. and cryptosporidiosis. Microbiol Rev 50:458–483, 1986

2 Soave R, Armstrong D: *Cryptosporidium* and cryptosporidiosis. Rev Infect Dis 8:1012–1023, 1986

3 Janoff EN, Barth Reller L: *Cryptosporidium* species, a protean protozoan. J. Clin Microbiol 25:967–975, 1987

4 Tyzzer EE: A sporozoan found in the peptic glands of the common mouse. Proc Soc Exp Bio Med 5:12–13, 1907

5 Slavin D: *Cryptosporidium meleagridis* (sp. nor). J Comp Pathol 65:262–266, 1955

6 Tzipori S: Cryptosporidiosis in animals and humans. Microbiol Rev 47:84–96, 1983

7 Current WL, Reese NC, Ernst JV, et al: Human cryptosporidiosis in immunocompetent and immunodeficient persons. N Engl J Med 308:1252–1257, 1983

8 Jokipii L, Pohjola S, Jokipii AM: Cryptosporidiosis associated with traveling and giardiasis. Gastroenterology 89:838–842, 1985

9 Soave R, Ma P: Cryptosporidiosis: Traveler's diarrhea in two families. Arch Intern Med 145:70–72, 1985

10 Levine ND: Taxonomy and review of the coccidian genus *Cryptosporidium* (Protozoa, Apicomplexa). J Protozool 31:94–98, 1984

11 Tzipori S, Angus KW, Campbell I, et al: *Cryptosporidium*: Evidence for a single-species genus. Infect Immun 30:884–886, 1980

12 Upton SJ, Current WL: The species of *Cryptosporidium* (Apicomplexa: Cryptosporidiidae) infecting mammals. J Parasitol 71:625–629, 1985

13 Current WL, Haynes TB: Complete development of *Cryptosporidium* in cell culture. Science 224:603–605, 1984

14 Soave R, Danner RL, Honig CL, et al: Cryptosporidiosis in homosexual men. Ann Intern Med 100:504–511, 1984

15 Guarda LA, Stein SA, Cleary KA, et al: Human cryptosporidiosis in the acquired immune deficiency syndrome. Arch Pathol Lab Med 107:562–566, 1983

16 Blumberg RS, Kelsey P, Perrone T, et al: Cytomegalovirus- and *Cryptosporidium*-associated acalculous gangrenous cholecystitis. Am J Med 76: 1118–1123, 1984

17 Forgacs P, Tarshis A, Ma P, et al: Intestinal and bronchial cryptosporidiosis in an immunodeficient homosexual man. Ann Intern Med 99:793–794, 1983

18 Heine J, Pohlenz JFL, Moon HW, et al: Enteric lesions and diarrhea in gnotobiotic calves monoinfected with *Cryptosporidium* species. J Infect Dis 150:768–775, 1984

19 Wolfson JS, Richter JM, Waldron MA, et al: Cryptosporidiosis in immunocompetent patients. N Engl J Med 321:1278–1282, 1985

20 Jokipii L, Jokipii AMM: Timing of symptoms and oocyst excretion in human cryptosporidiosis. N Engl J Med 315:1643–1647, 1986

21 Henricksen SA, Pohlenz, JFL: Staining of cryptosporidia by a modified Ziehl-Neelsen technique. Acta Vet Scand 22:594–596, 1981

22 Ma P, Soave R: Three-step stool examination for cryptosporidiosis in 10 homosexual men with protracted watery diarrhea. J Infect Dis 147:824–828, 1983

23 Sterling CR, Arrowood MJ: Detection of *Cryptosporidium* sp. infections using a direct immunofluorescent assay. Pediatr Infect Dis 5:139–142, 1986

24 Garcia LS, Brewer TC, Bruckner DA: Fluorescence detection of *Cryptosporidium* oocysts in human fecal specimens by using monoclonal antibodies. J Clin Microbiol 25:119–121, 1987

25 Ungar BLP, Soave R, Fayer R, et al: Enzyme immunoassay detection of immunoglobulin M and G antibodies to *Cryptosporidium* in immunocompetent and immunocompromised persons. J Infect Dis 153:570–578, 1986

26 Navin TR: Cryptosporidiosis in humans: Review of recent epidemiologic studies. Eur J Epidemiol 1:77–83, 1985

27 D'Antonio RG, Winn RE: A waterborne outbreak of cryptosporidiosis in normal hosts. Ann Intern Med 103:886–888, 1985

28 Ongerth JE, Stibbs HH: Identification of *Cryptosporidium* oocysts in river water. Appl Environ Microbiol 53:672–676, 1987

29 Madore MS, Rose JB, Gerba CP, et al: Occurrence of *Cryptosporidium* oocysts in sewage effluents and select surface waters. J Parasitol 73:702–705, 1987

30 Rose JB, Cifrino A, Madore MS, et al: Detection of *Cryptosporidium* from wastewater and freshwater environments. Wat Sci Tech 18:233–239, 1986

31 Brandborg LL, Goldberg SB, Briedenbach WC: Human coccidiosis—a possible cause of malabsorption: The life cycle in small-bowel mucosal biopsies as a diagnostic feature. N Engl J Med 283:1306–1313, 1970

32 Trier JS, Moxey PC, Schimmel EM, et al: Chronic intestinal coccidiosis in man: Intestinal morphology and response to treatment. Gastroenterology 66:923–935, 1974

33 Webster BH: Human isosporiasis: A report of three cases with necropsy findings in one case. Am J Trop Med 6:86–89, 1957

34 Liebman WM, Thaler MM, DeLorimier A, et al: Intractable diarrhea of infancy due to intestinal coccidiosis. Gastroenterology 78:579, 1980

35 Dubey JP, Frenkel JK: Extra-intestinal stages of *Isospora felis I. rivolta* (Protozoa: Eimeridiae) in cats. J Protozool 19:89–92, 1972

36 Restrepo C, Macher AM, Radany EH: Disseminated extraintestinal isosporiasis in a patient with acquired immune deficiency syndrome. Am J Clin Pathol 87:536, 1987

37 DeHovitz JA, Pape JW, Boncy M, et al: Clinical manifestations and therapy of *Isospora belli* infection in patients with acquired immunodeficiency syndrome. N Engl J Med 315:87, 1986

38 Forthal DN, Guest SS: *Isospora belli* enteritis in three homosexual men. Am J Trop Med Hyg 33:1060, 1984

39 Faria JA, Brust MB: Human isosporiasis caused by *Isospora belli*, Wenyon 1923, Salvador-Bahia. Rev Inst Med Trop Sao Paulo 251:47–49, 1983

40 Faust EC, Giraldo LE, Caicedo G, et al: Human isosporosis in the Western Hemisphere. Am J Trop Med 10:343, 1983

CHAPTER 41 / *Trichomoniasis* · Thomas C. Quinn · John N. Krieger

Trichomonas vaginalis is a pathogenic protozoan commonly found in the human genitourinary tract. Transmitted primarily by sexual intercourse, this organism causes vaginitis in women and nongonococcal urethritis in men. More than 200 million people worldwide are infected with this parasite annually [*1*]. In the developed countries, *T. vaginalis* is perhaps the most common pathogenic protozoan of humans with estimates of trichomoniasis of 3 to 4 million cases annually in the United States [*2,3*] and over 1.5 million cases in Great Britain [*2*].

PARASITE

BIOLOGY

Trichomonads are flagellated eukaryotic organisms belonging to the protozoan order Trichomonadida. Over 100 separate species have been reported. Most trichomonads are commensal organisms of the intestinal tract of mammals and birds. Of the three species found in humans, *T. vaginalis* is a parasite of the genitourinary tract, and *T. tenax* and *Pentatrichomonas hominis* are nonpathogenic trichomonads found in the oral cavity and large intestine, respectively.

The size and shape of *T. vaginalis* are variable depending on culture conditions and the vaginal microenvironment. Typically, the organism has an oval or fusiform shape with a mean length of 15 μm and mean width of 7 μm (size of a leukocyte). Trichomonads demonstrate a characteristic twitching erratic motility as they are propelled by four anterior flagella which originate in an anterior kinetosomal complex (Fig. 41-1). A fifth flagellum is attached to the undulating membrane which originates from the kinetosomal complex and extends halfway down the organism. Within the organism there is an anterior nucleus containing five chromosomes, a parabasal apparatus, a Golgi complex, and an axostyle, which runs centrally through the cell to eventually form a posterior pointed tail or "projection." Parallel to the axostyle and costa are three rows of large chromatic granules, which are believed to be hydrogenosomes because of their biochemical nature [*4*]. Reproduction, which can occur every 8 to 12 h under optimal conditions, is by mitotic division and longitudinal fission. *T. vaginalis* is believed to exist only in trophozoite form since a cyst form has never been described.

Cells of *T. vaginalis* are capable of phagocytosis, and vacuoles, particles, bacteria, and, rarely, leukocytes and erythrocytes are found within the cytoplasm. Particle recognition and phagocytosis by *T. vaginalis* appear to be mediated by non-immunological means and by specific immunological cell surface receptors which may be similar to the Fc and complement receptors of polymorphonuclear leukocytes [*5*]. Older literature suggested that some treatment failures in patients with gonorrhea resulted from protection of viable gonococci within trichomonads. However, when *T. vaginalis* were mixed with suspensions of *Neisseria gonorrhoeae*, *Mycoplasma hominis*, or *Chlamydia trachomatis* in vitro, most gonococci were killed within 6 h, and all mycoplasmas were killed within 3 h. Electron-microscopic studies revealed phagocytic uptake and destruction within the trichomonads. There was no evidence that

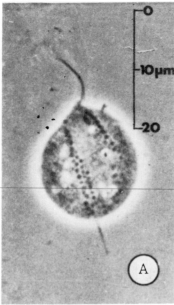

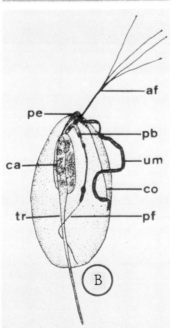

Figure 41-1. *Trichomonas vaginalis*. *A*. Dark phase-contrast photomicrograph of living organisms. *B*. Line diagrams prepared with the aid of camera lucida. af = anterior flagella; pe = pelta; pb = parabasal body; um = undulating membrane; ca = capitulum; co = costa; tr = trunle of the axostyle; pf = parabasal filament. (*From* [7].)

C. trachomatis organisms persisted in mixed culture with *T. vaginalis* [6].

T. vaginalis is basically an aerotolerant anaerobe: growth is inhibited at high oxygen tensions due to deficiency of catalase [7], but some multiplication can be observed in media equilibrated with air. This aerotolerance is attributed to the presence of active superoxide dismutase. The trichomonal energy metabolism appears rather unique, involving the metabolism of pyruvate to lactate in the hydrogenosomes. These organelles contain pyruvate oxidizing enzyme (pyruvate-ferredoxin oxidoreductase) and hydrogenase which are linked by an electron transport protein of low redox potential. Although more information is required, this low-redox-potential protein appears to play a critical role in the action of antitrichomonal nitroimidazoles.

In common with most other parasitic protozoa, trichomonads are unable to synthesize purine ring structures or to interconvert purine nucleotides. However, washed cell suspensions are capable of salvaging the purine bases adenine and guanine, and their nucleosides. Trichomonad nucleoside phosphorylase and nucleoside kinase activities appear to be responsible for conversion of the purine bases and nucleosides to nucleoside monophosphates.

Macromolecules derived from the host may be important in the metabolism and pathogenicity of trichomoniasis, either through biological mimicry or through accumulation of nutrients from the host. These molecules include 1-antitrypsin, iron, lactoferrin, low-density lipoproteins, and lipids [8]. Some evidence suggests that 1-antitrypsin, the major serine protease inhibitor in plasma, binds to specific receptors on the parasite cell surface where it may protect the parasites from host degradative enzymes [9]. Low-density lipoproteins derived from the host appear to be necessary for assembly of new parasite membranes [8]. Several observations suggest that acquisition of iron from the host may be important in the pathogenesis of trichomoniasis. Iron uptake and increased intracellular enzyme activity follow host lactoferrin binding by receptors on the parasites [9]. *T. vaginalis* also possesses hemolytic activity that may be important for destruction of erythrocytes in menstrual blood with release of iron [10]. Isoenzyme patterns of *T. vaginalis* have been evaluated in an attempt to characterize differences among isolates. The isoenzyme patterns of four enzymes (lactate dehydrogenase, malate dehydrogenase, hexokinase, and glucose phosphate isomerase) proved useful in classifying 32 isolates into five groups.

Growth and multiplication of *T. vaginalis* is optimal in a moist milieu with temperature between 35 and 37°C and pH between 4.9 and 7.5. The organisms can be easily cultivated axenically in nutrient media designed to provide optimum Eh, pH, and antibiotics to suppress other microorganisms [11]. The pH is a critical growth-limiting factor since the more robust and smaller organisms are observed in pH ranges of 5.5 to 5.8, whereas the less motile, enlarged organisms are encountered at pH levels lower or higher than optimum. The vaginal pH in trichomonal vaginitis is usually 5.5 to 6.0 [3]. Clinical signs and symptoms are less prominent at lower pH levels when trichomonads are found. Winston [12] has suggested that smaller oval organisms are found in symptomatic women, and larger more rounded organisms are found in asymptomatic women, reflecting growth conditions within the vagina.

The influence of the normal vaginal flora and of local non-specific environmental factors on the growth and pathogenicity of *T. vaginalis* requires further study. In most studies the great majority of women with trichomoniasis are simultaneously infected with other urogenital organisms with pathogenic potential, including *Ureaplasma urealyticum* and/or *M. hominis* in over 90 percent, *Gardnerella vaginalis* in about 90 percent, *N. gonorrhoeae* in approximately 30 percent, yeasts in approximately 20 percent, and *C. trachomatis* in approximately 15 percent. In addition a 5.5-kb double-stranded RNA has been described in *T. vaginalis* [13]. On electron microscopy this RNA appears to be a linear structure 1.5 μm in length without hairpins or loops. Purification revealed the presence of icosahedral viruslike particles. This viruslike material has been isolated from 40 of 43 *T. vaginalis* isolates tested, at densities ranging from 280 to 1380 copies per cell [13]. It has also been suggested that the presence of viral RNA is related to the ability of some isolates to undergo phenotypic variation [13]. The importance of these concomitant infections in the susceptibility of the host to trichomonal infection and the clinical presentation of urogenital trichomoniasis, however, remains unclear.

ANTIGENIC ANALYSIS

Considerable variation in the cell surface of *T. vaginalis* has made it difficult to define strain differences or serogroups of the protozoa. Variations in surface saccharides have been demonstrated by differential binding of fluorescein-conjugated plant lectins. Other reports identified type-specific antigens of *T. vaginalis* using polyclonal antisera in hemagglutination, complement fixation assays, and by the immunoblot technique [7,12]. By such methods estimates of the number of serotypes have ranged from two to eight in selected areas of Europe. Antigenic distinctions among *T. vaginalis* isolates were also demonstrated using polyclonal antisera. Recent investigations using monoclonal antibodies in indirect immunofluorescence assays confirmed the presence of antigenic variation among isolates of *T. vaginalis* [14]. Significant variation has also been described among isolates from diverse geographical areas of North America.

There appears to be considerable plasticity in the antigenic composition of the parasite cell surface. This phenomenon was characterized using a monoclonal antibody that recognized a prominent, high-molecular-weight, immunogenic molecule which appeared to be either present or absent from trichomonal membranes [15]. A single laboratory strain was fractionated to obtain subpopulations of trichomonads either reactive or nonreactive with serum immunoglobulin G from patients with trichomoniasis. Phenotypic variation among trichomonads was also observed during in vitro growth. Enhanced parasitism and killing of HeLa cells in monolayer cultures were observed for subpopulations that were nonreactive with the patient serum. These data support the idea that phenotypic variation of *T. vaginalis* may be coordinated for a repertoire of trichomonad immunogens and that such variation may influence expression of virulence of the protozoa.

PATIENT

PATHOPHYSIOLOGY

Despite extensive studies, little is known regarding the pathogenesis of *T. vaginalis* infection. Human beings are the only known hosts of *T. vaginalis*, and no animal reservoirs are known to exist. Absence of a completely satisfactory animal model has hindered efforts to define the pathogenetic mechanisms of *T. vaginalis*. A mouse subcutaneous abscess model has been the employed in many studies [7], but this model correlates imperfectly with clinical findings in patients and does not follow the natural routes of urogenital sites of infection. Intravaginal models have met with limited success. The best results have been reported using female squirrel monkeys (*Saimiri sciureus*), with intravaginal infections occurring in four of six animals for periods ranging up to 1 month [16]. Cost considerations and limited availability of nonhuman primates make routine use of this model unlikely.

The inherent pathogenicity of *T. vaginalis* in women has been demonstrated by the development of purulent, frothy vaginal discharge in women infected intravaginally with axenic cultures of *T. vaginalis* [17]. In contrast, it is surprising that the sites of colonization in the male genital tract are still not clearly determined, and the role of *T. vaginalis* in producing inflammation in the male genital tract remains unclear [10].

The mechanisms of disease by *T. vaginalis* have been investigated in vitro. Studies of the cytopathic effects of trichomonads on a number of different mammalian cell lines support the importance of contact-dependent extracellular killing of cells in tissue culture [18]. Ameboid morphology appears to facilitate direct contact and destruction of epithelial cells by virulent strains of the protozoa. Kinetic analysis of target cell killing by trichomonads has revealed that the probability of cell death was related to the probability of contact with *T. vaginalis* [18]. Simultaneous studies of [111]indium oxine label release from tissue culture cells and trypan blue dye exclusion demonstrated that *T. vaginalis* killed cells extracellularly without phagocytosis. Filtrates of trichomonad cultures or from media in which trichomonads were killing cells had no effect on tissue culture cell monolayers, implying that trichomonads did not kill cells by a cell-free or secreted cytotoxin. The microfilament inhibitor cytochalasin D inhibited trichomonad killing of cell monolayers, but microtubule inhibitors had little or no effect on killing of target cells. These findings support the concept that *T. vaginalis* kills tissue culture cells by direct contact without phagocytosis, an event that requires intact trichomonad microfilament function [18].

The importance of extracellular cytotoxins has been emphasized, however, in other studies [19]. A factor that caused detachment and clumping of susceptible tissue culture cells was identified in polyethylene glycol concentrates from *T. vaginalis* culture filtrates [19]. Virulence of recent human isolates was correlated with the presence of β-hemolytic activity and with the ability of certain strains to produce subcutaneous abscesses in mice [7,19]. These studies imply that *T. vaginalis* may possess a number of different virulence-associated characteristics. However, the relevance of these observations to the clinical presentation of disease in patients is still undefined. Further investigations are needed on factors influencing growth of *T. vaginalis* in the vagina, interactions of the protozoa with intact vaginal epithelium, cytotoxicity, interactions of the protozoa with local antibodies, phagocytes, and lymphocytes at the mucosal surface, and on the presence of microbial virulence factors.

HISTOPATHOLOGY

T. vaginalis is commonly associated with increased blood vessel dilatation in the surface epithelium and submucosa of the vagina and cervix. Grossly, this distension of blood vessels with local extravasation of blood (petechiae) produces an appearance of the exocervix, often referred to as a "strawberry cervix" [20]. Presence of the classical "strawberry cervix" occurs in only 2 percent of women with trichomoniasis; however, typical findings may be observed in over one-third of infected women on colposcopy (unpublished observation). This finding appears to be highly specific for trichomoniasis. There is edema of the squamous epithelium, and a significant degree of desquamation occurs together with an inflammatory exudate. Trichomonads are typically found adhering to epithelial cells of the vagina and free in pooled vaginal fluid, but rarely if ever inside intact host cells. Cellular changes noted in addition to an increased number of parabasal cells include binucleation, nuclear enlargement, nucler hyperchromasia, and perinuclear halos that may be confused with koilocytotic atypia due to human papilloma virus infection. The changes sometimes mimic those seen in mild dysplasia; however, no causal relationship has been established between cervical cancer and trichomonal vaginitis [7]. Studies which have suggested an association between these two entities, based primarily on the high prevalence rate of *T. vaginalis* (30 to 39 percent) of patients with cervical cancer [20], have not been carefully controlled for other genital pathogens such as herpes simplex virus or human papilloma virus.

Infected patients produce cellular, humoral, and secretory immune responses to the organism. The most prominent and obvious host response to *T. vaginalis* infection is the presence of polymorphonuclear leukocytes (PMNL) within the superficial epithelium and the intraluminal exudate of the vagina. The quantity of PMNL found in vaginal exudate correlates with the presence of symptoms [21]. Strains of *T. vaginalis* have been reported to differ in their ability to cause chemotaxis of PMNL. During in vitro and experimental in vivo studies, PMNL readily attack trichomonads, resulting in phagocytosis or fragmentation of the organism by groups of adherent PMNL. Similar studies have confirmed phagocytosis and killing of *T. vagini-*

alis by macrophages [22]. Cytoskeletal function of the host phagocytes appears to be important in natural cell-mediated cytotoxicity against *T. vaginalis* [23]. *T. vaginalis* also appears to activate the alternative complement pathway.

Although serum antibody has been demonstrated in human infections, no definitive correlation between levels of specific serum antibody and resistance to infection has been demonstrated except for a few experimental studies of intraperitoneal and subcutaneous injections of *T. vaginalis* in animals. An enzyme-linked immunosorbent assay that employed antihuman immunoglobulin and isotype-specific antisera was used to demonstrate an immune response in 21 to 23 infected women [24]. All 21 positive specimens contained IgG, 17 contained IgM, and 6 contained IgA antibodies against *T. vaginalis*. Western blot analysis revealed approximately 29 antigenic trichomonad polypeptides, and individual patients had different patterns of reactivity.

In studies of local antibody, Ackers et al. [25] demonstrated IgA antibody to *T. vaginalis* in vaginal secretions of 76 percent of 29 infected women and in 42 percent of 19 infected women. Higher levels of antitrichomonal antibody were seen in patients with a lower parasite load, suggesting some protection afforded by local antibody. However, no local antibody to *T. vaginalis* has been documented in the urethra of men with urethral trichomonal infection, and no correlation has been found between the presence or absence of local antibodies and the severity of inflammation or duration of symptoms [25].

Other factors may be important in protecting the male lower urogenital tract against infection by *T. vaginalis*. For example, the high zinc content in human prostatic secretions may be an important defense of the male lower urinary tract against infection by a wide variety of urogenital pathogens, including *T. vaginalis* [10]. Trichomonads were rapidly killed by zinc salts at concentrations similar to those in prostatic secretions of normal men. The minimal inhibitory concentration of zinc was 0.8 to 6.4 mM for 15 clinical isolates of *T. vaginalis*. A time-kill technique showed subtle differences in the kinetics of zinc killing of trichomonad strains and that it was possible to select relatively zinc-resistant substrains of *T. vaginalis*. When similar time-kill studies were carried out using canine prostatic secretions, it was found that the killing of *T. vaginalis* depended on the concentration of zinc, as well as other, undefined factors in prostatic secretions. Variations in the zinc sensitivity of infecting *T. vaginalis* strains or in the zinc content of host prostatic secretions may be important determinants of the natural history of *T. vaginalis* infection in men.

CLINICAL MANIFESTATIONS

Sites of infection

In women *T. vaginalis* primarily infects vaginal epithelium and is less commonly isolated from the endocervix of infected women [3]. The urethra, the Bartholin's gland, and Skene's gland are other common sites of infection, and cultures of the urethra are positive in up to 90 percent of infected women. It is still unclear whether these areas harbor low numbers of trichomonads asymptomatically and are a source of reinfection or relapse due to alterations in vaginal microenvironment or other host factors. Bladder infections due to *T. vaginalis* have also been reported, but actual differentiation from urethral infection has not been reliably demonstrated. Rare reports of extravaginal sites of infection include isolation of *T. vaginalis* from fallopian tubes of women with acute salpingitis, from a perinephric abscess, and from cerebrospinal fluid of a patient with polymicrobial meningitis. In men, the urethra is most commonly infected, but trichomonads have also been isolated from epididymal aspirates, prostatic secretions, seminal vesicles, and from lesions of the median raphe [10].

Infections in women

The clinical manifestations of vaginal trichomonal infection range from asymptomatic carriage to severe vaginitis. The percentage of women infected with *T. vaginalis* who have no symptoms varies from 20 to 50 percent, depending on the selection of the population and type of diagnostic methods employed [26]. Indeed, many studies have suggested that the presence of *T. vaginalis* correlates poorly with symptoms and physical examination (Table 41-1) [7,20,26]. Unfortunately, many of these studies have not carefully differentiated between patients with cervicitis and vaginitis, and they did not rule out coinfections with pathogens such as *N. gonorrhoeae*, *C. trachomatis*, nonspecific vaginitis, or herpes infection.

However, in most studies a consistent finding in trichomonal vaginitis is the presence of many PMNL in a homogeneous discharge, which typically gives the discharge a yellow-green color; this contrasts with the characteristic white floccular or clumped discharge of *Candida* vaginitis and the white or gray homogeneous discharge of *Gardnerella vaginalis*–associated vaginosis (bacterial vaginosis). Abnormal vaginal bleeding such as postcoital bleeding may be due to cervicitis caused by

Table 41-1. Presenting symptoms and signs in 400 women with and without vaginitis due to *Trichomonas vaginalis*

| | Percent with sign or symptom | |
| | Trichomonas | No Trichomonas |
Symptoms and signs	(n = 131)	(n = 269)
Dysuria	18	12
Discharge, total	56	51
Acute	41	36
Chronic	15	15
Discharge quality:		
Menses or no leukorrhea	19	23
Homogeneous leukorrhea	69	72
Frothy leukorrhea	12*	5
Spontaneous leukorrhea	9	6

*$0.020 \leq p \leq 0.025$.

Source: Data from [19].

T. vaginalis or associated pathogens. Abdominal pain, described in up to 12 percent of women [7,20], may reflect severe vaginitis, regional lymphadenopathy, or conceivably endometritis or salpingitis due to *T. vaginalis* or another concurrent infection.

In addition to the purulent discharge, the vulva is erythematous and edematous, and excoriations may be evident. The vagina and cervix are erythematous, and small punctate hemorrhages and ulcerations can sometimes be found [20]. When present on the cervix these lesions are referred to as "strawberry" cervix and are more often visible by colposcope. Tender lymphadenopathy and cervical tenderness have been described in a small number of patients. Infection with *C. trachomatis*, *N. gonorrhoeae*, herpes simplex virus (HSV), or *C. albicans* may potentiate or alter these findings [3,20]. If not treated, trichomonal vaginitis may develop into a chronic infection characterized by intermittent symptoms or signs of less severe vulvovaginitis.

The presence or absence of symptoms is clearly related to individual variation in the threshold of patient perception, as well as to other host factors, trichomonal virulence factors, and to the presence of coexisting infections. A vaginal discharge with evidence of vaginal inflammation may be present in many infected women who lack symptoms, although the amount of discharge and number of PMNL are usually less than are observed in symptomatic disease [21].

Infections in men

T. vaginalis has been isolated from the urethras of 70 percent of men who have had recent contact with an infected woman. The majority (50 to 90 percent) of these men are asymptomatic, and the infection often appears to be self-limited. Two weeks after contact only 33 percent of the men were culture-positive [20,21]. This may be due to specific or nonspecific host immune factors, such as the presence of zinc in prostatic fluid, which may have antitrichomonal properties. In some men *T. vaginalis* has been associated with urethritis characterized by the presence of a discharge, dysuria, and, rarely, superficial penile ulcerations [10]. In developed countries, *T. vaginalis* has been isolated from less than 15 percent of men with nongonococcal urethritis (NGU) and usually from less than 5 percent. However, in the Soviet Union and in some developing countries, where the prevalence of *T. vaginalis* remains very high, some researchers believe that a higher proportion of NGU is caused by this agent [27]. Additional reported complications in men include epididymitis and prostatitis.

Neonatal trichomonal infection

Between 2 and 17 percent of female infants born to infected women develop vaginal infections [28]. Neonatal vaginal epithelium is relatively mature epithelium due to the influence of maternal estrogen and is thus susceptible to *T. vaginalis* infection. A vaginal discharge may develop, but typically the infection is asymptomatic. Maternal estrogens are metabolized by 3 to 4 weeks of age, and the vaginal epithelium returns to a prepubescent state, which is relatively resistant to *T. vaginalis* infection. It is not clear whether a latent or asymptomatic state of *T. vaginalis* carriage can persist through childhood.

Diagnosis

Since the clinical manifestations of trichomoniasis are varied and coexisting infections are common, diagnostic criteria dependent on history and physical examination are neither sensitive nor specific. While several studies have shown that a purulent yellow-green vaginal discharge is characteristic of trichomonal vaginitis [20], it is absent in a varying percentage of cases. Thus, diagnosis of trichomonal infection is dependent upon the identification of *T. vaginalis* by either wet-mount preparations, cultures, pap smears, or special stains.

Cultures for *T. vaginalis* are far more sensitive and specific in identifying the presence of *T. vaginalis* in infected secretions than the other diagnostic tests [11,20], particularly in women who do not have symptoms or signs of vaginitis. For example, in one recent study 86 of 177 inner-city women attending a clinic for sexually transmitted disease had positive cultures or wet mounts for *T. vaginalis* [29]. Culture using Diamond's medium was more sensitive than the wet mount (98 versus 38 percent) and symptoms were not reliable for diagnosis of infection. Quantitative agar cultures showed that 70 percent of infected patients had $> 10^4$ colony-forming units per milliliter of *T. vaginalis*. Although the wet-mount preparation is less sensitive in asymptomatic patients who have a lower concentration of *T. vaginalis* in their vaginal secretions, the wet mount may be 80 to 90 percent sensitive in symptomatic patients in some populations [21]. It is rapid, inexpensive, and if positive, treatment can be instituted immediately. Therefore, in evaluating women with symptoms and signs suggestive of trichomonal vaginitis we recommend a microscopical examination of fresh vaginal or urethral secretions for typical motile organisms; if none are observed, the discharge should be inoculated into culture medium to exclude trichomonal infection. The combination of both techniques should increase the sensitivity of detecting trichomoniasis to 98 percent in women. The sensitivity in men is probably lower; optimally men should be examined early in the morning before urination by culturing anterior urethral secretions with a swab or wire loop.

Fixed and stained preparations utilizing Gram's stain, acridine orange, fluorescein, neutral red, and other dyes have also been used for identifying the parasite. Generally these stains have been less sensitive than culture [20,26]. Giemsa- and Papanicolaou-stained smears may be useful in detecting *T. vaginalis* in asymptomatic women who have routine pap smears [34,46]. However, most reports that compare this technique versus wet mount and culture suggest a high percentage of false-positive and false-negative results associated with pap smears.

A number of tests have been evaluated for clinical detection of trichomoniasis based on detection of the host immunological response by methods such as enzyme-linked immunosorbent assay, indirect hemagglutination, and direct immunofluorescence. None of these methods have proven sufficiently sensitive for accurate clinical diagnosis or adequately specific for current infection. Although such techniques may prove useful in epidemiological studies, they have little utility in routine clinical practice. In one study the conventional wet-mount examination was compared with cytology, two different culture media, and monoclonal antibody staining of direct clinical specimens in a high-risk population of 600 randomly selected women [30]. Use of Feinberg-Whittington or Diamond's medium resulted in diagnosis of 82 and 78 cases, respectively, while the combination of two cultures identified 88 women with trichomoniasis. The wet-mount examination detected only 53 of the 88 cases (60 percent). Papanicolaou-stained gynecological smears were interpreted as positive in 49 of the 88 cases (56 percent) but also resulted in seven false-positive smears, and specimens from 18 additional women were read as "suspicious" for *T. vaginalis* infections. Monoclonal antibody staining detected 76 of the 88 cases (77 pecent), including 27 of 35 wet-mount-negative cases. Thus, the wet-mount and cytological studies had low sensitivity, and cytology had the lowest specificity for diagnosis of trichomoniasis. Direct immunofluorescence using monoclonal antibodies is a promising alternative to cultures for rapid diagnosis of trichomoniasis.

MANAGEMENT

In 1958, Cosar and Julou demonstrated the in vitro antitrichomonal activity of metronidazole [31]. One year later Durel et al. proved the efficacy of systemic metronidazole in the treatment of human trichomonal vaginitis [31]. Since then, metronidazole and other 5-nitroimidazoles, such as tinidazole and nimorazole, have been used extensively in treating trichomoniasis. Although the vast majority of strains of *T. vaginalis* are sensitive to all the nitroimidazoles, several strains, which were isolated from patients who were not cured by metronidazole, have demonstrated in vitro and in vivo high levels of resistance to the drug. Minimum inhibitory concentrations were reported at greater than 100 µg/mL, and only large doses of metronidazole, at least 500 to 750 mg three times a day for 7 days, have been partially effective in the treatment of these cases. The mechanisms of resistance are not known.

Presently, the recommended dosage of metronidazole for initial treatment of trichomonal infection is 2 g orally as a single dose [31]. Cure rates of 95 percent are reported when sexual partners are simultaneously treated, since the asymptomatic male partner is the main source of reinfection and of alleged treatment failures [31]. Side effects of the 2-g dose are mild and include metallic taste and nausea in 10 percent of patients. Metronidazole blocks the metabolism of alcohol, and nausea, vomiting, and flushing are exhibited when alcohol is taken simultaneously or soon after metronidazole administration. Metronidazole has been regarded as a possible carcinogen, since it is mutagenic for certain bacteria [31] and capable of producing lung tumors in mice after long-term administration of the drug. However, extended follow-up studies of women who have taken metronidazole have not yet demonstrated an increased incidence of cancer [32].

The major contraindication to administration of metronidazole is pregnancy. However, in one study of pregnant women receiving the drug during the first trimester, 3.8 percent of pregnancies resulted in babies with developmental anomalies, which was slightly higher than expected, while another study demonstrated no defects. Until the safety of the drug can be determined, it is prudent, however, to avoid metronidazole during pregnancy, and for symptomatic trichomoniasis, local administration of clotrimazole is sometimes effective and safe to use during pregnancy. Alternatively, vinegar douches twice weekly can be utilized with some efficacy.

Other drugs in the nitroimidazole class are effective against *T. vaginalis*, but none of these drugs holds a clear advantage over metronidazole. In one study niridazole, a nitroimidazole derivative with activity against other protozoa, appeared to be more effective than metronidazole in inhibiting hydrogen production by a metronidazole-resistant isolate in vitro [33], but the clinical effectiveness of this agent in patients with metronidazole-resistant organisms is uncertain.

In Europe a lactobacillus vaccine (SolcoTricovac) has been used for immunization and treatment of women with trichomoniasis. The proposed basis for this mode of therapy is that vaccination leads to production of antibodies that cross-react with *T. vaginalis*. However, presence of such antibodies has not been demonstrated, and there is no convincing evidence of a therapeutic effect.

POPULATION

EPIDEMIOLOGY

The prevalence of trichomoniasis varies widely according to the type of population studied and the diagnostic technique utilized for identification of the organism. Prevalence rates range from 5 to 10 percent in healthy women to as high as 50 to 70 percent in prostitutes and female prison inmates. An increased risk of infection has been demonstrated in individuals with multiple sex partners, poor personal hygiene, and low socioeconomic status. Several investigations have also shown a greater prevalence of trichomoniasis in blacks, multiparous women, women married at an early age, and during pregnancy. Women at high risk of acquiring other sexually transmitted diseases are often found to have coexistent trichomoniasis. For example, 30 to 50 percent of women with gonorrhea have been found to have *T. vaginalis* infection [3,20].

The peak incidence of trichomonal infection is usually between 16 and 35 years of age. However, unlike other sexually transmitted diseases, a second peak incidence has been re-

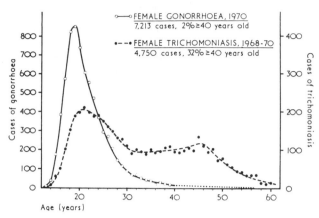

Figure 41-2. Number of women with trichomoniasis and with gonorrhea, by age group, detected in specimens examined at Statens Seruminstitut, Copenhagen. (*From* [34].)

ported in postmenopausal women (Fig. 41-2) [34]. The factors responsible for this second peak are poorly understand. Persistence of the organism in asymptomatic women and increased susceptibility or increased frequency of testing of older women can be postulated as possible explanations.

TRANSMISSION

As discussed above *T. vaginalis* is transmitted primarily by sexual intercourse. Seventy percent of men who have had sexual contact with infected women within the previous 48 h will harbor *T. vaginalis*. There is an increased cure rate with metronidazole when both partners are treated simultaneously. Furthermore, the sexual transmission of *T. vaginalis* has also been documented experimentally in human volunteers, and it is rarely, if ever, found in adult virgins [2].

Some experimental data suggest that *T. vaginalis* occasionally can be transmitted by contaminated articles, although transmission by fomites has not been well-documented in humans. Motile trichomonads have been demonstrated in secretions deposited on toilet seats up to 45 min after use by an infected individual. While nonvenereal transmission may be uncommon, it may be responsible for some cases of reinfection or for high prevalence rates in individuals with poor hygiene such as in prisons and other institutions.

CONTROL

The control of trichomonal infection can only be achieved through accurate diagnosis and treatment of infected individuals and of all recent sexual partners. Treatment of all recent sex partners of infected patients regardless of symptoms or identification of *T. vaginalis* in the partner(s) is warranted in order to be effective in prevention of reinfection. Follow-up with cultures and education of the patient regarding this infection is important in achieving compliance and optimum therapy.

REFERENCES

1 Brown MT: Trichomoniasis. Practitioner 209:639, 1972

2 Catterall RD: Trichomoniasis. Med Clin North Am 56:1203, 1972

3 Rein MF, Chapel TA: Trichomoniasis, candidiasis, and the minor venereal diseases. Clin Obstet Gynecol 18:73, 1975

4 Muller M: Biochemical cytology of trichomonad flagellates. I. Subcellular localization of hydrolases, dehydrogenases, and catalase in *Tritrichomonas foetus*, J Cell Biol 57:453, 1973

5 Soave R., Roberts RB: Phagocytosis by *Trichomonas vaginalis* compared to human neutrophils. Clin Res 30:372A, 1982, abstract

6 Street DA, Wells C, Taylor-Robinson D, et al: Interaction between *Trichomonas vaginalis* and other pathogenic microorganisms of the human genital tract. Br J Vener Dis 60:31–38, 1984

7 Honigberg B: Trichomonads of importance in human medicine, in Kreier JP (ed): *Parasitic Protozoa*. New York, Academic, 1978, vol 2, p 275

8 Peterson KM, Alderete JF: Selective acquisition of plasma proteins by *Trichomonas vaginalis* is dependent on uptake and degradation of human low density lipoproteins. J Exp Med 160:1261, 1984

9 Peterson KM, Alderete JF: Acquisition of 1-antitrypsin by a pathogenic strain of *Trichomonas vaginalis*. Infect Immunol 40:640, 1983

10 Krieger JN: Urological aspects of trichomoniasis. Invest Urol 18:411, 1981

11 Hess J: Review of current methods of the detection of *Trichomonas* in clinical material. J Clin Pathol 22:269, 1969

12 Winston RML: The relation between size and pathogenicity of *Trichomonas vaginalis*. J Obstet Gynecol Br Comm 81:399, 1974

13 Wang A, Wang CC, Alderete JF: *Trichomonas vaginalis* phenotypic variation occurs only among trichomonads infected with the double-stranded RNA virus. J Exp Med 166:142, 1987

14 Krieger JN, Holmes KK, Spence MR, et al: Geographic variation among isolates of *Trichomonas vaginalis*: Demonstration of antigenic heterogeneity by using monoclonal antibodies and the indirect immunofluorescence technique. J Infect Dis 152:979, 1985

15 Alderete JF, Demes P, Gombosova A, et al. Phenotypes and protein-epitope phenotypic variation among fresh isolates of *Trichomonas vaginalis*. Infect Immunol 55:28, 1988

16 Street DA, Taylor-Robinson D, Hetherington CM: Infection of female squirrel monkeys (*Saimiri sciureus*) with *Trichomonas vaginalis* as a model of trichomoniasis in women. Br J Vener Dis 59:249, 1983

17 Asami K, Nakamura M: Experimental inoculation of bacteria-free *Trichomonas vaginalis* into human vaginae and its effect on the glycogen content of vaginal epithelia. Am J Trop Med Hyg 4:254, 1955

18 Krieger JN, Ravdin JI, Rein MF: Contact-dependent cytopathogenic mechanisms of *Trichomonas vaginalis*. Infect Immunol 50:778, 1985

19 Pindak FF, Gardner WA Jr, de Pindak MM: Growth and cytopathogenicity of *Trichomonas vaginalis* in tissue cultures. J Clin Microbiol 23:672, 1986

20 Fouts AC, Kraus SJ: *Trichomonas vaginalis*: Reevaluation of its clinical presentation and laboratory diagnosis. J Infect Dis 141:137, 1980

21 Rein MF, Muller M: *Trichomonas vaginalis*, in Holmes KK, Mardh PA, Sparling PF (eds): *Sexually Transmitted Diseases*. New York, McGraw-Hill, 1981

22 Landolfo S, Giovanna M, Martinetto P, et al: Natural cell-mediated cytotoxicity against *Trichomonas vaginalis* in the mouse. J Immunol 124:508, 1980

23 Martonitti MG, Gallione MA, Martinetto P, et al: Role of cytoskeleton in natural cell-mediated cytotoxicity against *Trichomonas vaginalis*. Microbiol 5:389, 1982

24 Wos SM, Watt RM: Immunoglobulin isotypes of anti-*Trichomonas vaginalis* antibodies in patients with vaginal trichomoniasis. J Clin Microbiol 24:790, 1986

25 Ackers JP, Lumsden WHR, Catterall RD, et al: Antitrichomonal antibody in the vaginal secretions of women infected with *T. vaginalis*. Br J Vener Dis 51:319, 1975

26 Spence MR, Hollander DH, Smith J, et al: The clinical and laboratory diagnosis of *Trichomonas vaginalis* infection. Sex Transm Dis 7:168, 1980

27 Non-gonococcal urethritis and other sexually transmitted diseases. WHO Tech Rep Ser. Geneva, World Health Organization, 1981

28 Al-Salihi FL, Curran JP, Wang J-S: Neonatal *Trichomonas vaginalis* report of 3 cases and review of the literature. Pediatrics 53:196, 1974

29 Philip A, Carter-Scott P, Rogers C: An agar culture technique to quantitate *Trichomonas vaginalis* from women. J Infect Dis 155:304, 1987

30 Krieger JN, Tam MR, Stevens CE, et al: Diagnosis of trichomoniasis: comparison of conventional wet-mount examination with cytologic studies, cultures, and monoclonal antibody staining of direct specimens. JAMA 259:1223, 1988

31 Goldman P: Metronidazole. N Engl J Med 303:1212, 1980

32 Beard CM, Noller KL, O'Fallon WM, et al: Lack of evidence for cancer due to use of metronidazole. N Engl J Med 301:519, 1979

33 Yarlett N, Rowlands CC, Yarlett NC, et al: Reduction of niridazole by metronidazole resistant and susceptible strains of *Trichomonas vaginalis*. Parasitology 94:93, 1987

34 Nielsen R: *Trichomonas vaginalis*. II. Laboratory investigations in trichomoniasis. Br J Vener Dis 49:531, 1973

PART III Metazoan Diseases

CHAPTER 42

Introduction · Adel A. F. Mahmoud

Metazoa comprise a myriad of parasitic agents that are potentially pathogenic to humans; they fall into three major groups: worms, venomous animals, and arthropods. Parasitic metazoans are unique etiological agents of disease in humans because of their size, complex biology, and prevalence. Metazoa are multicellular organisms; their bodies have evolved from the relatively simple unicellular protozoan structure into multiple well-differentiated body organs and systems. The requirements for metazoan survival have in some cases necessitated a complicated set of developmental stages within two or more different hosts. It is partly because of the complex structure and life cycle of Metazoa that their host-parasite relationship is fundamentally different from that of most other infectious agents with respect to mechanisms of disease and immunity.

Worms are among the major parasites of human beings; they are divided into two phyla: Nematoda (round) and Platyhelminthes (flat). Of the latter, two classes are of particular importance, Trematoda and Cestoda [1]. Although each phylum has general biological characteristics and the two phyla share some epidemiological and pathogenetic features, the classification is unsatisfactory since it relies mainly on morphological or developmental criteria.

The epidemiology of worm infections in human populations has several unique and important features. The distribution of infections follows a negative binomial pattern whereby most infected individuals harbor low worm burden and only few show remarkable parasite load (see Chap. 10). It is this relatively small proportion of infected individuals with high intensity of infection who are of epidemiological and pathological significance.

Parasitic helminths generally invade humans by ingestion or by penetration of intact skin. The latter may be via the bite of an insect vector. Following a migratory pathway inside the mammalian host, almost all adult worms reach their final habitats in well-defined anatomical locations. There, they begin producing the next developmental stage, which has to leave the mammalian host in order to complete the organism's life cycle. The inability of worms to multiply within the mammalian host characterizes helminths and sets them apart from almost all other infectious agents. To increase the population of worms in a specific mammalian host, reexposure is necessary. The intensity of worm infections may, however, increase without further exposure to the parasites in strongyloidiasis and echinococcosis.

Another common feature of worms, particularly those that migrate in mammalian tissues, is the association with eosinophilia both in peripheral blood and in tissues. This long-known correlation of eosinophilia and tissue-dwelling worm infections has recently led to expansion of our understanding of the functional role of eosinophils. These cells have been shown to possess different antiparasite capabilities that result in destruction of helminths in vitro. Furthermore, depletion of eosinophils in vivo in experimental animals may result in abrogation of their resistance to worm infections [2].

This part of the text deals with the major global metazoan diseases. Nematode infections are covered in Chaps. 43 to 53, trematode infections in Chaps. 54 and 55, and cestode infections in Chaps. 56 and 57. Diseases due to arthropods and venomous animals are discussed in Chaps. 58 and 59. The prevalence and resulting morbidity and mortality rates of metazoan diseases contrast sharply with the modest worldwide control efforts. Our understanding of the biology of worms and arthropods remains sketchy. It is hoped, however, that the introduction of modern immunological and molecular tools to studies of metazoan diseases will lead to a leap forward in our ability to contain these infections.

REFERENCES

1 Schmidt GD, Roberts LS: *Foundations of Parasitology,* 2d ed. St. Louis, Mosby, 1981, p 795
2 Anderson RM, May RM: Helminthic infections of humans: Mathematical models, population dynamics, and control. Adv Parasitol 24:1–101, 1985

Nematode Infections

Ascariasis · Zbigniew S. Pawlowski

Ascaris lumbricoides is the largest nematode parasitizing the human intestine. *Ascaris* sp. is also one of the genera of nematodes which is most extensively studied in laboratories and of which the morphology, physiology, and biochemistry are well known, yet our knowledge of the ecology and of many medically important biological data related to this nematode is still inadequate in spite of growing interest in the subject [*1–3*].

Ascariasis is the most common intestinal parasitic infection, present in about 25 percent of the human population. Although mortality and morbidity due to ascariasis are both relatively low, the absolute number of fatal or diseased cases is high. The annual global mortality from ascariasis was calculated as 20,000 cases [*4*], due mainly to intestinal complications, and the annual morbidity as 1,000,000 cases [*4*], due mainly to abdominal or pulmonary manifestations and malnutrition. The hospitalization rate due to ascariasis in endemic areas varies from 0.02 to 0.9 per 1000 persons infected [*2*]. The global prevalence of ascariasis, which is a preventable fecal- and soil-transmitted infection, depends not so much on the regional ecological conditions as on local standards of social and economic development. With modern chemotherapy the control of ascariasis is feasible [*3*].

PARASITE

ASCARIS LUMBRICOIDES
AND OTHER ROUNDWORMS

The primary cause of human ascariasis is the large intestinal roundworm *Ascaris lumbricoides*, which is specific for humans and which has been only accidentally found in other hosts such as the orangutan, dog, cat, pig, and sheep. The parasite most closely related to *A. lumbricoides* is the pig roundworm—*Ascaris suum*. These two parasites definitely differ in host specificity: the natural host for *A. suum* is the pig. The larvae of *A. suum* can develop in humans [*5*], but without often reaching the mature, intestinal stage. Similarly, the other species of roundworms living in dogs and cats, *Toxocara canis* and *T. cati,* which are responsible for the visceral larva migrans syndrome in humans caused by their migrating larvae, only occasionally parasitize the human intestine as adult worms. *A. lumbricoides* and *A. suum* taxonomy and epidemiology have

seldom been studied in areas where humans and pigs still live in proximity.

LIFE CYCLE OF *ASCARIS LUMBRICOIDES*

Ascaris lumbricoides has a relatively simple life cycle (Fig. 43-1), with humans as the host for both the larval and adult stages and soil as the environment for development and a natural reservoir of eggs. Roundworms, together with hookworms and whipworms, belong to the soil-transmitted helminths or, in other words, to the geohelminths, having an essential part of their development on the ground.

The *Ascaris* eggs which leave their human host in the feces are undeveloped, and some are even unfertilized. Embryogenesis, i.e., development of the first larval stage in the fertilized eggs, takes 10 to 14 days in shaded soil at an optimal temperature of 28 to 32°C, at a moisture level of above 80 percent, and in the presence of oxygen. In lower temperatures the development is much slower (45 to 55 days at 16 to 18°C). The invasive *Ascaris* eggs, i.e., those containing an invasive larva, can survive for as long as 6 years in temperate zones but probably only for a few days in warm, arid zones. Since the eggshell is permeable to water, higher temperatures and desiccation readily kill the eggs. The *Ascaris* eggs can also be destroyed by some microorganisms, especially fungi.

When the *Ascaris* eggs are ingested and enter the human intestine, the second-stage larvae leave the eggshell and within a short time penetrate into the small-intestine mucosa, beginning an extraintestinal migration through lymphatics and/or blood vessels to the liver and lungs. On days 1 to 4 of infection, *Ascaris* larvae are present in the liver, and later on, up to 14 days following infection, in the lung tissue. They then penetrate the alveolar walls and, through the upper respiratory tract and throat, return again to the alimentary tract. The extraintestinal migration of the *Ascaris* larvae is reminiscent of a past multihostal evolutionary cycle. During the migration, which lasts about a fortnight, the larvae grow from 190 to 260 μm to about 2.2 mm and molt twice. The last molt takes place in the small intestine. It has been demonstrated that *A. lumbricoides* females grow more rapidly than males. In the first 2 to 3 months most of the growth is in length; later on the weight gain is more evident so that weight rather than length might

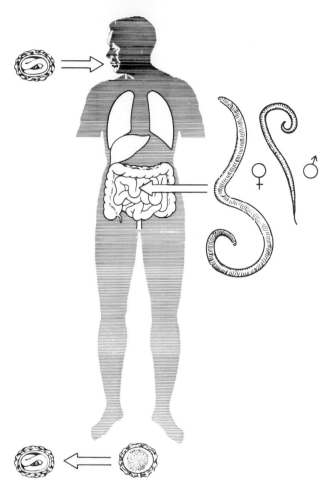

Figure 43-1. Life cycle of *Ascaris lumbricoides*.

MORPHOLOGY AND BIOLOGY OF ADULT *ASCARIS LUMBRICOIDES*

The sexual dimorphism between *A. lumbricoides* female and male adults is well expressed: female worms are 20 to 49 cm long and 3 to 6 mm in diameter; male worms are 15 to 30 cm long and 2 to 4 mm in diameter. This difference in size may depend on the age of the roundworms and on the worm load. The body of *A. lumbricoides* is rounded and tense due to the body cavity (pseudocoelom) being filled with fluid at a pressure of up to 225 mmHg (29.92 kPa). The cuticular surface of *Ascaris* is striated and flesh-colored with two whitish lateral lines in which the excretory canals are situated. There are three prominent lips in the anterior part, the vulvar opening on the ventral surface between the anterior and middle thirds of the body length in the females, and two copulatory spicules and numerous papillae at the ventrally curved posterior end of the males. Most of the inside of the *Ascaris* worm is taken up by an alimentary canal and a tubular reproductive organ, which is double in females and single in males.

The structure of the *Ascaris* alimentary tract is well adapted to the high pressure of the pseudocoelom fluid: the intestine is flat and collapsed unless it is filled with food. *Ascaris* feeds with limited selectivity on the intestinal contents of humans—it also ingests the barium contrast used for x-ray examination. *Ascaris* has its own battery of basic digestive enzymes, such as amylase, protease, and lipase, which are mainly excreted in the pharynx and anterior part of the intestine. Nutrients are absorbed and transferred by the enterocytes or through the intracellular space between them into the pseudocoelom, which distributes them further.

Ascaris adults are facultative anaerobic organisms with a high glycogen consumption—1.3 g per 100 grams of body weight per 24 h; glycogen constitutes 14 to 24 percent of the dry weight of *A. lumbricoides*. The carbohydrate metabolism is a combination of glycolysis by the Embden-Meyerhof pathway and oxidative decarboxylation with volatile fatty acids as the characteristic end products. The eggs and the first-, second-, and third-stage larvae have an aerobic metabolism and a rather active lipid metabolism; the invasive larvae within the eggs, being in a dormant state, have a minimal metabolism. The protein metabolism is extensive during the growth, molting, and egg production periods. Amino acids necessary for the production of *Ascaris* eggs are partly absorbed, partly synthesized in the ovaries. The enormous reproductive potential of *Ascaris*, expressed by the approximately 240,000 eggs produced daily by a single female [8], is one of the most important features of the biology of the parasite.

PATIENT

The human host response and the clinical picture in ascariasis differ in the tissue phase of infection, caused by migrating larvae, and in the intestinal infection with preadult and adult worms. The difference is mainly in the type of reaction and

be a better indicator of age in the later stage of development [6]. The first *Ascaris* eggs can be detected when the female worm is longer than 12.6 cm; egg production increases until the female is about 25 cm long, reaches a plateau, and then starts to decrease in female worms longer than 27.5 cm [7]. The age-dependent changing fecundity of the female worms is one of the factors influencing the variation in the number of eggs excreted with the feces. In general, the development into sexual maturity in the small intestine takes 45 to 60 days, i.e., the new *Ascaris* eggs are produced 60 to 75 days after the invasive eggs have been ingested. As the radiological observations have shown, most of the adult *Ascaris* live in the jejunum (87.2 percent); only a few (11.9 percent) were found in the ileum. The mean life span of *Ascaris* in humans is thought to be about a year, but there are few solid observations on this.

its intensity. In the tissue phase the inflammatory and immunological reactions prevail, whereas in the intestinal phase the host's intestinal functions seem to be most affected.

PATHOGENESIS OF THE TISSUE PHASE OF ASCARIASIS

During their migration *Ascaris* larvae meet several barriers provoking many specific and nonspecific host reactions. During the passage through the intestinal mucosa some *Ascaris* larvae may be immobilized, covered with eosinophils, enveloped in eosinophilic granulomas, and destroyed. In addition, in the liver sinusoids some larvae may degenerate in infiltrations of eosinophils, neutrophils, and histiocytes; many of these granulomas develop into pseudotubercles with epithelioid and multinucleated giant cells. The presence of masses of amorphous acidophilic material around the larvae (Splendore-Hoeppli phenomenon) suggests a hypersensitive type of host reaction. The hypersensitivity reactions are even more pronounced during the pulmonary migration of *Ascaris* larvae: the alveolar sacs are filled with a serous exudate, the peribronchial tissue is infiltrated with eosinophils, the production of mucus in the bronchi is increased, and bronchial spasms are not uncommon. The migrating *Ascaris* larvae are frequently surrounded by hemorrhage and/or exudate and later on are destroyed in eosinophilic granulomas.

The intensity of the host reaction to migrating *Ascaris* larvae varies greatly. The host reaction is usually proportional to the number of *Ascaris* larvae which are destroyed during migration, but some pulmonary signs and symptoms were observed in human experimental invasions with small numbers of eggs such as from 6 to 45. In individuals sensitized by seasonable exposure to the infection the reactions are usually strong, but the pulmonary symptoms may be infrequent in members of the communities desensitized by permanent exposure to the infection [9,10]. *A. suum* larvae are nonspecific to humans but seem to provoke much stronger reactions than *A. lumbricoides* [5].

During *Ascaris* migration local reactions are usually accompanied by general hypersensitivity reactions such as bronchial asthma, transient eosinophilic pulmonary infiltrates (Loeffler's syndrome), angioneurotic edema, and urticaria. These reactions can also be mediated by contact with *Ascaris* allergen without any actual infection. In experimental monkeys similar pulmonary reactions have been produced by *Ascaris* antigen, rabbit anti-IgE, histamine, and the mast cell degranulating compound 48-80. It has been suggested that IgE antibodies found in the serum of patients with ascariasis are responsible for bronchial asthma and urticaria; they may also mediate the release of vasoactive amines, increased vascular permeability, and the disposition of antigen-antibody complexes in lung parenchyma, which results in Loeffler's syndrome. Loeffler's syndrome is not specific for helminthic infection and has been observed also in rheumatoid polyarthritis and drug intoxications.

PATHOGENESIS OF INTESTINAL ASCARIASIS

The host usually shows a great deal of tolerance to intestinal infection with preadult and adult *A. lumbricoides*. Little is known about the reaction to *Ascaris* larvae reentering the small intestine after extraintestinal migration, except that the fourth-stage larvae are strongly immunogenic and some may not be able to settle in or survive for long in the human gut. Adult *Ascaris* worms are not greatly affected by normal peristaltic action because for most of the time they are braced against the intestinal wall; they can go forward by means of a spiral movement and show a tendency to enter small openings such as the ampulla of Vater. In the majority of patients with ascariasis, a coarsening of the mucosal folds of the jejunum can be observed during x-ray examination. This corresponds well with the observations made in pigs infected with *A. suum*, which showed a corrugated appearance of the intestinal mucosa, a shortening of the crypt depth, a diminished amount of mucus, and a highly significant hypertrophy of the intestinal muscle layers [11]. The latter could be responsible for a quicker intestinal passage or for intestinal obstruction which is not infrequently observed in ascariasis.

Strong inhibitors of pepsin, cathepsin E, trypsin, and chymotrypsin in the host were found to be produced by *A. suum*. It is unlikely that these antienzymes greatly disturb the digestive functions of the host intestine.

Diminished food intake and the synergistic effect of polyparasitism have recently been listed among the many factors which may have a negative influence on the nutritional status of the host. A lower food intake is also a common phenomenon in other intestinal parasitic infections.

The coexistence of ascariasis and protein-energy malnutrition has long been observed [1,12]. However, numerous field studies on the effect of ascariasis on malnutrition have given very controversial results, mainly due to inadequate study design which neglected such important variants as the worm load, the duration of infection, the nutritional status of the host before deworming, and past or coexisting diseases. Clinical studies performed in metabolic wards on the effect of deworming on nutrition showed that *Ascaris* can negatively affect the absorption of nutrients in children on a marginal diet and with a heavy parasite load. A mean total nitrogen loss to the host, which was calculated as 22.7 mg per worm per day, may be insignificant for a child on an adequate protein diet and with only a moderate infection. On the other hand, there have been some observations of a lactase insufficiency in humans and pigs infected with *Ascaris;* lactose is an important source of energy in children under 2 years of age [13]. The results of recent field studies in Indonesia have confirmed the opinion that a significant negative correlation between the *Ascaris* burden and the nutritional status is apparent only in the segment of the population characterized by lower nutritional intake and poor utilization of health care facilities [14]. The relationship between ascariasis and child nutrition, which depends upon the interaction of multiple biomedical and behavioral factors, needs far more study.

There is also the need for further study of the specific deficiencies related to ascariasis; functional pyridoxine deficiency and substandard levels of vitamins A and C in parasitized children have been reported. Some *Ascaris* metabolites are readily absorbed by humans, and some, such as volatile fatty acids, are excreted in easily detectable amounts in the urine of infected hosts; there is still little information on how the host tolerates *Ascaris* metabolites and whether they interfere with the host metabolism.

SYMPTOMATOLOGY OF ASCARIASIS

Ascariasis does not always cause any symptoms, but when symptoms are manifest, they may differ widely depending on the stage and intensity of the infection and the nature of the host reaction. The symptomatology of ascariasis can be categorized as follows: (1) pulmonary ascariasis; (2) intestinal ascariasis; (3) complications of ascariasis; and (4) allergy to *Ascaris*.

Pulmonary ascariasis

During the migration of *Ascaris* larvae abdominal symptoms and signs, including hepatomegaly, are rare; occasionally there is some biochemical evidence of transient hepatocellular damage. Pulmonary manifestation is the most frequent symptom and varies from a slight cough of a few days to a severe, seasonal, *Ascaris* pneumonitis. The clinical and laboratory characteristics of seasonable *Ascaris* pneumonitis, based on the report of 95 cases observed in Saudi Arabia [9], are as follows: brief (less than 5 days) history of illness; cough (rarely in paroxysm); dyspnea (but rarely cyanosis); substernal discomfort (mostly burning); subfebrile state rather than fever; frequent wheezing and rales at auscultation; occasionally, skin rash; *Ascaris* larvae in the sputum or gastric washings; negative bacteriological examination of the sputum; high eosinophilia in the later stage of the disease; in x-ray chest examination discrete soft bilateral densities, sometimes becoming confluent in the perihilar areas.

In moderate cases of pulmonary involvement the mild symptoms usually contrast with the intense, but transient, pathological changes in the lungs as detected by x-ray examination.

Intestinal ascariasis

The symptomatology of intestinal ascariasis differs from, on the one extreme, cases with vague occasional abdominal pains and without any other clinical signs, to the other extreme of complicated cases of ascariasis which could be characterized as follows: a child of 2 to 5 years old, listless, underweight, and somewhat anemic, with anorexia, vague abdominal pains, intermittent loose stools, and occasional vomiting; with face resembling the "moonface" of kwashiorkor, the hair dry and

somewhat light in color, with skin lusterless and scaly; and with abdomen full and/or distended with small-intestinal loops visible through the thin abdominal wall. In a case like this ascariasis is an important factor, though only one of many, responsible for the whole clinical picture; other factors are poor living conditions, inadequate nutrition, and coexistent or past parasitic or infectious diseases.

In less diseased cases of ascariasis the most frequent symptom is abdominal pain; in children it is often vague and is localized mainly in the area of the navel; in adults the pain is peptic ulcer–like or colicky and localized mainly in the epigastrum. Upper abdominal discomfort, nausea, or vomiting are not frequent manifestations; anorexia and restlessness have been reported occasionally, but their causal relationship to the *Ascaris* infection remains unclear.

Complications of ascariasis

The adult *Ascaris* worm is a relatively common cause of severe complications due to its characteristically large size and aggregating and/or migratory activities. The migration of adult *Ascaris* may be promoted by some drugs, including some antihelminthics and those used for anesthesia, but also by fever and peppery food.

Only few data are available on the frequency of migration or aggregation of adult *Ascaris*. In 580 cases observed in Poland, *Ascaris* worms were expelled orally in 3.3 percent of the patients and in one case had caused an intestinal obstruction [15]. In a rural area of the southeastern United States, the approximate rate of intestinal obstruction was 2 per 1000 children with ascariasis per year [16]. In endemic areas intestinal obstruction due to *Ascaris* is diagnosed and the patient hospitalized in up to 0.5 cases per 1000 infected; ascariasis causes 1 to 35 percent of all intestinal obstructions [2]. Laparotomies due to complicated ascariasis may constitute as much as 11 percent of all laparotomies carried out in pediatric wards in the tropics [2] (Figs. 43-2 and 43-3).

The clinical course of the intestinal obstructions differs from the relatively mild symptoms and signs to dramatic ones, depending on (1) the number of worms involved, which can be as high as 1063; (2) the localization of the obstruction, most commonly the terminal ileum; (3) the character of the obstruction, which can be complete or partial; (4) further complications, such as intussusception, volvulus, hemorrhagic infarction of the intestine, and perforation. The symptoms usually start suddenly with vomiting and colicky, recurring abdominal pain; constipation and passing worms from the rectum or the mouth are less common. Among the most common signs are abdominal distension and tenderness, abnormal abdominal sounds, and x-ray evidence of intestinal obstruction [16].

The next most common complication is biliary or hepatic ascariasis, which occurs most frequently in children; in some areas this condition is rare or not diagnosed properly [2,17,18]. It may be suspected in patients with ascariasis suffering from

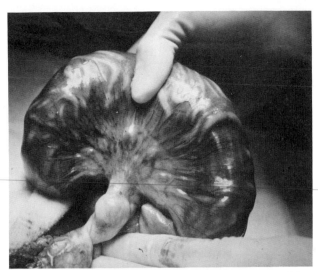

Figure 43-2. Intestinal volvulus caused by *Ascaris*. (*Courtesy of Professor J. Pinus.*)

right upper abdominal pain, which is characterized by a sudden onset, a paroxysmal course, and a very strong intensity which may be refractory to the usual analgesics; vomiting with bile-stained gastric contents frequently coexists with the pain. A typical sign is pain at the pressure point just below the xiphoid process. Fever, leukocytosis, and jaundice may occur later on as complications such as infection, common bile duct stricture, or penetration into the hepatic tissue occur. The *Ascaris* worm, which is one-third to one-half of the length of the extrahepatic biliary tree in children, may return to the intestine spontaneously, but it may also happen that several *Ascaris* adult worms invade the bile ducts or the liver tissue and cause the

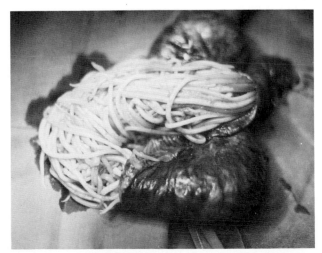

Figure 43-3. Conglomerate of *Ascaris* in resected small intestine. (*Courtesy of Professor J. Pinus.*)

formation of an abscess or granulomatous lesions. It has been observed that the left lobe is affected more frequently than the right one, possibly because the left hepatic duct is straighter [17]. Evidence is accumulating that in endemic areas *Ascaris* eggs or tissues are frequently responsible for formation of biliary stones [19].

The other abdominal complications of ascariasis, such as appendicitis, pancreatitis, volvulus, intussusception, and intestinal perforation and peritonitis, may cause severe clinical problems and are frequently fatal. Asphyxia due to obstruction of the upper respiratory tract by migrating *Ascaris* adult worms has occasionally been reported as the cause of death related to ascariasis.

Allergy to *Ascaris*

The *Ascaris* allergen is one of the most potent allergens of parasitic origin. Its physicochemical and biological properties are known. An increase in circulating IgE globulins in response to *Ascaris* infection is common, but only a small number of IgE globulins have antibodies specific for *Ascaris*. The impact of this nonspecific potentiation of IgE response on the health of whole populations living in areas endemic for ascariasis is controversial and requires further well-controlled studies [15].

Exposure to *Ascaris* allergen may cause hypersensitivity reactions in lungs, skin, conjunctiva, and intestinal mucosa. Asthmatic reactions to *Ascaris* allergen may occur not only in infected subjects but in most individuals who were found to be *Ascaris*-positive on skin testing or in a mother of an infected child. The most common skin change is urticaria. Repeated abdominal pain, heartburn, and diarrhea were described in an uninfected laboratory technician exposed to *Ascaris* antigen at work [1,20]; however, the most common reactions in individuals working with *Ascaris* worms are conjunctivitis and facial edema.

DIAGNOSIS OF ASCARIASIS

A direct diagnosis of ascariasis is possible by finding the adult parasite, larvae, or eggs.

Adult *Ascaris*, due to senility or host reaction or other factors promoting migration, are rather commonly expelled through the anus or mouth. They can also be easily diagnosed in the small intestine during abdominal surgery. *Ascaris* adults are occasionally found in the intestinal tract during x-ray examination. There is an increased use of endoscopy and sonography techniques for diagnosing intestinal or biliary ascariasis [21,22].

Ascaris larvae may be found in the sputum or gastric washings between the eighth and sixteenth day following exposure and are occasionally found in liver or lung biopsy material.

Ascaris eggs first appear in the feces 60 to 75 days after exposure. The *Ascaris* eggs found in feces may be fertile or infertile. The fertile eggs are ovoid and measure 45 to 70 μm by 35 to 50 μm. The shell is thick and consists of several layers; the outer protein coat is a spongelike structure, adhesive and highly protective against mechanical injuries; it is derived from *Ascaris* uterine secretion and stained brown by host bile pigments. The inner five layers are made of a structureless material or chitinous fibers, secreted by the developing egg itself. The ova are unsegmented in the eggs excreted with feces. Sometimes the fertilized eggs are decorticated, i.e., deprived of their outer coat. The infertile eggs are of irregular shape and usually longer and narrower (90 by 40 μm) than the fertile ones; they have a thinner mammillated shell and disorganized material instead of an ovum.

The most effective coprological techniques for diagnosis of *Ascaris* eggs are the Kato and Miura thick smear and simple sedimentation. Flotation techniques may not be effective for the detection of rather heavy unfertilized eggs. The rate of positive stool examinations may be low in those infections with only a few *Ascaris* worms. In a study in Korea false-negative results were found in 15 percent of ascariasis cases, due to the presence of male worms only (52 percent), too young or too old females only (33 percent), or the inadequacy of the examination technique (15 percent) [6]. A direct smear of 2 mg of fecal material normally has two to six eggs per female worm and is usually found to be negative in one-third of infections with a single female worm. The thick smear (after Kato and Miura) consists of between 30 and 70 mg of fecal material and has many more eggs per female worm.

Ascaris is sometimes neglected as a possible etiological factor of disease; out of 26 cases of *Ascaris* erraticism reported from the Philippines (23 of them fatal) no parasitological fecal examination was done in 15 cases; in 3 cases it was done but found negative, and in 6 cases it was done and found positive for *Ascaris*, but no antihelminthic treatment was given [23].

An indirect diagnosis of ascariasis is possible by immunological or biochemical procedures. Several immunological tests have been used in diagnosing the early migratory stage of ascariasis, e.g., agar-gel diffusion and immunoelectrophoretic analysis to detect the presence of IgM antibodies to the *Ascaris* antigen [5], solid-phase radioimmunoassay technique, indirect immunofluorescence test, and hemagglutination test with both larval and adult *Ascaris* antigen. The interpretation of these tests is always a problem because of the complex antigenic structure of the helminths, the possibility of heterologous reactions with blood group antibodies or host tissue components, and/or the presence of mixed infection of *Ascaris* and *Toxocara*. The skin test with purified *Ascaris* antigen is rather sensitive, but its widespread use is hazardous because of the possibility of severe reaction in some hypersensitive patients.

Eosinophilia may be high (30 to 50 percent) during the later migratory phase of ascariasis, but it decreases rapidly during the intestinal stage of the infection.

TREATMENT OF ASCARIASIS

No specific treatment for pulmonary ascariasis is available. In severe cases most of the symptoms, which are of a hypersensitivity type, respond well to corticosteroid therapy [5].

Intestinal ascariasis

Intestinal ascariasis should be treated whenever diagnosed or even simply suspected, since the presence of immature or male worms only cannot be diagnosed by laboratory examination and the risk of serious complications always exists even from an infection with a single worm. Modern antihelminthics such as piperazine, levamisole, pyrantel, and benzimidazole carbamates are highly effective and relatively safe and have successfully replaced the older drugs used against ascariasis such as chenopodium oil, santonin, kainic acid, papain enzyme preparation, bephenium, and thiabendazole.

Piperazine derivates (usually citrate or adipate) temporarily paralyze the *Ascaris* worms by producing neuromuscular blockage through an anticholinergic action at the myoneural junction; the paralyzed worms are easily evacuated by the peristaltic movement of the intestine. Piperazine, widely used for over 25 years in ascariasis and enterobiasis, is now being withdrawn from the market in the developed countries because of sporadic hypersensitive and neurotoxic reactions and also because better drugs have been introduced. In developing countries piperazine is still used because it is one of the cheapest drugs available. The daily dose is 75 mg per kilogram of body weight with a maximum individual dose of 4 g for adults and 2 g for children under 20 kg in weight. The efficacy of a single-dose treatment is 70 to 80 percent; treatment for two consecutive days is effective in over 90 percent of ascariasis cases [24].

Levamisole, a levorotatory *s*-isomer of tetramisole, is a potent inhibitor of fumarate reductase activity, which is an enzyme essential in the carbohydrate metabolism of *Ascaris*. Levamisole, practically devoid of toxicity for humans, shows nonspecific activation of macrophages and some immunomodulating activities. Used in a single dose of 150 mg for adults and 3 to 5 mg/kg in children, it is effective in 80 to 100 percent of cases of ascariasis [15,24].

Pyrantel, which is a cyclic amidine, acts on the neuromuscular transmission in *Ascaris* and causes a spastic acetylcholinelike paralysis of the worm. Pyrantel emboate is used in a single dose of about 100 mg per kilogram of body weight (maximum 750 mg in adults). The efficacy of a single-dose treatment in ascariasis is over 90 percent [15,24]. In control campaigns against ascariasis much lower doses (2.5 mg/kg) used periodically were found to be effective [6]. Mixed infections with *Ascaris* and hookworm need treatment for 2 to 4 days.

Mebendazole, a benzimidazole carbamate, inhibits phosphorylation in the *Ascaris* mitochondria and damages the tubular system of the intestinal cells, leading to the slow death of the worm. It has been observed that *Ascaris* are rather frequently expelled by mouth during therapy. The single dose of mebendazole is 200 mg irrespective of age. Mixed *Ascaris*, hookworm, and *Trichuris* infections need a higher dosage (in adults a single dose of 600 mg or up to 400 mg daily for 3 to 4 days). The efficacy of mebendazole in ascariasis is between 84 and 100 percent [15,24]. The other benzimidazole carbamates such as fenbendazole, flubendazole, and albendazole show a similar efficacy and good tolerance. Benzimidazole compounds, which are embryotoxic in some rodents, are contraindicated in pregnancy.

Complications of ascariasis

Complications due to intestinal ascariasis need conservative rather than surgical treatment, depending on the case.

In cases of intestinal obstruction due to *A. lumbricoides* conservative treatment consists of nasogastric suction for 12 to 24 h, repeated doses of piperazine citrate or pyrantel given through the nasogastric tube, and intravenous fluids. This form of therapy is usually decided on in the early stages of obstruction, which is frequently not complete. Surgical intervention has to be undertaken immediately in patients with definite clinical or radiological evidence of complete intestinal obstruction, with signs of acute abdominal surgical emergency, or complications such as perforation, peritonitis, or volvulus. The simplest operative procedure is to massage the worms from the ileum into the cecum if the intestinal wall is viable enough for this type of manipulation and if the bolus of worms can easily be dislodged. Resection of the obstructed segment of the intestine and end-to-end anastomosis usually give better results than enterotomy and extraction of the ascarids one by one, which frequently leads to peritonitis. Resection with double enterostomy is practiced in some acutely ill patients, especially infants and children, but has many disadvantages especially in tropical conditions. At the Medical University of South Carolina, out of 99 patients hospitalized for intestinal obstruction due to ascariasis, only 17 were operated upon, but 3 died [*16*].

In biliary ascariasis conservative treatment with antispasmodics and antihelminthics, as well as intestinal decompression and intravenous fluid, is appropriate in the early stage of disease. It may be ineffective due to duct stricture or due to *Ascaris* being numerous or dead, or invading the liver tissue; in these cases appropriate surgical intervention is necessary [*18*].

POPULATION

BASIC EPIDEMIOLOGICAL DATA AND A MATHEMATICAL MODEL FOR ASCARIASIS

Ascariasis can spread epidemically, as it did in 1947 to 1948 around the vast, sewage-irrigated fields at Griesheim in West Germany [*25*], but this is rare. Basically ascariasis is an endemic infection with rather stable prevalence rates due to the high reproductive potential of the parasite, intensive contamination of the environment, and easy reinfection. A single *A. lumbricoides* female worm produces daily about 240,000 eggs. In spite of heavy losses in viability and infectivity in the environment, 1 g of contaminated soil may contain as many as several hundred invasive *Ascaris* eggs. This makes reinfection easy, as does the fact that the host immunity is not fully protective.

Ascariasis is a soil-transmitted infection spread either directly by the not uncommon habit of eating soil (pica), or indirectly by soil-contaminated hands, food such as vegetables and fruits, and water. Contaminated soil may be carried for some distance on human feet or footwear, on the fur and feet of domesticated animals, by flies and other invertebrates, and by water or dust. However, the most contaminated areas are usually those directly polluted with human excreta (around households, in vegetable gardens fertilized with human feces).

In endemic areas the prevalence of ascariasis increases sharply during the first 2 to 3 years of age, remains at a maximum between the ages of 4 and 14 years, and either persists at a slightly lower level or declines in adults. The intensity of infection is maximal in children of preschool age. A slight difference in sex distribution in favor of women was observed in some areas where household transmission is common. Infections with *Ascaris* are frequently aggregated in families due to their specific modes of behavior or lower economic or educational position. Ascariasis is not an occupational infection but is nonetheless more common in agricultural than in industrialized societies.

The transmission of *Ascaris* eggs occurs all year round in many moist tropical areas or may show some seasonality due to winter, monsoon, or dry season. Seasonal fluctuations may also be provoked by the consumption of stored foods, i.e., pickled vegetables prepared for winter in Korea.

Much basic information is still needed (on the life span of adult *Ascaris*, the survival time of *Ascaris* eggs in the external environment, *Ascaris* infection turnover in humans) in order to understand fully the dynamic relationship between *Ascaris* and humans. Despite these limitations, the modern science of population dynamics tries to elucidate and measure those factors regulating the abundance of *Ascaris* and contributing to the observed stability of *Ascaris* populations. Endemic ascariasis is stable if each female parasite exactly replaces herself in the next generation, i.e., when R—the effective reproductive and transmission potential of the parasite—is equal to unity. The R parameter has recently been estimated for several helminthic infections in different parts of the world. The parameter R in conjunction with the life-expectancy of the adult *Ascaris* (A), the degree of worm aggregation (k), and the severity of density-dependent constraints on *Ascaris* population growth (z) acts to determine the average intensity (M) and prevalence (P) of ascariasis at equilibrium in a given community. Then

$$M = (R^{1/(k+1)} - 1)\left(\frac{k}{1-z}\right) \text{ and}$$

$$P = 1 - \left(1 + \frac{M}{k}\right)^{-k}$$

For ascariasis in an area in Iran the parameters were calculated as follows: $R = 4.3$, $A = 1$, $z = 0.96$, $K = 0.57$, $M = 22$ [*26,27*]. The proposed model shows that after a single chemotherapeutic intervention the prevalence would return to the level before treatment within 12 months. Although the mathematical model is helpful in understanding the basic relationship between the populations of humans and *Ascaris*, it is of a limited value because it could hardly take into consideration all the human, parasitic, and environmental factors responsible for the local transmission which act in nature and are closely interrelated.

DISTRIBUTION AND PREVALENCE OF ASCARIASIS

The distribution of ascariasis can be discussed from the global, regional, or community aspects.

In 1979 the global prevalence of ascariasis was between 800 million and 1 billion cases, as estimated from WHO data and from published studies performed in well-defined populations [3,4]. In other words, ascariasis, with every fourth person in the world being infected, is third among the 10 most common human infections. According to the studies supported by WHO 32.3 percent of people living in Africa, i.e., about 155 million, have ascariasis, 1 in 50 being heavily infected [28]. In Latin America, 1,796,235 people were found infected, i.e., 25.5 percent out of 7,024,685 examined in the years 1975–1987 [2].

The distribution of ascariasis in the world is, generally speaking, proportional to the density of the human population, standards of education, levels of sanitation and agricultural development, as well as regional geoclimatic conditions. The density of the human population is one of the critical factors facilitating the spread of ascariasis. Ascariasis, as a fecal and soil-transmitted infection, is most prevalent in crowded, rural, and periurban areas, where sanitary facilities are lacking or not used because of ignorance and/or low standards of social infrastructure (e.g., small children left alone defecate anywhere). Primitive agricultural practices using fresh human night soil as a fertilizer, especially for the production of vegetables, are responsible for the high prevalence of ascariasis in certain regions of the world. The distribution of ascariasis reflects the local level of social and economic development in areas where the geoclimatic conditions permit the parasite to develop. *Ascaris* develops best in moist, noninsulated soil, not necessarily in tropical or subtropical areas. For examples, in Chile ascariasis is prevalent in a biogeographical forestry zone which is moderately cold and moist, and agriculturally developed; ascariasis is rare in the desert, steppes, brushwood, or very cold zones in Chile. In Africa ascariasis is rare in the arid savanna area. In the warm and arid regions of the Arabian peninsula *Ascaris* infection is only transmitted seasonally.

Several studies comparing the prevalence of ascariasis in different countries have shown substantial differences in prevalence in localities situated in similar biogeographical zones. One study performed in nine closely situated villages in the Caspian region of Iran showed that the socioagricultural factors greatly influenced the prevalence of intestinal parasitic infections: ascariasis was common (46 percent) only in an area where vegetables were cultivated; hookworm infections were prevalent in the rice-growing area; and taeniasis in the mountainous cattle-breeding area.

It is also known that in communities living in the same village the distribution of infection can be uneven: most people may have no, or only a few, parasites, but a few people carry excessive worm burdens. The pattern of distribution is aggregated, and in statistical terms is best described as a negative binomial. The uneven distribution may be a result of increased susceptibility, some behavioral or occupational traits, or just the superimposition of several random dispersions. The latter possibility was suggested to explain the situation in Jazin, Esfahan, Iran, where 5 out of 111 persons examined carried 16 percent of all the *Ascaris* worms found [26,30]. Some individual predisposition to heavy or light *Ascaris* infection has been confirmed in India [31]; however, more studies on genetic, spatial, and behavioral factors are needed to understand all these phenomena.

INTENSITY OF ASCARIASIS AND ITS REGULATING MECHANISMS

There are three principal mechanisms regulating the *Ascaris* population in humans: (1) infection pressure, (2) host immunity, and (3) age limitation of the parasite.

The term *infection pressure* means the number of possible human exposures in a certain area in a given time. The human exposure depends on the intensity of human contacts with contaminated material and the degree of contamination of this material. In hyperendemic areas, where the transmission of ascariasis is year-round, human beings are probably exposed to *Ascaris* eggs permanently in proportion to human behavioral patterns; small children are those most exposed to contact with contaminated soil. There is, however, one behavioral mechanism which can cause intensive infections, i.e., pica. This deviant habit of ingestion of nonfood substances may have a psychological or nutritional (iron deficiency) background. Pica is quite a common phenomenon among children below 6 years of age, and its definite association with *Toxocara* infections in humans has been confirmed. The number of invasive *Ascaris* eggs in the soil depends on the degree of fecal contamination (promiscuous defecation of small children around houses, inadequate sanitation, use of human night soil as a fertilizer) as well as on the various ecological factors affecting development and survival of *Ascaris* eggs in the environment. The degree of soil contamination may be quite high. For example, in Sawahlunto, west Sumatra (Indonesia), *Ascaris* eggs were found in 45 percent of 55 samples of soil (2 g each) collected around 9 farm houses. In some heavily infected areas some subsamples of soil may contain more eggs than others due to the nature of the soil and the scattering and sorting action of rain, as well as the activity of some invertebrates [32]. Ecological factors, therefore, may also be responsible for the nonuniform exposure of humans to *Ascaris*.

Humans are unable to develop a fully protective immunity

to reinfection with *Ascaris*, but immunological and nonspecific reactions to exposure to *Ascaris* larvae may greatly reduce the final number of parasites settled in humans. The immune response is effective mainly against migrating *Ascaris* larvae in the liver and lungs, also against fourth-stage larvae reentering the small intestine. In nonimmune hosts the first antibodies were detected on the sixth day of infection. The maximal level of circulating antibodies was observed in the third and fourth weeks. During the second and third months the circulating antibodies slowly decreased. As with other infections IgM antibodies appear first followed by those of the IgG classes, which prevail later. Experimental immune hosts responded almost immediately to inoculation with *Ascaris*. In patients infected with *A. suum*, the high titers of precipitating antibody of IgM class were well correlated with the final reduction in the worm burden. Cellular immunity also plays an important role in reducing the number of migrating larvae, but the effector mechanism remains unclear. The mechanisms of the nonspecific responses to invading *Ascaris* larvae may be mediated by the eosinophil chemotactic factor and neutrophil chemotactic factor and may have a cytotoxic character. From experimental infections with *A. suum* in piglets it is known that the number of worms found in the intestine was negatively proportional to the size of the inoculum: 0.013 percent at doses of between 1000 and 10,000 eggs, 2.9 percent at a dose of 500 eggs, and 64 percent at a dose of 50 eggs. The reduction in size of the inoculum (the larger the inoculum, the higher the reduction) was explained partially by the expulsion of fourth-stage larvae 10 days after inoculation and of immature worms after 4 weeks of infection [*33*].

The effect of the host immune and nonspecific responses on the final intensity of ascariasis as well as the effect of infection pressure cannot be measured separately in humans, but their combined effect is expressed as the reinfection rate, which is measurable. The reinfection rate, calculated after mass treatment against *Ascaris*, can, in some hyperendemic areas, be as high as 54.9 percent after 7 months [*34*]. Because the life span of *Ascaris* is limited to about 1 year, there are constant reinfections which keep ascariasis endemic and common in many parts of the world.

The intensity of ascariasis is usually related to the prevalence. Certain patterns were observed in Korea: the percentage of light infections (fewer than 4 *Ascaris*) was rather constant (33 to 41 percent of the population) and independent of the various prevalence rates (24 to 67 percent); only the number of moderate or heavy infections (over 10 *Ascaris*) was proportional to the prevalence [*6*]. In Kenya the mean intensity of ascariasis was calculated as 7 *Ascaris* per host at the overall prevalence of 25 percent [*29*]. In Jazin (Iran) the mean intensity was 22 *Ascaris* per host at the overall prevalence of 86 percent [*26*].

The intensity of infection in ascariasis can best be measured by the number of *Ascaris* expelled after successful treatment. Quantitative stool examination is not a precise method, irrespective of the techniques used, but is still used in practice to evaluate the approximate intensity of ascariasis, both in individual cases and in epidemiological surveys.

PREVENTION AND CONTROL OF ASCARIASIS

In theory ascariasis, as an infection spread by humans, is preventable. In fact, in many developed countries it is an infection which disappears with improved levels of sanitation only, without any specific control intervention; e.g., in the Poznan area (Poland) the prevalence of ascariasis among rural school children was 8 percent in 1955 to 1956 and 3 percent in 1970 to 1971. In an Iranian village, the installation of basic sanitary facilities (piped water, latrines) lowered the prevalence of ascariasis from 67 to 57 percent within 2 years. In areas with a hot and moist climate and where the people are less cooperative the effects of the improved sanitation may become visible only after several decades. When there is no time to wait and where the organizational facilities and economic potential are adequate enough to permit the control of intestinal parasitic infections, chemotherapy is the most potent tool, and one which offers more immediate results [*1–3,35*].

Control strategies based on chemotherapy should be adapted to the local conditions, but it is generally accepted that the treatment should be repeated every 3 months and continued for several years. Blanket treatment of the whole population is suggested when the prevalence of ascariasis is high; later on selective treatment is preferable, covering most of those who remain infected and have been detected by mass examination. In areas where mass examination is difficult, the best chemotherapeutic control strategy should be decided on after a basic epidemiological survey has been done, to define the prevalence, intensity, and distribution of ascariasis in the local population as well as the transmission characteristics in a given area. Target treatment repeatedly given to those most heavily infected, e.g., preschool and school children, has been seen to lower the prevalence of ascariasis effectively in the whole community [*36*].

In many areas medical treatment of individual cases of ascariasis or self-medication is practiced but does not have much effect on the prevalence of the infection. Effective control of ascariasis by chemotherapy has to be community-oriented, integrated where possible into existing health programs, and preferably carried out simultaneously with sanitation and education programs. Experience in southeast Asia has already shown that the control of ascariasis by chemotherapy is a good "entry point" to community participation in other health or social programs such as nutrition and family planning [*1,3*]. It has been calculated for Kenya that the annual cost of mass treatment would amount to only one-fifth of the losses due to human ascariasis [*29*].

The control of ascariasis in countries where waste water is used for agricultural purposes poses several technical problems [*25*]. The pesticides and mineral fertilizers affect the survival time and invasiveness of *Ascaris* eggs on the ground only to a rather moderate degree.

Individual prevention by washing hands, vegetables, and fruits or by boiling water only may not be fully protective, therefore ascariasis is occasionally detected in international travelers to hyperendemic areas.

REFERENCES

1 Crompton DWT, Nesheim MC, Pawlowski ZS (eds): *Ascariasis and its Public Health Significance*. London, Taylor and Francis, 1985

2 Crompton DWT, Nesheim MC, Pawlowski ZS (eds): *Prevention and Control of Ascariasis*. London, Taylor and Francis, in print

3 Prevention and Control of Intestinal Parasitic Infections: Report of a WHO Expert Committee. WHO Tech Rep Ser 749, Geneva, World Health Organization, 1987

4 Walsh JA, Warren KS: Selective primary health care: An interim strategy for disease control in developing countries. N Engl J Med 301:967–974, 1979

5 Phills JA, Harrold AJ, Whiteman GV, et al: Pulmonary infiltrates, asthma and eosinophilia due to *Ascaris suum* infestation in man. N Engl J Med 286:965–970, 1972

6 Seo BS: Ascariasis and its control problems in Korea. Seoul J Med 22:323–341, 1981

7 Chai JY, Hong ST, Lee SH, et al: Fluctuation of the egg production amounts according to worm burden and length of *Ascaris lumbricoides*. Korean J Parasitol 19:38–44, 1981

8 Sinniah B: Daily egg production of *Ascaris lumbricoides:* The distribution of eggs in the faeces and the variability of egg counts. Parasitology 84:167–175, 1982

9 Gelpi AP, Mustafa A: Seasonal pneumonitis with eosinophilia: A study of larval ascariasis in Saudi Arabia. Am J Trop Med Hyg 16:646–657, 1967

10 Spillman RK: Pulmonary ascariasis in tropical communities. Am J Trop Med Hyg 24:791–800, 1975

11 Stephenson LS, Pond WG, Nesheim MC et al: *Ascaris suum:* Nutrient absorption, growth and intestinal pathology in young pigs experimentally infected with 15-day-old larvae. Exp Parasitol 49:15–25, 1980

12 Stephenson LS: The contribution of *Ascaris lumbricoides* to malnutrition in children. Parasitology 81:221–233, 1980

13 Carrera E, Nesheim MC, Crompton DWT: Lactose maldigestion in *Ascaris* infected preschool children. Am J Clin Nutr 39:255–265, 1984

14 Cerf BJ, Rohde JE, Soesanto T: *Ascaris* and malnutrition in a Balinese village: A conditional relationship. Trop Geogr Med 33:367–373, 1981

15 Pawlowski ZS: Ascariasis. Clin Gastroenterol 7:157–178, 1978

16 Blumenthal DS, Schultz MG: Incidence of intestinal obstruction in children infected with *Ascaris lumbricoides*. Am J Trop Med Hyg 24:801–805, 1975

17 Maki T: Surgical diseases due to *Ascaris lumbricoides,* in Morishita K, Komiya Y, Matsubayashi H (eds): *Progress of Medical Parasitology in Japan*. Tokyo, Meguro Parasitological Museum, 1972, vol 4, pp 221–270

18 Davies MRQ, Rode H: Biliary ascariasis in children, in Rickham PP, Hecker WCh, Prévot J (eds): *Pediatric Surgery in Tropical Countries*. Baltimore-Munich, Urban & Schwarzenberg, 1982, pp 55–74

19 Schulman A: Non-western patterns of biliary stones and the role of ascariasis. Radiology 162:425–430, 1987

20 Coles GC: Gastro-intestinal allergy to nematodes. Trans R Soc Trop Med Hyg 69:362–363, 1975

21 Chen YS, Den BX, Huang BI, et al: Endoscopic diagnosis and management of *Ascaris*-induced acute pancreatitis. Endoscopy 18:127–128, 1986

22 Khuroo MS, Zargar SA, Mahajan R, et al: Sonographic appearances in biliary ascariasis. Gastroenterology 93:267–272, 1987

23 Chanco PP, Jr: *Ascaris lumbricoides*—its erraticism, in Abstracts of the Tenth International Congress on Tropical Medicine and Malaria. Manila, Philippines, November 9–15, 1980, pp 142–143

24 Janssens PG: Chemotherapy of gastrointestinal nematodiasis in man, in Vanden Bossche et al (eds): *Handbook of Experimental Pharmacology*. Berlin, Springer-Verlag, 77:183–406, 1985

25 Pawlowski ZS, Schultzberg K: Ascariasis and sewage in Europe, in Block JC et al (eds): *Epidemiological Studies of Risks Associated with the Agricultural Use of Sewage Sludge: Knowledge and Needs*. London, Elsevier, 1986, pp 83–93

26 Croll NA, Ghadirian E: Wormy persons: Contribution to the nature and patterns of overdispersion with *Ascaris lumbricoides, Ancylostoma duodenale, Necator americanus,* and *Trichuris trichiura*. Trop Geogr Med 33:241–248, 1981

27 Anderson RM, May RM: Population dynamics of human helminth infections: Control by chemotherapy. Nature 297:557–563, 1982

28 Crompton DWT, Tulley JJ: How much ascariasis is there in Africa? Parasitol Today 3:123–127, 1987

29 Stephenson LS, Lathan MC, Oduori ML: Costs, prevalence and approaches for control of *Ascaris* infection in Kenya. J Trop Pediatr 26:246–263, 1980

30 Croll NA, Anderson RM, Gyorkos TW, et al: The population biology and control of *Ascaris lumbricoides* in a rural community in Iran. Trans R Soc Trop Med Hyg 76:187–197, 1982

31 Haswell-Elkins MR, Elkins DB, Anderson RM: Evidence for predisposition in humans to infection with *Ascaris*, hookworm, *Enterobius,* and *Trichuris* in a South Indian fishing community. Parasitology 95:323–337, 1987

32 Beaver PC: Biology of soil-transmitted helminths: The massive infection. Health Lab Sci 12:116–125, 1975

33 Andersen S, Jørgensen RJ, Nansen P, et al: Experimental *Ascaris suum* infection in piglets. Acta Pathol Microbiol Scand (B) 81:650–656, 1973

34 Hayashi S: A model for the evaluation and assessment of the effect of control of the soil-transmitted helminthiases, in *Collected Papers on the Control of Soil-Transmitted Helminthiases*. Tokyo, Asian Parasite Control Organization, 1980, vol 1, pp 265–273

35 Pawlowski ZS: Strategies for the control of ascariasis. Ann Soc Belge Med Trop 64:125–134, 1984

36 Cabrera BD, Cruz AC: A comparative study on the effect of mass treatment of the entire community and selective treatment of children on the total prevalence of soil-transmitted helminthiasis in two communities, Mindoro, Philippines, in Yokogawa G, Hayashi S, Kobayashi A, et al (eds): *Collected Papers on the Control of Soil-transmitted Helminthiases*. Tokyo, Asian Parasite Control Organization, 1982, vol 2, pp 266–287

Hookworms · *Gerhard A. Schad* · *John G. Banwell*

PARASITE

The hookworms parasitizing humans form two groups, one that normally develops and matures, and another, constituted of zoophilic species, which rarely, or never, matures in humans. The first includes *Ancylostoma duodenale* and *Necator americanus,* misleadingly named the "old" and "new" world hookworms, respectively. Both species are widely distributed in tropical and subtropical Asia and Africa, but *A. duodenale* occurs alone in the Middle East, north Africa, and southern Europe. In the new world, *N. americanus* is the predominant species, but *A. duodenale* does occur focally in the Caribbean Islands and in Central and South America [1,2]. The second group includes several hookworms of cats and dogs that invade humans in whom they migrate and develop to differing degrees. *A. ceylanicum* infections are rare, and parasitized individuals harbor very few adult worms, but in restricted parts of its range (e.g., New Guinea) adult worms are common in humans. Other species (e.g., *A. braziliense, Uncinaria stenocephala*), although capable of penetrating the skin, generally fail to migrate to deeper tissues and do not mature.

The adult hookworm is a voracious blood-sucking nematode that normally resides in the small intestine, particularly the jejunum. In excessively heavy infections, it is less habitat specific and may invade the stomach and/or large intestine. It attaches to the intestinal wall by drawing a plug of mucosa into its large buccal capsule. Enzymes from the esophageal glands digest the plug. This process, coupled with the general boring of the worm, eventually leads to the rupture of a blood vessel. Once this occurs, the worm's boring ceases, but esophageal pumping accelerates, resulting in a rapid passage of blood through the worm [3–6].

Frequently cited estimates of egg output for *N. americanus* and *A. duodenale* are 10,000 to 20,000 and 25,000 or more eggs per female per day, respectively. Egg output is influenced by a number of factors, including the age of the worms, their number, and the immunological response of the host. Density-dependent effects are particularly well known, egg output being markedly depressed in heavy infections [7]. Density-dependent depression of egg output may even occur in light infections [8], but this conclusion has been challenged as an artifact of data analysis [9].

The eggs are discharged into the intestinal lumen, where they undergo a number of cell divisions before being passed in the stools. Given sufficient moisture, warmth, and oxygen, the eggs embryonate in the feces and hatch within 24 h [10]. The worm which emerges on hatching is a rhabditiform, first-stage (L_1) larva, with a rhabditiform esophagus (Fig. 44-1). The L_1 lives in the feces, or in fecally polluted soils, feeding

on microbes and other small organic particles. Bouts of feeding and growth are separated by intervals of rest and molting, so that during its life as a free-living organism the hookworm completes two rhabditiform larval stages (L_1 and L_2) separated by one molt, and comes to rest as a nonfeeding, ensheathed, infective third-stage (L_3) larva. At tropical soil temperatures, development from egg to L_3 takes 5 to 10 days, and during this time larvae are not infective. The mouth tube of the L_3 (Fig. 44-1), which will not feed until it penetrates the host, does not have the prominent lumen seen in the preceding stages. In fact, feeding is impossible because both the mouth and buccal tube are solidly plugged. The ensheathed L_3 is

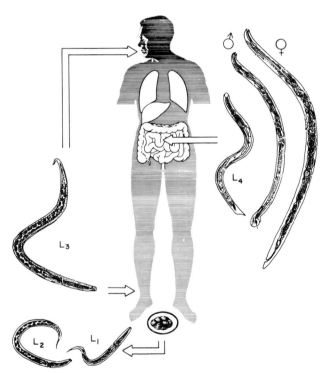

Figure 44-1. Life cycle of the hookworms *Ancylostoma duodenale* and *Necator americanus*. Both species infect percutaneously, whereas only *A. duodenale* is successful if ingested and swallowed. The free-living stages, eggs and larvae (L_1 and L_3), live in feces or fecally polluted soil. After penetrating the skin, infective filariform larvae (L_3) migrate to the gastrointestinal tract via the circulation, lung and respiratory tree. The final larval stage (L_4) and the adult worms occur in the small intestine (*Adapted from E.C. Faust, P.C. Beaver, and R.C. Jung: Animal Agents and Vectors of Human Disease, Philadelphia, Lea & Febiger, 1976; and A.C. Chandler, Hookworm Disease, New York, Macmillan, 1929.*)

adapted to migrate vertically and comes to the soil surface, where it rests, unless moisture films extend onto vegetation or surface debris, in which case it continues to migrate upward as far as the films extend. Since the larva is extremely vulnerable to desiccation, it must migrate up and down vertically in response to changing moisture conditions, but many are trapped and die above the soil surface when the environment dries and moisture films become disjunct. Furthermore, repeated migration in response to alternating conditions of moisture and drying rapidly exhausts the food reserves of this nonfeeding stage. Therefore, under tropical conditions of high temperature and periodic rainfall, larval life is short, most dying within 3 to 4 weeks.

Although the infective larva is particularly vulnerable to desiccation when on the surface, it must position itself there to facilitate host contact. It responds to stimuli from the host (e.g., carbon dioxide, warmth) and moves toward the source of such stimuli [2]. If contact is made, microscopic discontinuities in the epidermis (scales, fissures, hair follicles) are used to initiate skin penetration. This is facilitated by histolytic enzymes, boring movements, and perhaps also by the buccal tube, an oral spear which may be protrusible. The larvae exsheath as penetration begins.

Once within the host, the parasitic L_3 enters the circulation and is carried to the lungs where it breaks into the airspaces and moves via the respiratory tree to the pharynx. It is then swallowed and ultimately arrives in the small intestine where final development and maturation occur. The intestinal stages of the parasite (Fig. 44-1) include a fourth-stage larva (L_4) equipped with a temporary buccal capsule and capable of feeding on blood, and an adult stage, as already described. The provisional mouth capsule is shed with the cuticle during the molt separating the L_4 and the adult stage.

Depending on the species, the adult worms live for about a year (*A. duodenale*) or for 4 to 5 years (*N. americanus*) [11–13]. As judged by the passage of eggs in the feces of individuals who have left tropical endemic areas, the potential life span of hookworms in the absence of natural reinfection may be much longer, i.e., up to 15 years for *N. americanus* [1].

Eggs of *N. americanus* usually appear in the feces in 40 to 60 days. *A. duodenale* has a much more variable prepatent period, ranging from 43 to 105 days [14]. The longer periods include an interval of interrupted development, as deduced from epidemiological and experimental investigations [15–19].

Some *A. duodenale* larvae that enter humans do not develop immediately. Instead, they become arrested in their development for an extended period before resuming growth and maturing. The site of dormancy is uncertain, but it has been suggested that the larvae become latent in the intestine after completing tracheal migration [16,18], which is consistent with the recovery of parasitic third-stage larvae from the purged feces of patients long after they were hospitalized and removed from reinfection [18]. In addition, the larvae may become dormant in the muscles. *A. duodenale* larvae migrate and subsequently become dormant in the musculature of calves or swine in which they will not mature [19,20]. When raw meat from a 28-day old infection was fed to puppies, adult worms developed. Presumably human infections could be acquired similarly [20].

MORPHOLOGY

Adult hookworms are cylindrical, moderately stout nematodes, with males measuring 5 to 11 mm in length and females 9 to 13 mm, having more or less dorsally bent anterior ends. *N. americanus* is more definitely bent (hooked) and more strongly tapered anteriorly than is *A. duodenale*. These nematodes may be distinguished microscopically by characteristics of the oral opening and by the configuration of the rays supporting the copulatory bursa of the male. To examine the oral opening, a parasite is rolled under a coverslip to permit a view directly into the mouth. The ventral side (i.e., anterior end) of the opening is armed with a pair of curved cutting plates in *N. americanus* or with one or more pairs of teeth in the genus *Ancylostoma* (Fig. 44-2).

The species of hookworms are difficult to distinguish on the basis of egg size (60 × 40 μm) or structure. However, infective larvae from fecal cultures can be specifically identified by a number of morphological attributes [1].

BIOCHEMISTRY, PHYSIOLOGY, AND IN VITRO CULTIVATION

The biochemistry and physiology of *N. americanus* and *A. duodenale* are poorly known because without a good laboratory animal–host, these species have been unavailable in sufficient supply. Recent work to develop more useful host-parasite systems to supply parasitic stages is cited below under "Animal Models."

A. caninum is more available and has served as a model for investigating the physiology and biochemistry of hookworms generally. It is now certain that *A. caninum* is a blood-sucking nematode [3,6], the feeding of which is facilitated by the production of proteolytic enzymes and anticoagulants [21–24]. In vitro studies suggest that active feeding is triggered by unidentified constituents in serum because esophageal contractions cease in worms maintained in Ringer's solution, with glucose, but without blood or serum [3]. Oscilloscopic records of worms maintained in blood indicate that an actively sucking worm contracts its esophagus 120 to 200 times per minute. The transit time of blood through the worm is rapid, taking about 1 to 2 min [3]. In vivo the average worm sucks about 0.05 mL of blood per female per day, and clouds of red cells are explosively ejected from the worm's anus at frequent intervals. This rapid transit time, along with the ejection of intact red cells, led to the belief that erythrocytes were not digested. However, in vitro studies using ^{51}Cr-labeled cells suggest that 40 percent of ingested erythrocytes are used by the worm [3].

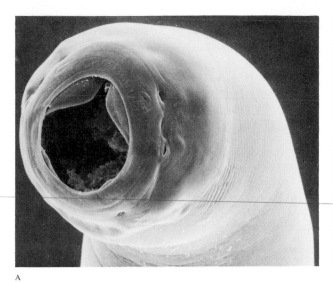

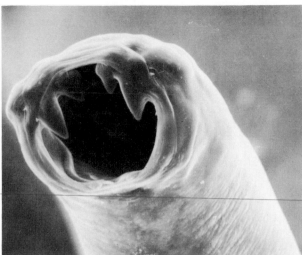

A   B

Figure 44-2. *A.* Anterior end of *N. americanus.* The pair of curved cutting plates in the oral opening distinguishes this species from *A. duodenale.* (*From E.K. Markell and M. Voge, Medical Parasitol-* *ogy, Philadelphia, W.B. Saunders, 1981.*) *B.* Anterior end of *A. duodenale.* The two pairs of equal-sized teeth distinguish this species from other hookworms of humans.

Why there is little visible evidence of cell destruction remains unclear. Possibly the cells are lysed and digested externally or in the worm's mouth capsule, and, therefore, little evidence of cell lysis may be visible in the worm's intestine. Electron-microscopic studies of adult *A. ceylanicum* fixed in situ indicate that exodigestion plays an important role in this species' feeding [*25,26*].

Oxygen consumption in vitro is relatively high, namely 38 and 53 μL per gram of wet weight per day in females and males, respectively. Based on an average blood consumption of 0.05 mL per female per day, Roche and Layrisse estimated that about 25 to 30 percent of the hookworm's needs are provided by blood; presumably the remainder is obtained via the cuticle from the relatively abundant supply adjacent to the mucosa [*3*].

In vitro, in the presence of serum, the worms use glucose for glycogenesis with the production of little pyruvate. They excrete acetate, proprionate, isobutyrate, and α-methylbutyrate. Both of the former result from glucose degradation and the latter from the degradation of amino acids [*27*]. Because aminotransferases (glutamic acid dehydrogenase and gluta-minic acid–pyruvate aminotransferase) have been demonstrated in *A. caninum,* it has been suggested that the adult worm can convert ammonia to glutamic acid for use in protein synthesis [*28*].

Recent studies of the structure and function of the anterior sense organs of *N. americanus* [*29*] demonstrate that the amphids, lateral pitlike chemosensory structures at the cephalic end of the worm, also have a secretory function. Huge secretory cells, the ''amphidial glands'' of previous generations of microscopists, extending one-fourth the length of the worm,

were found to be closely associated anteriorly with the terminal, cilialike endings of the amphidial axons and were shown to secrete large amounts of acetylcholinesterase to the exterior through the amphidial pores. The function of this abundantly produced enzyme remains uncertain, but it has been suggested that it acts as a ''chemical holdfast,'' enabling the worm to maintain position in the intestine [*30*]. Alternatively, the enzyme's primary function may be to lyse the abundant mucus produced by sensitized hosts that might otherwise coat the worms and dislodge them [*30*].

Hookworms can be maintained in sterile saline with glucose for up to 15 days, and with serum and glucose for up to 82 days. In some of these systems the worms feed, copulate, and lay viable eggs [*3,14*]. However, development from adult to adult in axenic culture has yet to be reported.

ANIMAL MODELS

Hookworm research has been seriously impeded by a lack of suitable animals for the laboratory maintenance and experimental study of *N. americanus* and *A. duodenale.* Worms will develop to maturity in pups, and recently long-term maintenance has been achieved using laboratory-raised, young, hookworm-naive, prednisolone-treated pups [*31,32*].

N. americanus has been adapted to hamsters by serial passage under cortisone [*33*], but this model has not had wide acceptance as an experimental system. It has, however, emerged as a valuable source of parasitic stages [*34*]. Other models still under development include *A. americanus* and *A. duodenale* in rabbits and *A. ceylanicum* in mice [*35–37*]. In the absence of a convenient host-parasite system involving either *A. duodenale* or *N. americanus*, *A. caninum* (the probable ancestor of *A. duodenale*) has been used as model for both parasites of human beings [*38*]. More recently, *A. ceylanicum* has served the same purpose [*24–26,39*]. The dog is used as the laboratory host for both species.

PARATENIC HOSTS

In rodents, *A. duodenale* migrates to the musculature, where the larvae become dormant. Recent investigations have shown that the larvae will also migrate in pigs, calves, rabbits, and to a lesser extent in sheep. To test the ability of these larvae to develop to adulthood, the dog-model system was used. It showed that the muscle larvae remain infective for at least 28 days and will resume development and mature in a suitable definitive host [*31,32*]. These observations indicate that meatborne *A. duodenale* infection of humans is possible, although no work has been done to explore its importance in nature [*20*].

PATIENT

INFECTION AND DISEASE

Because hookworms, like most other helminths, cannot multiply within the body, it is essential to distinguish between mere infection and disease. Hookworm infection includes a number of clinical entities, but generally, hookworm disease is an iron-deficiency anemia due to simple blood loss with an attendant depletion of the host's iron reserves. Worm populations of insufficient size to compromise the host's ability to compensate for iron loss result in subclinical carrier states which do not usually cause symptoms or merit treatment, unless parasite transmission is a concern.

The significance of different levels of infection depends on a variety of host and parasite factors, namely the iron reserves of the host, pregnancy and the general need for iron, adequacy of iron intake, and the state of the patient's health. With reference to the parasite, the number and species of the worm present are of particular importance [*38,40*].

Grades of infection based on fecal egg count have been established as follows: heavy, more than 5000 eggs per gram (EPG) of feces; moderately heavy, 2000 to 5000 EPG; moderately light, 500 to 2000 EPG; and light, less than 500 EPG. It is thought that infections constituted of 150 *N. americanus,* represented by less than 2000 EPG, do not necessarily require treatment provided that the intake of dietary iron is adequate and there are no other mitigating circumstances [*41*].

ROUTES OF INFECTION

Dermal

Both *A. duodenale* and *N. americanus* have been successfully transmitted to humans by the *dermal* route with successful penetration of the skin and infection being achieved in 40 to 60 percent of instances [*38*]. Variable success in achieving infection may have been attributable to infectivity of larvae and to conditions of the experiments rather than true resistance.

Oral

The *oral* route of infection has, in general, been less easy to achieve experimentally. Techniques by which oral infection was attempted as well as the state of the larvae utilized may have been crucial factors in success. *A. duodenale* is well adapted for oral infection [*13*]. In addition, it is known that invasion also occurs via the buccal or esophageal mucosa [*14*].

Transmammary

The overall significance of the *transmammary* route of infection in humans remains uncertain [*11,42–44*]. The evidence for transmammary transmission of human hookworms, specifically, *A. duodenale,* is indirect, hookworm larvae never having been demonstrated in breast milk [*42–44*]. However, *A. duodenale* infects nursing infants with no apparent exposure to other routes of infection [*42,45*]. Furthermore, when the species composition of the hookworm burden is assessed in surveys of children, *A. duodenale* is the species characteristically present in the youngest children (see ''Ecology'' for references).

Cutaneous and visceral larva migrans

In some types of hookworm disease, larvae invade and migrate in the skin, causing symptoms primarily at this site, and do not appear to complete their migration cycle. Only in rare instances do true visceral symptoms of tissue involvement occur and then usually only with massive infections. *Cutaneous larva migrans* has been described with three species of hookworm, *A. braziliense, U. stenocephala,* and *Bunostomum phlebotomum* [*38*]. The incidence would appear to be much higher with *A. braziliense* than with other species. Early lesions resemble the creeping eruption seen with early stages of the human infection, but cutaneous larva migrans patients develop a characteristic clinical picture with tortuous inflammatory areas in the dermis associated with swelling, erythema, papular dermatitis, and pruritus. Accurate proof of the nature of the infecting worm is very difficult even with skin biopsies [*46,47*], so that evidence is usually by association. *Visceral larva migrans* is rare with hookworm disease. Features of pulmonary inflammation, with symptoms of cough, wheezing, and patchy infiltrate visible on chest x-ray, may occur but are much less common than in other parasitic infections. It is unclear whether such symptoms are the response to the migration of the larvae, perhaps in larger numbers due to an overwhelming acute infection, or to abnormal responsiveness of the tissue associated with acquired resistance to the migration.

Hyperacute syndrome

Severe early morbidity has been described in the response to massive infection with larvae in unusual circumstances. Rapid development of acute illness and gastrointestinal bleeding after heavy exposure has been described [47–49]. Young, predominantly male worms were detected on vermifugation in these studies, and (perhaps significantly) reports have involved *A. duodenale* predominantly.

Autoreinfection

An interesting circumvention of the classical parasitic life cycle of *A. duodenale, A. ceylanicum,* and *N. americanus* has been described in which adult worms develop in closed cystic spaces in the human intestine. These cysts contained eggs and first- and second-stage larvae, but the missing third-stage larvae presumably could have migrated into the mucosa to complete an autoreinfection life cycle without having left the host. There have been several records of this phenomenon, and its relatively high frequency in autopsy reports would suggest its development as a disordered balance between parasite and host in favor of the parasitic cycle [50].

RESISTANCE TO HOOKWORM INFECTION

Protective immunity

Immunity with protective features is typical of hookworm infection in the dog and other animals, but there is little *direct* evidence that protective immunity to hookworm develops in humans [38,57]. This is an inadequately explored area which requires study by modern immunological techniques. Repeated experimental infection of volunteers or patients with polycythemia vera fails to cause resistance. Studies of a single volunteer [52] demonstrated the course of infection following repeated challenge. No larval migration in the skin was observed on the first infection, but after later infections larvae gave rise to creeping eruptions which suggested that local immune factors in the skin may have been important. The significance of these observations for hookworm in an holoendemic area is uncertain. Repeated infections with small inocula of *N. americanus* produce repetitive infections with no reduction in overall worm load and a rise in specific IgG and IgE antibody. Since intestinal secretions were not examined, the presence of specific secretory IgA is not known [53].

Epidemiological evidence has suggested that immunity may develop. Worms are acquired steadily during early life, but during the second to fifth decade, the level of infection remains remarkably stable at a slightly higher level in men than women. After the fifth decade the infection increases again [54]. Several authors attribute the static worm population during the second and fifth decades to acquired immunity. In the absence of immunity a steady increase in the worm burden would be expected. Additional support for this concept is the low level of reinfection with adult worms following application of a vermifuge [55].

Much better evidence for protective resistance can be observed in the dog exposed to *A. caninum* and *ceylanicum.* Specific immunity was acquired by dogs exposed to repeated infection with larvae [38,54]. Resistance was general and independent of the subsequent route of exposure to larvae. In addition, a canine hookworm vaccine provides active immunity for dogs of all ages [56]. A cDNA clone encoding a specific antigenic protease may be a candidate immunogen [22,23] in human beings. Recent studies in human volunteers, however, have demonstrated only meager IgG, IgE, and lymphocyte blastogenesis responses to low-dose *Necator* challenge [53].

Genetic factors

Distribution of hookworm infection is worldwide and is primarily influenced by climatic and environmental factors. Females appear to be inherently more resistant to infection than males, and non-Caucasians are more resistant than Caucasians [3,55,83,85]. The most heavily infected individuals in populations at risk appear to be predisposed to heavy infection not by chance but by as yet undefined genetic, ecological, behavioral, or social factors [46,57].

The role of nutrition in resistance to infection

The impact of host nutritional status on worm infection has been imperfectly defined. Malnourished children develop more serious consequences from acute hookworm anemia [49]. Nutritional repletion of human hookworm patients with high protein diets did not alter quantitative egg counts, intestinal blood loss, or number of spontaneously expelled worms, but there was no documentation of weight gain or increase in body mass in this study [58,59].

PATHOPHYSIOLOGY

Intestinal mucosal injury

The most important pathophysiological features of hookworm infection are due to the attachment of the worms by their buccal capsule to the mucosa of the upper intestine. Blood is then sucked and passed through the worm as well as being spilled around the feeding worms, leading to iron-deficiency anemia and the clinical features of hookworm disease.

Attachment and Feeding of Hookworms. Hookworms attach to the mucosa of the upper intestine by their buccal capsules and in heavy infections may be present throughout the intestine and distributed as low as the ileum [3–6,25,26,60]. Attachment of the worm results in bleeding into the GI tract. The mechanisms for this have been derived from direct observations of *A. caninum*–infected dogs [4,5]. Worms were found to change their site of attachment every 4 to 6 h to seek out new feeding sites in addition to less frequent movement for

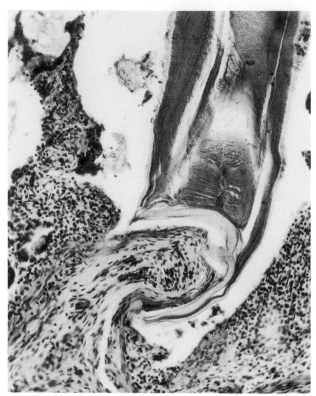

Figure 44-3. Hookworm attached to intestinal mucosa. (*With acknowledgment, Armed Forces Institute of Pathology, Photo no. N33818, Washington, D.C.*)

purposes of mating. The buccal capsule orifice of the worms was apposed to one or two villi or to the upper crypt region of the mucosal surface, and with attachment and suction, a plug of the host tissue was drawn into the buccal capsule (Fig. 44-3). The mucosal cells of the tissue plug were pulled free from the lamina propria, and villous capillary loops burst and allowed blood to flow out. Continuous or intermittent suction by the worms caused tissue stroma and blood to be drawn into the worm's intestinal tract. Successive plugs of tissue were ingested as the area of tissue destruction increased in size, and in less than 2 h an inflammatory exudate composed of polymorphonuclear leukocytes developed around the worm. The muscularis mucosa defined the maximum depth of penetration of the worm prior to its detachment and fixation at another site [5]. A maximally developed mucosal lesion would usually involve about nine villi, and an individual worm might cause as many as six such lesions per day. Although blood loss occurred by passage through the worm's intestinal tract, bleeding from damaged mucosa adjacent to the worm during and after feeding was a significant secondary cause of blood loss [3,5]. Blood was of only secondary importance as a food source for the worm since intact erythrocytes were found at all levels in the worm's midgut surrounded by remains of partially digested mucosal tissue [5,6]. Anticoagulant material produced in the

buccal capsule of the worm may enhance the blood loss [24]. Bleeding is ultimately dependent on the worm load since bleeding ceases after deworming. After detachment of the worm, histological changes in intestinal mucosa are minimal and consist of evidence of increased crypt mitotic activity and for presence of immature cells further up the villi [5].

Blood Loss Associated with Hookworm Infection. Recorded blood loss is of the order of 0.03 mL/day per worm for *N. americanus,* and attains 0.26 mL/day per worm for *A. duodenale* infections when measured utilizing ^{51}Cr-tagged red blood cells [3,55,58,62]. Although blood loss may be of little nutritional importance to the worm, cumulatively it has momentous implications for the host. Some of the iron lost as hemoglobin into the intestine may be reabsorbed, but it only amounts, on average, to 40 to 60 percent; fecal iron loss is increased in hookworm patients commensurate with the worm load. Even so, patients with hookworm disease retain an ability to absorb orally administered elemental or organic-bound iron as well as do control subjects with a similar degree of anemia.

Studies of several different populations have demonstrated an association between anemia and the severity of the hookworm load. However, it has always been puzzling to clinicians that heavy infections might occur without anemia and conversely that anemia might develop in association with very light infections. Roche and Layrisse [3] have emphasized that these apparent discrepancies are readily understood in the light of variations in available dietary iron stores, and the duration and severity of the hookworm infections. In persons with adequate iron stores, anemia may never develop. Blood loss associated with a light infection of *A. duodenale* may be 8.0 mL/day, with heavy infection 60 to 100 mL/day. In areas of the world endemic for hookworm, dietary iron intake is seldom low but may not be available for absorption or may be reduced by associated intestinal diseases [59].

Anemia associated with hookworm disease responds rapidly (within several weeks) to the administration of iron salts. In addition, in most populations, it is possible to treat patients by administration of a vermifuge without a change in diet. In such cases, however, the anemia responds slowly, with hemoglobin levels only returning to normal 15 to 20 months after removal of the worm load [3]. Although this approach is not a practical step toward management, it serves to emphasize that in most areas endemic for hookworm disease, dietary iron intake is capable eventually of repleting iron stores. Decreased red cell survival time and loss of iron via sweat are other incidental factors of only very limited importance in the pathogenesis of hookworm anemia [59].

Intestinal Injury and Absorption of Nutrients. The relationship between hookworm infection and impaired iron absorption may be complicated by severe malnutrition and hypoproteinemia and an enteropathy endemic to tropical regions. This has caused difficulty in defining the exact role the mucosal injury (caused by hookworm attachment) might have in reducing intestinal absorptive capacity. Careful balance studies were performed in Uganda which showed an impairment of nitrogen balance in severe hookworm infection [61], which might be interpreted as resulting from increased gastrointestinal protein loss rather than diminished absorptive capacity for dietary proteins. Later studies from this same geographical region (in which tropical sprue is rarely encountered) confirmed an impression that hookworm infection rarely caused clinical malabsorption and did not significantly contribute to the steatorrhea of other malabsorptive states, such as exocrine pancreatic disease [62,63]. To document the effect of impaired nutritional status on the absorptive capacity of patients with hookworm anemia, protein "refeeding" experiments lasting 52 to 247 days were performed [64]. Fecal fat excretion and folic acid and vitamin A absorption returned to normal in hookworm patients solely by improvement in their nutritional status without recourse to administration of a vermifuge. It is possible, albeit not verified in humans, that an absorptive defect may be present in the duodenum and jejunum (at the major site of hookworm attachment), but owing to the reserve absorptive capacity of the distal small intestine, overall absorption of dietary nutrients remains adequate [65].

In general, hookworm patients are no more malnourished than uninfected subjects. Impairment of appetite and pica are described with severe anemia [3,59].

Role of Altered Small-Bowel Motility. Segmenting and peristaltic activity of the upper intestine is increased in the disease [66]. Changes in motility might contribute to disordered absorption of nutrients for the host or alter the ability of the worm to maintain its location in the bowel.

Intestinal Protein Loss due to Hookworm Infection. Hypoproteinemia with hypoalbuminemia is characteristic of hookworm infection [3,59]. Although low dietary protein intake due to poverty and diminished appetite are frequent contributory factors, loss of protein into the intestinal tract (protein-losing enteropathy) in the form of plasma or tissue protein is well described. Methods utilized to demonstrate this have ranged from the use of ^{131}I-labeled albumin with an ion-exchange resin to ^{51}Cr-labeled albumin. Several studies [55,65,67,68] were able to correlate the worm loads with the degree of plasma loss, but it is likely that these only provide a gross measure of protein loss due to the inherent inaccuracies of the ^{131}I-labeled albumin method they utilized. Serum and tissue protein extravasated into the jejunal lumen during hookworm infection may be digested by proteolysis and undergo reabsorption in the distal small intestine.

PATHOLOGY

Intestinal mucosal morphology

Small hemorrhagic erosive lesions of the mucosa with engorgement of local capillaries and associated tissue edema are a common finding in experimental hookworm infection and can be observed in human small-bowel biopsies [55,64]. These lesions heal rapidly after migration of the worm or vermifugation. Severe jejunoileitis may develop with overwhelming infections [47].

Morphological features of an associated tropical enteropathy with loss of villus height, increased crypt-villus ratio and increased chronic inflammatory cell infiltrate in the lumina propria are most probably unrelated to the infection. Several discussions of this problem are available [38,59].

In other body organs remote from hookworm infection, pathological changes occur (1) in the bone marrow in response to chronic blood loss, (2) in enlargement of retroperitoneal lymph nodes due to antigenic stimulation, and (3) in fatty deterioration of heart, liver, and kidneys associated with anemia and anoxia [3,38,47].

CLINICAL FEATURES

The clinical features of hookworm infection (Table 44-1) are readily understood in relation to the life cycle. The major clinical features of disease result directly from attachment of adult

Table 44-1. Clinical features of hookworm disease

Site	Cause	Clinical features
Dermal	Cutaneous invasion and subcutaneous migration of filariform larvae	Local erythema, macules, papules ("ground itch"); features more prominent on reinfection
Respiratory tract	Migration of larvae through lungs, bronchi, and trachea to the esophagus	Bronchitis, pneumonitis, eosinophilia relatively uncommon except during reinfection or severe hyperacute infection
Gastrointestinal	Attachment of adult worms to upper intestinal mucosa; traumatic injury to mucosal surface	Anorexia, pica, epigastric pain and tenderness, peptic ulcer symptoms, gastrointestinal hemorrhage, diarrhea during acute invasion
Hematological	Chronic intestinal blood loss due to sucking of worms	Iron-deficiency anemia, protein-losing enteropathy, hypoproteinemia, edema
Cardiac	Chronic iron-deficiency anemia	High-output cardiac failure, exertional dyspnea, edema
Nutritional and metabolic	Loss of nutrients into intestine. Iron deficiency	Hypoalbuminemia, edema. Growth retardation, impaired work productivity. Adverse effects on learning and cognitive development.

hookworms to the duodenal and jejunal mucosa and the subsequent effects on host nutrition occasioned by anorexia, intestinal blood loss, and anemia. These features are best considered in relation to the organ system involved.

Dermatological

Penetration of the skin by larvae causes a stinging sensation. Skin reactions vary from erythematous papules lasting 7 to 10 days, to vesiculation and edema. Secondary bacterial infection is common.

Respiratory

Features of cough and wheezing associated with bronchitis and pneumonitis are uncommon and only readily recognized following experimental infection. Patchy, fluffy opacities representing areas of pneumonitis may be seen on chest x-rays. Occasionally, severe acute reactions may follow exposure to infective larvae. Wakana disease in Japan, due to oral ingestion of fecally contaminated radishes, will cause the acute onset of pharyngeal itching, coughing, dyspnea, wheezing, urticaria, nausea, and vomiting [47].

Gastrointestinal

Light infections usually produce no symptoms. Epigastric discomfort and tenderness occur with heavy infections in 20 to 50 percent of persons and may be confused with peptic ulcer disease. The appetite is usually impaired, especially in the later stages of anemia and congestive heart failure. Nausea and vomiting are unusual. Abnormal perverted taste—pica and geophagia—may develop. Should serious disease develop during childhood, growth and development may be stunted. Alteration in bowel habit (constipation) occurs as a result of a change in dietary intake.

Hematological

After a variable time, depending on the worm load and dietary iron intake, anemia develops with symptoms of lassitude, breathlessness, palpitations, tinnitus, mental apathy, depression, and syncope. Physical performance of workers is impaired by anemia [69]. The mucous membranes and skin become pallid, the face puffy, and ankles swollen from associated hypoproteinemia. Physical examination may reveal angular stomatitis, cheilosis, and retinal hemorrhages. Since the disease is usually chronic, anemia is the major clinical feature. In severe cases hemoglobin values of 3 to 8 g/dL are not uncommon [3]. Marked microcytosis and hypochromia are the rule. The reticulocyte count is usually normal. There is loss of iron from bone marrow stores, low to absent serum iron levels, and low serum albumin levels. Megaloblastic changes are rare but may be seen when an associated folate deficiency occurs. The white cell count is usually normal except for a mild eosinophilia (7 to 14 percent) in the established disease.

Acute onset of anemia due to gastrointestinal bleeding is rare [49].

Severe anemia has a deleterious influence on pregnancy. Maternal and fetal mortality are high on this account in regions in which hookworm disease is prevalent [47].

Cardiological

Cardiac symptoms include dyspnea, palpitations, and cardiac pain. Dyspnea is extremely common and is most often occasioned by exertion. It is usually the result of increased ventilatory work resulting from peripheral anoxia, but in late stages, dyspnea may be of cardiac origin associated with heart failure. Palpitations are usually due to the increased force of myocardial contraction and increased stroke volume rather than due to specific tachyarrhythmias. Precordial chest pain may be the result of coronary insufficiency and can develop in the absence of significant coronary artery disease. (Coronary artery disease is uncommon in most populations in which hookworm disease is endemic.) Physical findings are those of a high output state with a widened peripheral pulse pressure, a decreased diastolic pressure and collapsing pulse, peripheral bruits, hemic systolic ejection murmur in the pulmonic areas, raised jugular venous pressure, and cardiomegaly. On exertion, cardiac output, already greatly increased, is usually increased by heart rate but not by an increase in stroke volume. Peripheral edema is usually a manifestation of hypoproteinemia but may also develop with features of congestive cardiac failure. Cardiomegaly is present on x-ray and nonspecific ST and T wave changes on electrocardiogram. Cardiac failure is reversible on treatment of anemia [3,51].

Nutritional and Metabolic

Edema is usually the consequence of hypoproteinemia and hypoalbuminemia. Total plasma protein less than 5 g/dL and albumin of less than 3 g/dL are associated with edema [55,59]. Edema may be dependent but is often present as generalized anasarca and may be associated with pleural effusions and ascites. Other effects of plasma loss on minerals and micronutrients are unknown.

Evidence derived from several studies has emphasized that severe metabolic sequelae of hookworm disease occur in childhood. There is persuasive evidence at this age that iron deficiency adversely affects behavior through metabolic effects on the nervous system. Impairment of cognitive function, disturbances of noncognitive behavior, as well as limitations in physical activity and work capacity, have been identified to occur more frequently in iron-deficient and anemic patients in several recent well-controlled population studies [69,92]. [P. Hotez, personal communication, as well as 11,12,48,49].

MORBIDITY AND MORTALITY

International figures for morbidity for hookworm disease are unavailable, but its widespread prevalence has been emphasized [1,3,47]. The second most common cause for admission to the adult medical wards in Kampala, Uganda, in 1958, was hookworm disease; its incidence was unchanged 13 years later [38]. Anemia may account for 5 to 9 percent of heart failure in Uganda and Nigeria. In some regions of the world (Puerto Rico), changes in sanitation have dramatically reduced incidence; in contrast, where social conditions had deteriorated, a 50 percent mortality rate was observed in a childhood population [49].

DIAGNOSIS

Egg identification and counting [3,7,8,38,70]

Accurate diagnosis is dependent on the identification of hookworm eggs in the feces. A direct fecal film on a microscope slide mounted in saline or iodine solution is suitable for detection of moderate and severe infections, but in light infections (< 400 eggs per gram of feces) concentration techniques will be required to demonstrate the eggs. The *zinc sulfate flotation technique* is effective and permits the hookworm eggs, which are of lower specific gravity than the solution, to rise to the surface and the fecal debris to sink to the bottom. The *formalin-ether technique*, or one of its modifications, is a sedimentation method and may be useful also. In this technique, eggs are heavier than the solution and can be centrifuged to form a pellet.

To distinguish between *N. americanus* and *A. duodenale* infections, *filariform larvae* may be reared in a fecal smear on a moist filter paper strip. The smear is confined to the middle of the strip so that the ends remain clean. The paper is incubated in a test tube containing a small amount of water. Filariform larvae develop in 5 to 7 days and collect in the reservoir of water at the bottom of the tube.

Occasionally, it is necessary to distinguish between the *rhabditiform larvae* of the hookworm and of *Strongyloides stercoralis*. The former can be distinguished by the presence of a buccal tube extending from the mouth to the esophagus.

Worm burdens are usually estimated by counting eggs in fecal samples. There are several methods available [1,7,11]. These estimates are used in population surveys, control programs, and antihelminthic trials. Fecal egg counts do not indicate the exact number of adult worms in a patient, but many authorities have found that they furnish a reasonable approximation of worm burden and are indicative of the severity of hookworm infection (2000 eggs per gram, light; 2600 to 13,000, moderate; >13,000, heavy). The accuracy of these procedures must be accepted with caution because there is no general agreement as to the number of eggs laid per female per day [70,71], and, furthermore, there may be a significant density-dependent depression of egg output [8,9].

A measure of the adult worm load in any patient can be obtained after treatment by vermifuge and the use of a purge, sieving out of the worms from the fecal specimen, and direct counting of adult worms passed. Methods are described in detail in standard texts. Probably 85 to 90 percent of adult worms can be recovered by this technique.

Diagnostic immunology

Accumulated and de novo synthesized antigens expressed by L3, L4, and adult *N. americanus* can be identified in the serum by immunoblotting [72]. A few of these antigens are shared between developmental stages and the several adult epitopes recognized. Utilizing recombinant DNA procedures, such molecules may prove useful in immunological assays for species-specific and stage-specific diagnostic tests [73,90]. Binding of IgG antibody to *A. caninum* larvae has been demonstrated in vitro [74]. However, surface-specific cross-reactivity is a common occurrence in multiple helminthic infections in humans [73]. Patients with hookworm express antibody activity against *Schistosoma mansoni* and *Ascaris,* which presents a problem for serodiagnosis. IgE levels are increased in serum of hookworm patients. [53].

MANAGEMENT AND TREATMENT OF HOOKWORM DISEASES

Control of hookworm infection comprises four principles: (1) sanitary disposal of feces, (2) health education with community participation, (3) chemotherapy with antihelminthics, and (4) correction of anemia [75]. The first two subjects are discussed under "Prevention and Control."

Chemotherapy

Several general principles govern chemotherapy of hookworm disease:

1. Single-dose treatment of *A. duodenale* and *N. americanus* infections is moderately less effective in curing the infection than repeated doses. Repeated treatments may be necessary to obtain high cure rates (>90 percent) except with light infections.
2. A drug which has a better effect on one species usually has some effect on the other species and can, therefore, be used to treat mixed infections.
3. Many satisfactory antihelminthics, active against both species of hookworm, are inexpensive and nontoxic. Tetrachlorethylene, widely used because of its very low cost and established efficacy, does have toxicity.
4. Tetrachlorethylene stimulates ascarid migration to cause intestinal obstruction: Ascariasis should be treated first before tetrachlorethylene is given.

Table 44-2 describes major therapeutic agents available at the present time. All these agents have received study in a variety of geographical areas [1,75,76]. The individual choice of drug will depend on (1) whether it is to be used for mass treatment or individual use; (2) the species of hookworm and whether other intestinal parasites are present; and (3) the severity of the worm load and likelihood of reinfection after

Table 44-2. Hookworm: antihelminthics available for treatment

Drugs	Therapeutic effect	Dosage	Mode of action	Unwanted effect	Comments
Mebendazole	N.a., A.d.	300 mg single dose; 100 mg bid—3 days	Direct action on worm with inhibition of glucose uptake	Mild, occasional abdominal pain, diarrhea, vomiting	Well tolerated. Also has marked ovicidal properties. A very useful drug for multiple infections.
Pyrantel pamoate	A.d., (N.a.)	10–20 mg/kg as a single dose	Neuromuscular blockage and immobilization of worm	Mild, occasional diarrhea, vomiting and abdominal pain. Poorly absorbed from GI tract	Almost equally effective against both species. Very useful for combined infection with *Ascaris*. Effective for infants.
Bephenium hydroxynaphthoate	A.d., (N.a.)	5 g tid for 1 day taken with water before breakfast	Uncertain	Nausea, vomiting, diarrhea	When combined with tetrachlorethylene is very effective against *N. americanus* as well. Combined therapy should be reserved for patients in good health.
Albendazole	N.a., A.d.	400–600 mg single dose	Similar action to mebendazole	Nausea, vomiting, diarrhea (<5%)	Active against pre- and intestinal stages. Useful in combined helminth infections.
Tetrachlorethylene	N.a., (A.d.)	0.1 mg/kg (max 5 mL) taken when fasting in capsules. Allow food 3 h later. Repeat at 4-day interval 2 ×.	Neuromuscular blockage	Burning epigastric pain, nausea, vomiting, drowsiness; rarely syncope, hypotension, and collapse	Necessary to treat *Ascaris* infection first. Purging unnecessary and harmful. Avoid heavy exercise immediately following therapy.
Thiabendazole	Cutaneous larva migrans, A.b.	Topical 15% ointment applied for 3–5 days. 25 mg/kg bid for 2 days, PO	Unknown	Nausea, vomiting, vertigo, drowsiness with systemic administration	The most effective agent for this condition.

N.a. = *Necator americanus;* A.d. = *Ancylostoma duodenale;* A.b. = *Ancylostoma braziliensis;* (   ) = lesser effect.

administration of the vermifuge. As a general rule, the treatment of individuals with light infections is unlikely to be useful in endemic areas in which reinfection is frequent. Discretion should be used in the treatment of light infections in individuals who have returned to the United States or Europe. Those with good sanitary conditions and good diet may not require treatment. Certain individuals may require treatment even for light infections, because the infection may remain present for many years causing continued iron loss, and such individuals may represent a potential public health problem if their employment (mining, for instance) would permit infection of others.

Demonstration of arrested development in *A. duodenale* infections has implications for the treatment of this species [15,40]. During hypobiosis larvae are resistant or, at least, only responsive to doses of antihelminthics which are greatly in excess of those customarily used therapeutically. Thiabendazole is effective against migratory larvae and might also be effective against dormant larvae, but effective dosage regimens have not been defined to date for the arrested stages. This phenomenon of arrested development may explain apparent treatment failures as discussed previously.

Thiabendazole and mebendazole have larvicidal activity. Unlike other therapeutic agents, mebendazole also has a marked ovicidal effect [38,75]. Levimasole may be useful for multiple infections [75]. Albendazole, a new agent, is effective in preintestinal and intestinal phases of infection [77]. The effectiveness, if any, against arrested larvae of *A. duodenale* remains to be determined.

Iron therapy

Hematological improvement will occur slowly after antihelminthic drugs, but rapid correction is best achieved by supplementation of dietary iron with ferrous sulfate (300 mg) administered between meals three times a day. Hemoglobin will rise at a rate of 1 g/(L·week) even without deworming. In pregnant women, iron-deficiency anemia should be treated with ferrous sulfate alone and antihelminthic use delayed until after delivery. Treatment should be sustained for 3 months after restoration of normal hemoglobin levels to replete iron stores.

Blood transfusion and heart disease

The management of anemic heart disease is best accomplished by treatment of the anemia with antihelminthics and iron. Chronic anemia of a severe degree may be tolerated for years. However, myocardial reserve is reduced after prolonged anemia, which has implications for treatment of anemia with blood replacement. Blood transfusion by administration of packed cells administered slowly *should only be employed with great care in very severely anemic patients* (hemaglobin < 4 g/dL). The volume load of whole blood transfusions may readily precipitate failure and circulatory congestion. It is a wise precaution, therefore, to digitalize the patient prior to transfusion and, in addition, to transfuse packed cells, rather than whole blood. Simultaneous removal by phlebotomy of an equivalent volume of the patient's (anemic) blood may be useful. Monitoring central venous blood pressure via an intravenous catheter in the great veins provides excellent control in a seriously ill patient. Administration of a diuretic prior to transfusion may be of value. It is undesirable to administer diuretics to treat edema since this may reduce cardiac output. Although there is controversy over the effectiveness of digitalis in anemic heart disease, it should be considered a useful measure for supporting myocardial function during treatment [51].

POPULATION

ECOLOGY

The population ecology of the hookworms of humans is complicated by the common occurrence of two species that differ in several characteristics influencing their number and distribution [78]. Their relative abundance varies geographically and with age, sex, and other factors. In Bengal, A. duodenale predominates in infants and young children, N. americanus becoming increasingly numerous later in childhood. In the population generally it is twice as abundant as A. duodenale [11,12]. A similar predominance of A. duodenale in infants in Taiwan [79] and elsewhere prompted us to suggest that A. duodenale may be transmitted via the transmammary route [51]. Lactogenic infection occurs in the closely related species A. caninum, which normally infects pups via colostrum and

milk. There is no evidence for milkborne infection with N. americanus [51].

A. duodenale has a number of the attributes of an opportunistic species, namely, rapid colonization of hosts, intensive exploitation of host-provided resources (blood), short adult life span, and diverse routes of transmission to new hosts. Like opportunists generally, it has a particularly high egg output. In contrast, N. americanus produces fewer eggs, uses host resources in a less profligate manner, has a longer adult life span, and uses fewer transmission pathways [78].

Parasite fecundities are such that even low-grade infections will produce dense populations of free-living infective larvae if the rates of hatch, development, and survival are high. In endemic areas fecal egg counts of 1000 eggs per gram (EPG) are frequent as are large bulky stools. In eastern India, in a low intensity–high prevalence area, stools containing 200,000 eggs are commonplace. If all of these developed, larval populations would number in the order of 1075 cm^{-2}, but because few survive to infectivity and because they continue to die rapidly thereafter, natural populations are much smaller than theoretically possible [80]. Larval abundance also varies during the course of the rainy season, but the distribution of larvae remains aggregated even in the most rainy months of the year when dispersal in surface water might be expected. For example, the frequency distributions of monthly rainy season counts of infective larvae recovered from the soil surface in defecation sites in eastern India were well-described by the negative binomial probability distribution, with the value of k (an inverse measure of aggregation) remaining small and remarkably constant (0.01 to 0.08) for each of 10 sets of counts made during an 18-month period, despite variation in the monthly mean larval recovery.

In great regions of the vast tropical and subtropical belt in which hookworms are endemic, rainfall is seasonal, resulting in an attendant seasonal variation in the presence of infective larvae on the soil surface [81]. Until recently it was thought adult hookworms were long-lived and that, therefore, intensity of infection would not reflect seasonal variation in transmission. However, intensity of infection does vary seasonally where A. duodenale, a short-lived species, represents a substantial fraction of the parasite population [15,54].

Investigations in rural West Bengal have demonstrated that the species-specific frequency distributions of the adult hookworms are also well-described by the negative binomial probability distribution [40]. These distributions showed marked aggregation of both adult A. duodenale and N. americanus in individual villagers, more than 60 percent of the total adult hookworm population occurring in less than 10 percent of the people ($k = 0.618$ and 0.627, respectively). These estimates were based on counts of worms expelled after antihelminthic treatment. Nine rounds of fecal egg counts representing the mixed worm burdens of an untreated sample of the same population were also well-described by this probability distribution, and again the counts were highly aggregated and the measure of aggregation, k, was stable (0.78 to 0.85) over all rounds, while mean egg counts varied moderately (2440 to 3500 eggs per gram).

Recent investigations of the aggregation of hookworms in individuals have indicated that the heavily infected persons are predisposed to such levels of infection [40,82]. The basis for this predisposition, whether genetic, ecological, behavioral, or social, remains uncertain, although immunoparsitologists suspect it may have a largely genetic basis [57]. Regardless of its basis, predisposition has important implications for parasite control, as is discussed below.

EPIDEMIOLOGY

Hookworms parasitize more than 900 million people. Thus, almost one-quarter of the world's population is infected, and ancylostomiasis is second only to ascariasis as the most common helminth parasitism.

Prevalence and intensity of infection

The prevalence of hookworm infection varies from 80 to 90 precent in unsanitated, rural areas of the moist tropics (e.g., West Bengal) to 10 to 20 percent in relatively dry unsanitated areas (e.g., Iraq, Pakistan [81]). In other places (e.g., southern United States, Japan) where parasitism was once highly prevalent, it is now uncommon due, in part, to planned public efforts and, in part, to a general increase in the standard of living, including the widespread desire for indoor plumbing.

The occurrence of hookworm disease depends largely on the number of worms present; therefore, both intensity and prevalence of infection are important parameters. However, qualitative fecal examinations continue to prevail, even though they provide insufficient information to judge the importance of hookworm infection in a given population [81]. Although the intensity of infection tends to vary directly with prevalence, there can be a high prevalence of light infections, and, alternatively, certain families may be foci of heavy infection in larger areas of low prevalence. Indeed foci of heavy infection can occur within regions generally free of hookworms, i.e., in moist, temperate confines of mines in arid or cold areas of the world [83].

AGE, SEX, AND RACE

The prevalence and intensity of hookworm infection generally increases with age, but often levels off or declines in adulthood. The change in the rate of worm gain occurring in adulthood is usually attributed to the increased use of shoes, or to a decreased interaction with fecally polluted soils [84]. These explanations became entrenched in the 1920s before it was generally believed that resistance to hookworms could be acquired. While direct evidence for immunity in humans is still lacking, since the worm burden fails to increase into adulthood and there is no evidence for a change in the rate of exposure,

it is likely that the host's immune response limits the hookworm populations [54].

Sex-associated effects also have been attributed to differences in exposure to infection; i.e., it was thought that the less active female segment of the population made fewer contacts with polluted soil and, therefore, was exposed to less infection [85]. Exceptions to this generalization included certain groups of female laborers who, by the special nature of their work, were particularly exposed to fecally polluted soils.

Natural resistance to hookworms has also been reported in blacks, but the basis for this resistance is unknown. The evidence for racial natural immunity arises from observations made in the American south, where rural blacks and whites, of similar socioeconomic status, were differentially parasitized, the latter harboring many more hookworms than the former [85].

Ancylostomiasis is often considered an agricultural disease, but as Chandler has indicated repeatedly [85], it is not that hookworm infection is necessarily associated with farming, but with rural conditions permitting defecation in the open. It is only directly associated with agriculture when crops are fecally polluted either intentionally (night soil) or unintentionally (lack of sanitary facilities). Any close association with polluted ground increases the risk of infection. Thus, when as in the past, mines and tunnels lacked sanitary facilities, ancylostomiasis was also a disease of underground workers. Differences in the prevalence and intensity of hookworm infection are also associated with caste and religion [83,85,86]. Cultural attitudinal differences toward human excreta have a powerful influence on the occurrence of fecally transmitted diseases in general and on hookworm infection in particular. Heavy infections attributable to the use of night soil as manure in China, where it is valued and extensively used [83], contrast with the generally lighter infections of India, where Hindu culture makes its general use as a manure difficult, if not impossible [83,86].

PREVENTION AND CONTROL

In warm rural areas where soil pollution is the norm, prevention of infection is impractical, if not impossible, until rural sanitation becomes available and accepted. In fecally polluted areas where it would be of most benefit, the use of footwear is also likely to be rejected, because mud is more readily washed from bare feet than from a pair of shoes, an expensive luxury in the poor rural tropics [75]. Vaccination is theoretically possible but remains impractical at this time [57].

Control, aimed at the free-living stages (eggs and larvae), is largely dependent upon the safe disposal of feces and, hence, is determined by the availability and acceptance of rural sanitation. In many so-called soil pollution countries, habits, customs, and/or beliefs concerned with cleanliness and personal hygiene are major obstacles to the regular use of latrines, even if cost is not a prohibitive factor. Once the feces enter the environment, little can be done to limit the free-living hookworm population given favorable microenvironmental conditions, since there are no practical ovicides or larvicides [87].

Defecation in places where free-living stages will find conditions unfavorable for development or survival is beneficial. Thus, defecation on saline soils, on open, dry, fallow land, or in flooded fields limits hookworm abundance and should be encouraged by health education [87,88].

Mass chemotherapy is a long-established form of hookworm control. It has the great advantage that it immediately benefits those treated, and by reducing the number of eggs entering the environment it contributes to control. It has the disadvantage that in most endemic areas, reinfection is rapid, and therefore, unless repeated community-wide treatment is possible, the value of chemotherapy is transitory. For economic reasons, repeated treatment has rarely been feasible, and it has become even less practical due to the high cost of modern antihelminthics [75,88]. It has been suggested that mass treatment be timed to coincide with seasons when external environmental conditions are unfavorable for larval hookworms, i.e., a dry season in warm regions, when reinfection will be minimal. This suggestion remains valid for the control of *N. americanus*. Unfortunately, however, arrested development in *A. duodenale,* an adaptation for dry season survival, will decrease the value of strategically timed mass treatment because dormant larvae resist most antihelminthics.

In parts of the southern United States control was made relatively cost effective by targeting for detection and control programs only that fraction of the population having a high prevalence of clinical infections [81,87,88].

The observation that persons heavily infected with hookworms are predisposed to infection has increased the interest in selective chemotherapy, because, in theory at least, *individuals* can now be targeted for repetitive chemotherapy [40, 89]. Once these persons are identified, treatment can be focused on them repeatedly, and this will eliminate the necessity of repeated detection of the most heavily infected individuals. Elimination of the need for fecal egg counts preceding each round of community-based chemotherapy will make selective chemotherapy most cost-effective. As we indicated previously, when 60 percent of the total worm population is harbored by less than 10 percent of the community, successful treatment of these heavily infected people should make a major contribution to hookworm control.

REFERENCES

1 Intestinal Protozoan and Helminthic Infections. Report of a WHO Scientific Group. WHO Tech Rep Ser 666, Geneva, World Health Organization, 1981

2 Expert Committee on Helminthiasis: Soil Transmitted Helminths. WHO Tech Rep Ser 277, Geneva, World Health Organization, 1964

3 Roche M, Layrisse M: The nature and causes of "hookworm anemia." Am J Trop Med Hyg 15(6) part 2, 1966

4 Kalkofen UP: Attachment and feeding behavior of *Ancylostoma caninum*. Z Parasitenkd 33:339–354, 1970

5 Kalkofen UP: Intestinal trauma resulting from feeding activities of *Ancylostoma caninum*. Am J Trop Med Hyg 23:1046–1053, 1974

6 Wells HS: Observations on the blood sucking activities of the hookworm *Ancylostoma caninum*. J Parasitol 17:167–182, 1931

7 Hill RB: The estimation of the numbers of hookworms harbored by the use of the dilution egg count method. Am J Hyg 6(suppl 2):19–41, 1926

8 Anderson RM, Schad GA: Hookworm burdens and fecal egg counts: The basis of variation. Trans R Soc Trop Med Hyg 79: 743–884, 1985

9 Keymer AE, Slater EF: Helminth fecundity: Density dependence or statistical delusion? Parasitol Today 3:56–58, 1987

10 Smith G, Schad GA: *Ancylostoma duodenale* and *Necator americanus:* Effect of temperature on development and mortality of eggs. Parasitology, in press

11 Nawalinski TA, Schad GA, Chowdhury AB: Population biology of hookworms in children in rural West Bengal. I. General parasitological observations. Am J Trop Med Hyg 27:1152–1161, 1978

12 Nawalinski TA, Schad GA, Chowdhury AB: Population biology of hookworms in children in rural West Bengal. II. Acquisition and loss of hookworms. Am J Trop Med Hyg 27:1162–1173, 1978

13 Kendrick JF: The length of life and the rate of loss of the hookworms, *Ancylostoma duodenale* and *Necator americanus*. Am J Trop Med 14:363–379, 1934

14 Komiya Y, Yasuraoka K: The biology of hookworms, in Morishita K, et al (eds): *Progress of Medical Parasitology in Japan*. Tokyo, Meguro Parasitological Museum, 1966, vol 2, pp 5–114

15 Schad GA, Chowdhury AB, Dean CG, et al: Arrested development in human hookworm infection: An adaptation to a seasonally unfavorable external environment. Science 180:502–504, 1973

16 Nawalinski TA, Schad GA: Arrested development in *Ancylostoma duodenale:* Course of a self-induced infection in man. Am J Trop Med Hyg 23:1974

17 Wang MP, Hu YF, Peng JM, et al: Persistent migration of *Ancylostoma duodenale* larvae in human infection. Chin Med J 97:147–149, 1984

18 Brumpt LC, Sang HT: Diapause des ankylostomes chez les grande anemiques. C R Soc Biol (Paris) 147:1064–1066, 1953

19 Koshy A, Raina V, Sharma MP, et al: An unusual outbreak of hookworm disease in North India. Am J Trop Med Hyg 27:225–233, 1978

20 Schad GA, Murrell KD, Murr KD, Fayer R, et al: Paratenesis in *Ancylostoma duodenale* suggests possible meat toxic infection. Trans R Soc Med Hyg 78:203–204, 1984

21 Thorson RE: The effect of extracts of amphidial glands, excretory glands and esophagus of adults of *A. caninum* on coagulation of dog's blood. J Parasitol 72:26–30, 1956

22 Hotez PJ, LeTrang N, McKerrow JH, et al: Isolation and characterization of a proteolytic enzyme from the adult hookworm, *Ancylostoma caninum*. J Biol Chem 260:7343–7348, 1985

23 Hotez PJ, LeTrang N, Cerami A: Hookworm antigens: The potential for vaccination. Parasitol Today 3:247–249, 1987

24 Carroll SM, Howse DJ, Grove DI: The anticoagulant effects of the hookworm, *Ancylostoma ceylancium*. Thromb Haemostas 51:222–227, 1984

25 Carroll SM, Robertson T, Papadimitriou J, et al: Transmission electron microscopial studies of attachment of *Ancylostoma ceylanicum* to the small bowel mucosa of the dog. J Helminth 58: 313–320

26 Carroll SM, Robertson T, Papdimitriou J, et al: Scanning electron microscopy of *Ancylostoma ceylanicum* and its site of attachment for the intestinal mucosa of the dog. Z Parasitenk 71:79–85, 1985

27 Barrett J: Energy metabolism in nematodes, in Croll NA (ed): *The Organization of Nematodes.* New York, Academic, 1976, pp 11–70

28 Lee DL, Atkinson HG: *Physiology of Nematodes.* Columbia University Press, New York, 1977

29 McLaren DJ: Sense organs and their secretions, in Croll NA (ed): *The Organization of Nematodes.* New York, Academic, 1976, pp 139–161

30 Phillip M: Acetylcholinesterase secreted by intestinal nematodes: A reinterpretation of its putative role as a "biochemical holdfast." Trans R Soc Trop Med Hyg 78:138–139, 1984

31 Schad GA: *Ancylostoma duodenale:* Maintenance through six generations in helminth-naive pups. Exp Parasitol 47:246–253, 1979

32 Leiby D, El Naggar H, Schad GA: Thirty generations of *Ancylostoma duodenale* in laboratory reared beagles. J Parasitol 70:844–848, 1987

33 Sen HG: *Necator americanus:* Behavior in hamsters. Exp Parasitol 32:26–32, 1975

34 Behnke JM, Paul V, Rajasekariah G: The growth and migration of *Necator americanus* in neonatal hamsters. Trans R Soc Trop Med Hyg 80:146–149, 1986

35 Bhopale MK, Menon S: Complete development of human hookworm, *Ancylostoma duodenale* (Dubini, in 1843) in infant rabbits. Experientia 35:463, 1979

36 Bhopale MK, Menon S, Kulkarni L: *Necator americanus* in infant rabbits: Complete development, humoral antibody, leukocyte response and serum protein changes following infection. J Helminthol 54:97–104, 1980

37 Ray DK, Bhopale KK, Shrivastava VB: Development of *Ancylostoma ceylanicum* Looss, 1911 (Hamster Strain) in the albino mouse, *Mus musculus,* with and without cortisone. Parasitology 71:193–197, 1975

38 Miller TA: Hookworm infection in man. Adv Parasitol 17:315–383, 1979

39 Carroll SM, Grove D: Parasitological, hematological and immunologic response in acute and chronic infections of dogs with *Ancylostoma ceylanicum:* A model of human hookworm infection. J Infect Dis 150:284–294, 1984

40 Schad GA, Anderson RM: Predisposition to hookworm infection in humans. Science 228:1537–1540, 1985

41 Yanagisawa R: The epidemiology of hookworm disease, in Morishita K, et al (eds): *Progress of Medical Parasitology in Japan.* Tokyo, Meguro Parasitological Museum, 1966, vol 2, pp 287–370

42 Nwosu ABC: Human neonatal infections with hookworms in an endemic area of Southern Nigeria. Trop Geogr Med 33:105–111, 1981

43 Donges J, Madecki O: The possibility of hookworm infection through breast milk. German Med Monthly 13:391–392, 1968

44 Brown RC, Girardeau MHF: Transmammary passage of *Strongyloides* sp. larvae in the human host. Am J Trop Med Hyg 26:215–219, 1976

45 Lambotte C, Bayoka S, Mulunda LE, Basilo P: L'hydroxynaphthoate et bephenium dans l'ankylostomose du nourrison et de l'enfant. Ann Soc Belge Med Trop 40:771–781, 1960

46 White GF, Dove WE: The causation of creeping eruption. JAMA 90:1701–1704, 1928

47 Matsusaki G: Hookworm diseases and prevention, in Morishita K, et al (eds): *Progress of Medical Parasitology in Japan* 3:187–282, 1966. Meguro Parasitological Museum, Tokyo, Japan.

48 Hollander M, Takingo R, Stankewich WR: Successful treatment of massive intestinal hemorrhage due to hookworm infection in a neonate. J Pediatr 82:332–334, 1973

49 Zimmerman HM: Fatal hookworm disease in infancy and childhood on Guam. Am J Pathol 22:1081–1100, 1946

50 Whipple GH: Uncinariasis in Panama. Am J Med Sci 138:40–48, 1909

51 Banwell JG, Schad GA: Hookworm, in Marsden P (ed): *Intestinal Parasites,* in Clin Gastroenterol 7:129–156, 1978

52 Ball PAJ, Bartlett A: Serological reactions to infection with *Necator americanus.* Trans R Soc Trop Med Hyg 63:362–369, 1969

53 Maxwell C, Hussain R, Nutman TB, et al: The clinical and immunologic responses of normal human volunteers to low dose hookworm (*Necator americanus*) infection. Am J Trop Med Hyg 37:126–134, 1987

54 Schad GA, Soulsby EJL, Chowdhury AB, et al: Epidemiological and serological studies of hookworm infection in endemic areas in India and West Africa, in *Nuclear Techniques in Helminthology Research.* Vienna, International Atomic Energy Agency, 1975, pp 41–54

55 Gilles HM, Watson-Williams EJ, Ball P: Hookworm infection and anemia. Q J Med 33:1–24, 1964

56 Otto GF, Kerr KB: I. The immunization of dogs against hookworm *Ancylostoma caninum* by subcutaneous injection of graded doses of living larvae. Am J Hyg 29D:25–45, 1939

57 Behnke JM: Do hookworms elicit protective immunity in man? Parasitol Today 3:200–206, 1987

58 Tripathy K, Garcia FT, Lotero H: Effect of nutritional repletion on human hookworm infection. Am J Trop Med Hyg 20:219–223, 1971

59 Variyam EP, Banwell JG: Nutrition implications of hookworm infection. Rev Infect Dis 4:830–835, 1982

60 Mettrick DF, Podesta RB: Ecological and physiological aspects of helminth-host interaction in the mammalian gastrointestinal canal. Adv Parasitol 23:183–278, 1974

61 Darke ST: Malnutrition in African adults. 5. Effects of hookworm infection on absorption of foodstuffs. Br J Nutr 13:278–282, 1959

62 Banwell JG, Marsden PD, Blackman V, et al: Hookworm infection and intestinal absorption amongst Africans in Uganda. Am J Trop Med Hyg 16:304–308, 1967

63 Tandon BW, Kohle RK, Saraya AK, et al: Role of parasites in the pathogenesis of intestinal malabsorption in hookworm disease. Gut 10:293–298, 1969

64 Mayoral LG, Tripathy K, Garcia FT, et al: Malabsorption in the tropics: A second look. I. The role of protein malnutrition. Am J Clin Nutr 20:866–883, 1967

65 Migesena S, Gilles HM, Maegraith BG: Studies of *Ancylostoma caninum* infection in dogs. I: Absorption for the small intestine of amino acids, carbohydrates and fats. Ann Trop Med Parasitol 66:107–128, 1972

66 Hodes PJ, Keefer GP: Hookworm disease. A small intestinal study. Am J Roentgenol Radium Ther Nuc Med 54:728–742, 1945

67 Blackman V, Marsden P, Banwell JG, et al: Albumin metabolism in hookworm anemia. Trans R Soc Trop Med Hyg 59:472–482, 1965

68 Arrekul S, Radomyos P, Viraran C: Experimental infection with *Ancylostoma ceylanicum.* J Med Assoc Thailand 53:190–194, 1970

69 Basta SS, Soerkirman KD, Scrimshaw NS: Iron deficiency anemia and the productivity of adult males in Indonesia. Am J Clin Nutr 32:916–925, 1979

70 Martin LK, Beaver PC: Evaluation of Kato thick-smear technique for quantitative diagnosis of helminth infections. Am J Med Hyg 17:382–391, 1968

71 Villarejos VM, Argueda JA, Vargas C, et al: Evaluation of the skin test for hookworm as an epidemiological tool. Am J Trop Med Hyg 24:250–255, 1975

72 Carr A, Pritchard DI: Antigen expression during development of the human hookworm, *Necator americanus* (Nematoda). Parasite Immunol 9:219–234, 1987

73 Correa-Oliveira R, Dusse LMS, Viana IRC, et al: Human antibody responses against schistosomal antigens. Am J Trop Med Hyg 38:348–355, 1988

74 Klaver-Wesseling JCM, Vetter JCM, Schoeman EN: The *in vitro* interaction between several components of the canine immune system and infective larvae of *Ancylostoma canium*. Parasite Immunol 4:227–232, 1981

75 Gilles HM: Selective primary health care: Strategies for control of disease in the developing world. XVII. Hookworm infection and anemia. Rev Infect Dis 7:111–118, 1985

76 Lozoff B, Warren KS, Mahmoud AAF: Algorithms in the diagnosis and management of exotic diseases. VIII. Hookworm. J Infect Dis 132:606–610, 1975

77 Cline BL, Little MD, Baltholomew RK, et al: Larvicidal activity of albendazole against *Necator americanus* in human volunteers. Am J Trop Med Hyg 33:387–394, 1984

78 Hoagland KE, Schad GA: *Necator americanus* and *Ancylostoma duodenale:* Life history parameters and epidemiological implications of two sympatic hookworms of humans. Exp Parasitol 44:36–49, 1978

79 Hsieh HC: Studies on endemic hookworm. I. Survey and longitudinal observations in Taiwan. Jpn J Parasitol 19:508–522, 1970

80 Hominick WM, Dean CG, Schad GA: Population biology of hookworms in West Bengal: Analysis of numbers of infective larvae recovered from damp pads applied to the soil surface at defecation time. Trans R Soc Trop Med Hyg 81:978–986, 1987

81 Beaver PC: *Control of Soil-transmitted Helminths*. WHO Public Health Pap 10, Geneva, World Health Organization, p 44, 1961

82 Haswell-Elkins M, Elkins D, Anderson RM: Evidence for predisposition in humans to infection with *Ascaris,* hookworm, *Enterobius,* and *Trichuris* in a South Indian fishing community. Parasitology 95:323–337, 1987

83 Schad GA, Nawalinski T, Kochar V: Human ecology and the distribution and abundance of hookworm populations, in Croll N, Cross J (eds): *Human Ecology and Infectious Disease*. New York, Academic, 1984, pp 187–223

84 Chandler AC: The review of recent work on the rate of acquisitions and loss of hookworms. Am J Trop Med Hyg 15:357–370, 1935

85 Chandler AC: *Hookworm Disease. Its Distribution, Biology, Epidemiology, Pathology, Diagnosis, Treatment and Control.* New York, Macmillan, 1929, p 494

86 Kochar V, Schad GA, et al: Human factors in regulation of parasitic infectious cultural ecology of hookworm populations in rural West Bengal, in Grolling FX, Haley HB (eds): *Medical Anthropology*. Mouton Hague, 1976, pp 287–312

87 Schad GA, Rozeboom LE: Integrated control of helminths in human populations. Ann Rev Ecol Syst 7:393–420, 1976

88 Schad GA: Control, in Cox FEG (ed): *Modern Parasitology*. Oxford, Blackwell, 1982, pp 252–286

89 Anderson RM, Medley GF: Community control of helminth infections of many by mass and selective chemotherapy. Parasitology 90:629–660, 1988

90 Crompton DWT: Hookworm disease: Current status and new directions. Parasitol Today 5:1–2, 1989

91 Keymer A, Bundy D: Seventy-five years of solicitude. Nature 337:91, 1989

92 Lozoff B, Brittenham GM: Behavioral alterations in iron deficiency. Hematol/Oncol Clin N Am I:449–463, 1987

CHAPTER 45 / *Strongyloidiasis* · David I. Grove

Strongyloidiasis is one of the major human intestinal nematode infections. It is usually due to *Strongyloides stercoralis,* which is distributed widely in the tropics and subtropics. The infection is most commonly acquired when infective larvae penetrate the intact skin. This parasitic helminth is unusual because multiplication and autoinfection occur within the infected person; this accounts for the persistence of infection for many years. The major clinical features are abdominal pain, diarrhea, and urticaria. In immunosuppressed persons, host defenses break down and larvae disseminate throughout the body. The diagnosis is confirmed by finding larvae in feces or other fluids. Treatment is with thiabendazole, although this is not always successful. Occasionally, strongyloidiasis is caused by *S. fuelleborni.*

PARASITE

LIFE HISTORY

S. stercoralis has a complex life history (Fig. 45-1). Complete cycles of development may occur both within the host and in the external environment.

The parasitic cycle

Primary Infection. Infective (third-stage, or filariform) larvae in soil contaminated with feces penetrate the intact skin and pass to the lungs, where they enter the alveolar spaces. They then ascend the airways to the mouth, are swallowed, and reach the small intestines.

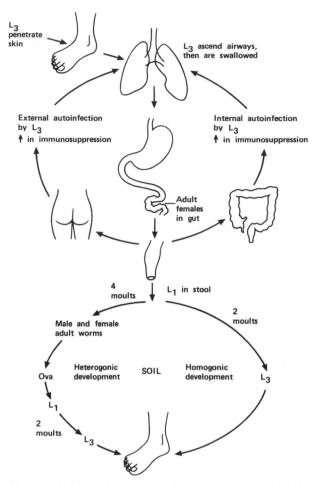

Figure 45-1. Life cycle of *Strongyloides stercoralis*. L₁ = rhabditiform larvae; L₃ = infective, filariform larvae; ↑ = increased.

The precise details of migration and development, however, are controversial. It is uncertain whether infective larvae enter through the hair follicles or penetrate the stratum corneum directly. It is presumed that larvae reach the lungs via the bloodstream, although larvae may migrate through the connective tissues with transitory lodgment in other tissues, especially the muscles. In the small bowel, infective larvae molt twice, becoming adolescent, then adult female worms. These worms live in tunnels between the enterocytes. The life span of these parasitic female worms is unknown. They produce eggs by parthenogenesis which then rapidly transform into first-stage (rhabditiform) larvae. These rhabditiform larvae may then either be passed in the feces or enter the autoinfective cycle. The period from exposure until the appearance of larvae in the stool is nearly 3 weeks.

Autoinfection. A proportion of rhabditiform larvae develop into infective larvae within the intestinal lumen. They penetrate either the mucous membrane of the bowel (internal autoinfection) or the perianal skin (external autoinfection) and then follow the same pathway as described earlier. This capacity to replicate within the host is most unusual among human helminth infections and is the basis of both the persistence of infection for many years and the hyperinfection that is seen in overwhelming strongyloidiasis.

The free-living cycle

Rhabditiform larvae passed in the stool and deposited on moist soil may develop in one of two ways.

Direct (Homogonic) Development. Some or all of the first-stage larvae molt twice and become infective larvae within several days. Depending upon environmental conditions, they may remain viable for a few days to several weeks.

Indirect (Heterogonic) Development. Some first-stage larvae may molt four times to become free-living male and female adult worms. These mate, and large numbers of rhabditiform larvae appear within a week or so. These larvae then develop either into infective larvae or into new free-living adult worms. This mode of development gives two advantages to the parasite: multiplication of organisms, thus improving the chances of infecting a new definitive host, and maintenance of the worm in the external environment.

MORPHOLOGY

The free-living adult female worm is approximately 1 mm long and 60 μm in diameter, while the adult male worm measures 750 by 45 μm. The parasitic female is 2.2 mm long and 50 μm in diameter. The anterior one-third of the worm contains the long, cylindrical esphophagus, while the posterior two-thirds holds the intestinal and reproductive organs. Eggs are oval, thin-shelled, and embryonated when laid and measure 55 by 30 μm. Rhabditiform larvae measure 250 by 15 μm (Fig. 45-2); they have a short buccal capsule and an esophagus which occupies one-fifth the length of the larva and has a prominent posterior bulb. Filariform larvae measure 500 by 15 μm (Fig. 45-2); the nonbulbous esophagus measures one-third the length of the worm, and the tail is notched.

RESERVOIR HOSTS

Humans are the major hosts of *S. stercoralis,* although it has been found in a number of nonhuman primates including the chimpanzee, gibbon, and orangutan, as well as in dogs and cats. Galliard considered that there are "geographical" races of *S. stercoralis* which differ in their infectivity for different hosts [1]. For example, *S. stercoralis* from humans in Indochina easily infected dogs while that from Calcutta infected cats. The prevalence of strongyloidiasis in dogs and cats in various geographical areas has not been intensively investi-

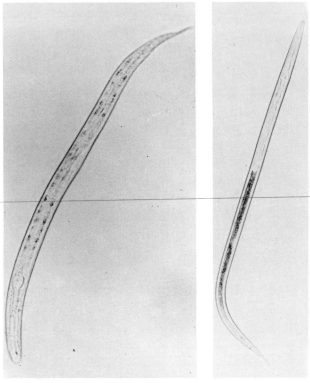

Figure 45-2. Photomicrograph of a rhabditiform larva approximately 250 μm in length (*left*) and a filariform larva approximately 600 μm long (*right*).

gated; approximately 1 percent of dogs in the eastern United States appear to be infected.

ANIMAL MODELS

Many studies of the host-parasite relationship in strongyloidiasis have been undertaken with *S. ratti* in rats and inbred mice. Unfortunately, this parasite does not autoinfect. Consequently, models have been developed utilizing *S. stercoralis* infections of immunocompetent [2] and immunosuppressed [3] dogs. Disseminated infections develop in the latter as well as in normal *Erythrocebus patas* monkeys [4].

PATIENT

PATHOGENESIS

The factors determining host susceptibility and resistance to infection are poorly understood [5]. A feature which sets strongyloidiasis apart from almost all other human helminth infections is the ability of *S. stercoralis* to replicate within the host. In chronic strongyloidiasis, a balance is reached between parasite and host whereby worms are restricted in number and confined principally to the skin and gut, but the host is unable to eradicate the organism. When host defenses break down in

immunosuppressed persons, worms multiply rapidly and disseminate throughout the body. Thus, the means by which the host contains the infection appear to be immunologically based, although the precise mechanisms are unknown. Similarly, the ways in which worms evade total destruction by these immune processes are unclear. It seems unlikely that all people are equally prone to chronic infection. For example, despite intense exposure over several years, less than one-third of Caucasian prisoners of war in southeast Asia during World War II were infected when investigated 35 years later [6]. Thus, genetic influences may be important in controlling host resistance to infection. Whether or not prior exposure increases resistance to subsequent infection is not known.

Although it has not yet been proven, the characteristic cutaneous lesions seen in strongyloidiasis are almost certainly mediated by immediate hypersensitivity reactions to migrating worms or their products. The enteritis which sometimes occurs may be the result of direct mechanical trauma, the inflammatory reaction which develops against worms, and secondary bacterial colonization of ulcerative lesions. In mild infections, diarrhea occurs, but in heavy infections, a malabsorption syndrome may develop. In disseminated strongyloidiasis, not only may migrating larvae damage tissues directly, but widespread secondary bacterial infection complicates the illness. These bacteria may either be carried by migrating larvae or enter the bloodstream through gut lesions.

PATHOLOGY

Chronic strongyloidiasis

Gross lesions of the small intestine are usually absent although some fibrosis may be seen in patients with long-standing infections. Histologically, adult worms are found in the crypts of Lieberkühn, and eggs or larvae may be seen. Inflammatory cell infiltration is usually minimal, as is partial villous atrophy. The nature of any pathological reactions which may occur around larvae migrating through the skin or lungs is unknown.

Overwhelming strongyloidiasis

Pathological changes may be found in the gut either in persons who are exposed to very heavy infections or in immunosuppressed patients with disseminated infection. Macroscopically, the bowel is edematous and congested, and the mucosal surface may be ulcerated and covered with abundant mucus. Histologically, filariform larvae with surrounding inflammation are found in the walls of both the small and large intestine. In disseminated infections, filariform larvae may invade any organ. Presumably, depending upon the degree of immunosuppression, there may be no reaction, or the larvae may provoke a mixed inflammatory cell infiltrate of lymphocytes, histiocytes, giant cells, plasma cells, eosinophils, and neutrophils. Granulomas may surround degenerating larvae. The appearances may be complicated by secondary bacterial infection.

CLINICAL MANIFESTATIONS

Acute strongyloidiasis

The symptoms and signs of recently acquired infections have not been well documented but presumably reflect the intensity of infection. It is probable that only occasional persons with heavy worm burdens have significant clinical manifestations. Passage of larvae through the lungs may produce Loeffler's syndrome (pulmonary infiltrates with eosinophilia), but this does not appear to be common; patients complain of cough, shortness of breath, wheezing, and fever, while transient pulmonary opacities are seen on chest x-ray, and a peripheral eosinophilia is found. Lodgment of worms in the gut may cause abdominal pain and diarrhea which is often difficult to differentiate from other gastrointestinal infections. A dull ache or cramping pains are frequently located in the epigastrium. In heavy infections, malabsorption sometimes develops with the appearance of steatorrheic stools, weight loss, and edema [7].

Chronic strongyloidiasis

Patients with *Strongyloides* infections persisting for more than 35 years have been described. Although many people are asymptomatic, cutaneous and gastrointestinal symptoms are common [6]. The classic triad consists of abdominal pain, diarrhea, and urticaria. Respiratory complaints are not prominent. Rarely, immune complex deposition causes a reactive arthritis.

Cutaneous manifestations are the most characteristic feature and are present in two-thirds of patients. Many people have urticarial eruptions in which crops of stationary wheals lasting 1 to 2 days and recurring at irregular intervals appear, particularly on the buttocks and around the waist. Less commonly, the pathognomonic larva currens is found (Fig. 45-3); this urticarial rash may migrate in a serpiginous fashion at the rate of several centimeters per hour and last for up to 1 to 2 days [8].

A variety of nonspecific gastrointestinal symptoms is seen in patients with chronic strongyloidiasis more commonly than in the general population. These include indigestion, cramping lower abdominal pains, intermittent or persistent diarrhea, pruritus ani, and weight loss.

Disseminated strongyloidiasis

Overwhelming strongyloidiasis with dissemination of larvae throughout the body is being recognized increasingly in patients who are immunosuppressed either as a result of disease, because of the administration of immunosuppressive agents, or both [9,10]. Occasionally, dissemination occurs for no apparent reason. Disseminated strongyloidiasis has been seen in children with protein-calorie malnutrition and patients with burns, chronic infections such as tuberculosis and syphilis, irradiation, and a variety of lymphomas. It has also been described in the acquired immune deficiency syndrome [11] but

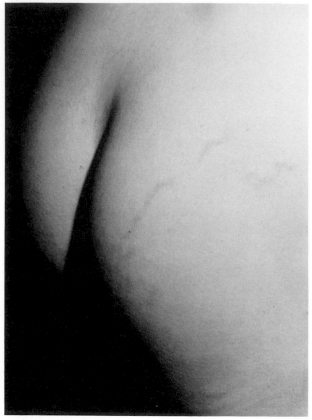

Figure 45-3. Larva currens.

much less commonly than might be predicted from the relative frequencies of both conditions in Africa. More frequent reports have described this syndrome in patients who have received systemic corticosteroid therapy for asthma, carcinoma, cerebral edema, eye disease, idiopathic thrombocytopenic purpura, leprosy, leukemia, lymphoma, polymyositis, renal transplantation, skin disorders, systemic lupus erythematosus, and ulcerative colitis.

Patients commonly present with severe, generalized abdominal pain, abdominal distension, and shock. Ileus and edema lead to small-bowel obstruction which may culminate in a fatal necrotizing jejunitis. Jaundice may appear. Massive larval invasion of the lungs may result in cough, wheezing, and dyspnea. A variety of neurological signs ranging from mild changes in mental status to coma indicate cerebral involvement. A high fever develops frequently, and gram-negative septicemia which may lead to pneumonia or meningitis is often found.

DIAGNOSIS

Strongyloidiasis should be suspected in someone with abdominal pain, diarrhea, or urticaria, particularly if they have lived at some time in their lives in an endemic area. Sudden deterioration in an immunosuppressed patient suggests the possibility of disseminated strongyloidiasis.

An increase in the blood eosinophils or an elevated serum IgE level may be useful indicators of infection in patients who do not have concurrent infections with other tissue helminths, although neither feature is invariable in chronic strongyloidiasis. Similarly, the blood eosinophil count is frequently normal in people with depressed cell-mediated immunity and disseminated strongyloidiasis.

Radiology

The predominance of gastrointestinal symptoms often initiates radiodiagnostic procedures [12]. In mild infections, a barium meal is usually normal but may show duodenal and jejunal dilatation, rigidity, and mucosal edema. In severe chronic infections, strictures may be found. Abnormalities of the colon are unusual. In overwhelming strongyloidiasis, a plain x-ray of the abdomen may disclose multiple loops of dilated small bowel containing fluid levels.

Parasitology

The definitive diagnosis is made by finding larvae of *S. stercoralis*. Rhabditiform or, occasionally, filariform larvae may be seen in the stool or in duodenal contents. Examination of the feces is simplest and most reliable. Feces may be examined by direct microscopy, after concentration by the formalin-ether technique, or after culture. *Strongyloides* larvae do not float in saturated salt solutions. In chronic strongyloidiasis, larvae are often present in very low numbers and may be difficult to detect, even after repeated examination of specimens.

Alternatively, larvae may be sought in duodenal fluid. The simplest method for obtaining this is by use of the Enterotest capsule, in which is packed a white nylon thread. The capsule is swallowed by the patient, and the free end of line is secured to the face. After several hours, the string is withdrawn and attached mucus examined under the microscope. Larvae are occasionally found in fluid obtained by aspiration through a duodenoscope, but this technique is less reliable. Duodenal biopsy is usually not helpful. In suspected disseminated strongyloidiasis, concentrated specimens of sputum should also be examined for filariform larvae.

Serology

Immunodiagnostic assays are particularly useful for the diagnosis of chronic strongyloidiasis where it may be difficult to demonstrate the presence of larvae. Immunofluorescent [13] and enzyme-linked immunosorbent [14] assays have been described. A major difficulty with these tests is that they do not differentiate between past and current infection. This drawback may be overcome if an assay to detect antigen in blood, urine, or feces is developed.

MANAGEMENT

Uncomplicated strongyloidiasis

All infected patients should be treated. Since worms are able to multiply and an asymptomatic infected person has the potential for becoming ill in the future, the aim of therapy is eradication of worms since any remaining parasites may produce autoinfection, resulting in persistent disease. The antihelminthic most commonly used is thiabendazole, 25 mg/kg orally twice daily for 3 days. Unfortunately, this drug is both toxic and not always effective. Most patients complain of side effects, particularly nausea, vomiting, malaise, dizziness, feelings of disembodiment, and smelly urine [15]. Confirmation of effective therapy may be difficult since worm burdens are often low before treatment, and a partial reduction in worm numbers may make it almost impossible to detect any remaining parasites. One recent study suggests that up to one-third of patients may not be cured with a single course of thiabendazole [15]. Ideally, patients should be reassessed 6 and 12 months after treatment.

Mebandazole has been used for the treatment of strongyloidiasis but its efficacy is uncertain. Cambendazole has been used with apparent success in a number of human clinical studies [16], although long-term assessment of its efficacy has not been made. Experimental studies in murine strongyloidiasis [17] and in immunocompetent and immunosuppressed dogs infected with *S. stercoralis* [18] have suggested that cambendazole is much more effective than both thiabendazole and mebandazole. Cambendazole, however, is not recommended by the manufacturers for the treatment of human strongyloidiasis.

Albendazole has been used with limited success in human strongyloidiasis [19]. Experimental studies in animals have confirmed that this drug has some efficacy but suggest that relatively large doses may be necessary [20]. Drugs that are currently undergoing investigation and may eventually prove to have something to offer in the treatment of strongyloidiasis include ivermectin and cyclosporin A.

Disseminated strongyloidiasis

Thiabendazole treatment is mandatory in all patients who are at risk from systemic strongyloidiasis. This applies particularly to infected patients who are going to be given immunosuppressive doses of corticosteroids [21]. The treatment of established disseminated strongyloidiasis may be difficult, and some patients die despite intensive therapy. Patients should be given thiabendazole, 25 mg/kg twice daily for up to 1 week. Patients with intestinal obstruction may require intravenous fluids and suction plus intermittent administration of thiabendazole suspension via a nasogastric tube. If possible, the dose of immunosuppressive agents should be reduced, at least temporarily. The administration of thiabendazole to patients undergoing hemodialysis has been described by Schumaker et al. [22]. Septicemia and other bacterial infections should be sought carefully and treated rigorously with appropriate antibiotics. Patients who recover should be followed carefully, and, if necessary, given repeated courses of thiabendazole, 25 mg/kg twice daily for 2 days at monthly intervals.

POPULATION

EPIDEMIOLOGY

Strongyloidiasis is widespread throughout the tropics and subtropics, but occasional patients have been described who have never left cold or temperate zones. The prevalence of infection is uncertain, although it has been estimated that 50 to 100 million people are infected. The age and sex distribution of S. stercoralis in different populations has not been documented. In addition to infection being endemic in many rural areas of the tropics, high infection rates have also been recorded among residents of some institutions for the mentally retarded.

Humans are the primary reservoir of infection although other primates and dogs have been found naturally infected. The infection has been acquired occasionally as a zoonosis. The presence of a free-living cycle ensures perpetuation of the parasite during the absence of a suitable host.

Infection is acquired most commonly when infective larvae in the soil come in contact with the skin. Since transmission of S. stercoralis is facilitated by poor personal and public hygiene, the prevalence of infection is greatest in areas where socioeconomic status is lowest. Under optimal conditions of warmth, light, moisture, and oxygen, filariform larvae develop in the soil and may remain viable for several weeks. It has been demonstrated recently that infective larvae may sometimes be transmitted in breast milk, but the relative importance of transmammary transmission in determining the prevalence of infection in endemic areas has not been quantitated. The proportion of patients in such areas who suffer ill health as a result of infection with S. stercoralis is unclear. Indeed, it may never be possible to delineate the burden of disease since concurrent infections of the gastrointestinal tract with other agents are almost always present. Nevertheless, since this parasite can replicate within the human host, all infected people are at risk for developing potentially fatal overwhelming strongyloidiasis.

CONTROL

The control of strongyloidiasis is dependent primarily upon improved standards of living with installation of effective waste disposal facilities. These may range from pit latrines to extensive sewage systems. If these become available, then health education must be pressed vigorously and continually to persuade people to use them constantly and properly. If human feces is to be used as a fertilizer for crops, it should be composted with vegetable refuse so that the temperature is raised above the thermal death point of the larvae. It is unlikely that physical measures for the control of strongyloidiasis will ever be pursued in isolation. Rather, they should be viewed in the context of measures designed to control a wide range of gastrointestinal infections. The place of mass administration of antihelminthics in the control of strongyloidiasis is uncertain.

INFECTIONS WITH OTHER *STRONGYLOIDES* SPECIES

Human infections with S. fuelleborni are common in parts of Africa [23]. The parasite is often found in primates, and human infection may be acquired as a zoonosis. In some of these locations, the organism appears to be endemic in the human population and transmitted from person to person. It is unknown whether S. fuelleborni is prone to autoinfection. Experimental studies in human volunteers have indicated that eggs appear in the feces by 4 weeks after infection. On second exposure, a rash appeared at the site of infection and was followed by lymphangitis. A cough was noted on the fifth day, and anorexia, malaise, abdominal pain, and bouts of diarrhea appeared after 3 weeks. An eosinophilia was present between the fourth and tenth weeks of infection. The diagnosis is made by finding embryonated eggs measuring 55 by 30 μm in the feces. Treatment is with thiabendazole.

In Papua New Guinea where there are no nonhuman primates, infections with a S. fuelleborni-like organism have been described. This parasite has been associated with a fatal illness in infants who develop abdominal distension, respiratory distress, and generalized edema [24].

REFERENCES

1 Galliard H: Pathogenesis of *Strongyloides*. Helminthol Abst 36:247–260, 1967
2 Grove DI, Northern C: Infection and immunity in dogs infected with a human strain of *Strongyloides stercoralis*. Trans R Soc Trop Med Hyg 76:833–838, 1982
3 Grove DI, Heenan PJ, Northern C: Persistent and disseminated infections with *Strongyloides stercoralis* in immunosuppressed dogs. Int J Parasitol 13:483–490, 1983
4 Harper JS III, Genta RM, Gam A, et al: Experimental disseminated strongyloidiasis in *Erythrocebus patas*. I. Pathology. Am J Trop Med Hyg 33:431–443, 1984
5 Genta RM: *Strongyloides stercoralis:* Immunobiological considerations on an unusual worm. Parasitol Today 2:241–246, 1986
6 Grove DI: Strongyloidiasis in Allied ex-prisoners of war in Southeast Asia. Br Med J 280:598–601, 1980
7 Milner PF, Irvine RA, Barton CJ, et al: Intestinal malabsorption in *Strongyloides stercoralis* infection. Gut 6:574–581, 1965
8 Smith JD, Goette DK, Odom RB: Larva currens: Cutaneous strongyloidiasis. Arch Dermatol 112:1161–1163, 1976
9 Scowden EB, Schaffner W, Stone WJ: Overwhelming strongyloidiasis: An unappreciated opportunistic infection. Medicine (Baltimore) 57:527–544, 1978
10 Igra-Siegman Y, Kapila R, Sen P, et al: Syndrome of hyperinfection with *Strongyloides stercoralis*. Rev Infect Dis 3:397–407, 1981
11 Mayaan S, Wormser GP, Widerhorn J, et al: *Strongyloides stercoralis* hyperinfection in a patient with the acquired immune deficiency syndrome. Am J Med 83:945–948, 1987

12 Louisy CL, Barton CJ: The radiological diagnosis of *Strongyloides stercoralis* enteritis. Radiology 98:535–541, 1971

13 Grove DI, Blair AJ: Diagnosis of human strongyloidiasis by immunofluorescence using *S. ratti* and *S. stercoralis* larvae. Am J Trop Med Hyg 30:344–349, 1981

14 Gam AA, Neva FA, Krotoski WA: Comparative sensitivity and specificity of ELISA and IHA for serodiagnosis of strongyloidiasis with larval antigens. Am J Trop Med Hyg 37:157–161, 1987

15 Grove DI: Treatment of strongyloidiasis with thiabendazole: An analysis of toxicity and effectiveness. Trans R Soc Trop Med Hyg 76:114–118, 1982

16 Bicalho SA, Leão OJ, Pena Q Jr: Cambendazole in the treatment of human strongyloidiasis. Am J Trop Med Hyg 32:1181–1183, 1983

17 Grove DI: *Strongyloides ratti* and *S. stercoralis:* The effects of thiabendazole, mebendazole and cambendazole in infected mice. Am J Trop Med Hyg 31:469–476, 1982

18 Grove DI, Northern C: The effects of thiabendazole, mebendazole and cambendazole in normal and immunosuppressed dogs infected with a human strain of *Strongyloides stercoralis*. Trans R Soc Trop Med Hyg 82:146–149, 1988

19 Rossignol JF, Maisonneuve H: Albendazole: Placebo-controlled study in 870 patients with intestinal helminthiasis. Trans R Soc Trop Med Hyg 77:707–711, 1983

20 Grove DI, Lumsden J, Northern C: Efficacy of albendazole against *Strongyloides ratti* and *S. stercoralis in vitro,* in mice, and in normal and immunosuppressed dogs. J Antimicrob Ther 21:75–84, 1988

21 Morgan JS, Schaffner W, Stone WJ: Opportunistic strongyloidiasis in renal transplant recipients. Transplantation 42:518–524, 1986

22 Schumaker JD, Band JD, Lensmeyer GL, et al: Thiabendazole treatment of severe strongyloidiasis in a hemodialysed patient. Ann Intern Med 89:644–645, 1978

23 Hira PR, Patel BG: Human strongyloidiasis due to the primate species *Strongyloides fuelleborni*. Trop Geogr Med 32:23–29, 1980

24 Vince JD, Ashford RW, Gratten MJ, et al: *Strongyloides* species infestation in young infants of Papua New Guinea: Association with generalized oedema. Papua New Guinea Med J 22:120–127, 1979

CHAPTER 46 / *Trichuriasis* · D. A. P. Bundy · E. S. Cooper

Trichuriasis describes infection with the whipworm *Trichuris*. In some parts of the world *Trichocephalus* is used as a synonym for this genus, although *Trichuris* has been afforded priority by the Nomenclature Committee of the American Society of Parasitologists.

Trichuris is a parasite of the large bowel of mammals. The species *T. trichiura* is almost exclusively a human parasite, with rare records of occurrence in other primates. Human zoonotic infection may occur with the swine whipworm, *T. suis*, and rarely with that of the dog, *T. vulpis*.

Human infection with *T. trichiura* differs from that with the other major geohelminths (*Ascaris lumbricoides* and the hookworms) in three important ways: (1) there is no pulmonary migration by the larvae; (2) the adult is located in the cecum, not the small intestine; and (3) the adult parasite is in continuous and intimate tissue contact and at no stage is free in the lumen. Intense infection in children is associated with a severe disease simulating ulcerative colitis, while recent evidence indicates that even moderate infection may result in significant pathology.

PARASITE

LIFE CYCLE

Developmental stages

Female worms in the human cecum shed between 3000 and 20,000 eggs per day, the fecundity of each worm declining as the number of worms increases. Embryonation occurs externally to the host over a period of 15 to 30 days at tropical temperatures. On average, an infective egg survives for less than a year, although individual eggs may survive for several years. The eggs hatch on ingestion to release a larva whose fate during the first 5 to 10 days of development is controversial. Contradictory evidence from studies of animal parasites have led to the suggestion that there is a transient development within the duodenal mucosa before the larvae migrate to their adult location in the cecum, although there is equally persuasive evidence that larvae migrate directly to, or hatch directly in, the cecum without a histotrophic phase [1,2].

Postembryonic development occurs only in the cecum or colon, where the larvae penetrate the columnar epithelium at the base of the crypts of Lieberkühn and then migrate up the crypt walls to the luminal surface. The larvae remain within the epithelium throughout this migration and move by tunneling through the enterocyte membranes.

Adult

Inside the luminal epithelium the worm matures through four larval stages to the adult. The body differentiates into a long, threadlike anterior stichosome and a thick, blunt, posterior region containing the intestine and reproductive organs. The thickened posterior region continues to grow until it breaks out of the epithelium and protrudes into the cecal lumen. In the adult stage the short posterior end is free in the lumen for

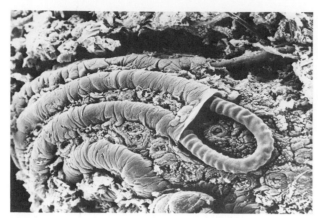

Figure 46-1. Scanning electron micrograph of the anterior region of *Trichuris trichiura* threaded through the epithelium of the human cecum. (*From V. Zaman: Proceedings of the Southeast Asian Parasitology Symposium, Hong Kong, 1983.*)

defecation, copulation, and egg release, while the anterior end—almost three-quarters the length of the worm—remains entirely within the superficial mucosa (Fig. 46-1). The period from infection to egg-laying is approximately 60 to 70 days. The mean expected life span of the fecund adult is approximately 1 year, although maximum longevity may be several years. The adults are about 4 cm in length and weigh up to 10 mg.

Feeding activity is restricted to the epithelium and lamina propria; the anterior end of the worm does not enter the lumen or penetrate beyond the muscularis mucosa. Observations on animal trichuroids indicate that probing movements of the mouth of the worm, armed with a stylet, create a cytoplasmic syncytium resembling the feeding syncytia of other tissue nematodes [3]. Blood may also form part of the diet: the stylet has been observed to penetrate capillaries, and blood products have been identified in the esophagus of *Trichuris* spp. It is unclear to what extent blood is an important nutrient for the worms, but it is certain that they do not feed on blood with the avidity of hookworms.

PATIENT

PATHOLOGY AND IMMUNOLOGY

The adult worms are found mainly in the cecum and ascending colon, but may be present from the terminal ileum to the rectum in intense infection. The major pathology resembles that of inflammatory bowel disease. The recent introduction of fiber-optic colonoscopy has allowed biopsy of the mucosa of the entire large bowel (Fig. 46-2). Histology reveals a generally normal crypt and gland architecture, with no increase in lymphocyte number in the lamina propria. In contrast to ulcerative colitis, there is no general decrease in goblet cell number; in fact goblet cells are generally more numerous, although there are some foci of depletion around worms. In these areas the

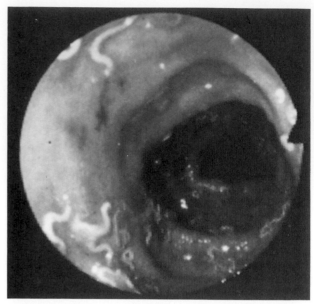

Figure 46-2. Fiber-optic colonoscopy of the cecum of a child with clinical trichuriasis. (*From E.S. Cooper, D.A.P. Bundy: Bailliere's Clin Trop Med Commum Dis 2:629–643, 1987.*)

crypts themselves may be elongated, and infiltration of both eosinophils and neutrophils occurs in the areas of epithelial denudation.

Despite the different histopathology, the growth stunting that may occur in chronic trichuriasis parallels that seen in other forms of large bowel disease, notably ulcerative colitis. Why inflammation of the colon should produce this effect is deserving of further study.

The anemia associated with intense trichuriasis is attributable to a combination of blood loss, both from the inflamed mucosa and by worm ingestion, and compromised iron balance.

The pathogenesis of the colitis is unknown. Some epidemiological studies indicate an association with intestinal protozoa and bacteria, and studies in animals suggest that such secondary invasion produces the inflammatory lesion [2].

The immune response in human trichuriasis is uncharacterized. Infection evokes a specific antibody response, although there is no evidence that this is effective. Murine infection with *T. muris* evokes an effective immune response, involving both humoral and cellular components, which results in worm expulsion [4]. Chronic murine trichuriasis, mimicking human infection, can be artificially achieved by ablating the immune response with corticosteroids, suggesting that the immune response has a limited role in human trichuriasis.

CLINICAL PICTURE

A form of dysentery, associated with signs of acute malnutrition, is ascribable to intense *Trichuris* infection involving the whole colon from the cecum to the rectum [5]. It may be indistinguishable from bacterial or amebic dysentery on clinical grounds, although a carefully taken history will nearly always reveal a history of the frequent passage of stools with mucus going back at least a year before the acute presentation. Children aged 2 to 10 years are most frequently affected, corresponding to the age of the intensity peak of the infection in human communities. Varying intensities of *Trichuris* infection are thus associated with varying degrees of colitis. We have found it convenient to divide the clinical picture into two descriptions, the "classical" dysenteric form [5,6] and the milder form corresponding to a lower intensity of infection.

Classical *Trichuris* dysentery syndrome

The child is likely to be both stunted (short for age) and wasted (underweight even allowing for the short stature). Secondary signs of malnutrition or biochemical indexes of metabolic de-

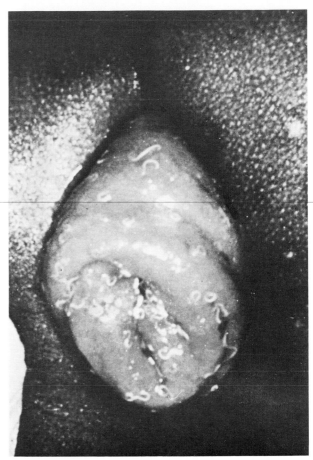

Figure 46-4. Full-thickness rectal prolapse in classical trichuriasis. Note the numerous worms attached to the mucosa.

compensation are likely to be in proportion to the wasting (Fig. 46-3). The stool is unformed rather than watery, with visible mucus and, usually, frank blood. There may be sand, gravel, or pebbles, since these children tend to be habitual eaters of earth. On defecation there is often a mucosal or full-thickness prolapse of the rectum, which is easily reduced (Fig. 46-4). Worms may be seen on the bloody, edematous surface. There is often tenesmus and variable abdominal pain. The extraintestinal effects, apart from malnutrition, include anemia, which may be extremely severe and associated with high-output heart failure, and finger clubbing. Shigellosis and amebiasis often coexist with the *Trichuris* dysentery syndrome. The *Trichuris* burden is in excess of 500 and can reach 5000 or more.

Chronic *Trichuris* colitis with growth retardation

There is no sharp demarcation from the more severe features described above, but the child is more likely to be brought to medical attention because of short stature or pica than because of chronic diarrhea. The stool frequency may be no more than

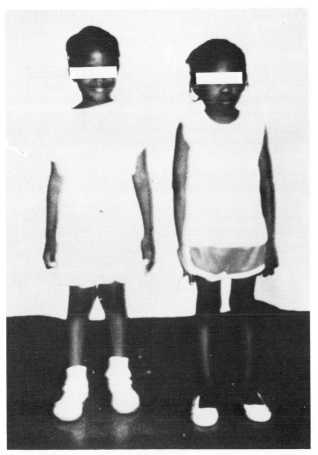

Figure 46-3. Linear growth stunting due to trichuriasis. The child on the left is a healthy 5-year-old, the other is a 9-year-old with a history of chronic trichuriasis. The stunted child grew at a height velocity of 12 cm/year (twice the average at that age) following mebendazole treatment.

three per day, soft or loose with mucus and only occasional blood, although enquiry often reveals that the child awakes from nocturnal sleep to defecate, a habit that is otherwise unusual. The appetite for food is usually depressed, but there is no consistent history of abdominal pain or nausea, and vomiting is rare. There may occasionally be an intermittent mucosal rectal prolapse. Anemia is inconstant, and finger clubbing is minimal or absent. Although linear growth is retarded, there may be no wasting and no secondary signs of malnutrition. The condition may continue for years, sometimes evolving into the classical picture of dysentery. Stature may fall far below the third percentile with a worm burden no greater than 200.

Following therapy to expel *Trichuris* from the colon, combined with the correction of iron deficiency, rapid catch-up growth in height can proceed even against a background of general poverty and deprivation, suggesting that the relationship between chronic colitis and growth retardation is specific.

DIAGNOSIS

The presence of the characteristic barrel-shaped eggs in stool is evidence of infection. The association between pathology and worm burden requires that the intensity of infection also be assessed, most conveniently using the Kato technique. The severe syndrome is usually associated with egg densities in excess of 20,000 to 30,000 eggs per gram of stool. In intense infection adult worms may be seen on proctoscopy or attached to the mucosa of the prolapsed rectum.

TREATMENT

The long-standing difficulty in treating trichuriasis has been resolved by the availability of the following anthelmintics:

1. Albendazole,* 200-mg tablets or 100 mg per 5 mL suspension. It is most often used as a single dose of 400 mg. The dosage for symptomatic infection is 400 mg daily for 3 days.
2. Mebendazole, 100-mg tablets or 100 mg per 5 mL suspension. The usual dose is 100 mg twice daily for 3 days. The tablets are chewable and suitable for young children. Mebendazole is also formulated as a 500-mg tablet for single-dose treatment.
3. Flubendazole*, 100-mg tablets or 100 mg per 5 mL suspension, is used in the same dosage as mebendazole.

The above drugs are closely related benzimidazole carbamates. They are broad-spectrum anthelmintics. They should not be given to pregnant women or to infants less than 1 year old without careful consideration, as their safety for these groups is unproven. For children and adults in general side effects of any kind are very few: the main one reported is the emergence of roundworms via abnormal routes, e.g., the mouth.

*This drug has not been approved by the U.S. Food and Drug Administration at the time of publication.

Single-dose therapy is convenient for treating asymptomatic infection and for use in chemotherapeutic control programs. For symptomatic infection, therapy over several days will increase the probability of complete cure and is to be preferred.

One other drug is useful against *Trichuris*: oxantel*, a membrane-depolarizing drug which is a close analogue of pyrantel. The two are formulated in combination as a broad-spectrum anthelmintic. The suspension contains 50 mg of oxantel and 50 mg pyrantel per milliliter. A single dose of 10 mg per kilogram of body weight of oxantel is recommended for whipworm expulsion; but in symptomatic infection the dose should be repeated, e.g., for a total of 3 consecutive days.

POPULATION

GEOGRAPHICAL DISTRIBUTION

The whipworm has had a long association with humans and was probably acquired from the original primate ancestor. Archeological evidence confirms that *T. trichiura* was already present throughout Eurasia more than 2000 years ago, and was in the Americas in pre-Columbian times.

Recent estimates suggest that 800 million people are infected worldwide, the majority living in tropical regions [7]. *T. trichiura* is not exclusively a tropical parasite: infection was prevalent in northern Europe until this century, and is today endemic in many temperate regions. There are an estimated 2.2 million infections in the United States. The present, largely tropical, distribution appears to be a consequence of socioeconomic rather than ecological factors; infection is likely to be prevalent wherever sanitation is compromised. Climate does have a role, however, in excluding the parasite from areas of extreme cold or aridity.

T. trichiura and *A. lumbricoides* tend to have cointensive distributions, although there is a trend for the former to be more common in some areas (Far East, Caribbean) and the latter in others (Africa).

T. trichiura is particularly prevalent in insanitary and overcrowded communities, whether rural villages or urban slums. High rates of population increase and rural-urban migration are likely to substantially increase the prevalence of this infection in developing countries.

POPULATION BIOLOGY

In an endemic area, most children are likely to be infected by the age of 2 years, and to be continuously reinfected for the rest of their lives. The intensity of infection reaches a maximum value in children between 5 and 10 years old and declines substantially in adulthood. Thus, although a similar proportion of children and adults are infected, adults tend to harbor significantly fewer worms.

Within any age group of the population there is considerable variation in the number of worms harbored by each individual.

The worm burdens are highly aggregated in certain individuals, such that most people have few worms, while a few individuals have disproportionately large worm burdens. The population mean burden is usually less than 100 worms whereas intensely infected individuals harbor several thousand. Typically, more than 65 percent of all the worms in a population are found in less than 15 percent of the people. Such heavily infected individuals tend to reacquire heavier than average *T. trichiura* worm burdens even after successful treatment. These intense infections tend to occur in family groups, such that all the members of a household are likely to be heavily infected. Whatever the reasons, and they remain unresolved at present, the distribution of intense infection has implications for both morbidity and control: the most heavily infected individuals, households, and age groups are not only at increased risk of disease but are also the major source of environmental contamination with infective stages [8].

PREVALENCE OF DISEASE

The population biology of *T. trichiura* infection has important implications for the distribution of disease. Since intense infection predominantly occurs in the 5- to 10-year-old age group, disease is also most likely to occur in children. Since the distribution of worm burdens in children is highly aggregated, well-defined symptoms of trichuriasis are most likely to occur in that small proportion of the population which is most heavily infected. It does not follow, however, that disease is rare: a significant minority of children have worm burdens likely to cause intermediate levels of disease, such as growth stunting. On a global scale, several million children are likely to be in this category.

A community-based study in the Caribbean [9] calculated a morbidity rate (based on observed signs) of 100 per 1000 infected children, and a rate as assessed by self-presentation to medical services of less than 10 per 1000. In that community, 3.5 percent of 6-month to 6-year-old children had recurrent rectal prolapse. These observations contrast with estimates based on case reports which suggest that the global morbidity rate of trichuriasis is only 0.2 cases per 1000 infected. Detailed morbidity studies from other geographical areas are required to determine whether trichuriasis is similarly underreported on a global scale.

CONTROL

Procedures for the control of *T. trichiura* are essentially similar to those required for the control of *A. lumbricoides*.

Sanitation

Fecal contamination of the environment is the only source of infection. Infective eggs may be ingested from contaminated soil either directly, through the common practice of geophagia, or indirectly from contaminated hands and utensils if hygiene is inadequate. Contamination of food may occur due to disseminating agents such as houseflies, or through fertilizing of crops with human excreta.

Sanitary disposal of feces will prevent transmission, but community-wide programs are necessary, as improvements to an individual dwelling do not protect the inhabitants from sources of infection elsewhere in the community. Infrastructural programs need also to be supported by health education to encourage hygienic practices. Decades of sanitational improvement may be required to achieve a significant reduction in infection.

Vaccination

There is no vaccine available and little prospect of vaccine development. Not only is the human immune response in trichuriasis uncharacterized, but the epidemiological evidence suggests that the natural targets for vaccination—the heavily infected individuals—rapidly reacquire intense infection despite their substantial prior exposure.

Chemotherapy

Chemotherapy is the most commonly used means of control. The available anthelmintics have a broad spectrum of activity and will simultaneously control for all the major geohelminthiases. Single-dose therapy is adequate for this role, but treatment must be repeated at 4- to 6-month intervals due to the rapidity of reinfection. Identification and treatment of infected individuals is not generally necessary due to the low risk associated with available therapy.

Mass treatment may be inappropriate to the resources of an endemic area, and a more rational strategy is to target treatment at 2- to 10-year old children [10]. This age group has the highest intensity of infection (usually 90 percent of intensely infected individuals are in this age group), the highest incidence of disease, and the highest density of infective eggs in their stools. Children are also one of the most accessible groups for treatment. Their treatment will result in an immediate reduction in community morbidity and transmission.

The disadvantage of chemotherapy is that alone it does not provide a permanent solution; the gains of chemotherapy have only been consolidated where they have been accompanied by a general improvement in living standards. It seems likely that the future development of trichuriasis control programs will require a closer integration of the immediate, and affordable, gains of chemotherapy with longer term, and costly, improvements in sanitation.

REFERENCES

1 Panesar TS, Croll NA: The location of parasites within their hosts: Site selection by *Trichuris muris* in the laboratory mouse. Int J Parasitol 10:261–274, 1980

2 Beer RJS: Whipworms of domestic animals. Vet Bull 41:343–349, 1971

3 Lee TDG, Wright KA: The morphology of the attachment and probable feeding site of the nematode *Trichuris muris* (Schrank, 1788) Hall, 1916. Can J Zool 56:1889–1905, 1978

4 Wakelin D: Immune expulsion of *Trichuris muris* from mice during a primary infection: Analysis of the components involved. Parasitology 70:397–406, 1975

5 Gilman RH, Chong YH, Davis C, et al: The adverse consequences of heavy *Trichuris* infection. Trans R Soc Trop Med Hyg 77:432–438, 1983

6 Jung RC, Beaver PC: Clinical observations on *Trichocephalus trichiurus* (whipworm) infestation in children. Pediatrics 8:548–557, 1951

7 Bundy DAP, Cooper ES: Human *Trichuris* and trichuriasis. Adv Parasitol, vol 28, 1989, in press

8 Bundy DAP: Epidemiological aspects of *Trichuris* and trichuriasis in Caribbean communities. Trans R Soc Trop Med Hyg 80:706–718, 1986

9 Cooper ES, Bundy DAP: Trichuriasis in St. Lucia, in McNeish AS, Walker-Smith JA (eds): *Diarrhoea and Malnutrition in Childhood*. London, Butterworths, 1986, pp 91–96

10 Anderson RM, May RM: The population dynamics and control of human helminth infections: Control by chemotherapy. Nature 297:557–563, 1982

C H A P T E R **47** / *Enterobiasis* · Zbigniew S. Pawlowski

Enterobius species are parasites of the human large intestine, highly prevalent throughout the world, and infrequently the cause of any severe clinical problems. Enterobiasis belongs to the group of infections least studied, understood, and controlled.

PARASITE

LIFE CYCLE AND ECOLOGY

Humans are practically the only hosts of *Enterobius* (formerly *Oxyuris*) *vermicularis*—the pinworm—although a few cases of enterobiasis have been reported in zoo monkeys. As a rule the Oxyuridae other than *Enterobius vermicularis* occur in herbivorous or omnivorous mammals only. Most of the gravid female pinworms, detached from the colonic mucosa, actively pass out of the anus and lay sticky eggs while crawling over the perianal and perineal skin for a few or up to 60 min. The eggs are either expelled by uterine contractions or liberated by the rupture of the desiccating worm. The number of eggs produced by a single female is about 11,000. They are ovoid but asymmetrically flattened on one side, measuring 56 to 58 by 27 to 29 μm; a colorless, thick shell covers the larva (Fig. 47-1). The final development process of *E. vermicularis* larvae is initiated by contact with atmospheric oxygen, and is quickly continued in temperatures of 30 to 40°C and a humidity of over 40 percent. Under optimal conditions (36 to 37°C) the larva inside the egg becomes fully developed and invasive within 4 h after oviposition. The survival of the larvae depends on their glycogen and water reserves and on an undisturbed excretion of the metabolic products, especially CO_2. Some larvae can survive indoors for about 2 weeks, but they start to lose their infectivity early on—1 or 2 days after completion of the larval development, especially in warm (27 to 29°C) and dry (under 50 percent humidity) conditions. The maximum survival time observed in vitro was 19 weeks. Humans acquire the infection by ingesting *E. vermicularis* eggs. The invasive larvae hatch in the jejunum and develop in the ileum. The final habitat of the adult worm is the cecum and adjacent parts of the colon. There is some confusion about the life span of the female *E. vermicularis*, which lies between 37 and 93 days with an average of 49 to 51 days. The earliest oviposition observed was at the forth-fifth day. The intensity of the infection is usually light or moderate, between just a few and some hundreds of worms; the most pinworms ever reported in a human being was over 10,000.

MORPHOLOGY OF THE ADULT

There is marked sexual dimorphism between adult *E. vermicularis*. The female worm is 8 to 13 mm long and up to 0.5 mm wide; the anterior part of the body is blunted by a pair of cuticular alae, and the posterior, the last third of the body, is pointed and transparent since it contains neither intestine nor reproductive organ. The esophagus has a typical muscular posterior bulb; the intestine opens just before the pointed posterior part. There is a double reproductive tube; two saclike uteri when gravid distend the middle part of the body; the vulva opening is between the anterior and the middle portions. The male worm is much smaller, with a length of between 2 and 5 mm, and has a curved posterior part of the body; it has two

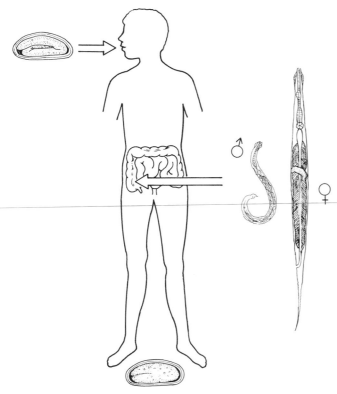

Figure 47-1. Life cycle of *Enterobius vermicularis*.

alae, an esophagus typical for Oxyuridae, a single reproductive tube, and a single copulatory spicule (Fig. 47–1).

PATIENT

PATHOGENESIS AND CLINICAL PATHOLOGY

As a self-limiting infection enterobiasis sometimes occurs as a sporadic and sometimes as a recurrent phenomenon. A continuous infection is the result of frequent exposure to invasive eggs either by autoinfection, infection from family members, or extrafamilial sources. Continuous infections are usually intensive and can cause clinical problems, yet the intensity of the infection has rarely been taken into account in the studies of clinical pathology of enterobiasis.

Enterobius causes little mechanical injury to the colonic mucosa. The toxemic or allergic action is disputable. Children exhibiting emotional instability and hyperactivity are frequently found to be infected, but their behavior may be a result as well as a cause of intensive infection. *E. vermicularis* has no potent IgE-stimulating effect; in one study the prevalence of enterobiasis in children with allergic asthma was not found to be statistically significant. However, the presence of dermal sensitivity to *E. vermicularis* antigen has been demonstrated. Most of the evident pathological changes due to enterobiasis

are caused in the appendix, in the anal region, and by ectopic localization of the parasite. Surgically removed appendixes were found to be invaded by *Enterobius* at a rate varying widely from 1 to 38 percent. In a study in Tunis, one to ten *Enterobius* worms were found in 368 (7.4 percent) out of 5000 appendixes. *E. vermicularis* may cause acute apendicitis, but subacute or chronic appendicitis is more common. In a number of cases there was no inflammatory reaction at all to *Enterobius* present in the appendix [1,2]. Pruritus ani is generally accepted as being pathognomonic for enterobiasis, but it may also be caused by several other diseases (proctitis, diabetes, etc.). This syndrome, reported only by one-quarter of infected people, varies greatly in intensity owing to individual sensitivity and possibly to an allergic component. A perianal eczematous dermatitis, secondarily infected by pyogenic bacteria, is not uncommon.

It has been demonstrated that *E. vermicularis* eggs transmit trophozoites of *Dientamoeba fragilis* from one human host to another [3].

NONINTESTINAL ENTEROBIASIS

The most commonly reported abnormal migration of *E. vermicularis* is that along the female reproductive passages. Enterobiasis is one of the important causes of vulvovaginitis in children and adolescents. Endometriosis and lesions of the fallopian tubes have been reported to be associated with the migration of *Enterobius* female worms. There have also been several reports of granulomatous lesions due to *E. vermicularis* females or eggs mainly in the peritoneal cavity; chronic pelvic peritonitis can occur in some cases.

There is some evidence that *E. vermicularis* worms may enter the urinary tract of both male and female hosts; *Enterobius* eggs have been found in the prostate gland. Secondary enuresis can be associated with enterobiasis but often disappears after antihelminthic therapy [2,4].

The observation that girls with urinary tract infection also more commonly have enterobiasis (57 versus 10 percent in the control subjects) needs further confirmation [2,5].

SYMPTOMATOLOGY

Most *E. vermicularis* infections are light and asymptomatic [6]. In one study the following symptoms were found to have a significant frequency: abdominal pain (54 percent), anal pruritus (29 percent), cephalalgia (35 percent), pallor (26 percent), and dysentery (11 percent) and tenesmus (11 percent). Most statistical evaluations of the symptomatology of enterobiasis have not taken into account the intensity and duration of the infection or the individual host factors such as age, concomitant diseases, etc., which determine the clinical expression. There are enough observations in practice to show that in some individuals enterobiasis constitutes an important clinical or psychological problem and can cause severe complications (skin lesions, vulvovaginitis in children, appendicopathia oxyurica, peritonitis). The clinical importance of these cases is lost in the statistics, which evaluate only two groups: infected and noninfected.

DIAGNOSIS

The diagnosis of enterobiasis can be made by finding adult worms or eggs. The adult worms—mostly females, as the males are rather small—can be seen in the perianal area or during anoscopy, proctoscopy, and vaginoscopy, and also in the feces during diarrhea or after antihelminthic therapy. *Enterobius* eggs can be found by coproscopical examination only in 10 to 15 percent of those infected. Sometimes *E. vermicularis* eggs are found in the urine or on vaginal smears.

The only effective laboratory examination for enterobiasis is the use of anal swabs or prints. The most popular method is prints made in the morning, with Scotch tape pressed for awhile on the perianal skin and then placed on a microscopic slide. It is agreed that one examination can detect more than half of the infections—and four examinations, the majority of cases—yet seven examinations every second day are needed in order to exclude enterobiasis. There are many different types of anal swab using glass, plastic, or wooden applicators, cellophane (NIH), wax, or cotton; they differ little in efficiency.

TREATMENT

The chemotherapy of enterobiasis does not pose many problems as there are a number of drugs available with a cure rate of over 90 percent; the responsible factors in a few unsuccessfully treated cases have rarely been studied.

The dosage of antihelminthics used in enterobiasis is usually lower than that against other intestinal helminthiases. Mebendazole is recommended in a single 100-mg tablet for all ages. Pyrantel pamoate is used in a single dose of 10 mg/kg (maximal dose 500 mg). Pyrvinium pamoate is used in a single dose of 5 mg/kg (maximal dose 250 mg). How often the antihelminthic treatment should be repeated depends on the type of infection: in sporadic enterobiasis only one single treatment is recommended; nonintensive infections under constant exposure (schoolchildren) require treatment every 3 to 4 months to keep the intensity of the enterobiasis low; in intensive and symptomatic cases therapy is to be repeated after 2 weeks and every 2 months thereafter to prevent early reinfection from the contaminated environment [6].

Any decision regarding the possible treatment of other family members or members of an institution should respect the specific individual situation; in heavily infected families all the members are usually treated simultaneously at least twice; this is not necessary for a sporadic infection in one member of a family comprised of adults only.

Specific measures of hygiene are daily change of pajamas and/or underwear, and early-morning shower or washing of the perianal region; these would eliminate over 90 percent of the *Enterobius* eggs laid early in the night.

POPULATION

TRANSMISSION PATTERN

The active migration of female worms out of the human host, the early invasiveness of *E. vermicularis* eggs, and the short survival time of the eggs in the environment are all factors which favor direct transmission. Of these, the most direct is by transferring invasive eggs to the mouth from hands contaminated by scratching the anal region; this is common in children and is responsible for very intensive infections. Intensive infections can also be caused by handling the nightclothes or bed linen of infected people; the number of invasive eggs inhaled may be high, as has been shown, for example, by examination of the dust collected by a vacuum cleaner during the shaking out of bed linen. Dust as well as hands can easily contaminate food, toys, etc., and infect humans indirectly. Enterobiasis is usually acquired for the first time outside the home, but the infection becomes intensive and continuous by permanent indoor spread; this takes about half a year.

Family agglomerations and institutional epidemics are characteristic for enterobiasis. Retrofection, i.e., reinvasion with *Enterobius* larvae hatched in the perianal area and returning into the gut, first suggested in 1943 [7], does not play an important role in the epidemiology of enterobiasis. It has been demonstrated in a few adult human volunteers but has not been confirmed as a common phenomenon.

PREVALENCE OF ENTEROBIASIS

The spread of enterobiasis depends much on the population density and indoor environmental conditions, such as overcrowding of flats, artificial climatization, etc. Therefore, *E. vermicularis* infections are quite common in developed countries in the temperate zone; with about 42 million people infected, enterobiasis is by far the most common of all helminthic infections in the United States, but the prevalence shows a decreasing tendency [8]. For a long time enterobiasis was believed to be rare in the tropics, but this is not so, at least not in overpopulated urban areas. The prevalence of enterobiasis in children in kindergartens in Shanghai was 66 percent; in orphanages in Taipei, 74 percent; among child patients in Singapore, 21 percent; among children in Kuala Lumpur University Hospital, 25 percent; in children attending kindergartens in Teheran, 63 percent; and among schoolchildren in a rural village north of Cairo, 96 percent. The results of fecal examinations in rural populations in the tropics showed that enterobiasis exists in many of them. Counting worms expelled following mass antihelminthic therapy confirmed that enterobiasis is common and highly aggregated in some communities in the tropics [9].

Enterobiasis is most common in schoolchildren. Where preschool institutions are popular, the highest prevalence may be in younger children. People of an advanced age are also more frequently infected than adults.

PREVENTION AND CONTROL

In the United States, enterobiasis, together with gonorrhea, scabies, and pediculosis, has been included in the class of childhood "social diseases" [10]; there are many more such social diseases among the populations living in the tropics, where enterobiasis has never been taken seriously. Therefore, most of the experience in prevention and control of enterobiasis has come from the developed countries. [1,11].

The prevention or control measures differ depending on whether the *E. vermicularis* infection is causing problems in individuals, families, or institutions [6].

In preschools and schools there are usually some wormy children who contribute most to the spread of infection. Identifying wormy individuals by repeated examination or questioning is difficult but not impossible. The education of children and their parents with regard to sanitation may help a great deal, but even more effective is the control of enterobiasis in such institutions by periodic chemotherapy, general and specific hygiene, and preventive treatment for all infected newcomers to the institution.

In the tropics the prevalence of enterobiasis is reduced by using certain antihelminthics (piperazine, pyrantel, albendazole, or mebendazole) against ascariasis.

REFERENCES

1 Akagi K: *Enterobius vermicularis* and enterobiasis, in Morishita K et al (eds): *Progress in Medical Parasitology in Japan,* vol V. Tokyo, Meguro Parasitological Museum, 1973

2 Mayers CP, Purvis RJ: Manifestations of pinworms. Can Med Assoc J 103:489–493, 1970

3 Ockert G: Zur Epidemiologie von *Dientamoeba fragilis*. III. Weitere Versuche zur Übertragung mit Enterobius-Eiern. J Hyg Epidemiol Microbiol Immunol (Praha), 19:17–21, 1975

4 Sachdev YV, Howards SS: *Enterobius vermicularis* infestation and secondary enuresis. J Urol 113:143–144, 1975

5 Simon RD: Pinworm infestation and urinary tract infection in young girls. Am J Dis Child 128:21–22, 1974

6 Pawlowski ZS: Enterobiasis, in Pawlowski ZS (ed): *Intestinal Helminthic Infections*. Baillière's Clinical Tropical Medicine and Communicable Diseases. London, Baillière Tindall. 2(3):667–676, 1987.

7 Schüffner W, Swellengrebel NH: Retrofection in oxyuriasis. A newly discovered mode of infection with *Enterobius vermicularis*. J Parasitol 35:138–146, 1943

8 Wagner ED, Eby WC: Pinworm prevalence in California elementary school children, and diagnostic methods. *Am J Trop Med Hyg* 32:998–1001, 1983

9 Haswell-Elkins M, Elkins DB, Manjula K, et al: The distribution and abundance of *Enterobius vermicularis* in a South Indian fishing community. Parasitology 95:339–354, 1987

10 Welsh NM: Recent insights into the childhood "social diseases"— gonorrhea, scabies, pediculosis, pinworms. Clin Pediatr 17:318–322, 1978

11 Cram EB: Studies on oxyuriasis. XXVIII. Summary and Conclusions. Am J Dis Child 65:46–59, 1943

CHAPTER 48 | *The Filariases and Tropical Eosinophilia* · Eric A. Ottesen

Though eight filarial parasites commonly infect humans (Table 48-1), three species account for most of the pathology associated with these infections. They are the lymphatic-dwelling filariae *Wuchereria bancrofti* and *Brugia malayi* and the subcutaneous filarid *Onchocerca volvulus* (see Chap. 49).

All eight parasites, however, have important features in common. Each is transmitted by biting arthropods (mosquitoes, flies, or midges), and each goes through a complex life cycle (Fig. 48-1) that includes a slow maturation (often 3 to 12 months) from the infective larval stage carried by the insects to the adult worm (generally 3 to 10 cm long but up to 60 cm for female *O. volvulus*) which resides either in the lymph nodes and adjacent lymphatics or in the subcutaneous tissue. The

offspring of the adults, the microfilariae, are 200 to 350 μm in length and either circulate in the blood or migrate through the skin awaiting ingestion by the insect vectors. Patent infection is generally not established unless exposure to infective larvae is intense and prolonged, a situation distinctly different from that in malaria, where the bite of a single infectious mosquito often leads to patent infection. Furthermore, the manifestations of disease often develop slowly. Diagnosis of infection can be extremely difficult, since it relies almost exclusively on parasitological techniques to demonstrate microfilariae in blood or tissue specimens; as yet there are no completely satisfactory means for making a definitive diagnosis of states of "amicrofilaremic filariasis" (see below). Finally,

Table 48-1. The common filarial parasites of humans

Species	Distribution	Vector	Primary pathology
Wuchereria bancrofti	Tropics worldwide	Mosquitoes	Lymphatic, pulmonary
Brugia malayi	Southeast Asia	Mosquitoes	Lymphatic, pulmonary
Brugia timori	Indonesia	Mosquitoes	Lymphatic
Onchocerca volvulus	Africa, Central and South America	Blackfly	Skin, eye, lymphatic
Loa loa	Africa	Horsefly	Dermal, renal
Mansonella perstans	Africa, South America	Midge	? Allergic
Mansonella streptocerca	Africa	Midge	Dermal
Mansonella ozzardi	Central and South America	Midge	Vague

though drug sensitivities of these filariae do differ, none of the parasites has yet been practically controlled by the currently available chemotherapy regimens.

LYMPHATIC FILARIASIS

PARASITE

Wuchereria bancrofti

(Synonyms: *Filaria sanguinis hominis, Filaria bancrofti, Filaria nocturna, Filaria philippinensis, Wuchereria pacifica,* and *Wuchereria vauceli.*) Adult *W. bancrofti* (Cobbold, 1877) are found in the lymph nodes and lymphatic channels of humans. Male worms, about 40 mm in length and 0.1 mm in width, are less than half the size of the females, which measure 80 to 100 by 0.24 to 0.3 mm. Both are creamy white, cylindrical, bluntly tapering, threadlike nematodes with smooth cuticular surfaces and unarmed mouths. The vulva of the female opens just 0.8 to 0.9 mm from the anterior tip of the worm

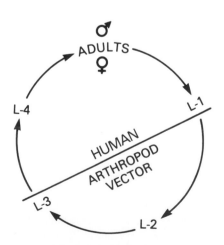

Figure 48-1. Life cycle of the filarial parasites of humans. Vectors for each species of filariae are listed in Table 48-1 and discussed in the text.

but extends posteriorly to the vagina and the bilateral coiled uterus that runs the full length of the adult female. In this uterus microfilarial embryos (about 3.8 by 25 μm in size) develop within individual membranes or "shells." These are retained after the microfilariae have been discharged from the female and are recognized as the microfilarial sheaths. Mature microfilariae found in the blood or occasionally in hydrocele fluid or chylous urine average 260 by 7.5 to 10 μm when the specimens are measured fresh, rapidly dried, or fixed in 5% formalin. They have characteristic morphological features helpful in differentiating one species' microfilariae from another's [1], but the most helpful of these for *W. bancrofti* are the presence of a sheath and the absence of caudal nuclei (see Fig. 48-2 and Table 48-2).

After the microfilariae are ingested by the mosquito during the blood meal, they exsheath, penetrate the wall of the midgut to reach the mosquito's body cavity and, within a few hours, its flight muscles. There they develop into short, thick sausagelike forms (250 by 15 μm) and over the next 10 to 14 days undergo two molts to become filariform, infective third-stage larvae (L_3) that are approximately 1.5 mm long and 20 μm wide. These mature larvae migrate throughout the mosquito's body and exit from the mouthparts when the mosquito takes its blood meal. From the surface of the skin they penetrate the human host, probably through the puncture site made by the mosquito. Details of larval molting and development in humans are largely unavailable, but it is felt that almost a year is required for the adults to mature, mate, and produce microfilariae.

Though morphological differences have been difficult to define, it has been hypothesized on the basis of physiological criteria that there may be distinct races or even subspecies of *W. bancrofti*. One of these criteria is the periodicity of circulating microfilariae. Throughout most of the tropical and subtropical regions of the world nocturnally periodic parasites are found. Their microfilariae begin to appear in the blood late in the evening and reach maximum levels between 12 and 4 A.M. before receding from the peripheral circulation almost completely during the day. The major exception to this pattern is

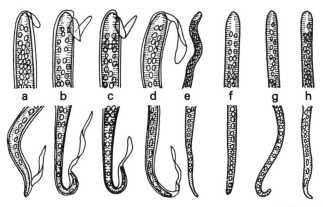

Figure 48-2. Differential characteristics of anterior or posterior ends of the microfilariae of *a*, *Wuchereria bancrofti*; *b*, *Brugia malayi*; *c*, *Brugia timori*; *d*, *Loa loa*; *e*, *Onchocerca volvulus*; *f*, *Mansonella perstans*; *g*, *Mansonella streptocerca*; and *h*, *Mansonella ozzardi*. Other characteristics of the microfilariae are listed in Table 48-2. (*Redrawn after Faust and Russell: Clinical Parasitology, 7th ed, Philadelphia, Lea & Febiger, 1964.*)

the nonperiodic (or slightly diurnally periodic) form of the parasite found in Polynesia and the New Caledonian region. These microfilariae circulate at reasonably constant levels throughout the day and night. Nocturnally subperiodic parasites described in western Thailand can be detected in the blood throughout the 24 h but at heightened levels during the night. Such differences in periodicity coupled, first, with the observations that microfilariae of *W. bancrofti* from different parts of the world are not equally infective for the different mosquitoes that serve as vectors of the ''same'' parasite in other parts of the world and, second, with the variable severity in

human pathology associated with *W. bancrofti* infection in different endemic regions serve to stimulate efforts to identify various subspecies of a *W. bancrofti* ''complex'' [*1*].

Probably the major impediment to progress in understanding so much of what remains unknown about *W. bancrofti* (including subspeciation, structure, biochemistry, pathogenicity, immunity, etc.) has been the inability to maintain the parasite in any animal model or, alternatively, to cultivate it completely in vitro. There is no natural or reservoir host for *W. bancrofti* other than humans and, until recently, no successful experimental infections except those in a few highly immunosuppressed macaques [*2*]. Recently, however, leaf monkeys (*Presbytis* species) from Indonesia and Malaysia have been experimentally infected with *W. bancrofti* and have produced both moderate microfilaremias and abundant adult worms [*3*]. It is hoped that this parasitological breakthrough can be exploited to address many problems of bancroftian filarias that have heretofore been unapproachable.

Brugia malayi

(Synonyms: *Filaria malayi, Wuchereria malayi*.) Adult *B. malayi* (Lichtenstein, 1927) live in human lymph nodes and lymphatics and share many features with *W. bancrofti*. Female worms (43 to 55 mm long and 0.13 to 0.17 mm wide) are morphologically indistinguishable from those of *W. bancrofti*, though they may not reach the same length. Male worms are smaller than the females, measuring 14 to 23 by 0.08 mm, and have copulatory spicules and caudal papillae that distinguish them from *W. bancrofti*. Microfilariae are sheathed, average 220 by 6 μm, and have a column of nuclei that extends into the caudal region with two terminal nuclei. These caudal nuclei along with a long cephalic space (distance from the anterior

Table 48-2. Characteristics of microfilariae in humans

Species	Location	Periodicity	Presence of sheath	Mean length (and range)	Presence of caudal nuclei
Wuchereria bancrofti	Blood, hydrocele fluid	Nocturnal, subperiodic	+	260 μm (244–296)	−
Brugia malayi	Blood	Nocturnal, subperiodic	+	220 μm (177–230)	+ (isolated)
Brugia timori	Blood	Nocturnal	+	287 μm (265–323)	+ (isolated)
Onchocerca volvulus	Skin	None or minimal	−	254 μm (221–287)	−
Loa loa	Blood	Diurnal	+	275 μm (250–300)	+ (terminal)
Mansonella perstans	Blood	None	−	195 μm (190–200)	+ (terminal)
Mansonella streptocerca	Skin	None	−	210 μm (180–240)	+ (terminal)
Mansonella ozzardi	Blood	None	−	200 μm (173–240)	−

tip to the beginning of the column of nuclei) that is approximately 1.6 or 1.7 times the width of the head are the most helpful characteristics distinguishing microfilariae of *B. malayi* from those of *W. bancrofti* (Table 48-2). Development in the mosquito takes 10 to 14 days during which the microfilaria first develops through the "sausage" stage and then elongates and undergoes two molts to become the filariform third-stage infective larva (L_3) capable of penetrating the host's skin following the mosquito "bite."

Two races of *B. malayi* have been defined on the basis of physiological differences. Microfilariae of the nocturnally periodic form of the parasite are rarely seen in the blood during the day. This periodic race is generally found in coastal rice fields and open swamps, is highly infectious for anopheline mosquitoes but poorly infectious for most mansonian mosquitoes, and generally develops poorly or not at all in experimental laboratory animals (cats, jirds, hamsters, rats). Its features contrast markedly with those of the semiperiodic race of *B. malayi*, in which in humans microfilaremia may show a nocturnal rise but generally persists throughout the day, and which is found in freshwater swamps and forests, is highly infective for mansonian mosquitoes but noninfective to anophelines, and readily infects felines in nature as well as cats and other experimental animals in the laboratory. Furthermore, while Giemsa-stained blood films consistently identify the sheaths of microfilariae of the subperiodic strain, about 60 percent of the periodic strain microfilariae shed their sheaths during the routine processing of blood films [1].

This ready infectivity by subperiodic *B. malayi* has both positive and negative implications. On the negative side, it means that *B. malayi* is a zoonosis in endemic regions with its reservoir hosts already demonstrated to include a number of wild and domestic animals like the leaf monkey, wild cat, civet cat, and pangolin. Thus, control measures are much more difficult than if the infection were restricted to human beings. On the other hand the ability to maintain the parasite in the laboratory (especially in jirds and cats) has been responsible for much of the recent increase in our understanding of the biology, biochemistry, structure, and genetic makeup and antigenic features of the brugian parasites. Though knowledge of their biochemistry is still rudimentary, they are recognized as being primarily anaerobic, homolactate-fermenting organisms with intact tricarboxylic acid cycles but with dependency on the host for certain aspects of folic acid metabolism [4]. These facts have been of practical importance in efforts to develop and screen new chemotherapeutic agents for treating the infection in humans. Furthermore, electron-microscopic and radioisotopic analyses of the parasite's surface antigens and its excretory-secretory products [5], along with molecular biological analyses of its genome [6], have been made possible by the ready availability of laboratory models of *Brugia* infections. The findings from these studies should prove applicable to issues such as species-specific immunodiagnosis, immunopathology, and protective immunity.

Brugia timori

(Synonym: *Timor filaria*.) *Brugia timori* is a relatively uncommon human filarial pathogen sharing many features with *B. malayi* [7]. Adult females average 26.7 mm by 99 μm while the males are smaller (16.9 mm × 72 μm). Subtle but distinct differences exist between the adult worms of *B. timori* and *B. malayi* (mainly the number, size, and location of papillae and spicules projecting from the surface) as well as in the infective L_3 forms of the parasites. However, the features that most distinguish *B. timori* from other *Brugia* species are found in the microfilariae; namely, the characteristically large cephalic space (ratio of cephalic space length to width of 2.7:1 compared with 1.7:1 for *B. malayi* microfilariae), greater overall body length, and the absence of staining of the sheath by Giemsa stain. Like the periodic strains of *B. malayi* about 60 percent of *B. timori* microfilariae are found to have shed their sheaths in blood film preparations. Microfilaremia in *B. timori* infections is also nocturnally periodic.

There appears to be no animal reservoir of *B. timori*. The jird (*Meriones unguiculatus*), which has proved to be an excellent host for a number of different filariae, will also accept *B. timori*. Recent studies have used surface labeling techniques to describe surface antigens specific to *B. timori* that are not shared with *B. malayi* or *W. bancrofti* [5]. Similarities between repeated DNA sequences in the genomes of *B. timori* and *B. malayi* have also been noted [6].

PATIENT

Pathogenesis

Studies of the mechanisms of pathogenesis in lymphatic filariasis must focus on two primary issues: namely, the means by which the parasites evade the host's immune system to persist and thrive for long periods of time and the ways in which actual damage is done to the host.

Immunological Determinants. While filarial infections unquestionably elicit immune responses of all types (e.g., T lymphocyte, B lymphocyte, humoral, and eosinophil) from their human hosts, recent studies leave little doubt but that the immune systems of infected individuals (particularly those with microfilaremia) can be characterized as being markedly hyporesponsive to parasite antigens [8]. This hyporesponsiveness appears to derive not from an inability of the host to recognize and react to the parasite but rather from the development of prominent immunoregulatory mechanisms acting to "contain" or limit normal responsiveness of the host to parasite antigens.

The "immunosuppressed" state of these individuals has been most clearly demonstrated in studies of in vitro lymphocyte function in which suppressor mononuclear cells (both T cells and monocytes) and suppressive serum factors inhibit lymphocyte responses to parasite antigens in patients with both bancroftian and brugian filariasis, especially the microfilaremic forms [8]. Similarly, although the parasites elicit high levels of specific IgE antibody that might be expected to lead to significant allergic responsiveness in infected individuals, these are generally not seen. Very high levels of IgG "blocking antibodies" directed against the parasite allergens likely account for the absence of clinically evident hypersensitivity responses [9]. Additionally, it is well recognized that patients who are microfilaremic have the lowest levels of circulating antibodies (IgG and IgM) against the parasite and these low levels may reflect B-cell immunoregulation in such infected individuals [10].

The origin of these immunoregulatory mechanisms has been little studied. The fact that disease expression among the population living in an endemic region is often very different (i.e., much less "virulent") from that in recent entrants to that same area [8] has led to the notion that the children born in endemic regions may become tolerant to parasite antigens in utero. Indeed, recent studies have provided clear evidence for prenatal and immediately postpartum sensitization to filaria antigens among babies born in endemic regions [11,12].

In the absence of these immunoregulatory mechanisms (either because they never developed or because they diminished in activity) a "peaceful state of parasitism" cannot be maintained. Immune-mediated inflammatory reactions to the parasite develop, causing local tissue damage and concomitant clinical pathology. Such is clearly the case for patients with the tropical eosinophilia syndrome in which profound humoral immune hyperresponsiveness results in the production of extremely high levels of IgE and IgG antibodies directed against the parasite, especially the microfilarial stage [13]. Microfilariae from the adult female worms in such patients presumably are rapidly cleared in the lungs or other reticuloendothelial system (RES) organs, probably by the high levels of IgG opsonins. As the microfilariae are destroyed, the released antigens trigger IgE-mediated inflammatory responses in the lung which are reflected clinically as the asthma, eosinophilic pulmonary infiltrates, and chronic interstitial lung disease that define this syndrome.

A second important situation where immunological hyperresponsiveness appears to translate into distinct immunopathology is in the lymphatic lesions. Patients with elephantiasis and filarial fevers (recurrent adenolymphangitis) generally are not microfilaremic. Their lymphocytes are significantly more reactive to parasite antigens than are those from people with asymptomatic microfilaremia [8] as are their IgG3 antibody responses to parasite antigens [14]. Furthermore, their ability to regulate immediate hypersensitivity responsiveness to parasite antigens via IgG blocking antibodies appears similarly impaired. Any of these mechanisms, as well as others, could be important initiators of the recurrent inflammatory episodes that lead to the lymphatic damage. Further studies are needed to resolve these important issues.

Nonimmunological Determinants. A number of nonimmunological factors have been suggested that may cause or ac-

celerate the development of lymphatic pathology in patients with filariasis. First among these is the simple physical upright posture of humans that results in increased hydrostatic pressure in the lymphatics of the lower extremities. Since the earliest stages of developing lymphatic pathology involve valvular incompetence [15], the additional hydrostatic pressure from the upright posture could exacerbate even minimal structural damage.

Bacterial lymphangitis, especially streptococcal, may also play a role in the etiology of lymphatic pathology. Experimental studies in animals have shown that lymphatics damaged either experimentally or during the course of *B. malayi* infection are more susceptible to a bacterial challenge than are normal lymphatics [16]. Though there are certainly documented instances in which bacterial infection has complicated filarial lymphatic pathology, no good data exist to substantiate the commonly held notion that filarial fever attacks are really the manifestation of bacterial superinfection of previously damaged lymphatics.

Indeed, the etiology of these attacks, which lead eventually to the chronic pathological changes, remains an important enigma that must be resolved before we understand the pathogenesis of lymphatic filarial damage. In addition to the multiple immune mechanisms already cited, it has also been suggested that developing L_3 and L_4 stage larvae or their molting fluids may induce these local lymphatic inflammatory responses. This suggestion was based both on experimental studies in dogs [17] and on epidemiological observations noting the decreased frequency of such attacks when affected individuals are removed from endemic regions [18]. Whether such molting fluids act in a nonimmunological (i.e., toxic) manner or, more likely, initiate immunologically mediated inflammatory responses has not been investigated.

One further nonimmunological factor that may also contribute to the elephantatic pathology of the lower extremities in bancroftian and brugian filariasis is the composition of the soil to which the barefoot individuals in endemic regions are exposed. It has been shown convincingly that there is one form of elephantiasis in the filaria-free highlands of Ethiopia and other east African countries that is geochemical in origin [19]. Repeated exposure to soil derived from volcanic lava that is rich in basalt and contains iron, aluminum, silica, and other metals leads to penetration of the skin by small colloid particles of the claylike soil. These elements ultimately deposit in the draining nodes and result in lymphatic obstruction and pathology. The occurrence of such changes even in the absence of lymphatic filarial infection makes it likely that similar toxic soil elements may enhance the severity of the lymphatic lesions in regions where filarial infections and such soils coexist.

Genetic Determinants. Genetic influences on the pathogenesis of filarial disease can relate either to parasite or to host. Clearly, strain differences exist among both *W. bancrofti* and *B. malayi*, as defined, for example, by different patterns of microfilarial periodicity and different degrees of pathogenicity associated with the same parasite in different parts of the world. No rigorous investigation, however, has thus far addressed this issue.

The familial clustering of patients with filariasis has been noted by numerous authors, but whether this clustering is genetically determined is still uncertain [20,21].

Pathology

Chronic Lymphatic Pathology. Most of the pathology associated with bancroftian and brugian filariasis derives from damage to the lymphatics which ultimately leads to chronic lymphedema, elephantiasis, or chyluria. The location of the damage determines the site and type of pathology expressed. Though such pathology has been recognized for millennia (elephantiasis having been documented in pharaonic paintings), only in the past 20 years has the development of lymphangiographic techniques permitted direct observation of the progression of the lymphatic lesions.

Normal lymph vessels are delicate endothelium-lined channels leading from an extensive network of peripheral lymph capillaries through a series of collecting vessels and intermediate lymph nodes to the large cisterna chyli and thoracic duct that empties into the vena cava. Lymph is propelled through these channels primarily by contraction of skeletal muscles in the presence of an extensive system of intraluminal valves. In infected individuals adult worms reside within these lymphatic vessels, generally in the afferent approaches or cortical sinuses of the lymph nodes. The parasites first cause dilatation of the lymphatic and then hypertrophy of the vessel wall. There is endothelial and connective tissue proliferation with polypoid growths protruding into the lumen, but so long as the worm remains alive, it appears that the vessel stays patent [22]. This patency, however, does not ensure normal lymphatic function, as lymphangiographic studies document clearly the development of tortuosity of the lymph vessels with loss of valvular function and lymph backflow even during this preobliterative phase of the lymphatic changes [15]. Thus, lymph stasis may occur while the worm is still alive and result in early lymphedematous changes in the affected limb, genitals, kidney, or breast.

It is uncertain what causes adult worms to die, but their deaths are associated with distinctive pathological changes [22]. An area of necrosis develops around the dead parasite, followed by a granulomatous reaction with the formation of foreign-body giant cells and a concomitant infiltration of plasma cells and eosinophils. Collagen deposition is seen and the usually fragmented parasite either is resorbed or becomes partially calcified. It is during these inflammatory reactions that lymphatic obstruction occurs, and an associated endophlebitis may further complicate the picture. Though there is subsequent formation of collateral lymphatics and some recanalization of obstructed vessels, lymphatic function remains compromised.

Funiculitis, epididymitis, and orchitis are also frequent concomitants of chronic filarial infection in the male. The inflammation at each of these sites occurs as a direct result of parasites in the associated lymphatics. The inflammatory response in these lymphatics ranges from infiltrative to granulomatous, and there is often an associated phlebitis [22]. Undoubtedly, the mechanisms underlying the inflammation of the genital lymphatics and the progression to obstructive pathology are similar to those responsible for the lymphatic inflammation and obstruction found elsewhere.

Acute Lymphatic Pathology. In endemic areas residents harboring parasites may have recurrent episodes of acute lymphangitis and adenolymphangitis ("filarial fevers") that play an important role in damaging the lymphatics. Despite their importance, however, there has been little study of the etiology or pathology of these acute episodes. Instead, our knowledge of the lymphatic changes during such acute inflammatory episodes comes largely from evaluation of the lesions acquired by American soldiers deployed during World War II in the Pacific region where bancroftian filariasis is endemic. As indicated below (see "Clinical Manifestations"), these previously unexposed individuals reacted to filarial infection much more vigorously than the native residents of the same endemic regions, so it is only a presumption that the findings in these soldiers are similar to those in chronically infected individuals who infrequently develop such recurrent inflammatory episodes.

In a study of biopsies from 64 of the affected soldiers, adult or preadult parasites were identified from about a quarter of the specimens [23]. It was clear that the marked lymphatic inflammation observed in these patients was being caused both by reactions to dying parasites, as previously described in chronically infected patients [22], and also by responses to living adult worms of both sexes. In addition to changes in the lymphatics such as endothelial thickening and varicosities, inflammation that appeared to result from release or secretion of material from the parasite developed around the worms and was characterized by infiltration of eosinophils, plasma cells, lymphocytes, and macrophages which tended to form into nodules. Necrosis was sometimes absent but was frequently extensive and accompanied by the precipitates of variable amounts of intensely eosinophilic-staining material (Splendore-Hoeppli phenomenon). In older lesions in which the worms were dead or had been present for a long time, macrophages and exudative cells were less conspicuous, and there were concentrically arranged layers of dense acellular collagen.

Microfilaria-Related Pathology. While it is possible that microfilariae also play a role in inducing the lymphatic inflammation described above, most of the recognized pathology associated with this stage of the parasite results from tissue reactions around parasites that have been cleared from the blood. In microfilaremic individuals where there is continual production of microfilariae, clearance of these worms presumably takes place constantly in the lungs, liver, and spleen, but this clearance appears to be unassociated with clinical symptoms. Occasionally aberrant microfilariae will be found in the breast, subcutaneous tissue, or other sites where they elicit a granulomatous response that can evoke a symptomatic clinical presentation (e.g., [24]), but generally the attrition of microfilariae from the blood takes place silently. It is likely that immunological regulatory mechanisms are responsible for the lack of overt responsiveness to the microfilarial stage of the parasite in most patients with filariasis, and some of these have been described above (see "Immunological Determinants").

The situation, however, is entirely different in patients with the tropical eosinophilia syndrome in which individuals appear to be immunologically hyperreactive to filarial antigens, especially those from microfilariae. Though the clinical presentation of these patients is often similar to that of asthmatics, the pulmonary pathology is much different, generally reflecting the prominence of restrictive rather than obstructive lung disease. Biopsies from a large series of patients [25] indicate that within the first weeks of illness early histiocytic infiltrates found initially in the alveolar spaces and interstitium give way to a picture of eosinophilic bronchopneumonia and eosinophilic abscesses apparently initiated by trapped microfilariae. After a period of several months mixed cell exudates often characterized by eosinophils, histiocytes, and lymphocytes organized in nodular patterns progressively evolved to predominantly histiocytic, granulomatous responses marked by increasing fibrosis. Such findings are in distinct contrast to the abnormalities found in patients with acute and chronic asthma; indeed, but for the blood eosinophils, the presentation of long-standing tropical eosinophilia has been likened rather to that of chronic pulmonary interstitial fibrosis [25].

When microfilariae have been found in lymph nodes of patients with tropical eosinophilia, the pathological picture has been one of prominent aggregates of eosinophils, foreign-body giant cells and eosinophilic precipitates (Meyers-Kouwenaar bodies [26]) around the degenerating microfilariae or worm fragments.

Clinical manifestations

Lymphatic filariasis is one of the great "spectrum diseases," producing in different patients a broad range of clinical manifestations for reasons that are still largely unknown. A major

cause of this lack of understanding is the fact that the techniques for diagnosing filarial infection are extremely inadequate, definitive diagnosis only being made parasitologically by detecting microfilariae in blood, hydrocele fluid, or, more rarely, tissues of the reticuloendothelial system (RES). Since many people with filariasis are amicrofilaremic, in these individuals diagnosis must either be made clinically or missed altogether.

Clinical Features of Filariasis in Patients Native to Endemic Areas. Figure 48-3 indicates the clinical syndromes of lymphatic filariasis currently recognized among individuals living in regions endemic for *W. bancrofti*, *B. malayi*, or *B. timori*. At one extreme are many individuals with no indication of filarial infection. These people's exposures to infective larvae are equivalent to those of patients with clinically definable filariasis. While it is likely that some are uninfected and, indeed, probably immune to the parasite, others probably do harbor the infection but remain clinically unaffected with parasites that are undetectable. There are two reasons for presuming the existence of such a group of "asymptomatic, infected" individuals: first, the fact that parallel situations exist in many of the animal models of filariasis; and second, that high levels of specific antifilarial antibodies and good lymphocyte responses to filarial antigens are found in many of these individuals. Only the development of more sensitive techniques to detect the presence of parasites in vivo (e.g., by sensitive antigen detection immunodiagnostic techniques) will permit further definition of these asymptomatic individuals.

Another asymptomatic clinical presentation is one defined by microfilaremia in persons who feel and appear otherwise perfectly normal. Such patients generally come to the physician's attention through an incidental finding of microfilariae in the peripheral blood smear or when blood eosinophilia leads to a diagnostic evaluation for filariasis. While some of these individuals remain asymptomatic for years (sometimes for their whole lives) and others likely clear their infections spontaneously, a third group of these patients progresses to develop symptomatic filarial disease. What it is that determines such changes in this group of patients is entirely unknown.

Most common of the symptomatic clinical syndromes are the recurrent episodes of "filarial fever." These febrile episodes are characterized by high fever (often with shaking chills), lymphadenitis, and often a distinctive lymphangitis that extends in a retrograde fashion *from* the affected nodes where the adult parasites reside. These attacks occur up to 6 to 10

Figure 48-3. Spectrum of clinical manifestation of filarial infection in regions endemic for the lymphatic filariases.

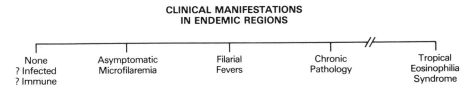

CLINICAL MANIFESTATIONS IN ENDEMIC REGIONS

None ? Infected ? Immune   Asymptomatic Microfilaremia   Filarial Fevers   Chronic Pathology   Tropical Eosinophilia Syndrome

times a year and usually last from 3 to 7 days before subsiding spontaneously for reasons that are as undefined as are the factors that initiate such episodes. Affected nodes are enlarged and painful, and the entire lymphatic often becomes indurated and inflamed. Concomitant local thrombophlebitis is common. Lymphedema frequently develops during these episodes but usually subsides after the acute phase. In some individuals, with brugian filariasis especially, the lymphatic inflammatory response becomes so great that a single local abscess may form along the inflamed lymphatic which subsequently ulcerates and eventually leaves a characteristic scar (Fig. 48-4) whose presence has been used epidemiologically as an indication of clinical "activity" of filarial infection in *Brugia* endemic regions [27]. The whole course of a filarial fever episode that is complicated by abscess formation and cicatrization may last 2 to 3 months, thereby resulting in prolonged disability. While the lymphadenitis and lymphangitis develop more commonly in the lower extremities than in the upper extremities in both bancroftian and brugian filariasis, involvement of the genital lymphatics is almost exclusively a feature of *W. bancrofti* in-

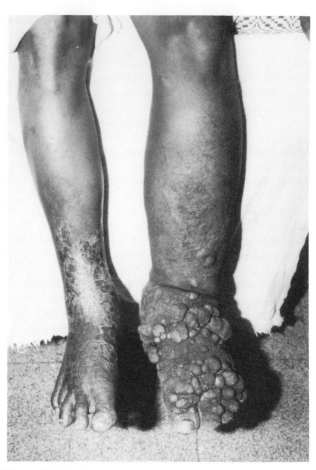

Figure 48-5. Left leg of a patient with chronic bancroftian filariasis shows thickened hyperkeratotic subcutaneous tissue with nodular, papillomatous hyperplastic changes. Right leg shows lichenified skin with evidence of desquamation, changes that reflect repeated transient episodes of edema associated with filarial fever episodes.

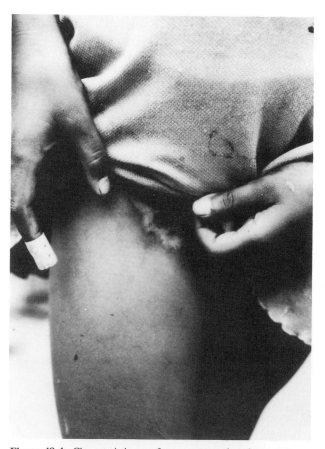

Figure 48-4. Characteristic scar from a suppurative abscess over an inflamed lymphatic tract in a patient with *Brugia timori* filariasis. (*Courtesy of Dr. James Palmieri.*)

fection. Thus, acute bancrofti episodes also frequently involve funiculitis, epididymitis, scrotal pain, and tenderness. Patients with these filarial fevers may be microfilaremic but more often are not.

With time (often measured in decades) and repeated lymphatic damage, the edema and anatomic distortion that were initially transient develop into the permanent changes of chronic lymphatic pathology. Pitting edema of the skin yields to brawny edema, and there is both thickening of subcutaneous tissue and hyperkeratosis. Fissuring of the skin develops along with nodular and papillomatous hyperplastic changes (Fig. 48-5), and superinfection becomes a problem. In bancroftian filariasis these changes may involve the leg(s), scrotum, arm(s), vulva, or breast(s), while in brugian filariasis the leg(s), especially below the knee, and the arm(s), especially below the elbow, are characteristically affected. In addition, for patients with bancroftian filariasis, obstructed genital lymphatics may lead to scrotal lymphedema or hydrocele, while obstruction of the retroperitoneal lymphatics can increase hydrostatic pressure in the renal lymphatics, causing them to rupture into the renal pelvis or tubules and lead to chyluria [28]. Characteristically the chyluria is intermittent, sometimes lasting days or weeks before abating spontaneously and then recurring. Often chyluria is most prominent in the morning after the patient first arises. Genital involvement has not been reported in brugian filariasis except in areas where it and bancroftian filariasis coexist.

Clinical Features of Filariasis in New Arrivals to Endemic Areas.

It is interesting that there are significant differences in the clinical manifestations of filarial infection, or at least in the time course over which they are acquired, between individuals who have recently entered endemic regions and those who have resided there their whole lives [8].

For whatever reason (perhaps inefficient mechanisms for transmitting infective larvae from vector to host, "innate resistance" of the host, etc.), in order for people entering endemic regions to acquire bancroftian or brugian infection, it is generally necessary for them to be exposed to infection for at least several months. After that, what happens can be inferred from the experiences of two large groups of such migrants. The best-documented occurrence was during World War II when tens of thousands of previously unexposed U.S. soldiers were deployed in the Pacific region where they were intensively exposed to bancroftian filariasis [18]. While fewer than 0.1 percent of these young men developed patent (i.e., microfilaremic) infections (in contrast to microfilaremia rates of 30 to 50 percent in the local populations), fully a third of those exposed (nearly 12,000 men) did become infected and symptomatic. Instead of developing microfilaremia, however, they presented with signs and symptoms of acute lymphatic or scrotal inflammation. Pain and erythema of the scrotum (56 percent), arms (38 percent), and legs (14 percent) were common as were urticaria and localized angioedema. Lymphadenitis of the inguinal, femoral, axillary, or epitrochlear nodes was often followed by lymphangitis which progressed in the characteristic retrograde fashion from the affected node. Attacks were nearly always short (3 to 5 days' duration at most) and, in contrast to the filarial fever episodes occurring in the endemic population, were generally unaccompanied by fever. Because of great concern that these men would develop the physical stigmata of chronic filariasis, they were usually evacuated rather promptly from the endemic regions after becoming symptomatic. When removed from continual exposure to the parasite, their acute signs and symptoms generally disappeared. Very few men continued to be acutely symptomatic, and very few went on to develop signs of chronic lymphatic obstruction.

A second well-documented migration of previously unexposed individuals into an endemic area has been described in Indonesians being resettled from overpopulated islands where no filariasis is present to less densely populated islands where brugian filariasis is endemic [29]. A large number of these "transmigrants" acquired filarial infection and soon showed signs and symptoms of lymphatic inflammation very similar to those seen among the American soldiers in the Pacific. The differences between these two groups, however, lie in the events that followed the initial episodes. Instead of being evacuated from the endemic region as the Americans had been, these transmigrants remained in their new homesteads, living under a constant attack of mosquito-borne infective filarial larvae. In these individuals the occurrence of acute episodes did not abate but, instead, continued with an increasingly severe character that led first to temporary and then to permanent lymphatic inflammatory obstruction. Elephantiasis developed not only among the adults but also in young children. While the pathogenesis of the lymphatic disease appears to be qualitatively similar to that found among the indigenous residents of the endemic area, the rate of progression of the disease in these transmigrants seems telescoped into a much shorter period of time. Interestingly, if such persons were removed from the endemic focus at any point in the development of their lymphatic pathology, progression of the lymphatic damage was usually halted, and those aspects of the pathology that were still reversible reverted toward normal.

From these two undesigned "experiments of nature" one can infer a number of things about the clinical aspects of lymphatic filarial infection in previously unexposed individuals. First, given sufficient exposure (generally 3 to 6 months), infection is common. Second, the manifestations are generally lymphatic-oriented and more acute and intense than those usually seen in natives of the endemic regions. (Probably, these patients have yet to develop the immunomodulatory mechanisms generally found among those with chronic infection. See "Immunological Determinants.") Third, early removal of patients from continued reexposure to the infection appears to hasten the end of clinical symptoms or at least to halt the progression of the clinical disease.

The Tropical Eosinophilia Syndrome.

"Tropical eosinophilia," though probably recognized earlier, was first described in the 1940s in patients from the tropics who presented with paroxysmal cough and wheezing that generally occurred at night, scanty sputum production, occasional weight loss, low-grade fever, adenopathy, and extreme blood eosinophilia (> 3000 mm^3) [30,31]. That this syndrome was of filarial etiology was not recognized until the 1950s and 1960s when it was noted that the antifilarial drug diethylcarbamazine (DEC) was effective in patients with this syndrome and that these patients had extremely high levels of antifilarial antibodies in their sera. Though circulating microfilariae were never found, prolonged search in lung and lymph node biopsies from several typical cases of this disorder revealed trapped, often degenerating, microfilariae [32,33]. It was then that attention was called to the earlier work of Dutch and French workers who had found degenerating microfilariae surrounded by eosinophilic deposits (Meyers-Kouwenaar bodies) in hyperplastic lymph nodes from hypereosinophilic patients who had presented with or without asthmatic pulmonary disease [*34*]. The general term *occult filariasis* was suggested to describe both the pulmonary and extrapulmonary manifestations of filarial disease characterized by extreme peripheral eosinophilia without microfilaremia.

Patients with this syndrome are most often male (4:1 predominance) and in their twenties or thirties. Most cases have been reported from India, Indonesia, Sri Lanka, Pakistan, and southeast Asia, but any area where human filariasis is transmitted is a potential source. The individuals are generally ill, often with bouts of cough, with or without wheezing, that occur characteristically at night. Dyspnea and occasionally chest pain or tightness accompany these episodes. X-ray films of the chest can be normal but generally show increased bronchovascular markings, diffuse miliary lesions 1 to 3 mm in size, or mottled opacities involving primarily the middle and basal regions of the lungs. The upper lung fields are less likely to be involved, hilar adenopathy is not common, and pleural effusions are rare. When pulmonary functions have been examined in these patients, airway obstruction, the hallmark of asthma, can be seen in only 25 to 30 percent of individuals, while the great majority have restrictive abnormalities such as diminished vital and total lung capacities and decreased residual volumes. If left untreated, the pulmonary lesions progress to a severely debilitating chronic interstitial lung disease. Whether or not pulmonary hypertension results from this chronic infection is uncertain, but it has been speculated that untreated tropical eosinophilia may be responsible for much chronic lung disease of unknown cause in endemic areas.

As indicated already, generalized adenopathy and eosinophilia may be the main presenting features in some patients, either with or without pulmonary symptoms. The reasons for these varied presentations are unclear but may relate to some still undefined factor such as the patient's age. In series describing adult cases of tropical eosinophilia the absence of general adenopathy and hepatosplenomegaly has been noted, but in series that include children moderate degrees of lymphadenopathy and hepatomegaly were common; even minimal splenomegaly was noted in some.

Other Syndromes of Uncertain Relationship to Lymphatic Filariasis. A variety of syndromes that coexist with filariasis are found in filarial endemic regions and that show some evidence of therapeutic response to the antifilarial drug DEC have been suggested as being manifestations of bancroftian or brugian filariasis. These include arthritis (typically monoarticular), endomyocardial fibrosis, tenosynovitis, thrombophlebitis, glomerulonephritis, dermatosis, lateral popliteal nerve palsy, and others. While future studies may strengthen the relationships, such syndromes at present cannot confidently be attributed to filarial infection.

Diagnosis

Definitive diagnosis can be made only by demonstration of the parasite—adult worms associated with the lymphatics (very rarely observed), microfilariae trapped in the tissues (as in the tropical eosinophilia syndrome), or microfilariae found in blood, hydrocele fluid, or urine.

Microfilaremic States. No periodicity has been reported for microfilariae in hydrocele fluid or urine, but blood collection should be timed to take into account the parasite's possible nocturnal periodicity. Optimal blood drawing times for nocturnally periodic brugia or bancrofti filariae are between 10 P.M. and 4 A.M.; for subperiodic strains any time is satisfactory, though there is often a late afternoon (about 4 P.M.) peak in the microfilaremia [*1*]. After it was found that DEC given during the daytime to patients with nocturnally periodic brugian and bancroftian parasites stimulated the release of microfilariae into the blood, the "DEC provocative test" was suggested to simplify diagnosis of nocturnally periodic filariasis [*35*]. This test, however, in which 50 to 100 mg of DEC is given during the day with blood being examined 45 min later, has a lower sensitivity than examination of night blood samples. Furthermore, in areas where *W. bancrofti* occurs together with *O. volvulus* or *Loa loa* the dose of DEC used for the provocative test may elicit very severe reactions in patients with double infections and thus should not be used indiscriminately.

The simplest technique for examining blood or other fluids is to spread 20 μL evenly over a clean slide that is dried and then stained with Giemsa or some similar stain. A wet smear may also be made by diluting 20 to 40 μL of anticoagulated blood with water or 2% saponin, which will lyse the red blood cells but allow the microfilariae to remain motile and thus more readily identifiable. The larger the blood volumes examined, the greater will be the likelihood of detecting low parasitemias. Knott's concentration technique has been used to examine 1-mL volumes of anticoagulated blood by mixing the blood with 10 mL of 2% formalin, centrifuging the preparation and examining the sediment either unstained or fixed and stained; the microfilariae are nonmotile and generally straight and can be easily missed if the viscous sediment is not searched diligently. More recently, membrane filtration has been advanced as the most sensitive technique for detecting and quantitating microfilariae in blood, urine, or other body fluid. Polycarbonate (Nuclepore) filters have proved most satisfactory, especially those with a 3-μm pore size. A known volume of anticoagulated blood or other fluid is passed through the filter followed by a large volume (about 35 mL) of prefiltered water that lyses the red blood cells. A volume of air then follows the water, and the filter is removed, placed on a slide, and stained. Morphology is much more difficult to assess than in specimens prepared initially on slides, but detection and quantification are very straightforward.

Amicrofilaremic States (Including Tropical Eosinophilia). Many of the lymphatic filarial syndromes are not associated with microfilaremia, and what is sorely needed for diagnosis of such conditions is a tool for sensitively detecting the presence of parasite material (e.g., antigen) in an infected individual's body fluids. Until these assays become available, however, diagnosis of these amicrofilaremic syndromes must be made "clinically" (i.e., on circumstantial evidence).

The most secure of these clinical diagnoses is that of the tropical eosinophilia syndrome. In addition to the distinctive clinical presentation patients have extraordinarily high levels of total serum immunoglobulin E, almost always in excess of 10,000 ng/mL and sometimes in the range of 200,000 ng/mL [*36*]. Their levels of specific antifilarial antibodies (both IgG and IgE antibodies) are extremely high, the absolute levels differing depending on the specific test used. Diagnosis depends primarily on distinguishing tropical eosinophila from other important eosinophilic syndromes with pulmonary involvement, particularly Loeffler's syndrome, chronic eosinophilic pneumonia, allergic aspergillosis, certain vasculitic syndromes, the idiopathic hypereosinophilia syndrome, drug allergies, and some helminth infections. Though there is no one clinical or laboratory criterion which will distinguish tropical eosinophilia from the other conditions (Table 48-3), a history of prolonged residence in the tropics, elevated antifilarial antibody and total IgE levels, and a therapeutic response to DEC are the most helpful differential points.

The acute lymphatic manifestations of filariasis can be confused primarily with thrombophlebitis, infection, and trauma, while the edema and other lymphatic obstructive changes associated with chronic filarial infection must be distinguished from manifestations of congestive heart failure, malignancy, trauma, postsurgical scarring, and a number of less common congenital and idiopathic abnormalities of the lymphatic system. Also the many disorders associated with serum IgE and blood eosinophil elevations must be considered in evaluating asymptomatic filarial infections. The following are several specific points that may help in this differential diagnosis: (1) exposure to filariae must be prolonged or intense (usually at least several months) before individuals become infected; (2) the finding or history of *retrograde* lymphangitis can often aid in distinguishing filarial from bacterial lymphangitis; (3) lymphadenopathy is characteristic but not diagnostic of filariasis; (4) lymphangiographic patterns of filarial elephantiasis and chyluria are well defined so that, even if not always diagnostic, lymphangiography can often be useful in distinguishing filarial from congenital or neoplastic lymphatic abnormalities; (5) though total serum IgE and blood eosinophil levels are almost always elevated in filarial infections, they cannot by themselves distinguish filarial from other helminth infections except in the case of the tropical eosinophilia syndrome; (6) positive immunodiagnostic tests based on serum antibody determinations or skin test results are of little diagnostic value except in patients *not* native to the endemic areas. This is because most residents of endemic regions will have positive reactions [*37*], presumably because they have been immunologically "sensitized" to filarial antigens through years of exposure to infected mosquitoes and because of the fact that filarial antigens may be cross-reactive with those of other nematode parasites also found in these areas. Thus, a positive immunodiagnostic test is a necessary but not sufficient prerequisite for the diagnosis of brugian or bancroftian filariasis.

Treatment

Chemotherapy. DEC is the mainstay of the current chemotherapy for bancroftian and brugian filariasis. A derivative of

Table 48-3. Features likely to distinguish tropical (filarial) eosinophilia from other eosinophilic syndromes with pulmonary involvement

Feature	Tropical eosinophilia	Loeffler's syndrome	Chronic eosinophilic pneumonia	Allergic aspergillosis	Vasculitis syndromes	Idiopathic hypereosinophilia	Drug allergies	Other helminthic infections
Wheezing	Often	Rare	Often	Often	Absent	Absent	Rare	Possible
Systemic symptoms	Often	Rare	Often	Often	Often	Often	Often	Variable
Eosinophil level	High	Moderate	Moderate to high	High	Low	High	Moderate to high	Variable
IgE level	High	Moderate	?	High	Low to moderate	Low to moderate	Moderate	Moderate to high
Filarial antibodies	High	?	Absent	Absent	Absent	Absent	Absent	Possible
Diethylcarbamazine response	Present	?	Absent	Absent	Absent	Absent	Absent	Possible

Source: See [*13*].

piperazine (l-diethylcarbamyl-4-methylpiperazine),

it was introduced in 1947 [38] and because of its much lower toxicity quickly superceded the antimonials and arsenicals that had been previously used for treating these infections. DEC is a remarkably effective microfilaricidal drug; while also capable of killing adult *Wuchereria* and *Brugia* worms, its effect on this stage of the parasite is much less dramatic, and extended periods of treatment are often required for therapeutic success [39]. Interestingly, despite more than 40 years of observation and study, its mode of action is still a mystery. In vitro it has no discernible effect on either microfilariae or adult worms, but in vivo it causes a rapid fall in the number of circulating microfilariae. In humans, for example, the microfilaremia of *W. bancrofti* infections decreases within 15 min of an oral dose of DEC, and by 1 h, greater than 90 percent of the circulating microfilariae have been cleared from the blood [40]. This "opsonic" activity of the drug likely involves a three-way interaction between DEC, the host's immune system, and the parasite, but evidence has also been presented recently that platelets may play a critical role in this clearance reaction [41]. DEC has other interesting pharmacological properties, including effects on mediator release from mast cells and basophils and effects on leukotriene–arachidonic acid metabolism [39].

In the field, numerous different treatment regimens have been tried to optimize DEC's antifilarial action. Dosages of 5 to 6 mg/(kg·day) given at daily, weekly, or even monthly intervals to a total dose of 72 mg/kg in bancroftian filariasis and 36 mg/kg in the brugian infections have all proved successful in decreasing the microfilaremia rate in a community by at least 90 percent when evaluated several months after treatment is stopped. Microfilaremia, however, reappeared in many treated individuals weeks or months following the last dose of a standard regimen such as 6 mg/(kg·day) for 12 days in *W. bancrofti* infection, and this finding led to doubts about DEC's ability to kill adult worms. Recent experience with both brugian [42] and bancroftian filariasis, however, has suggested that very prolonged administration of low-dose DEC [2 mg/(kg·day)] at weekly intervals for periods up to 1½ years can successfully eradicate adult worms as well as microfilariae. If these early observations are substantiated, it may be that this long-term regimen will be the optimal approach to treating these infections with DEC.

The side effects associated with DEC are of two types. At doses of 10 to 20 mg/(kg·day), as used in studies of single-dose therapy in China [38], gastrointestinal side effects (nausea and vomiting) are common. When given, however, at dosages of 2 to 10 mg/(kg·day) in single or divided doses, DEC is essentially free of direct toxic side effects. The side effects that occur are the result of the host's reaction to the dying microfilariae, and, as such, their intensity is directly proportional to the number of microfilariae in the host's circulation [43]. These adverse reactions include fever, headache, nausea, vomiting, arthralgia, chills, dizziness, and prostration, all developing generally within the first 24 to 36 h of therapy. The frequency of severe reactions is much greater in patients with *B. malayi* or *B. timori* infection than in those with *W. bancrofti*. To minimize these reactions in highly parasitemic individuals, one can initiate treatment with very small doses of DEC (e.g., 25 mg) or premedicate the patients with antihistamines or steroids as suggested for onchocerciasis. Later in the course of treatment (after the first couple of days), some patients, with or without microfilaremia, may develop typical filarial fever episodes apparently precipitated by chemotherapeutic intrusion on the normal host-parasite equilibrium. Additionally, some investigators have recorded the formation of inflammatory nodules surrounding dead or damaged adult worms that develop in the scrotum (or less frequently in the limbs) of a variable proportion of DEC-treated patients 2 to 14 days after treatment has begun [39]. Though most of the side effects occur early in treatment and generally subside with continued administration of DEC, their development often has profoundly negative effects on patient compliance towards completion of the full course of therapy.

Ivermectin, a remarkably effective antihelminthic agent shown initially to be extremely active in killing the microfilariae of *O. volvulus* without causing the marked side reactions induced by DEC (see Chap 49), has recently been shown to be also a potent microfilaricide for *W. bancrofti* in humans [44]. Though eliciting side reactions similar to those of DEC, ivermectin has the distinct advantage of achieving its almost equivalent microfilaricidal efficacy after only a *single* oral dose of drug (1 mg for an adult) that is one-sixth the dosage used to treat patients with onchocerciasis. Though ivermectin's effect on adult worms is not yet known, its potent microfilaricidal activity after single-oral dose therapy likely will make it the future drug of choice for this infection, at least for large-scale, mass treatment control programs.

MANAGEMENT OF CHRONIC LYMPHATIC PATHOLOGY

Elephantiasis and the other chronic manifestations of severe lymphatic damage in filariasis patients have recently been shown to have a surprising degree of reversibility [45]. Optimal management of such affected individuals should include long-term, low-dose DEC (to eradicate persistent or new filarial infections) as well as diligent attention to local care of the lymphedematous extremity through limb elevation, use of special massage techniques and elastic stockings, and prevention of superficial bacterial and fungal infection. More severely affected patients may benefit remarkably from surgical decompression of the lymphatic system through "nodovenous shunt" surgery followed by excision of redundant tissue. Hydroceles can be repeatedly drained or repaired surgically. Chyluria also can sometimes be corrected surgically; interestingly, however, diagnostic lymphangiography itself has been reported in many cases to terminate the leak of chyle into the urine, probably as a result of its sclerosing effects.

POPULATION

Transmission

The worldwide distribution of *W. bancrofti* and *B. malayi* filariasis is summarized in Fig. 48-6.

Though now sparing Europe and North America, *W. bancrofti* is widely distributed throughout the tropics and subtropics in regions of Central and South America, Africa, Asia, and the Pacific. The nocturnally periodic race—the most widely distributed ecological type—is transmitted by mosquitoes of the *Culex pipiens* complex and is often referred to as the "urban type" of bancroftian filariasis. These mosquitoes are highly domestic, breeding mainly in sewage pools and other polluted waters near human dwellings. They have nocturnal

biting habits and generally feed on individuals asleep in their dwellings. "Rural" bancroftian filariasis, found in Africa, China, Malaysia, the Philippines, and New Guinea, is transmitted by several species of *Anopheles* mosquitoes whose breeding places are located in rural environments. In many of these regions, these same mosquitoes also serve as the vectors of malaria. In the Pacific regions, these mosquitoes as well as certain species of *Aëdes* serve as the principal vectors of the subperiodic (and even in some instances the nocturnally periodic) forms of the parasite.

B. malayi is confined to areas of east and south Asia (Fig. 48-6). Of the two physiological races, the nocturnally subperiodic type found in Malaysia, Indonesia, and the Philippines is transmitted by mosquitoes of *Mansonia* species. The larvae of these mosquitoes have a siphon that is characteristically modified for piercing plant tissues (e.g., *Pistia* or water hyacinths) to gain access to air. Therefore, these mosquitoes breed in swamps and ponds attached to roots or stems of aquatic plants throughout the larval and pupal stages of development. The nocturnally periodic type of *B. malayi* found widely distributed in south and southeast Asia is primarily transmitted by the open swamp–breeding mosquitoes of *Mansonia uniformis* and related mansonian species. Various species of *Anopheles* mosquitoes, which breed mainly in rice paddies, open swamps, and ponds, may also serve as vectors of periodic

DISTRIBUTION OF THE LYMPHATIC FILARIASES

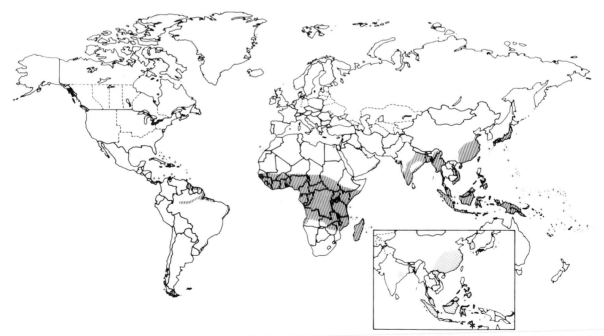

Figure 48-6. Distribution of *Wuchereria bancrofti* (world map) and *Brugia malayi* (insert) filariasis. The asterisk in the insert indicates the islands of Timor and Flores to which *Brugia timori* is restricted.

(*Drawn from data compiled by Dr. F. Hawking and distributed by the World Health Organization as WHO/Fil/71.94, 73.114, 71.124, and 75.136.*)

B. malayi in ecological habitats similar to those in which *M. uniformis* is a principal vector, but mosquitoes of the *Aëdes togoi* type have been found to be responsible for transmission of this type of *Brugia* in endemic regions in which villages lie near coastal beaches where rock pools serve as the mosquito breeding sites.

B. timori, reported only from the two Indonesian islands Timor and Flores, appears to be transmitted by *Anopheles barbirostris.* The epidemiology of these lymphatic filarial infections is an intimate weave of interactions among parasite, mosquito, and host [27]. Significant changes in the lifestyle of any one of these elements can drastically alter the balance among the others, and attempts to control filarial disease have continually focused on upsetting this delicate balance.

Control

The primary purpose of filarial control programs should be to reduce the morbidity of filariasis, not necessarily to eradicate the vectors or parasite. Some programs have concentrated only on altering one of the three components of the infection (parasite, vector, or host), but most have sought to affect at least two of these concurrently. In general, surveys of an area to determine the extent of filarial infection are followed by vector control measures in addition to either mass chemotherapy with DEC or selective treatment of microfilaremic individuals, in both cases to reduce the number of bloodborne microfilariae in a community to levels so low that transmission cannot occur. Depending on the type of transmission in the treatment area, these vector control measures may involve various combinations of residual (domestic) insecticides, larviciding, and abolition of mosquito breeding sites by either clean-up campaigns or changes in the construction or design of houses, latrines, etc. It is clear that while vector control by itself has caused the disappearance of filarial transmission in certain regions, because of the longevity of the parasite in the host, the most effective campaigns have been those that also involved treating infected individuals with DEC. In some instances this DEC has been targeted in single courses for microfilaremic patients; in others, short courses of DEC have been given at weekly or monthly intervals for longer periods of time; and in still others, DEC has been incorporated into the table salt for continuous, low-dose administration to the entire population. All three approaches can be successful. In fact, it has been demonstrated repeatedly in numerous areas throughout the world that a combined program of chemotherapy and vector control can be effective in reducing filarial transmission; the problem with such long-term control (i.e., the reason why many programs have failed) has been the difficulty in sustaining the commitment required for long-term vigilance and repeated vector and parasite control operations. As indicated above, the use of the new microfilaricidal agent ivermectin that requires only a single oral dose for effectiveness may help to make such operations easier (and thus more successful) in the future.

Prevention of filariasis by immunization is not yet feasible; in fact, there is disappointingly little information available even in animal models about the mechanisms of protective immunity in the lymphatic filariases. Protection of individuals entering endemic regions may, however, prove possible. Because DEC kills developing preadult forms of many filarial species, it is used routinely in veterinary practice as a prophylactic agent to prevent filarial infection of dogs. Moreover, its efficacy as a prophylactic for human *Loa loa* infections has recently been established (see below), and it is quite possible that DEC could be similarly effective for lymphatic filariasis as well; its potential in this regard remains to be evaluated.

LOA LOA

(Synonyms: *Filaria loa, Filaria oculi humani, F. lacrimalis, F. subconjunctivalis, Microfilaria diurna,* eyeworm.)

PARASITE [1]

L. loa (Cobbold, 1864) is a filiform semitransparent worm bluntly tapered at both extremities. Adults live wandering through the subcutaneous tissue in humans, occasionally appearing in the eye of the infected individuals as their wanderings take them to the subconjunctival region (Fig. 48-7). Females measure 50 to 70 mm in length by 0.5 mm in width, while male worms are smaller (30 to 34 mm long and 0.35 to

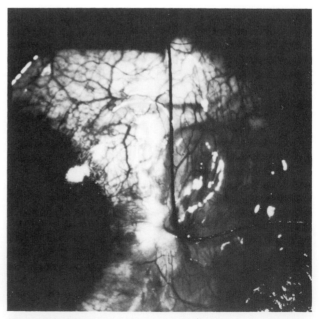

Figure 48-7. Subconjunctival adult *Loa loa* migrating across the sclera of the left eye of an African boy. The worm has been immobilized by a suture through the conjunctiva and around the parasite. Iris is at left and scleral margin, at right. (*Courtesy of Dr. David G. Cogan, National Eye Institute.*)

0.43 mm wide). The cuticle is covered with small bosses helpful in histologically distinguishing *L. loa* from other filarial parasites. Other characteristic morphological features include a unique clustering of perianal papillae in the caudal region of the male and a vulvar opening in the female that is about 2.5 mm from the anterior tip in the cervical region. From this vulva the vagina extends posteriorly to the bifurcated uterus that runs most of the length of the adult female and contains the microfilarial embryos that are extruded fully sheathed when mature. These mature microfilariae are 250 to 300 μm long and 6 to 8.5 μm wide. Nuclei extend caudally to the tip of the tail, but *Loa* microfilariae can be distinguished from those of *B. malayi* by the fact that their nuclei extend not as an isolated pair but rather as a column of nuclei into the tail and by the fact that the cephalic space is much shorter (Fig. 48-2).

The microfilariae of *L. loa* circulate in the blood of humans with a diurnal periodicity whose peak occurs at about noon. They are ingested by tabanid flies (deer- or horseflies) and develop in the fat body tissues of these flies over a period of about 10 days into mature, infective, third-stage larvae capable of infecting humans when they break out from the fly's head at the time of feeding. These mature L_3 forms are about 2 mm in length and 30 μm in width. They molt twice in the subcutaneous tissue of humans while becoming mature adults, and females shed microfilariae after a period of about 4 to 6 months.

There are probably two physiological races of *Loa*. One infects humans, has microfilariae with a diurnal periodicity, and is transmitted by day-biting species of *Chrysops* living near the ground; the other infects a number of African primates including the drill, the putty-nosed quenon, the mona monkey, and others. It has nocturnally periodic microfilariae and is transmitted by nocturnal or crepuscular biting *Chrysops* dwelling high in the forest canopy. Experimental infections in drills, patas monkeys, and baboons have shown that the human parasite readily infects these monkeys [46,47] and, interestingly, the diurnal periodicity of the human parasite persists in the animal host. However, though the parasites are morphologically indistinguishable and overlap in their geographical distribution, it is felt that their ecological differences are such that there is little or no cross-infection between the cycles of loa in humans and in nonhuman primates; i.e., the primates do not serve as a reservoir of human infection.

PATIENT

Pathogenesis and pathology

The most common pathology associated with *L. loa* infection in humans is the characteristic ''Calabar swelling'' named after the region in Africa where it was described. These are areas of angioedema that develop anywhere on the body but predominantly on the extremities, usually last for 1 to 3 days and are thought to reflect the host response to parasites or parasite antigens at the site of the swelling. Unfortunately little work has been done to define accurately the etiology, pathology, or pathogenesis of the lesions.

Less common pathological changes found associated with loiasis include nephropathy, cardiomyopathy, and encephalopathy. The nephropathy, generally presenting as proteinuria with or without mild hematuria, appears to be immune-complex-determined, but definitive studies are still lacking. Renal biopsies have shown chronic glomerulonephritis or membranous glomerulopathy. Following treatment with DEC, the proteinuria may increase transiently but subsequently has regressed in about half of the patients followed [48]. Encephalopathy, on the other hand, occurred only rarely in patients with loiasis before DEC became available for treatment. In its mildest form, the encephalopathy was manifested by psychoneurotic complaints such as insomnia, irritability, depression, and headache [49]. Though precise numbers are not available, more severe encephalitic complications leading to coma and death have been recorded after therapy with DEC in patients with very high microfilaremias (generally $> 50,000$ mL^{-1}). In such patients, microfilariae are often found in the cerebrospinal fluid, and in fatal cases studied at autopsy two distinct types of central nervous system (CNS) pathology have been noted. The first is a generalized acute cerebral edema thought to originate as an ''allergic'' reaction to the parasite and likely responsible for the coma and rapid demise of many of the patients. The second is a chronic or subacute encephalitis characterized by necrotizing granulomatous reactions around degenerating microfilariae found not only associated with the cerebral vessels but also extending into the parenchyma. Similar granulomatous lesions have been seen in the visceral organs as well.

Cardiomyopathy is related to loiasis more circumstantially than nephropathy or encephalopathy. Epidemologically, correlations have been made between the distribution of loiasis and the syndrome of endomyocardial fibrosis (EMF), a form of heart disease common in equatorial Africa in which there is fibrosis of the endocardium in one or both ventricles that affects the apex and inflow tracts by binding down the papillary muscles, the cords, and sometimes the posterior leaflets of the atrioventricular valves [50]. Also, clinically there have been reports of a number of Europeans or other non-Africans who lived for a time in *Loa* endemic regions and then developed the EMF syndrome [51]. They presented with characteristic cardiac abnormalities in addition to high levels of peripheral blood eosinophilia and usually had elevated antifilarial titers when these were evaluated. Though the relationship between EMF and loiasis is not yet clear, it is probably less the filariae themselves and more the eosinophilia they evoke that leads to the cardiac damage of EMF since the cardiac lesions found appear essentially identical to those of Loeffler's ''fibroplastic parietal endocarditis,'' the cardiopathology that characterizes the clinical disorder of eosinophil production known as the hypereosinophilic syndrome [52].

In primates, there is another form of pathology seen with

L. loa. These are granulomatous reactions around degenerating microfilariae in the spleens of animals with "repressed" microfilaremia. After the prepatent phase of infection in these primates microfilaremia develops progressively for about 3 to 4 months and then falls precipitously over 3 to 6 weeks to reach a low and fairly constant residual density. Thereafter, the level of microfilaremia remains low and little affected by subsequent superinfections. As production of microfilariae by the adult worms and the numbers of microfilariae in the pulmonary vasculature (the locus of the parasites when they do not circulate in the peripheral blood) can be shown to remain the same before and after the suppression of microfilaremia, the low counts found in the blood reflect clearance of the microfilariae by the spleen. It is not clear how much similar splenic pathology occurs in human infections.

Clinical manifestations

It is becoming increasingly clear that there are two major types of clinical presentation in loiasis, one more common among individuals native to the endemic regions and the other more common in "outsiders" who enter these areas and then acquire infection [*53*].

Among the natives, loiasis may be manifested only by an asymptomatic microfilaremia, with the infection being unrecognized until an adult worm moves subconjunctivally across the eye (Fig. 48-7). Others with microfilaremia may have occasional intermittent transient episodes of Calabar swellings, which are localized areas of erythema and angioedema that may be 5 to 10 cm or more in size. Often they occur in the extremities and last for several days before regressing spontaneously. If the inflammatory reaction extends to nearby joints or peripheral nerves, corresponding symptoms may develop. These swellings appear to be some form of hypersensitivity reaction to the adult worm, whose presence can also be detected in some individuals either by a crawling sensation subcutaneously or by the appearance of a fine, vermiform hive superficially in the skin. Routine x-rays on people in endemic areas often reveal calcified dead worms lying between the metacarpals. The rarer encephalopathic and renal presentations have been described above (see "Pathogenesis and Pathology").

The major difference between this presentation of loiasis and that seen in visitors to endemic regions is the greater predominance of allergic or hyperreactive symptoms in this latter group [*53*]. The episodes of recurrent angioedema (Calabar swellings) are likely to be more frequent and debilitating, and patients are much less likely to demonstrate microfilaremia. In addition, they very often have extremely high levels of peripheral blood eosinophilia, 30 to 60 percent of the total (elevated) white blood cell count not being uncommon. In these regards such patients resemble the hyperresponsive individuals with lymphatic filariasis who present either with acute inflammatory reactions after initial exposure to infection or with the tropical eosinophilia syndrome. The lack of microfilaremia

sometimes makes diagnosis difficult until one links the eosinophilia and angioedema with the patient's exposure history and elevated filarial antibody titers. The cardiomyopathy that some of these patients can develop, presumably as a result of the hypereosinophilia, has been described above.

Treatment

DEC is essentially the only drug used to treat loiasis. Its effectiveness against both microfilariae and adults is generally accepted on the basis of many complete cures after single courses of 8 to 10 mg/(kg·day) for 2 to 3 weeks. Microfilariae are cleared very rapidly from the blood, and evidence of adult worm destruction [nodules and local angioedema (Fig. 48-8)] has been found at various times within the first week of treatment. In some patients, however, multiple courses of DEC are required for cure [*53*]; the reason for the variable responsiveness to DEC among these patients is unclear.

Except in patients with heavy microfilaremia, side effects of DEC treatment in loiasis are few and limited primarily to the induction of angioedema episodes, pruritus, or hives. Microfilaremic individuals, however, frequently experience allergic and other inflammatory reactions similar to those seen in onchocerciasis (see Chap. 49, "Onchocerciasis") and lymphatic filariasis; in the most severe cases the CNS is also involved, leading to coma, meningoencephalitis, and retinal hemorrhage. Because of these severe complications, it has been recommended that heavily microfilaremic patients with loiasis should be managed as are those with heavy onchocerciasis, i.e., with low doses of DEC [such as 1 mg/(kg·day)] in the initial days of treatment and simultaneous administration of steroids.

Effective chemoprophylaxis with once-weekly DEC (300 mg) has recently been demonstrated in Peace Corps volunteers working in endemic regions of west Africa [*54*]. Such a regimen, with few or no associated side effects, would be appropriate for travelers likely to have significant exposure to this parasite.

POPULATION

Transmission

L. loa infection is confined to the rain forest belt of western and central Africa and equatorial Sudan (Fig. 48-9) where the *Chrysops* vectors (primarily *Chrysops silacea*) can easily find breeding spots. It is interesting that though several species of tabanid flies (horse- or deerflies) in the United States can serve very efficiently as vectors of *L. loa,* loiasis was never established in the Americas, as *W. bancrofti* was, following the massive influx of west Africans during the slave trade.

Control

Extensive programs to limit the spread of loiasis have not been carried out. Normal village growth automatically produces a degree of control of *L. loa* transmission by clearing adjacent forests for new farmland and thus destroying the *Chrysops'*

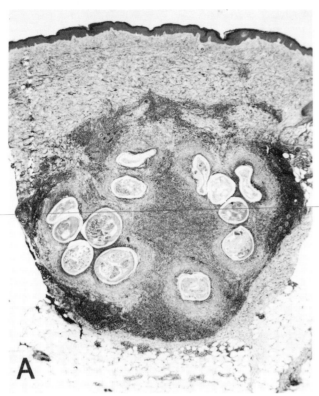

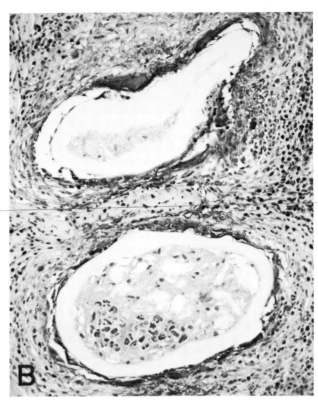

Figure 48-8. *A.* Cross section of a deep dermal inflammatory lesion containing a coiled, partially degenerated gravid adult female *Loa loa.* The nodule formed within 8 h after diethylcarbamazine was administered to a patient with amicrofilaremic loiasis; it was removed about 36 h later. The surrounding inflammatory reaction is comprised of granulomatous and scar tissue infiltrated by histiocytes, epithelioid cells, giant cells, plasma cells, eosinophils, and lymphocytes. (*Movat*

*stain, 25 ×; Armed Forces Institute of Pathology [AFIP] #82-11243; courtesy of Dr. Daniel H. Connor.) **B.** A higher magnification of tangential sections of the parasites in A.* Irregularly spaced cuticular bosses characteristic of *L. loa* are seen in the lower section. The cuticle is intact but the internal structures are degenerate. Nuclear fragments (lower left) are still recognizable as degenerating microfilariae. (*Movat stain, 160 ×; AFIP #82-11248; courtesy of Dr. Daniel H. Connor.*)

breeding sites in the forest mud. The spraying of such breeding sites with insecticides is also possible and biologically effective, but, in practice, the application of insecticides to control the horsefly population is extremely difficult because of the cost, labor requirements, and overall effectiveness.

Protection of individuals from loiasis by immunization has received almost no attention, but chemoprophylaxis with DEC (300 mg once weekly) has proven effective for uninfected individuals exposed to loiasis for the first time [*54*].

MANSONELLA PERSTANS

(Synonyms: *Filaria perstans, Acanthocheilonema perstans, Dipetalonema perstans, Tetrapetalonema perstans.*)

PARASITE

Adults of *M. perstans* (Manson, 1891) have only rarely been recovered in humans but appear to reside in the peritoneal, pleural, and pericardial cavities, mesentery and perirenal and retroperitoneal tissues. Females are 70 to 80 mm long, while the smaller males average 45 mm; both are about 60 μm wide. They are creamy white, cylindrical worms with smooth cuticles and various projecting papillae that distinguish them from other filarial parasites [*1*]. Microfilariae are liberated from the females *unsheathed* and circulate in the blood without regular periodicity. Their diagnostic morphological features are indicated in Fig. 48-2 and Table 48-2. Ingested by biting midges (*Culicoides* spp.) they develop from microfilariae (L_1) to mature infective L_3 larvae. Transmission occurs when these larvae reach the skin of humans as the biting midge feeds. The length of the prepatent period (i.e., the time required for the infective larvae to mature, mate, and produce circulating microfilariae) has not been well studied. A similar lack of information exists for questions such as the susceptibility of other animals to this parasite and the possibility of reservoir hosts.

DISTRIBUTION OF *L. LOA* AND *T. PERSTANS*

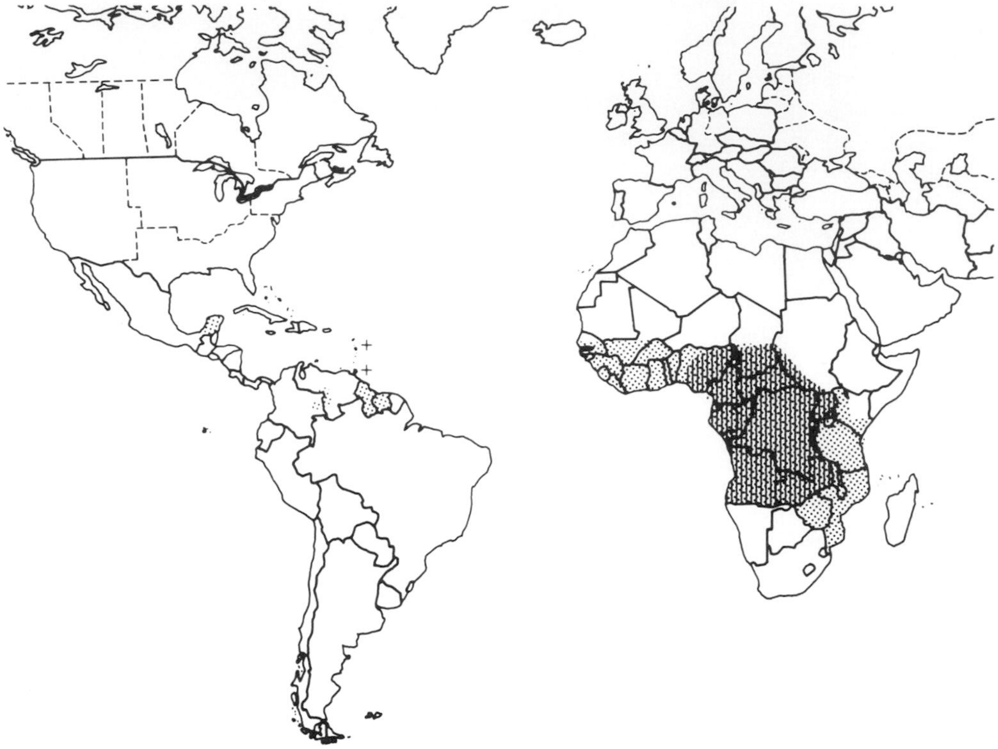

Figure 48-9. Distribution of *Loa loa* (vertical hatch) and *Mansonella perstans* (dotted area) filariasis. The +'s in the Caribbean indicate islands endemic for *M. perstans;* loiasis is only endemic to Africa. (*Drawn from data compiled by Dr. F. Hawking as described in legend to Fig. 48-6.*)

PATIENT

Pathogenesis, pathology, and clinical manifestations

The pathology of perstans filariasis is not well defined, both because the clinical features of the infection are incompletely characterized and because little pathological material has been available for study. Because up to 90 percent of individuals in certain regions could be found infected with *M. perstans* yet appeared to experience little or no difficulty from their infections, it was initially felt that the parasite could be regarded as an asymptomatic commensal. However, a number of subsequent reports [55,56] have indicated quite clearly that *M. perstans* infection can induce a variety of symptoms including the following: angioedematous swellings of the arms, face, and other parts of the body that usually last for 2 to 4 days and appear similar or identical to Calabar swellings; pruritus; fever; headache; pain or ache in bursae and/or joint synovia, in serous cavities, or in the liver region; neurological or psychological symptoms and extreme exhaustion. There is some evidence that the symptoms are more pronounced in individuals coming to endemic regions from areas where *M. perstans* does not occur [55,56]; but in no series, even

those evaluating Europeans or Americans who have acquired perstans filariasis, have all of the patients been symptomatic. In at least a quarter of infected individuals the infection remains entirely asymptomatic with microfilariae circulating generally both day and night in the blood.

At the other extreme, however, are those patients with disease manifestations that can be extremely debilitating (because of angioedema, joint pain, or neurological symptoms) or even fatal (e.g., from pericarditis or hepatitis [57]). While such life-threatening presentations are rare, the other symptoms as well as hives and eosinophilia are reasonably common and can be shown quite clearly to disappear after successful treatment. Though meningitis and encephalopathy have been attributed to *M. perstans* on the basis of finding perstans microfilariae in the spinal fluid, it has been suggested that the parasite found in such individuals is not really *M. perstans* but *Meningonema peruzzi,* a CNS filarid usually found in nonhuman primates [58]. Moreover, a study of 22 asymptomatic or minimally symptomatic patients with perstans filariasis failed to reveal any abnormality in the cerebrospinal fluid [59]. Thus, the relationship between *M. perstans* infection and meningoencephalitis needs further definition.

Diagnosis of the infection is made parasitologically by finding the unsheathed microfilariae (Fig. 48-2) in the blood, generally both day and night but occasionally *either* in the day *or* the night. When polycarbonate filters are used for screening blood, 3-μm-pore sizes are preferable to 5-μm ones because of the relatively smaller size of these microfilariae. Sometimes the microfilariae can be seen in other body fluids as well, such as in pericardial effusion. Perstans filariasis is often associated with an eosinophilia, which in some patients can be massive, and with elevated antifilarial antibody titers.

Treatment

In perstans, as in the other forms of filariasis, DEC is currently the drug of choice. Its effects, however, are not completely satisfactory. In some cases microfilaremia disappears after a single course of treatment with DEC [5 to 6 mg/(kg·day) for 10 to 20 days], but in many the microfilaremia persists and up to 8 or 10 such treatment regimens are required over the course of a year or so to effect cure. When cure is attained, patients characteristically lose their symptoms, their eosinophilia, and their general malaise.

The side reactions that accompany treatment of perstans infection with DEC are similar to those seen when treating other forms of filariasis. The drug itself has little toxicity, but when used to treat heavily infected individuals, it can cause systemic allergic-type reactions similar to those described following treatment of the lymphatic filariases or onchocerciasis (see Chap. 49). Also, it is not uncommon to induce angioedema episodes after DEC treatment is initiated, episodes perhaps reflecting local parasite damage and an allergic response to the worm products. Recently mebendazole has also been tried in the treatment of *M. perstans* with moderate success [60].

POPULATION

Transmission and control

M. perstans is distributed across the center of Africa from Senegal and Gambia on the west coast to Kenya, Zimbabwe, and Tanzania on the east. In South America it is localized to the northeast coast (Fig. 48-10). The vector, biting midges of *Culicoides* spp., thrives in the underbrush. While burning the underbrush and application of insecticides is effective in decreasing the *Culicoides* populations, no large-scale control pro-

DISTRIBUTION OF *M. OZZARDI* AND *T. STREPTOCERCA*

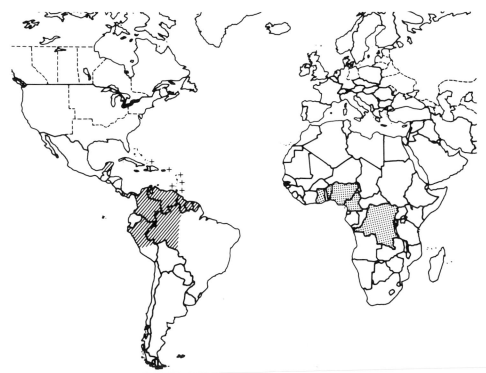

Figure 48-10. Distribution of *Mansonella ozzardi* (diagonally hatched area and +'s along Caribbean Islands) and *Mansonella streptocerca* (dotted area). (*Drawn from data compiled by Dr. F. Hawking as indicated in legend to Fig. 48-6.*)

grams aimed specifically at controlling these vectors of perstans filariasis have been carried out.

Though the implications of the observation are unclear, there is a distinct association between *M. perstans* infection and infection with *W. bancrofti* and *L. loa* in areas where the distributions of these parasites overlap [61,62]. Thus, a careful search for "polyparasitism" should be carried out in individuals identified as having perstans filariasis but whose exposure histories are compatible with these other filarial infections as well.

MANSONELLA STREPTOCERCA

(Synonyms: *Agamofilaria streptocerca, Dipetalonema streptocerca, Tetrapetalonema streptocerca.*)

PARASITE

Adult *M. streptocerca* (Macfie and Corson, 1922) live in the dermal collagen and subcutaneous tissue of humans. Females are about 27 mm in length, and both males and females are morphologically distinguishable from those of *O. volvulus* and *M. perstans* [63]. The microfilariae found in the skin are unsheathed (as are those of *O. volvulus*) but distinguished from *O. volvulus* by their being more slender, tapered at both ends, and having a shepherd's crook-shaped tail with nuclei extending to the very end (Fig. 48-2). They measure 180 to 240 μm in length by 3 μm in diameter. The microfilariae of *M. streptocerca* develop into infective larvae after 7 to 8 days in biting midges (*Culicoides* spp.). Information on the development of the L_3 to adult stage in humans is lacking, as are data to define the susceptibility of other animal species to the parasite. Since the parasite has been found in both chimpanzees and gorillas, it may be that these primates serve as reservoir hosts.

PATIENT

Pathogenesis and pathology

The pathology of streptocerciasis is dermal and lymphatic [63]. In the skin, grossly, there are hypopigmented macules and occasional papules; microscopically, microfilariae can be seen in the dermal collagen along with dermal fibrosis, phagocytized melanin in the upper dermis, dilated lymphatics, and perivascular collections of eosinophils and lymphocytes. Biopsied lymph nodes have shown chronic lymphadenitis with scarring, dilated lymphatics, reduced germinal activity, and an infiltration of plasma cells and eosinophils.

Clinical manifestations

The major clinical features of streptocerciasis are related to the skin, i.e., altered pigmentation, papules, and mild pruritus. Most individuals also show inguinal lymphadenopathy, and it has been suggested that *M. streptocerca* might be a cause of lymphedema and elephantiasis in some areas [63]. Many infected individuals, however, appear to remain asymptomatic.

Leprosy is the most important disease to be distinguished from streptocerciasis. Clinically, the hypopigmented macules of leprosy have decreased sensitivity for light-touch and for heat-cold discrimination, and histologically there are characteristic features. Granuloma multiforme is another condition resulting in hypopigmented macules, but it too has a characteristic histology. While streptocercal dermatitis may be similar to onchocercal dermatitis, the microfilariae in the skin can be readily differentiated; furthermore, the distribution of the parasites in the skin (generally across the shoulders and upper torso) is different from that in African onchocerciasis (see Chap. 49, "Onchocerciasis"). Also, clinical involvement of the eye is not a feature of streptocerciasis.

Treatment

DEC is particularly effective for treating streptocerciasis. Following doses of 2 to 4 mg/(kg·day) for 21 days, most patients develop intense pruritus with the subsequent development of papules, and in some there is urticaria, cutaneous edema, joint or muscular pains, headache, cough, and abdominal complaints—very similar to the Mazzotti reaction that follows treatment of onchocerciasis (see Chap. 49) but occurring somewhat more slowly. The papules are unique, however, in that they contain dying adult worms (in contrast to dying microfilariae in onchocerciasis) surrounded by a marked eosinophilic inflammatory reaction. These findings give assurance that DEC is an effective macrofilaricide, as well as microfilaricide, in streptocerciasis and suggest that prolonged treatment at this or a slightly higher dosage [e.g., 5 to 6 mg/(kg·day) for 21 days] should effect a radical cure of this filarial infection.

POPULATION

Transmission and control

M. streptocerca is found exclusively in the tropical rain forest zone of western and central Africa from Ghana to Zaire and Angola. Its distribution overlaps considerably with that of *L. loa, M. perstans,* and *O. volvulus.* Studies of polyparasitism in individuals living in such rain forest regions have indicated a strong association between the numbers of *M. perstans* and *M. streptocerca* in multiply infected persons [61].

There have been no control programs aimed specifically at streptocerca or its *Culicoides* vector. Simiarly, nothing is known about the potential of chemotherapeutic or vaccine prophylaxis for this infection.

MANSONELLA OZZARDI

(Synonyms: *Filaria demarquay, Filaria ozzardi, Filaria juncea.*)

PARASITE [1]

Adult worms of *M. ozzardi* (Manson, 1897) have been recovered from humans only twice, both times from the peritoneal cavity at autopsy. Females ranged from 65 to 81 mm in length by 0.21 to 0.25 mm in width, had smooth cuticles and a pair of fleshy flaps at the caudal extremity. A complete male has not yet been recovered. The microfilariae, 173 to 240 μm long and 5 μm broad, are unsheathed, lack caudal nuclei at the tip of the tail, and circulate in the blood with minimal (peak 8 A.M.) or no periodicity. Microfilariae develop in both biting midges (*Culicoides furens*) and blackflies (*Simulium amazonicum*), requiring 7 to 8 days to mature to infective third-stage larvae. The length of the prepatent period in humans is unknown. There is no evidence that *M. ozzardi* has an animal reservoir, but patas monkeys (in contrast to a number of other primates) acquire the infection experimentally [64].

PATIENT

Pathogenesis, pathology, and clinical manifestations

As with perstans filariasis, the pathology of *M. ozzardi* infection has been difficult to define because of the imprecise clinical descriptions of patients with this infection. Many consider these parasites to be nonpathogenic, but one of the fullest clinical studies of an affected population [65] asserts that the major clinical presentation of the infection is severe articular pain or dysfunction, especially in the arms and shoulders and more severe in patients older than 35 years. Headache, fever, pulmonary symptoms, adenopathy, hepatomegaly, and pruritic skin eruptions have also been described in a small number of patients with a frequency much greater than that of the nonparasitized individuals in the same population. Eosinophilia also seems a common concomitant of *M. ozzardi* infection.

Microfilariae can be demonstrated in the peripheral blood throughout the day and night, though there may be a slight diurnal character to their periodicity. They are unsheathed but distinguishable from the other sheathless microfilariae found in the blood of humans, *M. perstans,* by their pointed tails. Since skin snips, as used for diagnosis of *O. volvulus* infection, also detect up to a third of the patients with microfilaremic mansonellosis, the microfilariae in a positive "skin" snip must be differentiated in areas where the two infections overlap.

Treatment

DEC has little or no effect on patients with *M. ozzardi* infection, but a single dose of ivermectin (150 μg/kg) was recently reported to be effective for one infected individual [66].

POPULATION

Transmission and control

M. ozzardi is a parasite restricted to humans and limited in distribution to certain of the Caribbean Islands, the whole of Central America and South America from northern Argentina and Bolivia to the coast of Colombia, Guyana, and Brazil (Fig. 48-10). In the Caribbean and in Central America the midge *Culicoides furens* or *C. phlebotomus* transmits the infection from human to human but in the Amazonas of Brazil and Colombia blackflies, *S. amazonicum* and *S. sanguineum*, serve as vectors. Though these differing vector requirements might imply different strains or races of *M. ozzardi,* until adult parasites can be recovered from infected individuals in these two areas, no comparative evaluation of the parasites can be undertaken.

There have been no programs designed to control infection with *M. ozzardi,* largely because there is little agreement on the public health importance of mansonellosis; and this, despite the fact that in some populations of Amerindians in South America infection rates of up to 96 percent of the adult population have been recorded [65].

REFERENCES

1 Sasa M: *Human Filariasis. A Global Survey of Epidemiology and Control.* Baltimore, University Park Press, 1976, p 819
2 Cross JH, Partono F, Hsu MR, et al: Experimental transmission of *Wuchereria bancrofti* to monkeys. Am J Trop Med Hyg 28:56–66, 1979
3 Sucharit S, Harinasuta C, Choochote W: Experimental transmission of subperiodic *Wuchereria bancrofti* to the leaf monkey (*Presbytis melalophos*), and its periodicity. Am J Trop Med Hyg 31:599–601, 1982
4 Saz HJ: Biochemical aspects of filarial parasites. Trends Biochem Sci 6:117–119, 1981
5 Selkirk ME, Denham DA, Partono F, et al: Molecular characterization of antigens of lymphatic filarial parasites. Parasitology 92(suppl):S15–38, 1986
6 Piessens WF, McReynolds LA, Williams SA: Highly repeated DNA sequences as species-specific probes for *Brugia*. Immunol Today 3:378–379, 1987
7 Partono F, Purnomo, Dennis DT, et al: *Brugia timori* sp.n. (Nematoda: Filarioidea) from Flores Island, Indonesia. J Parasitol 63:540–546, 1977
8 Ottesen EA: Immunological aspects of lymphatic filariasis and onchocerciasis in humans. Trans R Soc Trop Med Hyg 78(suppl):9–18, 1984
9 Ottesen EA, Kumaraswami V, Paranjape R, et al: Naturally occurring blocking antibodies modulate immediate hypersensitivity responses in human filariasis. J Immunol 127:2014–2020, 1981
10 Nutman TB, Kumaraswami V, Pao L, et al: An analysis of in vitro B cell immune responsiveness in human lymphatic filariasis. J Immunol 138:3954–3959, 1987
11 Weil GJ, Hussain R, Kumaraswami V, et al: Prenatal allergic sensitization to helminth antigens in offspring of parasite-infected mothers. J Clin Invest 71:1124–1129, 1983
12 Petralanda I, Yarzabal L, Piessens WF: Parasite antigens in breast milk of women infected with *Onchocerca volvulus*. Am J Trop Med Hyg 38:372–379, 1988
13 Neva FA, Ottesen EA: Tropical (filarial) eosinophilia. N Engl J Med 298:1129–1131, 1978
14 Hussain R, Grogl M, Ottesen EA: IgG antibody subclasses in hu-

man filariasis: Differential subclass recognition of parasite antigens correlates with different clinical manifestations of infection. J Immunol 139:2794–2798, 1987

15 Cohen LB, Nelson G, Wood AM, et al: Lymphangiography in filarial lymphoedema and elephantiasis. Am J Trop Med Hyg 10: 843–848, 1961

16 Bosworth W, Ewert A, Bray J: The interaction of *Brugia malayi* and *Streptococcus* in an animal model. Am J Trop Med Hyg 22: 714–719, 1973

17 Schacher JF, Sahyoun PF: A chronological study of the histopathology of filarial disease in cats and dogs caused by *Brugia pahangi* (Buckley and Edeson, 1956). Trans R Soc Trop Med Hyg 61:234–243, 1967

18 Wartman WB: Filariasis in American armed forces in World War II. Medicine 26:334–394, 1947

19 Price EW: The association of endemic elephantiasis on the lower legs in East Africa with soil derived from volcanic rocks. Trans R Soc Trop Med Hyg 70:228–295, 1976

20 Ottesen EA, Mendell NR, MacQueen JM, et al: Familial predisposition to filarial infection—not linked to HLA-A or -B locus specificities. Acta Trop (Basel) 28:205–216, 1981

21 Chan SH, Dissanayake S, Mak JW, et al: HLA and filariasis in Sri Lankans and Indians. Southeast Asian J Trop Med Public Health 15:281–286, 1984

22 O'Connor FW: The etiology of the disease syndrome in *Wuchereria bancrofti* infections. Trans R Soc Trop Med Hyg 26:13–33, 1932

23 Michael P: Filariasis among Navy and Marine personnel. Report on laboratory investigations. US Navy Med Bull 42:1059–1074, 1974

24 Saxena H, Singh SN, Samuel KC, et al: Nodular breast lesions caused by filarial worms: Report of three cases. Am J Trop Med Hyg 24:894–896, 1975

25 Udwadia FE: *Pulmonary Eosinophilia: Progress in Respiration Research.* Basel, Karger, vol 7, 1975, p 286

26 Meyers FM, Kouwenaar W: Over hypereosinophilie en over un merkwaardigen vorm von filariasis. Geneesk Tijdschr Ned Indie 79:853–873, 1939

27 Dennis DT, Partono F, Purnomo, et al: Timor filariasis: Epidemiologic and clinical features in a defined community. Am J Trop Med Hyg 25:797–802, 1976

28 Gooneratne BWN: *Lymphangiography—Clinical and Experimental.* London, Butterworths, 1974, p 194

29 Partono F, Purnomo, Pribadi W, et al: Epidemiological and clinical features of *Brugia timori* in a newly established village, Karakuak, West Flores, Indonesia. Am J Trop Med Hyg 27:910–915, 1978

30 Frimodt-Möller C, Barton RM: Pseudo-tuberculous condition associated with eosinophilia. Indian Med Gaz 75:607–613, 1940

31 Weingarten RJ: Tropical eosinophilia. Lancet i:103–105, 1943

32 Webb JKG, Job CK, Gault EW: Tropical eosinophilia: Demonstration of microfilariae in lung, liver, and lymph-nodes. Lancet i:835–842, 1960

33 Danaraj TJ, Pacheco G, Shanmugaratnam K, et al: The etiology and pathology of eosinophilic lung (tropical eosinophilia). Am J Trop Med Hyg 15:183–189, 1966

34 Joe LK: Occult filariasis: Its relationship with tropical pulmonary eosinophilia. Am J Trop Med Hyg 11:646–652, 1962

35 Dennis DT, McConnell E, White GB: Bancroftian filariasis and

membrane filters: Are night surveys necessary? Am J Trop Med Hyg 25:257–262, 1976

36 Hussain R, Hamilton RG, Kumaraswami V, et al: IgE responses in human filariasis. I. Quantitation of filaria-specific IgE. J Immunol 27:1623–1629, 1981

37 Ottesen EA, Weller PF, Lunde MN, et al: Endemic filariasis on a Pacific island. II. Immunologic aspects: Immunoglobulin, complement and specific antifilarial IgG, IgM and IgE antibodies. Am J Trop Med Hyg 31:953–961, 1982

38 Hawking F: Diethylcarbamazine and new compounds for the treatment of filariasis. Adv Pharmacol Chemother 16:129–194, 1979

39 Ottesen EA: Efficacy of diethylcarbamazine in eradicating infection with lymphatic dwelling filariae in humans. Rev Infect Dis 7: 341–356, 1985

40 Weller PF, Ottesen EA: Failure of diethylcarbamazine as a provocative test in subperiodic *Wuchereria bancrofti* filariasis. Trans R Soc Trop Med Hyg 72:31–32, 1978

41 Cesbron J-Y, Capron A, Vargaftig BB: Platelets mediate the action of diethylcarbamazine on microfilariae. Nature 325:533–536, 1987

42 Partono F, Purnomo, Oemijati S, et al: The long term effects of repeated diethylcarbamazine administration with special reference to microfilaremia and elephantiasis. Acta Trop (Basel) 38:217–225, 1981

43 Ottesen EA: Description, mechanisms and control of post-treatment reactions in human filariasis, in *Filariasis.* Ciba Found Symp 127:265–283, 1987

44 Kumaraswami V, Ottesen EA, Vijayasekaran V et al: Ivermectin for treatment of *Wuchereria bancrofti* filariasis: Efficacy and adverse reactions. JAMA 259:3150–3153, 1988

45 World Health Organization: Lymphatic pathology and immunopathology in filariasis: Report of the Twelfth Meeting of the Scientific Working Group on Filariasis. TDR/FIL-SWG(12)/85.3, 1985

46 Duke BOL, Wijers DJB: Studies on loiasis in monkeys. I. The relationship between human and simian *Loa* in the rain-forest zone of the British Cameroons. Ann Trop Med Parasitol 52:158–173, 1958

47 Orihel TC, Moore PJ: *Loa loa:* Experimental infection in two species of African primates. Am J Trop Med Hyg 24:606–609, 1975

48 Zuidema PJ: Renal changes in loiasis. Folia Med Neerl 14:168–172, 1971

49 Van Bogaert L, Dubois A, Janssens PG, et al: Encephalitis in *Loa loa* filariasis. J Neurol Neurosurg Psychiatry 18:103–119, 1955

50 Ive FA, Willis AJP, Ikema AC, et al: Endomyocardial fibrosis and filariasis. Q J Med 36:495–516, 1967

51 Brockington IF, Olsen EGJ, Goodwin JF: Endomyocardial fibrosis in European residents in tropical Africa. Lancet i:583–588, 1967

52 Chusid MJ, Dale DC, West BC, et al: The hypereosinophilic syndrome: Analysis of fourteen cases with review of the literature. Medicine (Baltimore) 54:1–27, 1975

53 Nutman TB, Miller KD, Mulligan M, et al: *Loa loa* infection in temporary residents of endemic regions: Recognition of a hyperresponsive syndrome with characteristic clinical manifestations. J Infect Dis 154:10–18, 1986

54 Nutman TB, Miller KD, Mulligan M, et al: Diethylcarbamazine provides effective prophylaxis for human loiasis: Results of a double-blinded study. N Engl J Med 319:752–756, 1988

55 Adolph PE, Kagan IG, McQuay RM: Diagnosis and treatment of

Acanthocheilonema perstans filariasis. Am J Trop Med Hyg 11: 76–88, 1962

56 Clarke V deV, Harwin RM, MacDonald DF, et al: Filariasis: *Dipetalonema perstans* infections in Rhodesia. Cent Afr J Med 17:1–11, 1971

57 Gelfand M, Wessels P: *Acanthocheilonema perstans* in a European female. A discussion of its possible pathogenicity and a suggested new syndrome. Trans R Soc Trop Med Hyg 58:552–556, 1964

58 Orihel TC: Cerebral filariasis in Rhodesia–a zoonotic infection? Am J Trop Med Hyg 22:596–599, 1973

59 Holmes GKT, Gelfand M, Boyt W, et al: A study to investigate the pathogenicity of a parasite resembling *Acanthocheilonema perstans*. Trans R Soc Trop Med Hyg 63:479–484, 1969

60 Maertens K, Wery M: Effect of mebendazole and levamisole on *Onchocerca volvulus* and *Dipetalonema perstans*. Trans R Soc Trop Med Hyg 69:359–360, 1975

61 Buck AA, Anderson RI, MacRae AA, et al: Epidemiology of polyparasitism. II. Types of combinations, relative frequency and associations of multiple infections. Tropenmed Parasitol 29:137–144, 1978

62 Keita MF, Prost A, Balique H, et al: Associations of filarial infections in man in the Savannah zones of Mali and Upper Volta. Am J Trop Med Hyg 30:590–592, 1981

63 Meyers WM, Connor DH, Harman LE, et al: Human streptocerciasis: A clinico-pathologic study of 40 Africans (Zairians) including identification of the adult filaria. Am J Trop Med Hyg 21:528–545, 1972

64 Orihel TC, Lowrie RC, Eberhard ML, et al: Susceptibility of laboratory primates to infection with *Mansonella ozzardi* from man. Am J Trop Med Hyg 30:790–794, 1981

65 Marinkelle CJ, German E: Mansonelliasis in the comisaria del Vaupes of Colombia. Trop Geogr Med 22:101–111, 1970

66 Nutman TB, Nash TE, Ottesen EA: Ivermectin in the successful treatment of a patient with *Mansonella ozzardi* infection. J Infect Dis 156:662–665, 1987

Onchocerciasis · Bruce M. Greene

C H A P T E R
49

Onchocerciasis is caused by the filarial nematode *Onchocerca volvulus*. An estimated 20 million persons, located largely in equatorial Africa and Central America, are infected by *O. volvulus*. Onchocerciasis is one of the four leading causes of blindness worldwide; in addition, it causes great suffering and disfigurement from dermatitis. Furthermore, onchocercal blindness is associated with markedly increased mortality rates in adults. There is at present no suitable means of prevention or cure. *O. volvulus* infection is transmitted by the bite of female blackflies, *Simulium* species, which oviposit on to objects in freely flowing streams and rivers. The adult male and female *O. volvulus* worms live predominantly in the subcutaneous tissues, between intermuscular fascial planes, and in the deep tissues surrounding joints. Gravid females produce myriads of microfilariae which migrate throughout the tissues of the host. The predominant pathology in symptomatic onchocerciasis involves the eyes, skin, and lymph nodes. Although vector control has achieved considerable success in some endemic areas, adequate means of vector and parasite control to limit the worldwide impact of the disease are currently lacking.

PARASITE

LIFE CYCLE

Infection in humans (Fig. 49-1) begins with inoculation of infective larvae into the skin by the bite of the female blackfly (*Simulium* species). Infective larvae develop into adult worms over a period estimated at several months; the adult worms then coil up into roughly spherical bundles, typically containing two to three females and one to two males, but with wide variations in these numbers. The gravid female releases microfilariae which then migrate out of the nodule and throughout the tissues of the host, concentrating in the dermis. Microfilariae are found in the skin after a prepatent period of from 7 to 34 months following introduction of infective larvae [1]. Transmission of infection to other individuals is initiated by the bite of a female fly, which, along with a blood meal, ingests microfilariae from the host skin. Some of the ingested microfilariae migrate from the gut of the blackfly into the thoracic muscles and develop into infective larvae over a period of 6 to 8 days. These infective larvae then migrate to the head of the fly where they may be transmitted to a second host in the process of taking a blood meal.

MORPHOLOGY

Infective larvae are 440 to 700 μm in length (mean 600 μm) and 19 to 28 μm in width [2,3]. Features which are most helpful in distinguishing infective larvae of *O. volvulus* from those of other species include the length, the position of the anus (average 31.2 μm from the caudal extremity), and the morphology of the caudal extremity (narrowing behind the anus with a rounded caudal extremity) [3]. Adult *O. volvulus* females are 23 to 70 cm in length and 275 to 325 μm in width

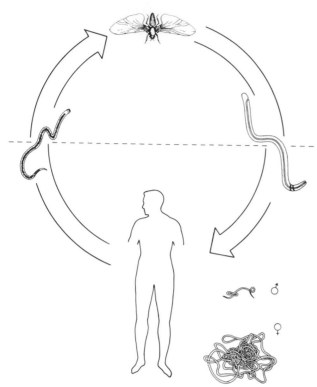

Figure 49-1. Life cycle of *Onchocerca volvulus*.

[*4*], with a mean weight of 36 mg [*5*]. Freshly isolated adult females exhibit prominent and regular annulations of the cuticle. The nerve ring is 170 μm and the vulva 940 μm from the anterior end. At the caudal end, the anus lies 210 μm from the posterior end of the worm. The reproductive system consists of a vagina and paired uteri, seminal receptacles, oviducts, and ovaries. Adult males are 3 to 6 cm in length and 130 to 150 μm in width [*4*], with a mean weight of 0.4 mg [*5*]. In nodules, males are usually found located superficially, coiled around the cephalad end of a female. Annulations are very closely spaced (5 μm), and quite inconspicuous relative to the female's. The nerve ring is 140 μm from the anterior end, and the anus is 65 μm from the posterior tip. The reproductive system consists of a testis, a vas deferens, an ejaculatory duct, and two copulatory spicules which can be projected out of the anus. *O. volvulus* microfilariae are unsheathed and measure 210 to 320 μm in length and 6 to 9 μm in width [*3,6*]. When freshly emergent from tissue they exhibit very rapid coiling and uncoiling movements. Morphological features of stained microfilariae which help to differentiate them from other filarial species include a cephalic space of 7 to 13 μm between the anterior end and first nucleus, a caudal space of 9 to 15 μm between the terminal nucleus and the posterior end, elongation of the terminal nuclei, and a sharply pointed tail [*7,8*].

VECTOR

Simulium damnosum and its subspecies represent the predominant vector in most of the endemic areas in Africa and in south Arabia. The *S. neavei* complex are vectors in eastern Zaire, Uganda, Ethiopia, Tanzania, Malawi, and in Kenya, where transmission was terminated as a result of an intensive campaign of DDT spraying in the 1950s. In Central America, *S. ochraceum* is the principal vector; *S. metallicum* and *S. calladium* are less important vector species [9].

In Africa, a number of subspecies of *S. damnosum* have been identified in different geographical locations. More importantly, vector-parasite complexes have been described in which transmission of a given strain of parasite is relatively restricted to a given subspecies of blackfly. For example, there is evidence that the forest strain of *O. volvulus* in west Africa is transmitted by *S. yahense*, *S. sanctipauli*, *S. soubrense*, and *S. squamosum*, while the savannah strain is transmitted by *S. damnosum sensu stricto* and *S. sirbanum* [10]. Although it is not certain that this relationship is based on vector refractoriness to certain parasite strains, there are data to support this hypothesis [*11*].

Simuliids (blackflies) oviposit into free-flowing rivers and streams, particularly in rapids. The gravid female deposits eggs on sticks, rocks, and trailing vegetation or other superficial debris. Eggs hatch into larvae in 2 days; these migrate downstream and develop into pupae in 8 to 10 days. Pupae remain fixed to some structure in the stream of water, and the adult fly emerges from the pupal shell in 2 days. Adult females are hematophagous, requiring a blood meal for initiation of a gonotrophic cycle, whereas males do not require blood and therefore do not transmit *O. volvulus* infection. The majority of microfilariae ingested as part of a blood meal are damaged by the buccopharyngeal apparatus of the fly. Others are carried to the stomach, and most of these pass on to the midgut where they die and disintegrate. A small proportion of the microfilariae, however, penetrate the gut wall and migrate into the thorax where they develop into infective larvae. They then pass to the head where they can be transmitted to humans in the process of obtaining a blood meal. Female blackflies generally restrict their flight to within a few kilometers of larval and pupal habitats (commonly termed *breeding sites*) and bite most intensely in the immediate vicinity. However, blackflies can be carried long distances, perhaps hundreds of kilometers, in association with monsoon winds.

PATIENT

HOST IMMUNE RESPONSE

The host develops a humoral immune response against the parasite, as evidenced by opsonizing antibodies directed against microfilariae and infective larvae [*12,13*]. In addition, antibodies, including IgE, against crude adult worm antigen have been found in sera from infected persons [*14,15*]. However, any possible significance of this antibody response in protective immunity remains to be established. High levels of IgG, IgM, and IgE, of unknown specificity, have also been found in *O. volvulus*–infected persons. In addition, increased levels of circulating immune complexes have been demonstrated by several techniques. With regard to cellular immunity, there is an increased prevalence of lepromatous leprosy in *O. volvulus*–infected persons [16], and skin reactivity against mycobacterial antigens is reduced [17]. Lymphocyte reactivity against *O. volvulus* antigens is reduced in the majority of infected persons [18–20]. However, reduced reactivity appears to be acquired since younger persons (ages 12 to 17) show a much higher frequency of responsiveness than do older persons [19].

PATHOLOGY AND PATHOGENESIS

The pathology of onchocerciasis [7,21–23] is manifested primarily in the skin, lymph nodes, and eye. Definition of pathological changes associated with *O. volvulus* infection remains incomplete, particularly for ocular lesions, as pathological material is very scarce and often shows end-stage disease.

In the skin, microfilariae are most frequently seen in the upper dermis, characteristically with no evidence of a surrounding tissue reaction. Aside from microfilariae in the dermis, early changes include localization of inflammatory cells around vessels and dermal appendages and an increase in dermal fibroblasts and mast cells. Subsequent changes include hyperkeratosis, focal parakeratosis, acanthosis with melanophores and increased mucin in the upper dermis, accompanied by dilated lymphatics and tortuous upper dermis vessels. This process ultimately leads to loss of elastic fibers and progressive fibrosis. End-state disease is characterized by advanced atrophy of the epidermis with loss of rete ridges; only very thin layers of epidermis and keratin remain overlying the dermis.

Over a period of months to years, adult worms become encased in a rim of host tissue, thus forming the characteristic subcutaneous nodules (onchocercomata). This rim is composed of hyalinized and vascularized scar tissues surrounding the adult worms and variable amounts of chronic inflammatory elements including fibrin, plasma cells, neutrophilic and eosinophilic granulocytes, lymphocytes, giant cells, and Russell bodies. Some nodules contain only necrotic material with liquefied and sometimes partially calcified remnants of adult worms.

The pathology of lymph nodes from Africans infected with *O. volvulus* consists of scarring of lymphoid areas, with sinus histiocytosis and infiltration with inflammatory cells. In contrast, lymph nodes from infected Yemenites show follicular hyperplasia.

In the ocular tissues, the bulbar conjunctiva shows an infiltrate of plasma cells, eosinophils, and mast cells with hyperemia and dilatation of vessels and some vessel thickening and perivascular fibrosis. Punctate keratitis has been shown on corneal biopsy to consist of a collection of inflammatory cells surrounding a degenerating microfilaria [24]. Sclerosing keratitis shows scarring, chronic inflammation, and vascularization. The pathology of anterior uveitis and chorioretinitis reflects a low-grade chronic nongranulomatous inflammatory process.

The pathogenesis of disease manifestations in onchocerciasis is largely unknown. The only exception, as alluded to above, is punctate keratitis, which on biopsy has been shown to represent an inflammatory focus surrounding dead or dying microfilariae. However, these lesions are transitory and resolve completely, and any direct relation of microfilariae to other tissue lesions remains speculative. Nevertheless, because of their vast numbers and wide distribution throughout the body, as well as the clinical correlation between microfilaria counts and complications, microfilariae are thought to cause, directly or indirectly, most of the disease manifestations. It is believed that the host immune response, including a contribution of immediate hypersensitivity, immune complex deposition, products of activated lymphoid cells, and perhaps autoantibodies and cytotoxic T cells, is largely responsible for the disease.

CLINICAL MANIFESTATIONS

The major disease manifestations are dermatitis, onchocercomata, lymphadenitis, and visual impairment or blindness. The frequency of these features varies according to duration and intensity of exposure and geographical location. However, comprehensive controlled surveys establishing the prevalence of onchocerciasis morbidity are not available.

Skin

The most frequent manifestation of onchocercal dermatitis is pruritus. In lightly infected persons, this may persist as the only symptom. The pruritus can be unrelenting and incapacitating, even through microfilariae in the skin may be very sparse or not detectable except by extensive skin snipping. In addition, transitory localized areas of edema and erythema may occur in any part of the body. Over a period of years, most persons with significant infections will develop premature and exaggerated wrinkling of the skin, which has been associated with accelerated loss of elastic fibers. Atrophy of the epidermis with loss of elastic fibers can lead to loose, redundant skin. Pronounced atrophy of the skin (Fig. 49-2) was seen in 13 and 22 percent of individuals with rain forest and savannah infection, respectively, in Cameroon [25]. Changes in pigmentation with hypo- or hyperpigmentation is another sign seen frequently in the absence of more serious changes. Skin depigmentation (Fig. 49-3) was seen in 20 percent of persons in the rain forest in Cameroon, but in only 1 percent or less with savannah-type infection [25]. In Central America, premature wrinkling of the superior aspect of the pinna of the ear is a frequent finding, and thickening of the skin of the face, par-

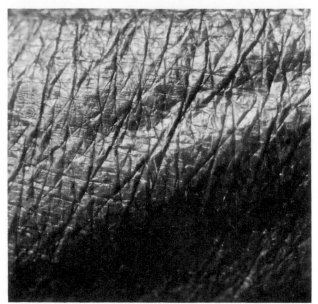

Figure 49-2. Premature atrophy of skin on the forearm in *O. volvulus* infection.

ticularly noticeable in the earlobes, or leonine facies is seen in long-standing infection.

A localized eczematoid dermatitis with hyperkeratosis, scaling, and pigmentary changes (Fig. 49-4) occurs with variable

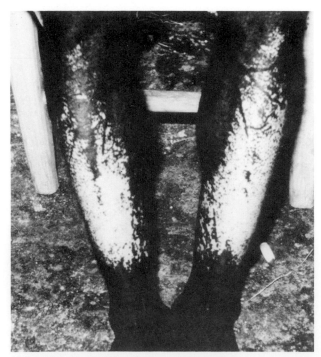

Figure 49-3. Depigmentation due to onchocerciasis.

severity. Such lesions are commonly seen in the lower extremities but in some cases are quite extensive. They can become superinfected, particularly with repeated trauma or excoriation.

Onchocercomata

These subcutaneous nodules, which may be visible or palpable, contain the adult worms. In Africa, these are found particularly over the coccyx and sacrum, the trochanter of the femur, and the lateral and anterior iliac crests. Other common locations include various bony prominences such as the skin overlying the bony thorax, the paraspinous areas, the medial and lateral aspects of the elbow or knee, and the head. In Central American onchocerciasis, nodules tend to be distributed preferentially about the head, neck, and shoulders, but when sought are also found frequently in other areas of the body, as in Africa. Nodules vary in size from a few millimeters and barely palpable to several centimeters in diameter. On palpation they are firm, nontender, and have variable mobility depending on degree of adherence to bony structures. Very young nodules may be soft and nondistinct owing to a lack of surrounding fibrous tissue; conversely, very old nodules may be fluctuant as a result of necrosis and liquefaction of contents.

Lymph nodes

Lymphadenopathy of a mild to moderate degree is frequent, particularly in the inguinal and femoral areas in Africans. For example, inguinal and/or femoral lymphadenopathy were grossly visible in 40 and 26 percent of persons with rain forest and savannah infection, respectively, in Cameroon [25]. Involved nodes are typically firm and nontender. Occasionally lymph node enlargement reaches massive proportions and can be associated with evidence of local lymphatic obstruction. Often this is associated with severe dermatitis in the edematous limb. Enlarged inguinal or femoral nodes and surrounding fluid may become dependent (''hanging groin'') (Fig. 49-5), and may predispose to hernia formation in the inguinal and femoral areas [26].

Ocular tissues

Visual impairment is the major complication of onchocerciasis, usually seen only in persons with moderate or heavy levels of infection. Lesions occur in all parts of the eye.

Conjunctiva. Conjunctivitis with photophobia is a common early finding, particularly in young persons. It does not lead to permanent sequelae.

Cornea. Punctate keratitis occurs as an acute inflammatory infiltrate surrounding dying microfilariae, manifest as ''snowflake'' opacities (Fig. 49-6). Such opacities were seen in 15 percent of persons with rain forest infection and 10 percent of those with the savannah type [25]. These lesions are most

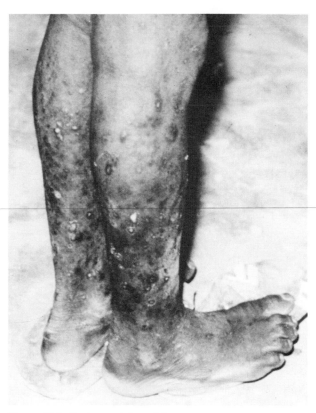

Figure 49-4. Onchocercal dermatitis.

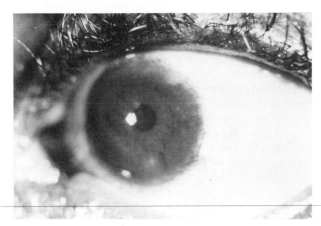

Figure 49-6. Punctate keratitis related to microfilarial invasion of the cornea. (*Courtesy of Dr. Hugh R. Taylor.*)

frequent in younger age groups and resolve without apparent sequelae. Sclerosing keratitis of a mild to moderate degree occurs in approximately 5 percent of persons with savannah-type infection and 1 percent of those with the forest strain, while severe sclerosing keratitis (Fig. 49-7) occurs in 1 to 4 percent of those with savannah strain but is less common in those infected with the forest strain [25]. It is the leading cause of onchocercal blindness in the savannah areas of Africa. Sclerosing keratitis begins at the limbus and progresses inward, leading to irreversible visual impairment.

Anterior Uveal Tract. Anterior uveitis and iridocyclitis occur in roughly 5 percent of all infected persons in Africa [25]. Complications of anterior uveal tract involvement (e.g., pupillary deformity) are particularly prominent relative to other causes of impaired vision in Central American onchocerciasis [27]. Uveal tract involvement can also lead to secondary glaucoma, although without this complication intraocular pres-

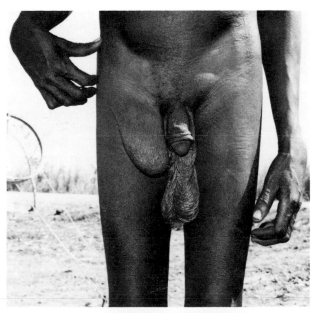

Figure 49-5. Onchocercal lymphadenitis in the femoral region with adenocele formation. (*AFIP negative no. 70-3172.*)

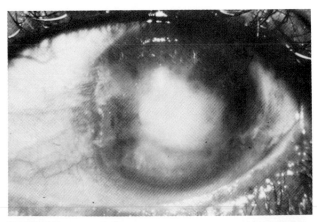

Figure 49-7. Advanced sclerosing keratitis in *O. volvulus* infection. (*Courtesy of Dr. Hugh R. Taylor.*)

sure in onchocerciasis is reported to be lower than in a control group [28].

Chorioretinal Lesions. Characteristic lesions have been described (Fig. 49-8), with atrophy of the retinal pigment epithelium and of the choriocapillaris and hyperpigmentation of the pigment epithelial layer [29]. These changes were seen in about 5 percent of infected persons in both the rain forest and savannah in Cameroon [25]. Chorioretinal lesions are more frequently a cause of blindness in the forest areas of Africa than is sclerosing keratitis.

Optic Nerve Lesions. Constriction of the visual fields and frank optic atrophy may occur as part of the natural disease process. Primary changes in the optic disk related to *O. volvulus* infection occur in about 2 percent of infected persons in Africa [25]. Therapy with diethylcarbamazine and possibly suramin may account for many instances of optic nerve damage [30,31].

SYSTEMIC MANIFESTATIONS

Some heavily infected individuals show wasting and generalized weakness, with loss of adipose tissue and muscle mass [32]. Such persons may be at increased risk of other infections such as tuberculosis. In persons who become blind, there is a three- to fourfold increased mortality rate in adults beyond the fourth decade [33]. Although microfilariae have been found in most major internal organs at autopsy, there is no convincing evidence that significant organ dysfunction occurs as a consequence of this widespread infestation.

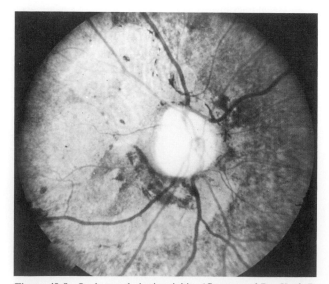

Figure 49-8. Onchocercal chorioretinitis. (*Courtesy of Dr. Hugh R. Taylor.*)

DIAGNOSIS

Diagnosis of onchocerciasis is based principally on parasitological techniques, particularly demonstration of microfilariae in the skin. Microfilariae in the cornea or anterior chamber may also reveal the diagnosis. The most convenient method for skin biopsy is to use a sclerocorneal punch, to obtain an essentially blood-free biopsy which extends just below the epidermis to the tips of the dermal papillae. Alternatively, a razor blade can be used to shave off the tip of a dome of skin created by elevation with straight pin. The biopsy specimen is gently blotted and weighed. The tissue fragment is then incubated in tissue-culture medium or in saline in a flat-bottom microtiter plate or on a glass slide, and the emergent microfilariae are counted after 2 to 4 h or overnight incubation. In Africa, it is customary to take biopsies from the scapular, gluteal, and calf areas, while in Central America the deltoids are substituted for the calves.

The value of the skin-snip examination lies in the fact that it can provide both a definitive diagnosis and some quantification of the intensity of infection. One hundred or more microfilariae per milligram of skin indicates heavy infection and implies a significant risk of serious complications. The disadvantages of the skin-snip examination include low sensitivity in lightly infected cases or those with severe dermatitis, its inherently cumbersome nature, and imprecision in defining intensity of infection. It is important to note that the much smaller microfilariae of *Dipetalonema streptocerca* can also be found in the skin in the African rain forest and can be confused with those of *O. volvulus* [8].

The reaction which persons with *O. volvulus* infection often experience subsequent to a single 50-mg dose of diethylcarbamazine (DEC), the Mazzotti reaction [34], has been proposed as a diagnostic test. While this provocative test is a highly sensitive means of detecting infected persons, false-negative reactions do occur and it may precipitate serious complications, particularly in heavily infected individuals. It cannot be recommended as a routine diagnostic procedure.

Histopathological examination of an excised nodule can yield the diagnosis, and a small percentage of individuals with negative skin biopsies will have palpable nodules which can be excised. In addition, several serodiagnostic tests for onchocerciasis have been described, including an indirect fluorescent antibody test using microfilariae as targets, and more recently enzyme-linked immunosorbent assays. However, the sensitivity and specificity of such serodiagnostic tests for clinical and epidemiological surveys remain to be established. Similarly, several antigen preparations for intradermal tests have been developed, but further evaluation of their potential utility is required.

MANAGEMENT

The major goals of therapy of infected individuals are to prevent irreversible ocular and skin lesions and to alleviate distressing symptoms, particularly pruritus. DEC and suramin, the two traditional drugs for treatment of onchocerciasis, can cause serious systemic complications and ocular damage, including optic atrophy. Ivermectin, a newly developed drug [35], is not associated with these complications and is now the drug of choice for onchocerciasis.

Ivermectin

Ivermectin, a semisynthetic macrocyclic lactone, has been extensively tested in human onchocerciasis over the past few years and is now considered the drug of choice [35–37]. The advantages of this drug over DEC are: (1) it can be given in a single dose orally; (2) it causes little or no systemic and ocular reaction; and (3) it appears to suppress microfilariae in the skin and eye for a more prolonged period of time than does DEC, and therefore can be given on a yearly basis.

Ivermectin is given orally on an empty stomach and at least 2 h before the next meal in a single dose of 150 μg/kg. Following treatment, most persons have little or no reaction. Approximately 1 to 10 percent of persons will develop cutaneous edema and pruritus, with or without a maculopapular rash characteristic of the Mazzotti reaction (*vide infra*), and rare individuals will develop bullous lesions over the extremities or in the groin area which carry the risk of septic complications if skin breakdown occurs. Symptomatic hypotension develops in about 1 person per 10,000, and rarely may require intravenous fluids and additional supportive measures. Significant ocular reactions are rare. The frequency and severity of reactions following ivermectin treatment appears to vary directly with the intensity of infection.

Contraindications to ivermectin treatment include pregnancy; breast feeding within the first 3 months following delivery; central nervous system disorders including, in particular, meningitis or other illnesses that may increase penetration of ivermectin into the central nervous system; allergy to the drug; and age less than 5 years.

Following treatment with ivermectin, it is recommended that skin-snips be taken on a 6-monthly to yearly basis in the individual patient to document the effect and establish the need for retreatment. The need for repeated ocular examination depends upon the type and extent of ocular involvement at the beginning of treatment. Ordinarily, ivermectin should be given yearly. In mass campaigns in which individual diagnosis will not be carried out, treatment on a yearly basis of all those likely to be infected is recommended.

Diethylcarbamazine (DEC)

DEC treatment results in rapid and massive killing of a majority of microfilariae over a period of a few days. In association with this microfilaricidal action, most individuals experience a number of adverse effects and, in some cases, serious complications. The early side effects include pruritus, painful swelling of lymph nodes (particularly femoral, inguinal, and axillary), rash, fever, headache, nausea and vomiting, and occasionally vertigo, arthralgias, and myalgias. Cardiovascular collapse has also been described. Frequent early ocular effects include conjunctivitis, punctate keratitis, limbitis, and anterior uveitis. These are usually accompanied by photophobia. The delayed complications which may result in permanently impaired vision include optic neuritis or optic atrophy and chorioretinal scars [30,38]. Although the frequency of delayed complications affecting vision is not precisely known, in one study optic atrophy or visual-field constriction was seen in 3 of 10 individuals with forest-strain infection [38], and in another study visual-field constriction was found in 5 of 18 persons with Sudan-savannah infection [39].

There are two means of reducing the severity of the DEC reaction. The first is to begin therapy with a test dose, e.g., 25 to 50 mg on the first day. If the test dose is tolerated, DEC is then continued for 2 weeks at 3 to 4 mg/(kg·day) in two daily doses. Secondly, the use of moderate doses of corticosteroids, when started 24 to 48 h before therapy, significantly blunts the reaction. Whether to use corticosteroids depends on the likelihood of a severe reaction, which can be predicted in part by the intensity of infection. Thus, individuals with heavy infections (100 or more microfilariae per milligram of skin) are at high risk and should receive corticosteroid pretreatment (e.g., dexamethazone 2 to 4 mg twice daily) and a 25-mg test dose of DEC. Steroids are tapered over 3 to 4 days after the reaction has waned, usually in 4 to 7 days. Aspirin can be very useful in the less severe reactions. Although the acute symptomatic reaction to DEC therapy can be minimized using these measures, it is not yet known whether the incidence of residual permanent complications, particularly optic nerve changes, is also reduced.

During the acute phase of the reaction, it is important to provide for adequate observation of the patient, including measurement of vital signs if the reaction is severe. Further, fluid and nutritional support must be maintained. A topical ophthalmic mydriatic and topical steroid may be necessary for anterior uveitis.

Treatment with DEC results in a profound decrease in microfilaria counts in the skin and usually in the cornea and anterior chamber. Unfortunately, this effect is short-lived, as repopulation with microfilariae occures over approximately 6 to 18 months. Further, efforts to avoid repopulation with chronic suppressive doses of DEC have been plagued by frequent adverse reactions, complications, and poor compliance. Thus, it is apparent that mass chemotherapy of onchocerciasis cannot rely on DEC alone unless a safe means of preventing the adverse effects and complications associated with DEC therapy can be found. In the individual, DEC should be given only if ivermectin is contraindicated or unavailable and there is a clear need for treatment.

Suramin

Suramin is a proven and potent macrofilaricidal agent, but it has major toxicity and must be given intravenously in repeated doses. Therefore, its use is restricted to the rare individual with moderate to heavy levels of infection who is leaving the endemic area and who cannot take repeated doses of ivermectin. Because suramin also has significant microfilaricidal action which can lead to adverse effects similar to those seen with DEC, it is suggested that a full course of DEC be given prior to suramin therapy in order to first eliminate microfilariae. It is now apparent that suramin can be given with good results and less toxicity in lower doses than previously thought necessary. Because of the rare occurrence of idiosyncratic anaphylactoid reactions, a test dose of 1 mg is given intravenously, then 50 mg after 1 min, and another 50 mg after another minute. Subsequently, weekly doses starting with 0.2 g and increasing by 0.2-g increments are given until a total of 60 to 70 mg/kg is given [40] For a complete cure, one or two additional weekly doses of 15 mg/kg each should be given.

Because of suramin's prominent nephrotoxicity, the urinalysis must be followed carefully, looking particularly for proteinuria and granular casts, and the serum creatinine level should be followed serially. Severe prostration, prolonged diarrhea, exfoliative dermatitis, and high fever may also necessitate cessation of therapy. Reactions similar to those described for DEC may occur as a consequence of microfilarial killing. In addition, swelling, as well as pain and occasionally abscess formation, may occur after death of the adult worms.

Nodulectomy

Surgical excision should be performed whenever nodules are detected in the head region. Although not mandatory, it is advisable to remove accessible nodules in other areas as well unless drug therapy designed to kill adult worms is to be employed.

POPULATION

EPIDEMIOLOGY

There are an estimated 20 million persons worldwide infected with *O. volvulus* [41]. The vast majority live in equatorial Africa in a belt that extends for more than 6000 km from a far western Atlantic coast to the Red Sea. The Guatemalan and Mexican foci of about 70,000 infected persons, located at altitudes of 500 to 1500 m on the Pacific slope of the Sierra Madre, and the Venezuelan focus of about 20,000, constitute the bulk of the remainder. Smaller foci have been found in Colombia, Brazil, Ecuador, Yemen, and Saudi Arabia.

A minority of persons with *O. volvulus* infection have demonstrable disease. The prevalence of blindness, the major complication, is estimated at 1 to 4 percent or less, though in some hyperendemic villages 30 percent or more of adults may be blinded. Although the adult worms of *O. volvulus* do not multiply in the host, with repeated exposure the adult worm burden and the microfilaria counts mount progressively over the years. Age-specific prevalence and intensity of infection

are greater in males than females, presumably reflecting greater exposure related to work habits.

Onchocerciasis occurs in foci which are determined by the relation of the population to *Simulium* breeding sites. The level of endemicity depends upon distance from larval and pupal habitats, the hyperendemic zones lying within a few kilometers. The risk of disease transmission in a given area is determined by the number of fly bites and the proportion of flies harboring infective larvae. This is established by observation of the number of bites an individual is subject to over an 11-h period, with dissection of trapped flies to determine infectivity. The exposure risk is expressed quantitatively as the annual transmission potential (ATP) [42] which is obtained by totaling the monthly results from the following formula:

$$\frac{\text{No. of flies caught} \times \text{no. of infective larvae}}{\text{No. of flies dissected}}$$
$$\times \frac{\text{no. of days in month}}{\text{no. of days worked}}$$

Similary, the annual biting rate (ABR) is the annual total of monthly biting rates obtained as follows:

$$\frac{\text{No. of flies caught} \times \text{no. of days in month}}{\text{No. of days worked}}$$

These indexes provide some quantification of the exposure risk in a given area, and this in turn relates to the level of endemicity and the prevalence of complications. For example, in one study in the savannah zone in west Africa, an ATP of 500 was associated with no blindness, while an ATP of 2900 was found in a village with a blindness rate of 10 percent [43]. In areas in which vector control is being attempted, the ATP and ABR are also utilized to measure effectiveness. In hyperendemic areas, the prevalence of ocular complications and blindness increases progressively from approximately age 20. The risk of ocular complications relates more closely to the intensity of infection, as measured by the ATP, than to the prevalence. That is, although the prevalence of infection tends to plateau beyond a given intensity of exposure, the risk of ocular complications continues to increase as the ATP increases [44].

CONTROL

There are two major means of control of onchocerciasis: (1) elimination of the vector, and (2) chemotherapy to reduce morbidity associated with infection in the human host. Other approaches worthy of mention include nodulectomy to reduce the adult worm burden and avoidance of the vector.

Vector control

The potential of vector control as a means of containment of onchocerciasis is dependent on a number of local factors. These include the size, number, and accessibility of larval and pupal habitats; the proximity of other foci of onchocerciasis which may serve as a source of reinvading flies; the topography and vegetation; rainfall patterns; and the dynamics of transmission. Such factors must be carefully assessed for each area or major focus if vector control is to be considered.

Vector control has been attempted in Africa over the past several decades with mixed results. Perhaps the most spectacular success was achieved in a program to eradicate onchocerciasis from Kenya which was begun in the early 1950s, relying on the use of DDT. This effort was aided by the fact that *S. neavei* has a limited flight range, as well as the association of larvae and pupae with riverine crabs, which simplified surveys of breeding sites. By far the most massive campaign against the fly vector is now ongoing in the Volta River Basin and surrounding areas, the Onchocerciasis Control Program (OCP) [45,46]. Vector control commenced in 1975, and by 1977 the entire originally designated control area, comprising 654,000 km^2, was involved. Since the maximum lifespan of adult worms is estimated at 15 to 18 years, the initial plan was to continue vector control for 20 years. Because of evidence of reinvasion from south of the control area by flies carried on monsoon winds, the area was extended in the years 1978 to 1979 to include another 110,000 km^2 in Ivory Coast, and a westward extension is underway. Control is based on the aerial distribution of the larvicide temephos on a 7-day cycle. It is important to note that aerial spraying would not have been feasible had it not been for the relatively large size of the waterways which constitute larval and pupal habitats. This represents a major advantage to the OCP, one which does not exist in a large proportion of the remaining onchocerciasis endemic areas in Africa or in the mountainous terrain of Central America. At the end of the first 5-year period the control program had achieved considerable success, with a reduction of the ATP and ABR to less than 100 and 1000, respectively, in 80 percent of the control area. These levels are associated with negligible risk of blindness, and ocular disease is indeed declining [46]. Nevertheless, there are major threats to the OCP including emerging resistance to temephos, requiring use of more expensive alternative agents, reinvasion from outside the control area, and excessive expense [10]. The lack of suitable means of mass chemotherapy has also frustrated the effort to control the infection in the human host, but the availability of ivermectin shows promise in this regard. Finally, although vector control may be quite beneficial over a period of time in areas of high endemicity with breeding sites which are vulnerable to attack, a large proportion of endemic areas are not suited to this means of control based on current technology.

Chemotherapy

Treatment to prevent or limit complications of onchocerciasis has been severely impeded by the lack of safe and effective chemotherapy. Although DEC combined with suramin can lead to a cure in the individual, proper administration of such a regimen is extremely time consuming and therefore not practical for mass therapy. Ivermectin in yearly single doses may prove a viable means of chemotherapeutic control of disease [37]. Furthermore, ivermectin may have an effect on transmission of infection [47]. No drug has yet been shown to be an effective prophylactic agent against infective larvae of *O. volvulus*.

Nodulectomy

Surgical extirpation of head nodules as a means of control has been practiced in Mexico and Guatemala since the 1930s. Although tthere is no evidence of a decrease in the prevalence of infection, it is possible that the nodulectomy program has reduced the prevalence of blindness from onchocerciasis [41]. In Africa, surgical removal of all accessible nodules resulted in a significant decrease in skin microfilaria counts 2 years later [49]. There may also be some long-term benefit to reducing the adult worm burden. However, as nodulectomy is extremely labor intensive and therefore costly, it cannot yet be recommended as a general method for control. Nevertheless, most authorities agree that any nodules in the head region, because of their proximity to the eyes, should be removed.

Avoidance of the vector

Even though in theory it is possible to minimize *Simulium* bites by avoiding fly-infested areas in the morning and evening and by wearing protective garments, it is unlikely that such measures will achieve significant success for the indigenous populations in the near future. Experience indicates that under present socioeconomic conditions, the population at risk cannot or will not alter their lifestyle to avoid being bitten and cannot afford, or will not wear, protective clothing. In some instances, relocation of entire villages to an area remote from breeding sites has been utilized as a last resort.

REFERENCES

1 Prost A: Latence parasitaire dans l'onchocercose. Bull WHO 58: 923–925, 1980
2 Nelson GS, Pester FRN: The identification of infective filarial larvae in Simuliidae. Bull WHO 27:473–481, 1962
3 Blacklock DB: The development of *Onchocerca volvulus* in *Simulium damnosum*. Ann Trop Med Parasitol 20:1–48, 1926
4 Neafie RC: Morpohology of *Onchocerca volvulus*. Am J Clin Pathol 57:574–586, 1972
5 Albiez EJ: Klinische und parasitologische untersuchungen der knoten bei der Onchozerkose in Westafrika. Dissertation dem Fachbereich Medizin der Universität Hamburg, 1978, p 66
6 Gibson CL: Comparative morphology of the skin-inhabiting microfilariae of man, cattle, and equines in Guatemala. Am J Trop Med Hyg 1:250–261, 1952
7 Gibson DW, Heggie C, Connor DH: Clinical and pathologic aspects of Onchocerciasis, in Somers SC, Rosen PP (eds): *Pathology Annual*, part 2, 15:195–240, 1980

8 Buck AA (ed): *Onchocerciasis.* Geneva, World Health Organization, 1974, p 19

9 Collins RC: Onchocerciasis transmission potentials of four species of Guatemalan Simuliidae. Am J Trop Med Hyg 28:72–75, 1979

10 Report of the WHO Independent Commission on the Long-term Prospects of the Onchocerciasis Control Programme. Geneva, World Health Organization, 1981, pp 1–77

11 Duke BOL, Lewis DJ, Moore PJ: *Onchocerca-Simulium* complexes. I. Transmission of forest and Sudan-savanna strains of *Onchocerca volvulus*, from Cameroon, by *Simulium damnosum* from various West African bioclimatic zones. Ann Trop Med 60:318–336, 1966

12 Mackenzie CD: Eosinophil leucocytes in filarial infections. Trans R Soc Trop Med Hyg 74(suppl):51–58, 1980

13 Greene BM, Taylor HR, Aikawa M: Cellular killing of microfilariae of *Onchocerca volvulus*: Eosinophil and neutrophil-mediated immune serum-dependent destruction. J Immunol 127:1611–1618, 1981

14 Greene BM, Gbakima AA, Albiez EJ, et al: The humoral and cellular immune response to *Onchocerca volvulus* in man. Rev Infect Dis 7:789–795, 1985

15 Ottesen EA: Immediate hypersensitivity responses in the immunopathogenesis of human onchocerciasis. Rev Infect Dis 7:796–801, 1985

16 Prost A, Nebout M, Rougemont A: Lepromatous leprosy and onchocerciasis. Br Med J 1:589–590, 1979

17 Buck AA, Anderson RI, Kawata K, et al: Onchocerciasis: Some new epidemiologic and clinical findings. Am J Trop Med Hyg 18:217–230, 1969

18 Greene BM, Fanning MM, Ellner JJ: Non-specific suppression of antigen-induced lymphocyte blastogenesis in *Onchocerca volvulus* infection in man. Clin Exp Immunol 52:259–265, 1983

19 Gallin M, Edmonds K, Ellner JJ, et al: Cell-mediated immune responses in human infection with *Onchocerca volvulus*. J Immunol 140:1999–2007, 1988

20 Ward DJ, Nutman TB, Zea-Flores G, et al: Onchocerciasis and immunity in humans: Enhanced T cell responsiveness to parasite antigen in putatively immune individuals. J Infect Dis 157:536–543, 1988

21 Connor DH, Neafie RC: Onchocerciasis, in Binford CH, Connor DH (ed): *Pathology of Tropical and Extraordinary Diseases*, vol 2, sect 8, 3:360–372, Washington, D.C., Armed Forces Institute of Pathology, 1976

22 Anderson J, Font RL: Ocular onchocerciasis, in Binford CH, Connor DH (eds): *Pathology of Tropical and Extraordinary Diseases*, vol 2, section 8, 3:373–381. Washington, D.C., Armed Forces Institute of Pathology, 1976

23 Connor DH, Goerge GH, Gibson DW: Pathologic changes of human onchocerciasis: implications for future research. Rev Infect Dis 7:809–819, 1985

24 Rodger FC: The dissolution of microfilariae of *Onchocerca volvulus* in the human eye and its effect on the tissues. Trans R Soc Trop Med Hyg 53:400–403, 1959

25 Anderson J, Fuglsang H, Hamilton PJS, et al: Studies on onchocerciasis in the United Cameroon Republic. I. Comparison of populations with and without *Onchocerca volvulus*. Trans R Soc Trop Med Hyg 68(3):190–208, 1974

26 Nelson GS: ''Hanging Groin'' and hernia, complications of onchocerciasis. Trans R Soc Trop Med Hyg 52:272–275, 1958

27 Choyce DP: Ocular onchocerciasis in Central American, Africa and British Isles. Trans R Soc Trop Med Hyg 58:11–36, 1964

28 Thylefors B, Duppenthaler JL: Epidemiological aspects of intraocular pressure in an onchocerciasis endemic area. Bull WHO 57:963–969, 1979

29 Bird AC, Anderson J, Fuglsang H: Morphology of posterior segment lesions of the eye in patients with onchocerciasis. Br J Ophthalmol 60:2–20, 1976

30 Anderson J, Fuglsang H: Effects of diethylcarbamazine on ocular onchocerciasis. Tropenmed Parasitol 27:263–278, 1976

31 Thylefors B, Rolland A: The risk of optic atrophy following suramin treatment of ocular onchocerciasis. Bull WHO 57:479–480, 1979

32 Buck AA, Anderson RI, Colston AC Jr: Microfilaruria in onchocerciasis. Bull WHO 45:353–369, 1971

33 Kirkwood B, Smith P, Marshall T, et al: Relationship between mortality, visual acuity and microfilarial load in the area of the Onchocerciasis Control Programme. Trans R Soc Trop Med Hyg 77:862–871, 1983

34 Mazzotti L: Posibilidad de utilizar como medio diagnostico auxiliar en la oncocercosis las reacciones alergicas consecutivas a la administracion del ''Hetrazan.'' Rev Inst Salub Enferm Trop 19:235–237, 1948

35 Greene BM, Taylor HR, Cupp EW, et al: Comparison of ivermectin and diethylcarbamazine in the treatment of onchocerciasis. N Engl J Med 313:133–138, 1985

36 White AT, Newland HS, Taylor HR, et al: Controlled trial and dose finding study of ivermectin for treatment of onchocerciasis. J Infect Dis 156:463–470, 1987

37 Greene BM, White AT, Newland HS, et al: Single dose therapy with ivermectin for onchocerciasis. Trans Assoc Am Phys, in press

38 Taylor HR, Greene BM: Ocular changes with oral and transepidermal diethylcarbamazine therapy of onchocerciasis. Br J Ophthalmol 65:494–502, 1981

39 Bird AC, Sheikh HE, Anderson J, et al: Changes in visual function and in the posterior segment of the eye during treatment of onchocerciasis with diethylcarbamazine citrate. Br J Ophthalmol 64:191–200, 1980

40 Rougemont A, Thylefors B, Duncan M, et al: Traitement de l'onchocercose par la suramine à faibles doses progressive dan les collectivités hyperendémiques d'Afrique occidentale. I. Résultats parasitologiques et surveillance ophtalmologique en zone transmission non interrompue. Bull WHO 58:917–922, 1980

41 WHO Expert Committee on Onchocerciasis: Third report. Geneva, World Health Organization, 1987

42 Duke BOL: Studies on factors influencing the transmission of onchocerciasis. IV. The biting cycles, infective biting density, and transmission potential of forest *Simulium damnosum*. Ann Trop Med Parasitol 62:95–106, 1968

43 Duke BOL, Anderson J, Fuglsang H: The *Onchocerca volvulus* transmission potentials and associated patterns of onchocerciasis at four Cameroon Sudan-savanna villages. Tropenmed Parasitol 16:143–154, 1975

44 Thylefors B, Philippon B, Prost A: Transmission potentials of *Onchocerca volvulus* and the associated intensity of onchocerciasis in a Sudan-savanna area. Tropenmed Parasitol 29:346–354, 1978

45 Walsh JF, Davies JB, LeBerre R: Entomological aspects of the first five years of the onchocerciasis control programme in the Volta River Basin. Tropenmed Parasitol 30:328–344, 1979

46 Dadzie KY, Remme J, Rolland A, et al: The effect of 7–8 years of vector control on the evolution of ocular onchocerciasis in West African savanna. Trop Med Parasitol 37:263–270, 1986

47 Cupp EW, Bernardo MJ, Kiszewski AE, et al: The effects of ivermectin on transmission of *Onchocerca volvulus*. Science 231:740–742, 1986

48 Marroquin HF: Robles' disease (American onchocerciasis) in Gua-temala, in *Research and Control of Onchocerciasis in the Western Hemisphere*, Proceedings of an International Symposium, Scientific Publication no. 298, Washington D.C., Pan American Health Organization, 1974, pp 100–104

49 Albiez EJ: Effects of a single complete nodulectomy on nodule burden and microfilarial density two years later. Trop Med Parasitol 36:17–20, 1985

CHAPTER 50 / *Dracunculiasis* · Donald R. Hopkins

The antiquity of this infection is attested to by the fact that evidence of the 2- to 3-foot-long guinea worms have been found in Egyptian mummies. Indeed, the time-honored practice of extracting the worm by slowly winding it around a stick is thought by some to be the origin of the caduceus and the staff of Aesculepius, the ancient symbols of the healing arts. Apart from the worm's dramatic appearance and the wretched status of its victims, however, this disease's contemporary significance derives from its severe adverse effects on agriculture in endemic areas, which effects are a direct result of the prolonged, painful incapacitation that the worm causes in large numbers of farmers at crucial times in the agricultural year. Since 1986, this disease has been targeted by the World Health Organization as the next disease to be eradicated after smallpox.

PARASITE

Dracunculiasis (dracontiasis, dracunculosis, guinea worm disease) is acquired only by drinking water containing small crustaceans called copepods, which themselves have been infected by the larval stage of the parasite. Once water containing the infected copepods has been ingested, the digestive juices of the human host kill the copepods, thereby liberating the larvae, which penetrate the stomach or intestine and enter the abdominal cavity, where they apparently mature. After about 3 months, the mature worms mate, after which the male worms die, leaving the females to grow to their full length of about 1 m. The adult female worms are about 0.2 cm in diameter. About 1 year after the contaminated water was drunk, the fully mature female worms raise a blister on the skin usually of the lower leg, ankle, or foot. When the affected part of the body is placed in cool water the blister ruptures, leaving an ulcer at its base, through which the worm ejects hundreds of thousands of larvae as it slowly emerges.

Larvae released by the worm into fresh water must be ingested by an appropriate carnivorous species of copepod (*Cy-clops*) in order to survive. In the copepod, the first-stage larvae undergo two molts within about 2 weeks at ambient tropical temperatures, after which they are infective to humans if their host copepod is ingested. The larvae themselves are too small to be seen by the naked eye, although the copepods can barely be seen as darting flecks if water containing them is held up to a strong light.

Cyclops are widely distributed in nature, worldwide, although the species of *Dracunculus* that infects humans does not appear to have any natural animal host or reservoir except humans. Dogs especially have been suspected of possibly being a reservoir host of the parasite, but even in areas such as the southern Soviet Union, where this disease was eliminated in the 1920s, *Dracunculus medinensis* has not sustained itself in dogs and reinfected humans. Other species of *Dracunculus* infect various wildlife such as raccoons and foxes. The parasite of humans, *D. medinensis,* has been maintained experimentally in rhesus monkeys. Recently, scientists have developed a more practical animal model by infecting ferrets with *D. insignis.*

Morphologically, the adult female worm is about 60 to 100 cm long and 1.5 to 2.0 mm in diameter. The worm's exterior cuticle is creamy-white, smooth, and round. The anterior end of the worm is rounded, with a triangular mouth connected to a small alimentary canal. The mouth is surrounded by two circles of papillae which are the source of the toxic secretion that causes a blister on the skin of the host when the worm begins to emerge. A narrow nerve ring surrounding the lower esophagus is followed externally by two lateral cervical papillae. Most of the worm's interior is taken up by a double uterus filled with millions of larvae, with a double ovary and oviducts at the rear end of the worm.

The male parasite is much smaller and does not live after mating. The tiny, cross-striated, rhabditiform larvae measure about 500 to 700 μm in length, and are flat, with a blunt, rounded anterior and narrow "tail." They contain an alimentary canal with a bulbous esophagus and an anus.

PATIENT

CLINICAL MANIFESTATIONS AND PATHOLOGY

Usually the first sign of the infection after the year-long incubation period is the painful blister which the female worm causes at the site where she is ready to emerge (Fig. 50-1). Patients in endemic areas know that they can relieve the pain from the blister by immersing the affected part of their body into cold fresh water—which of course is exactly what the worm wants them to do. Sometimes the adult worm is first manifest by appearing as a serpiginous line just under the skin. On other occasions, the worm appears at the center of an abscess.

Before the worm produces the blister, there is usually no histological reaction to the adult parasite. Once the worm begins to emerge, however, an infiltration of inflammatory cells may be observed around the body of the worm in the tissues. This inflammatory reaction is apparently the reason why the worm cannot just be pulled out of the body unless an incision is made down to a worm just under the skin before it begins to emerge on its own.

Some worms fail to emerge at all, in which case they die in the body, producing an abscess, or they are either resorbed or calcify. In the latter instance, the only sign that the individual has been infected will be a bizarre but characteristic appearance of the calcified worm(s) on x-ray.

Most patients have only one worm to emerge in any "guinea worm season." However, some especially unfortunate victims may have as many as two dozen worms or more emerge at the same time. And although most worms emerge through the skin on the lower leg, the parasites sometimes emerge from any part of the body—scalp, chest, breast, abdomen, scrotum, vagina, or wherever. Worms that find their way into the spinal cord, heart, or other vital organs will cause commensurably serious or even fatal complications.

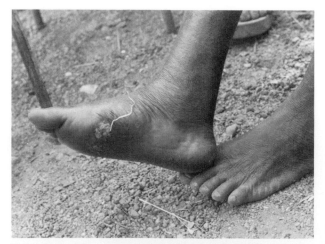

Figure 50-1. Guinea worm emerging from a victim's foot.

Ordinarily, each worm emerges over a period of about 4 weeks. In about half of the cases, however, the wound caused by the parasite becomes secondarily infected by bacteria, in which case the duration of painful incapacitation caused by the emergence of the parasite may be as long as 2 or 3 months or more. Inflammation associated with an emerging worm may manifest as arthritis in a nearby joint, even if the joint itself is not invaded by the worm, which also sometimes happens. One of the most serious complications arises when the wound of a susceptible person becomes secondarily infected with tetanus bacilli. Although dracunculiasis is not usually a fatal disease, secondary infections with tetanus are unfortunately not rare.

In less than half of 1 percent of cases, a permanent disability is sustained as a result of acute dracunculiasis, usually in the form of a frozen or ankylosed joint or muscle contracture.

No effective immunity is developed in response to this parasite, so persons in endemic communities are often infected repeatedly, year after year.

DIAGNOSIS AND MANAGEMENT

Patent dracunculiasis infections are easily diagnosed, without any kind of laboratory assistance, since few other diseases are likely to be confused with this one. In endemic areas, even the appearance of the blister when the worm is about to emerge is readily recognized as a sign of the infection. Only in cases of cutaneous larva migrans and *Loa loa* are relatively long worms seen to be beneath the skin or in the anterior chamber of the eye, respectively, that might be mistaken by an inexperienced observer for a guinea worm. The appearance of fly larvae, or maggots, in a wound has also sometimes been misdiagnosed as guinea worm. The ulcer produced by the emerging worm is not distinctive except when the emerging worm itself is visible.

No serological test is available to identify infected persons reliably during the long incubation period when there are no signs or symptoms of the infection. During the first several days after the worm begins to emerge, fluid discharged by the worm when immersed in cold water may be examined under a microscope to demonstrate living larvae, but such examination is hardly ever really necessary in order to know when one is dealing with a guinea worm.

The most effective treatment, once the worm has begun to emerge, is the time-honored method of winding the worm slowly around a small stick or twig, or tying a piece of string around the external part of the worm's body to prevent it from withdrawing into the human host. These techniques are intended to facilitate the extrusion of the worm without breaking it. Broken worms withdraw into the body and cause severe inflammatory reactions.

There is no anthelmintic or other drug to cure an infection with this parasite, although many have been tried. Niridazole, thiabendazole, and metronidazole have been reported to reduce inflammation associated with emerging worms, and thereby sometimes facilitate their removal or hasten their emergence.

Their mode of action may be mostly anti-inflammatory. Niridazole, given orally at 12.5 mg/(kg·day) for 1 week, may be the most useful chemotherapy. However, none of these drugs is suitable for effective mass treatment.

Aspirin can help relieve the pain associated with *Dracunculus* infections, and administration of antibiotics and cleansing and dressing of wounds are important for reducing the incidence of secondary infections. Administration of tetanus toxoid is also important to help prevent a potentially fatal complication.

Recently, some studies have been conducted to try to identify a drug which might act prophylactically, to kill immature worms if administered soon after the infection has begun in a person. This would be a very useful additional tool for attacking this parasite, but so far no such anthelmintic has been shown to be effective in that way, either.

POPULATION

EPIDEMIOLOGY

Although it was formerly much more widespread, dracunculiasis now is limited to India, Pakistan, Saudi Arabia, and Yemen in Asia, and 17 African countries (Benin, Burkina Faso, Cameroon, Central African Republic, Chad, Côte d'Ivoire, Ethiopia, Ghana, Kenya, Mali, Mauritania, Niger, Nigeria, Senegal, Sudan, Togo, Uganda). About 140 million persons are at risk of infection in these endemic countries, where some 10 million persons are thought to be actually infected each year. Reporting of dracunculiasis is especially poor, however, and the true extent of the disease is not known, except in India and Pakistan where national searches for cases have been conducted.

In Asian countries where dracunculiasis occurs, prevalence rates usually do not exceed 20 percent. In many affected African countries, more than 40 percent of the population in endemic communities is stricken at the peak of the guinea worm season. In all affected areas, the disease is very sporadically distributed and restricted to rural areas.

Persons between the ages of 5 and 50 years are the ones most heavily affected, with the brunt of the infection falling on the working age population. Males and females are both affected, although sometimes one or the other sex will suffer more, depending on the local propensity for drinking water from contaminated sources. Farmers, male and female, tend to suffer from the infection disproportionately, apparently because their occupation puts them at special risk of drinking large quantities of contaminated water. Since the task of collecting water for household use usually is the responsibility of women and girls, however, it is probable that they may be particularly important as contaminators of the drinking water.

This is a seasonal infection, the incidence of which is closely tied to the local pattern of rainfall. In the endemic countries of the Sahel, just below the Sahara in Africa, guinea worm is most prevalent during the brief rainy season, when surface water is available. In countries closer to the coast of west Africa, where the rainy season is more prolonged, transmission of the disease, and prevalence of the infection, are most common during the dry season, when drinking water sources are most polluted and scarce (during the rainy season, surface water is so abundant in this region that the likelihood of it being heavily contaminated is much reduced).

PREVENTION AND CONTROL

There are at least three ways to prevent dracunculiasis: provision of safe water sources, health education, and chemical control of the vector. Each of these has been shown to be extremely effective in stopping transmission of the infection. Provision of safe drinking water is the most expensive, and the most durable, intervention. It also has the advantage of providing other important benefits besides eliminating the guinea worm. When a village in Nigeria was provided safe drinking water in the 1960s, the incidence of dracunculiasis declined from 60 percent to zero in 2 years.

Health education is the least expensive intervention, and can also be very effective. The first message that needs to be conveyed to persons living in endemic communities is that this infection comes from their drinking water. The second message is that the infection can be prevented by dissuading persons who have worms emerging from entering the village's sources of drinking water and by filtering or boiling drinking water. Boiling water is usually impractical in the areas of concern because of the scarcity or high cost of wood or other fuel. Recent development of a monofilament nylon material has facilitated promotion of filtration of water to prevent guinea worm. Use of health education to promote use of such filters in Burkina Faso recently, without any other intervention, reduced the prevalence of dracunculiasis in three villages from 54, 37, and 24 percent, respectively, to zero, within two transmission seasons.

Vector control, using the chemical temephos (Abate) in a concentration of 1 part per million, applied at intervals of 4 to 6 weeks during the transmission season to the stagnant ponds that usually are the contaminated sources of drinking water, is another potentially effective intervention. This method, when used in a primary health care project in Mali, reduced the incidence of dracunculiasis by 87 percent in 1 year. In an Indian study, the efficacy of this intervention in 1 year was 97 percent.

Global attention to dracunculiasis, and increased efforts to prevent it, expanded significantly with the advent of the United Nations–sponsored International Drinking Water Supply and Sanitation Decade in 1981. Since one of the two main goals of that decade is to provide safe drinking water to persons in need of it by 1990, eradication of guinea worm disease was accepted as an official subgoal of the decade. In 1986, the World Health Assembly adopted a resolution calling for the eradication of dracunculiasis—the first such resolution since the successful smallpox eradication campaign.

By March 1988, when the Second Regional Workshop on Dracunculiasis in Africa was convened under the sponsorship of the World Health Organization, about half of the remaining dracunculiasis-endemic countries had begun active programs to eradicate the disease. India, which began its national Guinea Worm Eradication Program in 1980, reduced the annual number of cases found from 44,819 in 1983, to 17,031 cases in 1987, with one of the seven originally endemic states already having been freed of the infection. Another important benefit of the eradication efforts has been the increased documentation of the severe impact of dracunculiasis on school attendance and on agricultural production in endemic areas. This latter documentation is significant beyond dracunculiasis itself because it is a special opportunity to show the relevance of a parasitic disease to development in an unusually direct way.

REFERENCES

1 Muller R: *Dracunculus* and dracunculiasis, in Dawes B (ed): *Advances in Parasitology*. London, Academic, 1971, vol 9, pp 73–151
2 Hopkins DR: Dracunculiasis: An eradicable scourge. Epidemiol Rev 5:208–219, 1983
3 Hopkins DR: Dracunculiasis eradication: A mid-decade status report. Am J Trop Med Hyg 37:115–118, 1987
4 Watts SJ: Dracunculiasis in Africa in 1986: Its geographic extent, incidence, and at risk population. Am J Trop Med Hyg 37:119–125, 1987
5 World Health Organization: Dracunculiasis: Global surveillance summary—1986. Wkly Epidemiol Rec 62:337–339, 1987

CHAPTER 51 / *Trichinosis* · James W. Kazura

Trichinella spiralis is a nematode parasite of humans that is cosmopolitan in its geographical distribution. Humans are infected when parasite-infected meat (pork in most instances) is ingested. Clinical signs and symptoms are usually associated with exposure to a large inoculum of larvae and include fever, myalgia, periorbital edema, and eosinophilia.

PARASITE

LIFE HISTORY

T. spiralis infection is a zoonosis. Rats and other rodents are primarily responsible for the endemicity of this infection. The life cycle in nature is maintained by animals which are fed (e.g., pigs) or hunt (e.g., bears) other animals whose striated muscles contain infective larvae (e.g., rodents). Humans are infected incidentally when they eat the improperly processed meat of these carnivorous mammals. After exposure to the acid-pepsin environment of the stomach, the infective third-stage larvae are released from the acellular muscle cyst and pass into the small bowel, where they develop into adult female and male worms. These parasite stages, which lie coiled in the crypts of the duodenum and jejunum, copulate; newborn larvae are subsequently produced within the uterus of the fecund female. The adult parasites are expelled from the bowel over a 3-week period; however, newborn larvae are first released (approximately 1500 from each female worm) and pass through the intestinal mucosa. From this location, they migrate to

striated muscle via the lymphatics and bloodstream and penetrate the striated muscle cell membrane. The helminths subsequently molt and develop into an infective larva within a host-derived structure called the nurse cell. Encystment in muscle is completed in 4 to 5 weeks. *T. spiralis* can remain viable in this location for several years.

DESCRIPTION OF PARASITE

Morphology and biochemistry

Each stage of the *T. spiralis* life cycle has distinct morphological and biochemical features. Muscle larvae are the largest stage, measuring approximately 40 by 1200 μm. Because they are bound by a 1-μm-thick cuticle, they are resistant to physical damage, such as exposure to water or low temperatures. This stage of the organism remains viable after storage at 4°C and requires few nutrients to survive. The light-microscopic appearance of muscle larvae, apparent on crushed muscle preparations under low power ($\times$ 4 to 10), is characterized by a coiled, motile parasite within a muscle cell. Large amounts of glycogen are stored within the cells of muscle larvae; this is apparently a major energy source which may be broken down by aerobic or anaerobic glycolysis. In contrast to this developmental stage, newborn larvae are small (7 by 120 μm) and bound by a relatively thin cuticle. These forms die after 1 to 2 days of incubation at 37°C and cannot withstand low temperatures. Adult males and females measure 30 by 1300 μm and 36 by 2000 μm, respectively. Detailed studies of the biochemistry and energy metabolism of newborn larvae and adult parasites have not been performed.

Animal models

Mice and rats have most commonly been used for immunological studies of trichinosis. Investigations of the physiological responses of gut and muscle to infection have employed swine and rats as the experimental hosts.

Reservoir hosts

Pigs have been and are currently the primary source of infection for humans. However, as the practice of feeding garbage (which may contain rats or other *T. spiralis*–infected rodents) to swine declines, aquatic mammals (walruses) and wild game (bears and boars) have emerged as major sources (i.e., reservoirs) of human infection. Hyenas, jackals, leopards, and dogs have also been found to have *T. spiralis* in their muscles.

PATIENT

IMMUNOLOGY AND HOST DEFENSE MECHANISMS

T. spiralis infection of humans induces specific humoral and cell-mediated immune reactions. In 25 cases of human trichinosis recently reported, antibodies of the IgM, IgG, and IgA classes (measured by indirect immunofluorescence with intact muscle larvae as the target antigen) were detectable 10 to 20 days after the onset of disease. Twenty-five percent of the subjects still had anti-*Trichinella* antibodies 2 years after the acute illness [1]. Experimental studies in rodents suggest that host protective immunity is directed against gut-dwelling parasites and migratory newborn larvae. Acquired resistance in several strains of rats and mice is manifested by accelerated expulsion of enteric worms, a process mediated in part by anti-*Trichinella* homocytotropic (IgE) antibodies [2–4]. Stichocyte antigens of 48 and 50 to 55 kDa have been implicated as major immunogens in the induction of this response [5]. Opsonic antibodies to newborn larvae also may result in eosinophil-mediated elimination of this tissue migratory stage [6]. Examination of persons with parasitologically documented trichinosis substantiates the existence of this host defense mechanism in humans [7]. Toxic eosinophil proteins such as major basic protein and oxidative metabolites are important mediators of this aspect of host defense [8,9].

Blood eosinophilia (>500 cells per cubic millimeter of blood) is a major laboratory finding in trichinosis. Eosinophil counts are maximal 2 to 4 weeks after ingestion of infective larvae (coincidental with migration of newborn larvae through the tissues) and may last for several months. Experimental investigations of trichinosis in mice and rats suggest this hematological response to *T. spiralis* infection is T-lymphocyte-dependent and may be mediated by lymphocyte products.

PATHOLOGY AND PATHOPHYSIOLOGY

The gastrointestinal tract, blood, and striated muscle are the major tissue sites invaded by *T. spiralis;* pathological reactions to the parasite are thus most prominent in these locations. Studies in mice and rats indicate that an acute inflammatory response, consisting primarily of neutrophils, appears in areas of the gut mucosa adjacent to adult worms within 5 to 7 days of infection. These histopathological changes peak by 8 days and are followed by the appearance of a mixed cellular infiltrate consisting of eosinophils, macrophages, and plasma cells [4]. Third-stage larvae reside in muscle cells. The pathological response in this location in mice commences with the apposition of sarcolemmal surface membrane and larva. The organism is eventually surrounded by this membrane, which becomes part of the host-derived nurse cell. Large numbers of mononuclear cells and polymorphonuclear leukocytes then surround the muscle larvae. As the cyst wall develops between 4 and 6 weeks, the mixed cellular infiltrate in rodents and humans is replaced by granulomas containing Langhan's giant cells and eosinophils. The cysts may eventually calcify.

The physiological alterations associated with the presence of adult *T. spiralis* in the gut have been studied extensively in experimental animals but not in humans. A decrease in mucosal disaccharidase and increase in mucosal peroxidase precede expulsion of adult worms in rats infected with *T. spiralis* [2]. Experiments in rats relevant to the pathogenesis of diarrhea (occasionally observed in humans) indicate that *T. spiralis* induces net fluid secretion into the lumen of the gut. These physiological abnormalities are temporally associated with alterations of mucosal hexose absorption, increased small-intestinal myoelectric activity (segmental motility), and net secretion of chloride ion from serosa to mucosa [10].

CLINICAL MANIFESTATIONS

Description of the clinical manifestations of trichinosis is primarily dependent on reports of large outbreaks that are characterized by heavy parasite burdens. In this regard, the signs and symptoms (if any) associated with light infection have not been well characterized. The time from ingestion of *T. spiralis*–containing meat to onset of clinical manifestations is widely variable. In 29 cases reported to the Communicable Disease Centers in 1984, the mean period of time was 8 days with a range of 1 to 34 days [11].

Gastrointestinal signs and symptoms may be the first evidence of infection; however, many infected individuals report no gastrointestinal distress. Diarrhea, constipation, or abdominal cramps occurred in 6 to 58 percent of patients in outbreaks of trichinosis reported since 1865 (Table 51-1). In an outbreak in England in the year 1940–1941, for example, only 5 and 10 percent of 76 patients reported vomiting and diarrhea, respectively [2]. When these symptoms do occur, they appear between 2 and 10 days of ingesting larvae and are

Table 51-1. Major signs and symptoms of trichinosis

Clinical findings	Frequency (in percent)	
	Mean	Range
Abdominal discomfort	27	5–100
Fever	92	65–100
Headache	56	25–83
Myalgia	86	59–100
Subconjunctival hemorrhages and petechiae	42	25–58
Periorbital edema	84	57–100

Source: Compiled from [12,14–16,21].

coincidental with the presence of adult parasites in the small bowel. Prolonged diarrhea of 5 to 14 days' duration has been reported in outbreaks of trichinosis occurring in the Canadian Arctic [13]. It is not known if this unusual clinical manifestation results from peculiarities in host reactivity of the affected Inuit population or from parasite characteristics unique to Arctic strains of *T. spiralis.*

The most prominent and clinically significant phase of trichinosis is associated with tissue migration of the released newborn larvae and eventually their encystment in striated muscles and occasionally other sites. Myalgias, generalized weakness, fatigue, and headache have been estimated to occur in 60 to 100 percent of subjects in various outbreaks (Table 51-1) [12,14–16]. Muscle pain (particularly in the masseter and extraocular muscles) may be quite severe and is often the symptom that prompts the patient to seek medical attention. Signs at this stage include periorbital edema (60 to 100 percent of patients), conjunctivitis, and urticarial rashes (6 to 14 percent of patients) (Table 51-1). Fever of 38 to 40°C has been reported in almost all subjects in well-studied outbreaks of trichinosis. Central nervous system invasion and possibly hypersensitivity reactions in cerebral blood vessels are unusual but may occur in heavy infection. Manifestations of central nervous system involvement include seizures, meningitis, polyneuritis, and psychosis [17]. These may occur in the absence of myalgias and other characteristic signs of trichinosis. Other uncommon clinical signs and symptoms are heart failure, dysrhythmias, and cough (probably due to passage of newborn larvae through the lung). A polyarteritis nodosa–like illness with polyarthralgia, mononeuritis multiplex, abdominal pain, and hypertension has also been associated with *T. spiralis* infection [18]. Although the mortality in outbreaks of trichinosis has been reported to be as high as 10 to 25 percent, recent common-source infections have resulted in death rates of 0 to 10 percent. Death is generally due to invasion of the central nervous system or cardiac involvement. Trichinosis has also been observed in immunosuppressed patients. In this situation, clinical manifestations of infection and the host inflammatory response may be minimal, and the diagnosis depends on a high index of suspicion and demonstration of larvae in muscle [19].

Laboratory findings

Eosinophilia ranging from 4 percent to greater than 60 percent of the total white blood cell count has been reported in over 90 percent of subjects in well-documented outbreaks. Elevated eosinophil counts are first detected by 1 to 2 weeks of infection and persist for 4 to 5 weeks to several months. Muscle enzymes such as creatine phosphokinase (CPK) and lactate dehydrogenase (LDH) are elevated in at least 50 percent of patients and may correlate with abnormal electromyograms. Serum antibodies against *T. spiralis* (measurable by the bentonite flocculation assay) first become evident within 3 to 4 weeks of infection and may persist for several years. Titers of less than or equal to a ten- or fourfold rise over a period of several weeks are indicative of recent infection. Intradermal skin tests employing *Trichinella* antigens are not useful for diagnosis. A positive reaction may persist for years and will thus not distinguish between a recent and a remote infection [20].

DIAGNOSIS

Diagnosis of trichinosis depends on a combination of (1) clinical manifestations with a history of ingesting meat that may contain larvae, (2) confirmatory laboratory studies, and occasionally (3) muscle biopsy. The findings of myalgias, periorbital edema, fever, and eosinophilia in an individual who gives a history of eating improperly processed pork or carnivorous game make the diagnosis of trichinosis likely. A similar illness in family members or others who ingested the same food is also helpful. Positive serology (diagnostic titers in the bentonite flocculation assay) and/or muscle biopsy are confirmatory. These two tests are complementary; both may not give positive results. In documented cases of trichinosis in the United States in 1978, for example, 2 of 13 patients with positive serology had no larvae demonstrable in muscle specimens. Conversely, 6 of 11 subjects with larvae in muscle biopsies had negative serology [21]. Serology is most likely to be negative if done exclusively within the first 3 to 4 weeks of infection. Muscle biopsy need not always be done and should be performed only in selected situations. These circumstances include the presence of an equivocal history or physical examination and if serological testing cannot be performed rapidly. If done properly (tender muscle is biopsied and examined by an experienced observer), this procedure is confirmatory in greater than 90 percent of cases [21].

MANAGEMENT

Thiabendazole in a dosage of 25 mg per kilogram of body weight twice daily for 1 week is the current recommendation for treatment of trichinosis [22]. This drug appears to be ineffective against tissue-migrating or encysted muscle stages and thus is unsatisfactory after about the first week of infection, the period of time when the greatest numbers of susceptible gut-dwelling parasites are present. Most infected subjects, however, are asymptomatic at this stage and cannot be identified unless they are involved in a recognized outbreak. Studies in experimental animals and several infected humans suggest that mebendazole may have an antiparasitic effect against the invasive and encystment phases of *T. spiralis* [23–25]. Corticosteroids may be administered to critically ill patients such as those with myocarditis or central nervous system damage, but evidence of their beneficial effect is anecdotal.

POPULATION

EPIDEMIOLOGY

Human and animal infections of *T. spiralis* have been reported in the Arctic, temperate climates of Europe and North America, Latin America, Asia, and tropical Africa. The parasite does not exist in Australia and some islands of the South Pacific region. Over the past two decades, there has been a remarkable decrease in the United States in the prevalence of trichinosis. In 1973, for example, only 1.8 percent of diaphragms examined in Americans less than 45 years of age were found to contain larvae. This compares to a prevalence of 16.1 percent in the period 1936–1941 and 4.1 percent in 1966–1970 [26]. The decline in prevalence of human trichinosis parallels a similar decrease in infection in swine (from 9.5 per 1000 in the 1930s to 1.25 per 1000 in 1966–1970).

Some outbreaks of trichinosis have not clearly been associated with the consumption of pork products. Ingestion of the meat of herbivorous animals such as cattle or horses, for example, has been implicated in the United States and France [6]. In these situations, it was suspected that the meat was adulterated with small amounts of pork or that butcher knives contaminated with infested pork were used. Other recently appreciated sources of infection in outbreaks are black bears, wild boar, and walruses (particularly in Inuit populations).

INFECTION AND DISEASE

Although the prevalence of *T. spiralis* larvae in autopsy series had been reported to be as high as 2 to 4 percent, reports of clinical manifestations of this infection are largely limited to outbreaks and are not common in the general population. This contrast between the relatively high prevalence of infection and uncommon disease manifestations is most likely related to the number of larvae which eventually parasitize the host. Most individuals have light infections (less than 10 larvae per gram of muscle) and are presumably asymptomatic, while a few subjects have heavy infections (50 to 100 larvae per gram of muscle) and develop clinical signs and symptoms. The exact relationship of intensity of infection to morbidity cannot be clearly delineated because systematic studies of this nature have not been done.

PREVENTION AND CONTROL

Infection may be avoided by eating only properly processed meat products. Pork (or other meat products) should be cooked until there is no trace of pink fluid or flesh (this occurs at 55°C); storage in a freezer at −15°C for 3 weeks also kills the larvae. Arctic strains have been reported to be relatively more resistant to killing by exposure to low temperature for long periods of time [27]. Smoked or salted meat may still contain live parasites. Education on the risks of trichinosis should be directed at those who consume raw meat products.

Continued control of this infection can be implemented by strict adherence to the practice of not feeding raw garbage (which may contain infected rodents) to swine. Education of individuals or groups which consume such animals should focus on the potential hazard of this practice and proper methods to kill the larvae during the cooking process. Governmental inspection of meats specifically for *T. spiralis* is not currently practiced in many countries (including the United States). Its impact on the prevalence of infection would be difficult to measure in view of the low prevalence of clinically significant trichinosis.

REFERENCES

1 Ljungstrom I: Antibody response to *Trichinella spiralis,* in Kim C (ed): *Trichinellosis.* New York, Intext Medical Publishers, 1974, pp 449–460

2 Castro GA, Hessell JJ, Whalen GW: Altered intestinal fluid movement in response to *Trichinella spiralis* in immunized rats. Parasite Immunol 1:259–266, 1979

3 Bell RG, McGregor DD: Requirement for two discrete stimuli for the induction of the intestinal rapid expulsion response against *Trichinella spiralis* in rats. Infect Immun 29:186–195, 1980

4 Larsh JE Jr: Experimental trichiniasis. Adv Parasitol 1:213–286, 1963

5 Silberstein DS, Despommier DD: Antigens from *Trichinella spiralis* that induce a protective response in the mouse. J Immunol 142:898–904, 1984

6 Kazura JW, Aikawa M: Host defense mechanisms against *Trichinella spiralis* infection in the mouse: Eosinophil-mediated destruction of newborn larvae in vitro. J Immunol 124:355–361, 1980

7 Kazura JW: Host defense mechanisms against nematode parasites: Destruction of *Trichinella spiralis* newborn larvae by parasite stage–specific human antibody and granulocytes. J Infect Dis 143:712–718, 1981

8 Hamann KJ, Barker RL, Loegering, DA, et al: Comparative toxicity of purified human eosinophil granule proteins for newborn larvae of *Trichinella spiralis.* J Parasitol 73:523–529, 1986

9 Grove DI, Mahmoud AAF, Warren KS: Eosinophils and resistance to *Trichinella spiralis.* J Exp Med 145:755–759, 1977

10 Harari Y, Russell DA, Castro GA: Anaphylaxis-mediated epithelial C1$^-$ secretion and parasite rejection in rat intestine. J Immunol 138:1250–1255, 1987

11 Stehr-Green JK, Schantz PM, Chisolm EM: Trichinosis surveillance, 1984. MMWR 35(2SS):11SS–15SS, 1984

12 Sheldon JH: An outbreak of trichiniasis in Wolverhampton and district. Lancet i:203–205, 1941

13 Viallet J, MacLean JD, Goresky CA, et al: Arctic trichinosis presenting as prolonged diarrhea. Gastroenterology 91:938–946, 1986

14 Bouree P, Bouvier JB, Passeron J, et al: Outbreak of trichinosis near Paris. Lancet i:1047–1049, 1979

15 Wand M, Lyman D: Trichinosis from bear meat: Clinical and laboratory features. JAMA 220:245–246, 1972

16 Barrett-Connor E, Davis CF, Hamburger RN, et al: An epidemic of trichinosis after ingestion of wild pig in Hawaii. J Infect Dis 133:473–477, 1976

17 Dalessio DJ, Wolff HG: *Trichinella spiralis* infection of the central nervous system: Report of a case and review of the literature. Arch Neurol 4:407–417, 1960

18 Frayha RA: Trichinosis-related polyarteritis nodosa. Am J Med 71:307–312, 1981

19 Jacobson ES, Jacobson HG: Trichinosis in an immunosuppressed human host. Am J Clin Pathol 68:791–794, 1977

20 Cox MO, Schultz MG, Kagan IG, et al: Trichinosis—five year serologic and clinical follow-up. Am J Epidemiol 89:651–659, 1969

21 Centers for Disease Control: Trichinosis Surveillance Annual Summary, 1978. September, 1979

22 Drugs for parasitic infection. The Medical Letter 30 (issue 759): 15–24, 1988

23 Hess JA, Chandrasekar PH, Mortiere M, et al: Comparative efficacy of ketoconazole and mebendazole in experimental trichinosis. Antimicrob Agents Chemother 30:953–954, 1986

24 McCracken RO, Taylor DD: Mebendazole therapy of parenteral trichinosis. Science 207:1220–1222, 1980

25 Levin ML: Treatment of trichinosis with mebendazole. Am J Trop Med Hyg 32:980–983, 1983

26 Zimmerman WJ, Steele JH, Kagan I: Trichinosis in the U.S. population, 1966–1970. Public Health Rep 88:606–623, 1973

27 Eaton, RDP: Trichinosis in the Arctic. Can Med Assoc J 120:22, 1979

CHAPTER 52 / *Toxocariasis and Related Syndromes* · Lawrence T. Glickman

Several roundworm parasites of lower animals also infect humans. These include members of the genus *Toxocara*, namely *T. canis* and *T. cati*, the common dog and cat roundworm, respectively, and *Baylisascaris procyonis*, a roundworm of raccoons. However, only *T. canis* is commonly recognized as the cause of human disease. This may reflect either the more aggressive behavior of *T. canis* compared with *T. cati* larvae in host tissues or greater human contact with *T. canis* eggs compared with those of *B. procyonis*.

Human *T. canis* infection results from ingestion of soil contaminated with embryonated eggs. The spectrum of clinical manifestations is broad and a function of the dose and frequency of infection, migratory route of larvae in host tissues, and intensity of the inflammatory response. Signs range from a clinically inapparent and mild eosinophilia to a fulminating disease with multisystem involvement. Generalized infection is referred to as systemic toxocariasis or visceral larva migrans (VLM). Some individuals infected with *T. canis* have no systemic signs, but develop eye disease. This syndrome is known as ocular toxocariasis or ocular larva migrans (OLM). Only rarely does infection result in concurrent VLM and OLM.

PARASITE

MORPHOLOGY

T. canis adult worms live in the proximal small intestine of the fox and dog (Fig. 52-1). Adult male worms measure up to 10 cm in length and females up to 18 cm. Males can also be distinguished by a terminal appendage and caudal alae; the spicules measure 0.6 to 0.9 mm long. Female reproductive organs are prominent, and each worm may release up to 200,000 eggs per day. The eggs are subglobular, measure 90 by 75 μm, and have a thick, finely pitted shell. Eggs embryonate in 14 to 21 days under optimal environmental conditions. The infective-stage larvae within the egg measure 20 to 400 μm and are morphologically similar to larvae recovered from human tissues. Detailed descriptions of the developmental stages of *T. canis* have been published [1,2].

LIFE CYCLE AND ECOLOGY

Toxocariasis is classified as a *saprozoonosis* because a non-animal site is essential for development. Eggs are passed in

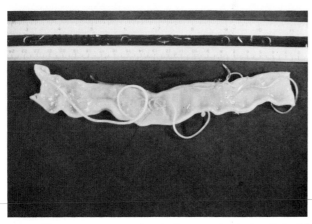

Figure 52-1. *Toxocara canis* female (larger) and male (smaller) adult worms in the small intestine of a 3-month-old puppy.

the feces of dogs and embryonate in the soil, where they may be ingested by the definitive host or by a variety of paratenic hosts. Paratenic hosts such as small rodents can also serve as transport hosts for *T. canis* if they are cannibalized.

In the dog, eggs hatch in the small intestine, and larvae enter the hepatic portal circulation where they are carried to the liver, heart, and lungs. The subsequent route of migration, either tracheal or somatic, is primarily determined by the age of the dog and the infective dose. In puppies less than 5 weeks of age, larvae usually penetrate pulmonary blood vessels, enter the alveoli, migrate up the bronchi and trachea, and are swallowed (tracheal migration). Adults develop in the small intestine and live an average of 4 months. In older dogs, some larvae are trapped in the liver and lungs while others migrate through the pulmonary veins and heart into the systemic circulation (somatic migration). Somatic larvae penetrate the capillaries of numerous tissues and remain encysted for years.

In the female dog, encysted larvae become active during the last trimester of pregnancy and cross the placenta. These larvae migrate through the uterine and umbilical circulation into the fetal liver and then follow the tracheal route previously described. In addition to transplacental transmission and ingestion of embryonated eggs, puppies can be infected by ingestion of larvae in tissues of smaller mammals or by ingestion of larvae and immature adults in the vomitus or feces of infected puppies.

Paratenic hosts including humans, are usually infected by ingestion of soil contaminated with embryonated eggs. Once swallowed the eggs hatch in the proximal small intestine and the larvae undergo extensive somatic migration. Larvae have been found in the liver, heart, lung, brain, muscle, and eyes of infected persons [3]. These migrating larvae produce tracks of hemorrhage, necrosis, and inflammation. Granuloma formation traps and destroys some larvae while others escape and remain viable for many years. In humans as in other paratenic

hosts, larvae undergo no further development and eggs are not found in the stool.

ANIMAL MODELS

A variety of experimentally infected paratenic hosts including the mouse, gerbil, guinea pig, rabbit, pig, monkey, baboon, and human have been used to investigate the pathogenesis of toxocariasis. Some of these models are more relevant to either VLM or OLM.

Models for VLM

In mice which have been infected orally with *T. canis* eggs, larvae are widely distributed in tissues but reach the brain in relatively larger numbers than do the larvae of other ascarid species [4]. *T. canis* larvae have an affinity for the cerebellum, with inoculum size and time elapsed since infection influencing their distribution in tissues [5,6]. Superinfection and multiple infection increase the relative number of encapsulated larvae located in the liver when compared with lower doses or single infections. In pregnant mice, the migration of larvae is influenced by the developmental stages of the placenta [7]. Similar effects have been observed in nonlactating females receiving daily injections of prolactin.

Central nervous system involvement in fatal human toxocariasis has been reported, but subclinical effects have been difficult to study. Experimental investigations suggest that *T. canis*–infected mice have marked disruptions of various behaviors including motor coordination, activity, exploration, and learning [8,9].

Toxocariasis in mice is characterized by peripheral eosinophilia and lymphocytosis; these occur within a few days after infection and are associated with lymphocytic infiltration of hepatic portal spaces and diffuse infiltration of the pulmonary parenchyma with eosinophils, lymphocytes, and polymorphonuclear leukocytes. Sequential histopathological studies indicate that *T. canis* elicits cell-mediated immunity that is manifested by eosinophil-rich granuloma formation [10]. However, there is inconclusive evidence that this process effectively destroys the larvae. Mice have also been used to study the development and distribution in tissues of excretory-secretory antigens of larval *T. canis* [11] and to assess the potential therapeutic value of antihelminthics, antihistamines, and corticosteroids.

Rabbits have been used primarily to characterize the serological response following *T. canis* infection and for development of immunodiagnostic tests. As few as 10 larvae per gram of body weight elicits antibody that is reactive with secretory antigens. Functional immunity was demonstrated by showing that previously infected rabbits could survive a challenge infection of 100,000 eggs, whereas naive rabbits died [12].

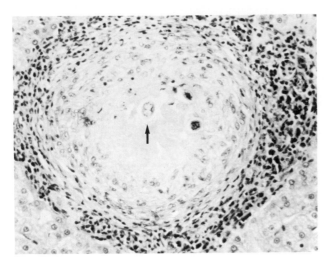

Figure 52-2. Characteristic histopathological lesion in the brain of a monkey (*Macaca fascicularis*) experimentally infected 75 days previously with 45,000 embryonated eggs of *Toxocara canis*. Note that a larva (arrow) is evident within the granuloma. (*From L.T. Glickman, F.S. Shofer: Vet Clin North Am 17:39–53, 1987.*)

Monkeys have been used to study the clinical, hematological, and serological response to oral infection with graded doses of *T. canis*. In one study of nine *Macaca* monkeys infected with 100,000 to 400,000 eggs of *T. canis*, six showed only mild and transient signs, including lack of appetite, depression, and cough, despite invasion of the central nervous system by larvae [13]. The three remaining animals developed severe neurological signs that terminated in paralysis. Hematological findings included transiently reduced erythrocyte counts and a marked eosinophilia that declined as the infection progressed. Serum changes included increased globulin concentrations, reduced albumin levels, and an elevated plasma transaminase. Postmortem examination in these and other infected monkeys generally revealed parasitic granuloma formation and focal necrosis in the brain and spinal cord (Fig. 52-2).

There are two reports in the literature of humans experimentally infected with small doses of *T. canis* [14,15]. In one instance an experimenter infected himself with 100 eggs and subsequently developed cough and eosinophilia. In another study two mentally retarded children were infected with 200 eggs, and each developed eosinophilia that persisted for as long as 13 months.

Models for OLM

Concurrent VLM and OLM have been produced in mice by oral administration of a large inoculum (1500 infective eggs) of *T. canis*. However, OLM in the absence of VLM has been successfully induced only by intraocular injection of small numbers of infective larvae using larger experimental animals.

Typical nematode endophthalmitis, including retinal hemorrhages and venous dilatation, was produced in owl monkeys by direct intravitreal infection with 15 or more *T. canis* larvae [16]. The intensity and timing of the intraocular reaction seemed to correlate with the size of the inoculum and the apparent disappearance of larvae from the eye. Only minimal or no intraocular changes were seen after nasogastric infection with 5000 eggs. Systemically infected animals developed serum antibodies to *Toxocara*, but intraocular fluids were negative for antibody in all monkeys including those infected systemically and/or intraocularly. This animal model appears particularly well suited for subsequent studies on the pathogenesis of OLM and for developing sensitive immunodiagnostic methods.

PATIENT

CLINICAL MANIFESTATIONS

Asymptomatic infection

Most humans infected by *T. canis* do not develop overt clinical disease. These individuals can usually be identified by the presence of a mild eosinophilia (2 to 5 percent) and low circulating levels of antibody to *Toxocara* (ELISA titer <1:32). Asymptomatic toxocariasis, however, will be identified with increasing frequency now that sensitive serodiagnostic tests are routinely available. While the long-term prognosis for these patients is unknown, eventual migration of a larva to the eye with development of OLM remains possible, since *T. canis* larvae can persist and migrate in the tissues of infected monkeys for up to 10 years [17]. Another concern is the finding that 29 percent of asthmatic children are serologically positive to *T. canis* antigens in comparison to only 6 percent of nonasthmatic children [18].

Over a 6-year period, Bass et al. [19] screened 153 Hispanic children attending a hospital-based primary care clinic in Massachusetts and found a 16 percent prevalence of asymptomatic toxocariasis. Follow-up of 20 asymptomatic children for periods of up to 7 years failed to demonstrate any clinical sequelae. However, these authors cautioned that longer periods would be necessary to entirely discount the possibility of latent ocular involvement.

Visceral larva migrans

In 1952, *T. canis* larvae were first identified in hepatic granulomas from a child with chronic extreme eosinophilia [20]. The term *visceral larva migrans* was proposed to describe this syndrome. The clinical signs were thought to be related to direct tissue damage caused by migrating larvae and to allergic responses to their products. Since that time until 1977, when a reliable serodiagnostic test was developed, most individuals with VLM have been characterized by persistent eosinophilia, leukocytosis, fever, hepatomegaly, and hypergammaglobulinemia. Clinical signs often include wheezing or coughing, and pulmonary infiltrates are evident in over one-third of patients [21]. Rare fatal cases of toxocariasis have resulted from extensive larval migration through the myocardium or central nervous system.

The mean age of VLM patients with serologically proven *T. canis* infection was reported as 4.6 ± 3.6 years [22]. Clinical findings included eosinophilia (>10 percent), leukocytosis (>10,000 cells per cubic millimeter), an increased anti-A (>1:400) or anti-B (>1:200) isohemagglutinin titer, and an elevated serum IgG level. However, hepatomegaly was present in only 25 percent of the patients.

A definitive diagnosis depends on microscopic identification of *T. canis* larva in infected tissues. Circumscribed granulomatous lesions composed primarily of epithelioid cells and lymphocytes are frequently found in the liver and lungs and often contain an intact larva or larval fragments.

Many children with VLM have a history of seizures, and there have been numerous reports of children with acute neurological disease who died and were found to have *T. canis* larvae in their brains at autopsy. However, a controlled epidemiological study found no association between *T. canis* infection and epilepsy in children [23].

Because of behavioral abnormalities in mice infected orally with *T. canis*, there has been concern that clinically inapparent infection in children may produce subtle neuropsychological damage. In one study, poor reading achievement, marked distractibility, and lower IQ scores were associated with *T. canis* infection [24]. However, when parental education, race, and sex were taken into account, the association was no longer statistically significant. Another study in New York City found that the rate of *T. canis* infection was approximately 5.5 percent in 4652 children 2 months to 14 years of age, and that 155 infected children when compared with age- and sex-matched noninfected controls performed significantly worse on several neuropsychological tests of motor and cognitive function [25].

Infection with *B. procyonis,* the common roundworm of raccoons, has caused epizootics of fatal central nervous system disease in domestic rabbits and caged birds. Experimentally, a fatal eosinophilic meningoencephalitis has been produced in monkeys. A recent report described a fatal case of VLM in a child in whom eosinophilic meningoencephalitis was the cause of death, and serological studies were negative for *T. canis*. Autopsy revealed a systemic larval infection with *B. procyonis,* and exposure to raccoon feces was thought to have been the source of infection [26].

VLM caused by *T. canis* has also been reported as an endemic disease of adults in the Midi-Pyrenees region of France [27]. The disease was characterized by weakness, pruritus, rash, difficulty breathing, abdominal pain, and pathologically by allergic manifestations including eosinophilia and increased serum immunoglobulin levels. Affected persons were significantly more likely to live in rural areas, to hunt or to live in a household with a hunter, or to own two or more dogs. A foodborne route of transmission for *T. canis* larvae has been suggested as one explanation for the unusual presentation of this VLM syndrome in French adults. *T. canis* larvae have not been identified in tissues from affected patients, but they consistently have diagnostic antibody titers to *T. canis* by ELISA and western blot tests and negative serological and coprological findings for other known causes of VLM.

Ocular larva migrans

T. canis was first recognized in 1950 to be a cause of ocular disease [28]. *Toxocara* larvae or larval fragments were identified in 24 of 46 eyes that had been enucleated because of endophthalmitis and presumed retinoblastoma. Ocular *Toxocara* infection in a child may resemble retinoblastoma by producing leukokoria, strabismus, failing vision, or a fundus mass [29].

Larvae usually produce unilateral posterior or peripheral granulomatous retinal lesions, but they also invade the iris. The site of the lesion is probably determined by chance migration of a larva, and the clinical form of the disease is the outcome of larval activity and host response. OLM typically affects the eye in three recognizable patterns, namely, a peripheral inflammatory mass in a quiet eye, a posterior pole granuloma, or painless endophthalmitis (Fig. 52-3).

Concurrent VLM and OLM are rare. Eosinophilia, which is both pronounced and persistent with VLM, is virtually absent with OLM. The average age of patients with OLM is higher than that of patients with VLM, and OLM also occurs in adults. OLM has been observed in two patients 4 and 10 years after an initial diagnosis of VLM. However, none of 20 children with asymptomatic toxocariasis with eosinophilia who were followed for periods of up to 7 years developed ocular disease caused by *T. canis* [19].

The characteristic lesion of OLM is an eosinophilic abscess surrounded by epithelioid cells and inflammatory granulation tissue containing eosinophils, lymphocytes, and plasma cells [28]. These abscesses are common in the retina and in the vitreous membrane. Not every abscess will contain a larva, and in those that do, many serial sections may be required to identify one.

A fourth pattern of OLM in children caused by *T. canis* has also been reported: periodic intraretinal meandering of larvae followed by quiescence with encapsulation, reemergence, and renewed migration [30]. The clinical course may extend over several years, and this confirms earlier experimental studies in monkeys concerning larval longevity. It also explains the disassociation in time between the clinical presentation of systemic toxocariasis and the rare sequelae of ocular involvement. The typical lesions and end results of meandering OLM are illustrated in Fig. 52-4.

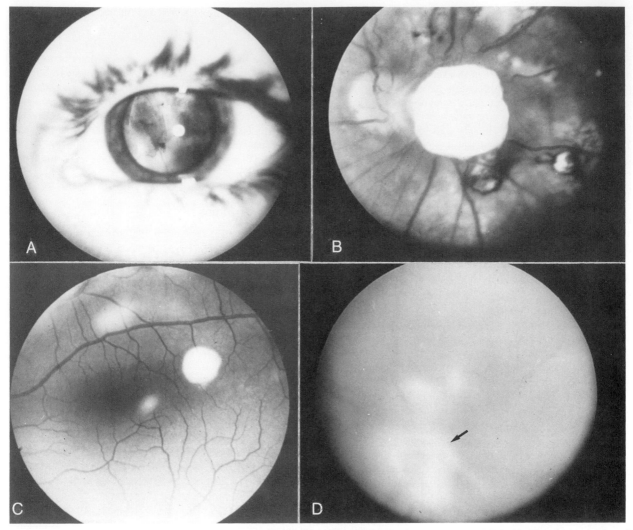

Figure 52-3. Typical clinical and pathological presentations in people with OLM. Leukokoria (*A*), posterior pole granuloma (*B*), and peripheral intraretinal granulomas (*C*) in a quiet eye as demonstrated by fluorescein angiography, and endophthalmitis (*D*) with suggestion of a posterior mass (arrow) through the vitreous haze. (*From L.T. Glickman, F.S. Shofer: Vet Clin North Am 17:39–53, 1987.*)

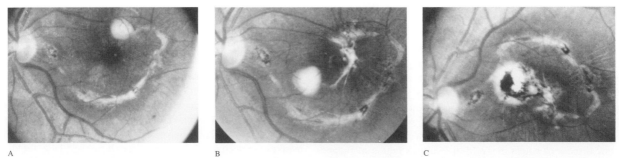

A   B   C

Figure 52-4. Appearance of the retina over a 2-year period in a 16-year-old boy with OLM. *A.* A subretinal tract leading to an equatorial nodule, presumably resulting from larval migration. Pigmentation within the tract marks sites of previous encapsulation. *B.* The larva has extended its migration and burrowed into the retinal pigment epithelium adjacent to the fovea, where new encystation has occurred. This photo was taken immediately after laser treatment. *C.* The ultimate scar following xenon photocoagulation (*From* [*30*].)

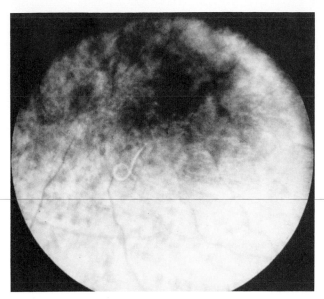

Figure 52-5. A subretinal ocular nematode in a patient with the diffuse unilateral subacute neuroretinitis syndrome. (*From* [*32*].)

Just as the raccoon ascarid *B. procyonis* is a rare cause of VLM, it also has the potential to invade the eye. Experimentally, OLM has been produced in cynomolgus and squirrel monkeys by oral infection with infective eggs, and the lesions produced resemble those caused by *T. canis* [*31*]. *B. procyonis* is one possible cause of an ocular syndrome in people called *diffuse unilateral subacute neuroretinitis* (DUSN) in which a larval nematode has been demonstrated in retinal photographs of 18 patients [*32*] (Fig. 52-5). These patients are uniformly negative for toxocaral antibodies, and the estimated size of the worms further suggests that they are not *T. canis*. Other candidate agents include ascarids, zoonotic hookworms, and filarids.

DIAGNOSIS

Visceral larva migrans

Determination of the exact etiology in individual cases of VLM presents a diagnostic challenge. In patients with VLM or OLM caused by *T. canis,* biopsy of tissues to identify larvae is rarely indicated. A presumptive diagnosis of VLM is based on clinical signs, laboratory findings, and a history of geophagia and exposure to puppies. The most consistent laboratory findings include chronic eosinophilia, leukocytosis, a decreased albumin-globulin ratio, an increase in serum levels of total IgG, IgM, and anti-A or anti-B isohemagglutinin titers. In the United States, *T. canis* is more likely to be associated with elevated isohemagglutinins than other parasites which cause eosinophilia [*23*].

A number of immunodiagnostic techniques and antigens have been used for toxocariasis in experimentally infected animals and in humans [*33*]. In general, tests that use larval-derived antigens are more sensitive and specific than those that use adult antigens. ELISA using larval antigens has been found superior (sensitivity = 78 percent; specificity = 93 percent) to the other serological methods if the serum is first absorbed with *Ascaris suum* antigens to remove cross-reacting antibodies.

Based on experimental murine infections, it may be possible to make an accurate histopathological diagnosis of larval toxocariasis in biopsy or autopsy specimens lacking an obvious etiological agent by staining the tissue with biotin-conjugated, rabbit anti-*Toxocara* excretory-secretory antigens [*11*].

It should be noted that children with VLM caused by *B. procyonis* do not react on serological tests using larval *T. canis* antigens, and an antemortem diagnosis may not be possible since routine serological tests for *B. procyonis* are not available.

Ocular larva migrans

Patients with OLM present an even greater diagnostic challenge than do those with VLM. Clinical signs are usually restricted to the eye and are difficult to distinguish from other childhood ocular diseases including retinoblastoma, Coat's disease, persistent hyperplastic primary vitreous, retinopathy or prematurity, toxoplasmosis, and histoplasmosis. Routine laboratory results are typically within normal limits, and a number of eyes with benign *Toxocara* inflammatory lesions have been unnecessarily enucleated because of suspected retinoblastoma. Aqueous cytology and enzyme determination may be informative in nematode ophthalmitis. An abnormal aqueous-plasma lactate dehydrogenase ratio and numerous eosinophils in the aqueous aspirate support a diagnosis of nematode ophthalmitis, but are not specific for *Toxocara* [*34*]. Clinical diagnostic approaches such as fluorescein angiography, radiography, ultrasonography, and computed tomography are also helpful in distinguishing OLM from retinoblastoma [*29*].

The ELISA for *Toxocara* has a sensitivity and specificity for OLM of 90 and 91 percent, respectively, at a diagnostic titer of 1:8. However, antibody titers to *Toxocara* are significantly lower in patients with OLM when compared to those with VLM. This raises the possibility that children with asymptomatic *Toxocara* infection and an inflammatory ocular disorder not associated with *Toxocara* (e.g., retinoblastoma) will be falsely labeled as having OLM if only serum titers are considered. As an adjunct to serum antibody determination, vitreous *Toxocara* antibody can be measured [*35*]. In five patients with a clinical diagnosis of nematode endophthalmitis thought to be caused by *T. canis,* the vitreous titer was equal to or greater than the serum titer. By comparison, vitreous from patients with no evidence of endophthalmitis did not contain antibody.

Similar results have been obtained by measuring *Toxocara* antibody titers in the aqueous and serum. Measurement of antibody in ocular fluids appears to increase the specificity of ELISA, and the increased risk to the patient may be warranted when a definitive diagnosis is crucial to management.

CLINICAL MANAGEMENT

Therapy of VLM and OLM is symptomatic and intended primarily to diminish the inflammatory responses to larvae or their metabolic products in tissues. Efficacy of specific antihelminthics against *T. canis* larvae has been evaluated in experimentally infected animals with mixed results.

Treatment of children with thiabendazole with a single 3-day course of 50 mg/kg in three divided doses or one 4-day course of 25 mg/kg in two divided doses [36] did not appear to alter the course of asymptomatic toxocariasis in a controlled 1-year trial as measured by eosinophil counts and specific *T. canis* antibody titers [19]. In contrast, children with acute VLM and profound eosinophilia (>80 percent) have responded clinically to treatment with thiabendazole at a dose of 20 to 50 mg/kg daily for 7 to 10 days and repeated after a 4-week interval [37,38]. The persistence of eosinophilia in some treated patients for months in spite of clinical improvement, however, may reflect the continued presence of viable *T. canis* larvae in tissues.

The types of drugs that have been used most frequently either alone or in combination with antihelminthics include corticosteroids, antibiotics, antihistamines, and bronchodilators. The use of anti-inflammatory drugs is indicated and may be lifesaving for acute allergic manifestations and in patients with extensive involvement of the myocardium or central nervous system.

Since only one larva in the eye may produce inflammation and severe visual loss, accurate diagnosis and prompt treatment of OLM is important. Modalities which have been used include those intended to directly destroy the larvae, e.g., antihelminthics and photocoagulation, as well as nonspecific interventions to prevent the severe ocular complications and to preserve or restore vision, e.g., cycloplegic drugs, corticosteroids, and various types of intraocular surgery [39].

PATHOGENESIS

VLM and OLM both result from tissue destruction caused by migrating *T. canis* larvae and an inflammatory response to the larvae or their metabolic products. Yet there are distinct clinical, pathological, and epidemiological differences between OLM and VLM in humans and animals. These differences may be related to the inoculum size. One hypothesis suggests that lower doses of *Toxocara* are associated with a higher probability of OLM than VLM [40]. As the number of larvae ingested increases, the probability of OLM decreases, and the chance of VLM increases. As the parasite load increases still

further, the likelihood of OLM (and concurrent VLM) once again increases, as does the severity of systemic signs. This would explain why most children with VLM have a history of pica and exposure to puppies, both of which are indicative of ingestion of large numbers of *Toxocara* eggs. In contrast, patients with OLM are usually older, lack systemic signs, and do not have pica. In these persons, infection with only small numbers of eggs is more likely. This would explain why *Toxocara* serum antibody titers are generally lower in persons with OLM than VLM.

HOST-PARASITE RELATIONSHIP

Host-*Toxocara* interactions are complex and comprise both host-protective and parasite-protective responses. A knowledge of both is important in formulating strategies for treatment and prevention. Of concern to physicians are the observations that (1) in experimentally infected monkeys larvae can live in the tissues for up to 9 or 10 years, (2) larvae in the tissue are well tolerated by children except when present in large numbers, and (3) a single larva can eventually migrate to the eye and cause extensive tissue damage. In vitro studies have shown that *T. canis* larvae have surface antigens that bind antiserum and that complete turnover of these antigens occurs within 3 h at 37°C [41]. If this happens in vivo, it could provide the larvae with an effective protective mechanism from the host's immune response.

Scanning and transmission electron-microscopic studies of larval-eosinophil interactions have shown that eosinophils adhere to a membranous sheath-like layer that was frequently detached from the larval epicuticle. The layers may be composed of surface antigens and antibody which protect larvae against antibody and eosinophil toxins by preventing their contact with the epicuticle. The release of surface antigens also may be important in allowing larvae to evade the host's immune response by facilitating the removal of antibody and eosinophils from the larval surface [42].

POPULATION

ECOLOGY

Prevalence in dogs

VLM and OLM probably occur wherever humans live in close proximity to dogs. The efficient life cycle of *T. canis*, including transplacental and transmammary transmission of larvae, ensures that nearly all puppies are infected by 6 weeks of age. The reported disparities in infection rates for dogs can be explained by regional differences in prevalence as well as by differences in the age, sex, and source of the dogs studied (e.g., privately owned versus strays), prior antihelminthic treatment, and the method used for determining infection status. For example, infection rates vary from nearly 100 percent in puppies to less than 10 percent in adult dogs. Twelve percent of puppies being sold in pet shops were found to be infected with *T. canis* despite the fact that 88 percent had received some form of antihelminthic treatment while at the store [*43*].

ENVIRONMENTAL SOURCES OF *T. CANIS*

Environmental contamination with *T. canis* eggs was recognized long before VLM or OLM was reported as a disease of humans. Since that time, most studies have consistently demonstrated high rates of soil contamination in parks, playgrounds, and other public places. *Toxocara* eggs may survive for years in the environment, depending on soil type and climatic conditions. Eggs have been found in sewage sludge samples collected from 27 municipal sewage treatment plants in the southern United States [*44*].

The whelping box represents a potentially important source of *T. canis* eggs for children. Feces from a litter of puppies may contaminate the home with millions of eggs per day, and these eggs may cling to the haircoat of puppies. However, unless the eggs are maintained under suitable conditions of temperature and humidity for 14 to 21 days, they will not be infective. With regular cleaning of the litter box and its contents, most eggs will probably undergo desiccation. This is unlike the situation when feces are deposited directly onto grass or soil.

EPIDEMIOLOGY

Frequency of human disease

There is no reliable information on the incidence or prevalence of VLM and OLM. Neither eggs nor worms are passed in the feces of humans and only recently have reliable serological tests become available. Therefore, human toxocariasis is greatly underdiagnosed.

More than 1900 cases of human toxocariasis have been reported from 50 countries around the world [*45*]. Of 780 detailed cases in the literature, 350 had VLM; 56 percent of these patients were less than 3 years of age. Among the 430 cases of OLM, 158 led to enucleation; in only a few cases were visceral and ocular signs associated. It has been estimated that 700 persons each year are diagnosed with toxocaral OLM in the United States.

Infection in humans

ELISA serology with a larval-secretory antigen has revealed that 2.6 percent of 922 British adults have elevated *Toxocara*-specific antibody levels. As with skin tests, positive reactions were more common for children with epilepsy (7.1 percent) [*46*]. Using an ELISA with larval antigens, the prevalence of human *Toxocara* infection in the United States was determined using more than 1400 samples collected as part of the Health and Nutrition Examination Survey in the period from 1971 to

1973 [*47*]. Seroprevalence ranged from 4.6 to 13 percent of children aged 1 to 11 years of age in different geographical regions. Seroprevalence was strongly associated with black race, rural residence, and low socioeconomic status. The rate was nearly 30 percent among black children ages 6 to 11 years of lower socioeconomic status. Within races, there was a strong negative correlation between total household income and toxocaral seroprevalence. Similar serological surveys have revealed infection rates in children of 7.1 percent in the Netherlands and 3.6 percent in Japan.

Risk factors for zoonotic transmission

Pica, especially geophagia, and a close association with puppies are two of the most important risk factors for human *Toxocara* infection. Clinical studies of patients with VLM have shown that almost all have a history of pica and an association with dogs or contaminated soil. For example, a case-control study of toxocaral infection in New York City found that children with a history of geophagia or having had a litter of puppies in their home were at 3.1 and 5.2 times greater risk, respectively, of developing toxocaral infection than were children without such a history. Children with a history of both geophagia and puppy contact had an approximately 16 times greater risk of infection [*25*]. These findings, however, are of limited diagnostic value, since dog ownership is common and from 20 to 30 percent of healthy children less than 5 years of age have a history of pica [*40*].

Clinical observations of patients with OLM have been inconsistent with regard to the importance of pica and dog exposure. This can be explained in part by the fact that patients with OLM are older than those with VLM, and often the clinical diagnosis has not been confirmed by serological tests. In contrast, a case-control epidemiological study of serologically proven OLM in which the age and sex of each patient was carefully controlled in the analysis found a significant association between OLM and the presence of puppies less than 3 months of age in the household within 1 year of clinical onset [*48*]. In this same study, 38 percent of OLM patients had a history of pica compared to 8 percent of controls with other ocular diseases.

PREVENTION AND CONTROL

Preventive programs for zoonotic toxocariasis should consider three interrelated problems: widespread environmental contamination with *T. canis* eggs, the high prevalence of infection in dogs, and conditions that favor transmission to humans. These efforts should involve public health and law enforcement officials, veterinarians, physicians, pet owners, dog breeders, pet stores, and humane societies. General recommendations for control of dog zoonoses have been developed at the National Conference on Dog and Cat Control [*49*] and by the World Health Organization [*50*].

Environment

The commonly used disinfectants will not kill *Toxocara* eggs in soil, and effective methods such as steam sterilization are not practical for general use. Therefore, contamination of public parks and playgrounds necessitates programs to reduce the number of stray and unsupervised pet dogs, local ordinances to exclude dogs from areas where children play, and laws requiring owners to remove feces deposited by their dogs. Children's sandboxes should be covered when not in use, and those already contaminated should be sterilized or replaced.

Infection in dogs

Roundworm infection in puppies cannot be entirely prevented because larvicidal drugs that block transplacental and transmammary transmission are not routinely available. However, adult roundworms can be eliminated from the small intestine of puppies before large numbers of eggs are shed into the feces. This requires that veterinarians, pet owners, and animal shelters treat all puppies with salts of piperazine at 2, 4, 6, and 8 weeks of age, and treat adult dogs as indicated by fecal examination or prophylactically once or twice a year. Dogs should not be sold or given as pets unless they have been properly treated for intestinal parasites and have had at least one negative stool examination for ova and parasites.

Zoonotic transmission

Both veterinarians and pet owners need to be educated about diseases transmitted from dogs to people. In one survey only 33 percent of practicing veterinarians thought that *T. canis* was a potential public health threat and only 54 percent said they routinely discussed the risk of toxocariasis and other zoonoses with their clients [51].

Pica in children is an important risk factor for several parasitic diseases and for lead poisoning. Research is needed on the physiological and sociological determinants of pica and the benefit versus the cost of intervention programs to treat for pica.

REFERENCES

1 Sprent JFA: Observations on the development of *Toxocara canis* in the dog. Parasitology 48:184–208, 1958
2 Nichols RL: The etiology of visceral larva migrans. J Parasitol 42:349–399, 1956
3 Dent JH, Nichols RL, Beaver PC, et al: Visceral larva migrans with a case report. Am J Pathol 32:777, 1956
4 Sprent JFA: On the invasion of the central nervous system by nematodes. II. Invasion of the nervous system in ascariasis. Parasitology 45:41–55, 1955
5 Burren CH: The distribution of *Toxocara* larvae in the central nervous system of the mouse. Trans R Soc Trop Med Hyg 65:450–453, 1971
6 Kayes, SG, Oaks JA: Effect of inoculum size and length of infection on the distribution of *Toxocara canis* larvae in the mouse. Am J Trop Med Hyg 25:573–580, 1976
7 Oshima T: Influence of pregnancy and lactation on migration of the larvae of *Toxocara canis* in mice. J Parasitol 47:657–660, 1961
8 Olson LJ, Rose JE: Effect of *Toxocara canis* infection on the ability of white rats to solve maze problems. Exp Parasitol 19:77–84, 1966
9 Dolinsky ZS, Burright RG, Donovick PJ, et al: Behavioral effects of lead and *Toxocara canis* in mice. Science 213:1142–1144, 1981
10 Kayes SG, Oaks JA: Development of the granulomatous response in murine toxocariasis. Am J Pathol 93:277–294, 1978
11 Parsons JC, Bowman DD, Grieve RB: Tissue localization of excretory-secretory antigens of larval *Toxocara canis* in acute and chronic murine toxocariasis. Am J Trop Med Hyg 35:974–981, 1986
12 Fernando ST: Immunological response of rabbits to *Toxocara canis* infection. Parasitology 58:91–103, 1968
13 Tomimura T, Yokota M, Takiguchi H: Experimental visceral larva migrans in monkeys. 1. Clinical, hematological, biochemical, and gross pathological observations on monkeys inoculated with embryonated eggs of the dog ascarid, *Toxocara canis*. Jpn J Vet Sci 38:533–548, 1976
14 Chadhuri RN, Saha TK: Tropical eosinophilia. Experiments with *Toxocara canis*. Lancet ii:493–495, 1959
15 Smith MHD, Beaver PC: Persistence and distribution of *Toxocara* larvae in tissues of children and mice. Pediatrics 12:491, 1953
16 Luxenberg MN: An experimental approach to the study of intraocular *Toxocara canis*. Trans Am Ophthalmol Soc 77:542–601, 1979
17 Beaver PC: Zoonoses with particular reference to parasites of veterinary importance, in Soulsby EJL (ed): *Biology of Parasites*. New York, Academic, 1966, pp 215–218
18 Desowitz RS, Rudoy R. Barnwell JW: Antibodies to canine helminth parasites in asthmatic and nonasthmatic children. Arch Allergy Appl Immunol 65:361–366, 1981
19 Bass JL, Mehta KA, Glickman LT, et al: Asymptomatic toxocariasis in children. Clin Pediatr 26:441–446, 1987
20 Beaver PC, Snyder CH, Carrera GM, et al: Chronic eosinophilia due to visceral larva migrans. Pediatrics 9:7–19, 1952
21 Mok CH: Visceral larva migrans—a discussion based on a review of the literature. Clin Pediatr 7:565–573, 1968
22 Glickman LT, Schantz PM, Cypess RH: Epidemiological characteristics and clinical findings in patients with serologically proven toxocariasis. Tran R Soc Trop Med Hyg 73:254–258, 1979
23 Glickman LT, Schantz PM, Cypess RH: Epidemiological characteristics and clinical findings in patients with serologically proven toxocariasis. Trans R Soc Trop Med Hyg 73:254–258, 1979
24 Worley G, Green JA, Frothingham TE, et al: *Toxocara canis* infection: Clinical and epidemiological associations in kindergarten children. J Infect Dis 149:591–597, 1984
25 Marmor M, Glickman L, Shofer F, et al: *Toxocara canis* infection of children: Epidemiologic and neuropsychologic findings. Am J Public Health 77:554–559, 1987
26 Huff D, Neafie R, Binder M, et al: The first fatal *Baylisascaris* infection in humans: An infant with eosinophilic meningitis. Pediatr Pathol 2:345–352, 1984
27 Glickman LT, Magnaval JF, Domanski LM, et al: Visceral larva

migrans in French adults: A new disease syndrome. Am J Epidemiol 125:1019–1034, 1987

28 Wilder HC; Nematode ophthalmitis. Trans Am Acad Ophthalmol Otolaryngol 55:99–109, 1950

29 Shields JA, Augsburger JJ: Current approaches to the diagnosis and management of retinoblastoma. Surv Ophthalmol 25:347–372, 1981

30 Sorr EM: Meandering ocular toxocariasis. Retina 4:90–96, 1984

31 Kazacos KR, Vestre WA, Kazacos EA: Raccoon ascarid larvae (*Baylisascaris procyonis*) as a cause of ocular larva migrans. Invest Ophthalmol Vis Sci 25:1177–1183, 1984

32 Gass JDM, Braunstein RA: Further observations concerning the diffuse unilateral subacute neuroretinitis syndrome. Arch Ophthalmol 101:1689–1697, 1983

33 Glickman LT, Schantz PM, Dombroske R, et al: Evaluation of serodiagnostic tests for visceral larva migrans. Am J Trop Med Hyg 27:492–498, 1978

34 Shields JA, Lerner HA, Felberg NT: Aqueous cytology and enzymes in nematode endophthalmitis. Am J Ophthalmol 84:319–322, 1972

35 Biglan AW, Glickman LT, Lokes LA: Serum and vitreous *Toxocara* antibody in nematode ophthalmitis. Am J Ophthalmol 88:898–901, 1979

36 American Academy Pediatrics Committee on Infectious Disease: Report of the Committee on Infectious Disease: Larva migrans, visceral (toxocariasis). Evanston, American Academy of Pediatrics, 1977, p 177

37 Aur RJA, Pratt CB, Johnson WW: Thiabendazole in visceral larva migrans. Am J Dis Child 121:226–229, 1971

38 Nelson JD, McConnell TH, Moore DV: Thiabendazole therapy of visceral larva migrans: A case report. Am J Trop Med Hyg 15:930–933, 1966

39 Shields JA: Ocular toxocariasis, a review. Survey Ophthalmol 28:361–381, 1984

40 Glickman LT, Schantz PM: Epidemiology and pathogenesis of zoonotic toxocariasis. Epidemiol Rev 3:230–250, 1981

41 Smith HV, Quinn R, Kusel JR, et al: The effect of temperature and antimetabolites on antibody binding to the outer surface of second stage *Toxocara canis* larvae. Mol Biochem Parasitol 4:183–193, 1981

42 Badley JE, Grieve RB, Rockey JH, et al: Immune-mediated adherence of eosinophils to *Toxocara canis* infective larvae: The role of excretory-secretory antigens. Parasite Immunol 9:133–143, 1987

43 Stehr-Green JK, Murray G, Schantz PM, et al: Intestinal parasites in pet store puppies in Atlanta. Am J Public Health 77:345–346, 1987

44 Reimers RS, Little MD, Englande AJ, et al: Parasites in southern sludges and disinfection by standard sludge treatment. U.S. Environmental Protection Agency, p 191

45 Ehrhard T, Kernbaum S: *Toxocara canis* et toxocarose humaine. Bull L'Institut Pasteur 77:225–227, 1979

46 DeSavigny DH, Voller A, Woodruff AW: Toxocariasis: Serological diagnosis by enzyme immunoassay. J Clin Pathol 32:284–288, 1979

47 Herrmann N, Glickman LT, Schantz PM, et al: Seroprevalence of zoonotic toxocariasis in the United States: 1971–1973. Am J Epidemiol 122:890–896, 1985

48 Schantz PM, Weiss PE, Pollard ZF, et al: Risk factors for toxocaral ocular larva migrans. Am J Public Health 70:1269–1272, 1980

49 Summary and conclusions: National conference on dog and cat control. J Am Vet Med Assoc 168:1125–1134, 1976

50 Action to reduce human health hazards arising from animals. WHO Chron 32:307–310, 1978

51 Kornblatt AN, Schantz PM: Veterinary and public health considerations in canine roundworm control: A survey of practicing veterinarians. J Am Vet Med Assoc 177:1212–1215, 1980

CHAPTER 53 / *Eosinophilic Meningitis* · Athasit Vejjajiva

Though inflammation of the meninges with eosinophilic pleocytosis in the cerebrospinal fluid may be of diverse etiology, the term *eosinophilic meningitis* has been used synonymously with central nervous system infection caused by the nematode *Angiostrongylus cantonensis*.

PARASITE

LIFE CYCLE [1,2,8]

Mature adult forms of *A. cantonensis* live in the pulmonary arteries of rats and related rodents. Eggs laid by fertilized females lodge in the terminal branches of the pulmonary arteries

and hatch into first-stage larvae, which migrate through the respiratory passages into the pharynx, are swallowed, and are subsequently excreted in the feces. Further development of the first-stage larvae takes place in one of several species of snails or slugs that serve as intermediate hosts. In the mollusk, the larvae grow and undergo two molts. The second-stage larva is immobile, while the third-stage larva is infective for the mammalian host. When infected mollusks are eaten by a rodent, liberated third-stage larvae migrate to the brain of the host to undergo two further stages of development. The young adult worms then migrate to the surface of the brain, enter the venous system, and eventually reach the pulmonary arteries, where they attain full sexual maturity. In humans, development of *A. cantonensis* almost always is arrested in the central nervous system, where the nematodes usually die, but the finding of adult worms in the pulmonary arteries at autopsy of fatal cases has been reported.

INTERMEDIATE AND PARATENIC HOSTS [3]

The natural intermediate hosts within which *A. cantonensis* larvae develop to the infective third stage are aquatic and terrestrial snails, notably the *Pila* spp., *Achatina fulica,* and slugs. Freshwater prawns, land crabs, and frogs have been found to harbor the third-stage larvae of the parasite as a result of eating infected intermediate hosts. Though the larvae are unable to continue their development in those animals, they remain infective for a certain period of time and are able to resume their development after ingestion of an infected paratenic (transport) host by a final host. Under specific conditions, paratenic hosts may have greater epidemiological significance than intermediate hosts.

PATIENT

PATHOGENESIS AND PATHOLOGY [4]

The ingested living third-stage larvae reach the central nervous system of the human host and cause damage because of their motility. In addition, inflammation and granulomatous reactions occur in the parenchyma of the brain and spinal cord and in the meninges from dead parasites. Autopsy findings of cases in which *A. cantonensis* was identified in the brain included the presence of tracklike lesions containing necrotic tissue debris, scattered inflammatory cells, mostly histiocytes and neutrophils, and generalized vascular congestion. Large numbers of Charcot-Leyden crystals were present in the meninges, indicating a massive response by eosinophils to the dead parasites.

CLINICAL MANIFESTATIONS [5–8]

The commonest presenting symptom occurring in almost all patients is headache, which is usually initially intermittent, throbbing or bursting in nature, and confined to the occipital or temporal region bilaterally. Headache soon becomes persistent and generalized when severe and is often associated with nausea and vomiting. Occasionally, stabbing pain in the head and paresthesia of the scalp are present. Disturbance of consciousness and seizure are uncommon except in children or in severely affected cases. Fever is uncommon and, when present, rarely exceeds 38°C and often lasts a few days. Examination reveals neck stiffness and Kernig's sign, but not invariably; in mild cases they are often absent. Cranial nerves, particularly the optic, the abducens, and the facial nerves, are sometimes affected. Paresthesias of the trunk or extremities are occasionally noted, but paralysis of the lower limbs is very rare. In the ocular form of *A. cantonensis,* young adult worms have been found in the anterior chamber of the eye or in the vitreous substance. Blepharospasm, ciliary injection, iritis, and increased ocular tension were noted in the affected eye. A patient with the parasite appearing in the eye 2 weeks after a mild attack of meningitis has also been reported. Respiratory symptoms and signs and radiographical features of pneumonitis have been encountered in some severe cases of nervous system angiostrongyliasis.

Laboratory findings [9,10]

The cerebrospinal fluid (CSF) is always abnormal, usually turbid in appearance (likened to coconut juice), and the pressure is often increased. The white cell count usually ranges from 500 to 5000 per cubic millimeter with eosinophils of 20 to 90 percent. The CSF protein is elevated but is usually less than 100 mg per 100 mL, while the glucose is normal or, rarely, is slightly decreased. A living fifth-stage *A. cantonensis,* measuring about 0.5 to 1.5 cm in length, has been isolated from CSF at lumbar puncture on very rare occasions. Blood leukocytosis, over 10,000 cells per cubic millimeter, is found in about one-half of cases, and eosinophilia of over 10 percent is present in the majority of patients. Serological examination using enzyme-linked immunosorbent assay (ELISA) is a helpful confirmatory test.

DIFFERENTIAL DIAGNOSIS [11,12]

Cerebral angiostrongyliasis should be considered in evaluation of patients with severe headache or paresthesia who live in, or have recently visited, areas where *A. cantonensis* is known to occur. Diagnosis is usually made on the history and clinical findings. Nervous system gnathostomiasis caused by the nematode *Gnathostoma spinigerum* prevalent in southeast Asia, particularly Thailand, usually has a different clinical presentation. Radiculomyelitis or myeloencephalitis with paralysis of limbs and often severe disabling sequelae are typical of gnathostomiasis. Rarely, it may present with headache and neck stiffness and thus mimics *A. cantonensis* infection, but the CSF in the former is usually bloodstained, unlike the turbid, coconut juice–like appearance of the latter.

TREATMENT AND OUTCOME

There is no specific treatment for the disease. Repeated lumbar punctures are often necessary for relief of headache. The efficacy of corticosteroid treatment is doubtful. The duration of the disease ranges from a few days to a month. Most patients recover completely. Permanent impairment of vision is occasionally seen in patients with ocular or optic nerve involvement. The mortality rate is less than 1 percent.

POPULATION

GEOGRAPHICAL DISTRIBUTION [8,13]

A. cantonensis is prevalent in many Asian-Pacific countries including Hawaii, Tahiti, Cook Island, Caroline Island, New Hebrides, American Samoa, New Caledonia, the Philippines, Indonesia, Malaysia, Thailand, Vietnam, Taiwan, Hong Kong, Japan, Papua New Guinea, and Australia. In addition the parasite has been found in Egypt and Cuba. Most of the clinically diagnosed cases, numbering thousands, and over 30 parasitologically proven cases were, however, reported from Thailand, Taiwan, and the south Pacific islands.

MODE OF HUMAN INFECTION

Humans are infected with *A. cantonensis* from eating raw or undercooked snails, slugs, freshwater prawns, or land crabs which are intermediate hosts carrying the third-stage larvae. In Thailand, *Pila* snails are the main source of infection. The disease often has seasonal occurrence, being more prevalent during the rainy season when *Pila* snails are readily available. It is commonly seen in epidemic extent or as several cases occurring together, both adults and children affected at the same time, a week or two after a common meal consisting of *Pila* snails, which are considered to be a great delicacy. The incubation period ranges from 3 days to 5 weeks, with an average of about 2 weeks.

PROPHYLAXIS

The most important means of prevention of infection in human beings is education about the nature and source of the disease, though admittedly, it is difficult to change the cultural factors affecting types of food consumed and methods of food preparation.

REFERENCES

1 Alicata JE, Jindrak K: *Angiostrongyliasis in the Pacific and Southeast Asia.* Springfield, Charles C Thomas, 1970
2 Yii C-Y, Chen C-Y, Fresh JW, et al: Human angiostrongyliasis involving lungs. Chin J Microbiol 1:148–150, 1968
3 Jindrak K: Angiostrongyliasis cantonensis (eosinophilic meningitis, Alicata's disease), in Hornabrook RW: *Topics in Tropical Neurology.* Philadelphia, Davis, 1975, pp 133–164
4 Tangchai P, Nye SW, Beaver PC: Eosinophilic meningoencephalitis caused by angiostrongyliasis in Thailand: Autopsy report. Am J Trop Med Hyg 16:454–461, 1967
5 Punyagupta S, Juttijudata P, Bunnag T: Eosinophilic meningitis in Thailand: Clinical studies of 484 typical cases probably caused by *Angiostrongylus cantonensis.* Am J Trop Med Hyg 24:921–931, 1975
6 Prommindaroj K, Leelawongs N, Pradatsundarasar A: Human angiostrongyliasis of the eye in Bangkok. Am J Trop Med Hyg 11: 759–761, 1962
7 Kanchanaranya C, Punyagupta S: Case of ocular angiostrongyliasis associated with eosinophilic meningitis. Am J Ophthalmol 71:931–934, 1971
8 Punyagupta S: Angiostrongyliasis, in Weatherall CJ, Ledingham JGG, Warrell DA: *Oxford Textbook of Medicine,* 2d ed. Oxford University Press, 1987, pp 5.555–5.558
9 Punyagupta S, Bunnag T, Juttijudata P, et al: Eosinophilic meningitis in Thailand: Epidemiologic studies of 484 typical cases and the etiologic role of *Angiostrongylus cantonensis.* Am J Trop Med Hyg 19:950–958, 1970
10 Ko RC, Chiu MC, Kum W, et al: First report of human angiostrongyliasis in Hong Kong diagnosed by computerized axial tomography (CAT) and enzyme linked immunosorbent assay. Trans R Soc Trop Med Hyg 78:354–355, 1984
11 Boongird P, Phuapradit P, Siridej N, et al: Neurological manifestations of gnathostomiasis. J Neurol Sci 31:279–291, 1977
12 Schmutzhard E, Boongird P, Vejjajiva A: Eosinophilic meningitis and radiculomyelitis in Thailand, caused by CNS invasion of *Gnathostoma spinigerum* and *Angiostrongylus cantonensis.* J Neurol Neurosurg Psychiatry 51:80–87, 1988
13 Rosen L, Loison G, Laigret J, et al: Studies on eosinophilic meningitis: 3.Epidemiologic and clinical observations on Pacific Islands and the possible etiologic role of *Angiostrongylus cantonensis.* Am J Epidemiol 85:17–44, 1967

Trematode Infections

Schistosomiasis · Adel A. F. Mahmoud
· M. Farid Abdel Wahab

The schistosomes are a group of digenetic dioecious trematodes which cause considerable morbidity and mortality in humans. Worms of the genus *Schistosoma* comprise several blood parasites of humans and other animals; they belong to the phylum Platyhelminthes and family Schistosomatidae. Humans may be infected by schistosome species of any of three groups:

1. Major human parasites including *Schistosoma haematobium*, *S. mansoni*, and *S. japonicum*
2. Less epidemiologically prevalent species such as *S. intercalatum* and *S. mekongi*
3. Certain species of avian and mammalian schistosomes that produce cercarial dermatitis

Schistosomiasis (bilharziasis) is a major human health problem in many parts of the developing world. Clinically, disease due to schistosomiasis affects mainly children and young adults; it has an insidious pathological course before its full features are manifested. Furthermore, animal schistosomes such as *S. bovis* cause economically important disease in cattle in some countries. Recently, an increase in prevalence of schistosomiasis has paralleled the economically essential land and irrigation development programs, particularly in Africa, thus complicating the magnitude and extent of this problem.

PARASITE

LIFE HISTORY

The genus *Schistosoma* includes several of the oldest human parasites known; *S. haematobium* eggs were found in the kidneys of twentieth-dynasty Egyptian mummies (1250–1000 B.C.). Adult schistosomes are obligatory parasites, but in contrast to all digenetic monoecious trematodes they exist as separate sexes (dioecious) in the definitive host [1]. The general pattern of life history of the schistosomes is similar for all species that cause patent infection in humans (Fig. 54-1). Adult schistosomes have elongate and slender bodies which are well suited for their habitat in the vesical and portal blood vessels. The exact location of adult worms in the human definitive host is determined by the parasite species: *S. haematobium* in vesical veins, *S. mansoni* in superior mesenteric veins, and *S. japonicum* in inferior mesenteric veins. This localization of adult worms is not absolute as parasites are occasionally found in other anatomical sites within the definitive host (e.g., *S. haematobium* worms in the mesenteric veins). A change in

the worm's final habitat in the mammalian host may reflect differences in the host-parasite relationship; for example, *S. haematobium* worms are mainly found in the mesenteric vessels of baboons. More importantly, worms may change their location according to the stage of infection and disease—e.g., the migration of *S. mansoni* adults toward the hepatic rather than the intestinal end of the portal circulation in patients with advanced hepatosplenic disease.

Sexual maturity of female schistosomes is dependent on the presence of living mature male worms. Egg deposition occurs in the small venules of the vesical or portal venous systems. When freshly deposited, *Schistosoma* ova are partially developed, and it takes approximately 10 days for the enclosed miracidia to mature. Oviposition occurs intravascularly; eggs thereafter work their way toward the lumen of ureters and urinary bladder (*S. haematobium*) or intestines (*S. mansoni*, *S. japonicum*) in order to be carried to the outside with urine or feces. Following release from the definitive host and under optimal environmental conditions, the schistosome eggs hatch, leading to liberation of actively swimming miracidia. The next phase of development occurs when miracidia find and penetrate the snail intermediate hosts. Within the mollusk, two generations of sporocysts develop which result in the emergence of furocercous cercariae. These infective forms are found in contaminated waters; they are capable of penetrating intact skin of definitive hosts, migrating through several tissues to reach their final habitat.

MORPHOLOGY

Although adult schistosomes are dioecious, they are usually found paired. The larger male has a ventral gynecophoric canal in which the slender female is held. The body of adult schistosomes is elongate, varying in length from 6 to 26 mm. The male is light gray, and the female is darker in color. Mature worms of both sexes have two suckers each, an oral and a ventral. The mouth is located in the center of the oral sucker and connects to forked, blind-ending intestinal ceca. Four to eight testes are found in adult males; they are situated dorsally and posterior to the ventral sucker. The number and size of testes may serve to differentiate schistosome species [2]. Adult female schistosomes are generally longer than males; they are cylindrical in shape and have a characteristic black color in their intestines from ingested erythrocytes. Characterization of

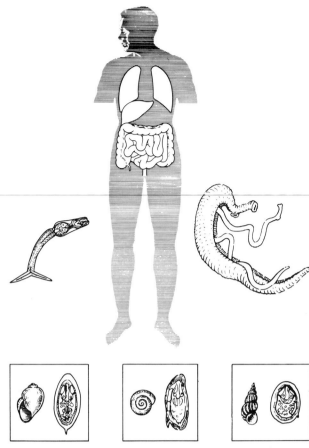

Figure 54-1. Schematic representation of the life cycle of the three schistosome species that commonly infect humans (*S. haematobium, S. mansoni,* and *S. japonicum*); the characteristic shapes of the snail intermediate host and parasite eggs are included.

which reach full maturity in approximately 10 days. Within humans or other mammalian hosts, eggs are incapable of hatching, but upon reaching suitable environmental conditions of temperature, pH, salt concentration, and light, the shell splits open along its long axis. The miracidium, an oval ciliated organism, escapes headfirst; this organism is capable of swimming forward and of avoiding obstacles. It is positively phototactic and negatively thermotactic. The internal organs of the miracidium are bilaterally symmetrical. They include a primitive digestive tract, anterior and lateral secretory glands, flame cells, a nerve center, and a posterior mass of germinal cells. Morphological differentiation of schistosome species during the miracidium stage is impossible. Once freed, the schistosome miracidia are infective to the intermediate mollusk hosts up to 32 h. The effective infective period under natural conditions is probably much shorter. Miracidia are attracted by the chemotactic action of the snail tissues. Following penetration of snails, miracidia lose their mobility, shed their ciliary membrane, and change into elongate, thin-walled sporocysts which are filled with germ cells. The sporocysts increase in size and finally rupture, liberating a second generation of 200 to 400 organisms. Cercariae form within these secondary sporocysts; they penetrate through the snail tissues and escape to water. Mature cercariae are elongate and have pear-shaped bodies and long bifurcated tails (Fig. 54-2). The large anterior

species of female worms depends on the position of the ovary, the length of the uterus, and the number of eggs within [2].

The integument of schistosomes is similar to that of many other blood flukes in that it has a characteristic and unique ultrastructural appearance [3]. It is made of two lipid bilayers, each approximately 7 nm in thickness; the entire membrane is approximately 18 nm thick. It is worth noting here that schistosome cercariae have a trilaminate membrane (one lipid bilayer) which changes to the characteristic adult heptalaminate membrane upon transformation of cercariae into schistosomula. Some of the factors involved in this membrane transformation, including the role of microtubules connecting subtegumental cells to the syncytial surface membrane, have recently been examined [3].

The generally ovoid eggs of schistosomes are nonoperculated and have spines in various positions characteristic of the species (Fig. 54-1). The eggshell is made of resistant protein material from the granules of the yolk sac. When freshly deposited, the schistosome eggs contain immature miracidia

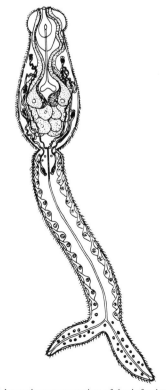

Figure 54-2. Schematic representation of the infective stage (cercaria) of *S. mansoni.*

sucker occupies the front end of the cercarial body, where the gut and ducts of cephalic glands open. The ventral sucker is a well-developed muscular organ situated on the posterior fourth of the body and serves, as does the anterior sucker, as an attachment organ.

Penetration of the definitive host is initiated by attachment of cercariae through their anterior or ventral suckers to skin. The vibratory movements of the cercarial body, the lashing of its tail, and the secretions of the cephalic penetration glands result in completion of penetration, usually within minutes. During this process, cercariae shake off their tails, lose most of their glycocalyx, and proceed to occupy tunnels in the stratum corneum parallel to the skin surface. These organisms are called *schistosomula* and correspond to the migrating metacercariae of other trematodes. Schistosomula have a double lipid bilayer membrane (heptalaminate) similar to that observed on adult worms. The internal organs of schistosomula undergo a maturational process along with their migration from the dermal sites of cercarial penetration through the lungs and finally to the liver.

BIOLOGY OF THE SCHISTOSOMES

The intermediary metabolism of the different maturational stages of schistosomes has not been examined in detail. Adult schistosomes have a very high rate of glycolysis; they utilize glucose at a rate of one-fifth of their body weight per hour. No Krebs cycle pathway was found in adult worms.

Studies of cercarial metabolism, however, have shown that cercariae possess a functional Krebs cycle; these organisms consume pyruvate rapidly and produce large quantities of CO_2. A great reduction of pyruvate catabolism occurs, however, once cercariae change into schistosomula. Perhaps the most biologically important changes that occur in the schistosomes from the point of view of parasitization of the definitive host are those associated with the change in schistosomula metabolism, antigenicity, and ability to survive the hostile environment of the host [4,5]. Within a few days of their penetration of a mammalian host, schistosomula exhibit increased mobility, their surface area increases dramatically because of added surface involutions, and the distribution of intramembranous particles is altered. In addition to the formation of the heptalaminate membrane, schistosomula acquire the ability to resist most in vitro effector killing mechanisms and exhibit multiple host proteins adsorbed on the membrane surface.

The nutritional needs of the different stages of schistosomes are not well understood. Adult worms ingest host erythrocytes but not to a degree that will result in manifest anemia. Adult worms also actively utilize glucose and perhaps amino acids. In vitro, it is possible to maintain male and female worms for several weeks; however, only eggs which were contained in the uterus will be deposited. No artificial medium has yet successfully supported in vitro vitellogenesis. In vitro culture of schistosome cells has not been developed to a stage where it will contribute to understanding schistosome biology [6]. In contrast, schistosomula have been maintained in culture to reach adult worm morphology and exhibit several of its nutritional features (e.g., ingestion of erythrocytes).

Early attempts to calculate the mean life span of adult schistosomes were based on examination of individuals who moved out of endemic areas. These reports suggest extreme limits of worm longevity of 20 to 30 years but fail to indicate the mean worm survival time. Using stochastic models, the mean life span of *S. mansoni* was calculated to vary from 1.5 to 18 years. In contrast, by evaluating the decline of egg counts in a group of Yemeni immigrants to California, the mean worm survival time was suggested to vary from 5 to 10 years [7]. Further support for a short rather than an extreme mean life span of *S. mansoni* was obtained by analyzing data from St. Lucia; worm longevity varied from 2.7 to 4.5 years. These values must be taken as approximations at best since such calculations assume that egg output is linearly related to worm burden and that the helminth survival in a specific host is independent of worm load.

Another controversial issue concerns the rate of egg production by adult schistosomes. All experimental studies are based on the assumption that egg production in infected animals proceeds at a regular rate. For example, the mean daily egg production by female worms has been calculated to be 239 in *S. haematobium,* 300 in *S. mansoni,* 3000 in *S. japonicum,* and 207 in *S. intercalatum.* Furthermore, the possibility that the rate of oviposition may vary with the immune status of the host has recently been suggested.

Utilization of molecular biological techniques to study the schistosomes is just beginning [8]. Furthermore, the karyotypes of *S. mansoni* have recently been reexamined; there are eight pairs of chromosomes ($2n = 16$), which can be divided into three groups according to size [9]. The presence of sex chromosomes was suggested by finding a heteromorphic pair in female worms (zw) and a homomorphic pair in males (zz). Recently, the use of monoclonal antibodies has resulted in isolation and characterization of several candidate schistosome protective antigens. Some of these molecules have been cloned, and the recombinant antigens are now being tested as potential vaccines [10–12].

INTERMEDIATE HOST

Schistosome development requires a phase in an intermediate molluscan host. During this phase the parasite undergoes asexual multiplication and differentiation. In addition, it uses the snail as a medium for transportation and dissemination. Recent studies on snail host-parasite relationships indicate the complex nature of the schistosome-snail interaction. The first difficulty concerns snail taxonomy [13]. Because of the multiplicity of snails involved in schistosomiasis transmission in different endemic areas, a sound taxonomy is vital. Morphological, biochemical, and genetic techniques are being used to identify snail species; there remains, however, a lot to explore in the snail-schistosome complex. Compatibility of the parasite and its specific snail intermediate host is controlled by several factors, although genetics seem to play a central role. For example, it is possible to breed *Biomphalaria glabrata* to produce susceptible and refractory snails; some may be susceptible as juveniles and become refractory as adults. Other important aspects concern snail cultivation, physiology, and acquisition of resistance to molluscicides, which may be of considerable significance in control programs.

The snail hosts of *S. haematobium* belong to the genus *Bulinus*, which has been divided into two subgenera: *Bulinus* and *Physopsis*. *Bulinus* snails have been further classified into three species groups: *B. forskalii*, *B. reticulatus*, and the *B. truncatus–B. tropicus* complex. The natural snail intermediate host of *S. intercalatum* is not clear. Experimental infections were successful in the *B. forskalii* and *B. reticulatus* groups. *S. mansoni* in the Americas is transmitted by snails of the genus *Biomphalaria*, of which *B. glabrata*, *B. straminea*, and *B. tenagophila* have been found naturally infected with the parasite. In Africa and the Middle East the biomphalarids are divided into four species groups: *B. pfeifferi*, *B. alexandrina*, *B. choanomphala*, and *B. sudanica*. It is felt, however, that the taxonomic status of the African species of *Biomphalaria* is not satisfactory and requires further investigation. In the Far East, *S. japonicum* is transmitted by the polytypic *Oncomelania hupensis*, of which there are six geographical strains that have been found naturally infected in China, Taiwan, Indonesia, Japan, and the Philippines. *S. mekongi* has been shown to be transmitted by *Tricula aperta*.

PATIENT

HOST-PARASITE INTERFACE

Schistosome infection of the definitive mammalian host is initiated by cercarial penetration of skin. The outcome of infection varies across a wide spectrum: cercariae may die as they attempt to penetrate skin; schistosomula may be killed in the subcutaneous tissues or en route to their final habitat. Nevertheless, patent infection may be established in humans or experimental animals. The dynamic interactions between a multitude of factors that influence the invader and the host and control their encounter spell the success of the schistosome's parasitic way of life for thousands of years.

Invasion of dermal tissues is followed by a series of changes that result in the transformation of cercariae into schistosomula. These include morphological, biochemical, antigenic, and particularly membrane changes. In *S. mansoni* the heptalaminate membrane begins to appear within 60 min of skin penetration and is complete by 3 h. The process is believed to involve fusion of the bounding membrane of the multilaminate vesicles with the surface plasma membrane of the integument. Furthermore, it has been shown that vesicle formation and fusion into integument is dependent on microtubule function

[3]. Detailed investigations of schistosomula membrane changes may be of biological relevance since these organisms quickly lose their susceptibility to antibody-dependent killing. Originally, it was thought that the acquired resistance of schistosomula was due to acquisition of host antigens on their surface. It was, however, realized that besides blood group substances several others, such as products of the major histocompatibility complex and serum proteins, can be demonstrated on the parasite surface. Further, the continuous turnover of the membrane may lead to loss of antigenic components that can be recognized by antibodies. The question of how the schistosomes evade the host immune response, though, has been the subject of considerable investigations and is still unanswered.

Controversy still exists concerning the route of migration of schistosomula from skin sites of infection to the lungs and finally to the portal and vesical veins. Recent evidence suggests that blood vessels are the most probable route that carries schistosomula to the lungs; how these organisms reach their final habitat is, however, unclear.

The chronic nature of schistosome infection and the multicellular and complex nature of the organisms expose the host immune and defense mechanisms to a myriad of challenges. The infective forms are capable of penetrating intact skin, but not all of them mature even in the most susceptible hosts known (mice and hamsters). Whether or not the proportion of lost cercariae under these circumstances represents innate resistance needs further evaluation [14]. During the course of maturation of the schistosomes within humans or experimental animals several classes and specifications of antibodies are formed as well as populations of sensitized lymphocytes. It is only under specific conditions in vivo or in vitro that a proportion of the host immune response (antibodies and/or cells) has been shown to participate in acquired resistance against subsequent challenge with the schistosomes [5]. Whereas several effector cells have been shown to lead to parasite damage in vitro [15], the eosinophils and mononuclear phagocytes appear as the most likely cells involved in host protection in vivo [16].

Another aspect of human response to schistosomiasis concerns the development of humoral and cellular immunity against the parasite eggs. These responses have been implicated as the major pathological lesions leading to granuloma formation with its space-occupying nature and subsequent fibrosis [17]. Extensive investigations in experimental animals showed that *S. mansoni* and *S. haematobium* eggs elicit a delayed hypersensitivity granulomatous response that is made mainly of lymphoctyes, macrophages, and eosinophils. Furthermore, the immune response to schistosome eggs involves modulatory mechanisms which ameliorate granuloma size and the subsequent clinicopathological effects in chronically infected animals [18].

In contrast to the detailed information on the mechanisms that elicit and modulate immunopathology of schistosomiasis in experimental animals, understanding of human responses is incomplete. Peripheral blood lymphocytes of infected individuals respond to various antigenic preparations obtained from worms or eggs. There seems to be an inverse correlation between the intensity of infection as determined by egg counting and immune responsiveness [19]. Several mechanisms, humoral and cellular, have been demonstrated which may contribute to suppression of lymphocyte reactivity. Furthermore, variability in disease manifestations and immune responsiveness in some areas where schistosomiasis is endemic, such as Egypt, Brazil, and Japan, has promoted examination of other host factors that might contribute to disease. In Brazil an association between severity of hepatosplenomegaly and blood groups or race has been suggested, whereas in Egypt the same manifestations of schistosomiasis mansoni have been correlated with certain haplotypes of the HLA system [20].

PATHOGENESIS

The etiology of disease that follows human infection with the schistosomes is related to multiple factors including stage of infection, previous exposures of host, worm load, and extent and magnitude of host responses. These factors are in turn influenced by epidemiological and genetic considerations. Basic to understanding pathogenesis in schistosomiasis is the realization that pathological sequelae of infection may occur in a considerable proportion of infected individuals (e.g., *S. haematobium*) or in a small but significant percentage (e.g., *S. mansoni* or *S. japonicum*).

The major disease syndromes associated with schistosomiasis are related to the stage of infection. Cercarial dermatitis is due to skin invasion and is likely a result of host sensitization. Indeed, both humoral and cellular immune responses to cercarial antigens have been demonstrated in infected humans and experimental animals [17]. What is not clear is why cercarial dermatitis has been reported with some (*S. haematobium* or *S. mansoni*) but not other species (*S. japonicum*) of human schistosomes, and why it is almost a constant feature of human infection with avian parasites. Death of cercariae in subcutaneous tissues is the major feature of human infection with nonhuman parasites; that may explain the regularity of observing cercarial dermatitis in its severe forms in this condition. While primary exposure to these parasites may be associated with a few clinical manifestations, the characteristic maculopapular itchy rash appears on subsequent encounters. Skin manifestations follow immediately and may be related to the development of reaginic antibodies that give rise to manifestations of immediate hypersensitivity at the sites of parasite invasion. Papular rash along with mononuclear and eosinophil infiltrate appears subsequently and suggests a role for cell-mediated hypersensitivity.

Acute schistosomiasis or Katayama fever is a clinical syndrome that has been described a few weeks following primary infection, particularly with *S. japonicum* or *S. mansoni*. The characteristic clinical features include fever, hepatosplenomegaly, lymphadenopathy, and peripheral eosinophilia. Katayama fever seems more frequently associated with heavy infections. Besides the clinical manifestations of acute schistosomiasis, the rise in IgG and IgE immunoglobulins and antischistosomal antibodies was positively correlated with egg output. Although the etiology of acute schistosomiasis is unknown, its manifestations and association with primary heavy infection have led to the suggestion that it is a form of serum sickness or antigen-antibody complex disease.

The established lesions in patent schistosomiasis are related to the eggs retained in tissues and the subsequent host responses. A considerable proportion of schistosome eggs is retained in the urinary tract or intestinal tissues; an estimated 33 percent reach the liver in individuals infected with the schistosomes of the portomesenteric system. It takes approximately 10 days for schistosome eggs trapped in the host tissues to complete maturation of the enclosed miracidia, which can survive further for 2 to 3 weeks. During this period several enzymes and antigenic materials are released, induce host sensitization, and contribute to the resulting pathological lesions. The host granulomatous response to the retained schistosome eggs has been demonstrated to be a form of immune reactiveness. Cell-mediated hypersensitivity plays the key role in granuloma formation around *S. haematobium* and *S. mansoni* eggs, while the mechanism of this response in schistosomiasis japonica is not yet clear. Granuloma formation leads to a compact cellular infiltrate surrounding the parasite eggs, made of lymphocytes, eosinophils, macrophages, and fibroblasts. The formation of these granulomas in the wall of the urinary or intestinal tracts is the major cause of pathological changes. In addition, the presence of granulomas may lead to mechanical obstruction of the urinary tract or portal circulation.

The transition from granuloma formation to fibrous tissue deposition marks the establishment of the permanent fibroobstructive lesions of schistosomiasis. In experimental schistosomiasis mansoni collagen synthesis and hepatic concentration of proline are increased. Similar studies also were performed on wedge biopsies from patients with hepatosplenomegaly and showed that collagen content was two- to fivefold higher than that of normal liver. While these studies have started to explore the initial steps in liver collagen synthesis in schistosomiasis, several other steps remain unknown. Specifically, what controls the switch from the localized granulomatous response around schistosome eggs to the massive claypipestem fibrosis, and what are the dynamic synthetic and degradative processes that determine the final outcome in schistosomal liver fibrosis?

There are several other chronic sequelae of schistosomiasis such as central nervous system infection and schistosomal cor pulmonale where the pathogenesis of disease is probably related to the chain of events described above, i.e., egg deposition, inflammation, and granuloma formation which leads to fibrosis. Central nervous system disease in schistosomiasis is related to the species of the parasite. Cord disease (e.g., transverse myelitis) has been described in *S. mansoni* or *S. haematobium* infection, while cerebral pathology is characteristic of *S. japonicum* infection [*21*]. While there are several clinical and pathological descriptions, most of these syndromes remain poorly defined. There are, however, some other manifestations that deserve special emphasis. Carcinoma of the bladder has been associated with chronic *S. haematobium* infection in Egypt, Zimbabwe, and Iraq. The lesions occur in persons who are a decade or two younger than the mean age of incidence of carcinoma of the bladder in the developed world. The majority of these cases are squamous cell carcinomas, which is in striking contrast to the transitional cell tumors seen in nonbilharzial cases. In a recent autopsy study ureteral hyperplasia, metaplasia, and dysplasia were shown to be more common in *S. haematobium*–infected patients than control subjects. The relevance of these lesions as precancerous and the exact etiology of malignancy associated with *S. haematobium* are, however, unknown.

SCHISTOSOMIASIS HAEMATOBIA

Among human schistosome infections, *S. haematobium* infection is the most pathogenic since urinary tract disease is present in a considerable proportion of infected individuals. Moreover, recent studies suggest that obstructive uropathy due to *S. haematobium* infection and its sequelae are progressive in nature.

Pathology

Adult *S. haematobium* worms migrate from the liver to the inferior mesenteric and finally to the vesical veins via the rectal, hemorrhoidal, and pudendal vessels. It takes 4 to 9 weeks from cercarial penetration to detection of eggs in urine. A considerable number of these eggs are retained in host tissues, particularly in the urinary bladder and lower ureters. Fewer eggs are detected in upper ureters, kidneys, seminal vesicles, prostate, and rectum. Furthermore, egg burdens in the lower right ureters have been observed to be significantly higher than in the left, which correlates with more right-sided disease in infected individuals. In autopsy materials, intensity of tissue egg counts was shown to correlate significantly with severity of urinary tract lesions and with the occurrence of obstructive uropathy manifesting as hydroureters and hydronephrosis. The gross pathological lesions ascribed to schistosomiasis haematobia are more frequently seen in heavily infected individuals. These lesions include sandy patches, polyposis, and bladder ulcers; less frequently seen are urinary tract calculi and ureteritis cystica calcinosa.

The association of urinary tract bacterial infections and schistosomiasis haematobia is not yet well established. Increased prevalence of bacteriuria in infected subjects in Egypt and Gambia has been demonstrated. In contrast, no such association was found in the Malumfashi area of Nigeria [*22*]. Whether the difference is simply due to the low intensity of *S. haematobium* infection in the latter study or to other factors is presently unclear. A more common association is that of pyelonephritis with schistosomal obstructive uropathy; it is significantly higher than its association with other etiologies of obstructive uropathy. Another epidemiological association of major clinical importance is that of *S. haematobium* infection and carcinoma of the bladder [*23*]. From the several published autopsy studies specific features of this complication can be outlined [*24*]. Bladder cancer occurs in a relatively younger age group (mean, 47 years). The majority of schistosomal bladder cancers are of the nodular fungating variety. Histopathologically, two-thirds of these tumors are of the squamous cell type and a fourth is classified as transitional cell carcinoma. Other differences worth noting concern the low rate of involvement of bladder trigone and prostate as compared with nonschistosomal bladder cancer.

Clinical manifestations

Symptoms due to penetration of human skin with *S. haematobium* cercariae (swimmer's itch) and during maturation of adult worms (acute schistosomiasis) have rarely been reported in urinary schistosomiasis. In contrast, once infection is established and ova deposition begins, frequent symptoms and signs have been reported. In several well-controlled studies of schoolage children and whole communities in endemic areas, *S. haematobium* infection was associated with dysuria, terminal or total hematuria, and frequency [*25–27*]. While the occurrence of these symptoms seems to be related to intensity of infection, as more than 90 percent of individuals with 1000 or more eggs per 10 mL urine complained of hematuria, almost half of lightly infected individuals gave a history of dysuria and hematuria. Urine examinations during this phase of uncomplicated urinary schistosomiasis demonstrate that the degree of proteinuria and hematuria is significantly correlated with intensity of infection. Other laboratory findings in urine of infected individuals may be seen once complications occur such as bacteriuria, casts, or changes in urine osmolality. In one cystoscopic study hyperemia was most common (33 percent) but more frequent in heavily infected subjects (60 percent). The frequency of other lesions was less: sandy patches (33 percent), tubercles (18 percent), ulcers (9 percent), and nodules and polyps (7 percent) [*28*]. Most of these lesions were again more frequent in heavily infected individuals. Radiological examination illustrates the extent of disease in the urinary tract including calcification of the bladder and lower ureters, obstructive uropathy with hydroureters and hydronephrosis (Fig. 54-3), calculi and irregularities of mucosa, and filling defects. More recently, the noninvasive ultrasonographic examination of individuals with *S. haematobium* infection has added to our understanding of its sequelae (Figs. 54-4 and 54-5) [*26*]. The natural history of urinary tract lesions in schistosomiasis haematobia is unknown although suggestive evidence indicates its progressive nature [*27*].

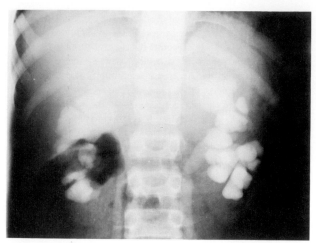

Figure 54-3. Intravenous pyelography showing extensive bilateral hydronephrosis and hydroureters in a 14-year-old Kenyan with *S. haematobium* infection.

The clinical presentation of patients with schistosomal bladder cancer does not differ markedly from those of uncomplicated schistosomiasis haematobia. In a recent series of 304 patients approximately two-thirds complained of painful micturition and frequency while hematuria was reported by half. Most of these tumors originate in the posterior bladder wall (45 percent).

Other clinical presentations attributable to *S. haematobium* infection such as cor pulmonale (Fig. 54-6) and transverse

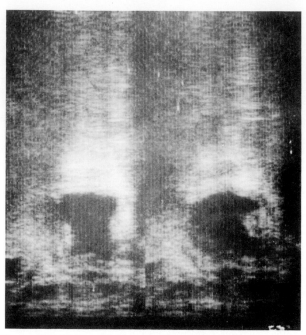

Figure 54-5. Urinary bladder ultrasonographic examination of a 10-year-old Kenyan infected with *S. haematobium*. Note the irregularities and thickening of bladder wall and the granulomas protruding into the organ cavity.

myelitis are less commonly seen than disease in the urinary tract. There is no convincing evidence that *S. haematobium* infection may lead to hepatosplenomegaly.

Diagnosis

Definitive diagnosis of schistosomiasis haematobia can be accomplished by demonstrating parasite eggs in urine samples. Peak egg excretion occurs between noon and 3 P.M. when samples should ideally be obtained [29], particularly if quantitative methods are to be used. Urine samples can be examined qualitatively by simple sedimentation or following centrifugation. The sediment is placed on a microscope slide and examined for parasite eggs. If quantitative information is needed, one of several methods may be used. The method of choice currently is nuclepore filtration in which a known volume of urine is filtered; the membrane can then be examined immediately or can be kept on a glass slide for later evaluation. The nuclepore filtration method has the added advantage of not requiring staining or special fixation procedures. In specific circumstances, particularly when new drugs are being evaluated, a hatching test may be necessary to evaluate viability of eggs. *S. haematobium* eggs also may be found in stool samples or biopsy material from the urinary bladder or rectum. The latter procedures are rarely needed for diagnostic purposes. Serological testing for *S. haematobium* infection is unsatisfac-

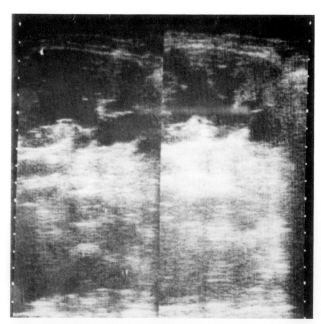

Figure 54-4. Renal ultrasonographic examination of a 12-year-old Kenyan infected with *S. haematobium*. Note the extensive hydronephrosis with destruction of kidney tissue.

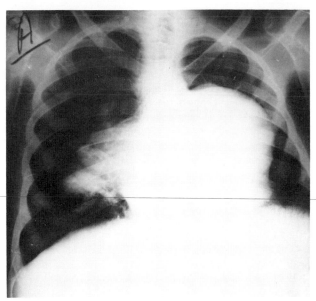

Figure 54-6. Schistosomal cor pulmonale in an Egyptian with hepatosplenic schistosomiasis mansoni.

tory because of the absence of specific antigens; schistosome serology may, however, be helpful in diagnosis of cases of transverse myelitis with low-intensity infection when eggs are rarely detected in excreta.

Other appropriate diagnostic investigations may be needed in some individuals infected with S. haematobium in order to assess the extent of disease and to plan therapeutic modalities. For example, the effects of obstructive uropathy or calculi need to be evaluated by ultrasonography; cytology and cytoscopic examination may be needed for patients suspected of having bladder cancer.

Management

The approach to individuals with S. haematobium infection should aim at elimination of parasites and reversal of pathological changes in the urinary tract. For infected populations where resources are limited the objective may be to achieve a marked reduction of egg counts. The current drugs of choice for treatment of S. haematobium infection are metrifonate or praziquantel. For individual patients three doses of metrifonate are recommended at weekly intervals; each dose is administered orally (7.5 mg per kilogram of body weight). This regimen will result in approximately 90 to 95 percent reduction of egg counts and parasitological cure in 40 to 90 percent of treated individuals. The antischistosomal effect of metrifonate seems to result in more parasitological cure in lightly infected individuals. Although the reduction in egg counts following metrifonate therapy is highly significant, the low cure rate obtained is poorly understood. Recently it has been reported that drug failure with metrifonate occurs in approximately 16 per-

cent of treated individuals. It is therefore essential to follow individual patients when treated with metrifonate by quantitative egg counts. In addition, the effect of metrifonate therapy on urinary tract disease, particularly obstructive uropathy, is not known. Previous experience with antimonials and niridazole indicates that some reversibility of lesions can be expected, but whether it is dependent on age, intensity of infection, and/or lesions and the drug used is not clear. Because of the safety and reliability of metrifonate and its moderate success in achieving parasitological cure in schistosomiasis haematobia, it has been used for mass chemotherapy in multiple or single doses [26].

Praziquantel has been evaluated against S. haematobium in several endemic areas and is the other drug of choice for treating this infection [26]. The recommended dose is 40 mg per kilogram of body weight.

Management of disease syndromes due to S. haematobium may necessitate further intervention. For example, patients with urinary tract calculi or permanent obstructive lesions may need surgical treatment. Early detection followed by surgical removal of the bladder cancer is the recommended procedure for this complication.

SCHISTOSOMIASIS MANSONI

Human infection with S. mansoni is endemic in geographically larger areas than with the other species infecting humans, but significant disease occurs in only a small proportion of infected individuals.

Pathology

Cercarial dermatitis following skin penetration by S. mansoni cercariae has been reported but does not seem to have the severity accompanied by exposure to nonhuman schistosomes. Acute schistosomiasis or Katayma fever, on the other hand, has been observed following exposure to S. mansoni, particularly in heavily infected individuals [30]. The incubation period varies from 18 to 58 days following exposure. While the pathogenesis of this syndrome is unknown, it manifests as fever, hepatosplenomegaly, lymphadenopathy, eosinophilia, and elevated immunoglobulins. These features may suggest a serum sickness–like syndrome.

Disease during established S. mansoni infection is usually seen in sites where a significant proportion of eggs are deposited. Intestinal lesions are usually confined to the colon and appendix. The mucosa may be granular and shows minute hemorrhages and ulcerations [31]. Nevertheless, the only intestinal lesion that seems to have clinical significance is diffuse colonic polyposis (Fig. 54-7). This lesion is particularly prevalent in Egypt but not in Brazilian individuals with the same intensity of infection. More than two-thirds of the polyps are found in the rectosigmoid. These lesions are made of an inflammatory mass associated with a much greater concentration of S. mansoni eggs than in the remainder of the mucosa and

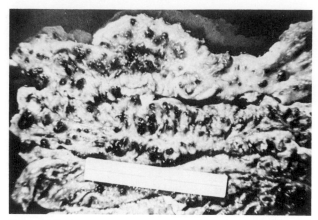

Figure 54-7. A postmortem specimen showing extensive colonic polyposis in an Egyptian patient infected with *S. mansoni.*

submucosa. Furthermore, most polyps show proliferation and distortion of glands but no adenomatous changes.

In contrast to the paucity of intestinal lesions in schistosomiasis mansoni, the liver usually shows consistent pathological changes. In mild cases, schistosome eggs with or without granulomatous lesions are seen as well as lymphocyte infiltration of portal tracts. In severe hepatic schistosomiasis mansoni, the liver is grossly enlarged, its external surface is uneven, and the cut surface may show the typical clay-pipestem fibrosis with thickened portal vein branches (Fig. 54-8). Histologically, egg granulomas, diffuse portal inflammation and fibrous tissue deposition are seen, but the liver parenchyma is usually well preserved [32]. A major effect of liver disease in schistosomiasis mansoni is the presinusoidal block in portal blood flow with subsequent portal hypertension (Fig. 54-9) and develop-

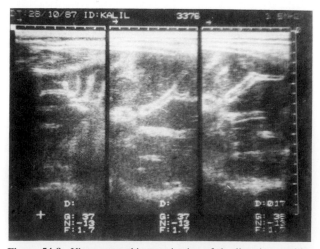

Figure 54-8. Ultrasonographic examination of the liver in a patient with advanced hepatosplenic schistosomiasis mansoni. Note the thickened portal vein branches.

ment of portosystemic collaterals (Fig. 54-10). Furthermore, portal hypertension adds a congestive element to the proliferative lesions seen in the splenic parenchyma, resulting in marked splenomegaly. With the development of collateral circulation, schistosomal eggs may enter the lungs, causing scattered granulomas, chronic obliterative arteritis, diffuse hypertensive arteriolar changes, and cor pulmonale. Schistosomal lung disease may be seen with all three species infecting humans: with *S. haematobium* the location of adult worms allows eggs to travel via the inferior vena cava, while with both *S. mansoni* and *S. japonicum,* eggs usually lodge in the lungs only after the development of portosystemic collaterals.

Clinical manifestations

The incidence of acute schistosomiasis in individuals infected with *S. mansoni* is unknown. Over 80 percent of symptomatic individuals from Puerto Rico presented with fever, anorexia, weight loss, abdominal pain, and headache [30]. More than two-thirds of these patients also complained of diaphoresis, myalgia, arthralgia, diarrhea, and dry cough. Hepatomegaly was found in 33 percent and enlargement of the spleen was reported in 20 percent. The most consistent laboratory observations were marked elevation of peripheral blood eosinophil counts and IgE levels. In this study, the severity of illness was significantly correlated to fecal egg counts.

The prevalence of clinical symptoms and signs during uncomplicated, established *S. mansoni* infection is surprisingly low. In several recent controlled observations of individuals living in endemic communities, infection was found to be correlated with higher incidence of crampy abdominal pain and bloody diarrhea in less than half of infected subjects. The most consistent clinical finding in those with uncomplicated schistosomiasis mansoni was hepatosplenomegaly. Again, significant organomegaly was not detected in more than 25 percent of infected individuals. In well-established hepatosplenic schistosomiasis, symptoms may still be lacking. Besides the nonspecific complaints of epigastric pain and distension, particularly following meals, the more consistent findings relate to right upper quadrant pain and a heavy feeling. There is usually no jaundice or other stigmata of liver disease. The liver in these individuals is enlarged; the organ is firm, not tender, with a smooth surface and a well-defined edge. The spleen in most of these patients is also enlarged, firm, and nontender. In late infection, the liver shrinks in size, becomes firmer, and its surface becomes granular. Huge enlargement of the spleen is noted, along with ascites and often manifestations of portal hypertension [33,34]. Esophagogastric varices are demonstrable in many patients who present with these chronic sequelae and may lead to hematemesis and malaria. Hematemesis usually recurs in portosystemic encephalopathy and is uncommon except in very advanced cases. Liver function tests remain relatively normal in most of those patients. Furthermore, a high frequency of coexisting hepatitis B infection is found in pa-

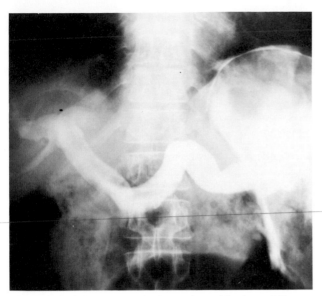

Figure 54-9. Splenoportography in a patient with advanced *S. mansoni* hepatosplenomegaly. Note the extensive dilatation of splenic and portal veins and the almost complete obstruction of portal circulation through the liver due to presinusoidal block.

tients hospitalized for decompensated hepatic schistosomiasis. This may be partly responsible for the liver pathology seen in these patients. The severity of symptoms and signs due to *S. mansoni* infection has been shown in several endemic areas to correlate with intensity of infection. This correlation does not, however, provide an explanation for all cases of hepatosplenomegaly seen in endemic areas. Because of the nature of age-specific intensity of *S. mansoni* infection, egg counts at certain ages might not reflect previous worm loads. Furthermore, it is possible that the immunological reactions of certain individuals are such that they are predisposed to organomegaly. For example, there is evidence that hepatosplenic disease in schistosomiasis mansoni is more severe in certain races, subjects with specific blood groups, or HLA haplotypes.

The major clinical complications in schistosomiasis mansoni relate to the hemodynamic changes in the portal system. Patients may present for the first time with hematemesis from esophageal varices. These individuals usually have normal liver function and can therefore, with conservative treatment, overcome the effects of blood loss. While there is no controlled observation on the final outcome in chronic schistosomiasis mansoni, most individuals proceed to develop repeated episodes of hematemesis and liver cell failure perhaps due to added insults, such as viral hepatitis or nutritional deficiencies.

Patients with advanced *S. mansoni* disease acquire salmonella infection with greater frequency. Similar observations have been reported in individuals infected with the other human schistosomes. The increased frequency of salmonella infection may be due to the immunological alterations associated with schistosomiasis or to bacterial attachment and proliferation on the surface or in the intestinal tract of adult worms. Clinically, patients with hepatosplenic schistosomiasis complicated with salmonella infection (usually *S. typhi* or *S. paratyphi* A or B) present with prolonged intermittent fever lasting months or years and leading to marked cachexia and severe refractory anemia. The spleen is markedly enlarged. Salmonella can be cultured from blood, but stool cultures are usually negative.

Other clinical manifestations of chronic schistosomiasis mansoni include cor pulmonale due to egg deposition in the lungs and subsequent development of pulmonary hypertension. With the exception of evidence of *S. mansoni* infection (or other human schistosomes), the clinical features are similar to other cases of pulmonary hypertension. These include easy fatiguability, palpitation, and dyspnea on exertion. Right ventricular hypertrophy and dilatation of pulmonary artery is observed. ECG may show right ventricular hypertrophy and strain. Some patients develop large aneurysmal dilatation of the pulmonary artery (Fig. 54-6). Cyanosis occurs only as a manifestation of cardiac decompensation. Most cases of pulmonary schistosomiasis occur in patients with advanced hepatic disease, which allows shunting of parasite eggs through portosystemic collaterals. In recent years, several case reports have been published describing patients with nephrotic syndrome associated with *S. mansoni* infection. Kidney biopsies demonstrate antigen-antibody complex deposition, but the origin of these antigens and their relation to the schistosomes are not yet known.

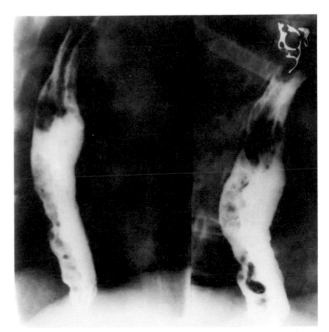

Figure 54-10. Barium swallow showing extensive esophageal varices in a patient with portal hypertension associated with hepatosplenic schistosomiasis mansoni.

Diagnosis

S. mansoni eggs can be detected in stools of infected individuals either by qualitative or quantitative techniques. A direct stool smear (1 to 2 mg feces) is a low-sensitivity procedure but may be useful for screening purposes. The Kato thick smear using either 20- or 50-mg fecal samples has been shown to be a reliable and easy quantitative procedure [29]. Note has to be taken, however, of the necessity of keeping slides long enough to clear fecal materials and of the differences in egg counts obtained by the Kato and other quantitative methods such as the Bell technique. In epidemiological surveys one method should be used throughout; the Kato thick smear has the added advantage of simplicity, adaptability to field conditions, and provision of a permanent record that needs no special fixation or staining. Diagnosis of the individual with light *S. mansoni* infection may pose a problem; in these cases a rectal biopsy examined by a competent pathologist to determine viability of eggs may be needed. Furthermore, in cases where eggs cannot be found, serological examination by any of many available techniques may be used as suggestive evidence of infection.

Management

Of the several new antischistosomal drugs, oxamniquine or praziquantel are the most appropriate for treatment of *S. mansoni* infection. Oxamniquine is given orally as a single dose of 15 to 20 mg per kilogram of body weight. Few reports from Africa indicate that a higher dose of up to 60 mg per kilogram of body weight is needed. Oxamniquine has been shown to reduce egg counts by 95 to 97 percent and results in 70 to 100 percent cure rates. Praziquantel has a broad range of activity against all human schistosome species [35]. It is given as a single oral dose of 40 mg per kilogram of body weight; egg counts have been reported to be reduced by 95 to 97 percent with cure rates of approximately 85 percent.

Patients with hepatosplenomegaly may benefit from antischistosomal therapy if instituted early, particularly in infected children and young adults. Similar trends have not been seen in adults, but antischistosomal therapy may still be beneficial in preventing further egg deposition. Patients presenting with the major complications of chronic schistosomiasis mansoni such as hematemesis, ascites, or cor pulmonale are to be treated conservatively. Shunting of portal blood by any of several surgical procedures is not recommended unless the recurrence or degree of bleeding becomes difficult to manage medically.

SCHISTOSOMIASIS JAPONICA

Infection with *S. japonicum* has several characteristics which distinguish it from other human schistosomes. The spectrum of definitive hosts is large; *S. japonicum* can infect several animal species in nature, thus compounding its epidemiology.

Another biological characteristic of these worms is that they are capable of producing 3000 eggs per worm per day, which led to suggestions that the ensuing disease syndromes may be more severe than those observed following *S. mansoni* infection. Nevertheless, the few recent controlled clinical studies in areas endemic for *S. japonicum* do not lend credence to these previous claims.

Pathology

Cercarial dermatitis has been reported only in newcomers to endemic areas and in only a small proportion of those exposed (2 to 4 percent). On the other hand, Katayama fever or acute schistosomiasis similar to that described in schistosomiasis mansoni occurs in a considerable proportion of *S. japonicum*–infected individuals (50 to 60 percent in one series).

In contrast to the detailed pathological studies on *S. mansoni*– and *S. haematobium*–infected individuals, the characteristic lesions in schistosomiasis japonica and their pathogenesis are less well defined. The most important pathological changes in the liver are noticed in the portal triads [36]. Eggs which sometimes are calcified are surrounded with varying stages of granulomas. Although the liver lobule architecture is preserved in cases of pure *S. japonicum* infection, widening of portal triads, fibrosis, and numerous new capillaries in the fibrous portal tissues are seen. Umbilical portography shows the typical presinusoidal block with abnormal narrowing of the secondary branches of the portal vein and lack of further branching in the liver lobes.

Cerebral schistosomiasis is a distinct syndrome which occurs in association with *S. japonicum* infection. The syndrome manifests as convulsive attacks, psychic seizures, or episodic disturbances of consciousness. Although worms have never been found in the brain, large aggregates of eggs have been seen.

Clinical manifestations

Symptoms and signs of acute schistosomiasis japonica or Katayama fever occur more frequently in infected individuals than those of cercarial dermatitis. While no more than 10 percent of American soldiers who contracted *S. japonicum* infection on landing in Leyte in the Philippines suffered from swimmer's itch, more than 80 percent showed features consistent with Katayama fever. In one series the prepatent period ranged from 42 to 52 days and two-thirds of infected individuals had hepatomegaly. Fatal cases have occurred from acute schistosomiasis japonica; the incidence of such complication is, however, unknown.

During chronic schistosomiasis japonica complaints such as abdominal pain and diarrhea are frequently reported, but in the few recent controlled cross-sectional studies no clear correlation to infection or its intensity has been found [37]. The major physical findings relate to organomegaly; in one large series (2540 infected individuals) 31 percent had mild hepatosplenomegaly, 9 percent had ascites, and 1.4 percent showed signs of severe portal hypertension. The progression of disease in schistosomiasis japonica seems to parallel that caused by *S. mansoni,* including pulmonary lesions. In contrast, cerebral schistosomiasis seems to be a unique clinical entity occurring in areas endemic for *S. japonicum* [38]. It has been reported to occur in 2 to 4 percent of infected individuals, although confirmation of such observations is lacking. In a recent study of 75 patients with cerebral schistosomiasis japonica in the Philippines the main clinical features were generalized convulsions, jacksonian epilepsy, or psychomotor epilepsy. Abnormal asymmetrical EEG findings were found in 68 percent.

Diagnosis

Eggs of *S. japonicum* can be detected in stool samples by qualitative or quantitative techniques as discussed under schistosomiasis mansoni. The most difficult diagnostic problem concerns cerebral schistosomiasis, as the nonspecificity of clinical presentation precludes an etiological diagnosis [38]. Furthermore, in endemic areas the presence of parasite eggs in fecal samples or positive serological evaluation cannot be equated with establishing etiological diagnosis for cerebral manifestations. The diagnosis of cerebral schistosomiasis japonica remains, therefore, a clinical decision based on elimination of other possible etiologies.

Management

The introduction of praziquantel as an antischistosomal agent has changed the chemotherapeutics of schistosomiasis japonica [35]. Praziquantel given orally as three doses of 20 mg per kilogram of body weight or as a single dose of 50 mg per kilogram of body weight results in an average parasitiological cure of 76 to 80 percent; the reduction in egg counts in those remaining positive was approximately 95 to 96 percent. In situations where praziquantel is not available, niridazole can be used as 25 mg per kilogram of body weight per day in divided doses for 2 weeks. Treatment of chronic sequelae of schistosomiasis japonica or its cerebral manifestations consists of antiparasite chemotherapy and conservative medical management.

OTHER SCHISTOSOME INFECTIONS OF HUMANS

S. intercalatum is a relatively new schistosome species which is endemic in some parts of west and central Africa [39]. Adult parasites obtained from experimentally infected hamsters are roughly comparable in length to *S. haematobium,* but the maximum number of uterine eggs seen in *S. intercalatum* is less than that seen in most *S. haematobium* strains. *S. intercalatum* eggs have terminal spines and average 167 to 172 μm in length by 58 to 59 μm in width. The most important characteristic feature of *S. intercalatum* eggs is the Ziehl-positive staining reaction of the shell in histological sections provided that initial fixation is performed in Bouin's fluid.

The life cycle of *S. intercalatum* is similar to that of other schistosomes; strains of *Bulinus forskalii* serve as intermediate hosts. The infection is endemic in several focuses in west Africa. Besides humans, natural infection was found in one species of mice, but several other laboratory animals can be experimentally infected. In humans, adult worms parasitize the mesenteric blood vessels and terminal-spine eggs break through into the intestinal lumen to be passed out in feces. Disease syndromes due to *S. intercalatum* are poorly defined. Abdominal pain, diarrhea, and blood in stools have been reported. Diagnosis is based on detection of characteristically stained eggs in stools. Praziquantel has been reported as an effective chemotherapeutic agent.

S. mekongi is a newly recognized species of schistosome which infects humans on the mainland in Indochina. The parasite is closely related to *S. japonicum* but can be differentiated on the basis of the smaller egg size and characteristic shape; the mean measurement of *S. mekongi* eggs is 66 by 57 μm. Another differentiating feature concerns the snail intermediate host of *S. mekongi, Tricula aperta.* Schistosomiasis mekongi is endemic along the Mekong River or its tributaries in Cambodia, Laos, and Thailand.

Clinical disease due to *S. mekongi* is only manifest in a relatively small proportion of infected individuals [40]. In symptomatic patients vague abdominal complaints and diarrhea may be noticed. On physical examination hepatosplenomegaly and its chronic sequelae may be found. Diagnosis is established by stool examination for the characteristic eggs; rectal biopsy may be rarely needed. Praziquantel is the drug of choice for schistosomiasis mekongi.

Cercarial dermatitis ("swimmer's itch")

Secondary exposure of human skin to cercariae of several schistosome species has been known to result in an itchy maculopapular rash. While the syndrome has been reported following exposure to human schistosomes, it is usually mild and may pass unnoticed. In contrast, exposure to cercariae of the genera *Trichobilharzia* and *Bilharziella,* which normally infect birds, is the most common cause of severe episodes of swimmer's itch. In presensitized persons maculopapular rash is followed by the development of erythema, vesicles, and edema. The condition usually subsides in a few days. Cercarial dermatitis is prevalent in many parts of both the developed and developing worlds. Detailed epidemiological information on its distribution is, however, lacking. Treatment of cercarial dermatitis is symptomatic, and avoiding exposure to contaminated waters is the only effective control measure.

POPULATION

Human schistosomiasis occurs in areas where opportunities exist for the parasites to propagate their life cycle between the definitive host and the snail intermediate host. Transmission requires the presence of a pool of infected individuals; their promiscuous urination and defecation disseminate parasite eggs into the environment, particularly freshwater bodies. A population of specific snails must be available for the hatching miracidia to penetrate and develop; subsequently a population of susceptible hosts is needed for cercarial infection. The schistosome life cycle has been maintained in spite of the various ecological hazards because of the nature of human social, cultural, and economic conditions in endemic areas. In areas where a fundamental change in the human-water relationship was introduced transmission was significantly reduced.

EPIDEMIOLOGY

The areas endemic for the three major human schistosomes are illustrated in Figs. 54-11 to 54-13. With the present political divisions these include 79 countries and areas of special sovereignty with an estimated total population of 3 billion people. This represents approximately 90 percent of the population of less-developed countries. It is projected that by the year 2000 the average increase in the population of these areas will be 50 percent. It has been very difficult to obtain reasonably reliable figures for schistosomiasis prevalence. Recently, the proportion of population at risk in 42 countries endemic for human schistosomiasis was estimated as 21 percent [41]. By using this percentage, the population at risk in the 79 endemic countries is approximately 600 million. While these estimates may serve as guidelines, data on prevalence are extremely variable; those based on proper sampling and surveys are almost nonexistent. A recent attempt to map schistosomiasis endemicity on a country-by-country basis has been published [42].

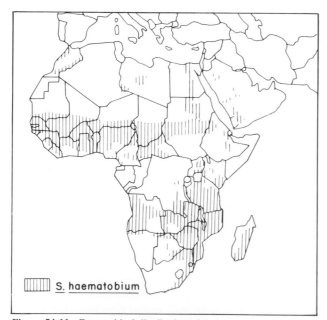

Figure 54-11. Geographical distribution of *S. haematobium.*

Prevalence and intensity of infection in areas where schistosomiasis is endemic show a characteristic relationship to age and sex. In most circumstances both prevalence and intensity increase gradually by age to peak approximately at 10 to 19 years of age. In some situations the peak prevalence may reach 100 percent, or it may vary according to the endemicity of infection. A similar trend is noted in intensity; egg counts in urine or feces peak at the same age range. Females may in some endemic communities show slightly less prevalence and intensity. By the beginning of the third decade of life, a slight or moderate decrease in prevalence may be noted in populations living in the endemic areas. The significant change occurs, however, in age-specific intensity curves; egg counts are markedly lower in those above 30 years of age [43]. This general pattern of slow buildup of infection followed by a remarkable decrease in egg counts has been extensively used as evidence for the occurrence of immunity in human schistosomiasis although water contact patterns may be an equally logical explanation. The third epidemiological parameter applicable to schistosomiasis transmission concerns incidence. Because of the nature of infection and the available diagnostic tests, it has only been possible to obtain reasonable estimates of schistosomiasis incidence in young children, using conversion rates rather than true incidence across all ages of a specific community. These rates have ranged from 2 to 4 percent and confirm the mathematically predicted low incidence rates. There are several factors that govern the outcome of the transmission process in areas where schistosomiasis is endemic. A small proportion of snails are infected at any one time, they shed at specific times of the day, cercariae are dispersed in huge water bodies, and they have limited effective duration of infectivity. Furthermore, chances of human-water contact at points of maximal cercarial concentration are dependent on many social and cultural habits of the populations of endemic areas. In fact, it has been calculated that individuals in some endemic areas in Egypt acquire no more than one worm pair per year. A corollary of this process can be seen in the distribution of worm loads as evaluated by egg counts in excreta in the population of any specific endemic area. Schistosome infection, like many other worm infections, has a characteristic negative binomial distribution; i.e., most infected individuals harbor low worm loads and a minority suffer from high-intensity infection. Most of the latter group are the young, who, therefore, suffer the burden of schistosomiasis and probably contribute most to its dissemination.

PREVENTION AND CONTROL

For the single individual living or traveling to endemic areas, avoiding contact with contaminated freshwater bodies is the only practical control measure. Infection in individuals or groups can also be controlled by administration of chemotherapy, and if it is given early (to infected children), both intensity of infection and disease manifestations are remarkably

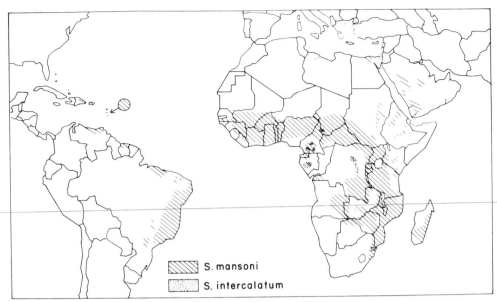

Figure 54-12. Geographical distribution of *S. mansoni* and *S. intercalatum.*

decreased [*44*]. The difficult choice is, however, related to strategies of control in endemic areas. Molluscicides, whether chemical or natural, played a prominent role previously. They necessitate frequent repeated applications and have a slow effect on infection in humans and no effect on disease. Chemotherapy, on the other hand, has been shown over the last decade or so to result in reduction of intensity of infection which lasts for several years (in *S. mansoni*–endemic areas) [*44*]. Drug treatment is also the only way to reduce the burden of schistosomal disease in endemic communities. With the introduction of new, safe, single-oral-dose antischistosomal agents, chemotherapy applied on a targeted basis to control disease and reduce transmission is the current recommended strategy [*45*]. This can, in specific situations, be supplemented by focal mollusciciding if certain transmission focuses can be delineated.

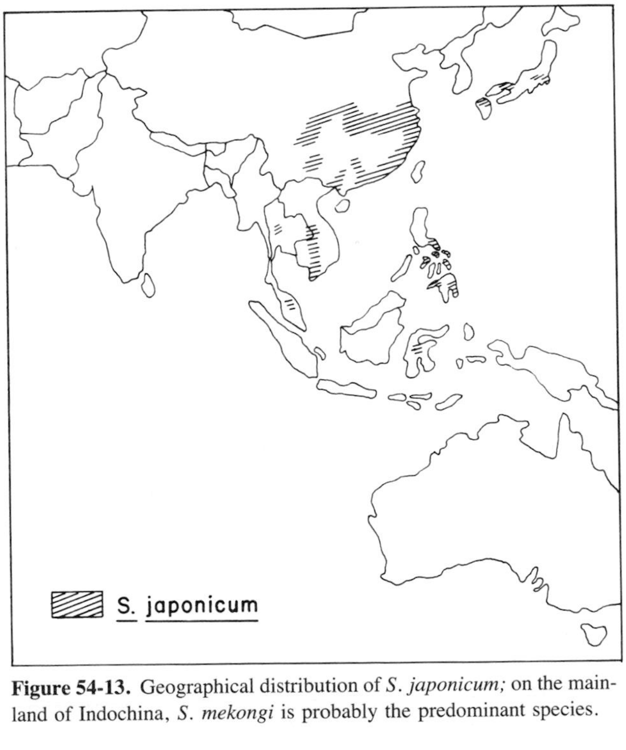

The role of cultural, social, economic, and political changes in schistosomiasis control has not been subjected to real evaluation except in Japan, where general development resulted in marked decrease in schistosomiasis. The ecology of this infection is such that it is intimately related to people's economic standards; the well-to-do have access to privies and clean water supply, and have no social or economic need to come in contact with contaminated fresh water. In contrast, the deprived and their children use these water bodies constantly for a multitude of purposes. Whether behavioral changes through health education alone may help play a role in schistosomiasis control is doubtful. Control must be based on economic change, which has eluded the people of the third world and endemic countries for several decades.

Prophylaxis against schistosomiasis is a strategy for the future. There are currently no chemotherapeutic agents that are protective on a prophylactic basis, and research on vaccine is in its infancy. One practical prophylactic measure concerns limiting the spread of schistosomiasis that parallels most of the new irrigation projects. Establishing tight screening, therapeutic, and monitoring procedures may help alleviate this most untoward result of land and irrigation development pro-

Figure 54-13. Geographical distribution of *S. japonicum;* on the mainland of Indochina, *S. mekongi* is probably the predominant species.

grams. Vaccination, though it may not be achievable in the immediate future, offers a rational approach to schistosomiasis control [46].

REFERENCES

1 Sturrock RF: Biology and ecology of human schistosomes, in Mahmoud AAF (ed): *Bailliere's Clinical Tropical Medicine and Communicable Diseases, Schistosomiasis,* vol 2, no 2. London, Bailliere Tindall, 1987, pp 249–266

2 Schmidt GD, Roberts LS: *Foundations of Parasitology,* 2d ed. St. Louis, Mosby, 1981, pp 275–296

3 Wiest PM, Tartakoff AM, Aikawa M, et al: Inhibition of heptalaminate surface membrane maturation in schistosomula of *Schistosoma mansoni.* Proc Natl Acad Sci USA 85:3825–3830, 1988

4 Sher A, Moser G: Schistosomiasis. Immunologic properties of developing schistosomula. Am J Pathol 102:121–126, 1981

5 Butterworth AE, Taylor DW, Veith MD, et al: Studies of the mechanisms of immunity in human schistosomiasis. Immunol Rev 61:5–39, 1982

6 Weller TH, Wheeldon SK: The cultivation in vitro of cells derived from adult *Schistosoma mansoni.* I. Methodology: Criteria for evaluation of cultures and development of media. Am J Trop Med Hyg 31:335–348, 1982

7 Warren KS, Mahmoud AAF, Cummings P, et al: Schistosomiasis mansoni in Yemeni in California: Duration of infection, presence of disease, therapeutic management. Am J Trop Med Hyg 23:902–929, 1974

8 Davis AH, Blanton R, Rottman F, et al: Isolation of cDNA clones for differentially expressed genes of the human parasite *Schistosoma mansoni.* Proc Natl Acad Sci USA 83:5534–5538, 1986

9 Short RB, Grossman AI: Conventional Giesmsa and C-banded karyotypes of *Schistosoma mansoni* and *S. rodhaini.* J Parasitol 67:661–671, 1981

10 Capron A, Dessaint JP, Capron M, et al: Immunity to schistosomes: Progress toward vaccine. Science 238:1065–1072, 1987

11 Butterworth AE: Potential for vaccines against human schistosomes, in Mahmoud AAF (ed): *Bailliere's Clinical Tropical Medicine and Communicable Diseases, Schistosomiasis,* vol 2, no 2. London, Bailliere Tindall, 1987, pp 465–483

12 King CJ, Lett RR, Nanduri J, et al: Isolation and characterization of a protective antigen for adjuvant-free immunization against *Schistosoma mansoni.* J Immunol 139:4218–4224, 1987

13 World Health Organization: The control of schistosomiasis. WHO Tech Rep Ser 728, 1985, p 113

14 Peck CA, Carpenter MD, Mahmoud AAF: Species-related innate resistance to schistosomiasis mansoni: Role of mononuclear phagocytes in schistosomula killing in vitro. J Clin Invest 71:66–72, 1983

15 Ellner JJ, Mahmoud AAF: Phagocytes and worms: David and Goliath, revisited. Rev Infect Dis 4:698–714, 1982

16 Mahmoud AAF: The ecology of eosinophils in schistosomiais. J Infect Dis 145:613–622, 1982

17 Colley DG: Dynamics of the human immune response to schistosomes, in Mahmoud AAF (ed): *Bailliere's Clinical Tropical Medicine and Communicable Diseases, Schistosomiasis,* vol 2, no 2. London, Bailliere Tindall, 1987, pp 315–332

18 Warren KS: Determinants of disease in human schistosomiasis, in Mahmoud AAF (ed): *Bailliere's Clinical Tropical Medicine and*

Communicable Diseases, Schistosomiasis, vol 2, no 2. London, Bailliere Tindall, 1987, pp 301–313.

19 Ellner JJ, Olds GR, Osman GS, et al: Dichotomies in the reactivity to worm antigen in human schistosomiasis mansoni. J Immunol 126:309–312, 1981

20 Abdel Salam E, et al: Association of HLA class I antigens (A1, B5, B8, and CW2) with disease manifestations and infection in human schistosomiasis mansoni in Egypt. Tissue Antigens 23:142–146, 1986

21 Scrimgeour EM, Gajdusek DC: Involvement of the central nervous system in *Schistosoma mansoni* and *Schistosoma haematobium* infection. A review. Brain 108:1023–1038, 1985

22 Pugh RNH, Gilles HM: Malumfashi endemic diseases research project. X. *Schistosoma haematobium* and bacteriuria in the Malumfashi area. Ann Trop Med Parasitol 73:349–354, 1979

23 Schwartz DH: Helminths in the induction of cancer. II. *Schistosoma haematobium* and bladder cancer. Trop Geogr Med 33:1–7, 1981

24 World Health Organization: Progress in assessment of morbidity due to *Schistosoma haematobium* infection: A review of recent literature. WHO/Schisto/87.91, World Health Organization, 1987

25 Wilkins A, Gilles H: Schistosomiasis haematobia, in Mahmoud AAF (ed): *Bailliere's Clinical Tropical Medicine and Communicable Diseases, Schistosomiasis,* vol 2, no 2. London, Bailliere Tindall, 1987, pp 333–348

26 King CH, Lombardi G, Lombardi C, et al: Chemotherapy-based control of schistosomiasis haematobia. I. Metrifonate versus praziquantel in control of intensity and prevalence of infection. Am J Trop Med Hyg 39:295–305, 1988

27 King CH, Keating CE, Muruka JF, et al: Urinary tract morbidity in schistosomiasis haematobia: Associations with age and intensity of infection in an endemic area of Coast Province, Kenya. Am J Trop Med Hyg 39:361–368, 1988

28 Abdel Salam E, Ehsan A: Cytoscopic picture of *Schistosoma haematobium* in Egyptian children correlated with intensity of infection and morbidity. Am J Trop Med Hyg 27:774–778, 1978

29 Peters PAS, Kazura JW: Update on diagnostic methods for schistosomiasis, in Mahmoud AAF (ed): *Bailliere's Clinical Tropical Medicine and Communicable Diseases, Schistosomiasis,* vol 2, no 2. London, Bailliere Tindall, 1987, pp 419–433

30 Hiatt RA, Sotomayor ZR, Sanchez G, et al: Factors in the pathogenesis of acute schistosomiasis mansoni. J Infect Dis 139:659–666, 1979

31 Cheever AW, Kamel IA, Elwi AM, et al: *Schistosoma mansoni* and *S. haematobium* infections in Egypt. III. Extrahepatic pathology. Am J Trop Med Hyg 27:55–75, 1978

32 Kamel IA, Elwi AM, Cheever AW, et al: *Schistosoma mansoni* and *S. haematobium* infections in Egypt. IV. Hepatic lesions. Am J Trop Med Hyg 27:939–943, 1978

33 Abdel Wahab MF, Mahmoud SS: Schistosomiasis mansoni in Egypt, in Mahmoud AAF (ed): *Bailliere's Clinical Tropical Medicine and Communicable Diseases, Schistosomiasis,* vol 2, no 2. London, Bailliere Tindall, 1987, pp 371–395

34 Prata A: Schistosomiasis mansoni in Brazil, in Mahmoud AAF (ed): *Bailliere's Clinical Tropical Medicine and Communicable Diseases, Schistosomiasis,* vol 2, no 2. London, Bailliere Tindall, 1987, pp 349–369

35 King CH, Mahmoud AAF: Drugs five years later: Praziquantel. Ann Intern Med, in press

36 Kurniawan AN, Hardjawidjaja L, Clark RT: A clinico-pathologic study of cases with *Schistosoma japonicum* infection in Indonesia. Southeast Asian J Trop Med Public Health 7:263–269, 1976

37 Domingo EO, Tiu E, Peters PA, et al: Morbidity in schistosomiasis japonica in relation to intensity of infection: Study of a community in Leyte, Philippines. Am J Trop Med Hyg 29:858–867, 1980

38 Olveda RM, Domingo EO: Schistosomiasis japonica, in Mahmoud AAF (ed): *Bailliere's Clinical Tropical Medicine and Communicable Diseases, Schistosomiasis,* vol 2, no 2. London, Bailliere Tindall, 1987, pp 397–417

39 Jordan P, Webbe J: *Schistosomiasis.* Heinemann, 1982

40 Hofstetter M, Nash TE, Cheever AW, et al: Infection with *Schistosoma mekongi* in Southeast Asian refugees. J Infect Dis 144:420–426, 1981

41 Iarotski LS, Davis A: The schistosomiasis problem in the world: Results of a WHO questionnaire survey. Bull WHO 59:114–127, 1981

42 World Health Organization: Atlas of the global distribution of schistosomiasis. Parasitic Diseases Programme. Geneva, World Health Organization, 1987

43 Anderson RM: Determinants of infection in human schistosomiasis, in Mahmoud AAF (ed): *Bailliere's Clinical Tropical Medicine and Communicable Diseases, Schistosomiasis,* vol 2, no 2. London, Bailliere Tindall, 1987, pp 279–300

44 Mahmoud AAF, Siongok TKA, Ouma J, et al: Effect of targeted mass treatment on intensity of infection and morbidity in schistosomiasis mansoni: Three-year follow up of a community in Machakos, Kenya. Lancet i:849–851, 1983

45 Cook JA: Strategies for control of human schistosomiasis, in Mahmoud AAF (ed): *Bailliere's Clinical Tropical Medicine and Communicable Diseases, Schistosomiasis,* vol 2, no 2. London, Bailliere Tindall, 1987, pp 449–463

46 Mahmoud AAF: Strategies for schistosomiasis vaccines. L.W. Frohlich Award Conference, The New York Academy of Sciences, 1989, in press

CHAPTER 55 / *Liver, Lung, and Intestinal Trematodiasis* · Tranakchit Harinasuta

· Danai Bunnag

The trematodes or flukes of human beings may be grouped according to the organ they inhabit, as blood flukes, liver flukes, intestinal flukes, and lung flukes. The disease of blood flukes, schistosomiasis, is dealt with in Chap. 54, and the three other groups of trematodes are discussed in this chapter.

Liver, intestinal, and lung flukes vary in size from less than 1 mm to 7 to 8 cm and are hermaphrodite. Their morphologies are similar: bilaterally symmetrical, leaflike, and flattened dorsoventrally. The body is covered with cuticle with or without spines. Certain external features are characteristic: an oral sucker at the anterior end and a ventral sucker on the ventral surface, posteriorly to the oral sucker, an excretory pore at the posterior end, and a genital pore near the ventral sucker. In some species the opening of Laurer's canal is present on the middorsal surface. The internal organs are a blind bifurcate intestinal tract, or cecum, an excretory system, male and female reproductive organs, and a primitive nervous system. The shape, size, arrangement, and location of these organs are characteristic by species.

The egg of human fluke infections is oval and possesses an operculum. Ova vary in size from the large (120 to 150 μm) eggs of *Fasciolopsis buski, Fasciola hepatica, F. gigantica,* and *Gastrodiscoides hominis,* to the medium-sized eggs (70 to 100 μm) of *Echinostoma* sp. and *Paragonimus* sp., to the small eggs (25 to 30 μm) of *Clonorchis sinensis, Opisthorchis* sp., *Heterophyes heterophyes, Metagonimus yokogawai, Haplor-*

chis sp., *Phaneropsolus bonnei, Prosthodendrium* sp., etc. When passed, the eggs are undeveloped except in some species, such as *Clonorchis sinensis, Opisthorchis* sp., and *Heterophyes heterophyes,* in which the eggs are fully developed and contain miracidia.

In life cycle flukes are similar. Fundamentally trematodes are parasites of animals. The eggs come out with feces or sputum (in the case of the lung fluke, *Paragonimus* sp.). Eggs or hatched miracidia must enter specific snail intermediate hosts. In the snail the miracidium undergoes asexual multiplication; it develops to sporocyst, rediae, and cercariae. The cercariae emerge and encyst on vegetation or within tissue of aquatic animals such as fish or crabs, except for *Dicrocoelium* sp., whose cercariae encyst in ants. The encysted cercaria develops to a metacercaria, which is the infective stage to definitive hosts, animal and human.

Humans acquire infection by ingestion of raw or improperly cooked plant or animal food in which metacercaria have encysted.

The diagnosis of these trematode infections depends on finding the characteristic eggs; however, many flukes produce similar eggs. It is difficult even for experts to correctly identify species of the parasite. Only the identification of adult worms recovered in stool [1] or in sputum after treatment, at surgery, or at autopsy will confirm the species.

More than 50 million people are infected by one or more

species of these trematodes; the highest prevalence is of the liver fluke, *Clonorchis sinensis, Opisthorchis felineus,* and *O. viverrini.*

Immunodiagnosis is helpful in the diagnosis and differential diagnosis of some trematode infections. However, it must be borne in mind that the reaction may remain positive for some time after the patient has been freed from the infection, and cross-reaction within the related species is common. Chemotherapy of fluke infection has long been a problem, as there has been no highly effective broad-spectrum antihelminthic. Recently praziquantel has been found to be very effective against all kinds of trematode infections. Thus, the prognosis of patients suffering from trematode infections has improved, as have control programs in which mass treatment can be instituted.

OPISTHORCHIASIS

Opisthorchiasis is caused by *Opisthorchis viverrini* or *Opisthorchis felineus.*

PARASITE

Opisthorchis viverrini is transparent and lanceolate in shape (5 to 10 by 1 to 2 mm) with an attenuated anterior end and rounded posterior end (Fig. 55-1).

The egg is yellowish brown in color and oval in shape, with an operculum resting on shoulders with, or without, a tubercle-like knob at the abopercular end. The average size is 28 μm in length and 16 μm in breadth (Fig. 55-1). The ratio of the length to the breadth of the egg is approximately 2:1, resembling that of *C. sinensis,* while that of *O. felineus* is around 3:1. The life cycle is similar to that of digenic trematodes (Fig. 55-2).

The adult worms live in the distal bile ducts and some in the gallbladder as well. The eggs produced are carried in the bile and passed out in feces. The snail intermediate hosts for *O. viverrini* are *Bithynia goniomphalus, B. funiculata,* and *B. leavis* (*B. siamensis*); and the host for *O. felineus* is *B. leechii.*

Many species of cyprinoid fish serve as second intermediate hosts in southeast Asia; in Thailand *Cyclochielicthus siaja* is the most predominant. In central, eastern, and southern Europe and Siberia many species of carp are second intermediate hosts.

Cats, dogs, and many fish-eating mammals are definitive hosts. In the laboratory, golden hamsters, mice, and guinea pigs are also found to be good laboratory models [2].

PATIENT

Pathogenesis, pathology, and pathophysiology

The pathological changes are more or less related to the intensity and the duration of the infection as commonly seen in older patients with large numbers of flukes [3]. The pathogen-

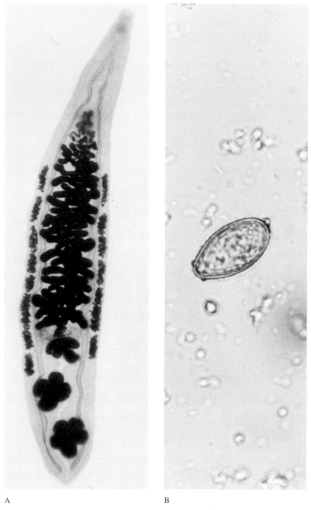

A   B

Figure 55-1. Photomicrograph of adult worm (*A*) and egg (*B*) of *Opisthorchis viverrini.*

esis results from mechanical irritation caused by the flukes and toxic substances that may be produced by them.

Lesions are mainly confined to the biliary system. There is hyperplasia of the epithelial cells lining the bile ducts, some of which are projected into the lumen, and the duct wall is thickened. In light infections there is no change in the liver parenchyma. In heavy and severe infections, there is obstruction of the biliary tract by the flukes, bile retention, hyperplasia of the biliary system with glandular proliferation of papillomatous and adenomatous type, cholangitis, periductal infiltration with eosinophils, round cells, and fibrosis in the portal areas, with necrosis and atrophy of hepatic cells. There is uniform dilatation of intrahepatic bile ducts with clubbing or cystic formation at the end, and in late cases these saccular or cystic formations may develop into large cysts. The gallbladder may enlarge from 10 to 20 cm in length and contain white

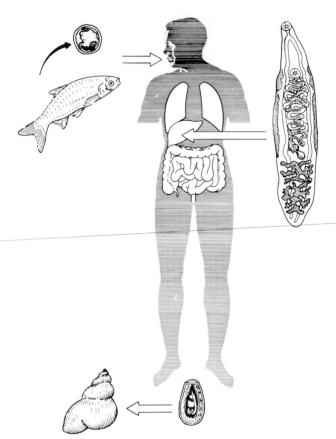

Figure 55-2. Life cycle of *Opisthorchis viverrini.*

bile. The epithelial lining is grossly hypertrophic and glandulous.

Autopsies have demonstrated that opisthorchiasis is often seen in association with obstructive jaundice, pancreatitis, cirrhosis, and cholangiocarcinoma [4]. It is, however, worth mentioning that hamsters fed with dimethylnitrosamine and metacercariae have developed cholangiocarcinoma and cholangiofibrosis, while those that were fed with only one or the other did not show pathogenicity [5].

In mild cases the liver biochemistry profile is generally normal; however, sera of asymptomatic carriers of *O. viverrini* that were subjected to acrylamide gel electrophoresis showed significant increases in the ceruloplasmin and hemopexin levels; one-third of cases had higher levels of haptoglobin.

Clinical manifestations

The majority of cases are symptomless and are diagnosed on routine stool examination. Clinical pictures of opisthorchiasis vary from mild to severe. The mild cases have symptoms of dyspepsia, flatulence, diarrhea or constipation, dull pain and discomfort in the right hypochondrium, sometimes spreading to the epigastrium and the left costal region, often lasting 1 to

2 h in the late afternoon. The duration varies, ranging from a few days to a few weeks and recurring for months or years. As the disease progresses, the duration of pain lengthens and becomes persistent over weeks and months, by which time the patient is unable to cope with work. A peculiar hot cutaneous sensation similar to "rubbing pounded chilies" on the skin, bearing no relationship to segmental nerve supplies, is commonly felt in a small area over the abdomen, or sometimes the whole abdomen, or the back. Other symptoms include lassitude, "loss of taste," anorexia, and weight loss. Urticarial rash is frequently recorded. The patients do not complain of this symptom because they get used to it. The physical signs tend to be well established in patients over 40 years of age in whom liver enlargement with a firm consistency is invariably present. On deep palpation there is a dull discomfort but never severe tenderness. This also applies to the epigastrium and the left costal region. The signs of weight loss and slight pedal edema which may be due to associated malnutrition are commonly seen. Although an enlarged gallbladder is a common radiological and sonographic finding, it is infrequently found on palpation.

In the minority, the manifestation is severe. There are symptoms and signs of relapsing cholangitis and calculous or acalculous cholecystitis. The patient is then seriously ill and may succumb to a septic shock. Cholangiocarcinoma, gallstones, and obstructive jaundice are usual associations.

In a few patients with long-standing infections laparoscopic examination reveals increased marking and dilatation of the biliary network under the surface of the liver. An enlarged, poorly functioning gallbladder may be detected through the use of a double dose of radiocontrast at oral cholecystography. The percutaneous, transhepatic cholangiographic technique will show dilatation and sacculation of the biliary tree (see Fig. 55-3) [6]. Ultrasonography will demonstrate dilatation of intrahepatic bile ducts with a honeycomblike appearance.

O. felineus is characterized by both acute and chronic forms. Migrants to endemic areas in the U.S.S.R. have presented with acute clinical manifestations which are not specific to opisthorchiasis but resemble Katayama fever. Generally, there is a 2- to 3-week prepatent period, with an irregular high fever, occasional edema of the face, enlargement of lymph nodes, myalgia, arthralgia, skin rash, and eosinophilia. In severe cases allergic hepatitis is also observed, the duration of illness lasting from 1 to 2 weeks, and occasionally from 4 to 6 months.

The chronic form presents a similar picture to *O. viverrini* infection, except that in some 30 percent of infected persons, flukes are also found in pancreatic ducts. Carcinoma of the pancreas and the stomach is also encountered [7].

Diagnosis. The characteristic ovum is the criterion for diagnosis. However, it is very difficult to differentiate the ova of *Opisthorchis* from those of the tiny intestinal flukes e.g., *Phaneropsolus bonnei* and *Prosthodendrium molenkampi*. In the mild form of opisthorchiasis peptic ulceration and gallstones

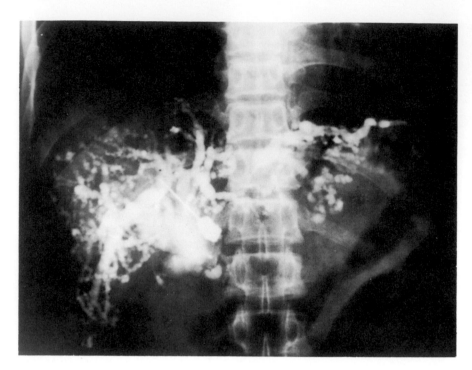

Figure 55-3. *Opisthorchiasis viverrini:* Percutaneous transhepatic cholangiography showing dilatation and sacculation of biliary tree. (*Courtesy of Tula Dhiensiri et al., Khon Kaen Hospital, Thailand.*)

should be excluded, while in its severe form, cholangitis from other causes should be differentiated.

Treatment. Praziquantel is the drug of choice. A 1-day regimen of 25 mg per kilogram of body weight three times after meals and a single dose of 40 or 50 mg per kilogram of body weight yielded 100 percent [8] and 91 and 96 percent cure rates [9], respectively. The flukes are expelled mostly dead and destroyed with peeling integument; those still viable are elongated. The eggs disappear in 1 week from the stool, while the clinical symptoms and the enlarged gallbladder take a few months to return to normal. Mebendazole, 30 mg/(kg·day) for 3 and 4 weeks, gave cure rates of 89 and 94 percent, respectively [10]. Albendazole, 400 mg twice daily for 3 and 7 days, yielded cure rates of 40 and 63 percent, respectively, while the percentage of egg reduction was 92 in both regimens [11]. Appropriate antibiotics should be prescribed for relapsing cholangitis.

A palliative surgical procedure is often required in the complicated cases with obstructive jaundice. A modified Longmire bypass operation is frequently used.

Prognosis. The majority of infected individuals do not suffer much. Only patients who have had relapsing cholangitis or superimposed cholangiocarcinoma have a grave prognosis. However, with the advent of the new effective antihelminthic, patients with relapsing cholangitis should now do well.

POPULATION

Epidemiology

O. viverrini in humans is found mainly in the northeast and northern parts of Thailand, and in Laos and Kampuchea, while *O. felineus* has been reported from the U.S.S.R. and central and eastern Europe.

The prevalence of *O. viverrini* infection in northeastern Thailand has risen from 3.5 million cases in 1965 to 5.4 million cases in 1981. This may principally be because of the high rate of population growth and an increase of the snail and fish intermediate hosts. Development of reservoirs and irrigation systems in the areas, lack of proper sanitation facilities, and the popular practice of consuming raw fish continue to provide suitable conditions for propagation of the infection.

There are probably a few million cases of *O. felineus* infection with a prevalence rate as high as 85 percent in some areas. It has been observed that the recent influx of immigrants to western Siberia has contributed to doubling the prevalence of *O. felineus* infection among the people of that region.

Rural populations in southeast Asia generally live in villages, each village comprised of 50 to 100 houses. In view of their heavy dependence on agricultural pursuits, such populations are concentrated in areas where water is readily available from ponds, lakes, or reservoirs and where the soil is fertile. In the absence of sanitary facilities humans, in addition to animals, perform their natural bodily functions in the open.

With the oncoming of the rains, the feces containing eggs are washed into the ponds and lakes and become food for the fish and snails.

In northeast Thailand a raw fish dish called *Koi Pla,* prepared from a chopped raw cyprinoid fish, is eaten regularly by almost everyone in the villages, from infants to the elders, whenever fish is available, which means daily in the rainy season. Infection is therefore not uncommon even among infants. The prevalence of the infection in some districts is well over 90 percent. The largest number of flukes is generally found in patients over 40 years of age owing to accumulation of flukes from repeated infections, lack of protective immunity, and the long life span of the flukes.

The people in the endemic areas of *O. felineus* infection are fond of eating raw freshwater fish and 1-day-old salted fish. In western Siberia, newly arrived immigrants acquired infections within the first year of arrival. Cats and fish intermediate hosts in some of these areas may all be infected.

CLONORCHIASIS

Clonorchiasis is an infection with *Clonorchis sinensis* of the bile ducts and, at times, the pancreatic duct. The parasite and the clinical manifestations, as well as the control of the infection, are similar to those of *Opisthorchis* and opisthorchiasis.

C. sinensis (Cobbold, 1875) Looss (1907) is also known as the Chinese or oriental liver fluke. Although *C. sinensis* should be included in the genus *Opisthorchis,* the genus *Clonorchis* is so well established that most parasitologists prefer to continue using this term. *C. sinensis* is larger than *O. felineus* and *O. viverrini* (10 to 24 by 3 to 5 mm) (Fig. 55-4). The egg (29 by 16 μm), resembles the egg of *O. viverrini,* but is broader than that of *O. felineus* (Fig. 55-4).

The life cycle of *C. sinensis* is similar to that of *Opisthorchis.* The intermediate hosts are slightly different. The first host is hydrobiid snails: *Parafossarulus manchouricus* in most endemic areas; *Bithynia fuchsiana* and *Alocinma longicornis* in other areas. The fish, the second intermediate host, is carp of the family Cyprinidae; 27 species in Japan, 29 in Korea, 15 in Taiwan, and 49 in China have been found with *C. sinensis* metacercariae [*12*].

The pathology and the clinical manifestations of clonorchiasis are similar to those of opisthorchiasis. Acute symptoms of anorexia, epigastric pain, diarrhea, and leukocytosis with eosinophilia occurred in two patients 10 to 26 days after the eating of fish with massive infections [*13*]. In long-term infection, cholangitis, cholelithiasis, pancreatitis, and cholangiocarcinoma are common complications and can be fatal. In Hong Kong, the mucin-secreting type of cholangiocarcinoma is associated with *C. sinensis* [*2*].

Praziquantel has been reported to be effective for clonorchiasis. Dosages of 25 mg per kilogram of body weight three

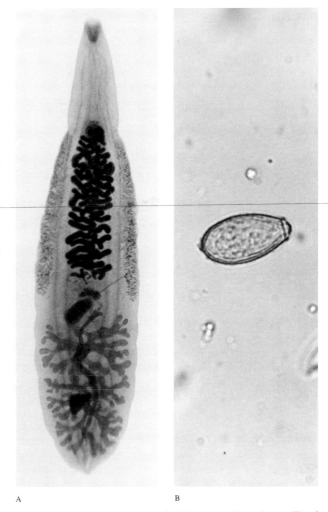

A   B

Figure 55-4. Photomicrograph of adult worm (*A*) and egg (*B*) of *Clonorchis sinesis.*

times daily for 1 and 2 days yielded cure rates of 86.8 and 100 percent, respectively [*14*].

Human clonorchiasis is endemic in Japan, Korea, China, Taiwan, and Vietnam, where the first and second intermediate hosts are found and where the population is accustomed to eating raw fish. In most areas, the fish are raised in fish ponds that are commonly fertilized with human and animal feces. This provides excellent nutrient for the growth of plant and animal life upon which the snails and fish feed, and also provides an opportunity for perpetuating the life cycle of the parasite.

It has been estimated that over 20 million persons in China have clonorchiasis in spite of concerted efforts to improve sanitation. The incidence of infection has been markedly reduced among the under-40 age group in Japan and Taiwan during the past few years. The decrease is attributed to the low snail population in these endemic areas due to industrialization, insecticide pollution of water, land reclamation, and health education.

The infection is known to be highly endemic in Hong Kong, but neither the snail nor fish intermediate hosts are indigenous to the area. Infected fish originate from China and are shipped in daily to provide the Hong Kong population with *Yu shun Chuk,* raw fish congee.

In recent years clonorchiasis has been reported in the United States and other countries where the infection is not considered endemic. All patients were immigrants from endemic areas.

Pigs, dogs, cats, and rats are also hosts for *C. sinensis,* and it is probable that other carnivorous animals are involved as reservoir hosts in nature.

FASCIOLIASIS

Fascioliasis is an infection caused by the sheep liver fluke, *Fasciola hepatica* or *F. gigantica.*

PARASITE

Fasciola hepatica (synonyms: *Distoma hepaticum, F. californica, F. hali,* etc.) is a brownish, large trematode (20 to 30 by 8 to 13 mm). A distinct cephalic cone gives a characteristic shouldered appearance (Fig. 55-5). The egg is large and ovoid (130 to 150 by 60 to 90 μm), with an inconspicuous operculum and is undeveloped when deposited (Fig. 55-5).

Adult *F. hepatica* live in the large biliary ducts, and eggs are passed in feces. The life cycle is similar to that of other digenic trematodes. Numerous species of snail, both amphibious and aquatic, serve as intermediate hosts. The cercariae encyst on various kinds of aquatic vegetation or even swim freely in the water and develop into metacercariae. Infections develop in the definitive hosts when they consume infected vegetation or ingest the encysted metacercariae in water. Metacercariae excyst in the duodenum and penetrate the intestinal wall to enter the peritoneal cavity. Then they invade the liver capsule and migrate through the parenchyma to the bile ducts. They mature in about 3 to 4 months. The life span of these flukes is 3 years in rabbits and at least 5 years in sheep.

The most important definitive hosts are sheep, but other herbivores, including goats, cattle, horses, camels, vicuna, hogs, rabbits, and deer, are commonly infected; even dogs may harbor the flukes.

F. gigantica (or *F. aegyptica*) may attain a length of 7.5 cm. It is more lanceolate and has a less distinct cephalic cone than *F. hepatica.* The eggs are larger (160 to 190 by 70 to 90 μm). The life cycle is similar, but the snail intermediate host is *Lymnaea natalensis* in Africa and *L. auricularia* and *L. acuminata* in Asia.

PATIENT

Pathology

In experimental animals the excysted metacercariae produce some necrosis of the hepatic parenchyma with fibrosis, cellular infiltration, and abscess formation. Sheep heavily infected with *F. hepatica* develop ''liver rot.'' Adult flukes may cause hyperplasia, desquamation, thickening, and dilation of the bile ducts. The amount of damage is correlated with worm load; in sheep, 600 flukes will cause death.

Human fascioliasis is usually mild but in rare cases of heavy infection, there is hyperplasia, necrosis, cystic dilation, leukocytic infiltration of the bile ducts, and subcapsular hematoma A fluke may rarely block the common bile duct. Wandering of flukes in the parenchyma may result in internal hemorrhage. Ectopic fascioliasis is also common. It is estimated that one fluke consumes 0.2 mL of blood per day.

Urticaria, granuloma, eosinophilia, and eosinophilic hyperplasia of the bone marrow may be provoked by the fluke's antigens. Various types of antibodies, precipitins, and hemagglutinins can be detected in the serum. Serum transpeptidases, alkaline phosphatase, bilirubin, thymol turbidity, cephalin flocculation, erythrocyte sedimentation rate, and γ-globulin concentrations may be abnormal.

Clinical manifestations

The clinical manifestations can be divided into two phases, i.e., larval migratory phase, or acute phase, and adult, or chronic, phase.

During the migration in which the immature flukes travel from gut lumen to bile ducts patients may develop acute dyspepsia, anorexia, nausea, vomiting, abdominal pain, especially in the epigastrium or right upper quadrant, fever, headache, liver enlargement and tenderness, and urticaria with marked

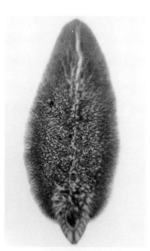
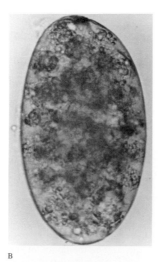

A   B

Figure 55-5. Photomicrograph of adult worm (*A*) and egg (*B*) of *Fasciola hepatica.*

eosinophilia. A variety of allergic symptoms may also occur. The symptoms may persist for several months.

When the flukes lodge in the biliary passages, there are usually few symptoms. Some patients have pain in the right hypochondrium and epigastrium, dyspepsia, diarrhea, nausea, vomiting, hepatomegaly, and jaundice. Eosinophilia, dysproteinemia, and altered liver function tests are frequent. If the extrahepatic bile ducts are occluded, the symptoms will be those of choledocholithiasis.

Flukes occasionally migrate to ectopic sites such as intestinal wall, lungs, heart, brain, and skin, where they may cause pruritic painful nodules or abscesses.

The acute nasopharyngitis known as *halzoun* in Lebanon or *marrara* in Sudan may be an allergic response to larval flukes eaten in raw sheep or goat liver.

Diagnosis

In enzootic areas, fascioliasis is suspected in patients suffering from fever, hepatomegaly, and eosinophilia with a history of consuming freshwater plants. Serological tests are particularly useful in the early phase of the illness while the flukes are still immature, before ova appear in the feces, and also in the ectopic type. Indirect hemagglutination, complement fixation, countercurrent electrophoresis, immunosorbent assay, and skin tests are used. Liver biopsy may be helpful in some cases.

Chronic fascioliasis is diagnosed by finding the characteristic eggs in stools or material obtained by duodenal or biliary drainage. Spurious infections should be ruled out by placing the patients on a liver-free diet for a few days and repeating the examination. Facioliasis can be excluded on geographical grounds. The eggs of *F. hepatica* and *F. buski* are difficult to distinguish. Recovery of adult flukes by surgical exploration, after antihelminthics, or at autopsy will confirm the diagnosis.

Treatment and prognosis

Praziquantel is effective at a dosage of 25 mg/kg t.i.d. after meals for 1 or 2 days.

The prognosis of human fascioliasis is good. Most patients recover spontaneously following evacuation of flukes through the intestinal tract.

POPULATION

Epidemiology

Fascioliasis is an important veterinary problem in sheep-raising areas. Because of the wide range of definitive and intermediate hosts the disease is geographically widespread. Human infection is most common where watercress is eaten. Sporadic human fascioliasis hepatica has been reported from many parts of the world including mainland United States and Hawaii, Europe, the Middle East, Asia, and Africa, with extensive outbreaks in France and Cuba. Human fascioliasis gigantica has been reported occasionally from Africa, Asia, and Hawaii.

Prevention and control

Human fascioliasis is prevented by not eating fresh aquatic plants, especially watercress, by boiling drinking water, and by thoroughly cooking sheep and goat liver. Long-range control measures are elimination of snail intermediate hosts by draining sheep pastures and treating with molluscicides (e.g., copper sulfate or Frescon) and eradication of the infection from definitive, herbivorous animals.

DICROCOELIASIS

Dicrocoeliasis is caused by *Dicrocoelium dendriticum* or *Dicrocoelium hospes*.

PARASITE

D. dendriticum (synonyms: *Fasciola lanceolata, Fasciola dendritica, Distomum lanceolatum,* etc.) is transparent, 5 to 15 by 1.5 to 2.5 mm, flat, and lanceolate. The eggs are dark brown (38 to 45 by 22 to 30 μm), slightly flattened on one side, thick-shelled with a large operculum, and contain a fully developed miracidium when laid. *D. hospes* is slender and shorter.

The adult flukes live in the biliary passages of sheep and cattle. The eggs are passed out in the feces and develop further to cercariae in the land snail. The cercariae are released in slime balls shed by the snail on vegetation as it crawls along and develop into infective metacercariae only if ingested by ants, the second intermediate hosts. Infected ants are eaten by grazing herbivores. The metacercariae excyst and migrate to the biliary tract. Humans also become infected by eating infected ants.

The land snails' first intermediate hosts are of the genus *Helicella,* whereas the ants' second intermediate hosts are *Formica fusca* and *F. rufibarbis,* etc.

PATIENT

Clinical manifestations

Symptoms of human dicrocoeliasis are mild. In heavy infections, vague biliary and gastrointestinal disturbances including abdominal distress, flatulence, biliary colic, vomiting, diarrhea, or constipation have been reported. The liver may be enlarged.

Diagnosis

Diagnosis is made by finding the characteristic ova in feces, bile, or duodenal fluid. Spurious infection must be ruled out. Recovery of adult flukes after antihelminthics, at surgery, or at autopsy may be necessary for specific diagnosis.

Treatment

Praziquantel in the same dose as for opisthorchiasis is recommended.

POPULATION

Epidemiology

Dicrocoeliasis is enzootic in sheep, goats, deer, and other herbivores. It is commonly seen in Europe, Turkey, North Africa, parts of Asia, and sometimes in America. Spurious human infections are common and are the consequence of consuming raw infected liver. True human infections are rare but have been reported from Europe, Egypt, Iran, Nigeria, Ivory Coast, and China.

Prevention and control

As the infection in humans is generally accidental, no preventive measures can be expected to be effective; however, raw vegetables should not be eaten in the endemic area.

PARAGONIMIASIS

Paragonimiasis is an infection caused by species of *Paragonimus*. The most common is the oriental lung fluke *P. westermani*.

Parasite

P. westermani (7 to 16 by 4 to 8 by 5 mm) (Kerbert, 1878) is a reddish-brown, plump, ovoid trematode with a rounded and broad anterior end (Fig. 55-6).

The operculated ova are immature when deposited (80 to 120 by 50 to 65 μm), ovoid, asymmetrical in shape, yellow-

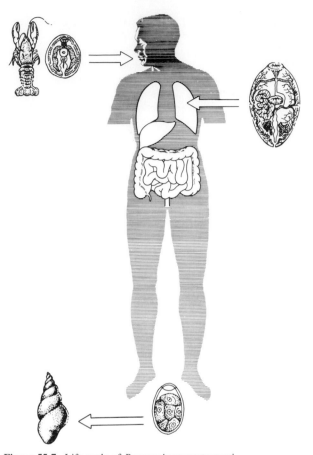

Figure 55-7. Life cycle of *Paragonimus westermani*.

brown in color, with the shell varying in thickness throughout (Fig. 55-6).

The life cycle is similar to that of digenic trematodes (Fig. 55-7).

The adult flukes are encysted in the lung. Ova are expectorated with the sputum or swallowed and passed in the feces.

There are several families of snails that serve as first intermediate hosts of *Paragonimus,* mainly belonging to Thiaridae, Pleuroceridae, and Hydrobilidae families.

The important second intermediate hosts are freshwater and brackish-water crabs; *Eriocheir japonicus, Potamon dehaani, P. ratbuni, P. smithianus,* and *Sundathelphusa philippina.* The crayfish *Procambarus alakii* is a second intermediate host in Korea.

Paragonimus is a parasite of humans and carnivores. More than 40 species have been reported, some of which are not valid. *P. westermani* had been considered to be the only species pathogenic to humans, until the last two decades when more than 10 species of *Paragonimus* have been reported as causing human paragonimiasis (Table 55-1) [*17*].

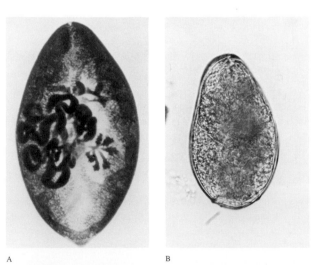

A   B

Figure 55-6. Photomicrograph of adult worm (*A*) and egg (*B*) of *Paragonimus westermani.*

Table 55-1. *Paragonimus* species reported to cause disease in humans

Paragonimus species	Country
P. westermani (Kerbert, 1878)	Far East, west Africa, and South America
P. westermani var. *szechuan* (Chung and Ts'ao, 1962)	China
P. westermani ichunensis (Chung et al., 1978)	China
P. philippinensis (Ito et al., 1978)	Philippines
*P. filipinus** (Miyazaki, 1978)	Philippines
P. pulmonalis (Baelz, 1880)	Japan, Korea, Taiwan
P. heterotremus (Chen and Hsia, 1964)	Thailand, Laos
P. tuanshanensis† (Chung et al., 1964)	China
P. africanus (Voelker and Vogel, 1965)	Cameroons
P. uterobilateralis (Voelker and Vogel, 1965)	Cameroons, Liberia, Nigeria
P. skrijabini (Chen, 1959)	China
P. szechuanensis‡ (Chung and Ts'ao, 1962)	China
P. miyazakii (Kamo et al., 1961)	Japan
P. hueitungensis (Chung et al., 1975)	China
P. kellicotti (Ward, 1908)	Peru, Ecuador, other Latin American countries
P. caliensis (Little, 1968)	Peru, Ecuador
P. mexicanus (Miyazaki and Ishii, 1968)	Mexico, Honduras, El Salvador, Ecuador, Peru, Costa Rica
P. peruvianus§ (Miyazaki et al., 1969)	Peru, Ecuador

*Same as *P. philippinensis*.
†Same as *P. heterotremus*.
‡Same as *P. skrijabini*.
§Same as *P. mexicanus*.

PATIENT

Pathogenesis, pathology, and pathophysiology

Young flukes lodge in the lung, cause hemorrhage and an inflammatory reaction with leukocytic infiltration and necrosis of lung parenchyma, and form a fibrous tissue capsule. "Worm cyst" or abscess cavities containing the fluke are then formed. In about 6 weeks the fluke matures and starts to produce eggs. The capsule swells and ruptures, usually into the bronchiole. The content of the cyst is expectorated in the sputum. Tunnels or burrows lined with fibrous tissue are also formed from the damaged and dilated bronchioles. The worm cysts are 1 to 2 cm in diameter; larger cysts are formed by the breakdown of adjacent cyst walls. The cysts are chocolate brown in color, often found in the right lung. There are one or two flukes in each cyst. Empty cysts are also occasionally encountered. It is unusual to find more than 20 flukes in the lungs. The wall of

a long-standing cyst is thick and fibrosclerotic, and some may be calcified. Granuloma or egg tubercles are frequently seen in the vicinity of the cyst. The bronchial arteries supplying the area may show hypertrophy and may cause hemoptysis when damaged.

In addition bronchopneumonia, interstitial pneumonia, bronchitis, bronchiectasis, atelectasis, fibrosis, pleural thickening, angiitis obliterans, and periphlebitis are encountered. These are not specific responses to the fluke or its ova, but may result from both allergic and toxic reactions plus superimposed bacterial infections.

Examination reveals lesions of various stages: early or acute reactions, or old or chronic changes which often coexist because of the migratory nature of the flukes.

Ectopic lesions, worm cysts, or abscesses may be detected in other organs such as the intestines, peritoneal cavity, mesenteric lymph nodes, liver, diaphragm, pleura, heart muscle, subcutaneous tissue, testes, uterus, brain, and spinal cord.

The worm cyst in the mucosa of the intestine may rupture, causing ulceration, resulting in passing of ova along with the feces. The pleura and pericardium when involved may produce an effusion with a high number of eosinophils.

Clinical manifestations

The clinical picture may be divided into an early or acute stage, and a late or chronic stage.

The early or acute stage corresponds to the period of invasion and migration of the young flukes and often passes without diagnosis; the incubation period is 2 to 20 days. The symptoms are diarrhea, abdominal pain, and urticaria, followed in a few days by fever, malaise, chest pain or tight sensation, cough, dyspnea, and night sweating [18].

The chronic manifestations may be divided into pulmonary and extrapulmonary. Generally the clinical picture of pulmonary paragonimiasis is mild and chronic. In light infection it is asymptomatic. The symptoms are chronic cough and vague respiratory discomfort, usually in the morning upon rising. Bouts of coughing produce mucoid, gelatinous, rusty-brown, "golden-flakes," blood-tinged sputum. Each expectoration is from 0.5 to 5 mL, totaling 10 to 50 mL daily. Microscopic examination reveals *Paragonimus* ova, necrotic tissue, blood, pus cells, and occasionally Charcot-Leyden crystals.

Attacks of hemoptysis, usually induced by heavy work, are the common presenting symptom of patients attending clinics or admitted to hospitals. On rare occasions, hemoptysis is so severe that it may endanger life. Pleural effusion, empyema, and pneumothorax may be present. Despite a long history of the infection, the patient looks well and may live for 50 years with it.

In the majority of cases, physical examinations show no abnormality, but in a few long-standing cases the picture is similar to that of other chronic lung diseases.

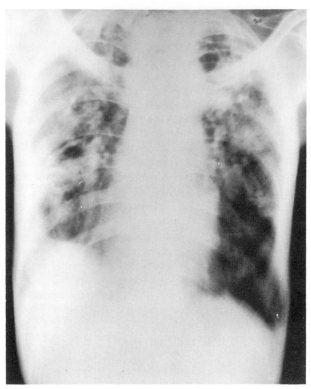

Figure 55-8. Chest x-ray showing generalized fibrosis, calcification, and cavitations in a lady of 79 years, who weighed 26 kg and had hemoptysis for 50 years.

Cerebral Paragonimiasis. Cerebral paragonimiasis is common in young age groups, 80 percent before the age of 20 and 52 percent before the age of 10. The disease may be acute or chronic. The symptoms of the acute stage are fever, headache, nausea, vomiting, visual disturbances, paralysis, and localized or generalized convulsions. There are papilledema, elevation of the cerebrospinal fluid pressure, and pleocytosis with a high eosinophil count. Death during the acute attack is not uncommon. Subarachnoid hemorrhage has also been recorded. In nonfatal cases there is spontaneous recovery in 1 or 2 months, but the symptom may recur within 2 years. The chronic stages are characterized mainly by epileptic seizures and paralysis. Occipital and temporal lobes are common sites of infestation. The pathological changes in the brain are granuloma or abscess formation. Occasionally both are present. The lesions vary in size from the size of a rice grain to that of a goose egg and may number from a few to as many as 100. Cerebral angiography or computed tomographic scan of the brain will locate the site of the lesion. In long-standing cases calcification is often seen. Mental retardation and subnormal intelligence have also been reported [20].

Abdominal Paragonimiasis. There are symptoms and signs of abscess formation in the liver, spleen, or abdominal cavity simulating other infections. In some instances there is ulceration of the intestine and *Paragonimus* eggs are present in the stool.

Ten to twenty percent of the chest x-rays are normal and two-thirds have two to three foci. The changes seen are patchy infiltration, cavitation, fibrosis, and pleural thickening (Fig. 55-8). A ring shadow (Fig. 55-9) with a crescent-shaped opacity along one side of the border "corona" is characteristic in paragonimiasis [19]. Tomography, bronchotomography, or computed tomographic scan of the lung are more effective in visualization of cavities and the tunnels or burrows joining them. Migratory lesions in the lung have been observed.

Extrapulmonary Paragonimiasis. It is not uncommon to find young flukes and even some of the mature flukes from the lung migrating to other areas and causing lesions in other organs. In such cases the disease is named after the organ affected, such as cerebral, spinal, abdominal, or cutaneous paragonimiasis.

Some species of *Paragonimus* other than *P. westermani,* such as *P. heterotremus* and *P. szechuanensis,* may be responsible for these ectopic lesions; the flukes are usually immature except in the brain. Trematode larva migrans is a clinical entity of *P. szechuanensis* infection [18].

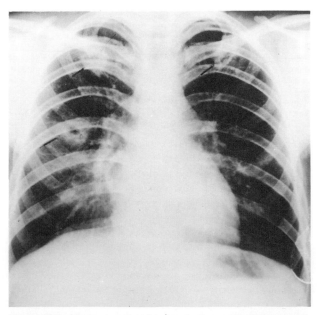

Figure 55-9. Chest x-ray showing ring shadows with thickened wall. (*Courtesy of Sirivan Vanijanonta, Hospital for Tropical Diseases, Bangkok.*)

Cutaneous Paragonimiasis. Subcutaneous migratory swelling with eosinophilia and subcutaneous nodules with the presence of immature or adult flukes [21] and ova have been observed.

Diagnosis

Paragonimiasis can be tentatively diagnosed by a history of having stayed in or been to the endemic area and eating raw crustaceans, together with blood spitting and the characteristic sputum. Correct diagnosis must, however, be confirmed by laboratory findings of ova.

Paragonimus ova are found in the sputum, feces, occasionally in the effusion fluid, pus, from biopsy of nodules or cysts, and at autopsy. The ova in the stool should be differentiated from those of *Diphyllobothrium latum* and the ova from nodules may be confused with eggs of *Achillurbainia nouveli*.

The recovery of an adult or immature fluke is the ideal for species identification; they are mostly found at autopsy, by biopsy of nodules, or, rarely, in the sputum [22].

Seroimmunodiagnostic tests are used for diagnosis of extrapulmonary paragonimiasis. Complement fixation test, countercurrent electrophoresis, and enzyme-linked immunosorbent assay (ELISA) are found to be highly sensitive and specific. Positive results are also obtained from cerebrospinal fluid.

The intradermal test is useful for screening a large population in an epidemiological survey [17].

Pulmonary paragonimiasis should always be differentiated from tuberculosis and other pulmonary diseases. The cerebral form must be differentiated from brain tumor and other parasitic cysts, especially cysticercosis, while the abdominal form must be differentiated from other abdominal or gastrointestinal diseases and the cutaneous form from cutaneous larva migrans such as gnathostomiasis.

Management

Praziquantel, in doses of 25 mg per kilogram of body weight three times daily after meals for 1, 2, and 3 days produced cure rates of 71.4, 89.5, and 100 percent, respectively. Side effects are mild and transient. With these drugs there is reduction in the amount of sputum within a few weeks after medication and the sputum becomes negative for eggs. The lesions in chest x-rays are cleared in a few months.

Management of chronic lung disease should include physiotherapy to improve pulmonary function.

POPULATION

Epidemiology

The prevalence of human paragonimiasis around the world is not known, but in all likelihood several million people are infected.

There are three main foci of the disease: in Asia endemic areas are China, Japan, Korea, Laos, the Philippines, Taiwan, and Thailand; in Africa, the Cameroons, the Congo Valley, Gambia, and Nigeria; and in South and Central America, Colombia, Costa Rica, Mexico, and Peru. The environment in these endemic areas is suitable for the fluke to complete its life cycle. Contributing factors include the presence of a large number of reservoir hosts among humans, felines, canines, and other animals; the presence of the first and second intermediate hosts; and social customs, such as spitting, and eating habits.

Raw or undercooked crab or crayfish are popular dishes: in China "drunken crab" (immersion of live crabs in wine), raw crab sauce, crab jam, raw crayfish, crayfish curd; in Thailand, *Kung Plah, Kung ten* (raw crayfish salad), *Nam Prik Poo* (crab sauce); in the Philippines, *Sinugba* (roast crab), *Kinilao* (raw crab); and in Korea, *Ke Jang* (crab in soy sauce).

Crustaceans are also used as medicine; in Korea and Japan, raw juice of crayfish or crab is used as an antipyretic for measles, diarrhea, and urticaria; some Africans eat raw crustaceans for fertility.

Another way of acquiring infection is through the contamination of utensils: chopping blocks and knives used in cutting crab, cloth used in squeezing crabs in the preparation of crab soup in Japan, and *Sinagang* in the Philippines.

In Taiwan, children often pull off crab legs and put them in the mouth just for fun [23].

Another means of transmission is eating the meat of a paratenic host containing immature flukes; for instance, wild boar meat.

Lack of food and the evacuation of people during wartime increased the prevalence of paragonimiasis in Japan during World War II and in Nigeria during the Nigerian civil war from 1967 to 1970 [24].

Prevention and control

In the control and eradication of these infections the epidemiology of the disease, the intermediate host, the parasite, the human host, and the environmental conditions all play important roles. Thus, preventive measures directed toward the interruption of the life cycle of the parasite can eliminate its spread. The snail intermediate hosts are difficult to control and are widespread. Molluscicides may destroy fish, which provide a dietary source of protein. Improvements in environmental sanitation can be achieved by extensive health education and compulsory use of latrines in the endemic areas. Specific measures to change the eating habits of the people are extremely difficult to implement since raw fish, crabs, and crayfish are delicacies that people are reluctant to give up. Effective chemotherapy, of course, remains one of the important measures of controlling these infections. It would, however, take decades to eradicate these infections.

INTESTINAL FLUKE INFECTIONS

Intestinal trematode infection is common in the Far East, southeast Asia, the Middle East, and north Africa. More than 50 species have been reported in humans, but only a few are known to cause morbidity. These include *Fasciolopsis buski, Heterophyes heterophyes, Metagonimus yokogawai,* and *Gastrodiscoides hominis. F. buski* is the most important.

FASCIOLOPSIASIS

Fasciolopsiasis is an infection with the giant intestinal fluke, *Fasciolopsis buski.*

PARASITE

F. buski (Lankester, 1857; Odhner, 1902) is the largest intestinal fluke (50 to 75 by 8 to 20 by 0.5 to 3 mm). It is fleshy, reddish-beef-colored, elongate, and ovoid in shape (Fig. 55-10). There is no cephalic cone. The egg is large (130 to 140 by 80 to 85 μm), shaped like a hen's egg and yellowish-brown, with a clear, thin shell and a small operculum at one end (Fig. 55-10). It is undeveloped when laid. The adult flukes inhabit the small intestine of pigs and humans. The eggs are passed with feces.

The life cycle is similar to that of *Fasciola hepatica;* the cercariae encyst on water plants. The snail hosts include *Segmentina, Hippeutis,* and *Gyraulus* spp. The edible water plants are water caltrop (*Trapa bicornis, T. natans*), water morning glory (*Ipomoea aquatica*), water chestnut (*Eliocharis tuberosa*, water bamboo (*Zizania aquatica*), and watercress (*Neptunia oleracea*). The life span of the fluke is only 1 year.

PATIENT

Pathology

The flukes attach to the mucosa of the duodenum and jejunum. Localized damage occurs at the sites of attachment, usually producing inflamed ulcerations, which are followed by deep

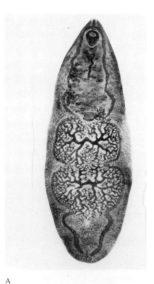 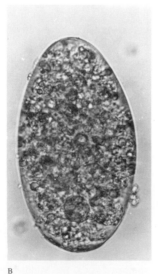

A   B

Figure 55-10. Photomicrograph of adult worm (*A*) and egg (*B*) of *Fasciolopsis buski.*

erosions and hemorrhage. The flukes provoke inflammation and hypersecretion with mucous discharge and in heavy worm loads may cause intestinal obstruction. In severe cases profound intoxication from absorption of the fluke metabolites and hypoalbuminemia secondary to malabsorption or protein-losing enteropathy may cause edema of the face and body. There is leukocytosis with eosinophilia.

Clinical manifestations

Most of the infections are light and asymptomatic. In heavy infections, the main symptom is diarrhea with hunger pains, simulating peptic ulcer. At first, diarrhea alternates with constipation, but later diarrhea becomes persistent. The stool is greenish yellow, foul-smelling, and contains undigested food. The appetite is moderate to excessive, but some patients are anorexic and nauseated and are vomiting. In severe cases, with heavy worm loads there are edema of face, trunk, and limbs, ascites, intestinal ileus and obstruction, dry and rough skin, and marked prostration. Death is rare.

Diagnosis

Specific diagnosis can be made by demonstrating the characteristic eggs and/or adult flukes in the feces or vomitus. The eggs must be distinguished from those of other species such as *Echinostoma* sp., *Fasciola hepatica,* and *F. gigantica.*

Treatment

The drug of choice is praziquantel, a single dose of 15 mg/kg after supper before retiring to bed. It is very effective; the flukes will be expelled on the following day. Niclosamide 150 mg/kg daily for 1 or 2 days or a single dose of tetrachloroethylene 0.1 mg/kg are less effective.

POPULATION

Epidemiology

The present prevalence of fasciolopsiasis is unknown. The disease is endemic in Taiwan, Thailand, Laos, Bangladesh, and India. Human infections have also been reported from Japan, the Philippines, Malaysia, and a number of western countries, but it is probable that these occurred in people who had migrated from endemic areas or that the eggs were misidentified.

Fasciolopsiasis seems to be restricted to areas where people raise water plants and pigs, and to populations that commonly eat freshwater plants. In many farms, pigs are kept near the ponds where water plants are grown. Pig excreta are washed into the ponds, where there are plenty of snail intermediate hosts. Water plants are fed to pigs, and the cycle of *F. buski* is continued.

Humans are infected by consuming raw stems, leaves and pods of water plants. Another means of acquiring the infection is by peeling with the teeth the outer layers of the plant where metacercariae are encysted. In central Thailand, where water caltrops are cultivated in canals along the side of the road, schoolchildren on their way to and from school enjoy picking and eating them fresh. This explains the high prevalence of fasciolopsiasis among children in these areas. Modifications in the local ecology through urbanization and industrialization have resulted in reduced prevalence rates in some areas of Thailand and Taiwan and eradication of some foci of infection.

Prevention

Water plants should be cooked or grown in ponds that are not contaminated with human or pig feces. Molluscicides could be used to eradicate the snail vectors.

ECHINOSTOMIASIS

Echinostomiasis is an infection by trematodes of the genus *Echinostoma* and its related genera.

PARASITE

Echinostomes are primarily intestinal worms of birds and a few mammals. There are more than 30 genera of the family Echinostomatidae (Poche, 1926), and about a dozen species have been reported from humans. The common species are *E. ilocanum, E. malayanum, E. revolutum,* and *Hypoderaeum conoideum.* Species less commonly recorded are *E. lindoense, E. recurvatum, E. melis (jassyense), E. macrochis, E. cinetorchis, Echinochasmus pertoliatus, Paryphostomum sufrartyfex,* and *Himasthla muehlensi.*

The echinostome flukes have a characteristic horseshoe-shaped collar of one or two rows of straight spines surrounding the dorsal and lateral sides of the oral sucker. The flukes are elongated, 5 to 15 by 1 to 2 mm, with slightly tapering, rounded ends (Fig. 55-11). The anterior portion of the body is covered by minute, scalelike spines that differ among species in their extent and distribution.

The egg is large, yellow to yellowish brown, thin-shelled, operculated, and ovoid and varies in size, being 83 to 154 by 53 to 95 μm. It is not embryonated when passed in the feces (Fig. 55-11). Eggs must be differentiated from those of *F. buski, F. hepatica, F. gigantica,* and possibly other spurious trematode infections.

The adult flukes are found in the small intestine of birds, mammals, and occasionally humans. The eggs are passed in the feces. The life cycle is similar to other digenic trematodes; planorbid snails are the first intermediate host and *Pila,* fishes, and tadpoles are second intermediate hosts. When humans and other definitive hosts ingest a second intermediate host improperly cooked, they become infected.

PATIENT

Pathology

The flukes attach to the small-bowel mucosa, producing shallow ulcers with a mild inflammatory response. Heavy infec-

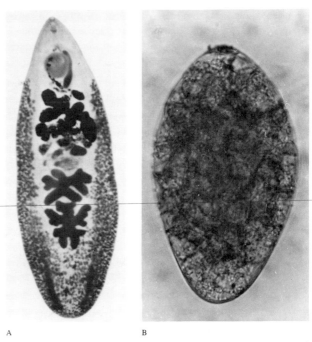

A   B

Figure 55-11. Photomicrograph of adult worm (**A**) and egg (**B**) of *Echinostoma malayanum.*

tions may produce necrosis and increased cellular infiltration in the intestinal mucosa.

Clinical manifestations

Definitive clinical manifestations associated with infection with echinostomes have not been recorded, and apparently little morbidity is produced by the infection. Heavy worm loads may cause vague abdominal complaints of flatulence and loose bowel movements. In children, diarrhea, abdominal pain, anemia, and edema, resembling infection with *F. buski,* have been reported.

Diagnosis

The diagnosis is made by recovering eggs from feces. However, it is impossible to differentiate between species except by examining adult worms recovered after treatment with antihelminthics or at autopsy.

Treatment

Drugs recommended for *F. buski* infection are effective. The prognosis is good.

POPULATION

Epidemiology

Echinostomiasis is common in Indonesia, Philippines, Thailand, and Taiwan, in places where there is an abundance of the intermediate hosts and lack of sanitary facilities. In some villages in northeastern Thailand, the prevalence rate is around 50 percent. *Echinostoma malayanum, Hypoderaeum conoideum, E. revolutum,* and *E. ilocanum* have been reported. A few decades ago, *E. lindoensis* was very common in Lindu Lake, Sulawesi (Celebes), and Indonesia, but it has now disappeared; this may be due to the introduction of *Tilapia mossambica* fish in 1951. The snail hosts have dwindled in numbers as there was competition for food with the fish.

Prevention

The infection could be prevented by thoroughly cooking and avoiding raw *Pila* snails and other second intermediate hosts.

HETEROPHYIASIS

Heterophyiasis is an infection by the tiny intestinal flukes of the genus *Heterophyes* which sometimes causes colicky and mucous diarrhea.

PARASITE

More than 10 species of minute heterophyid flukes have been found in humans. *Heterophyes heterophyes* (synonyms: *Distoma heterophyes, H. aegyptiaca, H. nocens,* etc.) is quite common.

Heterophyes heterophyes is a pyriform, gray, very small fluke (1.0 to 1.76 by 0.3 to 0.7 mm).

The egg is minute (28 to 30 by 15 to 17 μm), operculated, ovoid, and light brown, contains a mature miracidium, and is the size of opisthorchid species, but differs from *M. yokogawai* in having a thicker shell.

Life cycle

Adult *H. heterophyes* attach to the intestinal mucosa of the jejunum and upper ileum. The eggs come out with feces. The life cycle is similar to that of digenic trematode.

The proven snail first intermediate hosts are *Pironella conica* in the Middle East and *Cerithidea cingulata* and *Tympanotonus micropterus* in the Far East. The fish second intermediate hosts are the mullet (*Mugil cephalus*), minnow (*Gambusia affinis*), and *Acanthogubius* in Japan.

PATIENT

Pathology

Flukes attach to small-bowel mucosa producing shallow ulcers and a mild inflammatory response. Ova deposited in the bowel wall may enter blood vessels and embolize to the heart and central nervous system. In the Philippines severe cardiac damage was described in former times. The heart is dilated; there are subepicardial hemorrhages and myocardial damage caused by occlusion of vessels by the ova. Ova stick to the mitral valve, which becomes thickened and calcified.

Clinical features

Dyspepsia and gastroenterocolitis with mucous diarrhea are common. Cardiac involvement may produce chronic congestive cardiac failure, or there may be sudden death caused by massive coronary embolization. This disease was said to be responsible for more than 14 percent of cardiac deaths in the Philippines.

Diagnosis

Diagnosis is based on the recovery of characteristic eggs in the feces, but these are very difficult to differentiate from eggs of other heterophyid and opisthorchid trematodes.

Treatment

Praziquantel at a single dose of 15 to 25 mg/kg may be effective. The prognosis is good except when the brain and heart are involved.

POPULATION

Epidemiology

Human infection is common in Egypt, Iran, the Far East, Japan (*H. katsuradai*), South Korea, Taiwan, China, and the Philippines (*H. brevicaeca*). The fluke inhabits the small intestine of humans, cat, dog, fox, bird, and other fish-eating mammals. Humans are infected by eating infected raw fish. In Egypt the fish is eaten salted as ''fessikh''; the metacercariae are capable of living up to 7 days in the salted fish. The brackish-water fish *Mugil capito* caught off the coast of Israel have been found to be heavily infected.

Prevention and control

Efforts must focus on health education regarding the danger of eating raw, undercooked, or improperly salted or pickled fish and on the reduction of infection in the reservoir hosts (i.e., dogs, cats, and fish-eating animals).

METAGONIMIASIS

Metagonimiasis is caused by infection by *Metagonimus yokogawai*.

PARASITE

Matagonimus yokogawai (Katsurada, 1913) (synonyms: *Heterophyes yokogawai, Loxotrema ovatum, M. ovatus, Yokogawa yokogawai, Loossia romanica, L. parva, L. dobrogiensis, M. romanicus,* etc.) is the smallest human fluke (1 to 2.5 by 0.4 to 0.7 mm) and resembles *H. heterophyes* in size and shape (Fig. 55-12). The egg (27 by 16 μm) resembles that of *Clonorchis sinensis* but is more regularly ovoid. It is fully mature when laid (Fig. 55-12).

The life cycle is similar to *Heterophyes heterophyes*. The first intermediate hosts are *Semisulcospira libertina* and *Thiara*

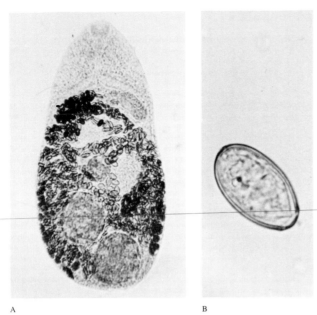

A   B

Figure 55-12. Photomicrograph of adult worm (**A**) and egg (**B**) of *Metagonimus yokogawai*.

granifera. The second intermediate hosts are salmonoid and cyprinoid fish. Sweet fish (*Plecoglossus altivelis*) and silver carp (*Carassius carassius*) are important hosts in Japan, Taiwan, and Korea. Metacercariae are usually found in scales, fins, and subcutaneous tissues of the fish.

PATIENT

Pathology

The flukes invade the mucosa of the small intestine, the duodenum, or the jejunum, causing inflammation, granulomatous infiltration, and ulceration. They ultimately become encapsulated. On rare occasions, eggs deposited in the tissues are carried by the bloodstream and deposited in other organs.

Clinical manifestations

The disease caused by *M. yokogawai* is similar to that of *H. heterophyes* infection.

Diagnosis

Diagnosis is confirmed by finding the ova in the feces; these are indistinguishable from ova of *H. heterophyes*. the definite diagnosis is made by identification of the adult fluke following antihelminthic therapy or at autopsy by scraping the intestinal mucosa.

Treatment

The treatment is the same as for heterophyiasis.

POPULATION

Epidemiology

M. yokogawai is believed to be the most common heterophyid fluke infection in the endemic areas of China, Japan, Korea, and Taiwan. It has also been reported from Siberia, Manchuria, Israel, the Balkans, and Spain. The prevalence of metagonimiasis in areas where there are clonorchiasis and other heterophyids is difficult to estimate as the eggs are similar.

Humans are infected by eating raw or undercooked fish.

Prevention and Control

Prevention and control of metagonimiasis are the same as for heterophyiasis.

GASTRODISCIASIS

Gastrodisciasis is caused by *Gastrodiscoides hominis*.

ETIOLOGY

Gastrodiscoides hominis (synonym: *Gastrodiscus hominis*) is an aspinous fluke. When alive it is bright-pinkish, very expansile (8 to 14 by 5 to 8 mm), and pyriform in outline, with a conical anterior and a discoidal posterior portion (Fig. 55-13). A huge acetabulum occupying the ventral posterior portion of the fluke bears a characteristic notch at its posterior extremity. The eggs are greenish brown and immature when laid (152 by 60 µm) (Fig. 55-13). The life cycle is not known, but it is probably similar to that of amphistomes. The cercariae probably encyst on vegetation.

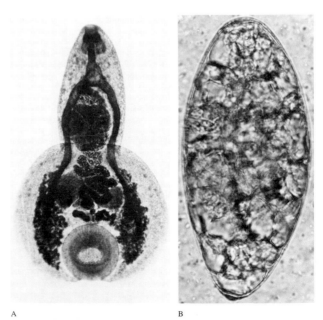

A   B

Figure 55-13. Photomicrograph of adult worm (**A**) and egg (**B**) of *Gastrodiscoides hominis*.

PATIENT

Pathology

G. hominis attaches to the mucosa of the cecum and ascending colon. The pathology in humans and pigs may be similar. At the site of attachment the mucosa is dragged out by the acetabulum forming a minute papilla in the sharply defined circular imprint made by the discoidal region of the fluke. There is surface desquamation of the mucosa. Both the mucosa and submucosa show infiltration with eosinophils, lymphocytes, and plasma cells.

Clinical Manifestation

The flukes live in the cecum in large numbers, usually producing no symptom. Mucous diarrhea associated with gastrodisciasis has been recorded.

Diagnosis

The diagnosis is based on the finding of characteristic ova or adult flukes after antihelminthic therapy. The ova resemble those of *F. buski* but are narrower and have a greenish-brown color. The adult fluke may be identified readily by its pyriform shape, bright-pinkish color, and huge, notched acetabulum.

Treatment

Praziquantel at the same dosage used in fasciolopsiasis may be effective.

POPULATION

Epidemiology

G. hominis is a common parasite in Assam, Bengal, Bihar, and Orissa in India. Human infections have also been reported from Burma, Malaysia, Vietnam, British Guyana, Kasakstan in the U.S.S.R., and Thailand.

Pigs are reservoir hosts in India, and the mouse deer is a reservoir host in Malaysia, while rats have been found to be hosts in Indonesia, Japan, and Thailand.

Prevention and Control

Improvement of sanitation may help in control of the disease.

OTHER INTESTINAL TREMATODIASES

Other intestinal trematode infections, including *Spelatrema brevicaeca, Plagiorchis philippinensis, P. javensis, Fibricola seoulensis, Phaneropsolus bonnei,* and *Prosthodendrium molenkampi,* have been reported from the Far East and southeast Asia. Praziquantel is the drug of choice. A primary health care delivery system could play an important role in any effort to control infection.

REFERENCES

1 Radomyos P, Bunnag D, Harinasuta T: Worms recovered in stools following praziquantel treatment. Arzneimittelforsch/Drug Res 34: 1215, 1984

2 Harinasuta C (ed): Clonorchiasis and Opisthorchiasis: Proceedings of the Fourth Southeast Asian Seminar on Parasitology and Tropical Medicine, Schistosomiasis and Other Snail Transmitted Helminthiases. Manila, February 24–27, 1969, pp 209–275

3 Upatham ES, Viyanant V, Kurathong S, et al: Morbidity in relation to intensity of infections in opisthorchiasis viverrini of a community in Khon Kaen, Thailand. Am J Trop Med Hyg 31:1156, 1982

4 Sonakul D, Koompirochana C, Chinda K, et al: Hepatic carcinoma with opisthorchiasis. Southeast Asian J Trop Med Pub Hlth 9:215–219, 1978

5 Thomavit W, Bhamarapravati N, Sahaphongs S, et al: Effects of dimethylnitrosamine on induction of cholangiocarcinoma in *Opisthorchis viverrini* infected Syrian golden hamsters. Cancer Res 38:4634–4639, 1978

6 Dhiensiri T, Eue-Ananta Y, Sinawat P: Obstructive jaundice in northeastern Thailand (in Thai). Bull Dept Med Serv 4:180–220, 1979

7 Ozeretskovskaya NN: The clinical features and treatment of opisthorchiasis in dependence on some endogenous and exogenous factors (in Russian, with English summary). Akademii Medicineskin Nauk 6:36–43, 1965

8 Bunnag D, Harinasuta T: Studies on the chemotherapy of human opisthorchiasis in Thailand: I. Clinical trial of praziquantel. Southeast Asian J Trop Med Pub Hlth 11:528–531, 1980

9 Bunnag D, Harinasuta T: Studies on the chemotherapy of human opisthorchiasis in Thailand: III. Minimum effective dose of praziquantel. Southeast Asian J Trop Med Pub Hlth 12:413–417, 1981

10 Jaroonvesama N, Charoenlarp K, Cross JH: Treatment of *Opisthorchis viverrini* with mebedazole. Southeast Asian J Trop Med Pub Hlth 12:595–597, 1981

11 Pungpark S, Bunnag D, Harinasuta T: Albendazole in treatment of opisthorchiasis and concomitant intestinal helminthic infections. Southeast Asian J Trop Med Pub Hlth 15:44, 1984

12 Komiya Y: *Clonorchis* and clonorchiasis. Adv Parasitol 4:53, 1966

13 Xu Z, Zhong H, Cao W: Acute chlonorchiasis: Report of 2 cases. Chin Med J 92:423, 1970

14 Rim HJ, Lyu KS, Lee JS, Joo KH: Clinical efficacy of praziquantel (EMBAY 8440) against *Clonorchis sinensis* infection in man. Ann Trop Med Parasitol 75:27, 1980

15 Hillyer GV: Fascioliasis in Puerto Rico: A review. Bol Asoc Med PR 73:94, 1981

16 Roche PJL: Human dicrocoeliasis in Nigeria. Trans R Soc Trop Med Hyg 41:819–820, 1948

17 Yokogawa M: *Paragonimus* and paragonimiasis. Adv Parasitol 3:99–158, 1965

18 Zhong Huilan (HL Chung), Ho Lianyin (LY Ho), et al: Recent progress in studies of *Paragonimus* and paragonimiasis control in China. Chinese Med J 94:483–494, 1981

19 Vanijanonta S, Bunnag D, Harinasuta T: Radiological findings in pulmonary paragonimiasis heterotremus. Southeast Asian J Trop Med Pub Hlth 15:122, 1984

20 Higashi K, Aoki H, Tatebayashi K, et al: Cerebral paragonimiasis. J Neurosurg 33:515–527, 1971

21 Miyazaki I, Harinasuta T: The first case of human paragonimiasis caused by *Paragonimus heterotremus* Chen et Hsia, 1964. Ann Trop Med Parasitol 60:509, 1966

22 Vanijanonta S, Radomyos P, Bunnag D, et al: Pulmonary para-gonimiasis with expectoration of worms: A case report. Southeast Asian J Trop Med Pub Hlth 12:104–106, 1981

23 Harinasuta C (ed): Paragonimiasis. Proceedings of the Fourth Southeast Asian Seminar on Parasitology and Tropical Medicine, Schistosomiasis and Other Snail-Transmitted Helminthiases, Manila, Feb 24–27, 1969, pp 277–320

24 Nwokolo C: Endemic paragonimiasis in eastern Nigeria. Trop Geogr Med 24:138–147, 1972

25 Bunnag D, Radomyos P, Harinasuta T: Field trial of the treatment of fasciolopsiasis with praziquantel. Southeast Asian J Trop Med Pub Hlth 14:216, 1983

26 Cross JH: Fasciolopsiasis in Southeast Asia and the Far East: A review. Proceedings of the Fourth Southeast Asian Seminar on Parasitology and Tropical Medicine: Schistosomiasis and Other Snail-Transmitted Helminthiasis, Manila, Feb. 24–27, 1969

27 Carney WP, Sodoma M, Purnomo: Echinostomiasis: A disease that disappeared. Trop Geogr Med 32:101, 1980

28 Africa CM, De Leon W, Garcia EY: Heterophyidiasis: II. Ova in sclerosed mitral valves with other chronic lesions in the myocardium. J Philipp Med Assn 15:583–592, 1935

SECTION C / Cestode Infections

CHAPTER 56 / Cestodiases: Taeniasis, Cysticercosis, Diphyllobothriasis, Hymenolepiasis, and Others · Zbigniew S. Pawlowski

The cestodes parasitizing humans constitute a very disparate group of parasites (Table 56-1). Taxonomically they belong to two distinct orders, Cyclo- and Pseudophyllidea, with essential differences in their morphology and life cycles. A human being may be the sole host and major disseminator of the infection or an accidental host of little or no importance in the further spread of the parasite. The majority of tapeworms cause intestinal infection, but cestode larvae can invade almost any internal organ in a human being. Many of the infections are clinically benign, but some, such as *Taenia solium* cysticercosis, are one of the major causes of death in certain countries. Human cestodiasis may be a feces, meat-, or fleaborne infection and can occur sporadically or in endemics or epidemics. Some cestodiases are prevalent in developed and some in developing countries. Most of the cestode infections are preventable, but, in spite of recent developments in immunology

Table 56-1. Cestodes parasitizing humans: hosts, habitat, and distribution

Taxonomic classification	Habitat in humans		Definitive hosts other than humans	Intermediate hosts	World distribution
	Adult worm	Larval stage			
Cyclophyllidea*					
Taenia saginata	Small intestine (jejunum)	No	No	Cattle and other Boviidae, reindeer	Cosmopolitan
T. solium	Small intestine (jejunum)	Cysticercus in muscle and internal organs (brain, eye)	Some monkeys	Pig, humans, and many other mammals	Central and South America, South and central Africa, India, Indonesia, Korea
T. multiceps		Coenurus in brain, eye	Dog and wild Canidae	Sheep, other ruminants, and rabbit	Several areas in the world
Echinococcus granulosus		Echinococcus (cystic) in liver, lungs, brain	Dog and wild carnivores	Sheep, cattle, pig, horse, camel, goat, and many wild mammals	Cosmopolitan
E. multilocularis		Echinococcus (alveolar) in liver	Fox, domestic cat, and wild Canidae	Wild rodent	Northern hemisphere
Hymenolepis nana	Ileum	Cysticercoid in intestinal villi	Full development in humans only		Cosmopolitan, warm countries
H. diminuta	Small intestine (jejunum)	No	Rat, mice, wild rodent	Fleas, flour beetles	Cosmopolitan
Pseudophyllidea					
Diphyllobothrium latum†	Small intestine (jejunum)	No	Cat, dog, and fish-eating carnivores	Planktonic copepods (*Cyclops* and *Diaptomus*) and freshwater fish	Lakes, rivers, and deltas in the northern hemisphere

*Some other Cyclophyllidea occasionally invade humans: e.g., the common dog tapeworm *Dipylidium caninum*.
†Several other species of *Diphyllobothrium* have been found in man, e.g., *D. pacificum*. Occasionally plerocercoid larvae of *Sparganum proliferum* or *Spirometra mansoni* invade human tissues.

and population studies related to cestodiases, only a few nationwide control activities have been undertaken [1,2].

Humans are parasitized by two major species of Taenia, i.e., *T. saginata* and *T. solium,* but probably other species as well. Recently a new species designation, *T. khavi?*, has been proposed for an armed tapeworm occurring in Taiwan aborigines; it has armed cysticerci developing in the liver of calves, goats, and certain strains of pigs [3]. Once a controversial species of a tapeworm was reported from the Philippines as well.

TAENIA SAGINATA TAENIASIS

PARASITE

Life cycle and ecology

T. saginata—the beef tapeworm—like many other tapeworms parasitizing humans belongs to the order Cyclophyllidea. A human being is the only definitive host of *T. saginata* and the only one in which the parasite multiplies. With *T. saginata* infection, about 6 gravid proglottids, each containing 80,000 to 103,000 eggs, pass daily through the anus. The eggs are globular, 35 μm in diameter; a thick, striated embryophore covers the usually well-developed hexacanth larva or oncosphere (Fig. 56-1). *T. saginata* eggs can survive in pastures for several months or years, being sensitive only to desiccation and temperatures higher than 56°C. The spread of the eggs in the environment is facilitated by water, wind, vertebrates (e.g., gull droppings) or invertebrates (e.g., coprophagous beetles). Field experiments with the sheep tapeworm have shown that an infected, kenneled dog can contaminate with *T. ovis* eggs

an area of about 10 ha within 10 days [4]. *T. saginata* eggs develop further when ingested by cattle. Some other Bovidae and antelopes as well as reindeer were also reported as intermediate hosts of *T. saginata*. The oncosphere leaves its embryophore in the cow's intestine and migrates to the muscles, where within 10 to 12 weeks the next larval stage—the cysticercus—develops. The cysticercus is an oval bladder (7 to 10 by 4 to 6 mm), filled with fluid and containing the invaginated scolex of the tapeworm. It can survive in the muscle of the cattle for 1 to 3 years and can infect humans when ingested with raw meat. The quadrangular scolex of the *T. saginata* then attaches itself to the jejunal mucosa, and within 3 to 3½ months a fully grown tapeworm is developed.

Morphology and biology of adult worm (Table 56-2)

The adult beef tapeworm is 4 to 10 m in length, depending on the number of proglottids (about 2000) and their degree of relaxation (Fig. 56-1). The scolex, less than 2 mm in diameter, is unarmed, has four strong hemispherical suckers, and is attached to the mucosa usually in the proximal jejunum. Behind the scolex and the undifferentiated but actively growing area there is a strobila consisting of sexually immature, mature, and gravid proglottids. The gravid proglottids, 20 to 30 mm long and 5 to 7 mm wide, each with a ramified uterus filled with eggs, become detached singly from the strobila and leave the host, usually passing actively through the anus. Occasionally a large part of the strobila is discharged and the excretion of proglottids is stopped for a time. Humans are more often infected with a single tapeworm, but multiple or mixed (with *T. solium*) infections do occur. *T. saginata* can live in humans for more than 30 years; self-cure is rare.

Table 56-2. Morphological differences between *T. solium* and *T. saginata*

	Taenia solium	*Taenia saginata*
Entire body		
Length (m)	2–8	4–12
Maximal breadth (mm)	7–10	12–14
Proglottids (number)	700–1000	≈ 2000
Scolex		
Diameter (mm)	0.6–1.0	1.5–2.0
Suckers (number)	4	4
Rostellum	Present	Absent
Hooks (number)	22–32	Absent
Mature proglottids		
Testes (number)	375–575	800–1200
Ovary (number of lobes)	3	2
Vaginal sphincter	Absent	Present
Gravid proglottids		
Uterus (number of branches each side)	7–12	18–32
Way of leaving host	In groups, passively	Single, spontaneously

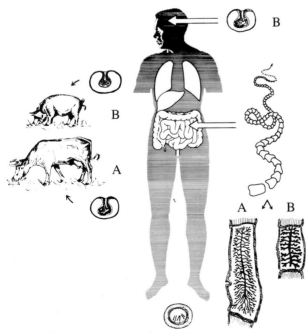

Figure 56-1. Life cycle of *T. saginata* (*A*) and *T. solium* (*B*).

T. saginata adult tapeworms have seldom been the object of biochemical or physiological studies since no animal model for this taeniasis exists. There is no protective immunity in human taeniasis, which as a rule provokes a weak immunological response. On the other hand, *T. saginata* cysticerci in cattle are much more immunogenic, especially when they degenerate and die.

PATIENT

Clinical pathology and symptomatology

T. saginata taeniasis more often causes changes in motility and secretion of the gastrointestinal tract than local pathological changes in the intestinal mucosa. In about 70 percent of the cases gastric secretion is reduced during the infection [5].

The presence of the tapeworm can hardly be overlooked by infected individuals as most of them feel some sensation in the perianal area when the proglottids are discharged. About one-third of patients with taeniasis claim vague abdominal pain, nausea, and increase or decrease of appetite and/or body weight. Abdominal discomfort and a feeling of weakness, insomnia, or irritability are sometimes reported; allergic signs are rare. Individual reactions to the infection differ widely and may be of a psychological nature as symptoms are often not reported until the patient becomes aware of being infected [5,6].

Sporadically straying *T. saginata* proglottids can cause acute or subacute appendicitis or cholangitis.

Diagnosis

Taeniasis is most difficult to diagnose in the first 3 months of infection, before the eggs are produced and the proglottids discharged. Serological tests are of little practical value for diagnosis. X-ray examination of the intestinal tract may sometimes show a ribbonlike contrast defect. Eosinophilia, when it does occur, is usually moderate. Serum IgE may be high. In endemic areas a history of eating raw beef may suggest the possibility of taeniasis.

Frequently the patient reports the discharge of a parasite or brings discharged proglottids for examination. The final diagnosis of *T. saginata* may not be easy as it is based on the parasitological examination of mature or gravid proglottids or the scolex of the tapeworm. The scolex is difficult to find after treatment with modern taeniacidal drugs, which cause the disintegration of the proximal part of the strobila. In some cases the differentiation between *T. saginata* and *T. solium* proglottids is uncertain (Table 56-2); counting the lateral uterine branches in the gravid proglottids, although used as a routine diagnostic technique for over a century, has recently been questioned as possibly having limited taxonomic value [7]. In routine laboratory practice if a proglottid has a doubtful characteristic, then other proglottids should be sought and examined. A helminthological taxonomist should be consulted in case of further doubt.

T. saginata eggs do not differ morphologically from *T. solium* eggs, and for this reason finding *Taenia* eggs in the feces or more frequently on anal swabs does not enable any final species diagnosis (Fig. 56-1). Differential laboratory diagnosis between *T. saginata* and *T. solium* is useful (see *T. solium* cysticercosis) for both clinical and epidemiological purposes.

Treatment

Praziquantel and niclosamide are now the best taeniacides. Older drugs such as mepacrine, tin compounds, and paromomycine are rarely used. Mebendazole and albendazole show some efficacy against taeniasis but are not "true" taeniaides [8].

Praziquantel is given in a single dose of 5 or 10 mg/kg, preferably after a light breakfast. The side effects are mostly mild and transient abdominal pain; dizziness and skin rashes are rare. Praziquantel in taeniasis has an efficacy of over 90 percent [8]. Treatment can be considered successful when no proglottids have appeared again within 4 months after therapy.

Niclosamide is given in a single dose of 2.0 g for adults (0.5 g is the dose for children 2 to 5 years old and 1.0g for older children). The tablets should be taken in the morning on an empty stomach and thoroughly chewed. The strobila is often evacuated within a few hours; if not, a purgative is recommended. Treatment is safe and effective in about 90 percent of cases. Niclosamide has no contraindications and can be used in pregnancy.

POPULATION

Factors related to epidemiology

Transmission dynamics of cestodiases depend mainly on tapeworm life span and biotic potential, on ecological factors affecting survival and spread of eggs, and on intermediate host immunity.

Recently some new categories of the dynamics of transmission have been proposed: hyperendemic state, where reproduction rate (R) of cestode population is much greater than 1.0; endemic state, where R is near to but greater than 1.0; and extinction state, where R is lower than 1.0 [9]. More studies are needed to confirm how much the rules based on observations in animals apply to tapeworms such as *T. saginata* and *T. solium*, having humans as the definite host. The very complex relationships, including social factors, between humans, cattle, and the environment can greatly complicate the dynamics of transmission. The role played by humans in this transmission is a crucial one, for only in a human being can the parasite multiply; humans are also important as disseminators of the eggs and lifelong reservoirs of the tapeworms. The environment (pastures, feedlots, silos, water) can serve as an egg reservoir and further spread the infection. Cattle are a reservoir for cysticerci, a source of infection for humans.

There are three main patterns of *T. saginata* transmission [*10*]: (1) Endemic, pastoral type, characteristic in Kenya, for example, where high prevalences of taeniasis in humans and cysticercosis in cattle are due to the close spatial and temporal contacts between nomadic, pastoral societies and their cattle. Some immunological mechanisms in cattle probably reduce the prevalence of bovine cysticercosis, which is usually less than 50 percent. (2) Endemic, urbanized type, characterized by the small number of human carriers, the wide dispersal of eggs in the environment, and a moderate prevalence of bovine cysticercosis, mostly of low intensity. This pattern is typical for European countries. (3) Epizootic type in feedlots (e.g., in the United States, Canada, and Czechoslovakia) can be caused by a single human carrier, frequently an immigrant from an endemically affected region, whose close contact with a herd of nonimmune cattle can result in an epidemic outbreak of bovine cysticercosis.

Prevalence of *T. saginata* infection

T. saginata is widespread in most cattle-breeding countries of the world [*1,5*]. It is highly endemic, with a prevalence exceeding 10 percent of the human population in some countries of central and east Africa, the Near East, and southern U.S.S.R. Moderate (below 5 percent) infection rates occur in many countries of Europe, southeast Asia, and South America. In the United States, Canada, and Australia the prevalence in the human population is less than 0.1 percent. It is estimated that the number of people in the world infected with *T. saginata* is 45 to 60 million.

In highly endemic areas the prevalence of bovine cysticercosis may be as high as 80 percent; in Europe it is between 1 and 5 percent.

Prevention and control

The best individual prophylaxis is to avoid eating raw or semiraw beef. Prevention at the national level, by means of meat inspection, does not detect some of the low-intensity cases of bovine cysticercosis. Carcasses with diagnosed intensive cysticercosis should be condemned or boiled; those with a light infection can be consumed after freezing at $-18°C$ for 5 days. Bovine cysticercosis may easily spread wherever sanitation, sewage disposal, and hygiene on cattle farms are inadequate.

Early detection and treatment of human taeniasis greatly helps to control the infection. On some feedlots all the workers are prophylactically treated every 3 months against eventual taeniasis. Trials to control bovine cysticercosis by vaccination or mass chemotherapy are being undertaken [*11*]. Artificial fertilizers, especially lime nitrogen, may substantially shorten the survival time of *T. saginata* eggs in the field [*12*].

TAENIA SOLIUM TAENIASIS AND CYSTICERCOSIS

PARASITE

Life cycle

T. solium—the pork tapeworm—is less specific in selecting its hosts than is *T. saginata*. The adult tapeworm develops not only in humans but also in some species of monkey and laboratory hamsters; the bladder larva cysticercus develops not only in pigs but also in humans, several species of monkey, wild boars, camels, bears, dogs, cats, and several other carnivores and rodents. However, the most important and common is the human-pig-human cycle.

T. solium produces up to 50,000 eggs per proglottid. The gravid proglottids become detached from the strobila, usually in groups of three to five, and are excreted passively in the human feces. The eggs are liberated from the proglottids which are damaged or macerated. The *T. solium* eggs can survive in the environment for several months. Pigs are infected after ingestion of a *T. solium* proglottid or eggs present in an environment contaminated by humans.

The oncosphere leaves the embryophore in the pig intestine and migrates to the tissue; the bladder larva cysticercus develops mainly in the muscle tissue and the myocardium but often also in the brain and liver. The cysticerci become fully grown and invasive for humans 2 months after ingestion of the eggs.

A human being acquires taeniasis by ingesting *T. solium* cysticerci in raw pork. In the human small intestine the evaginated scolex attaches itself to the mucosa and within 2 months develops into an adult tapeworm producing eggs.

Humans can also be infected by *T. solium* eggs, in which case human cysticercosis develops. There is some controversy about the mechanism of autoinfection, which is not uncommon. It is possible, but rather unlikely, that *T. solium* eggs or gravid proglottids enter the stomach during vomiting or reverse peristalsis, or during the medical treatment of taeniasis; only on these rare occasions can the embryophore of the invasive egg be digested and the oncosphere liberated, causing an internal autoinfection. External autoinfection is much more probable; some tapeworm carriers may easily ingest *T. solium* eggs from their hands or from food contaminated with fecal particles.

Morphology of *T. solium* tapeworm and cysticercus

The morphological differences between adult *T. solium* and *T. saginata* are presented in Table 56-2 and Fig. 56-1. Some specific protein bands have been demonstrated by polyacrylamide gel electrophoresis in the strobila of three taeniid species, but so far this technique has not been found useful as a means of differentiating *T. solium* from *T. saginata*. Enzyme electrophoresis studies have revealed some differences in glucose phosphate isomerase between *T. solium* and *T. saginata*.

T. solium cysticerci are in general larger (5 to 20 mm in diameter) than those of *T. saginata* (Fig. 56-2); the bladder is more transparent; and the scolex inside is smaller and has four delicate suckers and a rostellum armed with 22 to 32 hooks. When the scolex is not available, a differential diagnosis between *T. solium* and *T. saginata* can be made by analyzing the histological structure [*13*].

PATIENT

T. solium taeniasis

The pathology and symptomatology of *T. solium* taeniasis are usually less expressed than those of *T. saginata*. The *T. solium* tapeworms are smaller, their hooks do not do much damage to the mucosa, and their proglottids are less active and do not cause abdominal complications such as appendicitis or cholangitis. But *T. solium* taeniasis may remain unnoticed by the carrier because of the passive discharge of the proglottids, and thus may constitute a risk of cysticercosis for the carrier or for other people. About 25 percent of human cysticercosis cases were developed in *T. solium* tapeworm carriers.

T. solium infection is diagnosed by examination of the proglottids expelled either spontaneously or after provocative treatment with taeniacides. Finding the *Taenia* eggs in the feces in the absence of proglottids being discharged actively suggests *T. solium* infection. Since *T. solium* eggs may be scanty in the

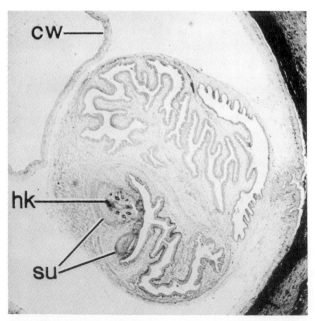

Figure 56-2. Human cysticercosis. *T. solium* cysticercus in the brain surrounded by fibrous tissue. In the invaginated scolex two suckers (su) are shown along with several hooks (hk). The scolex is surrounded by fluid and the cyst wall (cw). *(From ChH Binford and CH Conner: Pathology of Tropical and Extraordinary Diseases, vol 2, Armed Forces Institute of Pathology, Washington DC, 1976.)*

feces the laboratory examination should be repeated at least three times using the sediment concentration techniques. Any case diagnosed as, or suspected of being *T. solium* taeniasis is to be treated without delay because of the potential danger of cysticercosis. The taeniacides to be used are the same as for *T. saginata* taeniasis, i.e., praziquantel or niclosamide [*6,8*]. The efficacy of the treatment with both drugs is over 90 percent and should be evaluated by coproscopical examinations repeated weekly in the second and third months after therapy. Caution should be taken in handling the fecal material or discharged gravid proglottids of the parasite both at home and in the laboratory.

Human cysticercosis

Etiology. Human cysticercosis is mainly caused by *T. solium* larvae. In Mexico, South America, and South Africa several cases of racemose cysticercosis have been reported. The term *cysticercus racemosus* is used to describe translucent large vesicles, frequently lobulated or ramified, having no scolex, and usually located in the subarachnoid space or ventricles. The taxonomy of cysticercus racemosus is still a matter of controversy. It can be a cysticercus of *T. solium* which has degenerated or grown unobstructed by the surrounding tissue; it can also be a sterile coenurus-type larva of *T. multiceps*, *T. serialis* (both tapeworms parasitize dogs), or other *Taenia*. The answer will not be known until more basic studies have been made on the microstructure and the specific proteins or enzymes in the larval cestodes.

Infections with typical *T. multiceps* larvae, so-called coenurosis, are occasionally reported from different parts of the world. Subcutaneous and ocular coenurosis in Uganda is caused by *T. brauni*. Liver cysticercosis in humans caused by the larvae of *T. taeniaformis* or *T. crassiceps* has also been reported.

Clinical Pathology of Cerebral Cysticercosis. The clinical pathology of cerebral cysticercosis depends on the number, localization, and stage of development of the parasites and the individual host reaction [*14*].

The human brain can be invaded by one, by several, or even by more than two thousand cysticerci; in the majority of cases less than ten cysticerci are present. The cysticerci are localized mainly subarachnoidally in the cortex, in the cerebral ventricles, or in the basal cistern and also in the white matter of the cerebrum itself (Fig. 56-3). The presence of cysticerci on the surface of the brain may cause flattening or compression of the convolutions and inflammatory, or, later on, fibrotic, changes to the leptomeninges. The affected ventricles may be distended and deformed with signs of granular ependymitis. The lesions in the white matter are mechanical and inflammatory depending on the size and status of the cysticerci.

The cysticerci in the human brain may be of different sizes and stages of development: they can be juvenile, mature, or

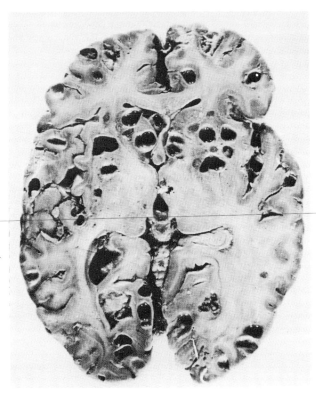

Figure 56-3. Human cysticercosis. Numerous *T. solium* cysticerci in the brain. *(From ChH Binford and CH Conner: Pathology of Tropical and Extraordinary Diseases, vol 2, Armed Forces Institute of Pathology, Washington DC, 1976.)*

old; each one can be intact, degenerating, or dead. Intact cysticerci do not usually provoke much host reaction since they are surrounded by a connective tissue membrane consisting of epithelial cells, collagen fibers, and slight cellular infiltration in which plasma cells and eosinophils prevail. This membrane enables the flow of nutrients, metabolites, and immunogenic substances. The dying and/or degenerating cysticerci provide a much more inflammatory reaction in the host; a granulomatous response composed of plasma cells, lymphocytes, eosinophils, and macrophages enclosed in a network of connective tissue is built up around the cysticerci. In later stages the host cells penetrate into the remnants of the parasite, which finally becomes transformed into a glial-connective scar or undergoes calcification; the latter is more characteristic for cysticerci with other than cerebral localization. The equilibrium between the biological potential of the cysticerci and the host reaction is unstable; usually some cysticerci degenerate earlier than others and intensify, in irregular periods of time, the host inflammatory and immunological response. Clinical improvement resulting from steroid treatment strongly suggests that allergic or inflammatory phenomena play an important role in cerebral cysticercosis.

There have been only a few basic studies on the immuno-

pathological phenomena of *T. solium* infections in humans [*15,16*]. The finding of immunoglobulinlike determinants on the surface of *T. solium* suggests that a surface antigen-antibody complex may be responsible for attracting the eosinophils around the parasite. The fact that eosinophils are frequently degranulated confirms their active role in the process of neutralization of the parasite metabolites, which may be either immunogenic or toxicogenic. The parasite integument itself is barely affected by cellular host reactions. The antigenic stimulation of the host is more intensive when cysticerci degenerate or die; this can be seen from higher titers in various serological tests, for example, after treatment of cysticerocosis with praziquantel. Endoarteritis and periarteritis in the vicinity of cysticerci is common and may be responsible for multifocal lesions and cerebral or cerebellar atrophy in the later stages of intensive cysticercosis [*17*].

Clinical Course and Manifestations of Cerebral Cysticercosis. The incubation period of human cysticercosis observed among British soldiers serving in India ranged from less than 1 year to 30 years, with an average of 4.8 years; it is usually shorter in infected children. The youngest child with cysticercosis was 14 months old. The onset is either insidious (intracranial hypertension) or abrupt (sudden block of cerebrospinal fluid by a floating cysticercus). The evolution of human cysticercosis is variable and unpredictable; there are shorter or longer remissions or a steady worsening of symptoms. Death, often unexpected, may occur at any moment of the disease. The prognosis in cerebral cysticercosis is always serious; the fatality rate in symptomatic untreated cases exceeds 50 percent. The survival time of human patients varies from a few hours to 35 years from the onset of the first symptoms.

The symptomatology of cerebral cysticercosis is characterized by three basic syndromes: convulsions, intracranial hypertension, and psychiatric disorders, occurring separately or in combination [*14*].

Convulsions may be focal (jacksonian type of epilepsy) or generalized, sporadic, or leading to status epilepticus, with a slow onset and steady progress or with sudden episodes at monthly or yearly intervals. Convulsions are common with a cortical localization of cysticerci. Intensive infections often cause convulsions plus mental disturbances. Cysticercosis is one of the most frequent causes of epilepsy in the tropics. Among adult Bantu people with epilepsy 15 percent had cerebral cysticercosis. Epilepsy due to cysticercosis frequently causes severe accidental burning, as observed in the Kapadoku people of Indonesia [*18*].

The syndrome of intracranial hypertension is manifested by vomiting, violent headache, and visual disturbances of an intermittent nature or, more frequently, steadily deteriorating. Intracranial hypertension occurs mostly in racemose cysticercosis or with intraventricular localization of the parasite, but may also develop in intensive brain infections.

Mental disturbances develop quite often either as an isolated syndrome or together with convulsions. The symptoms vary widely from simple hallucinations, slow-mindedness, and emotional disturbances, to mental confusion, apathy, global amnesia, and dementia. The mental disorders may be transient but often develop progressively.

Mixed clinical forms of cerebral cysticercosis are often observed in intensive infections with various localizations of the cysticerci or in advanced meningovascular lesions. Apart from these three main syndromes, various secondary or isolated symptoms and signs such as chiasmatic syndrome, ataxia, dysarthria, neck stiffness, clouding of consciousness, etc., may occur and simulate the most diverse neurological entities [14,17].

In addition to the progressive forms of neurocysticercosis there are common inactive forms such as parenchymal calcifications and hydrocephalus secondary to meningeal fibrosis [19]. The prognosis of cerebral cysticercosis is highly variable and unpredictable [20,21].

Cysticercosis Other Than Cerebral. Experiments in a monkey suggest that *T. solium* cysticerci are more or less uniformly disseminated within the internal organs. In pigs, *T. solium* cysticerci are concentrated in the muscle tissues and myocardium, which have a better blood supply. Autopsy studies in humans have confirmed the presence of *T. solium* cysticerci in many organs, including the spinal cord, eyes, muscle tissues, myocardium, lungs, peritoneal cavity, intestinal submucosa, thyroid glands, and subcutaneous tissues. Cysticercosis in the eyes, subcutaneous tissues, musculature, and spinal cord, in order of decreasing frequency, can be diagnosed by clinical examination.

Ocular cysticercosis constitutes about one-fifth of human neurocysticercosis cases. The most common localization is in the vitreous humor and subretinal tissue, but *T. solium* cysticerci may also invade the anterior chamber, conjunctiva, and other eye tissues. Host reactions to cysticerci vary from slight to severe inflammation with complications such as retinal detachment or atrophy, chorioretinitis, and iridocyclitis (Fig. 56-4).

Spinal cysticercosis constitutes about 5 percent of all cases of neurocysticercosis and is more frequently intramedullar than subarachnoidal. The main symptoms are motor or sensory disorders due to the compression of neural tissue.

Myocardial cysticercosis in humans is not uncommon in intensive infections but seldom causes clinical signs. Similarly, subcutaneous and/or muscle localization of cysticerci is usually of negligible clinical importance. Calcified changes in the muscles are frequently diagnosed purely by chance (Fig. 56-5). Subcutaneous nodules are usually asymptomatic.

Diagnosis of Human Cysticercosis. The final diagnosis of human *T. solium* cysticercosis is made parasitologically by finding a scolex, hooks, or fragments of the bladder walls. Therefore the easiest type to diagnose by biopsy is subcutaneous

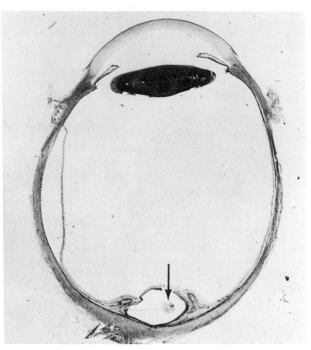

Figure 56-4. Ocular cysticercosis. The cysticercus (arrow) is between the retina and vitreous near the macula. *(From ChH Binford and DH Conner: Pathology of Tropical and Extraordinary Diseases, vol 2, Armed Forces Institute of Pathology, Washington, DC, 1976.)*

cysticercosis. However, a constellation of the clinical symptoms and signs plus x-ray, computed tomography (CT), serological tests, and laboratory examinations, if all positive, enables the diagnosis of neurocysticercosis with a high degree of accuracy. The differential clinical diagnosis with tumor, and vascular and inflammatory conditions (tuberculosis or fungal meningitis), especially in nonendemic areas, may be difficult. Coexistent ocular, subcutaneous, or muscle cysticercosis should always be looked for.

The radiological techniques used in cysticercosis are plain x-ray of the chest, neck, and arms (for calcified cysticerci) (Fig. 56-5) and skull x-ray (for calcifications or signs of intracranial hypertension). Cerebral angiography, pneumoencephalography, and ventriculography have been replaced by computed tomography, which if available is the most convenient and safe technique to identify space-occupying lesions in the internal organs, especially the brain. However, the interpretation of CT scanning may be uneasy; some lesions not visible at CT examination can be demonstrated by contrast-enhanced CT scans or by magnetic resonance imaging [22,23]. In the case of cerebral cysticercosis, examination of the cerebrospinal fluid (CSF) is most important; usually the pressure is low, the CSF clear, the glucose low, the protein level, especially γ-globulin fraction, raised, and there is a marked cellular reaction with a highly significant percentage of plasma

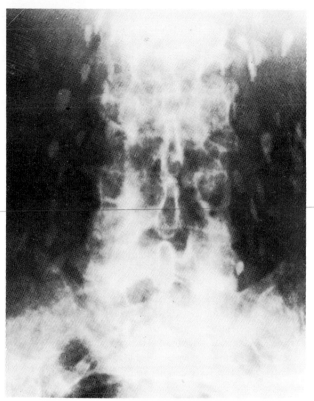

Figure 56-5. Human cysticercosis. X-ray reveals numerous calcified cysticerci. *(From ChH Binford and DH Conner: Pathology of Tropical and Extraordinary Diseases, vol 2, Armed Forces Institute of Pathology, Washington, DC, 1976.)*

cells and eosinophils. Blood eosinophilia is usually present. Also highly significant are certain immunological tests for CSF. The specificity and sensitivity of serological tests vary substantially, depending mainly on the techniques and antigens used. Two species-specific polypeptides which have recently been identified will probably greatly improve the specificity of the immunological tests with serum and CSF [24].

The diagnosis of human cysticercosis in the field causes several problems. Out of 200 adult Bantu tribesmen examined, 20 had *Taenia* eggs in the feces, 25 had positive serological tests, 9 showed x-ray signs of calcified cysticerci, and 4 had palpable subcutaneous cysts [25].

Treatment of Human Cysticercosis. For a long time surgery was the only possible treatment, and it still is necessary in some cases of obstructive hydrocephalus, infection of the IVth ventricle, and spinal and ocular cysticercosis. The introduction of steroids in the late 1950s somewhat reduced the rate of mortality from cysticercosis but often had only a temporary effect. Dexamethasone is indicated in acute parenchymatous forms with cerebral edema. Preliminary studies with metrifonate and albendazole have shown promising results, but so far

the only drug which has had an evident cysticercocidal effect in human patients is praziquantel.

Praziquantel (PZQ) is usually given in a daily dose of 50 mg/kg for 2 weeks [26]. Some clinicians prefer higher doses for a shorter time, e.g., 100 mg/kg for 4 days or 75 mg/kg for 3 to 7 days [27]. The praziquantel level in CSF is close to the level found in protein-free serum fraction and shows some individual variations according to absorption rate, liver first-pass effect, and changes in blood-brain barrier. For that reason it has been suggested that the optimal dose of praziquantel should be adapted individually according to the drug plasma level measured at the beginning of treatment [28]. Dermal cysticercosis usually needs lower doses [29]. In some patients with cysticercosis repetition of praziquantel treatment may be necessary. Steroids are frequently added to praziquantel therapy in order to prevent serious complications due to cerebral edema which may develop as reaction to damaged cysticerci. However, the use of steroids is still controversial because dexamethasone was shown to decrease praziquantel plasma level [30]. After several years of experience in chemotherapy of neurocysticercosis the indications for praziquantel treatment have been elaborated [31]. The majority of patients with parenchymal cysticercosis improves after praziquantel treatment, which is less effective in patients with arachnoiditis and usually not effective in nonactive forms of neurocysticercosis (see above). Treatment of ocular cysticercosis with praziquantel is not recommended as it may induce severe inflammatory and immunomediated reactions in ocular tissue.

POPULATION

Endemic and sporadic occurrence of human infections

While *T. saginata* infection occurs both in highly developed and developing countries, *T. solium* taeniasis and cysticercosis are prevalent in poor communities in which individuals live in close contact with pigs and eat raw pork.

Several factors facilitate the endemic spread of *T. solium* infection: (1) inadequate sanitation, which causes contamination of the human environment with fecal material and *Taenia* eggs; (2) breeding pigs in unsanitary conditions (e.g., deliberately feeding pigs human excrement, keeping pigs outdoors routing freely around human dwellings); (3) eating raw, uninspected pork, frequently on the occasion of a feast or pig slaughter.

When all three factors are present, as is often the case in the poor rural areas where humans and pigs live in proximity, an endemic focus of *T. solium* may easily develop and continue. Such focuses are characterized by a high prevalence of *T. solium* taeniasis and cysticercosis in the local population, heavy contamination of the environment with *Taenia* eggs, and a high prevalence of cysticercosis in pigs. However, the stability of transmission in these focuses is rather weak as is demonstrated by the spontaneous disappearance of *T. solium* infection in many European countries simply through the im-

provement of sanitation in rural areas and changing pig husbandry from an outdoor to an indoor type. On the other hand,
once the infection has been introduced into an area favorable
to it, it may easily develop into an epidemic, as has been the
case, for example, in the West Irian region of Indonesia.

Isolated cases of *T. solium* taeniasis or cysticercosis might
be found a long way from an endemic focus owing to (1)
human migration to and from the focus, (2) the wide spread
of *Taenia* eggs by food, water, or possibly wind, and (3) consumption of uninspected pork distributed from the focus. These
individual cases constitute an epidemiologically and clinically
distinct group (they are often infected with a single cysticercus).

World distribution of *T. solium* taeniasis and cysticercosis

The prevalence of *T. solium* infection varies greatly according
to the regional level of sanitation, the pig husbandry pattern,
and the eating habits. *T. solium* infection is practically nonexistent in Muslim countries.

It is very difficult to evaluate the prevalence of *T. solium*
taeniasis, as the coproscopical methods used for survey are
inadequate and do not differentiate between *T. solium* and
T. saginata infections. The prevalence of human cysticercosis
is in general high in several countries of Central and South
America, central and South Africa, and southeast Asia. The
prevalence of human cerebral cysticercosis in the general population in Latin America is estimated at 0.1 percent and ocular
cysticercosis at 0.025 percent; in human populations in Mexico, Ecuador, and Brazil the prevalence of neurocysticercosis
found by autopsy or biopsy exceeds 1 percent. In the 1970s in
Mexico, cysticercosis constituted 28 percent of all neurological
cases and about 1 percent of all causes of death. In a seroepidemiological survey in Mexico using the immunoelectrophoresis test, 0.45 percent of over 22,000 sera were positive,
which, after correction for false-negative results, means that 1
percent of examined Mexicans have, or have had, cysticercosis
[15]. In Africa both human and pig cysticercosis were reported
as common in the Republic of South Africa (e.g., Transkei
rural areas), Zimbabwe, Gambia, Guinea, Togo, Rwanda, Burundi, Malawi, Swaziland, Madagascar, Reunion, and Zaire.
The use by "witch" doctors of *Taenia* proglottids as a remedy
against some diseases in the Bantu tribes contributes a great
deal to the spread of cysticercosis. In Asia, human cysticercosis is common in northern India, where over 10 percent of
the human population in labor colonies and slums and 8 to 10
percent of pigs were infected with *T. solium,* and in China,
where, e.g., in 1980 in Jilin Province 10 to 20 percent of pigs
had cysticercosis and 1 percent of people had *T. solium* taeniasis [27]. An epidemic of human cysticercosis has been reported among the Kapadoku people in the West Irian region
of Indonesia. Taeniasis and cysticercosis are also common in
some areas of the Philippines, Thailand, Vietnam, Taiwan, and
South Korea. *T. solium* taeniasis and cysticercosis have been
eliminated in most of western and central Europe and are
slowly disappearing from eastern and southern Europe; they
are also rare in the United States. Several cases in Europe and
the United States were diagnosed in immigrants or in people
who had visited endemic areas in other continents.

T. solium taeniasis and cysticercosis are more common in
young adults (20 to 39 years of age); in some areas they are
more prevalent in males and in others more in females, depending on the eating habits.

Prevention and control of *T. solium* infection

The individual prophylaxis of *T. solium* taeniasis is simply to
avoid eating raw, uninspected pork. Prevention of human cysticercosis in individuals in endemically infected areas is more
difficult; the infections may occur despite scrupulous personal
hygiene and eating habits. Cysticercosis is not only fecesborne,
foodborne, and waterborne but is probably also airborne; the
possibility of *T. solium* eggs being spread by the wind has
recently been considered.

In many developed countries the inspection of meat has contributed much to the control of *T. solium* infection at the national level; meat inspection for pig cysticercosis is more effective than that for bovine cysticercosis. However in many
developing countries meat inspection is nonexistent or only
partially effective: for example, in Latin America only 15 percent of the pigs slaughtered are inspected. Trials with vaccination against pig cysticercosis are still at the experimental
stage.

Endemic focuses of *T. solium* taeniasis can easily be detected by the occurrence of cysticercosis in pigs. The control
of infection in such areas is possible by periodic community-
based chemotherapy with taeniacides. Studies in Ecuador demonstrated that low doses of praziquantel have successfully reduced the human reservoir of taeniasis and the incidence of
cysticercosis in pigs [32,33]. Improvement of local sanitation
and changing pig husbandry methods are effective, though
long-term, preventive measures. More emphasis should be
placed on the prevention of the spread to new areas of human
taeniasis and cysticercosis.

DIPHYLLOBOTHRIASIS

PARASITE

Life cycle and ecology

The life cycle and ecology of *Diphyllobothrium latum,* which
belongs to the order Pseudophyllidea, differ greatly from those
of other tapeworms invading human beings. Its larval stages
develop in water and in two intermediate hosts, i.e., freshwater
crustaceans and fish. About 1 million eggs are excreted every
day from mature proglottids into the intestinal lumen and feces.
The eggs are oval and measure approximately 65 by 45 μm;
the thin, yellowish shell has an operculum at one end and a

small knob at the other; inside the shell several yolk cells surround one zygote. The eggs need at least 12 days to embryonate. Under the effects of illumination (50 to 100 lx for 30 to 60 s) the first larval stage—coracidium—hatches through the opening left by the operculum. The coracidium, a ciliated oncosphere, 50 μm in diameter, dies within a few days if not swallowed by a specific freshwater copepod (*Diaptomus* spp., *Cyclops* spp.). It penetrates the body cavity of the copepod and within 2 to 3 weeks develops into an elongated, solid larva procercoid. The procercoid, about 500 μm long, when ingested by a fish penetrates into the muscles or viscera and within 4 weeks is then transformed into a plerocercoid. The plerocercoid has an elongated, wrinkled, and chalky body about 5 to 6 mm long and 1 mm wide, with an invaginated anterior portion. When a plankton-eating fish (Cyprinidae) is eaten by a carnivorous fish (pike, burbot, perch, ruff, and less frequently char, trout, or salmon entering fresh water for spawning) plerocercoids can penetrate and parasitize in the muscles and viscera of their new transport hosts. They can also develop in the tissues of some reptiles.

The ecological requirements of the developing larvae (water rich in oxygen, 8 to 12 mg of oxygen per liter, with a temperature below 22°C and a saline concentration of less than 0.9 percent) as well as the presence of the specific copepods put several limitations on the geographical distribution of the natural focuses of *D. latum*. They occur in shallow, brackish water full of vegetation, littoral marshes and deltas, slow-flowing rivers and inland lakes, as well as in water-power reservoirs situated in temperate and subarctic regions or in mountainous areas.

Morphology and biology of adult

D. latum is the longest tapeworm and may reach up to 25 m. It has an elongated scolex (2 to 3 mm long), with two sucking grooves, an unsegmented neck, and 3000 to 4000 proglottids. The proglottids are somewhat wider (up to 15 mm) than they are long, gray with a darker rosettelike spot in the center corresponding to the uterus filled with eggs. Most of the strobila consists of the mature proglottids, which periodically expel eggs through the uterine pore. The distal proglottids usually disintegrate; only occasionally does part of the strobila become detached and get evacuated with feces.

Single or multiple tapeworms parasitize the small intestine in humans; the greatest number ever recorded in a human being was 201 tapeworms (multiple tapeworms are usually much shorter). *D. latum* has enormous growth and reproductive potentials. The tapeworm grows about 5 cm/day and starts to produce eggs as early as 25 to 30 days after ingestion of the plerocercoid. In humans, *D. latum* can live for up to 40 years; in dogs, usually for less than 2 years.

The physiology and biochemistry of this parasite is relatively well studied, as it can be kept in several types of laboratory animal (e.g., hamsters, cats, and dogs). The surface of the *D. latum* integument is densely covered with microtrichia about 4 μm in length; they take nourishment from the host intestine. The integument itself, rich in mitochondria, is very active metabolically. The flame cells system controls the excretory and osmoregulatory functions. Most of the activities of the neck and proximal proglottids are aimed toward linear growth, the segmentation process, and building up the reproductive systems, which take up most of the space within each mature proglottid. The daily production of eggs from a single tapeworm is about 1 million.

Both plerocercoids and the adult tapeworms have a remarkable capacity to adapt. The plerocercoid withstands with relative ease the changes between the fish tissues (low temperature, low electrolyte concentration) and the intestinal tract of the mammals. *D. latum* plerocercoids and adult worms are less host-specific than, for example, members of the family Taeniidae; apart from pigs, dogs, and cats, over 20 species of wild fish-eating animals have been found to serve as the definitive host, e.g., foxes, wolves, minks, bears, walruses, seals, and sea lions. In nature the life cycle of *D. latum* can be maintained without a human host being involved; however, the longevity and high rate of reproductivity of the adult parasite in humans suggest that a human being is the most natural definitive host for *D. latum*.

PATIENT

Intestinal infection

Intestinal diphyllobothriasis is most frequent in adults, but it has been reported also in a 2-month-old child and in a 100-year-old man. It is a long-lasting infection which may continue for up to 40 years. The parasite is usually located in the lower jejunum or upper ileum [*34*].

In a well-controlled study in Finland, the following symptoms were found in 295 nonanemic *D. latum* carriers: fatigue and weakness (occurring in 66 percent of the carriers), craving for salt (62 percent), dizziness (53 percent), numbness of extremities (49 percent), and diarrhea (22 percent) [*35*]. The pathogenesis of these symptoms remains unclear; the possible mechanisms are response to mechanical or toxic irritation, allergic reactions, and nutrient deficiency. It is interesting to note that the lysolecithin which is transformed from lecithin released from the disintegrating strobila has a marked membrane toxicity; a hypersensitivity to lysolecithin has been observed in *D. latum*–infected patients [*35*].

The intestinal infection occasionally causes acute abdominal symptoms with vomiting and spastic abdominal pain. Intestinal obstruction, with or without perforation, and cholangitis or cholecystitis caused by migration of the proglottids may occur but are less common than in *T. saginata* taeniasis.

Diphyllobothrium pernicious anemia (DPA)

Diphyllobothrium pernicious anemia is the major, though not the only, manifestation of the general deficiency of vitamin

B$_{12}$ (cobalamin). On the other hand, the cobalamin deficiency is not the only one observed in diphyllobothriasis; impaired folate absorption and a lower serum level of ascorbic acid have also been described.

DPA usually develops in people over 40 of both sexes once the tissue stores have been depleted, i.e., 3 to 4 years after infection with *D. latum,* and is caused by an extensive absorption of vitamin B$_{12}$ by the adult worm as well as by interference with the absorption of cobalamins from the host intestine. The vitamin B$_{12}$ content in the adult tapeworm is constant and rather high, with a mean of 2.3 μg per gram of dry substance. DPA is manifest in only 2 percent of infected carriers in Finland [34] and even less than 2 percent in other parts of the world. The factors predisposing to DPA are inadequate supply of vitamin B$_{12}$ in the diet, intrinsic factor deficiency due to changes in the gastric mucosa, increased requirements for vitamin B$_{12}$, and, probably most important of all, multiple infection and the proximal localization of the tapeworm in the human intestine [36].

The diagnosis of DPA is based on (1) the presence of macrocytic, megaloblastic anemia with leukopenia, thrombocytopenia, and increased hemolysis; (2) the symptoms and signs of a subacute degeneration of the spinal cord and the peripheral nerves (paresthesia, impairment of the deep sensibility, disturbances of motility and coordination); (3) B$_{12}$ serum level below 100 pg/mL, which may, however, not be proportional to the degree of anemia. The mean level of vitamin B$_{12}$ in the sera of the control patients was 273.8 pg/100 mL, whereas in 366 *D. latum* carriers it was only 116.4 pg/100 mL; in 51.6 percent of the carriers it was less than 100 pg/mL; megaloblastic anemia was found in eight patients (1.9 percent).

Clinically, DPA is frequently accompanied by fever, glossitis, hemorrhage, edema due to hypoalbuminemia, and hemolytic jaundice of varying degrees of intensity. In DPA, the gastric secretion contains the intrinsic factor and often also free hydrochloric acid; this differentiates DPA from genuine pernicious anemia.

The course of DPA is frequently remittent [35]. Liver extracts, folic acid, and vitamin B$_{12}$ injections effectively promote a remission even without expulsion of the parasite.

Laboratory diagnosis

The laboratory diagnosis of *D. latum* infection by coproscopical examination is relatively easy because of the large number of characteristic eggs present in the feces. On the contrary, in 30 percent of the cases the proglottids escape detection, as they easily disintegrate in the human intestine. Other species of *Diphyllobothrium* parasitizing humans, usually smaller and less productive ones, may create some diagnostic problems. Eosinophilia, if it does occur in diphyllobothriasis, is usually moderate.

Treatment

In general, *D. latum* can easily be expelled by any taeniacide or taeniafuge. The drug of choice is praziquantel in a single dose of 25 mg/kg or niclosamide in a single dose of 2.0 g for adult patients. The proof of a successful cure is the expulsion of the tapeworm (or tapeworms) with the scolex or, better still, negative results from coproscopical examinations repeated once a week for 3 weeks, starting in the second month after the therapy has finished.

POPULATION

World distribution and prevalence

There are three main factors determining the endemicity of human diphyllobothriasis: ecology, human dietary habits, and improper disposal of human feces. The ecological factors (see "Life Cycle and Ecology") limit the occurrence of endemic focuses of *D. latum* mainly to the subarctic or temperate regions of the Eurasian continent. The oldest and largest endemic areas are found among the indigenous populations living close to water in Finland, northern areas of the U.S.S.R. (from the Kola Peninsula in the west to the Yenisey River in the east, and around the Volga River), Canada, and Alaska. In smaller endemic areas once reported in Romania (the Danube delta), Switzerland, and northern Italy (near the major alpine lakes), and in the United States (the Great Lakes), the infection seems to be in a state of extinction. The infection has become established in Uganda, in Chile, and in Japan (Hokkaido Island). In many other regions, sporadic cases have been reported either imported from other areas or acquired from the existing natural focuses of the infection. Human migration (as well as fish migration) plays an important role in the spread of diphyllobothriasis.

In 1973 approximately 9 million cases of *D. latum* infection in human beings were estimated: 5 million in Europe, 4 million in Asia, less than 0.1 million in North America and Africa. Now the number is probably much lower because of the various control campaigns undertaken in Finland and in some areas of the U.S.S.R. For example, the prevalence of diphyllobothriasis in Finland in the late 1970s was about one-tenth that of what it was in the 1950s [37]. On the other hand, new focuses of the infection are still reported, though only some are well documented.

Prevention and control of diphyllobothriasis

The best individual prophylaxis is to avoid eating raw or semiraw fish, salted hard roe, and fish livers originating from the endemic areas. Individual and community education and the imposing of adequate requirements for fish marketing are important measures. The plerocercoids can easily be killed by heating (above 54°C for only 5 minutes) or by freezing—for example, a fish weighing more than 5 kg should be frozen at −18°C for 24 h.

Early diagnosis and treatment of infected individuals and/or certain target groups (e.g., fishermen and their families) are essential control measures because of the chronicity of the infection. Human beings cannot have much influence on the transmission of *D. latum* in nature or on the reservoirs of infection in wild animals, but where human diphyllobothriasis is common, proper treatment of the sewage is important. Substances toxic for copepods can be periodically scattered around sewage outlets and landing stages as these may play a significant role in spreading the infection [*38*].

OTHER PSEUDOPHILLIDEA IN HUMANS

The genus *Diphyllobothrium* represents about 70 different species, some of them with an uncertain taxonomic position and unknown life cycle. The lack of species-characteristic morphological structures in the adult tapeworm creates several taxonomic problems [*39*]. Human beings have been reported to be parasitized by 12 species of *Diphyllobothrium*, 2 species of *Diploglonoporus*, and *Schistocephalus solidus* [*34,40*]. Among them *D. pacificum* is relatively common in Peru [*41*] and Chile. Seals are the main definitive hosts for *D. pacificum*. The adult *D. pacificum* is shorter than *D. latum*, being under 2 m in length; the uterus in the mature proglottids never forms a rosette; the *D. pacificum* eggs are also smaller (50 to 60 by 36 to 40 μm). Many intestinal infections are asymptomatic; pernicious anemia has not been reported in people infected with *D. pacificum*.

Humans can also be infected by the plerocercoid larva (*Sparganum*) of a diphyllobothrid tapeworm of the genus *Spirometra*, e.g., *S. mansoni* in the United States and the Far East and *S. mansonoides* in the United States and South America. The procercoids of *Spirometra* develop in copepods living in small ponds; the plerocercoids are found in amphibians, reptiles, and mammals. The adult tapeworms parasitize domestic cats and some wild carnivores in tropical and subtropical regions of America, Africa, Asia, and Australia. Many vertebrates, including humans, may serve as a paratenic host for the plerocercoids.

Humans can develop sparganosis by drinking water contaminated with an infected *Cyclops* (North America, east Africa), by putting the flesh of an infected frog on ulcers or on the eyes in order to heal them (Far East), or by eating the meat of infected snakes, birds, and mammals; in the latter two cases, plerocercoids are the infective stages and migrate to the human subcutaneous tissue, upper eyelids, or intestinal submucosa. A fibrous nodule about 2 cm in diameter is formed around the encysted plerocercoid; the latter has a typical diphyllobothrid scolex and a ribbonlike body several centimeters long. A differential diagnosis with dracunculosis should be made in the case of subcutaneous sparganosis. Ocular sparganosis may cause severe eye damage, especially during retrobulbar invasion. Surgery is the usual treatment for localized sparganosis. Sometimes the plerocercoid proliferates by lateral budding into the surrounding tissue and forms what is described as *Sparganum proliferum*. By producing metastases, the parasite larva can also invade the internal organs, including the brain, and cause a proliferative sparganosis. An attempt to treat this with mebendazole and praziquantel has been made [*42*].

HYMENOLEPIASIS

PARASITE

Taxonomy and life cycle

Hymenolepis nana, the dwarf tapeworm, is the only cestode parasitizing humans which does not require an intermediate host. Its present homoxeny has been acquired secondarily and the former diheteroxeny has become facultative as it can use insects as intermediate hosts in a similar way as does one of its subspecies—*H. nana* var. *fraterna*. *H. nana* var. *fraterna*, morphologically identical to *H. nana*, is a common parasite of rats and mice and uses fleas or beetles as an intermediate host. Although the infectivity of *H. nana* and *H. nana* var. *fraterna* is evidently higher in their typical hosts, a human being can sometimes be infected with the rodent subspecies or by *H. nana* which has developed in insects.

The eggs of *H. nana* leave the macerated gravid proglottids in the human ileum, by which time the oncosphere inside the eggs is already developed and invasive to the same or other hosts.

Autoinfection is a characteristic of hymenolepiasis: *H. nana* eggs, oncospheres, and the youngest tapeworm stages have been found in the ileum contents of an infected patient, confirming that internal autoinfection is possible; external self-infection from hands contaminated by eggs discharged with feces is common in children. *H. nana* eggs, 30 to 47 μm in diameter, have a delicate embryophore and cannot survive in an external environment for more than 10 days. When an egg is ingested the oncosphere is liberated in the small intestine and invades the villus, using its hooks and digestive secretions. After 4 days, a larva cysticercoid, 250 μm in diameter with one scolex, is developed. The cysticercoid is liberated by the rupture of the distended villus and the evaginated scolex attaches itself to the ileal mucosa. The tapeworm needs 10 to 12 days to mature and another 2 weeks to produce eggs. The life span of the adult *H. nana* has been estimated at 1 to 2½ months, but the simplicity of autoinfection keeps the infection, sometimes involving thousands of worms, going for several years.

Morphology of adult

H. nana is the smallest tapeworm parasitizing humans; it is 15 to 40 mm long and 0.5 to 1.0 mm wide. The scolex has four suckers and a retractable rostellum with a single row of 20 to 30 hooks. Behind a rather long neck there are about 200 proglottids, wide but short. In the mature proglottid there are three testes, one ovary, a vitelline gland, and a tubelike uterus. In the gravid proglottid, only the saclike uterus filled with 80 to 200 eggs is visible (Fig. 56-6).

H. nana var. *fraterna*, a common tapeworm in laboratory rodents, has been the object of many biochemical and immunological studies. The biochemical studies have little direct relation to the medical aspects of the infection.

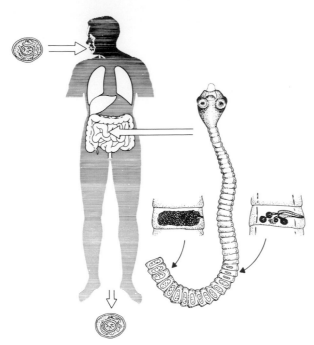

Figure 56-6. Life cycle of *H. nana.*

PATIENT

Immunology of *H. nana* infection

The immunological studies have shown that some degree of immunity against different stages of *H. nana* develops within a few weeks. It regulates the intensity of the parasite population, being almost fully protective. In laboratory mice there are two types of adult *H. nana:* that of long-term and that of short-term maturity; the latter are smaller, produce and release their eggs earlier, and are more likely to be expelled. The worm expulsion is a thymus-dependent phenomenon.

Little is known about a human being's immunity to hymenolepiasis. In many human cases, *H. nana* infection is spontaneously cured but can be acquired again later. In a study in the Punjab, 93 children were examined for hymenolepiasis 10 times within a 22-month period; 26 percent were positive all the time, 34 percent remained consistently negative, but as many as 39 percent either gained or lost the infection during the study period. The minimum length of time between infections was 7 months, and the average was 10 months. Very few studies have been made in regard to the factors which make hymenolepiasis an intensive and/or protracted infection.

In the ileum of mice deprived of T cells by preadult thymectomy and administration of anti-mouse thymocyte serum, thousands of adult worms and cysticerci can develop. The majority of the cysticerci do not contain scolices and are ballooned out by a large amount of fluid up to a size of 2 mm. Several cysts, similar to these cysticerci, have also been found in the lungs, mesenteric lymph nodes, and liver of immunosuppressed mice. An increasing number of human cases of dis-

seminated hymenolepiasis is reported in patients with Hodgkin's disease or severe malnutrition or in those treated with steroids [43]. Hymenolepiasis might be another opportunistic infection in humans, similar to, for example, strongyloidiasis.

Clinical pathology of the infection

Pathological changes due to hymenolepiasis greatly depend on the intensity of the infection, which in turn is regulated by the immune status of the host or by concomitant diseases. Intensive hymenolepiasis is common in immune-deficient and undernourished children, which makes it difficult to make an objective evaluation of the clinical pathology and symptomatology. Undoubtedly *H. nana* cysticercoids destroy the villi in the ileum and the growing or adult tapeworms do some mechanical damage to the mucosa.

Of interest are some of the findings on the intestinal functional disorders occurring in hymenolepiasis: protein losses from the small intestine, disturbances in protein digestion and absorption, and increased activity of intestinal enterokinase and phospholipase. The peroxidation of erythrocytic membranes has been found to increase in proportion to the duration and severity of the infection [44].

Some of the general symptoms ascribed to hymenolepiasis, such as pallor, weakness, and cephalalgia, were interpreted as being the result of a toxic or allergic action of *H. nana,* based only on the frequent association of these symptoms with the infection. It was found in Egypt that phlyctenular keratoconjunctivitis, which is known to be an allergic response of the corneal and conjunctival epithelium to the endogenous toxin, is strongly associated with hymenolepiasis; 57.4 percent of children with eye disease and 73.4 percent of those with multiple or recurrent phlyctens were infected with *H. nana,* whereas only 10.8 percent of the control children had hymenolepiasis [45]. The general and/or other than intestinal symptoms and signs in hymenolepiasis merit more attention and objective evaluation.

Symptomatology

The symptomatology of hymenolepiasis much depends on the intensity and longevity of the infection. It has been suggested that in the first year the infection is mainly subclinical, between 1 and 5 years there are usually some intestinal symptoms, and after 5 years the general symptoms, such as loss of weight and weakness, develop [46]. The infections with more than 3000 parasites were shown to be symptomatic, whereas those with less than 1000 may only have loose stools [47]. Symptoms which have been considered to be statistically significant are anorexia, cephalalgia, diarrhea, abdominal pain, and pallor. There is no clearcut understanding of the possible mechanisms involved.

Diagnosis

The diagnosis of *H. nana* infection is possible only by coproscopical examination. Light infections are better detected by flotation techniques, i.e., the Faust zinc-sulfate technique.

Because the egg output may be irregular a repeated examination is often needed. The eggs of *H. nana* are very fragile; they can easily be destroyed by pressure and desiccation, and disappear quickly in Kato thick smears.

Treatment

The treatment of hymenolepiasis was difficult until therapy with niclosamide was introduced in 1962. A dose of 60 to 80 mg/kg, with a maximum of 2 g daily, given for 5 to 7 days, is well tolerated and cures 90 percent of all infections. Treatment with praziquantel is even more effective and much simpler as it needs only a single dose of 25 mg/kg. Whether they are treated with praziquantel or niclosamide, heavy infections may require a repetition of the course after 10 days.

Follow-up fecal examinations, preferably by using the flotation technique, are suggested every second week for at least 3 months after treatment, as *H. nana* infections have shown a tendency to later recurrence. Contemporaneous treatment of all infected family members and institution inmates greatly diminishes the risk of reinfection from external sources.

POPULATION

Prevalence of hymenolepiasis

H. nana infection is the most common of all cestodiases. Its global prevalence has been calculated as between 45 and 50 million people, with two-thirds of those infected living in Asia. Hymenolepiasis is endemic in many tropical and subtropical countries; in those countries with an arid climate, where the spread of soil-transmitted helminthiases is limited, hymenolepiasis may be one of the most common intestinal parasitoses (Iran, Western Australia). In countries with a temperate climate hymenolepiasis is uncommon, but may occur epidemically in children and in mental institutions. In the Punjab, 26 percent of villagers were found to be infected with *H. nana*. In Tehran, 20.4 percent of kindergarten children were found to be infected; in Khuzestan (southwest Iran) the prevalence among the rural population was 9 percent and among the urban population 13 percent. Among 2431 outpatients in Ta'izz (Yemen) 13 percent had hymenolepiasis. A similar prevalence has been reported in children in Egypt and Zimbabwe. The infection rate in the aborigine population of Western Australia is 20.4 percent. The prevalence of *H. nana* infections was reported to be as high as 14 percent in some regions of Mexico; hymenolepiasis is also common in Peru, Chile, Colombia, and Brazil.

In developed countries with a temperate climate, individual cases of hymenolepiasis are reported occasionally, but several epidemic outbreaks have been described in orphanages and mental institutions [48].

Prevention and control of *H. nana* infections

Several epidemiological observations (epidemic outbreaks, family agglomerations) suggest that hymenolepiasis is easily transmitted from person to person. Since *H. nana* eggs are unable to survive for long in the environment, a more direct spread is probably by dirty hands or contaminated food. For example, in arid areas, where hymenolepiasis is most prevalent, it is a common practice among children to use hands and dirt to clean the perianal area following defecation.

Improved sanitation alone can effectively limit the endemic spread of hymenolepiasis, but epidemics can be better controlled by the use of mass chemotherapy. Several examples of successful control of hymenolepiasis in child institutions have been reported.

OTHER INTESTINAL CESTODIASES

Human beings can also occasionally be infected with several other species of cestodes which are natural parasites of animals. For example, infection from *Dipylidium caninum*, which is common in dogs and cats throughout the world, can be acquired by ingesting fleas containing *D. caninum* cysticercoids. Several hundred cases, mainly in children, have been reported. *Hymenolepis diminuta*, common in rodents, is also acquired by ingesting infected fleas or beetles. Human infections are not uncommon in poor communities plagued by rodents (Iran, Papua, New Guinea). Several species of *Raillietina*, a cestode infecting rats, have been reported in humans in southeast Asia and in South America. Another tapeworm common in rodents, *Inermicapsifer madagascariensis*, can infect humans in Africa as well as in Central and South America.

In Cuba and South America, sporadic human infections with *Bertiella studeri*, a tapeworm parasitizing monkeys, have been reported. A few human cases of *Mesocestoides variabilis*, a natural parasite of some carnivores, have been described from the United States, Rwanda, and Japan. Most of these intestinal cestodiases are benign and easily cured by praziquantel or niclosamide.

REFERENCES

1 Gemmel M, Matyas Z, Pawlowski ZS, et al. (eds): Guidelines for surveillance, prevention and control of taeniasis/cysticercosis. WHO, Geneva, 1983

2 Prevention and control of intestinal parasitic infections. Techn Rep Ser no 749, WHO, Geneva, 1987

3 Fan PC, Chung WC, Chan CH, et al: Studies on taeniasis in Taiwan. III. Preliminary report on experimental infections of Taiwan *Taenia* in domestic animals. Proceedings of the First Sino-American Symposium on Biotechnology and Parasitic Diseases, Taipei, Taiwan, Sept. 30–Oct. 4, 1985, vol 1, pp 119–125, 1987

4 Gemmell MA, Johnstone PD: Experimental epidemiology of hydatidosis and cysticercosis. Adv Parasitol 15:311–369, 1977

5 Pawlowski ZS, Schultz MG: Taeniasis and cysticercosis (*Taenia saginata*). Adv Parasitol 10:270–343, 1972

6 Kociecka W: Intestinal cestode infections, in Pawlowski Z (ed): *Intestinal Helminthic Infections*. Baillière Clinical Tropical Medicine and Communicable Diseases, 1987

7 Verster A: Redescription of *Taenia solium* Linnaeus, 1758 and *Taenia saginata* Goeze, 1782. Z. Parasitenkd 29:313–328, 1967

8 Groll E: Praziquantel for cestode infections in man. Acta Trop 37: 293–296, 1980

9 Gemmell M: A critical approach to the concept of control and eradication of echinococcosis/hydatidosis and taeniasis/cysticercosis, in Howell MJ (ed): *Parasitology—Quo vadit?* Proceedings of the Sixth International Congress of Parasitology, Canberra, Australian Academy of Sciences, pp 465–472, 1986

10 Pawlowski ZS: Epidemiology and prevention of *Taenia saginata* infection, in Flisser A et al (eds): *Cysticercosis: Present State of Knowledge and Perspectives.* New York, Academic, 1982, pp 69–85

11 Rickard MD, Arundel JH, Adolph AJ: A preliminary field trial to evaluate the use of immunisation for the control of naturally acquired *Taenia saginata* infection in cattle. Res Vet Sci 30:104–108, 1981

12 Jelenova I: Effects of fertilizers on eggs of *Taenia saginata* Goeze, 1782 under field conditions. Folia Parasitol (Praha) 28:285–287, 1981

13 Slais J: *The Morphology and Pathogenicity of the Bladder Worms:* Cysticercus cellulosae *and* Cysticercus bovis. Prague, Academia, 1970

14 Trelles JO, Trelles L: Cysticercosis of the nervous system, in Vinkin PJ et al (eds): *Infections of the Nervous System, Part III.* Amsterdam, North-Holland, 1978, pp 291–320

15 Flisser A: The immunology of human cysticercosis, in Larralde C et al (eds): *Molecules, Cells and Parasites in Immunology.* New York, Academic, 1980

16 Willms K, Merchant MT, Arcos L, et al: Immunopathology of cysticercosis, in Larralde C et al (eds): *Molecules, Cells and Parasites in Immunology.* New York, Academic, 1980

17 de Villiers JC: Cysticercosis of the nervous system. S Afr Med J 63:769–772, 1983

18 Subianto DB, Tumada LR, Margono SS: Burns and epileptic fits associated with cysticercosis in mountain people of Irian Jaya. Trop Geogr Med 30:275–278, 1978

19 Sotelo J, Marin C: Hydrocephalus secondary to cysticercotic arachnoiditis. A long-term follow-up review of 92 cases. J Neurosurg 66:686–689, 1987

20 Estanol B, Corona T, Abad P: A prognostic classification of cerebral cysticercosis: therapeutic implications. J Neurol Neurosurg Psychiatry 49:1131–1134, 1986

21 McCormick GF: Cysticercosis—review of 230 patients. Bull Clin Neurosci 50:76–101, 1985

22 Rodiek SO, Rupp N, von Einsiedel HG: MR and CT patterns of neurocysticercosis. ROFO 146:570–577, 1987

23 Suss RA, Maravilla KR, Thompson J: MR imaging of intracranial cysticercosis: comparison with CT and anatomopathologic features. AJNR 7:235–242, 1986

24 Gottstein B, Tsang VCW, Schantz PM: Demonstration of species-specific and cross-reactive components of *Taenia solium* metacestode antigens. Am J Trop Med Hyg 35:308–313, 1986

25 Heinz HJ, Klintworth GK: Cysticercosis in the aetiology of epilepsy. S Afr J Med Sci 30:32–36, 1965

26 Groll E: Chemotherapy of human cysticercosis with praziquantel, in Flisser A et al (eds): *Cysticercosis: Present State of Knowledge and Perspectives.* New York, Academic, 1982, pp 207–218

27 Jing JS, Wang PY: (Advance of studies on cysticercosis of man and pigs at home and abroad in recent years) (in Chinese). Chinese J Vet Sci Techn 6:33–36, 1985

28 Spina-Franca A, Machado LR, Nobrega JP, et al: Praziquantel in the cerebrospinal fluid in neurocysticercosis. Arq Neuropsiquiatr 43:243–259, 1985

29 Rim HJ, Won CR, Chu JW: Studies on the human cysticercosis

and its therapeutic trials with praziquantel (Embay 8440). Korea Univ Med J 17:459–472, 1980

30 Vazquez ML, Jung H, Sotelo J: Plasma levels of praziquantel decrease when dexamethasone is given simultaneously. Neurology 37:1561–1562, 1987

31 Vasconcelos D, Cruz-Segura H, Mateos-Gomez H, et al: Selective indications for the use of praziquantel in the treatment of brain cysticercosis. J Neurol Neurosurg Psychiatry 50:383–388, 1987

32 Cruz M, Davis A, Dixon H, et al: Operational studies on control of *Taenia solium* taeniasis/cysticercosis in Ecuador. Bull WHO (in press)

33 Pawlowski ZS: Large-scale use of chemotherapy of taeniasis as a control measure for *Taenia solium* infections, in Geerts S, Kumar V, Brandt J (eds): *Helminth Zoonoses.* Dordrecht, Martius Nijhoff, 1987, pp 100–105

34 Von Bonsdorff B: *Diphyllobothriasis in man.* London, Academic, 1977

35 Totterman G: On the pathogenesis of pernicious tapeworm anaemia. Ann Clin Res 8(suppl.18):7–48, 1976

36 Von Bonsdorff B, Gordin R: Castle's test (with vitamin B_{12} and normal gastric juice) in the ileum in patients with genuine and patients with tapeworm pernicious anaemia. Acta Med Scand 208:193–197, 1980

37 Von Bonsdorff B: The broad tapeworm story. Acta Med Scand 204:241–247, 1978

38 Razumova EP, Mikhailenko IYa: (Significance of landing stages in the spread of diphyllobothriasis in navigable waters) (in Russian). Med Parazitol (Mosk) 41(1):90–94, 1972

39 Vik R: The genus *Diphyllobothrium.* An example of the interdependence of systematics and experimental biology. Exp Parasitol 15:361–380, 1964

40 Rausch RL, Scott EM, Rausch VR: Helminths in Eskimos in Western Alaska with particular reference to *Diphyllobothrium* infection and anaemia. Trans R Soc Trop Med 61:351–357, 1967

41 Lumbreras H, Terashima A, Alvarez H, et al: Single dose treatment with praziquantel (Cesol R, EmBay 8440) of human cestodiasis caused by *Diphyllobothrium pacificum.* Tropenmed Parasitol 33:5–7, 1982

42 Torres JR, Noya OO, Noya BA, et al: Treatment of proliferative sparganosis with mebendazole and praziquantel. Trans R Soc Trop Med Hyg 75:846–847, 1981

43 Gamal-Eddin FM, Aboul-Atta AM, Hassounah OA: Extraintestinal nana cysticercoidiasis in asthmatic and filarised Egyptian patients. J Egypt Soc Parasitol 16:517–520, 1986

44 Kartasheva LD, Prokofieva MS, Lysakova LA, et al: (The functional activity of the gastrointestinal tract and the intensity of peroxidation of erythrocyte lipids in hymenolepidosis) (in Russian). Med Parazitol (Mosk) 49:32–37, 1980

45 Al-Hussaini MK, Khalifa R, Al-Ansary ATA, et al: Phlyctenular eye disease in association with *Hymenolepis nana* in Egypt. Br J Ophthalmol 63:627–631, 1979

46 Astafiev BA: (Results and prospects of the investigation of the pathogenesis, clinical course, treatment and organization of hymenolepidosis control) (in Russian). Med Parazitol (Mosk) 47(2):65–72, 1978

47 Chitchang S, Piamjinda T, Yodmanik B, et al: Relationship between severity of the symptom and the number of *Hymenolepis nana* after treatment. J Med Ass Thai 68:424–426, 1985

48 Plotkowiak J: Probleme der Hymenolepidose, hervorgerufen durch *Hymenolepis nana* im Bezirk Szczecin. Angew Parasitol 11:213–217, 1970

Echinococcosis (Hydatidosis)

· *Peter M. Schantz* · *G. B. A. Okelo*

Echinococcosis (hydatidosis) is a zoonotic infection caused by cestodes of the genus *Echinococcus* (Rudolphi, 1801). The parasites' definitive hosts are carnivores in whose intestines the adult-stage tapeworms occur. The larval stages proliferate by asexual budding in various mammalian intermediate hosts. The larval or metacestode forms are referred to as hydatid cysts and the diseases caused by them as hydatidosis or hydatid disease. Humans and intermediate hosts become infected by ingesting eggs passed in the feces of definitive hosts, whereas definitive hosts become infected by ingesting hydatid cysts in the organs of intermediate hosts. At present, four species are recognized: *Echinococcus granulosus* (Batsch, 1786), *Echinococcus multilocularis* Leuckart, 1862, *Echinococcus oligarthrus* (Diesing, 1862), and *Echinococcus vogeli* Rausch and Bernstein, 1972. *E. granulosus,* the cause of cystic hydatid disease, occurs worldwide and is of considerable public health and economic importance in some countries. *E. multilocularis* and *E. vogeli* cause the alveolar and polycystic forms of hydatid disease, respectively. *E. oligarthrus* has rarely caused disease in humans.

PARASITE

MORPHOLOGY AND DEVELOPMENT

Echinococcus spp. have three developmental stages. In sequence, they are (1) the oncosphere or true larva contained within the egg produced by the adult tapeworm, (2) the metacestode or hydatid cyst that, when fully developed, contains numerous protoscolices, and (3) the sexually mature adult.

Ovoid eggs (diameter 30 to 36 μm) containing single, fully differentiated oncospheres are shed with the feces of infected definitive hosts. When the eggs are ingested by a suitable intermediate host, digestive processes and other factors in the host's gut cause hatching and release of activated oncospheres. After penetration of the intestinal mucosa, oncospheres enter venous and lymphatic vessels and are distributed passively to other anatomic sites. Most larvae develop in the liver, but some may reach the lungs, and a few develop in the kidney, spleen, central nervous system, or other organs (Fig. 57-1).

Postoncospheral development involves degeneration of the oncospheral tissue, vesiculation, and production of protoscolices. Mechanisms of metacestode growth, asexual reproduction, and proliferation in tissues of the host are unique for each species of *Echinococcus* [1].

In its intermediate host the cyst of *E. granulosus* grows by concentric enlargement. The fully developed hydatid cyst is fluid-filled and typically unilocular; however, multilocular, or chambered, cysts may be found in sheep and some other hosts. Structurally, the cyst consists of an inner germinal layer of cells supported by an acellular "laminated" membrane of mu-

copolysaccharide material (Fig. 57-2). Together, these two membranes are referred to as the endocyst. Ultrastructural studies have described modifications of the membranous wall conducive to absorption and transport of nutritive substances into the cyst: cytoplasm of germinative cells unite to form a syncytium with microvillous extensions that project peripherally into the laminated layer toward the host tissues surrounding the cyst. Small secondary cysts, called *brood capsules,* develop internally from the germinal layer and produce multiple protoscolices by asexual budding. The protoscolex consists of a scolex invaginated into a small forebody (approximately 100 μm diameter), which is attached by a peduncle to the germinal membrane of the brood capsule. Protoscolices of *Echinococcus* spp. have the dual potential to develop into adult tapeworms within the gut of the definitive host or, by vesiculization, to differentiate into secondary hydatid cysts within the intermediate host when released after cyst rupture. Surrounding the cyst is a connective tissue adventitial reaction of variable intensity often referred to as the *ectocyst.* Hydatid cysts increase in diameter from 1 to 5 cm per year; protoscolex formation requires more than a year in sheep. In humans and other long-lived hosts the cysts may attain a volume of many liters and contain many thousands of protoscolices.

The larval *E. multilocularis* is more complex in structure. The alveolar arrangement of the metacestode is attained by extensions of germinal membrane that invade adjacent host tissues and gradually acquire a covering of laminated membrane; this process forms aggregates of small, contiguous chambers containing brood capsules (Fig. 57-3). In natural rodent hosts, growth of the larva from the single primary vesicle to the compound multivesicular stage with protoscolices

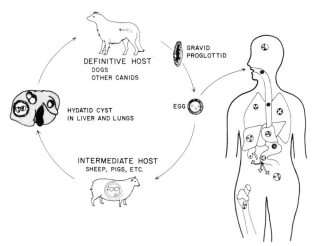

Figure 57-1. *Echinococcus granulosus* schematic life-cycle diagram and mode of infection for humans.

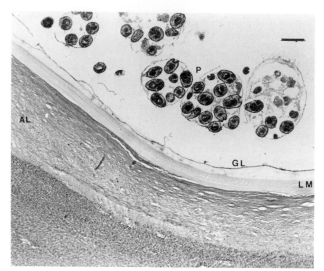

Figure 57-2. Hydatid cyst of *Echinococcus granulosus* in liver of sheep showing protoscolices (P) in brood capsules, germinative layer (GL), laminated membrane (LM), and adventitial layer (AL) or ectocyst. H and E. Bar = 100 μm.

may be completed in 4 to 7 months; the weight of the liver can exceed that of the remainder of the animal by about 50 days after infection.

The larval stage of *E. vogeli* exhibits developmental and structural characteristics considered intermediate between those of *E. granulosus* and *E. multilocularis* [1]. In the liver of the natural rodent host, the larval *E. vogeli* consists of a primary vesicle, within which endogenous proliferation of membranes is characteristic, resulting in formation of internal cavities. Brood capsules and protoscolices are formed in aggregations within the cavities. Observations on limited material available for *E. oligarthrus* suggested that the mature metacestode is morphologically similar to *E. vogeli* [1]. Whereas all primary *E. vogeli* larvae are located in the liver, *E. oligar-*

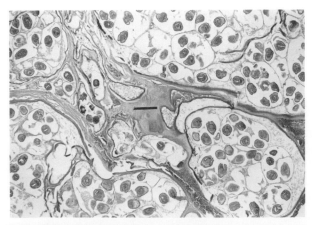

Figure 57-3. Larval *Echinococcus multilocularis* in liver of infected rodent showing alveolar-like microvesicles with protoscolices. H and E. Bar = 100 μm.

thrus larvae develop more commonly in extrahepatic sites, attached to the muscles. Larval stages of the two species, which may occur in the same host species, are distinguishable by differences in size and shape of rostellar hooks of protoscolices, dimensions of the protoscolices and brood capsules, and characteristics of the laminated membrane [1,2].

When metacestodes of *Echinococcus* spp. are ingested by suitable definitive hosts, the protoscolices, triggered by bile, pH, and presumably other factors in the host gut, evaginate in the upper part of the duodenum. They then make their way between villi and may enter the crypts of Lieberkuhn, achieving close contact with the host intestinal mucosa. Proglottid formation begins, and the worms reach the gravid adult stage in 32 to 80 days depending upon species and strain of parasite [3].

Adult *Echinococcus* spp. are small tapeworms, 2 to 11 mm long. The strobila consists of a scolex (with four suckers and a double row of rostellar hooks) and two to five proglottids. Morphological characteristics that, in combination, can be used for taxonomic discrimination in the genus *Echinococcus* include the form of the strobila, position of the genital pore in the mature and gravid proglottids, size of rostellar hooks, number and distribution of testes, and form of the gravid uterus [4].

HOST RANGE AND MAINTENANCE CYCLES

Under natural conditions, echinococcosis is transmitted to definitive hosts through carnivorism; therefore, host assemblages are linked together in predator-prey relationships. *E. granulosus* evolved and was maintained in cycles involving the wolf and wild ungulates [5]. As these hosts became domesticated, the cestode was dispersed widely and became adapted to a still wider variety of domestic and sylvatic host species. Throughout the greater parts of its range, the sheep appears to be the most important intermediate host. In some regions other domestic ungulates, including goats, swine, cattle, buffalo, horses, and camels, assume dominant importance. The occurrence of a parasite in a particular host assemblage (e.g., wolf/moose; dog/sheep; dog/horse) reflects a variable degree of host-parasite adaptation that may vary from one cestode population to another (see "Infraspecific Variation," below).

Host specificity is more strongly defined in adult-stage *E. granulosus*. Almost all known definitive hosts are members of the family Canidae, including the domestic dog, dingo, the wolf, the coyote, and the jackal. An exception is the lion (*Felis leo* L.) in Africa. Domestic cats are not suitable hosts for *E. granulosus*.

The natural definitive and intermediate hosts of *E. multilocularis* are foxes and small cricetid rodents (mainly of the subfamily Arvicolinae), respectively [5]. In the comparatively simple biotic conditions of the arctic tundra zone, the cestode is maintained in cycles involving the arctic fox, *Alopex alopex*, and several kinds of voles of the genera *Microtus* and *Clethrionomys*. In more complex biomes, a greater variety of host species is involved. The red fox, *Vulpes vulpes*, is the most important definitive host throughout most of the range of distribution outside the Arctic Circle. Other carnivores that have been found naturally infected are domestic dogs and cats, coyotes, and wolves.

The larval stages of *E. vogeli* and *E. oligarthrus* share some of the same intermediate hosts throughout much of their distribution in neotropical America. In regions investigated, the cycle of *E. vogeli* involves the bush dog, *Speothos venaticus*, and the paca, *Cuniculus paca*, as definitive and intermediate hosts, respectively [5]. *E. vogeli* larvae have also been found in agoutis (*Dasyprocta* spp.) and spiny rats (*Proechimys* spp.). Domestic dogs are also suitable definitive hosts.

E. oligarthrus is the only species that characteristically uses wild felids as definitive hosts. Naturally acquired infections have been demonstrated in the puma, the jaguarundi, the jaguar, the ocelot, the pampas cat, and Geoffroy's cat [5]. *E. oligarthrus* cysts have been described in pacas, agoutis, and spiny rats.

INFRASPECIFIC VARIATION

Echinococcus species exhibit considerable morphological variability and occur in a wide range of hosts; this had, until recently, led to taxonomic confusion and controversy [5,6]. The four species currently accepted as valid are distinguishable in both larval and adult stages, based on morphological and developmental characteristics. However, local populations of *E. granulosus*, the most widespread species, may vary intrinsically in morphological and biological features, and these infraspecific variants or strains may cause important local differences in the epidemiology and clinical characteristics of the disease. This is due to the infraspecific differences in (1) infectivity to various species of final and intermediate hosts, (2) transmission patterns, and (3) pathogenicity to humans [6].

One population, the indigenous form in arctic regions of North America and Eurasia, has been designated *E. granulosus canadensis*, or the northern sylvatic strain. This strain occurs in wolves and wild ungulates (moose and wild reindeer) and does not readily infect domestic sheep. Human infection is characterized by predominantly pulmonary localization, slower and more benign cyst growth, and a less frequent occurrence of clinical complications than reported for other forms [7].

E. granulosus in domestic sheep has been designated the nominate subspecies, *E. granulosus granulosus*; it is the most geographically widespread strain, and accounts for most human infections throughout the world. In Ireland, Great Britain and Western Europe a strain adapted to the dog/horse cycle is morphologically, biologically, and biochemically distinct from those recovered from the dog/sheep cycle. This strain is poorly, if at all, infective for humans. A study of *E. granulosus* populations in Australia using morphological, developmental, and comparative biochemical criteria suggested that three separate strains of *E. granulosus* occur. There are two "domestic" strains primarily perpetuated in a sheep/dog cycle; one is found throughout mainland Australia, whereas the other is peculiar to Tasmania. The third strain is a "sylvatic" strain restricted to wallabies and dingoes on the mainland of Australia [6]. In Europe and South Africa a strain of *E. granulosus* is uniquely adapted to dog/cattle cycles. In cattle, cysts are almost entirely confined to the lungs. The adult tapeworms are morphologically distinct and have a shorter maturation time (usually less than 40 days) than other strains.

E. granulosus metacestodes in Turkana tribesmen in east Africa appear to be highly virulent compared with other strains; the fact that infected human bodies are often scavenged by dogs and wild canids may have contributed to the development of this characteristic. Evidence exists that still other strains are adapted to host assemblages involving dog/pig (eastern Europe), dog/buffalo (Asia), dog/camel (Asia and Africa) and lion/warthogs (Africa). Additional work is required to clarify the validity and significance of these strains.

Although some evidence suggests variation in morphology, pathogenicity, developmental characteristics, and host specificity between different geographical populations of *E. multilocularis*, few comparative data are available and the existence of strains remains unconfirmed. *E. vogeli* and *E. oligarthrus* have restricted geographical distributions and host ranges, which may account for lack of reported variation within these species [6].

Because genetically determined variations in host specificity, pathogenesis, and other biological characteristics of the parasites may profoundly influence the local epidemiology and control of the disease, identification and evaluation of local strains are essential to developing a control strategy. For strain identification a wide spectrum of techniques is employed including morphological methods, infectivity trials, in vitro cultivation, isoenzyme and protein differentiation, immunological studies, and, most recently, molecular analysis involving DNA hybridization.

CYSTIC HYDATID DISEASE (*EHINOCOCCUS GRANULOSUS*)

PATIENT

Pathogenesis and pathology

In humans the most frequently reported site of hydatid cysts is the liver (50 to 70 percent), followed by the lungs (20 to 30 percent), and less frequently, the spleen, kidneys, heart, bones, central nervous system, and elsewhere. The slowly enlarging *E. granulosus* cyst is well tolerated by human hosts until it becomes large enough to cause pain or dysfunction. Cyst development is variable; in a group of infected (Kenya) nomads followed by ultrasound for one year, 66 percent of cysts grew, 20 percent remained static, and 14 percent collapsed or disappeared [8]. Rupture of a cyst with sudden release of large amounts of fluid can produce severe (occasionally fatal) allergic reactions. Ruptured cyst membranes may serve as a nidus for secondary bacterial infections. Death of the cyst may lead to complete calcification. Released protoscolices may be destroyed by the host response or undergo vesiculation to produce multiple secondary cysts. Cysts in bones grow abnormally, often producing vesicular masses, which erode the marrow cavities and cause extensive osteolysis.

Although cysts survive the lifetime of most intermediate hosts, the exact longevity is unknown. Most (>80 percent) are no longer viable in patients 60 years of age or older [9].

Clinical manifestations

Many human infections remain asymptomatic. In other instances, the severity and nature of the signs and symptoms produced by hydatid cysts are extremely variable and never pathognomonic. The particular manifestations are determined by the site of localization of the cysts, their size, and their condition.

It is rarely possible to ascertain when a patient's infection was first acquired, and the period before onset of signs and symptoms is highly variable and often lasts for several years. Most infections are diagnosed in patients between 10 and 50 years of age; however, infections may be acquired throughout the human life span. Persons of both sexes appear equally susceptible, but sex ratios may vary for epidemiological reasons.

Abrupt and sometimes intermittent, generalized urticaria and pruritus are believed to be associated with "leakage" of cyst fluid. Severe, and sometimes fatal, anaphylaxis may occur following cyst rupture.

Hydatid cysts of the liver may become relatively large before producing symptoms because of the large size of the organ and the distensible body area. A high proportion of liver cysts undergo endocyst detachment with resultant formation of internal septae and daughter cysts. Signs and symptoms may include hepatic enlargement with or without a palpable mass in the right upper quadrant, right epigastric pain, nausea, and vomiting. Rupture into the biliary tree can lead to bilary tract obstruction, and the patient can present initially with obstructive jaundice or cholangitis. Twenty-five percent of patients with hepatic cysts also had cysts in their lungs.

Intact hydatid cysts in the lungs may cause no symptoms, but leakage or rupture causes chest pain, coughing, dyspnea, and hemoptysis. Hydatid membranes may be coughed up, sometimes resulting in spontaneous cure. Complications, which may exist at the time of initial presentation, include cyst rupture and secondary bacterial infection. Nearly 40 percent of patients with pulmonary hydatidosis have liver involvement as well [9].

Five to ten percent of the cases involve organs other than the lungs or liver. The first symptom of cerebral cysts may be raised intracranial pressure or focal epilepsy, while kidney cysts may be manifested by loin pain or hematuria. Bone cysts are often asymptomatic until pathological fractures occur, and, because of resemblance, they are often misdiagnosed as tuberculous lesions.

Prognosis

The risks of anaphylactic reactions, of dissemination following rupture, and of relentless growth making later therapy more difficult or impossible, make a strong argument for therapy. Nevertheless, observations regarding the natural history of hydatid disease are largely anecdotal, and no controlled trials have been reported regarding the risks versus benefits of alternative methods of management.

Amir-Jahed and coworkers [10] in Iran reported death in 60 percent of 15 symptomatic hospital patients who did not have surgery. Of 27 Chinese patients wtih intrathoracic cysts who refused surgery, 6 (22 percent) died of their disease an average of 2.9 years after discharge, 9 (33 percent) spontaneously eliminated their cysts with no radiological evidence of recurrence after an average of 3.9 years, 5 (19 percent) returned for surgical treatment, and the remaining 7 had survived with their cysts for an average follow-up period of 8.1 years [11]. Cysts in the heart are especially dangerous because they may rupture and cause systemic dissemination of the protoscolices, anaphylaxis, or cardiac tamponade. The prognosis for hydatid disease of bones is poor, and amputation of the affected bone, if possible, is frequently necessary.

Diagnosis

Various sensitive imaging methods are available for identifying and characterizing mass lesions in internal organs. Plain roentgenography permits the detection of hydatid cysts in the lungs (Fig. 57-4), but usually only calcified cysts in other sites. Ultrasonic scanning (US), and computed tomography (CT) are useful for visualizing and characterizing the avascular cyst(s) in many organs (Figs. 57-5 and 57-6) [12,13]. Demonstration of internal septae or daughter cysts, which are present in approximately 50 percent of liver cysts, is virtually pathognomonic for hydatid cysts; in their absence such cysts are difficult

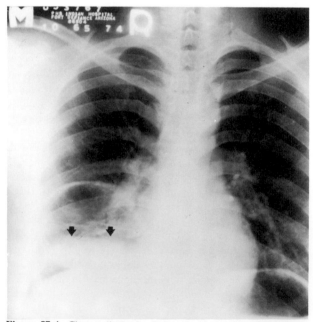

Figure 57-4. Chest radiograph of 19-year-old man showing ruptured hydatid cyst in right lung. Note fluid level (arrows).

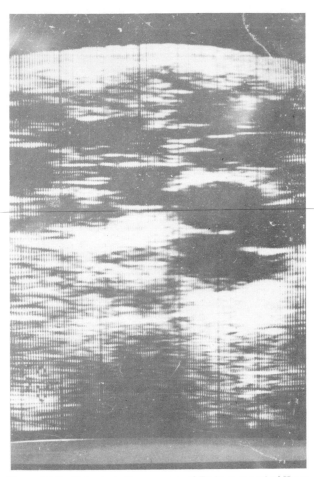

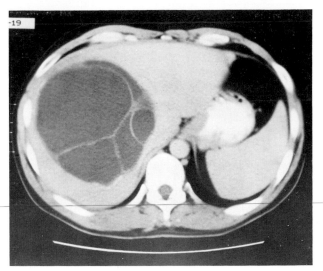

Figure 57-6. Abdominal CT scan showing large primary hydatid cyst (*Echinococcus granulosus*) in the right lobe of the liver. Note internal septations indicating secondary (daughter) cyst formation. (*Courtesy Dr. W. Tsionkas.*)

Figure 57-5. Abdominal ultrasonogram of Turkana nomad of Kenya revealing multiple hydatid cysts involving liver and peritoneal cavity.

to differentiate from simple (epithelial) cysts. Criteria for staging hydatid cysts that may be useful for determining appropriate management have been described [14,15]. Closed aspiration of hydatid cysts should not be attempted, because accidental spilling of the contents could cause secondary spread or anaphylaxis. Cyst membranes or protoscolices may sometimes be demonstrated in the sputum or bronchial washings; identification is facilitated by acid-fast staining of the hooklets. Intravenous pyelograms are helpful in visualizing renal cysts. Eosinophilia is present in one-third or fewer of cyst carriers.

Serodiagnostic tests can be useful if factors that can influence the results are understood [16]. Negative test results do not rule out echinococcosis, because some cyst carriers do not have detectable antibody. Detectable immune responses have been associated with the location, the integrity, and the vitality of the larval cyst. Cysts in the liver are more likely to elicit antibody response than cysts in the lungs, and regardless of localization, tests are least sensitive for diagnosing intact hyaline cysts. Such healthy metacestodes produce a low level of antigenic stimulation, and nearly 50 percent of carriers of this kind of cyst in the lungs may be serologically negative. Fis-

suration or rupture of the cyst is followed by an abrupt anamnestic stimulation of antibodies. Senescent or dead cysts apparently cease to stimulate the host, and such carriers may be seronegative.

Another cause of false-negative tests is antibody "mopping," in which antibody is bound with antigen in circulating immune complexes. Circulating antigen (CAg) was detectable in up to 50 percent of such serum specimens [17]. Therefore, tests for CAg provide a useful adjunct to antibody tests for diagnosis.

Indirect hemagglutination, indirect immunofluorescence, and enzyme-linked immunosorbent assay (ELISA) are highly sensitive tests for detecting circulating antibody in serum from patients with hydatid disease; diagnostic sensitivity varies from approximately 60 percent to 90 percent, depending upon the characteristics of the cases. Tests using whole *E. granulosus* antigens are not specific, however, and false positive reactions occur commonly in serum of persons with other helminth infections, liver cirrhosis, and cancer. Serodiagnostic tests based on the detection of antibody to the *Echinococcus* antigen 5 have the highest degree of specificity. Demonstration of the "arc 5" in a patient's serum may be considered diagnostic for hydatid disease with an important exception: Serum specimens from 5 percent to 10 percent of *Taenia solium* cysticercosis patients give false positive arc 5 reactions. However, this should not greatly confuse clinical diagnosis because cerebral cysticercosis is usually easily differentiated from hydatidosis (cerebral involvement in the latter is rare and, when it occurs, is usually characterized by fewer and larger cysts) [16].

Tests useful for the demonstration of arc 5 in serum specimens reactive in screening tests include immunoelectrophoresis, double diffusion, and counterimmunoelectrophoresis, the latter two tests being more sensitive than the first. Use of recently purified antigen 5 fractions in ELISA may further improve sensitivity.

Treatment

General Considerations. Until recently, treatment of cystic hydatid disease had been exclusively in the hands of surgeons, and there was little to offer patients with inoperable lesions or those who could not tolerate surgery. Experience with the benzimidazole carbamates, however, has established chemotherapy as a valid treatment alternative. The selection of the particular method(s) of treatment for individual patients depends on such factors as the number, location, and viability of the cysts, the severity of symptoms, and the general health status of the patient. At one extreme is the patient with large, potentially breakable, suppurated or otherwise complicated cyst(s) for whom surgery may be lifesaving or necessary to alleviate acute distress. At the other extreme is the patient with multiple organ involvement or otherwise inoperable cysts, or whose age or poor general condition makes surgery an unacceptable risk. Chemotherapy is indicated for the latter patient. For various reasons, some patients require a combination of surgery and chemotherapy. For example, cyst rupture or biliary obstruction requiring surgical intervention may occur in spite of, or perhaps because of, a positive response to chemotherapy. For fit patients with a solitary, uncomplicated cyst the low risk of surgery and prospects for rapid recovery must be balanced against the potential for adverse reactions to chemotherapy and the inconvenience of many months of treatment and follow-up.

Few viable cysts are found in patients older than 60 years [9]; therefore, these patients may be managed conservatively to avoid the risks of surgery or chemotherapy. Conservative management is generally employed for pulmonary infection with the more benign, northern sylvatic strain of *E. granulosus* [7].

Chemotherapy. In animal models and clinical trials both mebendazole and albendazole have been shown to be active against *E. granulosus* cysts [18,19]. Albendazole is the preferred drug because of its better absorption and efficacy. In vitro, albendazole sulfoxide, the principal active metabolite, kills protoscolices at concentrations likely to be achieved within cysts during treatment of patients [20,21]. The effects of benzimidazole carbamates are first evident on the tegumentary structure of protoscolices and the germinal layer: cyst material resected from patients treated with albendazole and examined by electron microscopy characteristically shows disrupted germinal membranes with only remnants of vesicles or necrotic tissue remaining in contact with the laminated layer (Fig. 57-7) [22,23]. Treatment of naturally infected sheep with albendazole for 30 days (10 to 20 mg/kg) killed most cysts [22].

Many human case reports indicate that therapy for 60 to 90 days with albendazole was followed by regression or collapse

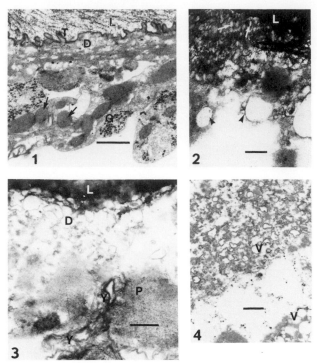

Figure 57-7. Transmission electron micrographs of normal-appearing *Echinococcus granulosus* germinal membrane (1) and those showing the effects of albendazole treatment (2,3,4). All cysts resected from infected humans. **1.** Germinal layer with mitochondria (arrows), glycogen reserves (G) and the truncated microtriches (T) of the distal cytoplasm (D) in contact with the laminated layer (L). Bar = 1 μm. **2.** Vesiculated remnants of the germinal layer (arrowheads) and distal cytoplasm (arrows) in contact with the laminated layer (L). Bar = 0.5 μm. **3.** Necrotic tissue in contact with the laminated layer (L). D, vesiculated distal cytoplasm; P, lipid droplet; Y, myelin figure. Bar = 0.5 μm. **4.** Fragments of vesiculated tissue (V) internal to the laminated layer. Bar = 1 μm. (*Courtesy Dr. K. Sylvia Richards.*)

of most cysts (Fig. 57-8) [23–27]. Of 22 albendazole-treated patients followed up for 4 years or more, 5 developed recurrence but 4 responded to further therapy [27a]. Even some cases involving bones, forms of hydatid disease not usually amenable to cure by surgery, responded to albendazole with no recurrence within 12 months [28]. Other reports were less favorable. Data provided by multiple clinical investigations to WHO on 54 patients treated with albendazole indicated only 27 percent were "successfully" treated [19]. Clinical trials have given mixed results partly because treated patients have often been the most complicated cases. Multiple cysts in diverse organ localizations, often with daughter cysts, hinder uniform penetration of drug to sites of viable metacestode tissue. The difficulty of ascertaining whether cysts were viable before chemotherapy further confounded the interpretation of many reports. Collectively, these experiences have demonstrated that, in the absence of controlled trials, it is easier to prove failure than success.

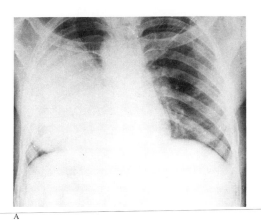
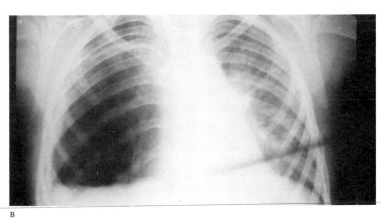

A   B

Figure 57-8. Chest radiograph of Turkana nomad in Kenya with *E. granulosus* hydatid cyst occupying most of right lung field, (*A*) before and (*B*) 6 months after completing 90 days of treatment with albendazole.

Evidence of mild liver toxicity appears in many treated patients and requires cessation of treatment in some [28,29]. Tests of liver function revert to normal when the drug is discontinued. Other reported adverse reactions include reversible neutropenia, alopecia, allergic conditions, and gastrointestinal symptoms [18,19].

Although clinical trials continue and the optimum treatment schedule has not been determined yet, experience to date suggests that patients selected for chemotherapy should receive albendazole, 10 mg/kg per day in divided doses, for 1 to 3 periods of 28 days with drug-free intervals of 14 days. Follow-up should continue for at least 12 months. In some cases, definite evidence of improvement has been seen after one course of therapy, but in others up to eight courses were required to effect improvement. Patients should receive strict

medical supervision and be monitored during therapy with weekly complete blood counts including platelets, liver function tests, and urinalysis.

Objective response to therapy is best assessed by repeated evaluation of cyst(s) size and consistency at 3-month intervals. Ultrasound is the least expensive imaging technique, but CT is more useful for detecting loss of tension, gradual shrinkage, and collapse of cysts (Fig. 57-9) [12]. Magnetic resonance imaging (MRI) achieves superior soft-tissue contrast and may permit differentiation of viable from dead cysts [31]. Cysts in the lungs and peritoneum appear to respond most promptly, possibly because of their thinner ectocysts which permit more rapid entry of the drug and early collapse of the degenerated cyst; in contrast, liver cysts, which usually have a more substantial adventitial layer surrounding them, may appear un-

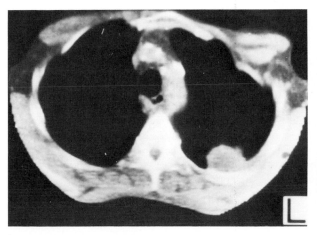
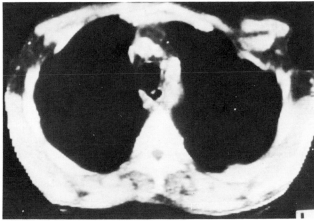

A   B

Figure 57-9. Thoracic CT of patient with single *Echinococcus granulosus* hydatid cyst adjacent to left posterior pleural surface, (*A*) before and (*B*) after completing 60 days treatment with albendazole. (*From* [23].)

changed by radiological assessment even after death of the metacestode.

Another indication for chemotherapy is prevention of recurrence or secondary hydatidosis which may occur in 2 to 10 percent of uncomplicated surgical patients [32,33] and in one-third of patients with known peritoneal spillage. The results of animal studies and limited clinical data suggest that administering albendazole, 10 mg/(kg · day), for 30 days starting immediately after known spillage may be effective in preventing establishment of secondary cysts from seeded protoscolices [20,34,35].

A second drug that may soon have a defined role in treating human hydatid disease is praziquantel, which is less toxic and better absorbed than the benzimidazoles. It is highly active against protoscolices in vitro [36], and when given to recipient rodents, it significantly reduces the number of cysts that become established after intraperitoneal inoculation of protoscolices. Conclusions regarding its effect on germinal membranes of established hydatid cysts have varied from none to limited; however, a recent study showed consistent praziquantel-induced changes in the ultrastructure of *E. granulosus* germinal membrane similar to those produced by long-term albendazole [37].

Surgery. The ideal result of surgery is enucleation of the entire cyst followed by obliteration of the cavity, both of which are often possible with intact, solitary, noncomplicated cysts. For liver cysts, cystectomy or partial hepatectomy and omentoplasty (filling the cavity with an omental pedicle) are superior to marsupialization or tube drainage, although the latter techniques are usually necessary in cases of suppuration [38,39]. For lung cysts a preferred technique is enucleation of the intact cyst; the cavity is then allowed to remain open or is closed by suture. Ruptured or infected cysts usually require resection techniques. Surgical risk varies with case selection, operative technique, and surgical skill. Reported operative mortality rates have ranged from 1 percent to 4 percent. Mortality for the first, second, or third operation was 2.6 percent, 6.0 percent, and 20.0 percent, respectively [10]. Postsurgical complications, the most frequent being secondary bacterial infection, may occur in 25 to 50 percent of operations. The possibility of anaphylaxis or dissemination of protoscolices during surgical manipulation of the cyst can be minimized by packing off the area around the cyst with pads saturated with 20% saline or 0.5% silver nitrate. Commonly, part of the cyst contents are aspirated and protoscolicidal solutions are injected to "sterilize" the cyst before resection or drainage. The efficacy of this procedure for preventing secondary hydatidosis from seeded protoscolices has not been evaluated, and it may be hazardous. The chemicals employed (hypertonic saline, silver nitrate, formalin, cetrimide) have all been associated with toxic reactions, and, if the fluid leaks into the biliary tree, it can cause sclerosing cholangitis [40–42]. In the event of cyst rupture or inadvertent spillage, a postoperative course of chemotherapy with albendazole or praziquantel as described above may reduce chances of recurrence.

POPULATION

Distribution and prevalence

The adaptability of *E. granulosus* to a wide variety of host species and the repeated introduction and movement of domestic animals throughout the world have made possible the present broad geographical distribution of this cestode and the disease it produces, from north of the Arctic Circle to as far south as Tierra del Fuego, Argentina, and Stewart Island, New Zealand (Fig. 57-10). Within this cosmopolitan distribution, the cestode occurs in all climates, in a wide variety of hosts, and at various levels of prevalence [43,44].

Crosshatched areas on the map (Fig. 57-10) are regions where *E. granulosus* infections are reported to be an important public health and economic problem. Reliable data are available from only a few countries. The most common index of the level of human infection in an area or region is the annual incidence of diagnosed or surgical cases. In Uruguay, three retrospective surveys of all medical and surgical centers determined the number of hospital cases diagnosed annually during the years between 1962 and 1971 [45]. The mean annual morbidity, whether expressed as the incidence of all hospital cases (20.7 cases per 100,000 population) or only new cases (17.7 per 100,000), gave Uruguay the highest echinococcosis national morbidity rate yet reported. In comparison, other high national figures at that time were 12.9 cases per 100,000 in Cyprus, 7.8 in Chile, 7.5 to 8.3 in Greece, 5.1 to 6.1 in Algeria, and 3.7 in Yugoslavia [43].

In most countries, hydatid disease is most prevalent in the rural areas. In Uruguay, for instance, the average annual incidence per 100,000 population was 123.0 for rural residents, but only 10.1 for urban and suburban residents [45]. In Argentina, the number of reported cases per year for the entire country varies from 1 to 2 per 100,000, but in several southern provinces the rate exceeds 150 per 100,000.

The use of diagnostic screening methods (radiology, ultrasonography, and serology) to detect asymptomatic cyst carriers indicates that symptomatic hospital cases represent only a tiny fraction of prevalent infections. For instance, in the province of Rio Negro, Argentina, where the annual incidence of hospital cases was 143 per 100,000, a mass miniature radiography survey of 15,000 persons demonstrated pulmonary hydatid infection in 460 per 100,000. These included only infections with pulmonary localization, representing only one-third or less of all infections. Ultrasound surveys detect even higher rates of asymptomatic infections: 1.4 percent infected in rural populations in Uruguay, 3.6 percent in central Tunisia, and 5.6 percent among Turkana nomads.

Epidemiology

Local differences in prevalence and patterns of transmission are determined by a multiplicity of factors concerning the host,

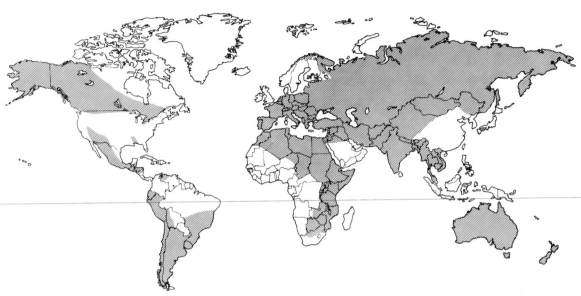

Figure 57-10. Geographical distribution of *Echinococcus granulosus* infection.

agent, environment, and human behavior [*43,46*]. Common practices in rural endemic areas of both advanced and developing countries are the widespread use of dogs for working livestock and the habit of feeding them on viscera of home-butchered sheep or other livestock. Thus, an artificial system that is more efficient than the natural systems in perpetuating the life cycle has been created. Under such conditions, canine infection occurs repeatedly, producing high prevalence rates and environmental contamination with cestode eggs.

There may be many thousands of *E. granulosus* adults in a heavily infected dog, and each worm sheds as many as 800 eggs every 2 weeks. Eggs require no further development and are immediately infective. Depending upon the conditions, eggs may survive only a few days or more than a year. High temperatures and desiccation are the most important factors limiting survival time of taeniid eggs in nature.

Human populations, sharing environments with infected dogs, are frequently exposed, and the probability that any given person will become infected depends, in part, upon such factors as personal hygiene and cleanliness. Direct contact with infected dogs, particularly the characteristic playful and intimate contact between children and their pets, may be the most important source of human infection. Cestode eggs adhere to hairs around the infected dog's anus and may also be found on their muzzle and paws. Indirect means of contact, via water and contaminated vegetables, or through the intermediary of flies and other arthropods, may also cause human infections [*47*].

Socioeconomic and cultural characteristics are among the best-defined risk factors for human infection [*43,46*]. A prevalence rate much greater than that of the local general population has been demonstrated for the Maori of New Zealand,

the Turkana of Kenya, persons of Basque origin, Navajo and Zuni Indians in the United States, and certain indigenous peoples of Argentina, Chile, and Peru. In many instances, the higher infection rates appear to be related to lower levels of education, hygiene, and sanitation, but specific cultural practices often contribute directly to parasite transmission.

Prevention and control

The principal objective of control of cystic hydatid disease is reduction in parasite prevalence in definitive and intermediate hosts below levels necessary for continued transmission. Several field trials and national control campaigns (New Zealand, Tasmania, Cyprus, Argentina, Chile) have shown that *E. granulosus* in domestic-animal life cycles is readily responsive to control [*48*] and, if control measures are maintained, may be eradicated. Measures employed in various circumstances include health education, control of livestock slaughtering in abattoirs and on farms, safe disposal of infected viscera, dog control, and periodic diagnostic testing and mass drug treatment of dogs. Praziquantel is highly effective in a single orally or intramuscularly administered dose (5 mg per kilogram of body weight) and appears particularly suitable for mass treatment. Repeated mass treatments of dogs at risk can rapidly reduce the rates of transmission to intermediate hosts. Developing a strategy for control appropriate for a given endemic region must take into account all the known epidemiological variables, including the local sociocultural factors related to transmission. Attention must also be given to the administrative structure of the control authority, the development of an ongoing surveillance program to monitor progress, and the commitment of adequate funds to insure completion of all phases of the program. WHO has sponsored the development of practical guidelines for the planning, development, implementation, and evaluation of hydatid disease control programs [*44*].

Practical immunization procedures have not yet been developed, although research indicates that they are theoretically feasible, and vaccination of sheep and other intermediate hosts may be possible as an adjunct control measure in the near future [*48*].

ALVEOLAR HYDATID DISEASE (ECHINOCOCCUS MULTILOCULARIS)

PATIENT

Pathogenesis and pathology

Compared with *E. granulosus*, larval *E. multilocularis* is more progressive and damaging to the host. Primary larval foci appear almost invariably in the liver. Growth in humans is different from that in the natural hosts in that the larval mass is inhibited from completing its development and remains in the proliferative stage indefinitely [*3*]. Thus, it continues to invade and destroy the hepatic parenchyma, and retrogressive changes within the mass result in necrosis of the central portion. Macroscopically, hepatic lesions usually appear as one or more firm to solid, whitish, rounded masses slightly elevated above the surrounding tissue of the surface of the liver. When transected, they display a central necrotic cavity surrounded by dense, pale tissue that lacks a clearly defined border with adjacent hepatic tissue (Fig. 57-11). In advanced cases, the cavity usually contains a turbid, yellowish to brown fluid with particles or fragments of necrotic tissue [*50*]. Microscopically, cysts of various sizes are scattered or closely aggregated in the matrix of connective tissues. Only rarely are brood capsules and calcareous corpuscles present, usually focally. Metastasis

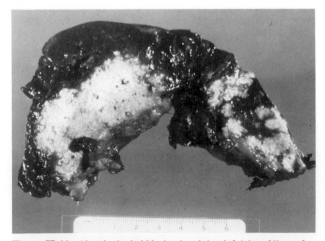

Figure 57-11. Alveolar hydatid lesion involving left lobe of liver after surgical resection. Note the extensive destruction of the hepatic parenchyma and the necrosis producing a central abscess.

by a hematogenous route is not uncommon, and secondary foci usually occur in the brain and lungs.

Clinical manifestations

Although some cases have been diagnosed in children, the clinical signs of the disease usually do not become evident until early adulthood or middle age [*50,51*].

Initial symptoms are generally vague. Mild upper quadrant and epigastric pain with hepatomegaly may progress to obstructive jaundice. Occasionally, the initial manifestations are related to metastasis to the lungs or brain. Patients eventually succumb to hepatic failure or invasion of contiguous structures.

Prognosis

Because alveolar hydatid disease is often not diagnosed until it is well advanced, the lesion is often inoperable; the percentage of surgically resectable cases has varied from 20 percent to 58 percent. Approximately 90 percent of patients with nonresectable disease die within 10 years [*52*], although survival time may be prolonged with chemotherapy (discussed below). Infection is not always progressive, however; recent findings indicate that a proportion of human *E. multilocularis* infections resolve spontaneously when the parasites die at an early age [*53*].

Diagnosis

The usual signs mimic hepatic carcinoma and cirrhosis, with which the disease is commonly confused. Plain roentgenography shows hepatomegaly and characteristic scattered radiolucencies outlined by calcific rings (2 to 8 mm). Where both cystic and alveolar hydatid disease occur together, the two can be distinguished by CT and by serology. The characteristic CT image in cystic hydatid disease shows sharply contoured cyst(s) (sometimes with internal daughter cysts) and marginal calcifications (Fig. 57-6). In contrast, the CT image of alveolar hydatid disease reveals uneven hyper- and hypodense areas with scattered calcifications (Fig. 57-12) [*13*]. Calcified lesions of small size (4 cm or less) may be inactive when adjacent hypodense areas cannot be discerned [*53*].

Purified *E. multilocularis* antigens (Em2) used in ELISA give positive serological reactions in more than 95 percent of cases [*54*]. Comparing serological reactivity to Em2 antigen with that to antigens containing components of both *E. multilocularis* and *E. granulosus* permits discrimination of patients with alveolar from cystic hydatid disease [*16*].

Exploratory laparotomy is sometimes performed to diagnose and delineate the extent of the lesion. The larval membranes can be demonstrated with periodic acid Schiff (PAS) stain, or the sterile larva can be reared to the adult stage after secondary passage in susceptible rodents.

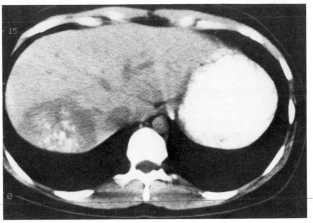

Figure 57-12. Abdominal CT scan of patient with *Echinococcus multilocularis* lesion in a lobe of the liver. Note irregular low-density zones alternating with scattered areas of calcification. (*Courtesy Dr. Joseph F. Wilson.*)

Treatment

Surgical resection of the entire larval mass is the only proven curative treatment for alveolar hydatid disease [*50–52*]. For hepatic and pulmonary lesions this usually requires removal of the entire affected lobe. When involvement is more extensive, wedge resections of the lesions may be attempted. Because alveolar hydatid disease is often nonresectable, partial resections and biliodigestive and hepatodigestive anastomoses are carried out as palliative measures, predominantly to ensure bile passage. Benzimidazole carbamate chemotherapy can alter the otherwise fatal outcome of nonresectable cases. Long-term continuous therapy with mebendazole (40 to 50 mg/(kg · day)) was associated with clinical improvement, significant regression of primary and metastatic lesions, no further progression of disease, and prolonged survival of most patients [*18,55,56*]. Mebendazole is parasitostatic rather than lethal to the parasite. Parasite tissue from some patients treated with mebendazole as long as 48 months survived and grew when injected into rodents [*56*]. Similarly good clinical responses have been observed in patients treated with albendazole (10 to 15 mg/(kg · day)) [*18,57*]. A parasitocidal effect on active alveolar hydatid disease was suggested from the findings in two recently reported cases treated preoperatively with albendazole for 58 and 84 days [*30*].

POPULATION

Distribution and prevalence

E. multilocularis has an extensive geographical range in the northern hemisphere (Fig. 57-13), including an endemic region in central Europe (central and southern Germany, western Austria, Switzerland, and southern France) and most of northern Eurasia, from Bulgaria and Turkey through the U.S.S.R., extending eastward to several of the Japanese islands (Rebun, Hokkaido, and Kuriles) [*5*]. Recent reports from Iran, India, China, Tunisia, and the United States have considerably extended the known southern limits of this cestode's range.

The distribution in North America appears to be discontinuous. This cestode is widely prevalent in the northern tundra zone, from the White Sea in the west to Hudson Bay in the east. There is no evidence that it occurs in the zone of boreal forest, south of the tundra zone, but recent studies have dem-

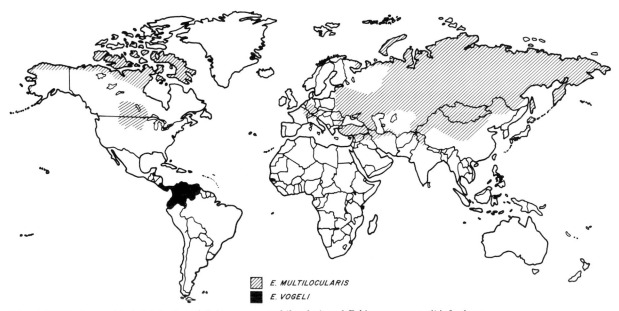

Figure 57-13. Geographical distribution of *Echinococcus multilocularis* and *Echinococcus vogeli* infections.

onstrated a large and increasing area of infection in south central Canada (Manitoba, Saskatchewan, and Alberta) and the north central United States (North Dakota, South Dakota, Minnesota, Iowa, Nebraska, Montana, and Wyoming) [5,46]. The first human case definitely associated with the central North American focus was diagnosed in 1977 in Minnesota. The availability of suitable hosts in adjacent areas presents a potential for further spread in North America.

Few data exist on the prevalence of human alveolar hydatid disease. Recent reviews indicate that cases occur frequently in parts of the U.S.S.R., northern Japan, western Alaska, and central Europe. Cases have been diagnosed in the population at risk in Alaska at an average annual rate of 28 per 100,000 [50].

Epidemiology

In the northern tundra zone, the arctic fox feeds almost exclusively on microtine rodents. In studies carried out at different times, infection rates in foxes and rodents ranged from 40 percent to 100 percent and from 2 percent to 16 percent, respectively. The variations seemed to correlate directly with fluctuations in the host populations. In biotically more complex zones, foxes feed upon a greater variety of animals, and infection rates are usually lower than those observed in the tundra zone.

E. multilocularis is largely restricted to wild animal hosts and is thereby separated ecologically from man. Human exposure is determined by occupational and avocational factors. Hunters, trappers, and persons who work with fox fur are most frequently exposed. Dogs that become infected by capturing and eating infected voles are even more important as a source of human infection [57]. When infected voles exist in villages as commensal rodents (as they do, for example, in some Eskimo villages of the tundra zone in North America), the cycle of the cestode is readily completed and a hyperendemic focus is produced. The poor sanitary conditions that usually exist in such villages permit extensive accumulation of dog feces and enhance the risk of human infection.

Prevention and control

Eliminating *E. multilocularis* from sylvatic animal hosts would be impractical under most circumstances. Personal preventive measures in areas where the infection is endemic include avoiding contact with foxes and other potentially infected final hosts. In areas where *E. multilocularis* occurs, pet dogs and cats must be prevented from preying on rodents. Patent infections in dogs and cats liable to eat infected rodents can be prevented by monthly prophylactic treatments with praziquantel (5 mg per kilogram of body weight). Potentially exposed human populations should be educated about the dangers so they practice better personal hygiene and sanitation and take effective measures to prevent their pets from eating rodents.

POLYCYSTIC HYDATID DISEASE (*ECHINOCOCCUS VOGELI*)

PATIENT

Pathogenesis and pathology

E. vogeli has been identified as the cause of a polycystic form of human hydatid disease with characteristics intermediate between cystic and alveolar hydatid disease [58]. The primary localization is in the liver, but cysts may spread to contiguous sites. These infections produced multiple fluid-filled vesicles (5 to 80 mm in diameter) with numerous brood capsules and protoscolices. Proliferation of vesicles sometimes destroys much of the liver, and involvement of adjacent structures is common.

Clinical manifestations

Among reported cases, age at onset of symptoms leading to diagnosis ranged from 13 to 74 years. Hepatomegaly or the presence of tumorlike masses in the liver have been typical findings (Fig. 57-14). Most of the reported cases were lost to follow-up, but prognosis is poor, because of the extensive nature of the disease.

Diagnosis

The diagnosis of hydatid disease was not considered preoperatively on most of the cases of polycystic hydatid disease thus far reported [58]. Techniques that can demonstrate cystic or alveolar hydatid disease should also be useful for diagnosing larval *E. vogeli* infections.

Treatment

Little has been reported concerning clinical aspects of polycystic hydatid disease, but management criteria similar to those for cystic and alveolar hydatid disease should apply. Animal

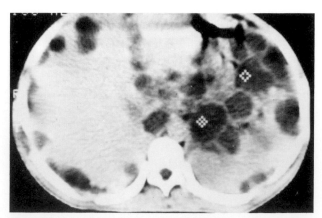

Figure 57-14. Abdominal CT scan showing multiple, oval hypodense areas in liver, spleen, and abdominal cavity of patient with *Echinococcus vogeli* infection. (*Courtesy Dr. U.G. Meneghelli.*)

studies and limited clinical experience indicate that *E. vogeli* cysts respond to albendazole treatment.

POPULATION

Distribution and prevalence

E. vogeli is known to occur within the range of its requisite hosts in Central and South America (Fig. 57-13). The presence of *E. vogeli* has been documented in human or lower animal intermediate hosts in Costa Rica, Panama, Colombia, Ecuador, Venezuela, Brazil, and Bolivia.

Epidemiology

E. vogeli appears to be maintained throughout its range in neotropical America in cycles involving bush dogs and pacas, and, to a lesser extent, agoutis and spiny rats [*5,15*]. In endemic areas, dogs are commonly fed viscera of paca, and human infections are probably acquired from the feces of infected hunting dogs. Bush dogs are rare and avoid humans, and, therefore, probably play little role in direct exposure of humans.

REFERENCES

1 Rausch RL, D'Allesandro A, Rausch VR: Characteristics of the larval *Echinococcus vogeli* Rausch and Bernstein, 1972 in the natural intermediate host, the paca, *Cuniculus paca* L. (Rodentia: Dasyproctidae). Am J Trop Med Hyg 30:1043–1052, 1981

2 Rausch RK. Rausch VR, D'Alessandro A: Discrimination of the larval stages of *Echinococcus oligarthrus* (Diesing, 1863) and *E. vogeli* Rausch and Bernstein, 1972 (Cestoda:Taeniidae). Am J Trop Med Hyg 27:1195–1199, 1978

3 Thompson RCA: Biology and systematics of Echinococcus, in Thompson RCA (ed): *The Biology of Echinococcus and Hydatid Disease*. London, George Allen & Unwin, 1986, pp 5–43

4 Rausch RL, Bernstein JJ: *Echinococcus vogeli* spp. n. (Cestoda: Taeniidae) from the bush dog, *Speothos venaticus* (Lund). Tropenmed Parasitol 23:25–34, 1972

5 Rausch RL: Life-cycle patterns and geographic distribution of *Echinococcus* species, in Thompson RCA (ed): *The Biology of Echinococcus and Hydatid Disease*. London, George Allen & Unwin, 1986, pp. 44–80

6 Thompson RCA, Lymberry AJ: The nature, extent and significance of variation within the genus *Echinococcus*. Adv Parasitol 27:210–263, 1988

7 Wilson JF, Diddams AC, Rausch RL: Cystic hydatid disease in Alaska. A review of 101 autochthonous cases of *Echinococcus granulosus* infection. Am Rev Respir Dis 98:1–15, 1968

8 Romig R, Zeyhle E, Macpherson CNL, et al: Cyst growth and spontaneous cure in hydatid disease. Lancet 1:861, 1986

9 Little JM: Hydatid disease at Royal Prince Alfred Hospital, 1964 to 1974. Med J Aust 1:903–908, 1976

10 Amir-Jahed AK, Fardin R, Farzad A, et al: Clinical echinococcosis. Ann Surg 182:541–546, 1975

11 Zhongxi Q, Shuyuan G, Guoxue T, et al: Immediate and long-term results of surgical treatment of intrathoracic hydatid cysts. Clin Med J 93:569–572, 1980

12 Beggs, I: The radiological appearances of hydatid disease of the liver. Clin Radiol 34:555–563, 1983

13 Didier D, Weiler S. Rohmer P, et al: Hepatic alveolar echinococcosis: Correlative US and Ct study. Radiology 154:179–186, 1985

14 Lewall DB, McCorkell SJ: Hepatic echinococcal cysts: Sonographic appearance and classification. Radiology 155:773–775, 1985

15 Kalovidouris A, Pissiotis C, Pontifex G, et al: CT characterization of multivesicular hydatid cysts. J Comput Assist Tomogr 10:428–431, 1986

16 Schantz PM, Gottstein B: Echinococcosis (Hydatidosis), in Walls KW, Schantz PM (eds): *Immunodiagnosis of Parasitic Diseases*. Orlando, Florida, Academic, 1986, pp 69–107

17 Craig PS: Detection of specific circulating antigen, immune complexes and antibodies in human hydatidosis from Turkana (Kenya) and Great Britain, by enzyme-immunoassay. Parasite Immunol 8:171–188, 1986

18 Davis A, Pawlowski ZS, Dixon H: Multicentre clinical trials of benzimidazolecarbamates in human echinococcosis. Bull WHO 64:383–388, 1986

19 Davis A, Dixon H, Pawlowski Z: Multicentre clinical trials of benzimidazole carbamates in human cystic echinococcosis (phase 2). Bull WHO (in press)

20 Chinnery J, Morris DL: Effect of albendazole sulphoxide on viability of hydatid protoscoleces. Trans R Soc Trop Med 80:815–817, 1986

21 Morris DL, Chinnery JB, Georgiou G, et al: Penetration of albendazole sulphoxide into hydatid cysts, Gut, 28:75–80, 1987

22 Morris DL, Clarkson MS, Stallbaumer MF, et al: Albendazole treatment of pulmonary hydatid cysts in naturally infected sheep: a study with relevance to man. Thorax 40:453–458, 1985

23 Morris DK, Dykes PW, Marriner, et al: Albendazole: objective evidence of response in human hydatid disease. JAMA 253:2053–2057, 1985

24 Saimot AG, Meulemans A, Cremieux AC, et al: Albendazole as a potential treatment for human hydatidosis. Lancet 2:652–656, 1983

25 Okelo GBA: Hydatid disease: Research and control in Turkana, III. Albendazole in the treatment of inoperable hydatid disease in Kenya—a report on 12 cases. Trans R Soc Trop Med Hyg 80:193–195, 1986

26 Rahemtulla A, Bryceson ADM, McManus DP, et al: Albendazole in the treatment of hydatid disease. J R Soc Med 80:119–120, 1987

27 Rowley AH, Shulman ST, Donaldson JS, Schantz PM: Albendazole treatment of recurrent echinococcosis. Pediatr Infect Dis 7:666–667, 1988

27a Morris DL: Personal communication

28 Szypryt EP, Morris DC, Mulholland RC: Combined chemotherapy and therapy for hydatid bone disease. J Bone Joint Surg 69B:141–144, 1987

29 Morris DL, Smith PG: Albendazole in hydatid disease—hepatocellular toxicity. Trans R Soc Trop Med Hyg 81:343–344, 1987

30 Wilson JF, Rausch RL, McMahon BJ, et al: Albendazole therapy in alveolar hydatid disease: A report of favorable results in two patients after short term therapy. Am J Trop Med 37:162–168, 1987

31 Morris DL, Buckley J, Gregson R, et al: Magnetic resonance imaging in hydatid disease. Clin Radiol 38:141–144, 1987

32 Mottaghian H, Saidi F: Postoperative recurrence of hydatid disease. Br J Surg 65:237–241, 1978

33 Quilici M, Dumon H, Delmont J: Les modalites de constitution des (recidives) postoperatoires de l'echinococcose à *Echinococcus granulosus*. Medecine Maladies Infect 6:12–16, 1976

34 Morris DL, Chinnery JB, Hardcastle JD: Can albendazole reduce the risk of implantation of spilled protoscoleces? An animal study. Trans R Soc Trop Med Hyg, 80:481–484, 1986

35 Morris DL, Taylor D: Sensitivity to albendazole sulfoxide of *Echinococcus granulosus* scoleces in man. Lancet II:1032, 1986

36 Morris DL, Richards KS, Chinnery JB: Protoscolicidal effect of praziquantel—in vitro and electron microscopy studies on *Echinococcus granulosus*. Antimicrob Chemother 18:681–691, 1986

37 Taylor DH, Morris DL, Richards RS: Combination chemotherapy of *Echinococcus granulosus:* the effects of praziquantel, *in vivo* and *in vitro,* on the ultrastructure of equine strain murine cysts. Parasitology 96:323–336, 1988

38 Barros JL: Hydatid disease of the liver. Am J Surg 135:596–600, 1978

39 Sayek I, Yalin R, Sanoc Y: Surgical treatment of hydatid disease of the liver. Arch Surg 115:847–850, 1980

40 Khodadadi DJ, Kurgon A, Schmidt B: Sclerosing cholangitis following the treatment of Echinococcus of the liver. Int Surg 66:361–362, 1981

41 Belghiti J, Benhamou JP, Perniceri T, et al: Sclerosing cholangitis. A complication of the surgical treatment of hydatid disease of the liver. Arch Surg 121:1162–1165, 1986

42 Teres J, Gomez-Moli J, Bruguera M: Sclerosing cholangitis after surgical treatment of hepatic echinococcal cysts—report of 3 cases. Am J Surg 147:694–697, 1984

43 Schantz PM: Echinococcosis/Hydatidosis, in Steele JH (ed): *Handbook of Zoonoses,* Series 3, *Parasitic Zoonoses*. Boca Raton, Fla, CRC Press (in press)

44 Eckert J, Gemmell MA, Soulsby EJL (eds): FAO/UNEP/WHO Guidelines for Surveillance, Prevention and Control of Echinococcosis/Hydatidosis. VPH/81.28, Geneva, 1981, 147 pp

45 Purriel P, Schantz PM, Beovide H, et al: Human echinococcosis (hydatidosis) in Uruguay: a comparison of indices of morbidity and mortality, 1962–71. Bull WHO 49:395–402, 1974

46 Schwabe CW: Current status of hydatid disease: a zoonosis of increasing importance, in Thompson RCA (ed): *The Biology of Echinococcus and Hydatid Disease*. London, George Allen & Unwin, 1986, pp 81–113

47 Lawson JR, Gemmell MA: Hydatidosis and cysticercosis: the dynamics of transmission, Adv Parasitol 22:261–308, 1983

48 Gemmell MA, Lawson JR, Roberts MG: Control of echinococcosis/hydatidosis: present status of world wide progress. Bull WHO 64:333–339, 1986

49 Rickard MD, Williams JF: Hydatidosis/Cysticercosis: Immune mechanisms and immunization against infection. Adv Parasitol 21:229–296, 1982

50 Wilson JF, Rausch RL: Alveolar hydatid disease. A review of clinical features of 33 indigenous cases of *Echinococcus multilocularis* infection in Alaskan Eskimos. Am J Trop Med Hyg 29:1340–1355, 1980

51 Kasai Y, Koshino I, Kawanishi N, et al: Alveolar echinococcosis of the liver. Ann Surg 191:145–152, 1980

52 Mosimann F: Is alveolar hydatid disease of the liver incurable? Ann Surg 192:118–123, 1980

53 Rausch RL, Wilson JF, Schantz PM, et al: Spontaneous death of *Echinococcus multilocularis:* Cases diagnosed serologically and clinical significance. Am J Trop Med Hyg 36:576–585, 1987

54 Gottstein B: Purification and characterization of a specific antigen from *Echinococcus multilocularis*. Parasite Immunol 7:201–212, 1985

55 Luder PJ, Robotti G, Meister FP, et al: High oral doses of mebendazole interfere with growth of larval *Echinococcus multilocularis* lesions. J Hepatol 1:369–377, 1985

56 Rausch RL, Wilson JF, McMahon BJ, et al: Consequences of continuous mebendazole therapy in alveolar hydatid disease—with a summary of a ten-year clinical trial. Ann Trop Med Parasitol 80:403–419, 1986

57 Stehr-Green JK, Stehr-Green PA, Schantz PM, et al: Risk factors for infection with *Echinococcus multilocularis* in Alaska. Am J Trop Med Hyg 38:380–385, 1988

58 D'Alessandro A, Rausch RL, Cuello C, et al: First observation of *Echinococcus vogeli* in man, with a review of human cases of polycystic hydatid disease in Colombia and neighboring countries. Am J Trop Med Hyg 28:303–317, 1979

CHAPTER 58 / *Arthropods Directly Causing Human Injury* · Philippe A. Rossignol · Fred M. Feinsod

Arthropods can act as direct agents of human disease and discomfort, causing a variety of clinical manifestations. Examples of pest arthropods are found in all human environments, occasionally producing severe injury. Physicians should be alert to arthropod-induced pathology, because treatment is generally available and subsequent patient-arthropod exposure can be minimized.

The patient's history is integral to the investigation of suspected arthropod-induced lesions. A general understanding of the patient's living and working conditions can suggest potential exposures to medically important arthropods. This includes personal exposures, pets or their recent removal, vacations, and travel history. The time course of the lesion may help to determine the environmental source. In addition, early lesion symptomatology and arthropod characterization provide vital clues. The physical examination can further expand the investigation by characterizing the lesion, finding additional lesions, and mapping out their distribution. Close scrutiny can sometimes locate the arthropod in question. Magnification is helpful, and a thorough examination of body hair and clothes, as well as skin scrapings, can be informative.

Injurious arthropods can be clinically separated into "arthroparasites" and "transient arthropod pests." This separation helps correlate suspected arthropods with the clinical presentation and natural history of the lesion. Arthroparasites remain in contact with the human body or a person's immediate environment for prolonged periods. Three classes of arthropods contain species which parasitize humans: insects (Insecta), arachnids (Arachnida), and tongue worms (Pentastomida). Insects include flies (Diptera), bugs (Hemiptera), fleas (Siphonaptera), and lice (Anoplura), while arachnids include ticks (Metastigmata) and mites (Mesostigmata). In contrast, transient pest arthropods are more elusive, injuring people during brief encounters. Four arthropod classes contain such species: Arachnids, insects, millipedes (Diplopoda), and centipedes (Chilopoda). Potential arachnid pests include scorpions (Scorpionida) and spiders (Araneeida). Insect pests include moths (Lepidoptera); flies (Diptera); beetles (Coleoptera); bees, wasps, and ants (Hymenoptera). Transient arthropod pests leave the host after inducing injury and, therefore, are less frequently caught by the patient.

This chapter provides an approach to the diagnosis, treatment, and epidemiology of arthropod-induced lesions. The lesion itself and its clinical history suggest general patterns of arthroparasitism or arthropod transience. Pictures of injurious arthropods are found in the reference books listed under "Recommended Reading."

ARTHROPARASITES OF HUMANS

Arthroparasites reside within or on the surface of humans or in their immediate environment for at least one stage in the arthropod life cycle. They can be invasive like larval flies or certain mites, or they can be hematophagous. Hematophagous parasites either remain in intimate contact with people (e.g., hard ticks) or reside on body hair or clothing (e.g., fleas and lice). Infestations are generally continuous or recurrent. Most arthroparasites primarily affect animals (zoophilic); they infest humans when people enter the animal-arthroparasite environment. On the other hand, several arthroparasites primarily infest humans (anthropophilic).

MYIASIS (TABLE 58-1)

Myiasis is due to infestation of human tissue by larvae of higher flies (Cyclorrhapha). In general, larvae are deposited by female adult flies as eggs or first-instar larvae. Larvae develop in host tissue and leave as mature, third-instar larvae to pupate away from the host. Fly larvae, or maggots, have been observed in festering wounds, ulcers, sores, and various body orifices; maggot infestations observed include nasal, aural, enteric, vaginal, and urinary tract infestations. Although certain species are noted for their ability to debride necrotic tissue, others can extend into and injure live tissue as well as induce secondary bacterial infection. Once removed, the wound is maggot-free unless fly eggs remain or adults deposit additional eggs or larvae.

There are three general patterns of myiasis dependency among flies. These patterns reflect larval conditions required for development and subsequent completion of a generation. One group requires the rich nutrient environment of animal tissue for larval development. Such flies generally feed poorly as adults so that the major nutritive intake is via the larva. Those flies which depend on myiasis (obligatory myiasis) include oestrids, cuterebrids, and gastrophilids as well as several

Table 58-1. Human myiasis

Lesion	Infesting fly	Clinical presentation	Complications
Furuncular myiasis	Human botfly (*Dermatobia hominis*)	Pruritic erythematous papule progressing to tender furuncles with draining central sinuses	Transient sharp pain, regional lymphadenopathy. CNS invasion in infants (rare)
	Tumbu fly (*Cordylobia anthropophaga*)	Erythematous and pruritic furuncles which may resemble impetigo, chickenpox, or scabies	Fever, malaise, ulceration in malnourished individuals, skin necrosis with numerous juxtaposed lesions
	Rodent and rabbit botflies (*Cuterebra* spp.)	Stinging or itching sensation. Papule evolving into a furuncle	
Migratory integumomyiasis	Horse botflies (*Gasterophilus intestinalis* and *G. haemorrhoidalis*)	Erythematous and pruritic cutaneous tracks which are distinctly serpiginous. Recurrent lesions can be nodular with pustular centers containing larvae.	Rare penetration into deeper structures such as pulmonary tissue where larvae can form coinlike lesions.
	Cattle botfly (*Hypoderma bovis*)	Migratory, localized swellings which are erythematous and painful. Migration is generally cephalad. Mature larvae cease migrating, inducing a furuncular swelling (warble) from which they emerge.	Rare invasion into CNS and eye tissue
Wound myiasis	Obligatory myiasis: 1. Primary or new world screwworm [(*Callitroga americana* or *Cochliomyia hominivorax*) Calliphoridae]	Pocketlike lesions of furuncles	Extensive local destruction. Secondary bacterial infection
	2. Old worm screwworm [(*Chrysomya bezziana*) Calliphoridae]	Shallow wounds produced by early instar maggots. Later instars are more invasive.	Same as above
	3. *Wohlfahrtia magnifica* (Sarcophagidae)	Invasive wound myiasis	Same as above
	Facultative myiasis: 1. Green bottle fly [(*Phaenicia-Lucilia sericata*) Calliphoridae]	Maggot-infested wounds	Occasional fistula formation. Secondary bacterial infection
	2. House fly [(*Musca domestica*) Muscidae]		
	3. Black blowfly [(*Phormia regina*) Calliphoridae] and others		

calliphorids and sarcophagids. In general, these larvae invade host tissues. Animals other than humans are the major hosts for this group of insects.

The most common human parasite is the human botfly (*Dermatobia hominis*). These large, neotropical flies oviposit onto other arthropods, typically mosquitoes. The botfly eggs hatch

Table 58-1. Human myiasis (*Continued*)

Treatment	Epidemiology	Prevention	Distribution
Apply animal fat to promote larva exit Surgical removal with care *not* to violate larval cuticle.	Gravid flies oviposit onto a second arthropod. Eggs hatch when the phoretic arthropod lands upon a human host. The resulting larvae enter the human skin via the phoretic arthropod's bite wound or by directly perforating the skin.	Phorid fly exposure reduced by insect repellent and nocturnal mosquito netting	Central America, North America, South America, Caribbean (visitors from above areas)
Mineral oil application to promote larval egress Gentle squeezing; surgical debridement may be necessary	Gravid flies oviposit onto urine-stained, sweat-stained, or wet clothing and urine-soaked earth. Newly hatched larvae penetrate host skin. Rodents are natural hosts.	Larvae exposure reduced by ironing clothes, drying clothes in screen-protected areas, and avoiding soil contact. Rodent control reduces fly population.	Africa
Manual expression or surgical evacuation of the larva	Flies oviposit onto vegetation or rocks near rabbit or rodent hosts. Human infestation results from accidental contact with contaminated objects.		North America
Excision of larva which is visualized beyond the erythematous tract by applying mineral oil	Gravid flies oviposit onto horse hair. Eggs or larvae transferred to people brushing against infested horse hair. Ranchers, equestrians at risk	Deet-sprayed, full-length pants and shirt sleeves worn around infested animals reduces larval transfer.	Widely dispersed
Excision	Gravid flies oviposit onto cattle hair. Eggs and larvae are transferred to people brushing against infested hair. Ranchers, dairy farmers at risk	Same as above	Widely dispersed
Larval removal and debridement. Wound exploration to locate all invading maggots	Gravid females oviposit near wounds on cattle and humans. Human patients tend to cluster around stockyards and ranches.	Cover wounds. Avoid sleeping outdoors in endemic areas.	South America, Central America, and southern North America
Same as above	Gravid flies oviposit inside the rim of wounds or onto unbroken skin above abscesses or hematomas. Infestations of head wounds most common. Cattle, peridomestic animals, as well as humans can be infested.	Same as above	Africa, southern Asia (especially India)
Same as above	Ground flies larviposit onto wounds	Same as above	Mediterranean region, central Europe, Asia
Same as above	Gravid flies oviposit onto wounds	Screen living quarters; wounds clean and covered	Widely dispersed

when the mosquito, or phoretic host, lands on a human host. The newly hatched larva then burrows into the human host's skin. The larva may be surgically removed, although care must be taken not to violate larval cuticle. Insect repellents reduce exposure to the phoretic arthropod.

A second form of myiasis requires less strict larval conditions. In this form, facultative myiasis, larvae can complete development in decaying animal or vegetable material or excrement, for adult flies generally ingest richer diets. However, these flies also ovi- or larviposit onto necrotic tissue, purulent sores, and open wounds. Indeed, facultative fly larvae can infest most skin insults including arthropod bites, malignancies, vascular-compromised skin, and surgically exposed areas such as tracheostomy sites. Although these maggots debride necrotic tissue, they can invade surrounding tissue, extending wounds and creating fissures. Larval infestations progress in wounds which are concealed such as those bandaged for prolonged periods, covered by necrotic tissue, or poorly visualized by the patient. Facultative myiasis is common among calliphorids, sarcophagids, and muscids. The third category of myiasis dependency, accidental myiasis, includes insects whose larvae are inadvertently introduced to areas of the body, such as the gastrointestinal tract, which do not generally support larval development.

Myiasis can be defined by the tissue affected or lesion produced (Table 58-1). In addition, maggot identification helps to establish the natural history of infestations, guiding the physician to limit further patient exposure. Maggots are usually identified by their posterior spiracles. Larval flies can also be reared on sheep blood agar and identified as adults. All stages of these flies may play an important role in forensic investigations [1].

ACARIASIS

Ticks and mites (Acarina) directly induce a variety of clinical manifestations in humans which can be uncomfortable and occasionally life-threatening. Injury-inducing acarines are generally located on the person or in the dwelling. However, it may be difficult to locate the infesting arthropods due to their minute size. A closely focused clinical history and skin examination, as well as home searches, may be necessary to locate infestations.

Tick bites

Hard ticks (Ixodidae) blood-feed for extended periods of time while soft ticks (Argasidae) feed faster. Although infrequent, hard ticks can induce systemic effects such as fever and paralysis, whereas soft ticks produce primarily local reactions.

Bites by hard ticks are generally innocuous and rarely reach the attention of physicians. Most individuals simply pull off attached ticks without complication. Prolonged feeding is made possible by painless attachment to the host. During tick attachment, host reaction is generally minimal, although small

pruritic and erythematous nodules occasionally form. Such nodules, which are characterized by local edema and an eosinophilic infiltrate, generally resolve without sequelae. Tick bite complications are generally rare but comprise the major portion of tick bites presented to physicians. Complications include cutaneous reaction to the bite, nonspecific cutaneous reaction to scratching, secondary infection, and systemic manifestations. Several types of cutaneous reactions may result. Minute eosinophilic nodules occasionally enlarge for extended periods following tick removal. Chronic nodules, or "tick granuloma," can be as wide as 3 cm in diameter. In certain cases, nodules may be darker than surrounding skin and contain central depressions. Hypostome removal does not alter nodule progression. More severe cutaneous reactions are vesicular in appearance and are characterized by an intense polymorphonuclear infiltration. Such reactions may be mediated in part by chemoattractant products derived from host complement [2]. Tick bites can precipitate secondary bacterial infection localized to the area of attachment or it may expand into cellulitis or lymphangitis.

Tick bites can also elicit systemic manifestations. One such reaction, tick-induced fever or tick pyrexia, is associated with malaise, headache, nausea, and vomiting. Symptoms resolve within $1\frac{1}{2}$ days after tick removal. Tick bites can also induce systemic anaphylaxis as well as regional edema. Paralysis is an extreme systemic manifestation of tick bite; it is an ascending symmetrical, flaccid paralysis which can progress to respiratory failure if not corrected [3]. Prodrome begins 5 to 7 days after tick attachment and includes general malaise, appetite loss, fever, headache, stomach cramps, and vomiting. This is followed by dyscoordination and reduced deep tendon reflexes in the lower extremities. Symptoms progress to weakness and subsequent paralysis of the lower extremities which evolve over several days to include upper limbs, torso, and cranial nerves. Ticks attached behind the ear may induce Bell's palsy. Time course for symptoms may be accelerated in children. Tick removal reverses paralysis, symptoms subsiding within an hour and complete recovery occurring over several days. Ticks tend to reside in hair-abundant body regions, obscuring their presence and requiring a thorough search. Tick-induced paralysis is a motor polyneuropathy with limited alteration in afferent pathways. The mechanism may involve compromised function in large motor nerves as well as at the neuromuscular junction [4].

Tick paralysis is most commonly associated with bites by females of several tick species. The American dog tick, *Dermacentor variabilis,* and the Rocky Mountain wood tick, *D. andersoni,* are most frequently associated with tick paralysis in North America. The lone star tick, *Amblyomma americanum,* and the black-legged tick, *Ixodes scapularis,* have induced bite-associated paralysis in southeastern United States. Bites by scrub ticks, *Ixodes holocyclus,* are associated with paralysis in Australia, while those of *Amblyomma ovale* are associated with paralysis in Central America.

Tick removal entails firmly retracting the tick from host skin [5]. Remaining mouthparts are usually walled off, presenting little problem to the host. Ticks should be removed by forceps rather than by hand to prevent possible rickettsial contact. Treating attached ticks with irritants or other chemicals is generally not helpful in promoting removal. In endemic areas, ticks should be searched for and removed daily. Long pants and sleeves reduce tick exposure. Deet (diethyltoluamide)-treated clothes may further diminish contact [6].

Soft tick or argasid bites are generally painless and lesions are time-limited. Initially, small macules appear. Papules, or bullae, which develop over a day, are circumscribed by erythema and hyperemia. Extensive bruising may also accompany bites. Although lesions are generally painless with minimal pruritus, certain soft tick species induce pain during biting. Histologically, lesions develop central necrotic foci and are characterized by edema and vascular congestion. Cellular infiltration is minimal. Grossly, lesions diminish in size over 2 weeks to small indurated macules. Sensitized individuals may experience systemic reactions and localized necrosis. Closely approximated bites may induce more extensive necrosis. Treatment for argasid bite lesions is conservative. Lesions should be kept clean and tetanus toxoid administered if needed. Systemic reactions may require antihistamine or, in extreme cases, epinephrine. Necrotic areas may require debridement, and secondary bacterial infection is contained with antibiotics.

Soft ticks exploit habitual activities of their hosts because they are nest or domicile parasites. Soft ticks frequent cracks in walls and floors as well as thatched roofs, biting occupants while they sleep. Argasids may be moved between dwellings via rugs or mats. Zoophilic argasids tend to concentrate in burrows, clearings, or caves frequented by various animals. People may be exposed by reposing near such areas. Attachment time is generally short. Although larvae may feed for a week, more mature forms feed for several minutes. Blood meals are small so that nymphs and adults feed frequently.

Mite infestation

Mites are ubiquitous acarines which are generally unobtrusive. However, there are several mite species which induce cutaneous discomfort. Particular species are unique to humans, such as the human scabies mite (*Sarcoptes scabiei f. scabiei*), while other mite species reside near or on animals and infest people incidentally. These include nest-acquired mites, field-acquired mites, food-acquired mites, and animal-transferred mites.

Scabies

Scabies is an infestation by the human scabies mite. This mite induces a pruritic skin eruption which occurs in two stages. The first is produced by burrowing female mites and is marked by blanched and tortuous, threadlike channels. Mite feces give a peppered appearance to the channels, while the burrowing mite itself is pearl-shaped and located at the channel terminus. Lesions tend to be symmetrical and localized to folds between fingers, on wrists and feet, at elbow extensor surfaces, in axillae, under breasts, and on the penis and scrotum. In bedridden individuals, lesions may be localized to sheet contact sites. Although there can be up to 15 burrowing females on hosts at a given time, the newly fertilized female is the infective form, spreading infestation between individuals. Mite infestations are diagnosed by skin scrapings. The second stage of the scabies rash is more obvious and extremely irritating. Small pruritic and erythematous papules and vesicles develop several weeks after the onset of initial symptoms. Lesions are edematous and tend to occur in areas separate from burrowing female mites such as the buttocks, scapulae, and abdomen. Pruritus is worse at night, and scratching induces secondary bacterial infection and eczematous skin changes. Occasionally, hypersensitive individuals develop pruritic nodules which persist. These nodules locate in covered areas such as the groin or axillae. Less commonly, a mite infestation becomes widespread [7]. Patients with this form of scabies, Norwegian scabies, develop thick crusted lesions containing numerous burrows and mites, rendering this condition highly contagious. Similar to the more common form of scabies, a diffuse papular rash develops in body regions separate from mite infestation. Pruritus tends to be minimal, but an eosinophilia may be present.

Treatment of choice is 10% crotamiton applied topically [8]. Initial bathing removes crusts and debris to permit more even distribution of crotamiton. Alternative treatments include lindane, benzyl benzoate, and sulfur in petroleum. All are applied topically; however, lindane is applied only once. Lindane can be neurotoxic and should be avoided in children and pregnant women. Simultaneous application of creams or oils with lindane should be avoided because they potentiate cutaneous penetration of lindane. All contacts should be treated. It is particularly important to treat recent contacts as they may harbor contagious mites without obvious skin lesions.

Scabies is distributed worldwide. Endemic areas tend to localize in population concentrations, especially where hygiene is minimal. Epidemics seem to occur in cycles which may reflect migrations, disasters, and/or changes in community immunity. Although the exact role of immunity is unclear in scabies, patients develop circulating immune complexes after infestation [9].

HEMIPTERAN INFESTATIONS

Bites by bedbugs (Cimicidae) and kissing bugs (Reduviidae) induce uncomfortable skin lesions. Human-biting species inhabit dwellings where nymphal forms and adults generally procure blood at night. These true bugs sequester in cracks and crevices, producing a sweet, musty odor.

Bedbug bites are generally annoying but rarely serious. Bites may elicit a slight tingling sensation and induce subsequent wheals or papules. However, most individuals experience minute erythematous spots. Delayed, erythematous papules are usually painless and may last for weeks. Lesions are generally clustered on the legs, buttocks, or shoulders. Flecks of blood may be observed on the bed linen. Bedbugs reside in bed mattresses and furniture as well as in floor and wall cracks near host-frequented areas. They spread to new dwellings via beds, couches, and mattresses. Bedbugs can also infest areas frequented by birds and bats. The common bedbug (*Cimex lectularius*) is distributed worldwide, while the tropical bedbug (*C. hemipterus*) inhabits warmer climates. *Leptocimex boueti* is restricted to west Africa.

Bedbug control is difficult over prolonged periods. Insecticides initially control bedbug populations; however, long-term control is made difficult by insecticide resistance.

Kissing bugs can produce more severe bite lesions than bedbugs. Bites are usually painless or accompanied by a tingling sensation. Early lesions induce little reaction or transient urticarial wheals; rarely, systemic anaphylaxis occurs. Delayed reactions can be severe. These lesions are usually vesicles or pruritic papules with central puncta. However, hemorrhagic bullae can also form, inducing localized edema and infection. These tend to occur on the feet or hands ("hand-foot syndrome") and may be accompanied by lymphangitis. Repeated bites by *Rhodnius prolixus* can induce skin necrosis. Bite lesions tend to be grouped and occur most frequently on the hands, arms, feet, head, and trunk. Reduviid bites are treated symptomatically. Antihistamines reduce swelling, although steroids or epinephrine may be indicated in extreme reactions. Hemorrhagic bullae are more difficult to treat, requiring bed rest, elevation, local heat, and antibiotics if infected.

Anthropophagic reduviids generally infest dwellings. Although certain species may have commensal and sylvian varieties, the major cause of discomfort are domestic reduviids. These insects thrive in mud and stick dwellings, feeding on both people and domestic animals. The walls of heavily infested dwellings are frequently stained by bug feces. Domestic reduviids are common in South and Central America and can be found as far north as southwestern United States. *Triatoma rubrofasciata* has been introduced in Africa, Asia, and Hawaii. Reduviid populations can be reduced temporarily by residual insecticides.

FLEA INFESTATIONS

Most human-biting fleas are nest-dwelling arthroparasites. They include zoophilic species which attack people in the absence of their usual host.

Nest-infesting fleas

Nest-infesting fleas generally bite the ankles and arms of their human hosts. Bites can be irritating but are seldom serious. There is usually an immediate urticaria and erythema which may evolve into papules marked by central puncta. Such papules remain pruritic for extended periods. Hypersensitive individuals may develop vesicles or bullae. Treatment is symptomatic. Antihistamines and corticosteroids reduce urticaria.

Nest-infesting fleas reside in the habitual resting places of their hosts as well as on the host. Dog and cat fleas (*Ctenocephalides canis* and *C. felis*) commonly infest domestic pets, while rat fleas (such as *Xenopsylla cheopis*) generally infest rodents. Larval fleas remain in the nest where they ingest host feces and debris but depend upon the added nutrient of host blood defecated into the nest by host-infesting adult fleas. Humans are bitten by animal-infesting fleas when entering an abandoned nest area where adult fleas are seeking an alternate blood source. The number of host-seeking fleas intensifies if the usual host is denied access to the nest. The human flea (*Pulex irritans*) infests human bedding or furniture as well as a variety of domestic animals. This flea can be a problem in dwellings where humidity remains adequate for flea development in bedding elevated above the ground. Human fleas, therefore, do poorly in houses with central heating, which tends to dry ambient air.

Flea control depends upon disrupting the nest environment. Both adult and larval fleas can be removed from animal bedding by frequent vacuuming or insecticide. Animals should be kept away from infested areas to prevent reintroduction. Insecticide-laden collars are most effective when worn by the host animals around infested nests. Similarly, human fleas can also be eliminated by insecticide treatment of infested areas.

Burrowing fleas

Chigoe fleas (*Tunga penetrans*) are hematophagous insects which procure blood by burrowing into host tissue. Human infestations frequently occur in the feet where fleas burrow under toenails, between toes, and in plantar surfaces [10]. Such infestations are referred to as tungiasis. Imbedded fleas frequently present as pruritic white papules with central black depressions. Fleas can expand to pea-size volumes while imbibing host blood and thereby produce painful subungual infestations. Prolonged infestations can induce bacterial infection, tetanus, and in extreme cases digital autoamputation. Chigoe fleas should be removed promptly. Early during attachment, fleas can be removed with a sterile needle. Later, lesions should be enlarged with a scalpel to expedite flea removal.

Chigoe fleas are found in tropical areas of Africa as well as South and Central America. The life cycle combines a soil habitat for immature forms with the adult parasitic-host relationship. Flea eggs are extruded by imbedded, gravid fleas onto soil where larvae develop and pupate. Larvae thrive in sandy soil or in the floor dust of human dwellings. Resultant adult fleas locate and attach to unprotected feet from which males detach soon after imbibing blood, but females burrow deeply into host tissues. Exposure can be minimized by wearing shoes.

LICE INFESTATIONS

The human louse (*Pediculus humanus*) has two varieties, each with its own particular niche. The body louse (*P. humanus humanus*) infests clothes, while the head louse (*P. humanus capitis*) infests the scalp (and other hair-abundant body areas during heavy infestations). A second species, the pubic louse (*Phthirus pubis*), generally resides in genital areas but may infest other body regions.

Body lice produce intensely irritating skin lesions. Pruritic wheals and macules result from louse-injected saliva and are easily infected by scratching. Prolonged infestations induce hardened, yellow macules referred to as vagabond's disease. Body lice are heat-sensitive and therefore reside in clothing. They are most common in clothing which remains close to the skin such as at the waistline, genital region, shoulders, and axillae. Lice contact the host body to procure blood. Mature females deposit about 7 to 10 eggs per day in clothing seams and occasionally on body hair. The nymphal stages are also hematophagous and reside in similar habitats as adults.

Body lice are found worldwide, occurring when clothes are worn continuously and bathing is infrequent. Lice transfer occurs when people are crowded and is potentiated by host fever. Infestations are eliminated by clothing sterilization and bathing. Clothes are deloused by heating or fumigation. Bathing removes most extraneous lice, whereas shaving the back and chest eliminates most of the eggs oviposited onto body hair. Residual insecticide may be necessary for widespread infestations.

Head lice induce scalp lesions which are morphologically similar to those produced by body lice. Infestations are characterized by pruritic wheals and macules, pustules, matted hair, nits (hair-attached eggs), and lice. In lighter manifestations, nits can be confused with other scalp and hair conditions [11]. School-aged girls experience the highest prevalence of head lice. Head lice are transferred by contact and are potentiated by long hair. Infestations are discouraged by frequent combing and eliminated by shampoos containing lindane, malathion, or pyrethrins [12].

Pubic lice produce intensely pruritic lesions which are characterized by hair-attached nits, minute lice, and crusted blood accumulated around lice and in underwear. Prolonged infestations can induce blue macules. Infestations occur in the perirectal or genital regions, although lice can also reside on eyelashes, axillary hair, and beards. Whereas body lice are mobile, pubic lice remain attached to body hair for extended periods. Infestations are eliminated by lindane preparations. Lice generally transfer between people during sexual contact.

FACE FLIES

Face flies (*Musca* spp.) and eye gnats (Chloropidae: *Siphunculina* spp., Asia; *Hippelates* spp., Americas) congregate around the head and open sores of people. They feed primarily on secretions and exudate; although rarely, they further ex-coriate existing lesions. Swatting does not deter these flies which, in many warmer regions, stud the heads of adults and children. Control is difficult.

PENTASTOMIASIS

Pentastomiasis is an infestation by tongue worms (Pentastomida, or Linguatulida). Tongue worms are mitelike organisms which also resemble annelids. However, they are generally referred to as a discrete group without definite affinity. Pentastomes are endoparasitic in animals and people, inducing in humans two general clinical entities, nasopharyngeal linguatulosis [13] and visceral porocephalosis (Table 58-2).

TRANSIENT ARTHROPOD PESTS

Arthropods can injure people during brief encounters. Attacks usually occur without warning, and the victim is generally unable to describe the arthropod attacker accurately. However, a victim's history may be informative, providing information about setting, time of day, and early tissue reaction. Previous reactions to arthropod-induced injury can be revealing. The lesion itself and its distribution may help incriminate an arthropod type. Serious attention should be given to arthropod-induced lesions because sequelae may ensue hours to several days following actual contact.

Transient arthropod-induced injury can be elicited via inhalant allergens, contact substances, and bite- or sting-injected toxins. Inhalant allergens include airborne fragments derived from arthropod bodies, whereas contact exposure transfers secretion directly or via arthropod spines. Arthropod bites can disrupt superficial skin as well as inject potentially irritating saliva. On the other hand, arthropod stings pierce victim skin via posterior station apparatus providing access to inject venom. Transferred toxins may injure tissue directly or initiate systemic reactions. Disrupted tissue can become secondarily infected.

INHALANT ALLERGENS

Arthropod-derived particles can become airborne and induce bronchospasm, conjunctival irritation, and rhinitis as well as pruritic skin eruptions. Such particles derive from arthropod scales, hairs (or setae), pulverized exuvia, and feces. These fragments can be extremely debilitating to sensitized individuals exposed to emergences of insects (such as mayflies), fluttering moths, or particle-laden dust. Prevention depends upon the allergenic source. Desensitization may be useful if the allergen is known. Insect control can be beneficial if allergens derive from certain household pests such as cockroaches. Dust control limits dust mite populations.

CONTACT IRRITANTS

Irritating substances can be transferred from arthropods to humans by direct contact, inducing localized as well as systemic

Table 58-2. Human pentastomiasis

Lesion	Infesting pentastomid	Clinical presentation	Complications
Nasopharyngeal linguatulosis	*Linguatula serrata*	Foreign body sensation in throat which may progress to lacerating pain. Coughing, sneezing, hoarseness, facial edema, nasal discharge. Occasional nasal discharge of white nymphs	Edema of the upper airway. Abscesses. Internal ophthalmomyiasis
Visceral porocephaliasis	*Armillifer armillatus* *Armillifer moniliformis*	Incidental findings at necropsy. Calcified crescent appearance radiographically (3–6 mm in length)	Abdominal adhesions, bronchial obstruction, and nerve compression

manifestations. Contact toxicants coat the bodies of certain millipedes, reside within setae of various moths, and may be contained within the bodies of beetles.

Millipede toxin causes a tingling sensation and slight skin darkening [14]. Skin color subsequently turns mahogany or purple, and blistering may occur within 1 to 2 days. Exfoliated blisters are easily infected. Millipede toxin which is transferred to the eyes causes a chemical conjunctivitis that is marked by periorbital edema and discharge and which may evolve to frank ulceration. Skin lesions should be washed with copious amounts of water or alcohol to remove residual toxin. Lesions should be kept clean to prevent secondary infection. Eye lesions should be irrigated with warm water and local anesthetic. Fluorescein dye localizes corneal ulcers to which atropine and an antibiotic are applied. Eye patching reduces further injury, and cold compresses diminish periorbital edema. Children are the most susceptible group, handling millipedes and transferring surface toxin to their eyes and face. Sleeping individuals may also be exposed during nocturnal forays by millipedes. One millipede species, *Rhinochrichus lethifer,* can project toxic secretions up to 50 cm. Millipedes generally reside in moist places, especially in superficial soil layers and forest litter where they feed on decaying vegetation.

Caterpillars and adult moths can possess irritating spines (setae or hair) which contain or are connected to specialized venom-producing tissue. Urticating setae induce injury by injecting irritant when embedded in skin. Exposure is usually by direct contact; however, spines can become airborne. The initial penetration of skin by urticating hairs is generally painful. Hair-injected toxin produces pruritic, erythematous patches which may be associated with small vesicles, papules, or edema. Lesions occasionally become petechial and may be accompanied by localized neuritis. Skin lesions are generally restricted to areas of direct contact; or in the case of airborne

contact, to the collar, abdominal flanks, axillae, inner thighs, and feet. Airborne contact may additionally induce pharyngitis and conjunctivitis. Systemic manifestations such as nausea, vomiting, lethargy, urticaria, muscle cramping, and headaches may result from urticating hair-induced injury. Adhesive tape will remove urticating hairs while alkaline compresses reduce initial symptoms [15]. Parenteral calcium gluconate temporarily relieves cramping, and antihistamines and steroids limit the reaction process. It is advisable to wash exposed clothes or bed linen which may harbor additional urticating hairs.

Caterpillar-induced injury is called *erucism,* while adult moth-induced injury is called *lepidopterism.* Both forms are widely dispersed. In warmer climates, agricultural workers are at risk. However, in temperate regions, setae may become airborne during major forest infestations. Occasionally caterpillars transfer urticating hairs onto pupae or cocoons and adults transfer hairs onto egg masses, rendering these forms urticating as well. Rarely, other arthropods such as spiders possess urticating hairs.

Members of several beetle families can induce vesicular lesions when crushed and smeared across human skin. Hemolymph and particular tissues of such insects contain irritating substances such as cantharidin (Meloidae, blister beetles) and pederin (Staphylinidae, *Paederus* spp.) which rapidly penetrate epidermis. Initially, tingling or burning occurs at the lesion site. The type of the subsequent skin reaction is dependent upon the family of the injury-inducing beetle. For example, the oedemerids (coconut beetles) can induce severe blistering, while crushed staphylinids induce urticaria and blistering. In extreme reactions, vesicles become painful and purulent within 2 days. Toxicant entering eyes produces a severe conjunctivitis. Lesion sites should be washed with copious amounts of water after initial exposure and subsequently kept clean. Early administration of steroids generally reduces reaction intensity.

Table 58-2. Human pentastomiasis (*Continued*)

Treatment	Epidemiology	Prevention	Distribution
Remove nymphal forms from nose and pharynx. Antihistamines to reduce pharyngeal and facial edema. Drainage of abcesses. Systemic antibiotics	Encysted nymphal forms reside in mesentery of intermediate host herbivores (sheep, cattle). Nymphs excyst when ingested by definitive hosts such as canines, felines, and humans. Nymphs ascend the esophagus and attach in the upper airway including nose and pharynx. Mature adults oviposit into oral and nasal secretion.	Cook liver and mesentery. Restrict raw viscera consumption by dogs.	Middle East: Lebanon—infestation referred to as ''halzoun'' Sudan—infestation referred to as ''marrara''
Symptomatic	Snakes probably harbor adult forms. When snake is ingested by humans, nymphs excyst and penetrate the intestine, encysting in the abdominal cavity.	Cook snake meat.	Central Africa, Asia, Malaysia

ARTHROPOD BITES

Arthropods can induce injury by biting. Bite injuries tend to be local, but they can expand to regional or systemic reactions (Figs. 58-1 and 58-2). Indeed, certain spider bites elicit limited local reactions but have potentially severe systemic effects. Bite lesions are induced by injected venom, as with spiders (Arachnida) and centipedes (Chilopoda); by injected saliva, as with biting flies (Diptera); or by skin excoriation, as with biting flies.

Spiders procure prey and defend themselves by injecting venom through adapted mouthparts, chelicerae. Only a few spider species can perforate human skin and thereby inject venom (Table 58-3). The most harmful of these include true spiders (suborder Labidognatha) such as widow spiders (*Lactrodectus* spp.), brown spiders (*Loxosceles* spp.), and the wandering or banana spider (*Phoneutria nigriventer*), as well as mygalomorphs (Mygalomorphae) like the funnel-web spiders (including *Atrax* spp.) and *Harpactirella* spp. Other spiders can induce more restricted lesions. Spider-injected venoms which produce systemic effects should be contained to the bite site. One effective method of containment has been demon-

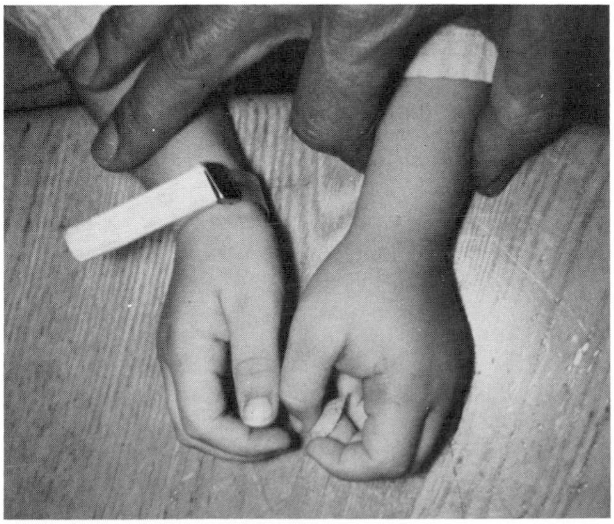

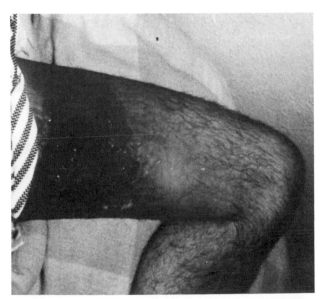

Figure 58-1. Swelling on the left hand of a child 4 h following the bite of a black widow spider, *Latrodectus mactans*. (*Courtesy of Dr. F. E. Russell, Univ. of Arizona.*)

Figure 58-2. Necrotic lesion on the thigh of an adult a week following the bite of a brown recluse spider, *Loxosceles* sp. (*Courtesy of Dr. F. E. Russell, Univ. of Arizona.*)

Table 58-3. Spider envenomation

Bite-induced syndrome	Spider species	Clinical manifestations	Complications	Treatment	Epidemiology	Distribution
Latrodectism	Widow spiders (6 species) such as black widow spiders (*Latrodectus mactans* sub spp.)	Painless bite followed by tender regional lymphadenopathy within several hours. Painful muscle rigidity, cramping of abdominal muscles, thighs, glutei, and back (mimics acute abdomen). Facies latrodectismica (diaphoretic erythema, periorbital edema, blepharoconjunctivitis, and painful grimace). Nausea, fever, sleeplessness, tachypnea, and hyperreflexia. Leukocytosis	Tachycardia, bradycardia, hypotension, ECG changes, albuminuria, scarlatiniform exanthum, death in small children and elderly or compromised adults	Antivenin 5 mL SC or IM with initial signs of systemic illness. A second dose 1 h later is given if symptoms progress. Systemic steroids or epinephrine may be necessary for anaphylaxis or serum sickness. Parenteral calcium gluconate reduces muscle spasm. Propranolol controls tachycardia and related arrhythmias	Only female widow spiders are poisonous. They are reclusive, residing in their webs. They are more aggressive if guarding an egg sac. Rural spiders locate webs beside stones, along trenches, in tree hollows and bushes. In North America, black widow spiders are more urbanized, inhabiting sheds, basements, privies	Worldwide
Loxoscelism	1. Brown spiders (*Loxosceles* spp.) 2. Brown recluse spider (*L. reclusa*) 3. South American brown recluse spider (*L. laeta*)	Several hours after envenomation, the bite becomes painful with development of erythema and a bite-localized blister. Lesion may ulcerate. Fever, chills, nausea, arthralgia	Skin sloughing. Destruction of adjacent tissues such as supporting ligaments or urethra after peroneal bites. Hemolysis; thrombocytopenia; renal failure. Severe reactions can be fatal.	Systemic steroids administered early in the first day. Heparin for disseminated intravascular coagulation	Outdoor spiders which frequently invade houses. They reside in lumber or brick piles, stored boxes, closets, and damp basements. Inactive during the day. Bites occur by disturbing secluded spiders during the day or by rolling onto foraging spiders at night. Dispersal widened when spiders sequester in boxes which are transported	1. Widely dispersed 2. Southern and eastern U.S. 3. South America, Central America, southern North America

Phoneutrism	Banana or wandering spider (*Phoneutria nigriventer*)	Painful bite. Salivation, visual disturbances, vertigo, diaphoresis, prostration. Priapism	Hypotension, hypothermia, respiratory paralysis	Antivenin	Spiders do not spin webs but forage at night for food. They commonly enter human dwellings and sequester themselves in shoes and clothes. People are bitten by rolling onto questing spiders or by failing to remove them from garments. Cornered spiders bite repeatedly.	South and Central America
Funnel-web envenomation	Sydney funnel-web spider (*Atrax robustus*)	Muscle fasciculation, salivation, lacrimation, diaphoresis, agitation	Pulmonary edema, hypotension	Antivenin, phenytoin	Spider bites occur most frequently during mating season when spiders wander and enter houses. Males are most voracious.	Sydney, Australia; New Zealand
Harpactirella envenomation	*Harpactirella lightfooti*	Burning pain at the bite area. Nausea, vomiting	Hypotension	*Latrodectus* antivenin protects experimentally bitten mice	Spiders forage actively for food and thereby enter houses. Webs are spun under logs, stones, and debris. People encounter spiders in dwellings or by disturbing webs.	South Africa
House spider bites	*Chiracanthium mildei*	Necrotizing skin lesions	Secondary infection	Keep wounds clean. Antibiotics for infection	Found in thickets in Europe; enter cars and houses in autumn in North America.	
Wolf sider bites	*Lycosa* spp.	Local pain, edema, short-term ischemia	Necrosis	Same	Found in gardens, fields, occasionally enter human dwellings	South, Central, and North America and Europe
Tarantism	"Tarantulas" or bird spiders (Therophosidae)	Usually none	Generally harmless		Usually large, haircovered, and ground-associated.	Widely distributed

strated for bites by Sydney funnel-web spiders [*16*]. Venom is restricted to the bite by applying a pressure bandage over the spider bite and immobilizing the affected extremity via splinting. This technique combined with antivenin administration should reduce envenomation morbidity. Contact with spiders can be reduced by shaking out clothing and boots and by examining bedding. In addition, clearing debris and wood or brick piles limits concealment. Furthermore, screened doors and windows discourage spider entry into houses.

Certain centipedes can pierce human skin with anterior poison claws or maxillipeds. Injected venom is intensely painful and may induce localized necrosis, lymphangitis, and regional edema. Limited generalized symptoms may occur such as headache, vertigo, and vomiting. Bites are usually not lethal, and treatment is palliative. Centipedes inhabit damp and secluded areas such as the undersurfaces of stones, in crevices, in forest litter, or under tree bark. Some reside in caves. Indoors, they are found in damp basements, under sinks, or in water closets. Since centipedes are nocturnal predators, they can be a nuisance to sleeping campers. Centipede exposure is reduced by mosquito netting and sleeping platforms or cots. Human envenomation has been reported from southern United States, Philippines, New Guinea, Crimea, and South America.

Biting flies can inflict painful bites and irritating skin lesions. Host reactions are usually limited to the bite site but may progress to include larger areas. Bites can also initiate systemic reactions. There are three medically important suborders of biting flies. Lower flies (Nematocera) are individually fragile insects whose adult females procure blood primarily for egg development. Lower flies include mosquitoes (Culicidae), sand flies (Phlebotomidae), biting midges (Ceratopogonidae), and blackflies (Simuliidae). Although bites are usually painless (with the exception of midge bites), they frequently induce pruritic skin eruptions. In contrast, bites by middle (Brachycera) and higher (Cyclorrhapha) flies are more painful and disruptive to host skin but less pruritic. Middle flies include horse- and deerflies (Tabanidae), while higher flies include tsetse and stable flies (Muscidae).

ARTHROPOD STINGS

Transient arthropod pests can injure people by injecting venom via a posterior sting. This sting pierces the victim's skin and transfers venom from sting-adjacent poison glands. Venom reactions are variable, depending upon the stinging arthropod and the size, health, and immunological status of the victim. Stinging arthropods include scorpions (Scorpionida), bees, vespid wasps, and ants (Hymenoptera).

Scorpion stings

Scorpion stings (Fig. 58-3) can cause local pain, hypesthesia, edema, and discoloration as well as a series of clinical manifestations leading to cardiovascular collapse. Early signs of systemic reaction include diaphoresis, pallor, salivation, con-

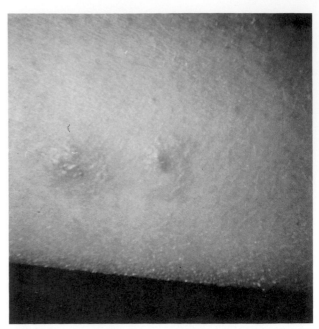

Figure 58-3. Local inflammatory reaction on the forearm of an adult 8 h following two repeated stings of a scorpion, *Vejovis spingerus.* (*Courtesy of Dr. F. E. Russell, Univ. of Arizona.*)

fusion, anxiety, nausea, abdominal cramps, and muscle fasciculations. Allergic reactions such as bronchial constriction may occur. A venom-induced catecholamine surge can induce hypertension and tachycardia with subsequent bradycardia. ECG may demonstrate infarctionlike patterns and conduction defects. In the most severe reactions, victims develop pulmonary edema and acute myocarditis. Hemolysis and acute renal failure may further complicate scorpion venom reactions. In a second type of scorpion envenomation, *Parabuthos* spp. can project venom toward a victim [*17*]. The severity of scorpion-induced reactions is dependent upon factors related to the victim as well as the arthropod. Adults in poor health and children tend to experience more life-threatening complications. Venom injected initially is less toxic than that subsequently injected [*18*]. Therefore, repeated stings are more dangerous because of increasing venom toxicity as well as a larger volume injected.

Initial treatment entails restricting venom to the bite area. Direct pressure bandage and extremity splinting would probably contain venom while lidocaine injection into the bite region will reduce pain. Antivenin, administered within several hours of the scorpion sting, reduces potential morbidity. However, antivenin is generally species specific. If the species is unknown, polyvalent preparations would be more useful. Serum sickness as well as anaphylaxis are hazards of antivenin use; concomitantly administered antihistamine could avert complications. Beta-adrenergic-blocking drugs control venom-induced, catecholamine-mediated manifestations. Eye envenomation is treated by washing the eye with scorpion antivenin diluted 10% in water. If not available, intensive saline washes should be used.

Dangerous scorpions are widely distributed in warmer climates. For example, three particularly venomous genera are found in southern Africa (*Parabuthos* spp., *Buthos* spp., and *Uroplectes* spp.) [*17*], while at least five (*Leiurus* spp., *Buthacus* spp., *Buthotus* spp., *Buthus* spp., and *Androctonus* spp.) are distributed in the Mediterranean region and Asia Minor; some extend further into southern Asia. One dangerous genus (*Tityus* spp.) is distributed in South America and Trinidad and another (*Centruroides* spp.) throughout central and southern North America.

Humans are most commonly exposed to scorpion stings when walking in infested areas without protective footwear. Scorpions are also encountered in shoes and clothes left exposed overnight. In addition, scorpions are generally nocturnal hunters and can enter low-level beds poorly protected by inadequate mosquito netting. Furthermore, individuals may be exposed to scorpion stings while lifting logs or rocks. Scorpions are occasionally trapped in empty bathtubs and showers. Scorpion encounters can be reduced by wearing boots, by shaking out footwear prior to use, by checking bed sheets at night before retiring, and by keeping mosquito netting well tucked.

Hymenoptera stings

Hymenoptera stings elicit reactions which are generally innocuous or localized; however, some allergic reactions can be systemic, rarely inducing severe morbidity and mortality due to allergic reactions. Sting sensitivity is more commonly observed after stings by honeybees (*Apis mellifera* sub spp.) and yellow jackets (*Vespula* spp. and *Dolichovespula* spp.) but may occur after stings by bumblebees (*Bombus* spp.), paper wasps (*Polistes* spp.), and hornets (*Vespa* spp.). Ant (Formicidae) stings tend to induce severe local reactions.

Honeybee stings generally induce transient local reactions (Fig. 58-4). The barbed stinger remains in the skin, thereby eviscerating the insect. Local reactions are usually painful and can be hyperemic and indurated. Dangerous reactions such as airway obstruction can result from stings to the neck and face. In addition, stings can induce anaphylaxis characterized by urticaria, malaise, weakness, chest tightness, nausea, vertigo, and cyanosis. Such reactions tend to be more severe in young adults and may occur without a previous systemic episode. Honeybee stings can also precipitate serum sickness, and multiple stings can be toxic.

The sting should be scraped from the lesion without squeezing the attached venom sac. Local pain can be reduced by cool compresses and local swelling can be reduced by topically applied antihistamine. Oral antihistamines reduce regional swelling, whereas both oral antihistamine and subcutaneous epinephrine should be administered promptly for airway ob-

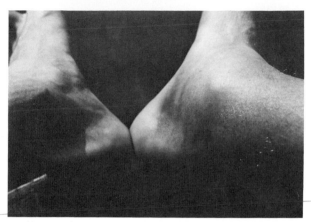

Figure 58-4. Edema and ecchymosis on the right ankle of an adult 24 h following the stings of three honeybees, *Apis mellifera*. (*Courtesy of D. Carmean, Oregon State Univ.*)

struction anaphylaxis. Patients do better when calm and resting in a cool area. Allergic individuals should be encouraged to carry beesting kits.

Bee venom contains at least two immunoreactive components, phospholipase A [*19*] and hyaluronidase [*20*]. In addition, three components—hyaluronidase, phospholipase A, and mast cell degranulation peptide—can disrupt mast cells. Mellitin, a major component of bee venom, induces local pain and inflammation. Bee venom also contains histamine, dopamine, and norepinephrine. Skin testing can be useful to identify sensitive individuals [*21*]. Desensitization using bee venom can be protective against subsequent stings; however, it can also induce anaphylaxis and should be performed with proper medical backup [*22*].

Honeybees comprise a complex of subspecies which are widely distributed and have varying aggressive natures. For example, the Carolina bee of eastern Europe (*A. m. carnica*) is nonaggressive, whereas African honeybees (*A. m. litorea* and *A. m. adansonii*) are ferocious. African honeybees were introduced into South America in 1957 and have retained their aggressive characteristics. They are successfully competing with indigenous bees as far north as Mexico.

Other hymenoptera, such as bumblebees, paper wasps, hornets, and yellow jackets, also sting people. These insects have pointed stings which are not retained in victim skin, so that individual insects can sting multiple times. Victim reactions and treatment are similar to those for honeybee stings. In addition, wasp stings can induce hemolysis. Bumblebees generally nest in the ground, stinging hikers or forest workers who walk near the nest. Paper wasps build nests in sheds, eaves, and bushes. Hornets construct nests in bushes, underground, and in houses. Their presence in orchards can interfere with harvesting. Yellow jackets generally nest underground or in logs. Although they usually seek other arthropods as food, some species scavenge and in this way come into contact with people. In late summer and fall, yellow jackets are particularly aggressive and elicit most of the hymenopteran-induced morbidity at that time. Vespid wasps sting humans when threatened. Nests are difficult to remove, although an effective method employs residual insecticide.

Ant stings can induce more protracted local reactions. Although a number of ant species sting, the fire ant (*Solenopsis* spp.) is especially voracious. Stings elicit sharp pain with transient wheal and flare reactions. This develops into an umbilicated papule. Secondary infection occasionally expands into cellulitis. Wounds are treated with elevation, daily cleaning and wrapping, and systemic antibiotics if infected. Anaphylaxis is rare.

Fire ants are distributed worldwide, adapting readily to a variety of ecological niches. They constitute a serious problem in agricultural areas where they attack humans and other animals. Fire ants attack individuals who walk near the nest. Exposure can be minimized by wearing boots and by walking where ground is not obscured by vegetation.

REFERENCES

1 Smith, KGV: *A Manual of Forensic Entomology.* Ithaca, New York, Cornell University Press, 1986, 205 pp
2 Berenber JL, Ward PA, Soneshine DE: Tick bite injury: Medication by a complement-derived chemotactic factor. J Immunol 109:451–456, 1972
3 Gothe R, Kunze K, Hoogstraal H: The mechanisms of pathogenicity in the tick paralyses. J Med Entomol 16:357–369, 1979
4 Swift TR, Ignacio OJ: Tick paralysis: Electrophysiologic studies. Neurology 25:1130–1133, 1975
5 Spielman A: How to diagnose and treat tick and mite infestations. Drug Therapy II:77–82, 88, 89, 1981
6 Gouck HK: Protection from ticks, fleas, chiggers, and leeches. Arch Dermatol 93:112, 113, 1966
7 Burks JW, Jung R, George WM: Norwegian scabies. Arch Dermatol 74:131–140, 1956.
8 Drugs for parasitic infections. *Med Lett Drugs Ther* 26:27–34, 1984
9 Van Neste D, Simon J: Circulating antigen antibody complexes in scabies. Dermatologica 157:221–224, 1978
10 Zalar GL, Walther RR: Infestation by *Tunga penetrans.* Arch Dermatol 116:80–81, 1980
11 Scott MJ Jr, Scott MJ Sr: Nits or not? Pseudonits—simple office diagnosis. JAMA 243:2325–2326, 1980
12 Taplin D, Castillero PM, Spiegel J, et al: Malathion for treatment of *Pediculus humanus* var *capitis* infestation. JAMA 247:3101–3105, 1982
13 Schacher JF, Saab S: The etiology of halzoun in Lebanon: Recovery of *Linguatula serrata* nymphs from two patients. Trans R Soc Trop Med Hyg 63:854–858, 1969
14 Radford AJ: Millipede burns in man. Trop Geogr Med 27:279–287, 1975
15 Pesce H, Delgado A: Poisoning from moths and caterpillars, in Bucher W, Buckley EE (eds): *Venomous Animals and Their Venoms,* III. New York, Academic, 1971, pp 119–156
16 Sutherland SK, Duncan AW, Tibballs J: Local inactivation of funnel-web spider (*Atrax robustus*) venom by first-aid measures. Med J Aust 2:435–437, 1980
17 Newlands G: Review of southern Africa scorpions and scorpionism. S Afr Med J 54:613–615, 1978
18 Yahel-Niv A, Zlotkin E: Comparative studies on venom obtained from individual scorpions by natural sting. Toxicon 17:435–446, 1979
19 Sabotka AK, Franklin RM, Adkinson NF, et al: Allergy to insect stings. II. Phospholipase A: The major allergen in honey bee venom. J Allergy Clin Immunol 57:29–40, 1976
20 Hoffman DR, Shipman WH: Allergens in bee venom. J Allergy Clin Immunol 58:551–562, 1976
21 Hunt KJ, Valentine MD, Sobotka AK, et al: Diagnosis of allergy to stinging insects by skin testing with Hymenoptera venom. Ann Intern Med 85:56–59, 1976
22 Hunt KJ, Valentine MD, Sobotka AK, et al: A controlled trial of immunotherapy in insect hypersensitivity. N Engl J Med 299:157–161, 1978

RECOMMENDED READING

Ebelig, W: *Urban Entomology,* Division of Agricultural Sciences, University of California at Berkeley, 1975
Harwood RF, James MT: *Entomology in Human and Animal Health,* 7th ed., New York, Macmillan, 1979
Smith, KGY (ed): *Insects and Other Arthropods of Medical Importance,* London, British Museum, 1973

Venomous and Poisonous Animals

• David A. Warrell

Some animals can inject their venom into prey or aggressors by a specialized venom apparatus: the fangs of snakes, chelicerae of spiders, stinging spines of fish, nematocysts of coelenterates, and radular teeth of cone shells. Venom may also be sprayed defensively onto sensitive or absorbent mucous membranes of the aggressor, from the fang tips of "spitting" cobras, and from the venom glands of some toads, whip scorpions, *Parabuthus* scorpions, and millipedes. The injected or parenteral venoms immobilize and digest the prey and warn off predators. The tissues of some other animals contain poisons which are either elaborated by the animal itself, as in the case of the skin of amphibians, or are acquired accidentally from the food chain, as in the case of marine animals such as fish, shellfish, and perhaps horseshoe crabs and turtles which take up toxin-containing dinoflagellates. *Envenoming* is the active injection of venom, whereas *poisoning* results from the absorption of a toxin from ingested animal material.

This chapter deals with clinical aspects of envenoming by snakes, lizards, fish, and a variety of marine and terrestrial invertebrates, and poisoning resulting from the ingestion of fish and other marine animals.

VENOMOUS SNAKES

CHARACTERISTICS OF VENOMOUS SNAKES

Morphology, taxonomy, and identification

There are more than 2700 species of snakes. Fewer than 500 belong to the families Atractaspididae, Viperidae, Elapidae, and Hydrophidae which are usually regarded as venomous. Less than 200 species have been reliably reported to have caused human deaths. Bites by more than 40 species of a fifth family, the Colubridae, formerly considered nonvenomous, have proved capable of envenoming humans [1]. Snake taxonomy is of medical importance, for it is possible to make some generalizations about clinical effects of venom within families and genera. All medically important species possess one or more pairs of enlarged teeth, the fangs, which penetrate the skin of the victim and conduct venom into the tissues along a groove or through a duct. Approximately 400 members of the family Colubridae possess short, immobile fangs situated at the posterior end of the maxilla. Bites by two African species, the boomslang *(Dispholidus typus)* and the vine, twig, or bird snake *(Thelotornis kirtlandi)* have caused several deaths in people who handled them. The Japanese yamakagashi *(Rhabdophis tigrinus)* was responsible for one reported death, while the southeast Asian red-necked keelback *(R. subminiatus)* has caused severe envenoming: snakes of this genus have enlarged posterior maxillary teeth—not fangs (Fig. 59-1). A

single genus of African snakes, the burrowing asps, also known as burrowing or mole vipers, adders, or false vipers *(Atractaspis),* have very long, hinged front fangs. Previously classified with the Viperidae, they are now regarded by many taxonomists as a separate family, Atractaspididae. Two species, *A. microlepidota* and *A. irregularis,* have caused human deaths and some other species have produced severe envenoming [2].

The fixed-front-fanged snakes, or Proteroglypha, comprise two families. The Elapidae include cobras, kraits, mambas, coral snakes, and sea snakes (sea kraits) of the genus *Laticauda* (Fig. 59-2). The family Hydrophidae includes all the medically important true sea snakes and all the terrestrial venomous Australasian snakes formerly classified with the Elapidae.

The group of movable-front-fanged snakes, or Solenoglypha, includes within the one family Viperidae the subfamilies Viperinae, the vipers and adders of the old world, and the Crotalinae, the rattlesnakes, moccasins, and lance-headed vipers of the Americas and the Asian pit vipers. The very long front fangs are curved and capable of a wide range of movement (Fig. 59-3). The crotaline snakes possess a heat-sensitive pit organ situated behind the nostrils for detecting their warm-blooded prey.

Table 59-1 lists the species which, in each continent, are responsible for most human deaths and severe morbidity. Some venomous species, such as the African night adders (genus

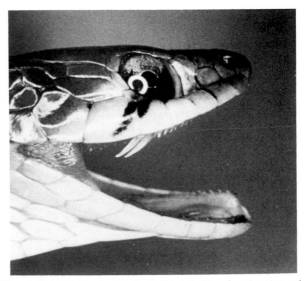

Figure 59-1. Red-necked keelback *(Rhabdophis subminiatus):* a colubrid snake with enlarged posterior maxillary teeth (not fangs) which is capable of causing severe envenoming in humans. *(Copyright D. A. Warrell.)*

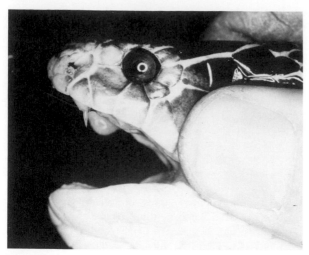

Figure 59-2. Monocellate Thai cobra *(Naja kaouthia):* showing small, relatively fixed front fang typical of elapid snakes. *(Copyright D. A. Warrell.)*

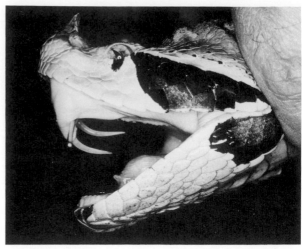

Figure 59-3. Gaboon viper *(Bitis gabonica):* one of the bulkiest of the Viperidae. Note the very long hinged front fangs. *(Photographed by courtesy of Zoological Society of London; copyright D. A. Warrell.)*

Table 59-1. Species responsible for most snakebite deaths and morbidity

Region	Scientific name*	Common name
North America	*Crotalus adamanteus*	Eastern diamondback rattlesnake
	C. atrox	Western diamondback rattlesnake
	C. viridis subspecies	Western rattlesnakes
Central America	*C. durissus durissus*	Central American rattlesnake
	Bothrops atrox asper	Terciopelo, Caissaca
South America	*B. atrox atrox*	''Fer de lance,'' Barba amarilla
	B. jararaca	Jararaca
	C. durissus terrificus	South American rattlesnake
Europe	*Vipera berus*	Viper, adder
	V. ammodytes	Long-nosed viper
Africa	*Echis carinatus*	Saw-scaled or carpet viper
	Bitis arietans	Puff adder
	Naja nigricollis	Black-necked spitting cobra
	N. haje	Egyptian cobra
	Dendroaspis species	Mambas
Asia, Middle East	*E. carinatus*	Saw-scaled or carpet viper
	Vipera lebetina	Levantine viper
	V. palaestinae	Palestine viper
Indian subcontinent and southeast Asia	*E. carinatus*	Saw-scaled or carpet viper
	Naja naja, N. kaouthia	Asian cobras
	Bungarus caeruleus	Indian krait
	V. russellii	Russell's viper
	Calloselasma (Agkistrodon) rhodostoma	Malayan pit viper
Far East	*N. naja*	Asian cobra
	Trimeresurus flavoviridis	Habu
	T. mucrosquamatus	Chinese habu
	Agkistrodon halys	Pallas' pit viper, mamushi
Australasia	*Acanthophis antarcticus*	Death adder
	Notechis scutatus	Tiger snake
	Pseudonaja textilis	Eastern brown snake

*Scientific names (Latin) are important because they are used internationally to describe the range of specificity of antivenoms.

Causus) and Asian green pit vipers (genus *Trimeresurus),* are responsible for many bites but rarely give rise to severe envenoming.

There is no absolutely reliable method for distinguishing venomous from nonvenomous snakes at a glance. The discovery of a pair of enlarged teeth, the fangs, at the front of the upper jaw strongly suggests that the snake is capable of envenoming, but these fangs may not be obvious. Fortunately, the most important species of venomous snake are easily recognized by their color, size, and characteristic behavior when aroused. For example, cobras rear up and spread a hood; rattlesnakes and saw-scaled vipers make a distinctive sound. Identification of the species of snake responsible for a bite is of the utmost importance in management. Herpetological books and papers have been published covering the identification of venomous snakes in most geographical areas [*3,4*].

Geographical distribution

Venomous species are widely distributed throughout the world. They are found at altitudes up to 5000 m *(Agkistrodon himalayanus).* The range of the ''European'' adder *(Vipera berus)* extends into the Arctic Circle. Regions free from venomous snakes include the Antarctic; Chile; most of the islands in the western Mediterranean, Atlantic, and Caribbean; Madagascar; New Zealand; New Caledonia, Hawaii, and some other Pacific islands; Ireland; Iceland; and most of the Arctic Circle. Sea snakes occur in tropical areas of the Indian and Pacific Oceans, from Southern Siberia to Tasmania *(Pelamis platurus)* and in rivers and freshwater lakes (e.g., *Enhydrina schistosa* in the Ramu River, Papua New Guinea; *Hydrophis semperi* in Lake Taal, Philippines).

Habits and ecology [5,6]

Venomous snakes have adapted to a large variety of habitats. Some, such as the *Atheris* vipers of Africa, green tree vipers (genus *Trimeresurus)* of Asia, some of the mambas (genus *Dendroaspis),* and many of the back-fanged Colubridae, lead an almost entirely arboreal existence. Many of the cobras enjoy a watery environment, for example, *Naja naja* in the paddy fields of Asia and particularly the lake-dwelling cobras (genus *Boulengerina)* of equatorial Africa. There are many desert species such as rattlesnakes, the small *Bitis* vipers of southwest Africa, and *Cerastes* vipers of north Africa. The tropical forests and savannas probably have the richest venomous snake fauna.

Snakes spend most of their lives inactive and invisible to humans by camouflage and concealment. Activity is determined by diurnal and seasonal rhythms. Many are strictly nocturnal. These habits conspire to make it impossible to assess the venomous snake population of an area merely by casual observation. The population dynamics of snakes are not understood, but the numbers of snakes seem to increase dramatically when there is flooding or destruction or invasion by a large

work force of the snake's environment. The numbers of small rodents which form the natural prey of most species of venomous snakes must be in some sort of balance with the size of the snake population.

Venom apparatus [7]

In the back-fanged members of the family Colubridae, the posterior part of the superior labial gland (Duvernoy's gland), present even in nonvenomous species, is contained in a separate capsule and discharges a venomous secretion which tracks down grooves in the anterior surfaces of the several enlarged posteriorly situated fangs. To inject sufficient venom into a human, using this rather unsophisticated apparatus, these snakes must grip and chew on their victim's finger. The opportunity for such a leisurely encounter arises only while snakes are being handled and explains why the victims are usually herpetologists. Venom glands of the Elapidae, Hydrophidae, and Viperidae are situated behind the eye (Fig. 59-4). Venom is squeezed out of the gland by compressor muscles, principally the adductor superficialis in Elapidae and Hydrophidae, and the compressor glandulae in Viperidae. Venom drains into a venom duct which, after passing through an accessory gland in some species, fuses with the mucosa of the fang sheath close to the opening of the venom canal in the anterior part of the pedestal of the fang. The fangs have partially closed grooves or completely closed canals through

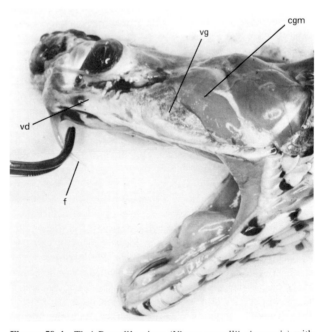

Figure 59-4. Thai Russell's viper *(Vipera russellii siamensis)* with skin removed to show the venom apparatus. vg = venom gland, cgm = compressor glandulae muscle, vd = venom duct, f = fang. *(Copyright D. A. Warrell.)*

which the venom travels to its exit point in the anterior part of the fang close to the tip. In four species of elapids the venom canal opens forward, above the tip of the fang, allowing venom to be ejected as a fine spray for a distance of 2 m or more into the eyes of an aggressor. This defensive behavior is shown by populations of the Asian cobra *(N. naja sputatrix)* in Burma, Thailand, Malaysia, Indonesia, Sri Lanka, and the Philippines, the spitting cobras of Africa *(N. nigricollis, N. katiensis, N. pallida,* and *N. mossambica),* and the ringhals of South Africa *(Hemachatus haemachatus).*

There is little evidence to support the idea that the snake can vary the amount of venom injected at a strike according to the size of the prey. In view of the high proportion of bites by some venomous species which result in little or no envenoming, it had been suggested that snakes might be capable of biting defensively without injecting venom. Some species, such as the Palestine viper, *Vipera palaestinae,* have been shown to inject doses of venom lethal to their natural prey at each of up to 10 or more consecutive strikes. The quantity of venom injected from strike to strike appears highly variable. *V. palaestinae* never injects more than half its total venom gland contents at a single strike and there is no support for the popular belief that snakes are less dangerous after they have eaten. Occasionally a snake has bitten two or more humans in rapid succession; the second or third victim was sometimes more severely envenomed than the first.

Venom composition

Snake venoms must not be thought of as single chemical compounds. They consist of a variety of enzymes, polypeptide toxins, glycoproteins, and low-molecular-weight substances. The similarities between the venoms of different species are generally proportional to their taxonomic relationships. Some species show a considerable degree of individual, seasonal, geographical, and age variation in their venom composition, and these variations are important in the selection of venoms for antivenom production. Most of the dry weight of venom is protein. Snake venoms are an exceptionally rich source of enzymes, but the role of many of these in envenoming is unknown or controversial. Examples of enzymes found in all snake venoms are L-amino acid oxidase, which may be digestive; phosphomono- and diesterases; hyaluronidase, which promotes the spread of venom through the tissues; and proteolytic enzymes, which may contribute to local changes in vascular permeability, hemorrhage, and necrosis. Phospholipase A2, the most widespread and extensively studied of venom enzymes has, under experimental conditions at least, damaging effects on mitochondria, red blood cells, leukocytes, platelets, skeletal muscle, nerve, vascular endothelium, and other membranes, and produces presynaptic neurotoxic activity and autopharmacological effects by releasing histamine. The venoms of Viperidae contain arginine esterhydrolases, which increase capillary permeability; kininogenase, which releases bradykinin from plasma kininogens causing hypotension; and coagulant enzymes. Ecarin, the prothrombin-activating enzyme of *E. carinatus* venom, is a zinc metalloprotein. Arvin, or ancrod, the coagulant of the Malayan pit viper *(Calloselasma rhodostoma,* formerly *Agkistrodon rhodostoma)* venom, is a glycoprotein, and the factor X–activating coagulant of Russell's viper *(Vipera russellii)* venom is an arginine esterhydrolase. Most elapid venoms contain acetylcholinesterase, which is no longer thought to contribute to their neurotoxicity.

Polypeptide toxins (neurotoxins) are found almost exclusively in the venoms of Elapidae and Hydrophidae. They are classified into two groups: those with 60 to 62 or 66 to 74 amino acid residues in a peptide chain cross-linked by four or five disulfides—which include the postsynaptic α neurotoxins and membrane toxins; and toxic phospholipases A₂—these include the presynaptic β neurotoxins and myonecrotic toxins [9]. Postsynaptic neurotoxins bind to the acetylcholine receptors on the motor end plate. Examples are α-bungarotoxin from the venom of the Chinese krait *(Bungarus multicinctus),* cobrotoxin from Chinese cobra venom *(Naja naja atra),* and erabutoxin b from the venom of the sea snake *Laticauda semifasciata.* Presynaptic neurotoxins such as β-bungarotoxin, also from the venom of *B. multicinctus,* notexin from the Australian tiger snake *(Notechis scutatus),* taipoxin from the Australian taipan *(Oxyuranus scutellatus),* and crotoxin from the South American rattlesnake *(Crotalus durissus terrificus)* inhibit release of acetylcholine at neuromuscular junctions. Most presynaptic neurotoxins exhibit some myonecrotic activity, and this is particularly marked in sea snakes such as the beaked sea snake *(Enhydrina schistosa),* some terrestrial Australasian snakes, and even some Viperidae (e.g., *C. durissus terrificus* and *Vipera russellii pulchella).* The amino acid sequence, three-dimensional structure, and structure-toxicity relationship have been established for many of the postsynaptic neurotoxins.

CLINICAL ASPECTS OF SNAKEBITE

Pathogenesis

Some snake venoms are absorbed to some extent when applied to mucosal membranes. For example, venoms of the spitting cobras can damage the conjunctival membrane and cornea and may sometimes be absorbed into the eye. Venom is nearly always injected through the skin and, depending on the length of fangs and efficiency of the strike, into deeper tissues. Absorption from the injection site depends on tissue-binding affinities of the various venom components and their molecular sizes, and local effects of the venom on tissue permeability and blood supply. The toxic polypeptides of Elapidae and Hydrophidae venoms are relatively small molecules which are absorbed rapidly into the bloodstream, whereas the much larger protein toxins of Viperidae are taken up more slowly through lymphatics. After systemic spread in the bloodstream, many venoms appear concentrated and bound in the kidney and much of the venom may be eliminated in the urine. There is great variation in the pattern of distribution and elimination of different venoms and their components. Thus the venom of *Agkistrodon piscivorus* is selectively bound in the lungs, some neurotoxins such as α-bungarotoxin are selectively bound at neuromuscular junctions, and a number of crotaline venoms are concentrated in the liver and eliminated to a large extent in the bile [*10*]. Most venoms penetrate the blood-brain barrier very poorly, but some have been shown to increase its permeability.

The pathogenesis of envenoming in humans is an aberration of the effects of venom in the much smaller amphibians, reptiles, and mammals which are the snake's natural prey. Thus human victims of *E. carinatus* may die a week or more after the bite from cerebral hemorrhage or hemorrhagic shock, whereas the natural prey of this snake, a small rodent, dies within minutes from massive intravascular coagulation. Similarly, the human victim of Russell's viper may survive the acute effects of envenoming but dies later of renal failure, and the patient bitten by *N. nigricollis* escapes the neurotoxic effects so dramatic in smaller mammals but may die of late complications of the locally necrotic effect of the venom. Large doses of hydrophid venoms kill animals by their neurotoxicity, whereas smaller doses given subcutaneously reveal the generalized rhabdomyolitic effect seen in human victims. The results of envenoming are explained partly by the direct action of the various venom components on tissues, partly by indirect effects such as complement activation and autopharmacological release of endogenous vasoactive substances, and partly by complications of the primary effects of venom such as secondary infections.

Pathology

Patients who die with clinical features of neurotoxic envenoming show no postmortem abnormalities in the central nervous system or elsewhere apart from those attributable to terminal respiratory failure. Fatalities from hemorrhagic and coagulant venoms usually show bleeding into the bitten limb, brain, serosal cavities, gastrointestinal tract, retroperitoneal tissues, and genitourinary tract. Venoms of sea snakes, some Australasian snakes (e.g., *Notechis scutatus*, *Oxyuranus scutellatus* and *Pseudechis australis*), *C. durissus* and some other rattlesnakes, and *V. russellii pulchella* cause scattered focuses of necrosis of muscle fibers, clogging of the renal tubules with myoglobin, and myoglobinuria. Renal histological changes in snakebite victims have attracted a great deal of attention, and a wide variety of changes has been reported, of which acute tubular necrosis is the most important [*11*]. It may be difficult to decide to what extent these appearances represent primary nephrotoxicity or result from secondary effects of ischemia and antivenom therapy, and to what extent they arise from pre-existing renal disease.

Clinical manifestations, pathophysiology, and pharmacology

General Clinical Features. The snake-bitten patient may present with symptoms resulting from fear, from prehospital treatment, and from the effects of the venom itself and complications of those effects. Snakebite is a terrifying experience for most people, especially for those who believe that all bites are rapidly fatal, so it is not surprising that physiological manifestations of anxiety, even hysteria, may dominate the clinical picture and interfere with rational management. The patient may feel flushed, dizzy, and breathless, with a sensation of constriction of the chest, and may notice a thumping pulse, palpitations, sweating, and effects of hyperventilation such as acroparesthesia and carpopedal spasm, even in the absence of envenoming. Such symptoms feature prominently in many accounts of snakebites written by the victim, usually a herpetologist, and are sometimes attributed to neurotoxicity. Misguided, prehospital treatment can lead to congestion, swelling, and ischemia of a limb whose circulation has been occluded by a tourniquet, persistent bleeding, pain or sensory loss at the site of local incisions, and vomiting and other side effects of herbal remedies. Exceptionally, the terror of snakebite may precipitate angina pectoris, myocardial infarction, or cardiac arrhythmia. The evolution of symptoms and signs of envenoming is determined by the nature, dose, and site of injection of the venom and by what the victim does after being bitten. Pain is a prominent feature of most Viperidae and some Elapidae bites and has been attributed to biogenic amines such as histamine and 5-hydroxytryptamine which occur in greater quantities in the venoms of Viperidae. Conversely, bites by kraits *(Bungarus)* and some other elapids may produce local anesthesia. Local swelling may become noticeable within minutes of the bite and the blood may be totally defibrinated in a half hour after bites by *C. rhodostoma* and *E. carinatus*. Respiratory paralysis may be evident within 30 min and deaths have occurred as early as 15 min after the bite (*Naja naja* and mambas, genus *Dendroaspis*). Anaphylactic shock can appear as early as minutes after bites by some Viperidae and other snakes, suggesting autopharmacological effects (see below), and one death, 15 min after Russell's viper bite, has been described. These early deaths are, however, unusual, the usual times to death being hours after an elapid or sea snake bite and days after viper bites [*12*]. Fever is a common manifestation of the systemic inflammatory response to snake venoms.

Although most victims of snakebite show features of several venom activities, reflecting the numerous toxic components of snake venoms, it is clinically useful to classify the manifestations of snakebite into a number of syndromes.

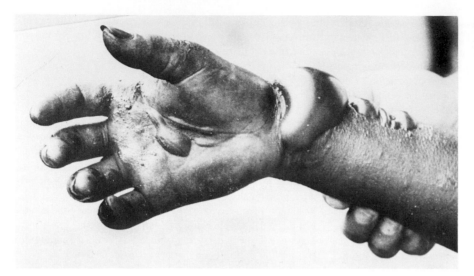

Figure 59-5. Serosanguinous bullae in a patient bitten by the Gaboon viper *(B. gabonica)* in Ivory Coast. *(Courtesy of Dr. J. Doucet and Acta Tropica, Basel.)*

Cytotoxicity. There is increased vascular permeability, inflammatory change, and tissue damage producing tender swelling spreading from the site of the bite and early tender enlargement of lymph nodes draining the bitten area. Within a few hours serosanguineous bullae may appear under the epidermis (Fig. 59-5). These effects are characteristic of bites by the Viperidae, including pit vipers of the subfamily Crotalinae, and cobras such as *N. nigricollis* and *N. mossambica* in Africa and *N. naja* in Asia. They have been attributed to basic polypeptides such as elapid cardiotoxin, to proteases of viperid venoms, and to release of autacoids such as histamine and 5-hydroxytryptamine. When blistering follows an elapid bite, tissue necrosis nearly always ensues; this is usually superficial but may be very extensive and extend up the fascial planes of the limb (Fig. 59-6), whereas in the case of bites by Viperidae the bullae may dry up and slough without the development of

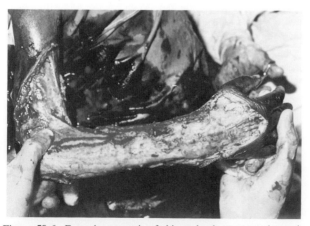

Figure 59-6. Extensive necrosis of skin and subcutaneous tissues in a Nigerian girl bitten on the forearm by a black-necked spitting cobra *(Naja nigricollis). (Copyright D. A. Warrell.)*

necrosis. A pale, demarcated, anesthetic area of skin with a characteristic odor of putrefaction signals the presence of necrosis (Fig. 59-7). This is a direct effect of the venom, but the gangrenous tissue is vulnerable to secondary bacterial infection especially by anaerobes.

With bites by most species of snakes, the appearance of local swelling is the best clinical evidence that venom has been injected. The bites of kraits *(Bungarus),* American coral snakes *(Micrurus* and *Micruroides),* and sea snakes cause negligible local reaction. The incidence of local necrosis in hospital cases of snakebite in northern Nigeria was 9 percent for *E. carinatus,* 36 percent for puff adder *(B. arietans),* and 71 percent for *N. nigricollis* [13]. Bites on the digits seem particularly likely to result in necrosis. This could be explained by a high local concentration of venom or by ischemia resulting from compression of the digital vessels in the pulp space as in the case of infective whitlow. In a tensely swollen limb there are two other mechanisms for necrosis other than direct cytotoxic effects of venom. A major artery could be compressed by tissue swelling within a tight fascial compartment, such as the anterior tibial compartment [14]. This problem appears particularly common with habu bites *(Trimeresurus flavoviridis)* in Okinawa. A major artery may thrombose because of a high local concentration of venom coagulant. An important consequence of increased vascular permeability and tissue damage in the bitten limb is the extravasation of blood with depletion of the circulating volume causing hypotension (see below).

Cardiovascular Toxicity. The most important sign of cardiovascular toxicity in snakebite victims is hypotension ("shock"). Possible mechanisms include hypovolemia resulting from extravasation of blood into a massively swollen limb, direct or autopharmacological effects of venom on blood vessels, increasing their permeability, and a direct effect on heart muscle. Hypotension may also develop in patients profoundly hypoxemic as a result of neurotoxic respiratory failure. Chapman has emphasized that liters of blood may be lost from the circulation into the swollen limb in patients bitten by the puff adder *(B. arietans)* [*15*]. Hypotension during early anaphylactic reactions following snakebites is clearly caused by histamine and other vasodilative autacoids (see below). In experimental animals, a variety of venoms produce hypotension by altering vascular caliber, for example, splanchnic vasodilatation. Direct myocardial activity has been demonstrated experimentally with some venoms. Human victims of *B. arietans,* like cats and dogs envenomed experimentally, develop hypotension and sinus bradycardia, and show ECG changes [*16*]. Changes in ST segments or T waves and tachy- or bradyarrhythmias have been observed in the ECGs of patients bitten by the European adder *(V. berus)*, *E. carinatus*, Burton's carpet viper *(E. coloratus)*, and *C. rhodostoma*. The venom of the burrowing asp *(Atractaspis engaddensis)* contains a cardiotoxin which causes coronary vasoconstriction.

Effects of Coagulants and Hemorrhagins.

In snakebite victims, spontaneous bleeding is most frequently detected in the gingival sulci, but epistaxis, subconjunctival hemorrhages, ecchymoses, and bleeding into the brain, retroperitoneal space, and the gastrointestinal and genitourinary tracts also occurs. The venom components responsible for spontaneous hemorrhage (hemorrhagins) have been demonstrated in some snake venoms and are separable from venom coagulants [*8*]. Coagulant activity is suspected in a patient when there is oozing of blood from sites of venipuncture or other recent trauma and is confirmed by demonstrating that the blood is incoagulable. The combination of coagulant and hemorrhagin activities is characteristic of venoms of vipers such as *V. russellii* and *E. carinatus,* pit vipers such as *C. rhodostoma, Trimeresurus* species, the western rattlesnake *(Crotalus viridis)*, the South American lance-headed vipers *(Bothrops)*, some terrestrial Australasian snakes such as *N. scutatus, O. scutellatus,* and some colubrid snakes such as *D. typus, T. kirtlandi,* and *Rhabdophis*. The mechanism of defibrination is gradual disseminated intravascular coagulation with fibrinolysis of the resulting fibrin. Bleeding resulting from hemorrhagin will be greatly exaggerated if the blood has been rendered incoagulable by a coagulant enzyme.

Neurotoxicity.

This is characteristic of envenoming by elapids, terrestrial Australasian snakes, and sea snakes. Venoms of some species of Viperidae also produce neurotoxic effects. These include the Eastern diamondback rattlesnake *(Crotalus adamanteus) C. durissus terrificus,* Pallas' pit viper *(Agkistrodon blomhoffi brevicaudus)*, berg adder *(Bitis atropos)*, and *V. russellii pulchella*. Early, preparalytic symptoms of neurotoxicity include vomiting, headache, abdominal pain, paresthesia especially around the mouth, dizziness or true vertigo, hyperacusis, and hypotensive collapse with loss of consciousness and signs of autonomic nervous system stimulation. Vomiting has proved a useful early sign of significant neurotoxic envenoming; it may start within minutes or hours of the bite. In tropical countries, the use of emetic herbal medicines for snakebite may cause misleading symptoms. The causes of early and transient loss of consciousness, convulsions, hypotension, and other signs are uncertain, but these may represent autopharmacological effects of venom. Paralytic effects may appear as early as 15 to 20 min after bites by cobras or mambas. In Papua New Guinea the average interval was $5\frac{1}{2}$ h, with a range from 1 to 10 h [*17*]. After krait bites there may be a delay of 10 h or more before paralysis develops. Early paralytic symptoms include heaviness of the eyelids, blurred vision, diplopia, and difficulty in speaking. The levator palpebrae superioris and extraocular muscles are the most sensitive to neuromuscular blockade, and in some patients the only evidence of neurotoxicity is ptosis and ophthalmoplegia. More serious effects are paralysis of the palate, jaws, tongue, vocal cords, neck muscles, and muscles of deglutition. Obstruction of the upper airways by the tongue or inhaled vomitus may precipitate respiratory arrest. The intercostal muscles are affected before the limbs, diaphragm, and superficial muscles. Objective sensory impairment is unusual. So far, central nervous system effects of neurotoxins have not been convincingly demonstrated in humans. Coma and convulsions could be secondary to the hypoxemia of respiratory paralysis or to the cardiovascular effects of elapid and other venoms. Intractable hypotension has been encountered in patients envenomed by Asian cobras and terrestrial Australasian snakes despite adequate respiratory support. Ptosis and physiological tiredness may sometimes be misinterpreted as coma. Neurotoxicity is completely reversible—in some cases acutely, in response to specific antivenom or anticholinesterase, in others slowly and spontaneously. In the absence of specific antivenom, patients sup-

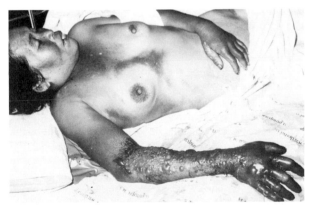

Figure 59-7. Coma, shock, extensive ecchymoses, blistering and gangrene in a Thai woman bitten on the hand 4 days previously by a Malayan pit viper *(Calloselasma rhodostoma)*. She went to a monastery for traditional treatment but was finally brought to hospital when her condition deteriorated. She recovered after antivenom treatment, but the gangrenous forearm was amputated. *(Copyright D. A. Warrell.)*

ported by artificial ventilation recover sufficient diaphragmatic movement to breathe adequately in 1 to 4 days. The ocular muscles recover in 2 to 4 days and there is usually full recovery of motor function in 3 to 7 days. These clinical effects are attributable to neurotoxins acting pre- and postsynaptically at the neuromuscular junction. Postsynaptic neurotoxins, such as cobrotoxin and α-bungarotoxin, act very like curare. In nerve muscle preparations, their effects can be reversed by anticholinesterases and by washing, implying loose binding of the neurotoxin. These observations provide a basis for the sometimes dramatic clinical effects of neostigmine and specific antivenom [18]. Presynaptic neurotoxins, such as β-bungarotoxin, notexin, crotoxin, and many sea snake neurotoxins, act like botulin and bind almost irreversibly at acetylcholine-releasing sites on the nerve ending. Some of these neurotoxins have a rhabdomyolytic effect contributing an additional group of clinical features (see below), and may be damaging to motor nerves.

Myotoxicity. Patients bitten by most species of true sea snakes, many species of terrestrial Australasian snakes (Hydrophidae), and some species of rattlesnake (e.g., *C. durissus terrificus, C. herridus atricaudatus*) and viper *(V. russellii pulchella)* may develop generalized rhabdomyolysis. This syndrome must be distinguished from the local muscle necrosis caused by cytotoxic venoms. In the case of sea snake bites, early symptoms include headache, a thick feeling of the tongue, thirst, sweating, and vomiting. Muscle aching, stiffness, and tenderness becomes noticeable between 30 min and $3\frac{1}{2}$ h after the bite and may become generalized. Trismus is a common feature. Later generalized flaccid paralysis develops, but consciousness is retained. Myoglobinuria appears 3 to 8 h after the bite. Serious consequences of generalized rhabdomyolysis include cardiac arrest and renal damage from hyperkalemia. Recovery may take many weeks or months [18a]. Rhabdomyolysis and myoglobinuria have been reported in patients bitten by several of the terrestrial Australasian hydrophids: *N. scutatus, O. scutellatus,* the king brown or mulga snake *(Pseudechis australis),* and the eastern small-eyed snake *(Cryptophis nigrescens).* These features may have been overlooked in patients bitten by other species.

Nephrotoxicity [11]. Renal failure has been described in patients severely envenomed by a variety of species, but it appears to be most frequent and severe in victims of *V. russellii, C. durissus terrificus,* the South American jararaca *(Bothrops jararaca),* and sea snakes. Many venoms are concentrated and bound in the kidney. Some appear to have a direct nephrotoxic effect (e.g., *V. russellii*), but, more often, acute renal failure is the result of ischemia from shock, microvascular occlusion by fibrin (DIC), or vasoconstriction. Myoglobinuria and hemoglobinuria may damage the kidney, but the associated hyperkalemia in sea snake and terrestrial Australasian snakebites might itself cause renal dysfunction. Antivenom may cause

immune-complex nephritis as part of the late reactions occurring 7 days or more after treatment.

Autopharmacological Effects. Patients bitten by *V. palaestinae* commonly develop abdominal colic, persistent watery diarrhea, sweating, hypotension, and angioedema of the tongue and lips within about 30 min of the bite. They may collapse unconscious with the appearance of anaphylactic shock within minutes of the bite. Similar symptoms have been described, less commonly, in patients bitten by *V. berus* and other European vipers, the burrowing asp *(A. engaddensis),* and some terrestrial Australasian snakes. These features could be explained by the release of autacoids such as histamine, 5-hydroxytryptamine, kinins, etc.

An alternative explanation for some of these early anaphylactic reactions would be hypersensitivity in people previously exposed to that particular venom.

Complement Activation. A variety of snake venoms, particularly those of elapids, contain cobra venom factor (which may be the cobra's own C3b) which activates complement by the alternative pathway [19]. Evidence of this activation has been found in humans bitten by *D. typus* and *N. nigricollis,* while the classical pathway is activated by Viperidae and other venoms. The complement system may also be activated by antivenoms (see below). The significance of complement in the pathogenesis of envenoming is unknown, but the effects could include vascular endothelial damage, necrosis, and coagulopathy [20].

Clinical Manifestations of Rattlesnake Envenoming [21]. The venoms of a number of species of rattlesnakes give rise to combinations of the above syndromes with some additional characteristic symptoms not easily ascribed to any of these activities. Pain at the site of the bite is variable. Swelling usually appears within 15 min of the bite and may spread rapidly. Bruising may appear within a few hours and may be extensive, especially with bites by *C. adamanteus, C. viridis,* and *C. horridus.* Early bruising may appear over the axillary lymph nodes and along the path of lymphatics. Blood-filled bullae are frequently seen, especially following bites by *C. adamanteus, C. atrox, C. horridus,* and *C. viridis.* Necrosis was frequently reported before the use of adequate doses of antivenom. Early symptoms of systemic envenoming include paresthesias of the tongue, lips, and scalp and an abnormal metallic taste, especially in patients bitten by *C. viridis.* Muscle fasciculation is a common and sometimes early sign of rattlesnake envenoming. Generalised rhabdomyolysis causing myoglobinuria has been described in victims of *C. durissus terrificus* and *C. horridus atricaudatus.* Other features include sweating and chills, dizziness, vomiting, tender and enlarged regional lymph nodes, weakness, spontaneous bleeding and blood coagulation disturbances, neurotoxic effects (especially from *C. adamanteus, C. durissus terrificus,* and *C. scutella-*

tus), hypotension, and ECG abnormalities. On occasions, bites by the Mojave rattlesnake *(C. scutellatus)* and *C. durissus terrificus* may produce little or no local swelling but severe systemic signs.

Venom Ophthalmia Caused by Spitting Cobras and the Ringhals [22].

If venom of the spitting snakes (see above) enters the eye, there is intense local pain, leukorrhea, blepharospasm, and palpebral edema. In more than half the patients spat at by *N. nigricollis,* slit-lamp or fluorescein examination reveals corneal erosions. Rarely, there is evidence of absorption of venom into the anterior chamber, producing hypopyon and anterior uveitis. Secondary infection of the corneal lesions may lead to corneal opacities or panophthalmitis.

Laboratory investigations

Neutrophil leukocytosis of more than about 20,000 cells per cubic millimeter indicates severe envenoming. Anemia is usually the result of bleeding. Although hemolysis is one of the best-known effects of snake venom in vitro, it is clinically significant in very few species, such as *V. russellii pulchella,* causing hemoglobinuria. Fragmented red blood cells and other evidence of microangiopathic hemolysis have been described in some patients envenomed by *E. carinatus* and other snakes whose venoms produce disseminated intravascular coagulation. Venoms containing coagulant may produce thrombocytopenia; this is common after bites by *C. rhodostoma* and *V. russellii,* but is seen only in severe envenoming by *E. carinatus.* Thrombocytopenia is also a feature of bites by *B. ar-*

ietans, although there are no other disturbances of hemostasis in human victims [*16*]. Simple bedside tests for venom-induced defibrination are equally appropriate in large urban centers and rural health stations.

Simple Whole Blood Clotting Tests.

A small amount of blood, taken by venipuncture, is placed in a clean, dry glass test tube, left undisturbed for 20 min, and then tipped to see if it has clotted. The tube is again examined after about 12 h to assess the size of the clot, which, in the absence of grossly increased fibrinolytic activity, is proportional to the fibrinogen concentration (Fig. 59-8).

A rapid test for fibrin-fibrinogen-related antigen, the latex slide test (Thrombo-Wellco test), is useful for detecting intravascular coagulation in patients whose blood is still coagulable. Serum potassium is elevated by the generalized rhabdomyolysis of sea snake envenoming. Serum enzymes such as aspartate and alanine aminotransferases and creatine phosphokinase are mildly elevated in patients with local tissue damage but are grossly raised in victims of sea snake and some terrestrial Australasian snakebites. Blood urea nitrogen and serum creatinine are elevated in many snakebite patients who have oliguria; in these cases, renal failure must be distinguished from simple dehydration (see below). Metabolic acidosis (lactic acidosis) has been reported in patients with severe cardiovascular disturbances from snakebite. The cerebrospinal fluid of patients with neurotoxic envenoming is normal. The urine of snakebite victims commonly contains red blood cells, leukocytes, granular casts, and protein. The finding of dark urine

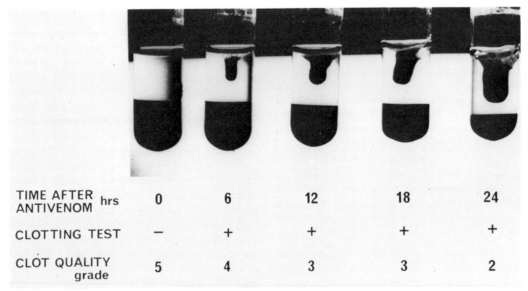

TIME AFTER ANTIVENOM hrs	0	6	12	18	24
CLOTTING TEST	−	+	+	+	+
CLOT QUALITY grade	5	4	3	3	2

Figure 59-8. Results of the simple whole blood clotting test and clot quality test in a patient envenomed by the saw-scaled or carpet viper *(Echis ocellatus).* Blood coagulability (clotting test: 0 = nonclotting, + = clotting) was restored 6 h after antivenom had been given, and there was progressive improvement of clot quality (reflecting increasing fibrinogen concentration) over the subsequent 18 h. *(Copyright D. A. Warrell.)*

which is positive for blood/hemoglobin on "stix" testing but lacks visible erythrocytes suggests the possibility of hemoglobinuria or myoglobinuria.

Immunodiagnosis of snakebite

Specific snake venom antigens have been detected in wound aspirate, wound biopsies, blood, urine, cerebrospinal fluid, and other body fluids by a variety of techniques. Immunological techniques have included precipitation, immunodiffusion, passive hemagglutination, lymphocyte transformation, countercurrent immunoelectrophoresis, radioimmunoassay, enzyme-linked immunoabsorbent assay (ELISA), and immunofluorescence. ELISA appears to be the simplest and most sensitive technique, but there may be some problems with cross reaction between related species and false positives [23]. The Commonwealth Serum Laboratories (CSL) in Australia have issued a snake venom detection kit employing the ELISA technique to distinguish venoms of the five most important Australian snakes in less than 30 min. Although in some cases these tests may give results quickly enough to guide clinical management, their main value may be in the investigation of the pathophysiology and epidemiology of snakebite, and for forensic purposes in people suspected of having died from snakebite.

MANAGEMENT OF SNAKEBITE

First aid

Although this subject has excited enormous speculation and controversy, only the following measures are generally accepted: reassure the frightened patient, immobilize the bitten limb as far as is practicable with a splint or sling, transport patients to a place where they may receive medical attention, and avoid harmful medicines and procedures. If possible, the dead snake should be taken along with the patient.

Muscular contraction promotes spread of higher-molecular-weight venom components which are absorbed mainly into lymphatics. In experimental animals immobilization of the injected limb delayed death and reduced symptoms of envenoming from some species. In restrained monkeys, splinting, combined with crepe bandaging of the injected limb, has also proved effective in delaying absorption of the venoms of the terrestrial Australasian snakes *C. atrox* and *N. naja* [23a].

Patients should be transported to the hospital or dispensary as rapidly and as comfortably as possible, in such a way as to spare them strenuous exercise. The following problems may arise en route:

Pain: Oral acetaminophen or intravenous meperidine are preferable to aspirin, which causes persistent gastric bleeding in patients with incoagulable blood.
Vomiting: Patients should lie on their side to avoid aspiration. Chlorpromazine (25 mg for adults, 1 mg/kg for children) by intravenous injection is given for persistent vomiting.

Anaphylactic shock with angioedema, abdominal colic, and diarrhea: These autopharmacological effects are treated with epinephrine (0.5 mL of 0.1%, solution for adults, 0.01 mL/kg for children) by subcutaneous or intramuscular injection and an antihistamine such as chlorpheniramine maleate (10 mg for adults, 0.2 mg/kg for children) by intravenous injection.
Airways obstruction from paralysis of the jaw and tongue: Patients are laid on their side, an oral airway is inserted, and the jaw elevated.
Respiratory or cardiac arrest: Mouth-to-mouth respiration and external cardiac massage should be attempted.

A variety of unproven and even potentially harmful first-aid methods have been suggested for the treatment of snakebite. These include cauterization; incisions at or excision of the bite site; amputation of the bitten digit; electric shocks; suction by mouth, vacuum pumps, or syringes or by the "venom-ex" apparatus which combines multiple incisions with suction; local injection or instillation of chemical compounds such as potassium permanganate and phenol; and cryotherapy. Local incisions carry a high risk of introducing infection; damaging nerves, blood vessels, or tendons; delaying wound healing; and, in patients with incoagulable blood, giving rise to uncontrolled bleeding from the wound. Powerful suction, chemicals, electric shocks, and cryotherapy may cause tissue necrosis in addition to that resulting from the venom itself. None of the methods aimed at removing venom from the bite site has received consistent support from results of animal experiments and the few clinical studies have been uncontrolled and inconclusive.

Potential dangers of ligatures, tourniquets and other occlusive methods such as pressure pads and crepe bandaging include ischemia, gangrene, damage to peripheral nerves (especially the lateral popliteal), increased fibrinolytic activity, congestion, swelling, increased bleeding, and increased local effects of venom in the bitten limb. Tourniquets of readily available materials are widely used in the rural tropics; they sometimes lead to horrifying complications and have not been shown to be beneficial. In Thai patients bitten by *C. rhodostoma* and Burmese patients bitten by *V. russellii* systemic venom antigen concentrations did not increase more rapidly after their tight tourniquets were released. However, envenoming by some elapid snakes, such as the black mamba, *Dendroaspis polylepis,* may develop so rapidly that fatal respiratory paralysis ensues within 30 min of the bite. Tight (arterial) tourniquets applied around the upper limb and firm crepe bandaging and splinting of the whole bitten limb can impede the systemic uptake of venom. These measures are recommended only after a bite by an identified dangerous elapid, terrestrial Australasian snake, or sea snake, if medical attention is likely to be delayed for 1 to 2 h and there is a risk that fatal respiratory paralysis might develop on the way to the hospital or dispensary. If the tourniquet or bandage is applied tightly enough to obliterate the distal arterial pulse, it must be released after an hour and, if reapplied, should be finally removed after two hours. Ideally, antivenom treatment should be started and facilities for cardiorespiratory resuscitation should be available before the tourniquet is finally released.

In the rural tropics the people who are likely to administer first aid are relatives, friends, or work mates of the snakebite victim who happen to be present when the bite occurs. First aid should therefore be taught to the community as a whole—in schools, on posters at clinics and in public buildings, and via the media.

Treatment by medically trained personnel

Because of the many uncertainties about the type, quantity, and quality of venom injected, and the variable time course for the development of signs of envenoming, all victims of snakebite should be kept under medical observation for at least 24 h at the hospital, dispensary, or other health care facility. Level of consciousness, blood pressure, pulse rate, and respiration should be measured frequently and the progression of local envenoming recorded.

Initial clinical assessment will determine whether the patient requires antivenom, additional supportive treatment, or merely reassurance supported by a placebo.

Antivenom treatment

Antivenom (also known as antivenin, antevenene, and anti-snakebite serum) is the only specific cure for envenoming. Most commercial antivenoms are produced in horses. Immunoglobulins are purified by techniques such as pepsin digestion, ammonium sulfate precipitation, adsorption on aluminum hydroxide gel, dialysis, and ultracentrifugation [24]. Various directories of antivenoms have been published [21,25–27].

Indications for Antivenom. Antivenom should not be used indiscriminately because of its high cost and limited supply in tropical countries and the danger of reactions. Unfortunately, in many hospitals around the world a standard small dose of antivenom is given intramuscularly to any patients who think they have been bitten by a snake, irrespective of signs of envenoming and the identity of the biting or stinging animal. This practice exposes the majority of these patients, who may have mild or no envenoming, to the small risk of potentially fatal antivenom reactions, and squanders valuable antivenom. Indications for specific antivenom are as follows:

1. *Systemic envenoming* indicated by any of the following:
   Hemostatic disturbances such as spontaneous systemic bleeding, prolonged clotting time or completely incoagulable blood, elevated FDP, thrombocytopenia
   Cardiovascular abnormalities such as shock, hypotension, abnormal electrocardiogram, cardiac arrhythmia, cardiac failure, pulmonary edema

Neurotoxicity
Generalised rhabdomyolysis
Impaired consciousness
In patients with definite signs of local envenoming, the following indicate significant systemic envenoming: neutrophil leucocytosis, elevated serum enzymes such as creatine phosphokinase and aminotransferases, hemoconcentration, uremia, hypercreatininemia, oliguria, hypoxemia, acidosis, and vomiting.

2. *Severe local envenoming* indicated by spread of local swelling to involve more than half the bitten limb or by extensive blistering or bruising, especially in patients bitten by species whose venom is known to cause local necrosis.

Much wider indications for antivenom are accepted in relatively wealthy countries such as the United States and Australia, where the incidence of bites is very much lower than in the rural tropics. For examples, in the case of bites by the more dangerous rattlesnakes (*C. atrox, C. adamanteus,* etc.) it is recommended that antivenom should be given early, before systemic envenoming has become obvious. In these cases rapid spread of local swelling is considered an indication for antivenom [21]. Antivenom is advocated for bites by North American coral snakes (*Micrurus* and *Micruroides*) if there is immediate pain and any other symptom or sign of envenoming [21]. In Australia, antivenom has been recommended if markedly tender regional lymph nodes develop after a bite from a highly venomous snake [28].

Contraindications to Antivenom. There is no absolute contraindication to antivenom treatment, but, because of the increased danger of severe reactions, atopic individuals and those known to be hypersensitive to equine serum should be treated only if effects of envenoming are thought to be life-threatening. In these cases epinephrine, antihistamine, and corticosteroids can be given beforehand, but rapid desensitization is not recommended.

Timing of Antivenom Treatment. Bearing in mind the average intervals between bite and death (see above), antivenom should be given as soon as the criteria of severe envenoming are fulfilled. But it is almost never too late to try antivenom treatment. Sea snake envenoming has been reversed up to 2 days after the bite [18], and blood coagulability has been restored 10 days or more after the bite in the case of saw-scaled or carpet viper (*E. carinatus*) bite [13]. If possible, antivenom treatment should be started before releasing the tourniquet.

Choice of Antivenom. Only specific antivenom should be used, that is, antivenom whose range of specificity includes the biting species. Some antivenoms raised against the venoms of only one or two species have displayed, in vitro at least, wide paraspecific activity [25]. For example, CSL "tiger-sea snake" antivenom raised against venoms of *Notechis scutatus* and *Enhydrina schistosa* neutralizes venoms of three terrestrial Australasian snakes and at least 12 different sea snakes.

Expiry dates marked on ampules of antivenom may be very conservative (for purely commercial reasons) if storage has been at 5°C ± 3°C [*25*]. Opaque solutions should always be rejected, as precipitation of protein indicates loss of activity and increased risk of antivenom reactions.

Route of Administration. In experimental animals the intravenous route has proved much more effective than any other. Intramuscular or subcutaneous injection has the added disadvantage that it may lead to hematoma formation in patients with incoagulable blood. Local injection of antivenom into tissue compartments such as in the digits may cause pressure necrosis. Reconstituted antivenom should be given by slow intravenous injection (for example, 5 mL/min) or diluted in an appropriate volume of isotonic fluid (e.g., 5 mL per kilogram of body weight) and infused over 30 to 60 min. There is no difference in the incidence or severity of antivenom reactions in patients treated by these two methods [*29*]. An intravenous infusion may be easier to control but, in the rural tropics, the intravenous push method has the advantage of requiring less expensive equipment, being quicker to initiate and of compelling someone to remain at the patient's side while the injection is being given. In an emergency, if there is no one capable of giving an intravenous injection, antivenom may be given by deep intramuscular injection at multiple sites in the anterior parts of the thigh, followed by massage to promote absorption. However, the volumes of antivenom normally required would make this route impracticable as would the risk of local bleeding in patients with incoagulable blood. It seems rational to inject antivenom as close as possible to the site of the bite, for example into the fang marks, but this may be difficult, painful, and hazardous (especially in the case of bites on digits or into other tight fascial compartments) and has not proved effective in animal studies.

Dosage. Children must be given at least as large a dose of antivenom as adults, because the same volume of venom is injected. The ideal regimen would be a single dose of antivenom capable of completely neutralizing the injected venom and sustaining adequate plasma concentrations of antivenom until absorption of venom is complete. Absorption of venom from the "depot" at the site of the bite may continue for several days, indicating that it is not accessible to circulating antivenom, perhaps because of constriction or thrombosis of local blood vessels [*30*]. The apparent serum elimination half-times of antivenoms in envenomed patients range from about 25 to 100 h depending on how the antivenom has been refined. Recurrent venom antigenemia and systemic envenoming may recur as serum antivenom concentrations fall, even after a good initial response to treatment (Fig. 59-9).

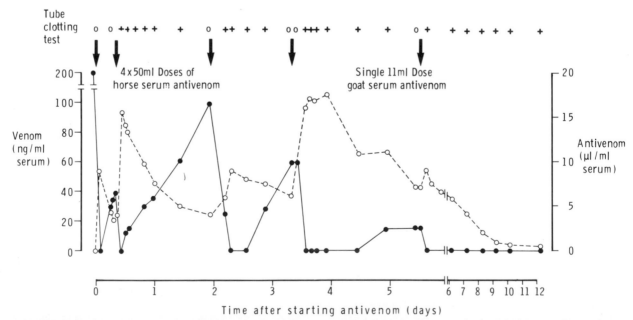

Figure 59-9. Serum venom antigen (filled circles) and equine antivenom (open circles) concentration during the treatment of systemic envenoming by the Malayan pit viper *(C. rhodostoma)*. At the top is the result of the simple whole blood clotting test as in Fig. 59-8 (0 = nonclotting, + = clotting). The arrows indicate the times of antivenom administration. The final dose was of caprine antivenom which was not detected in this assay using rabbit-anti-horse IgG conjugate. This case illustrates continued absorption of venom from the wound site with recurrent antigenemia and signs of systemic envenoming despite an initially satisfactory response to antivenom. *(Reproduced from [23] with permission.)*

The appropriate initial dose of antivenom for patients has been established experimentally in very few cases. For example, 20 mL of *Echis* antivenom from the South African Institute for Medical Research has proved effective in a large series of patients bitten by *E. carinatus* in Nigeria [*13*], while in India an average of 80 mL of Kasauli polyspecific *Naja, V. russellii, Bungarus caeruleus, Echis* antivenom was required for the same species. In Malaya, 50 mL of Thai Red Cross Society *C. rhodostoma* antivenom has proved effective in patients with systemic envenoming, while in Thailand, 100 mL of the same antivenom or 50 mL of Thai Government Pharmaceutical Organization monospecific antivenom was required [*31*]. Manufacturers' recommendations are usually based on mouse protection tests which cannot take into account species differences in response to venom and whose design may not reflect the real-life situation. These factors may explain the differences between clinical efficacy and potency in the mouse test.

Monitoring of Response to Antivenom. Responses may be dramatic. Patients often feel indefinably better soon after the infusion has started; this could well be placebo effect. Rapid correction of hypotension (e.g., in patients envenomed by *B. arietans* and *C. rhodostoma*) and respiratory paralysis (e.g., in those envenomed by Australasian death adders, genus *Acanthophis*) has been described. In the cases of *E. carinatus, V. russellii,* and *C. rhodostoma* envenoming, spontaneous systemic bleeding usually stops within 15 to 30 min and blood coagulability is restored within 1 to 6 h of an adequate neutralizing dose of antivenom. The simple clotting test (see above) repeated at 6-h intervals is a convenient method of monitoring the dose of antivenom when the venom contains a powerful coagulant [*13,31,32*].

In the case of bites by species with predominantly neurotoxic-myotoxic or cardiotoxic venoms, a further dose of antivenom should be given after 30 min if severe cardiorespiratory symptoms persist.

Antivenom Reactions. At least three kinds of reactions can occur. *Early anaphylactic reactions* usually develop within 10 to 20 min of starting intravenous injection or within 30 to 180 min of starting intravenous infusion of diluted antivenom [*29*]. Premonitory symptoms include restlessness, cough, itching of the scalp, nausea, vomiting, a feeling of heat, and palpitations. Later there is diffuse urticaria, generalized pruritus, fever, tachycardia, autonomic manifestations, and, in up to 40 percent of reactions, potentially fatal hypotension, airflow obstruction, and angioedema. The severe manifestations have been much publicized, leading to wholesale rejection of antivenom treatment in some countries where snakebite is uncommon. Fatal reactions are, however, rarely reported. In one series of 5000 snakebite patients who received antivenom in northwest Malaya during the years from 1955 to 1964, there was only one death doubtfully attributable to such a reaction,

and the mortality of anaphylaxis from other sera is reported as 0.1 percent. The incidence of reactions varies from about 3 to 54 percent [*29*]; incidence decreases with decreasing dose and increasing refinement of antivenom, and is greater when the intravenous rather than intramuscular route is used. The incidence also increases with the quality of observation during the first 2 h after initiating treatment. It is possible that some deaths attributed to snakebite may have been caused by severe early reactions.

Pyrogenic reactions may occur within 1 or 2 h of treatment and can precipitate febrile convulsions in children. They may be nonimmunological in nature. Pyrogenicity has been attributed to infusion equipment, the ammonium sulfate used for refinement, or to the horse protein itself.

Late serum sickness–type reactions may develop 5 to 24 days after antivenom in up to 75 percent of patients. As the dose of antivenom is increased, the incidence of late reactions increases, and the interval between treatment and appearance of symptoms decreases. The mechanism involves immune-complex formation.

Mechanism of Early Reactions. It had been assumed that all early reactions were type I IgE-mediated hypersensitivity reactions to equine serum proteins, but the prevalence of these reactions in communities unexposed to horses or their products and the lack of correlation with cutaneous hypersensitivity make this unlikely.

Some antivenoms activate complement in vitro. Anaphylactic reactions to homologous (human) immunoglobulin, which are clinically similar to early antivenom reactions, are associated with complement activation and immune complex formation in vivo. IgG aggregates are probably responsible for complement activation.

Prediction of Antivenom Reactions. Intradermal or conjunctival hypersensitivity tests do not reliably predict which patients will develop early or late reactions [*29*].

Treatment of Reactions. Epinephrine, 0.1%, 0.5 to 1.0 mL, given by subcutaneous injection is the most effective treatment for all symptoms of early reactions. The subcutaneous route is preferred to intramuscular injection because of the risk of inadvertent intravenous injection in the latter. An antihistamine such as promazine or chlorpheniramine should be given over the next 24 h to combat effects of histamine released during the reaction. Later reactions can be treated with a short course of antihistamine and corticosteroid in severe cases. Epinephrine is potentially too dangerous a drug to be given prophylactically to every patient receiving antivenom.

Supportive treatment

Neurotoxic Envenoming. Patients with bulbar or respiratory paralysis may die of airway obstruction resulting from inhalation or respiratory failure. Although artificial ventilation was first suggested for paralytic snakebite more than 100 years ago, there are still new reports in the literature of patients dying of untreated respiratory failure. Since all effects of neurotoxins are fully reversible in time, it is well worth ventilating patients by whatever means are available: mouth-to-mouth resuscitation, Ambubag, or respirator. Patients have recovered from respiratory paralysis after being manually ventilated by relays of relatives or nurses for up to 30 days. Since most patients with neurotoxic envenoming remain fully conscious, insertion of a cuffed tracheostomy tube under local anesthesia is preferred to endotracheal intubation.

Neostigmine and other anticholinesterases have been reported to improve, sometimes dramatically, neurotoxic symptoms induced by a variety of snake venoms [18]. The species include *N. naja*, *N. melanoleuca*, *B. caeruleus*, *B. candidus*, and *Dendroaspis viridis*. A test dose of rapidly acting edrophonium chloride (10 mg IV) after atropine (0.6 mg) is recommended in all cases of severe neurotoxic envenoming, as in the case of suspected myasthenia gravis. Patients who respond convincingly should be maintained on neostigmine methyl sulfate, 50 to 100 μg/kg, and atropine at least every 4 h, or by continuous infusion.

Circulatory Collapse. Circulatory collapse may respond to antivenom alone, but in patients who have leaked large amounts of blood and plasma into their swollen limbs hypovolemia must be corrected with a plasma expander, or preferably whole fresh blood. Hypotension in patients envenomed by *V. russellii* in Burma responded to dopamine infusion but not to methylprednisolone or naloxone [32]. Acute pituitary-adrenal failure may occur in patients bitten by *V. russellii* (Burma) and *Bothrops* species [33].

Renal Failure. Acute tubular necrosis is the most common cause of renal failure in snakebite victims. In patients bitten by sea snakes and other species whose venoms cause generalized rhabdomyolysis (see above), the urine should be alkalinized to prevent renal damage from myoglobin, and emergency treatment may be needed to control hyperkalemia. Renal failure can often be treated conservatively, but peritoneal dialysis and hemodialysis may be required.

Local Effects. The risk of local infection from pathogens on the snake's fangs is uncertain. Captive snakes develop a rich bacterial flora including anaerobes, but secondary infection of bite wounds is extremely rare in the absence of interference such as incision and suction, or necrosis. Antimicrobial treatment is unlikely to be harmful but is probably not necessary as a routine unless there has been interference, in which case tetanus prophylaxis should be considered as well. *Local necrosis* should be treated by surgical debridement, immediate split-skin grafting, and antimicrobials (including metronidazole for anaerobes) as soon as it is diagnosed. *Tense edema* of the

bitten limb raises the question of whether fasciotomy need be performed to relieve pressure in fascial compartments, especially the anterior tibial compartment [14]. Most people agree that fasciotomy is rarely if ever required if adequate antivenom is given, and that it is contraindicated in patients with incoagulable blood. It should not be undertaken without demonstrating raised tissue pressure in the compartment or severe narrowing of a major blood vessel by Doppler or angiography.

Other Drugs. *Corticosteroids* have been claimed to show beneficial effects in animals injected with *E. carinatus*, *N. naja*, and other venoms, but in patients they proved useless in *C. rhodostoma* envenoming in a controlled trial and against neurotoxic envenoming by *N. naja*. *Heparin* has been advocated for envenoming by *E. carinatus* and other species on the basis of animal studies and various uncontrolled clinical studies. A controlled trial in Nigeria, however, indicated that in the case of *E. carinatus* bites heparin offered no advantage over antivenom. In vitro the thrombins generated by venom procoagulants may be resistant to heparin. Heparin has exaggerated bleeding and contributed to the death of snakebite victims. Antihistamines, antifibrinolytic agents, clotting factors, local trypsin, and many other compounds and herbs have been suggested for the treatment of snakebite. Convincing clinical evidence in their support is universally lacking.

Management of snake venom ophthalmia

First aid for patients "spat" at by cobras consists of urgent liberal irrigation of the eye with water or any other bland liquid available. The eye should be examined using fluorescein staining or, preferably, a slit lamp, treated with a topical antimicrobial, and closed with a pad. The greatest danger is permanent blindness following secondary infection of corneal abrasions [22].

Prognosis

A proportion of bites by venomous snakes results in negligible or no envenoming. This important observation, emphasized by the work of H. A. Reid [18a,34], has an important bearing on prognosis and explains the apparent efficacy of a profusion of useless remedies. About 20 percent of patients bitten by North American rattlesnakes, Central American venomous snakes (mainly *Bothrops*), and *C. rhodostoma* [21] show no evidence of envenoming; and as many as 80 percent of patients bitten by sea snakes and 50 percent by *C. rhodostoma* and *V. russellii* have trivial or no envenoming [18a,32,34]. The mortality rates of untreated snakebite patients are hard to assess, as hospital admissions are biased in favor of severe cases and data for untreated patients are available only when supplies of antivenom run out. For bites by *C. durissus terrificus*, a reputed mortality rate of 74 percent for untreated patients has been reduced to 12 percent by antivenom [25], while for *E. cari-*

natus the mortality rate of about 20 percent for untreated patients can be reduced to around 3 percent with antivenom [*35*]. In Australia, reported mortalities before antivenom became available were 50 percent for *Acanthophis,* 45.5 percent for *N. scutatus,* and 18.7 percent for *Pseudonaja textilis* [*28*]. Prognosis is worst in young children and the elderly.

SNAKEBITE IN THE POPULATION

Incidence

The highest incidence of snakebite is in rural communities where the preference for traditional herbal treatment outside hospital, limited hospital and laboratory facilities, and shortage of capable investigators, make accurate data collection extremely difficult. As a result, "official" national statistics on snakebites, which depend largely on reported hospital admissions, have grossly underestimated the size of the problem and have led to the present situation where snakebite is the most neglected area of tropical medicine. For example, from 1947 to 1952, 166 cases of snakebite and 9 deaths were reported from the northern region of Nigeria, whereas during a similar period from 1964 to 1969, 953 bites and 50 deaths were recorded at a single mission hospital in the Muri division, a community of about a quarter of a million people within this region [*35*]. A recent survey from this same area of the Benue Valley obtained an incidence of 497 bites per 100,000 population per year with a 12.2 percent mortality rate. By visiting fishing villages along the northwest coast of Malaya, Reid and Lim [*36*] discovered details of 114 sea snake bites, only 18 of which had been treated in hospital. In the Malumfashi area of northern Nigeria, only 8.5 percent of people bitten by *N. nigricollis* had sought hospital treatment. The following examples, based on hospital returns, probably represent underestimates of the true incidence of mortality due to snakebite. In India, the reported annual number of deaths has exceeded 20,000 over the last 100 years, and in Maharashtra state alone there are more than 1000 deaths each year. In Sri Lanka there are more than 900 deaths each year among 60,000 bites. In Burma, snakebite, mainly by *V. russellii,* has been the fifth most important cause of death [*32*]. During the 1930s, when 2000 deaths were reported each year, the annual mortality rate in the Sagaing district near Mandalay was 36.8 per 100,000. In Brazil there are an estimated 2000 deaths due to snakebite per year. In Venezuela, between 1955 and 1968, an average of 973 bites occurred each year with 103 deaths; *B. atrox* was responsible for 38 percent and *C. durissus terrificus* for 24 percent of bites. In the Amami and Okinawa islands of Japan, the habu *(Tr. flavoviridis)* caused an average of 610 bites with 5.6 deaths per year during the 1960s.

The highest mortality rates from snakebite are suffered by some hunter-gatherer tribes. Snakebite is responsible for 2 percent of adult deaths among the Yanomamo of Amazonian Venezuela, and 5 percent among the Waorani of eastern Ecuador. The Phi Tong Luang of northeastern Thailand, the Hadza of Tanzania, some tribal groups in Papua New Guinea, and the aborigines of central Australia have also suffered high mortality rates from snakebite.

In the United States there are approximately 45,000 bites per year, 7000 of which are caused by venomous species, with 9 to 14 deaths [*21*]. Snakebite is an important cause of death among large grazing animals in some countries. In India in the 1880s almost 4000 cattle a year were reported to be killed by snakes. In South Africa *B. arietans* has been responsible for the deaths of many grazing animals, *V. lebetina* has killed horses and camels in the northwest frontier area of India and Cyprus, while a number of deaths, especially in foals, have been attributed to the brown snake *Pseudonaja textilis* in Queensland, Australia [*28*].

Epidemiology

Most snakebites occur on the lower limbs of farmers, herders, hunters, and children in the rural tropics. The incidence of bites by a particular species in a certain geographical region depends on the density of human and snake populations, the snake's irritability (its willingness to bite when trodden on or disturbed), the diurnal cycle of activity of humans and snakes, and the extent to which human activities encroach on the snake's habitat. There are few convincing reports of unprovoked aggression by snakes, even the notorious *D. polylepis* and *O. hannah,* and, in the tropics at least, snakebite is always the result of an inadvertent tread or touch. Many bites occur when farmers tread on snakes as they walk to or from their fields in the dark, while some species (*N. nigricollis* and the kraits *B. candidus* and *B. caeruleus*) seem particularly likely to bite people while they are asleep in their huts. In contrast, in the United States, 25 percent of bites result from snakes being handled or attacked; these bites are usually inflicted on the hands. Species which readily strike when disturbed include *V. russellii, E. carinatus, C. rhodostoma,* and most species of rattlesnakes and cobras; whereas kraits and the giant rain forest vipers, *B. gabonica* and *B. nasicornis,* seem reluctant to bite. In many regions there is a marked seasonal variation in the incidence of snakebite. For example, in west Africa, the peak incidence of *E. carinatus* bite coincides with the start of the rainy season around March to June, and in Burma there are peaks of incidence of *V. russellii* bite in June when the rice is planted and in November when it is harvested. Flooding may drive snakes from their retreats and increase contact with humans. This has resulted in epidemics of snakebite in areas such as Colombia, Pakistan, India, and Bangladesh. Development of snake-populated areas for new highways, irrigation, or hydroelectric projects has led to an increased incidence of snakebite in parts of Brazil and Sri Lanka. There are several reports of snake and other animal venoms being used as a means of suicide and murder.

Prevention

Snakebite is easily prevented by taking simple precautions. Snakes should never be disturbed, attacked, or handled even if they are said to be harmless species or appear to be dead. Venomous snakes should not be kept as pets or as performing animals. In snake-infested areas, boots, socks, and long trousers should be worn for walks in undergrowth or deep sand. A light should always be carried at night. Collecting firewood, dislodging logs and boulders with the bare hands, pushing sticks into burrows, holes, or crevices, climbing rocks and trees covered with dense foliage, and swimming in overgrown lakes and rivers are particularly dangerous activities. Unlit paths and roads are particularly dangerous after heavy rains. Unfortunately, these precautions are impracticable for the rural farmers and others exposed to the highest risk of snakebite. In Burma, attempts will be made to drive snakes from the paddy fields, in advance of the rice farmers, by beating on the ground and by driving cattle through the fields. In Thailand, the incidence of cobra bites among fish farmers has been reduced by wearing rubber boots. Efforts are being made to design protective clothing compatible with hard agricultural work in hot climates. The extermination of venomous species has been advocated for many years, but has not proved possible and would probably cause a population explosion among rodents, the natural prey of most species.

Vaccination against snakebite

The vaccination of high-risk populations using venom toxoids (venoids) has been pioneered by Y. Sawai in Japan. Formol venoids of HR1 and HR2 hemorrhagins from *T. flavoviridis* venom were used in large groups of volunteers in the Amami Islands. The degree of protection afforded by vaccination has not yet been established in humans, and local reactions to the venoid may be troublesome. Several other countries in Asia are carrying out preliminary studies with venoids [25].

VENOMOUS LIZARDS [37,21]

Two species of lizards possess inferior labial glands situated in the anterior half of the lower jaw which secrete a venomous saliva conducted along grooves in the lower teeth. The Gila monster *(Heloderma suspectum)*, which grows up to 60 cm in length, is found in the southwestern United States and adjacent parts of Mexico; and the Mexican beaded lizard or *escorpión (H. horridum)*, which reaches 80 cm, occurs in western Mexico and Central America (Fig. 59-10). The venom contains lethal toxins (gilatoxins) and shows various enzyme activities including phospholipase A, hyaluronidase, arginine esterase, and a kallikrein-like hypotensive enzyme (''helodermatine''). In experimental animals the venom causes hypotension, myocardial depression, respiratory arrhythmias and paralysis, autonomic stimulation, release of kinins and other mediators, and spontaneous hemorrhage in mice.

Most bites have resulted from handling pet heloderms but there have also been some accidental encounters. The bite is powerful and protracted. Severe local pain develops almost immediately with tender swelling and regional lymphadenopathy. Systemic symptoms include weakness, dizziness, hypotension, syncope, sweating, rigors, tinnitus, nausea, vomiting, and angioedema. Leukocytosis and ECG changes are reported. Deaths occurring in a few cases of *H. suspectum* bite reported up to the 1930s could not, with certainty, be attributed to envenoming.

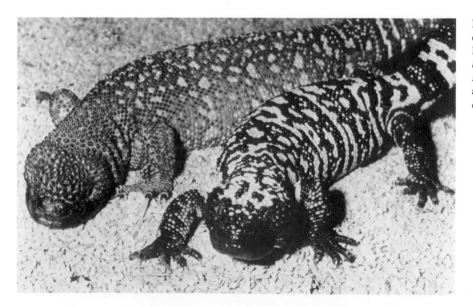

Figure 59-10. The two species of dangerously venomous lizards. Left: Mexican beaded lizard *(Heloderma horridum)*. Right: Gilamonster *(H. suspectum)*. Both specimens were approximately 50 cm long. *(Courtesy of the Zoological Society of London.)*

TREATMENT

The lizard should be pried off as soon as possible. The most effective and least inhumane method appears to be the application of a flame to the underside of the jaw. Multiple tooth punctures are produced, some containing shed teeth. Specific antivenom is not generally available. Strong analgesic may be required. Shock and anaphylactoid symptoms should be treated with epinephrine, antihistamine, and corticosteroid, bearing in mind the possible role of autacoids such as bradykinin and 5-hydroxytryptamine in their pathogenesis.

VENOMOUS FISH [38]

TAXONOMY

Of the approximately 250 species of fish which possess a defensive venom-injecting apparatus, more than 100 species have proved dangerous to humans. Fish sting by secreting venom around spines or barbs placed in front of dorsal fins or the tail, incorporated into dorsal and pectoral fins, or situated in the gill covers. The richest venomous fish fauna is around the coral reefs of tropical waters, particularly in the Indo-Pacific region, but venomous species such as sharks, chimeras, and weever fish also occur in temperate northern waters. Fatal stings by members of the following groups have been reported: Squaliformes (sharks and dogfish), Rajiformes (stingrays and mantas), Siluroidei (catfish), Trachinidae (weeverfish), Scorpaenidae (scorpionfish), Uranoscopidae (stargazers or stonelifters).

VENOM PROPERTIES [38,39]

Fish venoms are much less temperature-stable than the venoms of snakes and most other venomous animals. Stingray venom has been found to contain 5-hydroxytryptamine, 5-nucleotidase, phosphodiesterase, and three protein toxins. Stonefish venom contains at least 10 toxic proteins, one of which is lethal. Many fish venoms contain hyaluronidase. The principal pharmacological effects of fish venoms are direct effects on cardiac, skeletal, and smooth muscle, producing hypotension, ECG changes, and paralysis; and depression of the respiratory center and local necrotic effects.

VENOM APPARATUS, HABITS, AND CLINICAL EFFECTS OF SELECTED GROUPS OF STINGING FISH

The widely distributed stingrays (Rajiformes) are responsible for 750 to 1500 stings each year in the United States. They lie partly buried in sand or mud and are easily stepped upon by waders or bathers. Their response is to lash their tail against the intruding limb and stab with their barbed caudal spine, up to 30 cm long in some species, which can cause a deep lacerating wound, usually to the leg but occasionally penetrating body cavities, heart, or viscera when the swimmer falls or lies on the fish. The venom glands lie along the spine under a membrane or integument which is torn off as the spine enters the victim's flesh, releasing venom into the wound. Symptoms include severe pain, vomiting, diarrhea, hypotension, sweating, cardiac arrhythmias, and muscle contractions in response to pain. Local swelling and later necrosis is common, and there is a high risk of infection unless the broken spine and integument are removed from the wound. The mortality rate is said to be about 1 percent.

Weever fish (Trachinidae) occur in the temperate waters of the North Sea, the Mediterranean, and the coasts of north Africa. They are armed with dorsal and opercular spines and like stingrays lie in sand on the sea floor where they may be trodden on by bathers or caught and inadvertently handled by fishermen. Stings are common around the coasts of Britain in the summer months, and on the Adriatic coast of Yugoslavia. The symptoms are similar to those produced by stingrays but are rarely as severe, while the mechanical trauma is trivial in comparison.

The scorpion fish (Scorpaenidae) have the most highly evolved venom apparatus in 12 to 13 dorsal, 3 anal, and 2 pelvic spines. At least 300 stings each year are inflicted by *Scorpaena* species in the United States. The very ornate species of the genera *Pterois* and *Dendrochirus,* known as zebra, lion, turkey, or red fire fish or coral or fire cod, frequent tropical coral reefs and are increasingly popular aquarium pets. The most dangerous of all venomous fish are stonefish (genus *Synanceja*), which occur from the eastern coast of Africa across the Indian Ocean to the Pacific. They are very effectively camouflaged and live on the bottom of rock pools and in other shallow waters. Their short, thick spines contain bulky venom glands draining through paired venom ducts to the tips. Symptoms can be severe. Pain is excruciating and may persist for 2 days or more. Patients may lose consciousness rapidly and develop diarrhea, vomiting, signs of autonomic nervous system stimulation, hypotension, cardiac arrhythmias, respiratory distress, neurological signs, and convulsions. There is local swelling, blanching, cyanosis, and eventually necrosis. Although numbers of fatal cases have been reported, 81 cases of stings, mostly by *S. horrida,* seen at Pulau Bukom, an island south of Singapore, during a period of 4 years, had only mild symptoms. In former times there were many subsequent deaths from secondary infection.

TREATMENT [38,40,41]

Attention should be given to the wound. Bleeding should be controlled if there is severe trauma from a stingray dart. The venomous spine and associated membrane should be removed as soon as possible and the wound cleaned and irrigated. Immersion of the stung limb in water that is uncomfortably hot but not scalding (i.e., just under 50°C) has proved effective in relieving pain, presumably by inactivating the thermolabile venom. Temperature should be assessed by the unstung limb. One percent lignocaine can be injected, for example, as a ring block in the case of stung digits, but is less effective. However, local nerve block with 0.5% plain bupivacaine does seem to work. Antimicrobials and tetanus prophylaxis should be given. Injection of potassium permanganate and emetine hydrochloride and the application of cold packs may promote local necrosis. In patients with severe systemic symptoms, the airway should be kept clear and cardiopulmonary resuscitation used if necessary. Severe hypotension may respond to epinephrine and bradycardia to atropine.

Antivenom

The CSL of Australia manufacture an equine antivenom specific for *Synanceja trachynis*, but which also has some clinical effect with stings by the scorpion fish *(Scorpaena guttata)* and possibly with other members of the Scorpaenidae. The dose is calculated according to the number of sting punctures found on the victim (2 mL or 2000 U, the contents of one ampule, for each two punctures) or the severity of symptoms.

PREVENTION OF FISH STINGS

By shuffling rather than stepping, bathers and waders can reduce the risk of contact with stingrays, weever fish, stonefish, and other species which skulk in sand or mud. Footwear protects against most species but will not prevent penetration by stingray spines. Prodding with a stick in advance is also helpful. Skin divers, bathers, and fishermen should be aware of the danger of venomous fish and should avoid contact with them in nets, on lines, or where they are swimming freely.

POISONING BY INGESTION OF FISH, TURTLES, SHELLFISH, CRABS, AND OTHER MARINE ANIMALS [38,42]

Illness following ingestion of seafood may be caused by infections by *Vibrio parahaemolyticus* (after eating crustaceans, especially shrimps), *V. cholerae* (crabs and mollusks), non-01 *V. cholerae* (shellfish), *V. hollisae* (catfish), *Salmonella typhi* (mollusks), *Campylobacter jejuni* (clams), Hepatitis A virus (mollusks, especially clams and oysters), Norwalk agent (oysters and other mollusks), and "small, round viruses" (cockles and other mollusks). However, in some cases, toxins are involved. Clinical features of poisoning have now been described for a large number of different groups of fish, turtles, mollusks, crustaceans, and other marine animals. These can be resolved into two main clinical syndromes: a neurotoxic (paralytic) and gastrointestinal syndrome, which includes ciguatera and tetrodotoxin fish poisonings and paralytic and neurotoxic shellfish poisonings, and the histaminelike syndrome of scombrotoxin poisoning.

NEUROTOXIC AND GASTROINTESTINAL SYNDROME

Gastrointestinal symptoms including nausea, vomiting, colic, and tenesmus, and watery diarrhea may precede neurotoxic features. A dry mouth, metallic taste, and paresthesias of lips, tongue, throat, and extremities are often the earliest symptoms. Other neurotoxic manifestations are a distortion of temperature sensation so that cold objects feel hot (like dry ice) and vice versa, dizziness, myalgia, weakness starting with muscles of phonation and deglutition and progressing to respiratory paralysis and flaccid quadriplegia in some cases, ataxia, involuntary movements, convulsions, visual disturbances, hallucinations and psychoses, cranial nerve lesions, pupillary abnormalities, and hypersalivation. Cardiovascular abnormalities, including hypotension and bradycardia, and cutaneous lesions may develop. The following are selected important examples of this syndrome.

Ciguatera (fish) poisoning

Gastrointestinal or neurotoxic symptoms develop within 6 h (range of minutes to 30 h) after eating a wide range of tropical shore and reef fish such as red snapper, barracuda, grouper, amberjack, Moray eel, parrot fish, and more than 400 others occurring between latitudes 35° north and south. Symptoms may persist for a week or more. The mortality rate was 0.1 percent in New Caledonia [43]. The toxin, ultimately derived from planktonic or benthic dinoflagellates such as *Gambierdiscus toxicus,* is concentrated in the liver, viscera, and gonads especially of larger and older fish. Ciguatera toxin has a direct effect on excitable membranes, competing with calcium ions. The worldwide incidence of ciguatera poisoning is unknown. In New Caledonia between 20 and 90 cases are reported each month [43].

Chelonitoxication resulting from ingestion of marine turtles *(Chelonia)* has clinical features very similar to ciguatera poisoning. Most outbreaks have been in the Indo-Pacific area. The species usually implicated are green, hawksbill, and leathery turtles. The mortality rate among reported cases is 28 percent.

Tetrodotoxin (fish) poisoning

More than 50 species of scaleless toadfish, puffer fish, porcupine fish, boxfish, sunfish, and triggerfish (order Tetraodontiformes) occurring widely in tropical and subtropical oceans have proved poisonous. In Japan puffer fish (fugu) are relished, and despite government controls more than 250 cases of poisoning are reported each year with a 60 percent mortality rate. Paresthesia, dizziness, and ataxia become noticeable within 10 to 45 min of eating the fish. Generalized numbness, hypersalivation, sweating, and hypotension may develop. Gastrointestinal symptoms may occur early in the poisoning but are often completely absent. Death from respiratory paralysis usually occurs within the first 6 h. Erythema, petechiae, blistering, and desquamation may appear. Tetrodotoxin is found especially in the gonads, liver, and intestine. The origin of this toxin is unknown; it may derive from algae eaten by the fish. Its structure is now known. An identical toxin is found in some amphibians and octopuses. Its action is to block selectively the sodium pump of excitable membranes.

Paralytic shellfish and crustacean poisoning

Bivalve mollusks such as mussels, clams *(Saxidomus)*, oysters, cockles, and scallops; xanthid crabs; coconut crabs; and the eggs of horseshoe crabs may acquire neurotoxins such as saxitoxin from the dinoflagellates *Gonyaulax catenella, G. tamarensis,* and *G. excavata* which occur between latitudes 30° north and south. The dinoflagellates may be sufficiently abundant during the warmer months of May to October to produce a "red tide." The dangerous season is signaled by the discovery of unusual numbers of dead fish and sea birds. Symptoms develop within 30 min of ingestion. They include perioral paresthesia, gastrointestinal symptoms, ataxia, visual disturbances, and pareses progressing to respiratory paralysis within 12 h in 8 percent of cases. Milder gastrointestinal and neurotoxic symptoms without paralysis have been associated with ingestion of mollusks contaminated by neurotoxins from *Ptychodiscus brevis,* which also causes red tide.

HISTAMINELIKE SYNDROME [44]

The flesh of scombroid fish such as tuna, mackerel, bonito, and skipjack and of canned nonscombroid fish like sardines and pilchards may be decomposed by the action of bacteria such as *Proteus morgani* and *Klebsiella pneumoniae,* converting muscle histidine into saurine, histamine, and unidentified toxins. Between minutes and a few hours after ingestion flushing, burning, urticaria and pruritus of the skin, headache, abdominal colic, nausea, vomiting, diarrhea, and bronchial asthma may develop. Patients taking diamine oxidase inhibitors such as isoniazid are particualrly susceptible to histamine poisoning.

TREATMENT

The differential diagnosis includes bacterial food poisoning and allergic reactions. No specific treatments or antidotes are available. Gastrointestinal contents should be eliminated by emetics and purges. Activated charcoal adsorbs saxitoxin and other shellfish toxins. Atropine, anticholinesterases, and calcium gluconate have proved helpful in some cases of neurotoxic (paralytic) syndrome. In scombroid poisoning, antihistamines and bronchodilators should be used. In cases of respiratory paralysis, endotracheal intubation and mechanical ventilation have proved life-saving. Cardiac resuscitation may also be required.

PREVENTION

Ciguatera, tetrodotoxin, and the other toxins responsible are heat-stable, so cooking does not prevent poisoning. In tropical areas the flesh of fish should be separated from the skin, intestines, gonads, and other viscera which may have high con-

centrations of toxin. All scaleless fish should be regarded as potentially tetrodotoxic, while very large fish carry an increased risk of being ciguateratoxic. Moray eels should never be eaten. Some toxins are fairly water-soluble and may be leached out, so water in which fish are cooked should be thrown away. Scombroid poisoning can be prevented by prompt freezing or by eating the fish fresh. Shellfish should not be eaten during the dangerous seasons and when there are red tides.

VENOMOUS MARINE INVERTEBRATES [38]

COELENTERATES

Included in this group are jellyfish; cubomedusoids; sea wasps; Portuguese men-of-war, or bluebottles; polyps; hydroids; sea anemones; sea nettles; and corals.

The tentacles of coelenterates are armed with stinging capsules or nematocysts which can produce lines of painful irritant weals on the skin of swimmers unlucky enough to make contact with them. The venoms consist of peptides and also contain or release substances such as 5-hydroxytryptamine and histamine, prostaglandins, and kinins which cause immediate excruciating pain, inflammation, and urticaria. Rarely there are severe systemic effects including rigors, vomiting and diarrhea, hypotensive collapse, respiratory muscle paralysis, and convulsions. Local necrosis may develop. Dangerous species include *Chironex fleckeri* (box jellyfish, cubomedusoid, sea wasp, or indringa), which has caused at least 55 deaths in the Indo-Pacific region during the last 100 years [44a]; *Chiropsalmus* species (sea wasps); and *Carukia barnesi,* the cause of Irukandji sting in Australia. The Portuguese man-of-war, *Physalia* species, can also cause severe systemic symptoms but no deaths have been adequately documented. The imprint of nematocyst stings on the skin may have a diagnostic pattern. Many stings could be prevented if swimmers were particularly cautious during those seasons when jellyfish are swept inshore.

Treatment

The aim is to prevent further discharge of nematocysts on fragments of tentacles stuck to the skin. Methyl alcohol, the traditional remedy, has been shown to have the deleterious effect of causing massive discharge of nematocysts. Commercial vinegar or 4 to 6% acetic acid are, however, very effective for *Chironex* and *Physalia,* and baking soda and water (50% w/v) for *Chrysaora* [45]. Application of tourniquets proximal to the stung area may produce a useful delay in the absorption of venom. Specific "sea wasp" antivenom for *Chironex fleckeri* stings is made by the CSL in Australia. Cardiorespiratory resuscitation has proved effective.

ECHINODERMS

Starfish and sea urchins possess venomous spines and grapples (pedicellariae) which can cause local pain and swelling and rarely systemic effects such as paresthesia, cardiac arrhythmias, and respiratory paralysis which may prove fatal. The venoms include steroid glycosides and proteins. Spines and grapples should be removed from the wound after softening the skin with 2% salicylic acid ointment.

MOLLUSKS

The mollusks include snails, slugs, cones, and octopuses.

The venomous radula of the cone shell (Conidae), a kind of sea snail, produces local paresthesia and numbness and paralysis which progressed to fatal respiratory paralysis in 8 out of 30 reported cases. The blue-ringed octopuses *Hapalochlaena maculosa* and *H. lanulata* of the Australian region can cause serious systemic envenoming by introducing saliva containing tetrodotoxin, other toxins, and vasoactive amines into wounds inflicted by their beaks. The bite itself is painless, but generalized and fatal paralysis may develop within 15 min.

No specific treatment is available for mollusk envenoming. An arterial tourniquet may delay absorption until facilities for cardiorespiratory resuscitation are available.

VENOMOUS ARTHROPODS

HYMENOPTERA (BEES, WASPS, YELLOWJACKETS, AND HORNETS) [46–48]

In temperate countries, the prevalence of Type I IgE–mediated hypersensitivity to bee and wasp venoms is about 0.5 percent, and anaphylactic reactions, usually to single stings, cause more deaths than direct envenoming by snakes and other venomous animals. However, multiple hymenoptera stings can prove fatal even in nonallergic subjects. Only this direct toxicity of hymenoptera venoms will be discussed here.

Taxonomy

The commonest, and most severe, hymenoptera stings are caused by members of the families Apidae (e.g., *Apis mellifera*, honeybee) and Vespidae (e.g., *Paravespula* species, wasps; *Dolichovespula* species, yellowjackets; *Vespa* species, hornets). Particularly aggressive species are the Africanized "killer" bee *(A. mellifera scutellata)* and Asian hornets (*V. affinis*, *V. velutina*, and *V. mandarinia*).

Venom apparatus and composition

Venoms are injected through a barbed sting. Bees inject approximately 50 μg of venom, the total capacity of the venom sac, and leave the sting embedded in the skin, but wasps and hornets can sting repeatedly. Hymenoptera venoms contain biogenic amines (histamine, 5-hydroxytryptamine, acetylcholine), enzymes (such as phospholipase A2 and hyaluronidase) and other proteins, and toxic peptides or kinins [e.g., in Vespidae, wasp kinins; and in Apidae, a neurotoxin (apamin), a membrane lytic factor (melittin), and the mast cell degranu-

lating peptide "401"]. These toxins act by altering membrane ionic conductance. The high-molecular-weight enzymes phospholipase A2 and hyaluronidase are most important in inducing hypersensitivity, while the direct toxic effects of large doses of venom from multiple stings reflect histamine-releasing and direct toxic effects on skeletal muscle, erythrocytes, and perhaps the kidney.

Clinical features

In people who are not allergic to the venom, single or few stings usually produce only local effects attributable to the injected biogenic amines. For example, 5-hydroxytryptamine, wasp kinins, and protease are responsible for the pain of wasp stings. Pain, redness, swelling, whealing, and heat develop rapidly but rarely last for more than a few hours. Local effects are dangerous only if the airway is obstructed, for example following stings on the tongue.

In children, as few as 30 stings can cause fatal toxicity. Adults have survived more than 2000 stings by *A. mellifera*. The clinical picture is of histamine overdose—vasodilation, hypotension, vomiting, diarrhea, throbbing headache, and coma, together with the local effects of multiple stings. Rhabdomyolysis followed by myoglobinuria and renal failure can occur after multiple hornet stings *(V. affinis)*. Hemolysis, hemoglobinuria, thrombocytopenic purpura, myasthenia gravis, hepatic damage, and various renal glomerular lesions (for example mesangial proliferative nephritis) leading to nephrotic syndrome and acute tubular necrosis have been described after multiple stings by *V. orientalis* and other Asian vespids.

Treatment

The stings should be removed without squeezing, which will inject more venom. They should be scraped out with a blade or fingernail. Aspirin is an effective analgesic. In cases of severe systemic envenoming, life-threatening effects of biogenic amines can be treated with adrenaline and antihistamine. No specific antivenoms are available. Renal failure complicating myoglobinuria, hemoglobinuria, or a direct nephrotoxic effect may require peritoneal or hemodialysis.

Prevention

Nests should be avoided and not interfered with in any way. It is useful to know the appearance and most likely sites of nests of local species. Some hornets are so aggressive that their nests must be eradicated before their territory can safely be cultivated.

SCORPIONS [47,49–51]

Taxonomy

Scorpions (order Scorpionida) capable of inflicting fatal stings in humans are members of the families Buthidae and Scor-

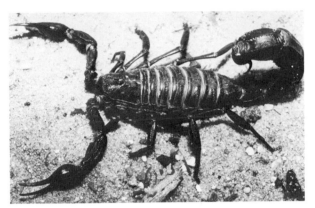

Figure 59-11. Dangerous north African scorpion (genus *Androctonus*). *(Photographed by courtesy of Zoological Society of London; copyright D. A. Warrell.)*

pionidae. Examples of the most deadly species are: *Androctonus australis* (north Africa and Middle East) (Fig. 59-11), *A. crassicauda* (Turkey, Middle East, and north Africa), *Buthus occitanus* (countries bordering the Mediterranean and Middle East), *Leiurus quinquestriatus* (north Africa and Middle East), *Hemiscorpion lepturus* (Iran and Iraq), *Parabuthus* species (South Africa), *Tityus trinitatis* (Trinidad and Venezuela), *T. serrulatus* and *T. bahiensis* (Brazil, Argentina), *Centruroides sculpturatus* (California, New Mexico, Arizona, and Baha California), *C. limpidus* and *C. suffusus* (Mexico), and *Buthotus* (formerly *Buthus*) *tamulus* (India).

Epidemiology

Painful scorpion stings are common throughout the tropics; however, fatal envenoming is frequent only in Mexico, Brazil, Trinidad, parts of north Africa and the Middle East, and in India. In southern Libya there were 900 stings with 7 deaths per 100,000 population in 1979. In Mexico there are between 1000 and 2000 deaths each year, with an incidence of 84 deaths per 100,000 per year in Colima State. Case mortality is about 50 percent in children up to 4 years old. In Trinidad, stings by *T. trinitatis* are an occupational hazard of sugar cane and cocoa farmers: there were 33 deaths in a group of 698 cases. Mortality was 25 percent among the children under 5 years compared to 0.25 percent in adults. In Brazil, mortality increases from around 1 percent in adults to 15 to 25 percent in children less than 6 years old. In Algeria there were an average of 1260 stings and 24 deaths per year. In India there are many cases of scorpion stings with fatalities in adults and children.

Clinical features

Rapidly developing, very intense local pain is the commonest symptom. Local signs such as swelling, redness, heat, and regional lymph node involvement are never extensive. Local necrosis is most unusual. Systemic symptoms may develop within minutes, but may be delayed for as much as 24 h. Features of autonomic nervous system excitation include dilated pupils, hypersalivation, profuse sweating, hyperthermia, vomiting, diarrhea, abdominal distension, loss of sphincter control, and priapism. Release of catecholamines, as in pheochromocytoma, produces hypertension and toxic myocarditis with arrhythmias (most commonly sinus bradycardia), cardiac failure, and acute pulmonary edema leading to cardiogenic shock with tachycardia and profound hypotension. These cardiovascular effects are particularly prominent following stings by *L. quinquestriatus* and *B. tamulus*. Neurotoxic effects such as fasciculation, spasms, and respiratory paralysis are a particular feature of stings by *C. sculpturatus*.

Hemiplegia and other neurological lesions have been attributed to fibrin deposition resulting from disseminated intravascular coagulation. Hyperglycemia and glycosuria are results of hypercatecholaminemia, but *T. trinitatis* venom also causes acute pancreatitis. Intravascular hemolysis and renal failure have also been described. Death can occur within minutes or up to 42 h after the sting.

Treatment

Pain may respond to local infiltration or ring block with local anesthetic. Local injection of emetine is said to relieve the pain but may cause necrosis. Parenteral opiate analgesics such as pethidine and morphine may be required but are said to be dangerous in victims of *C. sculpturatus*.

The treatment of choice for systemic envenoming is specific antivenom which should be given by intravenous injection (as described above for snakebite). Antivenom is manufactured in the United States, Britain, Germany, Mexico, Brazil, Turkey, Algeria, South Africa, Egypt, and Iran.

Many accessory treatments have been suggested. There is some clinical evidence to support the use of the following:

1. For patients with the hypercatecholaminemia syndrome (hypertension, bradycardia, and early pulmonary edema), rapid digitalization, potent loop diuretics, and alpha-blocking vasodilators such as prazosin hydrochloride. β-Blockers may be dangerous once cardiac failure has developed.
2. Atropine for patients with signs of parasympathetic nervous system stimulation such as bradycardia.
3. Anticonvulsants such as phenobarbitone for neurotoxic symptoms (*C. sculpturatus*).

No antivenom is commercially available for the treatment of *B. tamulus* stings in India. In this case, patients who develop priapism, dilated pupils, sweating, and bradycardia are at high risk of progressing to pulmonary edema. Early energetic treatment of cardiac failure may prevent this [*49*].

Prevention

High doorsteps and a row of ceramic tiles at the base of the outer wall may keep scorpions out of the house. Residual insecticides such as 1% lindane or dieldrin powders are effective. Prophylactic immunization with scorpion venom toxoid is under trial in Mexico.

SPIDERS (ARANEAE) [28,47,50,52]

More than 30,000 species of spiders have been named. However, only about 30 of these are known or suspected to be capable of dangerous envenoming in humans. Spiders bite with a pair of fangs, the *chelicerae*, to whose tips the venom glands are connected by a duct.

Epidemiology

Loxosceles species cause many bites in Central and South America, especially in Chile (*L. laeta*) where mortality ranges from 1 to 17 percent; the United States (*L. reclusa*); and the Mediterranean region, north Africa, and Israel (*L. rufescens*). Most people are bitten in their bedrooms while asleep or dressing, and in the United States men were bitten on the genitalia while they sat on outdoor lavatories in which the spiders had spun their webs.

  Latrodectus mactans tredecemguttatus ("tarantula") is common in Mediterranean countries and has been responsible for a series of bite epidemics (e.g., 946 cases between 1946 and 1951 in Italy). *L. m. hasselti*, the Australian red-backed spider, causes up to 340 bites each year in Australia; 20 deaths have been reported. *L. m. mactans* (Figure 59-12), the black widow spider, caused 63 deaths in the United States between 1950 and 1959. *Phoneutria nigriventer,* the banana spider, is an important cause of bites and deaths in South America. The aggressive male Sydney funnel web spider (*Atrax robustus*) caused at least 13 deaths between 1927 and 1980.

Clinical features

Of the four medically important genera of venomous spiders, *Loxosceles* causes necrotic araneism while *Latrodectus, Phoneutria,* and *Atrax* cause neurotoxic araneism.

Necrotic Araneism. There is burning pain at the site of the bite, which swells and, over a few days, develops a violaceous plaque which turns into a blackened eschar and sloughs in a few weeks, sometimes leaving a necrotic ulcer. These lesions may be extensive, rarely covering an entire limb. A generalized scarlatiniform desquamating rash may develop within 24 h of the bite. *L. reclusa* bites rarely cause skin necrosis but may give rise to a chronic pyoderma gangrenosum-like reaction. Less than one-fifth of cases have systemic symptoms such as jaundice and hemoglobinuria resulting from massive intravascular hemolysis, fever, respiratory distress, and shock. Mortality is about 6 percent in all reported cases and 30 percent in those with systemic envenoming.

Neurotoxic Araneism. The bite is very painful, but local signs are minimal (*L. m. mactans*) or moderate (*L. m. hasselti*).

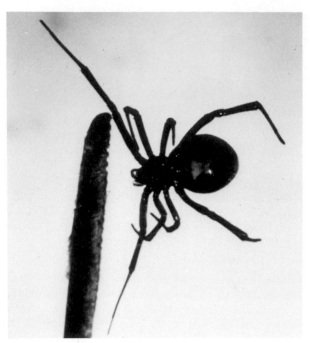

Figure 59-12. Black widow spider *(Latrodectus mactans mactans),* showing hourglass pattern on ventral surface of abdomen. *(Photographed by courtesy of Zoological Society of London; copyright D. A. Warrell.)*

Painful regional lymphadenopathy develops about 30 min after the bite. Patients complain of headache, nausea, vomiting, sweating, and painful muscle spasms and tremors which may be severe enough to embarrass respiration. Other features include tachycardia, hypertension, restlessness, irritability, psychosis, and priapism. *Facies latrodectismica* is a painful grimace caused by facial spasm and trismus associated with swollen eyelids, conjunctival congestion, flushing, and sweating associated particularly with bites by *L. m. tredecemguttatus, Phoneutria,* and *Atrax.*

Treatment

A. robustus can kill in 15 min and so a firm crepe bandage and splint or tight tourniquet should be applied as a first-aid measure to delay systemic spread of venom until the patient reaches hospital. Antivenoms for *Latrodectus* bites are made in Australia, the United States, the U.S.S.R., Italy, Yugoslavia, South Africa, and South America; for *Atrax* bites in Australia; for *Loxosceles* in Peru, Brazil, and Argentina; and for *Phoneutria* in Brazil. Neurotoxic araneism seems more responsive to antivenom than does the necrotic type. Oral dapsone (100 mg twice a day) is said to reduce the extent of necrotic lesions. Calcium gluconate (10 mL of 10% solution, given by slow intravenous injection) relieves the pain of muscle spasms caused by *Latrodectus* venom rapidly and more effectively than muscle relaxants such as diazepam or methocarbamol. Antihistamines, corticosteroids, β blockers, and atropine have also been advocated for bites of *Latrodectus*.

TICK-BITE PARALYSIS [47,53,54]

Paralysis has been reported after bites by adult females of about 30 species of hard tick (family Ixodidae) and six species of immature soft ticks (family Argasidae). Tick paralysis has been reported from all continents, but most cases have occurred in western North America (*Dermacentor andersoni*), the eastern United States (*D. variabilis*), and eastern Australia (*Ixodes holocyclus*). In British Columbia there were 305 cases with 10 percent mortality between 1900 and 1968. About 120 cases have been reported in the United States, and in New South Wales there were at least 20 deaths between 1900 and 1945.

Clinical features

Ticks are picked up in the countryside or from domestic animals, particularly dogs, in the home. A majority of patients and almost all fatal cases are children. After the tick has been attached for about 5 or 6 days a progressive ascending, lower motor neurone paralysis develops with paresthesiae. Often a child, who may have been irritable for the previous 24 h, falls on getting out of bed first thing in the morning, and is found to be weak. Paralysis increases over the next few days: death results from bulbar and respiratory paralysis and aspiration of stomach contents. Vomiting is a feature of the more acute course of *I. holocyclus* envenoming.

This clinical picture is often misinterpreted as poliomyelitis. Other neurological conditions including Guillain-Barré syndrome, myasthenia gravis, or botulism may also be suspected. Diagnosis depends on finding the tick, which is likely to be concealed in a crevice, orifice, or hairy area of the body. The scalp is the commonest place. Fatal tick paralysis has been caused by a tick attached to the tympanic membrane.

Treatment

The tick must be detached without being squeezed. It can be painted with ether, chloroform, paraffin, petrol, or turpentine, or prised out between the partially separated tips of a pair of small curved forceps. Following removal of the tick there is usually rapid and complete recovery; but in Australia, patients have died after the tick has been detached. An antivenom, raised in dogs or rabbits, is available in Australia. This is recommended for severely affected or very young patients; 20 to 30 mL are given intravenously.

CENTIPEDES [47,50]

Centipedes (Chilopoda) possess venom jaws. Many species can inflict painful bites producing local pain, swelling, inflammation, and lymphangitis. Systemic effects such as vomiting, headache, cardiac arrhythmias, and convulsions are extremely rare and the risk of mortality was probably greatly exaggerated in the older literature. The most important genus is *Scolopendra* which is distributed throughout tropical countries. Local

treatment is the same as for scorpion stings. No antivenom is available.

MILLIPEDES (DIPLOPIDA) [47,50,55]

Most species possess glands in each of their body segments which secrete, and in some cases squirt out, irritant liquids for defensive purposes. These contain hydrogen cyanide and a variety of aldehydes, esters, phenols, and quinonoids. Members of at least eight genera of millipedes have proved injurious to humans. Important genera are *Rhinocricus* (Caribbean), *Spirobolus* (Tanzania), *Spirostreptus* and *Iulus* (Indonesia), and *Polyceroconas* (Papua New Guinea). Children are particularly at risk when they handle or try to eat these large arthropods. When venom is squirted into the eye, intense conjunctivitis results and there may be corneal ulceration and even blindness. Skin lesions are initially stained brown or purple, blister after a few days, and then peel. First aid is generous irrigation with water. Eye injuries should be treated as for snake venom ophthalmia (see above).

REFERENCES

1 Minton SA: Beware: Nonpoisonous snakes. Clin Toxicol 15:259–265, 1979
2 Warrell DA, Ormerod LD, Davidson NMcD: Bites by the night adder *(Causus maculatus)* and burrowing vipers (genus *Atractaspis*) in Nigeria. Am J Trop Med Hyg 25:517–524, 1976
3 Minton SA, Dowling HG, Russell FE: *Poisonous Snakes of the World. A Manual for Use by U.S. Amphibious Forces.* Washington, DC, U.S. Govt Printing Office, 1965
4 Underwood G: Classification and distribution of venomous snakes in the world, in Lee C-Y (ed): *Snake Venoms.* Berlin, Springer-Verlag, 1979
5 Mendelssohn H: On the biology of the venomous snakes of Israel. Isr J Zool 12:143–170, 1963; 14:185–212, 1965
6 Klauber LM: *Rattlesnakes. Their Habits, Life Histories, and Influence on Mankind,* 2d ed. Berkeley, University of California Press, 1972
7 Kochva E: Oral glands of the reptilia. in Gans C, Gans KA (eds): *Biology of the Reptilia.* London, Academic, 1978, vol 8, pp 43–161
8 Kornalík F: The influence of snake venom enzymes on blood coagulation. Pharmacol Ther 29:353–405, 1985
9 Ménez A: Molecular immunology of snake toxins. Pharmacol Ther 30:91–113, 1985
10 Mebs D: Pharmacology of reptilian venoms, in Gans C, Gans KA (eds): *Biology of the Reptilia.* London, Academic, 1978, vol 8, pp 437–560
11 Sitprija V, Boonpucknavig V: Snake venoms and nephrotoxicity, in Lee C-Y (ed): *Snake Venoms.* Berlin, Springer-Verlag, 1979, pp 997–1018
12 Warrell DA: Animal poisons, in Manson-Bahr PEC, Bell DR (eds): *Manson's Tropical Diseases,* 19th ed. London, Bailliere Tindall, 1987, pp 855–898
13 Warrell DA: Clinical snake bite problems in the Nigerian savanna region. THD Schriftenreihe Wissenschaft u–Technik 14:31–60, 1979

14 Matsen FA: *Compartmental Syndromes*. New York, Grune & Stratton, 1980

15 Chapman DS: The symptomatology, pathology, and treatment of the bites of venomous snakes of Central and Southern Africa, in Bücherl W, Buckley EE, Deulofeu V (eds): *Venomous Animals and Their Venoms*. New York, Academic, 1968, vol I, pp 463–527

16 Warrell DA, Ormerod LD, Davidson NMcD: Bites by puff-adder *(Bitis arietans)* in Nigeria, and value of antivenom. Br Med J 4:697–700, 1975

17 Campbell CH: Venomous snake bite in Papua and its treatment with tracheostomy, artificial respiration and antivenene. Trans R Soc Trop Med Hyg 58:263–273, 1964

18 Watt G, Theakston RDG, Hayes CG, et al: Positive response to edrophonium in patients with neurotoxic envenoming by cobras *(Naja naja philippinensis)*. A placebo-controlled study. N Engl J Med 315:1444–1448, 1986

18a Reid HA: Symptomatology, pathology and treatment of the bites of sea snakes, in Lee C-Y (ed): *Snake Venoms*. Berlin, Springer-Verlag, 1979, pp 922–955

19 Birdsey V, Lindorfer J, Gewurz H: Interaction of toxic venoms with the complement system. Immunology 21:299–310, 1971

20 Warrell DA, Greenwood BM, Davidson NMcD, et al: Necrosis, haemorrhage and complement depletion following bites by the spitting cobra *(Naja nigricollis)*. Q J Med 45:1–22, 1976

21 Russell FE: *Snake Venom Poisoning*. Philadelphia, Lippincott, 1980

22 Warrell Da, Ormerod LD: Snake venom ophthalmia and blindness caused by the spitting cobra *(Naja nigricollis)* in Nigeria. Am J Trop Med Hyg 25:525–529, 1976

23 Ho M, Warrell MJ, Warrell DA, et al: A critical reappraisal of the use of ELISA in the study of snake bite. Toxicon 24:211–221, 1986

23a Sutherland SK, Coulter AR, Harris RD: Rationalisation of first-aid measures for elapid snakebite. Lancet i:183–186, 1979

24 Latifi M: Commercial production of anti-snakebite serum (anti-venom), in Gans C, Gans KA (eds): *Biology of the Reptilia*. London, Academic, 1978, vol 8, pp 561–588

25 World Health Organization: Progress in the characterization of venoms and antivenoms. WHO Publication No. 58, Geneva, WHO, 1981

26 Rappolt RT, Quinn H, Curtis L, et al: Medical toxicologist's notebook: Snakebite treatment and international antivenin index. Clin Toxicol 13:409–438, 1978

27 Chippaux JP, Goyffon M: Producers of antivenomous sera. Toxicon 21:739–752, 1983

28 Sutherland SK: *Australian Animal Toxins. The Creatures, Their Toxins and Care of the Poisoned Patient*. Melbourne, Oxford University Press, 1983, p 199

29 Malasit P, Warrell DA, Chanthavanich P, et al: Prediction, prevention and mechanism of early (anaphylactic) antivenom reactions in victims of snake bites. Br Med J 292:17–20, 1986

30 Ho M, Warrell DA, Looareesuwan S, et al: Clinical significance of venom antigen levels in patients envenomed by the Malayan pit viper *(Calloselasma rhodostoma)*. Am J Trop Med Hyg 35:579–587, 1986

31 Warrell DA, Looareesuwan S, Theakston RDG, et al: Randomized comparative trial of three monospecific antivenoms for bites by the Malayan pit viper *(Calloselasma rhodostoma)* in southern Thailand: clinical and laboratory correlations. Am J Trop Med Hyg, 35:1235–1247, 1986

32 Myint-Lwin, Warrell DA, Phillips RE, et al: Bites by Russell's viper *(Vipera russellii siamensis)* in Burma: haemostatic, vascular, and renal disturbances and response to treatment. Lancet ii:1259–1264, 1985

33 Tun-Pe, Phillips RE, Warrell DA, et al: Acute and chronic pituitary failure resembling Sheehan's syndrome following bites by Russell's viper in Burma. Lancet ii:763–767, 1987

34 Reid HA, Thean PC, Chan KE, et al: Clinical effects of bites by Malayan viper *(Ancistrodon rhodostoma)*. Lancet i:617, 1963

35 Warrell DA, Arnett C: The importance of bites by the saw-scaled or carpet viper *(Echis carinatus):* Epidemiological studies in Nigeria and a review of the world literature. Acta Trop (Basel) 33:307–341, 1976

36 Reid HA, Lim KJ: Sea-snake bite. A survey of fishing villages in north-west Malaya. Br Med J 2:1266–1272, 1957

37 Russell FE, Bogert CM: Gila monster: Its biology, venom and bite—a review. Toxicon 19:341–359, 1981

38 Halstead BW: *Poisonous and Venomous Marine Animals of the World* (rev ed). Princeton, Darwin Press, 1978

39 Russell FE: *Marine Toxins and Venomous and Poisonous Marine Animals*. New York, Academic, 1965

40 Edmonds C: *Dangerous Marine Animals of the Indo-Pacific Region*. Newport, Australia, Wedneil Publications, 1975

41 Williamson J, Exton D: *The Marine Stinger Book,* 3d ed. Brisbane, Surf Life Saving Assoc. Australia, 1985

42 Hughes JM, Merson MH: Fish and shellfish poisoning. N Engl J Med 295:117–1120, 1976

43 Bagnis R, Kuberski T, Laugier S: Clinical observations on 3009 cases of ciguatera (fish poisoning) in the South Pacific. Am J Trop Med Hyg 28:1067–1073, 1979

44 Russell FE, Maretić Z: Scombroid poisoning: mini-review with case histories. Toxicon 24:967–973, 1986

44a Williamson JA, Callanan VI, Hartwick RF: Serious envenomation by the Northern Australian box-jelly fish *(Chironex fleckeri)*. Med J Aust 1:13–15, 1980

45 Hartwick RF, Callanan VI, Williamson JA: Disarming the box-jelly fish. Nematocyst inhibition in *Chironex fleckeri*. Med J Aust 1:15–20, 1980

46 Akre RD, Davis Hg: Biology and pest status of venomous wasps. Ann Rev Entomol 23:215–238, 1978

47 Bettini S (ed): Arthropod venoms, in *Handbook of Experimental Pharmacology,* vol 48. Berlin, Springer-Verlag, 1978

48 Van der Vecht J: The vespinae of the Indo-Malaysian and Papuan areas (Hymenoptera, Vespidae). Zool Verh Leiden 34:1–83, 1957

49 Bawaskar HS: Diagnostic cardiac premonitory signs and symptoms of red scorpion sting. Lancet i:552–554, 1982

50 Bücherl W, Buckley EE: *Venomous Animals and Their Venoms,* vol III, *Venomous Invertebrates*. New York, Academic, 1971

51 Keegan HL: Scorpions of medical importance. University Press of Mississippi, 1980

52 Maretić Z, Lebez D: Araneism. Lancet, July 1980, 133–134

53 Gothe R, Kunze K, Hoogstraal H: The mechanism of pathogenicity in the tick paralysis. J Med Entomol 16:357–369, 1979

54 Pearn J: The clinical features of tick bite. Med J Austr 2:313, 1977

55 Radford AJ: Millipede burns in man. Trop Geogr Med 27:(3)279–287, 1975.

PART IV Viral and Chlamydial Diseases

CHAPTER 60 / *Introduction* · Scott B. Halstead

The viruses of tropical countries and their diseases continue to provide us with many surprises. Since the first edition of this book, as evidenced by the new titles of the chapters in this section, some viruses are on their way out, while others are rudely shouldering their way to unwanted prominence.

The success stories in the organized war against viruses require special mention. Most notable has been the campaign to immunize the world's children against measles and poliomyelitis led by the World Health Organization (WHO) and the United Nations Children's Fund (UNICEF). In June 1987 it was estimated that 45 percent of nearly 600 million children, aged 1 to 5 years, had received a potent measles vaccine at a time when maternal antibody levels were likely to permit seroconversion, and, further, that 54 percent of these children had received three or more doses of trivalent polio vaccines. UNICEF estimates that 800,000 measles deaths a year are being avoided as a result. The striking feat of raising global immunization percentages from 5 percent in 1980 to 50 percent in 1987 so emboldened the World Health Assembly that in 1987 it joined the Pan American Health Organization in calling for the global eradication of poliomyelitis before the end of the century.

Equally exciting has been the rapid deployment of plasma-derived and recombinant hepatitis B vaccines. When administered alone or with hepatitis B immune globulin, they prevented newborn infants from acquiring chronic hepatitis B infections from their chronically infected mothers. Outside the United States competing manufacturers of plasma-derived vaccines have reduced prices to the range where nationwide campaigns to eradicate hepatitis B can be contemplated. In the course of time, primary hepatocellular carcinoma will disappear from Asia, Africa, and Latin America, an historical event that will rank alongside the eradication of smallpox.

But there is more good news. New, efficacious live-attenuated vaccines are nearing the final stages of development and testing. Three of these have been developed by scientist-leaders from third world countries: an attenuated strain of Junin virus is in advanced phase III testing as a vaccine against Argentine hemorrhagic fever; three of four dengue serotypes serially passaged in dog kidney cells have been proven satisfactorily attenuated and immunogenic in adult volunteers studied in Thailand, and in large-scale trials in Chinese children a live-attenuated vaccine against Japanese encephalitis has proved safe and immunogenic. In the United States an attenuated rotavirus vaccine is in phase III efficacy trials, and killed and attenuated hepatitis A vaccines are nearing the final stages of laboratory development. Waiting in the wings are recombinant vaccinia-vectored Lassa and Epstein-Barr vaccines and a score of other antigens which might be delivered by one of several candidate vectors.

Meanwhile, using the more aggressive attenuated Edmonston-Zagreb measles strain, the age at which infants can be given measles vaccines without interference from maternal antibodies has been pushed back to 9 months. This development will narrow the age window when children can acquire severe and fatal measles infections.

This is not all. Solid evidence has been obtained for marked therapeutic efficacy of ribavirin in preventing deaths in Lassa fever. The drug is efficacious even when administered relatively late in the course of disease. Further, when given early in disease, ribavirin results in moderate reduction in severity and duration of illness and prevents about half of the expected deaths due to hemorrhagic fever with renal syndrome. Together with the proven effectiveness of immune serum in markedly reducing deaths due to Argentine hemorrhagic fever, a new chapter has been written in the effective and specific treatment of severe and fatal virus diseases of humankind.

Finally, new or improved killed rabies, polio, and hepatitis B vaccines have been shown to be satisfactorily immunogenic either by using a reduced dosage schedule or by intradermal injection of one-tenth volume of vaccine. These strategies reduce price and expand access by the world's poor to vaccines. Research on new vaccines, vaccine stability, adjuvants, and more antigenic vaccines is proceeding with reasonable support. In this regard the future holds much promise.

But the celebratory note of the past decade has been shattered by the emergence of viruses which are simultaneously invisible and lethal to the human immune system. HIV-1 and its virological cousins are the all-too-real Andromeda strain. Ground zero for the release of HIV-1 seems to be Lake Victoria, with infection rates declining linearly with distance from the lake in all directions. Unfortunately, there has been independent and widespread seeding of the virus so that AIDS is now a global catastrophe whose economic and demographical dimensions are as yet only dimly recognized. Without the emergence of a radical cure or a means of absolute prevention, illness and deaths just in those persons already infected threaten negative growth in some countries and place in jeopardy the public health gains described above.

If there is a lesson for tropical public health workers and microbiologists in this event and in the earlier emergence of Lassa, Marburg, and Ebola viruses, it is that as human populations expand in density and in geographical extent, chance adaptive encounters with microbial agents from other ecosystems are enhanced. The conclusion should be that these encounters will continue. It would be logical in the face of such experiences to strengthen global disease surveillance and to increase research resources for the study of the biology of parasitism. In fact, the proportion of research resources allocated to basic, laboratory research is increasing and field competence in disease biology is waning and could disappear. According to a 1987 report issued by the Board on Science and Technology for International Development of the National Research Council, the total U.S. government investment in tropical infectious diseases was only 1.5 percent of the national biomedical research budget (1984), and, further, other than for three overseas Defense Department facilities, no career path exists to train and sustain U.S. competence in the field aspects of tropical diseases. In most developing countries, resources allocated to support credible epidemiology surveillance or public health microbiology research are meager to the vanishing point.

Until the war on microbial agents is planned for the very long term, the diseases described in this chapter and their yet-to-be discovered successors may continue to plague the human race, standing firmly in the way of health for all.

C H A P T E R
61

Poliomyelitis · Joseph L. Melnick

Poliomyelitis is an acute infectious disease that in its serious form affects the central nervous system. The destruction of motor neurons in the spinal cord results in flaccid paralysis. However, most poliovirus infections are subclinical.

VIRUS

LIFE HISTORY AND ECOLOGY OF POLIOVIRUSES

Classification

Within the family Picornaviridae, poliovirus type I is the type species of the genus *Enterovirus,* which also includes coxsackieviruses, echoviruses, and the high-numbered enteroviruses.

There are three antigenic types of poliovirus, types I, II, and III, but even intratypic differences can now be distinguished by use of newly developed tools of molecular biology: highly strain-specific absorbed or monoclonal sera, oligonucleotide mapping, and sequencing of the bases of the viral genome. Poliovirus isolates should be identified by type, country (or city), strain number, and year of isolation. Thus, P1/Houston/23/62 designates a type I poliovirus strain, number 23, isolated in Houston in 1962.

Alimentary tract habitat

Polioviruses are transient inhabitants of the human alimentary tract, and may be isolated from the throat of patients (from just before onset to a week or less after onset), or from the lower intestine (from before onset to several weeks after onset).

Replicative cycle

Understanding the mode of replication of poliovirus provides useful insights into its transmission, its in vivo and in vitro host range, and its relation to other enteroviruses.

Polioviruses adsorb to cells at specific cell receptor sites. This is evidenced by the fact that intact poliovirus infects only primate cells in culture, whereas the viral RNA isolated from its surrounding capsid also infects nonprimate cells (rabbit, guinea pig, chick), where only one cycle of multiplication occurs. Multiple cycles of infection are not observed in nonprimate cells because the resulting progeny possess protein coats, and again will only attach to and infect primate cells.

After attachment, the virus particles are taken into the cell, and the viral RNA is uncoated. The single-stranded genomic RNA serves as its own messenger RNA (mRNA). This mRNA is translated, resulting in the formation of an enzyme, RNA polymerase. This enzyme is necessary for the formation of a replicative intermediate and then a replicative form, which is a double-stranded molecule consisting of a positive parental RNA strand and a complementary negative strand, and also for the formation of inhibitors that turn off the synthesis of cellular RNA and protein. Single-stranded viral RNA molecules—positive strands—are then synthesized from the replicative form. The newly synthesized positive-strand RNA molecules perform any of the following three functions: (1) serve as mRNA for synthesis of structural proteins; (2) serve as template for continued RNA replication; or (3) become encapsidated, resulting in mature progeny virions. The synthesis of viral capsid proteins is initiated at about the same time as RNA synthesis.

The entire poliovirus genome, acting as its own mRNA, is translated to form a single large polypeptide that is subsequently cleaved to produce the various viral capsid polypeptides. Thus, the poliovirus genome serves as a polycistronic messenger molecule. Completion of encapsidation produces mature virus particles that are then released when the cell undergoes lysis.

Polioviruses are included among the agents that during their replication produce deletion mutants called ''defective interfering'' particles that interfere with the growth of the normal virus from which they are derived. Defective interfering particles have potential clinical significance since they may play a role in limiting acute viral infections; furthermore, they are present in high concentrations in oral poliovaccines, suggesting the possibility that their presence may be a factor in attenuation [*1*].

Mutation

Like all living things, polioviruses can mutate, and this property presents both opportunities and problems in relation to human health. Pathogenic polioviruses, by propagation under manipulated conditions through many generations in cultured monkey kidney cells, were deliberately attenuated so as to be no longer neurovirulent for humans. By this means, attenuated live poliovirus vaccines were developed. However, the living vaccine viruses also may mutate, and their progeny may spread to persons not vaccinated [*2*], which has both advantages and disadvantages, as will be discussed below (see "Control of Poliomyelitis: Immunization with Inactivated Virus or Live Vaccine").

MORPHOLOGY, ULTRASTRUCTURE

Poliovirus particles are typical enteroviruses, 28 nm in diameter. The nucleocapsid, composed of 32 morphological subunits, possesses cubic symmetry. The virion has no envelope and contains a genome of single-stranded infectious ribonucleic acid (molecular weight 2.5×10^6). This size is equivalent to 7.5 kb, which is sufficient nucleic acid to encode 2500 amino acids. The complete sequence of poliovirus RNA has recently been determined. The molecular biology of poliovirus is being intensively studied [*3*], and the ultrastructure of the virus has been revealed by x-ray diffraction investigation [*4*].

Complement-fixing (CF) antigens for each of the three poliovirus types can be prepared from infected cell cultures. Two type-specific antigens can be detected by precipitin and CF tests. They are native (N) and heated (H) antigens. The N form can be converted to the H form by heating. The N form represents full particles containing RNA, and the H form, empty particles.

BIOCHEMISTRY, IN VITRO CULTURE

Like other enteroviruses, polioviruses are stable at acid pH levels (3.0 to 5.0). They are inactivated when heated at 55°C for 30 min, but molar magnesium chloride prevents this inactivation. While purified poliovirus is inactivated by chlorine (0.1 parts per million), much higher concentrations of chlorine are required to disinfect sewage containing the virus in fecal suspensions and in the presence of other organic matter.

The growth of polioviruses in monolayers of cultured cells is associated with a characteristic cytopathic effect [*5*]. Infected cells round up, show shrinkage and marked nuclear pyknosis, become refractive, and eventually degenerate and fall off the glass surface. In cell cultures covered by fluid nutrient medium, virus may spread via the fluid bathing the cells. Under agar overlay, which confines the spread of virus to a cell-to-adjoining-cell route, plaques of degenerating cells are formed

in the cultures. Methods that utilize plaque formation have provided very precise quantification of infective virus [*6*].

The factors underlying cell susceptibility to polioviruses are basic to understanding host susceptibility to infection. Human cells possess a receptor for poliovirus and can therefore be infected and killed by the virus. Rodent cells do not possess the receptor and cannot be infected by wild polioviruses. But in human-rodent hybrid cells, possession of a human gene for the poliovirus receptor is sufficient to enable the virus nucleic acid to gain entrance into the cell and replicate. The human chromosome carrying the gene concerned with poliovirus reception was identified by making use of human-rodent hybrid cells that differ in their complement of human chromosomes [*7*]. Only chromosome 19 was found to possess the information necessary for acceptance of poliovirus by a human cell, suggesting that only a single gene codes for the receptor protein.

Synthetic peptides from four separate (noncontiguous) regions of capsid protein VP1 of poliovirus type 1 have been shown to generate antisera with type-specific neutralizing activity [*3*]. The neutralization epitopes of the virus have been identified, since antisera against peptides from all other regions of VP1 fail to neutralize virus infectivity. These findings could lead to the designing of highly potent immunogens that could not possibly mutate towards virulence.

ANIMAL MODELS

Human polioviruses will infect only monkeys and chimpanzees, most readily by direct inoculation into the brain or spinal cord. Chimpanzees and cynomolgus monkeys can also be infected by the oral route. In chimpanzees, the infection thus produced is usually asymptomatic. The animals become intestinal carriers of the virus; they also develop a viremia that is quenched by the appearance of antibodies in the circulating blood. A few unusual strains have been transmitted to mice. Neurovirulence for monkeys remains the most sensitive and definitive test to determine the degree of attenuation, and consequently the safety, of a vaccine strain.

INTERMEDIATE HOSTS, RESERVOIR HOSTS

Human beings are the only known reservoir of poliovirus infection. During periods of wide prevalence of poliovirus in an area, houseflies become contaminated and may passively distribute virus to food. The role of flies in disease transmission is not fully understood, and they may play a more significant role in areas of poor sanitation. Virus may be present in urban sewage, which can serve as a source of contamination of flies or of water used for drinking, bathing, or irrigation [*8*].

PATIENT

HOST-VIRUS INTERFACE

Routes of transmission

With humans as the only reservoirs, close human contact is the primary avenue of spread. Virus can be recovered from the oropharynx and intestine of individuals infected either clinically or subclinically, and is generally shed for periods up to a month or two in stools—much longer than in secretions of the upper alimentary tract. Thus infectious feces spread by contaminated fingers constitute the usual source of infection. However, in the early stages of infection, droplets from coughing or sneezing can also be a source of contamination.

Warm weather favors the spread of virus by increasing human contacts, the susceptibility of the host, or the dissemination of virus. The viruses are most readily spread within the family, and the extent of intrafamilial infection appears to be closely related to duration of virus shedding, particularly by young children.

Immunity

Immunity is permanent to the type causing the infection. There may be a low degree of heterotypic resistance induced by infection, especially between type 1 and type 2 polioviruses. A passive transfer of neutralizing and CF antibodies from mother to infant occurs. Maternal antibodies gradually disappear during the first 6 months of life.

Antibody formation early in poliovirus infection is a result of virus multiplication in the intestinal tract and deep lymphatic structures before invasion of the nervous system. Since antibodies must be present in the blood to prevent the dissemination of virus to the brain and are not effective after this has already occurred, immunization is of value only if it precedes the onset of symptoms referable to the nervous system.

Circulating serum antibody against polioviruses is not the only source of protection against infection. Local or cellular immunity is important, as it protects against intestinal reinfection after recovery from a natural infection or after immunization with the live poliovirus vaccine. Local immunity may act through the production of secretory antibodies at the portal of entry [9].

It is being recognized increasingly that viral infections do carry an increased risk for persons with various immunodeficiencies in either humoral or cell-mediated immunity. In such persons, poliovirus infection—either by wild virus or by vaccine strains—may develop in an atypical manner, with an incubation period longer than 28 days, a high mortality rate after a long chronic illness, and unusual distribution of lesions in the central nervous system.

A decrease in resistance to poliovirus accompanies removal of tonsils and adenoids. Preexisting secretory antibody levels in the nasopharynx decrease sharply following operation (particularly in young male children) without any change in antibody levels in sera. Local antibody levels remain low or absent for as long as 7 months. In seronegative children, nasopharyngeal antibody response to poliovirus vaccine develops significantly later and to lower titers in children previously tonsillectomized than in those with intact tonsils. Thus, surgery of this type may eliminate a valuable source of immunocompetent tissue of importance in resistance to poliovirus.

PATHOGENESIS, PATHOLOGY

Virus implantation and multiplication occur in different tissues as the infectious agent travels to the target organ from the portal of entry. In the target organ, virus multiplication must reach a critical level before cell necrosis occurs and disease becomes manifest. Viruses call forth a different tissue response than do pathogenic bacteria, not only in the parenchymatous cells but also in cellular infiltration. Whereas polymorphonuclear leukocytes form the principal cellular response to the acute inflammation caused by pyogenic bacteria, infiltration with mononuclear cells and lymphocytes characterizes the inflammatory reaction in poliomyelitis [10].

The incubation period (defined as the time from exposure to onset of disease) is usually between 7 and 14 days, but may range from 2 to 35 days.

Poliovirus may be found in the blood of patients with the "abortive poliomyelitis" (minor-illness) manifestation of infection, and can be detected several days before onset of clinical signs of central nervous system (CNS) involvement in patients who develop "nonparalytic poliomyelitis" (aseptic meningitis) or the paralytic disease [10]. In orally infected monkeys and chimpanzees, viremia is also regularly present in the preparalytic phase of the disease. Antibodies to the virus appear early in the natural infection and also early in orally infected experimental animals. They are usually present by the time paralysis appears. In humans, viremia has been demonstrated regularly following ingestion of type II oral poliovaccine. Free virus is present in the serum between days 2 and 5 after vaccination, and virus bound to antibody can be detected for an additional few days [11]. Bound virus is detected by acid treatment, which inactivates the antibody and liberates active virus.

In the experimental infection in monkeys, poliovirus can spread along axons of peripheral nerves to the central nervous system, and there it continues to progress along the fibers of the lower motor neurons to increasingly involve the spinal cord or the brain. Neural spread to the brain may also occur in children who have nonapparent infections at the time of tonsillectomy. A similar mechanism of virus spread along neural pathways may be responsible for the rare instances of paralysis in a limb recently injected with an irritating material during a period of high poliovirus prevalence.

Poliovirus invades certain types of nerve cells, and in the process of its intracellular multiplication, it may damage or completely destroy these cells. The anterior horn cells of the spinal cord are most prominently involved, but in severe cases the intermediate gray ganglia and even the posterior horn and dorsal root ganglia are often affected. Lesions are found as far forward as the hypothalamus and thalamus. In the brain, the reticular formation, the vestibular nuclei, the cerebellar vermis, and the deep cerebellar nuclei are most often affected. The cortex is virtually spared, with the exception of the motor cortex along the precentral gyrus [10].

Although flaccid paralysis is the hallmark of poliomyelitis, poliovirus does not multiply in muscle in vivo. Its chief site of action is in the neuron, and the changes that occur in peripheral nerves and voluntary muscles are secondary to destruction of the nerve cell. Changes occur rapidly in nerve cells, from mild chromatolysis to neuronophagia and complete destruction. Cells that are not killed, but that lose their function temporarily as a result of edema, may recover completely. Inflammation occurs secondary to the attack on the nerve cells; the focal and perivascular infiltrations are chiefly lymphocytes, with some polymorphonuclear cells, plasma cells, and microglia. In addition to pathological changes in the nervous system, hyperplasia and inflammatory lesions of lymph nodes and of Peyer's patches and other lymph follicles in the intestinal tract are frequently observed; interstitial infiltration of the myocardium with leukocytes is common, but necrotizing myocarditis is rare.

CLINICAL MANIFESTATIONS

When an individual susceptible to infection is exposed to poliovirus, one of the following responses may occur: (1) inapparent infection without symptoms, (2) mild (minor) illness, (3) aseptic meningitis, (4) paralytic poliomyelitis. As the disease progresses, one response may merge with a more severe form, often resulting in a biphasic course: a minor illness, followed first by a few days free of symptoms and then by the major, severe illness. Only about 1 percent of infections result in recognized clinical illness.

Asymptomatic infections

By far the most common form of *infection* is asymptomatic, or is accompanied by no more than minor malaise.

Minor illness (abortive poliomyelitis)

In those instances where any *disease* occurs, the most common form is abortive poliomyelitis characterized by fever, malaise, drowsiness, headache, nausea, vomiting, constipation, or sore throat in various combinations. The patient recovers in a few days. Even during an epidemic, the diagnosis of abortive poliomyelitis cannot be made with assurance, except when the virus is isolated or antibody development is measured. Many other viruses may cause the same signs and symptoms.

Aseptic meningitis and/or transient mild paresis (nonparalytic poliomyelitis)

In addition to the aforementioned symptoms and signs, the patient with aseptic meningitis presents with stiffness and pain in the back and neck. The disease lasts 2 to 10 days. Occasionally, there may be mild muscle weakness or transient paralysis. Recovery is almost always complete, but, in a small percentage of cases, the disease advances to paralysis. Polioviruses are not the only viruses that produce aseptic meningitis. Many other agents, particularly other members of the enterovirus group, also produce this syndrome [12].

Paralytic poliomyelitis

The major illness may follow the minor illness previously described, particularly in young children, but it usually occurs without the antecedent first phase. The predominating sign is flaccid paralysis resulting from lower motor neuron damage. However, incoordination secondary to brainstem invasion and painful spasms of nonparalyzed muscles may also occur. The amount of damage and destruction varies from case to case. Muscle involvement is usually maximal within a few days after the paralytic phase begins. The maximal recovery usually occurs within 6 months, but may take longer.

LABORATORY DIAGNOSIS

Cerebrospinal fluid

The cerebrospinal fluid (CSF) contains an increased number of leukocytes—usually 10 to 200 per μL, seldom more than 500 per μL. In the early stage of the disease, the ratio of polymorphonuclear cells to lymphocytes is high, but within a few days the ratio is reversed. The total cell count slowly subsides to normal levels. The protein content of the CSF is elevated (average, about 40 to 50 mg/dL), but higher levels may occur and persist for weeks. The glucose content is normal.

Recovery of virus

Cultures of human or monkey cells may be used [6]. The virus may be recovered from throat swabs taken soon after onset of illness and, over longer periods, from rectal swabs or feces. The virus has been found in about 80 percent of patients during the first 2 weeks of illness but in only 25 percent by the third 2-week period. No permanent carriers are known. Recovery of poliovirus from the CSF is uncommon.

In fatal cases, the virus should be sought in the cervical and lumbar enlargements of the spinal cord, in the medulla, and in the colon contents. Histological examination of the spinal cord and parts of the brain should be made. If paralysis has lasted 4 to 5 days, it may be difficult to recover the virus from the cord.

Specimens should be kept frozen during transit to the laboratory and treated with antibiotics before inoculation of cell cultures. Cytopathic effects appear in 3 to 6 days. An isolated virus is identified and typed by neutralization with specific antiserum.

Serology

Neutralizing antibodies appear early and are usually already detectable at the time of hospitalization. If the first specimen is taken sufficiently early, a rise in titer can be demonstrated during the course of the disease by parallel testing of paired serum specimens (see Table 61-1).

During poliomyelitis infection, CF-H antibodies form before CF-N antibodies (see "Morphology, Ultrastructure" above). The level of H antibodies declines first. Early acute-stage sera

Table 61-1. Cell culture neutralization test with paired sera of patient infected with type I poliovirus

Virus*	Serum (day after onset)	Cellular degeneration (cytopathic effect): Final serum dilution					50% serum titer	
		1:2	1:10	1:50	1:250	1:1250	Logarithm	Antilog
Type I	1	000	+ + +	+ + +	+ + +	+ + +	0.7	5
	20	000	000	000	0 0 +	+ + +	2.5	320
Type II	1	000	+ + +	+ + +	+ + +	+ + +	0.7	5
	20	000	000	0 + +	+ + +	+ + +	1.5	32
Type III	1	+ + +	+ + +	+ + +	+ + +	+ + +	0	0
	20	+ + +	+ + +	+ + +	+ + +	+ + +	0	0
None	1	000						
	20	000						

*One hundred $TCID_{50}$ (50% tissue culture infectious doses) of each virus used in test. Three cultures were inoculated with each virus-serum mixture. A + indicates cytopathic change in a culture because of virus growth. A 0 indicates no growth of virus.

thus contain H antibodies only; 1 to 2 weeks later, both N and H antibodies are present; in late convalescent sera, the only CF antibodies present are the N type. Only first infection with a poliovirus induces strictly type-specific CF responses. Subsequent infections with heterotypic polioviruses recall or induce antibodies mostly against the heat-stable group antigen shared by all three types of poliovirus.

Interpretation of laboratory data

In Table 61-2 are summarized the various combinations of laboratory results that may be obtained. The last column indicates the interpretation in determining the presence and nature of a poliovirus infection.

MANAGEMENT

Treatment of patients with paralytic poliomyelitis involves reduction of pain and muscle spasm and maintenance of respiration and hydration. When the fever subsides, early mobilization and active exercise are begun. There is no role for antiserum [10].

POPULATION

Poliomyelitis occurs worldwide—year-round in the tropics and during summer and fall in the temperate zones. Winter outbreaks are rare. The prevalence of infection is highest among household contacts. By the time the first case is recognized in a family, all susceptible members of the family are already infected, the result of rapid dissemination of the virus. Rapid and extensive spread also occurs in other close associations such as those in children's institutions or in summer camps.

Age incidence

Poliovirus infections occur in all age groups, but children are usually more susceptible than adults because of the acquired immunity of the adult population. In isolated populations (e.g., Arctic Eskimos), poliovirus when introduced infects all ages equally. Poliovirus infection in older persons is more likely to produce serious illness. The fatality rate of paralytic polio is variable, being particularly high in older patients, where it may reach 5 to 10 percent. Historically there has been a trend toward upward shifts in the ages at which paralytic poliomyelitis has occurred, in parallel with rising standards of hygiene and sanitation. In some of the last paralytic polio outbreaks in the United States before the advent of poliovirus vaccines, parents of virus-shedding (but healthy) nursery-school children were especially vulnerable.

Relation to socioeconomic factors

Within a community, polioviruses generally spread horizontally via preschool children and circulate more widely and at earlier ages among families of lower socioeconomic level, where hygiene and sanitation are deficient. This is true in temperate-zone populations and also in developing countries with tropical climates.

Indeed, in some developing regions, even where oral poliovirus vaccine (OPV) may be used extensively, heavy exposure to virulent wild viruses may occur even in the first month or two of life, and thus unvaccinated infants in tropical countries are often the most frequent victims of paralytic polio.

EPIDEMIOLOGY

It is important to reemphasize that by far the most common form of infection with poliovirus is a mild or silent episode and that severe manifestations are rare. Paralytic poliomyelitis

Table 61-2. Interpretation of laboratory data in poliovirus infection

Virus isolation	Complement-fixing antibody	Neutralizing antibody	Antibody of IgM class	Interpretation of infection
−	−	−	−	None
+	−	−	−	Early
+	+	+	+	Current
−	+	+	+	Recent
−	−	+	−	Old

remained an epidemiological enigma until this concept was understood.

In warm countries and in families living under unsanitary and poor socioeconomic conditions in temperate zones, children are infected very early in life, and more than 90 percent may have already experienced infections with all three serotypes before the age of 5 years. In such settings, paralytic poliomyelitis is rarely recognized and epidemics generally do not occur. When infection is delayed to older childhood and young adult life, the reported incidence of paralytic poliomyelitis rises. The ratio of inapparent infections to paralytic cases is about 100:1 and may be higher among infants [13].

Poliomyelitis can be viewed as having three major epidemiological phases: endemic, epidemic, and vaccine-era. These phases have occurred sequentially in history, but they all coexist at the present time in different regions of the world. The first two can be termed *prevaccine,* whether in reference to the historical time before vaccines had been developed, or to the situation today in a region where vaccine has not been used or where coverage has been inadequate.

It appears that sporadic cases of paralytic poliomyelitis have occurred for at least as long as recorded history. From ancient times into the late 1800s, polioviruses became established throughout most of the world's populations and survived for many centuries in an endemic fashion, continuously infecting new susceptible infants born into the community. In this endemic pattern, with the almost universal presence of antibody to all three poliovirus types in women of childbearing age, passive immunity was transferred from mother to offspring, and many infants subsequently experienced their first poliovirus infections during the first few months of life while maternal antibodies still provided protection. Furthermore, because such a large proportion of poliovirus infections take an inapparent or subclinical form, the paralytic cases that did occur could go unnoted in populations faced with very high infant and child mortality rates.

Epidemiological patterns in developed nations in temperate zones

In the latter part of the nineteenth century and early in the twentieth century, the urban, industrialized parts of northern Europe and the United States began to suffer from epidemics of paralytic polio that became larger, more frequent, and more severe in more and more localities. The generally accepted explanation is that, with increased economic development and the corresponding resources for community and household hygiene, and with the additional factor of a temperate-zone climate, the opportunities for infection among infants and young children were reduced. Thus, increasing numbers of persons encountered poliovirus for the first time in later childhood or in adult life, at ages when poliovirus infections are more likely to take the paralytic form. Furthermore, the delay in exposure increased the pool of susceptible persons, opening the way for

rapid and explosive spread of the viruses once they did enter the population, in contrast to the steady endemic transmission of the preceding phase. This transition from the endemic phase to the epidemic phase sometimes took place abruptly and sometimes after gradual increases in the annual case rates of ''sporadic'' poliomyelitis.

In many developed countries, the vaccine era in poliomyelitis began after 1955 when inactivated poliovirus vaccine (IPV) was introduced, and notably after 1960 when live attenuated poliovaccine became available on a large scale. Rarely has a serious disease been controlled so quickly and dramatically as was poliomyelitis in these countries. In 1955, the U.S.S.R., 23 other European countries, the United States, Canada, Australia, and New Zealand experienced a total of more than 76,000 reported cases of poliomyelitis. Only 12 years later, in 1967, 1013 cases were recorded in these same countries, a reduction of almost 99 percent. Numbers of poliomyelitis cases continued to be reduced until now, in industrialized countries, poliomyelitis is a rare disease.

In the United States, before the inactivated virus vaccine became available, rates of the paralytic form of the disease were between 5 and 10 per 100,000 population (10,000 to 21,000 paralytic cases per year). After the inactivated virus vaccine came into use, cases were far fewer, in some years reaching incidence rates as low as 0.5 per 100,000 population. But this still meant that significant numbers of cases were occurring; in 1960, there were more than 2500. Concomitant with the use of inactivated virus vaccine in the United States and the decreasing number of cases as compared with the 1955 totals was the finding that some cases were occurring among the fully vaccinated. In a study of several thousand paralytic cases, 17 percent were in children who had received three injections of the vaccine. Some of the disappointing results were due to potency problems which have since been corrected in the few small countries (Holland, Sweden, Finland) that have used inactivated virus vaccines solely through most of the vaccine era.

After the introduction and widespread use of live attenuated vaccine in the United States, the numbers dropped precipitously, and from 1969 onward the largest number of cases in any year has been 32 in 1970. For the decade 1970–1979, the average annual number of cases was 17. For the period 1980–1988 the annual average was less than 10 per year. This has meant case rates consistently ranging from 0.02 down to 0.001 per 100,000 population [14].

The United States has for many years relied almost completely on live poliovirus vaccine, and it appears that there is no longer any endogenous reservoir of wild polioviruses within the country. Wild strains continue to be introduced, particularly from Mexico, but even such imported cases are sporadic and almost never result in secondary cases. It has been postulated [15] that the use of live poliovirus vaccine has achieved this result by establishing intestinal resistance extensively within the population, reducing the pool of susceptible individuals below the level required for perpetuation of wild polioviruses, and that a true break in the chain of infection has been achieved. Many other countries with extensive and continuing live vaccine programs also are reporting virtually no cases and few if any poliovirus isolates other than vaccinelike strains [15,16].

As mentioned, good results also have been obtained with inactivated virus vaccines, especially in Sweden, Finland, and the Netherlands, countries of relatively small populations (a total of only 26 million persons) which are culturally homogeneous and socially advanced. They have excellent public health services, and inactivated virus vaccine has been administered in intensive and regularly maintained immunization programs, achieving vaccine coverage among children that approaches 100 percent. Within these countries, wild polioviruses no longer circulate endemically.

However, even in the well-vaccinated countries that have achieved almost complete control of poliomyelitis, there may be important gaps in protection. This vulnerability was shown by the outbreaks of poliomyelitis among persons refusing vaccine on religious grounds in the Netherlands, Canada, and the United States in 1978 and 1979. The virulent epidemic strain was an imported one, now believed to have come from Turkey [17], and no cases occurred beyond these interconnected unvaccinated groups in any of the countries involved. There were no cases in the vaccinated Dutch population, but in nursery and primary schools in some of the affected communities 24 percent of the vaccinated and 71 percent of the nonvaccinated children tested were excreting the wild poliovirus [18].

In the IPV-vaccinated population of Finland—after 20 years of freedom from poliomyelitis—nine cases of paralytic polio and one nonparalytic case occurred between August 1984 and January 1985 [19,20]. On the basis of virus isolations from healthy individuals and from sewage, it is estimated that at least 100,000 persons in the general population were infected. Killed poliovirus vaccine (1.5 million extra doses) was administered to persons under 18 years of age, and OPV was widely offered in a mass campaign, covering about 95 percent of the entire population. The outbreak was halted in February 1985.

The epidemic strain of poliovirus (P3/Finland/84) was tested extensively by new molecular techniques in several laboratories, and was found to differ in both immunological and molecular properties from the type 3 vaccine strains. Analysis of sera collected before the outbreak indicated that prevalence of neutralizing antibodies against most of the new type 3 isolates was much lower than that of antibodies to the Saukett strain (the type 3 strain used in the killed vaccine). The precipitating factor in the outbreak was the appearance of a strain of poliovirus type 3 that was antigenically aberrant enough to break through low-grade herd immunity that resulted from the low immunogenicity of the type 3 component of the Finnish vaccine. After immunization with the new, potent IPV (van Wezel procedure) or with OPV, high serum antibody titers are produced against the Finnish epidemic type 3 strain. Thus, although differences among strains from various parts of the world have indeed been demonstrated for many years, the major neutralizing antigen of each poliovirus serotype is remarkably stable.

Another well-studied outbreak, which occurred in Israel in 1988, has yielded important information on immunological control. Israel began administration of OPV in 1961, and the continued widespread use of OPV in infancy, without further doses, has led to effective control in that country [20a]. However, an outbreak of 15 cases of paralytic polio caused by type 1 poliovirus occurred in 1988 [20b]. Most of the patients were 15 years and older. The focus of the outbreak (12 of the 15 cases) was an area where enhanced inactivated poliovirus vaccine (eIPV) had been the only poliovirus vaccine used for infants since 1982. Surveys of neutralizing antibodies carried out in recent years in Israel provided evidence of relatively low immunity to type 1 poliovirus in teenagers who had been immunized in the first year of life with trivalent OPV, but who had received no subsequent doses. A number of healthy infants tested at the onset of the 1988 outbreak were found to be excreting wild poliovirus.

A combination of factors appears to have been responsible for the outbreak: (1) lack of booster doses of OPV, which led to impaired immunity in the young adult population; (2) introduction of wild poliovirus from surrounding polio-endemic countries; and (3) transmission of wild poliovirus to susceptibles by eIPV-vaccinated infants, who were themselves protected from development of the paralytic disease, but who acquired intestinal infection and excreted the epidemic virus, thus spreading it to susceptibles in the community. The lesson from this outbreak is that exclusive use of inactivated poliovirus vaccine, even of enhanced potency, in infants is not adequate to protect other members of a partially susceptible population against paralytic poliomyelitis in the face of exposure to wild virus.

The outbreaks described above were unfortunate reminders that virulent polioviruses do indeed still exist and can readily circulate if given the right opportunity. Thus, importation of virulent wild polioviruses remains a clear danger against which no nation can be secure except by maintaining high levels of immunity through vaccination.

Epidemiological patterns in developing nations in tropical and subtropical zones

A prevaccine phase of polio epidemiology is of more than historical interest, for it is also a current situation that many nations face today. Worldwide, according to WHO, in the 1980s well over 300,000 cases of poliomyelitis are occurring each year. In India alone, about 200,000 cases were reported in 1985 and again in 1986 [21]. In Bombay alone, more than 1000 cases were reported each year from 1982 through 1986, with type 1 predominating. In 1986, 98 percent of the cases were in children under 5 years of age; 42 percent of the patients were infants in the first year of life, and 36 percent those in the second year of life. The age-specific incidence of paralytic polio was 265 per 100,000 infants below the age of 1 year. It is recognized (see below) that in many instances the reported cases may represent less than 10 percent of the actual number of cases that occurred [22,23]. Poliomyelitis clearly remains an urgent problem for many of the world's people.

In some crowded, developing countries, chiefly in the tropics, paralytic poliomyelitis has continued to be a disease of infancy that is seen only sporadically, i.e., in the endemic pattern. In the past, the rarity of reports of clinical poliomyelitis in the tropics had led many to believe that no poliovirus infections were occurring there, when in fact the reverse was true: polioviruses were highly endemic, but the infections were largely asymptomatic and cases were not being recognized and reported. Many of these countries are shifting toward the epidemic pattern in a far greater degree than had been recognized, despite the relatively low number of reported cases.

The contrast between relatively high frequency of poliomyelitic lameness and low numbers of reported cases was first described some 35 years ago [24]. A striking correlation was discovered between the early age at which clinical polio occurred and the similarly early acquisition of neutralizing antibodies among infants in Cairo, Egypt. As part of this study, the apparent rarity of polio among Egyptians was found to be due to a gross underreporting of the disease. During the 1940s, only 2 to 11 cases were being reported annually for all of Egypt; but when patients with persistent paralysis whose disease was never reported came for therapy and were counted along with the reported cases, it turned out that about 1500 cases had been occurring each year. Thus the annual incidence of polio in Egypt during the late 1940s was calculated to be about 7.8 per 100,000 population. In the United States during the epidemic years of 1932 to 1946, the average was 7.3 per 100,000 per year.

The findings reported in 1952 [24] have been confirmed repeatedly in recent studies utilizing surveys of residual lameness as an indication of past occurrences of paralytic poliomyelitis. Such data have been used to estimate the annual incidence of paralytic poliomyelitis during the years just prior to the surveys. For example, in Ghana, although no large epidemics had been reported, the incidence of poliomyelitis based on surveys of lameness in 1974 was estimated to have been 116 per 100,000 children 0 to 5 years of age during the 1960s, that is, about 23 per 100,000 total population [25]. This amounts to about 2100 cases annually, 10 to 20 times the number that had been diagnosed and reported. This incidence rate was higher than the rates of paralytic polio seen in the United States and Europe just before the poliovirus vaccines were introduced. About 91 percent of the children with poliomyelitic lameness in Ghana had experienced their acute disease during the first 4 years of life.

Similar lameness surveys [26,27] conducted in India in 1979 also indicated that the recent prevalence of paralytic polio-

Table 61-3. Mean annual reported incidence of poliomyelitis per 100,000 total population during the period 1976–1980*

Country	Reported incidence	Estimate from lameness survey
Burma	1.1	18
Egypt	1.8	7
Ghana	2.3	31
India	2.1	18
Indonesia	0.1	13
Ivory Coast	1.2	34
Malawi	1.2	28
Thailand	1.7	7
Cameroon	1.2	24
Yemen	3.3	14

*From [22]. Incidence estimated from surveys of lameness in selected countries.

myelitis had been 5 to 7 times higher than that shown in case reports. As indicated above, the actual situation became a national tragedy in the mid-1980s, with approximately 200,000 paralytic children being recorded annually [21].

Surveys in Africa, conducted in 1979 and 1980 in three different Ivory Coast school-age populations, yielded estimated annual incidence rates of 34 or more per 100,000 total population [28,29]. On the basis of these rates, the actual number of cases during the years when these children would have had their paralytic polio attacks (about 1965 to 1975) would have been at least 2300 annually (in this country of some 7 million population). The numbers reported officially to WHO varied from 90 to 270 each year [26,29]. Table 61-3 shows data from these and other surveys of residual paralysis, listing the reported incidence per 100,000 population during the period 1976–1980, as compared with the estimated incidence for the same period based on surveys of lameness [22]. The percentage of underreporting varies widely among the various countries and regions [30].

World variations in control of poliomyelitis

The worldwide trends in poliomyelitis, and also the magnitude of the problems that remain unresolved, are illustrated in Fig. 61-1, and in Tables 61-4, 61-5, and 61-6. The figure depicts on a world map the incidence of paralytic poliomyelitis reported to WHO for 1985 from various areas. The tables give examples of the reported numbers of poliomyelitis cases since 1951 in some parts of the world, comparing the countries or areas which now have controlled the disease and those countries in which control of polio is incomplete or only recently becoming established [22,26].

Table 61-4 includes countries of the western Pacific region that have the largest populations and for which recent data are available. In the top half of the table it can be seen that most of the countries of this region that now have succeeded in controlling polio were experiencing a very high incidence in the years from 1951 to 1955 before the advent of vaccines. By

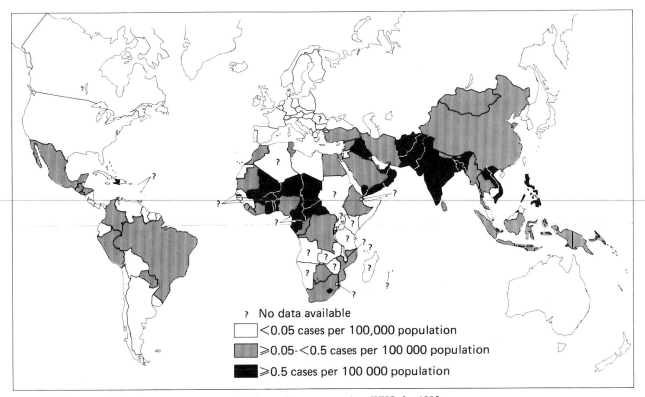

Figure 61-1. World map depicting occurrence of poliomyelitis as reported to WHO for 1985. Incidence is shown in cases per 100,000 population. (*From [23].*)

Table 61-4. Poliomyelitis in the western Pacific region: Comparison of countries in which the disease is controlled and those in which it is incompletely or only recently controlled*

	Population (millions) (est. 1985)	Average annual number of cases				Annual number of cases					
		1951–55	1966–70	1971–75	1976–80	1980	1981	1982	1983	1984	1985
Polio controlled[†]											
Australia	16	2187	1	2	1	0	0	0	0	0	0
Hong Kong	5	34	19	2	0	2	3	0	1	1	1
Japan	120	2414	21	5	0	2	2	1	0	1	1
Malaysia	15	124	97	349	36	5	2	5	2	2	4
New Zealand	3	413	1	0	0	N.A.[‡]	0	0	0	0	0
Singapore	3	61	3	1	0	1	0	1	2	2	0
Total[§]	162	5233	142	359	37	10	7	7	5	6	6
Polio incompletely or only recently controlled[†]											
China	1059	N.A.	N.A.	N.A.	7774	7442	4634	7741	3296	1626	1537
Laos	4	1	66	15	406	1166	N.A.	46	24	13	50
Papua New Guinea	3	N.A.	39	55	61	22	9	18	8	18	9
Philippines	54	221	556	880	894	790	353	256	355	740	533
Vietnam	60	54	85	142	785	1741	644	897	1109	1158	1600
Total[§]	1180	276	746	1092	9920	11161	5640	8958	4792	3555	3729

*Data compiled chiefly from reports made by national authorities to WHO [22,23,26].
[†]The countries selected as examples are, in general, those in which data were most complete, and which have the larger populations. A large number of other countries or areas in the region are in the "controlled" group, and virtually no cases are occurring in these smaller populations.
[‡]N.A. = data not available at the time of writing.
[§]The totals are those for the selected countries listed, and not for the entire western Pacific region.

1978 to 1980, some had almost eliminated the disease. For this entire "polio-controlled" group, with a total population of 162 million persons in 1985, there were only 10 cases in 1980, and only 5 to 7 cases each year since then—an incidence per 100,000 population of 0.003 to 0.004.

Australia, Japan, New Zealand, and Singapore accomplished control of polio very quickly, and have had relatively few cases since 1966 and virtually none for many recent years. In Hong Kong, full control was not achieved until the period 1971–1975. Malaysia, which had many years of difficulty, illustrates the transition from an endemic insidious pattern of poliomyelitis to an epidemic phase, followed finally by control of the disease through proper use of live poliovirus vaccine. Incidence fluctuated until there was a large outbreak in 1971–1972, with more than 1600 paralytic cases [26]. A rigorous immunization program begun in that year met with considerable success in containing outbreaks. A smaller outbreak in 1977 was found to indicate some flaws in the immunization program, chiefly problems in maintaining the vaccine in viable condition. Once these problems were corrected, the numbers of cases have greatly decreased, and control appears to have been achieved.

In the lower part of Table 61-4, the Philippines and Vietnam illustrate the contrasting trend in which, starting with relatively few cases in 1951 to 1955, increased numbers have been reported up to recent years. Polio clearly remains an important disease in these countries. From the recent data available, China, with more than 7700 cases in 1982, and twofold decreases for the next 2 years, has been making progress, despite the fact that in 1985 the reduction in cases was not as marked. It is the rural areas, particularly, where polio is not yet completely controlled.

In Table 61-5 are summarized the data for 41 countries or areas in the Americas. The 27 countries in this region that now have controlled polio are the ones that reported huge numbers of cases in the prevaccine period; with widespread use of vaccine, the incidence in these populations was greatly reduced over the decade 1966–1975. Since 1971 a number of areas

have had no cases or virtually none. Of the 53 cases reported for 1980 from this group, 41 were from Argentina, 9 from the United States, and 3 from Belize.

In contrast, the lower part of Table 61-5 shows that during 1951 to 1955 relatively few cases were reported from the countries now having problems; many of these countries were presumably in the insidious endemic phase of poliomyelitis. By 1966 to 1970, about five times as many cases were being reported. Some reduction was achieved in 1971 to 1975, but the number of cases occurring in this group of countries remained high through 1980. However, a large share of the recent cases come from only five countries, several of which have had many of the problems that hinder adequate vaccination coverage, that is, a large geographical area, rural regions difficult to reach, and growing urban fringe populations.

These countries (Bolivia, Brazil, Colombia, Honduras, and Mexico), with approximately 37 percent of the population of the American region, reported an annual average of 3409 cases during the period 1976–1980, 88 percent of the annual average of cases for the entire region during that period. Brazil, with 20 percent of the region's population, contributed 54 percent of the annual average numbers of cases. For 1980, the total in the "uncontrolled polio" group of countries had been reduced to 2895 cases, of which 1290 were in Brazil.

Table 61-6 indicates a great deal of progress in those 14 countries that in 1980 were considered not to have established control of polio. As can be noted, the incidence of polio has been greatly reduced in most of these countries, and several countries have reported no cases, or only one or two cases, in the last 3 or 4 years shown (1982 to 1985). Brazil and Mexico have made definite progress, but these countries—which, except for the United States, have by far the largest populations in the region—continue to have some difficulty in establishing complete control of polio [23,31].

However, the trend in cases clearly is downward in this group of countries, as in the American region as a whole, and it appears that a large majority of the countries in North, Central, and South America now belong in the "controlled" cate-

Table 61-5. Poliomyelitis in the American region as of 1980: Comparison of countries in which the disease was controlled and those in which it was incompletely controlled*

	Population (millions) (est. 1980)	Average annual number of cases			Annual number of cases				
		1951–1955	1966–1970	1971–1975	1976	1977	1978	1979	1980
Polio considered controlled as of 1980 (27 countries)†	305	44,391	470	221	24	34	28	64	53
Polio considered incompletely controlled as of 1980 (14 countries)‡	286	2202	14,454	10,249	3705	4592	3250	4664	2895

*Data compiled chiefly from reports made by national authorities to WHO [22,26].
†The countries or areas in the "controlled" group included Antigua, Argentina, Bahamas, Barbados, Belize, Bermuda, Canada, Canal Zone, Chile, Costa Rica, Cuba, Dominica, French Guiana, Grenada, Guadeloupe, Guyana, Jamaica, Martinique, Panama, Puerto Rico, Saint Kitts-Nevis-Anguilla, Saint Lucia, Saint Vincent, Surinam, Trinidad, Tobago, United States, and Uruguay.
‡The countries or areas in the "incompletely controlled" group are listed in Table 61-6.

Table 61-6. Poliomyelitis in the American region through 1985: Contrasting progress in countries in which the disease was considered in 1980 to be incompletely controlled*

	Population (millions) (est. 1985)	Average annual number of cases				Annual number of cases					
		1951–1955	1966–1970	1971–1975	1976–1980	1980	1981	1982	1983	1984	1985
Bolivia	6	4	31	59	125	48	15	10	7	0	0
Brazil	136	N.A.[†]	11688	8562	2100	1290	122	69	45	82	461
Colombia	29	103	463	396	401	129	576	187	88	18	36
Dominican Republic	6	4	31	60	74	148	71	68	7	0	2
Ecuador	9	42	334	100	14	11	11	11	5	0	0
El Salvador	5	49	72	86	30	55	52	16	88	19	10
Guatemala	8	103	147	122	84	287	40	136	208	17	29
Haiti	6	N.A.	5	11	27	20	35	34	62	63	90
Honduras	4	N.A.	47	37	100	3	18	8	8	76	4
Mexico	79	1365	1046	389	683	682	186	98	232	137	148
Nicaragua	3	81	129	68	32	21	46	0	0	0	0
Paraguay	4	58	58	107	20	7	53	4	11	3	3
Peru	20	107	188	131	127	182	245	215	111	102	67
Venezuela	17	286	214	121	20	11	68	30	9	9	8
Subtotals	332	2202	14453	10249	3837	2895	1538	884	881	526	855
Subtotals for countries with polio controlled in 1980	317	44391	470	221	34	53	9	79[b]	39	9	10
Totals for region	668	46593	14923	10470	3871	2948	1547	963	920	535	865

*Data compiled chiefly from reports made by national authorities to WHO [22,23,26] and from reports from the Centers for Disease Control [32].

[†]N.A. = data not available at time of this writing.

gory rather than in the "incompletely controlled" group. The Pan American Health Organization has indicated that 75 percent of children in the region less than 1 year old have now been immunized against polio, whereas before the Expanded Programme of Immunization (EPI) was launched in the Americas in 1978, the figure was only 25 percent immunized in this age group.

The Pan American Health Organization has also announced a plan to eradicate poliomyelitis from the entire American region by the year 1990, in the expectation that the goal can be achieved by using its staff and volunteers to coordinate separate national efforts to encourage immunization.

The total cost of this plan is estimated at $100 million, but in fact much of the infrastructure required is already in place, so that only about one-third of this sum seems to be needed in aid from developed countries, much of which is already committed.

It was in Europe that the classical huge poliomyelitis epidemics were first seen, with more than 50,000 cases reported annually from the U.S.S.R. and 26 other countries during 1951–1955. Once vaccines were developed, control was quickly established in most of the European region. In this large population (estimated at 824 million in 1985), cases were brought down to an annual average of 891 for the period 1966–1970, to 536 in 1971–1975, and to 387 in 1976–1979. In 1985, only 173 cases were reported to WHO for the entire region [23].

CONTROL OF POLIOMYELITIS

The prevention of poliomyelitis depends upon vaccination. Quarantine of patients or intimate contacts is ineffective in controlling the spread of the disease. This is understandable in view of the large number of inapparent infections that occur, and the fact that all susceptible members of a family will already have been infected by the time the disease has been diagnosed in one family member.

During epidemics children with fever should be given adequate bed rest. Undue exercise or fatigue, elective nose and throat operations, or dental extractions should be avoided. Food and human excrement should be protected from flies. Once the poliovirus type responsible for the epidemic is determined, live virus vaccine should be administered to susceptible persons in the population.

Patients with poliomyelitis can be admitted to general hospitals provided appropriate isolation precautions are employed. All pharyngeal and bowel discharges are considered infectious and should be disposed of quickly and safely.

Improved community and family sanitation and hygiene do limit the circulation of wild polioviruses, thus paradoxically "depriving" some unvaccinated infants of early immunizing infections (and hence postponing their poliovirus experience to a later, and possibly more severe, encounter). Nonetheless, limiting the circulation of these viruses has of course an overall positive effect, and when vaccination is combined with improvements in sanitation and hygiene the wild polioviruses can be virtually eliminated from an area.

Prophylaxis by passive immunization through administration of immune human serum globulin (γ-globulin) is seldom if ever used at present. Administration of immune human serum globulin in dosage of 0.3 mL per kilogram of body weight can provide protection for a few weeks against the paralytic disease but does not prevent subclinical infection. γ-Globulin is effective only if given shortly before infection; it is of no value after clinical symptoms develop.

Serological surveys have an important role in maintaining protection against resurgence of epidemic poliomyelitis, by making possible the surveillance of immunity levels. Continuing serological surveillance can answer such questions as the following: In the country under consideration, what age groups are most susceptible? Are significant proportions of the susceptible age group being reached and protected by vaccination? Do the results of serological surveys parallel the estimates from surveys of immunization history? How well do antibodies induced by vaccination persist over the years?

Immunization with inactivated virus or live vaccine

Recommended schedules for routine administration of poliovaccines to infants in the United States are shown in Table 61-7 [33]. However, since the early 1960s, OPV has been the only poliovirus vaccine in general use, and its use has led to the virtual elimination of paralytic polio.

Despite the availability of two effective poliomyelitis vaccines, there remain a number of developing countries, chiefly in tropical areas, in which vaccination is not adequately used.

Table 61-7. Recommended poliomyelitis immunization schedule for the United States*

Dose	Live poliovirus vaccine: Age, interval[†]	Killed poliovirus vaccine: Age, interval[‡]
Primary 1	6–12 weeks of age	6–12 weeks of age
Primary 2	After interval of 6–8 weeks	After interval of 4–8 weeks
Primary 3	After interval of more than 6 weeks, but before 18 months of age	After interval of 4–8 weeks
Primary 4		After interval of 6–12 months
Supplementary	4–6 years of age	4–6 years of age
Additional supplementary		Interval of every 5 years to age 18

*After recommendations of the Advisory Committee on Immunization Practices (ACIP), Centers for Disease Control [32].
[†]In tropical areas of high endemicity, an initial dose of monovalent type 1 vaccine is recommended soon after birth.
[‡]With the introduction of the van Wezel IPV in 1988, fewer booster doses will be required.

The primary immunization schedules in these countries not only should begin early, but in particular should be completed early in infancy; in some tropical areas a combined schedule should be considered [34,35].

Vaccine programs for regions—particularly in subtropical and tropical climates—where poliomyelitis remains uncontrolled may be more appropriately planned if the merits and problems associated with the use of inactivated and of live poliovirus vaccines are better understood. These are summarized in Tables 61-8 and 61-9 [36].

Properly prepared and administered, IPV can induce adequate levels of serum antibodies, conferring humoral immunity (see Table 61-7 for schedule). The inactivated virus vaccine, although it impedes pharyngeal shedding of virus, does not induce a high degree of intestinal immunity; therefore, wild polioviruses can still multiply in the intestinal tracts of such vaccinees. Although those adequately vaccinated are themselves protected by their serum antibodies so that even when infected they do not develop the paralytic disease, the virus

Table 61-8. Inactivated poliovirus vaccine: Advantages and disadvantages*

Advantages:
Confers humoral immunity in vaccinees if sufficient numbers of doses of potent vaccine are given.
Can be incorporated into regular pediatric immunization, with other vaccines (DPT).
Absence of living virus excludes potential for mutation and reversion to virulence.
Absence of living virus permits its use in immunodeficient or immunosuppressed individuals and their households.
Has greatly reduced the spread of polioviruses in three small northern European countries where it has been properly used (wide and frequent coverage).
May prove useful in certain tropical areas where live virus vaccine has failed to "take" in some young infants.
Disadvantages:
Early studies indicated a disappointing record in percentage of vaccinees developing antibodies after three doses, but more immunopotent antigens are now produced.
Generally, repeated boosters have been required to maintain detectable antibody levels.
Does not induce appreciable local intestinal immunity in the vaccinee; hence vaccinees do not serve as a block to transmission of wild polioviruses by the fecal-oral route.
More expensive than live virus vaccine.
Growing scarcity of monkeys for kidney tissue substrate. (Has been overcome by use of continuous-passage Vero monkey cells for vaccine production.)
Use of virulent polioviruses as vaccine seed creates potential for tragedy if a single failure in virus inactivation were to occur in a batch of released vaccine, especially since monkey neurovirulence tests are no longer required before release of inactivated virus vaccine. However, this problem can be overcome by use of attenuated strains for production.

*Modified from [36].

Table 61-9. Live poliovirus vaccine:
Advantages and disadvantages*

Advantages:
  Confers both humoral and intestinal immunity, like the natural
    infection.
  Immunity induced appears to be lifelong.
  Induces antibody very quickly in a large proportion of vaccinees.
  Oral administration is more acceptable to vaccinees than injection,
    and is easier to accomplish.
  Administration does not require use of highly trained personnel.
  When properly stabilized, can retain potency under difficult field
    conditions with little refrigeration and no freezers.
  Under epidemic conditions, not only induces antibody quickly but
    also rapidly infects the alimentary tract, blocking epidemic
    spread of the virus.
  Is relatively inexpensive, both to produce and to administer, and
    does not require continuing booster doses.
  Can be prepared in pretested human or monkey cells, thus is
    dependent on monkeys only for neurovirulence testing. Use of
    continuous cell lines eliminates the theoretical risk of including
    monkey virus contaminants in the vaccine.
Disadvantages:
  Vaccine viruses may mutate, and in very rare instances have
    reverted toward neurovirulence sufficient to cause paralytic polio
    in recipients or their contacts.
  Vaccine progeny virus spreads to household contacts.
  Vaccine virus also spreads to persons in the community. Some
    people consider this spread into the household and the
    community to be an advantage, but the progeny virus excreted
    and spread by vaccinees often is a mutated virus and obviously
    cannot be a safety-tested vaccine, licensed for use in the general
    population.
  In certain tropical countries, induction of antibodies in a
    satisfactorily high proportion of vaccinees has been difficult to
    accomplish.
  Contraindicated in those with immunodeficiency diseases, and in
    their household associates, as well as in persons undergoing
    immunosuppressive therapy, and their households.
  Requires monkeys for safety testing.

*Modified from [36].

they excrete can be a source of infection to others. Also, repeated booster injections have been required to maintain antibody levels; this adds to the higher cost of using inactivated virus vaccine. In developing countries, adequate use of such vaccine thus far has been difficult in view of the logistical problems posed by injection of several doses of vaccine at intervals into large numbers of infants and preschool children. Even in countries with highly developed health care systems and populations considered to be very well vaccinated with IPV, imported wild virus can spread not only in unvaccinated sectors of the population but also through those who have been vaccinated. The new, more concentrated and more potent IPVs prepared by the van Wezel procedure are proving to be more effective with fewer doses than the original Salk vaccine. Such

vaccines are now being used in northern Europe, and field trials are being conducted in some communities in developing tropical regions.

Hopes have been high that newer, enhanced IPV (eIPV) could provide long-lasting immunity after two doses [37], and that even a single dose could provide significant protection against paralytic polio by inducing an "immunological memory," whether or not antibody was induced [38]. Serological studies following immunization in several tropical areas had indicated seroconversion in 90 to 100 percent of vaccinees. However, direct evidence of clinical efficacy of eIPV in the field has been obtained only recently, in a field study conducted in Senegal.

Polio is endemic in Senegal but in 1986 an outbreak occurred throughout the country. A matched case-control study was conducted in the Kolda region, where considerable immunization efforts using eIPV have been made since 1980, and where 87 certified cases could be used in efficacy calculations. Two doses of eIPV were calculated to have an efficacy of 89 percent but one dose, only 36 percent. Thus, although the two-dose protection was encouraging, the hopes for single-dose induction of an effective "immunological memory" were not borne out [39,40].

Live, orally administered trivalent poliovirus vaccine (TOPV) has been more widely used, because of its greater ease of administration by the oral route, lower cost, ability to induce not only serum antibodies but also intestinal resistance, and the rapidity with which vaccinees develop long-lasting immunity (Table 61-9). Serological studies have indicated that the proportion of individuals found to possess antibodies is considerably greater than would appear to be explainable either by their vaccination histories or by the circulation of wild polioviruses in their communities. The spreading of vaccine-derived virus through the community with the resultant immunization of nonvaccinated persons is viewed by some as an advantage, despite the fact that such individuals may be infected with modified virus excreted by the vaccinees—a virus which has obviously not been tested for safety, as was the original vaccine administered.

Problems associated with live poliovirus vaccine relate chiefly to the fact that the vaccine consists of living viruses. Being alive, the vaccine viruses can mutate, and some poliovirus strains excreted by vaccinees—although still attenuated—are less attenuated than the vaccine viruses administered. There have been, in vaccine recipients and in close contacts of vaccinees, rare cases of paralytic poliomyelitis that are temporally and epidemiologically associated with vaccine administration. Among these vaccine-associated cases are cases in persons with immune deficiencies. An important caution that must be observed with live poliovirus vaccine, as with any other living infectious agent, is that it should not knowingly be given either to any such persons, or to their close contacts, whether the deficiency is long-term, or is temporarily induced in the course of cancer chemotherapy or organ transplantation.

The risks of paralytic polio associated with the live virus vaccine are exceedingly small, and by the 1980s such cases have decreased to an almost vanishing number. The latest figures available to WHO from four of the countries participating in its polio surveillance program (England, Hungary, Japan, and the United States) indicate that there is 1 recipient case and 1 contact case per 4 million doses of vaccine distributed [41]. These estimates are based on the maximum risk (that is, the risk calculated as though every "vaccine-associated" case were indeed vaccine-caused). In the most recent published evaluation of cases in the United States, covering the period 1973–1984, it has been estimated [14] that the overall frequency of vaccine-associated poliomyelitis was 1 case per 2.6 million vaccine doses distributed. However, the associated frequency of paralysis was 1 case per 520,000 first doses, versus 1 case per 12.3 million subsequent doses.

In West Germany, vaccine-associated cases are estimated to occur at a rate of 1 per 4.4 million among recipients, and 1 per 15.5 million among contacts. The comparatively low rate among contacts probably is the result of that country's policy of vaccinating families at the same time as their infants are vaccinated [42]. Israel once had epidemics of over 1000 paralytic cases per year, but since the introduction of oral vaccine only 1 vaccine-associated case has occurred every 2 years, and only 1 contact case every 7 years [43].

Three sequential 5-year studies of polio cases have been conducted collaboratively among 12 to 15 nations, under the auspices of WHO. In these and other studies, live poliovirus vaccine has been judged repeatedly to be an extraordinarily safe vaccine [41,44], with less than one reported case for every million babies vaccinated.

In some tropical countries live virus vaccines have not induced antibody production in a satisfactorily high percentage of vaccinees [45]. This lower rate of vaccine "takes" has been ascribed to various factors such as interference from other enteroviruses already present in the intestinal tract, the presence of antibody in breast milk, the presence of cellular resistance in the intestinal tract due to previous exposure to wild polioviruses (or perhaps to related viruses), and the presence of an inhibitor in the alimentary tract (saliva) of infants that acts against multiplication of the vaccine virus. Some feel that this low response, regardless of the reason, can be overcome by proper and repeated use of live virus vaccine.

The problems of controlling paralytic polio by use of vaccine are often exacerbated by the fact that in some areas the newborn infant has only a short time in which to acquire protective immunity because exposure comes so early, in their first months of life [46]. Various plans are now being pursued in different developing and tropical countries [47,48,49].

WHO's EPI Global Advisory Group [30] has concluded that immunization of the newborn with TOPV is a safe and effective means of improving protection against disease and that TOPV may be administered simultaneously with bacillus Calmette-Guérin (BCG) vaccine. Although the serological response to TOPV in the first week is less than that observed with immunization of older infants, 70 to 100 percent of neonates benefit by developing local immunity in the intestinal tract. In addition, 30 to 50 percent of the infants develop serum antibodies to one or more poliovirus types. Many of the remaining infants have been immunologically primed, and they respond promptly to additional doses later in life.

The EPI Advisory Group emphasizes that for those infants in many countries whose only encounter with preventive services is at the time of birth, this single dose of vaccine will offer some protection and they will be less likely to be a source of transmission of wild polioviruses during infancy and childhood. For the infants who receive only one or two additional doses of poliovirus vaccine, the initial dose at birth will help ensure higher levels of immunity. The EPI schedule designed to provide protection at the earliest possible age is: at birth, and then at 6, 10, and 14 weeks of age. If the antigens are not given at those ages, they should be given as soon as possible afterward. Intervals between doses greater than those listed do not require restarting the series.

Gradual Incorporation Into Routine Immunization Schedules. In many areas, live virus vaccines have been included in the regular childhood immunization programs, without there necessarily having been prior mass vaccination campaigns for poliomyelitis. This has meant that the increase in vaccine coverage—and the hoped for decrease in polio incidence—can be expected to be gradual. In a number of countries using this approach, reported polio cases have significantly declined since the early 1970s.

An example of recent progress can be seen in special programs conducted in three areas in tropical Africa that were experiencing incidence rates (as estimated from lameness surveys) ranging from 25 to 62 per 100,000 population in the mid- to late 1970s. The programs emphasized intensive and carefully targeted schedules of routine vaccination. Programs were instituted [50] in Yaounde, Cameroon; in The Gambia; and in Abidjan, Ivory Coast. They included administration of three doses of OPV during the first year of life, 1 month apart starting at 2 to 3 months of age. The vaccine coverage achieved was evaluated [51], and surveillance of poliomyelitis was conducted with care both before and after the vaccination program, using well-established methods [25,52,53,54]. Within a few years the proportion of the children who received three doses of the vaccine—which had been virtually zero except for some (low) coverage in Abidjan—was increased up to 50 to 70 percent. Even with this less than optimal vaccine coverage, the incidence of poliomyelitis has decreased significantly, in contrast to what has been reported from some other tropical countries, and OPV properly administered during the first year of life has been judged to be effective in controlling poliomyelitis in these localities. For example, in Yaounde by 1980, 50 percent of the children 12 to 13 months old had received three doses of vaccine, and from a preimmunization average of 62 cases per 100,000 in 1974 and 1975, the incidence of polio decreased 88 percent, to 7.5 per 100,000 in 1981. In a later report from Yaounde [55], of the children 12 to 23 months of age only 35 percent had received three doses of OPV, yet the incidence of paralytic polio decreased by 85 percent.

Maintaining a routine immunization schedule that reaches virtually all of the target population implies the ability to maintain a supply of viable vaccine constantly at the point of contact. This can be difficult in warm climates with limited cold-chain facilities, particularly if the vaccine has not been treated with a stabilizer equal or superior to molar $MgCl_2$ [56,57,58,59].

Mass Campaigns Repeated Annually. Sabin [47,48] has suggested that paralytic poliomyelitis in tropical countries might best be eliminated by repeated mass administration of OPV. He recommended annual campaigns that would include all age groups in which cases are occurring. All children from birth to 3, 4, or 5 years of age (depending on the epidemiological situation in a given country) should be given two doses of OPV twice each year regardless of how many doses of live virus vaccine they may have received previously. This mass administration would reach those missed in previous campaigns and would avoid the problems of recordkeeping, which often has been a barrier to full coverage in administering the vaccine.

Mass campaigns with OPV have been conducted successfully in a number of countries, not only bypassing the need for constantly maintaining refrigeration—as well as other logistical problems—but also providing a high level of coverage and at one time introducing massive quantities of live vaccine virus which may preempt the available hosts, thus blocking wild virus circulation. In Cuba since 1962, all children from birth to 3 or 5 years (depending on concurrent serosurvey findings), regardless of individual immunization history, have been given OPV on two Sundays each year, 2 months apart. Serosurveys show almost universal immunity by the age of 3, and since the end of the first campaign year, almost a quarter of a century ago, only six cases have been reported. Czechoslovakia, using the same strategy, has had similar success, with the total disappearance of paralytic poliomyelitis. High levels of public cooperation, discipline, and dedication seem to be vital factors in these successes—levels that may not necessarily be present in all situations.

This strategy of periodic mass campaigns, sometimes alone, sometimes combined with a constantly maintained schedule for immunizing infants, has been highly successful in some areas, although not yet in others. Brazil in 1980 instituted such a program, entailing a huge national effort in which, regardless of any vaccine history, each child in the selected age groups is given a dose of live virus vaccine twice each year, with a 2-month interval between doses [47,48]. Some 90,000 vaccination sites (10 times the number of permanent health stations) were established, and 400,000 volunteers were mobilized.

From several thousand cases annually in the late 1970s, polio cases in Brazil have been reduced dramatically, to an average of 80 annually during 1981 through 1984 [29,31,47,48,60]. However, there was an increase to 461 cases in 1985 [23] and to 612 in 1986, which seems to have been a temporary setback due to low potency of the type 3 component of the vaccine [31] (see Table 61-6). A significant improvement of seroconversion to type 3 has been reported in a field trial in Recife, Brazil, with a trivalent OPV containing an increased concentration of the type 3 vaccine strain [61]. It is suggested that this improvement was due to a relative reduction in the interference that is normally exerted by the type 2 component.

Important questions relative to such a program have been: Would developing nations be able and willing to make such an annual commitment of 2 days for each of two doses, with a 2-month interval between them? Would these nations have the resources to conduct such an annual, repetitive mass vaccination program? There also had been some misgivings as to whether the absence of recordkeeping could be detrimental to the program and whether concentration on OPV could detract from other needed health services. In practice in Brazil, the annual polio program has led to an increased awareness and activity for other immunizations.

Mexico likewise has had a long struggle to control polio through routine vaccinations, and still had an average of almost 700 cases reported annually in the period 1976–1980. In 1981, mass national immunization campaigns were instituted [62]. Monovalent type 1 vaccine—type 1 being the virus type that has long predominated in their paralytic cases—is used for the first dose, followed by trivalent vaccine 2 months later. Much fuller vaccination coverage is being achieved (more than 80 percent in 1982), and polio has been drastically reduced, to 186 cases in 1981, and 90 cases in 1987 [31].

"Pulsed" Mass Vaccination. In India, despite many efforts at controlling poliomyelitis, thousands of cases still occur, the highest incidence being in infants 6 to 18 months old [21]. It is estimated that more than 200,000 cases occur annually in that country alone [21,63]. John [63] advocates giving doses of OPV (along with diphtheria-pertussis-tetanus (DPT) and measles vaccines at appropriate intervals) to all the target children in each community at the same time, rather than following individual routine immunization schedules. His proposal would mean giving three doses of OPV before the first birthday, and three more between the first and second birthdays; a village would be visited three times in the course of the year at intervals of 4 to 6 weeks, and then no more vaccine would be given over a 9-month period.

"Insured" Immunization. An innovative approach to accomplishing better delivery of vaccine—not only of OPV but also of other pediatric immunizations—has proven productive in one area of China (Gaoyi County, Shijiazhuang Prefecture, Hebei Province—a county with a total population of 140,000 in 107 villages). To increase family cooperation in immunization programs and to encourage health staff members to enhance their preventive health efforts, the new plan, introduced in 1984, was expanded by early 1986 to include more than 12,000 children (62 percent of children under 7 years of age in the county) [64].

The average annual family income in Gaoyi is 438 yuan. The parents pay 10 yuan to the health center in the first year of their child's life, with a contract that "guarantees" that their child will not contract measles, pertussis, poliomyelitis, tetanus, or diphtheria if he or she receives the full recommended course of immunization. If the insured child suffers from measles or whooping cough, the parents receive an indemnity of 50 yuan; if poliomyelitis, diphtheria, or tetanus, 300 yuan.

The insurance premiums received (nearly 100,000 yuan as of 1985) are distributed among the village doctor, county health centers, and the county epidemic station, which expends them for immunization equipment and education, reserving funds to compensate parents when an enlisted child contracts any of the designated diseases. In turn, the village doctor and the county agencies share the costs of compensation. Up to the end of January 1986, a total of only 750 yuan had been paid in compensation, covering 15 cases of measles or whooping cough. There were no cases of poliomyelitis.

The advantages of the system have been described as follows:

1. It stimulates staff of health centres and village doctors to implement immunization activities.
2. Parents are enthusiastic to have their children immunized because they feel that they have paid a lot of money.
3. The primary health care setting has been strengthened because the staff can earn one-quarter to one-half more than their regular income.
4. Underreporting of cases has been reduced because parents are motivated to report a suspected case in order to receive compensation.
5. Wastage of vaccine has been minimized because the activities have been carried out strictly according to the schedule due to the enthusiasm of staff and parents. [64].

Combined Schedules Using Both Live and Killed Virus Vaccine. In some localities, it has been found advantageous to establish immunization schedules using both killed and live poliovirus vaccines. One type of situation in which this strategy has been successfully carried out has been the relatively recent addition of killed virus vaccine to supplement live virus vaccine immunization schedules, in some high-risk localities where there is very early and repeated exposure of infants to challenge by importations of wild, virulent viruses [33,46,20a].

A program using this approach was instituted in 1978 in Gaza and the West Bank, where some cases were occurring, particularly in infants, despite extensive campaigns of immunization with OPV. The combined schedule includes administration of OPV (type 1 monovalent) during the first month of an infant's life; then at $2\frac{1}{2}$ months and again at 4 months of age TOPV is given together with a quadruple vaccine consisting of DPT plus IPV; TOPV is given at $5\frac{1}{2}$ months, and again at 12 months. The rationale for the combined schedule was that, under conditions of regular and heavy importation of virus resulting in frequent challenge from virulent wild polioviruses early in infancy, features of both types of vaccine are needed. The OPV acts by inducing protective immunity both in the form of circulating humoral antibodies and in the form of intestinal immunity. Furthermore, the immunity that ensues is long-lasting, like that which follows the natural infection. The IPV, on the other hand, provides an immediate immunogenic stimulus that is not subject to the interfering or inhibiting factors described above, that may prevent live virus vaccine "takes" in some young infants. By administering both vaccines in a combined schedule, immediate protection can be provided in the critical first weeks or months of life, and long-lasting protection—both humoral and intestinal—also is provided.

Studies of the combined vaccine program described above indicate: (1) Protection provided by OPV alone was about 90 percent effective; that is, the case rate in those who received OPV alone was one-tenth the rate in those who were not vaccinated or were incompletely vaccinated (receiving only part of the series of live virus vaccine feedings). (2) The children who were fully vaccinated with OPV and had IPV in addition were even more effectively protected; virtually 100 percent protection was seen in those who received two doses of IPV plus three doses of OPV. Two serum surveys in children aged 9 to 36 months substantiated their protection [65].

Another type of combined program has been the addition of live virus vaccine in 1968 to supplement IPV in Denmark where, despite extensive coverage with IPV alone, epidemics still occurred, and antibody prevalence was less than desired [66]. The combined IPV-OPV program has resulted in the virtual elimination of poliomyelitis from that country.

CONCLUSION

Once considered a disease of the temperate zones, poliomyelitis is now far more prevalent in tropical countries. But excellent vaccines are available and sufficient knowledge now exists to allow the vaccines, usually alone but sometimes in combination, to be used with a high degree of effectiveness in a variety of settings. Thus those responsible for public health should consider the initiation or the intensification of well-targeted campaigns to decrease the numbers of cases of paralytic poliomyelitis. It is even possible at this writing to consider eradication of the disease from the world.

The question of whether, how, and where eradication of poliomyelitis can be achieved will be a focal point of international discussions in the next few years. The World Health Organization Expanded Programme on Immunization was initiated with the objective of reducing morbidity and mortality rates from six target diseases, including poliomyelitis, by providing immunization against them for every child in the world. The program depends heavily upon technical cooperation with and among developing countries, particularly those in tropical regions. Results are already being seen: increasing numbers of countries now participate in the WHO program or are otherwise enhancing their polio vaccination efforts. Better and more complete surveillance programs have been implemented to detect and assess cases. More information is being gathered on the epidemiology of poliomyelitis in specific regional and geographical settings. And—most crucial—better-informed and more determined national commitments to immunization are being made. As for the ultimate goal of reducing the incidence of poliomyelitis to the vanishing point, it is too early for accomplishment, but the coming years should bring significant progress.

REFERENCES

1 Cole CN: Defective interfering (DI) particles of poliovirus, in Melnick JL (ed): *Progress in Medical Virology,* vol 20. Basel, Karger, 1975, pp 180–207

2 Pan American Sanitary Bureau/Pan American Health Organization: *Live Poliovirus Vaccines, Papers Presented and Discussions Held at the First and Second International Conferences on Live Poliovirus Vaccines.* special publications No 44 and 50, Pan American Health Organization, Washington, DC, 1959

3 Nomoto A, Wimmer E: Genetic studies of the antigenicity and the attenuation phenotype of poliovirus, in Russell WD, Almond JW (eds): *Molecular Basis of Virus Disease.* Symposium 40, Society for General Microbiology. New York, Cambridge University Press, 1987, pp 107–134

4 Hogle JM, Chow M, Filman DJ: Three-dimensional structure of poliovirus at 2.9 Å resolution. Science 229:1358–1365, 1985

5 Reissig M, Howes D, Melnick JL: Sequence of morphological changes in epithelial cell cultures infected with poliovirus. J Exp Med 104:289–304, 1956

6 Melnick, JL, Wenner, HA, Phillips, CA: Enteroviruses, in Lennette EH, Schmidt NJ (eds): *Diagnostic Procedures for Viral, Rickettsial, and Chlamydial Infections,* 5th ed. Washington, DC, American Public Health Association, 1979, pp 471–534

7 Miller DA, Miller OJ, Vaithilingham GD, et al: Human chromosome 19 carries a poliovirus receptor gene. Cell 1:167–173, 1974

8 Rao VC, Metcalf TG, Melnick JL: Human viruses in sediments, sludges, and soils. Bull WHO 64:1–14, 1986 (Also in French, in Bull WHO 64:341–356, 1986)

9 Ogra PL, Fishaut M, Gallagher MR: Viral vaccination via the mucosal routes. Rev Infect Dis 2:352–369, 1980

10 Bodian D, Horstmann DM: Polioviruses, in Horsfall FL, Jr, Tamm I (eds): *Viral and Rickettsial Infections of Man,* 4th ed. Philadelphia, Lippincott, 1965, pp 430–473

11 Melnick JL, Proctor RO, Ocampo AR, et al: Free and bound virus in serum after administration of oral poliovirus vaccine. Am J Epidemiol 84:329–342, 1966

12 Cherry JD: Aseptic meningitis and viral meningitis, in Feigin RD, Cherry JD (eds): *Textbook of Pediatric Infectious Diseases,* 2d ed, vol I. Philadelphia, Saunders, 1987, pp 478–484

13 Melnick JL, Ledinko N: Development of neutralizing antibodies against the three types of poliomyelitis virus during an epidemic period. The ratio of inapparent infection to clinical poliomyelitis. Am J Hyg 58:207–222, 1953

14 Nkowane BM, Wassilak SGF, Orenstein WA, et al: Vaccine-associated paralytic poliomyelitis. United States: 1973 through 1984. JAMA 257:1335–1340, 1987

15 Yorke JA, Nathanson N, Pianigiani G, et al: Seasonality and the requirements for perpetuation and eradication of viruses in populations. Am J Epidemiol 109:103–123, 1979

16 *International Symposium on Poliomyelitis Control,* Horstmann DM, Quinn TC, Robbins FC (guest eds), held at Pan American Health Organization, Washington, DC, 1983. Rev Infect Dis 6(suppl 2):S301–S600, 1984

17 Rico-Hesse R, Pallansch MA, Nottay BK, et al: Geographic distribution of wild poliovirus type 1 genotypes. Virology 160:311–322, 1987

18 Schaap GJP, Bijkerk H, Coutinho RA, et al: The spread of wild poliovirus in the well-vaccinated Netherlands in connection with the 1978 epidemic. Prog Med Virol 29:124–149, 1984, (Basel, Karger)

19 Leinikki PO, Pasternack A, Mustonen J, et al: Paralytic poliomyelitis in Finland. Lancet ii:507, 1985 (Aug. 31)

20 Hovi T, Huovilainen A, Kuronen T, et al: Outbreak of paralytic poliomyelitis in Finland: Widespread circulation of antigenically altered poliovirus type 3 in a vaccinated population. Lancet i:1427–1432, 1986

20a Goldblum N, Swartz T, Gerichter CB, et al: The natural history of poliomyelitis in Israel, 1949–1982. Prog Med Virol 29:115–123, 1984 (Basel, Karger)

20b Slater PE, Orenstein W, Melnick JL, et al.: Outbreak of poliomyelitis in Israel, 1988. Manuscript in preparation, 1989

21 Dave KH: Report of Enterovirus Research Centre, Bombay, for 1986, published 1987

22 World Health Organization: Poliomyelitis in 1980 (parts 1 and 2). Weekly Epidemiological Record 56:329–336; 337–344, Oct 23 and Oct 30, 1981

23 World Health Organization: Poliomyelitis in 1985 (parts I and II). Weekly Epidemiological Record 62:273–280; 281–282. Sept 11 and Sept 18, 1987

24 Paul JR, Melnick JL, Barnett VH, et al: A survey of neutralizing antibodies to poliomyelitis in Cairo, Egypt. Am J Hyg 55:402–413, 1952

25 Ofosu-Amaah S, Kratzer JH, Nicholas DD: Is poliomyelitis a serious problem in developing countries? Lameness in Ghanaian schools. Br Med J i:1012–1014, 1977

26 World Health Organization: Poliomyelitis in 1979 (parts 1 and 2). Weekly Epidemiological Record 55:361–366, 369–376, Nov 21 and Nov 28, 1980

27 World Health Organization: Expanded programme on immunization (EPI): Poliomyelitis prevalence surveys. Tamil Nadu, India, 1979. Weekly Epidemiological Record 56:131–132, May 1, 1981

28 World Health Organization: Expanded programme on immunization (EPI): Poliomyelitis prevalence surveys, Ivory Coast. Weekly Epidemiological Record 55:401–403, Dec 23, 1980

29 World Health Organization: Poliomyelitis annual reports for 1974–1985. Weekly Epidemiological Records, 1976–1987

30 World Health Organization: Expanded programme on immuni-

zation Global Advisory Group: Summary of conclusions and recommendations. Weekly Epidemiological Record 60:13–16, 1985

31 Pan American Health Organization: Expanded Program on Immunization: Polio surveillance in the Americas. Weekly Bulletin vol II, No 50, for week ending Dec 19, 1987

32 Centers for Disease Control: Surveillance summaries through 1986, Atlanta, Centers for Disease Control, U.S. Department of Health and Human Services, Public Health Service (annual summaries published through 1987)

33 Advisory Committee on Immunization Practices (ACIP): Poliomyelitis prevention. CDC Morbidity and Mortality Weekly Report 31(no. 3, Jan 29, 1982):22–26, 31–33, 1982; and ACIP: Report of Meeting, October, 1985

34 Melnick JL: Combined use of live and killed vaccines to control poliomyelitis in tropical areas, in Hennessen W, van Wezel AL (eds): *Reassessment of Inactivated Poliomyelitis Vaccine: Developments in Biological Standardization,* vol 47. Basel, Karger, 1981, pp 265–273

35 Melnick JL: Recent developments in the worldwide control of poliomyelitis, in Kurstak E, Marusyk R (eds): *Control of Virus Diseases.* New York, Dekker, 1984, pp 3–31

36 Melnick JL: Advantages and disadvantages of killed and live poliomyelitis vaccines. Bull WHO 56:21–38, 1978

37 McBean AM, Thoms ML, Albrecht P, et al: Serological response to oral polio vaccine and enhanced-potency inactivated polio vaccines. Am J Epidemiol 128:615–628, 1988

38 Salk J: One-dose immunization against paralytic poliomyelitis using a non-infectious vaccine. Rev Infect Dis 6(suppl 2):S444–S450, 1984

39 Robertson SE, Traverso HP, Drucker JA, et al: Clinical efficacy of a new, enhanced-potency, inactivated poliovirus vaccine. Lancet i:897–899, 1988

40 Centers for Disease Control: Paralytic Poliomyelitis—Senegal, 1986–1987: Update on the N-IPV efficacy study. Morbidity and Mortality Weekly Report 37:257–259, 1988 (April 29, no 16)

41 World Health Organization Consultative Group on Poliomyelitis Vaccines: Report to WHO, Geneva. 1985

42 Maass G, Quast U: Acute spinal paralysis after the administration of oral poliomyelitis vaccine in the Federal Republic of Germany (1963–1984). J Biol Stand 15:185–191, 1987

43 Swartz TA, Handsher P, Goldblum N: Control of poliomyelitis in Israel, submitted for publication, 1988

44 Cockburn WC: The work of the WHO Consultative Group on Poliomyelitis Vaccines. Bull WHO 66:143–154, 1988

45 Domok I, Balayan MS, Fayinka OA, et al: Factors affecting the efficacy of live poliovirus vaccines in warm climates. Bull WHO 51:333–347, 1974

46 Lasch EE, Abed Y, Abdulla K, et al: Successful results of a program combining live and inactivated poliovirus vaccines to control poliomyelitis in Gaza. Rev Infect Dis 6(suppl 2)S467–S470, 1984

47 Sabin AB: Paralytic poliomyelitis: Old dogmas and new perspectives. Rev Infect Dis 3:543–564, 1981

48 Sabin AB: Oral poliovirus vaccine: History of its development and use and current challenge to eliminate poliomyelitis from the world. J Infect Dis 151:420–436, 1985

49 Robinson DA: Polio vaccination—a review of strategies. Trans R Soc Trop Med Hyg 76:575–581, 1982

50 Foster SO, Kesseng-Maben G, N'jie H, et al: Control of poliomyelitis in Africa. Rev Infect Dis 6:(suppl 2):S433–S437, 1984

51 Henderson RH, Sundaresan T: Cluster sampling to assess immunization coverage: a review of experience with a simplified sampling methodology. Bull WHO 60:253–260, 1982

52 Bernier RH: Prevalence survey techniques for paralytic polio: an update. Expanded Programme on Immunization Working Paper, EPI/GAG 83/10, Geneva, WHO, 1983

53 Heymann DL, Floyd VD, Luchnevski M, et al: Estimation of incidence of poliomyelitis by three survey methods in different regions of the United Republic of Cameroon. Bull WHO 61:501–507, 1983

54 LaForce FM, Lichnevski MS, Keja J, et al: Clinical survey techniques to estimate prevalence and annual incidence of poliomyelitis in developing countries. Bull WHO 58:609–620, 1980

55 Heymann DL, Murphy K, Brigaud M, et al: Oral poliovirus vaccine in tropical Africa: Bull WHO 65:495–501, 1987

56 Melnick JL, Ashkenazi A, Midulla VC, et al: Immunogenic potency of $MgCl_2$-stabilized oral poliovaccine. JAMA 185:406–408, 1963

57 Peetermans J, Colinet G, Stephenne J: Activity of attenuated poliomyelitis and measles vaccines exposed at different temperatures, in *Proceedings Symposium on Stability and Effectiveness of Measles, Poliomyelitis, and Pertussis Vaccines.* Zagreb, Yugoslav Academy of Sciences and Arts, 1976, pp 61–66

58 Finter NB, Ferris R, Kelly A, et al: Effects of adverse storage on live virus vaccines, in *Vaccinations in the Developing Countries: Developments in Biological Standardization,* vol 41. Basel, Karger, 1978, pp 61–66

59 Mirchamsy H, Shafyi A, Mahinpour M, et al: Stabilizing effect of magnesium chloride and sucrose on Sabin live polio vaccine, in *Vaccinations in the Developing Countries: Developments in Biological Standardization,* vol 41. Basel, Karger, 1978, pp 255–257

60 Risi JB, Jr: The control of poliomyelitis in Brazil. Rev Infect Dis 6:(suppl 2):S400–S403, 1984

61 Patriarca PA, Palmeira G, Filho JL, et al: Randomized trial of alternative formulations of oral poliovaccine in Brazil. Lancet i:429–433, 1988

62 Fernandez de Castro PJ: Comments on the geographic distribution of poliomyelitis in the Americas: Notes for a program on continental eradication of poliomyelitis (Translation). Revista Salud Publica de Mexico, vol 26, no 3, May–June 1984

63 John TJ: Poliomyelitis in India: Prospects and problems of control. Rev Infect Dis 6(suppl 2):S438–S441, 1984

64 World Health Organization: Expanded programme on immunization: Contract system tested. Weekly Epidemiological Record 62:142–143, May 15, 1987

65 Lasch EE, Abed Y, Marcus O, et al: Combined live and inactivated poliovirus vaccine to control poliomyelitis in a developing country—five years after, in *IABS Congress on Use and Standardization of Combined Vaccines, Developments in Biological Standardization,* vol 65. Basel, Karger, 1986, pp 137–143

66 von Magnus H, Petersen I: Vaccination with inactivated poliovirus vaccine and oral poliovirus vaccine in Denmark. Rev Infect Dis 6(suppl 2):S471–S474.

Rotavirus · Jorge Flores · Albert Z. Kapikian

Rotaviruses are the most frequently detected agents to be associated with severe infantile diarrhea. They annually cause over 125 million diarrheal episodes, which result in the death of approximately 1 million infants and young children in the developing world. In addition, these agents are also a frequent cause of morbidity and hospitalization in industrialized nations. The discovery of rotaviruses a decade and a half ago initiated a new era in the study of infantile diarrhea. The development of various techniques during the last few years has enabled a rapid accumulation of knowledge on the molecular biology, immunology, and pathogenesis of rotavirus disease. In addition, and most important, such information has been directly applied to the development of vaccine candidates.

AGENT

MORPHOLOGY AND STRUCTURE

Rotaviruses have a very distinctive appearance by negative stain electron microscopy (Fig. 62-1). Their wheellike appearance (*rota* means wheel) is due to the distinctive double capsid which possesses a sharply demarcated outer margin, reminiscent of the rim of a wheel, surrounding spokelike structures [*1*]. Recently, image processing electron microscopy has revealed certain finer details of rotavirus morphology: (1) the icosahedral structure has a triangulation number of 13; (2) 60 spikes not previously detected radiate from the surface of the outer capsid; and (3) large channels open up on the surface of the outer shell and appear to connect it with the inner shell.

Single-shelled 55-nm particles have a higher density (1.38 g/mL) than double-shelled viruses (1.36 g/mL) by centrifu-

gation in cesium chloride gradients. The inner capsid of the single-shelled particle is formed by at least four proteins: VP1, VP2, VP3, and VP6. Two proteins, VP4 and VP7 (a glycoprotein), form the outer shell. A schematic representation of the gene coding assignments and the location and molecular weights of viral proteins in the virion is shown in Fig. 62-2.

GENETIC STRUCTURE AND ANTIGENIC PROPERTIES

The rotavirus genome consists of 11 segments of double-stranded RNA. The segments range in size from about 680 to 3500 base pairs. Each segment acts as a discrete gene encoding one protein. A characteristic migration pattern is observed when the isolated genetic material is electrophoresed in acrylamide or agarose gels. The functional assignment of various genes continues to arouse considerable interest because of implications for vaccine development. As seen in Fig. 62-2, the fourth gene encodes VP4 (formerly designated VP3), the trypsin-sensitive outer capsid protein. Cleavage of VP4 activates the virus, and the two resulting peptides (VP5* and VP8*) remain attached to the virion. Gene 7, 8, or 9 (depending on the strain) encodes the VP7 glycoprotein, also located on the virus surface. The sixth gene encodes VP6, which is present in the inner capsid and is the most abundant structural protein [*2*].

Figure 62-2 summarizes the important antigenic properties of rotaviruses: (1) A group antigen is present on VP6; this antigen is common to all group A rotavirus and permits distinction of group A from other recently discovered groups (B to F). (2) A subgroup antigen also resides in the VP6 protein; group A rotaviruses have been classified into two subgroups, 1 and 2. (3) Neutralization antigens are present on both the VP7 and the VP4 proteins. At least nine different rotavirus serotypes based on VP7 have been described by neutralization assays and at least two different VP4 neutralization specificities have been described for human rotaviruses. Passively administered monoclonal antibodies against either VP4 or VP7 have been shown to protect animals from a rotavirus challenge.

Rotaviruses appear to undergo genetic variation by two mechanisms: genetic shift (by means of gene reassortment) and genetic drift (through point mutations) (Fig. 62-3). Due to their segmented genomes, rotaviruses may undergo gene reassortment (''shuffling of genes'') when a cell is infected simultaneously by two different strains; reassortment events appear to be common and result in strains with mixed genotypes. Various reassortants with combined properties from two viruses which are phenotypically different have been prepared experimentally [*2*]. In this way, the genes that encode particular viral functions

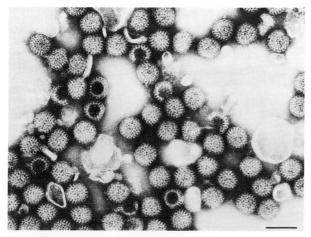

Figure 62-1. Negative stain electron microscopy.

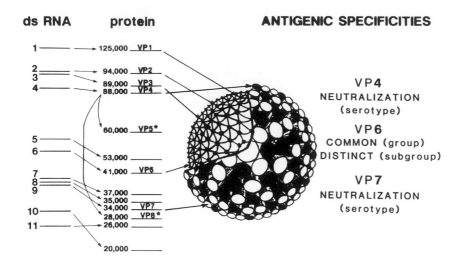

Figure 62-2. Rotavirus gene coding assignments.

unique to each parental strain have been identified. Figure 62-4 shows the genotype of a reassortant (strain 18-1) derived from coinfecting cells with a bovine virus (UK strain) and a human virus (Wa strain); in this reassortant only one gene segment is derived from the Wa parent. Since the neutralization specificity of this reassortant is similar to Wa, this phenotype can be assigned to the gene 9 product, the VP7 protein. This approach has also been used to recognize the functions of other genes.

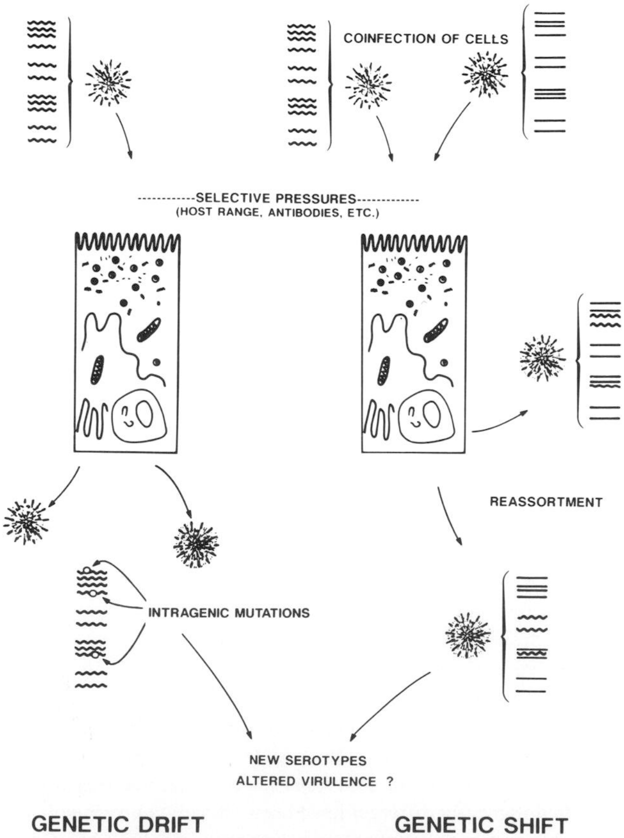

Although it is theoretically possible that rotavirus strains with many different combinations of subgroup VP4 serotype and VP7 serotype specificities could exist, it appears that a finite number of combinations currently circulate. For instance, the subgroup 1 specificity is uniformly associated with serotype 2 and with a specific VP4 serotype (no nomenclature has been agreed upon yet to design VP4 specificities). Most human rotaviruses are antigenically similar to the human prototype strains in their VP4, VP6, and VP7 specificities, suggesting the existence of gene linkages that select for particular gene combinations. Thus, human rotaviruses are classified into at least two genetic families: One, represented by prototype strain DS1, has a short electrophoretic migration pattern, belongs to subgroup 1, serotype 2 VP7, and has a specific VP4 gene. The other family, represented by prototype strain Wa, has a long electrophoretic migration pattern, belongs to subgroup 2, and has a VP4 shared by serotypes 1, 3, and 4 [3].

Gene sequencing studies alone or in combination with monoclonal antibody studies have allowed the detection of antigenic epitopes on both the VP4 and the VP7 proteins. Viruses belonging to different VP7 or VP4 serotypes exhibit a high degree of sequence divergence in discrete regions of their ninth and fourth gene respectively while the rest of the gene sequence is common to different serotypes. Furthermore, the sequence of the VP7 or VP4 genes from several strains of a given serotype is highly conserved. From these studies, it has been predicted that areas of high divergence in VP7 encode for neutralization specific epitopes; this has been confirmed by sequencing neutralization escape mutants selected with monoclonal antibodies to the VP7.

Studies on the molecular epidemiology of rotaviruses have revealed the existence of a considerable extent of genetic var-

Figure 62-3. Genetic variation in rotaviruses.

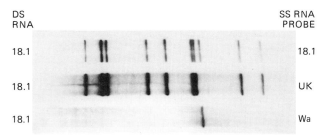

Figure 62-4. Genotype of a reassortant rotavirus as determined by RNA-RNA hybridization study.

iability as demonstrated by the marked polymorphism in the migration pattern of the viral RNA segments. Such variability has not yet been related to properties such as virulence, transmissibility, antigenic variation, etc. Analysis of gene sequences of rotaviruses belonging to the same serotype and isolated years apart from distant geographical locations as well as sequence analysis of strains from long-term nosocomial transmission studies suggest that the rotavirus genome is genetically more stable to drift mutations than influenza, polio, or other RNA viruses [4]. Indirectly, these observations suggest that the genetic polymorphism observed is the product of reassortment of a finite number of strains.

PATIENT "HOST"

IMMUNITY TO ROTAVIRUS

The presence of antibody in the intestinal lumen of animal models has been shown to play a major role in the prevention or control of rotavirus infection. Snodgrass et al. [5] have elegantly shown that rotavirus infection of newborn lambs is prevented if rotavirus antibody–containing colostrum is administered by the oral route concurrently with and several days after a rotavirus inoculum; however, if administration of colostral antibody precedes the inoculum by several hours, protection does not occur, since the antibodies in the colostrum enter the systemic circulation. However, because of marked differences in the local immune systems of animals and humans, it is difficult to extrapolate such data with certainty. In adult volunteers inoculated with a virulent rotavirus, circulating antibodies per se did not correlate with resistance to illness, but a level equal to or greater than 1:100 by plaque reduction neutralization afforded significant protection. Similarly, in Japan, Chiba et al. [6] showed that the presence of rotavirus-neutralizing antibody was not sufficient to protect children against homotypically induced illness, but a serum neutralization titer of at least 1:128 was associated with protection (Fig. 62-5).

While rotavirus infections occur at any time during infancy and early childhood, serum antibody responses are detected with greater consistency in infants over 6 months of age, a

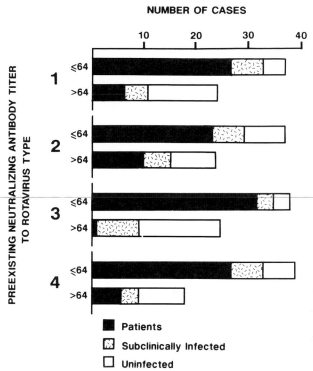

Figure 62-5. Relationship between rotavirus antibody levels and outcome of infections during a rotavirus serotype 3 outbreak. (*From* [6].)

time when the levels of maternally derived antibody are nil. Soon after infection, an IgM seroresponse is observed followed by both IgG and IgA responses. Antibody prevalence studies indicate that by the third year of life most individuals have acquired rotavirus antibody at levels comparable to those seen in adults; the latter are likely due to multiple reinfections, most of which are clinically silent [1].

A critical issue in the immunology of rotaviruses relates to the ability of natural rotavirus infection to confer either long-term (or even short-term) protection against reinfection or illness. Limited published data or anecdotal information suggests that characteristically only one severe diarrheal episode occurs during childhood. In most cases in which a second rotavirus illness has been documented, the two infecting viruses belonged to different serotypes, suggesting that homotypic immunity was important. However, recent vaccine studies have yielded conflicting information, since homotypic (via VP7) and heterotypic protection have been observed as well as failure to protect heterotypically (via VP7). Information on the potential role of VP4 in protective immunity is not yet available. Sequence data on the VP4 gene from several strains suggest that at least for human strains the number of different VP4 specificities is more limited than that of VP7. The relationship between the VP4s of the currently available vaccine candidates and those of human rotavirus strains is not known at present.

CLINICAL FEATURES

It is impossible to distinguish clinically a case of rotavirus gastroenteritis from those caused by other agents. Characteristically, after an incubation period of 2 to 3 days, children develop vomiting followed by profuse diarrhea which lasts longer than the vomiting; in many cases there is an abrupt onset which makes the parents seek medical attention. In a comparative study of children hospitalized in Washington, D.C., with either rotavirus or nonrotavirus diarrhea, 96 percent of the children with rotavirus had vomiting, 77 percent had fever, and 83 percent were dehydrated (Table 62-1). The mean duration of diarrhea or hospitalization was 5 days for both groups, with a range of 2- to 14-days hospitalization [7]. In most cases the resolution of the illness is rather benign, since the patients can be rehydrated within a few hours after admission.

Rotaviruses cause prolonged diarrhea in immunodeficient children, have been associated with severe and sometimes fatal diarrhea in adults and children receiving immunosuppressive therapy, and have been found in nurseries in association with neonatal hemorrhagic or necrotizing enterocolitis. The rotavirus literature contains case reports of single outbreaks of disease combining an unusual condition with naturally occurring rotavirus infections, such as Reye's syndrome, disseminated intravascular coagulation, exanthema subitum, sudden infant death syndrome, Kawasaki syndrome, and hepatic abscess.

A direct cause-effect relationship has not been established in any of these conditions, and most likely they were only coincidental.

DIAGNOSIS

Initially the direct electron-microscopic (EM) observation of diarrheal stools was the only method available for rotavirus detection. The distinctive morphology of the virus along with particle-rich stools observed during the acute phase enabled rapid, sensitive, and specific diagnosis by EM. The sensitivity of EM diagnosis may be further enhanced by centrifugation of stool preparations or by using immune electron microscopy (IEM). In addition, the EM may serve as the ''supreme court'' of rotavirus diagnosis when uncertain results are obtained in other assays.

More practical methods for diagnosis of rotavirus directly in stools are based on their recognition by specific antibody in enzyme-linked immunosorbent assays (ELISA) or agglutination tests. An array of ELISA variations has been described, and many of these are available commercially. What is most critical in this kind of assay (the sensitivity of which is adequate in most cases and superior to electron microscopy in some) is the need for either a blocking reaction or a confirmatory test, since false-positive reactions may occur. Enzyme immunoassays are particularly suitable when large numbers of samples are to be tested. Immunoassays are also available for

Table 62-1. Clinical characteristics of 150 children hospitalized with acute gastroenteritis

	Percent having each clinical finding	
Clinical finding	Rotavirus infection detected (72 patients)	Rotavirus infection not detected (78 patients)
Vomiting	96*	58*
Fever		
37.9–39°C	46	29
> 39°C	31	33
Total	77	61
Dehydration	83†	40†
Hypertonic	5	16
Isotonic	95	77
Hypotonic	0	6
Irritability	47	40
Lethargy	36	27
Pharyngeal erythema	49	32
Tonsillar exudate	3	3
Rhinitis	26	22
Red tympanic membrane with loss of landmarks	19	9
Rhonchi or wheezing	8	8
Palpable cervical lymph nodes	18	9

*$p < .01$ (two children not included).
†$p < .01$.

Source: From [7].

Table 62-2. Comparison of different methods for rotavirus diagnosis

Method	Sensitivity	Specificity	Practicality	Added advantages
Electron microscopy	+ + +	+ + + +	+	Fast, allows detection of non-group A rotaviruses
ELISA (confirmatory)	+ + + +	+ + + +	+ + +	Low cost, suitable for testing many samples simultaneously
Latex	+ +	+	+ + + +	Fast, simple to use, no need for any equipment
PAGE	+ +	+ + + +	+ +	RNA pattern is obtained, allows recognition of non-group A rotavirus
RNA hybridization	+ + + +	+ + +	+	Would allow recognition of specific sequences related to serotype, virulence, etc.

subgrouping and serotyping rotaviruses directly from stool specimens.

The latex agglutination test may be quite practical for bedside diagnosis; however, its sensitivity and specificity are lower than the confirmatory ELISA.

The enhanced sensitivity and specificity of assays that recognize the viral RNA by hybridization may be useful when only very small amounts of virus are shed. However, their application is limited to research laboratories because of the need for radioactive isotopes. A potential advantage of these assays is their ability to recognize discrete areas of the genome associated with known properties (for instance, serotype-specific sequences in the VP7 or VP4 genes). Substitution of the isotopic labeling by biotin or covalently linked enzymes might enable more widespread use of hybridization methods.

Table 62-2 compares these four approaches. Many other tests, most of which are variations on the four described above, have been developed for rotavirus diagnosis. The choice of a given method will finally depend on the specific needs and resources of the particular laboratory.

Tests have also been developed to investigate serological responses to rotavirus infections. Among them, the complement fixation (CF), ELISA, and immunoadherence tests are relatively easy to perform. Neutralization tests are important in determining the responses to specific rotavirus serotypes, but such assays are limited to research laboratories.

TREATMENT

Treatment of acute dehydrating diarrhea consists of prompt replacement of fluid and electrolyte loss and correction of acidosis, if present. Until recently, the standard therapy was intravenous fluid administration. However, oral rehydration, which is less costly, more practical, and requires only minimal training, has been replacing intravenous fluid administration in most settings. The efficacy of oral rehydration has been demonstrated in many studies. Figure 62-6 illustrates the rapidness with which rehydration was achieved in a group of 48 infants with rotavirus diarrhea in a study in Caracas. A positive fluid balance was reached promptly, and in over 90 percent of the infants the dehydration was corrected within 6 h after admission. Field studies in Egypt and Bangladesh have shown the

potential impact of oral rehydration therapy in decreasing mortality from diarrheal diseases.

The administration of human γ-globulin, human milk, and cow colostrum containing high titers of neutralizing antibody to rotavirus can be of prophylactic use in preventing symptomatic infection or diminishing the serious consequences of the disease in low-birth-weight human neonates and immunocompromised hosts. Conflicting evidence has been presented for a protective role of breast-feeding against rotavirus illness. Both breast-fed and not-breast-fed children develop illnesses at similar rates, although in at least one study the illness appeared to be milder in breast-fed babies.

POPULATION

EPIDEMIOLOGY

Shortly after their discovery in Australia [8], rotaviruses were found to be associated with severe infantile diarrhea in most

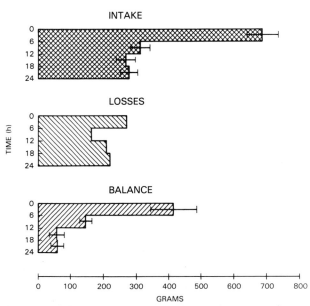

Figure 62-6. Effectiveness of oral rehydration therapy in children dehydrated by rotavirus gastroenteritis.

parts of the world, from the Far East to South America to northern Europe; at this time there is not one study of infantile diarrhea in which rotavirus has not been incriminated as a major etiological agent [1]. Rotavirus infections have been usually associated with 35 to 50 percent of the hospital admissions for diarrhea in children under 2 years of age. For instance, in long-term studies of diarrheal etiology in children admitted to hospitals in Washington, D.C., [9] (Fig. 62-7) and in Yamagata City, Japan [10], 35 and 45 percent of the patients, respectively, had rotavirus in their stool. In a prospective rotavirus vaccine study in Finland, 20 percent of infants under 6 months of age developed rotavirus illness during a single season, and 50 percent became infected. In investigations of diarrhea admissions at a treatment center in Bangladesh in which over 6000 individuals were studied, 46 percent of those under 2 years of age had rotavirus [11].

Areas with widely different levels of sanitation share similar rotavirus diarrheal incidence figures, suggesting that potable drinking water and adequate sewage may not have a major impact on the occurrence of rotavirus infections. This contrasts with the decrease in incidence of enteropathogenic bacteria and parasites that follows improvements in sanitary conditions.

Rotaviruses appear almost exclusively during the colder months of the year in countries where marked seasonal variations occur; in tropical countries they occur year-round. The most common risk factors for developing illness are age and perhaps, though this is not proven, the lack of a previous exposure. In developed countries most rotavirus episodes tend to occur after the age of 6 months, usually peaking between 9 and 15 months; in contrast, in developing countries, rotavirus illness is also commonly observed in children under 6 months

of age. The factors that may be responsible for this difference are not known. Suggestions include an increased environmental load of virus, the nutritional status of children, and hygienic habits. Since exposure to rotavirus infection extends over a longer period of the year in the developing countries, infants under 6 months are at greater risk of becoming infected. These differences, while not fully explained, are relevant to vaccination strategies.

Serological studies of adults in contact with rotavirus-positive infants have shown a high rate of asymptomatic reinfections. Although the frequency of asymptomatic infections in infants and young children has not been studied thoroughly, it is assumed that such infections occur often. Newborn infants in selected nurseries in several countries shed rotaviruses frequently but without, or with only mild, symptoms in most cases. Genetic studies of rotavirus strains isolated from such newborn infants suggest that the apparently low virulence and ease of transmission of the virus are properties that reside in the fourth gene segment [12]. Such "nursery" strains are of considerable interest because at least for one strain, neonatal infection resulted in protection against rotavirus illness later in life [13]. The four epidemiologically important VP7 serotypes have been isolated from asymptomatic newborns. Efforts are underway to test one of these serotypes in humans to determine if it retains its avirulent character and thus might be considered as a candidate for vaccine.

While the epidemiology of rotavirus serotypes could not be studied until recently, extensive analysis of the RNA migration patterns were carried out previously. In general, a limited number of rotavirus "electropherotypes" is observed at the beginning of the rotavirus season with the number of different pat-

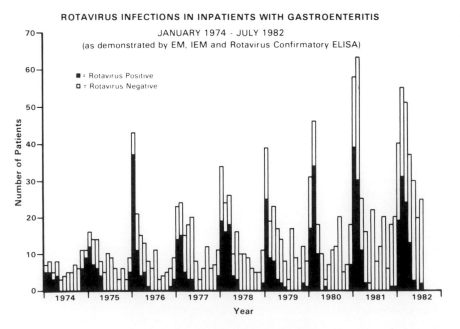

ROTAVIRUS INFECTIONS IN INPATIENTS WITH GASTROENTERITIS

JANUARY 1974 - JULY 1982
(as demonstrated by EM, IEM and Rotavirus Confirmatory ELISA)

■ = Rotavirus Positive
□ = Rotavirus Negative

Figure 62-7. Rotavirus infections in hospitalized patients with gastroenteritis. (*From* [9].)

Table 62-3. Relative frequency of rotavirus serotypes 1, 2, 3, and 4 in infants with gastroenteritis

No. tested	No. typed	Percent				Method of testing	Location, year
		Type 1	Type 2	Type 3	Type 4		
16	13	54	30	15	0	Fluorescent foci neutralization	Kenya, 1982–1983
30	30	56	7	NT	36	Solid phase IEM	Italy, 1981–1983
56	39	67	3	8	23	ELISA	Japan, 1981–1986
552	314	51	26	19	4	ELISA	Australia, 1975–1986
14	14	7	71	21	0	ELISA	China, 1982–1984
80	72	75	0	0	25	ELISA	Australia, 1983–1984
51	30	50	30	3	17	ELISA	Brazil
140	111	70	16	14	NT	ELISA	Bangui, 1983–1985
134	109	48	17	22	14	ELISA	Venezuela, 1981–1983

Note: NT = Not tested.

terns increasing gradually, suggesting either the entry of other strains or reassortment events between cocirculating strains. In developing countries where rotaviruses are present throughout the year, an even more marked degree of genetic polymorphism has been observed. While a particular pattern cannot provide more information than perhaps tracking chronologically or geographically the routes of transmission, one pattern has been associated with serotype 2 and subgroup 1 antigenic specificities, namely, the so-called short rotaviruses in which the migration of gene segments 10 and 11 is delayed with respect to that of the corresponding genes of most strains.

The recent development of solid phase serotyping assays will have an impact on prospective studies of the prevalence and virulence of different serotypes, and of the factors that may determine changes in their prevalence [14]. Such studies are of considerable importance in designing rotavirus vaccines. Table 62-3 presents a summary from different studies, mostly retrospective, of the association of VP7 serotypes 1 to 4 with human disease. Serotype 1 has been identified most frequently, followed by serotype 2. Serotypes 3 and 4 occur less often, but in certain time periods they predominate. The two recently described human rotavirus serotypes (8 and 9) have not been evaluated as extensively as serotypes 1 to 4. In Australia, the distribution of rotavirus serotypes 1 to 4 was investigated retrospectively in rotavirus specimens collected over a period of 11 years (Fig. 62-8). From these data it would appear that specific serotypes predominate in a given season rather than being uniformly distributed [15].

The ELISA typing assays are currently limited to VP7 serotypes, but since VP4-neutralizing monoclonal antibodies are now available, it is likely that serotyping tests will soon be expanded to assay for VP4 as well.

Rotaviruses have been detected in the stools of many animal species in association with diarrhea. Although some animal

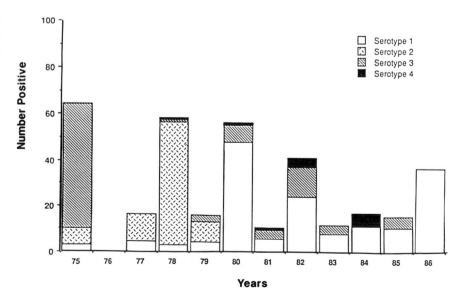

Figure 62-8. Distribution of rotavirus serotypes in a study of diarrheal illness in infants and young children in Australia. (*From [15].*)

strains share serotype specificity with human rotaviruses, transmission from the animal to the human host or vice versa has not been documented.

PREVENTION AND VACCINE DEVELOPMENT

While holistic approaches are necessary to improve the general quality of life and ameliorate the consequences of the diarrheal syndrome caused by rotaviruses and other agents, such improvements may not be totally adequate in the case of rotavirus infections since even in highly industrialized countries rotaviruses are an important cause of severe diarrheal disease. Specific interventions such as the use of oral rehydration solutions therapy at home are of extreme importance. However, parallel development of rotavirus vaccines is also essential since it should result in decreased morbidity and may ultimately result in diminished morbidity and mortality.

Table 62-4 summarizes a number of approaches currently being considered for the development of rotavirus vaccines. To date only the Jennerian and modified Jennerian approaches have undergone clinical evaluation [16]. The possibility that animal rotaviruses might induce attenuated, yet immunologically related infections in humans was initially suggested by observations that human rotavirus antibody reacted in CF as-

Table 62-4. Strategies for the development of rotavirus vaccines

The Jennerian approach
  Bovine rotavirus strains RIT 4237 UK WC 3
  Simian rotavirus strain MMU 18006 (RRV)
The modified Jennerian approach
  Rotavirus reassortants between human and animal strains
    RRV carrying VP7 gene from human rotavirus serotype 1, 2, or 4
    UK carrying VP7 gene from human rotavirus 1, 2, 3, or 4
    Other human or animal rotavirus reassortants with different gene combinations
Attenuated human rotavirus strains
  Attenuated by
    Cold adaptation
    Multiple passages in tissue culture
    Passage in heterologous hosts
  Naturally attenuated neonatal strains
    Serotype 1 M 37
    Serotype 2 1076
    Serotype 3 McN 13
    Serotype 4 ST 3
  Reassortants between different human strains
    VP7 gene from serotype 1, 2, 3, or 4 and 10 genes from neonatal strain
    VP7 gene from serotype 2 strain with 10 genes from cold-adapted rotavirus from serotype 1-3-4 family
Recombinant DNA technology
  Expression of VP7 and/or VP4 through recombination with adenovirus

says with animal rotavirus strains [17]. Further studies in pregnant cows demonstrated that the diarrheal illness caused by challenging newborn calves with the human strain Wa (a serotype 1 rotavirus) could be prevented by prior intrauterine inoculation with the bovine strain NCDV (a serotype 6 rotavirus) a few weeks before parturition [18]. The mechanism of protection is not known since Wa and NCDV present different serotype specificities when studied in tissue culture; however, most calves developed neutralizing antibodies to heterotypic rotavirus serotypes 1, 2, and 3. The possibility that "in vivo" infection with NCDV could induce protection against human rotaviruses in infants and young children was explored by the RIT Division of Smith, Kline & French. A cold-adapted high tissue culture passage of NCDV (RIT 4237) was evaluated in studies by Vesikari et al. [19]. Initially, very promising results were observed when over 80 percent protection against clinically significant diarrhea was found in children over the age of 6 months following vaccination. Further studies demonstrated that the vaccine (a serotype 6 strain) had induced protection against diarrhea caused by human rotavirus serotype 1. Unfortunately, when tested in younger infants in developing countries, the vaccine failed or was less effective in inducing protection [20]. It is possible that the strain is overattenuated for humans and may be unfavorably interfered with by enteroviruses commonly present in the intestine of infants of developing countries, or neutralized by the high levels of preexisting antibodies usually detected in the very young.

Another bovine rotavirus vaccine candidate (WC3) developed by the Wistar Institute (Philadelphia, PA) is being evaluated. Preliminary studies in 6- to 12-month infants showed this vaccine to be safe, immunogenic, and effective in preventing rotavirus diarrhea caused by serotype 1 rotavirus [21].

The rhesus rotavirus vaccine MMU 18006 developed at the National Institutes of Health (Bethesda, Maryland) has a few advantages: (1) it belongs to serotype 3, which has been isolated commonly from infants with diarrhea; and (2) it is more immunogenic (albeit more reactogenic) than the RIT 4237 vaccine. The RRV vaccine has been tested extensively in different clinical settings, in developed as well as in developing countries. At the dose employed in most of the studies (10^4 PFU), it is able to induce a seroresponse measurable by either neutralization assays or ELISA IgA in about 80 percent of the infants [22]. At this same dose, variable reactogenicity has been observed in different studies. In studies in Finland, Sweden, and Baltimore, up to one-third of the infants develop a transient febrile response lasting 1 to 2 days and in most cases not higher than 38.5°C; in addition 20 to 30 percent of the vaccinees develop loose stools, which usually last 1 day [22]. Lesser reactions have been observed using the same dose in studies in Venezuela, where vaccine has also been administered to newborn infants.

A phase II efficacy study conducted in Venezuela revealed an overall efficacy level of 68 percent in infants vaccinated at 1 to 10 months of age [23]. The level of protection against the

Table 62-5. Protective efficacy of rhesus rotavirus vaccine against rotavirus diarrhea according to the severity of diarrheal illness

Severity score of rotavirus diarrheal illness	No. of cases with indicated severity		% efficacy	Significance p*
	Controls $N = 124$	Vaccinees $N = 123$		
7 or more	9	2	77	.035
8 or more	7	1	86	.035
9 or more	6	0	100	.014
10 or more	5	0	100	.025

*By χ^2 analysis.

Note: 16 episodes of rotavirus diarrhea were observed in the 124 controls and 5 in the 123 vaccinees (68% efficacy; $p = .013$).
Source: From [23].

most severe episodes was higher. Furthermore, in the 1- to 4-month-old group the efficacy level reached 100 percent (Table 62-5). These promising results contrasted with parallel field trials of the RRV vaccine in Rochester and in an Indian reservation in Arizona. Although the same protocols and vaccine doses were used, no differences in the rate and severity of rotavirus diarrhea were detected between control and placebo groups. However, analysis of the rotavirus serotypes prevalent during these studies indicated that in the Venezuela study serotype 3 strains were prevalent, whereas in Rochester and Arizona other serotypes were predominant, suggesting that the vaccine was unable to induce protection against heterotypic (predominantly serotype 1) strains. Vaccine trials not yet completed in Finland and Sweden, on the other hand, suggest that varying grades of protection were induced by the vaccine against the serotype 1 strain; in these studies, however, older infants were tested, and it is possible that some of them had been primed by previous exposure to rotavirus. Thus, a rational explanation for such inconsistency appears to be the ability of the vaccine to induce homotypic but not heterotypic protection.

It thus appears that there is a need for a polyvalent vaccine corresponding to the four common human rotavirus serotypes. Studies with a quadrivalent preparation composed of RRV vaccine and three RRVx human rotavirus reassortants are currently being carried out. Single-gene substitution serotype 1, 2, and 4 reassortants carrying the VP7 gene of human rotaviruses D, DS1, and ST3 (VP7 serotypes 1, 2, and 4, respectively) and 10 genes from the RRV vaccine have been derived [24]. The individual reassortants have already been tested in infants for reactogenicity and antigenicity, and the results have warranted continuation with phase II efficacy studies which are currently being conducted in Rochester, Finland, and Peru. Ideally a quadrivalent vaccine comprising the three reassortants mentioned above plus the RRV vaccine itself could afford broad protection. Such a possibility is being tested in several studies. Phase I studies in Venezuela indicate that this quadrivalent combination does not induce unacceptable reactogenicity. Currently its immunogenicity is being evaluated.

Non-Jennerian alternative approaches to vaccine development are also being explored. The use of strains derived from human neonates is currently being subjected to clinical evaluation. Molecular engineering approaches include the production of rotavirus antigens by recombination of the corresponding genes with bacterial or viral expression vectors and evaluation of the potential antigenicity of synthetic peptides.

REFERENCES

1 Kapikian AZ, Chanock RM: Rotavirus, in Fields BN et al (eds): *Virology.* New York, Raven, 1985b, pp 863–906

2 Greenberg HB, Flores J, Kalica AR, et al: Gene coding assignments for growth restriction neutralization and subgroup specificities of the W and DS-1 strains of human rotavirus. J Gen Virol 64:313–320, 1983

3 Flores J, Perez I, White L, et al: Genetic relatedness among human rotaviruses as determined by RNA hybridization. Infect Immun 37:648–655, 1982

4 Flores J, Sears J, Green KY, et al: Genetic stability of rotaviruses recovered from asymptomatic neonatal infections. J Virol 12:4778–4781, 1988

5 Snodgrass DR, Wells PW: Passive immunity in rotaviral infections. J Am Vet Med Assoc 173:565–568, 1978

6 Chiba S, Yokoyama T, Nakata S, et al: Protective effect of naturally acquired homotypic and heterotypic rotavirus antibodies. Lancet ii:417–421, 1986

7 Rodriguez WJ, Kim HW, Brandt CD, et al: Rotavirus gastroenteritis in the Washington, D.C., area. Am J Dis Child 134:777–779, 1980

8 Bishop RF, Davidson GP, Holmes IH, et al: Virus particles in epithelial cells of duodenal mucosa from children with acute gastroenteritis. Lancet ii:1281–1283, 1973

9 Brandt CD, Kim HW, Rodriguez WJ, et al: Pediatric viral gastroenteritis during eight years of study. J Clin Microbiol 18:71–78, 1983

10 Konno T, Suzuki H, Imai A, et al: A long term survey of rotavirus infection in Japanese children with acute gastroenteritis. J Infect Dis 138:569–576, 1978

11 Black RE, Merson MH, Mizanur R, et al: A 2 year study of bacterial, viral, and parasitic agents associated with diarrhea in rural Bangladesh. J Infect Dis 142:660–664, 1980

12 Flores J, Midthun K, Hoshino Y, et al: Conservation of the fourth gene among rotaviruses recovered from asymptomatic newborn infants and its possible role in attenuation. J Virol 60:972–979, 1986

13 Bishop RF, Barnes GL, Cipriani E, et al: Clinical immunity after neonatal rotavirus infection: A prospective longitudinal study in young children. N Engl J Med 309:72–76, 1983

14 Taniguchi K, Urasawa S, Morita HB, et al: Direct serotyping of human rotavirus in stools by an enzyme-linked immunosorbent assay using serotype 1-, 2-, 3-, and 4-specific monoclonal antibodies to VP7. J Infect Dis 155:1159–1166, 1987

15 Birch CJ, Health RL, Gust ID: Use of serotype-specific monoclonal antibodies to study the epidemiology of rotavirus infection. J Med Virol 24:45–53, 1988

16 Kapikian AZ, Cline WL, Mebus CA, et al: New complement-fixation test for the human reovirus-like agent of infantile gastroenteritis: Nebraska calf diarrhea virus used as antigen. Lancet i:1056–1069, 1975

17 Kapikian AZ, Flores J, Hoshino Y, et al: Rotavirus: the major etiologic agent of severe infantile diarrhea may be controllable by a "Jennerian" approach to vaccination. J Infect Dis 153:815–822, 1986

18 Wyatt RG, Mebus CA, Yolken RH, et al: Rotaviral immunity in gnotobiotic calves: Heterologous resistance to human virus induced by bovine virus. Science 203:548–550, 1975

19 Vesikari T, Isolauri E, Delem A, et al: Clinical efficacy of the RIT 4237 live attenuated bovine rotavirus vaccine in infants vaccinated before a rotavirus epidemic. J Pediatr 107:189–194, 1985

20 DeMol P, Zissis G, Butzler JP, et al: Failure of live, attenuated oral rotavirus vaccine. Lancet ii:108, 1986

21 Clark HF, Borian FE, Bell LM: Protective effect of WC3 vaccine against rotavirus diarrhea in infants during a predominantly serotype 1 rotavirus season. J Infect Dis 158:570–587, 1988

22 Kapikian AZ, Flores J, Midthun K, et al: Development of a rotavirus vaccine by a "Jennerian" and a modified "Jennerian" approach, in Chanock RM, Lerner R (eds): Vaccines 1988. Cold Spring Harbor Laboratory, 1988

23 Flores J, Perez-Schael I, Gonzalez M, et al: Protection against severe rotavirus diarrhoea by rhesus rotavirus vaccine in Venezuelan children. Lancet i:882–884, 1987

24 Midthun K, Greenberg HB, Hoshino Y, et al: Reassortant rotaviruses as potential live rotavirus vaccine candidates. J Virol 53:949–954, 1985

CHAPTER 63 / *Hepatitis A and B* · Ian D. Gust

HEPATITIS A

Hepatitis A is an ancient and ubiquitous disease of humans. Although it has proved possible to transmit infection to various primates, there is no convincing evidence that natural infection occurs in the wild.

VIRUS

Morphology and ultrastructure

The disease is caused by a virus whose physical and biochemical characteristics are similar to members of the enterovirus group. Hepatitis A virus (HAV) has icosahedral symmetry, measures from 27 to 32 nm, and is made up of 32 apparently identical capsomers (see Fig. 63-1). Studies on the buoyant density of HAV have produced variable findings [1]. The simplest explanation is to assume that, as with other picornaviruses, three different virion structures are present: intact or mature particles with a buoyant density of 1.33 to 1.34 g/cm^3, empty particles with a buoyant density of 1.29 to 1.31 g/cm^3, and superdense particles with a buoyant density of 1.40 to 1.48 g/cm^3. Sedimentation analysis of HAV has also revealed three populations of particles with sedimentation coefficients

of 230 S, 160 S, and 50 to 90 S, which is consistent with the existence of three alternative virion structures.

Analysis of radiolabeled HAV has shown that the virus has four structural proteins with molecular weights of 33,000 (VP1), 26,500 (VP2), 22,500 (VP3), and 7000 (VP4).

Provost et al. [2] were first to postulate that the genetic material of HAV was RNA, because of the intracytoplasmic location of virus particles in infected marmoset liver cells, the pattern of staining with acridine orange, and the reduction of infectivity by treatment with RNase. Bradley et al. [3] provided further indirect evidence by demonstrating that, after pretreatment at alkaline pH, the sedimentation rate of the virus could be affected by treatment with RNase but not DNase.

Siegl and Frosner [4] extracted the nucleic acid released from HAV and demonstrated that it was sensitive to alkaline hydrolysis. Final proof was obtained by Coulepis et al. [5], who radiolabeled nucleic acid released from purified HAV and found that it was composed of a single piece of single-stranded RNA (ssRNA) with a sedimentation coefficient of 33 S, a buoyant density of 1.64 g/cm^3, and a molecular weight of 2.24×10^6. Further analysis of the genome revealed the presence of polyadenylic acid sequences.

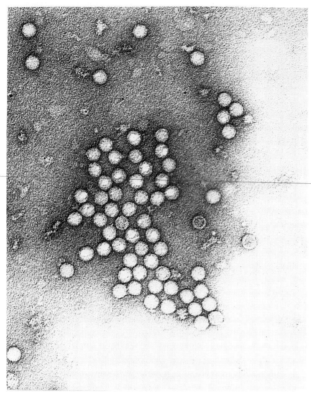

Figure 63-1. Electron micrograph of hepatitis A virus purified from the feces of a patient with acute hepatitis A. (*Courtesy of Dr. John Marshall.*)

The number and molecular weights of the virion polypeptides, together with evidence that the genome is ssRNA and is acid- and ether-stable, indicates that HAV is a picornavirus. The essential property of picornaviruses, the infectivity of genomic RNA, has also recently been demonstrated [6]. HAV has a number of unusual features, however, such as heat stability, a high degree of secondary structure of its genome, and the ability to establish persistent, nonlytic infections. These features, together with some aspects of its molecular biology (little nucleotide homology, distinct cleavage sites, and smaller VP4), suggest that HAV belongs in a separate genus.

In vitro cultivation

Isolation of HAV in cell culture was first reported in 1979 by Provost and Hilleman, who used a strain of virus, CR.326, which had been passaged five times in *Saguinus mystax* and 26 times in *Saguinus labiatus* marmosets, then inoculated into a cloned line of fetal rhesus monkey kidney cells [7]. Viral antigen could be detected in the cytoplasm of infected cells within 3 days of inoculation and increased in titer for 3 to 4 weeks. On passage the titer of antigen increased and the time

taken for peak levels to be achieved declined. While the virus was largely cell-associated, significant amounts appeared in the supernatant fluid and passages could be made with both cell lysate or supernatant fluid. Cell culture–derived virus retained the ability to infect marmosets and produce disease. At higher passage levels, the ability to produce disease was diminished. This group has now adapted CR.326 to growth in other cell lines, including diploid fibroblasts, and has succeeded in isolating HAV directly from fecal specimens.

In recent years several other groups have succeeded in isolating strains of HAV in cell culture. Daemer et al. [8] reported the isolation of an Australian strain, HM.175, in primary African green monkey kidney cells. Repeated passage of HM.175 also appears to result in a reduced capacity of the virus to produce disease in marmosets or chimpanzees. Additional strains have been isolated in FRhK-4, a hepatoma cell line known to be chronically infected with hepatitis B virus (HBV), in a variety of cells of monkey kidney origin and in diploid human fibroblasts. The optimal conditions for adaptation of virus to cell culture and for obtaining high yields of virus remain to be determined.

Replicative cycle

This is a little studied area, except for the work of Locarnini et al., who have compared the effects of HAV and poliovirus in Vero cells [6]. They found that while poliovirus rapidly inhibits protein synthesis in host cells, HAV does not. At least 11 viral-coded proteins were detected in HAV-infected cells, with molecular masses of 160, 110, 70, 51, 42, 39, 34, 29, 26, 24, and 14 kilodaltons. Peak levels of incorporation of labeled amino acids occurred within the 3- to 6-h postinfection period, and while incorporation was still taking place 48 h later, it was at a much reduced rate.

Infected Vero cells were also studied for evidence of synthesis of viral RNA. Whereas poliovirus nucleic acid formed a sharp peak at 35 S, HAV nucleic acid was found in a broad band from 30 to 37 S. Both zones were sensitive to RNase, but not to DNase. In poliovirus- and HAV-infected cells, a second peak of radioactivity with a sedimentation coefficient of 22 to 28 S was detected. These peaks were RNase-resistant and probably represent the double-stranded replicative form of the virus.

While the Vero cell system offers important insights into the mode of replication of HAV and a model for studying factors involved in replication, additional studies are required in cells such as AGMK or BGMK in which the virus has been shown to grow readily.

Animal models

A number of species of monkeys has been tested for susceptibility to infection with HAV, of which chimpanzees, owl monkeys, stump-tailed monkeys, and marmosets have proved to be useful models of the infection in humans [9].

Seronegative juvenile chimpanzees can be infected with HAV either by introducing the virus via a nasogastric tube or injecting it intravenously. Infected animals fail to develop clinical symptoms; however, after an incubation period of 3 to 4 weeks, they develop biochemical evidence of hepatitis. Hepatitis A antigen (HAAg) can be detected in the feces about 1 week prior to the development of hepatitis, with increases in titer for several days, then declines to undetectable levels over the next week. The average length of fecal shedding is about 7 days (range of 2 to 15 days).

Viral antigen can be detected in the cytoplasm of infected liver cells up to 10 days prior to the onset of abnormalities in liver function and may persist for weeks or months after the cells return to normal. Specific antibody usually appears early in the illness and rises rapidly, reaching peak titers 4 to 6 weeks later. Experimentally infected animals appear to be refractory when challenged with the same or other strains of HAV. Because chimpanzees are expensive and in relatively short supply, they have a limited role to play in studies of hepatitis A although they will clearly be important in the testing of vaccines.

Because of their more convenient size, shorter gestation period, greater availability, and lower cost, marmosets of the *Saguinus, Callithrix,* and *Rufiventer* genera have been widely used. The pattern of infection is similar to that described in chimpanzees. Marmosets have been extensively used to define the physical characteristics of HAV, to search for strain differences, to test tissue culture–derived strains for infectivity and virulence, and to study the pathogenesis of the disease.

There are many gaps in our knowledge of the pathogenesis of hepatitis A. From epidemiological investigations and human volunteer studies, it appears that patients are most infectious late in the incubation period and that the principal mode of spread is fecal-oral. By analogy with other enteroviruses, it is assumed that the primary site of replication is in the gastrointestinal tract. Some support has been given to this theory by the detection of hepatitis A–specific IgA in the feces of patients during the acute phase of the disease [10]. Experimental studies in chimpanzees and marmosets have, however, consistently failed to detect evidence of replication in the gut [11,12], although HAAg has been regularly detected in the liver and bile, and occasionally in the germinal centers of the spleen, abdominal lymph nodes, and the glomeruli.

Intermediate hosts or reservoirs

Despite their susceptibility to infection in the laboratory, there is no good evidence that monkeys provide a natural reservoir of infection. HAV has not been isolated from wild animals until some weeks after their capture, and the prevalence of antibody among jungle-caught animals appears to be related to the duration of captivity.

Apparently specific anti-HAV has been detected in the sera of several domestic dogs living in villages on the Pacific islands of Efate and Rarotonga [13]. Since dogs play a role in the disposal of human feces, it is possible that they occasionally become infected and spread the virus to susceptible children with whom they are in close contact. Alternatively the antibody which has been detected may be directed against a cross-reacting canine virus. Clearly the possibility of animal reservoirs of infection has not been adequately explored and requires further study.

PATIENT

Host-parasite relationship

Serological surveys indicate that in most communities from 75 to 100 percent of subjects over the age of 50 years have serological evidence of infection, yet relatively few can recall a previous episode of hepatitis or jaundice. Clearly infection must often occur without any obvious clinical signs. The frequency of subclinical infection has been estimated during epidemics by looking for evidence of biochemical abnormalities in persons without jaundice. Although such calculations omit subjects in whom the infection is completely silent, the ratio of anicteric to icteric cases may be as high as 12:1, with the highest ratios being observed in children [14]. Anicteric subjects may be completely symptomless or may have mild influenzalike symptoms with fever, anorexia, nausea, fatigue, and upper abdominal tenderness. Such people are infectious, and because they are unrecognized, they probably play an important role in spread of the virus.

The outcome of infection with HAV seems to depend upon the age at which infection occurs and perhaps upon the infecting dose. Studies in marmosets have shown a linear relationship between the infecting dose and the incubation period of the disease. As the clinical-subclinical ratio varies from outbreak to outbreak, other as yet unidentified factors such as susceptibility to infection and strain of virus may be involved.

HAV infection may occasionally cause acute fulminating disease. Because serological testing has only been available for a few years, it is difficult to get a precise estimate of its prevalence. During epidemics the frequency of fulminant hepatitis varies from 1 per 100 to 1 per 1000 patients with clinical disease. Among hospital patients with sporadic hepatitis A, the figures vary from 1 to 8 per 1000. A higher frequency has been reported in pregnant women in Asia and the Middle East, but these cases have not been serologically confirmed. Studies from Europe and the United States have not shown an association with pregnancy [14]. The factors which determine why some people develop fulminant disease are unknown.

Clinical manifestations

The infection is frequently mild especially among children. In adolescents and adults it is usually associated with symptoms such as loss of appetite, a loss of interest in cigarettes, nausea, and occasionally vomiting or diarrhea. Upper abdominal discomfort or pain under the right costal margin may also occur. These symptoms are often associated with a fever of up to 38.5°C and are followed after days or weeks by the onset of dark urine and jaundice. The course of the disease is variable. The general symptoms tend to disappear at the time that jaundice appears, while gastrointestinal symptoms become more severe for a week or so. Over the ensuing 3 to 4 weeks the patient's jaundice fades, the liver and spleen return to normal size, and the patient's appetite returns. A full recovery is usual, and long-term sequelae are unknown. A few patients have a relapse of symptoms within 2 months of the illness, usually associated with increased alcohol intake or violent exercise. Relapses are usually followed by a complete recovery.

Diagnosis

A clinical diagnosis can usually be made on the basis of the patient's history and clinical findings supported by liver function tests. The characteristic feature of patients with viral hepatitis is marked elevation of serum aspartate and alanine aminotransferase (AST, ALT) levels. Measurement of alkaline phosphatase may be useful in differentiating hepatitis from obstructive jaundice, as low levels are unusual in the latter condition.

Leukopenia is common in the early stage of hepatitis and atypical lymphocytes may be seen in up to 25 percent of cases. Confusion may occur with glandular fever; however, in this case the Paul-Bunnell test is usually positive. In many tropical regions the disease may be confused with leptospirosis, although the latter condition is usually associated with leukocytosis, muscle pain, reddened conjunctivas, and a petechial rash.

In recent years laboratory tests have been developed which can assist a clinician in establishing the diagnosis of hepatitis. These tests, originally restricted to research laboratories, are now available commercially but are not widely used in tropical areas because they are relatively expensive. In many regions of the world, these assays are available through a network of WHO Collaborating Centers for Viral Hepatitis.[1] Of the tests currently available, three are of particular value: the detection of HAAg in patient's feces, the detection of rising titers of anti-HAV, and the detection of hepatitis A–specific IgM (see Fig. 63-2).

Detection of virus particles or specific viral antigens in the feces confirms that a patient is infected with HAV, but since peak shedding of virus occurs during the late incubation period, the process may be over by the time the patient seeks attention. HAV can be detected in the feces of about 45 percent of pa-

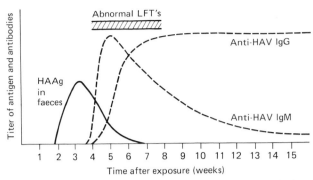

Figure 63-2. Diagrammatic representation of the shedding of virus and development of IgM and IgG antibody in a patient with hepatitis A.

tients admitted to the hospital within a week of the onset of dark urine. The detection rate falls dramatically in the second week, and particles or specific antigens are rarely detected for more than 21 days [15].

Rising titers of anti-HAV can be detected in serum specimens collected 10 to 14 days apart, provided that the first specimen is obtained early in the illness. Antibody is almost always present by the time the patient seeks medical attention and may already have reached peak or almost peak titer. Thus, although the absence of anti-HAV in a patient's sera precludes a diagnosis of hepatitis A, the absence of a rising titer does not.

To overcome this difficulty, assays have been developed for detection of hepatitis A–specific IgM [16]. Some of these assays are so sensitive that traces of antibody can be detected for 1 to 2 years after the onset of illness; however, it is possible to adjust the sensitivity of the test so that it will only detect antibody produced in the past 2 to 3 months.

Of the diagnostic methods currently available, the detection of hepatitis A–specific IgM is the most reliable, as it is invariably positive during the acute stage and early convalescent phase of the illness and requires only a single serum specimen collected at the time the patient seeks medical attention. By using sensitive assay systems, it is possible to provide a result within 24 h of the serum reaching the laboratory.

Management

Patients may be managed at home provided that adequate care is available. Hospital treatment may be required for special reasons (for example, if a mother and several children become ill and there is nobody capable of looking after them), because of the severity of the illness, or if the diagnosis is uncertain. Patients should be barrier nursed and special care taken in the disposal of feces. Attending staff and visitors should wear gowns if possible, and should wash their hands after touching the patient.

[1]Details of this network can be obtained from Dr. G. Torrigiani, Chief, Microbiology and Immunology Unit, World Health Organization, Geneva, Switzerland.

There is no specific treatment for the disease, which responds well to rest in bed. Occasionally deep jaundice may be associated with severe itching and require treatment with antipruritics or sedatives. For discussion of the value of γ-globulin see "Control."

POPULATION

Ecology

Information on the occurrence of hepatitis A can be obtained by analyzing reports from clinics, hospitals, and national health authorities or by serological surveys. In many countries, the data are difficult to interpret because of the inadequacy of national health statistics and the absence of reliable laboratory results.

Hepatitis A appears to be endemic throughout the world and to be responsible for both sporadic and epidemic disease. Some of the best data come from WHO's western Pacific region, where a number of serological studies have been performed [13]. This region, which comprises some 32 countries or territories, is of special interest as it includes populations ranging in size from several hundred millions to less than 10,000 and includes populations in areas which are highly developed, poorly developed, or developing rapidly.

Although hepatitis A appears to be endemic in the region, there is good evidence that in three of the most developed countries, Australia, New Zealand, and Japan, its prevalence is declining. This pattern is well documented in Australia where it is reflected in a decline in notifications and hospital admissions, a decline in the prevalence of antibody among children and young adults, and a change in the age at which the disease is most commonly seen. Whereas a decade ago hepatitis A was a disease of young children, the peak prevalence is now among the 15- to 29-year age group. This pattern is similar to that observed with poliomyelitis in the 1950s and 1960s and presumably reflects a steady improvement in hygiene and sanitation.

In the majority of the remaining countries, most children are infected in the first 10 years of life and virtually all the adult population have circulating antibodies. This pattern is characteristic of enteric infections in areas with overcrowding and poor standards of hygiene and personal sanitation. Under such circumstances, the clinical disease is relatively uncommon except among visitors, such as tourists, diplomats, missionaries, and Peace Corps workers. Epidemics of hepatitis occurring in these populations and apparently associated with ingestion of fecally contaminated water are unlikely to be due to HAV.

A third pattern has been recognized but is extremely uncommon. It occurs in isolated populations following outbreaks in which virtually all susceptible members are infected. While every person in the population alive at the time of the outbreak is found to have antibodies, children born subsequent to the outbreak are invariably seronegative. A relatively large number of isolated populations in the Pacific have been investigated, and surprisingly this pattern has only been encountered on one occasion, in the island of Ponape [17].

As there is some evidence that HAV is endemic in a number of these islands, it is interesting to postulate how the virus is able to survive. Almost 30 years ago, it was reported that hepatitis A had been transmitted to volunteers with fecal extracts collected from two patients 5 and 15 months after the onset of illness, suggesting the possibility of a chronic carrier state. Since no specimens remain from this study, there is no way of ascertaining whether the disease which was transmitted was hepatitis A or non-A non-B hepatitis. Against these data, scientists in many countries have examined the feces of patients with naturally acquired hepatitis A and have been consistently unable to detect virus particles or specific viral antigen for more than 3 to 4 weeks after the onset of illness. Thus, if a carrier state exists, it must be extremely rare.

In some islands fecal contamination of water supplies is relatively common and it is possible that HAV may persist in the polluted water. In some coral atolls untreated sewage is dumped into the central lagoon, stimulating a profuse growth of marine life and shellfish, which are then collected and eaten raw. HAV may accumulate in the shellfish and this could be a factor in persistence of infection in the population.

Apparently specific antibody has been detected in dogs, so that it is possible that under certain conditions dogs may provide an extrahuman reservoir of infection.

Perhaps the most logical explanation is to consider the Pacific Islands as a single epidemiological entity, rather like the suburbs of a large city. Even though the virus may be temporarily absent from an island, it is likely to be reintroduced within a very short period.

Strain Differences. There is no good evidence for the occurrence of different strains of HAV. In human beings second infections are unknown and attempts to reinfect laboratory animals with the same strain of HAV or strains obtained from other countries have been unsuccessful. Supportive evidence comes from the universal value of normal immunoglobulin in prophylaxis, regardless of the country of origin of the antibody, and from the ability of serological tests employing local reagents to detect infections acquired in any part of the world.

Epidemiology

Age and Distribution. Although infection may occur at any age, hepatitis A has traditionally been a disease of childhood, with the highest rates among preschool and school-age children. While this pattern still holds true in developing countries, in developed countries where the infection rate is declining, an increasing proportion of cases is now being seen among young adults.

Seasonal Pattern. The disease may occur at any time of the year. A seasonal peak in autumn and winter has been described in temperate zones but has been less prominent in the last decade, perhaps due to increased opportunities for travel. In temperate zones a cyclic pattern, with peaks every 6 to 10 years, has also been described.

Epidemics. Common source epidemics may be a particular problem following wars or natural disasters which result in damage to water supplies and sanitation services. Water- and foodborne epidemics have been reported when water supplies have become contaminated with human excreta or uncooked food has been prepared by a food-handler with poor personal hygiene. Most of these outbreaks have occurred in developed countries where a large proportion of the population is susceptible to infection.

Eating raw or partly cooked shellfish harvested from water which is subject to fecal contamination is associated with an increased risk of acquiring hepatitis A. Mollusks are able to concentrate HAV from large volumes of water, and the virus may remain viable for several days.

Control

General. Paradoxically, as the standards of hygiene and sanitation improve, hepatitis A may emerge as a public health problem because an increasing proportion of infections are delayed until adult life, at which time they are more likely to be associated with clinical symptoms. This is a temporary phenomenon and with sustained improvements in living conditions, the incidence of disease gradually declines.

Immunization. *Passive.* Numerous studies have shown the protective effects of pooled γ-globulin (immune serum globulin) if it is given prior to exposure or during the incubation period of the disease. When given in doses of 0.02 to 0.12 mL/kg within 1 to 2 weeks of exposure, this treatment is capable of preventing illness in more than 80 percent of subjects. Immunoglobulin is often administered to close contacts of an index case and prophylactically to travellers or troops about to enter an endemic area. If a prolonged stay is contemplated, the dose should be repeated every 4 to 6 months.

Because of the reduced incidence of hepatitis A in developed countries, there has been a decline in the titer of anti-HAV in some lots of globulin. To ensure that batches are of adequate potency, manufacturers are being encouraged to express the titer of their preparations in international units determined by reference to an International Reference Preparation.

Active. Isolation of HAV in cell culture has opened the door to the development of both killed virus and live virus vaccines. Several groups have prepared experimental batches of formalin-inactivated virus, which have been demonstrated to be safe, antigenic, and protective in nonhuman primates. Not all the substrates which have been used would be acceptable to licensing authorities. To overcome this problem, some strains of HAV have been adapted to growth in diploid human fibroblasts. Candidate vaccines produced in these cells are undergoing clinical trial and are likely to be licensed in the next 2 to 3 years.

In addition several attenuated strains of HAV, produced by prolonged passage in cell culture, are now available, and will shortly be tested in humans. The major manufacturers are working toward the development of a live attenuated vaccine which could be administered orally either as a single vaccine or in combination with oral poliovaccines.

HEPATITIS B

Hepatitis B is one of the commonest and most widespread infections of human beings. The disease was first recognized in Germany in 1885 when a large outbreak of jaundice occurred in shipyard workers who had been immunized against smallpox with a vaccine stabilized with human serum. Subsequently numerous cases were reported following the administration of pooled human serum, reuse of syringes contaminated with human blood, or as a late complication of blood transfusion. Because of its unusual epidemiology, it was suggested that hepatitis B was a new disease whose spread was dependent on modern medical practices.

Studies in recent years have altered this view. Hepatitis B appears to be an ancient and ubiquitous disease, capable of surviving in even the most isolated populations. Although infection can be transmitted to chimpanzees and certain other animals, there is no convincing evidence for the existence of an animal reservoir.

VIRUS

Morphology and ultrastructure

Three morphologically distinct particles can be visualized in infected sera—spherical particles measuring 20 to 22 nm in diameter, tubules of a similar diameter but of variable length, and 42-nm double-shelled structures (Dane particles) which are the mature hepatitis B virions (HBV) (see Figs. 63-3 and 63-4). The surfaces of all these particles possess a characteristic antigen, the hepatitis B surface antigen (HBsAg). The Dane particle has an outer coat approximately 7 nm thick and a central core. The core possesses two antigens, the hepatitis B core antigen (HBcAg), which is found on its surface, and the hepatitis B e antigen (HBeAg), whose location is still uncertain. Purified cores contain an HBV-specific, DNA-dependent DNA polymerase which appears to be involved in the synthesis of new DNA. The genetic material of the virus is circular, double-stranded DNA, with a molecular weight of approximately 2.0×10^4. Approximately 30 percent of the

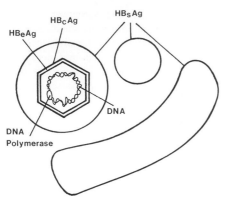

Figure 63-3. Diagrammatic representation of the three types of particle seen in the sera of patients infected with HBV.

circular DNA molecule is single-stranded, and it appears that the complementary strand of this segment is synthesized by the polymerase in vitro. The 22-nm spherical forms and tubules are normally present in great excess and probably represent coat material which is produced during a relatively inefficient replicative cycle and never assembled. These structures contain no internal components and are hence noninfectious. The surface of all three morphological forms possesses a group of antigens—the HBsAg—which are remarkably heterogeneous and can be used to divide hepatitis B viruses into a number of major subtypes.

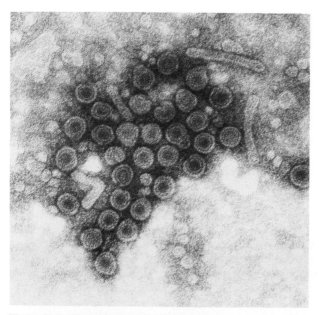

Figure 63-4. Electron micrograph of hepatitis B virus and associated particles in the serum of a chronic carrier of HBV. (*Courtesy of Dr. John Marshall.*)

Because antibodies directed against the surface antigens are responsible for resistance to reinfection, considerable attention has been devoted to a detailed analysis of the structure of HBsAg and the location of its antigenic sites. Purified preparations of HBsAg have been shown to consist of at least seven polypeptides, with molecular weights ranging from 23,000 to 97,000. Immunochemical studies show that the proteins share common determinants, suggesting that the physical differences reflect different degrees of glycosylation and aggregation. The amino acid sequences of HBsAg can be deduced from knowledge of the nucleotide sequence of its genome and the likely positions of the antigenic sites deduced. The relevant sequences can then be synthesized in the laboratory and tested for their ability to induce antibody to HBsAg (anti-HBs) in animals. To date, of 13 peptides synthesized, 7 have been found to be antigenic. These observations have important implications for vaccine production [19].

Antigenic subtypes

The surface of HBsAg contains a group-specific determinant designated *a* and two pairs of determinants *d* and *y*, and *w* and *r*, which behave as alleles and are present on the three morphological forms of HBsAg. They specify four major subtypes of the virus (*adw, adr, ayw,* and *ayr*) which represent the phenotypic expression of four distinct genotypes of the virus. While the subtypes are useful epidemiological markers, there is no evidence that they produce different types of disease; for practical purposes, infection with one type produces immunity to all.

Delta Antigen. Another antigen designated *delta* (HDAg) has been detected in liver biopsies obtained from some chronic carriers of HBV. This antigen is associated with a novel infectious agent [20] which is described in greater detail in Chap. 64.

In vitro culture

Despite numerous attempts, HBV has never been isolated in cell culture. Cell lines have been established from liver tissue obtained from patients with primary hepatocellular carcinoma, who were also chronic carriers of HBsAG [21]. These lines appear to be chronically infected with HBV and secrete 22-nm HBsAg particles into supernatant fluid. Mature HBV is not produced and the supernatant fluid is not infectious. HBV DNA has been detected in the tumor cells (with approximately four copies per cell) and appears to be integrated into cellular DNA [22,23]. It has been suggested that the integration of viral DNA may be the basis of oncogenic transformation.

Animal models

Primates. Chimpanzees and gibbons are highly susceptible to infection with HBV [9]; rhesus monkeys and woolly monkeys can also be infected but are less sensitive. Chimpanzees have been infected with each of the four major subtypes of HBsAg and have developed mild hepatitis with serological, histological, and biochemical changes which resemble natural infections in humans. These animals have proved invaluable for titrating preparations of HBsAg and studying the pathogenesis of the disease, as well as testing the safety and efficacy of vaccines and assessing the value of immune serum globulin and antiviral substances in the prevention and treatment of infection.

Other Species. Although HBV has not been detected in species other than humans and some nonhuman primates, viruses with a similar morphology to HBV and sharing antigenic features and genetic homology have been recognized to occur naturally in woodchucks (WHV), Beechy ground squirrels (GSHV), and Pekin ducks (DHV) [24–26]. The viruses all appear to infect hepatocytes and commonly cause persistent infection with high levels of morphologically similar particles being found in the blood. In woodchucks, chronic infection is also associated with hepatocellular carcinoma.

The existence of animal analogues of HBV infection of humans provides an opportunity to study aspects of pathogenesis and mode of spread of the disease and to define factors responsible for the development of long-term sequelae, such as chronic hepatitis and liver cell cancer.

Intermediate hosts or reservoirs

Hepatitis B has been reported in several nonhuman primates [9], and HBsAg has been detected in chimpanzeès, gibbons, and orangutans after capture. The prevalence of markers of infection appears to be related to the length of captivity, suggesting that infection is acquired by contact with human beings, not in the wild.

PATIENT

Host-parasite relationship

Infection with HBV may be completely silent, accompanied by a recognizable attack of acute viral hepatitis or associated with fulminant liver disease resulting in coma and death.

The most important factors determining the outcome of HBV infections are the age of the subject and the infecting dose. Infections acquired early in life are usually subclinical. In many developing countries, particularly those in tropical zones, more than 50 percent of children are infected before the age of 5 years, yet clinical disease is almost unknown. Infections acquired after the age of 15 years are more likely to be associated with symptoms.

The severity of the disease appears to be largely dose-dependent and is graphically illustrated by the difference in the case fatality rate of patients who acquire hepatitis B by blood transfusion (10 to 20 percent) or by other means (0.1 percent)

[27]. By contrast with many other viral infections, hepatitis B tends to be less severe in the immunocompromised or immunosuppressed subject than in normal subjects.

Carrier State. A proportion of people exposed to the virus become chronically infected and continue to harbor it for years. These people are known as chronic carriers and constitute an important reservoir of HBV infection.

It has been estimated that there are more than 200 million carriers in the world, although enormous differences in prevalence occur; for example, in most Anglo-Saxon populations it is less than 0.1 percent, whereas in certain Pacific islands it is greater than 50 percent. Several factors have been shown to influence the risk of an individual becoming a chronic carrier, of which the most important is the age of infection. While the risk of an adult becoming a carrier is between 5 and 10 percent, in babies it is greater than 50 percent.

Patients with lymphoproliferative disorders and those on immunosuppressive treatment are more likely to become carriers of HBsAg, as are subjects with Down's syndrome or patients with leprosy. In chronic carriers the titers of HBsAg usually decline with increasing age, and many people eventually eliminate the virus from their body and develop protective antibodies.

Higher carrier rates are observed among males than females. This has been shown to be because of a more rapid decline in HBsAg titer in women, resulting in a shorter duration of the carrier state.

Pathogenesis and pathology

The pathogenesis of hepatitis B is poorly understood. Liver cell damage is believed to be the result of elements of the cellular immune response acting on novel antigens synthesized in infected hepatocytes.

The incubation period of the disease varies from 2 weeks to 6 months (mean, 12 to 14 weeks) and is inversely related to the infecting dose. The first objective evidence of infection is the development of HBsAg and HBcAg in the cytoplasm and nuclei of infected liver cells and the appearance of HBsAg in the blood (see Fig. 63-5). The titer of HBsAg rises steadily over the next few weeks and is accompanied by the development of histological evidence of acute viral hepatitis and characteristic biochemical changes. Circulating anti-HBc appears about the time HBsAg reaches peak titer and reaches maximum titer in 4 to 6 weeks, thereafter declining slowly. Detectable levels of anti-HBc persist for many years. Liver function tests usually return to normal within 3 to 4 weeks as the titer of HBsAg in the blood declines. It is not unusual for HBsAg to remain detectable for several weeks after the liver function tests have become normal. Surprisingly, free circulating anti-HBs may not be detected for several months after HBsAg has been eliminated from the body. It persists for many years but is usually not as long-lasting as anti-HBc.

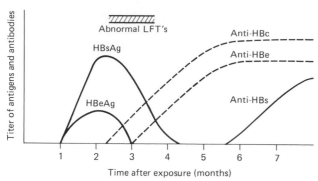

Figure 63-5. Diagrammatic representation of the presence of various antigens and antibodies in the sera of a patient with hepatitis B.

During the early part of the infection, when virus replication is at its peak and levels of HBsAg are increasing, HBeAg and HBV-specific, DNA-dependent DNA polymerase can be detected in the blood. HBeAg disappears rapidly and is replaced by anti-HBe.

In chronic carriers, the sequence of events differs considerably. First, after reaching peak levels, HBsAg remains at high levels for many years. Second, anti-HBc titers tend to be much higher than are found in acute uncomplicated infections and, third, free circulating anti-HBs is never detected. Chronic carriers' blood can be divided into two groups according to whether that blood contains either HBeAg or anti-HBe. The presence of HBeAg in a chronic carrier is a marker of active viral replication and the sera of such people is highly infectious.

Clinical manifestations

The clinical manifestations of hepatitis B are similar to those reported for hepatitis A, with the exception that extrahepatic manifestations, such as arthralgia and skin rashes, are more common. Periarteritis nodosa, glomerulonephritis, and acrodermatosis are rare complications. Approximately 5 to 10 percent of infections in adults progress to chronicity. Chronic carriage of HBV is frequently associated with normal health and a normal life expectancy. A proportion of chronic carriers however, develop chronic persistent or chronic active hepatitis, and some eventually develop primary hepatocellular carcinoma. The incidence of these complications varies from country to country and is highest in China, Japan, and southeast Asia and sub-Saharan Africa, where hepatocellular carcinoma is one of the leading causes of death. Whether HBV infection is the sole cause of this malignancy or whether other factors contribute remains unknown.

Diagnosis

Sensitive serological tests have been developed for the three antigens regularly associated with HBV infection—HBsAg, HBcAg, HBeAg—plus δ Ag and the antibodies directed against them. Most of these tests are expensive (radioimmunoassays are most commonly employed) and are not available in developing countries other than through reference laboratories or the WHO network. The most widely available test is for detection of HBsAg. The presence of HBsAg in the blood is evidence of active HBV infection, either acute or chronic; detection of anti-HBs is evidence of recovery from infection and, for practical purposes, indicates that the subject is immune to reinfection. Anti-HBc may be detected during active infection and during the convalescent phase. A rising titer of anti-HBc is evidence of recent infection.

Management

Management of patients with hepatitis B is essentially the same as for those with hepatitis A, with the exception that special care should be taken to prevent infection caused by contact with the patient's blood or secretions. Although infection may be transmitted to the patient's sexual partners, in practice there is little one can do to prevent this. Blood samples should be obtained at regular intervals to determine whether the patient has recovered or become chronically infected.

In countries where HBV infection is common and high numbers of the population are carriers, there is little advice that one can give an individual carrier. Transfusion services in such countries have adopted different practices according to the availability of blood and the funds available. Where blood is difficult to obtain and only administered in life-threatening situations, the donors are usually not screened for HBsAg except when the recipient is a visitor or migrant from a country with a low rate of HBV infection. In countries which find it easier to attract donors and where adequate funds are available, all donors are screened for HBsAg and only HBsAg-negative blood is used for transfusion.

In countries where HBV infection is relatively uncommon, carriers should be counseled as to the risk of transmitting the disease by direct contact with their blood. Such people should not become blood donors or share common toothbrushes or other articles which could transmit blood or secretions to another person. Provided that carrier has adequate standards of personal hygiene, little alteration of activity is needed. In most developed countries medical or nursing staff who are known to be HBsAg-positive are restricted from working in dialysis and oncology units on the grounds that if they infect a patient, the disease is likely to spread rapidly and become endemic in the unit.

POPULATION

Ecology

Hepatitis B has a worldwide distribution, and evidence of acute and chronic infection has been obtained in even the most isolated populations.

The prevalence of infection varies greatly from country to country and depends upon a complex mix of behavioral, environmental, and host factors. In general, it is lowest in countries with high standards of living (e.g., the United States, Canada, Australia, Scandinavia, Great Britain, etc.) and highest in countries which are poor and overcrowded (e.g., China, Indonesia, the Philippines, parts of Africa and South America, etc.). Intermediate rates of infection are found in the U.S.S.R., southern and eastern Europe, and some parts of Africa and Asia.

Within individual countries major differences in the prevalence of HBV infection exist between different ethnic groups. For example, in New Zealand the HBsAg carrier rate among Maoris is 9.5 percent compared with 0.1 to 0.2 percent among the white population. Even within an apparently homogenous population marked differences in infection and carrier rate may occur. In the tiny Pacific island of Nauru, 3500 Micronesians live in a series of villages dotted along the coast. Although approximately 80 percent of the people in each village show evidence of infection, the carriage rates vary from 5 to 28 percent [28]. The reason for these differences is not understood.

Epidemiology

Hepatitis B is a notifiable disease in many countries; however, attempts to define its epidemiology on a global basis have been hampered by the inadequacy of most reporting schemes. Not only are the basic data poorly collected, but clinical diagnoses are rarely supported by laboratory confirmation.

Reliable information on the incidence and long-term trend of hepatitis is only available from a few of the more affluent countries. In several, e.g., the United States, Scandinavia, and Australia, there has been a dramatic increase in HBV infection over the past decade, although there is some evidence that this trend has begun to reach a plateau.

This pattern parallels the epidemiology of intravenous drug use in these countries and is dramatic evidence of the importance of the disease in this group.

Mode of Spread. In developed countries hepatitis B has traditionally been a hazard of blood transfusion, the use of shared syringes, and exposure to infected blood. For these reasons high rates of infection occur in certain occupational groups such as dentists, staff and patients in dialysis units, biochemists, and hematologists. Transmission can occur in the family setting and tends to be related to the degree of crowding of the household and the intimacy of each person to the case or carrier. It may occur as a result of accidental percutaneous inoculation following the use of shared razors, toothbrushes, bath brushes, or towels, or by close contact. HBV has been detected in a variety of body secretions and excretions, including saliva, semen, and vaginal fluid, so that infection may be transmitted by kissing or by sexual intercourse. Hepatitis B does not appear

to be transmitted by the fecal-oral route and urine is probably not infectious unless contaminated with blood. There is no convincing evidence that airborne infections occur.

The high prevalence of hepatitis B infection in many tropical countries led to the suggestion that mosquitoes and other bloodsucking insects might be important in transmission of the disease; however, there is no convincing evidence to support this suggestion.

Transmission from chronic carrier mothers to their babies appears to be the single most important factor in determining the prevalence of HBV infection in some areas. The risk of infection depends upon the proportion of HBeAg-positive carrier mothers, which may be as high as 40 percent in some countries. Although HBV can infect the fetus in utero, this rarely happens, and most infections appear to occur at birth due to either a leak of maternal blood into the baby's circulation, ingestion, or accidental inoculation.

Age and Sex Distribution. Two different patterns of infection are recognized. In populations in which HBV is hyperendemic, infection is usually acquired early in life. The highest infection rates and carrier rates are seen among children and young adults. The carrier rate declines with increasing age, as does the prevalence of specific antibody.

In populations in which HBV is relatively uncommon, the majority of infections and the peak prevalence of HBsAg and specific antibody are in the 15- to 29-year age group. The highest rates of infection are found among groups who have a high risk of contact with blood or blood products. Prominent among these are health workers (particularly laboratory staff, dentists, and surgeons), patients and staff in institutions for the mentally retarded, intravenous drug users, and male homosexuals.

Seasonal Variations. Hepatitis B has no seasonal pattern and the long-term trend is not clear. Cyclical peaks which have been a feature of the epidemiology of hepatitis A have not been observed, and epidemics due to the widespread use of contaminated blood or blood products are increasingly rare.

Prevention

In developed countries infection with HBV can be reduced by avoiding exposure to potentially contaminated blood. The rate of posttransfusion hepatitis has fallen dramatically as a result of screening donor blood for HBsAg, and this procedure coupled with regular screening of staff and patients has reduced the incidence of hepatitis B in dialysis units. Improved understanding of the mode of spread of HBV and attention to personal hygiene and techniques of handling blood has reduced the incidence of the disease among laboratory workers.

Hepatitis B may occur following the use of blood products prepared by fractionating large pools of plasma collected from volunteer donors. All individual units of blood used in such procedures and the end products should be screened for HBsAg and positive units or batches destroyed. Transmission by inoculation of infected blood can be reduced by avoiding the practice of multiple usage of syringes and needles, and sterilizing needles used for tattooing, acupuncture, or ear piercing after each use.

In developing countries the majority of infections occur early in life. The best hope of controlling infection lies with immunization.

Control

Immunization. *Passive.* The availability of sensitive assays has made it possible to select units of plasma and produce batches of immunoglobulin with high titers of anti-HBs (hepatitis B immunoglobulin, or HBIG).

When administered prior to exposure, HBIG has been found to reduce the incidence of hepatitis B in both mentally retarded children and patients and staff working in dialysis units. Repeated doses are necessary to maintain protection. Despite its efficacy in these situations, HBIG is unlikely to be widely used for preexposure prophylaxis because of the development of a suitable vaccine.

The major indication for the use of HBIG is a single acute exposure to the virus, e.g., after accidental inoculation, contamination of the conjunctiva, or swallowing HBsAg-positive material. Doses of 0.04 to 0.07 mL/kg are usually administered. There is some evidence that greater protection is obtained by giving two doses 30 days apart. The value of HBIG depends on how soon it can be administered after the accident. It should be given as rapidly as possible, preferably within 48 h. Repeated doses of HBIG have also been shown to be capable of reducing the incidence of infection of babies born to HBsAg-positive mothers.

Active. Subunit vaccines take advantage of the fact that the sera of chronic carriers of HBV may contain from 10^{10} to 10^{12} 22-nm particles per milliliter and that these particles, while noninfectious, carry HBsAg on their surface and can be purified by a variety of biophysical and biochemical techniques. Vaccines produced in this way are usually treated with heat and/or formalin to destroy any residual virus and tested in chimpanzees.

Several subunit vaccines have been licensed for use in humans and have been demonstrated to be safe and effective [29,30]. The purification and inactivation procedures which are involved have been demonstrated to render the product free of the risk of transmission of AIDS. More than 20 million doses of subunit HBV vaccines have been administered, without any serious side effects being reported. The existence of multiple suppliers plus tendering for large-scale orders has led to a major reduction in the price of HBV vaccine. This vaccine is likely to be the next immunogen added to the WHO Expanded Programme on Immunization.

In developed countries HBV vaccine is used mainly in selected groups in whom the greatest benefit can be expected. In developing countries mass immunization campaigns are being developed in an attempt to reduce the long-term sequelae of chronic liver disease and hepatocellular carcinoma.

Because of the limited number of donor carriers available and the relatively low yield of vaccine per unit of blood, scientists have developed alternative means of producing the vaccine. Recent developments in recombinant DNA technology show that it is possible to produce either complete HBsAg or antigenically active fragments in the laboratory. HBV vaccines derived by expressing HBsAg in yeast are now licensed and vaccines produced in mammalian cells are undergoing clinical evaluation.

REFERENCES

1 Coulepis AG, Locarnini SA, Westaway EG, et al: The biophysical and biochemical characterization of hepatitis A virus. Intervirology 18:107–127, 1982

2 Provost PJ, Wolanski BS, Miller WJ, et al: Physical, chemical and morphological dimensions of human hepatitis A virus strain CR.326. Proc Soc Exp Biol Med 148:537–539, 1975

3 Bradley DW, Fields HA, McCaustland KA, et al: Biochemical and biophysical characterization of light and heavy hepatitis A virus particles: Evidence HAV is an RNA virus. J Med Virol 2:175–187, 1978

4 Siegl G, Frosner GG: Characterization and classification of virus particles associated with hepatitis A. II. Type and configuration of nucleic acid. J Virol 26:48–53, 1978

5 Coulepis AG, Tannock GA, Locarnini SA, et al: Evidence that the genome of hepatitis A virus consists of single-stranded RNA. J Virol 37:473–477, 1981

6 Locarnini SA, Coulepis AG, Westaway EG, et al: Restricted replication of human hepatitis A virus in cell culture: Intracellular biochemical studies. J Virol 37:216–225, 1981

7 Provost PJ, Hilleman MR: Propagation of human hepatitis A virus in cell culture in vitro. Proc Soc Exp Biol Med 160:213–221, 1979

8 Daemer RJ, Feinstone SM, Gust ID, et al: Propagation of human hepatitis A virus in African green monkey cell culture: Primary isolation and serial passage. Infect Immun 32:388–393, 1981

9 Reviewed by Deinhardt F: Hepatitis in primates, in Lauffer MA (ed): *Advances in Virus Research,* Academic, vol 20. New York, 1976, pp 113–157

10 Locarnini SA, Coulepis AG, Gust ID: Coproantibodies in Hepatitis A: Detection by enzyme-linked immunosorbent assay and immune electron microscopy. J Clin Micro 11:710–716, 1980

11 Mathieson LR, Drucker J, Lorenz D, et al: Localization of hepatitis A antigen in marmoset organs during acute infection with hepatitis A virus. J Infect Dis 138:369–377, 1978

12 Krzystof K, Krawczynski MD, Bradley DW, et al: Pathogenic aspects of hepatitis A virus infection in enterally inoculated marmosets. Am J Clin Pathol 76:698–706, 1981

13 Gust ID: A comparison of the epidemiology of hepatitis A and B, in Szmuness W, Maynard J, and Alter H (eds): *1981 International Symposium on Viral Hepatitis.* Philadelphia, Franklin Institute Press 18:129–143, 1982

14 Reviewed by Mathieson LR: The hepatitis A virus infection. Liver 1:81–109, 1981

15 Coulepis AG, Locarnini SA, Lehmann NI, et al: Detection of hepatitis A virus in the faeces of patients with naturally acquired infections. J Infect Dis 141:151–156, 1980

16 Locarnini SA, Coulepis AG, Stratton AM, et al: Solid-phase enzyme-linked immunosorbent assay for the detection of hepatitis A specific immunoglobulin M. J Clin Micro 9:459–465, 1979

17 Wong D, Purcell RH, Rosen L: Prevalence of antibody to hepatitis A and hepatitis B viruses in selected populations in the South Pacific. Am J Epidemiol 110:227–236, 1979

18 Advances in Viral Hepatitis. Report of the WHO Expert Committee on Viral Hepatitis. WHO Tech Rep Ser 602, Geneva, World Health Organization, pp 19–20, 1977

19 Lerner RA, Green N, Alexander H, et al: Chemically synthesized peptides predicted from the nucleotide sequence of the hepatitis B virus genome elicit antibodies reactive with the native envelope protein of Dane particles. Proc Natl Acad Sci 78:3403–3407, 1981

20 Rizzetto M, Canese MG, Gerin J, et al: Transmission of the hepatitis B virus-associated Delta antigen to chimpanzees. J Infect Dis 141:590–602, 1980

21 MacNab G, Alexander J, Lecatsas G, et al: Hepatitis B surface antigen produced by a human hepatoma cell line. Br J Cancer 34:509–515, 1976

22 Edman JC, Gray P, Valenzuela P, et al: Integration of hepatitis B virus sequences and their expression in a human hepatoma cell. Nature 286:535–538, 1980

23 Marion PL, Salazar FH, Alexander JJ, et al: State of hepatitis B viral DNA in a human hepatoma cell line. J Virol 33:795–806, 1980

24 Summers J, Smolec JM, Snyder RL: A virus similar to human hepatitis B virus associated with hepatitis and hepatoma in woodchucks. Proc Natl Acad Sci USA 75:4533–4537, 1978

25 Marion PL, Oshiro L, Regnery DC, et al: A virus in Beechy ground squirrels which is related to hepatitis B virus in man. Proc Natl Acad Sci USA 77:2941–2945, 1980

26 Mason WS, Seal G, Summers J: A virus of Pekin ducks with structural and biological relatedness to human hepatitis B virus. J Virol 36:829–836, 1980

27 Gust ID, Lucas CR: Post-transfusion hepatitis in Australia, in Japan Medical Research Foundation (eds): *Hepatitis Viruses.* Tokyo, University of Tokyo Press, 1978, pp 323–330

28 Gust ID, Dimitrakakis M, Zimmet P: Studies in hepatitis B surface antigen and antibody in Nauru. I. Distribution in Nauruans. Am J Trop Med Hyg 27:1030–1036, 1978

29 Maupas P, Barin F, Chiron JP, et al: Efficacy of hepatitis B vaccine in prevention of early HBsAg carrier state in children. Lancet 1:289–292, 1981

30 Szmuness W, Stevens CE, Harley EJ, et al: A hepatitis B vaccine: Demonstration of efficacy in a controlled clinical trial in a high risk population in the United States. N Engl J Med 303:833–841, 1980.

CHAPTER 64 / *Hepatitis D* · Ian D. Gust

Hepatitis delta virus (HDV) is a newly recognized agent which is capable of replicating only in the presence of hepatitis B virus (HBV). HDV may complicate acute or chronic infection with HBV and is an important cause of both acute and chronic hepatitis [1].

VIRUS

Morphology and ultrastructure

Hepatitis D is caused by an unusual virus (HDV) which has some of the characteristics of a chimera. The virion is spherical, measures 36 nm in diameter, and is made up of an outer coat of HBsAg surrounding a novel protein, delta antigen (HDAg). The genome is a small piece of single-stranded RNA, with a molecular weight of approximately 1700 (usually expressed as 1.7 kD) and a high degree of secondary structure. The RNA does not have a 3′ poly-A tail, nor does the virion contain reverse transcriptase [2].

Analysis of HDAg shows it to be composed of two major proteins with molecular weights of 27,000 and 29,000, respectively (p27 and p29) [3]. Complementary DNA fragments of the HDV genome have been cloned, and the entire nucleotide sequence is now known. In addition, HDAg has been expressed in yeast.

Hybridization of HDV RNA with libraries of RNA from normal and HBV-infected individuals has failed to reveal homologies, while computerized comparisons with the genome of other viruses have failed to reveal similarities. A cDNA fragment of HDV RNA has been cloned and analyzed, revealing 63 percent GC pairs and a high protein content in the derived amino acid. Fragments of cDNA failed to hybridize with HBV DNA. It is not yet known how the two major HDV proteins are coded or how HDAg and HDV RNA are packaged with HBsAg [2].

The molecular weight of the HDV genome is smaller than that of any known animal RNA virus and resembles certain plant viruses which are also encapsidated by material derived from a helper virus. Synthesis of HDV can be supported by animal hepadnaviruses—for example, woodchuck HBV and duck HBV—the resultant HDV being coated with either WHBsAg or DHBsAg [4].

In vitro cultivation

Despite numerous attempts, it has not proved possible to adapt HBV or HDV to growth in cell culture.

Animal models

HBV is a member of a recently identified group of viruses, the hepadnaviruses, which cause acute or chronic infection in a variety of species. The group includes the woodchuck hepatitis virus (WHBV) [5], ground squirrel hepatitis virus (GSHBV) [6], and Pekin duck hepatitis virus (DHBV) [7]. HDV has been transmitted to hepadnavirus-infected woodchucks and Pekin ducks; synthesis of HDV is supported by the animal virus, resulting in the production of novel delta viruses coated in either WHBsAg or DHBsAg. Replication of HDV appears to inhibit replication of the helper viruses.

HDV infection can also be transmitted to chimpanzees acutely or chronically infected with HBV. These animals have proved to be extremely useful models for studying the pathogenesis of HDV infection and the kinetics of antibody formation.

Intermediate host reservoirs

Despite their susceptibility to infection, there is no evidence that animals which harbor their own hepadnaviruses provide a natural reservoir of HDV infection, nor have naturally occurring HDV-like agents been identified in these species.

PATIENT

Host-parasite relationship

Infection with HDV can occur only in an individual who is already infected with HBV. The infection may be completely silent, may be accompanied by a typical attack of acute viral hepatitis, or may cause fulminant liver disease with coma and death. Chronic HDV infection in chronic carriers of HBsAg may result in the development of chronic liver disease and/or cirrhosis.

Two essentially different forms of infection are recognized when HDV complicates acute or chronic HBV invection—situations which are referred to as *coinfection* and *superinfection*. The severity of the disease varies widely in different parts of the world. The reasons for these differences are not known.

Coinfection

Coinfection occurs when a person or experimental animal is simultaneously infected with HBV and HDV. The usual outcome of this situation is an attack of acute hepatitis, which is usually indistinguishable on clinical or biochemical grounds from acute hepatitis B. Occasionally, the illness may be biphasic, with two peaks of elevated liver enzymes separated by several weeks. Coinfection is quite common and may account for up to 40 percent of viral hepatitis in some parts of the world, especially cities with a large population of intravenous drug users. Because of the similarity of the clinical illness to hepatitis B, coinfection can be recognized only if appropriate laboratory tests are available. Occasionally, coinfection of HBV and HDV is associated with severe or fulminant hepatitis—many of these episodes have occurred among intravenous drug users, suggesting that either (1) rapid passage of HBV has selected mutants with different properties or (2) some other infection is present.

Superinfection

Superinfection occurs when HDV infection takes place in an existing chronic carrier of HBV. Superinfections are usually more serious than coinfection as the virus has a large number of infected hepatocytes in which to multiply. Superinfection is usually recognized as an acute episode of hepatitis in a known carrier of HBV—These episodes may be severe and are recognized to be responsible for between 30 percent and 60 percent of episodes of fulminant HBsAg-positive hepatitis around the world [8].

Superinfection may resolve with clearance of and immunity to HDV (and occasionally HBV), or persist. Persistence of HDV infection appears to be quite common, and individuals with persistent HDV infection become chronically infected with HBV and HDV and act as reservoirs of both agents. In many countries chronic HDV infection carries a significant risk that the patient will develop chronic hepatitis and/or cirrhosis [9]. Studies in Italy suggest that up to 50 percent of subjects with chronic HBV infection who develop chronic liver disease do so due to superinfection with HDV. The course of the disease may be rapidly progressive—more than 90 percent of patients who develop cirrhosis within 12 months of an apparent HBV infection have been subsequently shown to be superinfected with HDV [8].

Pathogenesis

HDV appears to be a defective virus dependent upon helper functions provided by HBV. The virus is incapable of replication alone or in individuals who are immune to HBV infection. Knowledge of the pathogenesis of coinfection and superinfection has been obtained from studies in humans and from transmission studies in chimpanzees [10].

In coinfection, replication of HBV enables the rescue of HDV, which overwhelms the synthesis of HBV and causes an acute attack of hepatitis. When these events occur rapidly, only a single attack of hepatitis is seen. In some patients rescue of HDV is delayed by several weeks, resulting in a second episode of hepatitis and a biphasic illness. The outcome of both types of disease is usually benign: the infected cells are eliminated, markers of infection with both viruses are lost, and both anti-HBs and anti-HD develop.

In chronic carriers of HBV, infection with HDV results in vigorous replication and an acute attack of hepatitis. In a high proportion of cases, infection with HDV results in the development of a carrier state. For reasons which are not understood, carriers in whom HBV infection is quiescent (as indicated by absence of circulating HBV DNA and the presence of anti-HBc) are more likely to develop chronic hepatitis.

The outcome of infection appears to be influenced by the presence of preexisting liver disease—carriers with prior HBV-induced liver disease tend to develop chronic hepatitis or cirrhosis more rapidly. Unfortunately, the corollary is not true, and progressive liver disease may occur in previously healthy carriers of HBsAg.

Progression to chronic liver disease may be rapid—the case fatality rate of patients with chronic HDV infection followed for 3 years was three times higher (15 percent compared with 5 percent) than for matched patients with HBsAg-positive liver disease alone.

Very high titers of HDV (10^{10} or greater) may be found in the blood of infected individuals. The ability to detect low levels of HDV depends on the presence of large numbers of HBV-infected cells which are capable of amplifying the infection; e.g., while an inoculum containing both HBV and HDV was able to transmit infection to susceptible chimpanzees to maximum dilution of 10^{-7}, the same serum induced hepatitis in an HBsAg carrier animal when diluted 10^{-11}.

Carriers of HBsAg who are also infected with HDV do not have an increased risk of developing primary hepatocellular carcinoma.

Clinical manifestations

Coinfection. Coinfection of HBV and HDV usually results in an attack of hepatitis that is clinically indistinguishable from hepatitis B. Sometimes the illness is characterized by a biphasic hepatitis, with two peaks of elevated transaminases 2 or 3 weeks apart. Experimental infections in animals suggest that the first peak is due to the elimination of HDV-infected cells, and the second to elimination of cells infected with HBV. The attack usually resolves spontaneously, and the subject becomes immune to reinfection with either agent.

Occasionally (especially in intravenous drug users) coinfection may result in fulminating hepatitis. The frequency with which this occurs varies from country to country. Overall, coinfection is estimated to be responsible for between 6 and 30 percent of fulminant hepatitis B in the world [8].

The clinical picture of coinfection is usually insufficiently characteristic for recognition in the absence of specific laboratory tests.

Superinfection. The normal presentation is an attack of acute viral hepatitis in a person who is either known to be a carrier

of HBsAg or subsequently demonstrated to be one. In the past, these episodes were regarded either as relapses of HBV infection or attacks of non-A non-B hepatitis.

Although outbreaks of fulminant hepatitis are documented, they are usually mild; however, such attacks have a tendency to progress to chronicity and eventually cirrhosis. This process can be quite rapid, with biopsy evidence of impending cirrhosis developing within 2 months or so.

The outcome of delta infection depends upon a number of factors, including the previous state of the subject's liver—in carriers with preexisting liver disease, chronic HDV infection causes additional damage and hastens the development of chronic liver disease and cirrhosis. Progression is common and may be rapid; in one series, 23 of 152 (15 percent) patients with chronic HDV hepatitis died within 3 years, compared with 5 of 101 (5 percent) of matched carriers of HBV who were not infected with HDV [8].

Chronic delta hepatitis is characterized by progressive deterioration in liver function, splenomegaly, and autoimmune phenomena. Liver biopsy reveals severe lobular damage, eosinophilic degeneration of hepatocytes, and the presence of HDAg in infected cells.

Diagnosis

A range of diagnostic tests are now available. These include assays for HDAg and HDV, and for anti-HD IgM and HDV RNA. Although some are now available commercially, testing for HDV infection is still largely the province of reference laboratories.

Coinfection may be confirmed by the detection of HDAg in sera collected early in the illness, or by demonstrating a rising titer of anti-HD or the presence of specific IgM. Antigenemia is usually brief and easily missed. Of 52 patients with coinfection studied by enzyme-linked immunosorbent assay, only 15 (29 percent) had detectable levels of HDAg. The antibody response in coinfection is variable, with the most reliable marker being detection of anti-HDV IgM. These antibodies usually appear in the second or third week after the onset of dark urine, but are short lived, rarely being detected for more than 8 weeks after the onset of symptoms [11].

Blocking antibodies to HDV are detected in only about half the patients in whom an IgM response occurs. These antibodies are long lived.

A diagnosis of superinfection with HDV can be made by demonstrating a seroconversion to anti-HDV, detecting rising levels of anti-HD, or presence of HDAg in acute-phase sera. Anti-HDV IgM levels persist for many years, but may fluctuate in titer, with elevations tending to correspond with episodes of abnormal liver function.

Management

As there is no specific treatment for HDV infection, the management is essentially the same as for other types of viral hepatitis. Progress in the treatment of chronic delta hepatitis has been slow; a variety of substances, including corticosteroids, levamasole, and immunostimulants, have been tried without success. α-Interferon and some antiviral compounds appear to inhibit replication of the virus and are being assessed in clinical trials.

POPULATION

Ecology

When it was discovered, HDV was thought to be an unusual agent largely restricted to some parts of Italy. The development and wide-scale use of diagnostic tests has demonstrated that HDV infection is worldwide, but that there are wide differences in its prevalence and distribution [12].

In Europe, delta infection is widespread, and it appears to be endemic in many Mediterranean countries where HBV infection is also common. By contrast, it is rare and appears to be recently introduced in northern Europe, where HBV infection is uncommon (except among intravenous drug users). Infection is common in some parts of the Middle East, tropical Africa, some countries in the north of South America, and a number of Pacific Islands [13].

In developing countries transmission of HDV usually occurs by exposure to infected body fluids. Transfer requires intimate contact, such as occurs between sexual partners or members of a family group, and is facilitated by overcrowding, poor hygiene, and open skin wounds.

In developed countries, HDV is largely confined to migrants from areas of high prevalence and their families, and to intravenous drug users.

Perinatal transmission is rare and appears to be of no epidemiological importance. In keeping with HBV transmission, infection with HDV is uncommon in infants but increases sharply in the second decade of life, peaking in the third [14].

Strain differences

There is no evidence that HDVs from different parts of the world differ antigenically. Occasional outbreaks of disease associated with an unusually high mortality raise the possibility that strains with increased virulence may exist. To date, this has not been demonstrated in laboratory animals, suggesting that host factors or perhaps dose may be more important in determining outcome.

Some of these differences may be more apparent than real because of the limited amount of testing which has been undertaken and the selective nature of the populations which have been studied.

Epidemiology

As HDV is a bloodborne viral infection requiring the presence of HBV as a helper, its epidemiology is determined by patterns of HBV infection.

In areas in which HDV is endemic, infection appears to occur as a result of direct contact, presumably by exposure to infected body fluids. In a cross-sectional study of an island population in which both HBV and HDV are hyperendemic, HBV infections are found to occur in the first decade of life, whereas HDV infection reaches its peak in the second decade, coinciding with the onset of sexual activity [14].

Infection is more common in countries where there is overcrowding, standards of hygiene are poor, and open skin wounds are common.

In developed countries, HDV infection is largely restricted to migrants from endemic areas (or their close contacts), intravenous drug users, and people with hemophilia. There is evidence that HDV was introduced into drug users during the 1960s and has spread rapidly [15]. Perinatal transmission has been documented, but appears to be of little epidemiological importance. Household studies indicate that infection is predominantly horizontal and is most common among sexual partners.

The risk of posttransfusion HDV infection when HBsAg-screened blood is used is extremely low and in practical terms is probably only a risk in carriers of HBsAg who can rescue minute quantities of HDV.

Control

The development and widespread use of hepatitis B vaccine has the potential to reduce or even eliminate coinfection between HBV and HDV, provided groups at increased risk of infection have access to the vaccine. This effect does not apply to the large pool of chronic carriers of HBsAg estimated at more than 250 million worldwide, who remain susceptible to the risk of infection with HDV. Fortunately, despite careful study, there is no evidence that HDV is spreading through southeast Asia, where the largest number of carriers live. Work is underway to develop and test vaccines to prevent superinfection of HBsAg carriers. Whether these attempts will be successful remains to be seen.

REFERENCES

1 Rizzetto M, Canese MG, Arico S, et al: Immunofluorescence detection of a new antigen-antibody system (δ/anti-δ) associated to the hepatitis B virus in the liver and in the serum of HBsAg carriers. Gut 18:997–1003, 1977

2 Hoyer, BH, Bonino F, Ponzetta A., et al: Properties of delta-associated ribonucleic acid. Prog Clin Biol Res 113:91–97, 1983

3 Bonino F, Hoyer BH, Shih JW-K, et al: Delta hepatitis agent; structural and antigenic properties of the delta associated particle. Infect Immun 43:1000–1008, 1984

4 Ponzetto A, Cote PJ, Popper H, et al: Transmission of the hepatitis B virus associated δ agent to the eastern woodchuck. Proc Natl Acad Sci USA 81:2208–2212, 1984

5 Summers J, Smolec JM, Synder R: A virus similar to human hepatitis B virus associated with hepatitis and hepatoma in woodchucks. Proc Natl Acad Sci 75:4533–4537, 1978

6 Marion PL, Oshiro L, Regnery DC, et al: A virus in Beechy ground squirrels that is related to hepatitis B virus of man. Proc Natl Acad Sci USA 77:2941–2945, 1980

7 Mason WS, Seal G, Summers J: Virus of Pekin duck with structural and biological relatedness to human hepatitis B virus. J Virol 36:829–836, 1980

8 Bonino, F, Smedile A: Delta agent (type D) hepatitis. Semin Liver Dis 6:28–33, 1986

9 Rizzetto M, Verme G, Recchia S, et al: Chronic hepatitis in carriers of hepatitis B surface antigen, with intrahepatic expression of the delta antigen. An active and progressive disease unresponsive to immunosuppressive treatment. Ann Intern Med 98:437–441, 1983

10 Rizzetto M, Canese MG, Gerin LJ: Transmission of the hepatitis B virus associated δ antigen to chimpanzees. J Infect Dis 141:590–601, 1980

11 Gust ID, Dimitrakakis M: Epidemiology of HDV infection in Australia and the Western Pacific Region, in Rizzetto M et al (eds): *The Hepatitis Delta Virus and Its Infection*. New York, Alan R. Liss, 1987, pp 521–532

12 Purcell RH, Gerin JL: Epidemiology of the delta agent: An introduction. Prog Clin Biol Res 143:113–119, 1983

13 Dimitrakakis M, Crowe S, Gust ID: The prevalence of delta infection in the Western Pacific Region. J Med Virol 18:335–339, 1986

14 Gust ID, Speed B, Thoma K, et al: Control of HBV and HDV infection in an isolated Pacific Island. Submitted for publication.

15 Dimitrakakis M, Waters MJ, Wootton et al: Epidemiology of hepatitis D virus (delta) infection in Melbourne over a 15-year period. Med J Aust 145:125–130, 1986

CHAPTER 65

Hepatitis Non-A Non-B · Ian D. Gust

A considerable proportion of viral hepatitis is caused neither by HAV nor HBV, nor by infection with other occasionally hepatotropic agents, such as cytomegalovirus (CMV) and Epstein-Barr virus (EBV). This disease, which is referred to as *non-A non-B (NANB) hepatitis*, occurs in two epidemiologically distinct forms which are named after their predominant mode of transmission: enterically transmitted NANB hepatitis and parenterally transmitted NANB hepatitis.

Although candidate etiological agents have only recently been identified [1,2] and diagnostic tests are not generally available, a considerable amount of information is available on the epidemiology and natural history of both diseases.

ENTERICALLY TRANSMITTED NANB HEPATITIS

Although only recently recognized, this disease is probably ancient and widespread [3]. In the past 10 years, sporadic cases and epidemics have been reported from many countries.

AGENT

Morphology and ultrastructure

The candidate agent is a viruslike particle which can be recovered from the feces of patients during the acute phase of their illness and from the feces of experimentally infected cynomolgus monkeys [4]. The particles are variously described as being between 27 and 34 nm in diameter, with a mean of 32 nm. These differences may be technical or may reflect partial digestion of the virus as it passes down the alimentary tract.

The agent has an RNA genome and a sedimentation coefficient of 183 S, consistent with it being a member of the calicivirus group.

In vitro cultivation

The etiological agent has not been adapted to cell culture, nor is anything known of its replicative strategy.

Animal models

On two occasions, transmission of enterically transmitted NANB hepatitis to human volunteers has been reported with inocula (filtrates of feces from patients with the disease) from different outbreaks. In the first study the volunteer (who was immune to hepatitis A) developed viral hepatitis about 6 weeks after ingesting the inoculum [5].

Fecal specimens obtained from these patients during the acute phase of their illness and single specimens or pools of specimens obtained during outbreaks in several countries have been inoculated into a wide range of nonhuman primates (including marmosets, rhesus, African green, saimiri, and cynomolgus monkeys and chimpanzees).

A variety of markers have been used to determine whether the animal has been infected, and no agreed criteria exist. To date, most ''infections'' in nonhuman primates have been diagnosed on the basis of mild, transient elevations in serum transaminase or dehydrogenase levels.

Enterically transmitted NANB hepatitis has been transmitted to chimpanzees [2], tamarins (*Saguinus mystax*), and cynomolgus macaques (*Macaca fasicularis*). The virus has been passaged three times in cynomolgus monkeys, which develop biochemical and histological evidence of hepatitis and shed 27- to 34-nm particles in their feces [4]. These animals currently offer the best model of human infection.

Intermediate hosts or reservoirs

As specific laboratory tests are not widely available, little is known about the ecology of enterically transmitted NANB hepatitis or the existence of intermediate hosts. The occurrence of epidemics of the disease in refugee camps, where humans and animals live in close proximity and hygiene is poor, has led some workers to postulate that the virus may have a reservoir in nature.

PATIENT

Host-parasite relationship

The ratio of subclinical to clinical infections is not yet known, but is probably relatively high. Studies during epidemics have shown that for each person with clinical hepatitis, there may be an additional 8 to 10 people who have short-lived abnormalities of liver function, but no jaundice [6].

There is some evidence that enterically transmitted NANB hepatitis is more common among lower socioeconomic groups, and that a higher proportion are immune to infection. For example, when outbreaks of NANB hepatitis have occurred in military populations, the prevalence of disease has been higher among troops than among officers. Expatriate medical personnel who have investigated outbreaks in refugee camps where standards of hygiene and sanitation are poor have had very high attack rates. On the other hand, embassy staff living through waterborne epidemics who consumed only boiled water have been spared.

Perhaps the most striking difference between epidemics of enterically transmitted NANB hepatitis and epidemics of hepatitis A is the case fatality rate. Whereas the case fatality rate among patients with hepatitis A who are sufficiently ill to be admitted to hospital is 1 to 2 per 1000, in most epidemics of NANB hepatitis the overall case fatality rate has been 1 to 2 percent. The most severe form of the disease occurs among pregnant women, especially those in the third trimester. In virtually every outbreak, the case fatality rate in this group has been between 10 percent and 20 percent, and it appears to be a characteristic of the disease [7].

Apart from an increased incidence of fulminant hepatitis, acute NANB hepatitis appears to be self-limiting—long-term follow-up of patients involved in several outbreaks has failed to demonstrate an increased incidence of chronic liver disease or other chronic sequelae [8].

Similarly, there is no clinical or epidemiological evidence of the existence of a chronic carrier state.

Pathogenesis and pathology

Little is known about the pathogenesis of enterically transmitted NANB hepatitis—it is generally assumed to be an enteric infection with a primary site of replication in the gut and secondary site of replication in the liver. Whether liver cell damage is virus-induced or cell-mediated is unknown.

The consensus among pathologists familiar with the histology of other forms of viral hepatitis in humans and experimentally infected animals is that the histological changes in the liver of patients with enterically transmitted NANB hepatitis are quite characteristic and differ from the parenterally transmitted form.

The typical changes observed in tissue obtained from patients with the disease include portal inflammation; large numbers of Kupffer cells and polymorphonuclear leukocytes (but relatively few lymphocytes); canalicular cholestasis; and focal "toxic" changes in hepatocytes, which show ballooning, cytoplasmic cholestasis, and cytolytic necrosis. Similar changes have been observed in some experimentally infected nonhuman primates [9].

Diagnosis

To date diagnosis of enterically transmitted NANB hepatitis has been made on the basis of compatible epidemiological and clinical features, and exclusion of HAV, HBV, CMV, and EBV infection. Virological confirmation is now possible either by demonstration of 27- to 34-nm viruslike particles in fecal specimens collected during the acute phase of the illness, or by demonstrating a specific antibody response by immune electron microscopy. As commercial assays are not yet available, confirmation of diagnosis is restricted to a handful of research laboratories.

Clinical manifestations

Enterically transmitted NANB hepatitis is usually an acute self-limiting disease which resolves without sequelae. During large epidemics in developing countries, a significant mortality has been observed among cases sufficiently severe to require hospitalization. The most severe disease is seen among pregnant women, especially those in the third trimester of pregnancy, where case fatality rates are commonly 10 to 20 percent.

Management

As with other forms of viral hepatitis, management of enterically transmitted NANB hepatitis is basically supportive. The value of immune serum globulin for protection of close contacts is unknown.

EPIDEMIOLOGY

Enterically transmitted NANB hepatitis has been recognized in many countries in Asia, Africa, the Middle East, and Central

America. Although the first well-documented outbreak was the New Delhi epidemic of 1955–1956 [*10*], there is evidence that outbreaks with similar features occurred in Europe at the turn of the century [*3*].

Although the disease appears to occur in both epidemic and sporadic forms, the epidemic form is better documented. Over the past 30 years, numerous outbreaks have been recognized, mostly in Asia in a wide area extending from Mongolia and western China to Afghanistan (including the Indochinese peninsula, Burma, Thailand, India, Kashmir, Nepal, Burma, Pakistan, the central Asian republics of the U.S.S.R., and Indonesia). A number of outbreaks have been documented in Africa (Algeria, Tunisia, Ethiopia, Sudan, Somalia, and the Ivory Coast), and at least one has occurred in Central America (Mexico). Most outbreaks, but not all, have been associated with gross contamination of drinking water with fecal material (both human and animal), and have usually occurred during the rainy season or after flooding.

Two types of epidemics have been observed: short, sharp outbreaks lasting for several weeks, usually after a transient contamination of the water supply, and prolonged outbreaks lasting for several months, in which spread appears to be from person to person either directly or via contamination of the environment. Outbreaks of this type have recently been observed in some refugee camps in which there is extreme overcrowding and no adequate means of disposal of feces. The disease usually becomes apparent several weeks after the onset of the rainy season, when the surrounding land becomes a mixture of mud and excrement.

The incubation period of enterically transmitted NANB hepatitis ranges from 2 to 9 weeks with a mean of 6 weeks, although mean incubation periods as short as 2 weeks have been recorded in some epidemics. Whether these differences reflect degrees of exposure (dose) or are due to different agents involved is not clear. Although relatively few secondary cases are recognized, when household contacts of the index case are examined and serial liver function tests performed (e.g., in the Kashmir outbreaks of 1978–1979 [*11*]) at least 20 percent have elevated levels of serum transaminase.

During point source epidemics, the clinical attack rate is highest among young adults (15 to 39 years of age) with lower rates being observed among children and the elderly. For example, in the New Delhi outbreak, the prevalence of jaundice in the population was 1.3 percent in children less than 14 years of age, 2.9 percent in young adults 15 to 39 years of age, and 2 percent in those older than 40 years of age [*10*]. Higher attack rates have been observed in refugee camps where there is extreme overcrowding, inadequate sanitation, and increased opportunities for person-to-person spread.

The epidemiology of epidemic NANB hepatitis suggests that the source of infection is feces, either human or animal. The higher attack rate among people from higher socioeconomic groups suggests that the agent circulates in the population between epidemics and that infections (presumably acquired early in life) are associated with long-lasting immunity. If this scenario is correct, one would predict that sporadic cases of enterically transmitted NANB hepatitis could be detected in the period between epidemics. Evidence for the existence of sporadic NANB hepatitis has been obtained in several locations, especially in the Indian subcontinent [*12*]. A study of patients with viral hepatitis admitted to hospital in southeast Asia shows that from 25 percent to 50 percent of cases of sporadic hepatitis are the NANB form. Although no tests exist for differentiating the parenterally and enterically transmitted forms of the disease, the high case fatality rate of sporadic NANB hepatitis (especially in pregnant women) and the absence of evidence of chronic liver disease in survivors suggest that the enterically transmitted form is the major cause of NANB hepatitis in this region. If this is so, NANB hepatitis may be the most common cause of acute viral hepatitis in developing countries.

Neither epidemic nor sporadic cases of enterically transmitted NANB hepatitis have been reported in developed countries, except among travelers returning from endemic areas.

In some areas of the Indian subcontinent, enterically transmitted NANB hepatitis appears to be endemic and large numbers of cases are seen every year. To date there is no documented evidence of a second attack of NANB hepatitis. On several occasions during epidemics, acute viral hepatitis has been observed in both a mother and her child. In each instance, although the mother's illness has been NANB hepatitis, the baby's has been hepatitis A. Although some people have interpreted these data (and the fact that enterically transmitted NANB hepatitis has been seen almost exclusively among people with preexisting antibody to hepatitis A virus) to indicate that this form of NANB hepatitis is an atypical response to reinfection with hepatitis A virus, it is more likely that these observations reflect the result of exposure to both agents—with NANB hepatitis occurring in the mother, who is already immune to hepatitis A virus, and hepatitis A occurring in the child, who is susceptible to both.

CONTROL

Passive immunization

Several attempts have been made to protect populations at risk by administering immune serum globulin (ISG). Lots of ISG prepared in France had no effect on the incidence of NANB hepatitis among French troops in Algeria [*13*]. Conflicting claims exist for the value of locally produced ISG in reducing the incidence of NANB hepatitis in recipients when the material has been administered during an outbreak. A controlled study during an outbreak in India failed to demonstrate a statistically significant difference in the incidence of disease among subjects who did or did not receive ISG [*14*]. In a second, uncontrolled study, ISG was administered to 200 pregnant women during an outbreak in Kashmir. Although no cases of hepatitis were observed in this group, it is difficult to conclude that this was due to the ISG, as most infections had probably occurred by the time the material was administered and no more than one or two cases of disease would have been expected in the group.

Because of the high case fatality rate of enterically transmitted NANB hepatitis, especially among pregnant women, prospective studies of the value of locally produced ISG are urgently needed and consideration should be given to the production of hyperimmune globulin from plasma collected from patients convalescing from the disease.

Active immunization

The discovery of the etiological agent makes it possible to begin to develop vaccines against enterically transmitted NANB hepatitis. It is likely that these vaccines will be administered together with HAV vaccine to provide protection against both enterically transmitted forms of viral hepatitis.

PARENTERALLY TRANSMITTED NANB HEPATITIS

Although originally recognized as a complication of blood transfusion [15], parenterally transmitted NANB hepatitis appears to be an anicteric and widespread infection of humans which has a number of features in common with hepatitis B.

AGENT

Morphology and ultrastructure

At the time of writing, the etiological agent has not been visualized; however, several lines of evidence suggest that the agent is a single-stranded RNA virus, measuring about 50 nm in diameter, with a lipid-soluble envelope—suggesting that it may be a non-arthropod-borne togavirus.

Infectivity associated with one particular inoculum has been destroyed by treatment with chloroform, 1:1000 formalin, β-propiolactone, UV irradiation, or heating at 100°C for 60 min or 60°C for 10 h [16].

In vitro cultivation and replicative strategy

As the etiological agent(s) have not yet been isolated in cell culture, little is known of their replicative strategy. There is indirect evidence that the most important agent is an RNA virus which replicates in the cytoplasm of infected hepatocytes.

Animal models

NANB hepatitis has been transmitted to chimpanzees with a variety of inocula including sera or plasma from patients with acute or chronic hepatitis, whole blood from asymptomatic blood donors, and batches of clotting factor VIII implicated in transmission of NANB hepatitis [17,18].

Infected animals develop biochemical and histological hepa-

titis about 6 to 8 weeks after inoculation. Many of these animals develop fluctuating abnormalities of liver function and remain infectious for many years. Although chimpanzees infected with parenterally transmitted NANB hepatitis remain susceptible to HAV and HBV, they may develop another attack of hepatitis when challenged with a second inoculum containing parentally transmitted NANB hepatitis. For example, chimpanzees infected with one lot of factor XVIII complex, implicated in several cases of parenterally transmitted NANB hepatitis in humans, have developed a second attack of hepatitis when challenged with infected factor XVIII concentrate [19]. Several other studies have suggested that it is possible to have two separate attacks of parenterally transmitted NANB hepatitis. However, whether this is due to the existence of two different etiological agents or to reactivation of the original infection is unknown [15].

Intermediate hosts or reservoirs

There is no epidemiological evidence which speaks either for or against the possibility of an animal reservoir of parenterally transmitted NANB hepatitis.

PATIENT

Host-parasite relationship

Infection with parenterally transmitted NANB hepatitis usually results in a mild illness which would be overlooked if routine tests of liver function were not performed. Although at least 75 percent of infections are anicteric, the disease is characterized by prolonged fluctuating elevations of alanine aminotransferase (ALT) and a tendency to chronicity. Most infections are mild; however, acute, fulminating parenterally transmitted NANB hepatitis has been described, especially after blood transfusion.

Chronic carrier state

Several studies (reviewed by Bradley in [16]) suggest that parenterally transmitted NANB hepatitis is associated with a chronic carrier state and that in some countries, chronic carriers of this form of the disease may be several times more common than chronic carriers of HBV. In the United States the frequency of posttransfusion NANB hepatitis suggests that the prevalence of chronic carriers of the parentally transmitted form among the blood donor population is between 3 and 4 per 1000. Similar findings have been reported from a number of other countries.

Pathogenesis and pathology

Experimental infection of chimpanzees results in the development of biochemical and histological evidence of acute hepatitis, which may have distinctive ultrastructural features.

Histologically the most commonly reported features are eosinophilic clumping of cytoplasm, microvascular steotosis, activation of sinusoidal cells, mild inflammation, and piling up of bile duct cells.

At the ultrastructural level, the most commonly recorded changes are confined to the hepatocyte cytoplasm and include formation of distinctive convoluted membranes which appear to originate from a proliferation of the smooth endoplasmic reticulum. Bundles of granular microtubules and intranuclear particles have been demonstrated in some infected hepatocytes. As each of these structures has been reported in other diseases, they probably represent a nonspecific response to infection with parenterally transmitted NANB hepatitis.

Clinical manifestations

Parenterally transmitted NANB hepatitis is usually a mild illness, with an incubation period ranging from 2 to 26 weeks (mean of 7 to 9 weeks). The reason for the variation is unknown, but may be related to dose.

The majority of infections (more than 75 percent) are anicteric and go unrecognized. Compared with acute hepatitis B, patients with parenterally transmitted NANB hepatitis have lower peak ALT levels, which are more likely to fluctuate over a prolonged period, so that it is difficult to determine when and if recovery has taken place.

Fulminant hepatitis can occur, and although rare, parenterally transmitted NANB hepatitis appears to be an important cause of potential hepatitis, accounting for 25 to 44 percent of cases in most countries [21].

Prospective studies of individuals who have had an attack of parenterally transmitted NANB hepatitis indicate that a significant number develop evidence of chronic liver disease. In a review of 17 studies, ALT elevations lasting for more than 6 months were noted in 43 percent of 653 patients. Similar data were obtained when seven studies in which 339 patients were followed for more than 1 year were analyzed. When biopsies are performed on subjects with persistently abnormal liver function tests, the most common diagnoses are chronic active and chronic persistent hepatitis [21].

Chronic NANB hepatitis tends to be clinically mild and tends to progress slowly. The likelihood of progression to chronic liver disease does not appear to be influenced by the severity of the acute illness. Because of the asymptomatic nature of such chronic NANB hepatitis and its fluctuating course, it is difficult to predict what proportion of infections will progress to chronicity: the best estimate is probably 40 to 50 percent.

Diagnosis

At present a diagnosis of parenterally transmitted NANB hepatitis is made on the basis of a typical clinical picture, relevant epidemiological data, and exclusion of other causes of viral hepatitis, such as infection with HAV, HBV, CMV, or EBV.

It seems likely that the recent assay described by scientists at the Chiron Corporation and their colleagues at the Centers for Disease Control will prove to be a specific and sensitive marker of infection.

Management

The management of patients with parenterally transmitted NANB hepatitis is unremarkable and essentially symptomatic. Continued care and assessment are often required to identify those patients who will develop chronic liver disease. Because a significant number of people who have been infected with this form of hepatitis become chronic carriers of the disease, these people should refrain from blood donation. Although there are no definitive studies linking chronic parenterally transmitted NANB hepatitis and primary hepatocellular carcinoma, there is some indirect evidence of an association, especially in Japan.

EPIDEMIOLOGY

Originally described as a complication of blood transfusion, parenterally transmitted NANB hepatitis is now recognized in a number of other settings. Like hepatitis B, the disease is spread primarily by inoculation of blood and blood products.

Percutaneous transmission

In the 1970s, prospective studies of U.S. patients who had received multiple units of donor blood indicated that some 6 to 12 percent developed abnormal liver function tests consistent with a diagnosis of posttransfusion hepatitis (PTH). The introduction of routine HBsAg tests for donors did not appreciably alter the situation, and it was estimated that prior to the introduction of donor deferral and routine screening for AIDS antibodies, 7 to 10 percent of recipients of large volumes of donor blood developed PTH (a rate of 3 to 6 cases per 1000 units of blood transfused [20]. In the United States and most other developed countries, the parenterally transmitted NANB form of the disease is responsible for more than 90 percent of all cases of transfusion-associated hepatitis.

NANB hepatitis has been reported in people with a variety of coagulation diseases requiring regular infusions of clotting factors (reviewed by Dienstag and Alter in [21]). The risk appears to be highest with commercial factor VIII concentrates and has been described with antihemophiliac factor, factor IX, cryoprecipitate, or fibrinogen.

Annual attack rates of 2 to 6 percent have been reported in patients with hemophilia [22]: in one study of patients with hemophilia and von Willebrand's disease treated for the first time with factor VIII or IX concentrates, two-thirds developed abnormal liver function tests within 3 months of infusion. Chronic liver disease is common among hemophiliacs; much of this is probably due to chronic NANB hepatitis.

Discrete outbreaks and sporadic cases of NANB hepatitis

have been reported from dialysis units in many countries, and this disease has replaced hepatitis B as the major risk to patients and staff [23]. Cross-sectional studies in dialysis patients in several countries suggest that some 15 percent have persistently elevated levels of ALT consistent with NANB hepatitis and that the annual incidence of infection is 3 to 6 percent in patients and 10 percent in staff [24].

Recipients of organ transplants are also at increased risk of infection. In one study, 6.5 percent of renal transplant patients developed NANB hepatitis—most of these people subsequently developed chronic hepatitis [25]. Patients who developed hepatitis were more likely to die of sepsis during the first 3 years after transplantation and had a higher risk of developing severe liver disease within 5 to 10 years.

Parenterally transmitted NANB, hepatitis has also been observed among health care workers after penetrating injuries with bloodstained needles or other objects. The exact frequency of the disease and groups at greatest risk will not be determined until specific diagnostic tests become available.

Other

As with hepatitis B, parenterally transmitted NANB hepatitis can probably be transmitted by sexual intercourse and by infected mothers to their newborn babies. NANB hepatitis is well recognized among homosexual men, although the attack rate appears to be lower than for hepatitis B [12]. This, and the low rate of infection among heterosexual partners of patients with acute or chronic parenterally transmitted NANB hepatitis, suggests that sexual transmission, while possible, is relatively uncommon.

While transmission of infection from mothers to their babies has been demonstrated in women who developed acute NANB hepatitis during the third trimester of pregnancy, the importance and extent of perinatal transmission is unknown.

A substantial proportion of cases of NANB hepatitis which are seen by general practitioners or result in hospital admission have no recognizable source of infection. NANB hepatitis appears to account for 6 to 46 percent of sporadic cases of hepatitis worldwide [21]. The mechanism of infection in these patients remains unknown.

CONTROL

General measures

In the absence of specific diagnostic tests, it has been proved possible to reduce the incidence of parenterally transmitted NANB hepatitis by certain simple public health measures.

In the United States, the incidence of posttransfusion hepatitis fell threefold when paid donors were excluded from donor panels, and fell further after the introduction of donor referral and routine testing for AIDS antibodies. Similarly, the introduction of heat-treated clotting factors has reduced the incidence of parenterally transmitted NANB hepatitis among hemophiliacs and patients with other clotting disorders. The risk of acquiring parenterally transmitted NANB hepatitis occupationally can be reduced by careful attention to personal hygiene—especially wearing gowns and gloves when in contact with blood, tissue, or body fluids—and by avoidance of penetrating injuries.

A variety of tests have been described which claim to detect the etiological agent responsible for the disease. These tests have involved detection of a variety of antigens, antibodies, enzymes, or particles in the patient's blood or in infected hepatocytes. None of these assays has proved to be specific [21]. Recently, a new assay has been described which utilizes antigens expressed from cloned nucleic acid obtained from the blood of patients with proven parenterally transmitted NANB hepatitis. Early studies with this test suggest that it is specific, but further work will be required before it can be introduced into clinical practice.

In the absence of specific assays, some blood-transfusion services have introduced surrogate markers to detect carriers of parenterally transmitted NANB hepatitis. The two most commonly used markers have been elevated levels of ALT and/or the presence of anti-HBc [27,28]. Several studies have shown an association between elevated levels of ALT and the presence of anti-HBc in blood donors and the incidence of PTH. However, exclusion of all donors with these markers does not entirely remove the risk; e.g., exclusion of donors with abnormal ALTs (1 to 3 percent of most donor populations) resulted in only a 30 percent reduction in the incidence of PTH.

Passive immunization

Several placebo-controlled trials have been undertaken to evaluate normal immune globulin in prevention of posttransfusion hepatitis. No convincing evidence for efficacy has been obtained [21]. While hepatitis B immune globulin appeared to reduce the incidence of NANB hepatitis in dialysis units [29], a placebo-controlled trial in cardiac surgery patients failed to demonstrate protection.

REFERENCES

1 Bradley D, Andjaparidze A, Cook EH, et al: Aetiological agent of enterically transmitted non-A non-B hepatitis. J Gen Virol 69: 731–738, 1988

2 Arankalle WA, Ticehurst J, Sreenivasan, MA, et al: Aetiological association of a virus-like particle with enterically transmitted non-A non-B hepatitis. Lancet i:550–553, 1988

3 Cockayne EA: Catarrhal jaundice, sporadic and epidemic, and its relation to acute yellow atrophy of the liver. QJ Med 6:1–29, 1962

4 Bradley DW, Krawczynski K, Cook EH, et al: Enterically transmitted non-A non-B hepatitis: Serial passage of disease in cynomolgus macaques and tamarins and recovery of disease-associated 27–34 nm virus-like particles. Proc Nat Acad Sci USA 84:6277–6281, 1987

5 Balayan MS, Andjaparidze AC, Sarinskaya SS, et al: Evidence for

a virus in non-A non-B hepatitis transmitted via the fecal-oral route. Intervirology 20:23–31, 1983

6 Khuroo MS, Duermeyer W, Zargar SA, et al: Acute sporadic non-A non-B hepatitis in India. Am J Epidemiol 118:360–364, 1983

7 Khuroo MS, Teli MR, Skidmore S, et al: Incidence and severity of viral hepatitis in pregnancy. Am J Med 70:252–258, 1981

8 Khuroo MS, Saleem M, Teli MR, et al: Failure to detect chronic liver disease after epidemic non-A non-B hepatitis. Lancet ii: 97–98, 1980

9 Gust ID, Purcell RH: Waterborne non-A non-B hepatitis. J Infect Dis 156:630–635, 1987

10 Viswanathan R: Epidemiology. Am J Med Res Supp. 1:1–29, 1987

11 Khuroo, MS: Study of an epidemic of non-A non-B hepatitis: Possibility of another human virus distinct from post-transfusion non-A non-B. Am J Med 68:818–823, 1980

12 Khuroo MS, Duermeyer W, Zargar, SA, et al: Acute sporadic non-A non-B hepatitis in India. Am J Epidemiol 118:360–364, 1983

13 Belabbes H, Benatallha A, Bourgemouh A: Non-A non-B epidemic viral hepatitis in Algeria: Strong evidence for its water-spread, in Vyas GN et al (eds): *Viral Hepatitis and Liver Disease*. Orlando, Grune and Stratton, 1985, p. 637

14 Josh YK, Babu S, Sarkin S., et al: Immunoprophylaxis of epidemic non-A non-B hepatitis. Indian J Med Res 81:18–19, 1988

15 Feinstone SM, Kapikian AZ, Purcell RH, et al: Transfusion associated hepatitis not due to viral hepatitis type A or B. N Engl J Med 292:747–770, 1975

16 Bradley DW, Maynard JE: Etiology and natural history of post-transfusion and enterically-transmitted non-A non-B hepatitis. Semin Liver Dis 6:56–66, 1986

17 Alter HJ, Purcell, RH, Holland PV, et al: Transmissible agent in non-A non-B hepatitis. Lancet 1:459–463, 1978

18 Tabor E, Gerety RJ, Drucker JA, et al: Transmission of non-A non-B hepatitis from man to chimpanzee. Lancet i:463–466, 1978

19 Bradley DW, Maynard JE, Cook EH, et al: Non-A non-B hepatitis in experimentally infected chimpanzees: Cross-challenge and electron microscopic studies. J Med Virol 6:185–201, 1980

20 Alter HJ, Purcell RH, Holland PV, et al: Clinical and serological analysis of transfusion-associated hepatitis. Lancet ii:838–841, 1975.

21 Dienstag JL, Alter HJ, Non-A non-B hepatitis: Evolving epidemiologic and clinical perspective. Semin Liver Dis 6:67–81, 1986

22 Richard KA, Batey RG, Dority P, et al: Hepatitis and haemophilia therapy in Australia. Lancet ii:146–148, 1982

23 Seaworth BT, Garret LE, Stead WW, et al: Non-A non-B hepatitis and chronic dialysis—another dilemma. Am J Nephrol 4:235–237, 1984

24 Deinstag JL, Stevens CE, Szmuness W: The epidemiology of non-A non-B hepatitis: Emerging patterns, in: Gerety RJ, (ed): *Non-A Non-B Hepatitis*. New York, Academic 1981, pp 119–137

25 La Quaglia MP, Tolkoff-Rubin NE, Deinstag JL, et al: The impact of hepatitis on renal transplantation. Transplantation 32:504–507, 1981

26 Szmuness W, Stevens CE, Harley EJ, et al: Hepatitis B vaccine: Demonstration of efficacy in a controlled clinical trial in a high risk population in the United States. N Engl J Med 303:833–841, 1980

27 Aach RD, Szmuness W, Mosley JW, et al: Serum alanine aminotransferase of donors in relation to the risk of non-A non-B hepatitis in recipients: The transfusion-transmitted viruses study. N Engl J Med 304:989–994, 1981

28 Stevens CE, Aach RD, Hollinger FB, et al: Hepatitis B virus antibody in blood donors and the occurrence of non-A non-B hepatitis in transfusion recipients. Ann Intern Med 101:732–738, 1984

29 Simon, N: Prevention of non-A non-B hepatitis in haemodialysis patients by hepatitis B immune globulin. Lancet ii:1047, 1984

30 Sugg U, Schneider W, Hoffmeister HE, et al: Hepatitis B immune globulin to prevent non-A non-B post-transfusion hepatitis. Lancet i:405–406, 1985

CHAPTER **66** / *Measles* · *Neal A. Halsey* · *J. S. Job*

Measles is a cause of more than 2,000,000 preventable childhood deaths per year [1]. Although there are no significant differences in virus strains circulating throughout the world, the severity of disease is increased in developing countries, where case fatality rates are 10 to 1000 times higher than the rates observed in industrialized countries. Although effective vaccines have been available for more than 25 years, 50 percent or fewer of the children in developing countries receive the vaccine before they contract the disease. Large-scale global efforts are being coordinated by the World Health Organization (WHO) to minimize or eliminate measles as a major cause of disease and death.

VIRUS

Measles is a single-stranded, six-protein RNA virus classified as a member of the genus *Morbillivirus* in the family Paramyxoviridae. The genotype appears to be stable with no evidence of geographical variation in the antigens. Although minor strain differences have been developed in laboratories for development of vaccines, no major strain variations have been documented in isolates obtained from clinical specimens. Three of the six proteins or glycoproteins produced by the virus play important roles in pathogenesis. The hemagglutinin (H) which projects from the virion aids in the attachment to cell surfaces; the F protein facilitates intercellular spread; and the M protein appears to be necessary to generate intact viral particles.

The virus is sensitive to ultraviolet light, heat, pH changes, and drying. However, properly lyophilized measles virus and vaccines can be stored at 2 to 8°C for prolonged periods of time. Lyophilized virus stored at −20°C has remained stable for over 20 years.

Culture of the virus from clinical specimens has been difficult but has been accomplished most frequently on primary monkey kidney, human-infant kidney, or human-fetal tissue. Routine diagnosis by viral isolation is not practical. Several tissue-culture-adapted strains are available and utilized for development of diagnostic reagents. Viral culture in tissue lines should be confirmed by immunofluorescence, as other viral agents can mimic some of the characteristic cytopathic effects (CPE). Measles causes formation of multinucleated syncytia (Warthin-Finkeldey cells) which can be seen in swabs from tonsillar or other lymphoid material obtained from patients with clinical measles.

Modified forms of the virus appear in brain tissue with cell-to-cell passage of defective viral particles in the disease subacute sclerosing panencephalitis (SSPE). This virus cannot be isolated directly with the routinely used cell lines. However, cocultivations of brain tissue with laboratory-adapted cell lines have been successful in isolating the virus from SSPE patients.

PATHOGENESIS

Measles is highly contagious. The virus is transmitted by droplets or aerosol from the respiratory tract to mucous membranes on the upper respiratory tract or the conjunctiva. After primary multiplication in epithelial cells, a low-grade primary viremia develops 2 to 3 days after exposure with spread of the virus to regional lymph nodes and reticuloendothelial cells throughout the body. Further replication in these cells is followed by a high-grade secondary viremia beginning 7 to 9 days after exposure with infection of epithelial cells throughout the body and other multiple organs. Individuals are infectious beginning approximately 7 days after exposure and continuing through the first few days of rash onset, the most contagious period occurring during the 3 to 5 days prior to rash onset.

Cell-mediated immune responses are impaired during measles. Individuals with positive skin tests to tuberculin often revert to negative, wound healing is delayed, and hypersensitivity-mediated diseases such as glomerulonephritis and rheumatoid arthritis often go into remission. In severe disease, the degree to which total lymphocytes are depressed correlates with mortality.

PATIENT

CLINICAL MANIFESTATIONS

The terminology for measles has been a source of some confusion. The proper English scientific term is *rubeola*. How-

ever, in Spanish, rubeola means German measles (or rubella). Alternative Spanish terms are *sarampion comun* for measles and *sarampion alemon* for rubella. The French term is *rougeole*.

Nine to ten days following exposure, infected individuals develop the characteristic prodromal (prerash) manifestations of measles consisting of cough, coryza (rhinorrhea), conjunctivitis, and fever. The symptoms increase in intensity over 2 to 4 days prior to the onset of rash. In uncomplicated cases, the illness peaks on the first or second day of the rash and symptoms gradually resolve over 3 to 7 days. Koplik's spots (Fig. 66-1) are seen on the buccal mucosa in 60 to 80 percent of individuals with measles but are probably present in all patients if careful daily examinations are performed. The lesions are slightly raised 2- to 3-mm-diameter bluish-white dots on an erythematous base, and there is an irregular or blotchy enanthem on the entire buccal mucosa [2]. Koplik's spots appear about 24 h prior to the onset of rash and persist for only 1 to 3 days. The number of lesions varies from 1 to 5 to several hundred, and they are occasionally seen in other mucous membranes including the conjunctiva and vaginal mucosa. Although Koplik's spots are considered pathognomonic for measles, several other viral agents including enteroviruses cause buccal lesions that have been confused with Koplik's spots (Fig. 66-2).

Generalized lymphadenopathy occurs commonly in young children. Older children will usually complain of photophobia and occasionally of arthralgias.

The characteristic rash (Fig. 66-3) is usually noticed first on the face and posterior hairline and consists of discrete erythematous patches 2 to 6 mm in diamter. The rash peaks 2 to 3 days after onset and is most concentrated in the trunk and proximal portions of the upper extremities.

Discrete lesions can be seen on the palms of 25 to 50 percent of patients. The density of the lesions varies with the severity of the disease, but young infants who have had intensive exposure to the virus tend to have confluent lesions over the face and trunk (Figs. 66-4 and 66-5). In uncomplicated cases, the

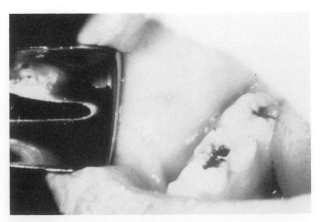

Figure 66-1. Koplik's spots on the buccal mucosa.

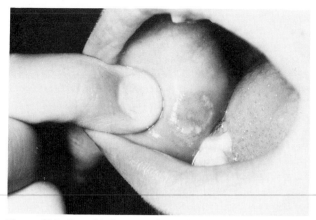

Figure 66-2. Buccal lesions associated with coxsackie A16 infection.

rash persists for 4 to 7 days. In many patients, a fine desquamation of the rash can be noted 7 to 8 days after onset which is often exaggerated in malnourished children living in developing countries (Fig. 66-6). Some children develop severe exfoliation of the skin [3]. This enhancement of the desquamation

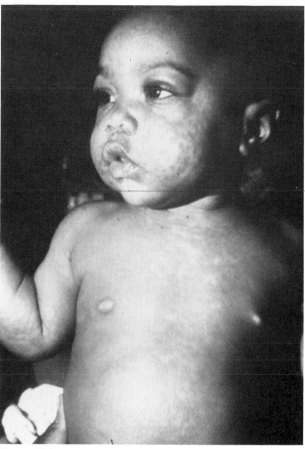

Figure 66-4. Day 2 of measles rash in a 6-month-old black infant. Note confluent lesions on the chest.

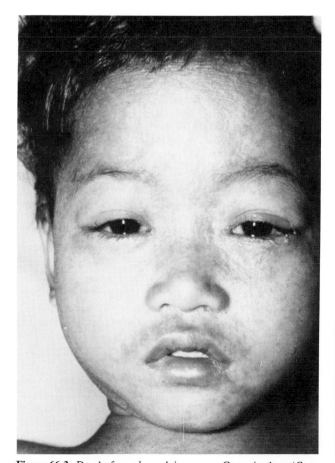

Figure 66-3. Day 1 of measles rash in a young Caucasian boy. (*Courtesy of WHO Expanded Programme on Immunization.*)

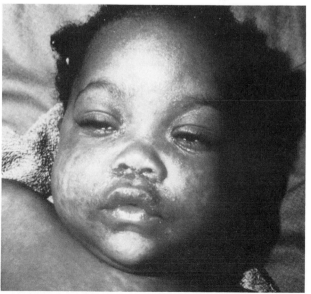

Figure 66-5. Conjunctivitis and rhinorrhea in a 6-month-old infant with measles.

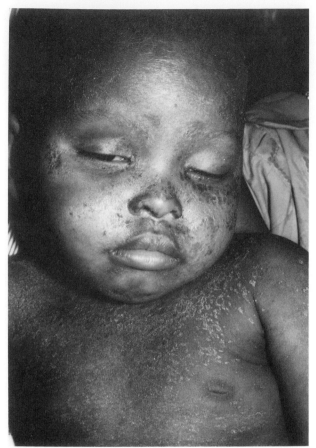

Figure 66-6. Desquamation on day 7 of measles rash in a Haitian infant.

may be caused by deficiencies of vitamin A, pyridoxine, or other factors that have not yet been established. A harsh, non-productive cough is present throughout the febrile period, persists for 1 to 2 weeks in uncomplicated cases of measles, and is often the last symptom to disappear.

Differential diagnosis

Establishing the clinical diagnosis of measles is not difficult in populations where measles has not been controlled by immunization programs. Some diseases that have been confused with measles include dengue, adenovirus infections, and Rocky Mountain spotted fever and other rickettsial diseases. Scarlet fever caused by group A streptococcal infections can be distinguished from measles by the nature and timing of the rash and the absence of a cough. In scarlet fever, the rash onset is usually on the same day as the fever and the rash is generalized, erythematous, and without discrete lesions. Rubella has been mistaken for measles, particularly in older adolescents. Rubella is a milder illness with low-grade fever, but 10 to 15 percent of adolescents may have moderate or high fever accompanied

by mild conjunctivitis or cough. It may be difficult to distinguish the two diseases, particularly if measles has been modified by passive antibody or prior immunization. Kawasaki's disease is a disorder of unknown etiology that is associated with high fever and a variable rash that can mimic the rash of measles. Other clinical features in Kawasaki's disease such as diffuse involvement of mucous membranes with cracking and peeling of the lips, exaggeration of the rash on the knees and elbows, the bright-red appearance of palms and soles and the absence of a cough help differentiate this disease from measles. Toxic shock syndrome occurs rarely in children with staphylococcal infections. The erythrodermal rash is generalized but may have some morbilliform components. Peeling of skin over the fingers and toes occurs 7 to 14 days after the onset of toxic shock syndrome. Occasionally, cases of staphylococcal scalded skin syndrome or drug eruptions including erythema multiforme and toxic epidermal necrolysis have been misdiagnosed as measles. Enteroviruses are common causes of mild illness associated with rashes that sometimes show a morbilliform distribution. Some enteroviruses, particularly the Coxsackie viruses, may cause an enanthem (Fig. 66-2) that has been confused with that of measles, but these viruses usually do not cause cough, coryza, or conjunctivitis.

Mild or "modified" forms of measles with variable symptoms occur in persons with partial protection from transplacentally acquired maternal antibody or from immunoglobulin preparations administered after exposure to measles. A small percentage of children who have received measles vaccine are not fully protected against disease following exposure, but the severity of clinical symptoms is often reduced as compared to measles in children who have not been vaccinated [4].

Laboratory methods

The most common technique for confirming the diagnosis of measles is by demonstrating a fourfold or greater rise in serum antibody titer in acute and convalescent serum specimens [5]. Available antibody detection methods include hemagglutination-inhibition (HI), complement fixation (CF), neutralization, or enzyme-linked immunosorbent assay (ELISA). The HI test has been traditionally used in assays to detect antibody, although the plaque reduction neutralization test is regarded as the most sensitive. A commercially available ELISA is rapidly becoming popular because it is as or more sensitive than HI, convenient, and easy to perform. Neutralization assays provide a direct measurement of the serum antibody that is probably responsible for protection against measles.

Serum should be collected at the time of the first visit and 2 to 4 weeks later. The acute and convalescent specimens should be run simultaneously in the same laboratory. Single sera obtained from 1 to 4 weeks after rash onset have been utilized to confirm the diagnosis if facilities are available to detect measles-specific IgM antibody.

Although the virus can be cultured during the prerash phase

of the disease, culture methods are difficult and not entirely reliable. Fluorescent antibody staining of infected respiratory epithelial cells has been performed, but the technique is not generally available. Smears obtained from tonsillar tissue during the acute phase have been stained with Papanicolau and other tissue-staining methodologies. The characteristic Warthin-Finkeldey cells are often present during the first few days of rash illness. Children with malnutrition may have these cells and shed virus for a more prolonged period of time [6].

Lymphocytopenia may occur during the acute illness, and a total lymphocyte count of less than 2000 has been associated with increased complication and fatality rates. The platelet count generally decreases during the acute illness and in rare instances manifests as thrombocytopenic purpura or disseminated intravascular coagulation (black measles). Black measles has a high case-fatality rate, and contributing factors such as secondary bacterial sepsis have not been ruled out in many cases.

COMPLICATIONS

Complications associated with measles have been reported to affect virtually all organ systems of the body (Table 66-1). Respiratory infections are the most common cause of significant morbidity and mortality in children with clinical measles. Otitis media occurs primarily in children under 10 years of age and is probably the most common respiratory complication. Laryngotracheobronchitis (or croup) can cause severe airway obstruction. Pneumonia may be due to the measles virus alone or to secondary infection with other viral agents, especially herpes simplex and adenoviruses, or bacterial organisms including pneumococci, *Haemophilus influenzae,* staphylococci, *Klebsiella,* and *Escherichia coli.* In several populations, measles has been demonstrated to be a significant factor associated with a high percentage of lower respiratory tract illnesses in hospitalized children over 6 months of age.

Table 66-1. Complications associated with measles infections by organ system

Respiratory:	Neurological:
Otitis media/mastoiditis	Convulsions
Pneumonia	Encephalitis
Laryngotracheobronchitis	Postinfectious encephalopathy
(croup)	Subacute sclerosing
Gastrointestinal:	panencephalitis (SSPE)
Mesenteric adenitis/	Reye's syndrome
appendicitis	Guillain-Barré syndrome
Enteritis	Transverse myelitis
Hepatitis	Dermatological:
Malnutrition	Severe desquamation
Mouth sores	Cardiovascular:
Hematological:	Myocarditis
Thrombocytopenic purpura	
Disseminated intravascular	
coagulation (black measles)	

Children with measles usually have mild irregularities of the cornea and iridocyclitis detectable by slit-lamp examination [8]. Children with vitamin A deficiency are at high risk of developing blindness due to severe keratitis and subsequent corneal scarring. Although the measles virus alone can probably cause sufficient damage to lead to scarring, there is some evidence to indicate that secondary herpes simplex infections contribute to the severe damage. In some areas, postmeasles keratitis has been the most common cause of blindness.

Measles infects the intestinal tract and is commonly associated with diarrhea in developing countries [7]. Some children have a protein-losing enteropathy and may lose 6 to 9 percent of their plasma protein in a single 24-h period. Secondary infections with bacterial enteric pathogens probably contribute to prolonged diarrhea, but studies have usually not revealed increased rates of particular bacterial pathogens as compared to children without measles in the same populations with diarrhea. Diarrhea is one of the major factors contributing to the well-documented adverse impact of measles on nutritional status [7]. Other contributing factors include decreased food intake because of malaise, sores in the mouth, increased metabolic requirements in the presence of fever, and inappropriate withholding of food during acute illness by parents and health care practitioners [3]. Secondary skin infections associated with staphylococcal or streptococcal infections occur occasionally in malnourished children.

Case-fatality rates for measles have ranged from as low as 1 per 10,000 reported cases in the United States in recent years to as high as 30 or 40 percent in infants under 1 year of age in selected populations. In all populations, the highest case-fatality rate has occurred in infants 6 to 11 months of age, and it decreases with increasing age until 20 years of age. The overall case-fatality rate for measles has been estimated at 3 to 6 percent in developing countries but is much higher in some countries (Table 66-2). These data probably underestimate the overall impact of measles on all childhood mortality because many children who die following measles are incorrectly classified as victims of respiratory disease or diarrhea. Increased mortality rates in children who have had measles as compared to children who have not have been demonstrated in Guinea-Bissau, Gambia, Bangladesh, and Haiti for up to 9 months after the onset of disease (Table 66-3). This increased mortality is probably due to the adverse effect of measles on nutritional status and the immune system which predisposes children to increased severity of disease due to respiratory and enteric pathogens. Other investigations have revealed that measles vaccine could prevent the majority of all deaths occurring from 9 months to 5 years of age.

Factors associating with increased severity of measles include young age at the time of measles, lower socioeconomic status, crowding, lack of access to health care, probably malnutrition, especially with specific nutrient deficiencies (vitamin A), and underlying immunodeficiency [9,10]. Respiratory complication rates are inversely associated with age (Table

Table 66-2. Measles case fatality rates as determined from prospective community studies in developing countries

Country	Author	Year published	0–4 years		All ages	
			No. cases	Case fatality rate, %	No. cases	Case fatality rate, %
Africa:						
Guinea-Bissau (rural)	Asby	1984	101	34	162	24
Guinea-Bissau (urban)	Asby	1984	124	15	161	14
Gambia	McGregor	1964	259	22		
Senegal	Pison	1988	537	18		
Nigeria	Morley	1967	222	7		
Kenya	Muller	1977	863	4	1089	4
Asia:						
Bangladesh (rural)	Koster	1981	510	4	896	4
Bangladesh (rural)	Bhuiya	1987	3458	2		
India (rural)	Sinha	1977	72	2	181	1
India (urban)	Reddy	1986	318	0		
Latin America:						
Guatemala	Gordon	1965	292	5	449	4
Guatemala	Mata	1978	231	4	276	3

Source: Adapted from P. Asby, and J. Clements; World Health Organization Expanded Programme on Immunization.

66-4) and directly contribute to the highest age-specific case fatality rates in infants between 6 and 12 months of age. This pattern has held for industrialized and developing countries throughout the world. The case-fatality rates in lower socio-economic populations of industrialized countries in the late 1800s were similar to those observed in developing countries today [3].

Studies on the role of preexisting malnutrition have yielded inconsistent results. During times of famine in industrialized countries, the measles case fatality rate has increased two- to fourfold. Malnutrition adversely affects the immune response as measured by the function of polymorphonuclear cells and cell-mediated immunity. Also, malnourished children have prolonged excretion of measles virus in their respiratory tract as compared to well-nourished children. However, in recent studies in Guinea-Bissau and Bangladesh, the preexposure nutritional status of children who died from measles was not significantly different from that of children who survived [7,9].

Vitamin A is essential for maintenance of the integrity of epithelial cells, and measles affects epithelial surfaces in the respiratory and gastrointestinal tracts. In a study by Sommer et al. [11], children with clinical signs of vitamin A deficiency had increased mortality rates as compared with the rates observed in normal children, but measles-associated deaths were not distinguished from respiratory-disease- and diarrhea-associated deaths in this study. Supplementation with vitamin A at

Table 66-3. Mortality during 9 months of follow-up for measles patients and community controls, The Gambia

Age at infection	Mortality of measles cases		Mortality of community controls 0–9 mo later	OR*	CI$_{95\%}$[†]
	Acute	Delayed 1–9 mo later			
3–11 mos	18% (2/11)	56% (5/9)	3% (3/94)	37.9	10.6–135.3
1–2 yrs	9% (3/35)	13% (4/32)	2% (3/190)	8.9	2.4–33.0
3–4 yrs	6% (2/31)	7% (2/29)	1% (1/182)	13.4	2.0–89.1
5–6 yrs	0% (0/36)	6% (2/36)	1% (2/188)	5.5	0.9–32.9

*Odds ratio (OR) for delayed mortality of measles cases compared with mortality of controls.
[†]95% confidence interval.

Source: Adapted from [33] P. Asby and J. Clements (World Health Organization).

Table 66-4. Complications noted in 306 cases of measles by age group, Chicago, Illinois

| | Age group in years | | | | | | | | | |
| | 0–4 | | 5–9 | | 10–14 | | 15+ | | Totals | |
	No.	%	No.	%	No.	%	No.	%	No.	%
Otitis media	43	(21.4)	11	(12.6)	2	(13.3)	0	(0)	56	(18.3)
Pneumonia	22	(10.9)	6	(6.9)	0	(01)	0	(0)	28	(9.2)
Total in age group	201		87		15		3		306	

the time of acute measles for children in Tanzania with clinical signs of vitamin A deficiency was associated with a reduction in mortality during the following month [12]. However, high case fatality rates following measles are well documented in populations without recognized vitamin A deficiency. The role of vitamin A supplementation for children with measles warrants further study in these populations.

Crowding has been demonstrated to be a factor associated with increased case fatality rates in children in Guinea-Bissau in studies by Asby et al. [9]. The probable biological explanation for this phenomenon is higher virus inocula in children exposed within households. An inoculum effect on severity of disease has been observed with several other viral infections. This phenomenon may explain the increased case fatality rates in lower socioeconomic status populations without malnutrition.

The presence of primary or acquired cell-mediated immunodeficiency disorders increases the risk of severe complications and mortality from measles. Children with agammaglobulinemia have developed clinical measles, but they did not have a rash and they usually recovered without increased complication rates. Children with T-cell deficiency disorders including leukemia and HIV-1 infections have had very high case fatality rates from acute measles.

Neurological complications from measles occur in 1 to 4 per 1000 infected children [13,14]. The most common manifestation is febrile seizures, which are not associated with persistent residua. Encephalitis or postinfectious encephalopathy occurs in approximately 1 in every 1000 infected children and is commonly associated with severe neurological deficits. Recent studies have revealed that measles antigen cannot be demonstrated in the central nervous system in most cases of encephalitis and that the etiology is most likely due to an abnormal immune response [15].

SSPE is a chronic neurological degenerative disorder associated with persistence of the measles virus in the central nervous system. The initial manifestations of SSPE are often misdiagnosed, since children present with gradually evolving behavioral disorders, declining school performance, and, eventually, myoclonic seizures. Characteristic electroencephalograms reveal a burst-suppression pattern, and the diagnosis can be made by demonstration of measles-specific antibody in cerebrospinal fluid or characteristic histopatholgy on brain bi-opsy or postmortem specimens. Factors associated with SSPE in controlled studies in the United States have included young age of measles infection, close exposure to birds, and failure to receive measles vaccine [16]. Unusual patterns of geographical clustering of SSPE have been observed in several countries and remain unexplained.

SSPE occurred in 5 to 20 children per 1,000,000 infected with measles in the United States [17]. The rate is probably higher in most developing countries because of the higher rates of infection in young children.

Measles infection during pregnancy has been associated with delivery of low-birth-weight infants and increased rates of miscarriages, but no increase in congenital malformations has been observed.

TREATMENT

For uncomplicated cases, supportive fluid and nutritional therapy are the only treatment indicated. In developing countries, maintenance of nutrition is critically important. Many children require 4 to 8 weeks to recover their premeasles nutritional status, and studies by Koster et al. [7] reveal that children with diarrhea and measles have decreased weight gain as compared with children without measles for 6 to 12 months (Fig. 66–7). Recent studies confirm that feeding non-lactose-containing foods during measles with or without diarrhea is not harmful and will help maintain nutritional status while diminishing duration of diarrhea. Breast feeding should be continued during the course of illness, but overcoming cultural beliefs and practices may be difficult in some countries. Most children with acute measles have loss of appetite, and the presence of oral lesions is usually associated with decreased food intake. Since malnutrition is an important complication of measles, parents should be encouraged to provide food even in the presence of diarrhea. If children become dehydrated, oral rehydration solution should be administered and may be alternated with breast milk and other foods during the acute phase of diarrhea.

Children with pneumonia should receive antibacterial agents effective against the most common organisms, pneumococci, *H. influenzae,* and staphylococci. However, opinions differ as to whether penicillin, ampicillin, trimethoprim-sulfamethoxazole, or other specific agents should be employed. When diagnostic facilities are available, blood cultures should be obtained prior to therapy and appropriate treatment initiated.

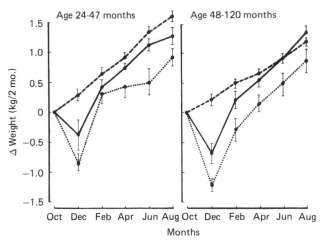

Figure 66-7. Changes in the mean body weight (± SE) in children of village M who had measles between October and 15 December. Dotted line, measles + ≥ 7-day diarrhea; solid line, measles + 0- to 6-day diarrhea; dashed line, controls. Minimum of 22 children per point. There were insufficient data for the children aged 7 to 23 months. (*From [7], with permission.*)

In populations where vitamin A deficiency is a recognized problem, the World Health Organization recommends that all infants receive a single high-dose supplement at the time of clinical measles [*18*]. For children over 1 year of age, the dose is 200,000 international units (IU) as a one-time dose, and it is 100,000 IU for children under 1 year of age. The recommendation to administer vitamin A to children in all countries where the measles case fatality rates exceed 1 percent needs to be further evaluated, since high case fatality rates continue to occur in some developing country populations in the absence of recognized vitamin A deficiency. It is not known whether vitamin A will have a beneficial effect in these populations.

Otitis media is often undiagnosed in countries where otoscopes are not readily available to examine the tympanic membranes. When diagnosed, antimicrobial agents (ampicillin or trimethoprim-sulfamethoxazole) should be administered for 10 days.

Laryngotracheobronchitis or croup can be severe. Although no specific therapy can reverse the primary process, humidified mist may minimize the severity, and aerosolized racemic epinephrine has been widely utilized in children with croup of other viral etiologies.

No specific therapy is available for treatment of neurological complications. To date, no drugs have proved to be effective for treatment of SSPE.

POPULATION

EPIDEMIOLOGY

Human beings are the principal but not the exclusive host infected by the measles virus. Monkeys in zoos are commonly infected, and the virus has persisted in populations of monkeys with rapid turnover, as observed during importation into the United States during the 1960s. However, transmission among monkeys in the wild does not appear to be an important source for persistence of the virus in nature.

Measles is highly contagious and spreads from person to person. The virus is excreted in high concentrations in respiratory secretions during the prodromal phase of disease and is transmitted by droplets. Airborne transmission has been well documented, and the virus can persist in the air for several hours, as evidenced in outbreaks of measles in medical care facilities. The efficiency of transmission is high. Outbreaks of measles have occurred in populations where only 3 to 7 percent of the individuals were susceptible, but contact rates were high enough to ensure exposure of susceptible individuals.

In unimmunized groups, 98 to 100 percent of the population acquires immunity prior to reaching 18 years of age. Prior to the introduction of vaccines in industrialized countries, the transmission rates were highest in children 4 to 10 years of age. The widespread use of measles vaccine in several industrialized countries has led to significant reductions in disease incidence (Fig. 66-8). In the United States, a more than 99 percent reduction in incidence of reported disease has been observed [*19*]. However, efforts to eradicate measles from this population have been unsuccessful due to continuing transmission among high school and college-age persons, especially during sporting events. Also, transmission has continued in urban settings where immunization rates for children under 2 years of age have been relatively low and contact rates are very high. In all countries, measles has occurred at an earlier age in major cities. In urban settings, measles is often endemic throughout the year, although there is some seasonality to the disease transmission rates. In several developing countries, 30 to 35 percent of infants have developed serological evidence of measles by 11 to 12 months of age and 80 percent or more of the children have been infected by the time they are 3 years old [*20–22*]. Age-specific attack rates for children living in rural areas are lower in the first few years of life. Most coun-

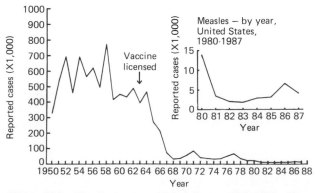

Figure 66-8. Measles by year, United States, 1950–1987. (*From* [*19*].)

tries have demonstrated 2- or 3-year cycles of peak measles activity. With the widespread use of measles vaccine and decreasing overall incidence of measles, the intervals between peaks have expanded in the United States, Canada, and other countries to 4 to 6 years.

The seasonal pattern of measles in the temperate zones is characterized by a late winter–early spring peak. In the northern hemisphere, this corresponds with February to May, and in the southern hemisphere, August to December. In tropical climates, measles often follows the pattern of rainfall, with peak activity shortly after the onset of rainy season (Fig. 66-9).

PREVENTION AND CONTROL

Passive Antibodies

Measles may be prevented by passively acquired antibodies. Since almost all children acquire some antibodies from their mother, infants are protected for the first 5 to 9 months of life. The administration of human immunoglobulin (γ-globulin or immune serum globulin) in doses of 0.25 mL/kg given within a few days after exposure has been demonstrated to prevent clinical manifestations of measles. Some treated children will develop subclinical cases of measles and long-term immunity. Lower doses of immunoglobulin preparations (0.1 mL/kg) will modify the disease. Intravenous immunoglobulin preparations are more expensive but provide equivalent or better levels of protection. The equivalent of a protective dose of standard immunoglobulin is 40 to 50 mg protein per kilogram. Immunoglobulins are primarily given to immunocompromised individuals in industrialized countries for whom live measles vaccines are contraindicated. Immunoglobulin preparations are too costly for routine use in developing country settings and play little role in the overall control of measles. Measles vaccines should be administered to all susceptible individuals during outbreaks.

Measles Vaccines

The original measles vaccines that were approved for use in children in 1963 were attenuated (Edmonston B) and inactivated vaccines. Since these vaccines are no longer in use, they will not be reviewed here. The vaccines currently in use throughout the world are further attenuated live measles virus vaccines. Several different vaccine strains have been prepared, but most were derived from the original Edmonston strain isolated in tissue culture in 1954 by Enders and Peebles [23] (Table 66-5). Serological studies have revealed that these vaccines induced seroconversion in 95 to 98 percent of recipients who were old enough to have lost all maternal antibody.

The standard dose of measles vaccine is at least 10^3 TCID$_{50}$ (50 percent tissue culture infective doses). Although seroconversion can be induced by giving smaller doses of vaccine to children without interfering maternal antibodies, this practice is not recommended. Measles vaccines are heat-labile, and some deterioration may have occurred between the time of manufacture and the time of administration at clinics. Manufacturers usually allow for some loss in titer and prepare the vaccine in doses of $10^{3.3}$ to $10^{4.2}$ TCID$_{50}$ to be administered in a volume of 0.5 mL.

The vaccine is usually lyophilized and reconstituted with sterile distilled water immediately prior to administration. Measles vaccine is generally administered subcutaneously in the upper arm but can be administered in the anterolateral thigh. Equivalent seroconversion rates have been demonstrated when the vaccine is given intramuscularly. Although two investigations have revealed that measles vaccine can be reconstituted with diphtheria and tetanus toxoids and pertussis vaccine combined (DTP), this practice is not recommended, as there are variations between manufacturers and stability studies have not been performed [24].

The lyophilized vaccine can be safely frozen at −20°C without loss of potency. The enhanced stabilizers in use for most, but not all, vaccines have resulted in maintenance of potency at 37°C for 7 days. The optimal maintenance of the "cold

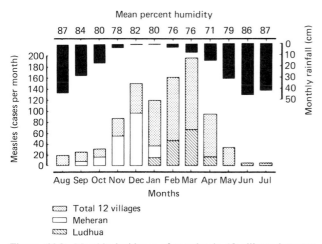

Figure 66-9. Monthly incidence of measles in 12 villages between August 1975 and July 1976, compared with monthly 10-year means for relative humidity (%) and rainfall (cm). (*From [7], with permission.*)

Table 66-5. Measles vaccines and source strains

Vaccine strain	Original source strain
AIK-C	Edmonston
Schwarz	Edmonston A
FF-8	Edmonston A
Connaught	Edmonston B
Edmonston-Zagreb	Edmonston B
Moraten	Edmonston B
Cam-70	Tanabe
Leningrad-16	Leningrad strain
Shanghai 191	?

chain'' from the manufacturing site to the time of administration of vaccine is of paramount importance, especially in the warm climate countries. The World Health Organization recommends that measles vaccine be maintained at 4 to 8°C at all times.

WHO recommends that measles vaccine be administered to children in developing countries at 9 months of age or as soon thereafter as possible. In Canada and several Scandinavian and European countries, the recommended age is 12 months. In the United States, advisory groups have recommended postponement of immunization to 15 months of age to ensure that all maternal antibody has disappeared from the body. Several studies in the United States demonstrated that small amounts of maternal antibody may persist until 12 or more months of age and modify or inhibit the antibody response to measles vaccine [25]. However, in developing countries, infants lose passively acquired maternal antibodies at a faster rate than infants in industrialized countries. The mechanism for this enhanced rate of loss of passively acquired antibody has not yet been determined, but it is most likely related to repeated infections and perhaps loss of antibody through the intestinal tract during episodes of diarrhea. Studies by Black et al. [26] have demonstrated that the average amount of antibody transmitted from mothers to infants appears to be relatively constant from population to population.

Since passively acquired maternal antibodies are lost at a more rapid rate in developing countries, seroconversion rates following measles vaccine are higher than those observed in industrialized countries when measles vaccine is administered at 9 months of age (Fig. 66-10). Although variation exists in age-specific seroconversion rates following measles vaccination, immunization at 9 months appears to be a reasonable compromise (Fig. 66-11). Unfortunately, immunization of 50 percent or more of infants between 9 and 12 months of age in densely populated urban centers has not had a significant impact on the transmission of measles in some communities [21,22]. The inability to successfully vaccinate a high proportion of infants under 9 months of age is the largest impediment to the effective control of measles in developing countries.

Recent studies in several developing country populations have revealed that increasing the dose of measles vaccine for infants under 9 months of age could elevate serological response rates in spite of the presence of low levels of maternal antibody [27,28]. For many years it was believed that all attenuated and further attenuated measles vaccines were similar. The Edmonston-Zagreb strain of measles vaccine produced in Yugoslavia and Mexico appears to be more effective in immunizing infants in the presence of maternal antibodies than the Schwarz strain used in many countries. Although several studies are in progress and the data are incomplete, the accumulated evidence suggests that infants might be effectively immunized at 6 months of age or even younger with doses of Edmonston-Zagreb vaccine of $10^{4.5}$ to $10^{5.5}$ $TCID_{50}$ [29]. No increased rates of adverse effects have been observed in the

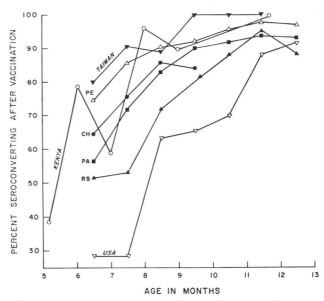

Figure 66-10. Seroconversion rates after vaccination at various ages between 6 and 13 months. Sources: United States, Kenya; Taiwan; Pernambuco (PE), Para (PA), and Rio Grande do Sul (RS), states of Brazil, and Santiago, Chile (CH). (*From Black FL, Measles: In Warren KS and Mahmoud AAF (eds): Tropical and Geographical Medicine, 1st ed. New York, McGraw-Hill, 1984, with permission.*)

infants who received these high-titer vaccines as compared to infants who received lower-titer measles vaccines. The data are inadequate to determine whether use of the Edmonston-Zagreb vaccine should become standard practice in developing countries and whether sufficient quantities of this strain of vaccine can be made available for all countries. Additional studies are in progress to evaluate other strains of vaccine that might be equally or more effective in young infants.

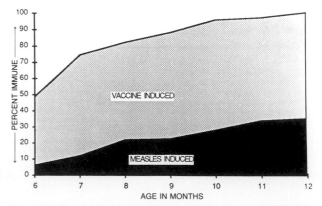

Figure 66-11. Immunity among Haitian infants after measles infection (measles-induced) or vaccination against measles (vaccine-induced). (*From Halsey NA, et al: N Engl J Med, Feb. 27, 1986, with permission.*)

Approximately 10 to 15 percent of infants immunized with standard vaccines have developed fever, and 10 to 20 percent have had a generalized rash lasting for 1 to 3 days beginning 5 to 7 days after vaccination. The reactions are generally mild and well tolerated. Immunoglobulins should not be given with measles vaccines to modify these reactions as this could interfere with the serological responses. Other complications from measles vaccines are relatively rare. Although neurological complications may occur following vaccination in less than 1 in 1,000,000 vaccinees, the risk is 1000-fold less than the rate of complications following measles in unvaccinated children (Table 66-6). Concurrent respiratory and gastrointestinal infections and skin infections have not interfered with the serological response with measles vaccine and do not constitute a contraindication to the vaccine [30,31]. Although measles vaccine has been demonstrated to depress the delayed hypersensitivity response to purified protein derivative (PPD), measles vaccine does not exacerbate tuberculosis, and it is not necessary to skin-test children before providing the vaccine. In developing countries where measles has not been controlled, measles vaccine should be given to all infants, since unvaccinated children will undoubtedly develop natural measles. Since measles is easily transmitted in hospital settings, hospitalized infants should be vaccinated. More than 200 children with HIV-1 infection have safely received measles vaccines, and advisory groups recommend that HIV-seropositive infants should be vaccinated.

Measles vaccine is commonly combined with rubella and mumps vaccines in industrialized countries throughout the world. Other live and inactivated bacterial and viral vaccines can be administered simultaneously without interference.

IMMUNITY

Natural infection provides lifelong immunity to measles, and children who responded to measles vaccine have been pro-

tected against disease for more than 16 years [32]. Excellent correlation has been demonstrated between the presence of serum neutralization or HI antibodies and protection against clinical measles. Complement-fixing antibodies are also produced following infection or vaccination, but titers decrease to undetectable levels in many individuals within a year, and the assay is less sensitive than HI. Enzyme immunoassays that are equally or more sensitive than the HI test have been developed and are in common use in many laboratories, but nonspecific activity may interfere with the ability to detect low levels of antibody. A WHO reference serum is available from the Statens Seruminstitut in Copenhagen, Denmark, for standardization of antibody assays. The results of antibody assays can be expressed in millinternational units per milliliter (mIU/mL). The precise level of antibody that correlates with protection against disease has not been definitely determined. Preliminary data from studies of neutralization antibody suggest that levels below 200 mIU/mL may not be protective against disease.

The development and persistence of serum antibodies following measles vaccines have been lower but parallel to the response following natural measles. Peak antibody responses occur 6 to 8 weeks after infection or vaccination. In populations isolated from repeat exposure to natural measles, the serum antibody responses after receiving vaccination may wane after 12 to 14 years to levels that are undetectable by HI, but low levels of neutralizing antibody persist. When these children were given additional doses of measles vaccine, they developed secondary antibody responses, suggesting the presence of some persisting immunity in spite of the absence of measurable antibodies [32]. These data suggest that measles vaccine produces immunity for at least 12 to 15 years and may provide lifelong protection. Occasional cases of clinical disease associated with serological responses to measles have been demonstrated in children who initially developed a serum antibody response after receiving measles vaccine. The importance

Table 66-6. Adverse reactions associated with measles vaccines and natural measles

Adverse effect	Estimated rate associated with vaccination	Rate associated with disease	Relative risk, natural disease/vaccine
Fever ≥ 39.4°C	1/16–1/6	1/2–1	3–16
Rash	1/100–1/5	1	5–15
Febrile convulsions	1/2500	1/500–1/100	5–25
Encephalitis/encephalopathy (and other neurological disorders)	<1/1,000,000	1/1000	>1000
Pneumonia	——	1/100–1/10	+ + +*
Subacute sclerosing panencephalitis (SSPE)	<1/1,000,000†	1/200,000–1/50,000	5–20
Thrombocytopenia	Occasional	Common	+*
Thrombocytopenic purpura	Very rare	Rare	+*

*From + to + + + = relative ratio; precise ratio uncertain.
†No cases of SSPE have been documented to be caused by measles vaccine.

Source: Adapted from [30].

of these observations in the context of measles control in developing countries is negligible. Most children who have developed rises in serum measles antibodies after exposure to disease many years after vaccination do not have clinical signs or symptoms of measles.

The use of a two-dose measles vaccine schedule to minimize the vaccine failure rate has been the subject of some debate. Although adopted by several developed countries, this practice has not been endorsed for routine use in developing countries because the increased costs of measles vaccines and delivery programs could be prohibitive. The second dose of measles vaccine would protect only 10 percent or fewer of those children who had already received a single dose. To achieve measles control, it may not be necessary to administer two doses of measles vaccine. However, to achieve measles eradication, a two-dose measles vaccine strategy may be imperative.

Clinical studies of measles vaccine have demonstrated an 85 to 95 percent protective efficacy in children who are immunized after 9 months of age in developing countries and efficacy of 95 percent or more in children in industrialized countries where children have been immunized after 12 months of age.

Several investigations have revealed that children who are vaccinated under 9 months of age with standard vaccine doses have lower seroconversion rates and vaccine efficacy [33]. For children who respond to vaccines, the geometric mean antibody titers were lower in children vaccinated under 9 months of age than in children who were vaccinated at older ages. Therefore, maternal antibodies not only prevented some children from developing an antibody response, but also blunted the response of some children who did respond. Of the children who failed to respond to measles vaccine because of interference by maternal antibody, some failed to develop an HI antibody response following a second dose of measles vaccine administered after 12 months of age [34]. Further investigation revealed that these children had low levels of neutralizing antibodies after the first dose of measles vaccine. These antibodies were sufficient to inhibit an HI response following the second dose of vaccine. Most investigators believe that these children are protected against clinical measles, but more studies and long-term follow-up of these children are necessary.

Measles vaccine is one of the most cost-effective methods of preventing morbidity and mortality in early childhood. The estimates of benefit-to-cost ratio have demonstrated a saving in health care expenditures of 5 to 15 times the investment. If the technical barriers to developing an effective vaccine for children at 6 months of age or younger are overcome successfully, then it may be possible to consider global eradication of measles. The largest challenge in achieving this goal will be to develop effective means to deliver measles vaccine to large numbers of children at an early enough age to prevent the clinical disease and subsequent transmission. In 1988, WHO reported that only 50 percent of the children living in developing countries had received measles vaccine.

REFERENCES

1 Walsh JA: Selective primary health care: Strategies for control of disease in the developing world. IV. Measles. Rev Infect Dis 5:330–340, 1983

2 Koplik HT: The diagnosis of the invasion of measles from a study of the exanthema as it appears on the buccal mucous membrane. Arch Pediatr 13:918–922, 1986

3 Morley DC: Measles in the developing world. Proc R Soc Med 67:1112–1115, 1974

4 Cherry JD: Measles: In Feigin RD and Cherry JD (eds): *Textbook of Pediatric Infectious Diseases*, 2d ed. Philadelphia, Saunders, 1987, pp 1607–1628

5 Norrby E: Measles virus, in Lennette EH, Balous A, Hauster WJ, et al (eds): *Manual of Clinical Microbiology*, 4th ed. Washington DC, American Society for Microbiology, 1985

6 Scheifele DW, Forbes CE: The biology of measles in African children. East Afr Med J 50:169–173, 1973

7 Koster F, Curlin G, Aziz KMA, et al: Synergistic impact of measles and diarrhoea in nutrition and mortality in Bangladesh. Bull WHO 59:309–311, 1986

8 Foster A, Sommer A: Childhood blindness from corneal ulceration in Africa: Causes, prevention, and treatment. Bull WHO 64: 619–23, 1986

9 Asby P, Coovadia II, Bukh J, et al: Severe measles: A reappraisal of the role of nutrition, overcrowding and virus dose. Med Hypoth 18:93–112, 1985

10 Bhuiya A, Wojtyniak B, D'Souza S, et al: Measles case-fatality among under fives: A multivariate analysis of risk factors in rural areas of Bangladesh. Soc Sci Med 24:439–443, 1987

11 Sommer A, Djunaedi E, Loeden AA, et al: Impact of vitamin A supplementation on childhood mortality: A randomized controlled community trial. Lancet i:1169–1173, 1986

12 Barclay AJG, Foster A, Sommer A: Vitamin A supplements and mortality related to measles: A randomized clinical trial. Br Med J 294:294–296, 1987

13 Miller DL: Frequency of complications of measles, 1963. Report on a national inquiry by the Public Health Laboratory Service in collaboration with the Society of Medical Officers of Health. Br Med J 2:75–78, 1964

14 CDC: Measles Surveillance Report No 11, 1977–1981. Issued in September 1982

15 Moench TR, Griffin DE, Obriecht CR, et al: Acute measles virus antigen and RNA. J Infect Dis 158:433–442, 1988

16 Halsey NA, Modlin JF, Jabbour JT, et al: Risk factors in subacute sclerosing panencephalitis: A case control study. Am J Epidemiol 3:415–420, 1980

17 Modlin JF, Jabbour JT, Witte JJ, et al: Epidemiologic studies of measles, measles vaccine, and subacute sclerosing panencephalitis. Pediatrics 59:505–512, 1977

18 Munro I: Vitamin A for measles. Lancet i:1067–68, 1987 (editorial)

19 Centers for Disease Control: Measles 1987. MMWR 36 (54): Sept. 16, 1988

20 Halsey NA, Boulos R, Mode F, et al: Responses to measles vaccine in Haitian infants 6 to 12 months old. Influence of maternal antibodies, malnutrition, and concurrent illnesses. N Engl J Med 313: 544–549, 1985

21 Dabis F, Sow A, Waldman RJ, et al: The epidemiology of measles

in a partially vaccinated population in an African city: Implications for immunization programs. Am J Epidemiol 127:171–178, 1988

22 Taylor WR, Ruti-Kalisa, Ma-Disu M, et al: Measles control in urban Africa complicated by high incidence of measles in the first year of life. Am J Epidemiol 127:788–794, 1988

23 Preblud SR, Katz SL: Measles vaccines, in Plotkin S, Mortimer E (eds): *Vaccine*. Philadelphia, Saunders, 1988

24 John TJ, Selvakumar R, Balraj V, et al: Antibody response to measles vaccine with DTPP. Am J Dis Child 141, 1987

25 Albrecht P, Ennis FA, Saltzman EJ, et al: Persistence of maternal antibody in infants beyond 12 months: Mechanism of measles vaccine failure. J Pediatr 91:715–718, 1977

26 Black FL, Berman LL, Borgono JM, et al: Geographic variation in infant loss of maternal measles antibody and in prevalence of rubella antibody. Am J Epidemiol 124:442–452, 1986

27 Markowitz LE, Bernier RH: Immunization of young infants with Edmonston-Zagreb measles vaccine. Pediatr Infect Dis J 6:804–12, 1987

28 Whittle HC, Mann G, Eccles M, et al: Effects of dose and strain of vaccine on success of measles vaccination of infants aged 4–5 months. Lancet i:963–966, 1988

29 Job JS, Halsey NA, Boulos R, et al: Comparison of Schwarz and Edmonston-Zagreb measles vaccines in Haitian infants. Presented at Workshop on Alternative Strategies for Measles Vaccination, Washington, DC, September 19, 1988.

30 Halsey NA, Stetler HC: Adverse reactions associated with vaccines administered in Expanded Program on Immunization projects, in Halsey NA and de Quadros C (eds): *Recent Advances in Immunization*. Washington, DC, Pan American Health Organization, 1983, pp 90–102

31 Galazka AM, Lauer BA, Henderson RH, et al: Indications and contra-indications for vaccines used in the Expanded Programme on Immunization. Bull WHO 62:357–66, 1984

32 Krugman S: Further-attenuated measles vaccine: Characteristics and use. Rev Infect Dis 5:477–481, 1983

33 Hull HF, Williams PJ, Oldfield F: Measles mortality and vaccine efficacy in rural West Africa. Lancet i:972–975, 1983

34 Stetler HC, Orenstein WA, Bernier RH, et al: Impact of revaccinating children who initially received measles vaccine before 10 months of age. Pediatrics 77:471–476, 1986

CHAPTER 67 / *Poxviruses* · Joel G. Breman

The poxviruses (family Poxviridae) are DNA-containing viruses classed according to morphological and antigenic similarities [*1*]. The genus *Orthopoxvirus* includes variola, monkeypox, and vaccinia viruses; the following discussion will focus on these viruses as they are most important for humans. Variola virus caused smallpox, an acute febrile eruptive disease that in its most severe form (variola major) killed up to 20 percent or more of patients. Smallpox has been eradicated, the last endemic case having occurred in Somalia in 1977, and the world was declared free of this disease in 1980 [*2*].

DEFINITION AND CHARACTERIZATION

The orthopoxviruses are brick-shaped, approximately 300 nm by 200 nm by 250 nm. Their genomes are a single molecule of double-stranded DNA. They are indistinguishable by electron microscopy, cross-react with antivaccinia serum, and produce a soluble hemagglutinin. The orthopoxviruses grow best on the chorioallantoic membrane (CAM) of embryonated chicken eggs. Each species can be identified by pock morphology and by optimal growth at certain temperatures and pH range [*1,3*]; they also grow in tissue culture. With the development of genome mapping using site-specific restriction endonucleases, strain and variant characterization of the poxviruses can now be done [*4,5*]. This powerful technique has demonstrated distinct differences in the genetic makeup of orthopoxviruses, particularly in the nucleotide sequences at the end segments of the genomes.

PATIENT

PATHOGENESIS AND PATHOLOGY

Knowledge of the pathogenesis of smallpox (and other orthopoxviruses) comes mainly from studies of mousepox [*6*] and rabbitpox [*7*]. The disease is usually spread by respiratory droplets; virus enters the upper respiratory tract of a newly contaminated individual, seeds the mucous membranes, and passes rapidly into local lymph nodes where primary multiplication occurs. A short viremia ensues, followed by a 4- to 14-day latent period during which time virus is removed and multiplies in the reticuloendothelial system. A second viremia occurs just before, or with, the prodrome onset. The mucous membranes of the mouth and pharynx become heavily infected at this time. Virus is usually undetectable in the blood after the 2- to 3-day prodome unless the disease is fulminant.

The skin is the major organ affected by the poxviruses, although the spleen, lymph nodes, liver, bone marrow, kidneys, and other viscera may also have large quantities of virus during the secondary multiplication phase. The virus invades the capillary epithelium of the corium leading to the evolution of macules, papules, vesicles, pustules, and crusts, the typical poxvirus lesions.

Neutralizing (neut) antibodies appear toward the end of the first week of illness but may be delayed in severe infections. Hemagglutination-inhibition (HI) and complement-fixing (CF) antibodies are detectable by the end of the second week. Neutralizing antibodies remain for many years while levels of HI and CF antibodies are variable, not reliable diagnostically, and begin to decrease after 1 year.

CLINICAL MANIFESTATIONS

The incubation period of smallpox varied from 7 to 17 days, with a mean of 10 to 12 days. Headache, backache, and fever began abruptly, coupled with muscle pain, severe malaise, and prostration. The temperature often rose to greater than 40°C (104°F) and decreased to normal over the 2- to 3-day prodrome. During this preeruptive period an initial transient erythematous or petechial rash was seen rarely over the inguinal, flank, and axillary areas. This rash faded before onset of the focal eruption. With severe cases of variola major the temperature often remained elevated throughout the prodrome and early eruption. Conversely, all signs and symptoms were milder with variola minor.

Red or dark brown macules were first noted predominantly over the face and extremities, although the whole body was covered in severe cases. The macules evolved over 1 to 2 days to firm 2- to 3-mm papules. After 1 to 2 days these became discrete 2- to 4-mm vesicles that remained for 2 to 3 days. Pustules of 4 to 6 mm formed about the end of the first week of the eruption, 9 to 10 days after clinical disease onset. These were pearly hard and well-fixed in the dermis. They remained for 5 to 8 days, when crusting began. The patient may have had a low-grade fever during the eruption and a second temperature elevation often occurred throughout the pustular phase, especially if there was secondary bacterial infection. Crusts began to separate by the end of the second week of the eruption and all crusts had usually fallen by 21 days [8]. Hypopigmented areas became hyperpigmented after several months.

Smallpox lesions had a peripheral (centrifugal) distribution (Fig. 67-1). Those over the body evolved usually through the same stages; however, pustules and crusts were frequently seen together. Facial, palm, and sole lesions persisted longer.

Skin lesions usually contained abundant viral particles throughout the acute illness. Virus was present in the throat, urine, and conjunctival secretions but diminished as convalescence progressed [9]. Infection with smallpox probably conferred lifelong immunity.

Pock-marking or pitting lesions of the face were seen commonly. These tended to disappear with time, particularly in children. It is disputed as to how often secondary bacterial infections occurred; when associated with pneumonia and bacteremia they were a substantial cause of mortality. Panophthalmitis and blindness from viral keratitis or secondary infection of the eye occurred in about 1 percent of infections due to variola major.

Useful classifications of smallpox according to evolution of the lesions and severity of clinical disease have been proposed by Dixon [8] and the World Health Organization. The WHO classification is more simplified and includes four recognizable clinical types [10]. The "ordinary" form, described above, constituted about 90 percent of cases. The disease severity and infectivity paralleled the extent of the eruption. The case fatality rate varied from 8 to 40 percent with variola major; variola minor, occurring mainly in South America and south and east Africa, caused death in less than 1 percent of cases. A "modified" type, comprising 5 to 7 percent of cases, occurred in persons previously vaccinated. It was characterized by a milder prodrome and fewer skin lesions, which were often smaller, more superficial, evolved more rapidly than ordinary lesions, and resulted in few deaths. Five to seven percent of the cases were of the "flat" type. Lesions evolved more slowly and the vesicles and papules were flat, generalized over the body, and often coalesced. The case fatality rate was above 50 percent. "Hemorrhagic" smallpox comprised less than 1 percent of cases and diagnosis was most difficult. This form was almost invariably fatal and patients usually died between the fifth and seventh day of illness.

Another variety of smallpox was *variola sine eruptione* seen in previously vaccinated close contacts of patients or in young infants with maternal antibody. This mild or modified illness was characterized by brief temperature elevation, headache, and influenzalike symptoms; likewise, the patient could be entirely asymptomatic. This form was postulated to have affected at least 41 percent of household contacts of overt cases [11]. There is no evidence that asymptomatic but infected patients transmitted the disease.

DIAGNOSIS

Varicella, or chickenpox, provides over 95 percent of the diagnostic dilemmas although any papulovesicular disease may be confused with one caused by a poxvirus. A patient with chickenpox is frequently exposed to a typical case about 2 weeks before onset of illness. The disease is usually mild. The eruption has a centripetal (central) concentration over the torso. Lesions occur in clusters ("crops") over different areas, and evolve from macule to crusting state in 4 to 6 days. Different stages of lesion evolution are seen over the body and desquamation is usual by 7 to 10 days. The differences between smallpox or monkeypox and chickenpox are seen in Table 67-1. (The differences between smallpox and monkeypox are described later.)

Drug rashes, including erythema multiforme exudativum (Stevens-Johnson syndrome), can be diagnosed best by careful interrogation and observation of the eruption evolution. A prodrome is unusual. Drugs containing sulfonamides cause more severe vesicular and bullous rashes than other drugs. A morbilliform rash on the face due to measles virus or coxsackie virus may, in the early stages, be confused with smallpox. The

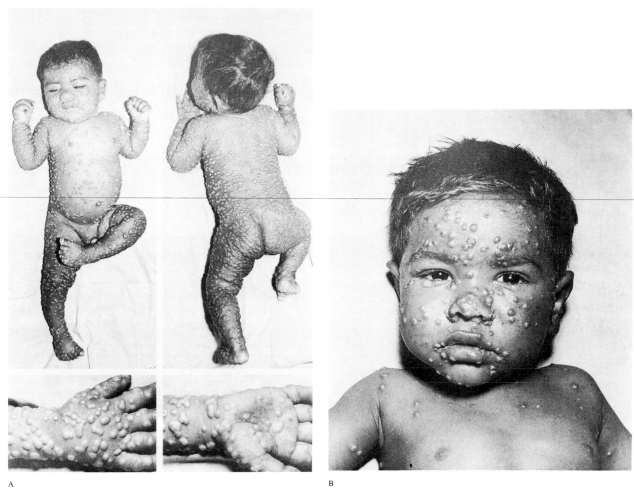

A   B

Figure 67-1. *A, B.* Smallpox on about day 8 of eruption. (*Courtesy of WHO.*)

typical measles prodrome, presence of Koplik's spots, and disease evolution reveal the diagnosis. Insect bites are often linear and may have a peripheral distribution over areas unprotected by clothing. Occasionally, there is an allergic response to the bites and they can become secondarily infected.

A single case of suspected smallpox is of utmost international concern. Therefore, the diagnosis must be confirmed. If it is in doubt national authorities and WHO must be contacted immediately. Scrapings of skin lesions and serum specimens should be sent to a WHO Collaborating Center (Viral Exanthems and Herpesvirus Branch, Division of Viral Diseases, Center for Infectious Diseases, Centers for Disease Control, Atlanta, Georgia 30333, U.S.A.; Laboratory of Smallpox Prophylaxis, Research Institute of Viral Preparations, Moscow, U.S.S.R.). Collection, preparation, and shipment of specimens should follow special recommendations [*12*].

In addition to electron microscopy and culture on chorioallantoic membrane (CAM) and on various cell cultures, serological (neut, HI, and CF) tests can be done. The radioim-

munoassay test has shown promise for identifying specific antibodies to variola, monkeypox, and vaccina viruses when sera have been suitably absorbed [*13*].

TREATMENT

As there is no specific treatment for the poxviruses, supportive care is required to minimize skin infections and ensure survival of severely ill patients. Systemic penicillins or other antibiotics should be used if lesions are dense, widespread, and secondarily infected, and if bacterial infection endangers the eyes. Daily rinsing of the eyes with sterile eyewash or saline is usually needed in severe cases. Patients require adequate nutrition and hydration because substantial fluid and protein can be lost from febrile persons with dense weeping lesions. Topical idoxuridine (IUDR-Dendrid, Herplex, Stoxil) should be used for corneal lesions. Antiviral agents, such as the thiosemicarbazone compounds or cytosine arabinoside, are not effective once the symptoms or signs of smallpox have begun.

Table 67-1. Differential diagnosis of smallpox or monkeypox and chickenpox

Evaluation criteria	Smallpox or monkeypox	Chickenpox
History		
Recent residence in smallpox or monkeypox endemic zone	+ + +	±
Contact with poxvirus	+ + +	−
Contact with chickenpox	−	+ + +
Prior vaccination*	−	±
Incubation period	10–12 days (7–17)	14–16 days
Prodrome	2–4 days	0–2 days
Fever	+ + +	±
Headache, backache	+ + +	+
Muscle pain, malaise	+ +	+
Pallor, transient rash	±	−
Physical Examination		
Vaccination scar*	−	±
Eruption		
Distribution	Peripheral	Central
Peak	7–10 days	3–5 days
Lesion stages	Same	Different
Size	4–6 mm	2–4 mm
Shape	Round	Oval
Depth	Deep	Superficial
Desquamation	14–21 days	6–14 days
Complications		
Skin infection	±	±
Facial scarring	+ +	±
Pneumonia	+	+
Blindness	+	−
Encephalitis	±	±
Case Fatality Rate		<1%
Asia	20%	
Africa†	15%	
South America	0.5%	
Children <1 year	40–60%	20%‡
Laboratory Diagnosis		
Electron microscope	Poxvirus particles	Herpes-varicella particles
Culture on chorioallantoic membrane	Characteristic pocks	Does not grow
Serology	Rise in antibody to *Orthopoxvirus*	Rise in antibody to varicella virus

*Less than 10 percent of patients with smallpox or monkeypox have given a history of prior vaccination or have a vaccination scar; as smallpox vaccination is no longer required, patients with chickenpox may not have a vaccination scar.
†Monkeypox with a 10 percent case fatality rate (CFR) has been observed only in west and central Africa; some countries in east Africa had variola minor with a CFR of <1 percent.
‡Neonatal chickenpox has a 20 percent CFR.

POPULATION

HISTORY AND EPIDEMIOLOGY OF SMALLPOX

Smallpox has been known since at least 1160 B.C when it probably killed the Egyptian Pharaoh Ramses V. The disease decimated large populations throughout the globe, up to the mid-twentieth century [2,8,14]. In 1959, a global eradication program began under the aegis of WHO, but this faltered because of lack of support. In 1967, a well-coordinated intensified eradication program began. Eleven years later transmission of smallpox had been interrupted throughout the world [2,15].

The unvaccinated, usually young children, had the highest attack rates. The mode of transmission was by aerosolized, virus-laden, respiratory droplets transmitted during face to face contact. Periodic epidemics occurred every 5 to 10 years in many endemic countries due to the buildup of susceptible individuals. The disease was most prevalent in the tropics in the dry season. This was ascribed to increased virus survival in low humidity [16] as well as to travel and other sociocultural patterns.

In the 1960s and 1970s smallpox was no longer viewed as an explosive disease. This was due to the relatively low rate of secondary spread (25 to 40 percent) and the 10- to 12-day incubation period. Measles, chickenpox, and influenza, for example, all have secondary attack rates of about 90 percent among susceptible persons.

PREVENTION

Vaccination

Variolation, or inoculation of material from smallpox lesions into the skin or nose of susceptible persons to protect by causing a mild illness, had been practiced in many areas of the world for centuries, but the disease was often severe in recipients and other contacts. Experimental inoculation of material from cowpox lesions was known in England and Germany since 1760, but the first scientific report proving the protection of cowpox against smallpox is attributed to Edward Jenner in 1796 [17]. Jenner, a British country physician, first inoculated young James Phipps in 1796 with cowpox taken from the hand of milkmaid Sara Nelmes and found him immune to smallpox when challenged 6 weeks later. Thus was launched the medical practice of immunoprophylaxis.

The major technical difficulties during the 160 years following Jenner's epochal discovery were related to vaccine production, potency, and stability. Production problems were partially resolved when injection of seed virus into the cleansed skin of calves proved commercially feasible. More recently, rigid requirements for vaccine production and standardization were developed by WHO to ensure potency. The use of lyophilization assured vaccine stability for long periods at high temperatures [18], allowing potent smallpox vaccine to be taken to every corner of the globe.

Invention of the bifurcated needle for administering smallpox vaccination during the intensified eradication program also gave great impetus to field activities. This simple, lightweight device virtually replaced less efficient vaccination instruments, although the needleless jet injector gun has been used in some mass campaigns.

History is unclear on the origin of vaccinia virus (smallpox vaccine), but it is thought to derive from Jenner's virus, the "cowpoxing" agent. By DNA mapping, cowpox isolates are clearly distinguishable from vaccinia. Vaccinia virus multiplies in the basilar epithelium causing a local cellular reaction at the vaccination site. A small, red, hard papule with an erythematous areola appears within 3 days. The lesion is a grayish-white, loculated, 1- to 2-cm-diameter vesicle by 6 days. On about the seventh day central umbilication begins. A lesion having this appearance at 6 to 8 days following vaccination is called a *Jennerian vesicle*. Crusting begins in the center of the lesion and spreads peripherally in the next 3 to 5 days. Local edema and a dark crust remain to the third week. Induration and congestion at the vaccination site between 6 and 8 days after inoculation signal successful revaccination.

A "major" vaccination reaction in primary vaccinees causes a Jennerian vesicle, and revaccinees have evidence of inflammation 6 to 8 days following vaccination. All other reactions are termed *equivocal* and indicate that virus multiplication may not have occurred and another vaccination should be given unless the level of neutralizing antibody is satisfactory. A successful primary vaccination confers immunity to smallpox and probably to other orthopoxviruses in over 95 percent of persons for at least 5 years, and revaccination probably protects for at least 10 to 20 years.

Complications from smallpox vaccination in the United States have undergone close scrutiny [19,20]. Abandonment of smallpox vaccination throughout the world was recommended by WHO following certification of eradication in 1980 [2]. This was because the risks from the procedure (postvaccinal encephalitis, eczema vaccinatum, progressive vaccinia, generalized vaccinia, ocular vaccinia, etc.) outweighed the nonexistent threat from endemic smallpox. Vaccination is advised now only as an occupational safety precaution, e.g., for laboratory workers in direct contact with human orthopoxviruses.

Vaccinia immune globulin (VIG) is used for severe vaccination complications (e.g., eczema vaccinatum, generalized vaccinia, or sight-threatening eye lesions) at a dose of 0.6 mL per kilogram of body weight. Except for the use of IUDR for autoinoculation of the eye, other drugs are not helpful.

The WHO smallpox eradication program

Of all the infectious diseases smallpox was, perhaps, the easiest to eliminate. Humans are the only hosts, and there is no carrier state, cases of epidemiological importance present a typical clinical syndrome, transmission is relatively slow and requires close contact with an active case, and there is an effective, stable vaccine that protects for several years. The disease was universally feared because of periodic epidemics, the scarring that commonly affected the face, and the high case fatality rates from variola major.

When the intensified WHO-coordinated smallpox eradication program began in 1966, endemic disease was widespread in Brazil, virtually all sub-Saharan Africa, the southern Asian subcontinent, and Indonesia; 33 countries had endemic smallpox, 14 countries had importations, and the remainder of the world was at risk. Of the factors that led to success, perhaps the most important was a simultaneous commitment from all nations—those with endemic disease and those at risk from importation—to work toward the common goal of interrupting transmission within 10 years; this goal was reached, albeit 1 year late. The last cases of endemic smallpox occurred in South America (Brazil) in 1971, and in Asia (Bangladesh) in 1975. In the horn of Africa, Ethiopia reported its last cases in 1976, and Somalia and Kenya (with importations) followed in 1977.

Programs in each geographical area benefited from the successes and failures of other programs. Two of these experiences are worth citing. First, at the start of the global program it was found that less than one-third of all lots of vaccine used met WHO standards and measures were taken to change this intolerable situation [21]; this meant that less than 10 percent of the actual vaccine then in use in endemic countries met accepted standards. Second, selective epidemiological surveillance for rapid identification and control of outbreaks, an important contribution from the west and central African program [*22*], became the modus operandi throughout the world. This strategy replaced the previously widespread inefficient approach of mass vaccination, used previously even in areas of low epidemiological priority.

Certification of eradication

Early in the global program it was recognized that a mechanism had to be developed to confirm that smallpox had been eradicated in one country or in a group of countries forming an epidemiological unit. Basic criteria for certification of smallpox eradication had been established by a WHO expert committee [*10*]; these include (1) an absence of patients with smallpox (e.g., interruption of transmission) for at least 2 years—excluding well-defined and contained importations; (2) an effective surveillance system to detect cases; (3) adequate documentation of the eradication activities, including results of special surveys; and (4) certification by an independent international commission that made a 1- to 3-week visit to the country or area to be certified. Investigations, including collection of specimens from suspected cases, were especially emphasized in areas considered most likely to have persisting infections, e.g., where health units were sparse or where routine notification was incomplete; where the last cases had occurred; along borders with recently endemic countries; among special groups such as nomads, refugees, and immigrant workers; in areas where variola minor had been prevalent (because this form of the disease could be confused with chickenpox and other eruptive diseases); and in geographically remote areas and places that were relatively inaccessible due to security problems.

Since 1973, 79 recently endemic or high-risk countries with populations totaling over 3 billion were certified free from smallpox by 21 international commissions and a global commission convened by WHO. The remaining 121 countries and areas in the world submitted statements to WHO attesting to their freedom from smallpox. In these countries smallpox had not been endemic for at least 10 years and surveillance systems were judged sufficiently sensitive [*2*].

The benefits of smallpox eradication have been measured in economic as well as medical terms. It has been estimated that $1 to $2 billion will be saved globally each year. This is mainly for costs related to the vaccination (production, administration, complications, treatment), for quarantine checks at international boundaries, and for lost productivity due to premature deaths.

MAINTENANCE OF ERADICATION

Laboratory infections

Laboratories now remain the only known source of variola virus. Laboratory-associated outbreaks of smallpox occurred in Great Britain in 1973 and 1978 [*23*]. These episodes demonstrate the need to ensure that strains of variola virus in laboratories do not cause reestablishment of endemic smallpox. Since 1975, WHO has contacted all laboratories that might be storing variola virus. In total, 76 such laboratories were identified and 74 have voluntarily transferred or destroyed their stocks upon request of WHO; only WHO Collaborating Poxvirus laboratories in the United States and the Soviet Union specified above maintain variola virus, and culture with live virus ceased in 1985. Strict physical and administrative security requirements for these laboratories have been formulated and visits by WHO biosafety teams began in 1978 to ensure compliance with the recommendations. In 1986, a WHO advisory orthopoxvirus group suggested that WHO should request destruction of all variola virus stocks. This was based on the rationale that cloned variola virus DNA can be used for future comparative studies; a fraction of the scientific community still supports retention of secured live virus stocks.

Smallpox from other sources

Apart from the laboratory, there has been speculation that variola virus might resurface from the following sources: inanimate objects, including variolation material, reactivation from a dormant biological state, mutant monkeypox virus, and other animal sources. The evidence weighs against any of these as sources for the reappearance of smallpox.

During the global eradication program, samples of materials were collected from variolators in Afghanistan, Ethiopia, and Pakistan. In no instance was live virus found more than 9 months after being taken from a patient. Variolators reported that material stored for more than 2 years was ineffective. A recent report indicated that variolation-associated smallpox had continued in two remote areas of China until 1965 [*24*], although in 1961 China reported to WHO that smallpox had been eradicated in 1959. The discrepancy is ascribed to a reporting deficiency. The outbreaks ceased after variolation was banned and when free vaccine was provided.

Reactivation of heat-inactivated orthopoxviruses by coinfection of cells with active poxvirus has been shown but occurs only under special laboratory conditions [*25*]. Moreover, the virus causing smallpox does not exist in humans either in a latent or otherwise quiescent state.

Monkeypox

Monkeypox virus has generated great interest since the first human monkeypox case was discovered in Zaire in 1970. The virus had previously caused 10 laboratory-associated outbreaks of disease in primates in Europe and North America between 1958 and 1968 (hence the name monkeypox) [*26,27*]. Since 1970 more than 400 cases of human monkeypox have been reported from west and central Africa, and over 95 percent of them have occurred in Zaire [*28*]. The clinical and epidemiological characteristics of these cases have been reviewed recently [*29–31*].

The noteworthy features of these cases are:

Monkeypox is clinically similar to smallpox as it was seen in the same areas of Africa, including a case fatality rate of 10 percent.

Lymphadenopathy is more prominent in monkeypox, and although very mild cases do occur, they are the exception.

Patients come mainly from small, remote forest villages where the residents have abundant contact with wild animals. Recent evidence suggests that squirrels may be part of the natural cycle of monkeypox virus [32].

There is poor interhuman transmission; relatively few secondary cases, occurring 7 to 24 days after the first case, have been observed among unvaccinated persons, and spread to a fourth generation is rare [33]. The rate of secondary spread, about 10 percent in susceptible family members and less than 5 percent in the general population, does not permit sustained interhuman transmission [34].

Smallpox vaccine affords protection against monkeypox.

Monkeypox virus is a separate species of *Orthopoxvirus* with biological properties and a genome map distinct from other *Orthopoxvirus* species, including variola virus. The question arises as to whether monkeypox infections of humans will occur more frequently and transmit more readily in a wider geographical area now that vaccination is stopping. Recent studies carried out by WHO and national teams in Zaire have shown that transmission of monkeypox virus is uncommon in endemic disease areas, even where vaccination levels are very low [28–33]. Undoubtedly, cases will continue to occur, but there is no evidence that monkeypox will become a public health problem.

Whitepox virus and white variants from monkeypox virus

Although only one isolate of monkeypox virus has been made from an animal in the wild [2] captured near human monkeypox cases, four virus isolates termed *whitepox virus* had been characterized in one laboratory, which suggested there was a possible animal reservoir for variola virus. The four isolates had been called whitepox because they produced variolalike pocks on CAMs of chicken embryos and had DNA maps like variola virus. These strains were from organs of animals (one chimpanzee, one monkey, and two rodents) captured in the wild in Zaire between 1971 and 1975. Two other cultured strains of whitepox virus also had been characterized in 1964 from the kidney tissue of monkeys. The importance of these six isolates was that they resembled variola virus in their biological properties and genome structure. However, their relevance must be interpreted with caution as variola virus was being handled in these laboratories at about the time these strains were being isolated [2,15]. Indeed, recent DNA comparative evidence indicated that the two strains isolated from monkey kidney tissue in 1964 were definite contaminants [2,35]. Moreover, epidemiological evidence weighs strongly against the existence of variola virus in nature. Field surveillance has not detected any apparently "spontaneous" outbreaks of smallpox in these areas, while many human monkeypox cases have been found.

In addition to the isolates of whitepox virus from animal specimens, there have been reports from the same laboratory that monkeypox virus gives rise to whitepox (variolalike) strains in both in vitro and animal experiments. These findings have not been confirmed in other laboratories suggesting that these were also instances of culture cross-contamination in the laboratory.

The modern techniques of genome analysis have helped greatly in defining the relatedness of monkeypox to other orthopoxviruses and to variola virus; clearly monkeypox virus cannot give rise to variola virus by one or several spontaneous mutational steps [2,36,37].

Vaccine issues

All countries had stopped smallpox vaccination of the general public by 1984. Military personnel in some countries still receive vaccination, despite the recommendation of WHO that such vaccination be terminated because of the inherent risks.

Extensive research with vaccinia virus as a vector for expressing genes of other organisms [38] offers promise that vaccinia can be used to deliver the antigenic and protective responses of future veterinary and human live virus vaccines [39]. One of the major issues in this evaluation will be that of complications following immunization.

Other poxviruses

Other poxviruses that occasionally cause disease in humans include those that cause cowpox, molluscum contagiosum, tanapox, milker's nodule, and contagious pustular dermatitis (orf); except for cowpox, none of these is an *Orthopoxvirus*. Cowpox, usually an occupational hazard of farm and dairy workers, causes vesicles on the hands from contact with the lesions of infected animals. Recent evidence indicates that rodents may be a reservoir of infection.

Molluscum contagiosum presents clusters of thick-walled vesiculopustular lesions on the face, lips, genitals, and buttocks; these may persist for months without discomfort and spread by direct contact or by fomites; poor hygiene promotes transmission. Tanapox manifests in one or two large, thick-walled papulovesicular lesions on the extremities. The lesions have only been reported in the Tana River Valley of Kenya and from Zaire. Milker's nodule resembles the lesion of cowpox. Contagious pustular dermatitis is seen in farmers, shepherds, and others handling sheep. A typical papulovesicular lesion develops with a central ulcer forming usually on the hand, arm, or eyelid. In lambs the disease is called *orf*. Orf and milker's nodule are due to two different members of the genus *Parapoxvirus*. Molluscum contagiosum (genus *Molluscivirus* proposed) have not been grown in culture. All of these diseases are usually distinguished by clinical and epidemiological features.

REFERENCES

1 Fenner F, Wittek R, Dumbell KR: *The Orthopoxviruses.* Orlando, FL, Academic, 1989

2 Fenner F, Henderson DA, Arita I, et al: *Smallpox and its Eradication.* Geneva, World Health Organization, 1988

3 Nakano JH: Smallpox, monkeypox, vaccinia and whitepox viruses, in Lennette EH et al (eds): *Manual of Clinical Microbiology*, 3d ed. Washington, DC, American Society for Microbiology, 1980, pp 810–822

4 Esposito JJ, Obijeski JF, Nakano JH: Orthopoxvirus DNA: strain differentiation by electrophoresis of restriction endonuclease fragmented virion DNA. Virology 89:53–66, 1978

5 Mackett M, Archard LC: Conservation and variation in orthopoxvirus genome structure. J Gen Virol 45:683–701, 1979

6 Roberts JA: Histopathogenesis of mousepox I respiratory infection. Br J Exp Pathol 43:451–461, 1961

7 Bedson HS, Duckworth MJ: Rabbitpox: An experimental study of the pathways of infection in rabbits. J Pathol Bacteriol 85:1–20, 1963

8 Dixon CW: *Smallpox*, London, J & A Churchill Ltd, 1962

9 Sarkar JK, Mitra AC, Mukherjee MK, et al: Virus excretion in smallpox: (i) Excretion in the throat, urine and conjunctiva of patients. Bull WHO 48:517–522, 1973

10 WHO Expert Committee on Smallpox Eradication, Second Report, Tech Rep Ser 493:20–23, 1972

11 Heiner GG, Fatima N, Daniel RW, et al: A study of inapparent infection in smallpox. Am J Epidemiol, 94:252–262, 1971

12 Nakano JH: Poxviruses, in Lennette EH, Schmidt NJ (eds): *Diagnostic Procedures for Viral, Rickettsial and Chlamydial Infections,* 5th ed. Washington, D.C., American Public Health Association, pp. 257–308, 1979

13 Walls HH, Ziegler DW, Nakano JH: A study of the specificities of sequential antisera to variola and monkeypox viruses by radioimmunoassay. Bull WHO 58:131–138, 1980

14 Hopkins, DH: *Princes and Peasants: Smallpox in History.* Chicago, University of Chicago Press, 1983

15 Breman JG, Arita I: The confirmation and maintenance of smallpox eradication. N Engl J Med. 303:1263–1273, 1980

16 Harper GJ: Airborne micro-organisms: Survival tests with 4 viruses. J Hyg (Camb) 59:479–484, 1961

17 Jenner E: *An Inquiry into the Causes and Effects of the Variolae Vaccinae, A Disease, Discovered in some of the Western Countries of England, Particularly Gloucestershire, and Known by the Name of Cowpox.* London, Sampson-low, reprinted by Cassel and Company, Ltd, London, 1896. No. 4 in Pamphlet Vol. 4232, National Library of Medicine, Bethesda, Maryland, 1798

18 Collier LH: The development of a stable smallpox vaccine. J Hyg (Camb) 53:76–101, 1955

19 Lane JM, Ruben FL, Neff JM, et al: Complications of smallpox vaccination, 1968. National Surveillance in the United States. N Engl J Med 281:1201–1207, 1969

20 Lane JM, Ruben FL, Millar JD: Complications of smallpox vaccination in the United States, 1968. Results of ten statewide surveys. J Infect Dis 122:303–309, 1970

21 Arita I: The control of vaccine quality in the Smallpox Eradication Programme, in *International Symposium on Smallpox Vaccine.* Symposium Series in Immunobiological Standardization, Basel, Karger, 1972, vol. 19, pp 79–87

22 Foege WH, Millar JD, Lane JM: Selective epidemiologic control in smallpox eradication. Am J Epidemiol 94:311–315, 1971

23 Hawkes N: Smallpox death in Britain challenges presumption of laboratory safety; peer review failed dismally. Science 203:855–856, 1979

24 Yutu J, Ma J, Guang X: Outbreaks of smallpox due to variation in China, 1962–1965. Am J Epidemiol 128:39–45, 1988

25 Fenner F, Holmes IH, Joklik WK, et al: Reactivation of heat-inactivated poxviruses: a general phenomenon which includes the fibroma-myxoma virus transformation of Berry and Dedrick. Nature 182:1340–1341, 1959

26 Arita I, Henderson DA: Smallpox and monkeypox in non-human primates. Bull WHO 39:277–283, 1968

27 Arita I, Henderson DA: Monkeypox and whitepox viruses in West and Central Africa. Bull WHO 53:347–353, 1976

28 Jezek Z, Khodakevich LN, Wickett JF: Smallpox and its post-eradication surveillance. Bull WHO 65:425–434, 1987

29 Breman JG, Kalisa-Ruti, Steniowski MV, et al: Human monkeypox, 1970–1979. Bull WHO 58:165–182, 1980

30 Arita, I, Jezek Z, Khodakevich LN, et al: Human monkeypox: a newly emerged orthopoxvirus zoonosis in the tropical rain forests of Africa. Am J Trop Med Hyg 34:781–789, 1985

31 Jezek Z, Szczeniowski M, Paluku KM, et al: Human monkeypox: clinical features of 282 patients. J Infect Dis 156:293–298, 1987

32 Khodakevich L, Szczeniowski M, Mambu-ma-Disu, et al: The role of squirrels in sustaining monkeypox virus transmission. Trop Geogr Med 39:115–122, 1987

33 Jezek Z, Arita I, Mutombo M, et al: Four generations of probable person-to-person transmission of human monkeypox. Am J Epidemiol 123:1004–1012, 1986

34 Jezek Z, Grab B, Dixon H: Stochastic model for interhuman spread of monkeypox. Am J Epidemiol 126:1082–1092, 1987

35 Dumbell KR, Kapsenberg JG: Laboratory investigation of two "whitepox" viruses and comparison with two variola strains from southern India. Bull WHO 60:381–387, 1982

36 Fenner F, Dumbell KR, Marennikova SS, et al: Monkeypox virus as a potential source of variola virus. Geneva, World Health Organization, WHO/SE/80–154, 1980

37 Esposito JJ, Nakano JH, Obijeski JF: Can variola-like viruses be derived from monkeypox virus? An investigation based on DNA mapping. Bull WHO 63:695–703, 1985

38 Moss B, Flexner C: Vaccinia virus expression vectors. Ann Rev Immunol 5:305–324, 1987

39 Esposito JJ, Murphy FA: Infectious recombinant vectored virus vaccines, in Bittle JL, Murphy FA (eds): *Vaccine Biotechnology. Advances in Veterinary Science,* Vol. 33. Orlando, FL, Academic, 1988

Epstein-Barr Virus · *Ben Z. Katz* · *George Miller*

Epstein-Barr virus (EBV) is a herpes virus of humans. Related viruses infect all old world primates and great apes but do not seem to infect new world monkeys [*1*]. The virus is distributed throughout the world in all climates and in all geographical areas. Isolated tribes living along the Amazon Basin or in the highlands of New Guinea have serological evidence of past infection with EBV, a finding which suggests that the virus is regularly transmitted in small groups and does not require reintroduction [*2*].

AGENT

LIFE HISTORY AND ECOLOGY

Two routes of transmission in humans are known—by saliva and by blood transfusion. Salivary transmission probably occurs both by intimate oral contact as well as by salivary residues left on drinking vessels, toys, and other objects. Blood transfusion of EBV has been documented infrequently. Although transmission by arthropod vectors is theoretically possible, there is no evidence for this pathway. Once transmission has occurred the virus probably persists for the life of the infected individuals. Two sites of persistent infection have been recognized, the lymphoid system and the salivary glands. In lymphoid cells the virus persists as a latent viral genome with little or no synthesis of mature virions. In the salivary glands and possibly other sites in the oropharynx mature virions, which are infectious, replicate. At least 20 percent of normal, seropositive persons excrete the virus in their saliva; in persons who are immunosuppressed, the rate of excretion may be as high as 50 percent.

MORPHOLOGY AND ANTIGENIC STRUCTURE

By electron microscopy EBV has a typical herpes virus morphology which is indistinguishable from other members of this group (Fig. 68-1). The diameter of the mature extracellular particle is about 150 to 180 nm. There is a lipoprotein envelope which contains at least four proteins, three of which are glycosylated. Within the envelope is a nucleocapsid which exhibits icosahedral symmetry and is thought to contain 162 capsomeres. Within the nucleocapsid is located a large genome of double-stranded DNA, approximately 170,000 base pairs.

The virion envelope contains antigens in common with antigens found on the cytoplasmic membrane of cells which are producing virions, though the virion envelope itself is thought to be acquired as the virus passes through the outer nuclear membrane. These so-called membrane antigens (MA) are responsible for eliciting virus neutralizing antibody [*3*]. The MA complex consists of three different gene products [*4*]. A murine

monoclonal antibody that recognizes epitopes on the largest component of the MA complex neutralizes immortalization. Whether the other proteins of the MA complex elicit virus neutralizing activity is not yet known.

The other structural antigen found within cells which are actively synthesizing virions is termed *viral capsid antigen* (VCA). Individuals with past exposure to EBV develop IgG antibody to capsid antigen which persists for life (Fig. 68-5). Antibody to VCA, detectable by immunofluorescence, has been the major tool in study of the seroepidemiology of EBV infections [*5*].

A nonstructural antigen complex found in cells which are activated toward the productive life cycle is termed *early antigen* (EA) because its synthesis does not depend on viral DNA synthesis. EA probably consists of a number of different polypeptides. At least two components of EA [D (diffuse) and R (restricted)] have been defined on the basis of their distribution in the cell and according to their differential solubility in methanol [*6*]. The functions of the proteins represented by the EA complex are not completely known, but it is likely that

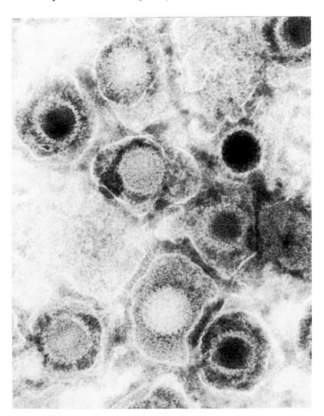

Figure 68-1. Epstein-Barr virus.

they include enzymes which are needed for viral DNA replication and transactivation. Three virion-encoded enzymatic activities have been identified—a DNA polymerase, a thymidine kinase, and an exonuclease. Recently, an early antigen has been identified which activates EBV replication in certain latently infected lymphoblastoid cell lines [7].

MA, VCA, and EA are all antigen systems which are associated with a productive phase of the virus's life cycle. In most lymphoid cells, this phase of the life cycle is inhibited; there are nonetheless two nonstructural antigens found in each cell which harbors EBV genomes in a nonproductive state. One is a nuclear antigen, Epstein-Barr nuclear antigen (EBNA). This antigen is found in every cell which contains EBV DNA. EBNA is now known to consist of a complex of the proteins of at least six different gene products, one of which is bound to chromosomes and appears to be required for maintenance of the virus as an episome, while another may play a role in lymphocyte immortalization. Another nonstructural antigen is found on the surface of cells with latent EBV genomes. This antigen, lymphocyte-determined membrane antigen (LYDMA), is evident by cell-mediated cytotoxicity but has not yet been demonstrated serologically. However, monoclonal antibodies have been raised which appear to react with antigens found on the surface of cells with latent EBV [8], some of which are virally encoded, and some of which are encoded by the cell.

EBV GENOME

Two different forms of the EBV genome exist. Inside the virion the genome is a linear double-stranded DNA which is not highly associated with chromosomal proteins. When the virus is in a latent state, the genome is circular and there is a nucleosomal structure, as revealed by micrococcal nuclease digestion.

Considerable information is available about the structure of EBV DNA found in virions. The entire genome has been cloned both as a set of overlapping restriction endonuclease fragments with the enzymes *Bam*HI, *Eco*RI, *Hind* III, and *Sal* I and as sheared fragments, and detailed physical maps are available (Fig. 68-2). The entire nucleotide sequence is also available for one strain of the virus [4]. At the ends of the genome are repeated sequences about 0.5 kilobase in length. These permit circularization of the genome. Within the genome is a series of repeats of a sequence of about 3000 base pairs. Strains differ in the number of these internal repeat units, which vary between 6 and 12 units per genome. Within the genome there are several regions which are homologous to other stretches of DNA at some distance away.

Only a few functions have been assigned to specific regions of EBV DNA. The genome encodes two small nuclear RNAs about 160 base pairs long, which become complexed with host-cell protein. The genes encoding these RNAs are located in the *Eco*RI J fragment. On the basis of gene-transfer experiments it has been found that nuclear antigens are encoded by the *Bam*HI E, K, and WYH fragments, and early antigens by the *Bam*HI H, M, R, and Z fragments [4,7]. The single EBV strain available which is unable to immortalize lymphocytes (see "Biological Properties") has a 2.4-kilobase deletion in *Bam*HI fragments Y and H, a region which must encode functions which play a role in the immortalization process.

Restriction enzyme analyses of DNAs obtained from virions from different ecological niches have shown variations. Each strain from epidemiologically unrelated individuals appears distinguishable on the basis of DNA polymorphisms [9]. Therefore, it is unlikely that these genomic differences underlie the spectrum of EBV-associated diseases (see "Patient").

BIOLOGICAL PROPERTIES OF THE VIRUS IN VITRO

The principal biological activity of EBV which underlies the pathogenesis of EBV-associated lymphoproliferative diseases and which is amenable to study in cell-culture systems is the ability of the virus to cause the indefinite proliferation of lym-

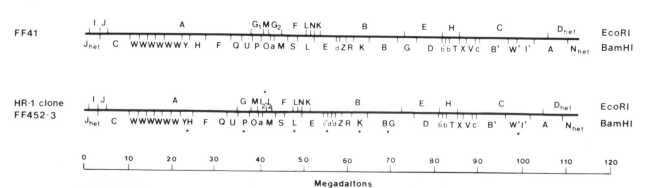

Figure 68-2. Physical maps of two strains of EBV with the restriction endonucleases *Eco*RI and *Bam*HI. Strain FF41 was originally isolated from saliva of a patient with mononucleosis. It is capable of immortalizing lymphocytes. Strain HR-1 was originally derived from a Burk-itt's lymphoma, Jijoye. Through laboratory passage it has lost the capacity to transform lymphocytes. Asterisks indicate regions of differences in restriction fragments of the two strains. (*Courtesy of M. Rabson.*)

phocytes which it has infected, a process termed *immortalization*. EB virions have been found to infect only lymphocytes which contain a receptor for the virus, the C3d receptor. Susceptible B lymphocytes are mainly well-differentiated cells which are programmed to synthesize all classes of immunoglobulin heavy chains and light chains. Following infection there is an orderly progression of events, starting with the synthesis of EBNA about 6 h after infection, followed by stimulation of cellular DNA synthesis about 20 h after infection. The first mitoses of virus-infected lymphocytes are seen about 36 h after infection.

At some point during the immortalization reaction the EBV genome is amplified, for every immortalized cell contains many copies of the viral genome, even though small numbers of virus were used to initiate infection. The majority of these genomes exist as circular plasmids which are not covalently attached to cellular chromosomal DNA. There is evidence that EBV DNA is integrated into the cellular chromosome in some cell lines, but not others. The presence of many EBV DNA copies within cells has facilitated the detection of EBV genomes in clinical material by nucleic hybridization methods.

Epstein-Barr virus DNA and RNA have been found in the epithelial cells of nasopharyngeal carcinoma [10]. Recently, epithelial cells from the uterine ectocervix have been directly infected with the EBV present in throat washings [11]. There is, to date, only a single, unconfirmed report of epithelial cells that were immortalized following transfection with a portion of the EBV genome [12].

Since lymphocytes are the only readily available in vitro hosts for EB viral replication at present, and since lymphocytes are generally restrictive of viral replication, it has been difficult to grow large amounts of virus in the laboratory. Viral growth has relied upon the spontaneous shedding of virus by producer lines of transformed lymphocytes. The lymphocytes of certain species of new world primate, especially cotton-top marmosets, permit synthesis of the largest quantities of virus. These cells have served as a source of virus for comparison of strains.

ANIMAL MODELS

Although old world primates and apes harbor EBV, little work has been done to study the pathogenesis of the natural infection in these species. Human EBV is able to infect cotton-top and some other species of marmosets, owl monkeys, and squirrel monkeys. In about one-fourth of cotton-top marmosets the virus induces a diffuse malignant lymphoma with a latent period of 5 weeks to 6 months [13].

PATIENT

PATTERNS OF HOST RESPONSE

It is convenient to consider the host response to EBV in two phases—those which are associated with the initial encounter with the virus, i.e., primary infection, and those which result from reactivated or recurrent infection. In tropical areas it is generally true that primary EBV infection is acquired at a young age, often before 2 years. Most of these primary infections are asymptomatic. When primary infection is delayed to older childhood or adulthood, as it is under conditions of improved sanitation, then the syndrome of infectious mononucleosis is seen in about one-third to one-half of primary infections. Infectious mononucleosis is not often recognized in tropical pediatric medicine. It is now evident that primary infection in certain immunodeficient patients which initially appears to be infectious mononucleosis may progress to immunoblastic sarcoma or lymphoma. Primary infection in childhood may also be evident as pneumonitis, thrombocytopenia, hepatitis, or rarely aseptic meningitis.

Intrauterine or perinatal infection is a special case of primary infection which has special clinical significance for all human herpes viruses except EBV. Although occasional case reports have suggested the possibility of congenital EBV disease, this pattern of host response does not seem to occur often.

Reactivated EBV infection is also asymptomatic in the majority of individuals. The two EBV-associated diseases of interest to geographical medicine, namely Burkitt's lymphoma (BL) and nasopharyngeal carcinoma (NPC), occur many years after primary infection.

PATHOLOGY AND PATHOGENESIS

BL is a diffuse undifferentiated malignant lymphoma which is thought to arise in a precursor in the B-cell series. The evidence of its B-cell origin is that nearly all BL have surface immunoglobulins, usually IgM. The lymphoid elements of the tumor are often heavily infiltrated with histiocytes or macrophages, which are also readily seen in imprints made from tumor cells, giving the tumor its characteristic "starry sky" appearance (Fig. 68-3). These phagocytic cells are probably reacting to cell death brought about by rapid tumor cell growth or immune cytolytic mechanisms.

NPC arise from nasopharyngeal epithelium and are, thus, variants of squamous-cell carcinomas. Electron microscopy reveals markers of epithelial cells in most of the histological variants. NPC are often heavily infiltrated with lymphocytes; in some instances the malignant epithelial cells may be difficult to visualize against the background of stroma and lymphocytes.

The pathogenesis of the malignant tumors associated with EBV is speculative. In the course of oropharyngeal replication of EBV, some lymphoid cells in the vicinity are thought to be immortalized, i.e., their growth potential is increased. Following this event there are thought to be additional events which confer upon one clone of immortalized cells the potential for autonomous growth. There is evidence that Burkitt's tumors are monoclonal. They contain only one immunoglobulin heavy chain, usually IgM, and one light chain. When BL arises in G6PD heterozygotes, only one enzyme phenotype is expressed in the tumor. Burkitt's tumors are also characterized by chromosomal translocations between the cellular-*myc* (c-*myc*) on-

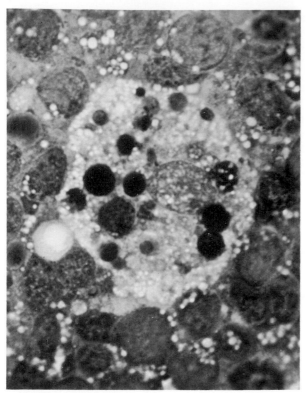

Figure 68-3. An imprint of a Burkitt's lymphoma, stained with Giemsa. In the center of the tumor cells is a large phagocytic cell filled with pyknotic nuclei.

lymphoid cells which harbor the EBV genome with infected epithelial cells. There are also cytoplasmic bridges between epithelial and lymphoid cells in the nasopharynx which could permit virus traverse.

Genetic factors undoubtedly play a role in susceptibility to NPC, since the incidence in persons of southern Chinese origin is so much higher than expected. However, the nature of the genetic defect, or even clear markers for it, are not available. The possibility of an environmental carcinogen playing a role in pathogenesis of NPC has also been considered. The one carcinogen for which there is some evidence is ingestion of salt fish cured with nitrosamines. Unlike cancer elsewhere in the mouth and pharynx, tobacco use does not seem to present an increased risk [*15*].

CLINICAL MANIFESTATIONS

In more than half the children BL presents as a unilateral swelling of the jaw (Fig. 68-4). Characteristically, jaw tumors are the presenting sign in younger children and abdominal masses

cogene on chromosome 8 and the immunoglobulin gene loci on chromosomes 2, 14, or 22. Because of the consistency of this observation and the presence of analogous recombinations in tumors that are *not* EBV-associated, this translocation is felt to be a key factor in the pathogenesis of BL [*14*].

It has been speculated that somehow the pathogenesis of BL may be related to coinfection with malaria. There are two theories about the way in which malaria might act as a promoter in BL. First, by inducing reticuloendothelial and immune hyperplasia secondary to reactions involved in the disposal of malaria parasites and products of hemolysis, there may be more, or different, lymphoid subpopulations available for transformation. Possibly viral genome integration may occur more readily in certain B-lymphoid subtypes. Alternatively, malaria may induce a degree of immunological paralysis and allow a small number of virus-transformed cells to multiply beyond the point where they can be eliminated by immune mechanisms.

The principal question about the pathogenesis of NPC as it relates to EBV is how the virus gains access to the epithelial cells. Several theories have been proposed. The nasopharyngeal epithelial cells of persons with certain genetic constitution may have virus receptors. Other viruses present in the nasopharynx, such as parainfluenza virus, may cause fusion of

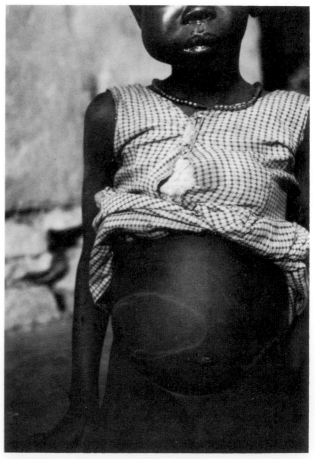

Figure 68-4. A child with a Burkitt's lymphoma. Note the masses in the jaw and in the right ovary. From a field study of Burkitt's lymphoma in the West Nile district of Uganda. (*Courtesy of A. Dean.*)

in older children. The disease is often multifocal at the time of diagnosis; there are usually additional sites of tumor involvement in abdominal viscera, kidney, liver, and lymphatic tissue of the gastrointestinal tract. Other favored sites for the tumor are the exocrine and endocrine glands, such as the thyroid, pancreas, ovary, and salivary glands [16]. The anatomical distribution of the disease characteristically spares the peripheral lymph nodes and the lung, and although the tumor is thought to arise in the trabecular marrow of the mandible, it does not generally involve the distal bone marrow and leukemia is not a feature of the disease. BL are very rapidly growing tumors which may appear suddenly. Because of rapid growth there is extensive cellular destruction and release of cellular breakdown products. One serious complication is acute renal failure due to urate nephropathy.

The presenting symptoms of NPC depend on the location of the primary tumor within the nasopharynx. In about half the cases the presenting sign is a cervical mass due to spread to regional lymph nodes. Other symptoms may include nasal obstruction, postnasal discharge, epistaxis, or those referable to obstruction of the eustachian tube such as impairment of hearing, tinnitus, or otitis media. If there has been local invasion within the head, the patient may present with cranial nerve involvement, headache, or trismus due to invasion of jaw muscles, or symptoms resultant from invasion of the paranasal sinuses. NPC may metastasize to the skeleton, especially the spine, and to liver, lung, and skin, as well as to peripheral lymph nodes.

Clinical manifestations of infectious mononucleosis (IM), which usually occurs in adolescents and young adults, is characterized by an incubation period of 30 to 50 days followed by a 3- to 5-day prodrome of mild headache, malaise, and fatigue. The acute illness is characterized by tonsillitis with an accompanying gray exudate, fever, generalized lymphadenopathy and splenomegaly. Occasionally hepatomegaly, hepatic tenderness and/or jaundice are seen. Rarely central nervous system and hematological syndromes can occur.

Diffuse, fatal lymphoproliferative disorders seen in immunocompromised patients commonly present with generalized lymphadenopathy and fever. Thus, they are indistinguishable from acute IM initially, but instead of gradual diminution of symptoms and recovery, there is a relentless course ending in death.

Burkitt-like lymphomas can also occur in the immunosuppressed, usually in the central nervous system. Rarely, previously healthy individuals can develop similar lesions [17].

IMMUNE RESPONSE

During primary infection with EBV the normal serological response includes production of antibodies against a variety of EBV-associated antigens—the capsid, the envelope or membrane, EA, and the nuclear antigen. These antibody responses occur in an orderly pattern (Fig. 68-5). IgM antibody to the

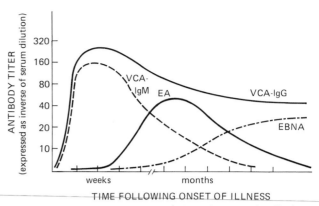

Figure 68-5. Scheme of time course of development of antibody to different EBV antigens following primary infection with the virus. VCA = viral capsid antigen, EA = early antigen, EBNA = nuclear antigen.

capsid is usually detected early after infection and an IgG antibody persists thereafter for life. Antibodies to EA are transient in the normal individual and often disappear soon after primary infection. Antibody to EBNA appears somewhat later but persists. Since EBNA is the only antigen found inside latently infected growing cells, it is thought that cell destruction must occur to liberate the antigen before antibody can be produced.

Patients with EBV-associated tumors do not have antibodies to any unique antigens which have been identified so far. However, certain serological reactions are either heightened or more persistent in patients with EBV-associated tumors. Patients with EBV-associated BL and NPC have elevated antibody titers to EBV capsid and EA. From the prospective study of BL in Uganda it appears that the elevated antibody titers precede the appearance of the clinically evident tumors [18]. Patients with tumors also have increased frequency of antibody to EA. These antibodies are thought to represent evidence of ongoing active EBV infection. In BL the antibodies are directed against the R component, and in NPC against the D component. Nearly all patients with NPC have serum antibodies to viral capsid antigen and EA of the IgA isotype, whereas only 5 percent of healthy controls have IgA anti-VCA and none have IgA anti-EA. Furthermore, NPC patients have in their saliva secretory IgA antibodies directed against EBV antigens.

The cell-mediated immune response to EBV-infected and -transformed cells is complex. The identity of the antigens which call forth the cell-mediated reactions is not clear. One seems to be LYDMA, which should not be confused with the MA found on cells producing virus. On the surface of EBV-transformed cells another antigen has recently been defined with monoclonal antibodies. A variety of effector cells contribute to the detection and elimination of EBV-infected cells in vitro. These include natural killer cells and cytotoxic memory T cells. The latter cells can be demonstrated by cytotoxic reactions between autologous T cells and continuous B-lymphocyte cell lines. Alternatively, the cytotoxic T cells may be measured by their ability to induce "regression" of the immortalization reaction in vitro. It appears that some of the inhibitory effects of T cells on lymphocyte immortalization are due to release of soluble mediators, of which immune interferon appears to be one.

DIAGNOSIS

The laboratory diagnosis of an EBV infection rests on two general techniques—demonstration of the virus, viral antigens, or viral DNA and serological responses. Biologically active virus can be isolated from saliva, blood, or lymphoid tissue by means of its ability to immortalize cultured human lymphocytes, usually from umbilical cord blood. This assay is time-consuming and requires specialized tissue culture facilities which are not generally available in the tropics. Viral antigens, particularly the nuclear antigen, can be found in lymphoid tissues and occasionally in a rare cell in peripheral blood, if the level of leukoviremia is high enough. Theoretically this technique should be applicable to rapid diagnosis in the field, particularly when monoclonal antibody to nuclear antigen becomes available and when the assays are converted to enzyme-linked immunosorbent assay (ELISA) or other techniques which can employ conventional microscopy. Finally EBV DNA can be found in tumors and other tissue by methods of nucleic acid hybridization. The probes are now made by recombinant DNA techniques. The methods of labeling the probes and detecting their hybridization for the present rely on ^{32}P or biotinylation, the latter of which should be applicable in the field because it is nonradioactive.

Serological tests are an aid to diagnosis of EBV infections but require some interpretation. The presence of IgG antibody to capsid antigen indicates past infection. Current infection is usually detected by presence of anticapsid antibody of the IgM type, or by showing a rise in antibody titer to one of the several EBV antigen systems. Since antibodies to EBNA appear late during primary infection, a rise in this antigen is most likely to be useful in the diagnosis of primary infection. Elevated and persistent antibody to EA is thought to be evidence of ongoing viral infection. The presence of serum antibody of the IgA type to EB VCA is the basis of a screening test for the early detection of NPC in high-incidence areas, such as China.

MANAGEMENT

NPC is treated by surgery in combination with local high-voltage radiotherapy. Success of therapy and survival in NPC is dependent on the stage of disease at the time of diagnosis. For tumors clinically confined to the nasopharynx (stage I), 5-year survival is about 80 percent. If the disease has spread along the cervical lymph nodes to the supraclavicular fossa (stage IV) distant metastases occur rapidly, and fewer than 20 percent of patients survive for 5 years. Nearly all patients are dead within 2 years if distant metastases are evident at the time of diagnosis.

Usually BL is multifocal at the time of diagnosis: therefore systemic chemotherapy is the chief mode of treatment with surgery and radiotherapy used as adjuncts. BL is particularly susceptible to cytotoxic agents. Attempts are made to induce remission with three to six cycles of cytotoxic agents. Cyclophosphamide is the mainstay of therapy. Single doses of 40 mg/kg are given at close intervals, usually every 2 to 3 weeks, allowing time for recovery of the peripheral granulocyte count to 1500 cells per millimeter. Most protocols include other agents to induce remission, such as vincristine, methotrexate, and prednisolone. A remission can be induced in about 80 to 90 percent of patients with African type of BL. Long-term survival figures of the African type of BL vary from 20 to 70 percent. The prognosis for Burkitt's tumor outside the endemic area and for EBV-negative B-cell lymphoma is much graver. Maintenance chemotherapy is not generally given in BL. However, the patients are followed frequently with examinations of the bone marrow and cerebral spinal fluid for evidence of tumor relapse. Some oncologists use prophylactic intrathecal methotrexate and CNS irradiation; others employ these modalities only if there is evidence of CNS relapse.

One important complication of therapy, particularly during the first week in patients with large tumor bulk, is the so-called acute tumor lysis syndrome. This is the result of rapid tumor cell breakdown and death. Patients develop metabolic acidosis, hyperuricemia, hyperphosphaturia (and hyperphosphatemia if renal function is abnormal), hyperproteinemia, and hyperkalemia. Such patients may die suddenly of cardiac arrhythmias. Others may develop acute renal failure probably secondary to uric acid nephropathy; this is managed by hemo- or peritoneal dialysis. It is recommended that uricosuric agents such as allopurinol be used before and during chemotherapy.

Infectious mononucleosis is rarely recognized in the tropics. At any event, therapy is usually symptomatic, especially bed rest. Antibiotics, particularly penicillin, may be given for the secondary pharyngeal infection with group A β-hemolytic streptococci which occasionally occurs. Ampicillin usually causes a rash in mononucleosis patients and is not recommended. In some rare complications of mononucleosis corticosteroids are indicated. These include respiratory obstruction and immune hemolytic anemia. The role of antiviral chemotherapy, with drugs such as acycloguanosine (acyclovir) which have activity against replicating (but not latent) virus in vitro, in the management of IM in a normal host requires further evaluation; in the immunocompromised patient, however, EBV-associated lymphomas and lymphoproliferative disorders have been reported to regress with such therapy [17].

POPULATION

POPULATION ECOLOGY

EBV infections are universal. Ultimately 80 to 90 percent or more of adults demonstrate serological evidence of past infection. No particular geographical or cultural setting spares one exposure to and infection by EBV. Antibodies to EBV have been found in every population thus far tested including very isolated peoples in Brazil and Alaska.

However, in certain populations there appears to be an increased risk to the development of severe forms of EBV-associated diseases, especially tumors. In the case of BL, the risks are increased in populations living in the hot wet lowlands of equatorial Africa, where BL is the commonest childhood cancer. The exact nature of the ecological factors associated with increased risk of BL in these areas (and in New Guinea) is not known, but the favored hypothesis is that malaria plays a role. In NPC, the risk appears to be immunogenetic in nature. Persons of southern Chinese origin and those with genetic similarities, e.g., the Malays, are at increased risk to the development of NPC, wherever they live. This is particularly notable in a place such as Singapore where persons of southern Chinese origin are noted to develop NPC considerably more frequently than Indians and Caucasians.

Among those who develop diffuse polyclonal B-cell lymphoma after EBV infection, the risk factor appears to be immune deficiency. That defect may be highly specific, such as occurs in certain families whose male members develop fatal B-cell lymphomas, or it may be a more generalized immunodeficiency such as occurs in patients who are immunosuppressed by chemotherapy for malignancy or organ transplantation, or by AIDS.

EPIDEMIOLOGY OF INFECTION WITH EBV

Infection with EBV knows no geographical limitations or season. This is in keeping with what is known about its modes of transmission. The virus is transmitted by salivary exchange, presumably between parents and children and siblings in a household. Infectious virus may also be acquired from saliva deposited on objects such as toys or cups. The rate of shedding of EBV by asymptomatic individuals is very high—about 20 percent of normal persons in the United States and 40 to 50 percent of healthy children in Africa were found to have infectious EBV in their saliva [19]. This large reservoir of shedders is thought to be responsible for continued ongoing transmission of virus in all parts of the world. Although old world primates and apes have their own EBV, there is no evidence for transmission of these viruses to humans, either directly or via arthropod vectors. Despite its ubiquity, there do seem to be certain environmental, social, or cultural factors which influence the transmission of EBV. This is seen most clearly in the relationship between socioeconomic class and the age at which EBV infection first occurs. In well-developed countries it is not unusual for the infection to be delayed until adolescence or early adulthood. By contrast, in tropical countries the infection is generally acquired at a very early age. Once maternal antibodies disappear, infants become susceptible to infection, which takes place rapidly over the next 12 months. In Ghana and in east Africa about 80 percent of 2-year-olds are EBV-seropositive. Exactly what accounts for these differences in the age of acquisition of EBV is not defined. It is not likely to be a geographical or climatic factor, as similar differences

in the rate of transmission among persons of different socioeconomic class in Philadelphia also have been noted. Variations either in the frequency or amounts of virus excreted or in personal hygienic customs are probably involved.

INFECTION AND DISEASE

The epidemiological patterns of viral transmission just described strongly influence the patterns of expression of EBV-associated disease. There is a formidable effect of the age at which primary infection is acquired on the clinical syndrome. Infectious mononucleosis, the classic manifestation of primary EBV infection, is more often seen in the older child, adolescent, or adult than in the young child. In developed countries between one-third and one-half of infections in this age group are clinically evident. Since infection with EBV occurs so early in the tropics, infectious mononucleosis is rarely, if ever, recognized. Most EBV infections are thought to be initially asymptomatic when the infection is acquired in infancy or early childhood. Recently, infections in the young child have been found to be associated with different clinical syndromes such as pneumonias and thrombocytopenia [20]. Whether these are part of the clinical picture of initial EBV infection in the tropics remains to be studied.

Once EBV infection has been established it persists in lymphoid cells and salivary glands for the remainder of life. In most instances this persistent infection is asymptomatic. The two EBV-associated tumors are events associated with persistent, not acute infection. In a recent prospective study of BL in Uganda, de The and his colleagues found that antibodies to EBV were present for many months before the clinical recognition of the tumor. In a significant proportion of BL patients, the EBV titers were elevated as compared with controls [18].

One important unanswered question concerns the possible relationship between age at the time of initial infection with the virus and the risk of development of an EBV-associated tumor. It seems clear that Burkitt's tumor is more common in those tropical countries where infection is acquired early than in other parts of the world where infection is delayed. Burkitt's tumor is an unusual lymphoma outside the endemic area. In fact, the majority of histologically classified BL tumors occurring outside the endemic areas of the tropics lack evidence of EBV DNA, but do contain the translocation involving c-*myc* previously discussed. Thus, while the translocation shows a better correlation with BL than infection with EBV, in areas of the world where EBV infection occurs early in life, EBV may permit the cells with the translocation to expand more readily, leading to the development of lymphoma. Other cofactors such as malaria may also play a role in the pathogenesis of BL [14].

PREVENTION OF INFECTION

Given the usual route of transmission of EBV, by salivary exchange or salivary droplets, it seems highly unlikely that prevention of infection can be achieved by interruption of the usual route of spread. Any vaccine which is contemplated must be active in providing immunity at the portal of entry in the oropharynx. It is doubtful that a subunit vaccine given parenterally would be likely to achieve this goal. A classic live virus vaccine would be unacceptable, given the known oncogenic potential of the virus. Two general strategies of vaccine production might be considered. One is a vaccine produced from the MA glycoprotein which induces virus neutralizing antibodies. Such a glycoprotein has been made by a variety of techniques, and has been tested in nonhuman primates with mixed results [21]. Another strategy is to construct viral mutants whose genomes are deleted in those regions which code for products involved in cell immortalization. It may perhaps be possible to cripple an EBV in such genes, while permitting the virus to replicate and immunize.

CONTROL OF EBV-ASSOCIATED DISEASE

Two methods of control of the common EBV-associated tumors of the tropics have been considered. In the case of BL, efforts have been directed toward control of malaria as a possible crucial cofactor. BL is endemic in areas of the world where malaria is either hyper- or holoendemic. In these areas malaria infection is universal, occurs very early in life, and is transmitted throughout the year. Conversely, endemic BL has not been encountered in nonmalarious areas of the world. Of great interest is the low incidence of disease in certain isolated areas—for example, the islands of Zanzibar and Pemba, which are only 32 km from the coast of Tanzania where the tumor is endemic; on these islands there is a very low incidence of malaria as the result of malaria eradication campaigns. The decreasing incidence of disease in Uganda and in Natal, as well as in New Guinea, can be correlated with programs of malaria eradication. A prospective field trial to reduce malaria prevalence in Tanzania through chloroquine prophylaxis is in progress. The effect on the incidence of BL will be studied. The control of NPC, a major public health problem in south China, Malaysia, and other parts of southeast Asia, increasingly relies on EBV serology as an adjunct. Persons found to have serum IgA antibodies to EB viral capsid are followed closely with clinical and radiological examinations. Some of these individuals have been shown to develop NPC 3 to 5 years after the first serological evidence of elevated IgA anti-VCA activity. This method has led to early diagnosis and treatment of NPC as well as the recognition of some putatively premalignant lesions.

REFERENCES

1 Frank A, Andiman W, Miller G: Epstein-Barr virus and non-human primates: Natural and experimental infection, in Klein G, Weinhouse S (eds): *Advances in Cancer Research,* vol 23. New York, Academic, 1976, pp 171–210

2 Black L, Hierholzer WJ, Pinheiro F, et al: Evidence for persistence of infectious agents in isolated human populations. Am J Epidemiol 100:230–250, 1974

3 Pearson GR: Epstein-Barr virus: Immunology, in Klein G (ed): *Viral Oncology.* New York, Raven, 1980, pp 739–767

4 Baer R, Bankier A, Biggin M, et al: DNA sequence and expression of the B95-8 Epstein-Barr virus genome. Nature 310:207–211, 1984

5 Henle G, Henle W: Immunofluorescence in cells derived from Burkitt's lymphoma. J Bacteriol 91:1248–1256, 1966

6 Henle G, Henle W, Klein G: Demonstration of two distinct components in the early antigen complex of Epstein-Barr virus-infected cells. Int J Cancer 8:272–282, 1971

7 Countryman J, Jenson H, Seibl R, et al: Polymorphic proteins encoded within BZLF1 of defective and standard Epstein-Barr viruses disrupt latency. J Virol 61:3672–3679, 1987

8 Kinter C, Sugden B: Identification of antigenic determinants unique to the surfaces of cells transformed by Epstein-Barr virus. Nature 294:458–460, 1981

9 Katz BZ, Niederman J, Olson B, et al: Fragment length polymorphisms among independent isolates of Epstein-Barr virus from immunocompromised and normal hosts. J Infect Dis 157:299–308, 1988

10 Raab-Traub N, Hood R, Yang C, et al: Epstein-Barr virus transcription in nasopharyngeal carcinoma. J Virol 48:580–590, 1983

11 Sixbey J, Vesterinen E, Nedrud J, et al: Replication of Epstein-Barr virus in human epithelial cells infected in vitro. Nature 306:480–483, 1983

12 Griffin B, Karran L: Immortalization of monkey epithelial cells by specific fragments of Epstein-Barr virus DNA. Nature 309:78–82, 1984

13 Miller G, Shope T, Coope D, et al: Lymphoma in cotton-top marmosets after inoculation with Epstein-Barr virus: Tumor incidence, histologic spectrum, antibody responses, demonstration of viral DNA, and characterization of viruses. J Exp Med 145:948–967, 1977

14 Pelicci P, Knowless D, Magrath I, et al: Chromosomal breakpoints and structural alterations of the c-myc locus differ in endemic and sporadic forms of Burkitt lymphoma. Proc Natl Acad Sci USA 83:2984–2988, 1986

15 de The G, Ho JNC, Muir CS: Nasopharyngeal carcinoma, in Evans AS (ed): *Viral Infections of Humans, Epidemiology and Control.* New York, Plenum, 1982, chap 25

16 Burkitt DP, Wright DH (eds): *Burkitt's Lymphoma.* Edinburgh, Livingstone, 1970

17 Starzl TE, Nalesnik MA, Porter KA, et al: Reversibility of lymphomas and lymphoproliferative lesions developing under cyclosporin-steroid therapy. Lancet i:583–587, 1984

18 de The G, Geser A, Day NE, et al: Epidemiological evidence for causal relationship between Epstein-Barr virus and Burkitt's lymphoma from Ugandan prospective study. Nature 274:756–761, 1978

19 Miller G: Epidemiology of Burkitt lymphoma, in Evans AS (ed): *Viral Infections of Humans, Epidemiology and Control.* New York, Plenum, 1982, chap 24

20 Andiman WA: Medical progress: The Epstein-Barr virus and EB virus infections in childhood. J Pediatr 95:171–182, 1979

21 Epstein MA: Vaccination against Epstein-Barr virus: Current progress and future strategies. Lancet i:1425–1427, 1986

Rabies · David A. Warrell · Robert E. Shope

Rabies is a major human viral disease of the tropics. It is characterized by meningoencephalitis which is nearly always fatal. The virus is transmitted to humans by the bite of dogs and cats or, in some places, by the bite of wild animals, especially bats and carnivores. The disease is distributed throughout the world except for areas which are free of rabies through isolation, eradication, and/or quarantine.

The incubation in humans and animals is usually at least 2 weeks and sometimes as long as 6 months or more. Hence animals incubating rabies have time to move for long distances as seemingly healthy animals. Pasteur developed postexposure prophylaxis. He first successfully vaccinated Joseph Meister in 1885 after the boy was bitten by a rabid dog. Since then advances in diagnosis, vaccination, passive antibody therapy, and regulation of animal hosts have led to effective control of rabies in most of the temperate parts of the world. In the tropics, however, bat-, cat-, and especially dog-transmitted disease continues in major proportions. Local social customs and the paucity of resources work against control. Nevertheless, prevention of rabies and limiting its spread in the tropics is currently a worthwhile and practical goal of tropical nations and of the World Health Organization.

PARASITE

MORPHOLOGY AND ULTRASTRUCTURE

Rabies virus belongs to the family Rhabdoviridae, from *rhabdos* meaning rod. The particles are bacilliform, rounded on one end and flat or concave on the other, 180 nm long, and 75 nm wide. They contain a central axial channel which houses the single-stranded RNA attached to a nucleoprotein. The coiled ribonucleoprotein confers the appearance of striations in electron micrographs (see Fig. 69-1). The virions also have a lipid envelope through which protrude 6- to 8-nm knoblike glycoprotein projections.

Particles are formed in the cytoplasm of neurons or other cells in the infected animal. The virions are sometimes associated with inclusions of massed nucleoprotein which produces a granular or linear matrix and which stains cherry red with aniline dyes such as in Seller's stain, accounting for the diagnostic Negri body (Fig. 69-2). When adapted by passage in laboratory animals, the virus becomes fixed in its incubation period. This fixed virus has a shorter incubation than wild virus (''street virus''). Virus particles are relatively sparse in naturally infected nerve cells in most animals; however, particles of salivary gland cells are characteristically found in large numbers in the acini, a remarkable adaptation of rabies virus to favor its transmission.

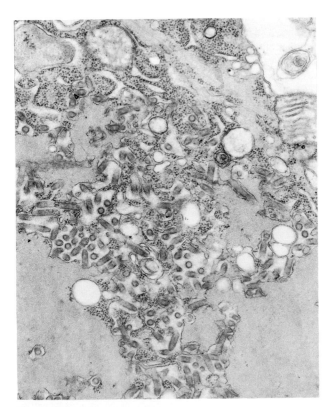

Figure 69-1. Rabies.

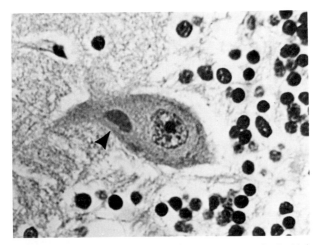

Figure 69-2. Negri body (arrowhead) in the cytoplasm of a Purkinje cell, human cerebellum × 4,000 (*Courtesy of Dr. Frederick A. Murphy.*)

BIOCHEMISTRY

It is generally accepted that the virus attaches at the plasma membrane, to which the virus envelope fuses, and the ribonucleoprotein enters the cytoplasm. Rabies virion RNA is not infectious; it requires a virion-associated RNA transcriptase to produce complementary-stranded messenger RNA. Translation results in a glycoprotein, a matrix protein, a phosphorylated (NS) protein, and a nucleoprotein. The glycoprotein induces neutralizing antibody and is responsible for the properties of attachment and hemagglutination. The nucleoprotein is usually produced in excess and is the major antigen detected in the immunofluorescence and complement fixation tests. This protein, in addition to the glycoprotein, plays a role in immunity [1]. There is also a large protein that may be the transcriptase.

The rabies RNA has been cloned and sequenced, and the cDNA representing the glycoprotein has been inserted into a vaccinia vector. The glycoprotein expressed by the vaccinia vector immunized experimental animals against rabies infection [2] and is an excellent candidate for a new rabies vaccine.

ANIMAL MODELS

Virtually all vertebrate animals can be infected with rabies virus, although the dose needed to infect is both strain-dependent and host-dependent. Experimental studies are usually carried out in mice, rats, rabbits, guinea pigs, dogs, foxes, monkeys, bats, or chickens. The baby hamster is sensitive to infection with very small doses of virus. The mouse, because of its small size, ready availability, and ease of handling, has been used extensively as a model. The disease in the mouse mimicks very closely that in dogs and humans. Indeed it was possible to use unpassaged rabies virus from fox salivary gland and reproduce the disease in mice after incubation periods of 1 to 3 months as seen in humans. The mouse thus can serve as a model for studying pathogenesis, for measuring vaccine potency, and, in challenge experiments, for testing vaccine efficacy.

RESERVOIR

Dogs and cats serve as the primary reservoir of rabies transmission to humans in the tropics; however, as is evident in places such as the United States where dog and cat rabies is under control, wildlife reservoirs also occur in most rabies-prevalent areas of the world. Rabies virus is able to maintain itself in dogs because of a combination of circumstances:

1. The incubation period in dogs is relatively long—between 2 weeks and 6 months usually—thus infected free-ranging dogs may appear normal.
2. In many tropical countries, dogs, although they may have an owner, roam freely and uncontrolled in packs. Thus, a rabid dog transmits easily to others in the pack and maintains the reservoir.
3. Saliva of dogs is infective for at least 2 days before illness, and the virus infects, among other CNS areas, the limbic system, which may drive the animal to bite and attack viciously.
4. In many parts of the tropics, dogs are not regularly vaccinated for rabies.
5. Asymptomatic dogs on rare occasions shed virus over periods of years [3].

Rabies of wild carnivores such as skunks, wolves, raccoons, and meerkats is primarily a problem of temperate zones. In the tropics, the major wildlife reservoir is the bat, especially the vampire bat (*Desmodus rotundus*) in Latin America. These bats transmit to their offspring and siblings through grooming and biting. They also transmit on a grand scale to cattle, but cattle are dead-end hosts, i.e., they do not maintain the cycle.

RABIES-RELATED VIRUSES

Five viruses related antigenically to rabies are indigenous to tropical Africa. Rabies and the related viruses Mokola, Duvenhage, and Lagos bat form the genus *Lyssavirus*. Two other viruses, Kotonkan and Obodhiang, are not known to infect people and have only a distant antigenic relationship to rabies. Mokola virus was recovered in 1968 from *Crocidura* spp. shrews in Ibadan, Nigeria. Shortly after, two human patients were diagnosed in Nigeria. One of these presented with poliomyelitis and recovered; the other presented with encephalitis and died. Duvenhage virus was isolated in South Africa from the brain of a patient who had been bitten on the lip by a bat. A variant of Duvenhage virus, called European bat lyssa virus, was responsible for the death of a zoologist in Finland and is enzootic in European bats. Lagos bat virus was found in fruit bats in Lagos, Nigeria, and since has been isolated from bats in Central African Republic and South Africa. It is not associated with human illness.

Rabies-related viruses were originally thought to be restricted to wildlife and to Africa. These viruses, however, have been isolated in Africa from cats and a dog in Zimbabwe [4] and from a variety of bats in Europe. From a practical point of view it is incumbent on physicians dealing with patients from Africa and Europe suspected of having rabies to consider in their diagnosis the rabies-related viruses. Rabies vaccine as tested in animals offers marginal if any protection to challenge with rabies-related viruses.

PATIENT

HOST-PARASITE INTERFACE

Rabies is a truly zoonotic virus. The host may be a human or a lower animal such as a bat, cow, cat, or dog. The virus commonly enters the host by bite, and infected saliva contaminates wound tissues. In experimental infections it has been shown that primary replication takes place in muscle cells, although it is also possible that the virus enters the nervous system directly through nerve endings. The best evidence indicates that rabies virus is indeed neurotropic and that the neuromuscular junctions have specific receptor sites for the virus, perhaps the acetylcholine receptors [5]. Other receptors on myocytes and neurons almost certainly also are involved in virus uptake. Under some conditions the virus may be sequestered at the site of introduction for long periods. Using a strain of rabies virus with an incubation of 1 to 3 months, rabies was prevented in mice by amputation of the sciatic nerve as long as 18 days after virus was introduced into the ipsilateral footpad [6].

Rabies virus may also cause infection after exposure of the host to aerosol or to oral inoculation. The precise anatomical site of virus entry by these routes—presumably nerve endings—is not known. Several cases of rabies have followed corneal transplants when rabies virus was surgically introduced directly into the eye [7].

PATHOLOGY [8]

Rabies virus causes an acute nonsuppurative meningoencephalitis. The brain is grossly normal except for slight congestion of the meningeal vessels. At the time of death lesions are widespread throughout the nervous system. The brain, spinal cord, and peripheral nerves show ganglion cell degeneration, perineural and perivascular mononuclear cell infiltration, neuronophagia, and glial nodules. In furious rabies, inflammatory changes are most marked in the midbrain and medulla, and in paralytic rabies, in the spinal cord. Negri bodies, found in up to 80 percent of human cases, are diagnostic intracytoplasmic inclusions consisting of masses of viral ribonucleoprotein (Fig. 69-2). They are most numerous in the pyramidal cells of Ammon's horn in the hippocampus, in cerebellar Purkinje cells, and in the medulla and ganglia. They can be demonstrated by direct immunofluorescence or Seller's stain in acetone-fixed specimens, and by Schleiften's or Gordon-Smith's stains in histological sections of gray matter. In the absence of Negri bodies there are no histological features that distinguish rabies from poliomyelitis or other forms of viral encephalitis. In view of the appalling prognosis of rabies encephalitis, neuronolysis is surprisingly mild and patchy, but functional disturbances such as defective cholinergic neurotransmission are not revealed by histopathology. The brainstem, limbic system, and hypothalamus appear to be most severely affected. A spongiform encephalopathy, probably an indirect immunological effect of infection, has been demonstrated in skunks and foxes [9]. Extraneural changes include focal degeneration of salivary and lacrimal glands, pancreas, adrenal medulla, and lymph nodes with an interstitial myocarditis with round cell infiltration in approximately 25 percent of cases. The brain of a fatal human case of Mokola virus encephalitis showed perivascular cuffing with lymphocytes and lymphoblastoid cells. Neurons contained large numbers of cytoplasmic inclusion bodies which were quite different in size and appearance from Negri bodies [10].

PATHOGENESIS

After the virus enters the neuron, it spreads via the axoplasm to the central nervous system. Antigen is first detected in the ipsilateral neurons serving the site of inoculation; it then spreads to the contralateral neurons. The infection then progresses rapidly through the spinal cord and brain, and antigen is localized in nerves throughout the brain. Finally, infection spreads centrifugally through nerves to the motor, sensory, and autonomic nerve termini and other cells of most organs of the body. At this stage the virus is in high titer in the exocrine tissue such as the pancreas and salivary glands. The saliva contains large amounts of infectious virus. Antigen is also easily demonstrated in the nerve endings of the skin and cornea. These sites are especially useful for diagnosis by corneal smear or skin biopsy.

CLINICAL MANIFESTATIONS [11]

The incubation period is between 20 and 90 days in more than two-thirds of cases, with an extreme range from 4 days to many years. Facial and severe multiple bites (Fig. 69-3), transmission by corneal transplant and accidental inoculation of live virus (rage de laboratoire) are associated with a short incubation period.

A few days of vague feverish symptoms commonly precede the development of definite signs of rabies encephalitis, but in more than one-third of cases itching, pain, or paresthesia at the site of the healed bite wound is a specific prodromal symptom (Fig. 69-4). The two distinct clinical types of rabies, furious (agitated) and paralytic (dumb), may reflect differences

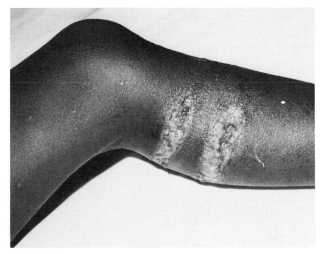

Figure 69-3. Severe bite wounds on the calf of a Nigerian child bitten by a rabid dog. (*Copyright D.A. Warrell.*)

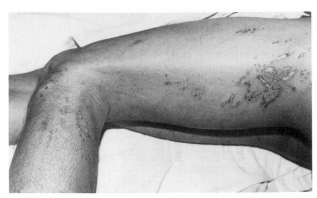

Figure 69-4. Intense itching developed eight weeks after a bite by a dog in the same limb. The patient developed furious rabies and died 3 days later. (*Courtesy of Dr. Sornchai Looareesuwan.*)

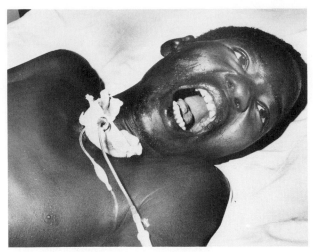

Figure 69-6. Nigerian man with furious rabies: generalized excitation, hallucinations, and shouting interspersed with periods of lucidity. (*Copyright D.A. Warrell.*)

in the infecting strain of rabies virus or in the host's immune response. Furious rabies, the more common presentation in humans, is characterized by hydrophobia and aerophobia, episodic generalized arousal, with sudden death or rapid progression to coma and generalized flaccid paralysis within the space of 48 to 72 h in the absence of intensive care. *Hydrophobia* is reflex, jerky inspiratory muscle spasm associated with inexplicable terror provoked by attempts to drink water (Fig. 69-5). A draught of air on the skin produces a similar reflex response, called *aerophobia*. These spasms may progress to opisthotonos and end in generalized convulsions with cardiac or respiratory arrest. Periods of generalized excitation (Fig. 69-6), during which the patient becomes wild, hallucinated, and sometimes aggressive, alternate with lucid intervals. These dramatic symptoms are probably explained by selective encephalitis involving the brainstem and limbic system [*12*]. Hypersalivation, lacrimation (Fig. 69-7), sweating,

and fluctuating blood pressure and body temperature result from disturbances of hypothalamic or autonomic nervous system function. Conventional neurological examination may be surprisingly normal, but there may be meningism, cranial nerve and upper motor neuron lesions, muscle fasciculation, and involuntary movements. Increased libido, priapism, and spontaneous orgasm suggests involvement of the amygdaloid nuclei.

Paralytic rabies is much less common than the furious form but is undoubtedly underdiagnosed. All cases of rabies transmitted by vampire bats in Latin America are of this type [*13*]. After the usual prodromal symptoms, there is flaccid paralysis and altered sensation starting usually in the bitten limb and

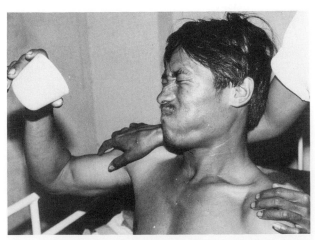

Figure 69-5. Hydrophobia: jerky spasms of sternocleidomastoid and other inspiratory muscles associated with terror prompted by attempts to drink water. (*Courtesy of Dr. Sornchai Looareesuwan.*)

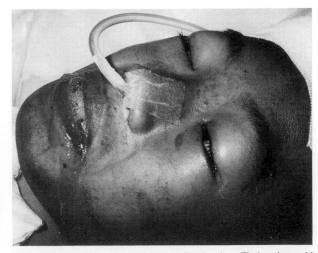

Figure 69-7. Lacrimation and hypersalivation in a Thai patient with furious rabies. (*Copyright D.A. Warrell.*)

ascending symmetrically or asymmetrically with pain, fasciculation, and mild sensory disturbances. Paraplegia and sphincter involvement then develop and finally quadriparesis and fatal paralysis of deglutitive and respiratory muscles. In the terminal phase hydrophobia may be represented by spontaneous inspiratory spasms. Patients may survive for several weeks even without intensive care.

Of the rabies-related viruses, Mokola virus infection was associated with upper respiratory tract symptoms in one patient and with fatal viral encephalitis with no distinguishing features in another patient, while Duvenhage virus infection causes an illness indistinguishable from furious rabies [14].

Differential diagnosis

Rabies must be considered in patients who develop appropriate neurological symptoms after being bitten by a mammal in the endemic area and in travelers who have been in an endemic area during the past few years. Not all patients can recall a mammal bite. Hydrophobia is a pathognomonic sign: characteristic jerky inspiratory spasms and intense anxiety are provoked by attempts to swallow or by directing a draught of air onto the patient's face. Furious rabies must be distinguished from other encephalitides, tetanus, intoxications, delirium tremens, laryngeal conditions, rabies phobia, and other psychoses. Paralytic rabies has been confused with postvaccinal encephalomyelitis (including Landry's ascending paralysis and Guillain-Barré syndrome) which can complicate vaccination with nervous tissue rabies vaccines [15], with poliomyelitis, and with simian herpes encephalomyelitis.

CLINICAL FEATURES OF RABIES IN MAMMALS

In domestic dogs the incubation period is usually 3 to 12 weeks (range 5 days to 14 months). A common prodromal sign is intense irritation at the site of the infecting bite. Seventy-five percent of infected animals present with paralytic (dumb) signs including dysphagia, ptosis, altered bark, paralysis of the jaw, neck, and hind limbs (Fig. 69-8), hypersalivation, congested conjunctivae, pruritis, shivering, trembling, snapping at imaginary objects, pica, and extreme restlessness and desire to wander away from home. The minority, which develop furious rabies, are aggressive and attack and may swallow inanimate objects, often seriously injuring their mouths in the process. On average, virus is excreted in the saliva for 3 days before signs appear and the animal dies within the next several days, providing a basis for the traditional 10-day observation period for dogs suspected of suffering from rabies. However, chronic excretion of virus in the saliva of apparently healthy dogs has been reported, although rarely, from India, Ethiopia, and elsewhere.

Among other species, signs are usually furious in horses, cats, mustelidae, and viverridae and usually paralytic in foxes and bovines.

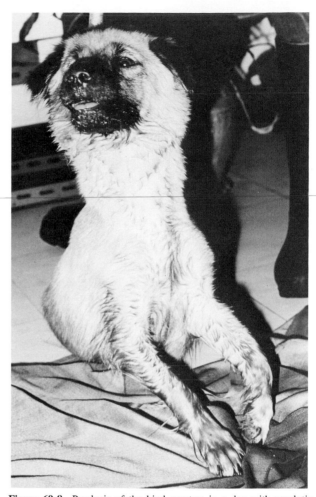

Figure 69-8. Paralysis of the hind quarters in a dog with paralytic rabies. (*Copyright D.A. Warrell.*)

LABORATORY DIAGNOSIS

Rabies should be suspected in any case of encephalitis, with or without a history of animal bite. The bite may have been completely forgotten, especially in instances where the incubation is several months long.

Immunofluorescence of brain or spinal cord is now the most widely used test to confirm rabies in the mammal responsible for the bite. This technique is more specific than the demonstration of Negri bodies. A simpler ELISA test and a very sensitive avidin-biotin peroxidase system, which can be used on formalin-fixed histological sections, have recently been developed. In patients, rabies can be confirmed during life by immunofluorescence of skin (Fig. 69-9) and brain biopsies and, rarely, also of corneal impression smears. Early in the illness rabies virus may be isolated from saliva, brain, cerebrospinal fluid (CSF), and even spun urine. Use of neuroblastoma cell cultures for virus isolation can produce a positive result in 2

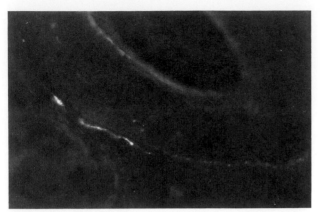

Figure 69-9. Rabies-specific immunofluorescence of nerve twiglets in a hair follicle. (*Courtesy of Dr. M.J. Warrell.*)

to 4 days instead of the 2 to 3 weeks required for the traditional intracerebral inoculation of mice [*16*]. Appearance of rabies antibodies in serum and CSF is usually delayed until after the first week of illness. In patients who have not received vaccine and immune globulin, rabies antibody in the serum and especially in the CSF is diagnostic. However, rabies-neutralizing antibody leaks into the CSF in patients with postvaccinal encephalomyelitis, although a very high titer suggests a diagnosis of rabies. The best way of distinguishing rabies from postvaccinal encephalomyelitis is by the immunofluorescence of skin biopsies [*17*]. Lymphocyte pleocytosis rarely exceeds a few hundred cells per microliter. A peripheral neutrophil leukocytosis is common.

The laboratory results should be interpreted with full knowledge of the field circumstances. If the person was bitten by a clinically rabid dog in a rabies-enzootic area, treatment should usually be initiated even if the laboratory results are not conclusive.

TREATMENT OF RABIES ENCEPHALITIS

There is no specific treatment, but life may be prolonged and in very rare instances even saved by intensive care [*18*]. Problems arising during intensive care include a variety of respiratory complications, including aspiration pneumonia, pneumothorax, and respiratory arrest; cardiac arrhythmias, hypotension, pulmonary edema, and effects of myocarditis; generalized convulsions, cerebral edema, diffuse neuropathy, and hematemesis associated with upper gastrointestinal tract ulceration. Adequate sedation and analgesia must be given to relieve the agonizing symptoms of rabies encephalitis. Antiviral agents, hyperimmune serum, α-interferon, and immunosuppressants have not proved useful.

POPULATION

Rabies can maintain a transmission cycle in any part of the tropics where carnivores exist. Areas free of rabies include the British Isles, Scandinavia (including Iceland but excluding Denmark and Greenland), Cyprus, Australia, Borneo, New Guinea, Bali, New Zealand, Antarctica, Oceania, Peninsular Malaysia, Singapore, Japan, Taiwan, and the Caribbean (except Cuba, Dominican Republic, Grenada, Haiti, and Trinidad and Tobago).

METHODS OF SPREAD

Long-range spread of rabies is facilitated by rapid transport in the modern era and by the long incubation period, which allows domestic animals to be taken abroad by their owners in the absence of signs of disease.

A more complex rabies problem is the short-range spread which plagues zones with effective control programs adjacent to highly enzootic areas. The Rio Grande Valley of Texas has consistently recorded dog rabies adjacent to the high-prevalence region in Matamoros, Mexico. The same phenomenon holds true in Malaysia where transmission originated across the border in Thailand. The area of spread is regulated by the range of young dogs and does not extend more than a few kilometers per year.

Rabies in vampire bats can move over much wider areas. Outbreaks in cattle in Latin America can be expected wherever vampire bats range. For example, vampire bat-transmitted cattle rabies occurred suddenly in Surinam in 1979 after being absent there since 1972.

Mountains, bodies of water, and deserts form natural barriers to the movements of wild animals and, to some extent, domestic animals. Advantage can be taken of these natural barriers to plan rabies control projects in the tropics. Once the disease is controlled on an island or in a valley surrounded by the mountains, it is relatively easier to maintain the area free than it is in zones without barriers.

POPULATION ECOLOGY

Rabies in the tropics is more prevalent in the urban population centers because of large concentrations of dogs in and around the cities. It is estimated that the ratio of dogs to persons is between 1:13 to 1:8 [*19*] and the incidence of rabies in dogs between 0 and 793/100,000. As human populations increase, so do dog populations. Dogs in Latin America account for more than 96 percent of the reported animal rabies and for nearly all the exposure of the human population [*20*]. The common practice in the tropics is for the family to maintain one or more dogs which eat at home but run loose, often completely free to roam, sometimes in packs. Thus a dog may be attacked by rabid animals out of sight of its owners, and later when the dog in turn develops rabies, it may return to completely familiar surroundings to expose family members, especially children.

The other major reservoir of rabies in the new world tropics is the common vampire bat (*Desmodus rotundus*). This species feeds primarily on the blood of cattle but also appears to feed indiscriminantly on other available animals including humans. Populations of vampire bats have increased over the last century, probably because of the increased food supply represented by larger herds of cattle in the tropics. The bats live in caves, trees, mines, and abandoned buildings in colonies of 50 to 1000 or more. They are common where cattle are abundant.

The vampire bat feeds only on the blood of animals and is thus ideally suited to transmit rabies. Cattle are usually dead-end hosts. The bat becomes sick and dies after infection but may transmit through its saliva for several days or even weeks prior to death.

EPIDEMIOLOGY

Age and sex

Rabies is a disease of all age groups; nearly 100 percent of the human population is susceptible. The disease, however, is more common in children between 1 and 14 years old and especially in young males. Children are more likely to play around sick dogs and are an easier target for a biting animal. There is experimental evidence, also, that younger animals are more susceptible to rabies virus infection.

Types of epidemics

Rabies epidemics are of two types. Small outbreaks result from the multiple attacks of a single rabid animal. Larger epidemics occur when rabies is uncontrolled in an area and multiple biting animals during the same time period expose the human population.

Prevalence

Rabies is an underreported disease and therefore the actual prevalence of rabies in the tropics is unknown. In parts of Asia such as India, it is a common cause of encephalitis. It is less common in the new world tropics, where between 1970 and 1979 there were 2696 reported human rabies cases. The Pan American Health Organization estimated that during the same period there were 2,600,000 persons who received postexposure prophylaxis in the Americas. Thirty percent completed the course. The treatment figure may give a better idea of the magnitude of the rabies problem than the number of cases reported.

INFECTION AND DISEASE

Whether or not rabies virus causes inapparent infection and chronic or persistent infections is an important, incompletely answered question. Attenuated strains of rabies can infect animals without causing disease and with development of full immunity. This is the basis for the live attenuated rabies vaccines for dogs and cats. Wild or street rabies characteristically causes central nervous system disease which is fatal.

Vampire bats were originally reported to shed rabies virus in saliva while the bats were asymptomatic [21]. More recent observations [22] cast doubt on the early work and indicate that bats do not develop a true carrier state.

In contrast, apparently healthy dogs have been confirmed on rare occasions to shed rabies virus in saliva periodically over several months. While this observation offers an important mechanism by which rabies may persist in an area, it does not negate the overwhelming evidence that rabies can be effectively controlled by vaccination of dogs and by leash regulations.

PREVENTION

Preexposure vaccination

The advent of safe tissue culture vaccines has made possible the recommendation of preexposure immunization for people at high risk living in rabies-endemic areas, such as veterinarians, most health care personnel, public health laboratory workers, and dog catchers; for those in nonendemic areas who come in contact with imported mammals in quarantine; for those who work with rabies virus in laboratories; and for those who intend to travel to rabies-endemic areas. Travelers at particular risk of exposure to rabies are zoologists and other fieldworkers, forest rangers, cave explorers, and those whose work involves walking and bicycling in urban and rural areas of India, southeast Asia, and Latin America. Any of the reputable tissue culture vaccines (see below) can be given either as 1 mL injected intramuscularly into the deltoid (not in the gluteal region) or 0.1 mL intradermally on days 0, 7, and 28. Booster doses are given every 2 years if the neutralizing antibody level falls and continued protection is needed. Laboratory personnel working with rabies virus should have their antibody titer checked every 6 months. Weekly chloroquine taken as malarial prophylaxis can suppress the response to preexposure vaccination with intradermal human diploid cell strain vaccine (HDCSV, see below) in tropical endemic countries. The intradermal course should therefore be completed well before departure or the vaccine given intramuscularly.

Postexposure prophylaxis [23]

Rabies virus inoculated by a bite can be neutralized by topical virucidal agents and by active and passive immunization until it enters the relative sanctuary of the peripheral and central nervous system. In Thailand, 45 percent of unvaccinated patients died of rabies after severe dog bites [24] and in other countries about 15 percent died after bites on the hands and fingers. This mortality can be prevented by modern postexposure prophylaxis. Postexposure prophylaxis is most likely to be effective if it can be instituted within the first 24 h after exposure. Wound cleaning is essential first aid for all animal bites and is particularly effective for superficial wounds. The wound should be scrubbed with soap or detergent under a

Table 69-1. Specific postexposure prophylaxis for use in a rabies-endemic area

Nature of exposure	Circumstances of bite and species involved	Treatment
Minor exposure Licks of the skin Scratches or abrasions Minor bites	(1) Unprovoked attack by cat or dog	Start vaccine: stop treatment if animal remains healthy for 5 days or if brain fluorescent antibody test proves negative; administer serum upon positive diagnosis and complete the course of vaccine.
	(2) Attack by wild animal or domestic cat or dog unavailable for observation	Serum and vaccine.
Major exposure Licks of mucosa Major bites (multiple or on face, head, finger, or neck)	(1) or (2) above	Serum and vaccine: stop if domestic cat or dog remains healthy for 5 days, or if any animal's brain fluorescent antibody test proves negative.

running tap for at least 5 min, and any foreign material should be removed. Effective virucidal agents include soap, povidone iodine, 0.1% aqueous iodine, or 40 to 70% alcohol. Quaternary ammonium compounds are no longer recommended. Deep wounds should be surgically debrided and irrigated under local or general anesthesia. Rabies virus is one of a number of pathogens associated with mammal bites: these include *Pasteurella multocida, Clostridium tetani,* other aerobic and anaerobic bacteria, spirochetes, viruses, and fungi. Suturing of wounds should be avoided or delayed at least until after rabies immune globulin has been infiltrated (see below). Indications for specific rabies prophylaxis are given in Table 69-1.

Active immunization

Nervous tissue vaccines (Semple and suckling mouse brain) are still the most widely used worldwide but are of variable potency and may be associated with severe neuroparalytic reactions. A number of tissue culture vaccines are now in large-scale production: these include the well-established human diploid cell strain vaccine (HDCSV) (Institut Mérieux) and the more recent and less expensive purified vero cell rabies vaccine (PVRV) (Institut Mérieux) and purified chicken embryo cell vaccine (PCEC) (Behringwerke). These vaccines are potent and carry a negligible risk of serious reactions. The recommended regimen is five or six 1-mL intramuscular or subcutaneous doses on days 0, 3, 7, 14, 30, and optionally on day 90. An abbreviated regimen consists of two 1-mL injections at different sites on day 0, followed by single 1-mL injections on days 7 and 21. The most economical regimen with proven efficacy consists of intradermal injections of 0.1 mL given at eight sites (deltoids, suprascapular, abdominal, and thighs) on day 0, four sites on day 7, and single sites on days 28 and 90 [25]. The initial dose of vaccine should be increased if there

has been delay of more than 48 h in starting postexposure prophylaxis, if passive immunization was given 24 h or more before active immunization, in elderly patients, in those with chronic diseases such as cirrhosis, and in those likely to be immunosuppressed and severely malnourished. *Intramuscular injections must never be given in the gluteal region* because the antibody response may be poor. Tissue culture vaccines cause mild local symptoms in about 15 percent of vaccinees, but intradermal injection causes local irritation in 35 percent. Systemic effects appear in approximately 7 percent of patients and include headache, fever, and a "flulike illness" but all symptoms are short-lived. In the United States, 10 percent of booster injections have been associated with mild immune complex disease 3 to 13 days later. This reaction is directed against protein components altered by β-propiolactone, the viral inactivator in the virus.

Passive immunization

Combined vaccination and administration of hyperimmune serum has proved effective in preventing rabies after severe head bites by rabid wolves in several natural experiments in Iran, U.S.S.R., and China. In unvaccinated people exposed to rabies, hyperimmune serum (equine antirabies serum or human rabies immune globulin) is indicated to neutralize rabies virus before the appearance of vaccine-induced antibody. It is particularly important in cases of severe multiple bites on the face, neck, and extremities. Most cases of apparent "failure" of tissue culture vaccination have been attributable to delayed, inadequate, or absent passive immunization [26]. Passive immunization should be given at the same time as the first dose of vaccine but in a different site. The dose of equine antirabies serum is 40 IU/kg and of human rabies immune globulin, 20 IU/kg. Approximately half the dose is infiltrated around the bite wound, and the rest is given intramuscularly at a site distant from the vaccine (*but not in the gluteal region*). The incidence of serum reactions to refined preparations of equine antirabies globulin is less than 5 percent. Skin testing does not predict reactions and should not be performed. Passive immunization may cause partial suppression of the response to vaccines, and so the recommended dose should not be exceeded.

Someone who has received a full preexposure course of tissue culture vaccine does not require passive immunization if subsequently bitten by a rabid animal. However, a short booster course of tissue culture vaccine is imperative, such as 1 mL of HDCSV by intramuscular injection on days 0, 3, and 7.

Failures of rabies prophylaxis

The recommended pre- and postexposure prophylaxis may not be effective against the rabies-related viruses Duvenhage, European bat lyssa virus (Duvenhage 4), and Mokola, because of their great antigenic differences from rabies [27–28,29]. In addition, there is experimental evidence for minor antigenic variation among rabies strains which might result in vaccine failures. However, since the HDCSV and immune globulin regimen has proved highly successful up until now, this possibility remains hypothetical. Postexposure prophylaxis may fail if vaccines of low potency are used (for example, some batches of nervous tissue vaccine), if the start of the vaccination is delayed for more than about a week, if wound cleaning and passive immunization are omitted, and if the immune responsiveness of the vaccinee is decreased.

CONTROL

Dogs and cats

The control of human rabies in the tropics depends on prevention in dogs and to a lesser extent in cats. In the past, when resources have been allocated for control of rabies in dogs, and campaigns instituted, transmission to humans has diminished or disappeared. Some areas, such as Japan and Malaysia, have remained free of rabies; others, such as parts of Colombia and east Africa, have suffered resurgence of disease when control measures have been relaxed.

Research on control of rabies in temperate regions where wildlife rabies is the prevalent form may prove applicable to control of dog rabies in the tropics. For instance oral live attenuated rabies vaccines in baits (chicken heads and fishmeal) have been successful in virtually eradicating fox rabies in parts of Switzerland and West Germany; experimental trials in raccoons in the United States also offer evidence of efficacy. A similar approach may be useful in the tropics to immunize stray dogs instead of trying to reduce or muzzle the dog population.

Control programs in both temperate and tropical countries need more information about the prevalence and host range of rabies in domestic and wild animals. Laboratory facilities for diagnosis are critically important. The human population should to be instructed to avoid contact with potentially rabid animals and not to keep wild carnivores (skunks, raccoons, coatimundis, and mongooses) as pets.

The World Health Organization and national governments in Africa have embarked on carefully conceived campaigns which serve as models for other tropical areas. These campaigns are based on a phased control of rabies in dogs, beginning with small geographical areas and extending to countrywide programs. The programs involve revision and enforcement of existing laws, education of the public to the need of control of stray dogs, improved surveillance and veterinary diagnostic facilities, canine vaccine production and distribution, and control of stray dogs.

About 90 percent of rabies patients and of those persons receiving rabies prophylaxis in the tropics have been exposed to dogs. Therefore successful dog rabies control is the single most effective measure for control of human rabies in the tropics.

REFERENCES

1 Dietzschold B, Wang H, Rupprecht C, et al: Induction of protective immunity against rabies by immunization with rabies virus ribonucleoprotein. Proc Natl Acad Sci USA 84:9165–9169, 1987

2 Wiktor TJ, MacFarlan RI, Reagan KJ, et al: Protection from rabies by a vaccinia virus recombinant containing the rabies virus glycoprotein gene. Proc Natl Acad Sci USA 81:7194–7198, 1984

3 Fekadu M, Shaddock JH, Baer GM: Intermittent excretion of rabies virus in the saliva of a dog two and six months after it had recovered from experimental rabies. Am J Trop Med Hyg 30:1113–1115, 1981

4 Foggin CM: Atypical rabies virus in cats and a dog in Zimbabwe. Vet Rec 110:338, 1982

5 Lentz TL, Burrage TH, Smith AL, et al: Is the acetylcholine receptor a rabies virus receptor? Science 215:182–184, 1982

6 Baer GM, Cleary WF: A model in mice for the pathogenesis and treatment of rabies. J Infect Dis 125:520–527, 1972

7 US Public Health Service: Human-to-human transmission of rabies via corneal transplant—Thailand. MMWR 30:473–474, 1981

8 Perl DP: The pathology of rabies in the central nervous system, in Baer GM (ed): *The Natural History of Rabies.* New York, Academic, 1975, vol 1, chap 13, pp 236–272

9 Charlton KM, Casey GA, Webster WA, et al: Experimental rabies in skunks and foxes. Pathogenesis of the spongiform lesions. Lab Invest 57:634–645, 1987

10 Familusi JB, Osunkoya BO, Moore DL, et al: A fatal human infection with Mokola virus. Am J Trop Med Hyg 21:959–963, 1972

11 Kaplan C, Turner GS, Warrell DA: *Rabies: The Facts,* 2d ed. Oxford University Press, 1986

12 Warrell DA, Davidson NMcD, Pope HM, et al: Pathophysiologic studies in human rabies. Am J Med 60:180–190, 1976

13 Pawan JL: Paralysis as a clinical manifestation in human rabies. Ann Trop Med Parasitol 33:21–29, 1939

14 Meredith CD, Rossouw AP, Van Fraag Koch H: An unusual case of human rabies thought to be of chiropteran origin. S Afr Med J 45:767–769, 1971

15 Alvord EC, Jahnke U, Fischer EH: The causes of the syndromes of Landry (1859) and of Guillain, Barré, and Strohl. Rev Neurol (Paris) 143:571–579, 1987

16 Smith AL, Tignor GH, Emmons RW, et al: Isolation of field rabies virus strains in CER and murine neuroblastoma cell cultures. Intervirology 9:359–361, 1978

17 Warrell MJ, Looareesuwan S, Manatsathit S, et al: Rapid diagnosis of rabies and post-vaccine encephalitides. Clin Exp Immunol 71: 229–234, 1988

18 Hattwick MAW, Gregg MB: The disease in man, in Baer GM (ed): *The Natural History of Rabies*. New York, Academic, 1975, vol 1, chap 19, pp 373–400

19 Escobar Cifuentes E: Animals and zoonoses—general bases for zoonoses control, in *Animal Health in the Americas, 1980. Animals in Human Life*. PAHO scientific publication 404, Washington, DC, 1981, pp 32–44

20 Acha P: A review of rabies prevention and control in the Americas, 1970–1980. Overall status of rabies. Bull Off Int Epiz 93:9–52, 1981

21 Pawan JL: An unusual strain of rabies virus in a vampire bat. Ann Trop Med Parasitol 82:35–38, 1938

22 Moreno JA, Baer GM: Experimental rabies virus in a vampire bat. Am J Trop Med Hyg 29:254–259, 1980

23 Centers for Disease Control Advisory Committee on Immunization Practices: Rabies prevention—United States. MMWR 33:393–408, 1984

24 Sitthi-Amorn C, Jiratanavattana V, Keoyoo J, et al: The diagnostic properties of laboratory tests for rabies. Int J Epidemiol 16:602–605, 1987

25 Warrell MJ, Nicholson KG, Warrell DA, et al: Economical multisite intradermal immunization with human diploid cell strain vaccine is effective for post-exposure rabies prophylaxis. Lancet i:1059–1062, 1985

26 Anonymous: Rabies vaccine failures. Lancet i:917–918, 1988 (editorial)

27 Tignor GH, Murphy FA, Clark HF, et al: Duvenhage virus: Morphological, biochemical, histopathological and antigenic relationships to the rabies serogroup. J Gen Virol 37:595–611, 1977

28 Tignor GH, Shope RE: Vaccination and challenge of mice with viruses of the rabies serogroup. J Infect Dis 125:322–324, 1972

29 Wiktor TJ: Is a special vaccine required against rabies-related viruses and variants of rabies? in Vodopija I, Nicholson KG, Smerdel S, et al (eds): *Improvements in Rabies Post-Exposure Treatment*. Zagreb Institute of Public Health, 1985

C H A P T E R 70 / *Chlamydia* · Cho-chou Kuo · J. Thomas Grayston

Chlamydia organisms cause diverse infection in birds, in humans, and in other mammals. Trachoma is almost exclusively tropical. Genital *Chlamydia trachomatis* infection is worldwide. It is a prevalent sexually transmitted disease in tropical countries. Lymphogranuloma venereum (LGV) is endemic in parts of Africa (e.g., Ethiopia and Nigeria). A newly recognized *Chlamydia, Chlamydia pneumoniae,* strain TWAR, may cause pneumonia and other acute respiratory diseases and may infect at an earlier age in the tropics. The *Chlamydia* agents are nonmotile, gram-negative, small coccoid bacteria [1]. Although they are obligate intracellular parasites of small size (0.2 to 0.4 μm), they are distinct from viruses in several aspects. They have a cell wall and a cell membrane, contain both RNA and DNA, most have a plasmid, multiply by binary fission without losing their morphological integrity at any time during the multiplication, and contain portions of enzyme systems that generate metabolically useful energy. Their growth is susceptible to antibiotics. The genome is among the smallest of all prokaryotes, MW 4 to 6 × 10⁸. The molar percent of guanine plus cytosine (G + C) is 39 to 45 by thermal denaturation (Tm). They can be separated from other genera of bacteria on the basis of their identifiable morphology, a common group antigen, and a distinctive developmental cycle of multiplication in the host cells.

AGENTS

The organisms, previously known as psittacosis-lymphogranuloma venereum-trachoma (PLT); Bedsonia (after Bedson, and English scientist, noted for his work in psittacosis); and Miyagawanella (after Miyagawa, a Japanese bacteriologist, for his work in lymphogranuloma venereum), are now placed in the genus *Chlamydia* (from the Greek *chlamys,* "cloak") in the family Chlamydiaceae, both of which are in the order Rickettsiales [2]. Two species are recognized [3]. *C. trachomatis* includes human pathogens which cause trachoma and various genital tract infections, and one mouse pneumonitis strain. *C. psittaci* includes pathogens in birds and lower mammals. Humans are an accidental host. Differentiation of these two species is most easily done by observing the inclusion morphology (Fig. 70-1) and iodine staining in cell culture [4]. *C. trachomatis* is further separated into three biovars (trachoma, LGV, mouse) on the basis of their behavior in laboratory animals and in cell culture [1].

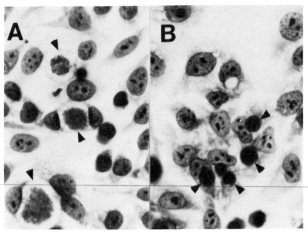

Figure 70-1. Illustration of two kinds of inclusions (arrowheads) in Giemsa stain of HeLa cell culture. *A.* Vacuolar and glycogen positive by iodine stain (*C. trachomatis*). *B.* Dense and glycogen negative (*C. psittaci* and *C. pneumoniae*). × 820.

A third species, *Chlamydia pneumoniae* [5], has been established for the newly identified *Chlamydia* agent called TWAR [6]. TWAR is primarily a respiratory pathogen of human origin. The elementary body has a unique morphology [7]. It is pleomorphic but typically pear-shaped (Fig. 70-2). The inclusions are round and dense in appearance and contain no glycogen. TWAR shares the *Chlamydia* genus-specific complement-fixation antigen, but can be identified by a monoclonal antibody specific to strain TWAR. Properties and characteristics of *Chlamydia* species and biovars are presented in Table 70-1.

MORPHOLOGY AND DEVELOPMENTAL CYCLE

Infection is initiated by an infectious particle called the *elementary body* (EB) (0.2 to 0.4 μm) which enters cells by a phagocytic mechanism [1]. The ingested EBs enter mammalian cells inside *phagosomes*, which are cytoplastic vacuoles surrounded by membranes derived from the plasma membrane of host cells and are protected by the inclusion membrane from destruction by the host's lysosomal enzymes. The EB is reorganized into a larger (0.5 to 1.0 μm) noninfectious, vege-

Table 70-1. Properties of the genus *Chlamydia*

| Property | C. trachomatis | | C. psittaci | C. pneumoniae |
	Trachoma	LGV		
Natural host	Human	Human	Bird, lower mammals	Human
Preferred site of infection	Squamocolumnar epithelium	Lymph nodes	Multiple sites	Respiratory
Laboratory animals:				
Intracerebral lethality for mice	−	+	+	−
Follicular conjunctivitis in nonhuman primates	+	−	−	−
Elementary body	Round	Round	Round	Pear-shaped
Inclusions in cell culture:				
Morphology, Giemsa stain	Oval, vacuolar	Oval, vacuolar	Variable shape, dense	Oval, dense
Glycogen content, iodine stain	+	+	−	−
Plaques in L cell	−	+	+	n.a.*
Cell culture infection enhanced by:				
Centrifugation of inoculum onto monolayer	+	−	−	+
Treatment of host cells with DEAE-dextran	+	−	±	±
Serotypes	12 (A through K, plus Ba)	3 (L$_1$, L$_2$, L$_3$)	n.a.*	1
DNA homology				
With trachoma biovar	100%	100%	10%	10%
With *C. pneumoniae*	10%	10%	10%	100%
Shared 1.55 × 10^5 cross-reacting antigen	+	+	−	−
Genus-specific CF antigen	+	+	+	+

*n.a. = not available.

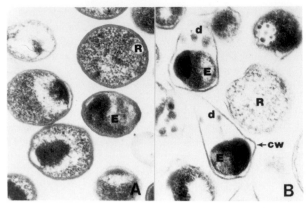

Figure 70-2. Illustration of two ultrastructural morphologies in elementary bodies (E): *A.* Round (*C. trachomatis* and *C. psittaci*); *B.* Pear-shaped (*C. pneumoniae*). Note no or little periplasmic space in *A* versus large periplasmic space and presence of electron-dense miniature bodies (d) in *B.* Reticulate bodies (R) are all round. cw = cell wall. × 80,000.

tative, multiplying form called the *reticulate body* (RB). The RB multiplies by repeated binary fission within the expanding membrane-bound vacuole. The developmental cycle is completed by reorganization of RB into EB in 19 to 36 h. The vacuole containing the particles is called an *inclusion body,* and has a characteristic morphology in Giemsa stain (Fig. 70-1). When the host cell is damaged, the infectious EB particles are released to repeat the cycle in other cells.

CULTURES

All known strains of *Chlamydia* grow in the yolk sacs of chicken embryos [8,9]. Most strains of *C. psittaci* and the LGV biovars of *C. trachomatis* multiply well in a variety of cell cultures. However, growth of the trachoma biovar of *C. trachomatis* and TWAR is best achieved with the aid of infection-promoting procedures such as centrifugation of the inoculum onto host-cell monolayers, pretreatment of host cells with polycations, and inhibition of the host cell's macromolecular synthesis. Mice are readily infected with many *C. psittaci* strains of avian origin and LGV biovars of *C. trachomatis,* and less effectively with most mammalian strains of *C. psittaci,* trachoma biovars of *C. trachomatis,* and TWAR [1,6].

Isolation in cell culture is the most commonly used method for *C. trachomatis.* A swab specimen is usually suspended in sucrose-phosphate buffer containing a suitable antimicrobial drug, streptomycin (or gentamicin), vancomycin, and amphotericin B (or nystatin). The cell lines most commonly used are McCoy cells (a heteroploid mouse line) and HeLa 229 cells (derived from a human cervical adenocarcinoma). The McCoy cells are infected by centrifuging the inoculum onto the monolayer at 1000 to 3000 × g for 1 h at 20 to 35°C. They are treated by x irradiation [10], cyclohexamide [11], iododeoxy-

uridine [12], or cytochalasin B [13] to inhibit host macromolecular synthesis either before or immediately after inoculation. When HeLa 229 cells are used, they are treated before infection with diethylaminoethyl dextran [14]. The inoculum is centrifuged onto the monolayer, and inhibitor of host macromolecular synthesis may or not be added. The monolayers are incubated for 2 to 3 days at 35 to 37°C and examined for the presence of chlamydial inclusions by stain with iodine (*C. trachomatis* only), Giemsa, or fluorescent antibody. If the results are negative or inconclusive, additional passage may be made.

TWAR has been isolated in chick embryos and in HeLa 229 cell culture [6]. The organisms grow better at 35°C than at 37°C in cell culture. Cell culture growth is enhanced by treatment of HeLa cells with DEAE-dextran before inoculation; centrifugation of inoculum onto cell monolayers; and incorporation of antimetabolites, such as cycloheximide, in the Eagle's minimum essential medium containing 10% fetal calf serum. After 3 days of incubation, inoculated cells are stained by fluorescent antibody using genus-specific, or TWAR-specific, monoclonal antibody. Serial passage in cell culture is difficult.

STRAIN CLASSIFICATION

Immunotyping of trachoma and LGV biovars of *C. trachomatis* is done by the indirect microimmunofluorescence (micro-IF) test of Wang and Grayston [15]. Twelve trachoma and three LGV immunotypes are now recognized [15–18]. The immunotypes are designated alphabetically from types A through K, plus Ba for trachoma and L_1, L_2, and L_3 for LGV. Serological cross-reaction is observed between some immunotypes and between trachoma and LGV biovars. No unified classification for *C. psittaci* has been adopted. Psittacosis strains have been classified according to their host origin by Meyer et al. [8]. Isolates from a common source often are similar antigenically. Only a single serotype has so far been found for TWAR [6].

SEROLOGY

Indirect immunofluorescence and complement-fixation (CF) tests are the two commonly used serological tests. The specificity of the indirect immunofluorescence test depends on the antigen used. It is type-specific when EBs are used in the indirect fluorescent antibody test as in Wang's micro-IF test [19] and is group specific (detects *C. trachomatis, C. psittaci,* and TWAR antibodies) when infected cells (inclusion stain) [20] or RBs [21] are used. Early (IgM) as well as late (IgG) antibody can be detected by using immunoglobulin-specific fluorescein conjugates.

A boiled, phenolized, or ether-extracted, group-specific antigen is used in the CF test [8,9]. The CF test is less sensitive than the micro-IF test and not specific. The CF test is not useful for trachoma or for most *Chlamydia*-caused sexually transmitted diseases. CF antibody is present in LGV infection. This test is most useful for psittacosis and TWAR infections but does not differentiate between them.

DELAYED HYPERSENSITIVITY

Chlamydial infection leads to the development of delayed hypersensitivity in the host. This was first demonstrated with the LGV skin test by Frei in 1925 [22]. Dermal hypersensitivity to *Chlamydia* is a delayed reaction of the tuberculin type with group specificity. The test is lacking in both sensitivity and specificity and is no longer recommended.

ANIMAL MODELS

Nonhuman primates are susceptible to human strains of *C. trachomatis* [23]. Many diseases including eye, respiratory, and genitourinary tract infection have been reproduced by the appropriate route of inoculation. Mice are useful small laboratory animals for studying the immunopathology and biological characteristics of *Chlamydia*. The susceptibility of mice to *Chlamydia* varies with the strains and the route of inoculation.

ANTIBIOTIC SENSITIVITY

The growth of chlamydiae in the yolk-sac cells of chicken embryos and in cell culture is inhibited by tetracyclines, erythromycin, chloramphenicol, rifampin, and clindamycin [24–27]. Chlamydial multiplication is not blocked by aminoglycosides, bacitracin, vancomycin, ristocetin, or nystatin, thus making these antibiotics useful in isolation of chlamydiae from contaminated specimens. Sulfonamides inhibit most *C. trachomatis* strains, but most *C. psittaci* strains and TWAR are not susceptible. Penicillins prevent the maturation of RBs into EBs. When penicillins are removed, the cycle resumes. Sulfonamides, tetracyclines, and erythromycin are recommended for treatment of *C. trachomatis*, and tetracyclines and erythromycin for *C. psittaci* and TWAR infections.

RESISTANCE AND IMMUNITY

Chlamydiae are successful parasites in natural hosts. Chronic or latent infections occur frequently. Immunity produced in the host is usually incomplete and short lived. Although chlamydial infection induces humoral (antibody) and cell-mediated (delayed-type skin reaction and in vitro lymphocyte transformation and leukocyte migration inhibition) immune responses, the host's resistance against *Chlamydia* is not well understood. Mouse experiments showed that mice recovered from intranasal or intravenous inoculation with *C. trachomatis* develop acquired immunity [28]. Immunity can be transferred to nascent mice by transfusion of immune spleen cells but not immune serum. Interferons have been shown to have a bacteriostatic effect by suppressing the development of *Chlamydia* in both nonphagocytic and phagocytic cells [29,30]. As most antibiotics effective against chlamydiae are bacteriostatic rather than bactericidal, and the organisms are located intracellularly,

drug administration often fails to eradicate the infecting agent. Prolonged antimicrobial therapy with a long period of observation of the patients is desirable.

PATIENT

There are two biovars of human *C. trachomatis* strains. These are the trachoma and LGV biovars. Trachoma biovar strains cause a variety of diseases involving many organ systems. The LGV biovar causes a distinctive sexually transmitted disease. Diseases that can be caused by *C. trachomatis* are listed in Table 70-2.

CHLAMYDIA TRACHOMATIS: TRACHOMA BIOVAR

Eye infection

The eye syndromes caused by *C. trachomatis* are trachoma and inclusion conjunctivitis. *Trachoma* has been defined as a chronic keratoconjunctivitis characterized by follicles, papillary hyperplasia, pannus (superficial vascularization of the cornea with infiltration of granulation tissue), and scar formation [31]. It is a potentially blinding disease. *Inclusion conjunctivitis* manifests clinically as an acute follicular conjunctivitis in children and adults and as a mucopurulent conjunctivitis with papillary hyperplasia in the newborn [32]. It is usually benign and self-limiting. In trachoma-endemic areas eye-to-eye transmission of *C. trachomatis* organisms occurs. In areas without endemic trachoma, transmission is from genital tract to eye usually resulting in the inclusion conjunctivitis syndrome. Less commonly the clinical characteristics of trachoma develop and

Table 70-2. Human diseases caused by *C. trachomatis*

Biovar	Disease or syndrome
Trachoma	Trachoma
	Inclusion conjunctivitis in newborn children and adults
	Pneumonia in infants
	Noncatarrhal rhinitis in infants
	Otitis media (?)
	Endocarditis (?), myocarditis (?)
	Nongonococcal urethritis in men
	Epididymitis
	Urethral syndrome in women
	Mucopurulent cervicitis
	Endometritis
	Salpingitis and sequelae of tubal infertility and ectopic pregnancy
	Proctitis
	Perihepatitis and peritonitis (Fitz-Hugh-Curtis syndrome) in women
	Bartholinitis (?)
Lymphogranuloma venereum	Lymphogranuloma venereum
Mouse	None

the disease may be referred to as *paratrachoma* [33]. Epidemiological studies [*23,34,35*] and experimental eye infection in monkeys [*36*] have shown that trachoma and inclusion conjunctivitis are not different diseases. Instead they represent a broad spectrum of clinical response to trachoma biovar strains of *C. trachomatis*. The inclusion conjunctivitis syndrome is seen after initial infection or first reinfection with trachoma organisms, while the chronic trachoma syndrome follows repeated reinfection. Any trachoma immunotype, whether from the eye or the genitourinary tract, can cause eye infection with clinical manifestations defined above. The effect of neonatal chlamydial conjunctivitis (birth canal infection) on the pathogenesis of trachoma (postnatal infection) is not known.

History. *C. trachomatis* eye infection is one of the oldest diseases known. A description of trachoma appeared as early as 1500 B.C. in the Ebers Papyrus [*37*]. A Greek physician, Pedanius Dioscorides, first used the term *trachoma* (Greek for "roughness") in A.D. 60. Halberstadter and von Prowazek discovered the cytoplasmic inclusion bodies that bear their names in conjunctival epithelial cells of human trachoma and experimentally infected apes in Java in 1907 [*38*]. Similar inclusions were discovered in nongonococcal conjunctivitis of the newborn by Lindner in 1910 [*39*], suggesting the etiological relationship of trachoma and inclusion conjunctivitis. The etiological agent of trachoma was first isolated by inoculation of the yolk sac of chicken embryos by T'ang et al. in Peking in 1957 [*40*]. The important role of *C. trachomatis* in sexually transmitted diseases was finally realized in the 1970s.

Epidemiology. Trachoma has been most prevalent in countries with hot and arid climates. The incidence and severity of trachoma have decreased greatly throughout the world during the past 30 years in areas with improving hygienic conditions and living standards. At the present time, endemic trachoma is the major cause of preventable blindness in north and sub-Saharan Africa and the Middle East. Pockets of blinding trachoma still exist in other parts of Africa, north India, parts of Asia, Australia, the Pacific Islands, and Latin America (WHO statistics, 1971) [*41*]. Nonblinding trachoma is present more broadly but in these same subtropical and tropical countries.

In endemic areas, trachoma is a familial disease perpetuated by eye-to-eye transmission. Almost all members of a family are infected during childhood. Because of frequent reinfection, the disease usually runs a course of recurrence and remission and may eventually progress to blindness. The serovars associated with endemic trachoma are types A, B, Ba, C, and D [*42*]. Types B, Ba, and D are also common causes of genital tract infection.

In Europe and North America, clinical trachoma is rare. Instead, another pattern of epidemiology is seen. *C. trachomatis* infection is the most common cause of sexually transmitted diseases in western countries [*43,44*]. The incidence of *C. trachomatis* infection is highest in young adults during the period of maximum sexual activity. It may be transferred to the eye. If a pregnant woman has cervical *C. trachomatis* infection, the newborn often acquires the infection during birth and may develop conjunctivitis or pneumonia. In the United States, it is estimated that 5 to 10 percent of pregnant women have *C. trachomatis* in their cervices. The rate is higher in young, poor, black women and lower in older white women. Of the babies born from infected mothers, 70 percent acquire clinical or subclinical infection, 25 to 35 percent develop conjunctivitis, and 10 to 20 percent pneumonia. Eye infection from the genital tract usually produces the inclusion conjunctivitis syndrome which tends to run a benign and self-limited course and heals without sequelae. Eye-to-eye infection with the genital strains is less common, not because of a decreased microbial virulence but because of the unsuitable environmental conditions for that mode of transmission. The predominant genital immunotype strains are types B and D through K [*42*].

Inclusion conjunctivitis of the newborn occurs in tropical and developing countries both with and without endemic trachoma. Whether the incidence is the same in countries with and without endemic trachoma and how it compares to that in western countries is unknown. No studies of incidence have been performed.

In a trachoma-endemic area of Egypt it has been shown that *C. trachomatis* can be isolated from one-third of randomly selected children beyond the neonatal period up to 2 years of age [*45*]. While the most common site for isolation was the conjunctiva, isolations were also obtained from swabs of the nasopharynx and rectum. Some of the isolations from the latter two sites were in the absence of conjunctival disease or isolation. The disease significance of these isolations is as yet unknown. The findings suggest that at least in young children trachoma may be systemic disease, a finding of significance for both transmission and treatment.

Laboratory Diagnosis. *Detection of Inclusion Bodies.* Detection of inclusion bodies in the conjunctival smear by Giemsa stain is the simplest method of laboratory diagnosis [*46*]. However, because of a lack of sensitivity it is recommended only for neonatal inclusion conjunctivitis or in trachoma-endemic areas where no other laboratory tests are available. A conjunctival scraping is usually taken with a blunt spatula or a cotton swab. A sufficient amount of epithelial cells should be taken from the site of maximum inflammation and spread in a small area of microscope slide. Gram stain should also be done with a duplicate smear for other bacteria.

Antigen and DNA Detection. The direct detection of organisms in conjunctival and nasopharyngeal smears by the *C. trachomatis* species-specific monoclonal antibody has become available commercially [*47*]. The test demonstrates a favorable degree of sensitivity and specificity [*48,49*]. The direct tests require less than an hour to perform. Enzyme-linked immunosorbent assay (ELISA) of antigens in swab specimens using polyclonal antibodies has been applied in genital and eye infection [*50,51*]. The test is genus-specific. Diagnosis of *C. trachomatis* by DNA hybridization is still experimental. Its usefulness has yet to be determined [*52*].

Isolation. Isolation is best done by inoculation of conjunctival swab material onto cell cultures [*10–14*]. Inoculation of the yolk sac of chicken embryos is a more cumbersome procedure [*8,9*] and is less sensitive than cell culture isolation especially for genital strains which may grow poorly in egg culture. Specimens for isolation should be kept at refrigerator temperature or frozen at −65°C if inoculation cannot be done within 24 h.

Serology. The only sensitive serological test for *C. trachomatis* is the indirect immunofluorescent antibody (IFA) test [*19*]. However, the predictive value of antibody is variable because of frequent high prevalence of serum antibody in persons who live in trachoma-endemic areas or in patients who frequent clinics that treat sexually transmitted disease. The disease activity of the eye infection is correlated better with antibody in eye secretions (tears) than in serum. Eye secretion is easily collected by inserting a small piece of sterile filter paper (5 by 20 mm) into the lower conjunctival sac, letting it saturate with eye secretion, and placing the filter paper in a vial containing a small (0.2 mL) amount of saline.

Eye infection: Trachoma

Epidemiology. Trachoma is present in many tropical and subtropical areas (see above). It affects all races.

Epidemiological studies in Taiwan [*34*], Saudi Arabia [*53*], and South Africa [*54*] showed that trachoma is a family disease. Although two or more types may be active in the community, all members in the same household usually have the same immunotype. Trachoma continues in the family by infection of susceptible young children. In endemic areas the highest rate of active infection is found among children under 10 years of age. This active childhood disease forms the reservoir in the community. Some older children and adults may continue to excrete the organisms with minimal evidence of active disease. While the younger children with active disease appear to be responsible for most transmission of the organism, mothers may serve as reservoirs and repeatedly reinfect their children. Transmission is from eye to eye by means of hands, fomites, or flies. Overcrowding, close family grouping, inadequate water supply, low standards of hygiene, and segregation in institutions favor the spread, increase the frequency of reinfection, and enhance the severity of the disease. Face washing has been shown to be associated with a lower frequency and lessens severity of trachoma.

Clinical Manifestations. Age of onset depends on the degree of endemicity. The greater the endemicity the lower the age of onset. The incubation period is usually 7 to 10 days but may be longer. Onset may be insidious or acute. Signs include

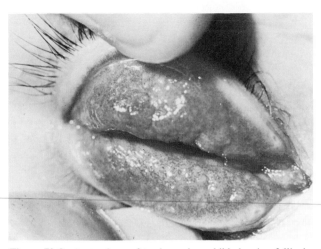

Figure 70-3. Acute phase of trachoma in a child showing follicular hypertrophy of the conjunctiva. (*Courtesy of Dr. San-pin Wang.*)

hyperemia, mucopurulent discharge, and lacrimation. Characteristic findings are follicular and papillary hypertrophy (most marked on the upper tarsus), pannus, and conjunctival scarring. Trachomatous follicles (Fig. 70-3) become necrotic and heal by scarring. The scar in the limbus, a characteristic dimple (Herbert's pit), is diagnostic for trachoma. Deformity of the tarsal plate due to scarring causes inward curvature of the eyelid (entropion) and eyelashes turned inward (trichiasis). Destruction of the conjunctival goblet cells, lacrimal ducts, and lacrimal glands may produce a "dry-eye" syndrome with resultant corneal opacity due to drying (xerosis) or secondary bacterial corneal ulcers. Corneal lesions are epithelial or subepithelial keratitis and cellular infiltration, most marked in the upper third of the cornea. Pannus (ingrowth of new blood vessels) (Fig. 70-4) is most marked superiorly. It progresses

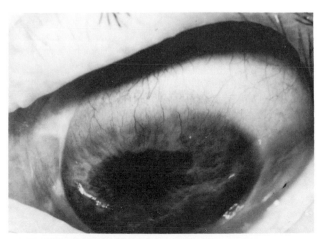

Figure 70-4. Trachomatous pannus showing neovascularization extending from the upper bulbar conjunctiva toward the cornea. (*Courtesy of Dr. Chandler R. Dawson.*)

Table 70-3. A simple system recommended by WHO for assessing trachoma*

Trachoma inflammation—follicular (TF):
  Presence of five or more follicles, at least 0.5 mm in diameter, in the upper tarsal conjunctiva; *presence of inflammatory trachoma.*
Trachoma inflammation—intense (TI):
  Pronounced inflammatory thickening of the upper tarsal conjunctiva that obscures more than half of the normal deep tarsal vessels; *severe intensity of inflammation.*
Trachomatous scarring (TS):
  The presence of scarring in the tarsal conjunctiva; *presence of cicatrical trachoma.*
Trachomatous trichiasis (TT):
  At least one eyelash rubs on the eyeball; *potentially disabling lesion.*
Corneal opacity (CO):
  Easily visible corneal opacity over the pupil; *visually disabling lesion.*

*From [*57*].

from the limbus toward the cornea and extends gradually across the cornea over a period of months or years. Secondary bacterial conjunctivitis particularly due to a variant of *Haemophilus influenzae,* known as Koch-Weeks bacillus or *H. aegypticus,* is an aggravating factor [*55*].

Diagnosis. Trachoma is diagnosed by clinical examination. It has been classified into stages according to the McCallum-WHO scheme [*31,56*], but recently a simplified scheme [*57*] has been recommended (Table 70-3). The simplified scheme, which is based on five key signs, is designed for nonspecialist health personnel to assess trachoma and its severity at the community level. The clinical examination should be performed by binocular loupes ($\times$ 2.5) under adequate lighting.

The diagnosis of trachoma is made in the presence of at least two of the following signs: (1) follicles on the upper tarsal conjunctiva, limbal follicles, or their sequelae (Herbert's pits); (2) epithelial or subepithelial keratitis, most marked in the upper third of the cornea; (3) pannus, most marked superiorly; (4) scars of characteristic configuration. In most of the persons converting to new trachoma disease during a period of observation, laboratory evidence of infection tended to occur simultaneously with the clinical changes. The first clinical signs of disease were often accompanied by rises in both tear and serum antibody and by isolation of trachoma organisms. In chronic or recurrent cases the disease activity is correlated better with tear antibody and isolation than serum antibody [*34*]. Isolation rates of trachoma organisms in cell culture from the eye have been most closely correlated with signs of acute inflammation [*58*].

Course and Prognosis. A full-blown trachomatous condition usually appears after recurrent bouts of follicular conjunctivitis. The main cause of blindness is opacification of the cornea

due to pannus, corneal abrasion caused by trichiasis, or injury to the unprotected cornea due to lid deformity. A complicating bacterial conjunctivitis may result in corneal ulceration with total loss of sight.

C. trachomatis eye infection does not necessarily progress to chronic disease. Even in endemic areas with severe trachoma and recurring seasonal bacterial conjunctivitis, great individual variations in severity exist, and only a small percentage of patients (less than 10 percent) progress to partial or complete blindness.

Pathogenesis. Trachoma is a reinfection disease. The greater the pressure of reinfection, the more severe the clinical course. After initial *C. trachomatis* eye infection, limited clinical disease is seen with only transient antibody response. Persistent eye disease and serum antibody follow reinfections. While inactive trachoma may relapse (e.g., in old age after cortisone eye ointment treatment, or spontaneously), such reactivation is much less important than is reinfection in the pathogenesis of chronic active disease and loss of sight. Persons with established active disease who move from an endemic to a nonendemic area lose their active disease in a few years. The exact process by which reinfection causes chronic disease is not understood but presumably involves an immunopathological mechanism.

Treatment. Sulfonamide, tetracycline, and erythromycin are effective drugs. Most sporadic or mild endemic trachoma responds to 3 to 6 weeks of full courses of systemic therapy with these chemotherapeutic agents. When trachoma is made more severe and complicated by secondary bacterial conjunctivitis, local treatment with tetracycline or erythromycin ointment twice daily 6 days a week for 10 consecutive weeks has produced satisfactory clinical improvement. Since it takes time for trachomatous hyperplasia to disappear even after the microorganism has been eliminated, a lapse time of 3 months or preferably 6 months after the end of treatment should be allowed before the treatment results are assessed. Unfortunately, in endemic areas reinfection will occur by 6 months after adequate therapy. Simultaneous treatment of active cases in household units offers a better chance for success.

Surgical repair of entropion, trichiasis, and stricture of the lacrimal duct should be introduced as soon as possible following or accompanying the medical treatment. It may reduce complications and prevent later visual loss.

Prevention. Improved hygienic conditions and living standards have produced a dramatic decline in the incidence and severity of trachoma. Adequate water supply for personal cleanliness may be a key factor. Face washing has been shown to favorably affect trachoma incidence and severity. In some areas the reduction of flies in the household is important.

No effective vaccines are available. The mass chemotherapy campaigns by WHO for the control of trachoma in endemic areas in the past have not proved effective. Progress toward blindness may be minimized by treatment of all active tra-choma in a family to prevent reinfection since the blinding sequelae usually appear only after several cycles of relapse or reinfection.

Eye infection in the newborn

Synonyms include *inclusion blenorrhea, inclusion conjunctiv-itis of the newborn,* and *ophthalmia neonatorum.* The disease is contracted at birth during delivery through an infected birth canal [*59*].

Clinical Manifestations. The incubation period is between 5 and 14 days. Onset before 3 days is rare but possible. Either one or both eyes may be affected. Inflammation varies from mild with scanty discharge, moderate reddening of the con-junctiva, and negligible lid edema to severe ophthalmia with swelling and redness of the lid, intense redness of the con-junctiva, and profuse purulent discharge with occasional pseu-domembrane formation. Papillary hypertrophy of the conjunc-tiva is a late manifestation and is most severe in the lower lid. Follicles are not seen unless conjunctivitis lasts longer than 3 months because lymphoid tissue is deficient in the newborn's conjunctiva. Corneal lesions, keratitis, and pannus are rare. There are no systemic symptoms except preauricular lymph-adenopathy and slight mucopurulent rhinitis. Vulvovaginitis may occur in baby girls. Without treatment, acute inflamma-tion lasts 1 to 3 weeks. Inflammation and infiltration regress gradually over a period of several months to a year. Conjunc-tival scarring and pannus are rare but do occur. With appro-priate antibiotic treatment, acute inflammation usually subsides in a few days. Swelling, redness, and discharge improve con-siderably, but redness may persist for weeks.

Diagnosis. Other bacteria are common causes of conjunctivitis in the newborn. These pathogens are *Neisseria gonorrhoeae, Staphylococcus aureus, Streptococcus pneumoniae,* and *H. in-fluenzae* [*60,61*]. Gram stain and bacterial cultures should be done routinely. Gonococcal conjunctivitis is of great concern because of its fulminant course, involvement of cornea, and potential for causing blindness. The incubation period is 1 to 3 days, shorter than that of chlamydial conjunctivitis. The dis-ease is characterized by severe conjunctivitis with chemosis and purulent discharge. Immediate treatment with local and systemic antibiotics is imperative. Penicillin is the drug of choice. However, emergence of penicillin-resistant (β-lecta-mase-producing) *N. gonorrhoeae* has been reported in some areas.

Treatment. Erythromycin ethyl succinate or estolate [40 mg/ (kg·day)] for 10 days is recommended. However, failure of erythromycin to eradicate nasopharyngeal, anal, and vaginal carriage of *Chlamydia* has been reported. Infants older than 2 months may be treated with sulfonamide [0.1 mg/(kg·day)] for 14 days. Local treatment alone is not recommended.

Prevention. Application of 1% silver nitrate eye drops (Crede's method) or erythromycin ophthalmic ointment at the time of delivery may not prevent *C. trachomatis* conjunctivitis [*62,63*]. Treatment of pregnant women with erythromycin (250 mg qid for 10 days) has been shown to be partially effective in preventing neonatal chlamydial infection.

Eye infection: Inclusion conjunctivitis after infancy

Transmission. Transmission is commonly due to autotransfer or heterotransfer of genitourinary material to the eye.

Clinical Manifestations. The eye disease is similar to one of the first cycles of eye-to-eye trachoma infection. The incuba-tion period is 7 to 14 days. Onset is either acute or subacute. Initial symptoms are sensation of foreign body, itching, burn-ing, lacrimation, and redness. Clinical findings are mucopu-rulent discharge; follicles most marked in the lower fornix and on the lower lid, less severe in the upper fornix, and relatively absent on the upper tarsus; diffuse hyperemia, edema, and infiltration of the conjunctivas. Keratitis and micropannus are occasionally seen. Extraocular manifestations are preauricular lymphadenitis, rhinopharyngitis, and occasionally otitis media. Symptoms related to genitourinary tract infection should al-ways be looked for, such as discharge, frequency of urination, miction pain, and pruritus. Conjunctivitis may be a manifes-tation of *Reiter's syndrome* (urethritis, conjunctivitis, arthritis, and mucocutaneous lesions in the genitalia). Reiter's syndrome is seen in patients with certain genetic disposition (HLA-B27 positive) who have *C. trachomatis* genital infection.

Prognosis. Prognosis is good if properly treated. The disease usually resolves without conjunctival scarring, pannus, or other corneal abnormality. However, it may run a chronic and re-current course and eventually lead to classic trachomatous changes which may be called *paratrachoma* to differentiate from endemic trachoma [*33,35*]. The unusual chronic disease may follow reinfection or improper treatment with inade-quate or ineffective antibiotics (chloramphenicol) or cortico-steroids [*35*].

Diagnosis. Other causes of conjunctivitis are bacteria, viruses, chemical and traumatic irritation, and allergy.

Frequent bacterial pathogens are *H. influenzae, Strep. pneu-moniae, N. gonorrhoeae, Corynebacterium diphtheriae,* staphylococci, and other streptococci. Bacterial conjunctivitis involves the bulbar conjunctiva more than palpebral conjunc-tiva. Membranous or pseudomembranous conjunctivitis may suggest *C. diphtheriae* and streptococcal etiology.

Follicular conjunctivitis due to adenovirus is usually more prominent in the lower than in the upper tarsus. Other systemic symptoms are usually present. Adenoviruses (especially types 3 and 7) cause pharyngoconjunctival fever. The disease often occurs in epidemics, as in "swimming pool conjunctivitis." Adenovirus types 8 and 19 are the cause of keratoconjunctivitis characterized by small round discrete infiltrates with rare systemic manifestation. The adenovirus inclusion is intranuclear which is in contrast to the intracytoplasmic nature of *C. trachomatis*.

Herpes simplex virus causes keratoconjunctivitis. The characteristic corneal lesions are dendritic ulcers. *Newcastle disease viruses,* which primarily affect fowls, can cause follicular conjunctivitis. A picornavirus, *enterovirus 70,* has been implicated in acute hemorrhagic conjunctivitis. This disease was first described in 1969 in epidemics in Ghana. The epidemics swept other countries in Africa, the Indian subcontinent, Asia, and some European countries from 1969 to 1974. The disease is manifested as an acute conjunctivitis with numerous punctate hemorrhages on the bulbar conjunctiva which become confluent within 24 h. There is also minor involvement of the cornea. The inflammation subsides in 4 to 7 days, but the hemorrhages do not resolve for 7 to 10 days. Other viruses associated with acute hemorrhagic conjunctivitis are coxsackievirus A24 and adenovirus 19.

Vernal conjunctivitis (spring catarrh), a recurrent bilateral conjunctivitis accompanied by eosinophilia, is a hypersensitivity reaction to exogenous allergens. It commonly occurs in young children. The primary manifestations are burning, itching, photophobia, and lacrimation. The characteristic findings are white ropy secretion and cobblestone appearance of the palpebral conjunctivas. Differential diagnosis from *C. trachomatis* conjunctivitis is important from the standpoint of treatment. Topical application of corticosteroids, a contraindication for *C. trachomatis* conjunctivitis, will result in prompt symptomatic relief for vernal conjunctivitis.

Treatment. To treat chlamydial inclusion conjunctivitis, a full dose of systemic tetracyclines or sulfonamides for 14 days is recommended. Erythromycin is substituted for tetracyclines in children. Topical antibiotic ointment alone is not adequate. Corticosteroids are contraindicated.

Prevention. Treatment for *C. trachomatis* genital infection in sexual partners in cases of adolescent or adult infection, and parents in the case of infection of children, should be considered mandatory.

Respiratory and other infection in infants

C. trachomatis may cause rhinitis and pneumonia in infants. Infantile *C. trachomatis* pneumonia is a distinctive pneumonia syndrome in infants less than 4 to 6 months of age [64,65]. It is characterized by a prolonged *afebrile* illness with congestion, cough, tachypnea, rales, hyperinflation with diffuse interstitial and patchy alveolar infiltrates, peripheral eosinophilia, and increased serum immunoglobulins. Although *C. trachomatis* pneumonia in immunosuppressed adults has been reported [66], chlamydia pneumonia in normal children and adults is due to the TWAR strain. (See under "*Chlamydia pneumoniae*" below.)

Transmission. Infection of the infant is acquired from the infected cervix of the mother. Eyes and nasopharynx are the initial colonization sites. Ninety percent of the cases of pneumonia have tear antibody and half of the cases have a history of conjunctivitis prior to or during respiratory illness.

Clinical Manifestations. Pneumonitis. Onset is gradual and diagnosis of pneumonia is usually not made until 6 weeks or later. Careful history usually reveals that symptoms began in the second or third week of life. Initial symptoms are nasal obstruction and/or discharge, tachypnea, and cough. The paroxysmal cough has been described as a staccato cough. The tempo of the cough is closely spaced. Each cough is separated by a brief inspiration. There is no posttussic inspiratory whoop.

On auscultation of the lungs, there are good breath sounds throughout the chest with crepitant inspiratory rales not uniformly distributed. Expiratory wheezing is unusual. Chest x-ray usually shows bilateral and symmetrical interstitial-type pulmonary infiltrates with hyperinflation and scattered areas of density representing atelectasis and alveolar infiltrate. Other physical findings are underweight, conjunctivitis, and ear abnormalities.

Noncatarrhal Rhinitis. Noncatarrhal rhinitis is a mild form of neonatal *C. trachomatis* disease. Onset is from 1 to 6 weeks of age. The disease manifestation is rhonchorus nasal congestion without rhinorrhea. Pus may be detected in the posterior nasopharynx with a swab. Conjunctivitis is present before or at the time of rhinitis in a quarter of the cases. The rhinitis may last from weeks to months. It rarely develops into pneumonia.

Subclinical Infection. C. trachomatis may colonize sites other than the conjunctiva and nasopharynx, such as the rectum and vagina. Colonization of the rectum and vagina is usually asymptomatic, and of the nasopharynx often subclinical. Duration of shedding from the nasopharynx, rectum, and vagina may be from a half year to two years [67].

Laboratory Findings. In infant *C. trachomatis* pneumonitis, routine blood counts are within normal limits except for an elevated absolute eosinophil value ($\geq$400 cells per cubic millimeter). Elevation of one or more of serum immunoglobulins A, G, and M is usually noted (IgA $\geq$ 30 mg/dL, IgG $\geq$ 500 mg/dL, and IgM > 110 mg/dL).

Diagnosis. Diagnosis is aided by positive maternal history of sexually transmitted disease. The diagnosis can be confirmed by isolation of *C. trachomatis* or detection of organisms in smears by the direct fluorescent antibody stain. Demonstration of *C. trachomatis* antibody with the immunofluorescence test is also used for diagnosis. Serum IgM antibody is found in 86 percent of infants with conjunctivitis, 70 percent with pneumonia, and 60 percent with rhinitis, and tear antibody which appears after 3 to 5 weeks of age is found in 83 percent of infants with conjunctivitis, 100 percent with pneumonia, and 83 percent with rhinitis [68]. The paroxysmal cough of C. trachomatis pneumonia may resemble pertussis. However, in C. trachomatis pneumonia there is no posttussic inspiratory whoop or lymphocytosis, both of which are typical for pertussis. Some viruses are frequent causes of upper and lower respiratory infection in infants. These are respiratory syncytial virus, parainfluenza virus, adeno- and rhinoviruses. These viral agents have been isolated concomitantly with C. trachomatis.

Treatment. Systemic administration of erythromycin ethyl succinate [40 mg/(kg·day)] or sulfisoxazole [150 mg/(kg·day)] for 2 to 3 weeks is recommended. Symptomatic improvement is usually seen in 5 to 7 days, and respiratory shedding of C. trachomatis is eliminated in 2 to 3 weeks.

Genital infection (see also Chap. 96, "Sexually Transmitted Diseases")

Epidemiology. Veneral infection due to trachoma biovars of C. trachomatis has taken over from N. gonorrhoeae as the leading cause of sexually transmitted disease in western countries [23,43,69]. C. trachomatis genital infection is also prevalent among sexually transmitted diseases in tropical countries. [70–72].

Clinical Manifestations. In males, strains of the trachoma biovar of C. trachomatis are the leading cause of *nongonococcal urethritis* (NGU) [73], a syndrome characterized by frequency of and burning sensation at urination, purulent discharge, and pyuria. Ascending infection may cause *epididymitis* [74]. These organisms also cause proctitis in homosexuals [75]. In females, the most common site of colonization is the endocervical mucosa. Infection may cause *mucopurulent cervicitis* [76]. However, many cases are asymptomatic [77]. C. trachomatis has been related to cervical dysplasia [78]. Urethral infection often accompanies the cervical infection and causes the *urethral syndrome* [79]. A serious complication of cervical infection is ascending infection of the endometrium (*endometritis*) [80] and the fallopian tubes leading to *salpingitis* or pelvic inflammatory disease (PID) [81]. This may also lead to a rare but serious complication in young women: peritonitis and perihepatitis (Fitz-Hugh-Curtis syndrome) [82]. C. trachomatis salpingitis is often unrecognized because it tends to be asymptomatic, but it results in tubal infertility, which is now a leading cause of preventable infertility [83]. Ectopic pregnancy [84], postpartum endometritis [85], and fetal wastage [86] have also been implicated as complications associated with C. trachomatis genital infection in pregnant women.

Laboratory Diagnosis. Isolation of the organism is the most helpful diagnostic procedure. Multiple infections with other bacteria, viruses, and protozoa are common in sexually promiscuous persons. Urethral and cervical swabs are inoculated in cell cultures. It is important to rub the swab sufficiently to obtain epithelial cells. Cell-free secretions such as mucus and urine are not good specimens for isolation. Many diagnostic kits for direct antigen detection in clinical specimens using IFA techniques or ELISA are available. Although the tests have been shown to give favorable sensitivity and specificity under ideal conditions, their claims may be hard to duplicate in laboratory and field conditions in tropical countries. The recommended serology is the indirect IFA test. Titer rises and IgM antibody may be seen in the acute stage. However, prevalence of serum IgG antibody in sexually promiscuous persons is generally high (60 to 80 percent); therefore, the presence of antibody alone is not diagnostic. On the other hand, cervical secretory antibody is a good indicator of active infection. Serum antibodies are usually higher in women than in men and are often very high in certain disease syndromes such as salpingitis and Fitz-Hugh-Curtis syndrome.

Treatment. Tetracyclines (2 g/day for 7 days) are recommended. Alternate drugs are erythromycin and sulfonamides.

CHLAMYDIA TRACHOMATIS: LGV BIOVAR

Lymphogranuloma venereum

LGV is a clinical syndrome characterized by acute inguinal lymphadenitis (bubo) and other local and systemic manifestations. It is a sexually transmitted disease caused by LGV biovars (immunotypes L_1, L_2, and L_3) of C. trachomatis. More evidence is needed to determine whether trachoma biovars can cause the LGV syndrome.

History. The disease was described as early as 1833 by Wallace [87] and was defined by Durand, Nicholas, and Favre in 1913 [88]. Frei in 1925 established LVG as a disease syndrome distinct from other bubo-forming diseases by introducing the skin test known as the *Frei test* [22]. The causative agent was first isolated by intracerebral inoculation of a monkey with pus from inguinal bubo by Hellerstrom and Wassen in 1930 [89]. EBs of the LGV agent were first identified in monocytes, leukocytes, and glial cells of intracerebrally infected monkeys and mice by Miyagawa et al. in 1935 [90,91]. Successful culture of LGV agents in the yolk sac of chick embryo was reported by Rake, McKee, and Shaffer in 1940 [92]. A comprehensive review of LGV can be found in Koteen's article [93].

Epidemiology. Distribution is worldwide. The incidence appears to be highest in tropical and subtropical countries. Recent studies showed that the disease is endemic in certain areas of Africa such as Ethiopia [94], Nigeria [95], and Swaziland [96]. In other countries, sporadic cases are found most often in seaport cities. In western countries LGV is usually found in homosexuals and prostitutes, or in sailors, travelers, and military personnel returning from areas where the disease is highly

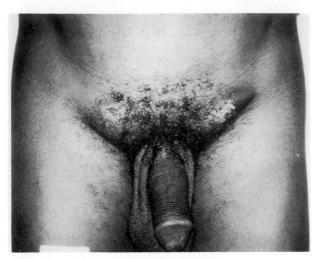

Figure 70-5. Bilateral inguinal lymph node enlargement (bubo) in a lymphogranuloma venereum patient. (*Courtesy of Dr. Peter L. Perine.*)

endemic. The incidence of clinical disease is higher in males than in females; the ratio is 6:1. Epidemiological and serological studies suggested that asymptomatic carriers of LGV exist and may serve as a reservoir of infection [97].

Clinical Manifestations. The primary lesion usually develops 12 days after the infective coitus and the inguinal bubo 10 to 30 days or as late as 6 months after the exposure.

The primary genital lesion appears as a small erosion, infiltrated papule, herpetiform vesicle, or ulcer in the coronal sulcus, prepuce, glans, or urethra in the male and in any part of the external genitalia in the female. It is painless, usually unnoticed, and heals spontaneously within a few days without scar formation. A bubo usually appears at the time the primary lesion disappears.

Inguinal bubo (Fig. 70-5) is the most frequent manifestation in the male. It is painful and is bilateral in one third of the cases. Enlarged lymph nodes above and below the groin give a groove appearance which is regarded as pathognomonic for LGV. If untreated the bubo becomes fluctuant and ruptures spontaneously. The anorectal syndrome or proctitis is the predominant manifestation in females and homosexual males. It is characterized by a bloody mucopurulent anal discharge, often associated with constipation or diarrhea, tenesmus, and abdominal pain. Proctoscopic findings are hyperemic mucosa, ulceration, granulation, and, in late stages, scar formation.

Systemic symptoms are noted during the acute stage of lymph node involvement. These are fever, headache, malaise, anorexia, nausea, vomiting, chills, and sweats. Skin manifestations include photosensitivity, erythema nodosum, erythema multiforme, and scarlatiniform eruption. Other rare manifestations are conjunctivitis, urethritis, arthritis, hepatitis, pruritus, and meningitis.

Laboratory Findings. Routine laboratory tests including blood counts, blood chemistry, urinalysis, and stool examinations are nonspecific. Abnormal findings are leukocytosis, elevated erythrocyte sedimentation rate (ESR), elevated serum globulin, false-positive serological test for syphilis (STS), pyuria, microscopic hematuria, and occult blood in the stool.

Specific tests for LGV are the Frei skin test, serology, and isolation of the organism. A positive skin test has been found in from 36 to 95 percent of known LGV cases [98,99]. CF antibody usually appears within 4 weeks after infection. A CF titer of 1:10 or greater is present in more than 80 percent of the cases [98]. Antibody in the micro-IF test is invariably present and the titer is usually high, greater than 1:512 in almost all cases during the acute stage [94]. Isolation of LGV organisms is done by inoculation of bubo aspirate and swab material from urethra, cervix, rectum, and ulcer into cell culture, chick embryo yolk sac, or mice intracerebrally. The positive isolation rate in cell culture and chick embryo yolk sac culture is 30 to 50 percent [94,98]. Isolation is usually not possible after the patient has received antibiotics. Organisms may be detected in swab and biopsy specimens by the fluorescent antibody stain using the *C. trachomatis* species-specific monoclonal antibody. [100].

Diagnosis. In the presence of inguinal bubo, diagnosis is made by specific serology or isolation. Inguinal bubo has been misdiagnosed as *inguinal hernia* resulting in unnecessary surgery. Genital ulcer and inguinal lymphadenopathy are the common manifestations of other sexually transmitted diseases. These are genital herpes, syphilis, chancroid, and granuloma inguinale. The proctitis of LGV may be mistaken for other lower GI disorders and infections, such as ulcerative colitis, and amebic or bacillary dysentery.

Treatment. A full systemic dose of sulfonamides or tetracyclines for 2 to 3 weeks is recommended. Longer therapy (30 days or more) is required for proctitis which may respond better to tetracyclines because of better control of secondary infection. Bubos should be aspirated when they become fluctuant to relieve pain and prevent rupture. Surgical correction is required for rectal strictures, fistula, and lymphatic obstruction.

Course and Sequelae. With proper antibiotic treatment, rapid abatement of fever and prompt relief of bubo pain, anorexia, headache, and malaise are noted. However, it may take several days to a few weeks for enlarged lymph nodes to resolve and heal. Late sequelae are genital elephantiasis or esthiomene, rectal strictures, lymphorrhoid fistula, and perirectal abcess.

Prevention. There are no vaccines or other means of prophylaxis. The only effective preventive measures are case identification, treatment of sexual contacts, distribution of information, and education in personal hygiene.

CHLAMYDIA PSITTACI

C. psittaci are natural pathogens for avians and lower mammals. Human infection is almost always acquired from contact with infected birds or sick animals. *Psittacosis* and *ornithosis* are equivalent terms for human infection with *C. psittaci* [101]. The mammalian *C. psittaci* do not readily infect humans.

PSITTACOSIS (ORNITHOSIS)

History and epidemiology

Human illness resulting from a disease of birds was first recorded by Jurgesson in 1874. Ritter in 1880 described a small outbreak of seven pneumotyphus cases in Ulster, Switzerland. The first extensive outbreak of psittacosis occurred in Paris between 1891 and 1892 [102,103]. Fifty-one human cases with sixteen deaths were reported. The outbreak was related to parrots shipped from Buenos Aires, Argentina, in which 300 of 500 parrots died on the voyage. Sporadic outbreaks of psittacosis were reported in continental Europe and in the United States in the next 30 years. A pandemic in 1929 led to the discovery of the organism by Bedson, Western, and Simpson [104]. This major outbreak was traced to an epidemic of psittacosis among the parrot population in Argentina. At least 350 human cases occurred with a mortality rate of 35 to 40 percent. This prompted many governments to ban the importation of psittacine birds.

For many years after the isolation of psittacosis agents from parrots, parakeets, and humans, it was believed that psittacine species imported from natural tropical habitat were the only source of infection. However, continuous investigations revealed that the hazard did not lie exclusively with imported birds and that in both continents infection was widespread in domestic aviaries [105]. Burnet in 1935 [106] reported that psittacosis is a native disease of budgerigars and cockatoos in Australia. Rasmussen-Ejde [107], and Haagen and Mauer [108] in 1938 discovered that fulmar petrels in the Faroe Islands were also infected and caused human cases among the islanders who hunted them for food. By 1940 it was established that racing and fancy pigeons were a potential source of human disease [109]. It was soon recognized that poultry, ducks, chickens, and turkeys can spread the infection to humans. Other wild and caged birds that have been found to be infected are canaries, finches, pheasants, and sea gulls.

By 1956 experimentation with an inexpensive medicated feed was begun in the Unied States [109]. Later this feed was commercially produced by impregnating 1 g of hulled millet seeds with 0.5 mg (0.5%) of crude tetracycline. In several field trials, acute infections were promptly arrested and latent infections eliminated after 15 days of treatment in 98 to 99 percent of the parakeets in breeding establishments and aviaries. However, it was later shown that holding imported psittacine birds in quarantine for 30 days in accordance with government regulation contributes to the spread of infection in crowded unsanitary conditions. The incidence of infection in psittacine birds caught in the bush is usually from less than 1 to 5 percent, but may increase to 30 to 40 percent during the quarantine period. Therefore modification of quarantine procedures and preventive antimicrobial therapy before and during shipment are recommended. These control measures have resulted in a decrease of human cases due to psittacine birds since the 1950s. The biggest and most important reservoirs of infection in Europe and North America have been pigeons [102,110], ducks [111,112], and more recently turkeys [113–115]. Poultry infection causes economic losses and involves risk for poultry breeders and processing workers.

Transmission

Transmission is by the airborne route, either by direct contact with infected birds or humans or indirectly by inhalation of dust contaminated with excreta of infected birds. The organisms resist drying and remain viable for a month at room temperature. Psittacosis strains are more virulent than ornithosis strains and the wild psittacosis strains are intrinsically more virulent than those from aviary-reared pets. The organism is destroyed within 3.5 to 5 min at 56°C; therefore, the risk of infection is eliminated by proper cooking of poultry. Although the disease has been contracted by poultry processing workers, no report of spread of the disease from processed birds to consumers has yet appeared.

Clinical manifestations

The incubation period is usually 7 to 14 days. However, it can range from 4 to 28 days. The primary site of human infection is the lung, although in severe cases the infection is generalized. The clinical picture varies from inapparent infection to febrile illness without localization to a fulminant pneumonia.

Respiratory symptoms include cough, dyspnea, pleuritic chest pain, epistaxis, sore throat, and hemoptysis. Systemic symptoms are fever, malaise, anorexia, shaking chills, sweats, nausea and vomiting, myalgia and arthralgia, headache, and abdominal pain.

Physical signs include rales, pulmonary consolidation, pleural friction rub, pulse-temperature deficit (relative bradycardia in spite of elevated temperature), pharyngeal erythema, hepatomegaly, splenomegaly, meningeal signs, and mental disturbance. Chest x-ray often reveals a picture of atypical pneumonia. The infiltration is usually unilateral, less commonly bilateral, and has been described as bandlike, reticular, and transparent with hilifugal distribution and as a fan-shaped shadow. Pleural reactions and hilar gland hyperplasia are common. Resolution of lung infiltration is usually delayed even after clinical improvement. It may take as long as 6 to 9 weeks to resolve.

Other rare primary manifestations are endocarditis [116,117] and myocarditis [118]. Chronic pulmonary infection with shedding of the organism has occurred.

Deaths due to psittacosis were not unusual in the preantibiotic era. The mortality rate was 20 percent or higher in some epidemics. Deaths have been reported in sporadic cases improperly treated. Cause of death is pulmonary insufficiency, generalized toxemia, or cardiac involvement.

Differential diagnosis from other forms of pneumonia due to viruses, *Mycoplasma pneumoniae*, and other bacteria should be sought by appropriate bacteriological and serological tests.

Laboratory findings

Routine laboratory tests are of little help for diagnosis. Abnormal findings include increased blood sedimentation rate, leukocytosis or leukopenia, anemia, proteinuria, abnormal liver function tests such as elevated serum alkaline phosphatase and glutamic oxaloacetic transaminase, and positive cephalin-cholesterol flocculation and thymol turbidity tests.

Diagnosis

A definite diagnosis cannot be made on clinical data alone. Isolation of psittacosis organisms from the sputum, throat swab, or blood of the patients or from the tissue of the animal viscera (lung, spleen, and intestine) coming to necropsy is diagnostic. The only available serological test is the CF test. Both acute and convalescent (2 to 3 weeks later) serum should be obtained. Criteria of positive CF test are seroconversion, fourfold rise or fall in titers, and high titers without increase or fall. CF antibody response may be masked in the patient receiving a large dose of tetracycline. Since isolation and serology are often not available or the test results won't be known early enough to institute the specific therapy, the single most valuable diagnostic clue is a history of exposure to birds, especially parrots and parakeets. Inquiries about contact with pet birds, pigeons, and poultry should be made in case of pneumonia and fever of unknown origin. Psittacosis in birds may be asymptomatic: a history of exposure to a bird should be sufficient to arouse the suspicion of the physician. Illness or death of pet birds is especially suggestive and provides a presumptive diagnosis. Treatment should be initiated as soon as psittaocosis is suspected.

Treatment

Tetracyclines are the drugs of choice. Treatment must be started early in the disease and be given in high doses for a long period to ensure successful eradication of the agent. A full systemic dose, 500 mg every 6 h by mouth [20 to 40 mg/(kg·day) for children], for 14 days or at least 7 days after clinical recovery is recommended. In severe cases a longer period of medication is recommended. Inadequate treatment may lead to relapse and establishment of a carrier state.

Control

An effective vaccine for animals is not available. Quarantine of imported birds in combination with preventive antibiotic treatment has been effective [109,119]. However, the success of this measure depends on law enforcement [120].

MAMMALIAN PSITTACOSIS

C. psittaci agents also cause disease and latent infection in large and small mammals other than humans [121]. Both domesticated (cattle, sheep, goats, hogs, dogs, guinea pigs, and mice) and wild (rodents, hares, koala, and seals) animals are involved. Each animal species has its own species-specific chlamydial infection. The common manifestations are pneumonitis, enteritis, conjunctivitis, polyarthritis, encephalitis, and abortion (involvement of placenta and fetus). These diseases may present serious problems in animal husbandry. Human infection due to mammalian *C. psittaci* infection is rare. It has been reported only in laboratory personnel or animal farmers. A feline pneumonitis agent [122], an agent of enzootic abortion of ewes [123], and a bovine abortion agent [124] have been reported to cause pneumonitis in humans. A case of keratoconjunctivitis in humans due to a feline pneumonitis agent [125] and two cases of pregnancy complicated by psittacosis acquired from sheep [126] have also been reported.

CHLAMYDIA PNEUMONIAE

Epidemiology

Seroepidemiological studies have shown that *C. pneumoniae*, strain TWAR, infections are very common worldwide. Prevalence antibody rates in adults are from 30 to 60 percent with somewhat higher rates in men than women [127]. This compares with *C. trachomatis* antibody in the same populations of 4 percent in males and 10 percent in females. There is a tendency for TWAR antibody rates to be higher in tropical countries and lower in countries in more northern climates.

In temperate zone countries, TWAR infection under the age of 5 years has been very uncommon; however, in a tropical country TWAR has been shown to be an important cause of acute lower respiratory tract infection in children 1 to 4 years of age.

A number of TWAR epidemics have been identified, usually involving young adults, particularly in military training [128,129]. Transmission of the organism appears to be human to human without any intervening animal or bird host.

Clinical manifestations

The TWAR organism has been identified most frequently in cases of pneumonia, usually with single pneumonic lesions [128–130]. Although it is uncommon, a severe spreading TWAR pneumonitis that is life threatening can occur [131]. TWAR also may be involved in serious pneumonia in older persons, especially those with chronic cardiopulmonary disease. These pneumonias may be complicated by bacterial infection and deaths have occurred.

Most TWAR pneumonias, particularly in younger persons, are mild and do not require hospitalization. They do require bed rest at home and loss of activity. Many of the patients fail to promptly recover from their infection, and many not treated with appropriate antibiotics have persistent cough for 1 or 2 months with some malaise. A biphasic illness that may be unique to TWAR infection has been identified. The first phase consists of severe pharyngitis often with hoarseness, followed in 1 to 3 weeks by pneumonia or bronchitis.

Patients with TWAR infections without pneumonia are usually diagnosed as having bronchitis, sinusitis, or pharyngitis [130]. In addition, a febrile "influenzalike" illness has been associated with TWAR infection. A wide range of severity has been observed with some TWAR infections being asymptomatic. Some of the asymptomatic patients have been demonstrated on chest radiograph to have pneumonitis.

Laboratory findings and diagnosis

TWAR infection is specifically diagnosed by use of the micro-IF serological test with TWAR antigen or by isolation of the organism from a throat swab or other respiratory tract secretions [130]. Unfortunately, these tests are available only in specialized laboratories.

Routine laboratory findings are not pathognomonic [129,130]. White blood cell counts are either normal or slightly elevated. The sedimentation rate is usually elevated. Cold agglutinins may or may not be present.

The standard *Chlamydia* CF test may give an indication of TWAR infection. Patients with acute respiratory disease who have not had a clear exposure to an ill psittacine bird or a turkey or duck processing plant, and do have *Chlamydia* CF antibodies, are most apt to have been infected by TWAR. Unfortunately, TWAR infections in most older patients and most hospitalized patients are reinfections, and *Chlamydia* CF antibody is usually not present.

Therapy

While both clinical experience [129,130] and laboratory studies [27] have shown that tetracycline and erythromycin are effective drugs against the TWAR organism, intensive and prolonged therapy is recommended. Until careful comparative clinical studies of TWAR are performed, our current recommendation for treatment is similar to that for *C. psittaci* infection: 2 g/day of tetracycline or erythromycin for 10 days to 2 weeks. An alternative therapy schedule could be 1 g/day for 21 days. Sulfa drugs are not effective against TWAR.

Prevention

There is no known method of prevention. However, complications and persistent illness can be avoided if the patient is treated with tetracycline or erythromycin, rather than a β-lactam antibiotic so often used in pneumonia.

REFERENCES

1 Moulder JW, Hatch TP, Kuo CC, et al: Genus Chlamydia Jones, Rake, and Stearns 1945, 55, in Krieg NR (ed): *Bergey's Manual of Systematic Bacteriology,* vol I. Baltimore, Williams & Wilkins, 1983, pp 729–739

2 Page LA: Revision of the family *Chlamydiaceae* Rake (Rickettsiales): Unification of the psittacosis-lymphogranuloma venereum-trachoma group of organisms in the genus *Chlamydia* Jones, Rake and Stearns, 1945. Int J Syst Bacteriol 16:223–252, 1966

3 Page LA: Proposal for the recognition of two species in the genus *Chlamydia* Jones, Rake and Stearns, 1945. Int J Syst Bacateriol 18:51–66, 1968

4 Gordon FB, Quan AL: Occurrence of glycogen in inclusions of the psittacosis-lymphogranuloma venereum-trachoma agents. J Infect Dis 115:186–196, 1965

5 Grayston JT, Kuo CC, Campbell LA, et al: *Chlamydia pneumoniae* sp. nov. for *Chlamydia* sp. strain TWAR. Int J Syst Bacteriol 39:88–90, 1989

6 Kuo CC, Chen HH, Wang SP, et al: Identification of a new group of *Chlamydia psittaci* strains called TWAR. J Clin Microbiol 24:1034–1037, 1986

7 Chi EY, Kuo CC, Grayston JT: Unique ultrastructure in the elementary body of *Chlamydia* sp. strain TWAR. J Microbiol 169:3757–3763, 1987

8 Meyer KF, Eddie B, Schachter J: Psittacosis-lymphogranuloma venereum agents, in Lennette EH et al (eds): *Diagnostic Procedures for Viral and Rickettsial Infections.* New York, American Public Health Association, 1969, pp 869–903

9 Thygeson P, Hanna L: TRIC agents, in Lennette EH et al (eds): *Diagnostic Procedures for Viral and Rickettsial Infections.* New York, American Public Health Association, 1969, pp 904–930

10 Gordon FB, Quan AL: Isolation of the trachoma agent in cell culture. Proc Soc Exp Biol Med 118:354–359, 1965

11 Rippa KT, Mardh PA: Cultivation of *Chlamydia trachomatis* in cyclohexamide-treated McCoy cells. J Clin Microbiol 6:328–331, 1977

12 Wentworth BB, Alexander ER: Isolation of *Chlamydia trachomatis* by use of 5-iodo-2-deoxyuridine-treated cells. Appl Microbiol 27:912–916, 1974

13 Sompolinsky D, Richmond S: Growth of *Chlamydia trachomatis* in McCoy cells treated with cytochalasin B. Appl Microbiol 28:912–914, 1974

14 Kuo CC, Wang SP, Wentworth BB, et al: Primary isolation of TRIC organisms in HeLa 229 cells treated with DEAE-dextran. J Infect Dis 125:665–668, 1972

15 Wang SP, Grayston JT: Classification of TRIC and related strains with micro immunofluorescence, in Nichols RL (ed): *Trachoma and Related Disorders Caused by Chlamydial Agents.* Amsterdam, Excerpta Medica, 1971, pp 305–321

16 Wang SP, Grayston JT, Gale JL: Three new immunologic types of trachoma-inclusion conjunctivitis organisms. J Immunol 110:873–879, 1973

17 Kuo CC, Wang SP, Grayston JT, et al: TRIC type K, a new immunologic type of *Chlamydia trachomatis.* J Immunol 113:591–596, 1974

18 Wang SP, Grayston JT: *Chlamydia trachomatis* immunotype J. J Immunol 115:1711–1716, 1975

19 Wang SP, Grayston JT: Immunologic relationship between genital TRIC, lymphogranuloma venereum, and related organisms in a

new micro-titer indirect immunofluorescence test. Am J Ophthalmol 70:367–374, 1970

20 Richmond SJ, Caul EO: Fluorescent antibody studies in chlamydial infection. J Clin Microbiol 1:345–352, 1975

21 Yong EC, Chinn JS, Caldwell HD, et al: Reticulate bodies as single antigen in *Chlamydia trachomatis* serology with micro-immunofluorescence. J Clin Microbiol 10:351–356, 1979

22 Frei W: Eine neue Hautreaktion bei "Lymphogranuloma inguinale." Klin Wochenschr 4:2148–2149, 1925

23 Grayston JT, Wang SP: New knowledge of chlamydiae and the disease they cause. J Infect Dis 132:82–89, 1975

24 Jawetz E: Chemotherapy of chlamydial infections. Adv Pharmacol Chemother 7:253–282, 1969

25 Becker Y: Antitrachoma activity of rifamycin B and 8-O-acetyl-rifamycin S. Nature 231:115–116, 1971

26 Ridgway GL, Owen JM, Oriel JD: The antimicrobial susceptibility of *Chlamydia trachomatis* in cell culture. Br J Vener Dis 54:103–106, 1978

27 Kuo CC, Grayston JT: In vitro drug susceptibility of *Chlamydia* sp. strain TWAR. Antimicrob Agents Chemother 32:257–258, 1988

28 Kuo CC, Chen WJ, Brunham RC, et al: A mouse model of *Chlamydia trachomatis* infection, in Mardh P-A et al (eds): *Chlamydial Infections*. Amsterdam, Elsevier Biomedical, 1982, pp 379–382

29 Byrne GI, Kruger DA: Lymphokine-mediated inhibition of *Chlamydia* replication in mouse fibroblasts is neutralized by anti-gamma interferon immunoglobulin. Infect Immun 42:1152–1158, 1983

30 Rothermel CD, Rubin BY, Murray HW: Gamma-interferon is the factor in lymphokine that activates human macrophages to inhibit intracellular *Chlamydia psittaci* replication. J Immunol 131:2542–2544, 1983

31 Tarizzo ML (ed): *Field Methods for the Control of Trachoma*. Geneva, World Health Organization, 1973

32 Jones BR: Ocular syndromes of TRIC virus infection and their possible genital significance. Br J Vener Dis 40:3–15, 1964

33 Jones BR: The prevention of blindness from trachoma. Trans Ophthalmol Soc UK 95:16–33, 1975

34 Grayston JT, Yeh JL, Wang SP, et al: Pathogenesis of ocular *Chlamydia trachomatis* infections in humans, in Hobson D, Holmes KK (eds): *Nongonococcal Urethritis and Related Disorders*. Washington, DC, American Society for Microbiology, 1977, pp 113–125

35 Mordhorst CH, Wang SP, Grayston JT: Childhood trachoma in a nonendemic area: Danish trachoma patients and their close contacts, 1963 to 1973. JAMA 239:1765–1771, 1978

36 Wang SP, Grayston JT: Pannus with experimental trachoma and inclusion conjunctivitis agent infection of Taiwan monkeys. Am J Ophthalmol 63:1133–1145, 1967

37 Thygeson P: Trachoma virus: Historical background and review of isolates. Ann NY Acad Sci 98:6–13, 1962

38 Halberstadter L, von Prowazek S: Uber Zelleinschlusse parasitarer Natur beim Trachom. Arb Gesundheitsamte 26:44–47, 1907

39 Lindner K: Zur Aetiologie der gonokokkenfreien Urethritis. Wien Klin Wochenschr 23:283–284, 1910

40 T'ang F, Chang H, Huang Y, et al: Studies on the etiology of trachoma with special reference to isolation of the virus in chick embryo. Chin Med J 75:429–447, 1957

41 World Health Organization Statistics Report (Rapport de Statistiques Sanitaires Mondiales) 24:248–329, 1971

42 Wang SP, Grayston JT, Kuo CC, et al: Serodiagnosis of *Chlamydia trachomatis* infection with the micro-immunofluorescence test, in Hobson D, Holmes KK (eds): *Nongonococcal Urethritis and Related Disorders*. Washington, DC, American Society for Microbiology, 1977, pp 237–248

43 Schachter, J: Chlamydia infections. N Engl J Med 298:428–435; 490–495; 540–549; 1978

44 Schachter J, Dawson CR: Chlamydial infections, a worldwide problem: Epidemiology and implications for trachoma therapy. Sex Transm Dis 8:167–174, 1981

45 Malaty R, Zaki S, Said ME, et al: Extraocular infections in children in areas with endemic trachoma. J Infect Dis 143:835, 1981

46 World Health Organization Symposium: *Guide to the Laboratory Diagnosis of Trachoma*. Geneva, World Health Organization, 1975

47 Kuo CC, Tam MR: Immunological diagnosis of *Chlamydia trachomatis* infection, in Young H, McMillan A (eds): *Immunological Diagnosis of Sexually Transmitted Diseases*. New York, Marcel Dekker, 1987, pp 191–211

48 Tam MR, Stamm WG, Handsfield HH, et al: Culture-independent diagnosis of *Chlamydia trachomatis* using monoclonal antibodies. N Engl J Med 310:1146–1150, 1984

49 Bell TA, Kuo CC, Stamm WE, et al: Direct fluorescent antibody stain for rapid detection of infant *Chlamydia trachomatis* infections. Pediatrics 74:224–228, 1984

50 Jones MF, Smith TF, Houghlum AJ, et al: Detection of *Chlamydia trachomatis* in genital specimens by the Chlamydiazyme test. J Clin Microbiol 20:465–467, 1984

51 Hammerschlag MR, Roblin PM, Cummings C, et al: Comparison of enzyme immunoassay and culture for diagnosis of Chlamydial conjunctivitis and respiratory infection in infants. J Clin Microbiol 25:2306–2308, 1987

52 Horn JE, Hammer ML, Falkow S, et al: Detection of *Chlamydia trachomatis* in tissue culture and cervical scrapings by in situ DNA hybridization. J Infect Dis 153:1155–1159, 1986

53 Barenfanger J: Studies on the role of the family unit in the transmission of trachoma. Am J Trop Med Hyg 24:509–515, 1975

54 Ballard RC, Sutter EE, Fotheringham P: Trachoma in a rural South African community. Am J Trop Med Hyg 27:113–120, 1978

55 Vastine DW, Dawson CR, Daghfous T, et al: Severe endemic trachoma in Tunisia, I, Effect of topical chemotherapy on conjunctivitis and ocular bacteria. Br J Ophthalmol 58:833–842, 1974

56 Dawson CR, Jones BR, Darougar S: Blinding and nonblinding trachoma: Assessment of intensity of upper tarsal inflammatory disease and disabling lesions. Bull WHO 52:279–282, 1975

57 Thylefors B, Dawson CR, Jones BR, et al: A simple system for the assessment of trachoma and its complications. Bull WHO 65:477–483, 1987

58 Wang SP, Grayston JT: Micro immunofluorescence antibody responses in *Chlamydia trachomatis* infection, a review, in Mardh P-A et al (eds): *Chlamydial Infections*. Amsterdam, Elsevier/North-Holland, 1982, pp 301–316

59 Chandler JW, Alexander ER, Pheiffer TA, et al: Ophthalmia neonatorum associated with maternal chlamydial infections. Trans Am Acad Ophthalmol Otolaryngol 83:302–308, 1977

60 Rowe DS, Aicardi EZ, Dawson CR, et al: Purulent ocular discharge in neonates: Significance of *Chlamydia trachomatis*. Pediatrics 63:628–632, 1979

61 Gigliotti F, Williams WT, Hayden FG, et al: Etiology of acute conjunctivitis in children. J Pediatr 98:531–536, 1981

62 Hammerschlag MR, Chandler JW, Alexander ER, et al: Erythromycin ointment for ocular prophylaxis of neonatal chlamydial infection. JAMA 244:2291–2293, 1980

63 Bell TA, Sandstrom KI, Gravett MG, et al: Comparison of ophthalmic silver nitrate solution and erythromycin ointment for prevention of natally acquired *Chlamydia trachomatis*. Sex Transm Dis 14:195–200, 1987

64 Beem M, Saxon EM: Respiratory-tract colonization and a distinctive pneumonia syndrome in infants infected with *Chlamydia trachomatis*. N Engl J Med 296:306–310, 1977

65 Harrison HR, English MG, Lee CK, et al: *Chlamydia trachomatis* infant pneumonitis. Comparison with matched controls and other infant pneumonitis. N Engl J Med 298:702–708, 1978

66 Tack KJ, Peterson PK, Rasp FL, et al: Isolation of *Chlamydia trachomatis* from the lower respiratory tract of adults. Lancet 1:116–120, 1980

67 Bell TA, Stamm WE, Kuo CC, et al: Chronic *Chlamydia trachomatis* infections in infants, in Oriel D et al (eds): *Chlamydial Infections*. Cambridge, Cambridge University Press, 1986, pp 305–308

68 Wang SP, Grayston JT: Microimmunofluorescence serology of *Chlamydia trachomatis*, in de la Maza LM, Peterson EM (eds): *Medical Virology III*. New York, Elsevier, 1984, pp 87–118

69 Thompson SE, Washington AE: Epidemiology of sexually transmitted *Chlamydia trachomatis* infections. Epidemiol Rev 5:96–123, 1983

70 Osoba AO: Sexually transmitted diseases in tropical Africa. A review of the present situation. Br J Vener Dis 57:89–94, 1981

71 Forsey T, Darougar S, Dines RT, et al: Chlamydial genital infection in Addis Ababa, Ethiopia. Br J Vener Dis 58:370–373, 1982

72 Nsanze H, Waigwa SRN, Mirza N, et al: Chlamydial infections in selected populations in Kenya, in Mardh P-A et al (eds): *Chlamydial Infections*. Amsterdam, Elsevier Biomedical, 1982, pp 421–424

73 Holmes KK, Handsfield HH, Wang SP, et al: Etiology of nongonococcal urethritis. N Engl J Med 292:1199–1205, 1975

74 Berger RE, Alexander ER, Monda GD, et al: *Chlamydia trachomatis* as a cause of acute "idiopathic" epididymitis. N Engl J Med 298:301–304, 1978

75 Quinn TC, Goodell SE, Mkritchian E, et al: *Chlamydia trachomatis* proctitis. N Engl J Med 305:195–200, 1981

76 Brunham RC, Paavonen J, Stevens CE, et al: Mucopurulent cervicitis—the ignored counterpart in women of urethritis in men. N Engl J Med 311:1–6, 1984

77 McCormack WM, Alpert S, McComb DE, et al: Fifteen-month follow-up study of women infected with *Chlamydia trachomatis*. N Engl M Med 300:123–125, 1979

78 Schachter J, Hill EC, King EB, et al: Chlamydial infection in women with cervical dysplasia. Am J Obstet Gynecol 123:753–757, 1975

79 Stamm WE, Wagner KF, Amsel R, et al: Causes of the acute urethral syndrome in women. N Engl J Med 303:409–415, 1980

80 Paavonen J, Kiviat N, Brunham RC, et al: Prevalence and manifestations of endometritis among women with cervicitis. Am J Obstet Gynecol 152:280–286, 1985

81 Mardh P-A, Ripa T, Swenson L, et al: *Chlamydia trachomatis* infection in patients with acute salpingitis. N Engl J Med 296:1377–1379, 1977

82 Wolner-Hanssen P, Svensson L, Westrom L, et al: Isolation of *Chlamydia trachomatis* from the liver capsule in Fitz-Hugh-Curtis syndrome. N Engl J Med 306:113, 1982

83 Moore DE, Spadoni LR, Foy HM, et al: Increased frequency of serum antibodies to *Chlamydia trachomatis* in infertility due to distal tubal disease. Lancet 2:574–577, 1982

84 Svensson L, Mardh P-A, Ahlgren M, et al: Ectopic pregnancy and antibodies to *Chlamydia trachomatis*. Fert Steril 44:313–317, 1985

85 Wager GP, Martin DH, Koutsky L, et al: Puerperal infectious morbidity: Relationship to route of delivery and to antepartum *Chlamydia trachomatis* infection. Am J Obstet Gynecol 138:1028–1033, 1980

86 Martin DH, Koutsky L, Eschenbach DA, et al: Prematurity and perinatal mortality in pregnancies complicated by maternal *Chlamydia trachomatis* infections. JAMA 247:1585–1588, 1982

87 Wallace WP: *Treatise on Venereal Disease and Its Varieties*. London, Henry Renshaw, 1838.

88 Durand M, Nicolas J, Favre M: Lymphogranulomatose inguinale subaigue d'origine genitale probable. Peut-etre venerienne. Bull Soc Med des Hopit 35:274, 1913

89 Hellerstrom S, Wassen E: Meningoencephalitische Veranderungen bei Affen nach Intracerebraler Imptung mit Lymphogranuloma inguinale. Proc Verh 85h Internat Kongr Dermat u Syph 1147–1151, 1930

90 Miyagawa Y, Mitamura T, Yaoi H, et al: Studies on virus lymphogranuloma inguinale Nicolas, Favre and Durand. I. Jpn J Exp Med 13:1–18, 1935

91 Miyagawa Y, Mitamura T, Yaoi H, et al: Studies on virus of lymphogranuloma inguinale Nicolas, Favre and Durand. II. Experimental findings in mouse infection. Jpn J Exp Med 13:331–339, 1935

92 Rake G, McKee CM, Schaffer MF: Agent of lymphogranuloma venereum in the yolk sac of the developing chick embryo. Proc Soc Exp Biol Med 43:332–334, 1940

93 Koteen H: Lymphogranuloma venereum. Medicine 24:1–69, 1945

94 Perine PL, Andersen AJ, Krause DW, et al: Diagnosis and treatment of lymphogranuloma venereum in Ethiopia, in *Current Chemotherapy and Infectious Disease*. Proceedings of the 11th International Congress of Chemotherapy and the 19th Interscience Conference on Antimicrobial Agents and Chemotherapy. Washington, DC, American Society for Microbiology, 1980, vol 2, pp 1280–1282

95 Sogbetun AO, Alausa KO, Osoba AO: Sexually transmitted diseases in Ibadan, Nigeria. Br J Vener Dis 53:155–160, 1977

96 Meheus A, van Dycke E, Ursi JP, et al: Etiology of genital ulcerations in Swaziland. Sex Transm Dis 10:33–35, 1983

97 Greaves AB, Taggart SR: Serology, Frei reaction and epidemiology of lymphogranuloma venereum. Am J Syph 37:273–282, 1953

98 Schachter J, Smith DE, Dawson CR, et al: Lymphogranuloma venereum, I. Comparison of the Frei test, complement fixation test and isolation of the agent. J Infect Dis 120:372–375, 1969

99 Abram AJ: Lymphogranuloma venereum. JAMA 205:199–202, 1968

100 Klotz SA, Drutz DJ, Tam MR, et al: Hemorrhagic proctitis due to lymphogranuloma venereum serogroup L$_2$. N Engl J Med 308:1563–1565, 1983

101 Meyer KF: Some general remarks and new observations on psittacosis and ornithosis. Bull WHO 20:101–119, 1959

102 Westwood JCN: Ornithosis. Practitioner 191:610–614, 1963

103 Westwood JCN: Psittacosis: Recent epidemiological observations. Proc R Soc Med 46:814–816, 1953

104 Bedson SP, Western GT, Simpson SL: Further observations on the etiology of psittacosis. Lancet 1:345–346, 1930

105 Meyer KF, Eddie B: Spontaneous psittacosis infections of the canary and butterfly finch. Proc Soc Exp Biol Med 30:481–482, 1933

106 Burnet FM: Enzootic psittacosis amongst wild Australian parrots. J Hyg 35:412–420, 1935

107 von Rasmussen-Ejde RK: Ueber eine durch Sturmvogel ubertragbare Lungenerkrankung auf den Faroen. Zentralbl Bakteriol 143:89–93, 1938

108 von Haagen E, Mauer G: Ueber eine auf den Minschen ubertragbare Viruskrankheit bei Sturmvogeln und ihre Beziehung zur Psittakose. Zentralbl Bakteriol 143:81–88, 1938

109 Meyer KF: The present status of psittacosis-ornithosis. Arch Environ Health 19:461–466, 1969

110 Rehacek J, Brezina R: Ornithosis in domestic pigeons gone wild in Bratislava. J Hyg Epidemiol Microbiol Immunol (Praha) 20:252–253, 1976

111 Strauss J: Microbiologic and epidemiologic aspects of duck ornithosis in Czechoslovakia. Am J Ophthalmol 63:1246–1259, 1967

112 Andrews BE, Major R, Palmer SR: Ornithosis in poultry workers. Lancet 1:632–634, 1981

113 Durfee PT, Pullen MM, Currier RW II, et al: Human psittacosis associated with commercial processing of turkeys. J Am Vet Med Assoc 167:804–808, 1975

114 Walker JW, Hand KA, Glass SC, et al: Cooperative state-federal turkey ornithosis task force, Texas, 1974. Avian Dis 20:355–360, 1976

115 Anderson DC, Stoesz PA, Kaufmann AF: Psittacosis outbreak in employees of a turkey-processing plant. Am J Epidemiol 107:140–148, 1978

116 Levison DA, Guthrie W, Ward C, et al: Infective endocarditis as part of psittacosis. Lancet 2:844–847, 1971

117 Jones RB, Priest JB, Kuo CC: Subacute chlamydial endocarditis. JAMA 247:655–658, 1982

118 Jannach JR: Myocarditis in infancy with inclusion characteristic of psittacosis. Am J Dis Child 96:734–740, 1958

119 Wachendorfer JG: Epidemiology and control of psittacosis. J Am Vet Med Assoc 162:298–303, 1973

120 Schachter J, Sugg N, Sung M: Psittacosis: The reservoir persists. J Infect Dis 137:44–49, 1978

121 Meyer KF: The host spectrum of psittacosis-lymphogranuloma venereum agents. Am J Ophthalmol 63:1225–1246, 1967

122 Baker JA: A virus obtained from a pneumonia of cats and its possible relation to the cause of atypical pneumonia in man. Science 96:475–476, 1942

123 Barwell CF: Laboratory infection of man with virus of enzootic abortion of ewes. Lancet 2:1369–1371, 1955

124 Barnes MG, Brainered H: Pneumonitis with alveolar capillary block in a cattle rancher exposed to epizootic bovine abortion. N Engl J Med 271:981–985, 1964

125 Schachter J, Ostler HB, Meyer KF: Human infection with the agent of feline pneumonitis. Lancet 1:1063–1065, 1969

126 Beer RJ, Bradford WP, Hart RJC: Pregnancy complicated by psittacosis acquired from sheep. Br Med J 284:1156–1157, 1982

127 Wang SP, Grayston JT: Microimmunofluorescence serological studies with the TWAR organism, in Oriel D et al (eds): *Chlamydial Infections*. Cambridge, England, Cambridge University Press, 1986, pp 329–332

128 Saikku P, Wang SP, Kleemola M, et al: An epidemic of mild pneumonia due to an unusual *Chlamydia psittaci* strain. J Infect Dis 151:832–839, 1985

129 Kleemola M, Saikku P, Visakorpi R, et al: Pneumonia epidemics in military trainees in Finland caused by TWAR, a new chlamydia organism. J Infect Dis 157:230–236, 1988

130 Grayston JC, Kuo CC, Wang SP, et al: A new *Chlamydia psittaci* strain, TWAR, isolated in acute respiratory tract infections. N Engl J Med 315:116–168, 1986

131 Marrie TJ, Grayston JT, Wang SP, et al: Pneumonia associated with the TWAR strain of *Chlamydia*. Ann Intern Med 106:507–511, 1987

Yellow Fever · Thomas P. Monath

Yellow fever is an acute mosquito-borne infection caused by a flavivirus and characterized in its full-blown form by fever, jaundice, albuminuria, and hemorrhage. Classified as one of the viral hemorrhagic fevers, it is unique in the severity of the hepatic impairment produced. Two forms are distinguished on the basis of transmission: *urban* yellow fever in which the virus is spread from person to person by peridomestic *Aëdes aegypti* mosquitoes (as is dengue fever) and *jungle* (*sylvan*) yellow fever transmitted by wild (usually tree-hole breeding) mosquitoes between nonhuman primates and thence to (and sometimes between) people. These epidemiologically distinct disease patterns are, however, clinically and pathoanatomically similar. For 200 years after its recognition as a nosological entity in the seventeenth century, yellow fever was one of the great epidemic scourges of humankind. Despite major advances in the twentieth century, including the development and deployment of an effective vaccine, the disease today remains a significant public health problem. Yellow fever is endemic and epidemic in tropical areas of the Americas and Africa but has not appeared in Asia or the Pacific region.

PARASITE

LIFE HISTORY

Yellow fever virus is an obligatory, intracellular parasite of humans, nonhuman primates, and mosquitoes. The ecology and life history of the agent are entirely dependent upon these hosts (see ''Intermediate and Reservoir Hosts'').

MORPHOLOGY AND ULTRASTRUCTURE

Yellow fever is the prototype of the *Flavivirus* genus of the family Flaviviridae. The genus comprises a group of serologically related, RNA-containing viruses of small size (35 to 45 nm in diameter) and consisting of a core (nucleocapsid) approximately 30 nm in diameter, surrounded by a lipid bilayer envelope [1].

Mature virus particles accumulate intracellularly within the endoplasmic reticulum and are released either by host cell lysis or by fusion of virus-laden cytoplasmic vesicles with host cell plasma membrane and egestion of enclosed virus (reverse phagocytosis) (Fig. 71-1). The process whereby virions mature on internal membranes remains to be clarified. Unlike alphaviruses, preformed nucleocapsids are not observed, and a budding process has not been clearly demonstrated.

CHEMICAL AND ANTIGENIC STRUCTURE

Flaviviruses are inactivated by lipid solvents (ether, chloroform, and deoxycholate), proteases (e.g., trypsin), and lipase.

Stability with pH and temperature changes depends upon the medium within which the virus is suspended. In the presence of sufficient protein (e.g., 20% serum), the virus is stable for long periods at $-60°C$ when wet-frozen and at $-20°C$ when lyophilized. The virus is readily inactivated at $56°C$ for 30 min. Improvement in vaccine stability has been achieved. Some freeze-dried 17D yellow fever vaccine preparations containing stabilizers retain their potency for 2 months or more at temperatures as high as $37°C$. Stability of yellow fever virus is optimal at around pH 8.0 and decreases rapidly below pH 6.6. The virus is readily inactivated by ultraviolet and γ-irradiation. Yellow fever virus is relatively stable in an aerosol; 25 percent of the original material can be recovered after 1 h, and temperature and humidity do not markedly affect decay rates.

Flaviviruses contain RNA, protein, lipids, and carbohydrates. The single-stranded 42-S RNA genome is infectious and of positive polarity (serves as a messenger for translation of virus-specified polypeptides and as a template for transcription of replicative, negative-sense, RNA).

The linear yellow fever genome has been completely sequenced and shown to contain 10,862 nucleotides with a single long open reading frame (10,233 nucleotides) encoding, in order, the three structural proteins (C, capsid; M, membrane;

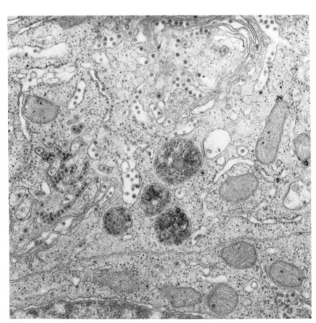

Figure 71-1. Flavivirus infection in mouse brain. Virus particles are present in distended endoplasmic reticulum. $\times$ 45,000. (*Courtesy of Alyne Harrison.*)

and E, envelope) and at least seven nonstructural proteins [2]. These final products result from proteolytic processing of a polyprotein precursor. From the medical point of view the most important gene products are the E protein (MW 54,000) and the first nonstructural (NS-1) protein (MW 46,000) to be synthesized downstream from E. The E glycoprotein is exposed on the surface of the mature virus particle and contains antigenic sites (epitopes) which have strain, type, complex, subgroup, and group specificity defined by monoclonal antibody analyses [3]. Epitopes are clustered in three spatially distinct domains on the glycoprotein spike and react with neutralization and hemagglutination-inhibiting antibodies.

The NS-1 glycoprotein, while not incorporated in the mature virion, is expressed on the surface of infected cells and incorporates both type-specific and group-reactive epitopes, some of which induce complement-fixing antibodies. Both neutralizing antibody induced by E antigens and complement-dependent cytolytic antibodies directed against NS-1 antigens appear to be important in protection against yellow fever infection [4].

The gene sequence of 17D vaccine virus differs from its parent Asibi virus at 32 amino acid positions [5] scattered throughout the genome; some of the 12 nonconservative changes in the E gene are likely to be responsible in part for the difference in virulence between these viruses.

The lipid portion of the viral envelope is derived from host cell rough endoplasmic reticulum; the specific lipoprotein content of virions varies with host cell source.

Flavivirus replication occurs entirely within the cytoplasm of infected cells. After adsorption, entry, and uncoating, the 40 S plus-strand genome is translated to yield viral replicases (including the NS-3 polypeptide) and serves as a template for transcription of minus-strand complementary RNA. In turn, progeny plus-strand RNAs are synthesized. These serve as mRNA for translation of viral proteins and incorporation into new virions on endoplasmic membranes in the perinuclear region of the infected cell.

Yellow fever is antigenically distinct, but appears to be more closely related to Banzi, Wesselsbron, Bouboui, Zika, and Uganda S viruses than to other flaviviruses [6]. Marked cross-protection between yellow fever and many flaviviruses can be demonstrated by use of the sensitive intraperitoneal test in infant mice. In more epidemiologically meaningful tests of cross-protection, prior immunization with Wesselsbron, Zika, and dengue viruses caused a significant reduction in viremias of monkeys challenged with virulent yellow fever virus [7,8]. Cross-reactions in antibody tests complicate survey and diagnostic serology (see below).

Antibody-dependent enhancement of flavivirus replication in Fc receptor–bearing leukocytes has been demonstrated in vitro and may explain the enhanced immunological response to attenuated dengue vaccines in persons previously vaccinated with yellow fever. Immune enhancement has been proposed

as a pathogenetic mechanism in dengue hemorrhagic fever (see Chap. 72). However, there is no evidence to suggest that prior exposure to heterologous flaviviruses enhances or exacerbates clinical yellow fever infection; instead, experimental and epidemiological studies suggest that cross-protection occurs. The early death in mice passively immunized with monoclonal antibodies prior to yellow fever challenge appears to depend on mechanisms other than immune enhancement of virus replication [9].

Antigenic differences have been shown between strains of yellow fever virus. By antibody-absorption techniques, strains from tropical America and Africa are distinguished [10]. Strains can also be differentiated on the basis of virulence characteristics for mice [11]. Monoclonal antibodies distinguish 17D vaccine virus from its virulent parent and even between substrains of vaccine virus. RNA oligonucleotide mapping has also shown African and neotropical virus strains to be different and has defined three genetically distinct geographical variants in Africa (1, Senegal-Gambia; 2, Ivory Coast–Burkina Faso–Nigeria; 3, central and east Africa) ([12] and Deubel, personal communication).

IN VITRO CULTURE AND INFECTIVITY ASSAYS

Yellow fever virus can be propagated in a wide variety of primary and continuous cell-culture systems. The 17D and French neurotropic vaccine strains are much easier to work with in the laboratory than wild virus strains and produce cytopathic effect and plaques in various continuous monkey kidney (MA-104, Vero, LLC-MK2), rabbit kidney (MA-111), baby hamster kidney (BHK), and porcine kidney (PS-2 and PK-15) cell lines as well as in primary chick and duck embryo fibroblast monolayers. Infectivity titers in many of the continuous cell lines are similar to the intracerebral LD_{50} for infant mice. Wild yellow fever virus strains can also be propagated in these cell cultures, but plaque formation is inconsistent and variable from strain to strain. Viral growth can be detected by immunofluorescence in advance of appearance of plaques.

Of considerable importance is the susceptibility of mosquito cell cultures to yellow fever viruses. These cultures, particularly the *Aëdes pseudoscutellaris* (AP61) cell line, may be conveniently used for primary isolation of yellow fever virus and are as or more sensitive for this purpose than Vero cells or infant mice. Unpassaged yellow fever virus grows in *Aëdes albopictus* cells without producing cytopathic effect, and infection must be assessed by immunofluorescence or subpassage to Vero cells or mice. The AP61 cell line responds to infection by forming cytopathic effect [13].

Intrathoracic inoculation of mosquitoes (*Toxorhynchites* or *A. aegypti*) is also useful for isolation or assay of yellow fever virus. After an appropriate incubation period, mosquitoes can be examined directly for virus by immunofluorescence or subpassaged to a susceptible host (e.g., suckling mice) [14].

ANIMAL MODELS

The susceptibility of vertebrate species depends largely on the strain and passage level of the infecting virus [15]. Yellow fever virus produces both neurotropic and viscerotropic patterns of infection; the predominant pattern produced is a function of the specific host species and inherent properties of the viral inoculum.

Viscerotropism reflects the pathogenicity of yellow fever virus for human or nonhuman primates infected by the peripheral route; disease is principally characterized by hepatic pathology. The viscerotropic pathogenicity of viral strains isolated in nature has not been extensively evaluated.

The neurotropic properties of yellow fever virus are most apparent in the mouse model; infant mice are highly susceptible to encephalitis after intraperitoneal or intracerebral inoculation. Considerable variation in neuropathogenicity for mice exists between viral strains [11]. Older mice are susceptible by the intracerebral route, as are guinea pigs. Monkeys develop mild encephalitis after intracerebral inoculation of viscerotropic virus and die of acute visceral yellow fever.

The rhesus monkey is an extremely susceptible species; the clinical illness and pathoanatomical changes in these animals are similar to those in humans (see "Pathogenesis and Pathophysiology"). Other monkey species are also highly susceptible to lethal infection (e.g., cynomolgus and howling monkeys).

The European hedgehog (*Erinaceus europaeus*) and Sudanese hedgehog (*E. pruneri*) are the only nonprimate experimental animals which develop severe visceral lesions in response to yellow fever infection [15]. Hamsters intraperitoneally inoculated with some virus strains are partially susceptible (scattered deaths), but they resist lethal infection with other virus strains. Rabbits resist intracerebral and peripheral challenge, but form antibodies. Newly hatched chickens develop viremic infection without disease.

INTERMEDIATE AND RESERVOIR HOSTS

Maintenance of yellow fever virus in nature depends upon cyclic transmission between vertebrate hosts and arthropod vectors. Both vertebrates and arthropods serve reservoir functions. When a proportion of the vertebrate host population sustains acute viremic infection, a pool of virus is accessible to blood-feeding arthropods. Although there is no evidence that chronic or relapsing viremic infections occur in vertebrate hosts, the arthropod vectors of yellow fever, once infected, remain so for life, thus constituting a natural reservoir of virus. Vertical transmission of virus in some arthropods adds to their capacity to provide a natural reservoir.

The specific intermediate host and vector species involved in viral transmission differ by geographical region. In both the old and the new world, monkeys are the principal wild vertebrate hosts; aedine mosquitoes in the Americas and in Africa are the principal vectors. Humans are also important intermediate hosts, where *A. aegypti* is responsible for transmission of urban yellow fever and where interhuman transmission is sustained by sylvatic vectors.

In South America, tamarins, marmosets, howling monkeys (*Alouatta* spp.), spider monkeys (*Ateles* sp.), squirrel monkeys (*Saimiri* sp.), and owl monkeys (*Aotus* sp.) are effective viremic hosts and commonly develop fatal infections. Die-offs in nature (particularly of howling monkeys) are an early sign of a yellow fever epizootic in progress. In contrast, capuchin monkeys (*Cebus* sp.) and wooly monkeys (*Lagothrix* sp.) are susceptible to viremic infection but usually do not develop clinical signs.

Other South American vertebrates including edentates, marsupials, and rodents are now believed to play a negligible role in the yellow fever transmission cycle, although further study of sloths appears warranted.

Mosquitoes of the genus *Haemagogus* are the principal vectors of jungle yellow fever in tropical America. *Haemagogus* breed in tree holes and feed in the forest canopy during the midday hours, but they have also been found biting humans in forest clearings and even inside houses in villages near the forest. The flight range of *Haemagogus* is quite far, a possible factor in virus dispersal. Experimental studies with a number of *Haemagogus* species have shown them capable of efficiently transmitting yellow fever virus.

Vertical transmission of yellow fever virus in *Haemagogus* has been experimentally demonstrated. This phenomenon may explain, in part, maintenance of the virus during prolonged dry seasons, when adult vector populations are diminished. The relatively drought resistant mosquito *Sabethes chloropterus* may also play a role in virus survival. This species has been shown experimentally to transmit yellow fever virus, but it is a relatively inefficient vector, requiring a blood meal containing a high concentration of virus and having a markedly prolonged extrinsic incubation period.

Primates are also the principal vertebrate hosts for yellow fever viruses in Africa. Where they are abundant, monkeys play an important part in the cycle of transmission. But in many areas of Africa, monkey populations have been reduced and their range increasingly restricted due to the expansion of human populations and modification of habitat. Humans play an increasingly important part in the natural history of yellow fever in Africa.

All species of cercopithecid and colobid monkeys tested have proved to be effective viremic hosts, circulating virus for several days or more at sufficient titers to infect mosquitoes. Infection infrequently results in illness or death, indicating a balanced host-parasite relationship. Among lemuroid primates, *Galago demidovii* is relatively refractory to yellow fever. *G. senegalensis,* a common and abundant animal in west African savannah habitats, develops high viremia but not illness; however, natural infections are quite rare, and this species does not figure importantly in the cycle of transmissions. *G. crassicaudatus* is highly susceptible to *fatal* infection.

Studies on the role of arthropods in the natural history of yellow fever in Africa have revealed complexity and regional variation. The virus-vector-host interrelationships have been reviewed by Germain and colleagues [*16*]. Excluding the contribution of *A. aegypti,* which is considered at the end of this section, the situation may be summarized as follows.

In the humid equatorial forests of central and west Africa, as well as in the high forests of Uganda, *A. africanus* is responsible for year-round virus transmission. Oviposition sites are tree holes, and biting activity is largely in the canopy. The level of viral activity in the enzootic high-forest zone is generally low, reflected by low immunity rates in human and monkey populations and absence of large epidemics. This is largely due to the extreme dilution of vectors and hosts in a continuous, uniformly favorable forest environment.

In zones bordering high forested areas of Uganda, *A. simpsoni* group mosquitoes play an important role in plantations in and around human habitations. They breed in plant axils, are strongly anthropophilic, and bite during the daytime. These mosquitoes link the forest cycle with humans and are responsible for intense interhuman spread during epidemics. Although *A. simpsoni* group mosquitoes are present in west Africa, they are not anthropophilic there.

The ecological zones bordering equatorial forest in west and central Africa have assumed extreme importance in yellow fever ecology. Appropriately named the *zone of emergence* by Germain and colleagues [*16*], the savannah-forest mosaic and Guinean and southern Sudan savannah vegetational zones, including riverine (gallery) forests, support large and *concentrated* populations of monkeys and vector mosquitoes. Viral activity intensifies during the rainy season and wanes during the dry season when vector populations virtually disappear. It now seems unlikely that the virus "retreats" into the high-forest enzootic zone during the dry season, since vertical transmission has been documented in vector species which survive the dry season in the egg stage. The principal species involved in sylvatic transmission and transmission to humans in the zone of emergence are *A. africanus, A. furcifer,* and *A. luteocephalus.* It is not unusual for these species to penetrate into villages and even to bite indoors. Human immunity rates are high; however, intense epidemic transmission may sometimes occur especially at the limits or fringe of the zone, where viral activity may subside for intervals of some years due to meteorological phenomena. Other vector species which play a secondary or accessory role in the zone of emergence are *A. opok, A. neoafricanus, A. vittatus,* and *A. metallicus.*

In areas subject to extreme drying, e.g., in the dry northern Sudan and Sahel savannah zones of west Africa, yellow fever occurs in intermittent epidemic form, and human immunity patterns indicate few or no infections during interepidemic periods. In these areas, domestic water storage is intensively practiced, domestic *A. aegypti* populations are high, and introduction of yellow fever virus may result in explosive outbreaks.

The role of *A. aegypti* in the transmission of yellow fever must be considered from historical, biological, and ecological perspectives. In the Americas, this species was responsible for large urban epidemics in North and South America until the early twentieth century. In large cities in tropical America, endemic interhuman transmission was maintained by this mosquito. The development of anti-*A. aegypti* campaigns, first in Cuba, then in Panama and elsewhere in Latin America during the twentieth century, culminated with eradication of the vector from most countries surrounding the Amazon Basin. The last example of urban transmission was in Trinidad (1954). However, within the last decade, *A. aegypti* has reinvaded many areas of Brazil, Bolivia, Ecuador, and Colombia. Infested towns and villages are now in juxtaposition with the jungle yellow fever cycle. The threat of urbanization of yellow fever in South America and potential for spread to the Caribbean, Central America, and the United States have significantly increased in the last decade.

In Africa, *A. aegypti* is widespread and abundant. As already mentioned, *A. aegypti*–borne epidemics have occurred in recent years in rural, dry-savannah areas where domestic water-storage jars, often buried in the ground, provide the principal breeding sites. High *A. aegypti* densities occur in towns and cities of sub-Saharan Africa, raising the possibility of urban epidemics. In 1987, yellow fever was introduced into large towns of western Nigeria from a remote area undergoing a sylvatic outbreak. An explosive *A. aegypti*–borne epidemic followed.

Experimental studies have demonstrated variation among geographical populations of *A. aegypti* in their ability to become infected with and to transmit yellow fever. Indeed, west African *A. aegypti* strains implicated in epidemic transmission have proved to be biologically poor vectors. It has been suggested that low vector competence may select virus strains capable of producing high viremias (and, perhaps, a high degree of virulence), but as yet no experimental evidence is available to support this hypothesis. A low level of vector competence in Asian *A. aegypti* has been put forth as an explanation for the absence of yellow fever from that continent, a hypothesis not clearly supported by experimental evidence or by the occurrence of epidemic spread by biologically poor vectors in west Africa.

Vertical transmission of yellow fever virus has been documented experimentally in *A. aegypti* and in natural populations of *A. furcifer-taylori* in Senegal (by isolation of the virus from field-collected males). The eggs of sylvatic *Aedes* species (and, thus, the virus) can survive desiccation during the long dry season when adult mosquito populations disappear.

The recent isolation of strains of yellow fever virus from *Amblyomma variegatum* ticks collected from cattle in the Central African Republic has raised the possibility that alternate vectors play a role in dispersal or dry-season maintenance of the virus. Yellow fever virus is transovarially transmitted in these ticks.

Yellow fever virus has been rarely isolated from other arthropods, including *A. dentatus, Coquilletidia fuscopennata,* and phlebotomine flies. In some areas (e.g., northern Nigeria and northern Kenya) *Mansonia africana* has been suspected to play a role in transmission. Virus has been isolated from a bat in Ethiopia. These observations are of interest but are either unimportant or peripheral to the ecology of yellow fever.

METHODS FOR STUDYING INTERMEDIATE HOSTS AND VECTORS

It is often important to determine the contribution of various host and vector species to the transmission of yellow fever virus, both during disease outbreaks and in research on interepidemic maintenance cycles. The techniques applicable for such studies are comprehensively reviewed in a recent guide [17]. In general, yellow fever vectors are not efficiently captured in traps and must be collected as they attempt to bite humans. Oviposition traps give valuable information about adult mosquito (especially *A. aegypti*) activity. Larval indexes are useful in assessing the distribution and density of peridomestic *A. aegypti*. A risk of epidemic yellow fever transmission by this vector is suggested by the finding of more than five containers positive for *A. aegypti* larvae per 100 houses.

PATIENT

FACTORS AFFECTING SUSCEPTIBILITY

Yellow fever affects all ages; the age-specific incidence of disease is largely determined on the basis of epidemiological factors (see ''Ecology and Epidemiology''). One study showed a lower mortality rate and milder disease syndrome in children. No clear sex difference in susceptibility has been documented.

Genetic factors are undoubtedly important in determining individual host responses to yellow fever infection, but have not been well defined. Older reports emphasize the severity of the disease in whites compared to blacks, but it is difficult to separate genetic from acquired resistance factors (e.g., immunity to yellow fever or heterologous flaviviruses). Descendants of Dutch colonists in Surinam who survived typhoid and yellow fever epidemics had significantly different gene frequencies from a large Dutch control group, possibly indicating selection through genetic control of survival.

PATHOGENESIS AND PATHOPHYSIOLOGY

Our present understanding of yellow fever pathogenesis and pathophysiology in humans is essentially nil, and we must rely heavily on experimental observations from the rhesus monkey model [18]. The hepatic parenchyma is the principal target organ, and hepatocellular damage is mediated directly by viral infection; the liver may also contribute significantly to viremia. Other sites of viral replication are less clear. However, several

lines of evidence suggest that mononuclear leukocytes play an important role. Serial examination of liver tissue from infected rhesus monkeys reveals the earliest cytopathological changes and appearance of immunofluorescent viral antigen within Kupffer cells. Lymphocytic necrosis in the germinal centers of the splenic periarteriolar lymphocytic sheath and necrosis of germinal centers in lymph node follicles are prominent findings in the rhesus monkey [19]. Yellow fever (17D) virus has been shown to replicate to high titer in human peripheral monocyte cultures and in peripheral blood lymphocytes stimulated by phytohemagglutinin. Macrophages and lymphocytes are important in containing and restricting yellow fever viral replication, but, in lethal infections, are apparently overwhelmed. These findings, as well as information from studies of dengue and other flaviviruses, suggest the following sequence of events: (1) after inoculation of the virus by a mosquito, the virus replicates in local tissues and regional lymph nodes; (2) with the ensuing viremia, other tissues, including lymphocyte-rich organs (lymph nodes, spleen, liver), smooth muscle, heart, pancreas, etc., become infected, produce virus, and feed the viremia; (3) infection reaches hepatic parenchyma by the hematogenous route and by direct spread from liver macrophages.

Hepatic injury in fatal human yellow fever is rarely as severe as in the rhesus monkey or as in fulminant viral hepatitis (acute yellow atrophy). In this sense, ''acute liver failure'' does not adequately describe either the clinical picture or mode of death in yellow fever. Nevertheless, the life-threatening pathophysiological events of the disease, including hemorrhage, renal failure, encephalopathy, shock, and electrolyte and acid-base disturbances, appear to be the result of hepatic injury, and one must suppose that the shock syndrome may represent a pathophysiological response to humoral agent(s) released from or inadequately inactivated by the diseased liver. Pathological changes in myocardial tissues, probably reflecting primary virus-mediated damage, accompanied by ventricular enlargement and arrhythmias may play a role in cardiovascular decompensation and shock. In the terminal stage of illness, decreased glycogenolysis and gluconeogenesis by the diseased liver produce hypoglycemia and contribute to metabolic acidosis. The terminal stage is also characterized by encephalopathic signs attributable to metabolic changes and cerebral edema.

Renal dysfunction manifested by albuminuria is an early feature of yellow fever, with onset in the period of infection (see ''Clinical Manifestations and Complications''). Dysfunction becomes more acute in the period of intoxication, with reduction in urine output and a rising blood urea nitrogen concentration. The contribution of renal disease to the course and outcome of infection in the individual case varies considerably, but it may be significant. The pathogenesis of the renal lesion is uncertain. Histopathological changes are classically those of acute tubular necrosis, without significant glomerular changes. However, glomerular lesions, difficult to observe with standard hematoxylin and eosin staining, have been revealed by other stains. In a large autopsy series, Schiff-positive transformation of the glomerular basement membrane was described and linked to altered permeability to proteins and albuminuria [20]. In experimentally infected rhesus monkeys, moreover, immunofluorescent viral antigen has been demonstrated in cells of the glomerular tuft. These observations suggest viral replication and/or immune-complex deposition and injury to the renal glomeruli as a basis for the albuminuria in yellow fever.

In the experimentally infected rhesus monkey, changes in renal function are most revealing during the interval between 36 and 12 h before death [19]. Diminishing urine output, rising serum creatinine level, proteinuria, and renal retention of Na$^+$ are found during this interval; arterial blood pressure remains normal, and renal biopsies show no histopathological changes. During the last 12 h before death, monkeys develop hypotension, anuria, acidosis, and hyperkalemia, and at death the kidneys show changes of acute tubular necrosis. The early oliguria was interpreted to reflect intrarenal changes in blood flow secondary to decreased effective blood volume, as postulated to occur in the hepatorenal syndrome, whereas the development of acute tubular necrosis late in the infection was the end result of the generalized circulatory collapse. If it occurs in humans, this *progression of prerenal failure to acute tubular necrosis* may be important in the management of patients (see ''Management'').

The pathogenesis of the bleeding diathesis in yellow fever is also complex. Decreased synthesis of vitamin K–dependent coagulation factors by the diseased liver is an important part of the hemorrhagic disorder. In some patients, disseminated intravascular coagulation may also be a significant factor [21,22].

IMMUNE RESPONSE

Neutralizing antibodies are usually detectable on the sixth or seventh day after onset of primary infection and are responsible for immune elimination of the virus. It is not unusual to demonstrate both infectious virus and antibody in serum, but the role of immune complexes in the pathogenesis of the disease remains uncertain. Antibody responses may be accelerated and broadened in individuals with prior flaviviral immunity (see ''Specific Diagnosis''). Depression of delayed hypersensitivity (tuberculin skin test reactivity) has been observed after administration of 17D vaccine. Whether the B-cell necrosis described in yellow fever of rhesus monkeys [19] is associated with suppression of antibody formation is not known.

PATHOLOGY

Gross pathological lesions include bile staining of tissues; cardiac enlargement; swelling and congestion of the kidneys; hemorrhages or petechiae of the mucous membranes, stomach, duodenum, renal capsule, and urinary bladder; and presence of small bloody pleural and peritoneal effusions. The liver is usually normal in size, red or yellow in color, and shows obliteration of normal lobular pattern and a greasy consistency.

Histopathological changes of the liver may be characteristic, but atypical cases are common. Conditions with which yellow fever may be confused on the basis of histopathology include Rift Valley fever, Crimean/Congo hemorrhagic fever, Marburg and Ebola virus diseases, viral hepatitis, and leptospirosis. The typical yellow fever lesion is marked by cloudy swelling, then by coagulative necrosis of hepatocytes in the midzone of the liver lobule, sparing cells bordering the central vein (Fig. 71-2A). Eosinophilic degeneration of hepatocytes results in the formation of Councilman bodies (Fig. 71-2B) and intranuclear eosinophilic granular inclusions (Torres bodies) (Fig. 71-2C). On an ultrastructural level, Councilman and Torres bodies consist of amorphous material without any viral structures. Multi- and microvacuolar fatty change is nearly always present, especially after the eighth day of illness. An inflammatory response is absent or mild. The reticulin framework is preserved, and healing is complete in recovered cases. Typical changes have been seen in biopsy specimens taken as early as the third day of illness; interpretation of biopsy or necropsy material obtained after the tenth day is often difficult. Biopsy is contraindicated, however, as a diagnostic procedure due to the high risk of hemorrhage. In cases in which death is delayed, partially disintegrated Councilman bodies, consisting of small, irregular, granular, ochre-colored bodies (Villela bodies) may be found in the midzone.

Renal glomerular changes are relatively insignificant compared to acute tubular necrosis and fatty metamorphosis, which may be marked. The myocardial fibers show cloudy swelling, degeneration, and fatty infiltration. The brain may show edema and petechial hemorrhages. Lymphocytic elements in the spleen and lymph nodes are depleted, and large mononuclear or histiocytic cells accumulate in the splenic follicles. These changes, although probably not specific for yellow fever, may be diagnostically helpful, and efforts should be made to obtain spleen and lymph nodes (as well as liver) from fatal human cases.

CLINICAL MANIFESTATIONS AND COMPLICATIONS

The incubation period is usually 3 to 6 days but may be longer. Yellow fever infection produces a spectrum from very mild, nonspecific, febrile illness to a fulminating sometimes fatal disease with pathognomonic features. The precise frequencies with which the various clinical forms occur is uncertain.

Abortive infections will not be suspected except possibly in the setting of an epidemic. In its mildest form, yellow fever is characterized by sudden onset of fever and headache, without other symptoms, lasting 48 h or less. In other patients, the fever is higher and the headache more severe and accompanied by myalgia, slight albuminuria, and bradycardia in relation to the height of fever (Faget's sign). The illness lasts several days, with uneventful recovery. Severe yellow fever begins abruptly

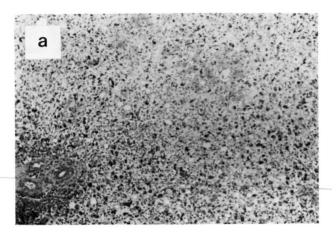

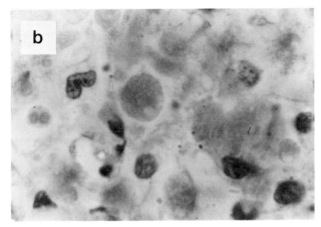

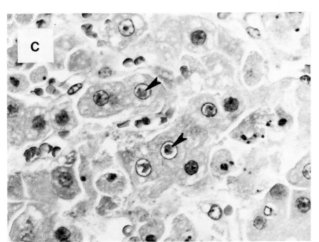

Figure 71-2. *A.* Liver of fatal human case of yellow fever, showing midzonal necrosis, sparing of cells bordering the central vein, and fatty change. *B.* Councilman body. *C.* Intranuclear inclusions [Torres bodies (arrows)].

with fever to 40°C, chills, severe headache, lumbosacral pain, and generalized myalgia. The patient appears distressed and anxious, the conjunctiva congested, the face and neck flushed, the tongue reddened at the tip and edges, the breath foul-smelling. Anorexia, nausea and vomiting, and minor gingival hemorrhages or epistaxes may occur. Despite a persistent or rising temperature, the pulse may decrease. This syndrome, lasting approximately 3 days, corresponds to the *period of infection,* during which yellow fever virus is present in the blood. It may be followed by a *period of remission,* with defervescence and mitigation of symptoms, usually lasting several to 24 h. Fever and symptoms reappear with more frequent vomiting, epigastric pain, prostration, and the appearance of jaundice (*period of intoxication*). Viremia is generally absent, and antibodies appear during this phase. The bleeding diathesis is manifested by hematemesis [coffee-grounds or black (*vomito negro*)], melena, metrorrhagia, petechiae, ecchymoses, and diffuse oozing from the mucous membranes. Bleeding is occasionally of life-threatening proportions. Dehydration results from vomiting and increased insensible losses. Renal dysfunction is marked by a sudden increase in albuminuria and by diminishing urine output. The pulse remains dissociated from fever but may weaken as the blood and pulse pressures decrease. The patient recovers either rapidly after a period of intoxication of 3 to 4 days or over a protracted course of up to 2 weeks. Death (in 20 to 50 percent of severe yellow fever cases) occurs usually on the seventh to tenth day of illness (occasionally as early as the fourth to sixth day) and is preceded by deepening jaundice, hemorrhages, rising pulse, hypotension, oliguria, and azotemia. Hypothermia, agitated delirium, intractable hiccup, stupor, and coma are terminal signs.

Physical findings during the period of intoxication include scleral and dermal icterus, hemorrhagic manifestations, epigastric (rarely hepatic) tenderness without enlargement, and the changes already noted in vital signs. Edema and ascites are not present.

The convalescent stage is sometimes prolonged, with profound weakness lasting 1 to 2 weeks. Late death, occurring at the end of convalescence or even weeks after complete recovery from the acute illness, is a rare phenomenon attributed to yellow fever myocardial damage and cardiac arrhythmia or failure. Suppurative parotitis (resulting from dehydration) and secondary bacterial pneumonia may complicate the disease. The duration of icterus in surviving cases is unknown; jaundice has been observed in African patients 2 to 3 months after recovery from serologically documented yellow fever, but the presence of unrelated hepatic disease was not investigated. Elevations of serum transaminase levels have been documented to persist for at least 2 months after onset of yellow fever.

CLINICAL LABORATORY FINDINGS

Leukopenia (white cell counts of 1.5 to 2.5 $\times$ 10^9 cells/L) occurs during the first week of illness. Differential counts show both an absolute neutropenia and lymphopenia, the former more severe than the latter. A marked leukocytosis may be present during the terminal stage of the disease. Prolongation of the clotting, prothrombin, and partial thromboplastin times is marked in cases with jaundice. The platelet count may be decreased, and fibrin-split products may be present in serum. In fatal cases, serum bilirubin elevations may be found as early as the third day and peak on the sixth to eighth day at average levels of 9 to 10 mg/dL, but may reach 48 mg/dL. Serum glutamic oxaloacetic and pyruvic transaminase levels are markedly elevated in all icteric (but inconstantly and to lower levels in anicteric) patients, with elevation on the second day and peak values between days 5 and 10 of the illness, and return toward normal by days 10 to 20; tests may remain abnormal for up to 2 months. The alkaline phosphatase level is generally normal. Hypoglycemia has been noted in patients with severe hepatic damage. Plasma protein (especially γ-globulin) concentration may fall during the acute illness.

During the period of infection, the urine may contain a small amount of albumin, which then increases on the fourth or fifth day, reaching levels of 3 to 5 g/L (rarely as high as 40 g/L). The urine contains bile; the cell sediment may be abnormal (granular casts) but is not diagnostically helpful. The cerebrospinal fluid is clear, without cells, but may be under increased pressure and may contain a mildly raised concentration of protein. Electrocardiographic (ST-T wave) abnormalities have been described.

PROGNOSIS

The case fatality rate of yellow fever with jaundice is 20 to 50 percent. Patients have been cared for under primitive conditions, however, and the prognosis may improve with availability of intensive hospital care facilities. The prognosis is guarded for the patient who, after a brief remission, enters a period of intoxication with rising fever and pulse rate and deepening jaundice.

Features which correlate with a poor prognosis include early onset of bilirubinemia and albuminuria, rising to high levels; marked elevations in the level of serum transaminases and marked prolongation of the prothrombin time (25 percent of normal); severe hemorrhage; and the appearance of shock, coma, hypothermia, and intractable hiccup.

DIFFERENTIAL DIAGNOSIS

Because the incubation period is sufficiently long to permit an infected person to travel a long distance, the diagnosis should be suspected in all unvaccinated patients with fever and jaundice residing in or traveling from the areas in tropical America and Africa shaded in Fig. 71-3.

Mild yellow fever cannot be clinically distinguished from a wide array of other infections. In the presence of jaundice and the other signs of severe yellow fever, conditions that must be differentiated include viral hepatitis, falciparum malaria,

spirochetal infections (tick-borne relapsing fever and Weil's disease), Rift Valley fever, typhoid, Q fever, typhus, and surgical, drug-induced, and toxic causes. The other viral hemorrhagic fevers, which usually present without jaundice, include dengue, Lassa, Marburg, and Ebola virus diseases, Bolivian and Argentine hemorrhagic fevers, and Crimean/Congo hemorrhagic fever.

SPECIFIC DIAGNOSIS

Specific diagnosis depends upon histopathological study, isolation of the virus, or demonstration of a specific antibody response. The virus is most readily isolated from serum obtained during the first 3 or 4 days of illness (period of infection), but it may be recovered from serum up to the twelfth day and occasionally from liver tissues at death. In the setting of a suspected outbreak, a search for patients with fever and generalized, nonspecific symptoms (i.e., those in the period of infection) may provide useful specimens for virus isolation attempts.

Proper handling of specimens is essential to avoid bacterial contamination and to preserve virus. Blood can be transported to the laboratory at ambient temperature for a few hours or on wet ice for 12 to 24 h, after which the serum should be aseptically removed and stored at the lowest possible temperature [preferably on dry ice, in an ultra-low-temperature mechanical freezer ($-70°C$), or in liquid nitrogen] until tested. Isolation attempts from clinical specimens can be made by intracerebral inoculation of infant mice or older mice (less sensitive) or by intrathoracic inoculation of *Toxorhynchites* mosquitoes. Various cell cultures can be used also, the most sensitive being AP61; cultures are observed for cytopathic effect and the virus identified by immunofluorescence. Type-specific monoclonal antibodies are available for this purpose. An antigen-capture enzyme immunoassay (ELISA) employing monoclonal antibodies provides a means of rapid, early diagnosis applicable under field conditions [23], but it is somewhat less sensitive than virus isolation [24]. An ELISA technique has also been adapted for detection of IgM-antigen complexes in serum.

Serological methods useful in the diagnosis of yellow fever include hemagglutination inhibition (HI), complement fixation (CF), neutralization (N), indirect immunofluorescence (IFA), and ELISA. The HI, IFA, and N antibodies appear within a week of onset; CF antibodies appear later. In many laboratories, the plaque-reduction N test has now largely replaced the less sensitive test in mice. Paired, acute, and convalescent phase specimens are required to establish the diagnosis by rise in antibody titer. Determination of IgM antibodies by ELISA is especially useful, both as a probable indicator of recent infection and as a means of arriving at a specific diagnosis in cases demonstrating extensive flavivirus cross-reactions by standard tests. The duration of IgM antibodies is uncertain and appears to be quite variable. In persons vaccinated with 17D virus, detectable IgM neutralizing antibodies are present as long as 18 months after immunization.

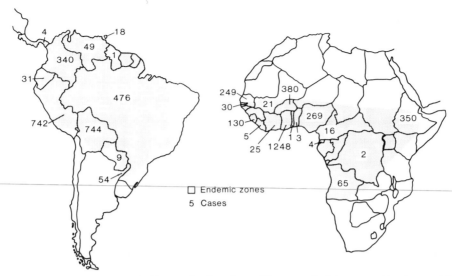

Figure 71-3. Distribution and incidence of yellow fever. The areas shaded are considered potentially endemic/enzootic, and travelers to these zones should be advised of risk of infection and immunized if potential exposure warrants (see text). Numbers indicate cases officially reported to WHO between 1965 and 1985.

Primary yellow fever infection is followed by the appearance of specific antibody responses by most test methods. In contrast, individuals with a prior flavivirus experience develop rapid and broadly cross-reactive responses. Antibody titers to the most recent infection may be higher than to heterologous titers, but occasionally the "doctrine of original antigenic sin" may dictate a higher rise in antibody to the remote than to the recent infecting agent. The N test provides more specific information than other techniques applied to whole serum. Measurement of IgM antibodies by the IFA test or ELISA provides a specific diagnosis of yellow fever in a high proportion of cases with cross-reactive superinfection patterns in tests on whole sera.

The use of yellow fever 17D vaccine may confound serodiagnosis. In persons without prior flavivirus exposures, the vaccine induces an N test seroconversion with a low titer (1:10 to 1:40) of HI antibodies and no detectable CF antibodies. However, in persons with preexisting flavivirus antibodies, vaccination may result in marked rises in yellow fever and heterologous HI and CF antibodies. The patterns produced may be broad or heterotypic, but in some cases homotypic responses are seen (a specific rise in yellow fever, HI, or CF antibodies), compatible with recent natural infection.

MANAGEMENT

In areas infected with *A. aegypti,* the patient should be protected from mosquito bites in a screened room or under a secure bed net. Bed rest and close monitoring of vital functions are essential. Temperature, pulse, blood pressure, respiratory rate, fluid intake, urine output, and other gastrointestinal losses should be monitored every 4 h. Analgesics (acetaminophen) may be used to control headache and myalgia.

Antiemetics (piperazine phenothiazines) may be used sparingly to control nausea and vomiting, but should be curtailed if hepatic dysfunction worsens or obtundation appears. Patients who enter the period of intoxication and who have signs of deepening hepatic dysfunction should be intensively monitored and treated, with careful initial and repeated evaluations of cardiovascular status, renal function, and electrolyte and acid-base balance. Oxygen should be administered, nutrition maintained, and 10 to 20% glucose solution given intravenously with care to avoid fluid overload. Nasogastric suction should be used to monitor hemorrhage, prevent gastric distension, and prevent aspiration. If severe bleeding occurs, fresh-frozen plasma or fresh whole blood should be administered to maintain an adequate blood volume. Administration of vitamin K is probably ineffective in cases of severe hepatic necrosis. Controversy exists regarding the role of disseminated intravascular coagulation (DIC) in yellow fever. Where strong laboratory evidence favors DIC, use of heparin may be considered, but patients must be closely monitored.

In patients who show signs of progressive acute renal failure, consideration may be given to dialysis. Unfortunately, no firm indications or guidelines can be formulated from experience. From animal experiments, the critical consideration is the differentiation between acute tubular necrosis and oliguria due to hypotension, reversible decrease in effective renal perfusion, and the hepatorenal syndrome. Thus, the finding of a urinary Na^+ (U_{Na+}) concentration less than 20 meq/L or a urine-plasma (U/P) creatinine ratio of 10 or more indicates prerenal azotemia. Such patients should be treated with supportive

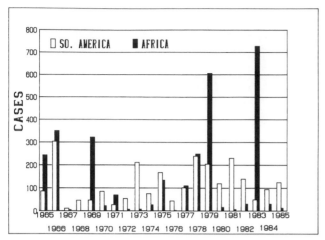

Figure 71-4. Annual incidence of reported cases of yellow fever in South America and Africa. The true incidence is undoubtedly much greater.

measures (volume expansion), whereas the presence of acute tubular necrosis (U_{Na+} greater than 20, U/P creatinine ratio less than 10), might be an indication for dialysis.

Secondary bacterial infections or concurrent infections (in particular, malaria) should be treated by the usual appropriate means. The possible benefits of antiviral chemotherapeutic agents such as ribavirin or human interferon remain unknown, but animal experiments suggest that these measures are unlikely to be of use once clinical illness is established. There is no indication for treatment with antibodies (or pooled γ-globulin), corticosteroids, or immunosuppressive agents. The value of techniques such as acrylonitrile dialysis, exchange transfusion, or cross-circulation remains to be determined.

POPULATION

ECOLOGY AND EPIDEMIOLOGY

Distribution and incidence

Yellow fever occurs through much of tropical South America and sub-Saharan Africa (shaded area, Fig. 71-3). Within this region, viral activity may be intermittent and quite localized. The exact location of viral activity in the vast tropical forests of South America, for example, is difficult to ascertain at any given time. The distribution of reported cases gives only a partial picture of the natural circulation of yellow fever virus and a misleading estimate of risk to travelers. High levels of vaccine-induced and natural immunity, inadequate reporting systems, low human population density, and other factors may result in an apparent absence of disease from areas with a high level of enzootic viral transmission.

The annual incidence of officially reported yellow fever cases is between 50 and 300 in tropical America, and between 5 and 500 in Africa. (Figs. 71-3 and 71-4). These data rep-

resent a significant underestimate of the true morbidity rate, as shown by investigations of various epidemics, especially in Africa (Table 71-1).

In South America, the reported incidence of jungle yellow fever is highest in the Amazon region of Brazil and in areas of eastern Bolivia, Peru, Ecuador, and Colombia which encircle the Amazon Basin (Fig. 71-3). In certain years, epizootic waves accompanied by human cases may sweep into areas such as Central America, northern Argentina and Paraguay, and southeastern Brazil (Minas Gerais, São Paulo, Paraná, Santa Catarina states) normally outside the enzootic zone.

Periodicity of jungle yellow fever activity is apparent (Fig. 71-5), with outbreaks occurring at rough intervals of 5 to 10 years. Human cases occur in rural areas, principally among persons living near and working in the forest. The opening of inaccessible forested areas to oil exploration, agricultural exploitation, and road construction has occasionally led to an influx of unvaccinated persons, with an ensuing epidemic.

In Africa, few sporadic cases are recognized annually, due to confusion with hyperendemic viral hepatitis, inadequate surveillance, and unavailability of diagnostic facilities. Where special efforts have been made to seek cases actively, they have been found, and it is probable that endemic yellow fever constitutes a considerable but unappreciated public health problem in many parts of Africa. Large epidemics have occurred at irregular intervals, principally in west Africa and in the southern Sudan and Ethiopia.

Seasonal incidence

In tropical America, the incidence of jungle yellow fever is highest during months with peak rainfall, humidity, and temperature (January to March in the Amazon Basin). In Africa,

Table 71-1. Example of discrepancies between the number of officially notified yellow fever cases and deaths and estimates of morbidity and mortality rates from direct investigations of epidemics

		Number of cases (deaths)	
Country	Year(s)	Officially notified	Determined by epidemiological investigation
Ethiopia	1960–1962	—*(3000)	100,000 (30,000)
Senegal	1965	243 (216)	2000–20,000 (200–2000)
Upper Volta	1969	87 (44)	3000 (100)
Nigeria	1969	208 (60)	100,000 (—*)
Nigeria	1970	4 (1)	786 (15–40)
The Gambia	1978–1979	30 (3)	5000–8000 (1000–1700)
Burkina Faso	1983	356 (286)	2500–3500 (1000–1400)

*No estimate available.

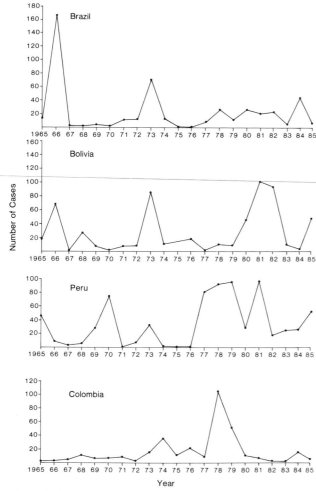

Figure 71-5. Incidence of jungle yellow fever in four neotropical countries showing asynchronous periodicity of the disease.

epidemics spread by tree-hole-breeding mosquitoes peak during the late rainy season and early dry season. Where *A. aegypti* is implicated, transmission may occur at any time of year, but is enhanced during the rainy season, when artificial containers around houses provide additional breeding sites for *A. aegypti*. With the advent of the long dry season, populations of wild (tree-hole-breeding) *Aëdes* decline rapidly, and yellow fever transmission by these vectors ceases, but domestic (water-jar) breeding may sustain *A. aegypti* populations sufficient for transmission to continue.

Age, sex, and occupation

In tropical America, jungle yellow fever principally affects young adult males. The male-female ratio is 10:1. The age-sex distribution reflects the higher incidence of exposure to *Haemagogus* vectors during wood-cutting and forest-clearing activities in the forest.

In Africa, background immunity (natural and vaccine-induced) is the principal factor determining the age distribution of cases. In outbreaks affecting immunologically virgin populations (e.g., in Ethiopia, 1960 to 1962), all ages were equally affected. A high level of naturally acquired immunity in adults was present in the Gambia (a region of hyperendemic flavivirus and intermittent yellow fever transmission at the fringe of the zone of emergence); with the reintroduction of yellow fever in 1978, the highest attack rate was in children [25]. Similarly, in the 1965 *A. aegypti*–borne epidemic in Senegal, young children were principally affected because vaccination of this age group had been suspended in 1960. An excess of cases in males has been observed in some outbreaks in which wild-breeding vectors were responsible for transmission. Exposure to mosquitoes may be greater in men and boys who tend to remain out of doors and outside village confines for longer periods after sundown than females. The excess of cases in males has not been as great as in tropical America. In one instance (Nigeria, 1969), despite a 4:1 male-female ratio of hospitalized cases, antibody surveys showed no sex difference in incidence of infection, indicating that males may have been more likely to utilize hospital facilities than females or that the disease is more severe in males.

Inapparent infection

Inapparent, abortive, or clinically mild infections with yellow fever are frequent. In endemic areas of west Africa subject to yearly wet season recrudescence and amplification of yellow fever, the annual incidence of infection may be as high as 1 to 5 percent; the prevalence of immunity in young adults in such areas reaches 50 to 90 percent. The N test provides the most specific information about cumulative past infection in a population, whereas the CF or IgM test can be used as a measure of recent infection. However, several factors must be kept in mind in interpreting serosurvey data. Cross-reactions with other flaviviruses frequently confound interpretation. Sera should be tested against yellow fever and *at least* several heterologous flaviviruses known to be present in the area sampled; determination of end-point titers and use of the more specific N test provide useful information. The prevalence of serological reactions specific for yellow fever provides a low estimate of the true prevalence of past yellow fever infections; the addition of individuals with yellow fever N antibodies but who have cross-reactive patterns, indicating multiple flavivirus exposures, provides a high estimate. Surveys utilizing nonspecific tests (HI, IFA) without inclusion of heterologous antigens provide little or no useful information about yellow fever immunity.

The ratio of inapparent to apparent yellow fever infection has not been definitely established. In one study [25], a low ratio (2:1) was found for persons (mainly children) who sustained primary yellow fever infections. Individuals with serological patterns indicating that they had sustained yellow fever infection on a background of prior exposure to one or more heterologous flaviviruses (of which Zika virus was the most prominent), an inapparent-apparent infection ratio of 22:1 was determined. As previously mentioned, experimental evidence in monkeys also indicates that prior infection with certain heterologous viruses (Zika, Wesselsbron, dengue) can ameliorate the response to yellow fever viral challenge. There is presently no evidence to suggest that prior heterologous flaviviral infection could ''sensitize'' the host to subsequent more severe yellow fever infection through a mechanism of immune enhancement (as postulated to occur in dengue hemorrhagic fever–shock syndrome) (see Chap. 72).

Vaccines

Travelers to endemic areas and persons working with yellow fever virus (wild strains or vaccine virus) in the laboratory should be immunized. The decision to immunize travelers should take into account both the national requirements for certification of vaccination and the risk of acquiring the infection. Travel within the areas shaded in Fig. 71-3 constitutes a risk of acquiring yellow fever. In general, the risk is greatest to travelers who visit rural or forested areas, and individuals who plan only brief visits (of several days) to large urban centers can be exempted from vaccination.

Yellow fever vaccine may be effectively employed as a prophylactic measure in populations within the endemic zone. In South America, many nations promulgate control through immunization; a high level of vaccine immunity has been achieved with the probable result that the disease incidence is low despite ample evidence for yellow fever transmission in the forest cycle. In Africa, however, the approach in most countries is to undertake mass immunization in response to the occurrence of disease outbreaks (see ''Control'').

As programs of multiple immunization for communicable diseases are developed for Africa and tropical America, consideration should be given to inclusion of yellow fever 17D vaccine.

Yellow fever 17D is the safest, most effective live viral vaccine in use. The vaccine is currently prepared from infected chicken embryos under standards developed by WHO [26]. The 0.5-mL dose, delivered subcutaneously by syringe and needle or jet injector, results in a demonstrable immune response in over 95 percent of vaccinees within 7 to 10 days. Intradermal inoculation by jet injector results in a significantly lower seroconversion rate. For the purposes of international certification, immunization is valid for 10 years, but various studies have shown persistence of antibodies for as long as 30 to 35 years, and immunity is probably lifelong.

Serious adverse reactions to 17D vaccine are extremely uncommon. No abnormalities in liver function tests are associated with 17D vaccination. Fewer than 10 percent of vaccinees experience headache and malaise. Allergic reactions, including skin rash, urticaria, and asthma, occur at a very low rate (approximately one in a million), predominantly in persons with an allergic history (especially to eggs). Neurological accidents are extremely uncommon; a single fatal case of encephalitis is reported in a 3-year-old child. In west Africa, at least four outbreaks have been recorded of severe bacterial (presumably clostridial or anaerobic streptococcal) infection at the inoculation site, leading in some cases to shock and death. These episodes underscore the need to handle and administer the vaccine with careful attention to recommended practices.

Vaccination results in a viremia lasting 1 to 5 days and beginning 3 to 4 days after inoculation. The low magnitude of viremia and the fact that A. aegypti is refractory to oral infection with 17D virus preclude the possibility of natural transmission (and possible reversion to virulence) of vaccine virus.

During mass vaccination campaigns, infants, young children, and pregnant women have been immunized without recognized untoward effects. On theoretical grounds, however, the vaccine should not be given to children under 6 months of age or to pregnant women unless there is a significant risk of acquiring yellow fever. Persons with known immunodeficiency states, including AIDS, or on immunosuppressive drugs should also not receive yellow fever vaccine.

Biological factors which may modulate seroconversion to the vaccine include (1) nutritional state, (2) simultaneous administration of other vaccines, and (3) preexisting heterologous flaviviral immunity. Children with kwashiorkor show marked impairment in antibody production after 17D vaccination. Persons administered 17D yellow fever and cholera vaccines simultaneously or 1 to 3 weeks apart showed reduced antibody responses to both vaccines. (Other vaccine combinations can be used without interference, including yellow fever and BCG, yellow fever and smallpox, yellow fever and measles [27], yellow fever and hepatitis B.) In persons given 17D chick embryo vaccine by the subcutaneous route, preexisting heterologous immunity did not interfere with rate of seroconversion or reduce N antibody titer.

At the present time, vaccines produced by some of the world's 12 manufacturing institutes are contaminated with avian leukosis virus (ALV). Although undesirable, this contaminant has not been associated with the development of leukemia, lymphoma, or other cancers.

The French neurotropic vaccine, produced from the brains of infected suckling mice, is no longer manufactured. This vaccine had the advantage of high stability and ease of administration (by scarification or multiple puncture). However, approximately 20 percent of vaccinees developed systemic symptoms, 3 to 4 percent meningeal signs, and 0.5 to 1.3 percent postvaccinal encephalitis. Neurological accidents were more frequent in children than adults.

Although production of 17D yellow fever vaccine could be stepped up rapidly, stocks of vaccine may be insufficient to meet demands posed by urbanization of the disease in the

Americas or its introduction into Asia. Efforts are underway to modernize vaccine production facilities and to develop vaccines in a cell culture substrate.

Other preventive measures

Areas infested with the domestic form of *A. aegypti* are at risk of the introduction and urbanization of yellow fever. This risk increases with close proximity to the enzootic cycle. The threat of urban yellow fever (as well as of epidemic dengue) has been the rationale for the *A. aegypti* eradication program of the Pan American Health Organization. The methods available for eliminating *A. aegypti* are beyond the scope of this book. Briefly, elimination of breeding sites (tires, artificial containers, etc.), treatment of potable water with temofos (Abate), perifocal spraying with organophosphorus insecticides, and use of larvivorous minnows are effective if applied in the context of a well-administered and continually supported program.

Control

The occurrence of epidemic yellow fever constitutes a major public health emergency, particularly in Africa where intense interhuman transmission and high attack rates are the rule.

Emergency mass vaccination has generally been the focus of control efforts. Such campaigns have been initiated after the epidemic peak, because of delays in recognition of the outbreak and in mobilization of resources necessary for mass vaccination. Significant problems are encountered in obtaining sufficient vaccine and jet injectors, in organizing trained teams to administer the vaccine, and in establishing and maintaining an adequate cold chain in remote areas. The effective use of mass vaccination to abort a yellow fever epidemic depends upon a high level of surveillance, early recognition, epidemiological assessment to judge the location of yellow fever activity and the expected patterns of spread, and rapid deployment and coordination of vaccinating teams.

Emergency vector control is aimed at rapid reduction of the adult female mosquito population. In the case of an outbreak of *A. aegypti*–borne yellow fever, ground or aerial ultra-low-volume (ULV) application of insecticides may theoretically be used [*28*]. Because they are not effective against immature stages, the adulticide applications must be repeated until the threat is over. In certain situations, it may be possible to augment the adulticide treatment by use of larvicides or source reduction to reduce the emergence of new adult mosquitoes which could perpetuate virus transmission by feeding on residually viremic persons. Attempts should be made to assess the effectiveness of spraying on reduction of the mosquito population and case incidence.

The control of yellow fever epidemics involving wild vector species requires aerial treatment of large forested areas and has not yet been shown capable of aborting an epidemic. In research trials, aerial ULV applications of malathion were shown to be effective for the control of the yellow fever vector *A. simpsoni* breeding in false banana (*Musa ensetta*) plantations in Ethiopia. Ground and aerial applications of malathion rapidly suppressed populations of *A. africanus* in forest habitats in west Africa for a period of time believed sufficient to interrupt virus transmission [*29*]. Aerial ULV was used to attempt control of *Haemagogus* vectors in forested areas in eastern Panama in 1974.

FUTURE PERSPECTIVES

Despite continuing expansion of human populations and environmental modifications in the developing world, the ecosystem supporting enzootic yellow fever in South America and Africa will remain viable for many years to come. In the absence of serious programs of mass immunization, epidemics of yellow fever transmitted by sylvan vectors will continue to threaten rural populations, particularly in Africa. In addition, the specter of reurbanization of the disease looms even larger. In the Americas, *A. aegypti* has reinvaded Brazil, Bolivia, Peru, and Ecuador. *A. aegypti* and epidemic dengue fever have invaded the Magdalena Valley of Colombia, the Amazon region of Brazil, and Rio de Janeiro. Jungle yellow fever has recently reappeared in Trinidad, an island infested with *A. aegypti* and prone to dengue outbreaks. In Africa, the growth of towns and cities and increasing economic development will augment the association of humans and *A. aegypti* vectors; the threat of urban outbreaks of *A. aegypti*–borne yellow fever, dengue, and chikungunya will increase in the decades to come. Indeed, an urban epidemic of yellow fever occurred in western Nigeria in 1987.

Notwithstanding a long record of accomplishments in yellow fever research, many questions about the disease remain unanswered. At the molecular level, advances in understanding the morphogenesis, replication strategy, mode of translation of viral polypeptides, structure and function of nonvirion proteins, genetic sequence, and gene-coding assignments of yellow fever have been reported. Some ultimate goals of such research include improved vaccine production by synthesis of immunogenic polypeptides, development of effective chemotherapeutic compounds, and improved diagnostic approaches. Oligonucleotide mapping, monoclonal antibodies, and other techniques applied to the geographical variation of yellow fever viral strains will provide molecular markers useful in epidemiological analyses of the origin and spread of epidemics. The variation in viscerotropism among yellow fever virus strains also requires further study. Quantitative data are needed on viremic responses in humans and monkeys, because viremia is the critical determinant of vector infection.

The commitment on the part of national and international agencies to support long-range field investigations of the ecology of yellow fever will be increasingly diluted by other funding priorities in the future. Nonetheless, continued research is urgently required on the basic biology of *A. aegypti* and sylvatic yellow fever vectors, including intraspecific variability in vector efficiency, vertical transmission, genetics, habitat preference, life cycles, longevity, biting habits, flight range, dispersal, and other factors relating to yellow fever transmission and recrudescence.

Surveillance of yellow fever is rudimentary or nonexistent in most areas. Improved surveillance, reporting, and laboratory diagnostic services are central to the development of preventive and control strategies.

The pathogenesis and pathophysiology of yellow fever are incompletely understood, and research priorities have been set forth in the body of this text. The need for more sophisticated clinical investigations of patients in future outbreaks has been underscored. Can clinical management of shock, renal dysfunction, disseminated intravascular coagulation, and other complications reduce mortality rates (as in dengue hemorrhagic fever)?

Efforts to modernize and standardize yellow fever vaccine production are now beginning. The need to utilize mass immunization as a preventive (rather than as an emergency control) measure will gain recognition in the future, possibly resulting in the eventual inclusion of yellow fever vaccine in expanded programs of childhood immunization.

Pressure will increase to employ emergency vector-control measures in future outbreaks; careful study will be required of the effectiveness of such measures, particularly in the setting of a sylvatic epidemic.

REFERENCES

1 Bergold GH, Weibel J: Demonstration of yellow fever virus with the electron microscope. Virology 17:554–562, 1962
2 Rice CM, Lenches EM, Eddy SR, et al: Nucleotide sequence of yellow fever virus: Implications for flavivirus gene expression and evolution. Science 229:726–733, 1985
3 Schlesinger JJ, Brandriss MW, Monath TP: Monoclonal antibodies distinguish between wild and vaccine strains of yellow fever virus by neutralization, hemagglutination inhibition, and immune precipitation of the virus envelope protein. Virology 125:8–17, 1983
4 Schlesinger JJ, Brandriss MW, Cropp CB, et al: Protection against yellow fever in monkeys by immunization with yellow fever virus nonstructural protein NS1. J Virol 60:1153–1155, 1986
5 Hahn CS, Dalrymple JM, Strauss JH, et al: Comparison of the virulent Asibi strain of yellow fever virus with the 17D vaccine strain derived from it. Proc Natl Acad Sci USA 84:2019–2023, 1987
6 Theiler M, Downs WG: *The Arthropod-borne Viruses of Vertebrates*. New Haven and London, Yale University Press, 1973
7 Theiler M, Anderson CR: The relative resistance of dengue-immune monkeys to yellow fever virus. Am J Trop Med Hyg 24:115–117, 1975
8 Henderson BE, Cheshire PP, Kirya GB, et al: Immunologic studies with yellow fever and selected African group B arboviruses in rhesus and vervet monkeys. Am J Trop Med Hyg 19:110–118, 1970
9 Gould EA, Buckley A, Groeger BK, et al: Immune enhancement of yellow fever virus neurovirulence for mice: Studies of mechanisms involved. J Gen Virol 68:3105–3112, 1987
10 Clarke DH: Antigenic analysis of certain group B arthropod-borne viruses by antibody absorption. J Exp Med 111:21–32, 1960
11 Fitzgeorge R, Bradish CJ: The in vivo differentiation of strains of yellow fever virus in mice. J Gen Virol 46:1–14, 1980
12 Deubel V, Digoutte JP, Monath TP, et al: Genetic heterogeneity of yellow fever virus strains from Africa and the Americas. J Gen Virol 67:209–213, 1986
13 Varma MGR, Pudney M, Leake CJ, et al: Isolation in a mosquito (*Aedes pseudoscutellaris*) cell line (Mos 61) of yellow fever strains from original field material. Intervirology 6:50–56, 1975–1976
14 Saluzzo JF, Gonzalez JP, Herve JP, et al: Isolements du virus de la fièvre jaune a partir de moustiques du groupe *Aedes (Stegomyia) africanus* (Theobold) en Republique Centrafrique au cours de l'année 1978. Ann Virol 131 E:313–321
15 Strode GK (ed): *Yellow Fever*. New York, McGraw-Hill, 1951
16 Germain M, Cornet M, Mouchet J, et al: La fièvre jaune selvatique en Afrique: Données récentes et conceptions actuelles. Med Trop (Marseilles) 41:31–43, 1981
17 Cordellier R, Germain M, Herve JP, et al: Guide practique pour l'études des vecteurs de fièvre jaune en Afrique et méthodes de lutte. Documentations Techniques ORSTOM, no 33, 1977
18 Monath TP: Yellow fever: A medically neglected disease. Report on a seminar. Rev Infect Dis 9:165–175, 1987
19 Monath TP, Brinker KR, Chandler FW, et al: Pathophysiologic correlations in a rhesus monkey model of yellow fever. Am J Trop Med Hyg 30:431–443, 1981
20 Barbareschi G: Glomerulosi tossica in febbre gialla. Rev Biol Trop 5:201–209, 1957
21 Dennis H, Reisberg BE, Crosbie J, et al: The original haemorrhagic fever: Yellow fever. Br J Haematol 17:455–462, 1969
22 Borges APA, Oliveira GSG, Almeida Netto JC: Estudo da coagulação sanguinea na febra amarela. Revta Patol Trop 2:143–149, 1973
23 Monath TP, Nystrom RR: Detection of yellow fever virus in serum by enzyme immunoassay. Am J Trop Med Hyg 33:151–157, 1984
24 Saluzzo JF, Monath TP, Cornet M, et al: Comparaison de différentes techniques pour la detection du virus de la fièvre jaune dans les prelèvements humains et les lots de moustiques: Intêret d'une methode rapide de diagnostique par ELISA. Ann Inst Pasteur/Virol 136E:115–129, 1985
25 Monath TP, Craven RB, Adjukiewicz A, et al: Yellow fever in the Gambia, 1978–1979: Epidemiologic aspects with observations on the occurrence of Orungo virus infections. Am J Trop Med Hyg 29:912–928, 1980
26 Smithburn KC, Durieux C, Koerber R, et al: Yellow fever vaccination. WHO Monogr Ser 30:1–238, 1956
27 Gateff C: Acquisitions récentes en matière d'associations vaccinales. Bull Soc Pathol Exot 65:784–794, 1972
28 Ribeiro H: The control of *Aedes aegypti* during the yellow fever epidemic in Luanda, Angola, in 1971. Bull WHO 48:504–505, 1973
29 Bang YH, Bown DN, Knudsen AB, et al: Ground application of malathion thermal fogs and cold mists for the control of sylvatic vectors of yellow fever in rural communities near Enugu, Nigeria. Mosq News 40:541–550, 1980

CHAPTER 72 / *Dengue* · Scott B. Halstead

Dengue viruses occur as four antigenically related but distinct serotypes transmitted to human beings in an urban cycle by *Aëdes aegypti* mosquitoes and to subhuman primates in a sylvan cycle by forest mosquitoes. Urban dengue occurs in nearly all tropical countries. In the American, African, and Indian regions, dengue transmission is associated with classical dengue fever, while in southeast Asia many children with dengue infection manifest a severe illness, dengue hemorrhagic fever–dengue shock syndrome (DHF–DSS). This syndrome may occur in infants born to dengue-immune mothers during initial infections and in children over the age of 1 year during secondary infections. A mechanism which explains this epidemiological paradox is the enhancement of dengue viral infection in mononuclear phagocytes mediated by subneutralizing concentrations of dengue antibody. DHF–DSS, an acute vascular permeability syndrome, may be treated by vigorous fluid and plasma replacement and by balancing electrolytes. Prevention of the infection is by avoidance of day-biting *A. aegypti* or by the eradication of this species from affected communities.

PARASITE

LIFE HISTORY, ECOLOGY

Dengue viruses survive in nature by two mechanisms: by transmission between infected vertebrates and mosquitoes and by vertical transmission in the mosquito. The first mechanism seems to involve as hosts species of primates, with a major urban cycle in which the only host is human beings and the vector is *A. aegypti* Linnaeus, and a sylvan cycle involving subhuman primates and forest mosquitoes. Stegomyia with relatively low anthropophilia such as *A. albopictus* Skuse, *A. scutellaris* Walk, and *A. polynesiensis* Marks may be important vectors of virus to human beings in certain locales [1,2]. The vast majority of adult monkeys living in southeast Asia at altitudes below 2000 feet above sea level are dengue-immune. In Malaysia, several species of feral monkeys have been shown to be infected with multiple types of dengue viruses. *A. niveus*, a canopy-feeding species, has been implicated as a vector [3]. It has been hypothesized that in this setting *A. albopictus* may bridge the urban and sylvan cycles by biting infected monkeys and transmitting the virus to susceptible humans.

Largely from experimental data it is known that dengue viruses can be transferred by infected females to their eggs or to the cells of the egg capsule, infecting reared progeny. The virus can also be passed from males to females by sexual contact [4]. Whether any of these mechanisms operate in nature and what their relative contribution is to virus survival is not

known. There have been reports of the recovery of dengue viruses from larval *A. aegypti* in Burma and Trinidad and from male *A. taylori* in Senegal, West Africa.

A. aegypti mosquitoes acquire dengue virus infection from viremic human beings. Virus replicates in gut tissues and is transferred via migratory infected coelomic cells to neuronal and salivary gland cells. Virus is shed in salivary exocrine secretions and injected intracutaneously through the proboscis during feeding.

MORPHOLOGY AND ANTIGENIC COMPOSITION

Dengue viruses are single-stranded enveloped RNA viruses of the family Flaviviridae (type species, yellow fever). The family comprises a group of 64 serologically related viruses of small size (35 to 45 nm in diameter) and consisting of a nucleocapsid core approximately 30 nm in diameter, surrounded by a lipoprotein envelope (E) [5]. The envelope, studded with poorly resolved projections, is composed of an E protein (MW 54,000) imbedded in a lipid bilayer. When assembled on the virion, the E protein bears epitopes which are specific to the virus serotype, to the dengue subgroup, and to the flavivirus family. An epitope is composed of discontinuous segments of the linear E protein. Very recently it has been possible to isolate or synthesize short-chain peptides which carry serotype specificity (B. Innis, personal communication). Interestingly, the nonstructural protein, NS-1 (MW 46,000), is inserted into the plasma membrane of flavivirus-infected cells. Immune responses directed against NS-1 antigens can abort and cure experimental yellow fever and dengue infections [6].

Using monoclonal antibodies or polyclonal neutralizing antibodies raised in human beings or subhuman primates, it has been possible to identify four distinct dengue viruses, types 1, 2, 3, and 4. Antigenic subtypes of dengue 3 and 4 viruses have been discovered. Dengue 3 viruses recovered in the Caribbean in 1963 and in Tahiti in 1969 differ from prototype dengue 3 and more recent isolates from southeast Asia. Antibody raised to this subtype poorly neutralizes southeast Asian dengue 3 viruses, but the subtype is well-neutralized by antibodies to southeast Asian type 3 strains [7]. A similar but reverse serological relationship was observed with a dengue 4 strain isolated in the Caribbean in 1981 [8].

Many evidences of genetic inhomogeneities exist. Electrophoretic analyses of large oligonucleotides (fingerprinting) demonstrate 50 to 75 percent variation of homology between dengue 1 and 2 viruses isolated in various geographical regions [9]. In general, viruses recovered from Africa, the Americas, and southeast Asia are genetically distinct from one another, while strains of the same serotypes recovered within regions

675

show greater homology. Viruses from the same region recovered 20 or more years apart also show greater homology than viruses recovered in different regions [9].

IN VITRO CULTURE AND INFECTIVITY ASSAYS

A wide range of animal and insect cells and cell lines support the replication of dengue viruses in vitro. In general, strains of dengue 2 enjoy the widest host range. The most-used systems for quantitating dengue viruses are plaque assays, employing either LLC-MK2 (continuous rhesus kidney), Vero (continuous grivet monkey kidney), BHK (continuous baby hamster kidney), or PS cells (continuous pig kidney), using agar, carboxymethyl cellulose, or tragacanth overlays. In most systems, dengue plaques form relatively slowly, circa 5 to 7 days, and often are not accompanied by death of cells or visible cytopathic changes. Dengue viruses replicate to relatively high titer in monolayer cultures of C6/36 (a selected clone of continuous *Aëdes albopictus*) [10]. Other cells used to study the replication of dengue viruses include HeLa, KB, *A. pseudoscutellaris,* primary rhesus kidney, African green monkey kidney, dog kidney, fetal human lung (WI-38), and fetal rhesus monkey (FRhL). Continuous subpassage in dog kidney cells results in selection of small-plaque, temperature-sensitive variants of reduced pathogenicity for subhuman primates, attributes of attenuation [11]. Although many cell systems can be used for recovery of dengue viruses from infected arthropods or human beings, the most widely used are C6/36 and *A. pseudoscutellaris* cells and delayed plaques on LLC-MK2 cells [12,13]. Presence of virus is identified by plaque formation, cytopathic changes, or visualization of antigen with fluorochrome or an enzyme-tagged antibody. Dengue viruses may also be quantitated in or recovered from infectious materials by inoculation of living mosquitoes, most commonly *Toxorhynchites* spp.

Dengue viruses also demonstrate growth in cultures of primate mononuclear phagocytes, in a human monocyte-like line (U 937) and a mouse macrophage-like line (P388D$_1$) with the important condition that nonneutralizing antibody must be added at the time of virus absorption [14,15]. The phenomenon of antibody-dependent enhancement of dengue virus infection receives fuller discussion below (see ''Patient'').

ANIMAL MODELS

Dengue viruses can infect only a restricted number of vertebrate species. Many species of subhuman primate can be infected by the peripheral inoculation of wild-type dengue strains. These animals do not appear to be ill. After a variable incubation period, animals are viremic for several days. The pathogenesis is quite well understood in rhesus monkeys [16]. Dengue viruses replicate in histiocyte-like cells at the inoculation site; next, virus is found in mononuclear cells in regional lymph nodes. Soon thereafter, virus can be recovered from lymphatic and reticuloendothelial organs—specifically in bone marrow cells, Kupffer cells, splenic macrophages, thymic macrophages, and mononuclear cells in Peyer's patches. Eventually virus can be found throughout the skin. Immediately preceding this final localization, virus-infected monocytes are found in the blood. Neither wild nor tissue-culture-passaged strains produce encephalitis or neurological signs following intracerebral inoculation of monkeys.

Many wild-type dengue viruses replicate in brain tissue following intracerebral inoculation of suckling mice or hamsters, resulting in lethal infection. Serial passage of virus in mouse brain results in a shortening of the incubation period to death, but increases virus yields resulting in useful laboratory reagents. Histological examination demonstrates infection of neurones. Wild-type dengue strains which do not kill mice following intracerebral inoculation, nonetheless produce protective immunity. Resistance of mice to challenge with virulent strains provides a sensitive method for detecting and isolating dengue viruses [16].

Dengue viruses readily replicate in various members of the subgenus *Stegomyia* after oral ingestion of virus. The range of arthropod species supporting dengue virus growth is enlarged by inoculating virus intrathoracically. Adults, often male *A. aegypti,* or *A. albopictus,* or *Toxorhynchitis,* are widely used as sensitive systems for dengue virus isolation [17]. Although the use of intrathoracic inoculation of mosquitoes often demonstrates up to 100 times more virus in suspensions which are quantitated by conventional tissue-culture assays, the sensitivity of mosquito inoculation for virus isolation is somewhat vitiated by the small inoculum size. In a comprehensive comparison of mosquito inoculation versus recovery of virus from buffy coat inoculated onto LLC-MK2 monolayers, the mosquito system yielded more isolates when serum hemagglutination-inhibiting (HI) antibody titers were 1:320 or below, but recovery rates of virus from mononuclear leukocytes were higher in the presence of high-titered antibody [18].

PATIENT

PATHOGENESIS

Following the deposit of dengue virus in the skin by the bite of mosquitoes there is a silent period with a mean duration of 4 days [19]. The first observable event is the onset of viremia, followed shortly thereafter by fever with a mean duration of 4 days. Termination of viremia, the beginning of a detectable antibody response, defervescence, and the occurrence of a terminal maculopapular rash signal the end of infection and of illness. While the pathogenic events underlying these visible manifestations are unknown, the similarity in type of cells which support dengue replication in rhesus monkeys and human beings suggests that fundamental pathogenetic events may also be the same *(vide supra)*. Dengue viruses appear to have evolved as parasites of mononuclear phagocytes (Table 72-1). Further, they have exploited antibody as a specific receptor for entry into these cells. Such antibodies are known as infection-

Table 72-1. Sites of dengue virus recovery or antigen detection in tissues from human beings

Method of study	Site	Patients, positive/studied	First author
Virus isolation from autopsy tissues	Recovery of virus from liver, heart, lymph node, lung, and bone marrow; fatal DSS secondary infections	7/199	A. Dasaneyavaja; A. Nisalak; Sumarmo
Virus isolation from autopsy tissues	Recovery of virus from liver, spleen, thymus, and lung; fatal DSS; primary infections in infants	2/2	S. Yoksan
Virus isolation from blood leukocytes	Recovery of virus from adherent peripheral blood leukocytes; DHF–DSS; secondary infections	76/322	R. McN. Scott
Fluorescent antibody test on skin biopsies	Dengue antigen in mononuclear phagocytes infiltrating dermal papillae; DHF–DSS; secondary infections	14/53	S. Boonpucknavig
Fluorescent antibody test on autopsy tissues	Dengue antigen in large lymphoid or reticulum cell in liver sinusoid; DHF–DSS; secondary infections	1/21	N. Bhamarapravati
Fluorescent antibody test on autopsy tissues	Dengue antigen in Kupffer cells or splenic, thymic, and pulmonary macrophages; fatal DSS; primary infections in infants	2/2	S. Yoksan
Electron microscopy on kidney biopsies	Crystalline arrays of dengue virion–like particles in cytoplasm of monocytes in renal biopsies; DHF–DSS; secondary infections	12/20	V. Boonpucknavig

Source: Modified from [20].

enhancing antibodies. Evidence that this is the case derives from four prospective population-based seroepidemiological studies in which children 1-year-old and above were always found to have detectable dengue antibody before acquiring the infection that resulted in their hospitalization for DHF–DSS [21–24]. In a heretofore unique pathogenetic phenomenon in human medicine, infants who acquire dengue antibody passively from their mothers are known to be at risk of developing DHF–DSS during their initial dengue infection [25]. This event occurs after the catabolism of protective antibody acquired at birth. Infants are hospitalized usually between 3 and 7 months after birth when infection-enhancing antibodies are at their peak of activity.

Studies in vitro and in vivo have shown that virus-antibody complexes play an important role in the infection of mononuclear phagocytes by dengue viruses. In cultures of human monocytes dengue replicates to higher titers in the presence of heterotypic flavivirus antibody or homotypic antibody at subneutralizing concentrations than in cultures treated similarly but without flavivirus antibody [26]. In vivo viremias were enhanced in rhesus monkeys initially infected with dengue virus types 1, 2, 3, or 4 and challenged 6 weeks to 6 months later with heterologous dengue type 2 [27]. Enhanced dengue 2 viremias have also been observed in rhesus monkeys injected intravenously with dengue antibody–positive human cord blood before infection with the virus. Control animals were injected with human cord blood without dengue antibodies.

Direct confirmation of enhanced infection during DHF–DSS has been technically difficult to achieve. Viremias during secondary dengue infection are depressed by rapid and early formation of effective neutralizing antibodies. However, several studies have shown that the quantity of dengue virus antigen, measured directly or indirectly, varies linearly with disease severity. Furthermore, complement consumed by the classical pathway, which provides a measure of antigen-antibody complexing, varies directly with disease severity (Table 72-2).

Epidemiological data suggest that such host factors as ethnicity, age, and sex influence the severity of dengue illness.

Table 72-2. Studies demonstrating a correlation between the concentration of circulating antigen-antibody complexes and severity of dengue disease

Test used	No. patients with immune complexes	First author
Clq precipitates (serum)	34	Memoranda, WHO
Raji cell assay (serum)	12	A. Theofilopoulos
Clq latex agglutination inhibition (serum)	67	W. Rongjirachaporn
Raji cell assay (serum)	56	W. Rongjirachaporn
Clq inhibition test (serum)	43	A. T. Sobel
C3 catabolism (serum)	17	V. A. Bokisch
Immune complexes observed in glomeruli by electron microscopy	10	V. Boonpucknavig

Source: Modified from [20].

In the Cuban outbreak of DHF–DSS of 1981, blacks were markedly underrepresented among severe cases, while a retrospective serological study demonstrated equal exposure of Cuban blacks and whites to dengue 1 in 1977 and to dengue 2 in 1981 [28]. In Cuba, where all individuals up to the age of 45 years shared the same dengue infection experience, classical dengue shock syndrome (for description, *vide infra*) was seldom seen in individuals above the age of 14 years. Data in Thailand indicate that females are at increased risk for DSS [29]. How these host-related attributes regulate disease severity is not known with certainty, but pathogenic interventions are possible at both the afferent and efferent stages of infection (Fig. 72-1). The presence of enhancing or neutralizing antibodies, concentrations of virus-antibody complexes, the number of mononuclear phagocytes, the phagocytic activity of these cells, and the permissiveness of these cells to dengue infection are examples of afferent phenomena that might regulate the number of infected mononuclear phagocytes. During the efferent stage, it seems likely that mediators of shock and hemorrhage are produced by dengue-infected mononuclear phagocytes when they come under attack by the immune elimination response. Epidemiological studies in Thailand show that low levels of heterotypic neutralizing antibodies from a single previous dengue infection prevented severe illness in children who acquire dengue 2 infections. By contrast, those children who circulated dengue-enhancing but not -neutralizing antibodies were at high risk of developing severe illness during a dengue 2 infection [30]. In experimental studies using monoclonal antibodies, infection could also be regulated when enhancing epitopes matched between successive infecting pairs of dengue viruses [31]. In this experiment antibody elicited in response to the first infection was capable of enhancing the infection of the second virus.

PATHOPHYSIOLOGY

DHF–DSS is accompanied by the simultaneous and parallel activation of the complement and hemostatic systems together with vascular permeability. The most abnormal values are found in the most severely ill patients. Blood levels of Clq, C3, C4, C5-8, and C3 proactivator may be depressed and C3 catabolic rates elevated [32]. These findings are compatible with activation of complement by both classic and alternative pathways. Hemostatic abnormalities, in order of frequency of occurrence, include thrombocytopenia; prolonged bleeding time; prolonged silicone clotting time; elevated prothrombin time; reductions in factors II, V, VII, and X; hypofibrinogenemia; and increased fibrin-split products.

Vascular permeability is characterized by elevated hematocrit, normal or low serum protein levels due to selective loss of albumin, and serous effusions. Radiographic evidence of pleural effusion, greater on the right than left, is seen in more than half of shock cases.

Severely ill patients demonstrate metabolic acidosis, hypoxia, and azotemia. The usual cause of death is not known but may be due to hyperkalemia and cardiac standstill. Severe and uncontrolled gastrointestinal hemorrhage is sometimes a problem, and when it occurs may be due to disseminated intravascular clotting. Intracerebral hemorrhage may occasionally cause localizing CNS signs and sometimes death.

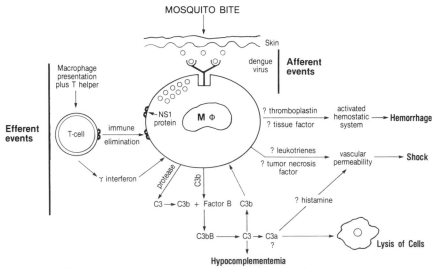

Antibody-Enhanced Infection

Figure 72-1. Model for pathogenetic events in dengue shock syndrome explaining consumption of complement, activation of hemostatic system, hemorrhage, shock, and marked lympholysis, which are the hallmarks of dengue.

Pathology

Published autopsy data are restricted to children dying of DSS. The usual observation in fatal dengue is the absence of sufficiently severe gross or microscopic lesions to explain the death of the individual [33]. Minimal to moderate hemorrhages are seen in the upper gastrointestinal tract, and petechial hemorrhages are frequent in the cardiac intraventricular septum, the atrium, pericardial surface, and on subserosal surfaces of major viscera. Focal hemorrhages are occasionally seen in lungs, liver, adrenals, and subarachnoid spaces. The liver is usually enlarged, often with fatty changes. Yellow, watery, at times blood-tinged effusions are present in serous cavities. Retroperitoneal tissues are markedly edematous.

Microscopically there is perivascular edema in soft tissues and widespread diapedesis of red blood cells. Bone marrow megakaryocytes in patients dying early in their disease show maturation arrest and increased numbers of them are seen in lung capillaries, renal glomeruli, and the sinusoids of liver and spleen. Marked lymphocytolysis or lymphatic atrophy is seen in the thymus and T-dependent areas of lymph nodes and spleen. In B-dependent areas of spleen and lymph nodes there is marked proliferation of lymphocytoid and plasmacytoid cells with central necrosis of germinal centers. In the spleen there is intensive lympho- and erythrophagocytosis. There is hyalin necrosis and cell hyperplasia of Kupffer cells, and the surrounding zone of hepatocytes show focal necrosis and fatty metamorphosis. In the spleen, reticulum cells show hyalin necrosis. There is a mild proliferative glomerulonephritis, presumably due to the deposition of dengue antigen, antibody, and complement. Biopsies of skin rash reveal round cell infiltration, swelling, and minimal necrosis of endothelial cells and subcutaneous deposits of fibrin. Endothelial cells fail to demonstrate ultrastructural lesions other than those seen in mild heat trauma [34].

There are no published comparisons of autopsy findings in individuals dying during primary versus secondary dengue infections. For this reason it is difficult to determine the changes in hemopoietic tissue which might result from a secondary-type antibody response versus those changes attributable to immune responses directed against virus-infected cells.

CLINICAL MANIFESTATIONS

Dengue fever

In the young child, dengue infection is usually unrecognizable. Although it is assumed that many dengue infections are completely inapparent, there is some evidence that a febrile illness occurs with virtually all infections [22]. These are most often characterized by pharyngeal reddening, mild rhinitis, cough, and mild gastrointestinal symptoms and are diagnosed as pharyngitis, influenza, or upper respiratory infections.

In the older child and adults, dengue produces a characteristic syndrome. It appears that primary dengue 2, 3, and 4 illnesses are generally milder than dengue 1. In the classical case, after an incubation period that varies between 2 to 7 days, there is sudden onset of fever which rises to 103 to 106°F (39.4 to 41°C). This is usually accompanied by a frontal or retroorbital headache, backache, pain in muscles and joints, chilliness, and a flushing of the face, puffiness of eyelids, and suffusion of conjunctival capillaries, often referred to as *dengue facies*. The patient often complains of pain on movement of the eyes. A transient macular, generalized rash which blanches under pressure may be seen during the first 24 h of fever. During the second to sixth day of fever, nausea and vomiting are apt to occur, and during this phase generalized lymphadenopathy, cutaneous hyperesthesia or hyperalgesia, palmar edema, taste aberrations, T-wave depression, pronounced anorexia, constipation, and feelings of anxiety or depression occur. Coincident with or 1 or 2 days after initial defervescence, a generalized morbilliform rash appears, which spares the palms and soles. It disappears in 1 to 5 days, often with some scaling. About the time of the appearance of this rash the body temperature may rise from previous values resulting in the classical biphasic temperature curve [19].

Epistaxis, petechiae, and purpuric lesions, although uncommon, may occur at any stage of disease. The frequency of such phenomena varies with outbreaks, with age and sex, and perhaps with dengue strains. Gastrointestinal bleeding, menometrorrhagia, and bleeding from other organs have been described, particularly in adults.

Pronounced bradycardia, often lasting for weeks, is common. In some outbreaks, post-illness depression may be quite severe.

Dengue hemorrhagic fever–dengue shock syndrome (DHF–DSS)

This syndrome has most often been observed in children. The essential pathophysiological features are increased capillary permeability and abnormal hemostasis, at least thrombocytopenia. When there is sufficient hypovolemia to produce hypotension or narrow pulse pressure, this subgroup is called DSS. Cases can be graded by severity and prognosis using criteria adopted by the World Health Organization (WHO) [35] (Table 72-3).

The incubation period of DHF–DSS is unknown but presumed to be that of dengue fever. In children, the progression of illness is characteristic. A relatively mild first phase with an abrupt onset of fever, malaise, vomiting, headache, anorexia, and cough is succeeded 2 to 5 days later by weakness and, sometimes, physical collapse. In this second phase the patient may manifest cold, clammy extremities, a warm trunk, a flushed face, and diaphoresis; is restless and irritable; and complains of midepigastric pain. Frequently, there are scattered petechiae on forehead and extremities and spontaneous ecchymoses, easy bruisability, and bleeding from sites of venipuncture. There may be circumoral and peripheral cyanosis.

Table 72-3. WHO system for classifying dengue syndromes (modified)

Syndrome	Clinical	Hemorrhage*	Laboratory†
Undifferentiated fever	Fever, mild respiratory or GI symptoms	T.T. + or −; bleeding signs + or −	plt NL hct NL
Dengue fever	Fever, headache, myalgia, leukopenia, usually rash	T.T. + or −; bleeding signs + or −	plt ↓ or NL hct NL
Dengue hemorrhagic fever			
Grade I	Fever, mild respiratory or GI symptoms	T.T. +; bleeding signs −	plt ↓ hct ↑
II	Fever, mild respiratory or GI symptoms	T.T. +; bleeding signs +	plt ↓ hct ↑
Dengue shock syndrome			
III	As in grade I or II. Cool, clammy skin, enlarged liver, hypotension or narrow pulse pressure‡	T.T. + or −; bleeding signs + or −	plt ↓ hct ↑
IV	As in grade III. Blood pressure unobtainable	T.T. usually −; bleeding signs + or −	plt ↓ hct ↑

*T.T. = tourniquet test, performed using blood pressure cuff inflated midway between systolic and diastolic for 5 min.
†plt = platelet count. Abnormal value = ≤100,000 platelets per cubic millimeter.
 hct = hematocrit. Abnormal value = 20 percent higher than recovery value.
‡Narrow pulse pressure = systolic-diastolic ≤20 mmHg.

Source: From [*35*].

Respirations are rapid and often labored. The pulse is weak, rapid, and thready. Patients may also present without the early signs of hypovolemia. Almost always patients have a positive tourniquet test. At this stage children develop leaky capillaries, most readily detected as pleural effusion on chest x-ray. To comply with the WHO criteria for DHF, the patient must have a hematocrit value which is 20 percent higher than convalescent value and thrombocytopenia (≤100,000 platelets per cubic millimeter). If the patient stabilizes at this point and does not become hypotensive or develop a narrow pulse pressure, the case is considered to be DHF without shock.

If the pulse pressure is narrow (≤20 mmHg) or the child is hypotensive for age, the case is considered to be DHF with shock or DSS. Usually within a day or two of hospital admission the liver becomes palpable two or three finger breadths below the costal margin; it is usually firm and nontender. Approximately 10 percent of patients manifest ecchymoses or gastrointestinal bleeding. Gross hematuria is almost never seen. After a 24 to 48-h period of crisis, convalescence is fairly rapid in children who have been appropriately treated.

DIAGNOSIS OF DENGUE INFECTION

Serological diagnosis

Etiological diagnosis can be made by the serological study of properly collected acute and convalescent serum samples or, when the IgM capture technique is used, by study of a single sample collected, usually, within 3 weeks of onset. For conventional serological studies, blood should be obtained during the febrile period, preferably before the fourth day after onset of illness, and a second sample should be taken 2 or more weeks after onset. When a secondary dengue infection is likely, paired sera can be collected during hospitalization at an interval of 1 or more days. Serological diagnosis depends on a fourfold or greater increase in antibody titer by the hemagglutination inhibition (HI), complement fixation (CF), enzyme-linked immunosorbent assay (ELISA), fluorescent antibody (FA), or neutralization (N) tests. IgM antibody with dengue specificity can be detected transiently (for 1 to 3 months) following both primary and secondary dengue infections. The presence of IgM dengue antibody is consistent with a recent infection. Differentiation of a primary from a secondary antibody response can be accomplished using the HI, CF, N, or IgM capture techniques [*35*]. In the HI test the evolution of a primary antibody response is relatively slow and the titer achieved is relatively low. Thus, the titer is generally less than 1:20 if measured before the fifth day and not more than 1:1280 2 weeks or more after onset. In a secondary response, the HI titer is generally greater than 1:20 before the fifth day after onset, with the titer rising to 1:2560 or greater, often so rapidly that high-fixed titers are observed. In the CF and N tests, primary infections result in relatively dengue type–specific responses in convalescent sera, while a broadly reactive response, usually involving all four types, characterizes a secondary-type antibody response. The second infecting agent may not be specifically discernible. However, it may be possible to identify the initial infecting dengue type by an "original antigen sin" antibody response measured by the N test [*36*]. In the IgM capture test the ratio of IgM to IgG is above 1 in acute phase of primary infections and below 1 in secondary infections [*37*].

Isolation of dengue viruses

Primary dengue illness is uniformly marked by viremia, and virus strains can be readily recovered by inoculation of serum or buffy-coat specimens into cell cultures or certain mosquito species (see ''In Vitro Culture and Infectivity Assays, Animal Models''). Serotypic identification is now reliably achieved by use of monoclonal antibodies in the IF test.

Blood should be obtained during the febrile period, preferably before the fifth day after onset of illness. The acute phase serum or plasma may be frozen, optimally at −65°C or colder. Because of large quantities of antibody, virus is only rarely isolated from blood during the acute phase of a secondary dengue infection. Results may be improved by the use of mosquito inoculation, fluid overlay cell cultures, or, possibly, macrophage cell lines as virus recovery systems.

TREATMENT

Dengue fever

Treatment is supportive. Bed rest is advised during the febrile period. Antipyretics or cold sponging should be used to keep the body temperature below 40°C. Salicylates should be avoided since dengue infections may be complicated by bleeding phenomena. Acetaminophen is preferable. Analgesics or mild sedation may be required to control pain. Fluid and electrolyte replacement therapy is required when there are deficits due to sweating, fasting, thirsting, vomiting, or diarrhea.

Dengue hemorrhagic fever–dengue shock syndrome

Despite its name, the critical clinical event requiring management in DHF–DSS is fluid loss and usually not hemorrhage. DHF–DSS is treated as if it were a diarrheal disease. Explicit recommendations for management of DSS have been made by a WHO expert committee [35]. In the face of an outbreak, the nearest WHO office should be contacted to purchase copies of the technical guide ''Dengue Haemorrhagic Fever: Diagnosis, Treatment and Control,'' published in Geneva, 1986 [35].

Treatment is directed at reversing physiological abnormalities and maintaining blood volume and blood pressure at near-normal levels until the capillary defect heals, usually within 12 to 48 h. Blood volume must be monitored frequently; a microhematocrit is the most useful test [19]. Figure 72-2 illustrates the use of hematocrit, serum proteins, and vital signs in management of severe shock syndrome.

Intravenous fluid replacement should be reduced as soon as there is evidence of repair of vascular defect to avoid heart failure secondary to hypervolemia from resorbed tissue fluid, which may be serious and life-threatening.

Patients without shock may be given oral fluids and water or juice as tolerated (oral rehydration solution: NaCl, 3.5 g; $NaHCO_3$, 2.5 g; KCl, 1.5 g; glucose, 20 g in 1 L water). When vomiting, acidosis, or hemoconcentration persist, parenteral fluid therapy is indicated. Approximately 1500 mL of fluid consisting of one-half 5% glucose in one-half lactated Ringer's may be given over a 24-h period. If the child seems severely dehydrated, half the volume is given in the first 8 h. Written orders should be explicit as to type of solution and the rate of administration.

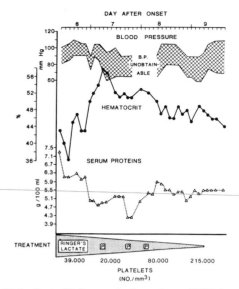

Figure 72-2. Grade IV dengue shock syndrome (DSS) in a 4-year-old Indonesian female, illustrating a stormy clinical course for approximately 56 h. Marked hemoconcentration, hypoproteinemia, and hypotension were treated with lactated Ringer's solution and intermittent plasma (P) transfusion. (*Courtesy of Dr. Yati Sunarto, Department of Child Health, Gadjah Mada University, Yogyakarta.*)

Shock is a medical emergency. Place patient in shock position, and provide oxygen therapy, blood matching, and immediate administration of fluid to expand plasma volume. Children may go into and out of shock for a 48-h period. Initial fluid therapy should consist of lactated Ringer's or isotonic saline, 20 mL/kg, run as rapidly as possible. In case of continued or profound shock, plasma or dextran, medium-sized MW, in normal saline, is given at an initial rate of 10 to 20 mL/(kg·h). In most cases not more than 20 to 30 mL/kg of plasma (or 10 to 15 mL/kg of dextran) is needed. Intravenous fluid is continued at 10 mL/(kg·h) even when there is definite improvement in vital signs and a declining hematocrit. During this period pulse, blood pressure, and respiratory rate should be taken every 15 to 30 min and hematocrit every 1 to 2 h.

Intravenous fluids should be discontinued when the hematocrit level drops to around 40 percent and the patient gains appetite. A good urine flow indicates sufficient circulating volume. Resorption of extravasated plasma produces a further drop in hematocrit which should not be interpreted as a sign of gastrointestinal bleeding if pulse is strong and pulse pressure wide or there is diuresis. Commonly, hyponatremia or metabolic acidosis occurs. Electrolytes and blood gases should be determined periodically in patients who do not respond as promptly as expected.

Blood transfusion is indicated in cases with significant clinical bleeding. Fresh whole blood is preferable and blood should be given up to a normal red blood cell mass. Concentrated platelets may be indicated when there is massive bleeding. If indicated by coagulation studies, heparin may be administered to counteract disseminated intravascular coagulation.

Use of sedatives may be needed to restrain an agitated child. Hepatotoxic drugs should be avoided. Chloral hydrate, 12.5 to 50 mg/kg, may be given as a single hypnotic dose, rectally, orally, or intramuscularly.

POPULATION

POPULATION ECOLOGY: THE URBAN CYCLE

The central facts in the epidemiology of dengue are that virus is transmitted only by certain species of day-biting *Aëdes* mosquitoes and that human beings, and in some regions monkeys, constitute the cycles of infection by which virus is perpetuated. *A. aegypti* Linnaeus, *A. albopictus* Skuse, and *A. scutellaris* Walk, are established vectors. Epidemiological evidence points to *A. polynesiensis* as vector on Tahiti.

A. aegypti mosquitoes can acquire the infection from patients 6 to 18 h before onset of fever and then for the duration of fever. A minimum extrinsic incubation period of 8 days, more usually 11 to 14 days, is required after an infective blood meal before the mosquito can transmit the infection. Once infected a mosquito can serve as a vector for the rest of its life. A high degree of anthropophilia, a habit of multiple and interrupted blood feedings, and the urban location of breeding make *A. aegypti* a highly efficient vector.

In most areas of the world, *A. aegypti* breeds indoors predominantly in clean, stored water in ceramic jars or metal drums, water-holding planters, and ant traps, and outdoors in natural or artificial containers which trap rain water, e.g., rubber tires, tin cans, plastic cups, roof drains, bamboo internodes, coconut husks, or leaf axils.

There is considerable evidence that *A. albopictus* serves as a secondary vector, although whether dengue viruses can survive endemically or whether large epidemics are transmitted by this species is less clear. The zoophilic *A. albopictus* predominantly bites and breeds outdoors in plant axils, cut bamboo stumps, and in natural or artificial water-holding containers.

Nonimmune populations support classical outbreaks of dengue fever, a large number of adult cases being a prerequisite for such an epidemic. DHF–DSS is usually confined to populations in which two or more dengue serotypes are sequentially or simultaneously epi-endemic. Most outbreaks of dengue and DHF–DSS occur at altitudes below 2000 feet, during warm and rainy weather. For most of the tropics increased dengue transmission accompanies the seasonal monsoon. Occasionally dengue outbreaks are seen during the dry, hot season, often as the result of increased water storage in and around human habitations. Frosts or sustained cold weather will usually destroy adult *Aëdes* mosquitoes. Epidemic transmission is seldom sustained at temperatures below 20°C. In Thailand, warmer than normal temperatures during the cool season are a predictor of a large epidemic during the succeeding hot, rainy season.

A. aegypti have a short flight range. The geographical dispersal of dengue viruses is almost entirely by the movement of viremic human beings. Under epidemic conditions, dengue usually spreads along major transportation arteries. Typically, dengue exhibits the epidemiological features of respiratory diseases. An infected index case introduces virus into a household infested with vector mosquitoes and, after the combined extrinsic (mosquito) and intrinsic (host) incubation periods, secondary cases occur. As a result, dengue transmission is often most intense in crowded urban areas, although in some countries, middle and upper income households provide more abundant breeding sites for *A. aegypti* than do the urban poor.

EPIDEMIOLOGY

During the twentieth century, numerous large outbreaks of dengue fever have occurred in tropical and temperate zones. Between 1 and 2 million people had dengue in Texas and Louisiana in 1922. The Queensland–New South Wales epidemics of 1925 to 1926 attacked 560,000 people, while more than 1 million cases were reported in Greece in 1928. Several million cases of dengue occurred in cities of the Inland Sea of Japan during the war years, 1942 to 1945. This outbreak reached most of the Pacific Islands, including Hawaii. While the situation has improved in temperate areas following World War II, *A. aegypti* is now almost universally distributed around the globe between 30°N and 20°S [38]. In these tropical and subtropical regions now live more than one-half of the world's human population. The ecological disturbances of World War II, the rapid postwar growth of population and urbanization, the deterioration of urban living environments, and recent global economic downturns have contributed collectively to the spread of *A. aegypti* and the epidemic or endemic dispersal of dengue viruses throughout this vast area.

Since World War II, large outbreaks of dengue 3 have occurred in the Caribbean, northern South America, and Central America beginning in 1963, dengue 2 from 1969, dengue 1 from 1977, and dengue 4 from 1981 [39]. A somewhat similar sequence has involved the Pacific Islands over the same time period. Since 1980, dengue epidemics have occurred repeatedly in South China and Hainan Island. In the past 10 years, epidemics of dengue fever have occurred in northern Australia, east Africa, much of coastal Brazil, northern Argentina, Paraguay, and Bolivia.

Epidemic DHF–DSS was recognized for the first time in 1954, although in retrospect, outbreaks probably occurred yearly in Bangkok from 1950, and there were historical outbreaks in Greece in 1928 and northern Australia as early as 1897 [40]. In 1981, a sharp outbreak of DHF–DSS occurred in Cuba involving 116,143 hospitalizations over approximately a 3-month period. This epidemic was associated with dengue 2 transmission in a population which had been exposed to dengue 1 4 years earlier. This was the only previous flavivirus experience in Cuba since before World War II. In 1981, nearly 24,000 cases of DHF occurred; 10,000 of these patients had

Table 72-4. Cases of dengue hemorrhagic fever reported to the World Health Organization regional offices, 1956–1986

Year	Philippines		Vietnam		China		Thailand		Burma		Malaysia	
	Cases	Deaths	Cases	Deaths	Cases	Deaths	Cases	Deaths	Cases	Deaths	Cases	Deaths
1956–1980	25,831	2,124	325,409	6,268	36,256	2,455	236,556	5,926	30,267	1,342	5,163	330
1981	324	8	35,323	408	———	———	25,670	198	1,524	90	486	14
1982	816	192	39,806	361	———	———	22,250	150	1,706	49	3,052	6
1983	1,684	305	149,519	1,798	85,293	51	30,025	229	2,856	83	790	10
1984	2,514	241	30,498	368	———	———	69,101	496	2,323	39	702	5
1985	2,096	210	45,107	399	10,000	200	79,450	320	2,666	134	354	11
1986	839	31	46,266	511	———	———	29,573	272	1,910	95	1,043	9
Subtotal	34,104	3,111	671,928	10,113	131,549	2,706	492,625	7,591	43,252	1,832	11,590	385

Year	Singapore		Indonesia		India		Sri Lanka		Cuba		Laos	
	Cases	Deaths	Cases	Deaths	Cases	Deaths	Cases	Deaths	Cases	Deaths	Cases	Deaths
1956–1980	5,240	51	48,982	2,676	1,500	156	79	17	———	———	———	———
1981	133	———	5,978	231	———	———	———	———	116,143	159	———	———
1982	216	———	5,451	255	———	———	———	———	———	———	———	———
1983	205	2	13,668	491	———	———	———	———	———	———	———	———
1984	86	———	12,710	382	———	———	———	———	———	———	———	———
1985	126	2	13,605	495	———	———	———	———	———	———	1,759	15
1986	354	———	16,529	608	———	———	———	———	———	———	———	———
Subtotal	6,360	55	116,923	5,138	1,500	156	79	17	116,143	159	1,759	15

Total cases = 1,630,812

Deaths = 31,178

shock, most of them children. Despite evidence that DHF–DSS can occur in the American region, *A. aegypti*-infested dengue-endemic countries in the Caribbean and in Latin America have not generated large-scale outbreaks. At present, DHF–DSS is endemic in the Philippines, Vietnam, Cambodia, Laos, Thailand, Malaysia, Indonesia, Burma, and South China. Over 1.5 million persons, predominantly children, have been hospitalized since the disease was first reported, and 31,000 have died. As shown in Table 72-4, the DHF–DSS situation in southeast Asia is steadily worsening.

INFECTION, DISEASE

Prospective seroepidemiological studies have resulted in ratios of hospitalized cases to secondary infection of between 1:50 and 1:200 [21–24]. However, in a study in Rayong, Thailand, where children were exposed to all four dengue serotypes, only dengue 2 produced DSS, and the sequence dengue 1–dengue 2 resulted in cases at a ratio of 1:5 [23]. More recently, Kliks and colleagues have shown that of nine children who circulated dengue 1, 3, or 4 antibodies but who lacked cross-reactive dengue 2–neutralizing antibodies, seven were hospitalized with a dengue 2 infection [30]. In contrast, none of 25 children with dengue antibodies 1, 3, or 4 which heterotypically neutralized dengue 2 virus became ill when infected with a dengue virus, predominantly type 2. Although dengue 2 viruses have played a major role in producing severe

secondary dengue infections in Thailand for nearly 30 years (from 1960), beginning in 1983 a lengthy dengue 3 and dengue 4 epidemic has been in progress. These viruses now contribute importantly to severe illness, but in the context of secondary infection. The mechanism explaining this changed pattern remains unknown.

CONTROL

Emergency control measures are based upon insecticide applications. Technical-grade malathion or fenitrothion can be applied by vehicle-mounted or portable ultra-low-volume aerosol generators at about 0.5 L/ha. Two adulticide treatments should be made at 10-day intervals [35].

Long-term control should be based upon comprehensive health education and community participation. Ideally, these measures should be supported by legislation against providing breeding sites for *A. aegypti* and by law enforcement. Health education should begin in schools and be directed at the community with simple and accurate information using all available media, e.g., books, newspapers, radio, television. More specific information should be directed at key educators, teachers, and public health staff. The aim is to reduce sites of *Aëdes* breeding to the absolute minimum. Central to effective control is the destruction of unnecessary water containers, the weekly emptying and cleaning of those containers which are essential, covering of tanks, filling tree holes with sand or cement, and plugging the tops of bamboo fences. Sand granules containing 1% temofos (Abate) can be applied to drinking and washing water. A dose of 1 ppm (10 g per 100 L of water) will be larvicidal for up to 6 months.

Personal protection involves avoidance of the bites of day-biting mosquitoes and the use of insect repellents. Provision of safe and ample supplies of piped water should in the long term reduce the breeding of *A. aegypti*.

At present there are no vaccines available for prevention of dengue fever or its severe complications. Candidate live attenuated vaccines for virus types 1, 2, and 4 are in an early phase of clinical testing [*41*].

REFERENCES

1 Gould DJ, Yuill TM, Moussa MA, et al: An insular outbreak of dengue hemorrhagic fever. III. Identification of vectors and observations on vector ecology. Am J Trop Med Hyg 17:609–618, 1968

2 Suzuki T, Hirshman JH: Distribution and density of *Aëdes aegypti* in the South Pacific. NZ Med J 85:374–380, 1977

3 Rudnick A: Ecology of dengue virus. Asian J Inf Dis 2:156–160, 1977

4 Rosen L, Shroyer DA, Tesh RB, et al: Transovarial transmission of dengue viruses by mosquitoes *Aëdes albopictus* and *Aëdes aegypti*. Am J Trop Med Hyg 32:1108–1119, 1983

5 Westaway EG, Brinton MA, Gaidamovich SYA, et al: Flaviviridae. Intervirology 24:183–192, 1985

6 Schlesinger JJ, Brandriss MW, Walsh EE, et al: Protection of mice against dengue 2 virus encephalitis by immunization with the dengue 2 virus non-structural glycoprotein NS1. J Gen Virol 68:853–857, 1987

7 Russell PK, McCown JM: Comparison of dengue-2 and dengue-3 virus strains by neutralization tests and identification of a subtype of dengue-3. Am J Trop Med Hyg 21:97–99, 1972

8 Henchal EA, Repik PM, McCown JM, et al: Identification of an antigenic and genetic variant of dengue-4 virus from the Caribbean. Am J Trop Med Hyg 35:393–400, 1986

9 Trent DW, Grant JA, Rosen L, et al: Genetic variation among dengue 2 viruses of different geographic origin. Virology 128:271–284, 1983

10 Igarashi A: Isolation of a Singh's *Aëdes albopictus* cell clone sensitive to dengue and chikungunya viruses. J Gen Virol 40:531–544, 1978

11 Halstead SB, Marchette NJ, Diwan AR, et al: Selection of attenuated dengue 4 viruses by serial passage in primary kidney cells. II. Attributes of virus cloned at different dog kidney passage levels. Am J Trop Med Hyg 33:666–671, 1984

12 Yuill TM, Sukhavachana P, Nisalak A, et al: Dengue virus recovery by direct and delayed plaques in LLC-MK2 cells. Am J Trop Med Hyg 17:441–448, 1968

13 Race MW, Fortune RAJ, Agostini C, et al: Isolation of dengue viruses in mosquito cell cultures under field conditions. Lancet i:48–49, 1978

14 Brandt WE, McCown JM, Gentry MK, et al: Infection enhancement of dengue 2 virus in the U-937 human monocyte cell line by antibodies to flavivirus cross-reactive determinants. Infect Immun 36:1036–1041, 1982

15 Halstead SB, Larsen K, Kliks S, et al: Comparison of P388D$_1$ mouse macrophage cell line and human monocytes for assay of dengue-2 infection-enhancing antibodies. Am J Trop Med Hyg 32:157–163, 1983

16 Hammon WMcD, Sather GE: Virological findings in the 1960 hemorrhagic fever epidemic (dengue) in Thailand. Am J Trop Med Hyg 13:629–641, 1964

17 Rosen L, Gubler D: The use of mosquitoes to detect and propagate dengue viruses. Am J Trop Med Hyg 23:1153–1160, 1974

18 Watts DM, Nisalak A, Burke DS, et al: Comparison of the mosquito inoculation technique with cell culture for isolating dengue viruses from patients. In preparation

19 Simmons JS, St John HH, Reynolds FHK: Experimental studies of dengue. Philip J Sci 44:1–251, 1931

20 Halstead SB: Pathogenesis of dengue: Challenges to molecular biology. Science 239:476–481, 1988

21 Russell PK, Yuill TM, Nisalak A, et al: An insular outbreak of dengue hemorrhagic fever. II. Virologic and serologic studies. Am J Trop Med Hyg 17:600–608, 1968

22 Halstead SB, Scanlon JE, Umpaivit P, et al: Dengue and chikungunya virus infection in man in Thailand, 1962–64. IV. Epidemiologic studies in the Bangkok metropolitan area. Am J Trop Med Hyg 18:997–1021, 1969

23 Sangkawibha N, Rojanasuphot S, Ahandvik S, et al: Risk factors in dengue shock syndrome. A prospective epidemiological study in Rayong, Thailand. I. The 1980 outbreak. Am J Epidemiol 120:653–669, 1984

24 Burke DS, Nisalak A, Johnson DE, et al: A prospective study of dengue infections in Bangkok. Am J Trop Med Hyg 38:172–180, 1988

25 Kliks S, Nimmannitya S, Nisalak A, et al: Evidence that maternal dengue antibodies are important in the development of dengue hemorrhagic fever in infants. Am J Trop Med Hyg 38:411–419, 1988

26 Halstead SB, O'Rourke EJ: Dengue viruses and mononuclear phagocytes. I. Infection enhancement by non-neutralizing antibody. J Exp Med 146:201–217, 1977

27 Halstead SB, Shotwell H, Casals J: Studies in the pathogenesis of dengue infection in monkeys. II. Clinical laboratory responses to heterologous infection. J Infect Dis 128:15–22, 1973

28 Guzman MG, Kouri G, Bravo J, et al: Retrospective seroepidemiological survey of dengue virus in El Cerro municipality, Havana-Cuba. In preparation

29 Halstead SB, Nimmannitya S, Cohen SN: Observations related to pathogenesis of dengue hemorrhagic fever. IV. Relation of disease severity to antibody response and virus recovered. Yale J Biol Med 42:311–328, 1970

30 Kliks S, Nisalak A, Brandt WE, et al: Antibody mediated enhancement as a risk factor in childhood dengue hemorrhagic fever. In preparation

31 Morens DM, Halstead SB: Disease severity–related antigenic differences in dengue 2 strains detected by dengue 4 monoclonal antibodies. J Med Virol 22:163–167, 1987

32 Memoranda: Pathogenetic mechanisms in dengue haemorrhagic fever. Report of an international collaborative study. Bull WHO 48:117–132, 1973

33 Bhamarapravati N, Tuchinda P, Boonyapaknavik V: Pathology of Thailand, haemorrhagic fever: A study of 100 autopsy cases. Ann Trop Med Parasitol 61:500–510, 1967

34 Sahaphong S, Riengrojpitak S, Bhamarapravati N, et al: Electron microscopic study of the vascular endothelial cell in dengue hemorrhagic fever. Southeast Asian J Trop Med Public Health 11: 194–204, 1980

35 Dengue Hemorrhagic Fever: Diagnosis, Treatment and Control. Geneva, WHO, 1986

36 Halstead SB, Rojanasuphot S, Sangkawibha N: Original antigenic sin in dengue. Am J Trop Med Hyg 32:154–156, 1983

37 Bundo K, Igarashi A: Antibody-capture ELISA for detection of immunoglobulin M antibodies in sera from Japanese encephalitis and dengue hemorrhagic fever patients. J Virol Meth 11:18–22, 1985

38 Brown AWA: Yellow fever, dengue and dengue haemorrhagic fever, in Howe GM (ed): *World Geography of Human Diseases.* London, Academic, 1977, pp 271–317

39 Halstead SB: Immunological parameters of Togavirus disease syndromes, in Schlesinger RW (ed): *The Togaviruses: Biology, Structure, Replication.* New York, Academic, 1980, pp 107–173

40 Halstead SB: Dengue haemorrhagic fever, a public health problem and a field for research. Bull WHO 58:1–21, 1980

41 Bhamarapravati N, Yoksan S, Chayaniyayothin T, et al: Immunization with a live attenuated dengue-2-virus candidate vaccine (16681-PDK 53): Clinical, immunological and biological responses in adult volunteers. Bull WHO 65:189–195, 1987

CHAPTER 73 / *Undifferentiated Arboviral Fevers*

· *Robert B. Tesh*

There are presently over 400 recognized arthropod-borne viruses of vertebrates. About 20 percent of these agents are known to infect humans. With the exception of those viruses commonly associated with encephalitis or hemorrhagic fever, most of the arboviruses infecting humans produce a self-limited, nonspecific febrile illness. Despite their similar symptoms, however, the natural history of each of these diseases is quite different. It is not possible to cover all of them, so this chapter will describe only six of the most common and representative undifferentiated arboviral fevers of humans.

WEST NILE FEVER

PARASITE

The etiological agent of West Nile fever is a mosquito-borne flavivirus (family Flaviviridae) which is closely related antigenically to Japanese B, Murray Valley, St. Louis, and Rocio encephalitis viruses [1]. West Nile virus also is more distantly related to dengue and yellow fever viruses. It was first isolated in 1937 from a febrile patient in the West Nile district of Uganda [1].

West Nile virus has a broad host range and infects a variety of mammalian and avian species [1]. It kills newborn mice by any route of inoculation. It also grows in a wide variety of tissue-culture lines (both vertebrate and invertebrate); thus, it is relatively easy to recover.

PATIENT

Clinical manifestations

West Nile fever begins suddenly after an incubation period of 3 to 6 days. The type of clinical illness produced by the virus is largely age dependent [2,3]. Infants and young children generally experience a mild, nonspecific febrile illness. Adolescents and adults usually develop a denguelike disease, characterized by fever, rash, severe frontal headache, orbital pain, backache, generalized myalgia, anorexia, lymphadenopathy, and leukopenia. The rash is nonpruritic and maculopapular in type, occurs mainly on the trunk, and clears without desquamation. Less frequent symptoms include sore throat, nausea, vomiting, and diarrhea. Occasionally patients in this age group also develop signs of meningeal irritation (stiff neck, positive Kernig's sign) during the acute phase of their illness. The cerebrospinal fluid in these cases usually shows a slight increase in cells and protein. In elderly and debilitated persons, West Nile virus infection sometimes produces meningoencephalitis and occasionally causes death [3]. Neurological symptoms in the latter patients may include depressed sensorium, somnolence, involuntary twitches, and coma.

West Nile fever is generally a self-limited disease, lasting 3 to 6 days, although general weakness and fatigue may persist for 1 to 2 weeks after the illness. In those cases which develop neurological involvement, the encephalitic signs do not usually appear until the fourth or fifth day of illness, after the temperature has returned to normal.

Diagnosis

Clinically this disease is very similar to dengue, phlebotomus fever, Rift Valley fever, and a number of other viral diseases. Therefore, laboratory tests are essential in establishing the diagnosis. Virus isolation is the best method; blood specimens obtained as late as the fourth symptomatic day may yield the agent when inoculated into newborn mice, embryonated eggs, or cell cultures. Serological diagnosis may also be attempted on paired sera, collected early in the illness and 2 or 3 weeks later during convalescence. However, previous infection with a related flavivirus, such as dengue or the 17D yellow fever vaccine strain, may make the interpretation of results extremely difficult due to the heterologous immune response which develops after a second flavivirus infection.

Management

Management of patients with this disease is symptomatic. Complications are uncommon.

POPULATION

Epidemiology

West Nile virus has a wide distribution. It occurs in rural areas of Africa, southern Europe, and central and south Asia [1]. Its eastern boundary is India. Millions of people living in this region have been infected with the virus. West Nile fever occurs in both endemic and epidemic forms. In areas where it is highly endemic, infection occurs early in childhood and most of the adult population is immune [4]. In regions where the virus is less active, sporadic epidemics of West Nile fever occur among persons of all ages [2]. Epidemics usually occur during the summer months and are correlated with seasonal peaks in populations of culicine mosquitoes. In Egypt, Israel, and South Africa, *Culex univittatus* is the principal vector, but other *Culex* species have also been implicated [2,4]. West Nile virus is thought to be maintained in nature by a mosquito–bird cycle, with humans serving as only an incidental host.

Prevention and control

Since there is no vaccine available, the only effective prevention of West Nile fever is to avoid mosquito bites. Mosquito control programs can reduce the vector population and thus the frequency of the disease. Visitors to areas where West Nile virus is endemic should use mosquito netting, screens, and insect repellent.

PHLEBOTOMUS (SANDFLY) FEVER

PARASITE

The phlebotomus fever group of arboviruses (family Bunyaviridae, genus *Phlebovirus*) currently consists of 44 distinct virus serotypes which have been isolated in Africa, southern Europe, central Asia, and the Americas [1]. By hemagglutination-inhibition (HI), complement-fixation (CF), and neutralization (N) tests, these viruses show varying degrees of antigenic relatedness [1]. A number of the phleboviruses cause human illness. With the exception of Rift Valley fever virus (covered separately in this chapter), the symptoms that they produce are similar and will be referred to here collectively as *phlebotomus fever*. Most of the viruses in this group kill newborn mice after intracerebral inoculation, but serial blind passage is sometimes necessary with original field isolates before they become pathogenic for mice [1]. All of the known phleboviruses grow in Vero cells, producing cytopathological effect in liquid cultures and plaques under agar.

PATIENT

Clinical manifestations

Available data suggest that phlebotomus fever is a relatively mild disease in children [5]. In adults, however, inapparent infections are uncommon, and most patients develop "classical" phlebotomus fever [6,7]. This disease is characterized by fever, headache, myalgia, photophobia, retroorbital pain, and marked conjunctival injection [6,7]. The illness has a 3- to 6-day incubation period and is usually sudden in onset. The skin may have an erythematous flush, but a true rash is absent. Nausea and vomiting occur, but other gastrointestinal and respiratory symptoms are uncommon. Most patients with phlebotomus fever develop a marked leukopenia, consisting of an initial lymphopenia followed by a protracted neutropenia [7]. The acute symptoms last only 2 to 4 days, but a general feeling of weakness and depression often persists for a week or more.

Diagnosis

An epidemiological or travel history represents the best clue to diagnosis. Virus isolation is difficult because of the short duration of viremia. Serological tests may be carried out but serve principally to exclude other possible causes such as Rift Valley fever, dengue, West Nile fever, and influenza. Phlebotomus fever is a self-limited disease. No deaths have been reported. Management is purely symptomatic. Infection with one phlebovirus usually results in lifelong immunity to that virus type but does not protect against the heterologous virus types [6,7]. Consequently, patients may have phlebotomus fever more than once.

POPULATION

Epidemiology

Phlebotomus fever is a public health problem mainly in rural areas of northern Africa, southern Europe, and central Asia, where it occurs in both endemic and epidemic forms [5]. In this geographical region, the principal sand-fly vectors are peridomestic and live in close association with humans. In endemic areas of the disease, most of the indigenous population is infected and acquires immunity early in life [5]. However, when groups of nonimmune adults (i.e., tourists, soldiers, technicians) enter an endemic area and are bitten by infected sand flies, epidemics of phlebotomus fever result. For this reason, the disease historically has been of some military importance. Phlebotomus fever also occurs in tropical America, but here the sand-fly vectors are mainly sylvan in distribution. Consequently the disease is sporadic in appearance and occurs mainly in adults who enter the forests for work or recreation [5].

Phlebotomine sand flies are tiny (2- to 3-mm) sand-colored midges which usually move in short hops and rarely travel more than a few hundred meters from their resting and breeding sites. The larvae develop in loose soil and organic debris in stone walls, wells, gardens, animal shelters, privies, tree buttresses, and leaf litter. Because of their limited flight range and special breeding requirements, sand flies are usually quite focal in their distribution. The adult females usually feed at night. Unlike mosquitoes, they are noiseless and bite by lacerating the skin with their mouth parts, leaving a small hemorrhagic spot surrounded by an area of erythema. In temperate climates, sand flies are active only during the summer months; thus, phlebotomus fever has the same seasonal pattern.

Available evidence suggests that many viruses in the phlebotomus fever group are maintained in the sand-fly population by transovarial (hereditary) transmission [5]. This mechanism ensures survival of the viruses during adverse climatic conditions and during periods when susceptible vertebrate hosts are not available.

Prevention and control

No vaccines are available for phlebotomus fever, but insecticides are highly effective in controlling the peridomestic sand-fly vectors. Using repellents and sleeping under fine-mesh nylon netting are also effective in avoiding sand-fly bites.

RIFT VALLEY FEVER

PARASITE

The agent causing Rift Valley fever (RVF) is included in the genus *Phlebovirus,* family Bunyaviridae. It is antigenically related to several viruses in the phlebotomus fever arbovirus serogroup [1]. Although RVF virus readily infects humans, it is primarily a pathogen of domestic ruminants. Epizootics of this disease cause heavy mortality and abortion rates among sheep and cattle [8]. The resulting loss of livestock can produce severe economic deprivation as well as malnutrition in an affected community. Consequently, RVF has both direct and indirect effects on human health.

RVF virus is relatively easy to recover, but it is highly infectious by aerosol, so extreme caution must be used in handling infected or potentially infected material. The virus is lethal to hamsters, mice, and rats when inoculated intracerebrally or intraperitoneally [8]. The virus also produces a cytopathological effect and plaques in Vero, LLC-MK2, and BHK-21 cells [8].

PATIENT

Clinical manifestations

Four different clinical syndromes have been described in humans infected with RVF virus: (1) a nonspecific febrile illness, (2) hemorrhagic fever with liver necrosis, (3) encephalitis, and (4) loss of vision [8,9]. A nonspecific febrile illness is by far the most common form of the disease. Clinically, it is indistinguishable from phlebotomus fever. After an incubation period of 2 to 6 days, the disease begins suddenly with fever, severe headache, retroorbital pain, photophobia, and generalized myalgia. Nausea, vomiting, and diarrhea may also occur.

Patients appear acutely ill, with flushed faces and marked conjunctival injection. The white count may be decreased, normal, or slightly elevated. In most patients the illness lasts 2 to 4 days, although sometimes a brief recrudescence of fever occurs, giving a biphasic temperature curve. Recovery in uncomplicated cases is complete, although convalescence may take several weeks.

A few patients (<1 percent) develop hemorrhagic manifestations [8,9]. These appear between the second and fourth day of illness, about the time the fever ends. The patient becomes progressively jaundiced and drowsy and develops petechiae, purpura, bleeding gums, hematemesis, and melena. Liver function tests also become abnormal. The prognosis in these cases is poor; death usually occurs within a week and is due to shock and hepatic failure. At autopsy, these patients have petechiae and hemorrhages throughout the gastrointestinal tract. The characteristic lesion is found in the liver and consists of diffuse central necrosis and hemorrhage. Affected hepatic cells show eosinophilic cytoplasmic degeneration similar to that seen in yellow fever (see Chap. 71).

Encephalitic complications of RVF occur 3 to 12 days after the acute febrile illness ends [8,9]. Neurological symptoms can include mental confusion, hallucinations, vertigo, meningismus, paresis, convulsions, and coma. A recrudescence of fever may also occur at this time. The cerebrospinal fluid shows increased protein levels, normal sugar levels, and pleocytosis with a predominance of lymphocytes. Most patients with this syndrome eventually recover, but convalescence may take several months and residual neurological damage is not uncommon.

About 1 percent of patients develop retinal lesions caused by vasculitis and edema following RVF [8,9]. Blurring of vision and loss of central visual acuity are the most common symptoms. These usually develop 1 to 3 weeks after the acute febrile illness. Fundoscopic examination reveals macular exudates, edema, and occasionally retinal hemorrhages. The prognosis is guarded; vision may gradually improve or there may be permanent visual damage.

Diagnosis

Uncomplicated RVF can mimic a variety of other nonspecific viral illnesses. Therefore, one must think of the disease in order to diagnose it. A thorough history is most helpful in suggesting the diagnosis, since most patients with RVF have a history of recent exposure to sick animals. The virus can usually be recovered from human blood during the febrile period and from the liver in fatal cases [8]. A serological diagnosis can also be made by demonstrating a fourfold or greater rise in antibody titer in paired sera taken early in the illness and 2 or 3 weeks later. HI, CF, and N antibodies appear in the serum within 5 to 10 days after infection. In interpreting results of serological tests, it should be remembered that RVF virus is antigenically related to a number of other phleboviruses; consequently cross-reactions among these agents may occur. This is important, because RVF occurs in some of the same areas where phlebotomus fever is endemic; thus, the two diseases could easily be confused.

Management

Despite occasional cases of liver necrosis and encephalitis, RVF in humans is generally a self-limited disease. The mortality rate is less than 1 percent. Unfortunately, however, there is no effective treatment for those individuals who develop the severe forms of the disease. Their management is entirely symptomatic (i.e., blood replacement for hemorrhage and sedation for convulsions). Although by no means proven, the apparent similarities in pathophysiology of RVF liver disease and yellow fever suggest that supportive measures outlined for the latter syndrome in Chap. 71 are worth a trial in the former.

POPULATION

Epidemiology

RVF currently occurs only in Africa; however, its recent appearance in Egypt suggests that it may be capable of spreading to other geographical regions, particularly the Middle East. Outbreaks of RVF in domestic animals are sporadic in occurrence. Transmission from animal to animal is presumed to occur mainly through the bite of infected mosquitoes, but the basic maintenance cycle of the virus between epizootics is unknown [8].

Humans usually acquire the virus by aerosol transmission or by direct contact with blood or tissues of infected animals [8]. It is uncertain what role, if any, mosquitoes play in the transmission of RVF to humans. Veterinarians, herders, slaughterhouse employees, and persons working in animal disease diagnostic laboratories are all at special risk during epizootics. RVF virus aerosols are highly infectious; cases of the disease have occurred in persons who have only been present in a room where a sick animal has been slaughtered or autopsied [9]. Because of the value of domestic animals in many economically depressed regions of Africa, animals are often housed in family compounds. Furthermore, sick and dying animals are usually killed to salvage their meat. Both of these practices greatly increase the risk of virus transmission to humans.

Control

During an epizootic of RVF, attempts should be made to control mosquito populations and to restrict the movement of susceptible animals. Vaccination of susceptible exposed animals is also important in control. Proper disposal and destruction of infected animal carcasses reduces the risk of secondary human infection. Because of the infectivity of RVF virus, extreme caution should be exercised in handling diseased animals or contaminated tissue samples. For this reason, diagnostic work with the virus should be done only in laboratories with high-security isolation facilities. A safe and effective formalin-in-

activated vaccine has been developed for humans and is available for investigational use. It should be given to veterinarians, laboratory workers, and other high-risk personnel.

OROPOUCHE FEVER

PARASITE

Oropouche virus, the etiological agent of Oropouche fever, is a member of the Simbu serogroup of the genus *Bunyavirus*, family Bunyaviridae [1]. It is transmitted by the bite of infected *Culicoides* midges. Oropouche virus is lethal to newborn mice and hamsters after intracerebral or intraperitoneal inoculation, causing death in 2 to 6 days [1]. It also grows in a variety of mammalian cell cultures, producing cytopathic effect in liquid medium and plaques under agar [1].

PATIENT

Clinical manifestations

The incubation period of Oropouche fever ranges from 4 to 8 days. The disease begins suddenly with chills, fever (up to 40°C), dizziness, headache, photophobia, generalized myalgia, arthralgia, anorexia, and prostration [10]. Nausea and vomiting also sometimes occur. The headache is often severe and may not be relieved by simple analgesics. There is no rash associated with this disease, nor are the liver, spleen, or lymph nodes enlarged. Leukopenia is a common feature of Oropouche fever. Clinical illness usually lasts 2 to 5 days, although a prolonged period of asthenia and occasionally dizziness may persist for up to a month [10]. Relapses with recurrence of clinical symptoms are not uncommon, particularly in persons who immediately resume strenuous physical activity. No fatalities have been reported with this disease; its management is entirely symptomatic.

Diagnosis

Oropouche virus can usually be recovered from blood during the acute phase of the illness [10]. This is the preferred method of diagnosis, since the virus is relatively easy to culture. Serological diagnosis can also be made on paired serum specimens taken early in the illness and 3 weeks later during convalescence. Most patients develop hemagglutination-inhibiting and neutralizing antibodies to Oropouche virus following infection [10].

POPULATION

Epidemiology

Oropouche virus has been recovered in Trinidad and in the Amazon River Basin of Brazil, but it probably occurs in other regions of northern South America [10]. Thousands of persons of all ages have been infected with this virus during epidemics in northern Brazil. Outbreaks have occurred in both rural and urban communities. Epidemics are sporadic in occurrence and usually occur during rainy seasons. Although Oropouche virus has been recovered in nature from both mosquitoes and *Culicoides* midges, epidemiological evidence points to *Culicoides paranensis* as the principal urban vector [*10*]. During urban outbreaks of the disease, Oropouche virus is thought to be transmitted from person to person by the bite of infected midges. The virus is probably maintained in a sylvan cycle involving wild vertebrates and an unknown arthropod.

Prevention

There is no treatment or vaccine available. The only prevention is to avoid *Culicoides* bites. This is difficult, since *C. paranensis* is active during daylight hours, readily passes through ordinary house screening, and often feeds indoors.

CHIKUNGUNYA FEVER

PARASITE

Chikungunya virus was first isolated during an epidemic in Tanzania (east Africa) in 1952 [*1*]. Its name comes from a description of the disease given by the local populace, meaning ''that which bends up,'' and refers to the characteristic posture assumed by patients afflicted with joint pains due to this illness. Chikungunya virus is a member of the genus *Alphavirus*, family Togaviridae. It is closely related antigenically to O'nyong-nyong virus, which also occurs in Africa, produces a similar illness, and is transmitted by *Anopheles* mosquitoes [*2*]. Chikungunya virus is more distantly related to Ross River and Mayaro and to eastern, western, and Venezuelan encephalitis viruses.

Chikungunya virus is lethal to newborn mice when inoculated intracerebrally or intraperitoneally [*1*]. It grows in a variety of vertebrate and mosquito cell lines. A number of mosquito species are susceptible to experimental infection with this agent and can transmit it by bite [*1*]. In nature, however, epidemics of the disease have usually been associated with *Aëdes aegypti* or with mosquitoes of the *A. furcifer-taylori* complex.

PATIENT

Clinical manifestations

The usual incubation period is 3 to 5 days. Typically, the disease begins abruptly with high fever (sometimes biphasic), headache, myalgia, arthralgia, weakness, and rash [*11*]. Joint pain is the most striking feature. The arthralgia affects persons of all ages but is generally more severe in adults. There is no marked sex difference. The arthralgia is usually bilateral and mainly affects joints in the extremities. Previously injured joints are especially susceptible. The severity varies from excruciating pain to vague weakness or stiffness. Affected joints are usually swollen and tender to touch, but other signs of inflammation are generally absent. The rash may appear with the initial symptoms, or it may occur several days later. It is maculopapular in type and is found mainly on the trunk and extremities, although the palms and soles can also be affected. The rash is nonpruritic and clears in 4 or 5 days without desquamation, leaving a brownish stain to the skin. Lymphadenopathy is also common, but the liver and spleen are not usually palpable. Most patients with this disease have a leukopenia with relative lymphocytosis during the first week of their illness. Rarely, hemorrhagic manifestations develop with chikungunya fever. Epistaxis, hematemesis, melena, petechiae, and purpura have all been reported in patients with this disease.

Treatment and prognosis

Treatment is symptomatic, and the prognosis is good. In most cases of chikungunya fever, symptoms persist for only a few days and complete recovery follows. However, in a small percentage of patients the joint symptoms persist for several months, resulting in prolonged disability. In these individuals, intermittent attacks of joint pain and swelling are common. The pathogenesis of the joint disease is unknown.

Diagnosis

The differential diagnosis would include other diseases producing fever, arthralgia, and rash, especially dengue fever. Chikungunya virus can usually be recovered from the patient's blood during the first 2 or 3 days of illness. This is the preferred method of diagnosis. Serological tests are the alternative. For the latter procedure, a first serum specimen should be obtained as early as possible during the acute illness, and a second drawn 14 to 21 days later. A fourfold rise in HI, CF, or N antibody titers between the paired serum specimens would indicate recent infection.

POPULATION

Epidemiology

The known geographical distribution of chikungunya virus includes most of Africa south of the Sahara, India, southeast Asia, the Indonesian archipelago, and the Philippine Islands [*1*]. Epidemiological studies suggest that in rural Africa the virus is maintained in a cycle involving wild primates and forest mosquitoes (*A. africanus* and *A. furcifer-taylori*), not unlike the sylvan cycle of yellow fever. Most urban outbreaks of chikungunya fever, however, have been associated with *A. aegypti*. In the latter situation, the virus is probably maintained in a human-mosquito-human cycle. Urban epidemics of chikungunya are sporadic in occurrence but explosive in character. Typically, the disease appears suddenly, infects a large percentage of the susceptible population, and then disappears. The survival mechanism of the virus between epidemics is poorly understood.

Prevention and control

There is no vaccine presently available against chikungunya fever. The only prevention is control of *A. aegypti* and avoiding their bites. Persons acutely ill with this disease should be kept in mosquito-free quarters, because they are a potential source of virus for *A. aegypti*.

ROSS RIVER FEVER

PARASITE

The etiological agent of Ross River fever (epidemic polyarthritis) is a mosquito-borne alphavirus, family Togaviridae [1,11]. It is closely related antigenically to chikungunya virus; in fact, the diseases produced by these two agents are very similar [11]. Although Ross River virus readily kills newborn mice and produces cytopathic effects in a variety of mammalian cell lines [1], relatively few isolates of this agent have been made from sick persons. Failure to recover the virus more frequently can probably be explained by the insidious onset of symptoms. Most patients with this disease do not consult a physician until they have been ill for several days, at which time they already have circulating antibodies and virus is no longer present in their blood [12].

PATIENT

Clinical manifestations

The incubation period of Ross River fever varies from 3 to 10 days [11,12]. The disease often begins insidiously with fatigue, anorexia, myalgia, headache, and low-grade fever. Arthralgia is the most prominent symptom; it may occur initially or develop 2 or 3 days later. The severity can vary from vague joint stiffness to excruciating pain. It is usually symmetrical and involves more than one joint. Fingers, wrists, elbows, toes, ankles, and knees are most commonly involved. Previously injured joints are often the most painful. The affected joints may be swollen and tender. Paresthesia in the skin covering the affected joints is not uncommon. Arthralgia due to Ross River fever occurs mainly in adults. In some patients, a fine nonpruritic maculopapular rash also develops about the third or fourth day of illness.

Ross River fever generally lasts about 7 days, although the arthralgia can persist for several weeks or months, causing considerable discomfort and disability. Treatment is symptomatic, and recovery is usually complete.

Diagnosis

Isolated cases of Ross River fever are difficult to diagnose because of the vague, nonspecific symptoms. Furthermore, there is a wide spectrum of clinical illness [11,12]. However, during an epidemic, one usually observes enough cases to see the full range of symptoms and the diagnosis is relatively easy.

Ross River virus can be recovered from the patient's blood during the first 2 or 3 days of illness [11]. The most sensitive isolation system for this agent is inoculation of live mosquitoes or mosquito cell cultures [12]. If virus isolation is not possible, a serological diagnosis can be made [11].

POPULATION

Epidemiology

Ross River virus has been recovered in Australia, New Guinea, the Solomon Islands, Fiji, American Samoa, and a number of other South Pacific islands [1,11,12]. The disease occurs in both endemic and epidemic forms. In Australia, the illness occurs mainly during the summer and autumn months among vacationers traveling in rural areas of the country. There the virus is thought to be maintained in a wild vertebrate–mosquito cycle, with *C. annulirostris* and *A. vigilax* serving as the principal vectors [11]. In contrast, recent epidemics occurring on smaller South Pacific islands have been explosive in character, involving 40 to 50 percent of the indigenous populations [11,12]. Epidemiological studies during these island outbreaks have incriminated *A. polynesiensis* as the probable vector and suggest that the virus is maintained in a human-mosquito-human cycle, analogous to urban epidemics of chikungunya fever [11,12].

Prevention and control

No vaccine is available against Ross River fever. Vector control and personal protection from mosquito bites are the only effective preventive measures.

REFERENCES

1 Karabatsos N: *International Catalogue of Arboviruses Including Certain Other Viruses of Vertebrates*. San Antonio, The American Society of Tropical Medicine and Hygiene, 1985

2 Goldblum N: West Nile fever in the Middle East. Proc 6th Int Congr Trop Med Malariol 5:112–125, 1959

3 Southam CM, Moore AE: Induced virus infections in man by the Egypt isolates of West Nile virus. Am J Trop Med Hyg 3:19–50, 1954

4 Taylor RM, Work TH, Hurlbut HS, et al: A study of the ecology of West Nile virus in Egypt. Am J Trop Med Hyg 5:579–620, 1956

5 Tesh RB, Saidi S, Gajdamovic JS, et al: Serological studies on the epidemiology of sandfly fever in the Old World. Bull WHO 54:663–674, 1976

6 Sabin AB: Experimental studies on phlebotomus (pappataci, sandfly) fever during World War II. Arch Gesamte Virusforsch 4:367–410, 1951

7 Bartelloni PJ, Tesh RB: Clinical and serological responses of volunteers infected with phlebotomus fever virus (Sicilian type). Am J Trop Med Hyg 25:456–462, 1976

8 Peters CJ, Meegan JM: Rift Valley fever, in Steele JH (ed): *Handbook Series in Zoonoses*, sect B, *Viral Zoonoses*, vol 1. Boca Raton, CRC Press, 1981, pp 403–420

9 Laughlin LW, Meegan JM, Strausbaugh LJ, et al: Epidemic Rift Valley fever in Egypt: Observations of the spectrum of human illness. Trans R Soc Trop Med Hyg 73:630–633, 1979

10 Pinheiro FP, Travassos da Rosa APA, Travassos da Rosa JFS, et al: Oropouche virus. 1. A review of clinical, epidemiological and ecological findings. Am J Trop Med Hyg 30:149–160, 1981

11 Tesh RB: Arthritides caused by mosquito-borne viruses. Ann Rev Med 33:31–40, 1982

12 Rosen L, Gubler DJ, Bennett PH: Epidemic polyarthritis (Ross River virus infection) in the Cook Islands. Am J Trop Med Hyg 53:921–925, 1981

CHAPTER 74 / *Arboviral Encephalitis* · *Richard T. Johnson*

Arthropod-borne viruses (arboviruses) are important causes of severe encephalitis in many areas of the world. Over 20 arboviruses cause encephalitis, but these agents are restricted to particular species of mosquitoes or ticks and to specific ecological systems. Therefore, the arboviral encephalitides show marked geographical restriction. In addition, they are seasonal diseases, corresponding to the major breeding and feeding seasons of the arthropod host.

Arboviruses are agents of several viral families that can replicate in both invertebrate and vertebrate cells. Dissemination by arthropods involves biological transmission; that is, replication and infection of the hematophagous host must occur prior to injection of the vertebrate host. This is in contrast to mechanical transmission, by which contaminated mouthparts or foreguts of biting flies transmit agents such as equine infectious anemia virus or the contaminated feet of flies and cockroaches spread enteric agents, for example.

The mosquito- and tickborne viruses that cause human encephalitis will be discussed in this chapter. The clinical disease and ecology are reviewed, with particular focus on Japanese encephalitis, the most important arboviral encephalitis.

PARASITE

TAXONOMY

Originally arbovirus was an official taxonomic family with subfamilies based on serological cross-reactions. But genetic structure and morphogenesis have taken a central role in taxonomy, and by these criteria the arboviruses that cause encephalitis belong to distinct virus families. The group A arboviruses are now alphaviruses, a genus of the family Togaviridae; the group B arboviruses now form Flaviviridae, a separate family; and most of group C and unclassified arboviruses make up the family Bunyaviridae, structurally a very distinct group (Table 74-1).

The nomenclature of specific strains of arboviruses demonstrates a long tradition of naming viruses for the geographical site of original isolation. This custom yields colorful names such as Bunyamwera, Bwamba, and Six Gun City. However, the names may not designate the site of major activity of the virus, as exemplified by California encephalitis, which is primarily a disease of the midwestern United States.

STRUCTURE AND REPLICATION

Both the alphaviruses and the flaviviruses contain a genome in the form of a single strand of positive RNA, but their strategies of replication are different. Alphaviruses specify a subgenomic 26-S mRNA corresponding to the 3' end of the genome that codes for structural proteins. This is then translated into a single polypeptide, with subsequent cleavage and processing. In contrast, the flaviviruses have no subgenomic mRNA; the 40-S genomic RNA appears to be the only message. Although flavivirus RNA is infectious, the RNA lacks the 3' poly(A) tract found in alphaviruses and usual mRNA (see Chap. 71). Bunyaviruses have a totally different mode of replication. They have a multisegmented genome of negative-stranded RNA and require a virion transcriptase to initiate replication. The diversity of viruses that can have biological cycles in arthropods is exemplified by the orbiviruses, naked viruses whose multisegmented genome is double-stranded RNA (Table 74-1). Although Colorado tick fever virus, a rare cause of encephalitis, is tentatively classified in the orbivirus genus of *Reoviridae*, unlike other reoviruses its genome is in 12 rather than 10 segments.

All arboviruses have a broad host range and a rapid replicative cycle; they induce cytopathology in a variety of human and other vertebrate cells. They all replicate in vitro in invertebrate cells but often without cytopathic effect. In cell culture alphaviruses enter cells by endocytosis via coated vesicles, and then fusion with cell membranes is triggered by the acid environment. Transcription and translation of alphaviruses, flaviviruses, and bunyaviruses occur in the cytoplasm. In alphavirus morphogenesis cytoplasmic assembly of the nucleocapsid is followed by budding of the mature virus from the cytoplasmic membrane; but flaviviruses and bunyaviruses acquire their envelopes by budding into endoplasmic reticu-

Table 74-1. Properties of virus families and genera that include arboviruses

Family Genus	Members of taxonomic group	Size, nm	Nucleic acid	Structure	Structural proteins	Morphogenesis	Major causes of human encephalitis
Togaviridae* *Alphavirus*	26	60–65	Single strand + RNA	Icosahedral capsid with envelope	2 or 3 surface glycoproteins; 1 capsid protein	Bud from plasma membrane	Western Eastern
Flaviviridae	60	40–45	Single strand + RNA	"Spherical" capsid with envelope	1 surface glycoprotein; 1 nonglycosylated protein; and 1 nucleoprotein	Bud through smooth endoplasmic reticulum	Japanese St. Louis Tickborne
Bunyaviridae	>200	80–120	3 circular segments; − RNA	Helical capsid with envelope	2 surface glycoproteins; 1 capsid protein; and transcriptase	Bud through smooth endoplasmic reticulum	California serogroup
Reoviridae* *Orbivirus*	12 serogroups	± 70	10 segments of double-stranded RNA	Icosahedral shell, spherical outershell, no envelope	5 core proteins; 2 outer capsid proteins	Complete cytoplasmic replication; release by cell lysis	None†

*These families have other genera of non-arthropod-borne viruses. Genera of Togaviridae include *Rubivirus* (rubella) and *Pestivirus* (bovine virus diarrhea), and genera of Reoviridae include enteric *Reovirus* and *Rotovirus* as well as genera that only infect plants and insects.
†Colorado tick fever, tentatively classified as an *Orbivirus*, rarely causes encephalitis.

lum, forming vacuoles; mature viruses are then released from cells by exocytosis or cell lysis. This may vary with host, since alphavirus morphogenesis can resemble flavivirus maturation in mosquito cells [*1*].

EXPERIMENTAL VERTEBRATE INFECTION

A wide range of animals are susceptible to infection, but mice have been the most widely studied experimental models. Newborn mice are susceptible to encephalitis after peripheral inoculation and adult mice usually only after intracerebral inoculation. In young mice after subcutaneous inoculation, analogous to infection by the arthropod, virus replicates in local tissues. Early replication in muscle has been shown with several alphaviruses. Flaviviruses often are carried to the regional lymphatics, where infection of lymphoid cells occurs, and virus seeds from the infected lymph nodes through the thoracic duct directly into the blood. In contrast, the alphaviruses and bunyaviruses have been shown to infect vascular endothelial cells—another efficient mechanism for seeding a plasma viremia.

Most arboviruses are small, and therefore they are cleared less efficiently by the reticuloendothelial system. Nevertheless, efficient replication is necessary to maintain a plasma viremia of a sufficient magnitude and duration to allow invasion of the central nervous system. In most experimental infections virus invades the brain via the cerebral capillaries; alphaviruses gen-

erally replicate in cerebrovascular endothelium and then in neural cells, whereas flaviviruses invade the neural parenchyma without infecting the vascular endothelium [*2*]. The possibility that arboviruses enter the brain across the olfactory mucosa, a historical hypothesis devised when the blood-brain barrier was considered impermeable to viruses, has been rekindled by recent experimental studies of St. Louis encephalitis virus in hamsters [*3*].

Because of the limited extracellular space, most viruses spread within the nervous system by direct cell-to-cell spread or by transport along dendritic and axonal processes. Arboviruses appear to spread extracellularly; they have been observed by electron microscopy in extracellular space and both alpha- and flavivirus encephalitis can be aborted by neutralizing antibodies even after the central nervous system is infected. In murine hosts, the arboviruses appear to infect predominantly neurons but also glial cells and ependyma [*2*].

Inflammatory response in animals is immunologically specific and dependent on T cells. The initial perivascular infiltrates are predominantly T helper-inducer cells with later entry of B cells and macrophages [*4*]. Intrathecal synthesis of antibody occurs in B cells, and macrophages clear infected cells, which may attenuate infection by destroying cells before they replicate with a full complement of progeny. In experimental arboviral encephalitis the role of immunopathological processes appears minimal; immunosuppression decreases inflammation but augments viral growth, shortens the course of disease, and increases lethality.

ARTHROPOD INFECTION

A susceptible arthropod is infected by ingestion of blood with a critical concentration of virus; the virus must penetrate the midgut and eventually infect the arthropod's salivary glands. The time from ingestion of the infected blood meal to the infection of the salivary glands is called the *extrinsic incubation period*, and its duration is highly dependent on ambient temperature. An increase in environmental temperature shortens the extrinsic incubation period, so high temperatures promote epidemics. Infection is noncytopathic in the arthropod, and it remains infected for life [5]. Mosquitoes can be maintained in the laboratory for many months, but in the wild, life is perilous, with about 10 percent mortality per day. This makes the length of the extrinsic incubation period very critical in nature. Ticks have longer survivals.

After experimental inoculation of Japanese encephalitis virus in its natural vector, *Culex tritaeniorhynchus,* virus infects the phagocytic hemolymph cells of the fat body within 2 days. Antigen never develops in the intervening muscle fibers. By the third to fifth day, cells of the nervous system are infected with consistent infection of all retinula cells in the compound eye and patchy involvement of neural cells in the cephalic, thoracic, and abdominal ganglia. Unlike the transient hemolymph infection, this pattern of neural infection persisted over subsequent weeks of observation. Neuronal infection precedes involvement of the salivary gland by several days, and the sequence is even more obvious when temperatures are lowered from 32 to 26°C where nervous system infection precedes salivary gland infection by 2 weeks. Whether neural infection is requisite to salivary gland infection remains unknown [6].

Japanese encephalitis virus is not only neurotropic in the mosquito, but highly selective in neuronal infection. There is consistent involvement of the neurons of the compound eye and a total absence of antigen in neurons of Johnston's organs that lie at the base of the antennae and form the auditory organs and probable synaptic sites of the chemoreceptors of the antennae. Concurrent field studies showed that a higher proportion (5:1) of infected mosquitoes are caught in light traps baited with CO_2 than in light traps without CO_2. This raises the intriguing possibility that persistent neural infection of the mosquito, although causing no disease or cytopathology, may modify behavior and bias the attraction of infected mosquitoes to CO_2-emitting targets such as humans [6]. The observation that mosquitoes infected with La Crosse virus have increased probing activity also demonstrates a behavioral effect of infection that may facilitate transmission to human beings [5].

PATIENT

PATHOGENESIS

In human beings infection begins when the infected feeding arthropod inoculates saliva containing virus into subcutaneous tissue or directly into blood. Aerosol spread of arboviruses has been reported in laboratory accidents and is suspected in the natural spread of Rift Valley fever, but, in general, infections occur only by inoculation. A viremia develops during the asymptomatic period, but in humans it is usually not of high titer or sustained duration.

The immune response is prompt. IgM antibodies are present in serum and spinal fluid of 60 to 80 percent of patients on the first day that they present with symptoms. At this time viremia is usually no longer detectable. Since the majority of persons infected with these viruses do not develop encephalitis (Table 74-2), viremia is presumably not of sufficient magnitude or virus is cleared before the central nervous system is infected. Siblings of patients with Japanese encephalitis who have serum IgM antibodies indicating recent infection show no intrathecal IgM to suggest nervous system infection [7]. Clinically inapparent infection of the central nervous system probably does not occur frequently, and mild forms of viral meningitis are seldom seen with Japanese encephalitis virus infections. When the central nervous system is invaded by Japanese encephalitis virus, clinical encephalitis usually ensues.

Encephalitis is slightly more common in males than in females. There are striking differences in frequency and severity of encephalitis with age. Japanese encephalitis is primarily a childhood disease in epidemic areas, but this is explained by almost universal antibody in adults. Movement of nonimmune adults into an epidemic area shows that adults are fully susceptible. In contrast, La Crosse virus infection occurs at all ages, but disease is limited almost exclusively to children. Eastern and western encephalitis viruses show a higher clinical-to-subclinical ratio in children and cause more severe disease in children. St. Louis encephalitis virus presents the opposite pattern, where larger numbers of cases and more serious disease correlate with increasing age (Table 74-2).

PATHOLOGY

In fatal cases, the brain shows congestion and swelling, but temporal lobe or cerebellar herniation is rare, suggesting that death is not usually secondary to cerebral edema. The meningeal inflammatory response is modest; inflammation is more marked in the parenchyma of the brain. Perivascular infiltrates of inflammatory cells, neuronophagia, and glial nodules are particularly prominent in gray matter (Fig. 74-1). Polymorphonuclear cells may be present in moderate numbers, and rod cells and microglia are abundant in the parenchyma. In Japanese encephalitis, a greater degree of inflammation and focal necrosis is found in the thalamus, basal ganglia, brainstem, and spinal cord [8].

Immunoperoxidase staining of brains of fatal cases of Japanese encephalitis shows that viral antigen is localized exclusively to neurons with larger numbers infected in the deep nuclei and the brainstem (Fig. 74-2). Inflammatory cells and the perivascular cuffs are predominantly T helper cells with a ratio of T4 to T8 cells of approximately 5:1 despite normal

Table 74-2. Examples of arboviral encephalitis with different epidemiological patterns and varying severity of human disease

Epidemiological pattern: Virus	Number of cases per year	Inapparent/apparent infection	Mortality rates	Sequelae
Annual epidemic disease:				
Japanese encephalitis	>10,000	1000:1	20–30%	30%
		As high as 50:1 (adults)	50% >50 years	
Annual endemic disease:				
Tickborne encephalitis	>2000	>30:1	East U.S.S.R 20%	30–60%
			Europe <5%	
California	± 100	26:1 under age 15	<1%	Mild
Annual endemic/intermittent epidemic disease:				
St. Louis encephalitis	Interepidemic years <50	19:1–470:1	8%	30–50% mild
	Epidemic years up to 2000		Young 2%	<10% severe
			Elderly >20%	
Western	Interepidemic years <50;	1000:1	10–20% < 1 year	55% age <1 month
	Epidemic years up to 1000		<3% adults	5% adults
Eastern	Interepidemic <5	20:1	50–80%	70% of young
	Outbreaks ± 10			
Intermittent epidemic disease:				
Murray Valley	Interepidemic 0	800:1	20%	40%
	Outbreaks 12 to 60			

ratios of about 2:1 in the peripheral blood. B cells are seen but are localized to the perivascular cuffs. Macrophages are abundant throughout the parenchyma, and they constitute the majority of cells in the areas of necrosis [8].

The paucity of pathology outside of the central nervous system fails to demonstrate sites of extraneuronal growth. In fatal Japanese encephalitis minor degrees of interstitial myocarditis and pulmonary interalveolitis with focal hemorrhages are found, as well as rather nonspecific perilobular fatty changes and cytoplasmic hyaline changes in the liver [9].

CLINICAL MANIFESTATIONS

The incubation period of arboviral encephalitis has been estimated at between 4 days and 3 weeks. Typically, there is a prodromal illness of 2 to 3 days with headache, fever, and malaise. In Venezuelan equine encephalitis and tickborne encephalitis, a diphasic disease usually occurs with an influenza-like illness followed by recovery and then the abrupt onset of neurological disease. Initial symptoms intensify with vomiting and confusion followed by obtundation and, frequently, coma.

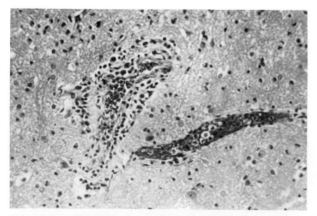

Figure 74-1. Histopathology of arboviral encephalitis is shown in brains of children who died of acute Japanese encephalitis. Hematoxylin and eosin. **A.** Perivascular inflammation in the pons. × 220.

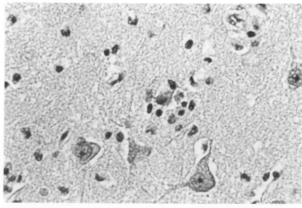

B. Neuronophagia with inflammatory cells around a pyknotic neuron (center) and normal adjacent neurons (below) in the thalamus. × 500.

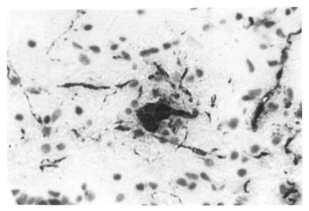

Figure 74-2. Selective neuronal infection in Japanese encephalitis. A neuron in the medulla shows viral antigen in cytoplasm and dendritic processes stained by immunoperoxidase method. Surrounding inflammatory and glial cells counterstained with hematoxylin show no viral antigen. × 550. (*Reproduced with permission from* [*8*].)

Generalized or focal seizures are common particularly in children.

On examination, depression of consciousness, general weakness, and hyperreflexia are evident. Japanese and tickborne encephalitides often show lower motor neuron disease with loss of tone, reflex loss, and sharply localized muscle weakness. These poliomyelitis-like findings are usually limited to the upper extremities, suggesting involvement of the gray matter of the cervical spinal cord. Severe coarse tremors are also seen, most notably in Japanese and St. Louis encephalitides. The syndrome of inappropriate secretions of antidiuretic hormone is common with St. Louis encephalitis [10].

Cerebrospinal fluid examination shows a pleocytosis composed predominantly of lymphocytes, except in fulminant Japanese or eastern encephalitides, where polymorphonuclear cells may predominate. Protein is usually modestly elevated; hypoglycorrhacia is rare. The electroencephalogram is usually diffusely abnormal and is nonspecific. Cerebral imaging may be normal or may show brain swelling and edema, but imaging usually fails to show any specific localization of disease.

The severity of the disease is highly variable. Twenty to 30 percent of patients with Japanese encephalitis die; over 50 percent of children infected with eastern encephalitis and less than 1 percent infected with California encephalitis die. St. Louis encephalitis shows very low mortality in the young but over 20 percent mortality in the elderly (Table 74-2).

Sequelae of varying severity are frequent after all forms of arboviral encephalitis. Intellectual impairment, memory loss, and personality changes are common. Following Japanese encephalitis approximately 30 percent of patients have sequelae, and these often include dystonic postures and parkinsonian features consistent with the localization of infection to the basal ganglia. Progressive atrophy of the upper extremities following tickborne encephalitis led to interest in the past in the possible relationship between this virus and amyotrophic lateral sclerosis. The only evidence of persistent infection related to sequelae is in patients with tickborne encephalitis who develop partial continuous epilepsy (Kozhevnikov's epilepsy). In two instances, cortical tissue resected during surgery for focal epilepsy long after encephalitis yielded tickborne encephalitis virus [11]. Similar North American patients with partial continuous epilepsy have had surgery, and tissue showed a chronic inflammatory encephalitis. No arbovirus or other agent has been recovered from these tissues [12].

DIAGNOSIS

Specific diagnosis requires the recovery of the virus or the demonstration of a significant increase in specific antibodies. At the time of encephalitis, virus isolation is usually not possible from blood and only rarely from spinal fluid. Virus can be isolated from brain or spinal cord tissue during the first week of disease but may not be recoverable thereafter.

Antibodies in serum can be quantitated using complement fixation, neutralization, hemagglutination inhibition, immunofluorescence, or enzyme-linked immunosorbent assays (ELISA). A fourfold or greater increase in antibodies between acute and convalescent phase sera is needed to document infection. Hemagglutination-inhibiting antibodies show the greatest degree of cross-reaction, and neutralizing antibodies are the most specific.

The development of the IgM antibody-capture ELISA has facilitated the early diagnosis of arboviral infections. Antiviral IgM is usually present in serum and spinal fluid within the first days of symptomatic disease. In areas where multiple related viruses are endemic, serum reactions may be ambiguous, but assays of cerebrospinal fluid are highly specific. Studies of Japanese encephalitis have found that 70 percent of children have IgM detectable in spinal fluid on the day of admission to the hospital, and this increases to nearly 100 percent by the fifth hospital day [7]. In addition, almost all children with spinal fluid antibody at the time of hospitalization survive. The absence of antibody correlates with the isolation of the virus from spinal fluid and the subsequent fatal outcome from the infection. Thus, this readily performed ELISA test can not only be used for diagnosis during the first days of hospitalization but also has prognostic value [13].

MANAGEMENT

No antiviral drugs are known to be effective in arboviral encephalitis. Since acyclovir is an effective drug in the treatment of herpesvirus encephalitis, the other most life-threatening form of viral encephalitis, this diagnosis must be excluded. A search for bacterial infections, cerebral malaria, and other treatable diseases is also important.

In arboviral encephalitis survival and the quality of recovery depend on supportive care. Patients with encephalitis are often comatose, but remarkable recoveries can occur after prolonged

Table 74-3. Arboviruses that cause encephalitis

Family Genus Complex Virus species	Vector	Animal reservoir	Geographical location	Importance in encephalitis*
Togaviridae				
Alphavirus[†]				
Eastern encephalitis	Mosquitoes (*Culiseta, Aëdes*)	Birds	Eastern and gulf coasts of U.S., Caribbean, and South America	+ +
Western encephalitis	Mosquitoes (*Culex*)	Birds	Widespread; but disease in western U.S. and Canada	+ +
Venezuelan equine encephalitis	Mosquitoes (*Aëdes, Culex, Mansonia*, et al.)	Horses and small mammals	South and Central America, Florida and southwest U.S.	+
Flaviviridae[‡]				
St. Louis complex				
St. Louis	Mosquitoes (*Culex*)	Birds	Widespread in U.S.	+ + +
Japanese	Mosquitoes (*Culex*)	Birds	Japan, China, SE Asia, and India	+ + + +
Murray Valley	Mosquitoes (*Culex*)	Birds	Australia and New Guinea	+ +
West Nile	Mosquitoes (*Culex*)	Birds	Africa and Middle East	+ +
Ilheus	Mosquitoes (*Psorophora*)	Birds	South and Central America	+
Rocio	Mosquitoes (?)	Birds	Brazil	+ +
Tickborne complex				
Far Eastern tickborne encephalitis[§]	Ticks (*Ixodes*)	Small mammals and birds	Eastern U.S.S.R	+ + +
Central European tickborne encephalitis	Ticks (*Ixodes*)	Small mammals and birds	Central Europe	+ + +
Kyasanur Forest	Ticks (*Haemophysalis*)	Small mammals and birds	India	+ +
Louping ill	Ticks (*Ixodes*)	Small mammals and birds	North England, Scotland, and North Ireland	+
Powassan	Ticks (*Ixodes*)	Small mammals and birds	Canada and northern U.S.	+
Negishi	Ticks (?)	Small mammals and birds	Japan	+
Bunyaviridae				
Bunyavirus				
California group				
California encephalitis	Mosquitoes (*Aëdes*)	Small mammals	Western U.S.	+
La Crosse	Mosquitoes (*Aëdes*)	Squirrels, chipmunks	Midwestern and eastern U.S.	+ + +
Jamestown Canyon	Mosquitoes (*Culiseta*)	Whitetailed deer	U.S. and Alaska	+
Snowshoe	Mosquitoes (*Culiseta*)	Snowshoe hare	Canada, Alaska, and northern U.S.	+
Tahyna	Mosquitoes (*Aëdes, Culiseta*)	Small mammals	Czechoslovakia, Yugoslavia, Italy, and southern France	+
Inkoo	Mosquitoes (?)	Reindeer, moose	Finland	+
Phlebovirus				
Rift Valley	Mosquitoes (*Culex, Aëdes*)	Sheep, cattle camels	East Africa	+
Reoviridae				
Orbivirus				
Colorado tick fever	Ticks (*Dermacentor*)	Small mammals	Rocky Mountain area	+

* + + + +, 10,000 cases/year; + + +, common outbreaks of >100 cases/year; + +, irregular outbreaks; +, rare occurrences.
[†]Formerly group A arboviruses.
[‡]Formerly group B arboviruses.
[§]Formerly Russian spring-summer encephalitis.

Source: Modified from [2].

coma, so vigorous supportive therapy and avoidance of complications are essential. The airway must be maintained; mechanical respiration may be necessary; and careful monitoring of fluids and electrolytes is essential because water, glucose, and salt control are frequently compromised during encephalitis. Infection of the respiratory tract, intravenous sites, urinary tract, and skin must be avoided. Seizures, if they develop, must be treated. Severe hyperthermia should be treated vigorously, but attempts to reduce temperature elevations to normal or subnormal levels may be ill-advised, because these viruses are thermolabile. Modest temperature elevations probably serve as a natural defense mechanism.

Mild increases in intracranial pressure can be treated with glycerol, and increased pressure over a prolonged period is best treated with corticosteroids. Routine use of corticosteroids must be balanced against the knowledge that herniation is not common in arboviral encephalitis and host defenses may be decreased by corticosteroids. In a limited placebo-controlled study of corticosteroids in patients with Japanese encephalitis, no differences in period of coma, morbidity, seizures, or survival were found between the groups receiving corticosteroids or placebo (unpublished data).

POPULATION

ECOLOGY AND EPIDEMIOLOGY

The arboviruses that cause encephalitis extend over wide geographical areas including the tropics, temperate zones, and the subarctic (Table 74-3). Viruses are of varying public health importance. Japanese encephalitis virus is most important; it extends across a wide area of Asia and causes the greatest mortality and morbidity, with many thousands of cases annually (Table 74-2). Several thousand human cases of tick-borne encephalitis are estimated to occur in the Soviet Union and Europe each year. Hundreds of cases occur at irregular intervals with St. Louis encephalitis virus or at relatively steady annual rates with California encephalitis viruses in the United States. Very infrequent outbreaks of Murray Valley encephalitis occur when the virus reaches the heavily populated areas of southern Australia. Rocio encephalitis virus caused over 400 cases of encephalitis and 61 deaths along the southern coast of Brazil in 1975. Small outbreaks of eastern encephalitis occur at irregular intervals in the United States. A number of viruses exist outside of the areas where they cause epidemic disease. Thus, sporadic cases of eastern encephalitis occur in Latin America as far south as Argentina, and sporadic cases of Japanese encephalitis occur in the Philippines and Indonesia where there is no epidemic disease.

Although the above viruses cause essentially subclinical infections unless encephalitis develops, a number of other arboviruses cause systemic illnesses in which encephalitis is a rare complication. Venezuelan equine encephalitis that kills horses generally causes an influenza-like disease in human beings, and only 3 percent of those persons with clinical disease develop encephalitis. Common arboviral fevers of human beings such as West Nile, Rift Valley, and Colorado tick fever (see Chap. 73) are rarely complicated with encephalitis. Louping ill is primarily an encephalitis of sheep, and only very rare cases of nonfatal human encephalitis have been reported.

The natural enzootic cycles of virus occur annually between animal reservoirs and arthropods. The density and habits of the vectors, the level of rainfall and groundwater, the temperature, the size of animal populations and the numbers of available nonimmunes to amplify the virus, and diverse human activities influence the spread of infection. The arthropod, once infected, is infected for life without disease. The amount of disease that occurs in wild animals and birds is uncertain. *Amplifying hosts* are animals which will develop high-titered and prolonged viremia, making them ideal for the infection of many other arthropods. Dead-end hosts such as humans generally do not provide a high-titered viremia, are not fed on by large numbers of mosquitoes, and therefore do not recycle virus back to the arthropod vector. The horse is usually a dead-end host except in the ecology of Venezuelan equine encephalitis, where horses can be an important amplifier during epidemics.

Japanese encephalitis

Japanese encephalitis is the most common cause of epidemic encephalitis worldwide. Epidemics have been recorded in Japan since the 1870s; the virus was initially isolated there in 1934. Since 1967, however, cases of encephalitis have declined in Japan. In contrast, the epidemic disease has been recognized with increasing frequency over a wider geographical area. It involves all but two of the provinces of China, and as many as 10,000 cases are reported there annually. At the present time Japanese encephalitis appears to be subsiding in China as well as in Japan and Korea, but it is increasing and spreading across parts of Bangladesh, Burma, India, Nepal, Thailand, and Vietnam [14]. Rice field–breeding mosquitoes, particularly *Culex tritaeniorhynchus,* are the major vectors. The natural cycle involves water birds, including herons and egrets (Fig. 74-3). The *Culex* mosquitoes feed at dusk, and among mammals they prefer water buffalos and pigs, biting human beings only as an alternative. Young pigs develop prolonged viremias and function as important amplifying hosts. The same is probably true during the first year of the life of water buffalos, but buffalos are kept for many years, and the immune mature buffalos serve as blocking hosts.

In southern China and southeast Asia, which are free of frost, mosquitoes and low levels of infection are present year-round. During the rainy season, however, mosquito density and numbers of viremic amplifying hosts increase, and epi-

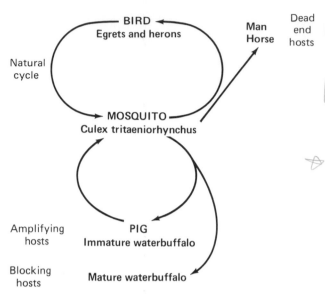

Figure 74-3. Schematic diagram of the enzootic, epizootic, and epidemic cycles of Japanese encephalitis virus.

demics occur regularly between mid-June and mid-August. In Thailand the virus is transmitted throughout the country, but cases of human encephalitis are concentrated in northern provinces. Disease is seen primarily in children, because antibody is virtually universal among adults, but adults moving from the mountains into the agricultural valleys or tourists venturing in the countryside are fully susceptible. By some estimates naive adults may be even more susceptible to encephalitis than children.

North American arboviral encephalitides

The arboviruses of North America have been studied extensively and exemplify the diversity of ecological cycles [15]. St. Louis encephalitis virus is closely related to Japanese encephalitis virus, and the western rural cycles of St. Louis and western encephalitis virus also have features in common with Japanese encephalitis virus. Both are found in small wild birds and are transmitted by culicine mosquitoes, primarily *Culex tarsalis,* a mosquito that breeds in fresh water, particularly in irrigated areas. On the other hand, the ecological cycle of St. Louis encephalitis virus in the eastern part of the United States is very different. In urban areas, virus cycles between the small birds and species of ''dirty breeding'' mosquitoes, such as *Culex pipiens,* that prefer water with high organic content, particularly inadequately drained sewage. Thus, paradoxically, in the west, St. Louis encephalitis epidemics occur in rural areas during years of high rainfall, while in the eastern United States, epidemics occur in urban areas during years of drought and poor drainage; such an epidemic occurred in over 30 states in 1975, involving over 2000 patients, with 171 deaths.

Eastern encephalitis is fortunately rare, since it is the most neuroinvasive and lethal encephalitis caused by any arbovirus. Small outbreaks occur at irregular intervals. This does not reflect an absence of the virus during intervening years, but the fact that the natural enzootic cycle is between marshland birds and *Culiseta melanura,* a mosquito that rarely bites human beings. When swamp water levels are high and bird populations and mosquito density increase, a spillover of virus can infect *Aëdes* mosquitoes, which serve as a vector to humans and other susceptible animals. Horse and pheasant deaths often precede human cases and serve as sentinels.

California encephalitis viruses differ from any other North American arboviruses in that birds are not involved in the natural cycle; indeed birds cannot be infected even experimentally with the California serogroup viruses. Although the prototype California virus has been associated with mild encephalitis, the majority of the cases of ''California encephalitis'' occur in the midwest caused by the related La Crosse virus, which appeared in the mid-1960s without historical or serological evidence of existence in prior years. The vertebrate hosts of La Crosse are small forest-dwelling animals including chipmunks and squirrels, and the vector mosquito is *Aëdes triseriatis,* which breeds in the tree holes of hardwood trees. In the California serogroup, transovarian transmission appears to be very important, and amplification occurs in nature by venereal transmission that occurs between transovarianly infected males and uninfected females. *A. triseriatis* has a short flight pattern, and, thus, La Crosse encephalitis usually occurs in children who venture into the woods or whose families keep old automobile tires in backyards, since tires provide a preferred alternative breeding site [16].

All North American mosquito-borne infections are strictly seasonal because of winter frost, which kills mosquitoes. Arboviral encephalitis occurs between June and October or as late as December in Florida. How viruses overwinter in temperate climates remains a mystery [15].

Venezuelan equine encephalitis

Venezuelan equine encephalitis is an interesting example of a virus in which different virus strains have very different epidemiological patterns and degrees of neurovirulence and in which different genera of mosquitoes may be involved. The endemic form is recognized in South America and Florida, where the enzootic cycle involves swamp mosquitoes and small rodents; human beings can occasionally be infected, but encephalitis is a rare occurrence. Epizootic and epidemic disease of horses and human beings was first recognized in western South America. This spread northward, and in 1971 the epidemic in Mexico caused many horse and 42 human deaths; it crossed the Rio Grande, causing over 100 horse deaths and over 100 nonfatal human illnesses in Texas with two cases of encephalitis [17].

Tickborne encephalitis

These viruses are spread by *Ixodes* ticks over a wide area of the northern temperate zone. In woodland areas across Siberia through Europe, hedgehogs, shrews, and small rodents are the natural hosts and the main reservoirs of the virus. Strains of the virus appear to be more virulent in the Far East and decrease in virulence across Russia and Europe; in Scotland and northern England, the looping ill virus very rarely causes human disease. The strains across the northern United States and Canada occasionally cause human encephalitis. Human infection occurs after exposure to ticks in rural wooded areas; disease is most frequent in May to June and September to October, when tick activity is greatest. An unusual mode of transmission has been described in Europe where goats are infected by the ticks; raw goat milk has apparently transmitted the virus to humans [*18*].

In 1957 monkey deaths suddenly occurred in the Kyasanur Forest of Mysore state of India. Initially there was fear that yellow fever had invaded the subcontinent, but the virus proved to be related to Far Eastern tickborne encephalitis virus. The vector was shown to be a tick, and it was postulated that the ticks had been carried on birds across the Himalayas into the Indian subcontinent. This virus usually causes a flulike illness with fever, headache, malaise, and hemorrhagic complications. Encephalitis is a rare late complication.

Murray Valley encephalitis

Another intriguing appearance and disappearance of virus occurs with Murray Valley encephalitis, previously called Australian X disease. Epidemics of encephalitis occurred in New South Wales in 1917 and 1918, only to disappear and reappear in 1922 and 1925 and again in 1957 and 1974. These irregular intervals have been explained by natural cycles of virus in the tropical sparsely inhabited areas of northern Australia. Birds migrating across the continent may sustain a viremia to transport the virus, or in the rare years when the dry riverbeds of the Australian outback contain fresh water, mosquitoes may breed and allow virus to cycle while they are en route to the heavily populated southeastern area of the continent. Overwintering of Murray Valley encephalitis virus in south Australia has been proposed, but no infections have been found there since 1974 [*15*].

VACCINES

Because of its public health importance Japanese encephalitis has been the major target of vaccine development. Two inactivated vaccines are used to protect against Japanese encephalitis; one is produced with virus grown in mouse brain, and the other with virus grown in primary baby hamster kidney cells. The mouse brain vaccine is highly purified, well-defined, and has been established to be effective and safe in a recent controlled clinical trial in Thailand [*19*]. Live vaccines have recently been tested in China using an attenuated strain of virus in primary baby hamster kidney cells. This strain has undergone field trials in children [*14*]. Unfortunately, neither type of vaccine is readily available in the United States. Adults or children from nonepidemic areas who will be spending time in rural areas of Asia, particularly during the rainy season, should be vaccinated.

Vaccines for tickborne encephalitis consisting of inactivated tissue-culture-grown virus are available in eastern Europe. Vaccines for eastern, western, and Venezuelan equine encephalitis are available for horses or for investigators working with these agents in the laboratory.

CONTROL

Vector control can be carried out in different ways. Control of the vectors of Japanese encephalitis and rural St. Louis encephalitis have been difficult because of the interference with the local agriculture. One cannot drain the rice fields of Asia or the vegetable fields of the San Joaquin Valley. Some control over irrigation, however, has been used. In contrast, for the eastern urban cycles of St. Louis encephalitis, urban spraying or better drainage for stagnant water can be effective. Some control of California encephalitis virus has involved the plugging of tree holes near inhabited areas, as well as the elimination of discarded tires and stagnant waters in the backyards of homes [*16*].

Amplifying hosts can potentially be blocked. To control Japanese encephalitis a live attenuated virus has been used to immunize young pigs to prevent viremia. Alternatively, pig breeding might be timed so that piglets are born with maternal antibodies during the buildup of mosquito populations. Although Japanese virus causes no disease in postnatal pigs, it causes abortion in pregnant sows, and farmers learned long ago to breed and deliver piglets in seasons of low virus dissemination. In turn, slaughter of young pigs for market removes immune, potentially blocking hosts and ensures a new amplifying population for the next epidemic. Immunization of horses may impede the cycle of epidemic Venezuelan equine encephalitis, but this strategy is ineffective in controlling eastern and western "equine" encephalitis viruses, in which the horse is not important in the amplification cycle.

Screening houses, placing netting over beds, covering the skin with clothing, and using repellents are additional protective measures. For example, education programs to net the bassinets of susceptible babies on summer evenings in California were introduced to decrease the risk of western encephalitis.

Control of arboviruses can thus employ a variety of strategies, including elimination of the arthropod, elimination or immunization of the natural amplifying host, and protection of human beings by immunization, netting, or repellents. Different strategies are needed with different enzootic and epizootic cycles, and any mode of effective control is dependent on the full knowledge of the natural ecology of the virus and its arthropod and vertebrate hosts.

REFERENCES

1 Schlesinger S, Schlesinger MJ (eds): *The Togaviridae and Flaviviridae.* New York, Plenum, 1986

2 Johnson RT: *Viral Infections of the Nervous System.* New York, Raven, 1982

3 Monath TP, Cropp CP, Harrison AK: Mode of entry of a neurotropic arbovirus into the central nervous system: Reinvestigation of an old controversy. Lab Invest 48:399–410, 1983

4 Moench TR, Griffin DE: Immunocytochemical identification and quantitation of the mononuclear cells in the cerebrospinal fluid, meninges, and brain during acute viral meningoencephalitis. J Exp Med 159:77–88, 1984

5 Grimstad PR: Mosquitoes and the incidence of encephalitis. Adv Virus Res 28:157–433, 1983

6 Leake CJ, Johnson RT: The pathogenesis of Japanese encephalitis virus in *Culex tritaeniorhynchus* mosquitoes. Trans R Soc Trop Med Hyg 81:681–685, 1987

7 Burke DS, Nisalak A, Ussery MA, et al: Kinetics of IgM and IgG responses to Japanese encephalitis virus in human serum and cerebrospinal fluid. J Infect Dis 151:1093–1099, 1985

8 Johnson RT, Burke DS, Elwell M, et al: Japanese encephalitis: Immunocytochemical studies of viral antigen and inflammatory cells in fatal cases. Ann Neurol 18:567–573, 1985

9 Miyake M: The pathology of Japanese encephalitis. Bull WHO 30:153–160, 1964

10 Monath TP (ed): *St. Louis Encephalitis.* Washington DC, American Public Health Association, 1980

11 Brody JA, Hadlow WJ, Hotchin J, et al: Soviet search for viruses that cause chronic neurologic disease in the USSR. Science 147:1114–1116, 1965

12 Asher DM: Persistent tick-borne encephalitis infection in man and monkeys. Relation to chronic neurologic disease, in Kurstak E (ed): *Arctic and Tropical Arboviruses.* New York, Academic, 1979, pp 179–195

13 Burke DS, Losomrudee W, Leake CJ, et al: Fatal outcome in Japanese encephalitis. Am J Trop Med Hyg 34:1203–1210, 1985

14 Umenai T, Krzysko R, Bektimirov TA, et al: Japanese encephalitis: Current worldwide status. Bull WHO 63:625–631, 1985

15 The epidemiology of Mosquito-Borne Virus Encephalitides in the United States, 1943–1987. Am J Trop Med Hyg 37(suppl):1–100 1987

16 Calisher CH, Thompson WH (eds): *California Serogroup Viruses.* New York, Alan R Liss, 1983

17 Ehrenkranz NJ, Ventura AK: Venezuelan equine encephalitis virus infection in man. Ann Rev Med 25:9–14, 1974

18 Gresikova M, Beran GW: Tick-borne encephalitis, in Geran GW (ed): *CRC Handbook Series in Zoonoses,* section B, *Viral Zoonoses,* vol 1. Boca Raton, CRC Press, 1981, pp 201–208

19 Hoke CH, Nisalak A, Sangawhipa N, et al: Protection against Japanese encephalitis by inactivated vaccines. N Engl J Med 319:608–614, 1988

CHAPTER
75

Viral Hemorrhagic Fevers

· Joseph B. McCormick · Susan Fisher-Hoch

Hemorrhagic fevers caused by viruses occur on every continent except Australia and North America. Responsible are membrane-bound RNA viruses that belong to four distinct families. Each is a zoonosis with distinct ecological and epidemiological features, including rodentborne, tickborne, and mosquitoborne transmission. Several also are transmissible from person to person, especially in hospitals, and many have a high case fatality. Their zoonotic character makes them primarily rural diseases, especially in Africa, and thus they tend to occur in areas with limited facilities for medical care, where they are often largely unrecognized. Each disease occurs as a result of a complex interaction of humans with their environment or with each other. Some of the more important variables associated with these interactions are found in Table 75-1. (For

other hemorrhagic fevers see Chap. 71 on yellow fever and Chap. 72 on dengue.)

ARENAVIRUSES

There are 13 recognized arenaviruses, 4 of which are known human pathogens [1]. These agents are principally parasites of wild rodents and are found in both the new and the old world [2]. Only the three major disease-producing members, Lassa, Junin, and Machupo will be treated in detail, although reference will be made in certain sections to lymphocytic choriomeningitis (LCM) virus because it is the most extensively studied virus in this family. The clinical diseases caused by these

Table 75-1. Viral hemorrhagic fevers: Epidemiologic features

Disease	Geography	Reservoir	Vector	Transmission	CF ratio	Comment
Argentine hemorrhagic fever	Moist, humid pampas	*Calomys, Mus, Akodon*	None	Rodent-human via urine	10–20% (1% if treated ≤ day 8)	Disease in harvesters
Bolivian hemorrhagic fever	Plains of Bolivia	*Calomys callosus*	None	Rodent-human via urine	10%	Associated with domestic rodent invasion
Lassa fever	Secondary forest and savannah of west Africa	*Mastomys natalensis*	None	1. Rodent-human via urine 2. Human-human via infected secretions	1–3% 20% in hospital patients (<5% if treated by day 7)	Focal distribution, most transmission in houses
Ebola, Marburg	Forest and savannah areas of east, central, and southern Africa	Unknown	Unknown if any	? to human, human-human	30–90%	Mortality varies with virus biotypes
HFRS-NE	Forest, grasslands of Asia and Europe; cities of Asia	Field mice, voles, rats	None	1. Rodent-human via urine 2. Also airborne	HFRS 3–5% NE <1%	Varies in pathogenicity and in rodent host by geographical area
CCHF	Africa, Asia, eastern Europe	Many mammals	>27 sp. Ixodid, Argasid ticks (vertical transmission)	1. Tick-human 2. Human-human via blood	15% in hospital 40% not in hospital	Higher rate in those working with domestic animals
RVF	Africa	Wild and domestic animals	Mosquito (*culex* sp.)	Mosquito-human; or animal-human, animal-animal, via blood	5–10% in hospital patients	Widely endemic & sporadically epidemic
KFD	Forest of Mysore, India	*Presbytis entollus, Macaca radiata*	*Hemophysalis* ticks, *Ixodes* sp.	Tick-human		
OHF	Steppe of western Siberia and southwest U.S.S.R.	Domestic animals, frogs, and (?) other reptiles	Ixodid ticks	Tick-human		

three arenaviruses are Lassa fever, Argentine hemorrhagic fever (AHF), and Bolivian hemorrhagic fever (BHF), respectively.

GENERAL ECOLOGY

A hallmark of the arenaviruses is their intimate biological relationship with rodents resulting in lifetime infection and chronic virus excretion. The encounter between humans and infected rodent is the critical factor resulting in human infection [2]. For many of the arenaviruses, contact between mouse and human rarely occurs (Tacaribe, Pichinde, Tamiami), or does not result in human infection (Latino), whereas for Lassa, Machupo, and Junin, the result may be a serious, even fatal, illness.

Many of the arenaviruses have more than one rodent host, although usually a single species will dominate as the reservoir in nature. The hosts of LCM have been many, including *Mus* sp., hamsters, and guinea pigs. The host of Machupo virus,

Calomys callosus (Fig. 75-1), is found in the plains of eastern Bolivia, northern Paraguay, and the western part of Mato Grosso, Brazil. Normally, the rodent is found in the grasslands and forest edges. In 1962 to 1964, the rodent population had markedly increased and had moved into the village houses of San Joaquin, Bolivia, and adapted to human habitations [3,4], creating a major epidemic. Latino virus, an arenavirus which has not been implicated in human infections, also has *C. callosus* as its host.

Junin virus has been isolated from cricetine rodents (*Calomys, Mus,* and *Akodon*) in Buenos Aires and Córdoba provinces of Argentina, where they are associated with grasslands and farming [5,6]. Although *Calomys* rodents rarely invade dwellings in this region, they achieve high population density in maize fields with the result that virus transmission occurs from March to June during the harvest of this important crop.

With the exception of Tacaribe virus, which was isolated from bats in Trinidad, all of the new world arenaviruses have cricetine rodent hosts.

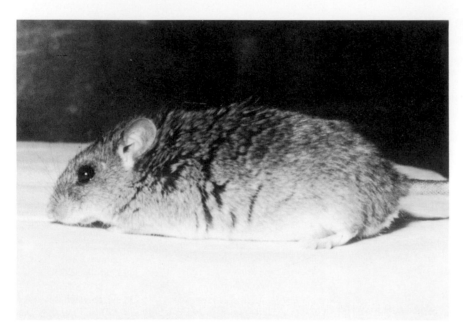

Figure 75-1. *Calomys callosus*, reservoir vector of Machupo virus.

Mastomys natalensis (Fig. 75-2), was identified in Sierra Leone in 1972 as a rodent reservoir of Lassa virus [7]. Since that time, three other related arenaviruses have been isolated from other parts of Africa including Mozambique, Zimbabwe, and Central African Republic.

In the highly endemic eastern region of Sierra Leone, the predominant *Mastomys* is a 32-chromosome rodent found al-most exclusively in association with human habitation. This area is secondary rain forest with 8 to 9 months of rainfall. In the drier savannah areas one finds 32- and 38-chromosome varieties of *Mastomys,* both of which carry Lassa virus. The 2N = 32 rodents tend to be found in houses, whereas the 2N = 38 is dominant in the surrounding bush areas [8].

The arenaviruses from Mozambique and Zimbabwe were isolated from wild *Mastomys* 2N = 36 rodents. This highly adaptable rodent is commonly found in savannah and agricul-tural areas throughout southern Africa. Its range includes areas with a substantial number of frost days and little rainfall as well as areas of mean temperature over 21°C and 400 cm of rainfall.

An arenavirus has also been isolated from *Paromys* sp. in the Central African Republic. None has been isolated from *Mastomys* of this area. The *Paromys* are found in gallery for-ests. The implications of these viruses for human disease are unknown.

MORPHOLOGY AND ULTRASTRUCTURE

Arenaviridae are morphologically indistinguishable viruses which appear as round, oval, or pleomorphic particles ranging from 50 to 300 nm with a mean of 100 to 130 nm [1]. There is a bilayer membrane with 10-nm regular surface projections. An internal nucleocapsid structure has not been identified but the particles contain variable numbers of electron-dense gran-ules about 20 nm in diameter which are host-cell ribosomes. These ribosomes somewhat resemble sand granules, providing the taxonomic designation (from the Latin *arena*, ''sand''). No function has yet been described for these ribosomes.

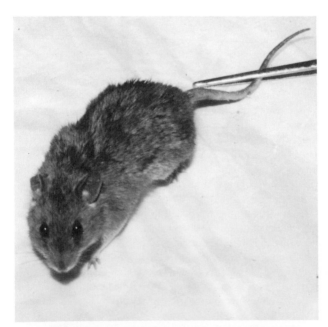

Figure 75-2. *Mastomys natalensis,* reservoir vector of Lassa virus.

BIOCHEMISTRY AND PROPAGATION

The arenaviruses possess two single strands of RNA [2]. The large (L) RNA ranges from 31 S to 37 S in size and encodes the viral RNA polymerase while the smaller (S) RNA ranges from 22 S to 25 S and encodes the nucleoprotein (N) corresponding to the 3' end of the viral RNA. The 5' half of the viral RNA encodes the glycoprotein gene. The glycoprotein is translated as a precursor and then cleaved into G1 and G2, both of which make up the virion surface [9,10]. The ambisense arrangement is thought to be associated with persistence of infection by allowing independent expression of N and GPC which may be important in viral regulation of the host's immune response. How this may occur is not understood.

Structural proteins of at least eight of the arenaviruses have been examined. Six of the viruses, including the human pathogens Lassa and Junin viruses, have three structural proteins. The largest ranges from 63,000 to 72,000 daltons for different viruses and is associated with the viral membrane as glycosylated protein. Except for Tacaribe and Tamiami which have only one, arenaviruses have a second glycosylated protein of 34,000 to 38,000 daltons.

Although the nucleoprotein is responsible for much of the immunological cross-reaction between arenaviruses from a given geographical area (e.g., South America), the most-conserved epitope of arenaviruses in South America and Africa resides on the G2.

Arenaviruses replicate in a rather broad variety of mammalian cells. Much of the detailed information is based on studies of LCM and Pichinde viruses and can presumably be generalized to other arenaviruses. Cellular penetration of LCM takes about 45 min following adsorption, which is maximized after 1.5 to 2 h. The genome is uncoated after 2 h and newly formed virus may be found after 7 to 8 h from infection. Unlike many other viruses, host-cell protein and RNA synthesis are not usually altered by arenavirus infection. The arenaviruses are not always lethal to host cells and chronically infected cell cultures can be produced [1,2].

ANIMAL MODELS

One of the first model animal systems to be studied was LCM infection in the mouse [2]. These studies led to the first observation of chronic viral infection and to the formulation of the concept of immune tolerance in immunology. Three basic responses have been observed in LCM-infected mice [2]. The first is the classical acute LCM resulting in the death of the adult mouse following intracerebral inoculation of a neurotropic virus strain. This response is mediated by a vigorous cytotoxic T-cell (CTL) response with infiltration and destruction of infected central nervous system cells [1,2]. Ablation of the T-cell response (by cyclophosphamide or anti-Thy1 serum) will result in persistent infection without disease. Similarly infection of mice in utero or within 5 to 7 days after birth will also result in persistent infection with a normal B-cell response and anti-LCM antibody but no T-cell response. Adoptive transfer of cytotoxic T cells from immune mice clears virus from these persistently infected animals, and produces lymphocytic choriomeningitis in animals with CNS infections. Thus, pathology is produced by the CTL response rather than by infection. The ability of the virus to establish persistent infection is common to all arenaviruses, but the effect on the rodent host varies with different arenaviruses. At least three of the viruses (LCM, Lassa, and Machupo) are transmitted in utero and thus establish immune tolerance and persistent infection even before birth.

Rhesus and cynomolgous monkeys are very susceptible to Machupo and Lassa viruses and develop illness similar to that observed in humans [2,11,12]. As in rodents, the viruses are highly lymphotropic; initial multiplication takes place in lymphoblasts, tissue macrophages, histiocytes, and perhaps megakaryocytes.

Monkeys become clinically ill by day 6 to 7 after subcutaneous inoculation with Machupo. The animals become anorexic by day 14 and 80 percent die by day 18 or 19 after inoculation. Diarrhea, an erythematous facial rash, and hemorrhagic nasal discharge are important signs. Most of the survivors develop CNS symptoms on days 26 to 40 after inoculation with severe tremors, nystagmus, incoordination, paresis, and coma leading to death. This late CNS syndrome, which occurs infrequently in humans, is marked by severe histological vasculitis and encephalitis.

Animals administered specific neutralizing antibodies as late as 7 days after Machupo virus infection survived acute infection although some animals subsequently developed the late neurological syndrome. Ribavirin at a dose of 5 mg/kg every 8 h for 10 days also prevented death of monkeys under identical conditions.

Most Lassa-infected rhesus or cynomolgous monkeys die 10 to 14 days following infection. There are two distinctive patterns of viremia highly correlated with outcome. In monkeys which die, the viremia rises 3 to 5 days after infection to levels of 10^4 to 10^5 TCID$_{50}$/mL[1] and is sustained until the monkeys die. Surviving monkeys achieve early viremia peaks of only 10^2 to 10^3 TCID$_{50}$/mL, which then decline. Anti-Lassa antibodies are produced nearly equally in all animals, beginning about 10 days after infection. Fatally infected monkeys also exhibit higher serum concentrations of serum glutamic-oxalacetic transaminases (SGOT) than survivors. The correlation between survival and dose of Lassa virus is not known.

Monkeys infected with Lassa virus survive if given ribavirin and/or plasma within 4 days after virus inoculation. The viremia pattern of treated monkeys was similar to that of untreated survivors. Cynomolgous monkeys treated with ribavirin or immune plasma on day 7 following infection were not pro-

---

[1]TCID$_{50}$ = tissue culture infectious dose$_{50}$.

tected from death whereas those treated by both regimens survived.

PATIENT

Infection and host response

Most human arenavirus infections probably occur as a result of viral contact with exposed membranes or skin abrasions. It is likely that the infectious dose is low, perhaps on the order of 10 to 100 infectious particles. The incubation periods range from 7 to as long as 20 days [6,8,17]. Patients with Lassa fever enter hospital 2 to 14 days after onset of symptoms. At this time viremia may be absent or present in widely different concentrations. Persistent high viremia is a significant predictor of outcome of illness (see "Clinical Description"). It is not unusual to encounter patients with viremia on admission to hospital who also have high levels of both IgM and IgG immunofluorescent antibody (IFA). In fact, there is no correlation between the viremia level and that of the IFA for Lassa fever [14]. Neutralizing antibodies to Lassa virus are almost never detectable in the serum of patients at the beginning of convalescence, and in most people they are never detectable. In a minority of patients some low-titer serum neutralizing activity may be observed but only several months after resolution of the disease and clearance of the virus [14].

Human response to Junin virus is quite different. The viremia, although detectable, appears to be lower. Antibody, especially neutralizing antibody, is detectable at the time the patient begins to recover from the acute illness. Indeed it has now been shown that the positive effect of immune plasma in patients with Junin infection is directly associated with the titer of neutralizing antibody, and that immediate reduction of viremia is associated with recovery from disease [15,16].

In some Lassa fever patients, small amounts of virus may be shed in urine for several weeks. No studies of tissue have been performed on humans after acute illness to evaluate persistence of virus in other organ systems. No such viral persistence occurs with the South American hemorrhagic fevers.

The role of antibody in Junin and Lassa viruses appears to be different. The antibody response to Junin virus may be sufficient, is probably necessary to clear virus during acute infection, and may also be sufficient to protect against future infections [15]. Although elements of a cell-mediated immune response to Junin virus have been shown, the importance of this response to virus clearance and subsequent protection are not known. The clearance of Lassa virus appears, on the other hand, to be independent of antibody formation, and thus to depend on a cell-mediated immune response. Although passive protection with antibody to Lassa virus has been demonstrated in animals, protection of humans has not. Thus the major immune response in human Lassa virus infection appears to be dependent on cell-mediated immune mechanisms, an observation supported by recent experience with Lassa vaccines.

Clinical description

Although there are some similarities in the clinical manifestations of AHF, BHF, and Lassa fever, there are enough differences to warrant separate descriptions (Table 75-2).

Lassa fever begins 7 to 18 days after the primary infection with subtle onset of fever, headache, and malaise [17]. Fever is sustained with peaks of 39 to 41°C, usually in early morning

Table 75-2. Viral hemorrhagic fevers: Significant clinical features

Feature	Lassa	Junin, Machupo	HFRS	Dengue	Marburg, Ebola	CCHF	YF
Case fatality, %	16	16	1–5	1–5	6–50	55–88	20–50
Hematological:							
Thrombocytopenia		+	+	+	+	+	+
Oozing	+	+	+	+	+	+	+
Petechiae			+	+			
Ecchymoses						+	
Circulatory:							
Shock	+	+	+	+	+	+	+
Edema	+		+	+	+		
ARDS	+		+		+		
Neurological:							
Encephalopathy	+	+					
Ataxia	+	+	+				
Deafness	+						
I/C Bleeding			+	+/−			
Organ failure:							
Renal			+				
Hepatic					+	+	+
Immune complex			+	+			

and early evening. Aching in the large joints and lower back pain develop in more than half of hospitalized patients by the third or fourth day of illness.

The physical examination shows these patients to be toxic and anxious. Unless the patient is in shock, the skin is usually moist from diaphoresis. There is an elevated respiratory rate, and the pulse is usually commensurate with the elevated body temperature. The systolic blood pressure ranges from >100 to >110 with a mean of 103. There is no characteristic skin rash. Petechiae and ecchymoses are not seen, nor is jaundice a feature of Lassa fever. Conjunctivitis occurs in about one-third of patients; conjunctival hemorrhages are occasionally seen and portend a poor prognosis. Seventy percent of patients have pharyngitis with diffusely inflamed and swollen posterior pharynx and tonsils, but few if any petechiae. In over half of the patients the pharyngitis is exudative, with yellow patches, primarily on the tonsils, and rarely with distinct ulcers. The pharyngeal pain associated with Lassa fever is extraordinarily severe, and it is common to see patients expectorate saliva in a cup because swallowing is so painful. Bleeding occurs in only 15 to 20 percent of all patients. It occurs most often in the gums and nose, but also occurs as GI or vaginal bleeding, and it is of course associated with severe disease. Edema of the face and neck are commonly seen also in severe disease, without peripheral edema—suggesting capillary leakage, rather than cardiac dysfunction and impaired venous return (Fig. 75-3A). Edema and bleeding may occur together or independently. About 20 percent of patients have pericardial or pleural rubs, presumably associated with effusions, which though rarely present on admission, develop in early convalescence occasionally in association with congestive cardiac failure. The ECG may be abnormal, primarily with elevated T waves, and evidence of pericarditis and myocarditis, but there does not appear to be any correlation between these T-wave abnormalities and the presence of a pericardial rub or other evidence of pericarditis. The abdomen is diffusely tender in just under half of the patients but there are no localizing signs and bowel signs are usually active.

Neurological manifestations may be absent in acute Lassa fever, or there may be a range of abnormalities from unilateral or bilateral deafness, with or without tinnitus, to moderate or severe diffuse encephalopathy with or without general seizures. The encephalopathic complications generally carry a poor prognosis, while the deafness usually occurs just as recovery is underway. Manifestations during the acute phase range from mild confusion and tremors to grand mal seizures and decerebrate coma. Focal fits are not seen. Cerebrospinal fluid specimens usually show a few lymphocytes but are otherwise normal, and virus titers are low. It is not clear whether cerebral infections or any other encephalopathy occurs without direct viral invasion.

Tremors are often seen in the hours just prior to death. Other than deafness, focal neurological signs rarely occur. Nerve

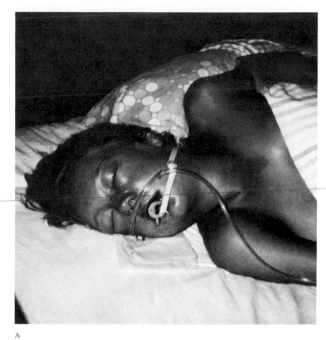

A

Figure 75-3. *A.* Patient with severe Lassa fever. Note edema of face and neck and decerebrate posture.

deafness, sometimes permanent, occurs in 25 percent of all Lassa infections.

The mean white blood cell count on admission is 6×10^9/L with early lymphopenia, relative thrombocytopenia, and in a few severe cases late neutrophilia [18]. A circulating inhibitor of platelet function has been detected in the plasma of severe cases both in humans and primates [19]. The hematocrit in Lassa fever patients is often elevated (mean 50.1) due to dehydration. Proteinuria is common, occurring in two-thirds of patients. The blood urea nitrogen may be moderately elevated probably due to dehydration.

Lassa fever is also a pediatric disease affecting children of all ages [8]. The disease appears to be difficult to diagnose in children because its manifestations are so general. In very young babies marked edema may be seen, associated with very severe disease. In older children the disease may manifest as diarrhea, as pneumonia, or simply as an unexplained prolonged fever. The case fatality rate in children is 12 to 14 percent. The clinical course of Lassa fever in children is as diverse as it is in adults, ranging from mild febrile illness to severe fulminating disease.

Lassa fever is a highly variable disease with a broad range of manifestations and many degrees of severity. This makes it difficult to distinguish clinically, especially in the early stages, from influenza or other upper or lower respiratory viral infections, as well as from other causes of general febrile illness or

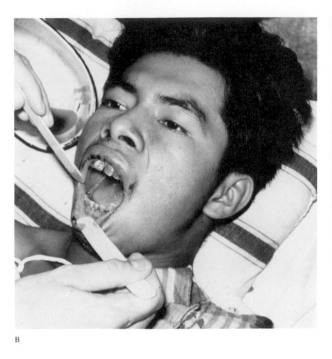

B

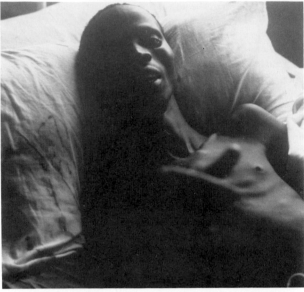

C

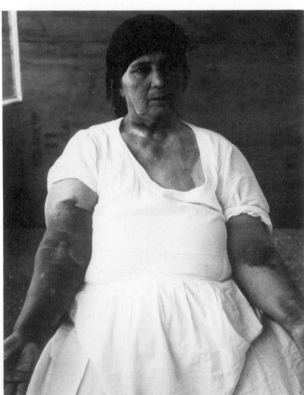

D

E

Figure 75-3 (Continued). *B.* Gingival hemorrhage in a patient with Bolivian hemorrhagic fever. *C.* Patient with Marburg virus infection. Note severe wasting of this previously robust 28-year-old man. *D.* Patient with hemorrhagic fever with renal syndrome. Note conjunctival hemorrhage, bleeding in nose, and petechiae. *E.* Patient with severe Crimean-Congo hemorrhagic fever. Note extensive ecchymoses.

from febrile gastroenteritis. Typhoid fever is a common misdiagnosis. There are no firm clinical predictors or pathognomonic signs of Lassa fever. Although it is classed as a hemorrhagic fever, it is not frequently a cause of overt bleeding.

A case-control study of the clinical manifestations of Lassa fever demonstrated the difficulty in making a firm clinical diagnosis or prognosis of the disease [17]. In this study fever with pharyngitis, proteinuria and retrosternal chest pain had a predictive value for Lassa fever of 81 percent and a specificity of 89 percent. Likewise a triad of pharyngitis, retrosternal chest pain, and proteinuria (in a febrile patient) correctly predicted Lassa fever 80 percent of the time (in an endemic area). However these triads had sensitivities of only 50 percent, illustrating the extreme difficulty of clinical diagnosis in Lassa fever. Bleeding and sore throat have a specificity for fatal outcome of 90 percent; however, these two criteria have a sensitivity of only 36 percent, so that the prognosis of many fatal patients would be misclassified (Table 75-3). There are two laboratory measures which are also associated with clinical outcome of acute Lassa fever. A serum aspartate transaminase (AST) level of >150 IU/L is associated with a case fatality of 50 percent, and there is a correlation between an ever increasing level and an increased risk of death. A second variable associated with outcome is the level of viremia; a viremia of $>1 \times 10^{3.0}$ TCID$_{50}$/mL is associated with an increasing case fatality (Fig. 75-4). Both factors together carry a risk of death of 80 percent.

There are several significant complications of Lassa fever which add to the overall burden of this disease in the poor rural populations of many west African countries. One of these is the adverse effect of Lassa fever during pregnancy [20].

Table 75-3. Predictive clinical variables for diagnosis and prognosis of Lassa fever

	Diagnosis		
Variable	**Predictive value**	**Sensitivity**	**Specificity**
Pharyngitis, retrosternal pain, proteinuria	.81	.46	.89
Pharyngitis, retrosternal pain, vomiting	.79	.51	.86
Sys. BP < 105 mmHg, hemoglobin <12 mg%	.72	.22	.91
Bleeding	.74	.17	.94
Exudative pharyngitis	.69	.43	.83
Conjunctivitis	.69	.39	.84
Pharyngitis, bleeding	.61	.70	.60

	Prognosis		
Variable	**Relative risk of death**	**Sensitivity**	**Specificity**
Sore throat and vomiting	5.5	.89	.47
Vomiting	4.6	.93	.30
Bleeding and sore throat	3.3	.36	.90
Fever > 39°C and vomiting	3.1	.51	.79

Limited data suggest that Lassa fever may be a common cause of maternal mortality in many areas of west Africa. Two studies have shown that the case fatality in pregnant women infected by Lassa virus is about 20 percent. However there is a nearly twofold increase in the number of third-trimester Lassa

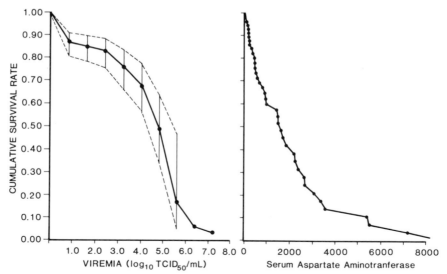

Figure 75-4. Survival rate of hospitalized patients with Lassa fever as a function of viremia levels and serum aspartate aminotransferase levels.

virus infections requiring hospitalization, compared to the first two trimesters, and a corresponding two- to threefold risk of maternal death from infection in the third trimester (30 percent). Very high levels of virus replication have been found in placental tissue in third-trimester patients. Drug therapy of these patients is currently under study but no data are yet available. An important observation is effect of evacuation of the uterus in the pregnant women [20]. A fourfold reduction was noted in case fatality among women who spontaneously or were therapeutically aborted compared to those who were not (odds ratio for fatality with pregnancy intact is 5.47 compared to those with uterine evacuation). Fetal loss is 87 percent, and does not seem to vary by trimester. Surviving children have not been studied for residual problems associated with their Lassa virus infection.

Another significant complication of Lassa fever is that of acute VIIIth nerve deafness [21]. Nearly 30 percent of patients with Lassa fever infection suffer an acute loss of hearing in one or both ears. The mean auditory threshold of these patients is 55 dB, and the mean disability is over 20 percent (Fig. 75-5).

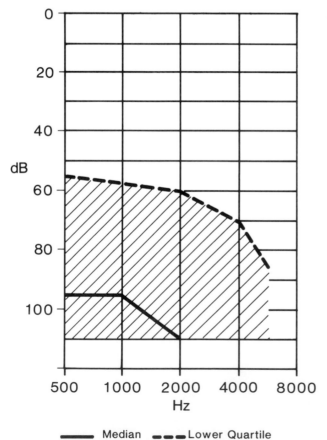

Figure 75-5. Audiogram depicting median hearing thresholds for a range of frequencies in a group of patients with deafness following Lassa virus infection. Normal threshold is < 25 dB.

About half of the patients show a near or complete recovery over the 3 to 4 months after onset, but the other half continue with significant sensorineural deafness. This degree of sensorineural deafness exceeds any previous report of deafness associated with any other postnatal infection, and appears to be larger than that reported from any other part of the world.

Other complications which appear to occur much less frequently are uveitis, pericarditis, orchitis, pleural effusion, and ascites [17]. Renal and hepatic failure are not seen.

Like that of Lassa fever, the onset of AHF or BHF is insidious, beginning with general malaise and fever for a 2- to 4-day period [2]. Also, as with Lassa, conjunctivitis is an important and frequent sign. Erythema of the face, neck, and upper thorax is often described and there is a relative bradycardia. Gastrointestinal symptoms are seen in less than half of the cases and respiratory symptoms are rare. Fever ranges from 38 to 40°C and is typically without much daily variation.

Unlike Lassa fever, hemorrhage is a frequent sign in AHF and BHF (30 percent with BHF), occurring between the fourth and sixth day of illness. This may be at many sites including skin of the upper trunk, oral mucous membrane (Fig. 75-3B), nose, bowel, and uterus. Hyperemia of the face and trunk, petechiae, and a macular enanthem are early signs which often herald clinical hemorrhage. Rarely is the loss of blood life-threatening. One-half (BHF) to two-thirds (AHF) of patients develop hypotension between 6 and 10 days of onset. In some patients, the hypotension is irreversible and results in death. Neurological symptoms such as intention tremors of the tongue and hands occur during the acute phase of illness in as many as 50 percent of cases. In many of these patients, the neurological symptoms progress to coarse tremors of the tongue and upper and lower extremities, delirium, facial grimacing, oculogyrus, and strabismus. These crises last only 2 to 4 days without sequelae. Convalescence may last several weeks with weakness, autonomic dysfunction, weight loss, and transient loss of scalp hair [2].

Leukopenia and thrombocytopenia occur more regularly with AHF and BHF than Lassa fever.

Two findings appear helpful in prognosis of AHF and BHF: increased hemoconcentration and increased urinary protein. Both are associated with a high risk of death for AHF and BHF and precede the onset of neurological symptoms or hypotension.

Pathophysiology and pathology

It seems likely that severe Lassa fever results from physiological dysfunction subsequent to infection of critical host-cell systems or the host response to infection rather than direct viral destruction of a particular organ system [11,22]. The clinical events associated with fatal disease appear to be intractable hypovolemic shock, and/or severe CNS involvement. Bleeding and edema of the face and neck are also highly associated with severe disease and death. The physiological correlates of this clinical picture are endothelial dysfunction demonstrated by alteration of the arachidonic acid pathway in endothelial cells and by platelet dysfunction [22]. The platelet dysfunction in the face of a normal platelet count is associated with a host-derived factor, as yet unidentified, other than that it is a protein and is found in quantity in serum (Fig. 75-6) [19].

Several clinical observations suggest that endothelial dysfunction and subsequent circulatory failure also occur in AHF and BHF. Proteinuria, petechial hemorrhage, and loss of intravascular volume without significant vomiting or diarrhea suggest alterations in endothelial function. That the shock is due to the loss of endothelial function and leakage of fluid into extravascular spaces is supported by the tissue edema frequently observed, and more directly by the pulmonary edema which may result from vigorous fluid therapy of shock. Proteinuria is significant, and dehydration with hemoconcentration appears to contribute to hypovolemia. Similar to Lassa fever, organ function, other than that of the endothelial system, ap-

pears to remain intact, and the critical period of shock lasts only 24 to 48 hours. Hepatitis is not seen, and renal function is well maintained. While bleeding is more pronounced with AHF and BHF than Lassa fever, it is not the cause of shock and death. The cause of the bleeding is poorly understood. It is not associated with evidence of disseminated intravascular coagulation (DIC) and even though there are petechiae suggesting some direct endothelial damage, no clear evidence of virus replication in and damage of endothelium has been demonstrated. It may be that a host factor is produced in the course of these infections, as one is for Lassa fever, which accounts for some of these changes, but no studies are available.

The neurological abnormalities also appear to be the result of metabolic and/or fluid changes (cerebral edema) rather than virus-induced inflammatory or necrotizing encephalitis [15]. The pathology of this syndrome is compatible with this interpretation. There is general absence of viral necrosis and inflammatory response. Tiny areas of eosinophilic necrosis may be observed in the liver. Scattered small hemorrhages are seen in mucosal membranes and occasionally in parenchymal tissues, but intravascular fibrin clots are generally absent. Tissue edema is generalized, but never as dramatic as that noted in rodentborne nephropathy (see below). There are no specific brain lesions and virus is not recovered from this organ. Virus titers obtained postmortem from lymphoid organs including spleen, nodes, and bone marrow are greater than those from other organs. These tissues may reveal evidence of lymphoid necrosis or of active regeneration and repair.

Like the South American hemorrhagic fevers, Lassa fever produces minimal histopathological changes [23]. The most obvious are in the liver where mild to occasional moderate focal necrosis may be seen. This necrosis is without inflammatory cells except for a few mononuclear cells (possibly macrophages), but no lymphocytes. Damage to other organs is certainly mild if present, since they do not manifest significant chemical or histological alterations. Despite clinical encephalopathy in some patients, brain pathology is minimal both in humans and in primates infected with Lassa virus. Virus replication occurs extensively in the adrenal glands, but no functional studies of the adrenal system have been done.

There are several key observations of clinical and laboratory nature in Lassa fever which together allow certain hypotheses to be entertained. First, there appears to be a brisk B-cell response to infection owing to the rather rapid appearance of antibodies to Lassa virus early in the illness (it must be remembered however that the incubation period is long relative to the viral illnesses) [14]. Second, histopathological lesions observed in the liver are without significant lymphocyte response, suggesting that some impairment may occur in the T-cell arm of the immune response, similar to that observed in LCM [23]. Indeed in primates the mixed lymphocyte response to nonspecific antigens is markedly reduced during the acute phase of fatal infection [22]. We do not have liver tissue from people who eventually recover from Lassa fever to com-

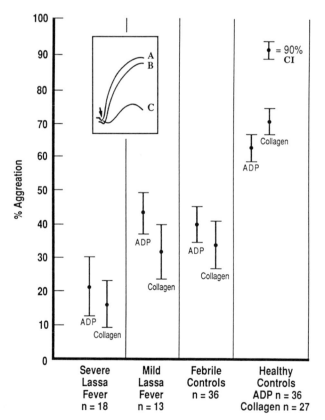

Figure 75-6. Platelet aggregation in patients with Lassa fever compared to fevers of other causes and to healthy people. Inset shows a typical aggregation response to ADP when platelets from healthy subjects are mixed with (**A**) normal platelet-poor plasma, (**B**) platelet-poor plasma from mild Lassa fever, and (**C**) platelet-poor plasma from severe Lassa fever illustrating the presence of an inhibitor of in vitro platelet aggregation.

pare with tissue of those who die. Perhaps such convalescent tissue would demonstrate a brisk lymphocyte response. Data from protection studies in primates coupled with the human observations suggest that the cell-mediated immune response to Lassa virus is in fact critical in virus clearance [24]. Furthermore the apparent paralysis of a part of the immune system could also be associated with the host-derived platelet inhibitory factor mentioned earlier. Perhaps this factor has very broad inhibitory effects on the immune system: a hypothesis now under study.

Diagnosis of arenaviruses

The simplest and most common methods of diagnosis are serological tests on paired sera by IFA or enzyme-linked immunosorbent assay (ELISA) to detect an increase in antibody titer or an elevated titer (at least 1:32), and presence of specific IgM [14,25]. The antigens are made from infected vero cell monolayers for IFA, or from infected cells, purified virus, or genetically engineered products for ELISA. All of the antigens are stable for many months at −20°C [25].

Virtually all of the known arenaviruses replicate well in cell culture [2]. Lassa virus produces sustained viremias so that virus isolation is reliable and may give a diagnosis in 2 or 3 days, depending on the level of viremia. More recent studies of South American hemorrhagic fever, particularly Junin infection, show that viremia is also a consistent feature, although probably not at the same levels as with Lassa fever [6]. Thus virus isolation is an alternative diagnostic method in the absence of paired sera.

Ideally, a method of rapid diagnosis would help with early identification and isolation of patients both for therapy and prevention of transmission; however, no such method has yet been developed. The diagnosis of Lassa fever by IFA on fixed tissue using monoclonal antibodies to Lassa virus makes possible postmortem diagnosis in situations where methods of collection and storage of specimens are limited [25].

For virus isolation, serum should be separated from a clotted specimen when possible, although whole blood may be used. Ideally, the specimen should be stored at −60°C but specimens stored at 4°C for several days still yielded virus. Lassa virus has been cultured from other sources, such as urine, spinal fluid, breast milk, pharyngeal secretions, and from tissues, especially liver, lymph node, and spleen. Specimens should be placed in dry ice or liquid nitrogen as soon as possible; −20°C storage will maintain virus viability for several days.

Management

Drugs and plasma. Although monkey studies suggest that Machupo infection in humans might be successfully treated with ribavirin or plasma, no such trials have been made. Conversely studies of the treatment of Junin virus infection in animals and humans show that convalescent-phase plasma is

very effective [16]. A randomized trial of patients with Argentine hemorrhagic fever demonstrated that convalescent-phase plasma reduced the mortality from 16 percent to 1 percent in the patients who were treated in the first 8 days of illness. Efficacy was directly related to the concentration of neutralizing antibodies. No data are available for ribavirin in Junin-infected patients. Late sequelae [15], e.g., neurological, were reported in 10 of 90 patients 2 to 3 weeks following successful immune plasma therapy. Although these signs were brief and, in most instances, completely reversed, one person died of acute ascending neurological paralysis.

Two randomized studies have evaluated the life-saving efficacy of convalescent plasma and ribavirin in patients with Lassa fever [26]. Patients were given a single unit (250 to 300 mL) of convalescent-phase plasma with an IFA titer of >128 or oral ribavirin in the first study, and either intravenous ribavirin alone or with convalescent plasma in the second study.

Patients given ribavirin who had elevated AST or viremia (risk factors for a fatal outcome—see under "Clinical Description") had significantly improved outcome compared with patients treated with plasma alone, or with patients who had not been treated. (Untreated patients were those with the same risk factors given supportive therapy at the same hospitals prior to the availability of ribavirin). Outcome also varied within each treatment group by day of illness on which treatment was begun.

Patients within the first 6 days of illness experienced a 5 to 9 percent case fatality (Table 75-4). Those with the same risk factors receiving treatment more than 6 days after the onset of illness had a case fatality of 20 to 47 percent. Case fatality was significantly less for ribavirin-treated patients in all categories than for either untreated patients or those treated with plasma. Furthermore patients treated with ribavirin had a significant reduction in viremia regardless of outcome whereas patients who were untreated or treated with plasma and who died showed no decrease in viremia. This suggests that survival is related to the amount of virus replication [25].

It appears that reduction in viremia later in disease course may not be accompanied by physiological improvement, sug-

Table 75-4. Case fatality in Lassa fever patients treated with ribavirin

		No treatment		Treated	
	Total	Lived	Died	Lived	Died
Group 1: Aspartate aminotransferase > 150 IU/L					
<7 days	38	7	11 (61%)	19	1 (5%)
>7 days	85	20	22 (52%)	32	11 (26%)
Total	123	27	33 (55%)	51	12 (19%)
Group 2: Viremia > $10^{3.6}$ TCID$_{50}$/mL					
<7 days	31	5	15 (75%)	10	1 (9%)
>7 days	39	6	21 (78%)	5	7 (58%)
Total	70	11	36 (77%)	15	8 (35%)

gesting that clinical management of physiological dysfunction is essential to improve the chances of survival in the late stages of disease.

Supportive Therapy. Supportive therapy is very similar for all of the arenaviral diseases. Many patients arrive in a moderately dehydrated state with elevated packed-cell volume (PCV), and require fluid replacement. No data are available on specific electrolyte or acid-base imbalances. The major crisis to be overcome is the sudden and profound hypotension which may occur between the fifth and the fourteenth day of illness. This crisis is difficult to manage in a rural setting. Acute pulmonary edema is a constant danger. For those patients with severe anemia, whole blood or packed cells may be helpful [27].

Whenever possible, fluid, electrolyte, and osmotic imbalances should be corrected in anticipation of the development of clinical shock, though it may be that even vigorous support of this kind may be insufficient to prevent fatal progression of disease.

Isolation. A prospective study has shown that in an endemic area Lassa virus infection occurs no more frequently in hospital personnel than in populations of neighboring villages, and this holds true for stratification by age, sex, patient contact, occupational exposure, and years working at the hospital [28]. These data indicate that simple protection measures (nondisposable gowns, gloves, and masks) used by the hospital personnel are effective in preventing excess risk of Lassa virus infection. Other observations also suggest that the risk of nosocomial transmission is low for Lassa fever. None of 159 hospital contacts of a severely ill Lassa fever patient in London seroconverted. None of nearly 100 other hospital contacts of Lassa fever in London had evidence of clinical disease. Thus available evidence suggests that nosocomial transmission is infrequent and that good hospital isolation and barrier nursing methods are sufficient to prevent transmission [29].

The degree to which patient isolation is accomplished depends on the hospital where the patient is admitted. The patient should be placed in a room with a single entrance, preferably through an adjoining room. This anteroom should contain the materials necessary for patient care and staff protection, including gowns, gloves, and masks. The entrance room should also contain hand-washing facilities and decontaminating solutions. An extra margin of assurance may be derived from a negative air pressure in the patient's room relative to the anteroom, and by single-pass air circulation, though in practice this may not be possible. Experience has shown that such air handling is not necessary when reasonable barrier nursing techniques are employed. Persons entering the patient's room should wear gowns, gloves, and masks (nondisposable ones may be decontaminated after use and reused). Feet should be covered, and protective eyewear should be worn by the staff if a patient is disoriented and combative or if procedures likely to produce vomiting or bleeding are performed (i.e., nasogas-

tric tube or arterial line). Protective clothing should be put on and removed in the entrance room, and only essential hospital personnel and immediate family members should be allowed in the room. More detailed procedures may be found elsewhere [29].

POPULATION

Ecology

The fundamental determinant of the ecology of arenaviral hemorrhagic fevers is the occurrence of persistent virus infection in rodents [1,2]. Infection of humans is a function of the behavior of the persistently infected rodent, plus the cultural and occupational patterns of human populations. The rodents that spread Lassa and Machupo viruses are peridomestic, and thus transmission to humans occurs as a result of human rodent interaction in rural houses. In contrast, *Calomys,* the reservoir of Junin virus, is found in maize fields, where it transmits the virus to agricultural workers primarily during the harvest season [30]. All three diseases are rural because none of the rodents is a successful inhabitant of large urban centers.

Epidemiology

Mode of Spread. The basic vehicle of spread of arenaviruses is thought to be infectious rodent urine; transmission occurs by aerosol or direct contact with skin abrasions or mucous membranes. In the case of AHF, skin abrasions among workers harvesting maize by hand were the most likely means of Junin virus entry. In recent years, however, aerosols created by, and bloody rodent tissues contaminating, modern harvesting machinery have likely contributed to a high infection rate among operators in the fields.

Recent studies suggest that person-to-person spread of Lassa virus is common, though it contributes less than rodent contacts to human infections [13]. Infection rates in families are significantly higher in households with rodents that have antibody to Lassa virus (undoubtedly reflecting persistent infection) and where food is stored indiscriminately. Spread of virus from rodents to humans is strongly associated with a large household rodent population as well as practices such as catching, cooking, and eating rodents. It is clear from a prospective study that extensive rodent trapping carried out in an entire village significantly reduced the frequency of seroconversion to Lassa virus. Person-to-person transmission in a household is associated with direct contact or care of someone with a febrile illness, as well as sexual contact with a partner during the incubation or convalescent phases of illnesses. No information is available on the presence of Lassa virus in semen during the acute or convalescent phases of illness.

Nosocomial transmission of Lassa virus was well described during the outbreaks that occasioned the discovery of the virus more than two decades ago. Recent data suggest that this is not a frequent event, and that basic barrier nursing methods (gloves, gowns, and masks) are highly effective in reducing the risk [28].

Nosocomial transmission of both Junin and Machupo viruses is a known but highly unusual phenomenon. The great difference in mean viremia induced by the respective agents may be crucial for the observed patterns in Lassa as compared to the American fevers.

Seasonality. Each of the three diseases has a distinctive pattern. AHF has a sharply circumscribed annual incidence during the harvest months of April to June in an austral temperature climate. Human contact and reservoir density are the important variables, and the latter accounts for long-term cycles of 3 to 5 years in annual fluctuation of human disease.

For BHF the transmission is endemic with a broad peak from March to July at the end of a 6-month rainy season in a tropical savannah biotope. Long-term fluctuations based on *Calomys* density also occur and may be explained by experimental studies which demonstrated that chronically infected rodents experience fatal infection and death with virtually complete reproductive infertility.

Lassa virus transmission is the most consistently endemic of the three arenaviruses. More patients are admitted to hospital during the dry season of February to May, but cases occur in every month of the year. *Mastomys* populations in villages do not vary temporally with this pattern, and it is perhaps significant that chronically infected animals gave birth to normal but Lassa-infected offspring in laboratory studies. It is possible that increased stability of Lassa virus at low relative humidity may account in part for the observed seasonality of transmission.

Incubation Period. The incubation periods of all the hemorrhagic fevers caused by arenaviruses are very similar, although all are based on estimates of the time of exposure, which is often difficult to ascertain. The estimates for AHF and BHF are about 2 weeks, with a lower limit of perhaps 10 days observed with AHF. For Lassa, the incubation period is estimated as 6 to 18 days based on observations of person-to-person transmission within hospitals.

Illness-to-Infection Ratio; Age, Sex, and Occupation. Illness-to-infection ratios vary widely almong the three major disease-causing arenaviruses. During the Machupo epidemic in San Joaquin, Bolivia, there was virtually a 100 percent illness-to-infection ratio based on human antibody prevalence and history of illness compatible with BHF. For AHF, few data are available concerning the illness-to-infection ratio, although serosurveys suggest that mild illness or perhaps no illness occurs in 10 percent of infections [2,6,30]. Seroconversion rates ranged from 5 to 20 percent in prospective studies of Lassa fever in susceptible (seronegative) populations of Sierra Leone villages [8,13]. The highest rates were in crowded, highly mobile populations with lower rates in tra-

ditional agricultural villages. These same studies demonstrated disease-to-infection ratios of 10 to 25 percent, and the proportion of febrile illness associated with seroconversion to Lassa virus was 5 to 14 percent. Hospitalization-to-infection ratios are 5 to 8 percent and the overall fatality-to-infection ratio is 1 to 2 percent (the fatality-to-illness ratio is probably 5 to 10 percent, while the hospitalized case fatality rate is 15 to 20 percent). The overall estimates of antibody prevalence range from 4 to 6 percent in Guinea to as high as 15 to 20 percent in Nigeria. Lassa fever is therefore more common than previously suspected and probably results in 200,000 to 300,000 infections per year in west Africa with 3000 to 5000 deaths. Careful examination shows disparity between seroconversion rates and antibody prevalence. There appears to be a loss of measurable IFA antibody over time, so that some of the apparent seroconversions observed in prospective studies are in fact reinfections in those who have lost antibody. Thus not all "seroconversions" are primary infections, and furthermore a new group of seronegative people is created each year by loss of detectable antibody, but these people are apparently susceptible only to infection, not to significant illness.

All age groups are affected by Lassa virus as shown by serological surveys as well as studies of hospitalized patients [17]. Age- and sex-specific antibody prevalence show that the proportion of the population with antibody increases with age, and there is no significant difference in antibody prevalence between sexes.

Because of the occupational nature of AHF, adult males are principally affected, although sporadic cases do occur in children and females. During the epidemic of BHF in San Joaquin, all ages and sexes were affected. However, the sporadic cases of BHF have a predominance in adult males who are engaged in agriculture.

AHF and BHF tend to affect persons of lower socioeconomic status such as farm laborers or families with poor housing which may be rodent-infested, as was observed with BHF during the San Joaquin epidemic. Lassa fever has not been associated with socioeconomic status. It is a rural village disease and affects the families of chiefs as well as those of ordinary persons. Housing differences are not often very marked in west African villages so that all houses are usually susceptible to rodent infestation.

Epidemic Investigation. Epidemic investigation of the three major arenavirus diseases should include assessment of rodent infestation and infection in conjunction with a careful history of the human disease. For Lassa, the role of human-to-human transmission is clearly more important than for the other two viruses and this must be kept in mind when investigating a case or cluster of cases in an endemic area. Investigations in a nonendemic area should center around possible human contacts or recent travel to an endemic Lassa area. For AHF and BHF cases, any case arising in a nonendemic area would be expected either to have a history of travel to an endemic area or to have had laboratory exposure.

Prevention

There are now two candidate vaccines for arenaviral diseases. A live attenuated virus vaccine against AHF has been extensively evaluated in monkeys, and is presently undergoing preliminary testing in field trials in Argentina. A vaccine against Lassa fever has been made by cloning and expressing the Lassa virus glycoprotein gene into vaccinia virus [24]. This vaccine has proven highly successful in preventing severe disease and death in challenged monkeys. Only the glycoprotein gene is protective in the two species of monkeys thus far tested. The nucleoprotein gene of Lassa virus expressed in vaccinia does not protect monkeys from a lethal Lassa virus challenge. The vaccinia–Lassa virus glycoprotein construct produces little detectable antibody by IFA after vaccination, and does not produce detectable neutralizing antibody, but is nevertheless protective, suggesting again that a vigorous cell-mediated immune response must play a part in its ability to protect. Thus far no system for consistently detecting such a response has been developed.

Based on available data, it could be predicted that passively administered antibodies are capable of preventing or aborting infection with Junin or Machupo viruses. For Lassa virus the evidence is less clear; but studies in monkeys suggest that higher concentrations of neutralizing antibodies will be required than those achieved by most convalescent patients. Ribavirin, at about 20 mg/(kg·day), alone or combined with antibody, also may be effective, although it is not clear how long this drug need be given to abort an infection [16,26].

Control

The manipulation of reservoir ecology has not been used in efforts to control any of the three major arenavirus diseases. This approach does not lend itself to control of these diseases with perhaps the exception of making houses rodentproof.

The major method of control, which has been used successfully for BHF and to a lesser degree for Lassa fever, is rodent trapping in villages. These is no doubt that rodent trapping in the village of San Joaquin in Bolivia eliminated BHF from the town. Within 1 incubation period of the trapping program, cases of BHF ceased to occur. It is also interesting to note that a large portion of the cat population in San Joaquin had been killed by malaria control–related DDT poisoning. The role this may have played in the subsequent epidemic is not clear but should not be ignored. For Lassa fever, two village trapping programs have been done with a reduction of sixfold in the transmission of virus after, compared to before, the campaign in one village, and a modest twofold reduction in another. From the point of view of cost and simplicity, this is by far the easiest method of disease control. For Lassa, more

experience with this approach is needed, especially in the savannah areas where rodents are found in the bush as well as the houses, and where rodent migration from bush to house may be more important. Elimination of rodents residing outside houses is clearly not feasible.

For AHF, such an approach is also not feasible because of the vast areas of rodent habitation. But unintentional ecological manipulation, the introduction of crop rotation using soybeans with corn, may be responsible for reduction of human disease during the past 5 years [30].

MARBURG AND EBOLA VIRUSES   Filoviridae

GENERAL ECOLOGY

Little is as yet known about these two African viruses, first isolated in 1967 and 1976 [31,32]. Both agents cause acute hemorrhagic fever in humans with very high mortality rates and the pattern of transmission in all outbreaks has been person-to-person. Although the initial Marburg outbreak occurred in Germany and was traced to infected green monkeys imported from Uganda, there is at present no solid evidence that African primates represent a significant reservoir or vector for the viruses. Sporadic clusters of cases have been reported from eastern, central, and southern Africa only.

MORPHOLOGY AND ULTRASTRUCTURE

These viruses are among the largest known, measuring 850 nm in length (Marburg) to 950 nm (Ebola), and 80 nm in diameter [33]. The nucleocapsid consists of a central axis which is 20 to 30 nm in diameter surrounded by a helical capsid of 40 to 50 nm in diameter and 5-nm cross-striation interval. There is a host-cell membrane-derived layer which surrounds the nucleocapsid and the terminal windings of nucleocapsid found at one end of the particle. The surface projections are 10-nm spikes seen in regular array. These viruses are tremendously pleomorphic and appear in negative stain preparations as torus-shaped, U-shaped, 6-shaped, and branched filamentous forms.

BIOCHEMISTRY AND REPLICATION

These viruses are the only members of a newly designated family known as the Filoviridae [33]. They are negative single-stranded RNA viruses with genomes ranging from 4×10^6 Da (Marburg virus) to 4.5×10^6 Da (Ebola virus). The RNA is a template for seven monocistronic messages which encode the seven virion proteins so far identified. Five proteins are virion structural proteins, one is the viral polymerase, and another is a nonstructural protein whose function is believed to be associated with transcription. The surface protein is heavily glycosylated. It appears that this may be the most important protein in the immune response. A second protein, VP40, is also associated with the membrane, but is poorly glycosylated.

The VP40 and nucleoprotein are both associated with the nucleocapsid, but specific functions are not yet known [34].

Oligonucleotide restriction mapping of viral RNA has shown that Marburg virus has 50 to 60 percent of its oligonucleotides distinct from Ebola virus. For Ebola virus, some 30 percent of the oligonucleotides of strains from Zaire are different from those of strains from Sudan. Mapping of strains isolated in different years from Zaire (1976, 1978) and Sudan (1976, 1979) showed geographical genetic stability over these intervals (Fig. 75-7). Marburg RNA obtained from viruses originating in Uganda, Kenya, and South Africa differed by about 20 to 30 percent of oligonucleotides. Marburg isolates representing different points in time from a single geographical area are not available for study.

Peptide maps show no similarities between Marburg strains and Ebola strains. Peptide maps of the strains of Ebola from Zaire and Sudan show two proteins to be significantly different, the nucleoprotein VP 2 and the glycoprotein 4.

Replication of viral RNA occurs in cellular cytoplasm where nucleocapsids are constructed. The nucleocapsids bud through the cell membrane where the envelopes and surface projections are added as the virus leaves the cell. This process appears to represent a variable extrusion of cell membrane rather than a discrete orderly budding, a phenomenon which may account for the great pleomorphism seen in virions.

ANIMAL MODELS

Difficulties in working with animals under laboratory conditions of maximum containment have limited the work done with animal models. The monkey has been the most successful animal used for the study of Marburg and Ebola viruses [35].

Rhesus monkeys inoculated intraperitoneally with 10^3 to 10^4 guinea pig infectious units of Ebola virus become febrile on the third to fifth day after inoculation. The monkeys develop a maculopapular rash on the forehead, face, limbs, and chest between the fourth and fifth days. Fever persists and severe prostration, sometimes with diarrhea occurs. Viremia is detectable by day 2 after inoculation and reaches a peak of $10^{5.5}$ to $10^{6.5}$ GPID$_{50}$* per milliliter on day 5. The monkeys all die by day 8 after a prolonged episode of hypovolemic shock, much like the human disease. Though little is known about the cause of the shock and hemorrhage, two important observations are disturbance in platelet function and dysfunction of vascular endothelium [35]. A decline in in vitro platelet aggregation begins 1 to 3 days prior to the onset of bleeding and shock progressing to virtually no aggregation at death. This is associated with an increase in platelet factor 4 (PF4) levels in plasma, and concomitant decrease in platelet-derived PF4, suggesting that platelets are being stimulated, but are unable to aggregate. Aortic endothelium taken at death has markedly reduced in vitro ability to produce prostacyclin compared with

*Guinea pig infectious dose.

endothelium from normal uninfected control animals, suggesting profound disturbance in its biochemical integrity (despite a normal histological appearance). Early in disease a significant lymphopenia is observed in the animals, but late in disease a marked neutrophilia occurs (reaching 20×10^9/L) in the absence of concurrent bacterial infection. This is an uncommon observation in viral diseases, and its significance is not understood, though it has been observed in other viral hemorrhagic fevers especially in severely sick patients.

Virus appears to replicate well in many organs (the brain being an exception). However, the histopathological changes are most marked in the liver where focal cellular necrosis occurs without significant inflammatory reaction. Hepatic enzyme levels do not suggest liver failure as a cause of hemorrhage, and this evidence is supported by the modest alterations in levels of liver-derived clotting factors.

Marburg virus and the two variants of Ebola also have been studied in guinea pigs and suckling mice. The ability of any of the viruses to kill guinea pigs is variable. The Zaire variant of Ebola kills guinea pigs consistently after several adaptive passages, the Sudan variant and Marburg virus do not. Only the Zaire virus was found to be lethal for suckling mice.

PATIENT

Infection and host responses

The precise portal of entry of Ebola virus infection is unknown, but studies of factors associated with person-to-person transmission suggest that the virus enters through mucous membranes or skin lesions, since very close contact with a patient is required. Early viral replication is thought to occur in the reticuloendothelial tissues and viremia is a constant feature of clinically apparent infection. Antibodies (IFA) appear in early convalescence (10 to 14 days). However neutralizing antibodies are not present in convalescent serum (from animals or humans). Similar to the experience with Lassa fever, it would appear that virus clearance is probably associated with the cell-mediated component of the immune response, though no direct evidence for this yet exists.

Clinical manifestations

Marburg and Ebola diseases usually have abrupt onset with fever, chills, headache, malaise, and weakness (Table 75-5) [31,36]. Myalgia and anorexia, together with abdominal pain and diarrhea, are established early in the clinical course, and the diarrhea, sometimes with vomiting, may persist until death. Stools and vomitus often contain blood. Sore throat is common; substantial chest or epigastric pain occurs frequently, as does conjunctivitis. Bleeding and diarrhea occur in about 80 percent, pharyngitis in 75 percent, vomiting in 65 percent, conjunctivitis in 60 percent, and cough in 35 percent of Ebola cases. A morbilliform rash on the trunk and back has been reported on many occasions but may be difficult to see in dark

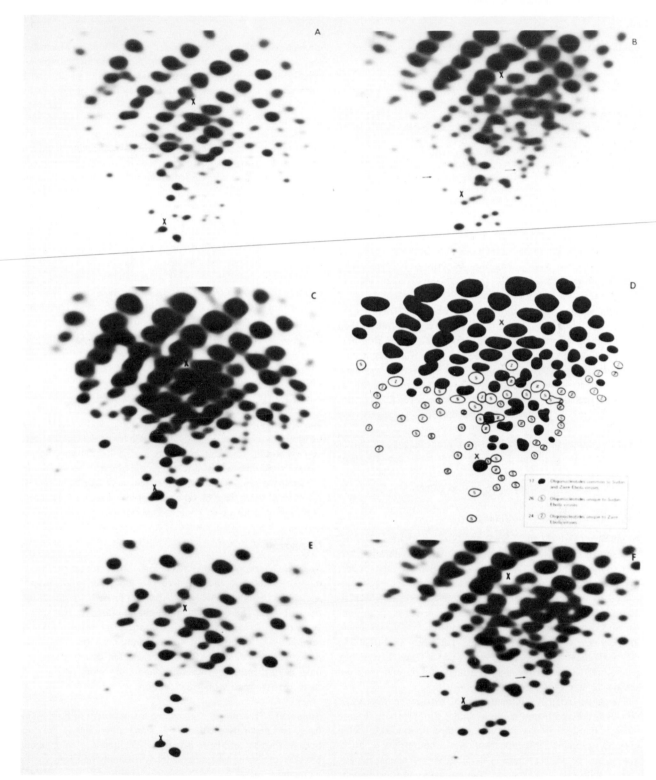

Figure 75-7. Oligonucleotide maps of RNA of strains of Ebola virus isolated in Zaire and Sudan. *A.* MAY, Zaire, 1976. *B.* BON, Sudan, 1976. *C.* ECK, Zaire, 1976. *D.* Mixture of MAY and BON. *E.* BND, Zaire, 1977. *F.* KUM, Sudan, 1979. Arrows indicate differences between strains BON and MAY. Upper and lower Xs denote positions of marker dyes. (*From [13].*)

Table 75-5. Symptoms and signs in fatal Ebola hemorrhagic fever patients, Zaire*

Symptoms	n[†]	%[‡]	Signs	n	%
Fever	231	98.1	Bleeding	223	77.6
Headache	210	96.2	Diarrhea	228	78.5
Abdominal pain	201	81.1	Oral-throat lesions	208	73.6
Sore throat	207	79.2	Vomiting	225	64.9
Myalgia	206	79.1	Conjunctivitis	208	58.2
Nausea	178	66.3	Cough	208	35.6
Arthritis	193	53.4	Abortion	73	24.7

*Fatality was 90 percent (288 deaths among 318 patients).
[†]n = respondents.
[‡]% = positive/respondents × 100.

skin. It often leads to desquamation. Proteinuria is uniformly present. Jaundice is not a feature of Marburg or Ebola disease. Complications include abortion and CNS involvement leading to hemiplegia and disorientation.

By the sixth to seventh day of Ebola illness, patients develop the typical "expressionless" face and severe prostration seen so frequently in patients who die. Most patients develop profound hypotension several hours before death. Bleeding occurs in nearly 100 percent of persons who die. Even in convalescence patients show prolonged weakness, severe weight loss, and in a few survivors there are serious but reversible personality changes including confusion, anxiety, and aggressive behavior.

The rapidity of onset and severity of clinical signs and symptoms and early death make these diseases truly fearsome. The occurrence of even a few cases in a community produces considerable anxiety and may even lead to panic.

Pathophysiology and pathology

At autopsy Marburg and Ebola infections are characterized by widespread hemorrhagic diathesis into skin, membranes, and soft tissues. There is focal necrosis in liver, lymph nodes, ovaries, and testis, with liver lesions most prominent, accompanied by eosinophilic hepatic cell inclusion bodies (Councilman-like), but significant inflammatory response is absent. Nonspecific, probably ischemic, encephalitic lesions are found in the brains of Marburg patients. Pathological differential diagnosis must include yellow fever, Lassa fever, Rift Valley fever, and Congo-Crimean hemorrhagic fever, and may not always be an easy task [32].

The most extensive human clinical experience with these viruses is derived from the initial outbreak of Marburg disease when a number of patients were studied in moderate detail [31]. Disseminated infection resulting in multiorgan dysfunction seems common. There is invariably evidence of hepatic disease with elevated aspartate transaminase and focal hepatic necrosis; however, this is not sufficiently extensive to invoke hepatic failure, evidenced by disproportionately low alanine transaminases (AST:ALT 7:1) and the lack of significant effect on liver-dependent hemostatic mechanisms. Gastroenteritis is

characteristic and may lead to dehydration, and to electrolyte and acid-base imbalance. Bleeding is prominent, though not usually of sufficient volume to induce shock in itself, and is furthermore not associated with solid evidence of DIC in the small number of animals or humans studied so far. The most profound physiological alteration, and that which is invariably associated with death, is shock, manifested by effusions and facial edema. The platelet and endothelial cell biochemical and physiological dysfunction described in animal experiments may underlie these clinical features, but the exact mechanisms are unknown [35].

Diagnosis

Marburg and the Zaire variant of Ebola virus are readily isolated from blood specimens taken in the first week of illness by inoculation of Vero or other mammalian cell cultures. Depending on blood concentration, identification can be made by IFA within 2 to 5 days after inoculation of cells. The Sudan variant of Ebola virus, however, is difficult to recover from blood or tissues of patients. Blind passages of cultured cells or use of guinea pigs which are monitored for febrile response are often necessary. Specimens including throat washing, urine, various soft-tissue effusates, semen, and anterior eye fluid may also contain virus. Specific identification is made generally by IFA. Although morphologically similar, Marburg and Ebola viruses are thus far immunologically distinct. A virus family diagnosis can also be made by detection of virions in postmortem formalin-fixed samples of liver tissue, an important technique where a reliable cold chain is not available. Under these circumstances, moreover, it is worth attempting isolation of virus from blood specimens because such materials unrefrigerated for up to 10 days have yielded virus strains.

Management

Specific Therapy. Temporal response after administration of passive antibodies and interferon to a worker who suffered accidental inoculation of Ebola virus led to early optimism that one or both of these treatments might be effective. But studies in monkeys have so far failed to confirm any significant antiviral activity for either substance. Many antiviral compounds have been tested against these viruses, but no effective ones have been identified. Therefore, laboratory work on these viruses is performed with great caution.

Supportive Treatment. Aggressive management of fluid, acid-base, and electrolyte balance is clearly important in the supportive therapy of these diseases. The inability to maintain intravascular volume is a particularly difficult challenge to clinical management. Although much has been written about DIC, particularly use of heparin, there is little evidence for the role of DIC in pathogenesis, and this drug remains controversial. The only experience has been the therapy of two individuals with Marburg disease in South Africa. However, both of these patients were secondary Marburg infections, and, curiously, none of eight known secondary patients with Marburg infection have died, and only those two received heparin therapy. Clinical judgment and fine-tuning of fluids and electrolytes along with blood, plasma, or platelet replacement are the approach to success in management of these diseases until more is understood of the disease processes, and until specific antiviral therapy becomes available.

Prevention of Human-to-Human Transmission. Epidemiological experience suggests that direct contact with blood, tissues, or secretions is the most common cause of secondary infection [*38*]. Therefore isolation of the patient with procedures described for Lassa fever, strict observations of barrier nursing techniques, and containment of clinical specimens are the most important means of preventing person-to-person transmission. Gowns, gloves, and masks and the liberal use of decontamination methods (chemical or heat) are essential in achieving this goal.

Suspect cases which occur in nonendemic areas may be managed more intensively [*29*]. The patients should be isolated in separate rooms. Hospital staff should be well trained in isolation techniques, and the number of persons attending should be limited to the requirement for good medical care. Disposable gowns, gloves, and masks should be used. Surveillance of hospital contacts and other close contacts of suspected cases should be done through daily interview by telephone, with fever as the primary measure of illness. Any contacts developing fever within 17 days of last contact with the case should be isolated and carefully studied for Marburg or Ebola disease.

POPULATION

Ecology

The ecological setting of Marburg and Ebola appears to center around central and south central Africa based on the origin of known outbreaks. The original outbreak of Marburg virus occurred following infections in monkeys imported from Uganda. Surveys of wild monkeys from the area in northern Uganda where the original Marburg-infected group originated failed to yield virus or definitive presence of antiviral antibodies. Cases of Marburg subsequently occurred in 1980 in western Kenya, on the border with Uganda, and in 1975 and 1982 in South Africa. Extensive studies of the area around the sugar cane–processing factory in western Kenya where a death from Marburg virus occurred in 1980 failed to reveal clues to the ecology of Marburg virus. Recently another fatal primary Marburg infection occurred in the same western area of Kenya as the case of 1980. The patient was a young boy who had spent considerable time in the same cave visited by the 1980 case. The cave contains large numbers of bats. The use of sentinel animals and other means of searching for the origin of virus have, however, failed to identify the bats (or any of a number

of wild mammals) as the ultimate source. Similarly, cases of Marburg disease were seen at two different times in South Africa. Both instances involved travelers from Zimbabwe to Johannesburg, South Africa. A thorough study of insects and mammals along the trail of the 1975 traveler did not produce evidence for virus infection.

Epidemiology

There have been five outbreaks of Marburg or Ebola diseases in Africa involving two or more cases [*31,36,37*]. In every instance the index case was fatal, and person-to-person spread, frequently in a hospital setting, was the cause of dissemination of disease to the community. In 1975, Marburg virus was spread from an index case admitted to a hospital in Johannesburg to a close contact of the patient and to a nurse. In 1980, a patient died 5 h after being admitted to a Nairobi hospital, and the attending doctor subsequently became ill with but survived Marburg infection. Both major epidemics of Ebola in 1976 and the one in 1979 involved person-to-person transmission in the family and hospital setting. Contaminated needles were important sources of infection in the Zaire outbreak. A study of risk factors for virus transmission in the Sudan epidemic in 1979 showed that caring for an ill patient carried a relative risk five times greater than persons with a lesser degree of physical contact and no cases occurred in persons who entered the room with an ill patient but had no contact. These data suggest that Ebola is not an airborne disease and depends on close contact probably with infected blood or secretions for its propagation.

The incubation period of Ebola in humans averages 6 days for instances of parenteral inoculation with a range of 1 to 15 days. The incubation period of Ebola for person-to-person spread is about 10 days with a range up to 3 weeks. The incubation for Marburg during the epidemic in 1967 was 4 to 9 days.

The illness-to-infection ratio for Marburg and Ebola seems very nearly 1 because during all the known epidemics few if any asymptomatic infections were provable. Serosurveys of village populations in epidemic areas have shown presence of low-titered Ebola and Marburg antibodies. If these reactions can be confirmed and extended by other methods and prospective studies, then infection without serious clinical disease is more common than presently realized.

The death-to-infection ratio for these viruses covers a wide range. Of the 37 known cases of Marburg, 29 were primary infections, of which the case fatality was 10 in 29 (35 percent), while no fatalities occurred among the 8 secondary cases. Whether this is due to infectious dose, or to virus modulation following primary human infection is not known [*31*]. The mortality ratios during the two epidemics of Ebola disease in Sudan were 55 and 65 percent, while that during the Zaire epidemic in 1976 was 88 percent.

Contact with patients ill with Ebola is the most important factor in determining risk of illness. During both of the major

Ebola epidemics, disease occurred in neonates, children, and adults. Too few data are available on Marburg in the African setting to draw any conclusion about its epidemiology.

The history of person-to-person transmission of Marburg and Ebola viruses dictates that any investigation of possible cases or epidemics of these diseases must focus on the primary role of this mode of spread. The important issues to be confronted are identification of active cases and of potential cases based on the type and degree of contact that have occurred with known cases. Identification of these two groups will allow safe and orderly care of the ill but will permit effective surveillance of high-risk contacts with prompt isolation if and when those people become ill. This will ensure rapid control of an epidemic and will prevent spread of virus through family or hospital contacts of acutely ill patients. Detailed study of the proximate activities of the index case is necessary in order to continue the search for clues to natural virus reservoirs.

Prevention

There is no vaccine against any of these diseases, and there is no clearly effective prophylaxis. Recent cloning and sequencing of the genes encoding the important surface glycoproteins of Ebola and Marburg viruses offer the best opportunity for development of effective vaccines [34]. Since the reservoir(s) of the viruses are not known, no specific precautions can be taken to avoid infections from the natural source of the viruses. The most important issue is that of awareness in the medical community that these diseases exist and they may result in extensive nosocomial spread if not recognized early and if appropriate isolation of the patient is not achieved.

There is no evidence for or against the use of passive antibody in preventing these diseases. The difficulty of collecting and storing human immune plasma will, for practical purposes, limit the supply of plasma and therefore the use of plasma in prevention will be severely curtailed.

Control

The identification of acutely ill patients and their isolation, along with careful surveillance of high-risk contacts, are the cornerstones of epidemic control. All epidemics have resulted from person-to-person spread of infection and this must be stopped in order to end the outbreak [29].

HANTAVIRUS INFECTIONS: HEMORRHAGIC FEVER WITH RENAL SYNDROME (HFRS) AND NEPHROPATHIA EPIDEMICA (NE)

GENERAL ECOLOGY

These widespread diseases have been recognized both in Europe and the Far East since the 1930s, but were first described in the international literature when epidemics occurred in United Nations troops stationed in Korea between 1951 and 1954 [39,40,41]. The cause of the epidemics became known as Korean hemorrhagic fever at that time, but similar clinical entities in different countries have been given many other names, such as *hemorrhagic nephrosonephritis* or *hemorrhagic fever with renal syndrome (HFRS)* in the U.S.S.R., *epidemic hemorrhagic fever (EHF)* in Japan and China, and *nephropathia epidemica (NE)* in Scandinavia [40,41]. As recognition of the disease complex became more widespread, other names proliferated. The suggested international appellation is now *hemorrhagic fever with renal syndrome (HFRS)*.

The viruses which cause HFRS persistently infect various rodent species throughout the world. They belong to the Bunyaviridae, and have recently been formed into a new genus, *Hantavirus* [42,43]. The range of rodent species infected is also wide, varying from region to region, so that the presence of the virus in a given area depends largely on the predominant rodent species in that area. Thus field mice and voles are important in rural areas and urban rats in cities. Human disease depends on intimate contact with rodents, such as may occur in agricultural areas with high human and rodent population densities, during military campaigns or exercises, or in crowded urban housing.

In the Soviet Far East, mainland China, and Korea, the best known rodent host is the Manchurian striped field mouse, *Apodemus agrarius,* but virus has now also been identified in *Clethrionomys* species, especially in the Soviet Union, and *Rattus* species in China, Korea, Japan, and southeast Asia. A specific correlation was made in 1961 when 129 employees of a scientific institute in the U.S.S.R. became ill following the introduction of a large number of wild-caught rodents, including some *Apodemus sylvaticus*. In Korea, virus has been isolated from *A. sylvaticus* in forests and *A. agrarius* in secondary and wet forests and in fields; *Microtus* in grasslands; and *Clethrionomys* in settings such as forests, domestic gardens, and agricultural areas. In Scandinavia the *Clethrionomys* species are the predominant hosts, which is probably true of most of the rest of Europe, with the exception of Greece and possibly also other Balkan countries, where *Apodemus* species have been primarily implicated [44].

In the United States viruses have been isolated from *Rattus* and *Microtus* species, but though virus-specific antibodies have been detected in human serum evidence of overt human disease is still lacking. Human infections from infected laboratory rat colonies, however, have been reported in Japan, Korea, Belgium, and the United Kingdom [39,45,46].

Virus characterization

A virus isolated from *Apodemus* in Korea in 1978 has now been suggested as the type species of a new genus, *Hantavirus,* of the Bunyaviridae family [47,48]. This genus now comprises several strains from rats, *Clethrionomys,* and *Microtus,* which are closely related to, but not identical with, the type species. In the main, isolates from single species resemble each other serologically, and presumably genetically, and differ from isolates from other species.

The hantaviruses are 80 to 115 nm in diameter, (average 92.5 nm), enveloped, with regular hollow surface projections [48]. They have no observable symmetry, a density of 1.15 to 1.19 g/mL, and are acid labile. By electron microscopy subtle structural differences distinguish them from other bunyaviridae. Like all bunyaviridae, hantaviruses possess a tripartite genome of negative polarity. The large (L), medium (M), and small (S) genome segments have relative molecular masses of approximately 2.7, 1.2, and 0.6×10^6, respectively, as estimated by agarose gel electrophoresis, and are enclosed in three separate nucleocapsid structures which are surrounded by a lipid envelope containing two virus-specified glycoproteins, designated G1 and G2 [42]. Their nucleocapsid is encoded in the S segment; envelope glycoproteins in the M segment; and the third, the L segment, is presumed to encode the viral polymerase. The nucleocapsid protein (N) has a molecular mass of 45,000, and there are two glycoproteins (G1 and G2) in the range of 64,000 and 53,700 respectively. Five potential asparagine-linked glycosylation sites are contained within the G1 amino acid sequence and two within the G2 sequence. Strain-specific epitopes exist on both N and G proteins, but sequence data available so far suggest greater variation on the glycoproteins, as might be expected.

Hantaan, like other viruses in the Bunyaviridae family, encodes its nucleocapsid protein in the S RNA segment; however, data suggest that this S segment differs considerably from the elaborate ambisense or overlapping reading frame strategies of phlebovirus and some bunyavirus S segments, allowing them to encode a nonstructural polypeptide for which there is no evidence in hantaviruses. Like those of other bunyaviridae, the M genome segment of Hantaan virus appears to encode polyprotein precursors which are processed into envelope glycoproteins. Mature G1 begins 18 amino acids beyond the first AUG of the open reading frame, preceded by a short, hydrophobic leader sequence. G2 begins at amino acid 649 and also follows a hydrophobic sequence. The absence of a nonstructural coding region between the signal sequence and G1 distinguishes Hantaan from the phleboviruses.

A possible small intergenic region (maximum 6K) is described between the carboxy terminus of G1 and the amino terminus of G2, similar to that predicted for Rift Valley fever virus. This sequence is hydrophobic, consistent with a membrane-spanning intergenic region, and a potential signal sequence has also been identified. The carboxy terminus of G2 is extremely hydrophobic, suggesting the presence of a membrane-anchoring protein region. Little is known of the functions of G1 and G2, except that a broadly cross-reactive monoclonal antibody to G2 can neutralize viral infectivity.

The viruses can be grown in tissue culture. *Apodemus'* and *Rattus*-derived viruses grow well in Vero-E6 cells, and maximum titers are achieved in about 7 to 10 days. The *Clethrionomys* viruses, on the other hand, grow only to low titer in tissue culture and are strictly cell associated, so that it is difficult to produce high-titer cell-free virus for laboratory studies. Suckling mouse or gerbil brain can also be used for antigen production. Gerbils have also been used for primary isolation. At present there is no useful animal model for pathogenesis, but laboratory rabbits can be productively infected, and low-titer viremia detected.

Currently the viruses are organized into four serological groups based on in vitro neutralization assays and monoclonal antibody reactivity. These are the *Apodemus* strains, with Hantaan virus as the prototype strain; the vole viruses such as Puumala; the rat viruses, with Seoul rat virus as the prime strain; and *Microtus*-type viruses such as Prospect Hill.

Natural hosts and animal models

The wide range of rodent hosts implicated in the transmission of hantaviruses suggests the potential for these or similar viruses to be found worldwide in different ecosystems [39,42]. In addition to mice, rats, and voles, virus has now been isolated from wild *Suncus murinus,* an insectivore, in China, where antibody and virus have been reported in cats. Although *Rattus* and *Apodemus* may sometimes occupy the same ecological niche, particularly in rural China, it is not known whether in these areas viral strains really have separate ecology, or whether intraspecies exchange of viral strains, or even reassortment, may occur in the wild, resulting in a mosaic of viral strains.

In two studies, adult *A. agrarius* and Wistar rats were infected with strains of *Hantavirus*. *Apodemus* mice developed transient viremia on the seventh day after intramuscular inoculation. Despite the subsequent formation of neutralizing antibodies, infectious virus was recovered from multiple sites including lung, kidney, salivary gland, and liver. Virus was excreted in saliva, urine, and feces for as long as 1 year after inoculation. Horizontal infection occurred in uninoculated cagemates, but vertical transmission has not been adequately studied. In Wistar rats, in which Hantaan virus was adapted after seven passages, specific antigen appeared in the lungs as early as 14 days and antibody developed after 3 weeks. Virus was also found in kidney, liver, spleen, and submaxillary and parotid glands. No data are presently available on excretion of virus by the Wistar rats. A strain of virus has now been adapted to suckling mice and appears to be pantropic after intraperitoneal or intracerebral inoculation. Titers in brain reach 10^8 tissue culture infectious doses $(TCID)_{50}/mL$, and mice are killed 11 to 17 days after inoculation.

Unfortunately neither the rabbit nor any other species yet tested, including a range of primates, develops a disease comparable in any way to human HFRS. This lack of a suitable animal model poses severe limitations on studies of vaccine protection in the laboratory.

PATIENT

Human disease

Details of viral invasion, replication, and host response to hantaviruses remain to be elucidated. There is evidence that infection is acquired from airborne virus, but direct inoculation via cuts or abrasions may also be important [*39*]. Sites of primary and secondary virus replication are unknown. The incubation period ranges from 12 to 21 days, but has been as little as 8 days or up to 5 weeks. By the time patients seek medical care, virus may be detected in whole blood in specimens taken early in disease, and both IgM- and IgG-specific antibodies are present in nearly all instances. Antigen-antibody complexes have been reported in blood of patients and in tissues, including renal tissue, and it is speculated that the tubular nephropathy unique among viruses causing HFRS may be an immunopathological phenomenon, presumably involving immune complex deposition. Mild or subclinical infection may occur, particularly in laboratory-rat-associated disease, but without data from prospective clinical and serological surveys we will not know how much inapparent disease results from *Apodemus*- or *Rattus*-derived infection. It is clear, however, that severity of disease is related to the originating strain, and in general infection from *Apodemus*-derived viruses is more severe, and more likely to produce hemorrhage and renal failure than infection from *Rattus*- or vole-derived viral strains.

Clinical manifestations

Classically the disease is divided into febrile, hypotensive, oliguric, diuretic, and convalescent phases (Fig. 75-8). In the first, febrile phase, there may be a vague prodromal stage, easily confused with a mild respiratory or gastrointestinal infection; nevertheless, onset is usually abrupt with chills, high fever, lethargy, and dizziness. Frontal or retroorbital headache may be accompanied by eye pain and photophobia, blurring of vision, mild myalgia, and generalized aching. Severe abdominal and back pain, anorexia, nausea, and vomiting are common, and laparotomy has been mistakenly performed in some cases. Diarrhea, when it occurs, may be severe. There may also be an unproductive cough [*39,40,44*].

On examination there is a typical erythematous flush of the face, especially extending to the supraorbital ridges, and spreading to the neck, shoulders, and upper thorax with blanching on pressure and dermatographia. There is periorbital and subscleral edema, and conjunctivas later may become injected with subconjunctival hemorrhages (Fig. 75-3*D*). Petechiae on the soft palate and axillae are almost invariable, and may spread to the face, neck, upper thorax, and axillary folds, as well as the hips and thighs. The characteristic triad of flushed face including the periorbital area, periorbital edema, and palatal and axillary petechiae is helpful and apparently specific in diagnosis in endemic areas. Injected soft palate and tonsils are not accompanied by sore throat, but some patients complain of pain on swallowing. The liver may occasionally be palpable, and the abdomen is soft, but commonly there is abdominal and renal angle tenderness.

Many patients make an uneventful though slow recovery after this phase, but some deteriorate, entering the hypotensive phase, which usually begins as the temperature falls toward

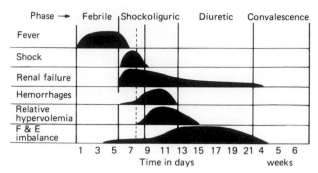

Figure 75-8. Clinical stages and course of illness of patients hospitalized with hemorrhagic fever with renal syndrome. F&E = fluid and electrolytes.

normal. If fever persists with hypotension, the prognosis is poor. Shock may occur by day 3, but usually not before day 5 or 6. This is mild and short-lived in most patients, but in some it can be severe. Bleeding and increased number of petechiae may be seen, and occasionally severe bleeding with convulsions and death. In practice the oliguric phase follows within 24 h of the onset of shock and often overlaps with the hypotensive phase. Renal function deteriorates, and the patient may become anuric and require dialysis. Recovery is then usually rapid, though hypertensive episodes may occur, and diuresis may be marked. Occasional deaths may still occur due to intracranial bleeding. Reports of case fatality range from 1 percent to 10 percent, but overall about 4 percent can be expected in *Apodemus* areas. Improvements in these rates usually result from physician experience in managing the particular problems associated with this disease.

The white blood cell count may be elevated, usually between 10,000 and 20,000, and immature granulocytes are seen at the end of the first week. Though lymphocytic cells become predominant during the second week of illness, a marked neutrophilia has also been reported. Thrombocytopenia, which may be drastic, is a uniform finding, with about half of the patients having less than 100,000 platelets per milliliter, with recovery of normal circulating counts by about the tenth day of illness. In addition it has recently been shown that the remaining circulating platelets do not function normally in in vitro aggregation tests in response to challenge with ADP and collagen. A raised hematocrit characterizes the hemoconcentration mainly during the shock/oliguric phase of the illness, and during the phase of uncontrolled diuresis. Proteinuria is profuse, and biochemical evidence of renal failure reflects the degree of oliguria/anuria. Liver function tests are only mildly affected, and there is no evidence of direct CNS involvement.

Urban disease acquired from rats is apparently less severe, and the disease in Scandinavia acquired from voles has traditionally been described as a separate entity, *nephropathia epidemica (NE)*, which is considered to be milder still. Hemorrhage and shock are unusual, oliguria is rarely severe enough to warrant dialysis, and fatal outcome is virtually unknown

[*39,44,46*]. However, severe cases have been reported from France and from Greece and the Balkan countries. In Greece another *Apodemus* species has been implicated. Currently the distinction between the Asian HFRS and European NE has become less clear. In North America viruses have been isolated, and serological evidence of human infection observed; however, human disease has not been reported, and the viruses may be silent in humans. It is possible that a mosaic of viruses with varying virulence exists, and prospective studies are needed to understand the true epidemiology of various strains and human disease.

Diagnosis

Laboratory diagnosis of *Hantavirus* infections can be made by demonstration of a rise in specific antibodies, demonstration of virus-specific IgM, and virus isolation. Serological assays include immunofluorescence, which though simple may produce false positives. Enzyme-linked immunoassays, including IgM capture assays, may supplant other serological assays. Antibodies persist for up to three decades. Sera react to highest titer with antigens from their own area, but in general sera from European cases react to higher titer with Asian strains than Asian sera with European strains. Virus neutralization is strain-specific, and though laborious is at present the only method available for obtaining some evidence of probable infecting strain. Several of the *Hantavirus* epitopes appear to be conformationally dependent, so that radioimmunoprecipitation, rather than Western blot, may be better in detecting antibody to individual viral proteins. Current efforts to obtain protein sequences are making possible the preparation of individual DNA probes and peptides which may eventually be helpful in determining strain differences both in serological tests, and when probing tissue specimens from wild-caught rodents.

Virus isolation requires careful handling, transport, and storage of specimens at −70°C and is labor-intensive. It should be attempted only under Biosafety Level P3 conditions. The E6 clone of Vero cells may be used, and for greater sensitivity, isolation may be made in young gerbils or by inoculation of suckling mouse or gerbil brain. A range of monoclonal antibodies is available for identification of isolates.

Pathology and pathophysiology

The clinical hallmark of severe HFRS and NE is extreme vascular instability with shock, oliguria/anuria, and bleeding [*40*]. There is widespread capillary leakage leading to extravasation of fluid and protein colloid far in excess of the loss of erythrocytes. This results in hypovolemic shock and, in severe cases, in adult respiratory distress syndrome. Endothelial cells do not appear histologically to be damaged. There is no evidence of direct invasion and lytic replication by the virus, though immunofluorescent studies in mice and humans show viral antigen on endothelium. It is possible that immune complexes or just virus may become adherent, or the virus may establish a nonlytic infection. In this way, or possibly indirectly via host-derived acute-phase cytokines, subtle damage results in biochemical and functional failure of these cells. The cause of the bleeding remains obscure, though reduction in platelet numbers and failure of platelet function must be important. There is little evidence for consumption coagulopathy or bleeding due to hepatic injury. DIC has been reported occasionally in fatal cases, but this is likely to be no more than a complicating terminal event, and not a feature of the primary bleeding disorder [*39,40*].

Pathological changes are reported from fatal cases, thus reflecting the severe end of the spectrum [*40*]. Vascular changes are very prominent and are characterized by capillary dilatation, erythrocyte diapedesis, focal hemorrhages, interstitial edema, and gross retroperitoneal edema. The capillary engorgement and focal hemorrhages are seen in the skin, several surface mucous membranes, and in many organs. Major findings include subendocardial hemorrhages, especially in the right atrium and atrial appendage, and hemorrhagic necrosis of the pituitary gland. These are especially prominent in those dying in the early phases of illness. Kidneys are large and edematous, with marked medullary hemorrhage. There is commonly interstitial edema of the cortex with distension of Bowman's capsule and renal tubules by homogeneous eosinophilic deposits. Electron microscopy shows intranuclear aggregates in renal tubular cells which may be viral. In about 30 percent of cases, mild focal hepatic necrosis is seen in the outer zonal portion of lobules. In the lungs, pulmonary edema is a frequent and prominent finding, but pulmonary hypertension is excluded by normal cardiac size. Occasionally cerebral edema and hemorrhages are seen.

Patient management and antiviral therapy

Recent studies have shown that intravenous ribavirin may also be useful in HFRS if given early in disease. Since the disease may be immunologically mediated, treatment with immune plasma would be inappropriate.

Management of the patient rests mainly on the fluid balance problems, which are notorious. Intravenous fluids during the febrile and shock phases will leak into the tissues, aggravating edema, particularly during the period of oliguria. Severe pulmonary edema may result in death. Patients may respond temporarily to vasopressors, but their use seems limited. In China cyclophosphamide has been used presumably to inhibit immune complex damage, and though reports are favorable, rigorous controlled clinical trials are needed. Diuretics are relatively ineffective, and peritoneal or hemodialysis may be lifesaving in rare cases. Most cases, with cautious management of circulatory volume, will make a spontaneous and complete recovery with no residual renal involvement. Uncontrolled hemorrhage remains the most intractable cause of death, but therapy such as use of heparin is probably dangerous and contraindicated.

POPULATION

Ecology and epidemiology

Reports of HFRS from the U.S.S.R., China, and Korea are generally of epidemic rural disease in agricultural or sylvatic settings, and/or sporadic and epidemic urban disease. Rural epidemics occur in early summer and late fall. These are thought to be temporally related to harvests, and migration of field rodents, particularly movement into houses at the onset of cold weather. Furthermore, the fall peak is apparently associated with *Apodemus* infections and the spring peak with *Rattus*. The disease was noted to be highly associated with dust production in a study of forest workers, and in France aerosol infection has also been implicated. During the numerous reports of epidemics during military campaigns, infections have been associated with trench warfare and bivouaks in the open.

Epidemics in the People's Republic of China have been increasing in size and can be massive in some rural areas, creating a major public health problem. In Korea, much of the disease is sporadic with fewer large clusters of cases. In Europe, especially Scandinavia, the disease is rural and associated with forestry or agricultural pursuits. The disease is sporadic, not epidemic, but most cases occur in winter.

Urban disease such as reported originally from Japan, and now from Korea and China, is sporadic and endemic, and is associated with crowded, rat-infested housing [39]. The disease is apparently milder. It is possible that the scale of this problem is not yet appreciated, especially in some densely populated Asian urban centers.

Institutional epidemics associated with laboratory rats have also been recorded in several countries, including the U.S.S.R., Japan, and Belgium, and persistently infected laboratory rodents, and indeed some continuous cell lines, may be a hazard [45,46].

There is no evidence for the spread of this virus from person to person, and no nosocomial transmission has been reported. The overwhelming evidence is that spread is from rodent to human through contact with infected rodent secretions or airborne transmission by infected dust particles.

It is clear that the diseases of this complex can be transmitted to persons of any age, and depending only on the ecological setting and opportunities for rodent-human contact. In rural areas mostly adult males are affected, especially forestry and agricultural workers, but in urban and densely populated rural areas both sexes and all age groups are involved, with increased risk associated with poor housing. In the U.S.S.R. those tending periurban gardens are exposed, and in Scandinavia individuals with summer homes, with rodent contact usually in sheds or barns [44].

Case fatalities vary widely, affected not only by the level of care given to the severely ill, but also by the particular infecting virus. However, the original distinctions are becoming less clear, and investigations are needed to focus on the details of association between the patient and the rodent reservoir. Trapping and identification of rodents from the patient's surroundings are essential elements in confirming the source of infection. Although the emergence of *Hantavirus* as a new genus of the Bunyaviridae might suggest vector transmission, there is now sufficient accumulated evidence to show that though mite transmission in particular remains conceivable, vector transmission is not the most important source of human infection, and is also unlikely to be of major importance in rodent-to-rodent spread.

Control

There are no rodentborne diseases for which completely effective control has been accomplished. Bolivian hemorrhagic fever is a disease that has been very sharply reduced by *Calomys* control, but this rodent host is not widespread. The variety of rodents and their ubiquity and success in many ecological settings make the control of hantaviruses by rodent control virtually impossible. Clearly, improvement of housing, and particularly food storage, will help prevent those cases caused by rodent invasion of houses. However, a large number of cases occur in rural settings associated with agricultural and forestry activities which are not so amenable to rodent exclusion. Education of populations to avoid rodents in these circumstances may only have marginal effect since the virus may be airborne.

Vaccination appears to be the best prospect for control. Use of a killed virus is feasible, and may be effective since long-lasting neutralizing antibodies result from natural infection, but the virus does not easily grow to high titer, so such a vaccine would be expensive to produce and supplies would probably be limited. In addition, it is not clear whether neutralizing antibodies alone would protect from aerosol spread. Genetic engineering techniques are being used to produce candidate recombinant vaccinia viruses, or to produce viral proteins. However, studies on the strain variation likely to be encountered in a target population and on the epitope recognition involved in protection are needed in order to design an effective, safe vaccine with broad enough specificity to protect against a variety of strains.

CONGO-CRIMEAN HEMORRHAGIC FEVER

AGENT

General ecology

Congo-Crimean hemorrhagic fever (CCHF) is a conspicuous clinical entity whose history dates to antiquity in south central Asia [49]. It emerged in the modern literature at the end of World War II when Soviet medical attention was drawn to outbreaks of disease which occurred in the wartorn Crimean peninsula. Clinically similar to the apparently more lethal central Asian hemorrhagic fever, this syndrome was observed to be associated with transmission to humans by ixodid ticks and was postulated to be a virus. When at length in 1966 the causative agent was isolated it was found to be immunologically virtually indistinguishable from Congo virus, previously recovered from humans in Zaire [50]. This virus was eventually named *Congo-Crimean hemorrhagic fever (CCHF) virus*. Its tickborne ecology has been amply confirmed [49].

Molecular viology and classification

The virion morphology of CCHF places it as a member of the Bunyaviridae, a very large family of related viruses, most of which are animal viruses and transmitted by insects [42]. It consists of a sphere of 85 to 100 nm in diameter with a unit membrane and regular surface projections. Subunit detail has not been resolved microscopically nor has the intracellular morphogenesis of this agent been elucidated, but it is likely that these properties are similar to those reported for other bunyaviruses such as the California encephalitis complex (see Chap. 71).

Because of the extreme biohazard involved in work with CCHF, most work has been done with closely related but less dangerous nairoviruses, to which genus it belongs, principally Hazara virus. Like all Bunyaviridae, the nairoviruses possess a tripartite RNA genome which is negative-sense, and thus inherently not infectious. However, they differ from other members of this large viral family in the molecular weights of the respective genomic segments which are approximately 4.3, 1.5, and 0.6×10^6 Da. The nucleocapsid core protein is about 50 kDa, and the two glycosylated surface and membrane proteins 75 and 30 kDa. In addition to recognized antigenic relationships, these properties are now used to distinguish the genus *Nairovirus* within the Bunyaviridae. The CCHF agent is the prototype of this taxon [42].

CCHF virions also contain lipids essential for infectivity as evidenced by the fact that CCHF is sensitive to organic lipid solvents. It is readily inactivated at pH of about 5 or lower, and is highly thermolabile unless suspended in a protein-rich menstruum.

The virus replicates in a variety of mammalian cell cultures, but is variably cytolytic, and does not shut off host-cell protein synthesis. It is difficult to achieve high infectious titers in tissue culture, but CCHF can also be grown in cell lines of tick origin, which appears to produce high-titer virus for laboratory studies. The virus is notorious for overproduction of nucleocapsid antigen and almost certainly defective interfering particles.

Animal models

No animal has yet been found which reproduces, even grossly, the clinical syndrome induced in humans by CCHF virus. Guinea pigs, rabbits, and several species of old world monkeys experience a transient fever following infection without overt signs of disease and subsequently develop virus-specific antibodies. A single baboon that was infected exhibited a morbilliform rash and was found on skin biopsy to have histological hemorrhage and inflammation. The virus produces fatal, predominantly encephalitic, disease in suckling, but not in adult albino mice.

Infection and host response

The route of infection of this virus in humans is not known, but there is strong circumstantial evidence that it may be transmitted by tick bite, handling or crushing ticks, or by contact with infected animal blood [49,51]. The agent replicates rapidly in a site or sites as yet unknown. Incubation periods can be as short as 3 days, suggesting hematogenous inoculation. Onset can be very sudden and dramatic with severe headache and prostration developing within a few hours, accompanied by high fever and incapacitating chills. Virus can easily be isolated from peripheral blood during the period of fever, and the disease runs a course of about 7 to 10 days, regardless of clinical severity of illness. Whether there is a direct relationship between quantitative viremia and disease severity is unknown. Virus is widely distributed in visceral tissues and its recovery at autopsy in particular organs appears to be related to temporal evolution of illness at time of death. IFA appear at about day 10, and neutralizing immunoglobulins are produced. If patients survive infection they are presumably immune for life. Persistence of antibodies over a 5-year period after infection is directly related to severity of clinical disease.

PATIENT

Clinical manifestations

The initial syndrome consists of severe headache, fever, chills, myalgia strongly localized to the lower back, joint pains, and epigastric pain. There may be associated conjunctivitis and a flushed tinge in the face and chest. Pharyngeal hyperemia and petechiae on the palate are frequent. Bradycardia is typical; occasional patients may exhibit diarrhea. The fever may be high (40°C). Patients are anorectic, irritable, or obtunded, and in evident great distress. Beginning 3 to 5 days after onset, signs of hemorrhagic diathesis may occur. Bleeding from the gums and epistaxis are common. Hematuria, proteinuria, and azotemia are common in severe forms of disease. If so, prognosis is poor. Bleeding may occur from virtually every orifice and from venipuncture sites, with development of sometimes spectacular, huge pressure-linked ecchymoses (Fig. 75-3*E*). There is biochemical evidence of hepatocellular damage, which may progress to severe hepatic impairment, particularly in those cases with uncontrolled bleeding. Pulmonary edema and hypovolemic shock, due to both leaky capillaries and blood loss, are the harbingers of fatal outcome. In severe cases the combination of very low platelet counts and hepatorenal failure may lead to DIC, but the relative importance in the bleeding phenomenon of this is at present unclear. Indeed, it may be different in different patients and at various stages of the disease. A variety of neurological signs has been described, but these bespeak encephalopathy rather than viral encephalitis, meningitis, or myelitis. Changes in affect and mood, including aggressive behavior, are described. Recovery after such massive generalized toxic insult may be slow. Results of serosurveys suggest that subclinical or asymptomatic infections occur.

Leukopenia may be profound with an early predominance of polymorphonuclear cells, giving way to a marked relative and absolute lymphopenia after 7 to 10 days. Drastic thrombocytopenia is common, with counts below 20,000 frequently encountered. Liver function tests may show marked hepatocellular dysfunction, and subsequent severe impairment of renal function.

Pathophysiology and pathology

Viremia, thrombocytopenia, lymphopenia, and eosinophilic necrosis of the liver (Councilman bodies are present) without inflammatory reaction are prominent. There is lymphoid depletion with necrosis of red and white pulp conspicuous in the spleen. Hemorrhages are widely distributed in many organs and death in this disease is often partially attributable to blood loss. The basic changes, however, most resemble those noted in Marburg and Ebola disease. Thus it seems highly possible that DIC is also important in the pathogenesis of CCHF although definitive hematological studies have not been reported and pathological evidence at autopsy for this syndrome is lacking [51].

Bacterial pneumonia and visceral sepsis may be present. This is the only finding which suggests immunological dysfunction and the available data point to direct viral damage rather than to immunopathology as the cause of clinical disease. CCHF virions were readily visualized by electron microscopy in hepatocytes of three patients studied in Iraq.

Diagnosis

Diagnosis of CCHF infection is made by identification of the agent in blood of acutely ill patients or by immunological methods. Suckling mice are highly susceptible to infection and antigens or virions can be recovered from brain 3 to 6 days following inoculation and identified by complement-fixation (CF), agar gel diffusion, hemagglutination-inhibition (HI), enzyme-linked immunoassay, neutralization, or immunofluorescence (IF) techniques. Several types of cultured cells may be used to isolate virus strains but in most cases infection is not cytolytic. The virus is fairly stable in blood for up to 10 days at 4°C, but transport at −50°C or less is important for virus isolation [51].

Acute and convalescent paired sera are used to demonstrate an increase in virus-specific antibodies. The IF method provides the earliest response (7 to 10 days after onset of illness). Neutralizing antibodies persist for many years.

Management

Specific Measures. Attempts by Soviet workers to treat acute CCHF with immune plasma have met with little success, with no difference in duration of viremia, fever, or in clinical outcome for 61 persons given 60 to 160 mL of plasma containing CCHF antibodies as compared to 88 subjects who received normal plasma. The virus is sensitive to ribavirin in vitro and at present it seems that intravenous therapy early in disease is a potential approach, but clinical trials are needed.

Supportive. In addition to the careful management of fluid and electrolyte dynamics during the acute stages of disease, CCHF is the hemorrhagic fever in which whole blood, platelets, and fresh plasma may be indicated.

Isolation. Together with Lassa, Marburg, and Ebola viruses, CCHF, especially outside Africa, is an agent known for its propensity to produce nosocomial and intrafamilial secondary infection. Infectious blood and vomitus are the most likely vehicles of such transmission. Thus strict isolation, restriction of attendant personnel, and observance of enteric precautions are the minimum essentials to limit exposure of patient caregivers (for details see "Management" under "Arenaviruses.")

POPULATION

Ecology and epidemiology

CCHF virus is a parasite of ixodid (hard) ticks [49]. These arthropods develop from eggs through three successive stages: larva, nymph, and adult. A blood meal is generally required at each postembryonic stage and both sexes actively seek vertebrate hosts for this purpose. Transovarial transmission of CCHF virus has been documented for a least one of the major tick vectors, and transstadial transmission for several others. Thus it is likely that ixodid ticks serve as both reservoir and vector of this agent.

Isolates of CCHF virus have been made from at least 24 species and subspecies of ixodid ticks, belonging to seven distinct genera. These in turn may be divided into arthropods having very distinct behavior, perhaps of importance in virus maintenance, but highly significant in terms of the natural ecology of infection of vertebrates, including humans. Thus CCHF virus can be found in ticks of one-, two-, or three-host types, and infects ticks with a wide host range.

The best-studied tick hosts are *Hyalomma marginatum marginatum* of southeastern Europe and the Caspian region, and *H. anatolicum anatolicum,* found in drier areas in south central Asia [49]. Each is a two-host species, the larva molting to nymph on the same animal, feeding, then falling away to molt to an adult which must find a new host animal. Immature stages of the former species generally parasitize ground-living or ground-feeding small vertebrates including birds, whereas adults prefer large domestic animals and avidly attack humans. In contrast, all stages of *H. a. anatolicum* feed predominantly on large domestic animals, even though nymphs leave the host to molt to adults. In each case it is presumably the adult tick which transmits infection to humans. Geographical differences in biological behavior have important consequences for the epidemiology of CCHF.

Tick behavior leads to many domestic and wild animals and birds becoming infected with CCHF virus. Certain birds such as rooks are not infected when bitten by infectious ticks and thus play no direct role in the cycle of viral maintenance, but tick transport on birds may account for the wide geographical distribution of the virus. Other animals, such as hares, cattle, sheep, and goats, become infected and develop viremia which may serve to amplify virus infection in tick populations. Since infected ticks can survive winter, unless periods of sustained freezing occur, and support transovarial passage they are the critical reservoirs as well as vectors of CCHF.

Human epidemiology

The incubation period is short, generally about 2 to 5 days, probably as a consequence of direct hematogenous infection from ticks or other means. The infectious dose of virus delivered by ticks is not known. Nosocomial infections may have a slightly longer incubation of 5 to 9 days.

The seasonality of CCHF depends on the region and the principal tick species involved [49,51,52]. In the lower Volga and Don river basins of the U.S.S.R. where *H. m. marginatum* is the main vector, the disease occurs almost exclusively in the spring months of April to June when adult ticks become active. In the Balkans, central Asia, and the Middle East, where *H. a. anatolicum* and other ticks which feed exclusively on domestic animals are the vectors, seasonality is much less pronounced, although more cases are generally registered in the warmer months. Autumnal sheep shearing has been noted to represent an activity of excess risk of infection. In Africa, human illness, usually nonhemorrhagic, has been documented only sporadically and no clear seasonal pattern has emerged. In the last few years, however, CCHF has emerged as an important sporadic disease in the arid farming areas favoring high tick populations, with peaks in the spring and fall coinciding with maximum tick infestation [51].

Few studies have addressed the question of illness-to-infection ratio. In the southern U.S.S.R. it was found that 1 in 5 infections resulted in clinical illness requiring medical attention. Data from a recent study in an endemic region of South Africa show that illness-to-infection ratios in this area are high (70 percent of those with evidence of past infection had a history of CCHF disease with hospitalization). These observations may be explained by differences in the ability to identify illness and or infections in given areas, or possibly differences in pathogenicity of viruses circulating. Mild or inapparent infection appears to be the rule for most mammalian species, with the exception of humans.

The case fatality in CCHF appears to vary widely but may actually depend in great part on the relative availability of medical and diagnostic services. It has been suggested, how-

ever, that there is marked strain difference in virulence, but there is no objective evidence for this or for the existence of more than one CCHF virus able to infect humans. In the southern U.S.S.R. where disease surveillance is good, milder disease forms are often noted and fatalities have rarely exceeded 5 to 10 percent in recent years. In South Africa where records have been kept since 1981, and good medical facilities and surveillance are available, up to 1986 the case fatality was 35 percent [51]. In central Asia and the Middle East reports are from 35 to 50 percent, and in nosocomial outbreaks the figure has been higher.

In the U.S.S.R., CCHF is a disease of adults of both sexes engaged in the handling and/or milking of cattle. Incidence is a function of sex division in agricultural practice. Milkmaids in some areas and sheep handlers in others appear to be at greatest risk. In central Asia and Iraq CCHF occurs nearly equally in males and females and among persons of all age groups. This is because the disease is "peridomestic" and may occur even in urban areas, where people live in very close daily proximity to sheep, goats, and camels and the associated infected ticks. The only case-control study of risk factors in human infections is in South Africa, and this did not show positive association with ticks or animal slaughter. It did, however, show association with handling of young sheep to vaccinate, castrate, cut ear notches, and dock tail, and with handling of goats. This study also showed that though antibody prevalence in domestic animals was high (15 percent of sheep, 39 percent of cattle, and 53 percent of goats), evidence of human infection was only 2.7 percent, and these were individuals such as farmers and farm laborers who handled animals daily.

Accumulated experience suggests that transmission of CCHF virus occurs through contamination by blood or infected material from animals or other humans, or through bites of infected ticks. The high prevalence in endemic areas of anti-CCHF antibodies in domestic animals and the relatively lower prevalence in humans show transmission from animals to humans (whatever the route) to be infrequent. It would appear that animal infection may be associated with brief and low viremia and therefore would only occasionally result in human infection, depending on the type of human-animal interaction. It may also be, based on this recent study in South Africa, that young animals (less than 6 months) attain higher and more prolonged viremia, presenting an increased hazard to humans. These studies need to be confirmed.

Missing from these studies are the correlations of animal infection, tick infestation, and population of ticks infected. It is clear that tick bites are frequent in persons living among domestic animals in CCHF endemic areas.

The relatively low prevalence of CCHF infection therefore suggests that relatively few of these bites result in infection, either because of low infection in ticks or inefficiency of virus transmission to humans. This latter point is especially poorly understood.

Epidemic investigations

The central issue begging for careful epidemiological investigations is that of virus transmission to humans and domestic animals. Such investigations therefore require a multidisciplinary approach, simultaneously examining infection in ticks, animals, and humans, by collecting materials suitable for virological and serological studies, as well as studies of the infectivity of the ticks. In addition detailed epidemiological studies of human, animal, and tick interaction must be conducted. Other important issues involve clinical epidemiological studies to elucidate the clinical course of disease and risk factors associated with severe disease and secondary human-to-human spread [53].

Prevention

Avoidance of tick bite is the most effective strategy for prevention of infection. Repellents applied to skin, or better, soaked into clothing prior to its use, are the methods of choice. Slaughter of potentially viremic animals is also a hazard, and care should be taken to avoid contamination of cuts or mucous membranes. Similarly, care of infected patients should avoid blood contact, and high-risk procedures such as mouth-to-mouth resuscitation are to be avoided [29].

A formalin-inactivated CCHF vaccine produced from brains of suckling mice has been reported and is currently used in Bulgaria in high-risk groups, such as farmers and border guards, but no efficacy data are available.

Control

Soviet scientists have employed 2 percent hypochlorite in efforts to control virus-transmitting tick species. When used for dipping dairy cattle, this material was said to reduce tick infestation and infection rates among milkmaids. When applied at the rate of 50 to 100 L/ha to pastures, reasonable control of adult ticks was achieved for about 6 weeks, and even better, longer-lasting results were achieved with immature stages that are the age class of virus transmitters for the following years. Nature itself may be an even more effective, if uncontrollable, weapon. In the Rostov region of the U.S.S.R., an exceptionally cold winter in 1968–1969 was followed by a fourfold reduction in disease in 1969 and the complete absence of human infection in 4 of the succeeding 5 years. *H. m. marginatum* virtually disappeared, but the cold-resistant *Rhipicephalus rossicus,* which rarely attacks humans, showed no such decline and continued to maintain CCHF. Since 1975 both *H. m. marginatum* and human disease have again increased.

OMSK HEMORRHAGIC FEVER

Caused by a flavivirus closely related to agents which cause tickborne encephalitis and Kyasanur Forest disease (KFD) (see Chap. 71), this tickborne syndrome was first recognized in 1943 and is limited to an area in northwestern Soviet Siberia

to and from which human travel is so strictly controlled that it is unlikely that non-Soviet physicians will ever encounter a case. The brief description here provided is thus for purposes of scientific documentation only [54].

AGENT

Little work of a basic nature has been reported for OHF virus. It almost certainly shares properties with other tickborne flaviviruses and possesses cross-reactive antigens with these agents. Indeed by the commonly used HI technique, OHF and tickborne encephalitis virus are virtually indistinguishable. Neutralization reactions in mice have been employed to distinguish these viruses, which occur in partially overlapping geographical areas of the U.S.S.R.

Adult and newborn mice, guinea pigs, and muskrats *(Ondatia zibethica)* are lethally infected by OHF virus. Mice experience encephalitic disease while muskrats develop hemorrhagic illness reminiscent of that observed in humans.

PATIENT

OHF is marked by sudden onset of high fever, chills, headache, myalgias, bradycardia, and facial flush after an incubation period of 2 to 9 days. Leukopenia, thrombocytopenia, and fine petechiae with occasional small hemorrhages from various sites are commonly observed. Hypotension is nearly always present, although frank shock is unusual and the mortality rate in this disease is less than 5 percent.

Several other features are distinctive. About half of patients experience a bimodal febrile course lasting up to 20 days. Meningeal signs are noteworthy in most of these patients. Additionally, about 40 percent of patients experience clinical bronchitis or interstitial pneumonia thought in most instances to be viral in origin. This pattern is virtually identical to the range of clinical findings reported for KFD in India.

Pathophysiology and pathology of OHF are poorly elucidated. Viremia is present for a few days early in the clinical course. Liver and kidney damage are minimal, although hemoconcentration, albuminuria, and microscopic hematuria may occur in the occasional severely ill patient. The few autopsy reports call attention to scattered focal hemorrhages, endothelial capillary damage, interstitial pneumonia, focal necrosis with mild inflammatory reaction in brain tissue, and the generally normal appearance of lymphoid tissues.

POPULATION

Ecology

The most important vector of OHF virus for humans is the tick *Dermacentor pictus.* Larvae and nymphs feed on small rodents, and adults, which have population peaks in spring and late summer, seek large animals, including humans, as hosts. Maintenance of the virus in nature is still uncertain. Transovarial transmission in ticks has not been reported. Soviet authors now believe in addition that another tick species, *Ixodes apronophorus,* which feeds exclusively on small rodents, may be important in continuous virus transmission. In addition, infected water voles, *Arvicola* sp., are thought to somehow transmit the virus to muskrats with whom they sometimes share "houses." Muskrats originally introduced into Siberia from Canada in 1929 experienced fatal epizootic infection with OHF virus.

Epidemiology

Although not a common disease, OHF has had two distinctive epidemiological patterns. The first is tickborne disease among agricultural workers with peaks in May and August corresponding well to those of *D. pictus* ticks. The second and more important is winter transmission among male muskrat trappers and skinners, transmission being by direct contact with blood of infected *Ondatra.* In recent years muskrat populations have been so low in the Omsk region that the fur industry based on this introduced species has virtually disappeared, and with it OHF as well. Little was ever learned regarding infection-to-morbidity ratios.

Prevention and control

Soviet workers have applied many of the measures used for tick control of CCHF virus with mixed results. Sparse human population in the region appears to be the most important factor in apparent absence of disease during the past decade. A formalin-inactivated suckling-mouse-brain vaccine was prepared, and it is stated that three injections of the material produced antibodies in most recipients. The product finds greater use in virological laboratories where OHF virus is highly infectious when aerosolized.

REFERENCES

1 Oldstone MBA (ed): *The Arenaviruses. Current Topics in Microbiology and Immunology,* vol 1 and vol 2. New York, Springer-Verlag, 1987

2 McCormick, JB: Arenaviruses. *Field's Virology,* in press, 1989

3 Johnson KM et al: Virus isolations from human cases of hemorrhagic fever in Bolivia. Proc Soc Exp Biol 118:113–118, 1965

4 Mackenzie RB, Beye HK, Valverde L, et al: Epidemic hemorrhagic fever in Bolivia. I. A preliminary report of the epidemiologic and clinical findings in a new epidemic area in South America. Am J Trop Med Hyg 13:620–625, 1964

5 Johnson KM, Halstead SB: Hemorrhagic fevers of Southeast Asia and South America: A comparative appraisal. Prog Med Virol 9:105–158, 1967

6 Maiztegui JI: Clinical and epidemiological patterns of Argentine haemorrhagic fever. Bull WHO 52:567–575, 1975

7 Monath TP, Newhouse VF, Kemp GE, et al: Cacciapouti. A Lassa virus isolation from *Mastomys natalensis* rodents during an epidemic in Sierra Leone. Science 185:263–265, 1974

8 McCormick JB: Epidemiology and Control of Lassa fever. Curr Top Microbiol Immunol 134:69–78, 1987

9 Auperin DD, Romanowski V, Galinski M, et al: Sequencing studies of Pichinde Arenavirus S RNA indicate a novel coding strategy, and ambisense viral S RNA. J Virol 52:897–904, 1984

10 Auperin DD, Sasso DR, McCormick JB: Nucleotide sequence of the glycoprotein gene and intergenic region of the Lassa virus S genome RNA. Virology 154:155–167, 1987

11 Fisher-Hoch SP, McCormick JB: Pathophysiology and treatment of Lassa fever. Curr Top Microbiol Immunol 134:231–240, 1988

12 Jahrling PB, Hesse RA, Eddy GA, et al: Lassa virus infection of rhesus monkeys: Pathogenesis and treatment with ribavirin. J Infect Dis 141:580–589, 1980

13 McCormick JB, Webb PA, Krebs JW, et al: A prospective study of the epidemiology and ecology of Lassa fever. J Infect Dis 155:437–444, 1987

14 Johnson KM, McCormick JB, King IJ, et al: Clinical virology of Lassa fever in hospitalized patients. J Infect Dis 155:456–464, 1987

15 Maiztegui JI, Fernandez NJ, de Damilano AJ: Efficacy of immune plasma in treatment of Argentine Haemorrhagic fever and association between treatment and a late neurological syndrome. Lancet 2:1216–1217, 1979

16 Enria DA, Franco SG, Ambrosio A, et al: Current status of the treatment of Argentine hemorrhagic fever. Med Microbiol Immunol (Berl) 175:173–176, 1986

17 McCormick JB, King IJ, Webb PA, et al: A case-control study of the clinical diagnosis and course of Lassa fever. J Infect Dis 155:445–455, 1987

18 Fisher-Hoch SP, McCormick JB, Sasso D, et al: Hematologic dysfunction in Lassa fever. J Med Virol 26:127–135, 1988

19 Cummins D, Fisher-Hoch SP, Walshe K, et al: A plasma inhibitor of platelet aggregation in patients with Lassa fever. Br J Hematol, in press

20 Price ME, Fisher-Hoch SP, Craven RB, et al: Prospective study of maternal and fetal outcome in acute Lassa fever during pregnancy. Br Med J 297:584–588, 1988

21 Cummins D, McCormick JB, Bennett D, et al: Acute sensorineural deafness in Lassa fever. Submitted for publication

22 Fisher-Hoch SP, Mitchell SW, Sasso DR, et al: Physiological and immunological disturbances associated with shock in a primate model of Lassa fever. J Infect Dis 155:465–474, 1987

23 Walker DH, McCormick JB, Johnson KM, et al: Pathologic and virologic study of fatal Lassa fever in man. Am J Pathol 107:349–356, 1982

24 Fisher-Hoch SP, McCormick JB, Auperin D, et al: Protection of rhesus monkeys from fatal Lassa fever by vaccination with a recombinant vaccinia virus containing the Lassa virus glycoprotein gene. Proc Natl Acad Sci USA 86:317–321, 1989

25 McCormick JB: Arenaviridae: The arenaviruses, in Balows A, Hausler Jr. WJ, Ohashi M, Twano A (eds): *Laboratory Diagnosis of Infectious Diseases. Principles and Practice,* vol 2. New York, Springer-Verlag, 1988, pp 647–662

26 McCormick JB, King IJ, Webb PA, et al: Lassa fever, Effective therapy with ribavirin. N Engl J Med 314:20–26, 1986

27 Fisher-Hoch SP, Price MJ, Craven RB, et al: Safe intensive care management of a severe case of Lassa fever using simple barrier nursing techniques. Lancet 2:1227–1229, 1985

28 Helmick CG, Webb PA, Scribner CL, et al: No evidence for increased risk of Lassa fever infection in hospital staff. Lancet 2:1202–1204, 1986

29 Centers for Disease Control: Management of patients with suspected viral hemorrhagic fevers. MMWR 37:(Suppl)3, 2/26/1988 pp. 1–16

30 Maiztegui JI, Feuillade M, Briggiler A: Progressive extension of the endemic area and changing incidence of Argentine Hemorrhagic Fever. Med Microbiol Immunol (Berl) 175:142–152, 1986

31 Martini GA, Siegert R (eds): *Marburg Virus Disease.* New York, Springer, 1971

32 Pattyn SR (ed): *Ebola Virus Hemorrhagic Fever.* Amsterdam, Elsevier/North Holland, 1978

33 Kiley MP, Cox NJ, Elliott LH, et al: Physicochemical properties of Marburg virus: Evidence for three distinct virus strains and their relationship to Ebola virus. J Gen Virol 69:1957–1967, 1988

34 Sanchez AS, Kiley MP, Auperin DA, et al: The nucleoprotein gene of Ebola virus: Cloning, sequencing, and in vitro expression. Submitted for publication

35 Fisher-Hoch SP, Platt GS, Neild GH, et al: Pathophysiology of shock and hemorrhage in a fulminating viral infection (Ebola). J Infect Dis 152:887–894, 1985

36 Report of an International Commission. Ebola haemorrhagic fever in Zaire, 1976. Bull WHO 56:271–293, 1978

37 Report of a WHO International Study Team. Ebola haemorrhagic fever in Sudan, 1976. Bull WHO 56:247–270, 1978

38 Baron RC, McCormick JB, Zubeir OA: Ebola virus disease in southern Sudan: Hospital dissemination and intrafamilial spread. Bull WHO 61:997–1003, 1983

39 Fisher-Hoch SP, McCormick JB: Hemorrhagic fever with renal syndrome: A review. Abstracts on Hygiene and Communicable Diseases 60:R1–R20, 1985

40 Symposium on epidemic fever. Am J Med 16:619–709, 1954

41 Smorodintsev AA, Chumakov VG, Churilov AV (trans Matthews): Excerpts from *Haemorrhagic Nephros-Nephritis,* New York, Pergamon, 1959, pp 27–119

42 Bishop DHL: Bunyaviridae. *Field's Virology,* 1989, in press

43 Schmaljohn CS, Hasty SE, Dalrymple JM, et al: Antigenic and genetic properties place viruses linked to hemorrhagic fever with renal syndrome into a newly-defined genus of Bunyaviridae. Science 227:1041–1044, 1985

44 Lahdevirta J: Nephropathia epidemica in Finland. A clinical histological and epidemiological study. Ann Clin Res 3(suppl)8:1–54, 1971

45 Kulagin SM, Fedorova NI, Ketiladze ES: A laboratory outbreak of haemorrhagic fever with renal syndrome (clinical-epidemiological functions). Zh Mikrobiol Epidemiol Immunobiol (Moscow) 33(10):121–126, 1962

46 Desmyter J, LeDuc JW, Johnson KM, et al: Laboratory rat associated outbreak of haemorrhagic fever with renal syndrome due to Hantaan-like virus in Belgium. Lancet 2:1445–1448, 1983

47 Lee HW, Lee PW, Johnson KM: Isolation of the etiologic agent of Korean hemorrhagic fever. J Infect Dis 137:298–308, 1978

48 McCormick JB, Sasso DR, Palmer EL, et al: Morphological identification of the agent of Korean hemorrhagic fever (Hantaan virus), as a member of the Bunyaviridae. Lancet 1:765–768, 1982

49 Hoogstraal H: The epidemiology of tick-borne Crimean-Congo hemorrhagic fever in Asia, Europe, and Africa. J Med Entomol 15:304–417, 1979

50 Simpson DIH, Knight EM, Courtois G, et al: Congo virus: A hitherto undescribed virus occurring in Africa. I. Human isolations—clinical notes. East Afr Med J 44:87–92, 1967

51 Swanepoel R, Shephard AJ, Leman PA, et al: Epidemiologic and clinical features of Crimean-Congo hemorrhagic fever in southern Africa. Am J Trop Med Hyg 36:120–132, 1987

52 Yu-Chen Y, Ling-Xiong K, Ling L, et al: Characteristics of Crimean-Congo hemorrhagic fever virus (Xinjiang strain) in China. Am J Trop Med Hyg 34:1179–1182, 1985

53 Burney MI, Ghafoor A, Saleen M, et al: Nosocomial outbreak of viral hemorrhagic fever caused by Crimean hemorrhagic fever-Congo virus in Pakistan, January 1976. Am J Trop Med Hyg 29:941–947, 1980

54 Mazhbich IB, Netsky GI: Three years of study of Omsk hemorrhagic fever (1946–1948). Trud Omsk Inst Epidemiol Mikrobiol Gigien 1:51–67, 1952 (NAMRU-3 Translation #333)

CHAPTER 76 / # Retroviruses and the Human Immunodeficiency Syndrome

· *Robert Colebunders* · *Thomas C. Quinn*

In 1981, physicians in the United States reported the unusual occurrence of opportunistic infections such as *Pneumocystis carinii* pneumonia and Kaposi's sarcoma in previously healthy homosexual men. Characteristic of these cases was an underlying severe cell-mediated immune suppression caused primarily by the loss of T helper (CD4+) lymphocytes. This condition was termed the *acquired immunodeficiency syndrome (AIDS).*

Since the original reports, there has been an extraordinary escalation in the number of reported cases of AIDS worldwide [1]. In March 1988, the World Health Organization (WHO) estimated that there were over 150,000 cases of AIDS, approximately 500,000 cases of AIDS-related complex (ARC), and 5 to 10 million persons infected with the etiological agent of this syndrome, the human immunodeficiency virus (HIV-1). While an estimated 2 to 3 million of these asymptomatic carriers are estimated to reside in the United States and Europe, the majority of asymptomatic carriers of HIV-1 are located in the countries of central Africa. It is from the human reservoir of asymptomatic people that HIV will be transmitted to other persons and in whom additional cases of AIDS will occur. Since many of these cases will be diagnosed among people in developing countries, AIDS will undoubtedly create an enormous social and political economic strain on these countries. With an 80 percent case-fatality rate 2 years from time of diagnosis and with the current lack of effective curative drugs or vaccines, AIDS has become an unprecedented major health problem of this century.

PARASITE

TAXONOMY

By 1984, intensive clinical, epidemiological, immunological, and virological investigations firmly established that the causative agent of AIDS was a retrovirus that infected T helper (CD4+) lymphocytes and mononuclear phagocytes and induced loss of immunological function due in part to a destruction of infected cells. Initially, the AIDS virus was referred to as *lymphadenopathy-associated virus (LAV)* [2], *human T-lymphotropic virus type III (HTLV-III)* [3], and *AIDS-related virus (ARV)* [4]. In May 1986, an international committee on viral nomenclature renamed the virus the *human immunodeficiency virus (HIV)*, since the above prototype viruses identified by individual scientists were shown to be essentially the same virus. In 1986, additional studies of AIDS patients from west Africa identified another closely related but distinct retrovirus associated with the clinical condition of AIDS [5]. Because it had greater than 50 percent heterogenicity, it was referred to as HIV-2, in comparison to the original AIDS virus, which was then renamed HIV-1. An additional retrovirus, identified in African green monkeys and captive macaques, is called the simian immunodeficiency virus (SIV or, previously, STLV-III). HIV-1, HIV-2, and SIV appear to be related in terms of morphology, cell tropism, in vitro cytopathic effect on CD4+ cells, and overall genetic organization. After cloning of these isolates, genomic analysis indicated that HIV-1 and HIV-2 share a similar genomic organization, suggesting a common evolutionary origin, but that they differ markedly in terms of nucleotide sequences. The more conserved *gag* and *pol* genes displayed a 56 and 66 percent nucleotide sequence homology, respectively, and less than 60 percent amino acid identity [6]. Calculation of nucleotide sequence homology for the other viral genes, particularly *env* genes, was even lower, making HIV-1 and HIV-2 only 42 percent homologous. Similar genomic studies carried out between HIV-2 and SIV demonstrated that although HIV-2 is more serologically cross-reactive to SIV than HIV-1, HIV-2 has distinct genomic differences from SIV with about 70 percent homology between the two viruses [7]. This suggests that HIV-2 may be evolutionarily more closely related to SIV than to HIV-1. It is highly likely

that a common ancestry—with similar properties and pathogenic potential—existed a long time ago and that divergence of HIV-1, HIV-2, and SIV occurred earlier than at the beginning of the present AIDS epidemic.

MORPHOLOGY

HIV-1 is slightly more than 100 nm in size and has a lipid envelope, a characteristic dense, cylindrical nucleoid containing genomic RNA and the enzyme reverse transcriptase, which makes HIV-1 a retrovirus. The term *retrovirus* denotes that the flow of biological information of the virus is the reverse of that in other cells. The RNA genome of the virus is copied via reverse transcriptase, or RNA-directed DNA polymerase, into a DNA "provirus."

The pathogenic human retroviruses are collectively known as the T-lymphotropic viruses because they preferentially infect T4 (CD4+) lymphocytes. However, these viruses now fall into two distinct taxonomic groups which include the human T-cell leukemia viruses (HTLV-I, HTLV-II) that are classified as oncoviruses, closely related to the bovine leukemia virus, and the lentiviruses. HIV-1 is classified as a lentivirus, because its ultrastructure and genomic organization are similar to those of visna virus, caprine arthritis encephalitis virus (CAEV), and equine infectious anemia virus (EIAV). Likewise, HIV-2 and SIV, because of their similarity to HIV-1, are included in the family of lentiviruses.

The structure of the HIV-1 genome is fundamentally similar to that of other retroviruses in that there are four major genes: group antigens (*gag*), polymerase (*pol*), envelope (*env*), and long terminal repeat (*LTR*) genes (Fig. 76-1). The *LTRs* act as promotors of gene expression and contain specific enhancer elements from which viral and cellular proteins react. The *gag* gene encodes for the 55-kDa precursor polypeptide (p55),

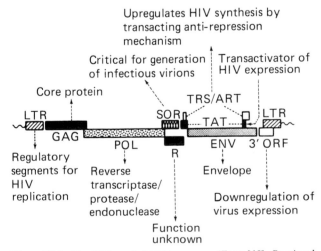

Figure 76-1. The HIV proviral DNA genome. (*From* [19]. *Reprinted with permission.*)

which is cleaved to form three core proteins, p15, p18, and p24. Each of these proteins is immunogenic, and antibodies to the three proteins are commonly detected in the serum of seropositive patients. The *pol* gene encodes for a precursor protein that is cleaved to form reverse transcriptase (p56 and p51), an endonuclease, and a protease that itself serves to cleave the *gag* p55 precursor. The *env* precursor, gp160, is cleaved to form two disulfide-linked envelope glycoproteins, the terminal gp120 and C-terminal gp41, both of which are glycosylated at multiple residues [8]. The gp41 protein is the transmembrane component, whereas gp120 serves as the external glycoprotein with binding specificity for the CD4 receptor on host cells [9].

Four other unique coding sequences include the short open reading frame (*sor*), the 3-prime open reading frame (*3'-orf*), transactivation of transcription (*tat*), and the antirepressor translocator (*art*) gene. Neither the *sor* gene nor the *3'-orf* gene appears to be absolutely necessary for HIV-1 replication in established CD4+ cell lines [10]. However, the *tat* gene appears to play one of the most important roles in viral replication. Viruses in which the *tat* gene has been completely deleted are unable to synthesize structural proteins sufficiently, to replicate, or to cause cytopathic effects, even when the *tat* protein was expressed at high levels from a molecular clone gene [11]. In contrast to *tat,* the *art* gene product will act only on HIV-1 *gag* and *env* messenger RNAs, and the two regulatory genes appear to be complementary. Small changes in these regulatory gene products could determine whether the provirus remains entirely latent in infected cells, shows low levels of antigen expression, or replicates sufficiently to induce cell fusion and other cytopathic effects.

LIFE CYCLE

HIV-1 can replicate in a limited number of cells in the human body, including lymphocytes, macrophages, and cells of the central nervous system. HIV-1 has a specific tropism for the CD4 receptor of the T helper lymphocyte by interaction with its viral envelope protein, gp120 [9]. After specific binding to the CD4 receptor, HIV-1 enters the cytoplasm of the cell via an unknown mechanism. Within the cytoplasm of the cell, the uncoated viral single-stranded RNA is transcribed into double-stranded DNA by the enzyme reverse transcriptase (Fig. 76-2). This double-stranded circular DNA enters the nucleus where it integrates into the host cell DNA. These viral genes may remain integrated for the lifetime of the cell, and hence infection of the individual is life-long. Stimulation of the infected lymphocyte activates viral replication, resulting in viral budding from the lymphocyte, cytolysis of the infected cell, and subsequent infection of other T4 lymphocytes. In vitro activation is achieved by mitogenic, antigenic, or allogeneic stimulation [12].

After replication of the virus during antigenic stimulation of the lymphocyte, syncytial formation and subsequent lysis of the cell occurs with gradual depletion of CD4+ lymphocytes

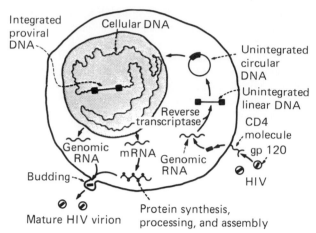

Figure 76-2. The life cycle of HIV. (*From [19]. Reprinted with permission.*)

from circulation. While an infected CD4+ lymphocyte shows a qualitative loss in immunological function, the major immunosuppression induced by HIV-1 is a quantitative effect resulting from the progressive loss of CD4+ lymphocytes. The mechanism for the cytopathic effect of HIV-1 is unknown, but it is hypothesized that the envelope glycoproteins are primarily responsible for the cytopathic effect not only in the cells they have infected but also in noninfected CD4+ cells. HIV-1 may induce cell fusion when virus or virus-infected cells are mixed with uninfected CD4-receptor-bearing cells and culture. The resulting syncytium, or formation of multinucleated giant cells, develops ballooning cytoplasm and lyses within a day. These syncytial cells are composed of both infected and uninfected cells. The uninfected cells are recruited into the syncytium because of the gp120 on the budding virions, which specifically binds to the CD4 molecules on uninfected cells [13]. The observation of large multinucleated cells in infected tissue, such as the brain of AIDS patients, suggests that syncytial induction plays a role in HIV-1 pathogenesis [14].

Another possibility responsible for the pathogenesis of HIV-1 infection is the secretion of gp120 *env* proteins, which bind to the CD4 receptor of noninfected cells, preventing them from functioning properly as helper cells. Autoantibodies may develop that block the function of CD4 antigens as a result of HIV-1 infection, in that coating of the cell with gp120 is recognized as a foreign protein and is cleared by the immune system. It has also been hypothesized that the transmembrane envelope glycoprotein gp41 may exert a direct immunosuppressive effect on the CD4+ cells. Lastly, HIV-1–infected lymphocytes may also become susceptible to the immunosuppressive effect of other antigens. If T cells are first infected with HIV-1 or transformed by HTLV-I, then productive CMV infection can occur in T cells. This type of enhancement, perhaps due to transactivator genes present in both HIV-1 and

HTLV-I, may result in faster depletion of the CD4 lymphocyte populations.

ANIMAL MODELS

The ideal animal model for AIDS would be one in which HIV-1 infects and induces AIDS-like disease in readily available laboratory animals. The only species that has so far reproducibly become infected after inoculation with HIV-1 is the chimpanzee [15]. After inoculation, these animals typically seroconvert with antibodies to HIV-1, and HIV-1 can be repeatedly recovered from the peripheral blood. This is an imperfect animal model in that no clinical disease has ever been demonstrated among these chimpanzees and they remain immunologically intact. However, because chimpanzees can be infected with HIV-1, they will remain a valuable animal model for the testing of HIV-1 vaccines. Unfortunately, there is a shortage of chimpanzees for AIDS research, and additional animal models as discussed below may be required for both immunopathogenic studies of retroviral infection and vaccine development.

The first primate retroviral infection was the Mason-Pfizer monkey virus (MPMV), described in 1970. This is a type D retrovirus that has been isolated from captive macaques in New England, California, Washington, and Oregon regional primate research centers [16]. The clinical disease caused by MPMV is often referred to as simian AIDS (SAIDS) and is characterized by a chronic wasting disease associated with immunological abnormalities, opportunistic infections, and tumors.

Since HIV-1 is classified as a lentivirus, recent attention has focused on other lentiviral infections of animals. The prototypic lentivirus is the maedi-visna virus (MVV), which causes a chronic, progressive interstitial pneumonia and severe demyelinating encephalomyelitis in sheep after an incubation period of months to years. Even though there is no dramatic evidence of immunosuppression, the neurotropism of MVV and its tendency to undergo continuous mutation and antigenic drift in persistently infected sheep provides an interesting animal model for studying these features of HIV-1 in humans [17]. Other lentiviral animal infections include caprine arthritis encephalitis virus (CAEV) and equine infectious anemia virus (EIAV).

Another nonhuman primate lentivirus identified, now called simian immunodeficiency virus (SIV), was isolated from captive rhesus macaques at the New England Regional Primate Center in 1984 [18]. Similar isolates have subsequently been obtained from African green monkeys, sooty mangabeys, and pigtailed macaques. SIV has growth properties and T4 cell tropism nearly identical to HIV-1, and there is a remarkable genomic similarity between SIV and HIV-2. After inoculation of SIV in macaques, the animals may develop diarrhea and profound wasting associated with a quantitative loss of T4 cells within 127 to 160 days. Encephalitis may also occur. In a second pattern of infection, the clinical disease is more chronic with the development of immunosuppression 25 to 68 weeks after inoculation associated with the development of lymphadenopathy.

PATIENT

IMMUNOPATHOGENESIS

Although a large number of immunological abnormalities that accompany HIV-1 infection have been described, all but a few can be attributed to the selective defect in the CD4 subset of T lymphocytes [19]. Since the CD4+ cells have a central role in the immune response, loss of the activity of the T helper subset will consequently compromise the function of other cell types. These defects include abnormalities of both cellular and humoral immunity that may vary in degree and frequency during different clinical stages of HIV-1 infection. There is a trend toward more severe immunological abnormalities, with clinical progression from an asymptomatic state to persistent generalized lymphadenopathy, ARC and AIDS.

Besides the cytopathic effect and possible autoimmune effects of HIV-1, other potential mechanisms of CD4 depletion may be responsible for the progressive depletion of CD4+ precursor or stem cells and may lead to lack of production in mature cells. In addition, HIV-1 might infect and selectively deplete a subset of CD4+ nonlymphoid cells that are critical to the propagation of the entire CD4+ cell pool. In this regard it is known that T4 lymphocytes elaborate factors, including interleukin 2 (IL-2), that are tropic for lymphocytes as well as for cells of the myeloid series. Another potential mechanism of T4 cell depletion is the induction by HIV-1 of soluble factors that are toxic to CD4+ lymphocytes.

In addition to the quantitative depletion of CD4+ lymphocytes, a qualitative or functional defect of a selective subset of CD4+ cells has also been shown [20]. The failure of purified CD4+ cell populations from patients with AIDS to respond to soluble antigens implies that a defect is intrinsic to these cells. Possible explanations for this defect include a selective loss of the subset of the CD4+ cell population. This selective defect in the antigen-reactive cell is supported by the observation that mitogenic responses to pokeweed mitogen are normal in patients with AIDS but that the response to specific soluble protein antigen, tetanus toxoid, is markedly reduced [21]. CD4 cell function may also be inhibited by HIV-1 in absence of infection of the cell. Alternatively, binding of HIV-1 envelope protein to the CD4 molecule of the T4 cell could readily block the critical interaction of this receptor with class II major histocompatibility complex (MHC) molecules. Responses of T4 cells to mitogens are not critically dependent on this CD4–class II MHC molecule interaction; therefore, mitogens might override the block seen with antigen responses [19].

Other immunological abnormalities may also be seen in HIV-1–infected persons. These abnormalities primarily include polyclonal activation with elevated immunoglobulin levels and a poor antibody response to novel antigens [*22*].

Mononuclear phagocytes also appear to be affected by HIV-1, possibly because of loss of T-helper-cell signals or possibly because of direct infection with HIV-1. Certain subsets of monocytes express the CD4 surface antigen and can therefore bind to the envelope of HIV-1. The virus has been isolated from monocytes obtained from the blood and from various organs of HIV-1 infected persons [*19*]. In the brain, the major cell type infected with HIV-1 appears to be the monocyte-macrophage, and this may have important consequences for the development of certain neuropsychiatric manifestations associated with HIV-1 infection [*23*]. Abnormalities of monocyte function in HIV-1–infected persons include defective intracellular killing, nonspecific cytotoxicity, depressed hydrogen peroxide release, and reduced levels of class II HLA antigens. Many of these abnormalities appear to result from a lack of interferon γ, but other reported abnormalities include spontaneous secretion of interleukin 1 (IL-1) and prostaglandin E2 or diminished responses to inducers of IL-1 release.

NATURAL HISTORY

Between 2 and 6 weeks after exposure to HIV-1 about 20 to 30 percent of patients will develop an acute illness [*24*]. Symptoms and signs include fever, sweating, fatigue, rash, swollen lymph nodes, and splenomegaly. An aseptic meningitis with recovery of the virus from the cerebrospinal fluid has also been reported during this acute phase [*25*]. Fever and rash are transitory, but the polyadenopathy and splenomegaly generally persist. Within 1 to 6 months after the acute infection, the infected person develops antibody to HIV-1, most prominently to *gag* and *env* proteins, and may then become asymptomatic for several months to more than 10 years. However, as the virus continues to replicate and selectively destroy and immunologically impair CD4+ lymphocytes, cellular immunosuppression progresses, and the patient eventually develops symptoms. Nearly all patients develop some immunological abnormalities after HIV-1 infection, and the virus can almost always be recovered from circulating lymphocytes during any given period after infection.

The length of time for clinically relevant immunosuppression to occur in an HIV-1–infected person depends on the rate of T-cell activation and subsequent viral replication, which can vary greatly from one person to another. In prospective studies of seropositive persons, factors that influence progression to AIDS include decreased numbers of T helper lymphocytes (less than 300 per cubic millimeter), low level of antibody to HIV-1 (particularly anti-p24), high titer of antibody to cytomegalovirus (CMV), and a history of sex with someone who developed AIDS [*26*]. The mean incubation period for developing AIDS is estimated to be 2 years in children and 8 years in adults [*27*]. Within an estimated 5 years of infection, 20 to 30 percent of HIV-1–infected persons will develop AIDS, and 25 to 50 percent will develop an AIDS-related illness [*28*].

CLINICAL FEATURES

Clinical manifestations of HIV-1 infection differ by geographical region and vary in severity from a healthy carrier state to the manifestations of potentially fatal opportunistic diseases. The clinical spectrum of AIDS in Africa is similar to that observed in the Caribbean but is different from that in the United States.

Different classification systems for HIV-1–related illnesses have been proposed, e.g., the Walter Reed classification system [*29*] and the Centers for Disease Control (CDC) classification system [*30*] (Table 76-1). Patients with ARC are included in groups III and IV of the CDC classification system. ARC patients have similar, but less severe, clinical and immunological abnormalities compared to AIDS patients, and they do not have opportunistic infections or HIV-1–related malignancies. AIDS is the most severe stage of the clinical spectrum of HIV-1 infection, characterized by life-threatening op-

Table 76-1. Centers for Disease Control (CDC) classification of HIV infection

Group I: Acute infection
Group II: Asymptomatic infection
Positive HIV antibody test or viral culture; may be subclassified on the basis of laboratory evaluation.
Group III: Persistent generalized lymphadenopathy
Lymphadenopathy (>1 cm) at 2 or more extrainguinal sites for more than 3 months in the absence of another illness to explain the findings.
Group IV: Other HIV disease
Subgroup A: Constitutional disease
One or more of the following: fever or diarrhea >1 month or involuntary weight loss >10 percent with no other illness to explain the findings.
Subgroup B: Neurological disease
Dementia, myelopathy, or peripheral neuropathy; no other illness to explain the findings.
Subgroup C1: Secondary infectious diseases
Symptomatic disease due to 1 of 12 specified diseases: *P. carinii* pneumonia, chronic cryptosporidiosis, toxoplasmosis, extraintestinal strongyloidiasis, isosporiasis, candidiasis (esophageal, bronchial, or pulmonary), cryptococcosis, histoplasmosis, mycobacterial infection, cytomegalovirus infection, chronic or disseminated herpes simplex virus infection, and progressive multifocal leukoencephalopathy.
Subgroup C2: Other infectious diseases
Symptomatic or invasive disease due to one of the following diseases: oral leukoplakia, multidermatomal herpes zoster, recurrent *Salmonella* bacteremia, nocardiosis, tuberculosis, and oral candidiasis.
Subgroup D: Secondary cancers
Kaposi's sarcoma, non-Hodgkin's lymphoma (small, noncleaved lymphoma or immunoblastic sarcoma), or primary CNS lymphoma.
Subgroup E: Other conditions
Patients with HIV-related illnesses not classifiable in previous groups (e.g., chronic lymphoid interstitial pneumonitis).

portunistic infections and malignancies; AIDS is included in group IV of the CDC classification scheme.

Progressive weight loss is often the first sign of HIV-1 infection. Weight loss, asthenia, anorexia, and intermittent or persistent fever or diarrhea are the most frequent symptoms. A diarrheal wasting syndrome occurs particularly often among AIDS patients in Africa [*31*]. Stools are generally liquid or semiliquid, and blood and mucus are rarely present. Diarrhea can be caused by various bacterial and viral agents, protozoa, and helminths, but in 30 to 50 percent of the cases no specific cause is identified [*32,33*].

A multitude of dermatological manifestations, including Kaposi's sarcoma, herpes zoster, herpes simplex, condyloma acuminata, bacterial folliculitis, onychomycosis, seborrheic dermatitis, and a generalized papular pruritic eruption, have been described among HIV-1–infected patients. In the tropics, a generalized papular pruritic eruption called *prurigo* is observed in approximately 20 percent of AIDS patients [*34*]. It frequently appears early in the infection. The initial skin lesion is a small (1 to 2 mm), firm, intensely pruritic papule. Once papules start appearing, this condition generally persists throughout the course of the patient's illness. Scratched papules later become hyperpigmented macules. These lesions (papules, excoriations, and hyperpigmented macules) are symmetrically distributed over the body but are most frequently found in extremities, especially the extensor surfaces and the backs of the hands, the ankles, and the dorsum of the feet (Fig. 76-3). The lesions are clinically and histologically similar to other forms of chronic prurigo.

HIV-1 can be isolated from brain tissue, spinal cord, peripheral nerves, and cerebrospinal fluid (CSF). Subacute encephalopathy, characterized by progressive mental changes associated with dementia (the AIDS dementia complex), is the most frequent neurological disorder in patients with HIV-1 infection [*35*]. It occurs in about one-third of American AIDS patients. The encephalopathy is insidious in most patients. Initially cognitive dysfunction predominates with loss of concentration and recent memory and mental slowing. Confusion, lack of coordination, social withdrawal, and apathy may also develop. Common early motor signs include tremor and slowness. The encephalopathy usually progresses to severe dementia. Ultimately the patient becomes bedridden, incontinent, and unresponsive. The CSF may be entirely normal or may show a few lymphocytes and an elevation in protein levels. Computed tomography shows cerebral atrophy with prominent sulci and ventricles. A vacuolar myelopathy develops in approximately 20 percent of AIDS patients and is characterized by paraparesis, which may be accompanied by paresthesia. Ataxia, paraplegia, and incontinence occur in severely affected patients. A symmetrical sensorimotor neuropathy with painful dysesthesia sometimes associated with weakness, distal atrophy, and autonomic nervous system involvement has also been described [*36*].

The opportunistic infections and malignancies frequently seen in AIDS patients are shown in Table 76-2. Oral candidiasis is often the first opportunistic infection in an HIV-1–infected person (Fig. 76-4). If oral candidiasis is accompanied by dysphagia, the patient probably has candidal esophagitis.

Cryptococcal meningitis occurs in 5 to 10 percent of AIDS patients with clinical features similar to those observed in other immunodepressed patients (see Chap. 21 [*37–39*]).

Pneumocystis carinii pneumonia (PCP) (see also Chap. 33) develops in 60 percent of American AIDS patients [*39*] but seems to occur less frequently in African AIDS patients [*40*]. PCP in AIDS patients generally has a subacute onset. Patients develop a nonproductive cough, often with shortness of breath. A chest x-ray can be normal in the early stages of the infection, with bilateral interstitial and alveolar infiltrates appearing later. Arterial blood gases generally show hypoxia. Severe shortness of breath can occur in a patient with a relatively normal chest x-ray. Cutaneous eruptions occur in 50 to 60 percent of the American AIDS patients with PCP treated with trimethoprim-sulfamethoxazole, but skin reactions occur only rarely during trimethoprim-sulfamethoxazole treatment in African AIDS patients [*41*].

Cryptosporidia and *Isospora belli* are the intestinal protozoa most frequently found as the cause of persistent diarrhea in AIDS cases (see also Chap. 32) [*32*].

Cerebral toxoplasmosis (see also Chap. 32) seems to occur more frequently in AIDS patients from developing countries. *Toxoplasma gondii* in AIDS patients generally causes brain abscesses. Serological tests are of limited value in diagnosing toxoplasma encephalitis in AIDS patients, since only 5 percent of patients with toxoplasma brain abscesses have IgM antibody to *T. gondii*. If cerebral toxoplasmosis is clinically suspected, a trial of antitoxoplasma treatment can be initiated.

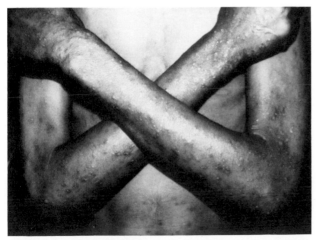

Figure 76-3. Generalized papulopruritic eruption in an HIV-1–infected patient. The lesions are particularly numerous on the extension surface of the arms.

Table 76-2. Opportunistic infections and malignancies in AIDS patients from Zaire, Haiti, and the United States

Opportunistic infections or malignancies	Zaire [37], % ($n = 196$)	Haiti [38], % ($n = 361$)	U.S.A. [39], % ($n = 30,632$)
Candida esophagitis	27	67	11
P. carinii pneumonia	17*	20	64
Persistent diarrhea with *Cryptosporidium* sp.	6	5	6
Persistent diarrhea with *Isospora belli*	1	NA	0.2
Cryptococcosis	5	3	7
Chronic herpes simplex ulcerations	3	8	4
Toxoplasma encephalitis	NA	3	3
Atypical mycobacterium infection	NA	NA	4
Generalized cytomegalovirus infection	NA	10	5
Progressive multifocal leukoencephalopathy	NA	2	0.6
Tuberculosis	13	24	3
Kaposi's sarcoma	4	26	21
Cerebral lymphoma	NA	0	0.7

Note: NA = information not available; * = a bilateral pulmonary infiltrate of unknown origin.

Disseminated *Mycobacterium avium-intracellulare* infection has been found in 4 to 10 percent of AIDS patients. *M. avium-intracellulare* has been isolated from lungs, liver, spleen, lymph nodes, brain, skin, and intestinal mucosa, and infection is diagnosed most efficiently by culturing blood or bone marrow.

Generally, severe cytomegalovirus (CMV) infection appears late in the course of AIDS. Clinical entities that may be caused by CMV are pneumonia, chorioretinitis, ulcerative colitis, esophagitis, adrenal gland necrosis, and encephalitis [42]. CMV chorioretinitis is characterized by bilateral exudates and hemorrhages and may lead to retinal infarction and necrosis, causing blindness [43]. Lesions need to be differentiated from cotton-wool spots of unknown etiology, which are commonly observed during funduscopy of AIDS patients.

Severe herpes simplex infections occur in about 5 percent of AIDS patients. Lesions are generally very painful. Initially,

herpes simplex ulcerations are often recurrent but later may become chronic. In heterosexual AIDS patients, lesions are generally localized in the genital area. Herpetic esophagitis and anorectal herpetic ulcerations are more often observed among American homosexuals with AIDS.

M. tuberculosis infection is a frequent complication of HIV-1 infection, particularly in developing countries [44]. Although pulmonary tuberculosis is the most common form seen in persons with HIV-1 infection, extrapulmonary involvement occurs more frequently among HIV-1–seropositive than HIV-1–seronegative tuberculosis patients. Tuberculous lymph nodes in AIDS patients frequently show no granulomas due to the inadequate cellular immune response. Tuberculosis in HIV-1–infected patients generally precedes other opportunistic infections by 1 to 17 months. In Africa, cutaneous anergy to tuberculin in a tuberculosis patient was strongly associated with HIV-1 infection. On the other hand, a positive tuberculin reaction in an AIDS patient in Africa may indicate active tuberculosis infection. Although there is some evidence that standard antituberculosis treatment is less effective in HIV-1–infected tuberculosis patients, most patients do respond well to treatment.

Herpes zoster may occur early in HIV-1 illness [44]. Herpes zoster is generally localized to two to three dermatomes (Fig. 76-5) and tends to recur.

In the tropics parasitic infections, such as malaria and amebiasis, do not seem to occur more frequently among HIV-1–infected persons [45]. In addition, the clinical presentation of these parasitic infections is similar for infected and uninfected patient groups, and the standard antiparasitic drug treatments are generally adequate.

Non-Hodgkin's lymphomas occur more frequently in AIDS patients than in other populations [46]. These lymphomas are generally of B-cell origin and include Burkitt's lymphoma. They are frequently localized at extranodal sites, including the

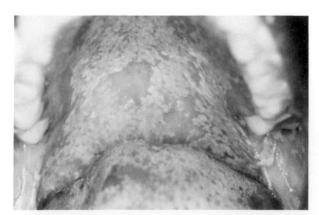

Figure 76-4. Oral candidiasis on the tongue and palatum of an HIV-1–infected patient.

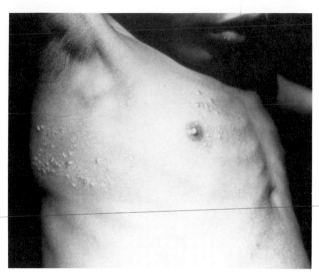

Figure 76-5. Thoracic herpes zoster in a 4-year-old HIV-1–infected boy.

central nervous system, the bone marrow, and the bowel. These lymphomas are generally high-grade malignancies and respond poorly to chemotherapy. Epstein-Barr virus (EBV), together with the immune deficiency associated with HIV-1 infection, probably plays a major role in the development of these B-cell lymphomas.

Kaposi's sarcoma, an angioproliferative disorder of endothelial origin, is observed in 48 percent of American homosexuals with AIDS and 5 percent of African AIDS patients. Among heterosexual AIDS patients, Kaposi's sarcoma occurs three to four times more often among males than females [47]. The classical form of Kaposi's sarcoma (Fig. 76-6), which is endemic in equatorial Africa, is unrelated to HIV infection and is not associated with immunosuppression. In HIV-1–infected patients, Kaposi's sarcoma occurs as a generalized disease with involvement of the skin, lymph nodes, and various organs, particularly the pulmonary and gastrointestinal systems (Figs. 76-7 to 76-11). This is in contrast with the classical endemic form of Kaposi's sarcoma, which is usually slowly progressive and limited to the skin mainly of the lower extremities. In the HIV-1–infected patient Kaposi's sarcoma lesions may develop on all parts of the body. Skin lesions are purple on white skin and hyperpigmented black on black skin. Lesions are mostly plaques or nodules but may be infiltrative or present as ulcerated tumors. When localized at the lower extremities, lesions are often surrounded by edema, as in the classical form. In the mouth, Kaposi's sarcoma lesions appear mainly on the hard palate. In 5 percent of patients with HIV-1–associated Kaposi's sarcoma, skin lesions are absent. Although internal organ involvement is frequent, overt clinical manifestations of visceral Kaposi's sarcoma occur in a comparatively small subset of patients early in their course. Gastrointestinal tract bleeding occurs only exceptionally. Pulmonary involvement may cause

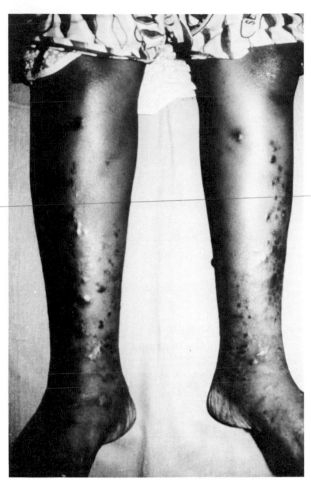

Figure 76-6. Kaposi's sarcoma lesions of the lower extremities in an HIV-1–infected woman.

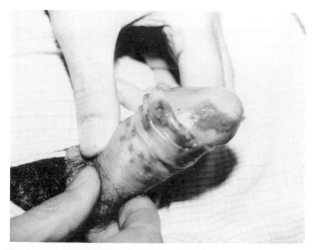

Figure 76-7. Kaposi's sarcoma on the penis of a white HIV-1–infected man.

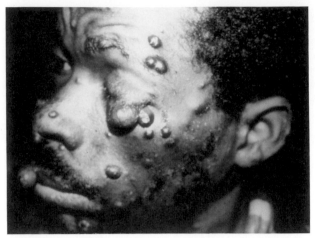

Figure 76-8. Nodular-tumoral Kaposi's sarcoma lesions on the face of an HIV-1–infected man.

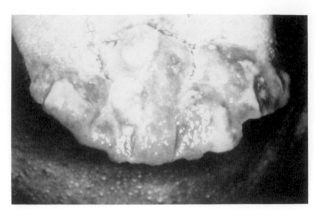

Figure 76-10. Kaposi's sarcoma and *Candida* infection of the tongue in an HIV-1–infected man.

intraalveolar hemorrhage and ventilatory failure. Involvement of the upper airway may result in obstruction. Histological features include interweaving bands of spindle cells and vascular structures embedded in a network of reticular and collagen fibers. The spindle cells may show a wide range of nuclear polymorphism. Histological characteristics of Kaposi's sarcoma lesions are similar in AIDS patients and patients with classical Kaposi's sarcoma. Neither chemotherapy nor radiotherapy has been able to produce disease-free remission rates for more than a few months. Since there is no evidence that effective treatment of Kaposi's sarcoma prolongs survival of AIDS patients, the management of Kaposi's sarcoma should be directed at palliating morbid lesions. AIDS patients with Kaposi's sarcoma generally die because of opportunistic infections and not because of Kaposi's sarcoma. Kaposi's sarcoma patients are more likely to develop other secondary cancers.

Oral hairy leukoplakia occurs as slightly raised, poorly demarcated lesions with corrugated or "hairy" surfaces that occur on the lateral borders of the tongue. The lesions range from a few millimeters to a few centimeters in size. They do not rub off and usually produce no symptoms. EBV has been found in the epithelial cells of hairy leukoplakia [48].

HIV-1 infection in children

HIV-1 illness is more rapid and severe in infants than in adults. Conditions reported in infants with congenitally acquired HIV infection include low birth weights and body lengths and smaller head circumferences for gestational age. Morbidity and mortality associated with perinatal HIV-1 infection appears to be higher in children born to mothers who already present symptomatic HIV-1–related illness. Most children born to asymptomatic HIV-seropositive mothers will appear clinically

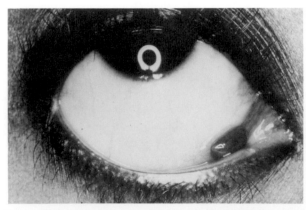

Figure 76-9. Kaposi's sarcoma lesion of the conjunctiva of an HIV-1–infected woman.

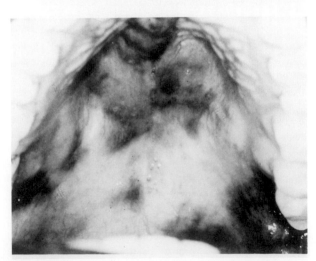

Figure 76-11. Kaposi's sarcoma lesion of the hard palate in an HIV-1–infected woman.

normal at birth. About 50 percent of perinatally infected children develop HIV-1–related symptoms and signs during the first months of life. Embryopathy, including facial malformations, has occasionally been described in children born to HIV-1–infected mothers in the United States. Clinical manifestations observed among HIV-1–infected children are similar to those observed among HIV-1–infected adults. In addition, children may fail to thrive and have abnormal psychomotor development. Bacterial infections, recurrent or chronic otitis, chronic parotid swelling, lymphoid interstitial pneumonitis, and hepatosplenomegaly are observed more often in children than in adults with HIV-1 infection. Lymphoid interstitial pneumonitis has been reported in 30 percent of pediatric AIDS cases and consists of a diffuse infiltration of the alveolar septa and peribronchiolar areas by lymphoid infiltrate. Its etiology and pathogenesis are unclear.

HIV-2 infection

HIV-2 has been isolated from the blood and CSF of asymptomatic persons and patients with AIDS and ARC who were not infected with HIV-1. The clinical expression and natural history of HIV-2 infection remains to be clarified. When AIDS develops as a result of HIV-2 infection, it seems to be similar to AIDS caused by HIV-1.

DIAGNOSIS

The laboratory diagnosis of retroviral infections is based on serology by enzyme-linked immunosorbent assay (ELISA) and a confirmatory test, such as Western blot or immunofluorescent antibody assays. Following infection with HIV-1, there is a brief period of antigenemia followed by a rise in IgM and IgG antibody to various viral antigenic components. Antibody to HIV-1 usually persists for the life of the infected person except during periods of marked immunosuppression, such as in AIDS patients when the antibody to p24 declines rapidly followed by decline in antibody to gp120. The decline of antibody to p24 is frequently associated with a rise in p24 antigen, and these serological changes are of prognostic value since they usually precede the development of opportunistic infection [49]. Highly sensitive and specific assays for HIV-1 were developed after the initial isolation of HIV-1 and have been commercially available since 1985. The ELISA test for antibody detection is highly sensitive and specific for detection of HIV-1 antibody, but because of occasional biological false positives, it may have a low predictive value in low-prevalence populations [50]. All serum samples repeatedly positive by ELISA must be confirmed by another serological test, such as Western blot. Antigen tests for circulating p24 antigen are also available and are useful during the early phase of infection when antibody is not yet detectable and during the late phases of HIV-1 infection [51]. HIV-1 antigenemia is frequently monitored during the late phase of disease to monitor the effectiveness of antiviral therapy. Culture of lymphocytes for HIV-1 is also available in research laboratories, but because

of its cost (greater than \$300) it is not practical for routine clinical use.

Diagnosis of HIV-2 infection also depends on serological confirmation. Unfortunately, the viral proteins of HIV-2, although divergent from HIV-1, have a 50 percent conservation for the *gag* and *pol* amino acids. Thus, HIV-2 antibody–positive serum recognizes the core proteins of HIV-1, but not the envelope proteins, in which there is greater than 70 percent divergence among amino acids. Serum from persons with antibody to HIV-2 may cross-react or be totally missed by the current serological assays for HIV-1, depending on the titer of antibody to *gag* and *pol* or envelope proteins. However, the recent development of specific polypeptide assays should enhance the specificity of HIV-1 and HIV-2 ELISA and Western blot tests.

Other laboratory abnormalities may be seen in HIV-1 infection, but they are usually dependent on the stage of disease. Lymphopenia, neutropenia, and thrombocytopenia may be observed in immunologically compromised persons. Lymphocyte subset determination typically reveals depressed T4 cells and initially elevated T suppressor (T8+, CD8+) cells, which subsequently decline in the latter phase of HIV-1 infection. The ratio of T helper to T suppressor cells is usually depressed below 0.9. Skin test reactivity to mitogens and specific antigens may be absent in the latter stages of HIV-1 infection. Anemia and pancytopenia may also be observed in ARC and AIDS patients [52]. Abnormalities of liver, renal function, and electrolytes may also occur but usually result from superimposed opportunistic infections.

For surveillance purposes in developing countries and to enable clinicians to diagnose AIDS in the absence of sophisticated diagnostic facilities, a clinical case definition of AIDS was proposed by the World Health Organization (WHO) (Table 76-3) [53]. Field evaluation in central Africa showed that this

Table 76-3. World Health Organization (WHO) clinical case definition of AIDS in adults when diagnostic resources are limited

AIDS in an adult is defined by the existence of at least two of the major signs associated with at least one of the minor signs, in the absence of known causes of immunosuppression, such as cancer or severe malnutrition, or other recognized etiologies.

1. Major signs
   a. Weight loss >10% of body weight
   b. Chronic diarrhea >1 month
   c. Prolonged fever >1 month
2. Minor signs
   a. Persistent cough for >1 month
   b. Generalized pruritic dermatitis
   c. Recurrent herpes zoster
   d. Oropharyngeal candidiasis
   e. Chronic progressive and disseminated herpes simplex infection
   f. Generalized lymphadenopathy

Generalized Kaposi's sarcoma and cryptococcal meningitis are sufficient by themselves for the diagnosis of AIDS.

definition was highly specific (94 percent) but relatively insensitive (62 percent) for HIV-1 infection [54]. Tuberculosis represents one of the major problems in differential diagnosis. The diagnosis of pediatric AIDS is often complex in developing countries, in part because of the prevalence of malnutrition and respiratory and gastrointestinal infections. Children with these conditions may have clinical manifestations similar to those observed among HIV-1–infected children. A major difficulty in diagnosing AIDS in newborns and infants through HIV-1-antibody testing is differentiating between passive antibodies transferred from the mother and antibodies actively produced by the infant. Maternal antibodies may remain with the infant for up to 15 months.

MANAGEMENT

Physicians treating AIDS patients face many medical, psychological, and social problems. Medical treatment includes support of symptoms, care of infectious and malignant complications of HIV-1 infection, and treatment of the HIV-1 infection itself. Treatment of these patients is particularly difficult. Indeed, AIDS remains an incurable disease, and several major symptoms and signs (e.g., persistent diarrhea and prurigo) rarely respond to treatment. Effective therapy is available for only a limited number of opportunistic infections (Table 76-4). In addition, opportunistic infections may reappear after treatment is stopped. Despite sequential treatment of different opportunistic infections, the clinical course of the AIDS patient is progressively downhill. Many antiviral drugs have been clinically tested. So far, zidovudine, formerly called azidothymidine, (AZT) is the only drug with clinically proven efficacy [55,56]. AZT is a competitive inhibitor of the reverse transcriptase.

Counseling is very important to managing the AIDS patient. Counselors need to explain to the patients the nature of their disease and the means of HIV-1 transmission so that the patients will know how to prevent the spread of HIV-1 to others. HIV-1–infected children may receive routine vaccination like uninfected children, except that inactivated polio virus vaccine is preferred over oral attenuated vaccine and bacillus Calmette-Guérin (BCG) vaccination is not indicated in symptomatic children [57].

POPULATION

EPIDEMIOLOGY

As of March 31, 1988, 136 countries from all continents reported at least one AIDS case to the WHO (Table 76-5). Of these, about 70 percent of AIDS cases have been reported from the United States [58]. However, reporting of AIDS cases from the developing world has in general been delayed and incomplete.

In the United States, AIDS is concentrated in cities with large numbers of high-risk individuals [homosexuals and intravenous (IV) drug abusers]: New York City, San Francisco,

Table 76-4. Therapy for infectious diseases in AIDS patients

Infections	Drug	Usual daily adult dose	Interval between divided doses	Route	Minimum duration*
Pneumocystis pneumonia	TMP-SMX†	20 mg/kg TMP with 100 mg/kg SMX	q 8 h	IV,PO	21 days
	Pentamidine isethionate	4 mg/kg	q d	IV	21 days
Toxoplasmosis	Pyrimethamine and sulfadiazine	75 mg pyrimethamine once, then 25 mg, with	q d	PO	28 days
		4 g sulfadiazine	q d	PO	28 days
Cryptosporidiosis	No drug known to be effective				
Isospora belli	TMP-SMX	10 mg/kg TMP 50 mg/kg SMX	q 6 h	PO	21 days
Oral candidiasis	Nystatin	3×10^5 units	q 4 h	PO	7–10 days
	or ketoconazole	200 mg	q 12 h	PO	7–10 days
Candida esophagitis	Ketoconazole	400 mg	q 12 h	PO	7–10 days
Cryptococcosis	Amphotericin	0.3 mg/kg	q d	IV	42 days
	and flucytosine	150 mg/kg	q 6 h	PO,IV	42 days
Mucocutaneous herpes simplex	Acyclovir	15 mg/kg	q 8 h	IV	7 days
Disseminated herpes zoster	Acyclovir	15–30 mg/kg	q 8 h	IV	7 days
Mycobacterium avium-intracellulare	Combination of amikacin, clofazimine, ethambutol, and rifampin?				?
Mycobacterium tuberculosis	Standard antituberculosis treatment				

*Optimal duration of therapy in AIDS patients is not well established.
†TMP-SMX = trimethoprim-sulfamethoxazole.

Table 76-5. AIDS reported to WHO as of March 21, 1988

Continent*	Number of cases	Number of countries reporting		
		Total	Zero cases	One or more cases
Africa	10,973	50	8	42
Americas	61,602	44	2	42
Asia	231	37	16	21
Europe	10,616	28	1	27
Oceania	834	14	10	4
Total	84,256	173	37	136

*By WHO region.

Los Angeles, and Miami. In the developing world, countries in central and eastern Africa are the most severely affected. In Africa the disease is mainly prevalent in the large urban centers and is generally absent in remote rural areas. In certain urban populations of central and east Africa, HIV-1 seroprevalence rates in the general population range from 3 to 20 percent [1], and the annual AIDS incidence has been estimated to be 500 to 1000 cases per million adults. Among hospital workers in Kinshasa, Zaire, the annual incidence of HIV-1 infection was found to be 1.8 percent. However, in a rural area of Zaire, HIV-1 seroprevalence remained stable at 0.8 percent over a 10-year period [59]. This observation suggests that the rate of HIV-1 transmission may remain stable in the absence of conditions that enhance its spread. Social changes with disruption of traditional lifestyles may have promoted the spread of HIV-1 infection in Africa. In Nairobi, the HIV-1 prevalence in selected prostitutes in a lower socioeconomic area rose from 8 percent in 1981 to 61 percent in 1985 [60].

While the male-to-female ratio of AIDS patients in the United States and Europe is over 10:1, in Africa it is approximately 1:1. In adults, HIV infection is most prevalent among persons 20 to 40 years old. HIV-1–infected women tend to be younger than HIV-infected men [1].

HIV-1 is transmitted through three major routes: sexual, parenteral, and perinatal. Despite the essential similarities in modes of transmission throughout the world, important regional variations exist.

In developed countries (e.g., United States, Canada, European countries, Australia), sexual transmission is predominantly homosexual. Serosurveys in the United States revealed infection rates among homosexuals of 20 to 50 percent [58]. In homosexual men, the number of sex partners and the frequency of receptive anal intercourse are important risk factors for acquiring HIV-1 infection. In addition, other practices that lead to rectal trauma increase the risk in receptive partners [28].

In developing countries, certainly in Africa, more than 80 percent of AIDS patients acquired the disease by heterosexual contact [1]. In South America, HIV-1 infection initially occurred mainly among homosexuals but is more and more frequently transmitted heterosexually.

HIV-1 has been isolated from semen as well as from cervical-vaginal secretions. That exposure of the female cervical and vaginal epithelium is sufficient for HIV-1 transmission was demonstrated by women who acquired HIV-1 infection as a result of artificial insemination with infected semen [61]. The risk of heterosexual transmission of HIV-1 per sexual contact remains unknown but has been estimated to be 1 per 500 to 1000 episodes of sexual contact. The main risk factors for heterosexual transmission of HIV-1 are sexual activity with multiple partners, with a person with HIV infection, and with persons of high-risk groups. Genital ulcers and other sexually transmitted diseases probably facilitate transmission of HIV-1 infection [1]. The clinical stage of HIV-1 infection may also influence infectivity. A decline in immune function is probably associated with increased virus replication, which may result in enhanced infectivity.

Parenteral transmission of HIV-1 in developed countries has involved blood transfusions, blood products (particularly factors VIII and IX), and needle or syringe sharing by IV drug users. IV drug abuse accounts for the second largest proportion of HIV-1 infections in the developed world. HIV-1 seroprevalence rates among IV drug abusers in the United States vary from 0 to 70 percent [1]. Receipt of blood from an HIV-1–infected donor probably always results in HIV-1 infection. Because blood donors in developed countries are screened for HIV-1, HIV-1 transmission by transfusions rarely occurs. In developing countries, however, it will take a long time before all blood units will be screened for HIV-1 antibodies in all transfusion centers. In many tropical countries, transfusion needs are very high, mainly among children, because of life-threatening anemia caused by malaria. Probably 30 percent of children in central Africa acquire HIV-1 infection through blood transfusion. Because of their transfusion requirements African patients with sickle cell disease are also at risk for acquiring HIV-1 infection. Most developing countries do not have an IV drug problem: however, in these countries, injection equipment and other skin-piercing instruments used by health care workers and by traditional practitioners are frequently insufficiently sterilized and could therefore transmit HIV-1. However, transmission of HIV-1 by this mode appears to be rare.

Perinatal HIV-1 transmission is mainly a problem in developing countries where an equal number of women and men are infected. In central and east Africa, 2 to 15 percent of pregnant women are HIV-1–infected. From 30 to 70 percent of infants born to HIV-1–infected mothers in Africa acquire HIV-1 infection perinatally. Acquisition in utero is probably the most frequent mechanism of HIV-1 transmission from mother to child. Mothers with more advanced stages of HIV-1 infection seem to transmit HIV-1 more efficiently to their offspring. HIV-1 has been cultured from breast milk, and case reports suggesting HIV-1 transmission by breast-feeding have been reported. However, the contribution of breast-feeding to perinatal transmission remains to be defined.

Risk of HIV-1 transmission from patients to health care workers is minimal but exists: 3 (0.03 percent) of 870 health care workers with documented parenteral exposure to blood of HIV-1–infected persons developed HIV-1 infection in association with a needlestick injury [62].

HIV-1 has been recovered from saliva, but the isolation rate is much lower than from blood. None of 48 health care workers became infected after parenteral or mucous membrane exposure to saliva of HIV-1–infected persons [62].

There is no evidence of HIV-1 transmission by casual contact within household and occupational settings or by arthropods.

HIV-2 transmission appears to occur principally in west Africa. Most AIDS cases caused by HIV-2 have been reported from Guinea-Bissau and Senegal. Serological surveys in the Ivory Coast found HIV-2 antibody prevalence rates of 0.3 percent among pregnant women and as high as 14 percent among female prostitutes [63]. In Guinea and Cape Verde Islands, 0.1 and 6.3 percent of various selected populations had HIV-2 antibodies. The spread of HIV-2 outside of west Africa seems to be limited so far [64].

Preliminary data suggest that HIV-2 infects populations similar to those infected by HIV-1, with heterosexual activity being the dominant mode of spread.

CONTROL

Control of HIV-1 infection has become a public health priority in many countries. With neither a treatment nor a vaccine in sight, primary prevention is the only tool to control HIV-1 infection and AIDS. As many as 80 percent of all new cases of HIV-1 infection in the world are acquired sexually; changing sexual behavior through health education would thus have the most impact on the further spread of AIDS. It is important to target this health education to persons exhibiting high-risk behavior and to adolescents. Whenever possible, AIDS education should be incorporated into existing health education programs. Reduction of risk of sexual transmission must be based on limiting of the number of sex partners, especially anonymous partners, and condom use. Spermicides have been shown in the laboratory to inactivate HIV-1 and may therefore provide additional protection. Every HIV-1–infected person needs to be considered currently infected with HIV-1 and presumably infectious. With increasing evidence that HIV-1 transmission is facilitated by genital ulcers, programs to diagnose and treat sexually transmitted diseases should be integrated into AIDS control efforts.

To prevent transmission of HIV-1 and related viruses through blood transfusions, transfusions should be given only when indicated, donors belonging to high-risk groups should be deferred, and all blood donors should be screened for HIV antibody. Sharing of syringes and needles among IV drug abusers needs to be discouraged. Needle exchange programs, providing free sterile needles and syringes to IV drug users when they return used ones, have been proposed to limit HIV transmission among IV drug abusers. In developing countries, efforts to promote proper sterilization of needles and syringes need to be initiated.

Preventing of perinatal transmission depends primarily on the success of prevention programs to limit the spread of HIV-1 infection to women of childbearing age. Reduction of perinatal transmission may also be achieved by counseling HIV-1–infected women on contraception. In the developed world, when a mother is HIV-1–infected, the known and potential benefits of breast-feeding for the child should be compared with the theoretical, but apparently small, incremental risk to the infant of becoming infected through breast-feeding. In developing countries, where safe and effective use of alternatives for breast-feeding are generally not available, breast-feeding by the biological mother should continue to be the feeding method of choice, irrespective of the mother's HIV-1-infection status.

Recommendations for infection-control practices among hospital workers do not differ from those for handling material from patients with any bloodborne infectious agent, such as hepatitis B [65]. HIV-1 seems to be less infectious and easier to kill than the hepatitis B virus. Most standard disinfectants and sterilization techniques kill HIV-1. A solution of 1 part of sodium hypochlorite (household bleach) in 10 parts of water is effective, as is alcohol. Needles, syringes, and other instruments must be sterilized by pressurized steam (in an autoclave or pressure cooker) at 121° C (250° F) for at least 20 min, or if that is not possible, by boiling water for 20 min. In general, hospitalized patients with AIDS do not have to be isolated in special wards. To minimize the risk of contagion, single rooms for AIDS patients may be indicated if patients are incontinent or psychotic or have communicable diseases such as tuberculosis or *Salmonella* infection. Bedclothes from patients infected with HIV-1 should be changed regularly and laundered in water heated to at least 70° C (160° F). Tubs and toilets should be frequently disinfected. Health care workers should follow strict infection control principles, not only when dealing with patients known to be infected with HIV-1 but also when interacting with all patients, since among them may be persons with unidentified HIV-1 infection.

REFERENCES

1 Piot P, Plummer FA, Mhalu FS, et al: AIDS: An international perspective. Science 239:573–579, 1988

2 Barre-Sinoussi F, Chermann JC, Rey F, et al: Isolation of a T-lymphotropic retrovirus from a patient at risk for acquired immunodeficiency syndrome (AIDS). Science 220:868–871, 1983

3 Gallo RC, Salahuddin SZ, Popovic M, et al: Frequent detection and isolation of cytopathic retroviruses (HTLV-III) from patients with AIDS and at risk for AIDS. Science 224:500–503, 1984

4 Levy JA, Hoffman AD, Kramer SM, et al: Isolation of lymphocytopathic retroviruses from San Francisco patients with AIDS. Science 225:840–842, 1984

5 Clavel F, Guetard D, Brun-Vezinet F, et al: Isolation of a new human retrovirus from West African patients with AIDS. Science 233:343–346, 1986

6 Guyader M, Emerman M, Sonigo P, et al: Genome organization and transactivation of the human immune deficiency virus type 2. Nature 326:662–669, 1987

7 Kestler HW, Li Y, Naidu YM, et al: Comparison of simian immunodeficiency virus isolates. Nature 331:619–622, 1988

8 Allan JS, Coligan JE, Lee T-H, et al: Major glycoprotein antigens that induce antibodies in AIDS patients are encoded by HTLV-III. Science 228:1091–1094, 1985

9 McDougal JS, Kennedy MS, Sligh JH, et al: Binding of HTLV-III/LAV to T4+ T cells by a complex of the 110K viral protein and the T4 molecule. Science 231:382–385, 1986

10 Arya SK, Gallo RC: Three novel genes of human T-lymphotropic virus type III: Immune reactivity of their products with sera from acquired immune deficiency syndrome patients. Proc Natl Acad Sci USA 83:2209–2213, 1986

11 Rosen C, Sodroski JG, Goh WC, et al: Post-transcriptional regulation accounts for the trans-activation of the human T-lymphotropic virus type III. Nature 319:555–559, 1986

12 Folks T, Powell DM, Lightfoote MM, et al: Induction of HTLV-III/LAV expression from a non-virus-producing T cell line: Implications for latent infection in man. Science 231:600, 1986

13 Lifson JD, Feinberg MB, Reyes GR, et al: Induction of CD4-dependent cell fusion by the HTLV-III/LAV envelope glycoprotein. Nature 323:725–728, 1986

14 Koenig S, Gendelman HE, Orenstein JM, et al: Detection of AIDS virus macrophages in brain tissue from AIDS patients with encephalopathy. Science 233:1089–1093, 1986

15 Desrosiers RC, Letvin NL: Animal models for acquired immunodeficiency syndrome. Rev Infect Dis 9:438, 1987

16 Daniel MD, King NW, Letvin NL, et al: A new type D retrovirus isolated from macaques with an immunodeficiency syndrome. Science 223:602–605, 1984

17 Gonda MA, Wong-Staal F, Gallo RC, et al: Sequence homology and morphologic similarity of HTLV-III and visna virus, a pathogenic lentivirus. Science 227:173–177, 1985

18 Daniel MD, Letvin NL, King NW, et al: Isolation of a T-cell tropic HTLV-III-like retrovirus from macaques. Science 228:1201–1204, 1985

19 Fauci AS: The human immunodeficiency virus: Infectivity and mechanisms of pathogenesis. Science 293:617–622, 1988

20 Lane HC, Depper JM, Greene WS et al: Qualitative analysis of immune function in patients with the acquired immunodeficiency syndrome: Evidence for a selective defect in soluble antigen recognition. N Engl J Med 313:79, 1985

21 Margolick JB, Volkman DJ, Folks TM, et al: Amplification of HTLV-III/LAV infection by antigen-induced activation of T cells and direct suppression by virus of lymphocyte blastogenic responses. J Immunol 138:1719–1723, 1987

22 Schnittman SM, Lane HC, Higgins SE, et al: Direct polyclonal activation of human B lymphocytes by the acquired immunodeficiency virus. Science 233:1084–1086, 1986

23 Ho DD, Pomerantz RJ, Kaplan JC: Pathogenesis of infection with human immunodeficiency virus. N Engl J Med 317:278–286, 1987

24 Fox R, Eldred LJ, Fuchs EJ, et al: Clinical manifestations of acute infection with human immunodeficiency virus in a cohort of gay men. AIDS 1:35–38, 1987

25 Carne CA, Tedder RS, Smith A, et al: Acute encephalopathy coincident with seroconversion for anti-HTLV-III. Lancet ii:1206–1208, 1985

26 Polk BF, Fox R, Brookmeyer R, et al: Predictors of the acquired immunodeficiency syndrome developing in a cohort of seropositive homosexual men. N Engl J Med 316:61–66, 1987

27 Medley GF, Anderson RM, Cox DR, et al: Incubation period of AIDS in patients infected via blood transfusion. Nature 328:719–721, 1987

28 Curran JW, Jaffe HW, Hardy AM, et al: Epidemiology of HIV-1 infection and AIDS in the United States. Science 239:610–616, 1988

29 Redfield RR, Wright DC, Tramont EC: The Walter Reed staging classification for HTLV-III/LAV infection. N Engl J Med 314:131–132, 1986

30 Centers for Disease Control: Classification system for human T-lymphotropic virus Type III/lymphadenopathy associated virus infection. Ann Intern Med 105:234–237, 1986

31 Serwada D, Mugerwa RD, Sewankambo NK, et al: Slim disease: A new disease in Uganda and its association with HTLV-III infection. Lancet ii:849–852, 1985

32 Colebunders R, Francis H, Mann JM, et al: Persistent diarrhea, strongly associated with HIV-1 infection in Kinshasa, Zaire. Am J Gastroenterol 82(9):859–864, 1987

33 Sewankambo N, Mugerwa RD, Goodgame R, et al: Enteropathic AIDS in Uganda: An endoscopic, histological and microbiological study. AIDS 1:9–13, 1987

34 Colebunders R, Mann JM, Francis H, et al: Generalised papular pruritic eruption: A manifestation of human immunodeficiency virus infection in African AIDS patients. AIDS 1:117–121, 1987

35 Price RW, Brew B, Sidtis T, et al: The brain in AIDS: Central nervous system HIV-1 infection and AIDS dementia complex. Science 239:586–592, 1988

36 Craddoch C, Pasvol G, Bull R, et al: Cardiorespiratory arrest and autonomic neuropathy in AIDS. Lancet i:16–18, 1987

37 Colebunders RL, Perriens J, Kapita B: Clinical manifestations and management of adults with HIV infection, in Piot P, Mann JM (eds): *Ballière's Clinical Medicine and Communicable Diseases: AIDS and HIV Infection in the Tropics.* London, Baillière 1988, pp 51–72

38 Pape JW, Liautaud B, Thomas F, et al: The acquired immunodeficiency syndrome in Haiti. Ann Intern Med 103:674–678, 1985

39 Selik RM, Starcher ET, Curran JW: Opportunistic diseases reported in AIDS patients: Frequencies, associations and trends. AIDS 1:175–182, 1987

40 Sonnet J, Taelman H: Clinical and biological profile of African AIDS: A study of 42 patients, in Stacquet M, Hemmer R, Baert A (eds): *Clinical Aspects of AIDS and AIDS-Related Complex.* New York, Oxford University Press, 1986, pp 78–89

41 Colebunders R, Lebughe I, Kapita B, et al: Cutaneous reactions to trimethoprim-sulfamethoxazole in African patients with the acquired immunodeficiency syndrome. Ann Intern Med 107:599–600, 1987

42 Jacobson MA, Mills J: Serious cytomegalovirus disease in the acquired immunodeficiency syndrome (AIDS). Ann Intern Med 108: 585–594, 1988

43 Mann JM, Snider DE, Francis H, et al: Association between HTLV-III/LAV infection and tuberculosis in Zaire. JAMA 3:346, 1986

44 Colebunders R, Mann JM, Francis H, et al: Herpes zoster and HIV-1 infection in Africa. J Infect Dis 157:314–318, 1988

45 Nguyen-Dinh P, Greenberg A, Ryder RW, et al: Absence of association between HIV-1 seropositivity and *Plasmodium falciparum* malaria in Kinshasa, Zaire. Bull WHO 65:607–613, 1987

46 Ziegler JL, Beckstead JA, Volberding PA, et al: Non-Hodgkins's lymphoma in 90 homosexual men. N Engl J Med 311:565, 1984

47 Bayley AC, Downing RG, Cheingsong-Popov R, et al: HTLV-III distinguishes atypical and endemic Kaposi's sarcoma in Africa. Lancet ii:359–361, 1985

48 Greenspan JS, Greenspan D, Lenette E, et al: Replication of Epstein-Barr virus within the epithelial cells of oral ''hairy'' leukoplakia, an AIDS-associated lesion. N Engl J Med 313:1564–1571, 1985

49 Weber JN, Clapham PR, Weiss RA, et al: Human immunodeficiency virus infection in two cohorts of homosexual men: Neutralizing sera and association of anti-*gag* antibody with prognosis. Lancet i:119–121, 1987

50 Denis F, Leonard G, Mounier M, et al: Efficacy of five enzyme immunoassays for antibody to HIV-1 in detecting antibody to HTLV-IV. Lancet i:324–325, 1987

51 Allain J-P, Laurian Y, Paul DA, et al: Serological markers in early stages of human immunodeficiency virus infection in haemophiliacs. Lancet ii:1233–1236, 1986

52 Spivak JL, Bender BS, Quinn TC: Hematologic abnormalities in the acquired immune deficiency syndrome. Am J Med 77:224–228, 1984

53 World Health Organization: Acquired immunodeficiency syndrome (AIDS). WHO/CDC case definition for AIDS. Wkly Epidemiol Rec 61:69–76, 1986

54 Colebunders RL, Mann JM, Francis H, et al: Evaluation of a clinical case definition of AIDS in Africa. Lancet i:492–494, 1987

55 Fischl Ma, Richman DD, Griego MH, et al: The efficacy of Azidothymidine in the treatment of patients with AIDS and AIDS-related complex. N Engl J Med 317:185–191, 1987

56 Declercq E: Chemotherapeutic approaches to the treatment of the acquired immune deficiency syndrome (AIDS). Am Chem Soc 29: 1561–1569, 1986

57 Centers for Disease Control: Immunization of children infected with human immunodeficiency virus. MMWR 37:181–183, 1988

58 Curran JW, Jaffe HW, Hardy AM, et al: Epidemiology of HIV-1 infection and AIDS in the United States. Science 239:610–616, 1988

59 Nzila N, De Cock KM, Forthal D, et al: Human immunodeficiency virus infection over 10 years in rural Zaire. N Engl J Med 318:276–279, 1988

60 Piot P, Plummer FA, Rey MA, et al: Retrospective epidemiology of HIV infection in Nairobi populations. J Infect Dis 155:1108–1112, 1987

61 Stewart GJ, Tyler JPP, Cunningham AL, et al: Transmission of human T-cell lymphotropic virus type III (HTLV-III) by artificial insemination by donor. Lancet ii:581–584, 1985

62 Centers for Disease Control: Update: Acquired immunodeficiency virus infection among health care workers. MMWR 37:229–234, 1988

63 Denis F, Barin FM, Gershy-Damet G, et al: Prevalence of human T-lymphotropic retroviruses type III(HIV) and type IV in Ivory Coast. Lancet i:408–411, 1987

64 Clavel F: HIV-2, the West African AIDS virus. AIDS 1:135–140, 1987

65 Centers for Disease Control: Recommendations for prevention of HIV transmission in the health-care settings. MMWR 36(suppl 2): 35–185, 1987

PART V Bacterial, Spirochetal, and Rickettsial Diseases

CHAPTER 77 / *Introduction* · *Charles C.J. Carpenter*

Those diseases for which specific cures are possible today and for which immunoprophylaxis is available are caused primarily by infectious agents. Throughout the developing world, acute infections, predominantly acute diarrheal illnesses and acute respiratory disease, are by far the leading causes of mortality. In the developed world, microbial disease processes remain the most common curable causes of both morbidity and mortality. Pneumococcal pneumonia, although curable by timely antimicrobial therapy and in large part preventable by immunization of susceptible population groups, remains among the 10 leading causes of death throughout the world. As a result of the global human immunodeficiency virus (HIV) pandemic, new infectious disease problems have appeared at a rapidly accelerating rate in immunocompromised individuals. The great number and variety of unusual infections occurring in immunodeficient patients, which have occurred in disproportionately large numbers in certain regions of the developing world, present rapidly expanding diagnostic and therapeutic challenges.

A positive effect of the current HIV pandemic is the recognition that control of infectious disease problems of the developing world is critical to the health of the industrialized nations as well—a delayed recognition of John Donne's statement that "any man's death diminishes me." This has led to a rapid increase in the application of the powerful tools of modern molecular biology to problems posed by the bacterial, spirochetal, and rickettsial diseases of the developing world.

While the global spread of the newly recognized HIV has created unprecedented challenges to the biomedical research community, rapid progress has continued in the development and application of vaccines effective against other major life-threatening illnesses; the utilization of recombinant deoxyribonucleic acid (DNA) technology and hybridoma-derived antibodies gives promise of yielding effective means of preventing additional bacterial and rickettsial infections.

The development of new vaccine strategies, in conjunction with the rapid progress achieved by the World Health Organization's Expanded Program on Immunization (EPI), with its emphasis on the protection of high-risk, susceptible women and young children, gives promise of major advances in our ability to prevent acute infectious diseases in the developing world in the next decade. This approach is critical in the most densely populated regions of the world, where time-honored approaches to the control of transmissible diseases (e.g., boiling water, pasteurizing milk, refrigerating food, washing hands before meals) are simply not possible.

In the face of rapid and sometimes bewildering changes, both in the nature of the infectious diseases with which clinicians are confronted and in the therapeutic armamentarium at their disposal, two basic principles continue to guide the physician's approach to patient management. When faced with a sick patient, the physician's primary responsibility is to determine whether or not the illness represents an acute infectious process. There is probably no situation in clinical medicine in which the thoughtful attention to all relevant details of a patient's medical history and a meticulous physical examination remain more important to the welfare of the patient. Once it is decided that a patient has an infectious process, the next responsibility is to determine whether or not the patient has a potentially fulminant, life-threatening illness that could cause death within the next few hours in the absence of prompt and appropriate therapy. Some life-threatening diseases are obvious, like acute bacterial meningitis, but they may also include such generally nonlethal illnesses as acute bacterial pneumonia. Because of the difficulty in determining which infectious processes are potentially death-dealing, it is incumbent upon the physician faced with a patient with an acute infectious process to establish a presumptive diagnosis and to initiate specific therapy for the presumed pathogen as rapidly as possible. In no other major group of illnesses is the rapid initiation of appropriate therapy so important as in acute infectious diseases. And in no other major group of illnesses is the physician better equipped to establish a working diagnosis and to initiate effective treatment without the use of sophisticated diagnostic techniques in the great majority of patients (e.g., individuals with acute diarrheal illnesses or with community-acquired pneumonia). This is a critically important issue, as sophisticated diagnostic equipment will not be available, in the next few decades, in the areas in which acute, potentially treatable infectious diseases take the greatest toll in human life and health.

Despite the prophylactic and therapeutic advances that have resulted from the rapid evolution of cellular and molecular biology, the microbial world continues to present the thoughtful physician with some of the most perplexing, and potentially rewarding, problems in the practice of medicine.

Cholera · Thomas Butler · David Sack

Cholera is an acute diarrheal disease caused by the bacterium *Vibrio cholerae* serogroup 01 and is characterized by frequent watery stools and vomiting. Cholera leads sometimes to profound isotonic dehydration, acidosis, and death within a few hours after the onset of diarrhea [1]. The disease is caused by cholera toxin, an enzyme secreted by *V. cholerae* which enters epithelial cells of the intestine and causes an increase in cyclic adenosine monophosphate (cAMP) leading to secretion of water and electrolytes into the intestinal lumen [2]. Rehydration of patients with isotonic intravenous fluid or oral rehydration solutions that employ glucose or other carbohydrate carriers of sodium is effective and can be lifesaving. Early antibiotic treatment shortens the illness significantly, whereas trials of antisecretory drugs have produced only small reductions in stool volume. An injectable cholera vaccine is available for travelers, and promising new oral vaccines are currently being tested.

PARASITE

CLASSIFICATION

V. cholerae was first isolated in pure culture by Robert Koch in 1883. It is a gram-negative comma-shaped bacillus with a unipolar flagellum that imparts a darting "shooting star" motility to the organism when examined with a dark-field microscope. The genus *Vibrio* contains several species, of which *V. cholerae* and *V. parahaemolyticus* are the most important pathogens in humans. On the basis of somatic (0) antigens *V. cholerae* is divided into more than 60 serovars. Cholera is caused by the serovar 01, which is subdivided into two serotypes, Inaba and Ogawa. A rare third type, *Hikojima*, cross-reacts with both Inaba and Ogawa antisera. *V. cholerae* 01 strains can be further divided into two biotypes: classical and El Tor. El Tor strains, in contrast to classical strains, are resistant to polymyxin B, cause agglutination of chicken erythrocytes, usually produce a hemolysin, and are Voges-Proskauer positive. Non-01 *V. cholerae,* and other vibrios (especially *V. mimicus*) may also cause diarrhea and may produce cholera toxin, but these other organisms do not cause epidemic cholera. Environmental *V. cholerae* 01 which do not produce cholera toxin have been found, but these have not been associated with epidemic cholera.

IDENTIFICATION

V. cholerae grows well on most bacteriological media but is inhibited on selective agars for fecal cultures such as MacConkey's agar. It ferments sucrose but not lactose. The preferred selective media for culturing stool include thiosulfate–citrate–bile salt–sucrose (TCBS) agar, on which the organism produces yellow colonies, and taurocholate tellurite gelatin agar (TTGA), on which the organism produces black colonies. Isolation of *V. cholerae* can be improved by inoculating the specimen in an enrichment medium (either alkaline peptone water or bile peptone water) and incubating for 6 h prior to inoculating a second TCBS or TTGA plate. Agglutination of bacteria in isolated colonies with 01 antiserum will identify an isolate as *V. cholerae* 01. *V. cholerae* is oxidase-positive, does not produce gas from carbohydrates, and possesses lysine and ornithine decarboxylase.

Rapid presumptive identification of *V. cholerae* can be accomplished by placing a drop of liquid stool on a microscope slide overlaid with a coverslip. Under a dark-field or phase-contrast microscope, rapid linear motility of the organism is characteristic. The addition of 01 antiserum (without preservative) to the stool preparation will result in a loss of this motility. Recently a coagglutination test has also been developed which may aid in the rapid identification of *V. cholerae* in stool [3].

CHOLERA TOXIN AND OTHER VIRULENCE FACTORS

The diarrhea of cholera is caused by an exotoxin called *cholera toxin* [4,5]. Cholera toxin was discovered by S. N. De in 1953 in Calcutta. He showed that supernatants of cultures of *V. cholerae* caused fluid secretion into the intestinal lumen of rabbits. This enterotoxin was subsequently shown to be a protein with a molecular weight of 84,000 and a subunit structure consisting of the A subunit (enzymatically active) and the B subunit (binding). The genes encoding cholera toxin are located on the chromosome of *V. cholerae*. Production of cholera toxin is regulated by a *tox* R gene which is stimulated by environmental changes in temperature, pH, osmolarity, and amino acids [6]. The action of cholera toxin is summarized in Fig. 78-1. The presence of normal bile acids in the small intestine enhances the enterotoxic activity of cholera toxin, as was shown in a mouse model by bile acids increasing the binding of cholera toxin to epithelial cells followed by increased fluid secretion [7]. Biological assays that are available in research laboratories include the rabbit ileal loop test, which shows accumulation of fluid after instillation of cholera toxin; the Y-1 adrenal cell test, in which cultured cells round up in response to the toxin; and the Chinese hamster ovary cells, which elongate after exposure to cholera toxin.

In addition to cholera toxin, *V. cholerae* also produces a number of other antigens which may contribute to its virulence.

1)

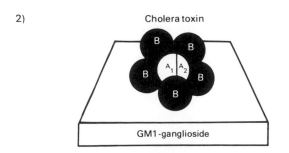

2)

Cholera toxin

GM1-ganglioside

3)

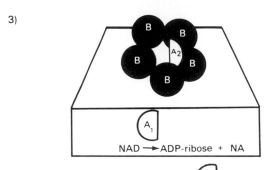

NAD $\longrightarrow$ ADP-ribose + NA

4) AC - RP - GTP + ADP-ribose $\longrightarrow$
AC - RP - GTP - ADP-ribose
(locked in active conformation)

5) ATP $\xrightarrow{\text{AC}}$ cAMP + Pi

6)

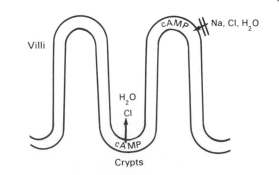

7) Isotonic dehydration and acidosis leading sometimes to fatal hypovolemic shock, lactic acidemia, renal failure, and hyperphosphatemia.

These include neuraminidase, mucinase, and chitinase. El tor strains may produce a hemolysin and some strains produce a shigalike toxin (verotoxin). Recently pili have been described which may be related to colonization of the vibrio [8].

ANTIBIOTIC RESISTANCE

V. cholerae strains are normally sensitive to tetracycline and other therapeutically useful antibiotics. Isolates of *V. cholerae* resistant to tetracycline and other antimicrobial drugs have been identified recently in patients in Bangladesh and in Tanzania [9]. Emergence of resistance was associated with widespread use of tetracycline in these countries. The resistance was mediated by plasmids that could be transferred to common enteric flora including *Escherichia coli*. Patients infected with resistant strains showed clinical evidence of failure to improve while receiving tetracycline.

BIOLOGICAL DIFFERENCES OF THE BIOTYPES

Virtually all cholera was caused by the classical biotype until 1961, when the El Tor strain spread from Sulawesi throughout endemic areas of Asia and Africa. This pandemic resulted in displacement of classical strains by El Tor strains which persists until today. In 1982 classical cholera reappeared in Bangladesh, but in subsequent years the two biotypes occurred there together with some predominance of El Tor strains. El Tor strains can survive longer in the environment than can classical strains, and El Tor strains are more likely than classical strains to cause asymptomatic infections.

PATIENT

CLINICAL MANIFESTATIONS

The clinical picture of cholera infection varies from asymptomatic excretion of *V. cholerae* to profuse watery diarrhea leading rapidly to dehydration and death. Following an incu-

⟵ **Figure 78-1.** Steps in the pathogenesis of cholera. 1. *Vibrio cholerae* colonizes the surface of small-intestinal epithelial cells and multiplies. 2. *V. cholerae* elaborates cholera toxin. Its B subunits bind to GM1-ganglioside receptors on the epithelial cell surface. 3. The A_1 portion of the A subunit is inserted into the epithelial cell membrane and enzymatically splits nicotinamide adenine dinucleotide (NAD) into adenosine diphosphate ribose (ADP-ribose) and nicotinamide (NA). 4. The A_1 portion of the A subunit ADP-ribosylates the regulatory protein–guanosine triphosphate complex (RP-GTP) of the enzyme adenyl cyclase (AC), locking AC into an active conformation. 5. Adenyl cyclase converts adenosine triphosphate (ATP) to cyclic adenosine monophosphate (cAMP) and phosphate (Pi). 6. Increased cAMP in small-intestinal epithelial cells leads to secretion of chloride and water in crypt cells and blockade of sodium, chloride, and water absorption by villus cells. 7. Potassium and bicarbonate are also secreted at increased rates. The colon participates by failing to absorb increased small intestinal secretions and by secreting additional potassium.

Table 78-1. Flow rates and composition of intestinal fluid in acute severe cholera*

	Flow rate (ml/h)	Concentrations (meq/L)			
		Sodium	**Potassium**	**Chloride**	**Bicarbonate**
Ileal fluid at ileocecal junction	472	145	5	110	45
Stool	457	120	24	95	52

*Mean values for 12 adults, adapted from [*10*].

bation period of 1 to 2 days, the typical history in severe cholera (cholera gravis) is the sudden onset of painless watery diarrhea. The diarrhea may be preceded momentarily by epigastric gurgling sounds and sensations of bloating, nausea, and vomiting. In some cases the vomiting is frequent and severe and accompanies the diarrhea. Muscle cramps, especially in the calves, is a common complaint. The watery diarrhea is passed frequently and often gives a sense of relief from sensations of abdominal bloating and cramping. Each bowel movement may amount to about a cupful of liquid, and this may be repeated several times an hour. In adults with severe cholera the rate of purging can average nearly half a liter per hour, with some patients purging more than a liter an hour (Table 78-1). Over a period of 4 to 12 h the typical patients develop severe dehydration and may die as soon as 6 h after the onset of diarrhea if not rehydrated.

For any given patient with cholera who has not received rehydration therapy, the clinical picture depends directly on the quantity of liquid stool that has been passed into the intestinal lumen from the body's extracellular space. As an estimate of clinical severity, the percent dehydration expressed as [(stool losses in liters/total body weight in kilograms) × 100] can be correlated with typical symptoms and signs of disease (Table 78-2). In the patient with severe dehydration, the mucous membranes of the eyes and mouth are dry, and the skin appears wrinkled. The eyes appear sunken (Figs. 78-2 and 78-3). Loss of skin turgor is demonstrable by grasping a fold

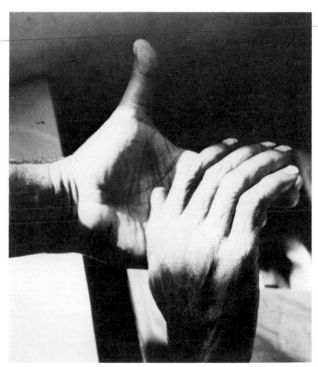

Figure 78-2. The skin of the hand in a patient with severe cholera is wrinkled and is called "washerwoman's hands."

Table 78-2. Symptoms and signs of cholera correlated with severity of dehydration

	Mild (1–4%)	**Moderate (5–7%)**	**Severe (≥8%)**
Symptoms	Thirst	Thirst, weakness, lethargy, shortness of breath	Prostration, obtundation, labored breathing
Signs of dehydration	None	Dry mucous membranes, loss of skin turgor	Marked dryness of mucous membranes, loss of skin turgor
Pulse rate	Normal	Increased	Very increased
Blood pressure	Normal	Diminished with orthostatic changes	More diminished or absent
Respiration	Normal	Hyperpnea	Kussmaul's respiration

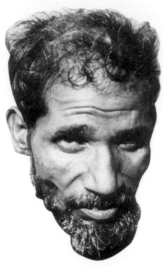

Figure 78-3. The eyes are sunken and mucous membranes are dry in severe cholera.

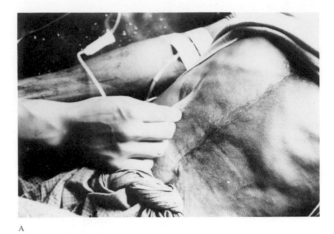

A

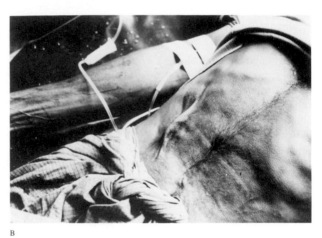

B

Figure 78-4. Diminished skin turgor in moderate or severe cholera is shown by (**A**) grasping a fold of skin over the abdomen and (**B**) observing retention of the ridged shape abnormally long.

of skin between one's fingers, releasing it, and seeing the skin retain its ridged shape abnormally long (Fig. 78-4*A* and 4*B*). The voice of the patient sounds faint or high pitched due to dryness of membranes in the respiratory tract. The breathing pattern is deep and rapid due to metabolic acidosis. The pulse is rapid and weak. The blood pressure may be unobtainable.

STOOL COMPOSITION AND BLOOD FINDINGS

The stool of cholera has been described as "rice water." It is liquid consisting of extracellular body fluid that has been secreted into the intestinal lumen and is nearly free of protein, red blood cells, and white blood cells. The "rice" part of cholera stool consists of light-colored flecks of mucus that are discharged from goblet cells of the small intestine. The electrolyte composition of the stool (Table 78-1) shows it is isotonic with serum but contains more potassium and bicarbonate than serum. Virtually all the fluid in cholera stool originates from the small intestine, especially from the duodenum and jejunum. During passage of the intestinal fluid through the colon, a small amount may be absorbed or a minor amount of fluid secreted by the colon [*10*]. The colon modifies the composition of cholera stool by absorbing some of the sodium and chloride and secreting additional potassium and bicarbonate (Table 78-1). The sodium concentration in cholera stool ranges from about 90 to 130 meq/L. The lowest concentrations of sodium occur in adults with low purging rates and in children. Stool potassium concentrations, on the other hand, vary inversely with purging rates, with somewhat lower concentrations found in patients with the highest purging rates.

The effects of severe cholera on the blood are marked hemoconcentration and metabolic acidosis. The acute contraction of extracellular fluid volume leads to hematocrits in excess of

55 percent and total serum protein concentrations of greater than 10g/100 mL. Accordingly, the serum-specific gravity increases from a normal value of around 1.025 to about 1.040 in severe cholera. The blood pH is reduced to around 7.2. Concentrations of sodium, potassium, and chloride are usually close to normal, but the bicarbonate can be reduced to 10 meq/L or lower (Table 78-3). An increased serum anion gap is due to increases in anionic protein concentration, lactic acidemia, and hyperphosphatemia [*11*]. The normal serum potassium concentration, despite great losses of potassium in stool, is attributable to a shift of potassium from cells into the extracellular fluid in a buffering exchange for hydrogen ion which enters cells. With correction of the acidosis, the serum potassium will decrease markedly, and potassium needs to be replaced while correcting the acidosis. The high serum phosphate is probably caused by a shift of intracellular phosphate into the extracellular space due to acidosis. The elevations in serum urea nitrogen and creatinine concentrations that occur during

Table 78-3. Values of serum electrolytes and other chemical measurements in patients with acute cholera during the initial severe dehydration and after recovery*

	Normal range	Acute dehydration	Recovery
Sodium	135–145	135	139
Potassium	3.5–5.5	4.6	4.0
Chloride	105–115	103	105
Bicarbonate	24–32	11.4	22.6
Anion gap			
[Na − (Cl + HCO$_3$)]	8–12	20.2	11.4
Protein	11.6–13.8	17.1	11.6
Lactate	0.7–1.8	4.1	1.6
Phosphate	1.8–2.6	4.4	1.9
Creatinine (mg/dL)	0.6–1.5	2.5	1.0
Calcium (mg/dL)	9.1–10.6	11.6	9.1
Magnesium (mg/dL)	1.6–2.6	3.1	2.1

*Mean values of 21 adult patients presenting with hypovolemic shock, adapted from [11]. Values in meq/L, or as stated.

severe cholera are usually mild and rapidly corrected after rehydration. Elevations of serum calcium and magnesium concentrations are likewise mild, and because total serum proteins are increased the concentrations of free ionic calcium and magnesium are likely to be normal.

SEROLOGY

Patients with cholera usually develop serum antibodies to the bacteria which can be detected in agglutination tests, complement-mediated vibriocidal assay, or enzyme-linked immunosorbent assay (ELISA) against the vibrio lipopolysaccharide. Although anticholera toxin antibodies also are stimulated following an episode, they are not specific for cholera because they cross-react with *E. coli* heat-labile enterotoxin.

TREATMENT

Without rehydration treatment, the case fatality rate for severe cholera exceeds 50 percent, but with treatment, no patient should die. Failure to provide adequate rehydration during an epidemic of cholera in Mali in 1984 resulted in a case fatality rate of 23 percent [12]. The cornerstone of therapy in cholera is prompt rehydration with isotonic fluid, followed by continued hydration to replace ongoing losses. Antibiotics are used to shorten the illness, but are not lifesaving [1,2].

Water and electrolyte replacement

Fluid and electrolyte replacement is divided into two phases: *rehydration* and *maintenance*. For rehydration, severely dehydrated patients will require intravenous fluids, while less severely dehydrated patients can usually be rehydrated with oral fluids (see under "Oral Rehydration" below). A single IV fluid can be used for all patients with cholera, and for these severe patients, the volume of fluid given initially should be

approximately 10 percent of the body weight. Ringer's lactate is the best commercially available intravenous solution, though fluids especially developed for severe diarrhea are optimal. One such fluid is "Dhaka solution" which contains (in milliequivalents per liter) sodium 133, potassium 13, chloride 98, and acetate 48. Normal saline is inferior to the polyelectrolyte solutions since it does not correct the acidosis nor does it replace the potassium, but can be used in emergency situations while replacing bicarbonate and potassium with oral fluids. Five percent dextrose and water (D5W) should not be used in cholera.

The parenteral fluids should be given by the intravenous route, not by the intraperitoneal or subcutaneous route, and should be given rapidly to completely correct the dehydration within about 4 h. IV fluids are generally needed only for initial rehydration; then oral fluids can be given to maintain hydration. If, because of very heavy purging, the patient again becomes dehydrated, intravenous fluids can again be given to rehydrate fully, followed by oral fluids once again.

Oral Rehydration. Less severely dehydrated patients (this includes many cholera patients as well as nearly all noncholera diarrhea patients) will not require intravenous fluids, but rather can be rehydrated orally. Mildly dehydrated patients will require 5 percent of their body weight replaced with oral fluids, and those who are moderately dehydrated will require about 7.5 percent. For infants a cup or spoon can be used to administer the fluid, and in rare situations where the patient is too weak to drink, it can be given by nasogastric tube.

Vomiting is common with cholera and during the initial phases of oral therapy, but in spite of the vomiting, oral therapy can be successful if frequent small feedings are given. If signs of dehydration reappear, however, intravenous fluids again should be administered to rehydrate. Then it is usually possible to resume oral therapy.

Maintenance Hydration. Following initial rehydration, additional oral rehydration solution should be given to match ongoing stool losses until the diarrhea stops. If possible, stool should be collected separately from urine so that an equal volume of oral solution can be provided. During the course of maintenance therapy, the hydration status of patients should be monitored frequently. The total fluid requirement (initial rehydration plus maintenance) for severe cholera in adults who receive appropriate antimicrobial therapy is usually 6 to 10 L.

The oral rehydration solution is not intended to provide replacement for usual sensible and insensible losses. Additional hypotonic fluids (e.g., water, breast milk) should be available for these normal fluid requirements, and water should not be restricted.

The oral rehydration solution recommended by WHO is shown in Table 78-4. This solution includes appropriate concentrations of electrolytes to replace the stool losses and also includes glucose to facilitate the absorption of sodium and water. Common table sugar (sucrose) is an adequate substitute for glucose. The citrate of trisodium citrate is converted by the liver to bicarbonate to allow correction of acidosis. Trisodium citrate is preferred to sodium bicarbonate because the dry ingredients in the packets before being mixed with water are more stable in the presence of the citrate salt, giving the packets a longer shelf life.

Alternate Formulations for Oral Rehydration Solution. Research is proceeding in hopes of improving and simplifying the formulation for oral rehydration solution. Rice starch (50 g/L) may be used in place of glucose if this is more suitable to the local situation. Patients treated with rice-based solutions have lower purging rates than comparable patients treated with the glucose solution. The addition of amino acids to glucose, especially alanine, also decreases the purging rate and may be associated with a decreased failure rate (i.e., percentage of patients who require additional intravenous fluids after starting oral maintenance therapy).

For cholera a "complete" formula should be used: i.e., the solution should contain the base and potassium. For less severe (noncholera) diarrheal illnesses, some have used a simple sugar-salt formula, but for cholera, this type of solution will result in hypokalemia and prolonged acidosis.

Cholera is a self-limited disease, and the rate of purging begins to decline on the first day after onset and usually stops within 5 days after onset even when antibiotics are not used.

Antibiotics

Antibiotics should be given to shorten the course of the disease and decrease the total purging volume. They will lessen the requirements for rehydration fluids, and this may be important in epidemic situations in developing countries where resources are scarce [13]. Antibiotics will eliminate the *Vibrio* from the stool, but this is of minimal public health significance in developing countries where only a few of those infected would be identified to receive antibiotics.

The antibiotic of choice is tetracycline 500 mg four times daily for 2 or 3 days [for children the dose is 50 mg/(kg · day) in four divided doses]. Doxycycline can also be used in a single dose of 300 mg for adults (4 to 6 mg/kg in children). For situations where tetracycline cannot be used, furazolidone 100 mg four times daily [5 mg/(kg · day) in four divided doses for children], or erythromycin 250 mg four times daily [30 mg/(kg · day) in four divided doses] can be used. Trimethoprim-sulfamethoxazole, 80 and 400 mg, respectively, twice daily [10 mg and 50 mg/(kg · day), in two divided doses for children] or chloramphenicol 500 mg four times daily is effective. All antibiotics can be given orally; there is no advantage to the parenteral route.

Prophylactic antibiotics are effective in preventing cholera in close family contacts; however, the use of prophylactic antibiotics is discouraged. In developing countries this would result in excessive antibiotic pressure in the community and would encourage resistant organisms. In developed countries, the disease is primarily foodborne and is not spread to family members.

Antisecretory agents

In addition to rehydration and antibiotics, considerable effort has been given to finding antisecretory therapies that will directly reduce purging rates in cholera. The first one to be effective in clinical trials was chlorpromazine. However, its sedative action and modest clinical efficacy when antibiotics are also used have limited the application of this therapy. Other

Table 78-4. Composition of oral rehydration solution

Ingredient	g/L	Resulting concentration	Meq or mmol/L
Sodium chloride	3.5	Sodium	90
Trisodium citrate	2.9	Potassium	20
(*or* sodium bicarbonate)	2.5	Chloride	80
Potassium chloride	1.5	Bicarbonate	30
Glucose	20	Glucose	111
(*or* sucrose)	40		

antisecretory drugs with some clinical efficacy include nicotinic acid and berberine sulfate, but trials with these agents also showed only a mild effect on stool volume, and they should not be used routinely [14]. Similarly, antiperistaltic drugs like diphenoxylate hydrochloride and loperamide hydrochloride should not be used in cholera because their action could have an adverse effect by causing intestinal pooling of secretions rather than prompt evacuation from the body. Kaolin, pectin, and activated charcoal have no value in the treatment of cholera.

Diet

Cholera patients can be fed a diet as soon as the initial vomiting ceases. There is no value in "resting the bowel."

COMPLICATIONS

Complications are rare if dehydration is corrected and hydration is maintained with a suitable polyelectrolyte solution. Most complications are the result of underhydration or use of inappropriate solutions. Persistent vomiting may be related to uncorrected acidosis. Acute renal failure can occur if rehydration was not adequate and occurs especially in patients who are given sufficient volumes to maintain life but not enough to restore circulation. Myocardial infarction and cerebrovascular thrombosis have been described as rare complications in adults due to circulatory insufficiency. Hypokalemia occurs if rehydration fluids do not contain sufficient potassium, and this may be manifest by abdominal distention, paralytic ileus, urinary retention, muscular weakness, cardiac arrhythmias, and even death. Acute pulmonary edema can occur with overreplacement of IV fluids, especially if the fluids have not corrected the acidosis (e.g., use of saline rather than Ringer's lactate). Periorbital edema occurs from excessive oral fluid replacement, but is easily corrected by decreasing the intake. Mild asymptomatic hypoglycemia occurs commonly in children during rehydration, and severe hypoglycemia occurs only occasionally. The latter is manifest by seizures and coma; if this should occur during therapy, IV glucose should be given immediately while awaiting a blood glucose determination. Pregnant women frequently abort if severely dehydrated; principles of treatment are the same as with other patients. Important determinants of mortality in children with cholera in Bangladesh following rehydration were shown to be preexisting malnutrition; concomitant pneumonia, shigellosis, or septicemia; and hypoglycemia [15].

POPULATION

INCIDENCE

The number of cholera cases reported to WHO in 1986 was 46,473. This is a gross underestimate of the incidence of cholera in the world because several countries with known cholera in excess of this number, such as Bangladesh, did not report any of their cases. African countries reported 40,626 cases, whereas Asian countries reported only 5,774. In some countries with endemic cholera, like Bangladesh, approximately 5 percent of all acute diarrheal episodes are due to cholera. In the Ganges delta area the incidence of cholera is about 1.5 per 1000 population per year suggesting that there may be more than 200,000 cases in this area alone. Thus, the annual incidence of cholera in the world can be estimated to be more than a million cases.

GEOGRAPHICAL DISTRIBUTION

Cholera infection is confined almost entirely to the tropical developing countries of Asia and Africa. In Asia, the countries with most cases are India, Bangladesh, Indonesia, Vietnam, and Thailand. In Africa, the countries with most cases are Somalia, Sierra Leone, Mauritania, Mali, Tanzania, and Zaire. In the Americas, South America and Central America are entirely free of cholera, but several cases have occurred in recent years in the United States along the Gulf Coast of Louisiana [16,17]. In European countries, small numbers of cases have been reported that were mostly imported in travelers returning from tropical areas. Small outbreaks have occurred in recent years in Italy, Spain, Portugal, and Israel.

TRANSMISSION

Cholera is transmitted by the fecal-oral route. This occurs usually by the ingestion of water contaminated with human feces. A person with cholera excretes about 10^8 cholera bacilli per milliliter of stool. These organisms can survive for an estimated 4 to 7 days in the environment. In countries with endemic cholera, most people do not have access to treated water and use outdoor makeshift latrines that lead to contamination of surface water. The use of surface water for drinking and bathing is commonplace and leads to the transmission of cholera. In addition to the fecal-oral spread, *V. cholerae* can survive for prolonged periods in surface estuarine waters without a human host; thus fecal contamination is not always necessary for transmission. Less common modes of cholera transmission include contaminated food and person-to-person spread within households. In Mali, an epidemic of cholera occurred in 1984 during a drought-related famine, and cases were linked to drinking water from a village well and eating leftover millet gruel [12]. There are no known animal hosts or reservoirs of *V. cholerae* in nature. In the United States, cholera has been recently acquired by ingestion of oysters, shrimp, and crabs [18]. These crustaceans appear to be effective in concentrating *V. cholerae* from water contaminated by human sewage, and they are occasionally eaten raw or partially cooked. Microflora (copepods and other plankton) may serve similar roles in the ecology of *V. cholerae* in some areas.

SEASONALITY

In countries with endemic cholera, well-defined epidemic peaks occur once or twice a year. In Bangladesh, the major peak in incidence occurs in November with a lesser rise occurring in April or May. In recent years in Bangladesh El Tor *V. cholerae* has predominantly caused the winter peak while classical *V. cholerae* has caused the spring peak, but this is the only area currently reporting classical cholera. In Calcutta, India, the major peak is in May. Although studies relating to patterns of water use and weather conditions have been carried out to clarify the reasons for the marked seasonality of cholera, the exact explanation for it remains unknown.

HOST FACTORS

All age groups and both sexes are susceptible to cholera infection, but there are certain groups that are more susceptible than others. Infants, especially those who are breast-feeding, are partially protected against cholera, and this protection has been correlated with levels of antibodies against *V. cholerae* in breast milk [19]. Children from 2 to 5 years and adult females show a greater incidence of cholera than adult males in certain endemic areas. This pattern of susceptibility has been related to mothers and children being closer to homes in which the use of the contaminated surface water is common. Following an episode of cholera infection, acquired immunity develops and protects against reinfection for 3 years or longer. Protection is correlated with the presence of IgA and IgG antibodies in the intestinal lumen directed against the lipopolysaccharide of *V. cholerae*. Immunization of travelers with cholera vaccine provides partial protection which lasts for only about 6 months. Reduced gastric acidity predisposes persons to cholera infection, and this factor may influence which individuals develop illness after exposure to infection. Neutralizing normal gastric acid in volunteers with sodium bicarbonate reduced dramatically the inoculum required for infection from about 10^{11} organisms to about 10^4. Thus, under natural conditions, the ingestion of milk or other foods before or with the ingestion of contaminated water may predispose to cholera infection. Individuals of blood group O are more susceptible to cholera than people of other blood groups.

VACCINATION

A parenteral vaccine has been available for nearly 100 years. Its use is not encouraged because of short-lasting immunity (6 months), significant side effects, and lack of efficacy in preventing spread. It is not generally recommended for travelers, although a few countries (primarily in Africa) still require it for travelers. Thus, to satisfy requirements of governments for entry into certain countries, immunization prior to travel may be needed. Travelers visiting countries with endemic cholera are placed at exceedingly low risk for acquiring cholera.

New oral vaccines made up of a mixture of killed whole vibrios (with or without the B subunit of cholera toxin) have been field tested. They are both safer and more effective than the old parenteral one, but these are not yet licensed [20]. Addition of the B subunit provides antitoxic immunity which increased the level of protective efficacy for the first 6 months but had little effect on long-term efficacy. The antitoxic immunity additionally provided short-term protection against *E. coli* diarrhea associated with bacteria producing heat-labile enterotoxin. New live attenuated bacterium vaccines are also being developed but have not yet been field tested.

PREVENTION

Since cholera is transmitted primarily through contaminated water and food, a major reduction in incidence will almost certainly occur when improved sanitation facilities are developed in endemic areas. In the meantime certain interventions seem practical now which decrease the risk. For travelers, the use of boiled or chemically pure water along with eating cooked foods will virtually eliminate the risk of cholera. For persons living in endemic areas, the use of safe water from tube wells (as opposed to surface water) decreases the risk of becoming infected. Though boiling water eliminates the *Vibrio,* this intervention is not always practical for many endemic areas. For infants, breast-feeding decreases the risk and should be encouraged as long as possible even while introducing other foods at the appropriate age [19].

In the United States the risk of cholera is very low, and the few cases that do occur all occur in the summer from undercooked seafood from the Gulf Coast. Hence, adequate cooking of crabs, oysters, and shrimp would eliminate these cases.

REFERENCES

1 Rabbani GH: Cholera. Clin Gastroenterol 15:507, 1986
2 Carpenter CCJ: The pathophysiology of secretory diarrheas. Med Clin North Amer 66:597, 1982
3 Rahman M, Sack DA, Mahmood S, et al: Rapid diagnosis of cholera by coagglutination test using 4 hour fecal enrichment cultures. J Clin Microbiol 25:2204, 1987
4 Holmgren J: Actions of cholera toxin and the prevention and treatment of cholera. Nature 292:413, 1981
5 Ribi HO, Ludwig DS, Mercer KL, et al: Three-dimensional structure of cholera toxin penetrating a lipid membrane. Science 239:1272, 1988
6 Miller VL, Mekalanos JJ: A novel suicide vector and its use in construction of insertion mutations: osmoregulation of outer membrane proteins and virulence determinants in *Vibrio cholerae* requires *tox* R. J Bacteriol 170:2575–2583, 1988
7 Lange S, Hansson HA, Lonnroth I: Influence of bile acids on cholera toxin-induced secretion in mouse jejunum. Acta Pathol Microbiol Immunol Scand [B] 91:215, 1983
8 Taylor RK, Miller VL, Furlong DB, et al: Use of phoA gene fusions to identify a pilus colonization factor coordinately regulated with cholera toxin. Proc Natl Acad Sci USA 84:2833, 1987

9 Glass RI, Huq MI, Alim ARMA, et al: Emergence of multiply antibiotic-resistant *Vibrio cholerae* in Bangladesh. J Infect Dis 142: 939, 1980

10 Speelman P, Butler T, Kabir I, et al: Colonic dysfunction during cholera infection. Gastroenterol 91:1164, 1986

11 Wang F, Butler T, Rabbani GH, et al: The acidosis of cholera. Contributions of hyperproteinemia, lactic acidemia, and hyperphosphatemia to an increased serum anion gap. N Engl J Med 315: 1591, 1986

12 Tauxe RV, Holmberg SD, Dodin A, et al: Epidemic cholera in Mali: high mortality and multiple routes of transmission. Epidem Inf 100:279, 1988

13 Islam MR: Single dose tetracycline in cholera. Gut 28:1029, 1987

14 Rabbani GH, Butler T, Knight J, et al: Randomized controlled trial of berberine sulfate therapy for diarrhea due to enterotoxigenic *Escherichia coli* and *Vibrio cholerae*. J Infect Dis 155:979, 1987

15 Butler T, Islam M, Azad AK, et al: Causes of death in diarrhoeal diseases after rehydration therapy: an autopsy study of 140 patients in Bangladesh. Bull WHO 65:317, 1987

16 Blake PA, Allegra DT, Snyder JD, et al: Cholera—a possible endemic focus in the United States. N Engl J Med 302:305, 1980

17 Johnston JM, Martin DL, Perdue J, et al: Cholera on a gulf coast oil rig. N Engl J Med 309:523, 1983

18 Klontz KC, Tauxe RV, Cook WL, et al: Cholera after the consumption of raw oysters. Ann Intern Med 107:846, 1987

19 Glass RI, Svennerholm A-M, Stoll BJ, et al: Protection against cholera in breast-fed children by antibodies in breast milk. N Engl J Med 308:1389, 1983

20 Clemens JD, Harris JR, Sack DA, et al: Field trial of oral cholera vaccines in Bangladesh: Results of one year follow-up. J Infect Dis 158:60, 1988

CHAPTER 79 / *Typhoid Fever* · Thomas Butler

Typhoid fever is a bacterial disease of humans caused by *Salmonella typhi*; it is characterized by prolonged fever, abdominal pain, diarrhea, delirium, rose spots, and splenomegaly and complicated sometimes by intestinal bleeding and perforation. The term *enteric fever* is synonymous with *typhoid fever,* which is occasionally caused also by *S. enteritidis* bioserotype Paratyphi A or B. Infection is transmitted by ingestion of bacteria via contaminated water and food, and chronic asymptomatic fecal carriers are an important reservoir of infection. Antimicrobial treatment reduces mortality to less than 5 percent of cases.

PARASITE

Gaffkey in Germany in 1884 first isolated *S. typhi* from patients. *S. typhi* is a motile gram-negative rod in the family Enterobacteriaceae and belongs to serogroup D_1. It possesses a cell wall (0) lipopolysaccharide antigen, a polysaccharide virulence (Vi) antigen located in the cell capsule, and a flagellar (H) antigen, with the overall antigenic formula 0 9,12 [Vi]: H d. The polysaccharide side chain of the 0 antigen confers serological specificity to the organism and is essential to virulence, as shown by the fact that *Salmonellae* other than *S. typhi* and *S. enteritidis* bioserotype Paratyphi A or B do not produce enteric fever in humans. These antigens play critical roles in permitting the organisms to invade lymphoid tissue from the gut lumen and to multiply within macrophages. Large numbers of bacteria in the lymphoid tissues of the intestine, liver, spleen, and bone marrow cause inflammation in these sites and result in the release of mediators of inflammation from macrophages, including interleukin 1 (endogenous pyrogen) and cachectin. Although the lipopolysaccharide endotoxin of *S. typhi* is pyrogenic in humans, this bacterial product does not circulate in measurable quantities during disease and does not seem to play a role in the pathogenesis of typhoid fever.

S. typhi is identified in the laboratory by an alkaline slant and acid butt without gas in triple sugar-iron agar, by failure to grow on Simmons' citrate, by a negative urease reaction, and by agglutination with group-specific antiserum. The typhoid bacillus survives well in the environment for prolonged periods while resisting desiccation and freezing. It is susceptible, however, to chlorination and temperatures achieved during pasteurization (63°C).

S. typhi and *S. paratyphi* are adapted only to humans and do not have animal reservoirs and do not cause disease in animals. The nontyphoid *Salmonellae*, on the other hand, have animal reservoirs and cause animal diseases, while in humans causing self-limited gastroenteritis without the capability of producing the characteristic prolonged enteric fever.

S. typhi is capable of acquiring R-factor plasmids that mediate multiple antibiotic resistance [1]. Epidemics of typhoid fever caused by chloramphenicol-resistant strains of *S. typhi* that carried a group H1 R factor occurred in the 1970s in Mexico and Vietnam. In the world today, a small minority of *S. typhi* strains carry R factors or other plasmids [2]. This low incidence of plasmid carriage by *S. typhi* has been attributed to the loss of acquired plasmids and to a slower growth rate of bacteria that have acquired plasmids.

Persons with typhoid fever develop serum antibodies against the several antigens of *S. typhi*. Additionally, cellular immunity can be demonstrated by a lymphocyte replication assay done with antigen from typhoid vaccine [*3*].

PATIENT

In 1829 in Paris, P. Louis described the clinical features of typhoid fever, including rose spots, ileal ulcers, and intestinal perforation.

After ingestion of *S. typhi,* part of the inoculum which survives passage through the acidity of the stomach enters the small intestine, where bacteria penetrate the mucosa and enter mononuclear phagocytes of ileal Peyer's patches and mesenteric lymph nodes. Inocula of at least 10^5 bacteria are necessary to initiate disease, and inocula of 10^7 and more will cause disease regularly. The incubation period ranges from 8 to 28 days, depending on inoculum size and immune status of the host [*4*]. Bacteria proliferate in mononuclear phagocytes and spread by way of the blood to the spleen, liver, and bone marrow, where further proliferation in macrophages occurs. The earliest symptoms of fever and chills (Table 79-1) are associated with bacteremia. Inflammatory reactions consisting of mononuclear cell infiltration, hyperplasia, and focal necrosis occur in the spleen, liver, bone marrow, Peyer's patches in mainly the terminal ileum, and skin. Focal collections of mononuclear leukocytes are called *typhoid nodules*. Intestinal manifestations are caused by hyperplasia of Peyer's patches with ulcerations of overlying mucosa (Fig. 79-1), resulting in pain, diarrhea, bleeding, or perforation.

In the first days of illness the nonspecific symptoms of fever, chills, and headache are mild and in the typical case build up in intensity stepwise during the first week, resulting in prostration [*5,6*]. The evolution of disease syndromes occurs stepwise over 1 to 3 weeks (Table 79-1) but may be variable in the time of appearance. The early symptoms of fever, abdominal pain, and prostration tend to persist throughout the illness, which in untreated cases lasts a month or longer. Abdominal pain occurs in more than half of patients and is frequently diffuse or located in the right lower quadrant over the

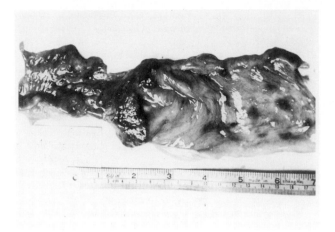

Figure 79-1. Mucosal surface of ileocecal junction in fatal typhoid fever showing deep hemorrhagic ulcers in terminal ileum (left) and proximal colon (right).

terminal ileum. Diarrhea occurs in about a third of patients and consists of either watery stools or semisolid stools described as being like "pea soup." Melena occurs less commonly. Rose spots (Fig. 79-2) occur in more than half of light-skinned individuals but are often not visible in dark-skinned patients. The rash is seen most commonly on the shoulders, thorax, and abdomen and rarely affects the extremities. The lesions are erythematous macules or papules about 1 to 5 mm in diameter, which typically blanch with pressure but may become hemorrhagic in nature. They fade quickly after a few days of treatment. Many patients display abnormal behavior or altered mental status that may be out of proportion to the severity of the systemic illness. Among the common presentations are "toxic" staring, delirium, aphonia, and coma. Seizures are common in children. Patients are infrequently jaundiced.

In about 5 percent of patients, the complications of intestinal bleeding and intestinal perforation will occur, usually after the second week of illness. These complications occur more often

Table 79-1. Evolution of typical symptoms and signs of typhoid fever

Disease period	Symptoms	Signs	Pathology
First week	Fever, chills gradually increasing and persisting; headache	Abdominal tenderness	Bacteremia
Second week	Rash, abdominal pain, diarrhea or constipation, delirium, prostration	Rose spots, splenomegaly, hepatomegaly	Mononuclear cell vasculitis of skin, hyperplasia of ileal Peyer's patches, typhoid nodules in spleen and liver
Third week	Complications of intestinal bleeding and perforation, shock	Melena, ileus, rigid abdomen, coma	Ulcerations over Peyer's patches, perforation with peritonitis
Fourth week and later	Resolution of symptoms, relapse, weight loss	Reappearance of acute disease, cachexia	Cholecystitis, chronic fecal carriage of bacteria

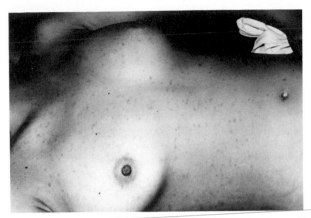

Figure 79-2. Rose spots on thorax and abdomen of patient with typhoid fever.

in adolescents and adults than in children [7]. Bleeding occurs from ileal ulcers and may present as melena or bright red blood in stools. Brisk bleeding develops rarely but is an occasional cause of death. Intestinal perforation presents as the sudden development of more severe abdominal pain, distention, and tenderness. Bowel sounds are diminished, and the abdominal x-ray usually reveals free air. Perforation most often occurs unexpectedly after a few days of treatment when a patient has started to improve. Other complications of typhoid fever include pneumonia, which develops as a superinfection due to other bacteria; myocarditis; acute cholecystitis; and acute meningitis.

Patients who have been ill for 3 weeks or longer often are cachectic because of anorexia and acute weight loss during this catabolic disease. Children who were malnourished before acquiring the infection can be expected to show more severe signs of illness [8].

Relapses occur in about 10 to 20 percent of patients treated with chloramphenicol. Patients with relapses experience the reappearance of typical symptoms about 7 to 14 days after the end of treatment. Relapses tend to be less severe than the initial episode.

DIAGNOSIS

The preferred method of diagnosis is isolation of *S. typhi* from a blood culture. The blood culture is positive in most patients during the first 2 weeks of illness. Urine and stool cultures are positive less frequently but should be taken to increase the diagnostic yield. The bone marrow culture is the most sensitive test, positive in nearly 90 percent of cases, and can be used when a bacteriological diagnosis is crucially needed or in patients who have been pretreated with antibiotics. The duodenal string test to culture bile has also been used with success in typhoid fever.

The Widal test for agglutinating antibodies against the so-matic (0) and flagellar (H) antigens of *S. typhi* is widely used for serodiagnosis. An 0 agglutinin titer of ≥1:80 or a fourfold rise supports a diagnosis of typhoid fever, whereas the H agglutinins are more often nonspecifically elevated by immunization or previous infections with other bacteria. Serodiagnosis should not be relied upon because false-positive results are often obtained in endemic areas and false-negative results occur in some cases of bacteriologically proven typhoid fever.

Other laboratory findings are anemia of variable severity and a white blood cell count that is normal or decreased with an increased percentage of band forms. Platelets are often diminished, and signs of disseminated intravascular coagulation are present. Liver function tests are frequently abnormal showing elevated aminotransferases and bilirubin concentrations. Renal failure is an infrequent complication. In patients with diarrhea, the stool shows fecal leukocytes [9].

The differential diagnosis depends on knowledge of which infections are endemic in the area where an individual contracted his or her infection. For returned travelers from developing countries, the common possibilities are malaria, hepatitis, typhus, amebic liver abscess, shigellosis, nontyphoid salmonellosis, and leptospirosis. In the United States, one must consider septicemia originating from the urinary tract, GI tract, or gallbladder as well as influenza, infectious mononucleosis, meningococcemia, miliary tuberculosis, and bacterial endocarditis.

TREATMENT

In 1948, T. Woodward first treated typhoid patients successfully using chloramphenicol in Malaysia. Chloramphenicol has remained the drug of choice since its introduction because no other drug has been demonstrated to cause more rapid or consistent improvement of disease. Resistance to chloramphenicol mediated by plasmid R factors has been reported only occasionally in patients who acquired infections in Mexico, India, and Thailand. Chloramphenicol is given orally in a dose of 50 to 60 mg per kilogram of body weight per day in four equal portions every 6 h. After defervescence and clinical improvement the dosage can be reduced to 30 mg/(kg·day) to complete a 14-day course. In patients unable to take oral medication the same dosage should be given intravenously until the patient can take capsules.

Alternative drugs should be considered when *S. typhi* resistant to chloramphenicol is isolated or strongly suspected. Since alternative drugs are nearly equal to chloramphenicol in clinical efficacy, a physician may choose to use another drug for a patient in whom bone marrow suppression is undesired. Trimethoprim-sulfamethoxazole is effective in a standard adult dose of 160 mg trimethoprim–800 mg sulfamethoxazole given orally or intravenously twice a day for 14 days. Other drugs that are effective include ampicillin (intravenously), amoxicillin, cefoperazone, and ceftriaxone.

Patients who are dehydrated, anorectic, or with diarrhea should receive intravenous saline with attention to electrolyte and acid-base disturbances. Patients with brisk intestinal bleeding will require blood transfusion. Patients with suspected perforation should have an abdominal x-ray to look for free air and peritoneal fluid. Laparotomy should be undertaken as early as possible to suture the perforation, and gentamicin should be added to broaden coverage for polymicrobial peritonitis.

In some high-risk patients with delirium, coma, or shock, high-dose dexamethasone in addition to antibiotics was shown to reduce mortality in Indonesia [10]. The dose should be 3 mg/kg initially followed by 1 mg/kg every 6 h for 48 h. One must be cautious with this therapy because signs and symptoms of perforation will be masked by the steroids. Antipyretic drugs such as aspirin should be avoided because they may produce reductions in blood pressure.

Patients with relapses of typhoid fever should be treated the same as patients with a first attack. Chronic fecal carriers (asymptomatic excretion for a year or longer) should be given high doses of ampicillin or amoxicillin, 100 mg/(kg·day), plus probenecid, 30 mg/(kg·day) for 4 to 6 weeks. Trimethoprim-sulfamethoxazole is also effective. Patients with gallstones or cholecystitis may require cholecystectomy for eradication of the carrier state. Chloramphenicol neither prevents nor can treat effectively the chronic carrier state.

PROGNOSIS

Typhoid fever carried a case fatality rate of about 12 percent in the preantibiotic era; that was reduced to about 4 percent after chloramphenicol came into use. Case fatality rates over 10 percent continue to be reported in developing countries despite availability of antibiotics, whereas developed countries show case fatality rates less than 1 percent. In Bangladesh, fatality rates in hospitalized patients were highest for infants (about 10 percent), lowest for children 2 to 10 years of age (about 2 percent), and intermediate in adolescents and adults (about 6 percent). After treatment with chloramphenicol or other effective drug, most patients become afebrile in 4 to 7 days. In the preantibiotic era, about 10 percent of recovered patients had relapses, and chloramphenicol treatment has not reduced this rate of relapses. The complications of intestinal bleeding or perforation occur in about 5 percent of patients and may not be prevented by antibiotic treatment. Thus, bleeding or perforation are occasionally detected after patients have defervesced during treatment. About 1 to 3 percent of patients become chronic fecal carriers after recovery from typhoid fever.

POPULATION

INCIDENCE AND PREVALENCE

Typhoid fever has been almost eliminated from developed countries because of sewage and water treatment facilities but remains a common disease in developing countries. In 1980, the number of cases occurring yearly was estimated as about 7 million in Asia, over 4 million in Africa, and 0.5 million in Latin America [1]. About 500 cases are diagnosed each year in the United States, and over half of these are in recently arrived travelers who contracted their infections abroad. American travelers face an overall risk of developing typhoid fever of less than 1 case in 10,000 trips, but travelers to high-risk countries like India and Pakistan have a probability of about 4 in 10,000 trips of getting typhoid fever.

TRANSMISSION

Adults and children of all ages and both sexes appear equally susceptible to infection. In developing countries, most cases occur in school-age children and young adults [11]. Although acquired immunity provides some protection, reinfections have been documented. Typhoid fever occurs during all seasons.

In 1873 W. Budd in England postulated that the disease was waterborne and originated from human fecal excretion. This view is still held today, with transmission occurring by the fecal-oral route through contaminated water or food. The main human sources of infection in the community are asymptomatic fecal carriers and cases either during disease or during convalescence. Studies of household contacts of typhoid cases in Chile revealed, however, a low frequency of chronic carriers in the homes and suggested that the cases acquired their infections from ingesting contaminated food and water outside the home [12].

Females and older males are prone to become chronic fecal carriers because underlying cholecystitis enables them to harbor chronic infection in the gallbladder. S. typhi is resistant to drying and cooling, thus allowing bacteria to survive prolonged periods in dried sewage, water, food, and ice.

Vi-phage typing of S. typhi is a useful epidemiological tool to trace cases of typhoid fever to a carrier or food source. Single-source outbreaks of typhoid fever are rare. In endemic situations, multiple Vi-phage types are present and several Vi-phage types may be responsible for an epidemic.

PREVENTION

The traditional method of controlling typhoid is to follow stool cultures of convalescent cases and to report positive cultures to the local health department. The health department investigates nonimported typhoid cases to identify possible food sources or contact with a chronic carrier. Outbreaks of typhoid fever are rare, but occasionally a restaurant can be identified as the source of infection and corrective action taken. If chronic carriers are identified, they should be treated and excluded from food-handling jobs. Travelers to developing countries should be advised to avoid drinking untreated water, drinks served with ice, peeled fruits, and other food that is not served hot. For inhabitants of developing countries, these same dietary precautions would prevent much of the typhoid fever. Additionally, more fundamental changes in sanitary habits and the provision of clean drinking water and methods of sewage disposal will be required.

Vaccination against typhoid fever is another important approach to prevention. The first typhoid vaccine was made in 1896 by Pfeiffer and Kalle. In the United States, the currently available typhoid vaccine, USP (Wyeth Laboratories, Philadelphia, PA) contains 10^9 killed *S. typhi* (Ty-2 strain) organisms per milliliter. It is administered as two subcutaneous injections of 0.5 mL each at intervals of 4 weeks with booster doses given every 3 years if needed. This vaccine results in local pain, fever, and constitutional symptoms on the first day after injection. Furthermore, the vaccine is only partially protective, necessitating that vaccinated persons also practice dietary constraints. Travelers going to endemic areas of Asia, Africa, and Central and South America should consider vaccination if they intend to be exposed to contaminated sources of water and food or will remain in the countries for several months or longer. In Bangkok, Thailand, annual immunization of school children with this vaccine has coincided with a sharp reduction of typhoid fever in that city [13]. A live virus oral vaccine of *S. typhi* Ty21a was developed by R. Germanier in 1975. Initial studies showed a protective efficacy of 94 percent for 3 years [14], but subsequent studies have yielded a lesser degree of protection. This vaccine is available commercially in Europe. Another new subcutaneous vaccine consisting of Vi capsular polysaccharide of *S. typhi* was given intramuscularly to a population at risk in Nepal and showed protective efficacy of about 75 percent [15]. Further testing of these new vaccines is required before they may be employed as alternatives to the standard killed virus vaccine.

REFERENCES

1 Edelman R, Levine MM: Summary of an international workshop on typhoid fever. Rev Infect Dis 8:329, 1986

2 Murray BE, Levine MM, Cordano AM, et al: Survey of plasmids in *Salmonella typhi* from Chile and Thailand. J Infect Dis 151:551, 1985

3 Murphy JR, Baqar S, Munoz C, et al: Characteristics of humoral and cellular immunity to *Salmonella typhi* in residents of typhoid-endemic and typhoid-free regions. J Infect Dis 156:1005, 1987

4 Naylor GRE: Incubation period and other features of food-borne and water-borne outbreaks of typhoid fever in relation to pathogenesis and genetics of resistance. Lancet 1:864, 1983

5 Thisyakorn U, Mansuwan P, Taylor DN: Typhoid and paratyphoid fever in 192 hospitalized children in Thailand. Am J Dis Child 141:862, 1987

6 Klotz SA, Jorgensen JH, Buckwold FJ, et al: Typhoid fever. An epidemic with remarkably few clinical signs and symptoms. Arch Intern Med 144:533, 1984

7 Butler T, Knight J, Nath SK, et al: Typhoid fever complicated by intestinal perforation: a persisting fatal disease requiring surgical management. Rev Infect Dis 7:244, 1985

8 Bradley SF, Kauffman CA: Effect of protein malnutrition on salmonellosis and fever. Infect Immun 56:1000–1002, 1988

9 Roy SK, Speelman P, Butler T, et al: Diarrhea associated with typhoid fever. J Infect Dis 151:1138, 1985

10 Hoffmann SL, Punjabi NH, Kumala S, et al: Reduction of mortality in chloramphenicol-treated typhoid fever by high dose dexamethasone. N Engl J Med 310:82, 1984

11 Hornick RB: Selective primary healthcare: strategies for control of disease in the developing world. XX. Typhoid fever. Rev Infect Dis 7:536, 1985

12 Morris JG, Ferreccio C, Garcia J, et al: Typhoid fever in Santiago, Chili: a study of household contacts of pediatric cases. Am J Trop Med Hyg 33:1198, 1984

13 Bodhidatta L, Taylor DN, Thisyakorn U, et al: Control of typhoid fever in Bangkok, Thailand, by annual immunization of school children with parenteral typhoid vaccine. Rev Infect Dis 9:841, 1987

14 Wahdan MH, Serie C, Cerisier Y, et al: A controlled field trial of live *Salmonella typhi* strain Ty21a oral vaccine against typhoid: Three-year results. J Infect Dis 145:292, 1982

15 Acharya IL, Lowe CW, Thapa R, et al: Prevention of typhoid fever in Nepal with the Vi capsular polysaccharide of *Salmonella typhi*. N Engl J Med 317:1101, 1987

C H A P T E R
80
Salmonellosis · Thomas Butler

Salmonellosis is an acute infection of the intestine and sometimes the blood and other extraintestinal sites with *Salmonella* species and serotypes. The term *Salmonellosis* is synonymous with *Salmonella diarrhea* and *nontyphoid Salmonella infection*. Clinical presentations include febrile enterocolitis, bacteremia, osteomyelitis in sickle cell disease, and infected arterial aneurysms. *Salmonella* other than *S. typhi* and *S. par-* *atyphi* have their natural reservoirs in animals. Humans acquire these infections primarily by eating contaminated meat, poultry, and dairy products. The widespread use of antibiotics in both animals and in humans has worsened this disease by promoting antibiotic resistance and increasing susceptibility of the host. Salmonellosis is one of the infections associated with the acquired immune deficiency syndrome (AIDS).

PARASITE

The salmonellae are motile gram-negative bacilli that belong to the family Enterobacteriaceae. There are three species of *Salmonella: S. typhi, S. choleraesuis,* and *S. enteritidis. S. typhi* is the cause of typhoid fever, *S. choleraesuis* causes diarrhea with a propensity to cause bacteremia, and *S. enteritidis* is the major species that causes disease of both humans and animals. *S. enteritidis* comprises more than 1000 different serotypes. The serotypes are properly written, for example, as *S. enteritidis* bioserotype Paratyphi A or *S. enteritidis* serotype Typhimurium. In common practice, however, they are written as *S. paratyphi* A and *S. typhimurium.*

The salmonellae grow well on agars containing bile salts and appear as gray lucent colonies on MacConkey's agar. They ferment glucose but not lactose. In triple sugar-iron agar they usually produce H_2S and gas. Identification is made by agglutination with antisera specific for serogroups and serotypes.

The species and serotypes of *Salmonella* other than *S. typhi* and *S. paratyphi,* which occur only in humans, are adapted to various animals with humans being an accidental host that plays no role in the maintenance of the organisms in nature. Certain serotypes have special animal preferences and are more pathogenic in humans. For example, in the United States, *S. typhimurium, S. newport,* and *S. dublin* are associated with bovine sources, including milk and beef. *S. hadar, S. heidelberg, S. pullorum,* and *S. enteritidis* are associated with the poultry products of chicken and eggs [1]. In recent years, *S. bredeney* infections have been associated with dried milk products in Australia and *S. ealing* with dried infant formula in England [2].

The nontyphoid salmonellae are susceptible to killing by acidity found in the stomach. At a pH of 3 or less, these organisms are rapidly killed, and this is why people with gastric achlorhydria or with gastric resections for peptic ulcer are prone to acquire salmonellosis. Similarly, volatile fatty acids produced by the normal bacterial flora of the lower intestine inhibit the growth of *Salmonella,* explaining the increased likelihood that persons and animals treated with antibiotics will acquire *Salmonella* infections [3].

The pathogenicity of *Salmonella* species depends on the lipopolysaccharide (0) antigen as shown by the fact that rough mutants with incomplete polysaccharide side chains are not virulent. Virulent strains of *Salmonella* are capable of penetrating the intestinal epithelium and eliciting an acute inflammatory reaction in the intestinal mucosa. Prostaglandins appear to participate in mediating the inflammation and diarrhea as shown by the fact that the inhibitor of prostaglandin synthesis, indomethacin, blocks *Salmonella*-induced diarrhea in an animal model. An enterotoxin that resembles the heat-labile enterotoxin of *Vibrio cholerae* has been described in some strains of *S. typhimurium,* but the role of the enterotoxin in causing *Salmonella* diarrhea is uncertain [4,5].

The nontyphoid salmonellae frequently acquire plasmids from other bacteria that mediate antibiotic resistance [6]. The frequency of plasmid-mediated antibiotic resistance in *Salmonella* strains isolated from humans in the United States rose from 16 percent in 1980 to 24 percent in 1985 [7]. To be fully virulent, nontyphoid salmonellae require the presence of a large (95-kilobase) plasmid. This plasmid is responsible for rendering the bacterium resistant to complement-dependent serum killing by encoding an outer membrane protein and a complete polysaccharide side chain of the lipopolysaccharide in the cell wall [8,9].

In animal infections, *Salmonella* causes widespread systemic infection with bacteremia and intracellular location of bacteria within macrophages of the spleen, liver, and bone marrow. In humans, these infections are usually limited to the intestinal mucosa. However, in patients with defective macrophage function, as occurs during the hemolysis of sickle cell disease, and in patients with hematological malignancies and HIV infections [10], who have defective cell-mediated immunity, *Salmonella* infections are likely to spread via the bloodstream to cause systemic and extraintestinal disease.

PATIENT

INOCULUM AND INCUBATION PERIOD

The first event in infection is the ingestion of contaminated food or water. The number of *Salmonella* required to initiate infection varies from about 10^2 in some outbreaks of naturally acquired illness to about 10^5 to 10^7 in experimentally induced typhoid fever [11]. Small inocula are probably adequate to produce illness in susceptible persons, such as infants and persons with altered intestinal factors including diminished gastric acid, rapid gastric emptying due to pyloroplasty or gastric resection, and medication with antacids or antibiotics [12]. In an outbreak of salmonellosis in the United States which was caused by contaminated milk, a survey showed that persons who had been taking antibiotics before their illnesses drank an average of 2.4 cups of milk, whereas persons who had not taken antibiotics drank an average of 3.6 cups of the milk [13]. During an incubation period of 6 to 48 h, ingested bacteria pass into the small intestine, multiply in the lumen, and penetrate the epithelial cell layer of the small intestine and colon. The incubation period is probably shorter in patients who ingest large inocula or have the altered intestinal factors that increase susceptibility to infection. An acute inflammatory response in the intestinal mucosa is evoked leading to diarrhea and fever. The intestine responds by showing mucosal edema, infiltration of the lamina propria by polymorphonuclear leukocytes and lymphocytes, superficial erosions and ulcerations, and crypt abscesses. The bacteria are present both in the lumen, from which they are excreted in feces, and in the intestinal mucosa, from which they may migrate to regional lymph nodes and circulate in the blood to reach extraintestinal sites.

In untreated patients the duration of fecal carriage is usually limited to 1 to 2 weeks, but some patients have colonization of the gallbladder with *Salmonella* and become chronic fecal carriers. Infants and young children excrete organisms longer than adults. An immune response develops with the formation of antibodies against O and H antigens. In patients with normal immune systems, these illnesses are self-limited and last for a week or less.

ENTEROCOLITIS

The illness begins abruptly with nausea, vomiting, fever, chills, headache, and myalgia (Table 80-1). Diarrhea is the cardinal feature and starts soon after the initial symptoms. The diarrhea is accompanied by abdominal cramping, which is often the most severe symptom and is located in the periumbilical region or the lower quadrants. The diarrhea varies from loose stools of low volume to high-volume watery stools like those of cholera. Occasionally gross blood and mucus are visible in the stools. Both the small intestine and colon are inflamed. Rectal biopsies frequently show erosions, ulceration, edema, cellular infiltrate of the lamina propria, and crypt abscesses. Fluid and electrolyte depletion is occasionally severe but hypovolemic shock is rare, except in small children and elderly individuals.

In most patients the disease is mild and limited to 1 to 4 days duration. Disease tends to be more severe and prolonged in young children, the elderly, and in patients with underlying diseases such as prior gastrectomy, other illnesses requiring antibiotic treatment, malignancies, liver disease, and immunodeficiency states.

The diagnostic approach is to obtain stool for culture on MacConkey's agar and Salmonella-shigella agar. Microscopic examination of stool with a drop of methylene blue reagent overlaid with a coverslip will reveal numerous leukocytes. The peripheral white blood cell count is usually normal but may

show an increase in band forms. The differential diagnosis includes food-poisoning syndromes, viral gastroenteritis, and other acute intestinal infections including shigellosis, diarrhea due to enterotoxigenic *Escherichia coli*, *Campylobacter* sp, *Yersinia enterocolitica*, *V. parahaemolyticus*, and *V. cholerae*.

In the treatment of uncomplicated enterocolitis, antibiotics are not helpful because they do not cause clinical improvement. Furthermore, antibiotic treatment has the unfavorable effect of prolonging fecal excretion of *Salmonella* and increasing the likelihood that a patient will excrete antibiotic-resistant organisms. Treatment should be to rehydrate the patient with isotonic intravenous fluids, when necessary, or with oral rehydration solution [*14*]. In patients with severe abdominal cramps, symptomatic relief may be obtained with diphenoxylate or loperamide.

BACTEREMIA

Blood cultures in patients with *Salmonella* enterocolitis are positive in about 5 percent of cases and usually represent transient bacteremia. In patients with underlying diseases, on the other hand, bacteremia often indicates defective cell-mediated immunity and a need for antibiotic treatment. Infection with *S. choleraesuis* causes bacteremia in the majority of cases. The overall incidence of bacteremia is bimodal by age with peaks in infancy and the elderly. Underlying diseases that predispose persons to *Salmonella* bacteremia are those that compromise reticuloendothelial cell function, such as lymphoma, leukemia, cancers, sickle cell disease and other hemoglobinopathies, collagen-vascular disease, acquired immunodeficiency (HIV infection), therapy with corticosteroids, and renal insufficiency managed by either hemodialysis or transplantation. In the 1960s at the Memorial Sloan-Kettering Cancer Center, *Sal-*

Table 80-1. *Salmonella* syndromes other than typhoid fever

Clinical manifestations	Predisposing factors	Relevant exposures
Acute diarrhea with fever, cramps, and vomiting	None or achlorhydria, gastrectomy, pyloroplasty, or antacid treatment. Antimicrobial treatment during preceding month.	Ingestion of incompletely cooked beef, chicken, or eggs. Ingestion of contaminated milk or dehydrated foods containing milk or eggs. Exposure to persons with diarrhea.
Bacteremia	Impaired cell-mediated immunity due to leukemia, lymphoma, other cancers, HIV infections, irradiation, or corticosteroid treatment. Hemolytic diseases or prior antimicrobial treatment.	None or same as above
Osteomyelitis	Sickle cell disease or other hemoglobinopathy. Trauma to bone or systemic lupus erythematosus.	None or same as above
Infected aneurysm	Increased age and atherosclerosis	None or same as above
Meningitis	Infancy	Infant formula or contaminated milk

monella bacteremia occurred in 35 percent of patients with salmonellosis.

The antimicrobials that are most effective against *Salmonella* bacteremia are ampicillin, amoxicillin, trimethoprim-sulfamethoxazole, and chloramphenicol. Antimicrobial resistance is common, and treatment must be selected accordingly. The newer cephalosporins including cefotaxime, ceftriaxone, and cefoperazone have shown promising results and can be considered as useful alternatives [*15*]. Treatment of salmonella bacteremia, in the absence of localizing signs, should be continued for about 14 days pending a satisfactory response. Patients with osteomyelitis or endocarditis will require treatment for 4 to 6 weeks or longer.

Salmonella bacteremia occurs also without clinically evident enterocolitis, and these patients may present with fever and no localizing signs of illness. They should be treated with an appropriate antibiotic. These patients with bacteremia may develop signs of local suppuration subsequently, and the physician must search carefully for any anatomical sites of localized inflammation. Chronic bacteremia with *Salmonella* has been described in patients with *Schistosoma mansoni* infection in Egypt, and this form of bacteremia occurs usually without symptoms.

In individuals infected by HIV, persistent *Salmonella* bacteremia has been reported throughout the world. About a third of these patients did not have symptoms of concurrent enterocolitis. Nearly half of them had one or more relapses of bacteremia following treatment. In many instances, *Salmonella* bacteremia occurred before other AIDS-defining opportunistic infections in this group of patients. The most common serotypes associated with HIV infection in the United States are *S. typhimurium* and *S. enteritidis*. The possible reasons for the association of HIV and *Salmonella* bacteremia are defective cell-mediated immunity, hemolysis, prior use of antibiotics, and increased exposure to infection [*10*]. The Centers for Disease Control list recurrent *Salmonella* bacteremia as one of the indicator diseases for AIDS. Therefore, any patient presenting with recurrent *Salmonella* bacteremia should be evaluated with serological tests for infection with the human immunodeficiency virus.

EXTRAINTESTINAL LOCALIZED INFECTION

Although the majority of patients with enterocolitis do not develop extraintestinal infection, there are several well-described diseases caused by *Salmonella* infection at various sites. Previous gastroenteritis is usually not described and stool cultures are negative, but the intestine is presumed to be the original site of entry of the infection. The extraintestinal diseases require antimicrobial treatment, as described for *Salmonella* bacteremia. In addition, surgical drainage or resection of the infected site is often needed.

Osteomyelitis or arthritis due to *Salmonella* may occur in normal bones but is more likely to develop in patients with sickle cell disease or other hemoglobinopathy, systemic lupus erythematosus, neoplasms, prior bone surgery or trauma, and cirrhosis of the liver. The bacteria are likely to localize in abnormal areas of bone, as occurs during infarction in sickle cell anemia. The long bones and vertebrae are common sites of osteomyelitis.

Meningitis due to *Salmonella* occurs almost exclusively in infants and carries a case fatality rate of about 85 percent. The clinical course is long, and there may be relapses. Neurological complications include cerebral abscess, subdural empyema, and hydrocephalus. Epidemics of *Salmonella* meningitis have been reported in hospital nurseries.

Arteritis occurs in patients over 50 years old who have atherosclerotic aneurysms. The bacteria localize in the aneurysm and produce acute inflammation. *S. choleraesuis* is the most common serotype in this infection. Mortality is high and early surgical intervention is often necessary.

Abscesses have been reported in the spleen, liver, surgical wounds, lung, and other tissues. Although the kidney is less commonly affected, *Salmonella* bacteriuria may occur in patients with structural defects in the urinary tract. Patients with chronic obstruction in the urinary tract due to *Schistosoma haematobium* are predisposed to be chronic urinary carriers of *Salmonella*.

POPULATION

INCIDENCE

Salmonella infection is one of the leading causes of acute diarrhea worldwide. It was the most common recognized cause of bacterial diarrhea in the United States until recent years when *Campylobacter* became more frequently identified. In the United States, 65,347 cases of human salmonellosis were reported to the Centers for Disease Control in 1985, representing about a threefold increase during the previous 10 years. The actual number of infections in the United States has been estimated at more than a million a year because of frequent failure to obtain cultures and underreporting [*16*]. In tropical countries with lower standards of hygiene, the incidence of salmonellosis is much higher, but lack of reporting makes it impossible to estimate the numbers of cases that occur.

TRANSMISSION

The most important means of acquiring *Salmonella* is by the ingestion of contaminated food. Contaminated water is rarely a source of infection in North America. The foods that are most likely to be contaminated with *Salmonella* are meats, especially beef and chicken, eggs, and milk. Because salmonellae survive for long periods in the environment and resist drying, contamination has been a problem with powdered milk, cake mixes, and other dehydrated products that contain either eggs or milk. The largest outbreak of salmonellosis in the United States occurred in 1985 in Illinois, affecting an estimated 168,000 people, and was caused by pasteurized milk that was contaminated in the plant by unpasteurized milk [*12*].

Eggs are a leading source of salmonellosis in the United States. Either the shell or the egg yolk may be contaminated. Foods containing raw eggs, such as eggnog and Hollandaise sauce, may be contaminated. Furthermore, the yolks of eggs that are served soft-boiled or fried "sunnyside up" may not reach adequate temperatures to kill bacteria and can transmit infection.

Person-to-person spread of *Salmonella* is possible because humans excrete organisms in their stool during disease and for varying periods during convalescence. This mode of transmission, however, appears to be relatively rare. Unlike typhoid fever, in which asymptomatic carriers working as food handlers have caused extensive infection, food handlers are not an important source of nontyphoid *Salmonella* infections. As infants are at high risk for salmonellosis, their mothers occasionally acquire infection from the handling of their children's stools. Other less frequent sources of infection are household pets, including turtles.

PERSONS AT RISK

Infants and the elderly, such as inhabitants of nursing homes, are more susceptible than other age groups. Patients with underlying diseases are more prone to salmonellosis. In particular, persons with achlorhydria or reduced stomach acid due to gastrectomy, vagotomy, or antacid therapy are at increased risk. Use of antibiotics in the month before infection may increase the risk of acquiring salmonellosis by fivefold or more.

Persons who eat institutional food that is prepared without optimal precautions taken in cooking, washing, and storage are at increased risk of acquiring salmonellosis. Similarly, attending group picnics may be associated with some risk. Travelers going to developing countries are at high risk of developing traveler's diarrhea, a part of which is attributable to *Salmonella* infection.

GEOGRAPHICAL DISTRIBUTION

Salmonellosis occurs in both developed and developing countries. In the least-developed countries, *Salmonella* is a much less frequent cause of diarrhea than shigellosis, enterotoxigenic *E. coli*, and rotavirus. This is probably because impoverished peoples eat relatively little meat, eggs, and milk. Furthermore, they cook food fresh and do not often store their food under refrigeration. In certain more developed countries, *Salmonella* becomes a more frequent cause of diarrhea because the use of meats and storage of meat under refrigeration is a common practice. Farmers in more-developed countries are likely to use antibiotics in the feed of chickens and cattle, thereby increasing susceptibility of these animals to acquiring *Salmonella* infections. Under conditions of antibiotic use, the *Salmonella* species will acquire antibiotic resistance plasmids [17]. In developed countries, the modern practice of large-scale food processing and the handling of unpasteurized milk in dairy plants has made widespread disease outbreaks possible.

PREVENTION

The prevention of salmonellosis requires attention to personal hygiene and governmental inspection of meat, eggs, milk, and food-processing facilities. Individuals can reduce the likelihood of infection by sanitary practices in the kitchen. When handling uncooked meats, it is important to wash one's hands and counter surfaces frequently so that potentially contaminated meat juices are not transferred to other foods such as salads or already cooked items. One should avoid eating incompletely cooked meats and foods containing raw eggs.

A more fundamental approach to reducing the problem of salmonellosis will require further regulation of farming and food production. Limiting the use of antibiotics for fattening animals would probably reduce the rate of contamination and the likelihood of propagating antibiotic-resistant organisms. To ensure that eggs are not contaminated, they may have to be pasteurized. Cows that show signs of illness and loss of weight should not be slaughtered to obtain lean beef. It has been proposed that any plant which processes dried milk should not allow any unpasteurized milk on the premises.

REFERENCES

1 St Louis ME, Morse DL, Potter ME, et al: The emergence of grade A eggs as a major source of *Salmonella enteritidis* infections. JAMA 259:2103, 1988

2 Rowe B, Begg NT, Hutchinson DN, et al: *Salmonella ealing* infections associated with consumption of infant dried milk. Lancet 2:900, 1987

3 Que JV, Casey SW, Hentges DJ: Factors responsible for increased susceptibility of mice to intestinal colonization after treatment with streptomycin. Infect Immun 53:116, 1986

4 Baloda SB, Popoff MY, Wadstrom T: Enterotoxigenicity among *Salmonella typhimurium* strains isolated in France. Eur J Microbiol 4:129, 1985

5 Molina NC, Peterson JW: A cholera toxin-like toxin released by *Salmonella* species in the presence of mitomycin C. Infect Immun 30:224, 1980

6 Frost JA, Rowe B, Ward LR, et al: Characterization of resistance plasmids and carried phages in an epidemic clone of multi-resistant *Salmonella typhimurium* in India. J Hyg Camb 88:193, 1982

7 MacDonald KL, Cohen ML, Hargrett-Bean NT, et al: Changes in antimicrobial resistance of Salmonella isolated from humans in the United States. JAMA 258:1496, 1987

8 Hackett J, Wyk P, Reeves P, et al: Mediation of serum resistance in *Salmonella typhimurium* by an 11-kilodalton polypeptide encoded by the cryptic plasmid. J Infect Dis 155:540, 1987

9 Vandenbosch JL, Rabert DK, Jones GW: Plasmid-associated resistance of *Salmonella typhimurium* to complement activated by the classical pathway. Infect Immun 55:2645, 1987

10 Sperber SJ, Schleupner CJ: Salmonellosis during infection with human immunodeficiency virus. Rev Infect Dis 9:925, 1987

11 Blaser MJ, Newman LS: A review of human salmonellosis: I. Infective dose. Rev Infect Dis 4:1096, 1982

12 Riley LW, Cohen ML, Seals JE, et al: Importance of host factors in human salmonellosis caused by multiresistant strains of *Salmonella*. J Infect Dis 149:878, 1984

13 Ryan CA, Nickels MK, Hargrett-Bean NT, et al: Massive outbreak of antimicrobial-resistant salmonellosis traced to pasteurized milk. JAMA 258:3269, 1987

14 Gorbach SL: Bacterial diarrhoea and its treatment. Lancet 2:1378, 1987

15 Soe GB, Overturf GD: Treatment of typhoid fever and other systemic salmonellosis with cefotaxime, ceftriaxone, cefoperazone, and other newer cephalosporins. Rev Infect Dis 9:719, 1987

16 Chalker RB, Blaser MJ: A review of human salmonellosis: III. Magnitude of salmonella infection in the United States. Rev Infect Dis 10:111, 1988

17 Spika JS, Waterman SH, Hoo GWS, et al: Chloramphenicol-resistant *Salmonella newport* traced through hamburger to dairy farms. N Engl J Med 316:565, 1987

CHAPTER 81 / *Shigellosis* · Gerald T. Keusch · Samuel B. Formal · Michael L. Bennish

Although shigellosis is an ancient affliction, described with clarity in the Old Testament; by Thucidydes; in medical texts of the seventeenth century; and elsewhere, the causative organism was only isolated and described by Kiyoshi Shiga in 1898 [*1*]. With Shiga's discovery, the etiological separation of bacillary (*shigellosis*) and amebic forms of dysentery became possible for the first time.

Throughout history, bacillary dysentery has been associated with high mortality rates. In the present century, social, environmental, and economic changes in industrialized countries have altered its epidemiological behavior and have made death in association with shigellosis a rare event [*2–5*]. In less-developed countries (LDCs), however, the infection continues to be prevalent, significantly associated with malnutrition, and an important contributing cause of death in the young with an estimated 140 million cases and 576,000 deaths occurring annually in children less than 5 years old (excluding China) [*6*].

PARASITE

Shigellae are classified in the family Enterobacteriaceae, tribe Eschericheae, and are thus closely related to *Escherichia coli*. Indeed, the two genera (*Escherichia* and *Shigella*) cannot be distinguished from one another on the basis of polynucleotide-sequence relatedness. The microorganism is a slender, nonmotile, gram-negative bacillus capable of cellular invasion and produces a protein toxin with potent biological activity. On the basis of biochemical and serological distinctions, four species have been defined: (*S. dysenteriae, S. flexneri, S. boydii, S. sonnei*) with multiple subtypes within each species (Table 81-1). There are also important clinical and epidemiological distinctions between the four species (Table 81-2), but the reasons for these differences are not well understood.

Shigella has a narrow host range, occurring exclusively in humans and subhuman primates [*7*]. Despite its host specificity, *Shigella* has not adapted for prolonged survival as a commensal organism in nature. It causes significant rates of morbidity and mortality and is not carried in the stools for more than a few weeks during convalescence in most individuals. Rather, shigellae depend upon frequent contact among susceptible persons for continued existence [*7*].

Rapid transmission is even more important because the genus is not hardy in the environment. The organisms are very susceptible to high ambient temperatures and especially to desiccation. In cooler, more moist environments, shigellae (especially *S. sonnei*) survive better, but not for very long [*8*]. These conditions may be found in and around toilets in more temperate climates and may in part explain the increasing prevalence of *S. sonnei* infection in the industrialized nations.

The delicate nature of the organism in the environment is also manifested in the rapid loss of viability in human excreta; the difficulty in obtaining a positive swab culture from the anus and perianal region even during clinical infection; and the improved yield of positive cultures from rapid, bedside plating of stool specimens on suitable bacteriological media [*7*]. The organism is rapidly overgrown by the fecal flora in acid stools.

Lacking flagella, shigellae are nonmotile and therefore do not have flagellar H antigens. While some strains in nature may possess surface fimbriae or pili, the virulence of strains completely lacking surface appendages indicates that these structures are not necessary for virulence.

The organization of *Shigella* lipopolysaccharides and cell membrane structures is typical for the Enterobacteriaceae. For several serotypes the nature of the somatic O-antigen repeat groups has been immunochemically characterized. These determinants are important for diagnostic serological reactions and may play a role in pathogenesis. Occasional isolates produce surface (K) antigens which may interfere with their ability to agglutinate; heating these organisms in a boiling-water bath for 1 to 2 h restores the O-agglutinability. In addition, virulent strains in general possess one or more plasmids that may carry information for the synthesis of key virulence factors, and for

Table 81-1. Usual laboratory characteristics of the genus *Shigella*

Species	Sero-group	Serotypes (subtypes)	Mannitol utilization	Lactose utilization	Gas production	Ornithine decarboxylase	Lysine decarboxylase	H$_2$S production	Motility
S. dysenteriae	A	10	−	−	−	−	−	−	−
S. flexneri	B	6(12)	+	−	−*	−	−	−	−
S. boydii	C	15	+	−	−	−	−	−	−
S. sonnei	D	1†	+	−	−	+	−	−	−
E. coli— noninvasive	NA‡	NA	+	+	+	±	±	−	+
E. coli— invasive	NA	NA	+	±	−	±	±	−	±
Salmonella sp.	NA	NA	+	−	+	+	+	+	+

*A few *S. flexneri* 6 produce gas.
†Form I and II are serotypically distinguishable and multiple subtypes can be identified by colicin typing.
‡NA = not applicable.

plasmid-mediated transferrable antibiotic resistance. An 80 million MW plasmid carrying multiple drug resistance (sulfonamide, tetracycline, streptomycin, chloramphenicol) and a 5.5 million MW plasmid containing the ampicillin-resistance transposon, TnA, are the most frequently encountered.

VIRULENCE FACTORS

One of the most important attributes of the dysentery bacilli is their ability to penetrate and multiply within epithelial cells [9,10]. Within cells the organism is protected from host antibacterial factors and can multiply without inhibition. It is presumed to be this property that confers high infectivity with low inoculum size, in the range of a few hundred to a few thousand viable bacilli [8]. However, invasion occurs primarily in the colon, and not proximally, and the organism still has to get from the mouth to the colon before it can be sequestered intracellularly. In experimental models, invasion per se is surprisingly innocuous for the cell, and cell lysis is not an early consequence [11]. Nonetheless, virulence is associated with early escape from the phagocytic vesicle to the cytoplasm, and with subsequent multiplication leading to cell damage and death. The ability to multiply within the epithelial cell is distinguishable from invasion. For example, conjugal transfer or transduction of *E. coli* chromosomal DNA from the *xyl-rha*, the *his*, and the *purE* loci to *Shigella* recipients results in invasive hybrids that are unable to multiply and survive [12]. These strains are avirulent. At least in *S. flexneri*, the *xyl-rha* locus codes for an iron-binding protein, aerobactin, and an iron-regulated outer-membrane protein which may be important for iron metabolism [12]. The *his* region regulates expression of the specific side chains of the somatic antigen, but it is not clear how this enhances intracellular survival.

Transfer of these genetic loci, even with much of the rest of the *Shigella* chromosome, to *E. coli* K-12 does not result in a virulent transconjugant [13]. Additional necessary viru-

Table 81-2. Epidemiological and clinical features of *Shigella* species

Species	Prevalence	Environmental survival	Convalescent carriage	Frequency of plasmid-mediated antibiotic resistance	Frequency of symptoms		
					Diarrhea	Dysentery	HUS*
S. dysenteriae	Low, except during epidemic spread	Poor	<4 weeks, but prolonged in malnourished	+ + +	+	+ + +	+ +
S. flexneri	High in developing countries	Poor	<4 weeks, but prolonged in malnourished	+ +	+ +	+ +	±
S. boydii	Low, except the Indian subcontinent	Poor	<3 weeks	+	+ + +	+	−
S. sonnei	High in industrialized nations	Best, especially in a cool, moist environment	<2 weeks	+ + +	+ + + +	uncommon	−

*Hemolytic-uremic syndrome.

lence properties have been found on large (120 to 140 MDa) plasmids in all *Shigella* species and in enteroinvasive *E. coli,* and on small (5 MDa) plasmids in *S. dysenteriae* type 1 [*12*]. The large plasmids are functionally equivalent, genetically conserved, and contain several virulence genes. One, known as the *ipa* locus (invasion-plasmid antigen), controls several outer-membrane proteins (OMPs) that appear to recognize surface structures on epithelial cells and initiate internalization of the organism [*14*]. A second locus, *inv* (invasion), may function in the insertion of the OMPs into the bacterial outer membrane [*15*]. Additional genes of importance are *virF,* which can be recognized by binding of the dye Congo red, a marker of surface charge [*16*]; and *virG,* recognized as a hemolysin but which may really function in the escape of the organism from the phagosome to the cytoplasm and in transfer from cell to cell in extending local infection [*17,18*].

A second property of apparent importance is the production of a highly potent cytotoxin known as *Shiga toxin* [*19*]. Although originally described only in *S. dysenteriae* type 1, the same or a biologically similar toxin is found in all *Shigella* species. Shiga toxin has two subunits, a larger enzymatically active A subunit (approximately 32,000 Da), and a smaller B subunit (MW = 7791) which is involved in binding to cellular targets [*20*]. The native toxin consists of 1 A subunit and 5 B subunits. The mechanism of action of the A subunit has recently been defined. It has a highly specific glycohydrolase activity, splitting the sugar from adenine 4624 in the 28 S rRNA of the 60 S ribosomal subunit [*21*]. This results in irreversible inhibition of protein synthesis in a manner identical to that of the toxic plant lectin ricin. Indeed, a region of significant sequence homology in the A subunits of the two toxins

has been detected [*22*]. The B subunit of Shiga toxin is a lectin that recognizes a specific sequence of sugars, galactose-α 1→4 galactose, linked to other sugars or directly to ceramide [*23,24*]. This same disaccharide is present in certain globoseries glycolipids of the P blood-group system. At least in rabbit small bowel, the specific toxin-binding glycolipid is Gb3, a galactose-α 1→4 galactose-β 1→4 glucose trisaccharide attached to lipid [*23*].

Gb3 appears to be a critical determinant of enterotoxicity in the small intestine, that is, net fluid accumulation in response to introduction of toxin into the bowel lumen. In rabbits, Gb3 is not present in large amounts in brush borders until after week 16 of life, and the animal is refractory to toxin effects until that age [*25*]. The mechanism of the net secretory response is also related to Gb3 and is a consequence of its presence in villus but not crypt cells [*26*]. As a result, crypt cells are unaffected by toxin, and chloride secretion by toxin-treated mucosa remains normal. In contrast, Shiga toxin inhibits protein synthesis specifically in villus cells leading to impaired sodium absorption by both neutral NaCl and glucose-facilitated pathways. The resulting accumulation of Na in the lumen causes retention of water and leads to isotonic fluid accumulation.

PATIENT

PATHOGENESIS

Pathogenesis of clinical disease, especially the colonic phase of illness, is a complex sequence of events. First, shigellae invade colonic epithelial cells, escape to the cytoplasm, multiply, and invade adjacent cells [*27–29*]. An inflammatory re-

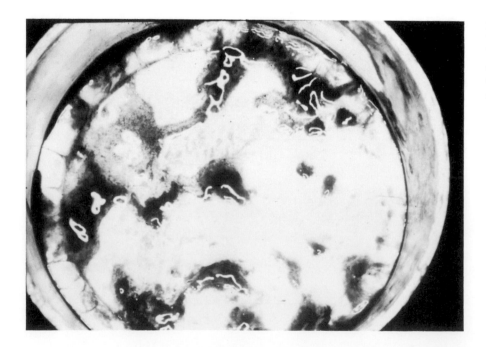

Figure 81-1. The classical stool of bacillary dysentery. Even in this black and white photo the scant quantities of bloody, mucoid excreta can be appreciated. (*Courtesy of Myron M. Levine.*)

sponse develops in the lamina propria, and there is damage and sloughing of epithelial cells [*29,30*], leading to microulcerations and a bloody inflammatory exudate (the dysenteric stool). The biological events which must occur include cell-cell contact of the bacteria and epithelial cells (possibly mediated by specific adhesins), rearrangement of the host cell's cytoskeleton leading to phagocytosis, rapid escape of the shigellae to the cytoplasm, distribution throughout the epithelial cell along actin filaments, and invasion of adjacent host cells [*16,18,31–33*].

The role of toxin in causing cell damage is still uncertain [*19*]. In experimental infections in the monkey, a phase of small-bowel involvement with fluid secretion and no epithelial cell invasion has been clearly demonstrated [*29*]. This secretory phase has been reproduced in rabbit small bowel with pure toxin [*25,26*]. Whether or not there is a small-bowel phase in human infection to account for the early watery diarrhea in shigellosis remains controversial. Toxin has been demonstrated by a specific enzyme-linked immunosorbent assay (ELISA) method in the stool of 80 percent of patients with *S. dysenteriae* type 1 infection, but in less than 20 percent of those with *S. flexneri* infection [*34*], possibly because many of the latter make antigenically distinct cytotoxins.

CLINICAL MANIFESTATIONS

There is a gradient in clinical shigellosis from mild to dehydrating watery diarrhea, and from blood-streaked diarrhea to dysentery [*35*], a syndrome comprising abdominal pain, tenesmus, and the frequent passage of stools composed largely of blood and mucus. Intestinal symptoms usually begin as watery diarrhea and progress within hours to a few days to dysentery, although *S. sonnei* (the predominant isolate in developed countries) ordinarily causes only watery diarrhea. In LDCs, where *S. dysenteriae* type 1 and *S. flexneri* infections predominate, dysentery is the symptom that usually prompts patients to seek medical attention.

Onset of the disease is heralded by fever, lethargy, and anorexia. Diarrhea usually follows within a day of the initial symptoms and is most often watery at the beginning. If dysentery occurs, it is likely within 24 to 48 h of the onset of illness, although in *S. dysenteriae* type 1 infections the disease progression can be so rapid that watery diarrhea is never apparent. In patients with more severe disease, the stools contain only blood and mucus, with no fecal material present (Fig. 81-1). Inflammation and ulceration is most extensive in the distal colon and rectum, becoming progressively more mild and less frequent in the transverse and ascending colon, respectively [*36*]. Ulceration can extend to the level of the lamina propria (Fig. 81-2), with an inflammatory infiltrate present in the submucosa as well as the surface epithelium [*37*]. Proctitis produces tenesmus, a painful straining during defecation that may be relieved only momentarily by the passage of stool. In younger children and infants, repeated episodes of tenesmus can result in rectal prolapse (Fig. 81-3). Stool frequency may

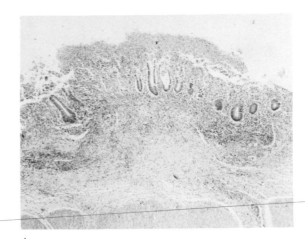

A

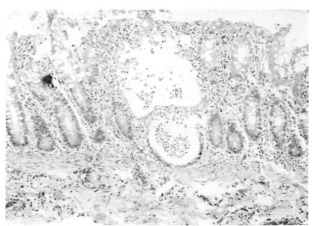

B

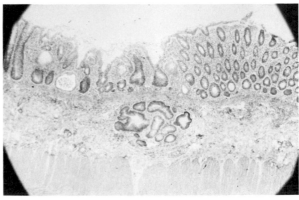

C

Figure 81-2. Histological examination of colonic tissue in patients with shigellosis. *A*. Acute ulceration with epithelial cell destruction, exudate, and crypt abscess. *B*. Large ulcer extending to the lamina propria and partially covered by a mucopurulent layer. *C*. Autopsy sample from a patient with prolonged disease which shows glandular regeneration below the lamina propria (colitis profunda). (*Courtesy of Dr. Moyenul Islam.*)

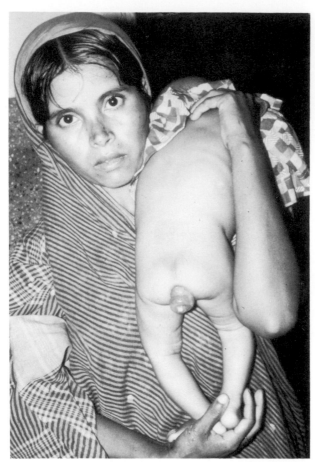

Figure 81-3. Rectal prolapse in a Bangladeshi child with acute shigellosis. The rectal mucosa was easily reduced by gentle manual manipulation, and the child made an uneventful recovery. (*Courtesy of Dr. Mujibur M. Rahaman.*)

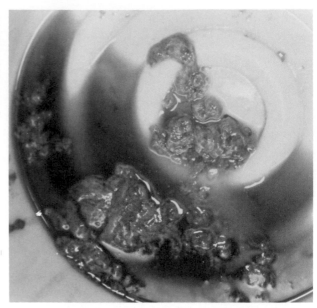

Figure 81-4. The typical stool of patients with shigellosis, showing a mixture of formed stool, blood, and mucus. In this patient, a sloughed pseudomembrane in the shape of the colon is evident in the center of the sample and is a consequence of extensive colonic inflammation (see Fig. 81-1).

be as much as 100 times a day, but the quantity passed is small, averaging less than 30 mL/(kg·day) [*38*], compared to 100 mL/(kg·day) or more in children with cholera or other watery diarrheas. Colitis can be so severe and extensive that the contiguous portions of the mucosal epithelium are shed along with a pseudomembrane consisting of a fibrinous exudate containing leukocytes, erythrocytes, and mucus (Fig. 81-4).

A variety of complications occur in association with shigellosis. These can be divided into colonic manifestations and systemic complications. Among the former, the most serious is *toxic megacolon* [*39*]. Patients develop a massively dilated colon (Fig. 81-5*A* and 81-5*B*), similar to toxic megacolon due to ulcerative colitis, with obtundation and often bizarre neurological manifestations (Fig. 81-5*C*). Pathogenesis remains obscure; however, this complication occurs most commonly in *S. dysenteriae* type 1 infection, and appears to be related to the intensity of the colitis rather than a direct effect of Shiga toxin on intestinal motility [*40*]. Colonic perforation is a sec-

ond, less common but potentially lethal complication [*41*]. The actual incidence of perforation is undoubtedly higher than reported because it can be difficult to distinguish perforation from the severe underlying colitis unless free peritoneal air is present on roentgenogram. A third colonic complication is a protein-losing enteropathy with severe infection [*42*]. Loss of protein from the gut contributes to the deterioration in nutritional status as well as host resistance to infection (see Chap. 23). Shigellosis may precipitate kwashiorkor in patients who are marginally nourished, as is often the case among infected patients in LDCs.

Systemic complications are seen most commonly, though not exclusively, in patients with *S. dysenteriae* type 1 infections. The most dramatic of these complications is the hemolytic-uremic syndrome (HUS) [*43*]. In developed countries, HUS is seen most commonly in association with infection by certain strains of *E. coli* that produce toxins related to Shiga toxin [*44*]. This complication usually develops at the end of the first week of illness when the dysentery is resolving. Patients will become oliguric, sometimes progressing to anuria, with azotemia. Hemolysis is often severe and rapid, with decreases in hematocrit of 10 percent or more within 24 h, and multiple blood transfusions may be required. The anuria presents a less immediate problem, as the rise in creatinine is gradual, and problems with hyperkalemia are uncommon since patients are often potassium depleted from preexisting malnutrition and from continuing potassium losses in the stool.

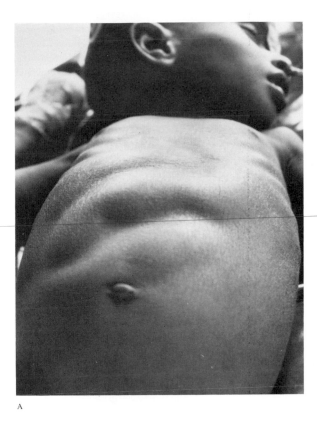

A

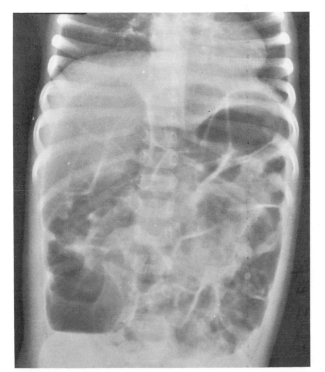

B

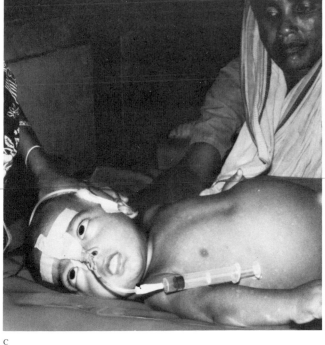

C

Figure 81-5. Toxic megacolon during shigellosis. *A.* A 3-year-old boy with marked colonic distention evident by visual inspection of the abdomen. *B.* Roentgenogram of the abdomen showing distention of the entire colon. There are also "mucosal islands" present in the ascending colon, indicating extensive ulceration and edema of the surrounding mucosa. *C.* A 15-month-old boy with toxic megacolon, obtundation and posturing. Lip smacking was one of a number of bizarre neurological findings in this patient.

Nonetheless, peritoneal dialysis, occasionally for periods of 3 weeks or longer, may be necessary. Thrombocytopenia is also part of this syndrome, is usually mild (30,000 to 100,000 per microliter) and uncommonly causes clinical manifestations such as purpura or hemorrhage. Any of the individual manifestations of HUS may occur alone.

Leukemoid reaction occurs primarily in Shiga bacillus dysentery, either in association with HUS or independently [45]. Patients with leukemoid reaction are at increased risk of death, but it is unclear if the increase in circulating neutrophils is in itself deleterious, or if other complications in association with leukocytosis are responsible for the increased mortality. Since the leukemoid reaction often occurs after treatment has been initiated, and *Shigella* have been eradicated from the gut, it may sustain the inflammatory reaction in the intestinal mucosa and contribute to the prolonged colitis that can be seen following infection.

Bacteremia with *Shigella* or other Enterobacteriaceae has been documented in 9 percent of severely ill, hospitalized patients in Bangladesh [46]. Malnourished patients are at highest risk and death is common (21 percent in the Bangladesh series). In addition, marked hyponatremia is frequently observed during either *S. dysenteriae* type 1 or *S. flexneri* infection, and does not appear to be related to stool water and sodium losses [*47*]. It too is associated with an increased risk of death. Although stool losses during shigellosis are modest compared with watery diarrhea due to *V. cholerae* or toxigenic *E. coli,* the frequency and severity of hyponatremia are more common in shigellosis. During a 1-year period in Bangladesh at the Treatment Centre of the International Centre for Diarrhoeal Disease Research (ICDDR), 29 percent of 154 patients infected with *S. dysenteriae* type 1 had admission serum sodiums of 120 mmol/L or less. These patients are generally obtunded or lethargic while severely hyponatremic, but rapidly become more alert following infusion of saline, even before full correction of serum sodium concentration (Fig. 81-6).

Seizures are the most common neurological complication in shigellosis [*48*], usually occurring in children during the early stages of illness. Seizures frequently develop before diarrhea begins, and are almost always accompanied by fever. Since

they are less commonly associated with other febrile diarrheas such as salmonellosis, precipitating factors in addition to fever may be present in shigellosis, but none have been identified. Seizures are most often generalized, usually do not recur, and are rarely complicated. If the patient recovers from the underlying illness there are almost never residual neurological deficits.

Reactive arthritis is described following *S. flexneri* infections, either alone or as part of a full-blown Reiter's syndrome (iritis, urethritis, arthritis) and is strongly associated with the HLA-B27 histocompatibility antigen [*49,50*]. The arthritis can be prolonged and destructive. It is not, to our knowledge, a commonly recognized problem in the developing world, in part because follow-up of patients is difficult or possibly because the necessary genetic predisposing factors are lacking.

The most important complication in terms of public health, however, is the effect of bacillary dysentery on the nutrition of children. Shigellosis can affect nutrition in at least four ways: (1) through the metabolic costs of infection, which in-

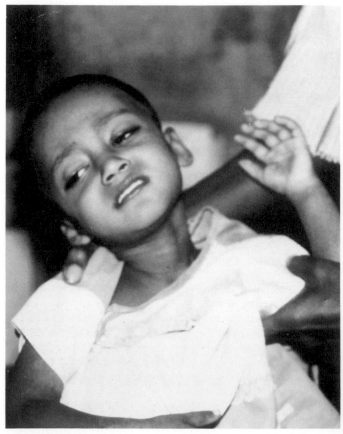

A

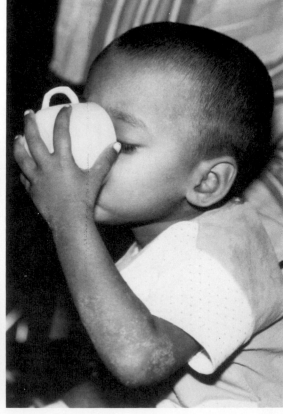

B

Figure 81-6. A 2-year-old child with *S. dysenteriae* type 1 infection and profound hyponatremia. *A.* The child prior to intravenous infusion of 3% NaCl when her serum sodium was 114 mmol/L, and she was markedly irritable and refused oral fluids. *B.* Following hypertonic saline infusion, the serum sodium concentration has risen to 123 mmol/L. Although still severely hyponatremic, she is alert, and extremely thirsty in spite of being well hydrated because of a high circulating level of antidiuretic hormone.

clude fever and catabolism associated with the host inflammatory response; (2) protein loss through an inflamed colonic mucosa; (3) decreased caloric intake because of anorexia; (4) diminished absorption of ingested nutrients (see Chap. 23). All of these effects contribute to the growth faltering that occurs in children in LDCs following shigellosis [51]. In otherwise healthy patients with access to adequate food, nutrient losses and growth faltering due to infection are quickly corrected during convalescence. In children subject to frequent infections with other pathogens, and who have limited access to food (which is usually bulky with low calorie density), these losses may never be overcome.

A variety of other complications have been seen during *Shigella* infection; among these are pneumonia, meningitis, vaginitis in prepubertal girls, keratoconjunctivitis, and a rash similar to the rose spots seen in typhoid fever. Some of these manifestations, especially pneumonia and meningitis, may be due to simultaneous infections with other pathogens, as isolation of *Shigella* from either sputum or cerebrospinal fluid rarely, if ever, occurs. The keratoconjunctivitis and vaginitis are probably direct infection with *Shigella*; however, neither is a common or important clinical problem.

In well-nourished persons, the disease is usually self-limited even without therapy, and symptoms last from a few days to a week or two. Duration depends in part on the infecting species, and perhaps to a larger degree on the nutritional status of the host [52]. Malnourished patients may have continued symptoms of colitis, and chronic changes in the colonic mucosa (Fig. 81-2C). Excretion of the organism in the stools usually persists for a few weeks without antibiotic treatment, although malnourished individuals may excrete the organism for prolonged periods of time [53].

Death in shigellosis is most common at the extremes of age, children under 5 years old (especially those less than 1 year old) and adults over 60. There is no one predominant cause of death in shigellosis, and most of the complications described can prove lethal. Although mortality in association with *S. dysenteriae* type 1 epidemics has received the most attention, in places where endemic shigellosis coexists with widespread childhood malnutrition, infection with any of the four species of *Shigella* may be fatal (Table 81-3). In these patients, the cause of death most commonly is progressive inanition and secondary infection. Mortality rates may also be higher for children discharged from the hospital after dysentery than for those who had watery diarrhea.

DIAGNOSIS

Definitive diagnosis of shigellosis is microbiological. Unfortunately, in LDCs (especially in the least developed of these countries, where shigellosis is most common), there are at least three major impediments to the routine use of microbiological diagnosis in the management of patients with shigellosis: (1) lack of proper laboratory facilities; (2) cost of media, other supplies, and equipment, which require expenditure of scarce foreign currency; (3) the time from culture to diagnosis is too long to have an impact in therapeutic decisions in nutritionally compromised patients, in whom early therapy appears critical.

In the field setting, then, diagnosis usually depends on the use of an algorithm based mainly on clinical features, aided by microscopic examination and culture of stool when facilities are available (Fig. 81-7). The most pathognomonic feature of shigellosis is bloody dysentery, and mothers in most LDCs are able to reliably describe this finding and to distinguish it from watery diarrhea [54]. Since etiology of the majority of cases of bloody dysentery in children is *Shigella* (and not *Entamoeba histolytica*, as is commonly believed and taught), a history of

Table 81-3. Fatality rates, by *Shigella* species, of patients with shigellosis admitted to a hospital in Dhaka, Bangladesh, during a 5-year period*

Species or serotype	Total admissions	Discharged alive	Left against advice	Transferred to other hospital	Died in hospital
S. flexneri	2319	1841 (79)[†]	211 (9)	37 (2)	230 (10)
S. dysenteriae type 1	1251	976 (78)	136 (11)	40 (3)	99 (8)
S. dysenteriae types 2–10	132	112 (85)	5 (4)	2 (2)	13 (10)
S. boydii	303	245 (81)	24 (8)	3 (1)	31 (10)
S. sonnei	145	119 (82)	12 (8)	2 (1)	12 (8)
Total	4150	3293 (79)	388 (9)	84 (2)	385 (9)

*Patients were admitted to the inpatient unit of the Dhaka Treatment Centre of the International Centre for Diarrhoeal Disease Research, Bangladesh. In this population, which contained a high percentage of malnourished patients, the fatality rates were high for all species, with the fatality rate in *S. flexneri*–infected patients actually slightly (and significantly) higher than for those with *S. dysenteriae* type 1.
[†]Percent is given in parenthesis.

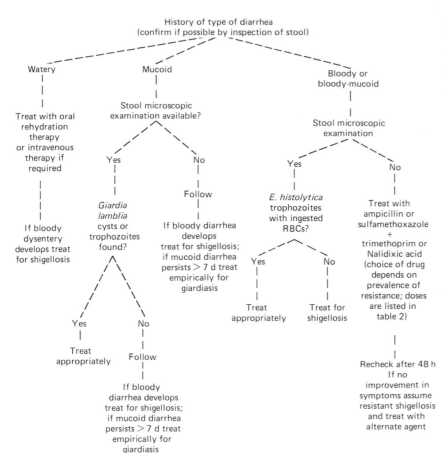

Figure 81-7. A simple algorithm for the management of acute shigellosis by community health workers in field situations, especially where *Shigella* infection is endemic and microbiological diagnosis is not available. If life-threatening complications are present initially or subsequently develop, patients should be referred to a regional health center, if possible.

acute bloody dysentery is a sufficient basis to initiate presumptive therapy for shigellosis [*54*]. Visual examination of the stool by a health worker will substantiate this finding. Microscopic examination, when available, is useful in excluding amebiasis by demonstrating no parasites and many leukocytes, especially in adults in whom amebiasis is a more common cause of dysentery than it is in children [*57a*].

Stool cultures are the only method to confirm the diagnosis and are useful in field surveys to establish the prevalence of the disease and the antibiotic resistance pattern in a particular community. Attention to four methodological details increases the chance of correct laboratory diagnosis: (1) Stool samples are preferable to rectal swab samples, and the material cultured should come from a mucoid portion of the sample [*55*]; (2) if a swab must be used to collect material, be certain that it passes beyond the anal sphincter into the rectum and that the swab is rubbed against the wall of the rectum; (3) inoculate specimens onto agar plates as soon as possible, preferably at the bedside, and if a delay is unavoidable, place them immediately in buffered glycerol-saline holding medium [*56*]; and (4) use more than one medium and *never* rely on *Salmonella-Shigella* (SS) agar alone because it is inhibitory to many shigellae [*55*]. A reasonable approach would be to use MacConkey's agar and

one or more of the following: xylose-lysine-deoxycholate (XLD), Hektoen enteric (HE), deoxycholate citrate (DCA), or tergitol-7-tetraphenyltetrazolium chloride (TTC). SS agar has an advantage for field laboratories since it is highly inhibitory to gram-positive bacteria and nonpathogenic enterobacteria and does not require autoclaving. However, the other culture media can be prepared and sterilized in the field using a kerosene or gas stove and an ordinary high-dome pressure cooker. All of these media should include an indicator dye to facilitate identification of lactose-negative colonies. These are picked and inoculated to a screening medium to determine fermentation and gas production from glucose, H_2S production, and inability to use lactose. Where *V. cholerae* is not endemic, the sucrose-containing triple sugar iron (TSI) agar can be used. Elsewhere, Kligler iron agar (KIA) is better because it facilitates identification of sucrose-fermenting vibrios. Subsequent biochemical testing follows standard procedures for Enterobacteriaceae. Presumptive diagnosis of any glucose-positive, nonmotile, non-gas-producing, H_2S-negative, lactose-negative organism may be rapidly done by serological agglutination with Shigella group-specific antisera. Unfortunately, commercial typing sera can be of poor quality, and are often too dilute or too cross-reactive to identify group- or type-specific antigens [*57*].

MANAGEMENT

The cornerstone of therapy of bacillary dysentery is early treatment with an effective antimicrobial agent. In contrast, watery diarrhea due to shigellosis in well-nourished patients will generally resolve in a few days without treatment. In the more severely ill patient, antimicrobial therapy can shorten the duration both of illness and of excretion of *Shigella* in the stool [58]. Almost all patients will become afebrile and have formed stools within 72 h of the initiation of appropriate therapy, and organisms are rarely recovered from stool after the first 48 h of treatment [59]. Many controlled comparative clinical trials have established the two basic principles of successful antimicrobial therapy: (1) The isolate must be susceptible in vitro, and (2) the drug must be present in both tissues and stool [60]. Nonabsorbable agents, such as furazolidone or neomycin, or highly absorbable agents, such as amoxycillin, will fail despite being effective in vitro, indicating that both the mucosal *and* the luminal populations of shigellae must be treated [60–62]. In addition, the following conditions must be met if a drug is to be of practical use in LDCs: (1) safe for use in children; (2) available in an oral formulation; (3) proven effective in controlled trials; (4) effective in vitro against the majority of strains of *Shigella* isolated in the community where it is to be used; (5) affordable. Three drugs, ampicillin, trimethoprim-sulfamethoxazole, and nalidixic acid, currently meet all of these criteria (see Table 81-4 for doses) [58,59,63]. Resistance to each drug exists, and may be highly prevalent in some places. Hence the choice of therapy will depend on the pattern of resistance in the community. Continuing surveillance of resistance patterns is required because antibiotic pressures and abuse in many countries permit rapid selection of resistance to agents in common use (Fig. 81-8). Where resistance to all three agents is common, options are limited. Pivamdinocillin, which selectively binds to penicillin-binding protein 2, has been used with success in treatment of some ampicillin-resistant strains [64]. The new fluoroquinolones are very active in vitro and in controlled clinical trials in adults have been found very effective [65,66]. However, their relatively greater cost, and concerns regarding their safety in childhood, currently limits their usefulness in LDCs.

Most treatment regimens have recommended multiple daily doses over 5 days. At least one study has found that ampicillin in a single dose of 4 g (or 100 mg/kg in children) is as effective in achieving clinical cure, although less effective in achieving bacteriological cure [67]. Single-dose therapy has particular advantages in LDCs, where, because of lack of compliance or concerns for cost, many patients fail to complete their course of therapy [68]. The new fluoroquinolones, if found safe for children, should be particularly attractive agents for single-dose therapy. Compared to ampicillin, they have a longer half-life, and in relation to their minimum inhibitory concentration for *Shigella* they achieve much higher stool concentrations. Single-dose therapy will reduce the cost of using these drugs as well.

Stool volumes in shigellosis are slight when compared to secretory diarrheas such as cholera, toxigenic *E. coli*, or rotavirus, and severe dehydration is not common. However, the stool losses, combined with increased insensible water loss secondary to fever, and decreased intake due to anorexia, often result in mild or moderate degrees of dehydration. This is treatable with standard WHO oral rehydration solution, which provides sufficient sodium (90 mmol/L) to replace the relatively high stool sodium losses (70 to 120 mmol/L) in shigellosis. The profound hyponatremia occurring in some patients with shigellosis is unlikely to be corrected with oral rehydration therapy alone, and intravenous infusions of saline can markedly improve the level of consciousness in such patients. Once volume is restored, free water intake should be restricted, as the problem appears to be due to resetting of the "osmostat"

Table 81-4. Options for antimicrobial therapy of shigellosis in less-developed countries*

Drug	Dose	
	Children	**Adults**
Ampicillin	100 mg/(kg · day) divided into four doses for 5 days	500 mg four times daily for 5 days *or* 4 g as a single dose
Trimethoprim-sulfamethoxazole	8 mg/(kg · day) trimethoprim, *plus* sulfamethoxazole 40 mg/(kg · day) divided into two doses for 5 days	160 mg trimethoprim *plus* 800 mg sulfamethoxazole twice daily for 5 days
Nalidixic acid	55 mg/(kg · day) divided into four doses for 5 days	500 mg four times daily for 5 days

*The choice of therapy depends on the prevalence of resistance to each agent in the community. All drugs should be given orally if possible. The newer quinolones are also effective. However, their cost, and the lack of information on safety in children, currently precludes their use as first-line agents in most LDCs.

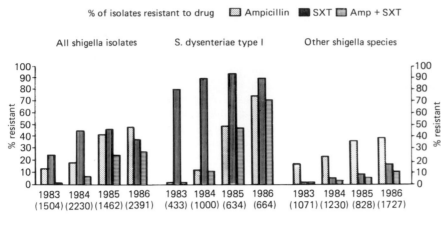

% of isolates resistant to drug ▨ Ampicillin ▩ SXT ▥ Amp + SXT

Figure 81-8. Antibiotic resistance pattern of *Shigella* isolated at the Dhaka Treatment Centre of the International Centre for Diarrhoeal Disease Research, Bangladesh, during the years 1983 through 1986. During this period of time, ampicillin and sulfamethoxazole-trimethoprim (SXT) were the drugs of choice and were heavily used. However, the percentage of isolates resistant to both drugs increased from less than 1 percent in 1983 to 24 percent in 1986 when nalidixic acid became the first choice for empirical treatment of presumed shigellosis. The increase in resistance was most dramatic for *S. dysenteriae* type 1, rising from 2 percent to 70 percent by 1986.

and hyponatremia may recur if patients are allowed unlimited access to water.

Mortality rates in shigellosis are highest in malnourished patients. Shigellosis itself can lead to growth faltering; hence nutritional support is a prime concern in the treatment of children. Feeding should be continued throughout the illness although anorexia often limits the quantity of food ingested, and therefore availability of calorie-dense food can be critical. If oral caloric intake is not adequate in severely ill malnourished children, nasogastric feedings should be initiated and continued until appetite returns. In patients with severe colitis, abdominal distension associated with diminished intestinal motility can occur. Most of these patients will tolerate enteral feedings anyway, and these should only be stopped if ileus is documented by gastric residuals prior to feeding.

With appropriate supportive care directed towards managing the renal failure and anemia, the hemolytic-uremic syndrome is a self-limited process, usually resolving within a few weeks of onset. Because hyperkalemia is generally not a major problem, the uremia can often be managed by careful attention to fluid intake. This obviates the need for peritoneal dialysis, with its associated risks, especially when it is carried out in less than ideal conditions. The anemia can also often be managed conservatively unless there is evidence of heart failure, thus avoiding blood transfusions and the associated risk of infection with human immunodeficiency or hepatitis B viruses.

Grand mal seizures occurring early in the course of shigellosis are usually resolved by the time that patients come to medical attention. Almost all affected patients are febrile, and acetaminophen should be provided along with other measures to reduce the body temperature. Anticonvulsants are reserved for patients who have prolonged, or recurrent, seizures.

Sepsis in the malnourished patient is suggested by poor peripheral perfusion, hypothermia, obtundation, and clotting abnormalities. Such patients require parenteral antimicrobial therapy with agents effective against Enterobacteriaceae. In LDCs, gentamicin is often the best choice, as it is widely available and inexpensive. The initiation of parenteral gentamicin therapy does not alter the need for oral antimicrobials to treat the primary *Shigella* infection, for although almost all strains of *Shigella* are susceptible to the drug in vitro, the efficacy of parenteral gentamicin in the treatment of shigellosis has not been established.

The optimal treatment for toxic megacolon has not been defined. In developed countries management often includes partial or total colectomy [69]. In poor children in the tropics the resultant permanent ileostomy would, in most cases, present an insurmountable problem in management. Therefore, treatment should be conservative, with antibiotic coverage expanded to include agents that are effective against large-bowel anaerobes (e.g., metronidazole) and Enterobacteriaceae (gentamicin). Surgery is reserved for patients who have clear evidence of perforation. Enteral feeding should be resumed as soon as possible.

In LDCs, where severe shigellosis is likely to be most prevalent, hospitals, clinics, treatment centers, physicians, nurses, and laboratory services are least likely to be available. Because early appropriate antibiotic therapy of shigellosis can reduce both the frequency of complications and number of deaths that occur, it is important to establish effective community-based treatment programs. These require a diagnostic and management algorithm based on clinical findings, such as is presented in Fig. 81-7. [54]. The choice of antimicrobial agent will depend on the prevalence of resistance in the community; however, in most situations no single agent will be effective against all strains. Therefore patients who are treated empirically must be reevaluated in 48 h, and if there has been no improvement in symptoms, treatment with an alternative antimicrobial agent should be initiated.

POPULATION

Shigellosis is a disease of underdevelopment, associated with crowding, poor levels of personal hygiene, inadequate water supplies, and malnutrition. These conditions may be present in selected populations in developed countries among the poor and disadvantaged, but they are most commonly found in LDCs. Everywhere, however, incidence rates are highest in children aged 1 to 5 years, and prospective studies conducted in Latin America, Africa, and Asia have found incidence rates of 750 to 2000 per 1000 children per year [53,70,71]. This compares with a reported incidence rate of 0.22 episodes of shigellosis per 1000 children per year in this age group in the United States [5]. Because of incomplete reporting, these data represent a gross underestimate, but even if the actual incidence were 100 times higher, it would still be less than one-thirtieth of the rate found in LDCs. Disease is less common in *Shigella*-infected infants under 6 months of age, but occurs even in neonates, and it is likely to be more severe among infants who are not being breast-fed [72].

Although *Shigella* are worldwide in distribution, developed countries and LDCs differ in the prevalence of the endemic species, with *S. sonnei* most common in developed countries and the more virulent *S. flexneri* predominating in LDCs. *S. dysenteriae* type 1 has characteristically been associated with epidemic disease, and during the 1980s major epidemics have been reported from the Indian subcontinent, Africa, and Thailand [54,73–75]. Disease due to *S. dysenteriae* type 1 in developed countries is almost always related to foreign travel [4]. Case fatality rates of 5 percent or more have been reported during recent *S. dysenteriae* type 1 epidemics [76,77]. These high fatality rates likely reflect some degree of selection bias of cases, with the most seriously ill patients coming to medical attention. In addition, there is no preexisting host immunity to moderate the disease. *S. dysenteriae* type 1 has also recently become endemic in certain countries, such as Bangladesh, where the presence of widespread childhood malnutrition results in fatalities during infection with any species of *Shigella* (Table 81-3). Indeed in such settings dysentery, primarily due to shigellosis, rather than watery diarrhea, accounts for the majority of all diarrhea-associated deaths and a substantial proportion of all childhood deaths, (Fig. 81-9).

Other than certain nonhuman primates, humans are the sole reservoir of *Shigella*. Although point-source outbreaks have been reported, in endemic settings the major mode of transmission is fecal-oral spread from person to person. Within families, attack rates are high, and rates of up to 35 percent have been reported [77–79]. Direct transmission is facilitated by the small infectious inoculum for *Shigella* (a few hundred to a few thousand organisms) and the large number (10^5 to 10^8 per gram) of organisms in feces in infected patients. In endemic settings disease occurs year-round, although seasonal variations may be found. The seasonal pattern varies from place to place. In both urban and rural Bangladesh, the disease peaks during the hot, dry season, when water availability for hand washing is limited [80]. This is similar to the seasonal pattern in Egypt [35,70,71]. In southern India, peak incidence is during the monsoon [81], while in Guatemala the peak is just before and during the early part of the rainy season [53]. The

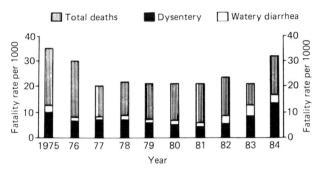

Figure 81-9. Death rates by type of diarrhea for children 1 to 4 years of age, living in Matlab, Bangladesh, a rural district with a population of 180,000 near Dhaka. Death rates were high in 1975 and 1976, reflecting the aftermath of the severe famine of 1974. The death rate rose again in 1984 due to epidemic *S. dysenteriae* type 1 infection. Of particular importance, however, is that in all years the dysentery deaths were far in excess of the deaths due to watery diarrhea.

reasons for these differences in temporal patterns are not clear.

Control of shigellosis currently depends on improvements in personal hygiene and public sanitation. Development of an effective vaccine may occur in the future. Economic and social development almost always brings with it improvement in the level of sanitation and a concomitant decrease in the incidence of shigellosis. This has been the experience not only of western countries, but more recently of Japan, where *Shigella* has gone from being a major killer in the post-World War II period to being a minor public health problem at present. It is clear that under controlled experimental conditions, specific interventions and educational efforts, such as providing soap and encouraging hand washing, can reduce the transmission of shigellosis [78]. Given the increasing impoverishment of many persons in LDCs, especially the landless who flock to the peri-urban slums that exist in most third world countries, and who often lack access to clean water or even the means to buy soap, it seems unlikely that educational efforts alone will effect substantial declines in the incidence of shigellosis.

REFERENCES

1 Shiga K: Ueber den dysenterie-bacillus (Bacillus dysenteriae). Zentralbl Bakteriol (orig) 24:913–918, 1898
2 Shiga K: The trend of prevention, the therapy and epidemiology of dysentery since the discovery of its causative organism. N Engl J Med 26:1205–1211, 1936
3 Kostrewski J, Stypulkowska-Misiurewicz H: Changes in the epidemiology of dysentery in Poland and the situation in Europe. Arch Immunol Ther Exp (Warz) 20:608–615, 1968
4 Gross RJ, Thomas LV, Rowe B: *Shigella dysenteriae, S. flexneri,* and *S. boydii* infections in England and Wales: The importance of foreign travel. Br Med J 2:744, 1979

5 Blaser MJ, Pollard RA, Feldman RA: Shigella infections in the United States, 1974–1980. J Infect Dis 147:771–775, 1983

6 The burden of disease resulting from diarrhea, in Katz SL (ed): *New Vaccine Development Establishing Priorities*. vol II, *Disease of Importance in Developing Countries*. Washington, DC, National Academy Press, 1986, p 165

7 Keusch GT, Bennish ML: Shigellosis, in Evans AS, Feldman H (eds): *Bacterial Infections of Humans. Epidemiology and Control*, 2nd ed. New York, Plenum, 1989

8 Christie AB: *Infectious Diseases. Epidemiology and Clinical Practice*, 3d ed. London, Churchill Livingstone, 1981, p 111

9 LaBrec EH, Schneider H, Magnani TJ, et al: Epithelial cell penetration as an essential step in the pathogenesis of bacillary dysentery. J Bacteriol 88:1503–1518, 1964

10 Formal SB, Hale TL, Sansonetti PJ: Invasive enteric pathogens. Rev Infect Dis 5:S702–S707, 1983

11 Takeuchi A, Sprinz H, LaBrec EH, et al: Experimental bacillary dysentery: An electron microscopic study of the response of the intestinal mucosa to bacterial invasion. Am J Pathol 47:1011–1044, 1965

12 Hale LH, Formal SB: Pathogenesis of Shigella infections. Pathol Immunopathol Res 6:117–127, 1987

13 Sansonetti PJ, Hale TL, Dammin GI, et al: Alterations in the pathogenicity of *Escherichia coli* K 12 after transfer of plasmids and chromosomal genes from *Shigella flexneri*. Infect Immun 39:1392–1402, 1983

14 Buysse J, Stover CK, Oaks EV, et al: Molecular cloning of invasion plasmid antigen (*ipa*) genes from *Shigella flexneri*: analysis of *ipa* gene products and genetic mapping. J Bacteriol 169:2561–2569, 1987

15 Watanabe H, Nakamura A: Identification of *Shigella sonnei* form I plasmid genes necessary for cell invasion and their conservation among *Shigella* species and enteroinvasive *Escherichia coli*. Infect Immun 53:352–358, 1986

16 Sakai T, Sasakawa C, Makino S, et al: DNA sequence and product analysis of the virF locus responsible for Congo red binding and cell invasion in *Shigella flexneri* za. Infect Immun 54:395–402, 1986

17 Makino S, Sasakawa C, Kamata K, et al: A genetic determinant required for continuous reinfection of adjacent cells on a large plasmid in *S. flexneri* za. Cell 46:551–555, 1986

18 Sansonetti PH, Ryter A, Clerc P, et al: Multiplication of *Shigella flexneri* with HeLa cells: lysis of the phagocytic vacuole and plasmid-mediated contact hemolysis. Infect Immun 51:461–469, 1986

19 Keusch GT, Donohue-Rolfe A, Jacewicz M: Shigella toxin and the pathogenesis of shigellosis, in Evered D, Whelan J (eds): *Microbial Toxins and Diarrhoeal Disease*. CIBA Foundation Symposium 112, London, Pitman, 1985, pp 193–214

20 Donohue-Rolfe A, Keusch GT, Edson C, et al: Pathogenesis of Shigella diarrhea. IX. Simplified high yield purification of Shigella toxin and characterization of subunit composition and function by the use of subunit specific monoclonal and polyclonal antibodies. J Exp Med 160:1767–1781, 1984

21 Endo Y, Tsurugi K, Yutsudo T, et al: Site of action of a Vero toxin (VT2) from *Escherichia coli* 0157:H7 and of Shiga toxin on eukaryotic ribosomes. RNA N-glycosidase activity of the toxins. Eur J Biochem 171:45–50, 1988

22 Calderwood SB, Auclair F, Donohue-Rolfe A, et al: Nucleotide

sequence of the iron-regulated Shiga-like toxin genes of *Escherichia coli*. Proc Natl Acad Sci USA 84:4364–4368, 1987

23 Jacewicz M, Clausen H, Nudelman E, et al: Pathogenesis of shigella diarrhea. XI. Isolation of a shigella toxin binding glycolipid from rabbit jejunum and HeLa cells and its identification as globotriasylceramide. J Exp Med 163:1391–1404, 1986

24 Lindberg AA, Brown JE, Stromberg N, et al: Identification of the carbohydrate receptor for Shiga toxin produced by *Shigella dysenteriae* Type 1. J Biol Chem 262:1779–1785, 1987

25 Mobassaleh M, Donohue-Rolfe A, Jacewicz M, et al: Pathogenesis of shigella diarrhea. XIII. Evidence for a developmentally regulated glycolipid receptor for shigella toxin involved in the fluid secretory response of rabbit small intestine. J Infect Dis 157:1023–1031, 1988

26 Kandel G, Donohue-Rolfe A, Donowitz M, et al: Pathogenesis of Shigella diarrhea. XV. Selective targetting of Shiga toxin to villus cells of rabbit jejunum explains the effect of the toxin on intestinal electrolyte transport. Submitted for publication

27 Levine MM, DuPont HL, Formal SB, et al: Pathogenesis of *Shigella dysenteriae* 1 (Shiga) dysentery. J Infect Dis 127:261–270, 1973

28 Mathan MM, Mathan VI: Ultrastructural pathology of the rectal mucosa in *Shigella* dysentery. Am J Pathol 123:25–38, 1986

29 Rout WR, Formal SB, Giannella RA, et al: Pathophysiology of *Shigella* diarrhea in the rhesus monkey: Intestinal transport, morphological, and bacteriological studies. Gastroenterology 68:270–278, 1975

30 Keenan KP, Sharpnack DD, Collins H, et al: Morphologic evaluation of the effects of Shiga toxin and *E. coli* Shiga-like toxin on the rabbit intestine. Am J Pathol 125:69–80, 1986

31 Clerc PL, Ryter A, Mounier J, et al: Plasmid-mediated early killing of eucaryotic cells by *Shigella flexerni* as studied by infection of J774 macrophages. Infect Immun 55:521–527, 1987

32 Clerc PL, Sansonetti PJ: Entry of *Shigella flexneri* into HeLa cells: evidence for directed phagocytosis involving actin polymerization and myosin accumulation. Infect Immun 55:2681–2688, 1987

33 Maurelli AT, Baudry B, d'Hauteville H, et al: Cloning of plasmid DNA sequences involved in invasion of HeLa cells by *Shigella flexneri*. Infect Immun 49:164–171, 1985

34 Donohue-Rolfe A, Kelley MA, Bennish M, et al: Enzyme-linked immunosorbent assay for *Shigella* toxin. J Clin Microbiol 24:65–68, 1986

35 Stoll BJ, Glass RI, Hug MI, et al: Epidemiologic and clinical features of patients infected with *Shigella* who attended a diarrheal disease hospital in Bangladesh. J Infect Dis 146:177–183, 1982

36 Speelman P, Kabir I, Islam M: Distribution and spread of colonic lesions in shigellosis: A colonoscopic study. J Infect Dis 150:899–903, 1984

37 Anand BS, Malhortra V, Bhattacharya SK, et al: Rectal histology in acute bacillary dysentery. Gastroenterology 90:654–660, 1986

38 Butler T, Speelman P, Kabir I, et al: Colonic dysfunction during shigellosis. J Infect Dis 154:817–824, 1986

39 Castro F, Rosal JE, Sanchez E: Hallazgos anatomopatologicos en 173 casos de disenteria bacilar. Simposio sobre disenteria Shiga en Centroamerica Washington, DC, Organization Panamericana de la Salud, Publicacion Cientifica 283:17–26, 1974

40 Fernandez A, Sninsky CA, O'Brien AD, et al: Purified *Shigella*

enterotoxin does not alter intestinal motility. Infect Immun 43: 477–481, 1984

41 Azad MAK, Islam M, Butler T: Colonic perforation in *Shigella dysenteriae* type 1 infection. Pediatr Infect Dis 5:103–104, 1986

42 Rahaman MM, Wahed MA: Direct nutrient loss and diarrhea, in Chen LC, Scrimshaw NS (eds): *Diarrhea and Malnutrition: Interactions, Mechanisms, and Interventions*. New York, Plenum, 1983, pp 269–286

43 Rahaman MM, Alam AKMJ, Islam MR, et al: Shiga bacillus dysentery associated with marked leukocytosis and erythrocyte fragmentation. Johns Hopkins Med J 135:65–70, 1975

44 Karmali MA, Petric M, Lim C, et al: The association between idiopathic hemolytic uremic syndrome and infection by verotoxin-producing *Escherichia coli*. J Infect Dis 151:775–782, 1985

45 Butler T, Islam MR, Bardhan PK: The leukemoid reaction in shigellosis. Am J Dis Child 138:162–165, 1984

46 Struelens MJ, Patte D, Kabir I, et al: Shigella septicemia: prevalence, presentation, risk factors, and outcome. J Infect Dis 152: 784–790, 1985

47 Samadi AR, Wahed MA, Islam MR, et al: Consequences of hyponatremia and hypernatremia in children with acute diarrhoea in Bangladesh. Br Med J 286:671–673, 1983

48 Askenazi S, Dinari G, Zevulunov A, et al: Convulsions in shigellosis: Evaluation of possible risk factors. Am J Dis Child 141: 208–210, 1987

49 Calin A, Fries JF: An "experimental" epidemic of Reiter's syndrome revisited: Follow-up evaluation on genetic and environmental factors. Ann Intern Med 84:564–566, 1976

50 Van Bohemen ChG, Lionarons RJ, van Bodegom P, et al: Susceptibility and HLA-B27 in post-dysenteric arthropathies. Immunology 56:377–379, 1985

51 Black RE, Brown KH, Becker S: Effects of diarrhea associated with specific enteropathogens on the growth of children in rural Bangladesh. Pediatrics 73:799–805, 1984

52 Black RE, Brown KH, Becker S: Malnutrition is a determining factor in diarrheal duration, but not incidence, among young children in a longitudinal study in rural Bangladesh. Am J Clin Nutr 39:87–94, 1984

53 Mata LJ: *The Children of Santa Maria Cauque: A Prospective Field Study of Health and Growth*. Cambridge, MA, The MIT Press, 1978

54 Ronsmans C, Bennish ML, Wierzba T: Diagnosis and management of shigellosis by community health workers. Lancet 2:552–555, 1988

55 Rahaman MM, Huq I, Dey CR: Superiority of MacConkey's agar over *Salmonella-Shigella* agar for isolation of *Shigella dysenteriae* type 1. J Infect Dis 131:700–703, 1975

56 Morris GK, Koehler JA, Gangarosa EJ, et al: Comparison of media for direct isolation and transport of shigellae from fecal specimens. Appl Microbiol 19:434–437, 1970

57 Evins GM, Gheesling LL, Tauxe RV: Quality of commercially produced *Shigella* serogrouping and serotyping antisera. J Clin Microbiol 26:438–442, 1988

57a Speelman P, McGlaughlin R, Kabir I, et al: Differential clinical features and stool findings in shigellosis and amoebic dysentery. Trans R Soc Trop Med Hyg 81:549–551, 1987

58 Haltalin KC, Nelson JD, Ring R, et al: Double-blind treatment study of shigellosis comparing ampicillin, sulfadiazine, and placebo. J Pediatr 70:970–981, 1967

59 Salam MA, Bennish ML: Therapy of shigellosis. I. Randomized, double blind trial of nalidixic acid in childhood shigellosis. J Pediatr 113:901–907, 1988

60 Haltalin KC, Nelson JD, Hinton LV, et al: Comparison of orally absorbable and nonabsorbable antibiotics in shigellosis. A double blind study with ampicillin and neomycin. J Pediatr 72:708–720, 1968

61 Haltalin KC, Nelson JD: Failure of furazolidone therapy in shigellosis. Am J Dis Child 123:40–44, 1972

62 Nelson JD, Haltalin KC: Amoxycillin less effective than ampicillin against *Shigella* in vitro and in vivo. Relationship of efficacy to activity in serum. J Infect Dis 129(suppl):S222–S227, 1974

63 Yunus M, Rahman ASMM, Farooque ASG, et al: Clinical trial of ampicillin v. trimethoprim-sulphamethoxazole in the treatment of *Shigella dysentery*. J Trop Med Hyg 85:195–199, 1982

64 Kabir I, Rahaman MM, Ahmed SM, et al: Comparative efficacies of pivmecillinam and ampicillin in acute shigellosis. Antimicrob Agents Chemother 25:643–645, 1984

65 Rogerie F, Ott D, Vandepitte J, et al: Comparison of norfloxacin and nalidixic acid for treatment of dysentery caused by *Shigella dysenteriae* type 1 in adults. Antimicrob Agents Chemother 29: 883–886, 1986

66 DeMol P, Mets T, Lagasse R, et al: Treatment of bacillary dysentery: A comparison between enoxacin and nalidixic acid. J Antimicrob Chemother 19:695–698, 1987

67 Gilman RR, Spira W, Rabbani H, et al: Single dose-ampicillin therapy for severe shigellosis in Bangladesh. J Infect Dis 143: 164–169, 1981

68 Hossain MM, Glass RL, Khan MR: Antibiotic use in a rural community in Bangladesh. Int J Epidemiol 11:402–405, 1982

69 Werlin SL, Grand RJ: Severe colitis in children and adolescents: Diagnosis, course, and treatment. Gastroenterology 73:828–832, 1977

70 Higgins AR, Floyd TM, Kader MA: Studies in shigellosis. II. Observations on incidence and etiology of diarrheal disease in Egyptian village children. Am J Trop Med Hyg 4:271–280, 1955

71 Black RE, Brown KH, Becker S, et al: Longitudinal studies of infectious diseases and physical growth of children in rural Bangladesh. Am J Epidemiol 115:315–324, 1982

72 Clemens JD, Stanton B, Stoll B, et al: Breast feeding as a determinant of severity in shigellosis. Am J Epidemiol 123:710–718, 1986

73 Pal SC: Epidemic bacillary dysentery in West Bengal, India, 1984. Lancet 1:1462, 1984

74 Malengreau M, Molima-Kaba, Gillieaux M, et al: Outbreak of *Shigella* dysentery in Eastern Zaire, 1980–1982. Ann Soc Belge Med Trop 63:59–67, 1983

75 Chatkaeomorakot A, Echeverria P, Taylor DN, et al: Trimethoprim-resistant *Shigella* and enterotoxigenic *Escherichia coli* strains in children in Thailand. Pediatr Infect Dis 6:735–739, 1987

76 Rahaman MM, Khan MM, Aziz KMS, et al: An outbreak of dysentery caused by *Shigella dysenteriae* type 1 on a coral island in the Bay of Bengal. J Infect Dis 132:15–19, 1975

77 Gangarosa EJ, Perera DR, Mata LJ, et al: Epidemic Shiga bacillus dysentery in Central America. II. Epidemiologic studies in 1969. J Infect Dis 122:181–190, 1970

78 Khan MU: Interruption of shigellosis by handwashing. Trans R Soc Trop Med Hyg 76:164–168, 1982

79 Boyce JM, Hughes JM, Alim ARMA, et al: Patterns of *Shigella* infection in families in Bangladesh. Am J Trop Med Hyg 31: 2015–2020, 1982

80 Blum D: The role of water supplies and sanitation in prevention of acute diarrhoeal diseases, in Gracey M (ed): *Diarrhoeal Disease and Malnutrition: A Clinical Update*. Edinburgh, Churchill Livingstone, 1985, pp 207–210

81 Feldman RA, Bhat P, Kamath KR: Infection and disease in a group of South Indian families. IV. Bacteriologic methods and a report of the frequency of enteric bacterial infection in preschool children. Am J Epidemiol 92:367–375, 1970

CHAPTER 82 / Escherichia coli *and Related Enteric Pathogens* · Richard L. Guerrant

Escherichia coli are widely recognized as common causes of urinary tract infections, bacteremia, and, in some settings, pneumonia or intravascular infection. However, the commonest infections by *E. coli* are those of the gastrointestinal tract. There, *E. coli* constitute one of the commonest, if not *the* commonest causes of diarrheal illness, especially in tropical climates and areas where sanitation facilities are limited [*1–3*]. As diarrheal illness constitutes the leading cause of death on a global scale [*4,5*] *E. coli* may well represent the single greatest cause of mortality. The morbidity of *E. coli* diarrhea, especially with its effects on childhood nutrition and development, may have an even greater impact. Thus, the importance of understanding and controlling *E. coli* enteric infections becomes paramount.

Within the species of *E. coli* is expressed much of the range of types of bacteria that cause enteric infection. In this chapter the current understanding of 7 (possibly 8) different types of *E. coli* is reviewed with respect to enteric pathogenesis, the in vitro and in vivo models used to detect their "virulence traits," and the nature of their genetic code. Still other organisms that may make toxins similar to those of *E. coli* are mentioned.

PARASITE

As *E. coli* may range from normal flora to one of the commonest life-threatening pathogens in the tropics, its virulence traits are especially important. Depending on these traits, *E. coli* may cause noninflammatory, small-bowel, secretory, cholera-like watery diarrhea or inflammatory, dysenteric colitis by totally different mechanisms.

E. coli are identified by their characteristic ability to ferment glucose and lactose as well as to produce catalase, reduce nitrates, and be oxidase-negative. Other biochemical characteristics include a positive methyl red reaction and negative reactions with Voges-Proskauer, urease, phenylalanine deaminase, and citrate reagents.

E. coli are further characterized by the lipopolysaccharide (LPS) in their cell walls. The lipid A and ketodeoxyoctonate constitute the core glycolipid, which is the basis for vaccine development to protect against endotoxemia. Smooth (S) forms of *E. coli* are characterized by 1 of 167 currently recognized O-specific LPS side chains (with subtypes a, b, c based on common or unshared cross-agglutinating antigens); often by one of over 80 different capsular polysaccharide (K) antigens [*6,7*]. Most K antigens are of the L (heat-labile) type; the B type having antibody-binding power that persists after heating to 100°C for $2\frac{1}{2}$ h. Another protein surface antigen group, the surface fimbriae or pili, endow certain strains (such as enterotoxigenic and colonizing *E. coli*) with specific adhering and hemagglutinating properties that allow them to colonize mucosal surfaces [*8*].

A few of the 167 O groups of *E. coli* are prevalent in the normal human gastrointestinal tract, and these are associated with a few predominant polysaccharide capsular antigens (Table 82-1) [*6*]. These same O and K antigenic groups of *E. coli* also tend to predominate in extraintestinal infections, including urinary tract infections, bacteremia, and meningitis. The K1 capsular polysaccharide antigen (α 2, O-linked *N*-acetylneuraminic acid polymer) is frequently found among *E. coli* isolated from the cerebrospinal fluid of infants with meningitis. K1 is also one of the commonest K antigens among *E. coli* that cause bacteremia, pyelonephritis, or other extraintestinal infections. The K1 antigen appears to be immunochemically identical to the meningococcal group B polysaccharide antigen.

E. COLI THAT CAUSE ENTERIC INFECTIONS AND DIARRHEA

E. coli (LTEC) and other Enterobacteriaceae that produce the cholera-like heat-labile enterotoxin (LT)

Although certain "enteropathogenic serotypes" of *E. coli* (the classical EPEC strains) had been recognized earlier in outbreaks of infantile diarrhea, the first clues to enterotox-producing *E. coli* came when De and others applied the ligated

Table 82-1. Types of *E. coli* grouped with respect to pathogenesis

	Mechanism	Model	Gene code	Predominant serogroups
Normal enteric flora	? Adherence traits	— —	— —	O groups 1,2,4,6,7,8,18 25,45,75,81
Genitourinary, bloodstream, or meningeal pathogens	? Capsular polysaccharide ± adherence pili	Several animals (mice, rabbits)	— —	O groups 1,2,4,6,7,8,9,11, 18,22,25,62,75 (K antigens 1,2,3,5,12,13)
E. coli that cause diarrhea: Enterotoxigenic *E. coli* (ETEC)				
LT-*E. coli* (LTEC)	Adenylate cyclase, like cholera toxin	Rabbit loops (all) CHO, V1 adrenal cells, immunoassay	Plasmid	LT:O6:K15,O8:K40 LT + ST:O11:H27,O15, O20:K79,O25:K7,O27, O63,O80,O85,O139
ST$_a$ *E. coli* (ST$_a$EC)	Guanylate cyclase	Suckling mice	Plasmid	ST:O groups 78,115,128:H7
ST$_b$ *E. coli* (ST$_b$EC)	Non-cyclic-nucleotide-dependent bicarbonate secretion	Piglet loops	Plasmid	O groups 148,149,153, 159,166,167
Enteroinvasive *E. coli* (EIEC)	Local mucosal invasion	Sereny test	Plasmid	O groups 28ac,29,112, 115,124,136,143,144, 147,152,164
Enteropathogenic *E. coli* (EPEC) [enteroadherent *E. coli* (EAEC)]				
Attaching and effacing *E. coli* (AEEC or "class I EPEC")	Attach to and efface brush border epithelium	Focal HEp-2 cell adherence	Plasmid (60 MDa, pMAR2)	O55:K59(B5):H⁻/H6/H7, O111ab:K58(B4)H⁻/H5/ H12,O119:K69(B14), O125ac:K70(B15)H21, O126:K71,(B16)H⁻/H27, O127a:K63(B8):H6*, O128ab:K67(B12) H12,O142,O158
"Class II EPEC"	? Close enteroadherence	Diffuse or no HEp-2 cell adherence	? Plasmid	O44:K74,086a:K61(B7), O144:H2
Autoagglutinating enteroadherent *E. coli*	? Cytotoxic	Aggregative pattern of HEp-2 cell adherence	Plasmid	? (Matthewson's 221)
Enterohemorrhagic *E. coli* (EHEC)	Shiga-like toxin 1 or 2 inhibits protein synthesis	HeLa cell cytotoxicity	Phage	O157:H7, O26:H11/H⁻, O128, O139, 053, 054 O111:K58:H8/H⁻, O113:K75:H7/H21, O121:H⁻, O145:H⁻, rough

*O127:H6 is the focally HEp-2 cell-adherent strain (E2348) from which the plasmid pMAR-2 was isolated.

rabbit ileal loop model that he had developed to study the pathogenesis of cholera to studies of *E. coli* [9,10]. Enterotoxigenic *E. coli* were also isolated from the upper small bowel of adults with diarrhea [11] in Bengal. Enterotoxigenic *E. coli* may produce one or more of at least three types of enterotoxin that cause intestinal fluid secretion: two different rapidly acting, reversible heat-stable enterotoxins and a long-lasting, heat-labile enterotoxin, LT. LT is remarkably similar to cholera toxin: antigenically, structurally, and mechanistically. However, unlike the chromosomally mediated cholera toxin, *E. coli* LT is encoded on transmissible plasmids [12], which may explain why other members of the Enterobacteriaceae family, including *Klebsiella*, *Citrobacter*, and *Salmonella*, as well as *Campylobacter jejuni*, have been reported to produce heat-labile entertoxins.

Mechanism of Action (Adenylate Cyclase Activation). Like cholera toxin, LT causes secretion by activating mucosal adenylate cyclase. LT is a polypeptide with binding (B) and active (A) subunits. The binding portion avidly binds the monologanglioside (G_{M1}) receptor, which is followed after a lag period by activation of intestinal adenylate cyclase. The active portion of the enterotoxin (A_1), then ADP-ribosylates the GTP-binding component (α subunit of the G-protein) of the regulatory portion of the adenylate cyclase enzyme in the intestinal mucosal cells. This blocks the normal "turn off" reaction for activated adenylate cyclase and results in the increased formation of cyclic AMP which may persist for the life of the cells. The increased cyclic AMP in intestinal mucosal cells appears to cause the net isotonic fluid secretion, apparently in two ways: by reducing the neutral sodium chloride absorption primarily in villus tips and by increasing the electrogenic secretory flux of chloride and possibly bicarbonate (presumably from crypt cells) [13]. This secretory effect of cholera toxin and LT leaves the glucose and neutral amino acid–coupled sodium transport mechanism intact, thus providing the basis for oral glucose-electrolyte therapy.

Animal and Tissue-Culture Models and Bioassays. In addition to dog, rabbit, mouse, and pig models [14–17], the capacity of LT and cholera toxin to activate adenylate cyclase in the many mammalian cell types has been used to develop tissue-culture bioassay methods, such as Chinese hamster ovary (CHO) cell, and the Y1 adrenal cell assays [18–20].

Immunological Assays. The antigenic similarity of *E. coli* and cholera toxin has facilitated the development of immunoassays. In addition to radioimmunoassay (RIA) and enzyme-linked immunosorbent assays (ELISA) [21], a passive immune hemolysis (PIH) test using LT-sensitized sheep erythrocytes with antitoxic antibody and complement has been developed for detection of LT and antiserum [22,23]. Modifications of the ELISA have been applied utilizing ganglioside as the base coat [24]. A special Biken agar has also been used in an Elek test in which single colonies, after polymyxin treatment, develop an Ochterlony precipitin line with antitoxic antiserum [25].

Gene Probe Assays. With the development of oligonucleotide gene probes, now available with nonradioactive alkaline phosphatase markers, these have become as simple, specific, and sensitive as many biological or immunological assays for enterotoxins including LT and ST_a [26].

Predominant Serotypes. The predominance of certain serotypes among enterotoxigenic *E. coli* has been noted as shown in Table 82-1 [6] and has been suggested as a possible screening tool [27]. However, because the capacity of an organism to produce LT may be transmitted via plasmid [12] or bacteriophage [28], the use of specially prepared antisera is of limited sensitivity and specificity, and may vary with the geographical region in which they are applied.

Heat-stable enterotoxigenic (ST_a) *E. coli*

Mechanism of Action (Guanylate Cyclase Activation). The concept that more than one type of secretory enterotoxin may be produced by *E. coli* was again developed by veterinary workers. In the early 1970s, a heat-stable enterotoxin (ST) was distinguished from the cholera-like, heat-labile enterotoxin LT [16]. Both LT and ST are separable, plasmid-encoded traits [16]. Furthermore, the enterotoxin traits may be spontaneously

transposable under selective pressure with antibiotic exposure. Cotransfer of enterotoxin and antibiotic resistance via plasmids has been demonstrated in vivo in piglets and suggested in several areas such as the Far East and Mexico among humans [29,30].

In contrast to the effects of cholera toxin and *E. coli* LT, ST effects are immediate and reversible and have no effect on nonintestinal tissue-culture systems [15,18,19]. Instead, the detection of ST requires the use of the in vivo suckling mouse assay [31,32]. Also in contrast to cholera toxin and *E. coli* LT, ST_a does not increase intestinal cyclic AMP concentrations [33,35] but activates the particulate fraction of intestinal mucosal guanylate cyclase to increase cyclic GMP concentrations. Like exogenous cyclic AMP, cyclic GMP analogues can mimic the secretory response seen with ST_a in the suckling mouse [33]. Because of the specificity of ST_a for only *intestinal* guanylate cyclase [35], nonintestinal bioassays and models have been much more difficult to develop for ST_a than for LT.

Animal Bioassays. The most widely used bioassay for ST is the suckling mouse assay. Remarkably reproducible increases in the intestine weight–body weight ratios occur 3 to 4 h after intragastric inoculation of ST-producing *E. coli* culture supernatants or filtrates [31,32]. Similar results are obtained with ligated rabbit, porcine, calf, and lamb jejunal or ileal segments and with perfused canine or rat jejunum [15,36]. In contrast to *E. coli* LT or cholera toxin, which require later observations for cumulative secretion (usually 15 to 18 h), ST is best detected at earlier times (usually 3 to 6 h for cumulative secretion). It now appears that different STs exist that are negative in the suckling mouse assay but that are detected by other animal loop assays (see discussion of ST_b below). *E. coli* ST has been reviewed in detail elsewhere [36].

Immunoassays. ST_a is a much smaller molecule than LT or cholera toxin, with 14 to 19 critical amino acids and three disulfide bonds, with a molecular weight ranging from 1500 to 10,000 [36]. ST is poorly antigenic and bears no recognized similarity to LT or cholera toxin. Consequently, immunoassays have been more difficult but have now been developed [37,38].

Predominant Serotypes. The majority (18) of the 20 *E. coli* serotypes that tend to be associated with enterotoxigenicity are those that usually make both ST and LT (9 strains) or ST alone (9 strains; see Table 82-1) [6,36,39]. As with other transmissible genetic traits, however, no specific serogroup is necessarily associated with enterotoxin production, and other strains, including previously unrecognized serotypes, may acquire the capacity to produce ST. The role of serotype (or associated traits) in an organism's ability to retain the enterotoxin or colonization factor plasmids or in contributing to virulence in other ways currently remains unclear.

ST Production by Other Microorganisms. In addition to *E. coli*, several other organisms have been reported to produce a heat-stable enterotoxin. The ST produced by *Yersinia enterocolitica* also activates guanylate cyclase [*40*]. Other low-molecular-weight heat-stable enterotoxins with similar biological activities have been reported from *Klebsiella pneumoniae, Enterobacter cloacae, Aeromonas* sp., and *Salmonella* sp. [*41*]; their roles in the diseases produced by these organisms remain unclear.

Heat-stable enterotoxigenic (ST$_b$) *E. coli*

Several workers have noted that heat-stable enterotoxic activity was detected from *E. coli* isolates from calves or piglets with diarrhea by using porcine, calf, or rabbit ligated intestinal segments, but not in the suckling mouse assay [*42*]. Other workers have reported similar experiences with perfused canine or rat intestinal loops that detected ST from certain *E. coli* that was not detected in the suckling mouse assay [*43,44*]. Different physical properties of this heat-stable enterotoxin have led to its separate identification as ST$_b$ [*45*]. ST$_b$ from porcine *E. coli* has been further separated from ST$_a$ or LT by the early secretory response in piglet loops that involves bicarbonate secretion by mechanisms that are not cyclic nucleotide–dependent [*46,47*]. ST$_b$ may not affect human tissue, and whether these strains might be important causes of diarrhea in humans is unknown at present [*48*].

Enteroinvasive *E. coli* (EIEC)

In addition to the noninflammatory or secretory diarrhea caused by the varied types of enterotoxigenic *E. coli*, other *E. coli* have the capacity to invade colonic mucosal tissue, much like *Shigella* species, and to cause an inflammatory colitis with fever and dysentery. In the mid-1940s, Ewing isolated a slow lactose-fermenting "*Shigella*-like" *E. coli* (subsequently identified as O124) in a U.S. Army laboratory in Italy from cases of enteritis in food handlers. This *E. coli* had some antigens that were identical to *Shigella dysenteriae* type 3. Other *Shigella*-like *E. coli* were recognized to be associated with inflammatory colitis and dysentery in Japan [*49*] and in Brazil [*2,50*]. Invasive *E. coli* have also been associated with a widespread outbreak in the United States that was associated with imported French Camembert cheese [*51*].

Biological Assays. A commonly used test for epithelial cell invasion is the Sereny test, in which purulent conjunctivitis and corneal invasion develop over 1 to 3 days after local inoculation of guinea pig eyes with invasive *E. coli* or *Shigella* [*17,50,52*]. Invasive *E. coli* or *Shigella* also infect opiate-treated animals and invade HeLa cells in tissue culture and multiply intracellularly [*17,53*]. Rabbit ileal loop mucosal destruction by whole cultures of invasive *E. coli* but not by culture filtrates suggests that the organism itself and not a cell-free toxin is responsible for this process [*17*].

Invasive* E. coli *Serotypes. Recognized invasive *E. coli* to date have been limited to a few serotypes. Although some invasive *E. coli* serotypes are included among the commercially available Difco grouping sera (groups B or C), there is a clear need for improved, widely available *E. coli* grouping sera, especially for the invasive *E. coli* serotypes.

In many respects, invasive *E. coli* resemble *Shigella* in terms of invasiveness, antigenicity, and metabolism. Ninety-seven invasive *E. coli* strains examined in Brazil were lysine decarboxylase–negative and often nonmotile and slow to ferment lactose [*54*].

Classical enteropathogenic *E. coli* (EPEC) serotypes

Since the 1930s, certain *E. coli* (recognized by slide agglutination with antiserum prepared in rabbits) have been associated with epidemic and sporadic diarrhea in infants. A serologically homogeneous strain of *E. coli* (O111) was isolated from 87.5 percent of infants with summer diarrhea in England (half of the cases were hospital-acquired) and from only 4 percent of asymptomatic controls [*55*]. Varela reported that this strain (*E. coli* "gomez") was associated with infantile diarrhea in Mexico as well. Several other serotypes of *E. coli* were identified that were clearly associated with infantile diarrhea, and these strains came to be recognized as *enteropathogenic E. coli* (EPEC). As seen in Table 82-1, these serotypes tend to be different from the enterotoxigenic or invasive *E. coli* and distinct from the predominant serotypes that invade the urinary tract, bloodstream, or cerebrospinal fluid, or those that inhabit the normal gastrointestinal tract. Although the majority of EPEC serotypes are included in commercially available typing sera (groups A and B), several cross-reactions with normal *E. coli* serotypes cause problems with "false-positive EPEC strains" when only a shortened serogrouping or typing procedure is used [*56*]. Because of the difficulty in performing the full procedure required and the relatively low yield, a thorough investigation for EPEC serotypes is often difficult or impossible except in collaboration with an experienced reference laboratory.

As shown in Table 82-1, enteropathogenic *E. coli* can now be divided into two groups [in addition to the *enteroinvasive (EIEC)* and *enterohemorrhagic (EHEC)* serotypes] that have been called *class I and class II EPEC*. Class I EPEC are distinguished by their ability to adhere in focal "microcolonies" to HEp-2 cells in tissue culture, a trait that is encoded by a 60 MDa plasmid, pMAR2 [*39*]. Class I EPEC include the most commonly and classically recognized serotypes including O55, O111, O119, O125, O126, O127, O128, O142, and O158. Class II EPEC contain the remainder of recognized EPEC serotypes and are characteristically capable of diffuse adherence to HEp-2 cells in tissue culture. An additional "aggregative" type of adherence may also be associated with diarrhea [*57*].

The mechanism by which EPEC serotypes cause diarrhea is least well understood among the types of enteric disease caused by *E. coli*. The EPEC serotypes usually do not make one of the enterotoxins (LT or ST) as recognized in standard tissue culture or animal models. Neither do EPEC usually cause an invasive colitis or a positive guinea pig conjunctivitis (Sereny) test. EPEC usually do not invade the bloodstream or cause disseminated infection. Most symptomatic infections are in infants, and infected adults are usually asymptomatic. Despite their negative reactions with the usual tests for enterotoxins, invasiveness, or Shiga-like (Vero) toxins, EPEC strains O142 or O127 still caused noninflammatory diarrhea in adult volunteers [58,59]. Heat-stable, low-molecular-weight and heat-labile, high-molecular-weight products that cause secretion in a rat jejunal perfusion model have been reported with EPEC serotypes O142, O114, O128, and O127. Current data suggest that the Vero cytotoxin and the ability to cause disease in adult volunteers and to cause rat jejunal secretion occur with different strains and involve at least two separate mechanisms.

The mechanism of close attachment and effacement of the brush border was suggested by the case report of Ulshen and Rollo which showed that EPEC O125 was isolated from an infant with protracted watery diarrhea [60]. This organism was shown to adhere closely to the small-bowel mucosal brush border where it was associated with local destruction of the microvillus brush border, villus blunting, crypt hypertrophy, histiocytic infiltration in the lamina propria, and reduction in brush border enzymes. Similar findings had been reported by Polotsky et al. with EPEC in rabbits [61], and also by Rothbaum et al. among several infants aged 3 weeks to 7 months with profuse watery diarrhea (often lasting over 7 days), who were infected with EPEC O119:B14 [62]. Close adherence of this latter organism to the intestinal mucosa was noted in case but not in control infants' biopsies. Cases also showed dissolution of the glycocalyx and flattened microvilli. This strain was negative in the traditional tests for LT and ST as well as Vero cytotoxin and exhibited no colonization factor antigen I or II. Whether these closely adhering and destructive EPEC serotypes are analogous to a rabbit diarrhea E. coli (RDEC) remains unclear [63,64]. The focal adherence of class I EPEC to HEp-2 cells in vitro not only provides a marker of this adherence trait, but it also appears morphologically similar to their adherence to the intestinal mucosa.

Enterohemorrhagic E. coli (EHEC)

Since 1977, several workers have demonstrated a Vero cell cytotoxin produced by certain serotypes of E. coli that were previously considered "enteropathogenic" serotypes, including serotypes O26:H11, O128, and O39 [59,65]. The Vero cell cytotoxin is heat-labile, is antigenically distinct from LT, and has a slight secretory effect in 18-h ligated rabbit ileal loops [66]. The capacity to produce this Vero toxin was then reported to be transferable to a recipient E. coli K 12 [59]. E. coli O26 has also been shown to adhere to the mucosa of human fetal small-intestinal tissue in vitro in a mannose-resistant fashion, a trait that is transmissible by a colicinogenic conjugative plasmid [67].

The role of this Vero cytotoxin in causing disease and its similarity (if not identity) to Shiga toxin (hence the name Shiga-like toxin) was further clarified following a multistate outbreak of hemorrhagic colitis in 1982 due to E. coli O157:H7 [68]. This organism had only been isolated several years before, from a similar case of noninflammatory, bloody diarrhea. Like strain O26:H11, E. coli O157:H7 has been shown to produce a phage-encoded, Shiga-like cytotoxin that is lethal for Vero cells and certain HeLa cell lines and is virtually identical to the neuro-cyto-enterotoxic Shiga toxin produced by Shigella dysenteriae. A second, antigenically distinct but biologically similar cytotoxin, Shiga-like toxin-2 (SLT-2) has recently been shown to be encoded by a different phage in E. coli O157:H7 [69,70].

Other enterotoxigenic organisms (besides Vibrio species)

As noted above, the genomes for LT, ST_a, and ST_b are on plasmids and can be transferred to other organisms by conjugation. In some instances, transposition of the enterotoxin code to other plasmids can also be demonstrated. Thus, organisms such as Klebsiella, Citrobacter, Aeromonas, Salmonella, and Y. enterocolitica may produce one or more of these enterotoxins [40,41,71–74], and outbreaks have even been associated with multiple different enterotoxigenic species at one time [71,73]. The roles of the enterotoxins of these organisms in causing disease remain unclear. Y. enterocolitica has been associated with inflammatory diarrhea or with mesenteric adenitis that may mimic appendicitis [75]. Most Yersinia infections have been in temperate climates, especially Finland, and they are not commonly recognized in the tropics.

Several other organisms, particularly those associated with food poisoning, may cause disease by producing secretory enterotoxins or cytotoxins. These include Bacillus cereus, Clostridium perfringens, Aeromonas sp., and now C. difficile (a cause of antibiotic-associated pseudomembranous colitis). B. cereus may produce a rapidly acting, heat-stable toxin like Staphylococcus aureus or a long-acting, heat-labile enterotoxin that may share the adenylate cyclase-activating mechanism with LT. Space does not permit detailed discussions of these organisms and their syndromes here, but discussion may be found elsewhere [76].

PATIENT

In the drama of enteric infection with E. coli, in addition to the microbial virulence traits, several critical host factors play major roles in determining who becomes symptomatically infected and how disease is manifested and controlled.

ENTERIC HOST DEFENSES

Host defenses such as intact skin; glottis; ciliary tracheal epithelium; intact urethral, bladder, and ureteropelvic systems;

and phagocytic and humoral immunity often determine when and where systemic, pulmonary, or genitourinary infections with *E. coli* occur. Several other host defenses are key determinants of enteric infections with *E. coli*. As these normal enteric host defenses may be overlooked or altered by medications, they deserve emphasis before considerations are given to drug or epidemiological control of *E. coli* infections.

Hygiene

As with other enteric pathogens, the chance of acquiring an *E. coli* enteric infection is typically by the fecal-oral route and is determined first by how many organisms one ingests from a fecally contaminated environment in food or water or by contact. As with most *Salmonella* and *Vibrio* infections, and unlike *Shigella*, LT- or ST-producing *E. coli*, invasive *E. coli*, and EPEC serotypes all appear to require ingestion of a relatively large number of organisms (10^6 to 10^{10}) for symptomatic infection in healthy adults [17,77]. Therefore, acquisition of these varied types of *E. coli* usually requires the ingestion of a large number of organisms in food or water, rather than by contact. Exceptions may occur in newborn special care units where spread of smaller inocula by contact may result in infection of the unique infant host with undeveloped or altered enteric defenses.

Gastric acidity

As with other enteric pathogens, gastric acidity provides a relative barrier to oral infection with *E. coli*. Neutralization of normal gastric acidity will reduce the infectious dose usually required and one would expect that patients with achlorhydria or gastrectomy would be at increased risk of acquiring an *E. coli* enteric infection.

Normal microbial flora

The role of normal flora is best defined in protecting against *Shigella* and *Salmonella* infection of the colon or distal small bowel. While normal, predominantly anaerobic, organisms may be less important in resisting upper small bowel than colonic infection, the tendency toward excessive, widespread use of prophylactic antimicrobial agents aimed primarily at enterotoxigenic *E. coli* infection deserves emphasis. From work with experimental animals and from experience with human infections, it is clear that normal flora provide an important host defense mechanism for some potentially serious enteric infections [76].

Normal intestinal motility

An often overlooked enteric host defense mechanism that also plays an important role in normal absorption of water and electrolytes, normal intestinal motility may be pharmacologically impaired to the detriment of the host with *E. coli* infection. Experimental animals are more susceptible to pathogens when motility is impaired. Furthermore, as documented with other inflammatory enteritides, infection with invasive *E. coli* might be worsened or prolonged by antimotility agents. Finally, inhibition of motility may reduce the absorption of fluids and electrolytes in the small bowel [78].

Gastrointestinal mucus

The constantly renewing fluid glycoprotein mucus coat produced by the intestinal surface provides the initial encounter of *E. coli* with the host. Motile *E. coli* have been shown to have a chemotactic capacity that enables them, like *V. cholerae*, to penetrate the mucus and adhere to the epithelial surface [79]. The nature and quantity of mucus flow and its biochemical, antibody, and microbial composition that may be altered with age, concomitant infections, or other individual differences all may influence the outcome of ingesting enterotoxigenic, invasive, or enteropathogenic *E. coli*.

Intestinal cell receptors

Intestinal receptors for attachment traits of enterotoxigenic *E. coli* are often species-specific. A genetic recessive strain of piglets is resistant to infection because it lacks the intestinal receptor for the K88 adhesin [80]. The number and availability of other receptors, such as ganglioside G_{M1} for LT or unknown receptors for enteropathogenic or invasive *E. coli*, may well help to explain the considerable individual variation in susceptibility to *E. coli* infection.

Local humoral and cellular immunity

In the intestinal tract, secretory and serum immunoglobulin as well as lymphocytic and phagocytic cellular immunity appear to be important in the lumen, the mucosa, and submucosa. Antibody may be directed toward colonizing microbial surface antigens, toward enterotoxic or cytotoxic products, or toward the organism itself.

Field studies suggest that prior infection with enterotoxigenic *E. coli* confers protection against subsequent infection. Volunteer studies have confirmed that enterotoxigenic *E. coli* infection confers protection against symptoms upon rechallenge with a homologous strain. Most (80 percent) of the volunteers developed antitoxic and antisomatic (O) antibody. However, the rechallenge of protected individuals did result in comparable colonization to that seen with controls [77], suggesting that protection was not related to bactericidal antibody. Antitoxic immunity, especially with the antigenically related cholera toxin and *E. coli* LT, was initially examined with great enthusiasm. However, studies with heterologous LT-producing *E. coli* showed that clinical disease was not protective against subsequent challenge with a different strain of *E. coli* that also produced LT [77]. Furthermore, the cholera toxoid vaccine trials likewise suggest that antitoxic immunity alone is not as effective as had been hoped, and that it will likely require local boosting in combination with other antiattachment or antisomatic immunity to be highly effective.

The smaller ST molecule is poorly antigenic, and adults living in endemic areas remain susceptible to reinfection with ST-producing E. coli [81,82]. Thus, antiattachment immunity has received considerable attention as a potential means of preventing small-bowel colonization by LT- or ST-producing E. coli where they cause disease. Local intestinal immunization against some of these adhesins has been demonstrated in animal models and is already in use in veterinary vaccines. The potential application of a vaccine to human enterotoxigenic E. coli will depend on the frequency with which a small group of adherence antigens occurs among enterotoxigenic E. coli that cause disease in humans (see ''Sites and Mechanisms of Adherence'').

Information on the nature and extent of protective immunity against invasive and classical enteropathogenic E. coli is incomplete. As with Shigella, protective immunity against invasive E. coli infections may relate to cell wall lipopolysaccharide antigens.

The role of immune mechanisms in limiting most symptomatic infections with EPEC to young infants is unclear. Although local antibody has been demonstrated, it does not protect against colonization [83]. Clinical relapse with the same strain and suprainfections with other EPEC strains also raise doubts about protective immunity for EPEC infections. However, mothers who carry EPEC asymptomatically may have high serum antibody and may passively transmit protective antibodies via either the placenta or colostrum [84].

Human milk

Many studies have documented the protection against diarrheal disease in infants afforded by breast-feeding [55,85,86], and ''weanling diarrhea'' is widely recognized [87]. Multiple immune and nonimmune factors are likely responsible for this protection. Increased exposure to a highly contaminated environment when solid food and other fluids are introduced during weaning may play a role, and the relationship of supplementary feeding to gastroenteritis has been noted in rural, urban, and hospital settings [88]. Changes in fecal flora and pH (from the bifidobacteria and low pH of breast-fed infants) may also play a role in creating an antagonistic environment in the bowel for E. coli [85]. Several nonspecific antibacterial factors such as lactoferrin, lysosomes, and phagocytes have also been reviewed [88]. Finally, sensitized lymphocytes and specific antienterotoxic secretory immunoglobulin [89] have been demonstrated. Although antibody is predominantly secretory IgA, IgG and IgM are also found in milk. Promising work shows passive protection of suckling animals against enterotoxigenic E. coli colonization antigens [90].

Age

The role of age in determining host susceptibility is complex and likely related to many factors, including changes in mucus,

microbial flora, cell types and products, and active and passive humoral and cellular immunity. The highest attack rates of E. coli enteric infections occur at the young age of greatest susceptibility to the complications of dehydration and undernutrition.

PATHOGENESIS AND PATHOLOGY

With its array of different virulence traits, E. coli may cause either noninflammatory or inflammatory diarrhea. Noninflammatory diarrhea arises in the upper small bowel, where an enterotoxin or other functional derangement shifts a delicate balance of massive bidirectional fluid and electrolyte fluxes toward decreased absorption or secretion. As shown in Table 82-2, this results in watery diarrhea without evidence of inflammation or fecal leukocytes. This type of diarrhea is caused by E. coli that produce LT, ST_a, or ST_b and by EPEC.

In contrast, inflammatory diarrhea arises from a mucosal invasive process, usually in the colon, to cause a dysenteric syndrome with sheets of distinct fecal polymorphonuclear neutrophils. Like Shigella, invasive E. coli cause inflammatory diarrhea or ''bacillary dysentery.'' The enterohemorrhagic E. coli are noninvasive, but produce Shiga-like toxin(s), and cause bloody, but noninflammatory, diarrhea.

Sites and mechanisms of adherence

E. coli must first adhere to the relevant site in the bowel, whether to deliver an enterotoxin or cytotoxin, to damage the brush border directly, or to invade the mucosa itself. For example, enterotoxigenic E. coli first colonize the upper small bowel where the enterotoxin has its secretory effect. A separable, plasmid-encoded colonization trait, the fimbriate K88 surface adhesin, was first recognized as a necessary prerequisite for enterotoxigenic E. coli to cause diarrhea in piglets [16]. While K88–positive, enterotoxigenic E. coli reproducibly colonize and cause disease, K88–negative strains (whether or not they were enterotoxigenic) fail to colonize or cause diarrhea. Even nonenterotoxigenic E. coli that had the K88 colonization antigen alone colonize and cause diarrhea in a third of animals. The intestinal receptor for this K88 adhesin is an autosomal dominant allele in the piglet. Homozygous recessive piglets

Table 82-2. Types of diarrhea caused by E. coli

	Noninflammatory	Inflammatory
Mechanism	Enterotoxin or decreased absorptive surface	Mucosal invasion
Principal sites	Small bowel	Colon
Type of diarrhea	Watery	Dysenteric
Presumptive diagnosis	No fecal leukocytes	Many fecal PMN
Examples	LT - E. coli	Enteroinvasive
	ST - E. coli	E. coli
	Enteropathogenic E. coli	

lack the K88 receptor and are resistant to "scours" caused by enterotoxigenic *E. coli* [80]. Several protein fimbriate surface adhesins have been described for *E. coli* that infect different species, including at least two that are important for human enterotoxigenic *E. coli:* the colonization factor antigen (CFA)/I and CFA/II [91,92]. As with the piglet studies, volunteers who ingested CFA/I-positive enterotoxigenic *E. coli* became ill, whereas none who ingested CFA/I-negative enterotoxigenic *E. coli* (LT$^+$, although this organism may have become ST$^-$) developed diarrhea or shed the organism for greater than 4 days [93]. The majority of those who ingested the CFA/I-positive strain developed serum antibody responses to the enterotoxin or somatic antigens.

Several antigenically distinct surface adhesins can be detected by a characteristic hemagglutination pattern, with most intestinal adhesins recognized to date exhibiting mannose-*resistant* hemagglutination (in contrast to the mannose-sensitive hemagglutination seen with the widely recognized type I pili) [8,91,94]. Recent reports suggest that CFA/I tends to be associated with *E. coli* in O serogroups 15, 125, 63, and 78, while CFA/II tends to occur among *E. coli* in O groups 6 and 8 [36].

Besides their importance for pathogenesis, the fimbriate attachment factors provide potential handles to control enterotoxigenic *E. coli* diarrhea by immunization and by biochemical means. Both passive and active local intestinal immunization with *E. coli* adhesins have been shown to be protective, and animal vaccines are already in use. However, protective immunity appears to be adhesin type-specific and the total number of antigenically and biologically different types of human *E. coli* surface adhesins remain unknown. While Evans et al. reported 86 percent of enterotoxigenic *E. coli* strains isolated from 29 adults with acute diarrhea in Mexico produced CFA/I, others find only 7 to 20 percent of human case isolates produce either CFA/I or CFA/II [91,94–96]. Likewise, the host species and age specificities of adhesin receptors remain poorly understood.

Finally, the nature of the lectin-like interaction of the protein surface, fimbriate bacterial adhesins with the carbohydrate (or glycoprotein or glycolipid) on the intestinal mucosal surface remains a fascinating area of potential exploitation for control of *E. coli* enteric infection. It now appears that a G_{M2} ganglioside-like glycoconjugate may be the erythrocyte receptor for CFA/I and K-99 hemagglutinins [97]. A general correlation has been made of the degree of hydrophobicity of bacterial adhesins with their adhesiveness [98]. Therefore, some carbohydrates like *N*-acetylneuraminic acid may nonspecifically inhibit adherence by increasing negative surface charges [94]. The actual receptors on red blood cells and intestinal epithelial cells, the glycocalyx, or mucus glycoprotein may be quite different and the carbohydrate blockers of hemagglutination may, therefore, not necessarily inhibit the adherence of these organisms to intestinal epithelial tissues [94].

Bacterial capsules may be involved in the close adherence of certain *E. coli*, such as EPEC and the rabbit diarrhea

E. coli (RDEC-1), to intestinal cells [60–64]. This close disruptive adherence occurs by mechanisms poorly understood at present.

Sites of enterotoxin action

The principal site of secretory derangement by enterotoxin appears to be the upper small bowel. The small intestinal mucosa constitutes a complex organ, the normal function of which determines the body's nutritional and hydration status. Constant massive bidirectional fluxes of electrolytes and water, probably exceeding 40 to 50 L/day of isotonic fluid, move in each direction across the normal human small bowel [99]. Complex regional epithelial specialization is involved in these secretory processes and their apparent regulation by cyclic nucleotides and enterotoxins. The cuboidal crypt cells multiply and provide a continuous supply of differentiating cells that migrate toward the villus tip as they specialize for absorption by developing microvillus brush borders and disaccharidase and other enzymes. Based in part on studies in short-circuit chambers using enterotoxin probes, it appears that villus tip cells are primarily absorptive while the crypts are primarily secretory. The serosal Na-K-activated ATPase-linked sodium pump may provide the driving force for both the electrically neutral sodium chloride absorption in villus tips and the electrogenic chloride secretion in crypts [13]. These different effects of pumping sodium out of cells can be explained by differences in the location of the neutral sodium chloride–coupled transport to the lumenal membrane in villus tips or to the serosal membrane in the crypts. Conversely, according to this postulate, the chloride permeability in villus tips would be primarily on the serosal side while in the crypts the chloride would leave the cell on the mucosal side, as shown.

Cholera toxin and presumably LT cause secretion by increasing unidirectional sodium secretion *and* by reducing unidirectional sodium absorption [99]. Several lines of evidence suggest that cholera toxin or cyclic AMP reduces neutral sodium chloride absorption primarily in villus tips and increases electrogenic chloride secretion from the crypt cells [13]. The prolonged activation of adenylate cyclase by *E. coli* LT or cholera toxin thus causes a persisting secretory response for which initiation and maintenance of replacement fluid therapy are imperative.

In contrast to the prolonged effect of *E. coli* LT and cholera toxin on adenylate cyclase in many tissues, the effect of ST is immediate, rinsable, and specific for intestinal mucosal particulate guanylate cyclase. The sequence of events leading to guanylate cyclase activation by ST is quite different from the events leading to adenylate cyclase activation by LT or cholera toxin. The smaller ST_a molecule does not bind to ganglioside or other recognized receptors [35]. Instead, free-radical formation may be involved in the activation of guanylate cyclase by ST, and membrane-active compounds such as indomethacin, quinacrine, and amodiaquine inhibit ST responses prior to guanylate cyclase activation [35,36].

In the small-intestinal mucosa, ST increases the short-circuit current and in rabbit ileal mucosa reduces the sodium and chloride absorption, the villus tips being where the greatest concentration of guanylate cyclase is found [34,36]. This concept of relative differences in villus tip and crypt cell function may also relate to the pathogenesis of viral infections of the small bowel which selectively infect and destroy the absorptive villus tip cells to cause net secretion. This effect may be important in worsened illnesses with mixed viral and enterotoxigenic *E. coli* (especially LT) infections.

Of potential importance in developing pharmacological agents to reverse or control the secretory derangements with *E. coli* LT or ST or cholera toxin, some final steps in the secretory effects of both cyclic AMP and cyclic GMP may be shared. Since chlorpromazine and lanthanum inhibit secretion induced by ST, cholera toxin, or the cyclic nucleotides themselves, a common step may involve dependence on calcium or calmodulin prior to secretion [36,100]. The apparent sharing of some final, calcium-dependent secretory pathways (possibly through protein kinases) in the small bowel by *E. coli* LT and ST and cholera toxin holds promise in designing antisecretory therapy.

Of great importance in therapy, the secretory effects of *E. coli* enterotoxins and cholera toxin leave the glucose and amino acid–coupled sodium transport mechanisms intact. Thus oral glucose-electrolyte solutions are highly effective rehydration therapy [101].

The pathological changes associated with enterotoxigenic *E. coli* infections are minimal. From animal experiments in which Thiry-Vella loops are infected and at a time when secretory and adenylate responses are maximal, only discharge of mucus from goblet cells and no other significant pathological changes are noted [102]. As with cholera, enterotoxigenic *E. coli* diarrhea is strictly an intralumenal infection and, unless complications of severe hypotension ensue, the organisms rarely disseminate beyond the intestine.

Sites of invasive *E. coli* infection

The dysentery-like syndrome reported with invasive *E. coli* is similar to that of acute shigellosis. There is a striking inflammatory exudate in the stool; the mucosal invasion spreads in the epithelium to cause a patchy, acute inflammation in the mucosa and submucosa, blunting and shortening of the villi, and focal denuding of the surface epithelium [17,53]. Rarely, however, does the organism penetrate to the submucosa or mesenteric nodes.

Site of Shiga-like toxin action (Enterohemorrhagic *E. coli*, EHEC)

The hemorrhagic colitis syndrome and possibly the occasional complication of hemolytic-uremic syndrome may relate to the production of Shiga-like toxin(s) produced in high levels by *E. coli* O157 and certain others. Like Shiga toxin, SLT has

binding and active subunits, is neutralized by anti-Shiga toxin antibody, and acts by inhibiting protein synthesis (much like the plant lectin, ricin) by cleaving an N-glycoside bond in the target cell 28 S ribosomal RNA. Some EHEC strains also produce a second cytotoxin (SLT-2) that is not neutralized by anti-Shiga toxin antibody [105,115].

CLINICAL MANIFESTATIONS

Enterotoxigenic *E. coli*

Since the early work that described enterotoxigenic *E. coli* in association with watery, cholera-like diarrhea in India and Brazil [9–11], considerable experience in outbreaks, among travelers and children in endemic tropical areas, and among human volunteers has revealed the types of illness caused by LT-, ST-, or LT + ST-producing *E. coli*. The diarrhea with enterotoxigenic *E. coli* tends to be mild and self-limited, except in small or undernourished children in whom the dehydration may constitute a major threat to life.

From studies of traveler's diarrhea in adults, the incubation period is 5 to 15 days and the illness typically involves malaise, anorexia, abdominal cramping, and often explosive, noninflammatory, watery diarrhea [3,103,104]. One-third of patients may experience a low-grade fever and one-fourth have nausea or vomiting. The diarrhea is nonbloody and contains no fecal leukocytes. The duration is usually 1 to 5 days but occasionally longer. From volunteer studies in adults, the incubation period may be as short as 14 h and the illness tends to be more severe with higher infecting doses [17,77]. The syndromes of LT- or ST-producing *E. coli* diarrhea are similar. In contrast to the protein-free fluid loss in classic cholera, studies from Bangladesh suggest that enterotoxigenic *E. coli* diarrhea may involve significant protein loss [105]. Therefore, the impact of enterotoxigenic *E. coli* diarrhea on the nutritional status, especially in young children, may be even greater than that of cholera.

Invasive *E. coli*

Illnesses due to invasive *E. coli* are similar clinically to *Shigella* dysentery, with predominant symptoms being fever, malaise, myalgias, tenesmus, and abdominal cramps. The incubation period is usually 1 to 3 days and the illness is usually self-limited, resolving within 7 to 10 days.

The disease caused in volunteers fed invasive *E. coli* began as a febrile illness within 48 h after ingestion of the organism (with temperatures as high as 40°C), with chills, myalgias, and abdominal cramps [17]. This was promptly followed by profuse diarrhea which was watery or dysenteric but usually contained fecal polymorphonuclear leukocytes. The febrile illness usually abated after 3 to 4 days and the diarrhea usually ceased within 1 week. However, in two instances in volunteers, systemic toxicity and transient hypotension necessitated ampicillin therapy which was followed by rapid resolution of symptoms and bacteriological cure. The median incubation period in an outbreak was 18 h [*51*]. One patient continued to excrete the organism for 8 weeks but cleared by 10 weeks. The median duration of illness was 2 days, but some patients had malaise for several weeks.

Enteropathogenic *E. coli*

EPEC serotypes cause diarrhea typically in young infants, especially in newborn nurseries. From reported outbreaks, the incubation period is 2 to 12 days and the syndrome ranges from mild, transient anorexia or failure to gain weight to explosive, fulminant diarrhea leading to death within 12 h [*55*]. The severity is worse in premature infants and in those with underlying disease or congenital abnormalities. EPEC rarely disseminate or cause infection elsewhere; *E. coli* O127 is said to produce nitrites that may lead to methemaglobinemia.

The duration of symptoms if untreated may exceed 2 weeks. For reasons that are not clear, the mortality rate of EPEC infection, which had been a very grave 50 percent before 1950, has been less than 3 percent in more recent outbreaks.

Enterohemorrhagic *E. coli* (EHEC)

A remarkable outbreak of bloody, noninflammatory diarrhea ("hemorrhagic colitis") was described in Oregon and in Michigan in February–March and in May–June, respectively, of 1982, that was traced to an unusual serotype of *E. coli*, O157:H7, an organism that had been reported only once, with a similar syndrome, 7 years before [*68*]. Since then, this organism has been shown to produce high levels of Shiga-like toxins [*69,70*] and to have a plasmid-encoded adhesin [*106*]. The clinical syndrome is distinguished from dysentery by the lack of fecal leukocytes or high fever. Since 1982, EHEC (O157, O26, and others) have emerged as significant causes of outbreaks and numerous sporadic cases of hemorrhagic colitis or (in children) hemolytic-uremic syndrome in schools, day care centers, nursing homes, and in the community [*68,106–109*].

DIAGNOSIS

The diagnosis of the various types of *E. coli* diarrhea is complicated by the need to separate the potential pathogens from normal flora. The noninflammatory or inflammatory nature of illnesses (the latter seen with enteroinvasive *E. coli* infections) can be easily distinguished by prompt examination for fecal leukocytes. The epidemiological setting of diarrhea during the summer or wet season in tropical areas with poor sanitation should lead one to a high suspicion of *E. coli* diarrhea. However, despite many recent advances, definitive demonstration of the enterotoxin, invasiveness, or serotype largely remains the tool of research or reference laboratories. Methods are further limited by the lack of a selective culture process for the pathogens (as routinely used for *Salmonella*, *Shigella*, and *Campylobacter*), and the need to examine a few randomly

selected coliform colonies. This process is insensitive at best. For example, enterotoxin testing of 10 isolates per patient identified enterotoxigenic *E. coli* in only 43 percent of documented cases in an outbreak in Oregon (36 percent had serum antitoxic antibody titer increases, 36 percent had neither) [*110*]. Many attempts at grouping strains for toxin testing or at direct examination of fecal specimens for enterotoxins have been even less sensitive. Recent application of recombinant DNA technology has used specific DNA sequences for *E. coli* ST and LT to probe isolated coliform colonies or even fecal specimens for the complementary enterotoxin genome by DNA hybridization [*111*]. The recent availability of oligonucleotide probes with nonradioactive alkaline phosphatase markers has provided a sensitive, specific tool for many laboratories. Serogrouping for predominant enterotoxigenic *E. coli* serotypes, as noted in Table 82-1, is of limited sensitivity and may vary with the geographical area. When antisera are available, immunoassay methods for enterotoxins (such as ELISA, RIA, PIH, and Biken tests) are easier than the tissue culture, suckling mouse, or animal loop bioassays.

Confirmation of invasive *E. coli* requires inoculation into guinea pig conjunctivae. Biotyping of nonmotile, lysine dicarboxylase–negative strains may also be helpful in screening for invasive *E. coli* [*54*]. In cases of inflammatory diarrhea, *Campylobacter*, *Shigella*, and *Salmonella*, and (when there is coastal or seafood exposure) *V. parahaemolyticus* should be excluded by special culture methods. Likewise, in cases of fulminant watery diarrhea, *V. cholerae* should be excluded by culture on thiosulfate–citrate–bile salt–sucrose (TCBS) agar.

Serogrouping for invasive *E. coli* and EPEC strains requires available grouping sera and specific sera for final identification [*6,50,56*]. In an outbreak, fluorescent antibody or slide agglutination of heated colonies using specific antisera may be helpful in the diagnosis of EPEC infection [*56*]. Gene probes for plasmids associated with EIEC, EPEC, and EHEC as well as ETEC have been developed.

MANAGEMENT

The mainstay of therapy of all diarrheal illnesses, including the various types of *E. coli* diarrheas, is rehydration. Fortunately, the secretory derangement by enterotoxigenic *E. coli* leaves the glucose-coupled sodium absorption intact. The World Health Organization–recommended oral glucose-electrolyte rehydration solution is, therefore, highly effective, especially if given early in illness. This major advance can be life-saving and can be applied early by mothers or healers at the village level, thus avoiding most needs for costly or inaccessible intravenous rehydration therapy [*101,112,113*]. It should be given with ad libitum free water and breast-feeding should be continued. Early refeeding is particularly important to minimize the potentially serious nutritional impact of *E. coli* diarrhea and should exceed normal intake for 1 week after illness.

As the diarrhea with enterotoxigenic *E. coli* is typically self-limited, rehydration therapy is usually sufficient. Data on the efficacy of antimicrobial agents for enterotoxigenic *E. coli* diarrhea came primarily from studies in travelers. Early treatment with agents such as sulfamethoxazole-trimethoprim will reduce a 3- to 5-day illness to 1 to 2 days in areas where the organisms remain susceptible [*103,114*]. Although prophylactic antibiotics have reduced the rates of traveler's diarrhea in several studies [*115*], their value is limited by the rapidly increasing emergence of resistance to antimicrobial agents in tropical, developing areas. Antibiotic resistance and enterotoxigenicity may even be cotransmissible [*29,30*]. Therefore, the limited efficacy, alteration of normal flora, and drug side effects pose potential risks that outweigh the benefits of widespread, indiscriminate use of prophylactic antimicrobial agents, and therefore most authorities do not use or recommend use of prophylactic antibiotics for enterotoxigenic *E. coli* diarrhea [*116*].

Appropriate absorbable antibiotics may be helpful in the treatment of invasive *E. coli* (as in *Shigella*) infections, but this remains unproven.

Because of the potential severity of EPEC infections, neomycin 100 mg/(kg·day) divided tid given orally for 3 to 10 days is recommended for EPEC diarrhea in infants [*114,117*]. However, even in an outbreak setting, prophylactic antibiotics are not recommended and only appear to increase resistance.

Antimotility agents, although widely used, should not be expected to reduce fluid losses and they are contraindicated in inflammatory enteritis. Bismuth subsalicylate has been shown to inhibit enterotoxin effects in an animal model, and has been of some therapeutic as well as prophylactic benefit in travelers [*118,119*]. Its value when used as recommended for treatment is unclear. Other antitoxic or antisecretory chemotherapy that might stop or reduce the secretory process, and thereby increase the efficacy of oral rehydration therapy, is under study.

POPULATION

POPULATION ECOLOGY

As noted at the outset, *E. coli* are the commonest cause of diarrhea, and diarrheal illnesses constitute the greatest cause of mortality on a global scale. In the first 5 years of life, 15 to 25 percent of live-born children die in some areas, over half of whom have diarrhea as the primary or associated cause of death [*4,5,99*]. As early infant deaths are often not recorded and traditional labels of diarrheal illnesses are overlooked, the mortality impact of diarrhea is likely even greater than indicated by published data from death records. With malnutrition and effects on childhood development, diarrheal illnesses, particularly those caused by *E. coli*, have a profound effect on the morbidity of many others who survive.

While enterotoxigenic and invasive *E. coli* are relatively rarely recognized causes of diarrhea in developed temperate climates, enterotoxigenic *E. coli* and, to a lesser extent, invasive *E. coli* are major causes of diarrhea throughout tropical areas where sanitation facilities are limited [*1,2,10,11,72*]. Nontoxigenic, noninvasive EPEC serotypes and enterohemorrhagic *E. coli* (EHEC) also remain a major cause of sporadic community-acquired and occasional institutional outbreaks of diarrheal illnesses in some areas [*85,108,109*].

The age-specific attack rate in carefully done prospective studies shows a striking predominance of diarrheal illnesses in children less than 5 years of age, with the maximum rate being up to 4 to 9 illnesses per child per year in infants less than 1 year of age [*1,85,86,99*]. Of these, the highest frequency of enterotoxigenic *E. coli* infections is in children under 3 years of age. Peaks of illness occur at younger ages when there is earlier weaning.

EPIDEMIOLOGY

Perhaps because of the relative species specificity of enterotoxigenic *E. coli* fimbriate adhesins or colonization factors, the principal recognized reservoir of human enterotoxigenic *E. coli* strains is the human gastrointestinal tract. Transmission takes place by the fecal-oral route in areas of poor sanitation whether in water, food, or by contact. Because the infectious doses are relatively high, contaminated food and water are likely important and have been documented to be highly contaminated and to be significant risk factors for travelers to tropical areas.

Like other bacterial enteritides, the seasonal pattern of enterotoxigenic *E. coli* infection shows a summer, wet seasonal peak, which is usually the peak of all diarrheal illnesses throughout tropical areas, including Africa [*72*], Brazil [*113*], Bengal [*1*], and the American Indian reservations [*81*]. This seasonal pattern of maximal risk of infection also applies to tourists who are most likely to experience traveler's diarrhea if they visit tropical areas during the indigenous peak of illnesses.

Documented risk factors for diarrheal illnesses in tropical areas are poor socioeconomic status (including poor or absent water supplies and sanitation facilities) and, in travelers, the degree of exposure to potentially contaminated food and water. In young children, for many complex reasons, breast-feeding is protective against weaning diarrheal illnesses that may increase well over tenfold at the time of weaning [*85–87,99*]. The further decrease in breast-feeding associated with institutionalization of childbirth and discordant development may actually worsen the already staggering morbidity and mortality due to diarrheal illnesses in coming years.

Data on the infection-to-case ratios with *E. coli* infections are limited because of the insensitivity of our culture methods and the relatively small number of studies of asymptomatic controls. Some data suggest that adults residing in endemic areas continue to acquire symptomatic infections with ST-producing *E. coli*, while they often carry LT-producing *E. coli* asymptomatically [*81,82*]. With the observation that all types of enterotoxigenic *E. coli* (LT, ST, or both) are associated with symptomatic illnesses in young children and in immunologically virgin travelers, these findings are consistent with a possible role for antitoxic immunity in the natural symptomatic protection of adults living in endemic areas against LT, but not against ST.

Limited data on invasive *E. coli* suggest that the infective doses are relatively high [17], but that such numbers may be spread in food with high attack rates [51]. EPEC gastroenteritis appears primarily in urban areas and particularly among hospitalized infants in the first 3 months of life, and relatively infrequently among sporadic cases in rural areas. Cross-infection has been incriminated primarily in hospital nursery populations, although community outbreaks of enteropathogenic *E. coli* are well recognized. Despite some geographical and temporal variation, certain serogroups tend to predominate in certain areas. While EPEC gastroenteritis was primarily associated with summer diarrhea, especially in poor or overcrowded conditions, more recent reports of nursery outbreaks have not demonstrated a seasonal pattern.

PREVENTION AND CONTROL

Rehydration therapy

Early delivery of oral glucose-electrolyte therapy is the most cost-effective, immediately available means of controlling the morbidity and mortality of *E. coli* and other diarrheal illnesses. Despite exciting developments in antisomatic, antitoxic, and antiadherence vaccines, treatment remains the most effective and least expensive means of preventing deaths due to noninflammatory diarrhea, including that due to enterotoxigenic *E. coli*. The limiting factor at present is on the culturally appropriate delivery of the oral rehydration solution, ideally at the home or village level. Although care must be taken to avoid preparations of hypertonic solutions, and available water may be highly contaminated, early delivery of the oral therapy solution by a network of traditional healers or village health workers is feasible and life-saving.

Epidemiological control

Interruption of fecal-oral transmission is key to the control of *E. coli* diarrhea. Although the value of improved water quantity (availability) and quality has been limited, significant reductions in diarrheal illness rates, as with population growth, have been consistently associated with overall development (with improved sanitation facilities, water quality and availability, housing, refrigeration, food handling, etc.) throughout history. In the meantime, several measures can and must be taken. Along with education and overall development, the trend toward decreasing frequency and duration of breast-feeding should be reversed by such measures as providing incentives or food supplements to lactating mothers. With early treatment, such measures should help substantially reduce the soaring rates of life-threatening diarrheal illnesses among the most susceptible infants and young children.

Travelers who are careful about water and food exposure can significantly reduce their risk of acquiring enterotoxigenic *E. coli* diarrhea. Finally, strict hand washing and isolating and cohorting of cases have controlled nursery outbreaks of EPEC diarrhea.

Immunological control

Exciting developments in potential vaccines directed toward protection against intestinal colonization are most promising. Such a vaccine might theoretically reduce the reservoir as well as protect the immunized individuals. As discussed in detail above, symptomatic infection with enterotoxigenic *E. coli* does protect against subsequent symptomatic infection with a homologous strain. In conjunction with vaccines that boost antiadherence or antisomatic immunity, toxoid vaccines may be developed. These would likely employ local boosting and possibly live derivative strains of nontoxigenic or toxoid-producing *E. coli* for optimal efficacy. The number of antigenically distinct colonization factors may be a limiting factor in the development of antiattachment vaccines.

Pharmacological control

The role of antimicrobial agents in treating or preventing *E. coli* diarrhea is limited by the increasing resistance, side effects, and cost. The concept of antisecretory agents, especially those that might inhibit late steps in the secretory pathways that may be common to several types of enterotoxin, is quite promising and worthy of further work. Finally, agents such as carbohydrates, lectins, or chemoattractants that might compete for the binding of organisms to the mucosa or prevent their penetration through the mucus coat are now on the horizon of new approaches to the control of the devastating *E. coli*, which quietly kill or intermittently incapacitate the majority of people on our planet.

REFERENCES

1 Black RE, Merson MH, Huq I, et al: Incidence and severity of rotavirus and *Escherichia coli* diarrhoea in rural Bangladesh. Implications for vaccine development. Lancet 1:141–143, 1981

2 Guerrant RL, Moore RA, Kirschenfeld PM, et al: Role of toxigenic and invasive bacteria in acute diarrhea of childhood. N Engl J Med 293:567–573, 1975

3 Merson MH, Mooris GK, Sack DA, et al: Traveler's diarrhea in Mexico: A prospective study of physicians and family members attending a congress. N Engl J Med 294:1299–1305, 1976

4 Puffer RR, Serrano CV: Patterns of mortality in childhood. Washington, D.C., Pan American Health Organization Scientific Publication No. 262, 1973

5 Walsh JA, Warren KS: Selective primary health care: An interim strategy for disease control in developing countries. N Engl J Med 301:967–974, 1979

6 Orskov I, Orskov F, Jann B, et al: Serology, chemistry and genetics of O and K antigens of *Escherichia coli*. Bacteriol 41:667–710, 1977

7 Edwards PR, Ewing WH: *Identification of Enterobacteriaceae,* 3d ed. Minneapolis, Burgess, 1972, pp 84–87

8 Jones GW: The attachment of bacteria to the surface of animal cells, in Reissig JL (ed): *Microbial Interactions: Receptors and Recognition,* series B. London, Chapman & Hall, 1977, pp 139–176

9 De SN, Bhathchaya K, Sakar JK: A study of the pathogenicity of strains of *Bacterium coli* from acute and chronic enteritis. J Pathol Bacteriol 71:201–209, 1956

10 Trabulsi LR: Revelacao de colibacilos associados as diarreias infantis pelo metodo da infeccao experimental de alca ligade do intestino do coelho. Rev Inst Med Trop São Paulo 6:197–203, 1964

11 Gorbach SL, Banwell JG, Chatterjee BD, et al: Acute undifferentiated human diarrhea in the tropics. I. Alterations in intestinal microflora. J Clin Invest 50:881–889, 1971

12 Skerman FJ, Formal SB, Falkow S: Plasmid-associated enterotoxin production in a strain of *Escherichia coli* isolated from humans. Infect Immun 5:622–624, 1972

13 Field M: Cholera toxin, adenylate cyclase, and the process of active secretion in the small intestine: the pathogenesis of diarrhea in cholera, in Andreoli TE et al (eds): *Physiology of Membrane Disorders,* New York, Plenum, 1978, pp 877–899

14 Guerrant RL, Chen LC, Sharp GWG: Intestinal adenyl-cyclase activity in canine cholera: Correlation with fluid accumulation. J Infect Dis 125:377–381, 1972

15 Evans DG, Evan DJ Jr, Pierce NF: Differences in the response of rabbit small intestine to heat-labile and heat-stable enterotoxins of *Escherichia coli*. Infect Immun 7:873–880, 1973

16 Smith HW, Linggood MA: Observations on the pathogenic properties of the K88, HLY, and ENT plasmids of *Escherichia coli* with particular reference to porcine diarrhea. J Med Microbiol 4:467–485, 1971

17 DuPont HL, Formal SB, Hornick RB, et al: Pathogenesis of *Escherichia coli* diarrhea. N Engl J Med 285:1–9, 1971

18 Guerrant RL, Brunton LL, Schnaitman TC, et al: Cyclic adenosine monophosphate and alteration of Chinese hamster ovary cell morphology. A rapid, sensitive in vitro assay for the enterotoxins of *Vibrio cholera* and *Escherichia coli*. Infect Immun 10:320–327, 1974

19 Donta ST, Moon HW, Whipp SC: Detection of heat-labile *Escherichia coli* enterotoxin with the use of adrenal cells in tissue culture. Science 183:334–335, 1974

20 Guerrant RL, Brunton LL: Characterization of the Chinese hamster ovary cell assay for the enterotoxins of *Vibrio cholerae* and *Escherichia coli* and for antitoxin: Differential inhibition by gangliosides, specific antisera, and toxoid. J Infect Dis 135:720–728, 1977

21 Yolken RH, Greenberg HB, Merson MH, et al: Enzyme-linked immunosorbent assay for detection of *Escherichia coli* heat-labile enterotoxin. J Clin Microbiol 6:439–444, 1977

22 Evans DJ, Evans DG: Direct serological assay for the heat-labile enterotoxin of *Escherichia coli,* using passive immune hemolysis. Infect Immun 16:604–609, 1977

23 Serafim MB, Pestana de Castro AF, Leonardo MB, et al: Single radial immune hemolysis test for detection of *Escherichia coli* thermolabile enterotoxin. J Clin Microbiol 14:473–478, 1981

24 Svennerholm A-M, Holmgren J: Identification of *Escherichia coli* heat-labile enterotoxin by means of a ganglioside immunosorbent assay (G_{M1}-ELISA) procedure. Curr Microbiol 1:19–23, 1978

25 Honda T, Tage S, Takeda Y, et al: Modified Elek test for detection of heat-labile enterotoxin of enterotoxigenic *Escherichia coli*. J Clin Microbiol 13:1–5, 1981

26 Sommerfelt H, Suennerhelm AM, Kalland KH, et al: Comparative study of colony hybridization with synthetic oligonucleotide probes and enzyme-linked immunosorbent assay for identification of *Escherichia coli*. J Clin Microbiol 26:530–534, 1988

27 Merson MH, Rowe B, Black RE, et al: Use of antisera for identification of enterotoxigenic *Escherichia coli*. Lancet 2:222–224, 1980

28 Takeda Y, Murphy JR: Bacteriophage conversion of heat-labile enterotoxin in *Escherichia coli*. J Bacteriol 133:172–177, 1978

29 Gyles CL, Falkow S, Rollins L: In vivo transfer of an *Escherichia coli* enterotoxin plasmid possessing genes for drug resistance. Am J Vet Res 39:1438–1441, 1978

30 Echeverria P, Ulyangco CV, Ho MT, et al: Antimicrobial resistance and enterotoxin production among isolates of *Escherichia coli* in the Far East. Lancet 2:589–592, 1978

31 Dean AG, Chiing Y, Williams RG, et al: Test for *Escherichia coli* enterotoxin using infant mice: Application in a study of diarrhea in children in Honolulu. J Infect Dis 125:407–411, 1972

32 Giannella RA: Suckling mouse model for detection of heat-stable *Escherichia coli* enterotoxin: Characteristics of the model. Infect Immun 14:95–99, 1976

33 Hughes JM, Murad F, Chang B, et al: Role of cyclic GMP in the action of heat-stable enterotoxin of *Escherichia Coli*. Nature 271:755–756, 1978

34 Field M, Graf LH Jr, Laird WJ, et al: Heat-stable enterotoxin of *Escherichia coli:* In vitro effects on guanylate cyclase activity, cyclic GMP concentration, and ion transport in small intestine. Proc Natl Acad Sci USA 75:2800–2804, 1978

35 Guerrant RL, Hughes JM, Chang B, et al: Activation of rat and rabbit intestinal guanylate cyclase by the heat-stable enterotoxin of *Escherichia coli:* Studies of tissue specificity, potential receptors and intermediates. J Infect Dis 142:220–228, 1980

36 Greenberg RN, Guerrant RL: *E. coli* heat-stable enterotoxin, chap 6 in Dorner F, Drews J (eds): *Pharmacology of Bacterial Toxins.* Oxford, Pergamon, 1986

37 Giannella RA, Drake KW, Luttrell MM: Development of a radioimmunoassay for *Escherichia coli* heat-stable enterotoxin: Comparison with the suckling mouse bioassay. Infect Immun 33:186–192, 1981

38 Frantz JC, Robertson DC: Immunological properties of *Escherichia coli* heat-stable enterotoxins: Development of a radioimmunoassay specific for heat-stable enterotoxins with suckling mouse activity. Infect Immun 33:193–198, 1981

39 Levine MM: *E. coli* that cause diarrhea: Enterotoxigenic, enteropathogenic, enteroinvasive, enterohemorrhagic, enteroadherent. J Infect Dis 155:377–388, 1987

40 Rao MC, Guandalini S, Laird WJ, et al: Effects of heat-stable enterotoxin of *Yersinia enterocolitica* on ion transport and cyclic guanosine $3',5'$-monophosphate metabolism in rabbit ileum. Infect Immun 26:875–878, 1979

41 Koupal LR, Deibel RH: Assay, characterization and localization of an enterotoxin produced by *Salmonella*. Infect Immun 11:14–22, 1975

42 Gyles CL: Limitations of the infant mouse test for *Escherichia coli* heat-stable enterotoxin. Can J Comp Med 43:371–379, 1979

43 Nalin DR, Levine MM, Young CR, et al: Increased *Escherichia coli* enterotoxin detection after concentrating culture supernatants: Possible new enterotoxin detectable in dogs but not in infant mice. J Clin Microbiol 8:700–703, 1978

44 Klipstein FA, Guerrant RL, Wells JG, et al: Comparison of assay of coliform enterotoxins by conventional techniques versus in vivo intestinal perfusion. Infect Immun 25:146–152, 1979

45 Burgess MN, Bywater RJ, Cowley CM, et al: Biological evaluation of a methanol soluble, heat-stable *Escherichia coli* enterotoxin in infant mice, pigs, rabbits and calves. Infect Immun 21:526–531, 1978

46 Kennedy DJ, Greenberg RN, Dunn JA, et al: Effects of *E. coli* heat stable enterotoxin STb on intestines of mice, rats, rabbits and piglets. Infect Immun 46:639–643, 1984

47 Weikel CS, Nellans HN, Guerrant RL: *In vivo* and *in vitro* effects of a novel enterotoxin, STb, produced by *E. coli*. J Infect Dis 153:893–901, 1986

48 Weikel CS, Tiemens KM, Moseley SL, et al: Species specificity and lack of production of STb enterotoxin by *E. coli* strains isolated from humans with diarrheal illness. Infect Immun 52:323–325, 1986

49 Sakazaki R, Tamura K, Saito M: Enteropathogenic *Escherichia coli* associated with diarrhea in children and adults. Jpn J Med Sci Biol 20:387–399, 1967

50 Trabulsi LR, Fernandes MFR, Zulianni ME: Novas bacterias patogenicas para o intestiuno do homen. Rev Inst Med Trop São Paulo 9:31, 1967

51 Marier R, Wells JG, Swanson RC, et al: An outbreak of enteropathogenic *Escherichia coli* foodborne disease traced to imported French cheese. Lancet 2:1376–1378, 1973

52 Sereny B: Experimental *Shigella* keratoconjunctivitis. A preliminary report. Acta Microbiol Acad Sci Hung 2:293–296, 1955

53 Formal SB, DuPont HL, Hornick R, et al: Experimental models in the investigation of the virulence of dysentery bacilli and *Escherichia coli*. Ann NY Acad Sci 176:190–196, 1971

54 Silva RM, Toledo MRF, Trabulsi LR: Biochemical and cultural characteristics of invasive *Escherichia coli*. J Clin Microbiol 11:441–444, 1980

55 Bray J: Isolation of antigenically homogeneous strains of *Bacterium coli neopolitanum* from summer diarrhea of infants. J Pathol Bacteriol 57:239–247, 1945

56 Farmer JJ, David BR, Cherry WB, et al: "Enteropathogenic serotypes" of *Escherichia coli* which really are not. J Pediatr 90:1047–1049, 1977

57 Nataro JP, Kaper JB, Robins-Browne R, et al: Patterns of adherence of diarrheagenic *E. coli* to HEp-2 cells. Pediatr Infect Dis 6:829–831, 1987

58 Levine MM, Bergquist EJ, Nalin DR, et al: *Escherichia coli* strains that cause diarrhoea but do not produce heat-labile or heat-stable enterotoxins and are non-invasive. Lancet 1:1119–1122, 1978

59 Scotland SM, Day NP, Willshaw GA, et al: Cytotoxic enteropathogenic *Escherichia coli*. Lancet 1:90, 1980

60 Ulshen MH, Rollo JL: Pathogenesis of *Escherichia coli* gastroenteritis in man—another mechanism. N Engl J Med 302:99, 1980

61 Polotosky Yu E, Dragunskaya EM, Seliverstova VG, et al: Pathogenic effect of enterotoxigenic *Escherichia coli* and *Escherichia coli* causing infantile diarrhea. Acta Microbiol Acad Sci Hung 24:221–236, 1977

62 Rothbaum RJ, Partin JC, McAdams AJ, et al: Enterocyte adherent *E. coli* O199:B14: A novel mechanism of infant diarrhea. Gastroenterology 80:1265, 1981

63 Cantey JR, Blake RK: Diarrhea due to *Escherichia coli* in the rabbit: A novel mechanism. J Infect Dis 135:454–462, 1977

64 Guerrant RL: Yet another pathogenic mechanism for *Escherichia coli* diarrhea? N Engl J Med 302:113–114, 1980

65 Konowalchuk J, Speirs JI, Stavric S: Vero response to a cytotoxin of *Escherichia coli*. Infect Immun 18:775–779, 1977

66 Konowalchuk J, Dickie N, Stavric S, et al: Properties of an *Escherichia coli* cytotoxin. Infect Immun 20:575–577, 1978

67 Williams PH, Sedgwick MI, Evans N, et al: Adherence of an enteropathogenic strain of *Escherichia coli* to human intestinal mucosa is mediated by a colicinogenic conjugative plasmid. Infect Immun 22:393–402, 1978

68 Riley LW, Remis RS, Helgerson SD, et al: Hemorrhagic colitis associated with a rare *E. coli* serotype. N Engl J Med 308:681–685, 1982

69 Scotland SM, Smith HR, Rowe B: Two distinct toxins active on Vero cells from *Escherichia coli* O157. Lancet 2:885–886, 1985

70 Strockbine NA, Marques LRM, Newland JW, et al: Two toxin-converting phages from *Escherichia coli* O157:H7 strain 933 encode antigenically distinct toxins with similar biologic activities. Infect Immun 53:135–140, 1986

71 Guerrant RL, Dickens MD, Wenzel RP, et al: Toxigenic bacterial diarrhea: Nursery outbreak involving multiple bacterial strains. J Pediatr 89:885–891, 1976

72 Wadstrom T, Aust-Kettis A, Habte D, et al: Enterotoxin-producing bacteria and parasites in stools of Ethiopian children with diarrhoeal disease. Arch Dis Child 51:865, 1976

73 Wachsmuth K, Wells J, Shipley P, et al: Heat-labile enterotoxin production in isolates from a shipboard outbreak of human diarrheal illness. Infect Immun 24:793–797, 1979

74 Sandefur PD, Peterson JW: Neutralization of *Salmonella* toxin-induced elongation of Chinese hamster ovary cells by cholera antitoxin. Infect Immun 15:988, 1977

75 Ahvonen P: Human yersiniosis in Finland. II. Clinical features. Ann Clin Res 4:39–44, 1972

76 Mandell GL, Douglas RG Jr, Bennett JE (eds): *Principles and Practice of Infectious Diseases*. New York, Wiley, 1979, chaps 70–74, pp 847–923

77 Levine MM, Nalin DR, Hoover DL, et al: Immunity to enterotoxigenic *Escherichia coli*. Infect Immun 23:729, 1979

78 Higgens JA, Code CF, Orvis AL: The influence of motility on the rate of absorption of sodium and water from the small intestine of healthy persons. Gastroenterology 31:708, 1956

79 Allweiss B, Dostal J, Carey KE, et al: The role of chemotaxis in the ecology of bacterial pathogenesis of mucosal surfaces. Nature 266:448, 1977

80 Sellwood R, Gibbons RA, Jones GW, et al: Adhesion of enteropathogenic *Escherichia coli* to pig intestinal brush borders: The

existence of two pig phenotypes. J Med Microbiol 8:405–411, 1975

81 Hughes JM, Rouse JD, Barada FA, et al: Etiology of summer diarrhea among the Navajo. Am J Trop Med Hyg 29:613–619, 1980

82 Korzenowski OM, Dantas W, Guerrant RL: Role of ST-producing *E. coli* in sporadic adult diarrhea in Brazil. Clin Res 26:400a, 1978

83 Kenny JF, Boesman MI, Michaels RH: Bacterial and viral co-proantibodies in breast-fed infants. Pediatrics 39:202, 1967

84 Sussman S: The passive transfer of antibodies to *Escherichia coli* O111:B4 from mother to offspring. Pediatrics 27:308, 1961

85 Mata LJ, Urrutia JJ: Intestinal colonization of breast-fed children in a rural area of low socioeconomic level. Ann NY Acad Sci 176:93, 1971

86 Guerrant RL, Kirchhoff LV, Shields DS, et al: Prospective study of diarrheal illnesses in Northeastern Brazil: Patterns of disease, nutrition impact, etiologies and risk factors. J Infect Dis 148:986–997, 1983

87 Gordon JE, Chitkara ID, Wyon JB: Weanling diarrhea. Am J Med Sci 245:345, 1963

88 Welsh JK, May JT: Anti-infective properties of breast milk. J Pediatr 94:1–9, 1979

89 Stoliar OA, Pelly RP, Kaniecki-Green E, et al: Secretory IgA against enterotoxins in breast-milk. Lancet 1:1258–1261, 1976

90 Nagy B: Vaccination of cows with a K99 extract to protect newborn calves against experimental enterotoxic colibacillosis. Infect Immun 27:21–24, 1980

91 Evans DG, Evans DJ Jr, Tjoa WS, et al: Detection and characterization of colonization factor of enterotoxigenic *Escherichia coli* isolated from adults with diarrhea. Infect Immun 19:727, 1978

92 Evans DG, Evans DJ Jr: New surface-associated heat-labile colonization factor antigen (CFA/II) produced by enterotoxigenic *Escherichia coli* serogroups of 06 to 08. Infect Immun 21:638, 1978

93 Satterwhite TK, Evans DG, DuPont HL, et al: Role of *Escherichia coli* colonization factor antigen in acute diarrhea. Lancet 2:181–184, 1978

94 Bergman MJ, Updike WS, Wood SJ, et al: Attachment factors among enterotoxigenic *Escherichia coli* from patients with acute diarrhea from diverse geographic areas. Infect Immun 32:881–888, 1981

95 Gross RJ, Cravioto A, Scotland SM, et al: The occurrence of colonization factor (CF) in enterotoxigenic *Escherichia coli*. FEMS Microbiol Letters 3:231, 1978

96 Levine MM, Rennels MB, Daya V, et al: Hemagglutination and colonization factors in enterotoxigenic and enteropathogenic *Escherichia coli* that cause diarrhea. J Infect Dis 141:733, 1980

97 Faris A, Lindahl M, Wadstrom T: GM2-like glycoconjugate as possible erythrocyte receptor for the CFA/I and K99 haemagglutinins of enterotoxigenic *Escherichia coli*. FEMS Microbiol Letters 7:265–269, 1980

98 Faris A, Wadstrom T, Freer JH: Hydrophobic absorptive and hemagglutinating properties of *Escherichia coli* possessing colonization factor antigens (CFA/I or CFA/II), type I Pili, or other Pili. Curr Microbiol 5:67–72, 1981

99 Guerrant RL: Pathophysiology of the enterotoxic and viral diarrheas. International Workshop on Interactions of Diarrhea and Malnutrition: Pathophysiology, Epidemiology and Interventions. Bellagio, Italy, Plenum, New York, 1982

100 Greenberg RN, Murad F, Guerrant RL: Lanthanum chloride inhibition of the secretory response to *Escherichia coli* heat-stable enterotoxin. Infect Immun 35:483–488, 1982

101 Hirschhorn N, Kinzie JL, Sachar DB, et al: Decrease in net stool output in cholera during intestinal perfusion with glucose containing solutions. N Engl J Med 279:176–180, 1968

102 Guerrant RL, Ganguly U, Casper AGT, et al: Effect of *Escherichia coli* on fluid transport across canine small bowel: Mechanism and time-course with enterotoxin and whole bacterial cells. J Clin Invest 52:1707–1714, 1973

103 DuPont HL, Reves RR, Galindo E, et al: Treatment of traveler's diarrhea with trimethoprim/sulfamethoxazole and with trimethoprim alone. N Engl J Med 307:841–844, 1982

104 Guerrant RL, Rouse JD, Hughes JM, et al: Turista among members of the Yale Glee Club in Latin America. Am J Trop Med Hyg 29:895–900, 1980

105 Rahaman MM, Wahed MA: Direct nutrient loss and diarrhoea. Interactions of diarrhea and malnutrition: Pathophysiology, Epidemiology, and Interventions. Bellagio, Italy, Plenum, New York, 1982

106 Levine MM, Xu J, Kaper JB, et al: A DNA probe to identify enterohemorrhagic *E. coli* of 0157:H7 and other serotypes that cause hemorrhagic colitis and hemolytic uremic syndrome. J Infect Dis 156:175–182, 1987

107 Karmali MA, Petric M, Lim C, et al: The association between idiopathic hemolytic uremic syndrome and infection by verotoxin-producing *E. coli*. J Infect Dis 151:775–782, 1985

108 Pai CH, Gordon R, Sims HV, et al: Sporadic cases of hemorrhagic colitis associated with *E. coli* 0157:H7. Ann Intern Med 101:738–742, 1984

109 Carter AO, Borczyk AA, Carlson AK, et al: A severe outbreak of *E. coli* 0157:H7-associated hemorrhagic colitis in a nursing home. N Engl J Med 317:1496–1500, 1987

110 Rosenberg ML, Koplan JP, Wachmuth IK, et al: Epidemic diarrhea at Crater Lake from enterotoxigenic *Escherichia coli*. A large, waterborne outbreak. Ann Intern Med 86:714, 1977

111 Moseley SL, Huq I, Alim ARMA, et al: Detection of enterotoxigenic *Escherichia coli* by DNA colony hybridization. J Infect Dis 142:892–898, 1980

112 Palmer DL, Koster FT, Islam AFRM, et al: A comparison of sucrose and glucose in oral electrolyte treatment of cholera and other severe diarrheas. N Engl J Med 297:1107, 1977

113 McLean M, Brennan R, Hughes JM, et al: Etiology of childhood diarrhea and oral rehydration therapy in northeastern Brazil. Bull PAHO 15(4):318–326, 1981

114 Levine MM: Antimicrobial therapy for infectious diarrhea. Rev Infect Dis 85(suppl):S207–S216, 1986

115 Sack RB: Antimicrobial prophylaxis of travelers' diarrhea: A selected summary. Rev Infect Dis 8S:S160–S166, 1986

116 Consensus development conference statement. Rev Infect Dis 8S:(suppl)S227–S233, 1986

117 Nelson JD: Duration of neomycin therapy for enteropathogenic *Escherichia coli* diarrheal disease: A comparative study of 113 cases. Pediatrics 48:248, 1971

118 Ericsson CD, DuPont HL, Johnson PC: Non antibiotic therapy for travelers' diarrhea. Rev Infect Dis 8(suppl):S202–S206, 1986

119 Steffan R, Heusser R, DuPont HL: Prevention of travelers' diarrhea by non antibiotic drugs. Rev Infect Dis 8(suppl):S152–S159, 1986

Campylobacter · David N. Taylor · Martin J. Blaser

In the 1950s, Elizabeth King found that *Campylobacter*, which she called the "closely related vibrio," was associated with diarrheal disease in humans [1]. The significance of this observation was not well understood until 1972 when Butzler and colleagues reported the isolation of *Campylobacter* by filtering fecal specimens from 5 percent of 800 Belgian children with diarrhea [2]. Soon after, Skirrow developed an antibiotic-containing, selective agar medium that could be used for the routine isolation of *Campylobacter* from feces [3]. The ability to isolate *Campylobacter* from fecal specimens led to literally thousands of publications on this organism over the ensuing decade. *Campylobacter* species now are recognized as organisms with a vast range of animal hosts, and as one of the most common causes of diarrheal illness in humans.

Although present in every environment, there are important geographical differences in the clinical and epidemiological features of *Campylobacter* infections. Chief among these differences is the reservoir of the organism in the environment and the age distribution of infected persons. In developed countries, the highest incidence of cases occurs in children, and a second peak occurs among young adults [4,5]. In developing countries, where the organism is more prevalent, *Campylobacter* causes diarrhea in young children, but rarely in adults [6].

In recent years the use of nonselective culture methods has led to the detection of a diverse group of *Campylobacter* species associated with diarrhea in humans [7]. There may be regional differences in the importance of these new *Campylobacter* species. Finally, there are also important differences in the clinical illnesses, complications, and species causing disease in immunocompromised hosts. In this chapter we will review what is currently known about the microbiology and pathogenesis of this pathogen, and discuss the possible reasons for the various epidemiological and clinical patterns.

PARASITE

Campylobacters are gram-negative, microaerophilic bacteria. *C. jejuni* is the species most commonly associated with diarrhea. Other species associated with diarrhea include *C. coli*, *C. laridis*, *C. hyointestinalis*, *C. fetus* spp. *fetus*, *C. cinaedi*, *C. fennelliae*, and *C. upsaliensis* [8–11]. These species can be distinguished from *C. jejuni* by their inability to hydrolyze hippurate. Beside the hippurate test, other biochemical tests may be useful in differentiating campylobacters or in biotyping strains [12]; however, there may be numerous exceptions to biochemical distinctions [13]. A more accurate method of classifying atypical strains is by determining DNA homology with well-characterized strains [7,13,14]. Hippurate-negative or

atypical hippurate-positive *Campylobacter* strains may account for 5 to 15 percent of the total *Campylobacter* isolated from patients with diarrhea. Since *C. jejuni* is the most common and best-studied *Campylobacter* species causing diarrheal illness, and because the clinical and epidemiological features associated with infection by other species, in general, are similar, our discussion will focus on *C. jejuni*.

C. fetus spp. *fetus* may also cause severe systemic infections in debilitated hosts. *C. cinaedi*, *C. fennelliae*, *C. hyointestinalis*, and *C. fetus* spp. *fetus* have been isolated from homosexuals with enteritis [9,15]. The newest *Campylobacter* of medical importance is *C. pylori*. This organism has been isolated from the stomach and duodenum, and is associated with gastritis, gastric and duodenal ulcer, and hypochlorhydria. Because it represents a separate clinical discussion and its taxonomic relationship to other *Campylobacter* species is uncertain [16], *C. pylori* will not be discussed in this chapter.

Most members of this genus are pathogens or commensals of a wide variety of mammalian and avian hosts [17]. Animals represent the most important reservoir for infection. Infection of animals may occur early in life and may be associated with morbidity. However, as the animals mature, long-term colonization and a commensal relationship develops. Detectable colonization may be intermittent, but once infected, animals appear to gain immunity to the consequences of reinfection. The continued fecal excretion of *C. jejuni* by infected animals represents an important source for transmission to humans either by direct contact or by contamination of food and water [18]. The animals with which humans are most frequently in contact, including cattle, sheep, swine, domesticated fowl, dogs, and cats, commonly carry *C. jejuni* in their intestinal contents. Saprophytic species of *Campylobacter* occur, but none of these have been shown to be pathogenic in animals or humans.

The term *Campylobacter* is derived from the Greek, meaning "curved rod." Organisms in young cultures are comma-shaped, spiral, or S-shaped (Fig. 83-1). Because of their small size (1.5 to 3.5 μm long and 0.2 to 0.4 μm wide), they can pass through a 0.65-μm filter. Campylobacters are motile with a single flagellum at one or both poles. As with other gram-negative organisms, the cell envelope of *Campylobacter* consists of an inner lipid bilayer cell membrane, a thin peptidoglycan cell wall, and an outer layer with a lipopolysaccharide (LPS) moiety, which has endotoxic activity, extending to the cell surface [19]. Interspersed in the outer layer are membrane proteins, some of which are exposed to the cell surface. Serum resistance in *C. jejuni* strains correlates with the carbohydrate content of the LPS produced, and long carbohydrate side chains may serve as a type of capsule that partially protects

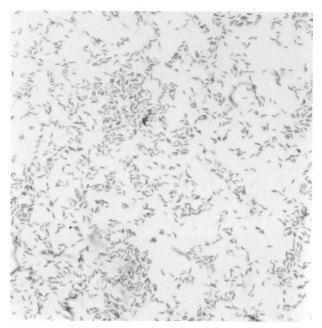

Figure 83-1. Gram stain of a pure culture of *Campylobacter jejuni.* The delicate comma- or S-shaped forms seen are nearly identical to those seen in cultures of *Vibrio cholerae,* but differences in growth and biochemical characteristics easily distinguish these organisms.

the organism from the killing activity of serum [20]. Most intestinal isolates of *C. jejuni* are killed by normal human serum while extraintestinal isolates may be either serum-sensitive or serum-resistant. Extraintestinal isolates from normal hosts are usually serum-resistant, whereas extraintestinal isolates from immunocompromised hosts resemble intestinal isolates.

The mechanism(s) by which *C. jejuni* causes disease are not known. There is evidence of cytotoxic, enterotoxic, invasive, and adherence properties in some isolates [21]. Although strains possess different pathogenic properties, there is as yet no well-defined association between specific clinical syndromes and any putative virulence characteristic. Furthermore, lack of serological response of infected hosts to several of the putative toxins argues against biological relevance in vivo.

The essential elements for isolating *C. jejuni* from fecal specimens are proper incubation atmosphere and temperature, and use of a selective isolation method. When these techniques are employed, isolation and identification of *C. jejuni* is not difficult [22]. Campylobacters are microaerophilic and will not grow in atmospheres with ambient oxygen or under anaerobic conditions. The optimal oxygen concentration for growth is 5%, but primary isolation of *C. jejuni* may be done using candle jars. Since campylobacters do not utilize carbohydrates and amino acids, Krebs cycle intermediates are their major energy sources.

Two serotyping systems are currently used. The Penner system is based on heat-stable somatic (O) antigens [23]. The Lior system is based on heat-labile surface (flagellar or capsular) antigens [24]. The two systems appear to be complementary. Strains of a single serotype in one system may belong to several serotypes in the other system [25]. Although both systems are reliable, the Lior system, which is based on slide agglutination, is more rapid to perform. At present there are 91 Lior serotypes of which 15 represent more than 75 percent of all human and animal isolates.

PATIENT

Campylobacters are susceptible to the bactericidal activity of gastric acid. Ingestion in vehicles with rapid wash-through such as water, or with high buffering capacity such as milk, aids in passage through the stomach. Data on the infectious dose are still limited. One human volunteer became ill after ingesting 500 organisms [26]. In volunteer trials, either of two strains of *C. jejuni* was ingested by adult volunteers [27]. At a dose of 10^6 to 10^8 organisms in milk, 59 percent of 17 persons became ill with one strain and 28 percent of 24 persons became ill with the second strain. Among those who were ill, the onset of fever and diarrhea began about 72 h (range, 53 to 88 h) after ingestion of the organism. In outbreaks, the incubation period has ranged from 1 to 7 days, with the majority between 2 and 4 days.

Once ingested, organisms multiply in the distal small intestine and colon. Ill persons excrete 10^6 to 10^9 *Campylobacter* per gram of feces. If left untreated, the median duration of excretion is 2 to 3 weeks [28,29]. Elimination of organisms coincides with the development of specific serum and intestinal antibodies. Persons with hypogammaglobulinemia have had recurrent infections, suggesting that one or more of the immunoglobulins are necessary for protection. Volunteers who developed illness with one strain were protected from illness, but not infection, when rechallenged with the same strain 1 month after recovery from the first infection [27].

The sites of injury include the distal small intestine and the colon. Among patients ill enough to seek medical attention, colonic involvement is frequent with hemorrhagic and exudative inflammation. Microscopic examination of rectal biopsy specimens shows infiltration of the lamina propria with neutrophils, eosinophils, and mononuclear cells, and degeneration of epithelial glands culminating in crypt abscess formation. These lesions may resemble those seen in other infectious colitides or those in idiopathic inflammatory bowel diseases such as chronic ulcerative colitis [30]. Despite signs of invasion, bacteremia is uncommon in normal hosts. None of the subjects in the volunteer studies had even transient bacteremia.

The clinical manifestations of *Campylobacter* infection may vary considerably, from watery diarrhea to dysentery with grossly bloody stools. The symptoms and signs of *Campylobacter* infection cannot be distinguished from illness caused by other enteric pathogens. Because of the selection of patients the symptoms reported in hospital-based surveys in developed countries probably represent the more severe end of the clinical spectrum. In the volunteer studies only half of the subjects developed symptoms with a dose of 10^6 to 10^8 organisms; however, fever, diarrhea, anorexia, malaise, and abdominal cramps were reported in the majority of those who became ill. Most ill persons also had blood in their stools, and all had fecal leukocytes. In outbreak situations, where case ascertainment was less selective, the spectrum of illness was broader and, on average, milder.

The most prominent features among patients presenting to medical attention are diarrhea, abdominal pain, and fever [28,29,31,32]. Grossly bloody stools are common and are often the reason for seeking medical attention. Abdominal pain is the most characteristic manifestation of illness and may be severe enough to mimic an acute abdomen. A prodrome of constitutional complaints, chiefly fever and myalgias, may precede the enteric symptoms by as much as 24 h, and occasionally may be the most pronounced symptoms. Most patients recover within 1 week, although up to 20 percent have either a relapse or a more prolonged illness. Some of these patients with persistent bloody diarrhea and high fevers may be misdiagnosed as having acute inflammatory bowel disease until Campylobacter infection is demonstrated. Rarer complications include toxic megacolon; massive lower gastrointestinal hemorrhage; and distant infections in the urinary tract, biliary tract, and central nervous system. Infection may be particularly severe in neonates and may be complicated by systemic infection [33]. Prolonged or unusually severe C. jejuni infections have been recognized in patients with hypogammaglobulinemia or acquired immunodeficiency syndrome [34]. Reactive arthritis is the most common postinfectious complication and in 60 percent of cases occurs in persons carrying the HLA-B27 histocompatibility antigen [35]. The Guillain-Barré syndrome may follow Campylobacter infection [36].

In developing countries, C. jejuni infection may also show a wide spectrum of presentations, but, in general, the illness recognized is milder than in patients in developed countries. The symptoms associated with Campylobacter infections in Bangladesh are seen in Table 83-1. Compared to patients with Campylobacter infections, patients with Shigella infections often had dysenteric symptoms, whereas those with enterotoxigenic Escherichia coli infections usually had watery diarrhea. In Thailand about one-third of C. jejuni infections in children were associated with bloody diarrhea [37]. Despite milder illnesses in indigenous populations, when western travelers to developing countries become infected with Campylobacter the symptoms resemble those seen in infections acquired in developed areas [38].

DIAGNOSIS

The diagnosis of Campylobacter infection is based on isolation of the organism from feces. Because campylobacters are sensitive to desiccation and to oxygen concentrations in ambient air, stool specimens or rectal swabs must be placed into a transport medium such as Cary-Blair if specimens cannot be plated within a short period of time. Since C. jejuni grows more slowly than the usual enteric flora, isolation from feces requires the use of a method of selection. The standard culture method from fecal specimens uses a blood-enriched, antibiotic-containing medium, a microaerobic atmosphere, and incubation at 42°C for 48 h. Three such media commonly used are the antibiotic-containing media of Skirrow [3], Butzler [22], and Blaser-Wang (Campy-BAP [31]). When incubations are

Table 83-1. Presenting complaints of patients with diarrhea associated with C. jejuni, Shigella, enterotoxigenic E. coli (ETEC), and any agent, Dhaka Hospital surveillance, 1980

	Percentage with complaint				
				C. jejuni	
Presenting complaint	All patients*, $N = 3350$	Shigella*, $N = 412$	ETEC*, $N = 624$	As only pathogen, $N = 164$	Total, $N = 436$
Watery diarrhea	65	30‡	78‡	66	69†
Abdominal pain	56	70‡	54	45†	43‡
Vomiting	58	37‡	67‡	66	64
Fever	46	52†	42	50	49
Stool with blood	20	55‡	10	17	19
Stool with mucus	60	86‡	46‡	61	57
Dehydration	20	13‡	26‡	20	20

*From Stoll BJ, Glass RI, Huq MI, et al: Epidemiologic and clinical features of patients infected with Shigella who attended a diarrheal disease hospital in Bangladesh. J Infect Dis 146:177–183, 1982. All patients' group includes Dec. 1, 1979 to Nov. 30, 1980. C. jejuni data begin March 1, 1980.

†$p < .05$ and ‡ $p < .01$; difference from all patients group.

done at 42°C, candle jars can be used in place of gas mixtures containing 5% oxygen. Blood-free media have also been shown to be useful [39]. Shortcomings of selective media include that some *Campylobacter* species are susceptible to antibiotics (especially cephalothin or colistin) in the media, and others do not grow at 42°C.

An alternative method uses a cellulose acetate filter (0.45-μm or 0.65-μm pore size) placed directly on a non-antibiotic-containing medium such as blood, chocolate, or *Brucella* agar [7,14,39]. A fecal suspension is applied onto the filter for 30 min, during which time campylobacters are able to pass through to the nonselective medium while virtually all other fecal organisms are excluded. The filter is removed, and the plate is incubated at 37°C in a microaerobic atmosphere for 48 h (Fig. 83-2). This technique must now be considered the method of choice for primary isolation of *Campylobacter* species from stools.

Another inexpensive diagnostic technique is direct microscopy of fecal specimens. Dark-field microscopy of stools within 2 h of passage may permit a presumptive diagnosis of *Campylobacter* enteritis if the characteristic darting motility is seen [40]. Similarly, Gram stain of stools may reveal the characteristic vibrio forms and also can be used to detect red blood cells and neutrophils. When compared to culture, direct microscopy is usually specific, but only 50 to 75 percent sensitive. Similarly, rapid presumptive identification of *Campylobacter* from culture can be done by observation of motility on dark-field microscopy, Gram stain showing gram-negative curved rods, and evidence of oxidase production on spot examination.

Serological assays to detect antibody response to *Campylobacter* infection are rarely clinically useful in patients with gastroenteritis. Serology may be useful as an epidemiological tool in determining the extent of outbreaks; demonstrating a relationship with late manifestations of *Campylobacter* infections, such as arthritis or Guillain-Barré syndrome; or determining the level of exposure to *Campylobacter* in various populations.

Many *Campylobacter* infections are asymptomatic, and a sizable proportion of clinically significant illnesses are self-limited and do not require specific antimicrobial treatment. However, with all diarrheal illnesses, fluid and electrolyte replacement are the cornerstones of treatment. Dehydration should be treated with intravenous fluids or oral rehydration solution, as appropriate. *Campylobacter* infections do not usually cause severe dehydrating diarrhea, even in infants.

Several clinical trials were not able to demonstrate clinical efficacy of erythromycin in altering the natural history of illness in unselected cases of *Campylobacter* infection [18]; in these studies, treatment usually began after diagnosis of infection, generally several days after onset of symptoms. In contrast, early administration of erythromycin was effective in improving the clinical course among Peruvian children with severe, dysenteric illness [41]. Anecdotal reports indicate rapid resolution of symptoms and fewer relapses after antimicrobial treatment. Clinical experience suggests that specific antimicrobial treatment is indicated in those patients in whom diarrhea is frequent or bloody, or in whom high fever or severe abdominal pain is present. In immunodeficient hosts, antibiotic resistance may develop in vivo [34].

Based on in vitro testing and in vivo responses, erythromycin is the drug of choice against campylobacters. In adults, 500 mg given orally twice a day for 5 to 7 days is usually sufficient; in children 30 to 50 mg/(kg·day) for 5 to 7 days is recommended. Erythromycin clears stools of campylobacters within 48 h. Alternative treatments include the 4-quinolones, tetracyclines, furazolidone, and clindamycin. The newer quinolones have not been released for use in children, and tetracyclines may stain teeth of children under 7 years old. Resistance to the tetracyclines and erythromycin may become clinically relevant especially in developing countries where these antibiotics are widely available [42]. In Bangkok 11 percent of *C. jejuni* and 46 percent of *C. coli* strains were resistant to erythromycin, and 65 percent of *C. jejuni* and 80 percent of *C. coli* strains were resistant to tetracycline. In animals and humans *C. coli* strains are more often resistant to tetracycline and erythromycin than *C. jejuni* strains.

POPULATION

Campylobacter infection is substantially more prevalent in developing areas than in industrialized countries. In developed countries, *Campylobacter* is isolated from about 5 percent of all persons with diarrheal disease, as often as *Salmonella* or *Shigella*, but it is rarely isolated from healthy persons [5,18,32]. Thus, only a small fraction of the population is infected and excreting the organism. In contrast, in developing countries it is not unusual to isolate *Campylobacter* from 10 percent of children with diarrheal disease, and from an equal proportion of healthy children without diarrhea [6,18]. The

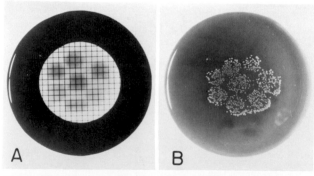

Figure 83-2. Membrane filtration culture method. *A.* Application of fecal suspension to membrane filter (0.45-μm pore size) on *Brucella* agar medium containing 5% sheep blood. *B. Campylobacter* colonies after incubation at 37°C for 48 h.

broad range in isolation rates (5 to 15 percent) reported in studies from developing countries reflects differing levels of hygiene and different age distributions of the populations studied. Nevertheless, these results contrast greatly with those derived in cross-sectional studies in developed countries, in which isolation rates from healthy persons are usually less than 1 percent [18].

In developed countries, isolation rates peak in infants and again in young adults [4,5]. Campylobacter isolations typically increase during the summer and fall months [4,5], and, while most cases appear to be sporadic, epidemics also occur [18]. Infections with multiple enteric pathogens are infrequent, and the mean duration of convalescent excretion of Campylobacter after an acute infection is 2 to 3 weeks [28,29].

In developing countries, Campylobacter infection is hyperendemic. In Thailand, for example, Campylobacter was isolated from 18 percent of children under 5 years old with diarrhea [37]. The highest isolation rate was in children 8 months of age. Cross-sectional surveys in Bangladesh indicate that a second peak does not occur in young adults (Table 83-2). In studies in Thailand, the mean duration of convalescent excretion of the same Campylobacter serotype was 14 days for children less than 1 year old and 8 days for children 1 to 5 years old. The rate of reinfection with another serotype in these children was 15 percent each week. There were an estimated 1.5 Campylobacter infections per year among children under 5 years old. In developing countries with tropical climates there is usually not a seasonal peak, and epidemics have not been reported. Infection may lead to mild illness or be asymptomatic and is less often associated with bloody diarrhea.

There is little evidence that strain differences can account for these markedly different clinical and epidemiological patterns. Campylobacter strains isolated in developing countries are biochemically and serotypically similar to strains isolated in developed countries [25,37]. Lior 4 and 36, which together accounted for about a third of the isolates in the United States, were also the most common serotypes in Thailand. One difference that may be important is the proportion of C. coli or other hippurate-negative strains isolated from infected persons in developing countries. In Thailand, C. coli strains were not associated with bloody diarrhea and were isolated more often from asymptomatic children than C. jejuni, features that suggest that C. coli infections may be milder than C. jejuni infections. In Europe and the United States, C. coli account for less than 5 percent of all Campylobacter infections. Thus Campylobacter infections may appear to be mild in areas where C. coli is frequently isolated, such as in Hong Kong and the Central African Republic, where C. coli accounted for 41 percent and 39 percent of isolates, respectively [43,44].

In developing countries, where Campylobacter infections are endemic, infections occur in the first year of life and are associated with a humoral response to cell-surface antigens of C. jejuni [37,45]. In Thailand, IgG antibodies to campylobacter peaked and rapidly fell before 2 years of age. In Thailand and Bangladesh, serum IgA levels to cell-surface antigens of C. jejuni rise progressively through life to much higher levels than in age-matched populations in the United States. The development of immunity to these or other antigens appears to play an important role in the age-related decreases in the case-to-infection ratio and the duration of convalescent excretion. Further exposure to Campylobacter probably continues to stimulate gut immunity and prevent tissue invasion and subsequent symptomatic infection, but has less effect on asymptomatic infections.

TRANSMISSION

In developed countries, the most commonly implicated modes or vehicles for transmission of Campylobacter infection include ingestion of contaminated food or water [18]. The largest outbreaks of Campylobacter enteritis have been associated with ingestion of contaminated milk and water. Direct transmission from dogs, cats, cattle, sheep, swine, and poultry has been documented. Many of these same animals are important food sources, and foodborne transmission from undercooked meats and unpasteurized milk has been reported. Ingestion of under-

Table 83-2. Age distribution of infections with C. jejuni in hospital patients with diarrhea and community controls, Dhaka, 1980

Age group, years	Hospital patients		Controls	
	No. examined	C. jejuni, %	No. examined	C. jejuni, %
< 1	607	24	4	25
1–2	663	17	—	—
3–4	276	13	24	4
5–9	246	9	36	6
10–19	145	8	36	0
20–39	373	4	53	0
≥40	157	6	18	0
Total	2467	13	171	2

Source: [6].

cooked chicken appears to be the most common cause of sporadic cases of *Campylobacter* enteritis [*46*]. Surface water can potentially become contaminated with feces from wild or domesticated animals, and if not properly treated, its consumption can lead to outbreaks of *Campylobacter* enteritis [*47*]. Person-to-person transmission appears to be uncommon except when the index case is a child who is not bowel-trained. In part the low person-to-person spread may also be due to the lack of a substantial human reservoir of infection in industrialized societies.

The vehicles for transmission of *Campylobacter* infection in developing areas are not well understood. In a survey of over 500 raw food samples from markets in Bangkok, *Campylobacter* was isolated from 41 percent of chickens, 5 percent of pork, and 1 percent of beef samples [*48*]. The serotypes of strains isolated from foods were similar to those from human isolates. Close direct contact with animals was reported as an important risk factor in rural areas [*5*]. Since campylobacters do not multiply at ambient temperatures and oxygen concentrations, recontamination of cooked foods should not, theoretically, be a problem. The population studies demonstrating a substantial reservoir of *Campylobacter* infections among humans suggest that person-to-person transmission could be more common. Family studies are needed to help elucidate the modes of transmission in the tropics.

Control of *C. jejuni* infections will ultimately be based on a better understanding of the reservoirs, epidemiology, and pathophysiology of the infection. Since the available evidence shows that household and farm animals constitute a major reservoir, interruption of transmission to humans from these sources should have a high priority. Awareness of the necessity for hand washing after contact with animals or animal products and the importance of proper cooking and storage of foods of animal origin is probably as important for preventing *C. jejuni* infections as it is for preventing other enteric infections. Pasteurization of milk, chlorination of water supplies, and thorough cooking of meat all readily kill *C. jejuni*. Consuming only treated water is another action that an individual can take to prevent illness from *Campylobacter* as well as other agents. While this recommendation is practical for travelers, it is hardly applicable to the rural populations in developing areas who must rely on grossly inadequate water supplies.

However, interrupting vehicleborne infection may be of little value if person-to-person transmission is frequent in developing countries. Under such circumstances, effective immunization may represent the only practical approach to interrupting transmission and diminishing the impact of infection. In general, with invasive organisms vaccines should be based on cell-surface moieties. No effective vaccine for preventing *C. jejuni* infection is presently available. Because of the wide diversity of somatic and heat-labile antigenic determinants of *C. jejuni,* a vaccine based on those characters would lack the broad specificity probably necessary. If possible, vaccine initiatives should be pursued using group antigens. For the traveler or the short-term visitor to developing areas, prophylaxis would be an attractive goal.

REFERENCES

1 King EO: Human infections with *Vibrio fetus* and a closely related vibrio. J Infect Dis 101:119–129, 1957

2 Butzler J-P, Dekeyser P, Detrain M, et al: Related vibrio in stools. J Pediatr 82:493–495, 1973

3 Skirrow MB: *Campylobacter* enteritis: A "new" disease. Br Med J 2:9–11, 1977

4 Finch MJ, Riley LW, et al: *Campylobacter* infections in the United States: results of an 11-state surveillance. Arch Intern Med 144:1610–1612, 1984

5 Skirrow MB: A demographic survey of *Campylobacter, Salmonella,* and *Shigella* infections in England. Epidem Infect 99:647–657, 1987

6 Glass RI, Stoll BJ, Huq MI, et al: Epidemiology and clinical features of endemic *Campylobacter jejuni* infection in Bangladesh. J Infect Dis 148:292–296, 1983

7 Steele TW, Sangster N, Lanser JA: DNA relatedness and biochemical features of *Campylobacter* spp isolated in Central and South Australia. J Clin Microbiol 22:71–74, 1985

8 Simor AE, Wilcox L: Enteritis associated with *Campylobacter laridis.* J Clin Microbiol 25:10–12, 1987

9 Totten PA, Fennell CL, Tenover FC, et al: *Campylobacter cinaedi* (sp nov) and *Campylobacter fennelliae* (sp nov): Two new *Campylobacter* species associated with enteric disease in homosexual men. J Infect Dis 151:131–139, 1985

10 Edmonds P, Patton CM, Griffin PM, et al: *Campylobacter hyointestinalis* associated with human gastrointestinal disease in the United States. J Clin Microbiol 25:685–691, 1987

11 Klein BS, Vergeront JM, Blaser MJ, et al: *Campylobacter* infection associated with raw milk: an outbreak of gastroenteritis due to *Campylobacter jejuni* and thermotolerant *Campylobacter fetus* subsp. *fetus.* JAMA 255:361–364, 1986

12 Lior H: New, extended biotyping scheme for *Campylobacter jejuni, Campylobacter coli,* and "Campylobacter laridis." J Clin Microbiol 20:636–640, 1984

13 Totten PA, Patton CM, Tenover FC, et al: Prevalence and characterization of hippurate-negative *Campylobacter jejuni* in King County, Washington. J Clin Microbiol 25:1747–1752, 1987

14 Tee W, Anderson BN, Ross BC, et al: Atypical campylobacters associated with gastroenteritis. J Clin Microbiol 25:1248–1252, 1987

15 Quinn TC, Goodell SE, Fennell C, et al: Infections with *Campylobacter jejuni* and *Campylobacter*-like organisms in homosexual men. Ann Intern Med 101:187–192, 1984

16 Romaniuk PJ, Zoltowska B, Trust TJ, et al: *Campylobacter pylori,* the spiral bacterium associated with human gastritis, is not a true *Campylobacter* sp. J Bacteriol 169:2137–2141, 1987

17 Smibert RM: The genus *Campylobacter.* Ann Rev Microbiol 32:700–773, 1978

18 Blaser MJ, Reller LB: *Campylobacter* enteritis. New Engl J Med 305:1444–1452, 1981

19 Perez GI, Blaser MJ: Lipopolysaccharide characteristics of pathogenic campylobacters. Infect Immun 47:353–359, 1985

20 Blaser MJ, Perez GP, Smith PF, et al: Extraintestinal *Campylobacter jejuni* and *Campylobacter coli* infections: Host factors and strain characteristics. J Infect Dis 153:552–559, 1986

21 Walker RI, Caldwell MB, Lee EC, et al: Pathophysiology of *Campylobacter* enteritis. Microbiol Rev 50:81–94, 1986

22 Morris GK, Patton CM: *Campylobacter*, in Lennette E, Balows A, Hausler WJ Jr, Shadomy HJ (eds): *Manual of Clinical Microbiology,* 4th ed. Washington, American Society for Microbiology, 1985, pp 302–308

23 Penner JL, Hennessey JN: Serotyping *Campylobacter fetus* subsp *jejuni* on the basis of somatic O antigens. J Clin Microbiol 12: 732–737, 1980

24 Lior H, Woodward DL, Edgar JA, et al: Serotyping of *Campylobacter jejuni* by slide agglutination based on heat-labile antigenic factors. J Clin Microbiol 15:761–768, 1982

25 Patton CM, Barrett TJ, Morris GK: Comparison of the Penner and Lior methods for serotyping *Campylobacter* spp. J Clin Microbiol 22:558–565, 1985

26 Robinson DA: Infective dose of *Campylobacter jejuni* in milk. Br Med J 282:1584, 1981

27 Black RE, Levine MM, Clements ML, et al: Experimental *Campylobacter jejuni* infection in humans. J Infect Dis 157:472–479, 1988

28 Karmali MA, Fleming PC: *Campylobacter* enteritis in children. J Pediatr 94:527–533, 1979

29 Svedhem A, Kaijser B: *Campylobacter fetus* subspecies jejuni: A common cause of diarrhea in Sweden. J Infect Dis 142:353–359, 1980

30 Blaser MJ, Parsons RB, Wang W-LL: Acute colitis caused by *Campylobacter fetus* ss *jejuni*. Gastroenterology 78:448–453, 1980

31 Blaser MJ, Berkowitz ID, LaForce FM, et al: *Campylobacter* enteritis: Clinical and epidemiological features. Ann Intern Med 91: 179–185, 1979

32 Blaser MJ, Wells JG, Feldman RA, et al: *Campylobacter* enteritis in the United States: A multicenter study. Ann Intern Med 98: 360–365, 1983

33 Goossens H, Henocque G, Kremp L, et al: Nosocomial outbreak of *Campylobacter jejuni* meningitis in newborn infants. Lancet 2:146–149, 1986

34 Perlman DM, Ampel NM, Schifman RB, et al: Persistent *Campylobacter jejuni* infections in patients infected with human immunodeficiency virus (HIV). Ann Intern Med 108:540–546, 1988

35 Schaad UB: Reactive arthritis associated with *Campylobacter* enteritis. Pediatr Infect Dis 1:328–332, 1982

36 Kaldor J, Speed BR: Guillain-Barré syndrome and *Campylobacter jejuni*: A serological study. Br Med J 288:1867–1870, 1984

37 Taylor DN, Echeverria P, Pitarangsi C, et al: Influence of strain characteristics and immunity on the epidemiology of *Campylobacter* infections in Thailand. J Clin Microbiol 26:863–868, 1988

38 Speelman P, Struelens MJ, Sanyal SC, et al: Detection of *Campylobacter jejuni* and other potential pathogens in travelers' diarrhoea in Bangladesh. Scand J Gastroenterol 18suppl84:19–23, 1983

39 Goossens H, De Boeck M, Coignau H, et al: Modified selective medium for isolation of *Campylobacter* spp. from feces: Comparison with Preston medium, a blood-free medium, and a filtration system. J Clin Microbiol 24:840–843, 1986

40 Paisley JW, Mirrett S, Lauer BA, et al: Dark-field microscopy of human feces for presumptive diagnosis of *Campylobacter fetus* subsp *jejuni* enteritis. J Clin Microbiol 15:61–63, 1982

41 Salazar-Lindo E, Sack RB, Chea-Woo E, et al: Early treatment with erythromycin of *Campylobacter jejuni*-associated dysentery in children. J Pediatr 109:355–360, 1986

42 Taylor DN, Blaser MJ, Echeverria P, et al: Erythromycin-resistant *Campylobacter* infections in Thailand. Antimicrob Agents Chemother 31:438–442, 1987

43 Ho DD, Wong WT: A one-year survey of *Campylobacter* enteritis and other forms of bacterial diarrhoea in Hong Kong. J Hyg (Camb) 94:55–60, 1985

44 Georges-Courbot MC, Baya C, Beraud AM, et al: Distribution and serotypes of *Campylobacter jejuni* and *Campylobacter coli* in enteric *Campylobacter* strains isolated from children in the Central African Republic. J Clin Microbiol 23:592–594, 1986

45 Blaser MJ, Taylor DN, Echeverria P: Immune response to *Campylobacter jejuni* in a rural community in Thailand. J Infect Dis 153:249–254, 1986

46 Deming MS, Tauxe RV, Blake PA, et al: *Campylobacter* enteritis at a university: Transmission from eating chicken and from cats. Am J Epidemiol 126:526–534, 1987

47 Blaser MJ, Taylor DN, Feldman RA: Epidemiology of *Campylobacter jejuni* infections. Epidemiol Rev 5:157–176, 1983

48 Rasrinaul L, Suthienkul O, Echeverria PD, et al: Foods as a source of enteropathogens causing childhood diarrhea in Thailand. Am J Trop Med Hyg 39:97–102, 1988

CHAPTER 84

Meningococcal Diseases · W. Michael Scheld

The meningitis syndrome has been recognized for centuries. Clinical descriptions of meningitis dating from the sixteenth century have been found. However, epidemic cerebrospinal meningitis with a purpuric rash was not identified until 1805 when Viesseux described an epidemic of "malignant purpuric fever" surrounding Geneva, the first clinical description of meningococcemia with meningitis. Autopsy reports documenting inflammation of the surface of the brain appeared the following year. The first accounts from the United States were those by Danielson and Mann of Massachusetts that appeared in 1806 and the descriptions collated in a treatise by Elisha North of Connecticut in 1811 (summarized in [1,2]). Then, as now, the syndrome was often dramatic and fulminant and the epidemic nature of the disease frightening. For example, Dr. Samuel Woodward of Torrington, Connecticut, wrote the following in the *American Mercury,* Hartford, in 1807:

> . . . The violent symptoms were great lassitude, with universal pains in the muscles, chills; heats, if any, were of short duration; unusual prostration of strength; delirium, with severe pain in the head; vomiting, with undescribable anxiety of stomach; eyes red and watery, and rolled up, and the head drawn back with spasm; pulse quick, weak, and irregular; petechiae and vibices all over the body, and a cadaverous countenance and smell: death often closed the scene in ten or fifteen hours after the first attack: . . . The body, near the fatal period, and soon after, became as spotted as an adder . . .

Similarly, the following account was written as a letter to the editor of the *Worcester Spy,* dated March 6, 1810, by Rev. Festus Foster of Petersham, Massachusetts:

> I hasten to give you a sketch of the spotted fever in this place. It made its first appearance about the beginning of January last; but the instances were few and distant from each other, until last week. Although it had proved fatal in most instances, seven only had died belonging to this town, previous to the 25th of February. Since that time the disorder has come upon us like a flood of mighty waters. We have buried eight persons within the last eight days. About twelve or fifteen new cases appeared on Thursday last; many of them very sudden and violent. This was the most melancholy and alarming day ever witnessed in this place. Seven or eight physicians were continually engaged in the neighborhood north of the meeting house, and I believe not one half hour passed in the forenoon without presenting a new case. Pale fear and extreme anxiety were visible in every countenance . . .

It is inconceivable that this entity had been previously unrecognized. One can only speculate on how the meningococcus changed to enhance its virulence for humans in the early nineteenth century. The etiological organism was first isolated in 1887 by Anton Weichselbaum in Vienna from the cerebrospinal fluid (CSF) of six patients and initially named *Diplococcus intracellularis meningitidis.*

Since these earliest accounts, meningococcal infections have continued as important problems on all continents. Although the definition of an "epidemic" is somewhat arbitrary, at least 30 countries worldwide experienced significant problems with meningococcal disease during the 1970s (Table 84-1). A few examples illustrate the magnitude of the problem. The meningitis belt of sub-Saharan Africa (Fig. 84-1) is a classic endemic area. Although the disease did not occur in the area until the 1880s, large outbreaks still occur regularly. The meningitis belt lies within the 300 mm and 1100 mm rainfall lines, but the precise influences of climatic conditions on the incidence of meningitis are unresolved (see under "Population" below). In the 10-year period 1951–1960 at least 390,000 cases with

Table 84-1. Countries in which epidemics of meningococcal disease occurred during the 1970s

Continent or region	Country or territory
Africa	Chad
	Federal Republic of Cameroun
	Ghana
	Mauritania
	Nigeria
	Senegal
	Togo
	Upper Volta (Burkina Faso)
Asia	Bahrain
	Jordan
	Lao Peoples Democratic Republic
	Mongolia
	Syrian Arab Republic
	Turkey
	Vietnam
Europe	Belgium
	Finland
	Great Britain
	Greece
	Iceland
	Netherlands
	Norway
	Romania
	Spain
	U.S.S.R.
North America	United States
Central America	Costa Rica
	Guatemala
South America	Argentina
	Brazil
	Uruguay
Oceania	New Caledonia
	New Hebrides

*Adapted from [3].

53,000 deaths occurred in the seven countries of the belt, and the average annual incidence since 1950 has been estimated as approximately 70 cases per 10^5 persons by WHO [3]. Similarly, within one month (October 1974), 4865 patients with meningitis were treated at the infectious diseases hospital in Sao Paulo, Brazil. The overall annual incidence of meningitis in Sao Paulo reached 370 cases per 10^5 population in 1974. The disease continues to occur in many other areas (Table 84-1).

Despite the introduction of new antimicrobials, the morbidity and mortality associated with meningococcal disease remain high. The sparsity of laboratory and medical facilities and/or supplies coupled with epidemiological features continue to ensure that meningococcal infections remain a serious problem in many developing countries, particularly in Africa.

PARASITE

IDENTIFICATION OF THE ETIOLOGICAL AGENT

Neisseria species are nonmotile, non-spore-forming, oxidase-positive, gram-negative cocci which usually appear as biscuit- or kidney-shaped diplococci on smears of infected fluids either extracellularly or within polymorphonuclear leukocytes. The individual cells are approximately 0.8 μm long by 0.6 μm

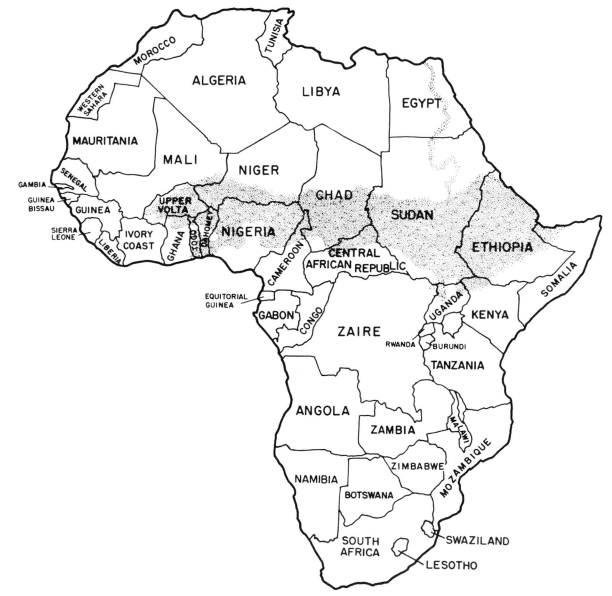

Figure 84-1. The ''meningitis belt'' of sub-Saharan Africa; areas of Africa endemic for serogroup A meningococcal meningitis.

wide. As other organisms (*Branhamella catarrhalis, Morax-ella* spp., etc.) are similar morphologically, identification rests on biochemical or immunological techniques. All *Neisseria* species are oxidase-positive. Sugar fermentation reactions are usually sufficient for speciation within the genus: *N. gonorrhoeae* ferments glucose (but not maltose or lactose) to acid, whereas *N. meningitidis* ferments both glucose and maltose. A related organism, *N. lactamica,* sometimes present in throat cultures, ferments glucose, maltose, and lactose. Occasionally, maltose-negative variants of *N. meningitidis* have been noted; these strains may be differentiated from *N. gonorrhoeae* (particularly when isolated from atypical locations such as the genital tract) by fluorescent antibody or coagglutination tests or electrophoretic analysis of hexokinase isoenzymes. These strains usually acquire the ability to ferment maltose on subculture; true maltose-negative strains are rare, but this property is linked genetically to sulfadiazine resistance.

IN VITRO CULTURE CHARACTERISTICS

Meningococci grow rapidly on blood, chocolate, gonococcal (Gc), or enriched Mueller-Hinton agar in a moist 3% to 10% CO_2 environment at 35° to 37° C. A modified Thayer-Martin medium is employed for isolation of meningococci from contaminated sites (e.g., detection of carriers, isolation from areas with complex indigenous flora). The colonies are smooth and gray in appearance and larger than gonococcal colonies. The specimens should be inoculated promptly due to the susceptibility of this organism to drying or chilling. The transoral approach for detection of the carrier state is more practical and at least as sensitive as older transnasal approaches. Inhibition of isolation of occasional *Neisseria* strains by sodium polyetholesulfonate, a frequent additive in commercial blood culture media, has been described.

ULTRASTRUCTURE AND CLASSIFICATION

Like other gram-negative bacteria, the ultrastructural characteristics of meningococci are complex (Figure 84-2). The surface components include capsular polysaccharide, pili, lipopolysaccharide (LPS), and outer-membrane proteins, and several of these structures are important pathogenically (see below). Meningococci are currently classified by serogroup (based on structural differences of the capsular polysaccharide and agglutination reactions with specific antisera) and further defined by serotype (based on analysis of the outer-membrane proteins). Thirteen serogroups are recognized: A, B, C, D, H, I, K, L, X, Y, Z, 29E, and W135 [4]. Most meningococcal disease is caused by organisms in serogroups A, B, C, or Y although the proportion due to W135 is increasing (see below). Capsular polysaccharide (i.e., positive agglutination with reference antisera) is uniform among invasive isolates; however 20 to 50 percent of isolates from carriers are nongroupable (unencapsulated). The serogroup has important epidemiological and prevention-related implications (see below).

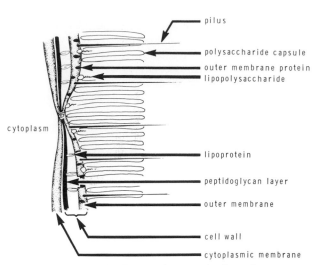

Figure 84-2. Schematic of the meningococcal cell envelope.

Serotypes within a serogroup of meningococci are classified largely on the basis of outer-membrane proteins in the cell envelope. At least 20 serotypes are now recognized, resulting in a classification scheme useful in epidemiological studies [5]. Physicochemical characterization of the four to five major outer-membrane proteins has led to the designation of five major classes. Class 2 and 3 proteins are the major porin proteins responsible for aqueous channels in the outer membrane. Class 5 proteins are surface-exposed and may have a role in virulence, but the functions of class 1 and 4 proteins are unknown. The designation of serotypes has important epidemiological uses and may identify virulence characteristics among meningococci. For example, serotype 2 (2a, 2b) strains are responsible for the majority (approximately 50 percent) of serogroup B disease (in which 15 serotypes have been described) followed by serotypes 15 and 9; in contrast serotypes 4 and 6 have been isolated only from carriers. Serotype 2 is also responsible for approximately 80 percent of group C serogroup strains causing disease and is an important marker for serogroup Y and W135 pathogenic strains [3,5]. All serogroup A meningococci, in contrast, are homogeneous with respect to outer-membrane proteins and show no homology to other serotypes within other serogroups. Serotype analysis has proven useful in delineating certain characteristics of the clinical syndrome [6], but this technique is, at present, only available in reference or research laboratories. In addition, at least eight immunotypes of meningococci are known to exist based on reactivity with LPS antigens, but their relation to pathogenesis and disease expression remains poorly defined. Nevertheless, LPS immunotypes may be useful in the further characterization of the epidemiology of meningococcal disease [3].

HOST RANGE

Neisseria meningitidis is a pathogen exclusive to humans. No intermediate or reservoir hosts, or animal-to-human transmission of meningococci, has ever been documented. Nevertheless, animal models of meningococcal infection have proven valuable in the delineation of certain pathogenetic events in humans.

PATIENT

As expected, the development of meningococcal disease in humans is dependent on a complex interaction of factors, some due to virulence properties of meningococci while others reflect the host's response. Thus, microbial virulence factors, the development of the carrier state, and humoral immunity (e.g., antibody, complement) are all important in the acquisition of meningococcal infections.

MICROBIAL VIRULENCE FACTORS

Putative meningococcal virulence characteristics are listed in Table 84-2. As noted above, all strains isolated from invasive meningococcal infections are encapsulated (serogroup-positive) whereas 20 to 50 percent of isolates from carriers are unencapsulated. The capsular polysaccharide appears essential for meningococcal virulence, probably by allowing the organism to escape host phagocytic clearance mechanisms within the bloodstream (and CSF). Pili are protein surface appendages composed of identical pilin repeating subunits. Meningococcal pili are morphologically and chemically related to gonococcal pili. Cross-reacting antibodies bind to a peptide sequence (residues 69–94) of gonococcal pili critical for receptor-binding function. Fresh isolates of meningococci from carriers or invasive infection contain 7 to 40 pili per diplococcus. Pili are important mediators of meningococcal adhesion to human nonciliated columnar nasopharyngeal cells, an essential early step in the development of the carrier state [7]. Pathogenic *Neisseria* (i.e., meningococci and gonococci) elaborate extracellular proteases that cleave IgA1 heavy chains in the hinge region. The role of IgA proteases in the pathogenesis of disease is debated, but they are produced only by a few organisms of importance to medicine (e.g., *N. meningitidis, N. gonorrhoeae, S. pneumoniae, H. influenzae, S. sanguis,* etc.), and intact IgA may have an important role in mucosal immunity at the pharyngeal portal of entry. Lipopolysaccharide (endotoxin) likely mediates many of the clinical features of fulminant meningococcemia including purpuric skin lesions, tissue injury, and disseminated intravascular coagulation (DIC). The meningococcal LPS differs from that of gram-negative bacilli (but resembles *H. influenzae* LPS) by a lack of O antigenic

Table 84-2. Potential meningococcal virulence factors

Capsular polysaccharide
Pili
IgA protease
Lipopolysaccharide (endotoxin)
Outer-membrane proteins
Outer-membrane vesicles (blebs)

polysaccharide side chains despite a smooth phenotype and proven virulence. Although a specific role for outer-membrane proteins in meningococcal virulence remains unproven, it is important to recognize that meningococci release substantial amounts of cell surface material (outer-membrane vesicles containing outer-membrane proteins and LPS) in the absence of cell lysis during growth in vitro and in vivo. These outer-membrane vesicles (blebs) likely represent vehicles for delivery of toxic moieties to host cells ([8]; see below). Tissue invasion may also be facilitated by the ability of meningococci to obtain iron from transferrin [9].

The natural reservoir for meningococci is the human nasopharynx, and transmission is facilitated by airborne droplets or close contact. Meningococcal infection may result in an asymptomatic carrier state (most common), or in endemic, hyperendemic, or epidemic disease. Although there is no clear relationship between carriage rate and overt disease, the development of the carrier state is crucial to conceptualizing the spread of meningococcal infection.

CARRIER STATE

Nasopharyngeal carriage rates of meningococci vary widely with age and the population under study. The rate is markedly influenced by age: 0.5 to 1 percent in children 3 to 48 months of age, approximately 5 percent in adolescents 14 to 17 years old, and 20 to 40 percent in young adults. During endemic periods, nasopharyngeal carriage usually persists for weeks to months. Carriage rates of 40 percent have been documented in close family contacts of meningococcal cases. In closed populations (e.g., military camps, especially during early training) carriage rates range from 20 to 60 percent and may approach 90 percent during epidemics. Spread of disease is usually carrier-mediated, not by case-to-case contacts. *N. meningitidis* is often introduced into the home by an adult family member with transmission to others, colonizing infants last. Containment of the infection to the nasopharynx versus dissemination is determined by host and environmental factors that are as yet uncharacterized, but host immunity plays an important role.

IMMUNITY

The age-specific incidence of meningococcal disease is inversely proportional to the presence of bactericidal antibodies (against serogroups A, B, C) in the serum. As a result of transplacental transfer, more than 50 percent of infants have bactericidal antibody at birth. However, the group B capsular polysaccharide is a polymer of 2 to 8 linked sialic acid residues and is immunologically identical to the oligosaccharides of several human glycoproteins, including brain gangliosides. Thus, immunological tolerance exists; although IgM antibody can be induced, the usual switch to IgG does not occur. As IgM does not cross the placenta, IgG bactericidal antibody to group B capsular polysaccharide is lacking in neonates, explaining the occurrence of group B disease in this patient population. In addition, the group B antigen is identical to the capsular polysaccharide of *E. coli* K1, a major cause (along with group B streptococci) of neonatal sepsis and meningitis. The prevalence of bactericidal antibodies is lowest between 6 and 24 months of age, thereafter increasing to early adulthood (70 percent with bactericidal activity). The relationship of bactericidal antibody to invasive disease was first documented during an outbreak of serogroup C meningitis among army recruits in 1968 [*10*]. In that study, the sera of only 5.6 percent of the recruits who developed meningococcal disease versus (82.2 percent of control sera) had bactericidal activity before illness. In addition, 5 out of 13 recruits (38.5 percent) without antibody developed illness after colonization with the group C strain.

Recovery from invasive meningococcal disease confers immunity against the homologous serogroup. This is not the major immunizing process, however. Nasopharyngeal colonization, particularly with serogroups B, C, and Y, may provoke the development of bactericidal activity (primarily against the colonizing strain but also to heterologous organisms) within 5 to 12 days of acquisition. Colonization with nongroupable meningococci may also induce immunity against groupable pathogenic strains. Cross-reactions with *N. lactamica* may produce protective immunity in young children. Nasopharyngeal carriage of (virtually always nonpathogenic) *N. lactamica* in children is highest (4 to 20 percent) between 3 months and 12 years of age versus an age-related prevalence of meningococcal carriage of only approximately 0.5 to 2 percent. In addition, the carriage rate of serogroups A and C is too low (especially in children) to account for antibody formation, and other cross-reacting bacteria have been proposed: *Bacillus pumilis* for group A polysaccharide, and *E. coli* for group C organisms.

Paradoxically, an exuberant IgA response to meningococci may actually favor the development of invasive disease. When a large proportion of antibodies within the individual directed against the capsular polysaccharide are of the IgA class, serum complement–mediated immune bacteriolysis by IgM is blocked, thus enhancing susceptibility. For example, meningococcal infections developed despite high levels of antibody to capsular polysaccharide in a Finnish study, but a large fraction (28.3 percent of antibodies) were of the IgA class [*11*]. This peculiar immunological phenomenon is transient (perhaps lasting only a few days) following asymptomatic nasopharyngeal carriage of *N. meningitidis* or closely related bacteria.

The complement cascade, in addition to antibody, is also important in host defense against meningococcal disease. Recurrent or chronic (chronic meningococcemia) infections with *N. meningitidis* or *N. gonorrhoeae* have been associated with rare isolated congenital deficiencies of late complement components (C5, C6, C7, or C8) occasionally in association with failure to make antimeningococcal antibodies. Recurrent episodes of meningococcal disease occur in these patients in the absence of susceptibility to other pathogens [*12,13*]. Since the course of the disease, response to therapy, and complications do not differ from other patients, screening for complement

defects by measuring total hemolytic complement activity is useful in patients with recurrent *Neisseria* infections. In addition, complement deficiency (congenital of late components) or depletion (C1, C3, or C4) due to underlying disease (e.g., systemic lupus erythematosus, hepatic failure [*14*], nephrotic syndrome, C3 nephritic factor, multiple myeloma) may predispose to the first episode of invasive meningococcal disease: 30 percent of 20 patients with invasive meningococcal disease displayed decreased complement function in one study. Properdin deficiency (or dysfunction despite normal concentrations) also predisposes to fulminant meningococcal disease, a defect reversible by vaccination [*15,16*]. Finally, splenectomy enhances susceptibility to infections with encapsulated bacteria particularly *S. pneumoniae* and *H. influenzae* but also including meningococci.

PATHOGENESIS

Although the above factors (microbial virulence characteristics, host immunity, etc.) undoubtedly contribute to the pathogenesis of meningococcal disease, the precise determinants leading to overt clinical illness (versus the usual outcome of infection-asymptomatic carriage) are poorly defined [*17*]. Various authors have estimated that only 1 in 1000 to 5000 infected patients developed disease [*3*], even during meningococcal epidemics. Overcrowding, lower socioeconomic status, and poor general health have all been considered predisposing factors to explain the increased incidence in blacks in the United States and among alcoholics in Finland or Alaska [*3*], but such conditions (e.g., the influence of overcrowding) have not been supported by other studies in Zaria, Nigeria. Since approximately one-third of meningococcal cases follow symptoms referable to the upper respiratory tract, an antecedent viral illness has been suggested as a predisposing factor. In 1981 an outbreak of meningococcal illness followed a large influenza epidemic in Texas, and simultaneous outbreaks of meningitis and influenza A2 have occurred in institutional settings. Meningococcal pneumonia has clearly followed influenza outbreaks (e.g., the 1918–1919 pandemic), but the role of upper respiratory viral infections in enhancing meningococcal dissemination is unproven.

Whatever the mechanism, the time from acquisition of nasopharyngeal infection to bloodstream invasion is short (usually less than or equal to 10 days). The incubation period may be quite short as household "secondary" cases often occur within 1 to 4 days of the index case. Furthermore, only 20 percent of prospectively studied recruits within 7 days of hospitalization for meningococcal disease actually carried the organism. Once bloodborne, over 90 percent of meningococcal disease is manifest as meningitis and/or meningococcemia.

PATHOPHYSIOLOGY

Once dissemination occurs, the clinical manifestations and/or tissue injury of meningococcal disease are likely due to LPS

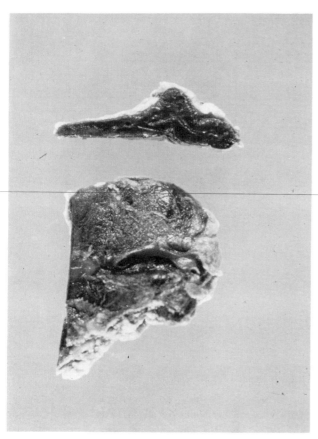

Figure 84-3. Hemorrhagic adrenal infarction (Waterhouse-Friderichsen syndrome) as a result of fulminant meningococcemia.

beyond the scope of this chapter. Nevertheless, there is a direct correlation between the presence of tumor necrosis factor in serum and a fatal outcome from meningococcal disease [21].

PATHOLOGY

The pathological alterations observed in acute meningococcemia occur when shock and DIC supervene. Fibrin thrombi and vasculitis of small blood vessels are seen in the skin lesions; meningococci may be visible in endothelial cells or within polymorphonuclear leukocytes surrounding damaged vessels. The purpura is thought to represent an LPS-mediated dermal Shwartzman reaction. Fulminant meningococcemia often leads to hemorrhagic adrenal infarction (Waterhouse-Friderichsen syndrome; Fig. 84-3), but the shock observed is due to sepsis, not adrenal failure since (1) fulminant meningococcemia does occur without adrenal hemorrhage; (2) serum cortisol concentrations are normal or elevated; (3) adrenal insufficiency does not develop in survivors. Most of the pathological findings of meningococcemia are probably related to LPS-mediated (or IL-1-mediated, TNF-mediated, etc.) events. Approximately 70 percent of fatal meningococcal cases have interstitial myocarditis evident at autopsy. The pathology of meningococcal meningitis is similar to that observed with pyogenic meningitis of other bacterial causes, except that a hemorrhagic ependymitis (Fig. 84-4) may be more prevalent with meningococcal disease.

CLINICAL MANIFESTATIONS

Illness supervenes when the initial asymptomatic nasopharyngeal (or, perhaps, other mucosal) colonization progresses to bloodstream invasion or pneumonia. The clinical picture may be mild or extremely fulminant, acute, or chronic, and is usually dominated by meningitis and/or meningococcemia.

(free, or in the form of outer-membrane vesicles). Although studies with meningococci have not been performed, analogous experiments with *H. influenzae* type b in rat models of meningitis have examined the cell surface factors relevant to the development of a CSF pleocytosis and increased blood-brain barrier permeability (BBBP) to exogenous protein (i.e., ^{125}I-albumin, normally excluded from the CSF). These studies support the following conclusions: (1) encapsulation with polyribosylribitol phosphate is not essential for BBB injury but facilitates its progression by allowing the organism to escape host clearance mechanisms; (2) LPS, in addition to capsule, is a separate virulence determinant for *H. influenzae;* (3) purified LPS increased BBBP in a dose- and time-dependent fashion, and inhibition studies suggest these effects are mediated by the lipid A portion of the molecule [18,20]. Furthermore, outer-membrane vesicles increase BBBP in a dose- and time-dependent manner virtually identical to purified *H. influenzae* LPS [20a]. Although meningococci were not examined, analogous conclusions are probably justified. Many of the phenomena may actually be mediated by a ''second messenger'' (e.g., interleukin 1, tumor necrosis factor), but this is conjectural and

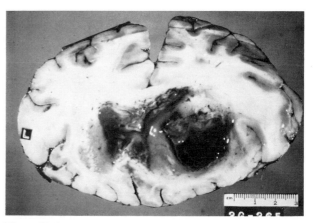

Figure 84-4. Hemorrhagic ependymitis in a gross specimen of a patient with fulminant meningococcemia and DIC. Note ventricular hemorrhage, periventricular white-matter edema, and massive right-to-left shift.

Meningitis

The majority of patients with meningococcal meningitis are 3 months to 15 years of age, but the median age shifts upward during epidemics. As 30 to 40 percent of cases are bacteremic, the clinical picture may be dominated by meningococcemia and/or meningitis. When the latter occurs, the history and physical findings are similar to those in other forms of pyogenic meningitis ([22]; Table 84-3). The abrupt onset of fever, generalized headache, stiff neck, and vomiting should suggest a meningeal syndrome. Many patients have had antecedent upper respiratory tract symptoms, but a preceding otitis media, mastoiditis, sinusitis, or pneumonia is less frequent than in meningitis due to *S. pneumoniae* or *H. influenzae* type b. Myalgias are, however, more common with meningococcal disease than with the other two major pathogens; backache and generalized weakness are frequent. The disease usually progresses rapidly with evidence of deteriorating higher cortical function from lethargy and confusion to obtundation and coma. The onset is, however, highly variable from a rapid course (24 h or less) without premonitory symptoms to a gradual evolution over several days with upper respiratory or nonlocalizing symptomatology. Rarely, the onset and clinical course may be indolent and suggest aseptic meningitis. CSF analysis in these cases usually reveals few (or no) cells, a negative Gram stain, but positive cultures for meningococci, indicating early meningeal involvement. An early delirium may be more common with meningococcal disease but is also present with temporal lobe abscess or encephalitis.

The patient is usually febrile with signs of meningeal irritation on examination (e.g., stiff neck, Kernig's and/or Brudzinski's signs, alterations in consciousness), but these findings may be subtle or absent in infants or obtunded or elderly patients. Fever and lethargy (or irritability in infants) should suggest meningitis in these patients, and whenever in doubt, prompt CSF analysis.

The presence of a petechial or purpuric rash in this setting should always suggest meningococcal disease. Many other conditions, however, may present with fever, altered sensorium, and a petechial rash including (1) rarely acute *S. pneumoniae* or *H. influenzae* meningitis; (2) acute *S. aureus* endocarditis, although a few lesions are actually pustular purpura and will reveal clumps of staphylococci on Gram stain; (3) rickettsial infections, prominently Rocky Mountain spotted fever in the United States (the season of the year is often helpful in differential diagnosis) and other agents in this group at other locales; (4) rarely viral aseptic meningitis (e.g., echovirus type 9); (5) various viral hemorrhagic fevers (dengue, etc.); and (6) other "noninfectious" causes including thrombotic thrombocytopenic purpura, hemolytic-uremic syndrome, leukocytoclastic vasculitis, etc.

It has been known since the earliest case examined pathologically that meningitis involves much more than just the meninges. For example, Danielson noted in 1806 in what is probably the first autopsy report of meningococcal meningitis in the United States: ". . . the substance of the brain itself remarkably soft, offering scarcely any resistance to the finger when thrust into it. . . ." Thus it is not surprising that some of the clinical features and/or sequelae of pyogenic meningitis may not be due to meningeal inflammation alone. For example, cranial nerve abnormalities (chiefly III, IV, VI, or VII) occur in 10 to 20 percent of patients with bacterial meningitis and usually resolve with recovery (Fig. 84-5). Persistent sensorineural hearing loss complicates approximately 10 percent of meningitis cases in children, and approximately another 15 percent develop transient conductive hearing loss. In children, permanent deafness complicates *S. pneumoniae* meningitis more often than disease due to *N. meningitidis* or *H. influenzae*. Deafness may rarely be the initial manifestation of meningococcal meningitis preceding all meningeal signs. Focal

Table 84-3. Symptoms and signs of pyogenic meningitis

Finding	Relative frequency (%)
Fever	≥90
Headache	80–90
Stiff neck	≥80
Brudzinski's sign	≈50
Kernig's sign	≈50
Myalgias	20–40*
Nausea, vomiting	≥80
Altered sensorium (lethargy to coma)	≥80
Cranial nerve palsy	10–15
Seizures	20–30
Focal cerebral signs	10–15
Papilledema	<1
Petechial rash	30–50*
Other suppurative focuses (otitis, sinusitis, pneumonia, endocarditis, arthritis, etc.)	0–30
Nonseptic arthritis-pericarditis during convalescence	2–10*

*Suggestive of meningococcal etiology (when compared to *S. pneumoniae*, *H. influenzae*, etc.)

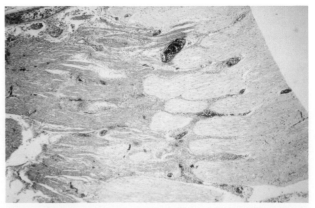

Figure 84-5. Necrosis of the central portion of the third cranial nerve as a result of meningococcal meningitis. The inflammation overlying the nerve (upper left) has extended into the nerve itself.

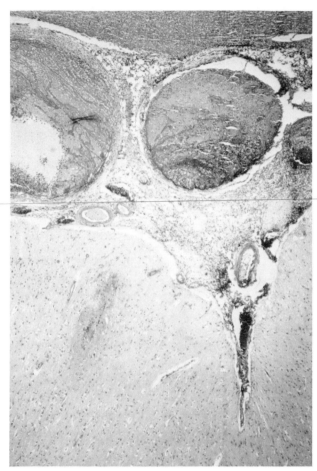

Figure 84-6. Thrombosis of two venules within the subarachnoid space, surrounded by inflammation and complicated by underlying brain infarction, as a result of meningitis.

cerebral findings (e.g., dysphasia, hemiparesis, visual field defects) occur in approximately 15 percent of meningitis patients. They may develop early or late in the course and often reflect vascular occlusive phenomena in the vessels that transverse the subarachnoid space (Fig. 84-6). Seizures occur in up to 30 percent of patients and may be due to fever alone (in infants), drug neurotoxicity, or focal cerebral injury due to an attendant encephalitis or vascular occlusion. They may occur early or late (approximately 7 to 10 days after onset) with focal findings due to cortical vein thrombophlebitis. Cerebral edema (probably reflecting vasogenic, cytotoxic, and interstitial mechanisms) is a uniform finding in fatal cases of meningitis examined at autopsy. The edema may increase intracranial pressure (ICP) with resultant seizures, IIId or VIth nerve palsy, abnormal reflexes, rapid onset of coma with hypertension and/or brachycardia. Nevertheless, papilledema is rare (less than 1 percent of cases) in meningitis and should suggest a space-occupying lesion (e.g., brain abscess, subdural empyema). The CSF acidosis associated with meningitis may induce central hyperventilation. A hemorrhagic ependymitis may complicate

meningococcal meningitis (usually with DIC) and is frequently fatal (Fig. 84-4).

Prompt and appropriate antimicrobial therapy usually leads to resolution of neurological deficits. Persistent or late-onset focal neurological signs, obtundation, or coma suggest cerebral edema and raised ICP, subdural effusions (in infants), loculated ventriculitis with or without hydrocephalus, cortical vein thrombophlebitis, sagittal sinus thrombosis, or, rarely, associated brain abscess (e.g., *C. diversus* meningitis in children). In addition, 10 to 20 percent of patients overall are left with permanent neurological sequelae after the acute state, including developmental delay or speech defects (each approximately 5 percent of cases) in children. Neurological sequelae are more common in infant survivors (30 to 50 percent). Overall, the clinical manifestations of meningococcal meningitis resemble those observed in other pyogenic meningitides (Table 84-3) except as noted.

Meningococcemia without meningitis accounts for approximately 20 percent of cases of meningococcal disease and may be acute (mild or fulminant) or chronic with an indolent, relapsing course that may persist for months.

Mild acute meningococcemia

This systemic illness is actually the most common form of meningococcemia and is characterized by the rapid onset of fever, chills, arthralgias, myalgias, and malaise, often following minor upper respiratory tract symptoms. Diarrhea may occur early in a minority of patients. The clinical course may evolve into

1. Resolution in 2 to 3 days, the diagnosis only established in retrospect from positive blood cultures.
2. Recurrent chills and the eruption of an erythematous macular rash, particularly on the extremities, often with scattered petechiae, which may progress to purpura and ecchymotic areas with gunmetal-gray necrotic centers in more severe disease (Figs. 84-7 and 84-8). Tachycardia and tachypnea

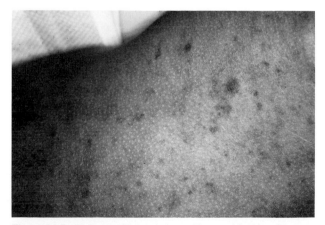

Figure 84-7. Early petechial rash in an 18-year-old male with acute mild meningococcemia.

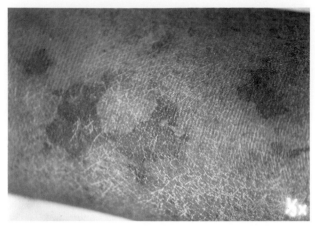

Figure 84-8. More extensive purpuric eruption in the same patient (as shown in Fig. 84-7) 3 h later. A portion of the forearm is shown.

are uniform and hypotension (and/or shock) may develop, resembling fulminant meningococcemia. An encephalitic presentation may dominate in approximately 15 percent of patients.

3. Persistence of the initial symptoms for approximately 1 week (with a few macular and petechial skin lesions) with the development of joint effusions.

Fulminant meningococcemia ("purpura fulminans")

This form constitutes about 10 percent of meningococcal infections and is the most dramatic, with rapid evolution to death (often in 10 h or less) unless properly treated (see opening section of chapter). High fever, true rigors, dizziness, headache, profound weakness, and generalized apprehension develop over a few hours. Diarrhea and abdominal pain may rarely be of sufficient severity to cause diagnostic delay. Petechiae appear in crops, initially on the extremities and may rapidly coalesce as new lesions appear in the buccal mucosa or conjunctivae. Purpura rapidly evolves (Figs. 84-6 through 84-10), and the patient may pass from a febrile state to hypothermia. Hypotension and shock supervene and are often accompanied by the clinical hallmarks of septic shock: altered sensorium (delirium progressing rapidly to obtundation and coma), respiratory alkalosis and hyperventilation, tachycardia (occasionally with heart failure due to myocarditis), DIC with enlarging hemorrhagic areas including mucosal and/or gastrointestinal bleeding, and the adult respiratory distress syndrome (ARDS; "shock lung"). Myocardial dysfunction has been documented by echocardiography in approximately 60 percent of children with meningococcemia and may be associated with a worse prognosis. Certain features (particularly when present as a constellation of findings) portend a poor prognosis: (1) petechiae for less than 12 h prior to hospitalization; (2) absence of meningitis; (3) shock; (4) fever 40°C or higher; (5) leukopenia; (6) thrombocytopenia or evidence of

DIC; (7) extremes of age. Laboratory evidence of DIC occurs in at least 25 percent of patients, and, in association with shock, often leads to large areas of hemorrhagic necrosis, acral cyanosis, or peripheral gangrene (Fig. 84-9) [24] which may require skin grafting or amputation [25]. Resolution is slow and distal areas may remain cold, cyanotic, and edematous showing lines of demarcation only after weeks. Late skeletal abnormalities (particularly epiphyseal-metaphyseal lesions) may be recognized months to years after recovery from meningococcemia and DIC in children [26].

Meningococcemia is not the sole cause of this syndrome noted above (sepsis with coagulopathy, purpura, and/or adrenal hemorrhage) as *S. pneumoniae* and *H. influenzae* sepsis in splenectomized hosts may be extremely fulminant. Of 42 febrile purpuric children analyzed over a 12-year period [27], 30 cases were due to meningococci versus 12 caused by *H. influenzae,* and similar cases continue to be reported [28]. The *H. influenzae* cases were more often lethargic or comatose on hospital admission when compared to meningococcemia patients. In addition, mortality was higher (9 out of 12 versus

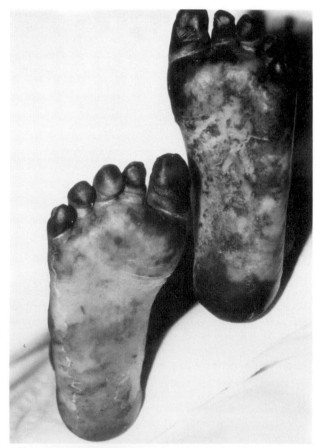

Figure 84-9. Fulminant meningococcemia with extensive purpura and peripheral gangrene in an 11-year-old Brazilian girl.

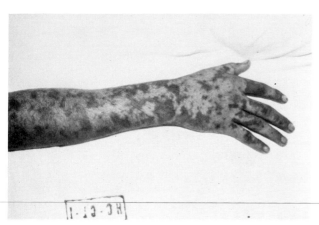

Figure 84-10. Extensive purpuric lesions in an adolescent with purpura fulminans due to serogroup B meningococci.

5 out of 30) and time to death shorter (approximately 20 versus approximately 120 h) when *H. influenzae* was the etiological agent. Septic shock due to other gram-negative organisms, group A streptococcal septicemia, and acute staphylococcal endocarditis may also simulate fulminant meningococcemia. In children at least, initial empirical therapy with penicillin alone may be inadvisable (see below).

Chronic meningococcemia

This unusual syndrome [23] is usually episodic with intermittent febrile periods of 1 to 6 days or (rarely) a sustained fever over weeks. The initial symptoms are fever, chills, migratory arthralgias (rarely frank arthritis), and headache with minimal toxicity which are then joined by a transient polymorphous rash (erythematous macules to purpuric nodules) that is negative by Gram stain. Skin biopsy reveals a leukocytoclastic vasculitis, thus raising confusion with various "allergic" vasculitis syndromes. Blood cultures are essential for diagnosis but are negative during afebrile periods and may not become positive until after several febrile episodes. Approximately 20 percent of patients develop splenomegaly and meningitis, respectively. Rarely, endocarditis or epididymitis may complicate the course. The nidus of colonization between recurrences is unclear (throat cultures are usually negative), but the syndrome is associated with deficiency of terminal complement components.

Arthritis

This complicates 2 to 16 percent of acute meningococcal disease and may present variably:

1. An isolated acute meningococcal arthritis resembling other forms of septic arthritis, in the absence of meningitis or meningococcemia (rarest type). Tenosynovitis and arthritis may coexist, thus simulating disseminated gonococcal infection, but this is very rare.

2. The most common type: early-onset (first 2 to 3 days) polyarthritis with small or absent effusions during meningitis or meningococcemia.
3. Late-onset (day 4 to later than day 10, when meningeal findings are waning) arthritis, commonly characterized as a mono- or oligoarthritis with prominent joint effusions, associated pleuropericarditis, recrudescence of fever, and new papulobullous skin lesions. The synovial and pericardial fluids are serosanguineous (or purulent) and sterile; immune complexes have been implicated in this syndrome by immunopathological techniques, secondary to local formation within the joint rather than deposition from serum. Treatment with anti-inflammatory agents (occasionally with joint aspiration) is sufficient.

Pericarditis

This may also present as three syndromes and complicates 2 to 20 percent of cases of meningococcal disease.

1. Isolated purulent pericarditis without meningitis or meningococcemia, usually manifest by a purulent pericardial effusion and the need for urgent surgical intervention due to tamponade (least common form). These patients tend to be older than the median age for all meningococcal diseases, and there is a strong association with serogroup C [29].
2. Early-onset purulent pericarditis due to meningococcal invasion during the first several days of meningitis and/or meningococcemia. Acute myopericarditis may rarely be the initial feature of meningococcemia.
3. Late-onset (4 days to more than 10 days into the illness) pericarditis with large, serosanguineous effusions and a favorable response to anti-inflammatory agents.

Upper respiratory tract infection

It is unknown how often meningococcal infection of the nasopharynx is symptomatic due to the frequent association with concurrent viral infection.

Pneumonia

Primary meningococcal pneumonia occurred frequently during the 1918 influenza pandemic but was rarely observed again until recently. The syndrome resembles other forms of community-acquired pneumonia, is bronchogenic (rather than hematogenous) in origin, and is usually caused by serogroup Y organisms. Group Y pneumonia is now the most frequent form of meningococcal disease encountered in military recruit populations. In contrast, group Y is almost never isolated from children under 5 years of age and causes meningococcemia (not pneumonia) in older children. The onset may be gradual or abrupt; is dominated by fever, chills, cough, and pleuritic pain; and may follow adenoviral or influenza infection. The process shows a predilection for the lower lobes and may be segmental, lobar, or bronchopneumonic in pattern. About 15 percent of cases are bacteremic, but the diagnosis is often suggested by sputum Gram stain (*B. catarrhalis* and other *Neisseria* spp. may be confused on smears). Meningitis or meningococcemia may be complicated by pneumonia during the course, but the former dominate the clinical picture.

Genital or anal infection

These occasionally are due to meningococci, the latter most commonly in homosexual males. The rate of rectal and nasopharyngeal carriage of meningococci in homosexual males approaches 2 percent and 45 percent, respectively. Some authorities assert that as many as 1 percent of "gonorrhea" cases are due to meningococci since full speciation is rarely performed. Female patients may exhibit asymptomatic or symptomatic cervical infections which may progress to salpingitis and/or dissemination. Urethritis is usually symptomatic.

Ocular infections

Less than 1 percent of patients with meningococcal disease develop panophthalmitis (which may be bilateral and/or lead to blindness) or conjunctivitis. Primary acute meningococcal conjunctivitis is even rarer, but systemic therapy (in addition to topical agents) is mandatory as approximately 10 percent of children with this condition develop disseminated disease.

DIAGNOSIS

The definitive bacteriological diagnosis of meningococcal disease requires cultural isolation of the organism from blood, CSF, or other body fluids. Alternatively, visualization on stained smears from an infected area in an appropriate clinical setting, or detection of capsular polysaccharide antigen (groups A, B, C, or Y) by immunological methods, is also satisfactory for diagnosis. Blood cultures are positive in approximately 30 to 40 percent of patients with meningococcal meningitis and

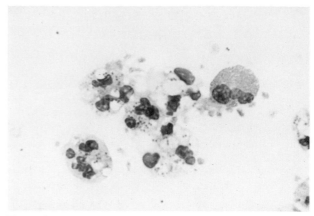

Figure 84-12. Smear of a petechial lesion from a patient with meningococcemia (Giemsa stain). Note cocci with vacuolated polymorphonuclear leukocytes.

in 50 to more than 75 percent of suspected meningococcemia cases, respectively. Stained smears (Gram or Wright stains) of blood or buffy coat occasionally reveal leukocyte-associated organisms in cases of fulminant meningococcemia (Fig 84-11). Although older reports from the 1940s suggested that stained smears (Gram, Wright, or Giemsa stains) of scrapings from skin lesions were positive in about 70 percent of cases, recent experience with this technique suggests a much lower sensitivity (Fig 84-12).

The overall sensitivity of the CSF culture in cases of pyogenic meningitis is approximately 80 to 90 percent, but this figure is lower in those receiving antimicrobial therapy prior to CSF evaluation [30]. The single most important rapid test on CSF is the Gram stain, which is positive in approximately 80 percent of patients, revealing characteristic biscuit-shaped gram-negative cocci (Fig 84-13). When the Gram stain is negative, various immunological methods, including latex agglu-

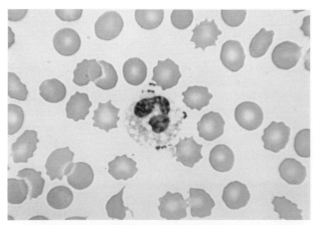

Figure 84-11. Peripheral-blood smear from a patient with fulminant meningococcemia (Wright's stain). Note diplococci associated with a vacuolated polymorphonuclear leukocyte.

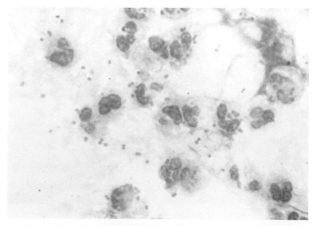

Figure 84-13. Gram-stained smear of CSF from a patient with meningococcal meningitis. Note typical "biscuit-shaped" gram-negative diplococci and polymorphonuclear leukocytes.

tination (LA), counterimmunoelectrophoresis (CIE), staphylococcal coagglutination, and enzyme-linked immunosorbent assay (ELISA) have been employed [31]. The overall sensitivity of these methods for detection of meningococcal capsular polysaccharide in CSF is approximately 70 percent, but cross-reactions between serogroup B and *E. coli* K1 antigen may cause diagnostic confusion. LA is preferred since it is simpler, less expensive, and more sensitive than CIE. Capsular antigen is detectable by these methods in 10 to 25 percent of patients with meningococcemia; its presence portends a poorer prognosis and a higher incidence of late-onset arthritis. The limulus lysate gelation assay for the detection of endotoxin in CSF is positive in nearly all patients with meningococcal meningitis but is rarely useful since similar results are obtained in patients with any form of gram-negative bacterial meningitis.

The sensitivity and specificity of the other tests done on CSF are beyond the scope of this chapter. The CSF analysis of patients with meningococcal meningitis is typical of findings present with other pyogenic forms: elevated opening pressure, a CSF pleocytosis (usually 10^2 to 10^4 cells per milliliter) with a polymorphonuclear predominance, hypoglycorrhachia, increased protein, and depressed lactate. Determination of CSF enzymes (e.g., LDH, CPK) or C-reactive protein is not helpful in differential diagnosis.

THERAPY

Meningococcal diseases are emergencies, and prompt initiation of therapy is essential. Respiratory isolation should be instituted for the first 24 to 48 h to minimize nosocomial spread of infection. These patients should be monitored, at least initially, in an intensive care unit setting (if available), as vigorous supportive care is mandatory in these critically ill patients.

Antimeningococcal antiserum was the first successful therapy employed in meningococcal disease. This technique was first employed by Dopter (as described by Delville) in France in 1907–1908 and widely publicized by Flexner in a series of 1300 patients in 1913. The mortality with serotherapy (including intrathecal injections) declined from 65 to 80 percent with no treatment to 15 to 30 percent with serum. Repeated lumbar punctures, ice bags, and other modalities were often employed in these patients. Serotherapy remained the mainstay of treatment for the next 20 years until the introduction of sulfonamides. The report by Schweutker and colleagues in 1937 [33a] was the first documenting cure with an antibiotic. Of 11 patients treated at the Johns Hopkins hospital with subcutaneous and intrathecal sulfonamide, only one died (9 percent mortality) despite a sterile CSF. The overall mortality from meingococcal meningitis was 5 to 12 percent during the sulfonamide era. Widespread sulfonamide resistance was first recognized in serogroup B organisms in 1963 in California. Sulfonamide resistance peaked in the United States in 1970 (67 percent of strains resistant) but had declined in 1980 to 12

percent (8 percent of group B, 30 percent of group C, 4 percent of group W135, 0 percent of group Y resistant [32]). If these trends continue and sulfonamide resistance declines to 10 percent or less, this class of agents may again be useful for prophylaxis. Nonetheless, sulfonamide resistance varies greatly by geographical locale and serogroup [33].

The efficacy of high-dose penicillin for the therapy of meningococcal disease was first conclusively reported in 1966. Penicillin remains the drug of choice in a regimen of 24 million units daily in the adult (in divided doses every 2 to 4 h or by continuous infusion) with meningococcal meningitis. Ampicillin (12 g daily in the adult in divided doses every 2 to 3 h) is equally effective. Although intramuscular administration of ampicillin appears comparable to the intravenous route [34], experience is scant and intramuscular injections should be avoided in patients with shock (poor absorption due to peripheral vasoconstriction) and/or DIC (bleeding into muscle). Although lower doses of penicillin (e.g., 8 to 12 million units daily) are sufficient to sterilize blood cultures promptly in meningococcemia, larger "meningitis" doses are commonly employed due to concerns regarding incipient meningitis and potential subtherapeutic concentrations in the CSF. Bactericidal concentrations in the CSF (i.e., 10- to 20-fold greater than the minimal bactericidal concentration for the pathogen) appear necessary for optimal therapy of meningitis [35]. Seven days of penicillin therapy is commonly used for meningococcal meningitis. Although some reports suggest that shorter courses (i.e., 4 days) are sufficient [36], this requires confirmation as no control group was included; only 50 patients were treated, and no children under age 7 were enrolled; no MICs or CSF drug concentrations are reported; and the results may not be applicable to developing countries. A Jarisch-Herxheimer type of reaction has rarely been reported after the initiation of penicillin therapy for meningococcal disease.

Due to recent developments, the recommendation of penicillin as the drug of choice for meningococcal disease may require future modification. Despite the widespread use of penicillin, the overall meningococcal carriage rate of 5 to 10 percent, and the poor penetration of penicillin into saliva, relatively penicillin-resistant meningococci have remained rare. The majority of meningococci are inhibited by concentration less than or equal to 0.06 µg/mL of penicillin. In 1980 in the United States, however, the MIC_{90} for penicillin was 0.12 µg/mL and the MIC_{100} was 0.5 µg/mL. This implies that rare strains require at least 0.12 µg/mL for inhibition. This situation may be changing. The first β-lactamase-producing *N. meningitidis,* apparently of urogenital origin, was reported in 1983 [37]. Of more concern, β-lactamase-producing strains from meningitis cases in South Africa were reported in 1988 [37a], but this mechanism of resistance remains rare. These isolates are absolutely resistant to penicillin (MIC > 250 µg/mL). In contrast, relatively penicillin-resistant meningococci are increasing in frequency. For example, only 1 of 3264 strains analyzed at the National Reference Laboratory in Spain between 1978 and 1985 was relatively resistant versus 15 out of 168 (9 percent) invasive isolates in the first 6 months of 1986 [38]. The mean penicillin MIC for these strains is 0.3 μg/mL (range, 0.1 to 0.7 μg/mL) [39], and most are in serogroup B (11 of 16) or serogroup C (4 of 16). The strains do not produce β-lactamase, and the relative resistance appears to be mediated by a reduced affinity for penicillin-binding protein 3 [38]. Similar trends have been reported from the United Kingdom ([40]; Table 84-4). As most patients harboring these strains received penicillin (or ampicillin) and recovered, their clinical significance is unclear. Nevertheless, susceptibility testing of CSF isolates with a 2-unit penicillin disc (versus the standard 10-unit disc) is recommended. It is also worrisome that meningococci resistant to both penicillin and chloramphenicol were recently (1988) reported from Malawi [40a].

Chloramphenicol is the recommended alternative for the therapy of meningococcal meningitis in the penicillin-allergic patient. In the developing world, it may represent the drug of choice. A single injection of chloramphenicol in an oily vehicle (Tifomycine) resulting in prolonged serum concentrations led to full recovery in 79 of 86 patients (92 percent) studied in Nigeria in 1979 [41]. The drug was administered during a meningitis outbreak in village dispensaries to both adults and children. This approach is cost-effective in developing countries, especially during large outbreaks in the meningitis belt. Third-generation cephalosporins are bactericidal at extremely low concentrations against meningococci in vitro. Cefotaxime and ceftriaxone have been studied most intensively. Seven days of ceftriaxone therapy is effective for meningococcal meningitis [42], but expense precludes this option in many areas worldwide.

Other supportive measures may be required in the individual patient, especially for fulminant meningococcemia. General measures employed in the therapy of septic shock are appropriate, including (1) monitoring mentation, vital signs, urine output, hemodynamics, and laboratory parameters frequently in an intensive care setting; (2) maintenance of tissue oxygenation ($P_{O_2} \geq 60$ mmHg) with supplemental oxygen and mechanical ventilation if necessary; (3) reversal of acidosis; (4) maintenance of intravascular volume with fluids and reversal of hypotension with vasopressors (dopamine) if necessary; (5) correction of heart failure with diuresis (digoxin is

rarely indicated); (6) reduction of raised ICP (monitor ICP, hyperventilation to a P_{CO_2} less than or equal to 25 mmHg, dexamethasone, mannitol, etc.); and (7) control of seizures (valium initially, then diphenylhydantoin, etc.). Corticosteroids have no proven benefit as adjunctive agents in septic shock [43] but may alleviate cerebral edema and raised ICP in meningitis patients. Recent evidence suggests that adjunctive dexamethasone (at a dosage of 0.6 mg/kg IV daily in four divided doses for 4 days) significantly reduces deafness following pyogenic meningitis in children without influencing mortality [44]. Use of this agent in meningococcal disease requires further study before routine administration can be recommended. As monoclonal antibodies directed against meningococcal capsular polysaccharide, outer-membrane proteins, or LPS are protective in animal models [45], specific passive immunotherapy may become possible in the future.

Laboratory evaluation for the detection of disseminated intravascular coagulation (DIC) should be performed in patients with meningococcemia (prothrombin time prolongation, hypofibrinogenemia, thrombocytopenia, elevated fibrin degradation products). The use of heparin in this setting is controversial, but heparin should not be administered on the basis of laboratory abnormalities alone. Some authorities suggest that DIC complicated by thrombosis or clinical bleeding into deep tissues or from mucosal surfaces is an indication for heparinization. Recent evidence suggests a more cautious approach. Purpura fulminans occurs in infants with homozygous protein C deficiency and in patients with heterozygous deficiency of protein C or S during the initial phase of warfarin therapy. In addition, patients with meningococcemia and purpura fulminans have profound reductions in both protein C anticoagulant activity and free protein S antigen early in the illness [46], an acquired deficiency which is not influenced by heparin despite an increase in the risk of bleeding. Repletion of proteins C and S with fresh-frozen plasma may be a more rational approach, but this area requires further study.

POPULATION

The epidemiology of meningococcal disease within a population has direct relevance to current prevention strategies. The incidence of disease is influenced by multiple factors including geographical locale, season, climate, meningococcal serogroup, and population demographics (e.g., age, sex) [3].

Although worldwide in distribution, the overall incidence of meningococcal disease is highly variable geographically. As outlined above, the average annual incidence since 1950 has been estimated at 70 cases per 10^5 population in the African meningitis belt but reached 370 cases per 10^5 persons in Sao Paulo in 1974. An attack rate of 517 cases per 10^5 inhabitants was reported during a group C epidemic in upper Volta (now Burkina Faso) in 1979, and recent studies from the Faroe Islands document an attack rate of 400 to 450 per 10^5 population in the 0- to 8-year-old group. In contrast, the mean annual

Table 84-4. Relatively penicillin-resistant meningococci (MIC ≥ 0.16 μg/mL) from infected patients in England and Wales*

Year	No. relatively resistant/No. tested (%)
1983	3/349 (0.86%)
1984	1/460
1985	1/583
1986	13/1016 (1.28%)
1987	36/1238 (2.91%)

*Modified from [40].

attack rate in the United States from 1975 to 1980 is approximately 1.2 per 10^5 persons (17.1 per 10^5 under 1 year of age, 5.2 per 10^5 in 1- to 4-year-olds, and 0.3 per 10^5 among adults). A similar overall figure (2.0 per 10^5) was reported from Finland for the period 1976–1980.

In industrialized nations, the peak incidence of meningococcal disease occurs in winter through early spring in both epidemic and endemic periods. Similar climatic factors appear important in the tropics. For example, both the group C and A epidemics in the Sao Paulo area in 1971–1974 began in May or June at the point of transition from the rainy to the dry season. Annual outbreaks in the African meningitis belt tend to peak in late April to early May when the dry desert wind (*harmattan*) has ceased and temperatures are high both day and night, only to terminate abruptly with the onset of the rainy season [3].

Meningococcal disease may be more prevalent in males but the reports are skewed by inclusion of military personnel and/or chronic alcoholics. In the United States and Finland, approximately 55 percent of meningococcal cases occur in children under age 5 during nonepidemic conditions, but the peak age affected in Zaria, Nigeria, is 5- to 9-year-olds. Epidemics are heralded by a shift to the right toward older age groups [3], a feature that may be useful in prediction of epidemics where prospective surveillance is feasible.

Serious epidemics due to serogroup A meningococci have occurred at 20- to 30-year intervals throughout the world in this century and at intervals of approximately 10 years in the meningitis belt, but these strains have rarely been isolated in the United States in the past decade. Nevertheless, serious outbreaks of group A, B, and C disease have occurred worldwide in the 1970s (Table 84-5). Groups B and C are now most commonly responsible for focal outbreaks and endemic disease in many countries. For example, in the United States for the period 1975–1980, the distribution of serogroups was as follows (n = 12,980 cases): B, 56 percent; C, 19 percent; Y, 11 percent; W135, 10 percent; A, 3 percent. Disease due to sero-

group W135, especially among adults, is increasing in the United States and appears to be increasing in Africa (e.g., Senegal) since 1981. Group B organisms (especially B:15:P1.16) have recently emerged as important pathogens in Northern Europe causing serious local outbreaks and, again, peaking in the 10- to 20-year-old group [47]. The continued prevalence of group B disease has important implications due to the current lack of an effective vaccine against this serogroup. An outbreak of group C disease occurred in Los Angeles in 1987, and serious group A disease continued during 1988 in Nepal and elsewhere. The exact reasons producing cyclical outbreaks of meningococcal disease within a defined population remain conjectural.

CHEMOPROPHYLAXIS

The risk of meningococcal disease among household contacts of an index case during nonepidemic periods is approximately 3 in 1000 (i.e., approximately 500-fold to more than 1000-fold higher than the background endemic rate) and is particularly increased in young children. Close contacts (e.g., household or day care center members that sleep and eat in the same dwelling, medical personnel performing mouth-to-mouth resuscitation) are at an increased risk of developing systemic meningococcal disease, often within 5 days. These contacts should receive chemoprophylaxis as soon as the primary case is identified, but the agent of choice remains controversial. Because resistance has developed, sulfadiazine is no longer used but may again prove effective as resistance rates continue to decline. Several agents have proven effective in eradication of *N. meningitidis* from the nasopharynx. Rifampin is currently recommended but has several shortcomings: (1) eradication rates are only approximately 80 percent and transient; (2) some adverse effects occur, and 2 days of administration are required; and (3) resistance has developed, and such resistant strains can cause disease. Minocycline is less expensive but associated with undesirable vestibular effects. Rifampin is

Table 84-5. Selected meningococcal epidemics during the 1970s: incidence and serogroups*

Serogroup, location, year	Maximal incidence/ (100,000 · year)	Minimal no. of cases
A		
Brazil (Sao Paulo area), 1974	370	30,555 per year
Finland, 1974	15	687 per year
Nigeria (Zaria), 1977	—	1257 in 3 months
B		
Norway, 1973	24	112 per year
Belgium, 1969–1976	5	519 per year
C		
Brazil (Sao Paulo area), 1971–1972	11	2005 in 2 years
Vietnam 1977–1978	20	>1000 per year

*Adapted from [3].

given in divided doses every 12 h for 2 days as follows: adults, 600 mg; children over 1 month of age, 10 mg/kg; neonates less than 1 month old, 5 mg/kg. More recently, a single 250-mg intramuscular injection of ceftriaxone eliminated the serogroup A carrier state in 97 percent of Saudi subjects at 2 weeks, but requires an injection [48]. Perhaps of more interest, a single oral dose of ciprofloxacin (500 or 750 mg to adults) will achieve the same result [49,50]. Large-scale prospective randomized studies are needed to settle this issue, but ciprofloxacin is the only agent proven effective after a single oral dose, and may be less prone to the emergence of resistance. Nevertheless, ciprofloxacin is relatively contraindicated in the highest-risk group (i.e., children). As high-dose penicillin does not reliably eliminate the nasopharyngeal carriage of the organism in patients with systemic meningococcal disease (4 out of 14 patients still positive 1 week after concluding therapy in one study [51]), chemoprophylaxis should be given (currently rifampin) to the index patient prior to hospital discharge. Widespread chemoprophylaxis to low-risk contacts should be strongly discouraged due to the emergence of resistance and future limitations on this approach. At any rate, chemoprophylaxis must be coupled with continued surveillance to detect resistance patterns, sources outside the household, coprimary cases, etc.

IMMUNOPROPHYLAXIS

Previous monovalent vaccines of purified serogroup A and C capsular polysaccharide have been shown to be immunogenic and safe in humans. The immunogenicity of both preparations increases with increasing molecular weight. Field trials in Europe and Africa with the group A vaccine document efficacy of approximately 85 to 95 percent and its usefulness in controlling epidemics. Similar results with the group C vaccine have been observed in military recruit populations and during an epidemic. Protection has been approximately 90 percent for at least 1 year in children older than 4 years of age and in young adults. Although the exact antibody concentration required for protection is unknown (some authorities suggest 2 μg/mL), the vaccines appear immunogenic in children above age 2; however, young infants do not mount an effective response. Similar results with the newly licensed quadrivalent (groups A, C, Y, and W135) vaccine have been documented in children [52], but bactericidal antibody responses are elicited in adults to each of the four polysaccharide antigens [53]. Unfortunately, a vaccine against serogroup B, the major cause of endemic meningococcal disease in many areas of the world, is not available. Current approaches with polysaccharide-protein conjugates or group B outer-membrane protein antigens show promise for the future. Nevertheless, the duration of protection is still short for all available preparations.

Routine immunization of the population against meningococcal disease is not recommended as the risk of disease is low in the absence of an outbreak. Immunization is currently recommended in industrialized countries for certain high-risk groups such as those with (1) terminal complement or properdin deficiencies; (2) asplenia; (3) travel to areas with epidemic meningococcal disease; and (4) close contacts of the primary case as an adjunct to chemoprophylaxis. However, the principal use of meningococcal vaccines is during outbreaks of disease due to the serogroups represented in the preparation. How to adapt this principle to developing countries with hyperendemic conditions is a difficult problem. The potentially susceptible population in certain areas (e.g., the meningitis belt) is huge and, since protection is of short duration, millions of doses would be required annually. Selective vaccination in affected villages has met with some success [54] but requires excellent surveillance systems, readily available vaccine, and trained vaccination teams. Mass immunization programs within four states of northern Nigeria between 1978 and 1981 to over 7.4 million persons have largely eliminated the yearly epidemics in the region [55], but the cost-effectiveness of this approach remains unknown. Significant progress toward eradication of meningococcal disease will be dependent on prophylactic strategies, not new antibiotics or diagnostic techniques. It is hoped that the rational and coordinated use of the tools available (e.g., chemo- and immunoprophylaxis) and the development of new reagents (e.g., an immunogenic, safe, and effective serogroup B vaccine) will lead to better control of meningococcal diseases.

REFERENCES

1 Danielson L, Mann E: The first American account of cerebrospinal meningitis. Reprinted from The Medical and Agricultural Register for the years 1806 and 1807, vol 1, no 5, edited by Daniel Adams, M.B., and printed in Boston by Manning and Loring. Rev Infect Dis 5:969–972, 1983

2 North E: Concerning the epidemic of spotted fever in New England. Rev Infect Dis 2:811–816, 1980

3 Peltola H: Meningococcal disease: Still with us. Rev Infect Dis 5:71–91, 1983

4 Ashton FE, Ryan A, Diena B, et al: A new serogroup (L) of *Neisseria meningitidis*. J Clin Microbiol 17:722–727, 1983

5 Frasch CE, Zollinger WE, Poolman JT: Serotype antigens of *Neisseria meningitidis* and a proposed scheme for designation of serotypes. Rev Infect Dis 7:504–510, 1985

6 Spanjaard L, Bol P, deMarie S, et al: Association of meningococcal serotypes with the course of disease: Serotypes 2a and 2b in the Netherlands, 1959–1981. J Infect Dis 155:277–282, 1987

7 Stephens DS, McGee ZA: Attachment of *Neisseria meningitidis* to human mucosal surfaces: Influence of pili and type of receptor cell. J Infect Dis 143:525–532, 1981

8 DeVoe IW, Gilchrist JE: Release of endotoxin in the form of cell wall blebs during in vitro growth of *Neisseria meningitidis*. J Exp Med 138:1156–1167, 1973

9 Mickelsen PA, Sparling PF: Ability of *Neisseria gonorrheae, Neisseria meningitidis* and commensal *Neisseria* species to obtain iron from transferrin and iron compounds. Infect Immun 33:555–564, 1981

10 Goldschneider I, Gotschlich EC, Artenstein MA: Human immunity to the meningococcus. I. The role of humoral antibodies. J Exp Med 129:1307–1326, 1969

11 Kayhty H, Jousimies-Somer H, Peltola H, et al: Antibody response to capsular polysaccharides of groups A and C *Neisseria meningitidis* and *Haemophilus influenzae* type b during bacteremic disease. J Infect Dis 143:32–41, 1981

12 Ross SC, Densen P: Complement deficiency states and infection: Epidemiology, pathogenesis and consequences of neisserial and other infections in an immune deficiency. Medicine 63:243–273, 1984

13 Rosen MS, Lorber B, Myers AR: Chronic meningococcal meningitis. An association with C5 deficiency. Arch Intern Med 148:1441–1442, 1988

14 Ellison RT III, Mason SR, Kohler PF, et al: Meningococcemia and acquired complement deficiency. Association in patients with hepatic failure. Arch Intern Med 146:1539–1540, 1986

15 Densen P, Weiler JM, Griffis JM, et al: Familial properdin deficiency and fatal meningococcemia. Correction of the bactericidal defect by vaccination. N Engl J Med 316:922–927, 1987

16 Sjoholm AG, Kuijper EJ, Tijssen CC, et al: Dysfunctional properdin in a Dutch family with meningococcal disease. N Engl J Med 319:33–37, 1988

17 DeVoe IW: The meningococcus and mechanisms of pathogenicity. Microbiol Rev 46:162–190, 1982

18 Quagliarello VJ, Long WJ, Scheld WM: Morphologic alterations of the blood-brain barrier with experimental meningitis in the rat: Temporal sequence and role of encapsulation. J Clin Invest 77:1084–1095, 1986

19 Lesse AJ, Moxon ER, Zwahlen A, et al: The role of cerebrospinal fluid pleocytosis and *Haemophilus influenzae* type b capsule on blood brain barrier permeability during experimental meningitis in the rat. J Clin Invest 82:102–109, 1988

20 Wispelwey B, Lesse AJ, Hansen EJ, et al: *Haemophilus influenzae* lipopolysaccharide induced blood brain barrier permeability during experimental meningitis in the rat. J Clin Invest, 82:1339–1346, 1988

20a Wispelwey B, Scheld WM: Unpublished data

21 Waage A, Halstensen A, Espevik T: Association between tumor necrosis factor in serum and fatal outcome in patients with meningococcal disease. Lancet 1:355–357, 1987

22 Feldman HA: Meningococcal infections. Adv Intern Med 18:117–140, 1972

23 Benoit FL: Chronic meningococcemia. Case report and review of the literature. Am J Med 35:103–118, 1963

24 Kingston ME, Mackey D: Skin clues in the diagnosis of life-threatening infections. Rev Infect Dis 8:1–11, 1986

25 Schaller RT Jr, Schaller JF: Surgical management of life-threatening and disfiguring sequelae of fulminant meningococcemia. Am J Surg 151:553–556, 1986

26 Robinow M, Johnson GF, Nanagas MT, et al: Skeletal lesions following meningococcemia and disseminated intravascular coagulation. A recognizable skeletal dystrophy. Am J Dis Child 137: 279–281, 1983

27 Jacobs RF, Hsi S, Wilson CB, et al: Apparent meningococcemia: Clinical features of disease due to *Haemophilus influenzae* and *Neisseria meningitidis*. Pediatrics 72:469–472, 1983

28 Muscat I, Curtis H, Shapiro D: Non-meningococcal purpuric sepsis. Lancet 2:51, 1988

29 Blaser MJ, Reingold AL, Alsever R, et al: Primary meningococcal pericarditis: A disease of adults associated with serogroup C *Neisseria meningitidis*. Rev Infect Dis 6:625–632, 1984

30 Talan DA, Hoffmann JR, Yoshikawa TT, et al: Role of empiric parenteral antibiotics prior to lumbar puncture in suspected bacterial meningitis: State of the art. Rev Infect Dis 10:365–376, 1988

31 Sippel JE: Meningococci. CRC Crit Rev Microbiol 8:267–302, 1981

32 Band JD, Chamberland ME, Platt T, et al: Trends in meningococcal disease in the United States, 1975–1980. J Infect Dis 148:754–758, 1983

33 Felman HA: The meningococcus: A twenty-year perspective. Rev Infect Dis 8:288–294, 1986

33a Schweutker et al: JAMA 108:1407, 1937

34 Girgis NI, Yassin W, Sippel JE, et al: Intramuscular compared with intravenous ampicillin in the treatment of meningococcal meningitis. Scand J Infect Dis 14:239–240, 1982

35 Scheld WM, Sande MA: Bactericidal versus bacteriostatic antibiotic therapy of experimental pneumococcal meningitis in rabbits. J Clin Invest 71:411–419, 1983

36 Viladrich PF, Pallares R, Ariza J, et al: Four days of penicillin therapy for meningococcal meningitis. Arch Intern Med 146:2380–2382, 1986

37 Dillon JR, Pauze M, Yeung K-H: Spread of penicillinase-producing and transfer plasmids from the gonococcus to *Neisseria meningitidis*. Lancet 1:779–781, 1983

37a Botha P: Lancet 1:54, 1988

38 Mendelman PM, Campos J, Chaffin DO, et al: Relative penicillin G resistance in *Neisseria meningitidis* and reduced affinity of penicillin-binding protein 3. Antimicrob Agents Chemother 32:706–709, 1988

39 Campos J, Mendelman PM, Sako MU, et al: Detection of relatively penicillin G resistant *Neisseria meningitidis* by disk susceptibility testing. Antimicrob Agents Chemother 31:1478–1482, 1987

40 Sutcliffe EM, Jones DM, El-Sheikh S, et al: Penicillin-insensitive meningococci in the U.K. Lancet 1:657, 1988

40a Round A, Hamilton W: Lancet 1:702, 1988

41 Puddicombe JB, Wali SS, Greenwood BM: A field trial of a single intramuscular injection of long-acting chloramphenicol in the treatment of meningococcal meningitis. Trans R Soc Trop Med Hyg 78:399–403, 1984

42 Lin T-Y Chrane DF, Nelson JD, et al: Seven days of ceftriaxone therapy is as effective as ten days' treatment for bacterial meningitis. JAMA 253:3559–3563, 1985

43 Sprung CL, Caralis PV, Marcial EH, et al: The effects of high-dose corticosteroids in patients with septic shock. A prospective, controlled study. N Engl J Med 311:1137–1143, 1984

44 Lebel MH, Freij BJ, Syrogiannopoulos GA, et al: Dexamethasone therapy for bacterial meningitis: Results of two double-blind, placebo controlled trials. N Engl J Med 319:964–971, 1988

45 Saukkonen K, Leinonen M, Kayhty H, et al: Monoclonal antibodies to the rough lipopolysaccharide of *Neisseria meningitidis* protect infant rats from meningococcal infection. J Infect Dis 158:209–211, 1988

46 Powars DR, Rogers ZR, Patch MJ, et al: Purpura fulminans in meningococcemia: Association with acquired deficiencies of proteins C and S. N Engl J Med 317:571–572, 1987

47 Editorial: Defences against meningococcal infections. Lancet 2:929, 1985

48 Schwartz B, Al-Ruwais A, A'ashi J, et al: Comparative efficacy of ceftriaxone and rifampicin in eradicating pharyngeal carriage of group A *Neisseria meningitidis*. Lancet 1:1239–1242, 1988

49 Pugsley MP, Dworzack, DL, Roccaforte JS, et al: An open study on the efficacy of a single dose of ciprofloxacin in eliminating the chronic nasopharyngeal carriage of *Neisseria meningitidis*. J Infect Dis 157:852–853, 1988

50 Gaunt PN, Lambert BE: Single dose ciprofloxacin for the eradication of pharyngeal carriage of *Neisseria meningitidis*. J Antimicrob Chemother 21:489–496, 1988

51 Abramson JS, Spika JS: Persistance of *Neisseria meningitidis* in the upper respiratory tract after intravenous antibiotic therapy for systemic meningococcal disease. J Infect Dis 151:370–371, 1985

52 Lepow ML, Beeler J, Randolph M, et al: Reactogenicity and immunogenicity of a quadrivalent combined meningococcal polysaccharide vaccine in children. J Infect Dis 154:1033–1036, 1986

53 Griffis JM, Brandt BL, Altieri PL, et al: Safety and immunogenicity of group Y and group W135 meningococcal capsular and polysaccharide vaccines in adults. Infect Immun 34:725–732, 1981

54 Greenwood BM, Wai SS: Control of meningococcal infection in the African meningitis belt by selective vaccination. Lancet 1:729–732, 1980

55 Mohammed I, Obineche EN, Onyemelukue GC, et al: Control of epidemic meningococcal meningitis by mass vaccination. I. Further epidemiologic evaluation of groups A and C vaccines in northern Nigeria. J Infect 9:190–196, 1984

CHAPTER 85 / *Pneumococcal Infections* · Robert M. Douglas

The pneumococcus (*Streptococcus pneumoniae*) is a gram-positive diplococcus which possesses a polysaccharide capsule that permits its classification into 84 distinct serotypes by means of typing sera. These organisms are normal inhabitants of the human upper respiratory tract but are also pathogenic in certain circumstances. Some pneumococcal serotypes are particularly invasive to human beings, and these types have been grown particularly commonly from the blood, cerebrospinal fluid, middle ear fluid, and lung fluid of patients suffering from pneumococcal bacteremia, meningitis, otitis media, and pneumonia. Pediatric infections are particularly associated with types 6, 14, 19, and 23 [1].

Precise estimates of the role of the pneumococcus in human morbidity are difficult to obtain, but it is probable that this organism remains the main cause of community-acquired bacterial pneumonia in most tropical countries. These illnesses are occasionally complicated by pleural effusion, empyema, and pericarditis. The pneumococcus is also the commonest cause of acute otitis media, accounting for 30 to 50 percent of bacterial isolates from middle ear fluid. It is the second commonest cause of purulent meningitis (after meningococcus) in adults and the third commonest (after meningococcus and *Haemophilus influenzae*) in children. Bacteremia with this organism is also often shown to be the cause of unexplained pyrexia in infants. Systemic invasion can lead to arthritis, peritonitis, and acute bacterial endocarditis. With *H. influenzae,* pneumococci play a role in many episodes of sinus infection and flare-ups of chronic bronchitis. The pneumococcus is also occasionally implicated as a cause of acute purulent conjunctivitis.

PARASITE

MORPHOLOGY

The pneumococcus is somewhat oval-shaped and usually grows in diplococcal pairs or short chains. Its diameter varies from 1.2 to 1.8 μm from tip to tip of the diplococcal pair, and its ''waist'' varies from 0.5 to 1.0 μm.

The capsule of the organism consists of a complex polysaccharide, the immunological identity of which forms the basis for serotype classification. For some types, especially type 3, the capsule is particularly prominent. When mixed with specific antiserum and viewed under the oil immersion lens of a light microscope, the capsule becomes more clearly outlined and apparently swollen (Fig. 85-1). This is known as the *quellung reaction*. Serotyping of pneumococci is carried out using a three-stage process. First, a suspension of the organism is mixed with each of eight *grouping sera*. A positive quellung reaction usually occurs with one of these grouping sera, and points to the need to test the suspension with from between 3 and 8 of the 46 *typing sera* (numbers 1 to 48 excepting 26 and 30) contained in that group. Most epidemiological studies of pneumococci stop at this second stage, but *factor sera* are available in special centers for distinguishing between the subtypes of 18 complex types (6, 7, 9, 10, 11, 12, 15, 17, 18, 19, 22, 23, 24, 28, 32, 33, 35, and 41). Grouping and typing sera are available from the State Serum Institute in Copenhagen, Denmark. Pneumococci that fail to give a positive quellung reaction and do not possess a capsular polysaccharide are

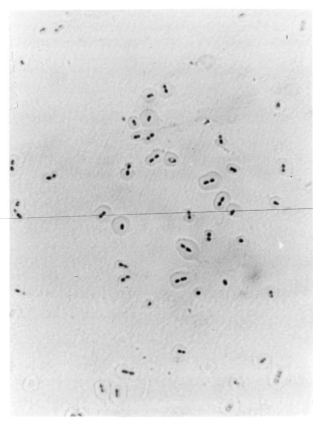

Figure 85-1. Pneumococci with positive quellung reaction.

called *"rough"* pneumococci and are nonpathogenic for humans.

Both rough and smooth (encapsulated) pneumococci possess a cell wall polysaccharide layer known as C polysaccharide. The cell wall is about 140 to 160 μm thick. In addition to the C polysaccharide, which is on the outermost surface of the cell wall, the wall is believed to contain several parallel layers of murein polymers.

Under the cell wall is the plasma membrane, about 75 μm thick, which is composed predominantly of lipid materials [2]. The plasma membrane forms a series of intracellular invaginations into the cell which are known as *mesosomes* or "chondroids," the number and complexity of which vary from cell to cell and the function and biochemistry of which are debated. Generally, the cytoplasmic constituents of pneumococci are poorly defined.

BIOCHEMISTRY

Many of the pneumococcal capsular polysaccharides have been chemically characterized, and their structure is known. The polysaccharides are cell-surface polymers consisting of repeating oligosaccharide units, some of which are linked to each other through phosphodiester bonds.

Considerable information is also available concerning the chemical composition and likely structure of the cell wall. Pneumococcal cell wall teichoic acid (C polysaccharide) is responsible for the interaction of pneumococci with C-reactive protein, which is a major acute phase reactant of human serum.

Most natural isolates of pneumococci are prone to autolysis in the stationary phase of their growth, and it is possible that the release of pneumococcal surface components into the environment of an infected host may result in release of serum components which are chemotactic, as well as having other local effects. It is known that large amounts of capsular polysaccharide are released into circulation, but this is nontoxic. A number of other breakdown products of the organism have been studied for their pathogenic effects, including a purpura-producing factor that is believed to be the consequence of the immune response to soluble pneumococcal cell wall components. Recent interest has centered on a pneumolysin that is known to have hemolytic effects and may be toxic in other ways [3].

CULTURE

The organism can be grown on either solid or liquid media. Suitable solid media include brain-heart infusion agar or trypticase soy agar enriched with 5% blood. The blood agar plates are incubated for 18 h in a candle jar or CO_2 incubator. If the material being cultured is likely to contain other microorganisms (e.g., sputum or nasopharyngeal swabs), gentamicin can be added to discourage overgrowth by other organisms.

On blood agar plates the organism forms round mucoid colonies with a surrounding area of pale-greenish α hemolysis. Colonies are often difficult to distinguish from those of other α-hemolytic streptococci. Young colonies are domed or hemispherical, but as the culture ages, autolysis results in sinking of the central portion of the colony to give rise to a flattened surface. The distinction from other α-hemolytic streptococci is made by the fact that pneumococci are sensitive to ethyl hydrocupreine hydrochloride (optichin) and other α-hemolytic streptococci are not (Fig. 85-2).

Liquid media include trypticase soy broth and brain-heart infusion broth. The addition of 5% defibrinated rabbit, sheep, horse, or human blood will permit longer survival of the culture. The addition of glucose to a final concentration of 1% ensures prolific growth of the organism. Pneumococci grow best at pH 7.6 and survive poorly outside the pH range 7 to 7.8. Cultures of pneumococci will remain viable for 6 to 8 weeks at 4°C if grown for 18 to 24 h in culture tubes to which defibrinated blood has been added.

The blood of any patient suspected of having a pneumococcal infection should be cultured in a liquid medium. The ratio of the amount of blood to the medium into which it is inoculated should approximate 1:10, and between 5 to 15 mL of blood should be used. The culture should be examined after 24 and 48 h of incubation at 37°C, and if turbid, subculture should be made on a blood agar plate.

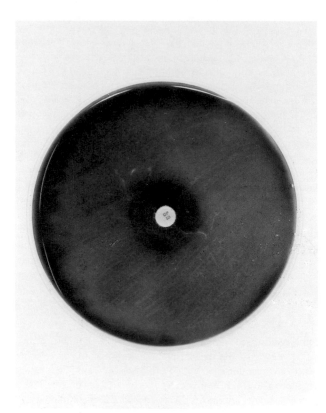

Figure 85-2. Culture showing inhibition of growth of pneumococci by an optichin disc.

ANIMAL MODELS

Experimental work has been done with the pneumococcus using mice, dogs, rabbits, and chinchillas to simulate human disease. Laboratory mice are particularly susceptible to pneumococcal infection, and intraperitoneal injection of as few as one or two encapsulated pneumococci usually results in death of the animals within 2 or 3 days. The organism can be cultured from heart's blood at autopsy of the animal and passage through mice is often used to maintain the invasive capacity of laboratory strains of pneumococcus. Intraperitoneal injection of putatively infected sputum or blood is also occasionally used as a method of in vivo culture. Mice have been used to study the pathogenesis of pneumococcal pneumonia and the nature of the immune response to capsular polysaccharides.

Rabbits have been used to produce high-concentration antisera to the capsular polysaccharides and also to study the pathogenesis of pneumonia and pneumococcal meningitis. The dog is another of the many experimental animals that have been studied in an endeavor to understand the mechanism by which pneumococci spread from the upper to the lower respiratory tract and the nature of the defense mechanisms that are called into play once alveolar infection has occurred.

Insights into the pathogenesis of otitis media have come from experiments involving chinchillas [4]. Influenza virus in-oculation alone simply leads to negative pressure in the middle ear, but if pneumococci are also present, the combination of pathogens results in the rapid appearance of a serous middle ear effusion which becomes culture-positive for *Streptococcus pneumoniae* in the second week after inoculation. Protection of chinchillas against experimental homotypic otitis media has been achieved by immunizing the animals with pneumococcal polysaccharide vaccine.

PATIENT "HOST"

THE HOST-PARASITE INTERFACE

Available information suggests that the human host depends primarily upon phagocytosis and mechanical factors to confine the pneumococcus to its normal habitat in the upper respiratory tract and to clear those organisms that stray into the lower respiratory tract or find their way into the bloodstream. Efficient phagocytosis depends in turn upon antibody, complement, adequate supplies of phagocytes, and a functioning spleen.

It follows, therefore, that patients with neutropenia, hyposplenia, hypogammaglobulinemia, and certain complement deficiencies are prime targets for systemic invasion by the pneumococcus. In addition to these factors, a number of mechanical defects are commonly associated with localized infections. Skull fracture is often followed by pneumoccal meningitis, presumably a result of mechanical access to the cerebrospinal space through the cribriform plate. Eustachian tube blockage appears to predispose to the pneumococcus establishing itself in the middle ear cleft. Decreased vascular perfusion, such as occurs in sickle cell infarction, congestive heart failure, and nephrotic syndrome, interferes with the efficiency of the humoral factors that are so essential to phagocytosis, and probably contributes to the high incidence of pneumococcal bacteremia. The incidence of pneumococcal peritonitis is especially high in patients with nephrotic syndrome. Pneumococcal pneumonia is particularly common among patients with prolonged and frequent ethanol intoxication. Alcoholism is associated with decreased ciliary activity, nutritional deficiencies, and decreased neutrophil chemotaxis.

Specific antibody to the capsular polysaccharide provides a most important opsonizing aid to phagocytosis. It is therefore not surprising that pneumococci, along with other pyogenic bacteria, are the organisms most commonly pathogenic in patients with hypogammaglobulinemia. Susceptibility can be partially corrected by administering γ-globulin to the patient, suggesting that the serum level of antibody is the important element in host defense.

Some subclasses of immunoglobulin seem to be more important than others in the humoral immune response to pneumococcal capsular polysaccharides. As with many other antigens, there is normally an early IgM response in the serum of mature adults followed later by a more sustained and perhaps more important IgG response. Growing evidence indicates that for many of the known capsular polysaccharides, IgG2 is a particularly important subclass [5] and that people with a deficiency in this subclass are particularly prone to pneumococcal infections. There is also some evidence that the predominant IgG subclass of the humoral response may vary at different ages and between pneumococcal serotypes [6].

The role of the spleen in clearing the blood of stray pneumococci is particularly important in host defense [7]. Approximately 50 percent of overwhelming postsplenectomy bacterial infections are caused by the pneumococcus. This syndrome occurs both in patients who have had their spleens removed and in those with nonfunctioning spleens, including patients with sickle cell disease, whose spleens usually become nonfunctional by the time they are 3 years old. It has been found that children with sickle cell disease experience a 600-fold increase in risk of developing pneumococcal disease compared with normal individuals. The spleen plays a role both in the provision of a phagocytic mass and in the production of antibody which facilitates opsonization. If the spleen is absent, both activities can take place elsewhere, but both are less efficient. When pneumococci are not opsonized by a specific antibody and/or complement, the spleen's role is vital. Thus, predisposition to overwhelming postsplenectomy infection is greatest in children younger than 2 years of age (whose specific antibody levels are relatively low).

The complement system also is vital [8] in both natural and acquired immunity to *S. pneumoniae*. Activation of the terminal components (C3 to C9) of the complement pathway can take place either through the classical pathway, which begins with an antigen-antibody reaction and the formation of an immune complex, or through an alternative pathway which does not require the presence of preexisting antibody. Once activated, the terminal components of complement become available to act as opsonins and thus facilitate phagocytosis. Certain activated complement components are also chemotactic and anaphylatoxic, and contribute to host defenses in these ways.

Studies of human sera have failed to show activation of the classical pathway by the pneumococcus. It seems more likely that in humans complement defenses against the pneumococcus are initiated via the alternative pathway. Different strains and serotypes differ in their capacity to activate the alternative pathway. The clinical importance of complement in defending patients against pneumococcal invasion is borne out by the fact that patients with isolated deficiencies of C2, C3, and C3b inactivator are particularly prone to pneumococcal infections.

In patients with inadequate numbers of circulating neutrophils (e.g., neutropenia, aplastic anemia) pneumococcal bacteremia has been reported to be relatively common. Patients with defects in phagocytic bactericidal activity (i.e., chronic granulomatous disease) are not unduly prone [9]. It seems that once the phagocyte has ingested the pneumococcus, it can deal with it—even when its own bactericidal functions are diminished.

The precise role played by nutritional defects in relation to defense against pneumococcal infections has been poorly documented but is highly relevant. Pneumococcal infection rates and pneumonia case fatality rates are particularly serious in areas where malnutrition is endemic. The propensity of chronic alcoholics to suffer from pneumococcal disease may relate partially to their impaired nutritional status.

PATHOGENESIS

Pneumonia

The passage of organisms from the upper to the lower respiratory tract is impeded by a series of natural defense mechanisms. They include the cough reflex, the action of cilia, the mucoid secretions of the respiratory tract, and the phagocytic activity of alveolar macrophages. Many bouts of pneumonia are preceded by an upper respiratory tract infection caused by a virus. At this time, the natural clearing mechanisms are impaired, and, therefore, upper respiratory secretions containing pneumococci are more likely to gain access to the lower respiratory tract. This bronchial embolization with infected mucinous secretions is followed shortly by an outpouring into the alveoli of a proteinaceous fluid which serves both as a nutrient for the pneumococci and as a vehicle for spread to adjacent alveoli. Subsequently, polymorphonuclear leukocytes appear on the scene, attracted by the products of the complement pathway, and phagocytosis begins in earnest. Specific anticapsular antibody increases the efficiency of phagocytosis approximately twofold and also contributes to pneumococcal agglutination.

At this early stage in the evolution of the infection, the affected area of lung is engorged, solid, and red due to the outpouring of erythrocytes, leukocytes, and fluid. Pneumococci are easily discernible at this time, but as the pathology moves toward gray hepatization (where the alveoli are packed with leukocytes), the bacteria are increasingly phagocytosed and difficult to demonstrate.

The outcome of the infection depends upon the efficacy of phagocytosis, which in turn depends at least partly on the availability of specific anticapsular antibody. In the absence of antibiotic therapy, approximately three-quarters of humans will make a spontaneous recovery from lobar pneumonia. As the natural and specific immune responses are called into play, specific antibody appears and macrophages are found in the alveoli, which return to normal over a period of 2 to 6 weeks.

Where phagocytosis fails to clear the organisms, pneumococci find their way to the hilar lymph nodes and the sinusoids of the lymph nodes where a similar process to that described in the alveoli occurs. If the infection is not checked at this point, organisms find their way via the thoracic duct into the circulation, and the spleen becomes the third line of defense.

Major lobar consolidation is particularly prone to occur in middle-aged patients rather than in the very young [10].

Meningitis

Pneumococcal meningitis in humans is a serious, frequently fatal condition characterized classically by dense purulent exudate in the subarachnoid, subdural, and extradural regions. Access to the central nervous system by pneumococci may result from a fracture of the cribriform plate, pneumococcal abscess formation in the mastoid air cells, or through bloodstream invasion. As a result of the intense inflammatory reaction, the meninges and subarachnoid space develop heavy fibrinous aggregations which tend to block the cisterns and may result in hydrocephalus.

Laboratory simulation of pneumococcal meningitis in animals [11] has produced two rather distinct models which may have clinical parallels among humans. The disease produced by instillation of pneumococci into the cerebrospinal space of nonimmune rabbits seems to mimic meningitis seen in young infants, in whom millions of organisms are found in the cerebrospinal fluid in the absence of any appreciable inflammatory response. In these cases there is a high mortality associated with rapid bacterial replication and septicemia. In contrast, experimental meningitis in the dog parallels cases of meningitis in older children or adults where a vigorous inflammatory response is effective in controlling the numbers of viable bacteria, but severe damage to the meninges and brain parenchyma still results.

Otitis media

The animal simulation of otitis media in the chinchilla [3] has permitted exploration of the role of locally produced and systemic antibody in this condition as well as a description of the morphological alterations of the middle ear cleft which occur in untreated episodes. The early inflammatory response is characterized by infiltration with polymorphonuclear leukocytes, together with capillary dilatation and extravasation of fluid into the subepithelial and middle ear spaces. Later, mononuclear leukocytes replace the neutrophils and the lining epithelium becomes metaplastic. In the experimental animal, the middle ear fluid becomes sterile after about 21 days and contains high concentrations of specific antibody relative to the serum.

CLINICAL MANIFESTATIONS

Pneumonia

The pneumococcus is the organism that is most commonly cultured from blood, lung aspirates, and upper respiratory secretions of adult patients who are suffering from community-acquired pneumonia, and the radiological picture ranges from one of patchy bronchopneumonia—a pattern often seen in the very young and the elderly—to the more classical picture of lobar or segmental consolidation which can affect patients in any age group. The clinical picture is not specific, however, and there is a marked overlap in the clinical presentation of pneumonia caused by the pneumococcus with that caused by many other respiratory pathogens. The clinical description that follows therefore may partially apply to pneumonia caused by other organisms. Furthermore, pneumococcal invasion of the lower respiratory tract can supervene on infection which has been initiated by other organisms such as influenza. Mixed infections by pneumococcus and *H. influenzae* are also quite common.

Many patients complain of a sudden shaking chill with a rapid rise in temperature and pulse rate. This may be followed by sharp pleuritic pain, cough, production of rusty sputum, and sustained fever. Often there is mild cyanosis as a result of reduced alveolar ventilation, and the patients may have dilated alae nasae and grunting respirations. Herpes labialis is commonly present. The patient is usually alert and his or her principal complaint, especially if the infection extends to the pleura, is of chest pain and dyspnea. In the early stages, sputum production is scanty. Rusty, mucoid sputum in the early stages is followed by deep, purulent and often thick, greenish expectorations as the condition progresses.

Physical findings vary considerably with the site and extent of consolidation. There will often be restricted motion of the infected hemithorax and localized percussion tenderness over the affected lung segment or lobe. The first hint of consolidation may be localized percussion tenderness, diminished air entry, or percussion dullness. In the early stages, localized rales, bronchial breathing, and pleural friction rubs may not appear. As the lesion evolves, breath sounds become increasingly tubular or bronchial in quality and fine rales are heard over the affected area.

In patients with major lobar consolidation or bacteremic infection, quite marked jaundice can accompany the condition. Jaundice has been a particular feature of lobar pneumonia in some tropical countries [12]. The mechanism is uncertain, although studies have indicated the presence of both prehepatic and hepatic factors. The jaundice tends to clear rapidly within days of instituting effective antipneumococcal therapy.

Occasionally, patients with severe pneumococcal pneumonia present *in extremis* with circulatory collapse, dyspnea, hypotension, and tachycardia. In patients whose disease is untreated for some days, there may be evidence of pleural effusion which sometimes becomes purulent. Pericarditis, arthritis, and/or acute bacterial endocarditis may supervene. Meningitis can also follow a primary pneumonia.

In most tropical countries, the diagnosis will depend on clinical findings, as laboratory and radiological investigations are often not available or affordable. Although the total white blood count is often elevated in pneumococcal pneumonia, it also may be normal, but with a striking increase in the proportion of very young ("band") leukocytes. Leukopenia is sometimes observed in patients with overwhelming infection and bacteremia. X-rays reveal either a homogeneous density (Fig. 85-3) in the infected area of the lung or a patchy bron-

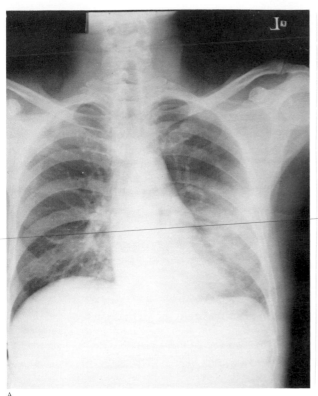

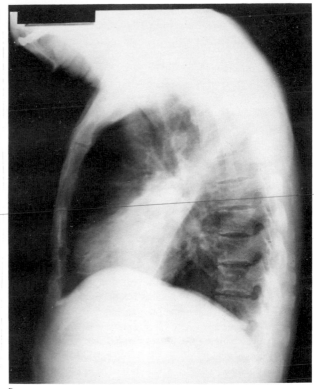

A   B

Figure 85-3. Lobar consolidation of the lung.

chopneumonic pattern which tends to affect the lower lobes. Where x-ray facilities are limited, routine radiography for patients suspected of suffering from pneumococcal pneumonia is not necessary except in patients with clinical evidence of complication, delayed response to antipneumococcal therapy, atelectasis, lung abscess, and/or pleural effusion.

In about 25 percent of cases of lobar pneumonia, the blood culture will be positive during the first 3 to 4 days of the illness. Sputum stained by Gram stain shows polymorphonuclear leukocytes and variable numbers of gram-positive cocci, which can be typed directly by the quellung reaction.

The clinical course following commencement of effective antipneumococcal therapy is usually dramatic. Temperature falls within the first 2 days and the patient, if previously young and healthy, rapidly recovers. Serum bilirubin and blood urea (which is also often elevated in severely toxic cases [12]) fall rapidly to normal over a period of 5 to 10 days. Auscultatory and radiological abnormalities in some cases may take up to 4 to 5 weeks to disappear. Untreated pneumococcal pneumonia has a 25 percent mortality in adults and, even with treatment, up to 20 percent of bacteremic cases may die despite vigorous antibiotic and supportive therapy [13].

Although the pneumococcus is the commonest cause of lobar pneumonia and the leading cause of bronchopneumonic consolidation in adults, a wide variety of other pathogenic agents can produce a similar clinical syndrome. They include *Mycoplasma pneumoniae*, a range of viruses (which can also predispose to pneumococcal invasion), tuberculosis, *Klebsiella pneumoniae*, and *Streptococcus pyogens*. Gram-negative organisms must also be considered, including *Escherichia coli*, *Proteus*, *Pseudomonas*, and *H. influenzae*. In patients with exposure to birds and animals, the possibility of psittacosis and Q fever must be borne in mind.

Pneumonia in early childhood

Acute infections of the respiratory tract are common at all ages and particularly in the first 5 years of life. Pneumonia is the most serious end of the spectrum of such infections, which are often life-threatening. Currently, it is estimated that about 4 million children die annually, especially in developing countries, as a consequence of unrecognized or inadequately treated pneumonia. The clinical pattern described above often applies to children, but the younger the child, the less the clinician can rely on the classical signs of alveolar consolidation.

For many young children who are suffering from pneumonia (whether the causative organism is pneumococcus or one of the others mentioned above), the predominant clinical evidence of the infection is a rapid respiratory rate, and there is little else to find on examination of the chest. Nor is the temperature always elevated. Sometimes there will be grunting respirations and indrawing of the intercostal muscles as the child breathes in. Lack of interest in feeding is often a sign that the infection is serious. These signs—rapid breathing, chest indrawing, and failure to feed—form the basis of a standard assessment and management plan for the care of undifferentiated acute respiratory infections and can be taught to parents and health workers at all levels of the health care system [*14*]. This plan is described below under "Treatment."

Meningitis

Clinically, pneumococcal meningitis is indistinguishable from acute pyogenic meningitis caused by other bacteria. The leading symptoms are headache and fever, with nausea, backache, neck stiffness, and photophobia as frequently associated complaints. On clinical examination, patients are usually febrile and toxic. Some impairment of consciousness is often present by the time the patient presents for clinical care, and the picture is often complicated by convulsions and cranial nerve palsies. Neck stiffness and a positive Kernig's sign can be elicited in adults and older children. There will often be evidence of raised intracranial pressure with a bulging fontanelle in young infants for whom the other features are less well developed or difficult to elucidate. The infection often spreads from a preexisting otitis media or pneumonia, and it may complicate damage to the base of the skull. Patients with damage to the base of the skull are prone to recurrent meningeal pneumococcal infections.

Diagnosis is confirmed by lumbar puncture. The cerebrospinal fluid is usually turbid and under increased pressure. Biochemical analysis reveals a high protein and a low glucose content. Gram stain reveals gram-positive diplococci, and the presence of pneumococci can be demonstrated by culture of the blood or the cerebrospinal fluid.

The prognosis for patients suffering from pneumococcal meningitis, especially when the picture is clinically advanced, is poor, with case fatality rates of the order of 30 to 50 percent despite immediate antimicrobial treatment. The reason for this failure of many cases to respond to treatment is not clear at present. These patients should be regarded as medical emergencies requiring urgent aggressive management under the most experienced available clinical supervision.

Otitis media

Pneumococcus and *H. influenzae* are the two major causes of otitis media in infancy and early childhood. Both are also common nasopharyngeal residents. Without culturing the middle ear fluid it is difficult to make a clinical distinction between them. Episodes of pneumococcal otitis tend to be associated with more fever and local ear pain than episodes caused by *Haemophilus*. The clinical picture is one of an irritable child, often wakeful at night and complaining of localized ear pain. There is frequently an antecedent history of upper respiratory tract infection. Clinical examination reveals a red, sometimes bulging drum which moves poorly on pneumatic otoscopy (Fig. 85-4) and is sometimes ruptured by the time of clinical examination. Systemic upset is variable but often includes temperature elevation or mild gastrointestinal disturbance. It is probable that many episodes of acute otitis media never receive care and that while some proceed to perforation and otorrhea, many settle spontaneously, passing through a phase of subacute otitis media with effusion which finally becomes sterile and is absorbed. The exact relationship between acute otitis media and chronic serous otitis (glue ear) is uncertain, but animal studies referred to above suggest that the two conditions are related.

Other pneumococcal infections

Pneumococci are frequently grown from the sinus washings of patients suffering from acute bacterial sinusitis, the sputum of patients sustaining acute flare-ups of bronchitis, and swabs of pus from patients with acute bacterial conjunctivitis. The exact role played in these conditions by the pneumococcus is uncertain. All three conditions are commonly treated with antibiotics to which they almost invariably respond rapidly.

DIAGNOSIS

The growth of a pneumococcus from a culture of blood, cerebrospinal fluid, middle ear fluid, pleural fluid, lung fluid, or peritoneal fluid leaves little doubt in the minds of clinicians or epidemiologists as to the pathogenic role played in the patient's illness. Because of the high incidence of carriage in the upper respiratory tract by normal individuals, however, isolation of a pneumococcus from respiratory tract secretions is no guarantee of that organism's pathogenic role. This problem of ascribing etiology to a pneumococcus cultured from the sputum or nasopharyngeal swab is particularly difficult in childhood, where carriage by normal individuals sometimes approaches 100 percent.

A variety of techniques aimed at improving the diagnostic usefulness of respiratory secretions, including quantitative colony counts, transtracheal aspirates, and direct examination of the sputum by means of omniserum, have been tried in an effort to circumvent this problem. None are entirely satisfactory, and, in view of the broad spectrum of coverage by antibiotic agents, many clinicians have become disenchanted with the value of sputum and nasopharyngeal culture in the diagnosis of pneumococcal disease of the respiratory tract. In fact, clinicians tend to choose their antibiotic therapy on the basis of clinical rather than laboratory findings, and the precise role played by the pneumococcus is very difficult to estimate except

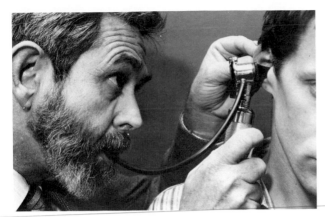

Figure 85-4. Pneumatic otoscopy. A simple method for testing the mobility of the tympanic membrane. Mobility is impeded by presence of fluid in the middle ear. This occurs both in serous otitis and acute otitis media.

where specially designed epidemiological studies with the full resources of the laboratory are brought to bear for epidemiological purposes.

Antecedent antibiotics often make it unlikely that a pneumococcus can be grown from blood cultures. In untreated patients, blood cultures tend to be positive in from 5 to 30 percent of cases of pneumococcal pneumonia.

Unfortunately, there is not at present an adequate species-specific serological test for the identification of pneumococcal infection. Even where paired convalescent sera are available, assuming a rising or falling antibody level to be adequate evidence of the organism's pathogenic role, the principal antibody involved is antibody to the capsular polysaccharide, which is, of course, type-specific. If the laboratory is to avoid running paired antibody assays to each of the 46 major serotypes, it needs information as to which serotype to concentrate upon. In these circumstances a typed nasopharyngeal or sputum isolate of pneumococcus provides a place to begin.

The problems with serological diagnosis of pneumococcal disease have led many investigators to approach the diagnosis from the perspective of antigen detection. This is theoretically an attractive approach, but the difficulty is that, so far, a species-specific antigen that is regularly released into the blood or bodily secretions of infected individuals has not been identified. The main antigens are the capsular polysaccharides, and these are detectable by a variety of methods of varying sensitivity. Counterimmunoelectrophoresis (CIE) has proved a useful method for the detection of antigen in the cerebrospinal fluid of patients suffering pneumococcal meningitis. For this, a pneumococcal omniserum is used as the antibody. The system generally works well for the detection of positively charged polysaccharides, but some of the invasive types, notably type 14, do not give a positive reaction with this test.

A variety of agglutination and other techniques have been developed in an attempt to increase the sensitivity of detection

of type-specific capsular polysaccharide in body fluids. The best estimates of antigen detection rates by the most sensitive assays in pneumococcal pneumonia are as follows: serum, 45 to 80 percent; urine, 50 to 64 percent; and sputum, 75 to 100 percent [15]. Thus, the early hope that these methods would be able to replace more laborious culture methods for identification of the causative organism have not been realized, though information from antigen testing can complement culture methods, especially where the patient has previously received antibiotic therapy.

A number of methods have been used to measure antibody to the capsular polysaccharide. The most commonly used radioimmunoassay [16] uses a labeled polysaccharide antigen which after incubation with the unknown serum provides a highly reproducible measure of antibody and can be adapted also to detect serum antigen. Its use tends to be restricted to specialist laboratories. Enzyme-linked immunosorbent assays have been developed for the detection of various immunoglobulin isotypes, and these have contributed to improved understanding of the character of the antibody response to capsular polysaccharides [17].

TREATMENT

Antimicrobial agents

Penicillin is still the antimicrobial agent of first choice in the treatment of all pneumococcal infections, but it is essential to be aware of the increasing role played by strains which display a degree of penicillin resistance. Until recently, pneumococci were exquisitely sensitive to penicillin, the cheapest of all antibiotics. The picture is changing, most dramatically in some areas where penicillin has remained almost the exclusive form of antibiotic therapy by primary health care workers. There have also been increasing numbers of reports of pneumococci resistant to other antimicrobial agents including tetracycline, sulfonamides, erythromycin, lincomycin, and chloramphenicol [18]. Most ominous in recent times, however, has been the report of isolation of pneumococci resistant to all β-lactam antibiotics (penicillins and cephalosporins), tetracycline, chloramphenicol, erythromycin, clindamycin, sulfonamides, rifampin, and streptomycin. For the most part, the level of penicillin resistance encountered has not been such as to invalidate the effectiveness of penicillin as a primary therapeutic agent in the treatment of pneumococcal disease. But the fact that outbreaks of serious disease caused by multiply resistant pneumococci have occurred gives cause for serious concern as to the future effectiveness of presently used antipneumococcal therapy. In association with outbreaks of multiply resistant strains, there has been evidence of dissemination of these strains among carriers. The mechanism of the increased resistance in these organisms is not at present clear [19]. An extensive search for a pneumococcal R plasmid has yielded negative results.

The implications of these findings are serious for clinicians and health care planners alike [20]. Local results of sensitivity testing of representative pneumococcal isolates from seriously ill patients and from carriers is an essential prerequisite to the prescription of rational antibiotic therapy.

The dosage and duration of penicillin therapy depends on the nature of the infection. Whereas patients with otitis media and pneumonia respond to relatively low dose, short courses of 5 to 7 days (for adults, an initial 24 h of crystalline penicillin 2 million units every 6 h followed by procaine penicillin 0.6 millions units every 12 h is an effective hospital regime, though it has been shown that a daily dose of 1.2 million units of procaine penicillin may be adequate for uncomplicated outpatients), those with bacteremia and/or meningitis require high dosage (e.g. 16 million units intravenously daily for the first 5 days and 3 million units intramuscularly every 6 h for the next 10 days), and those with endocarditis, empyema, or septic arthritis should have their high dosage maintained for a period ranging from 4 to 6 weeks.

Where penicillin or other β-lactam antibiotics, including the cephalosporins, are contraindicated either by the presence of known allergy or because of strong suspicion or knowledge of local prevalence of penicillin resistance, satisfactory alternatives are chloramphenicol (which has good penetration of the blood-brain barrier), erythromycin, and lincomycin. For outpatient situations where an oral antibiotic is desirable for management of otitis media, pneumonia, or sinusitis, ampicillin, amoxicillin, and cotrimoxazole are useful drugs because they also offer a spectrum of activity which includes a relatively high proportion of isolates of *H. influenzae* (though sensivity patterns for these drugs also are changing).

Patients with serious pneumococcal infections may suffer a variety of life-threatening complications which demand the resources of hospitals and intensive care units. These problems include dehydration, severe cardiovascular collapse, cardiac failure, respiratory failure, renal failure, metastatic abscesses, and disseminated intravascular coagulopathy.

Hospital case fatality rates for bacteremic pneumococcal infections are still high (10 to 50 percent) despite the widespread availability in hospital of antimicrobial therapy, and it is important to recognize that patients have often developed major cardiovascular, respiratory, or renal complications before admission which will require immediate attention and a high level of clinical awareness if these changes are to be successfully reversed.

Practical issues in management of undifferentiated acute respiratory infections in early childhood

The discussion in this chapter so far has centered around the pathology, clinical manifestations, and treatment of pneumococcal disease, but it has also emphasized that the clinical presentation of this type of infection is not specific. There is an overlap between pneumococcal pneumonia and pneumonia caused by other organisms, and there is also real clinical difficulty in distinguishing when a respiratory infection has extended from the upper respiratory tract to involve the lungs.

In fact, the main practical problem confronting primary health care workers is to decide whether a person with an acute respiratory infection needs antibiotic care and/or referral for further investigation and management. In developing countries millions of people, especially young children, die each year from pneumonia which remains totally untreated and unrecognized by families and by the health care system. The limited investigations that have been carried out on etiology suggest that pneumococci are the main bacterial causes of death together with *H. influenzae*.

In an effort to tackle this problem, especially among young children, there has been a major international effort in recent years, orchestrated by the World Health Organization, which aims to simplify clinical management decisions and to improve the identification of sick children in the community. The concept of a standard management plan for the clinical assessment and treatment of young children suffering from acute respiratory infections (ARI) has been promulgated as an attempt to deal with this problem, and pilot testing of this approach has been conspicuously successful in reducing mortality rates in areas where it has been introduced. The guidelines are shown in Fig. 85-5. They depend on the recognition of rapid breathing, chest indrawing, and inability to feed as critical decision points which can be widely taught to primary health care workers and to community leaders as well as to parents of young children. The guidelines have been derived from careful clinical studies of hospitalized cases, especially in developing countries, and have been validated in a number of settings where they have been shown to be relatively sensitive and specific. A summary of current guidelines for choice of antibiotic is shown in Table 85-1.

It is probable that similar schemes will be used in the future to improve primary assessment and management of adult patients with acute respiratory infections. The concept of a standard management plan is an important development in clinical care. It is no substitute for careful individual assessment by fully trained clinicians, but it involves a recognition that primary assessment of respiratory infections is almost invariably undertaken not by fully trained clinicians, but by relatively untrained members of the community.

POPULATION

ECOLOGY

Transmission of pneumococci among humans is probably by droplets and dust. No natural animal reservoirs are known to exist, although pneumococci are pathogenic to a number of laboratory species. The organism has been recovered from the dust of classrooms and hospitals but probably does not survive for long out of culture media.

The human nasopharynx is colonized by the pneumococcus from an early age—in some instances within hours of birth [21]. The organism can be grown from nasal or nasopharyngeal swabs, and in some tropical and underprivileged populations,

HOW TO MANAGE CHILD WITH A COUGH.

1.O. ASSESS THE CHILD

1. Ask:
   • can the child drink?
   • any fits or periods of not breathing?
   • how long has the child had cough?

2. Look for:
   • fast breathing
   • chest indrawing

3. Look and listen
   for wheeze

4. Listen for stridor

5. Look at the general condition for:
   • very sleepy and difficult to
     wake up (Admit)
   • severely undernourished (Admit)
   • dehydrated (Treat)

6. Assess the temperature

2.0 DECIDE HOW TO TREAT THE CHILD.

Is the child ABLE TO DRINK?
   Yes [ ] Go to next question
   No [ ] Refer for Admisson

Does the child have WHEEZE or STRIDOR?
   Yes, WHEEZE [ ] See CHILD WITH WHEEZE box below.
   Yes, STRIDOR [ ] See CHILD WITH STRIDOR box below.
   No [ ] Go to next question.

Does the child have CHEST INDRAWING?
   Yes [ ] Refer for Admission.
   No [ ] Go to next question.

Is the child BREATHING FAST?
   Yes [ ] Give Antibiotics and Homecare.
   No [ ] Go to next question.

Has the child had the COUGH FOR MORE THAN 30 DAYS?
   Yes [ ] Refer for Assessment.
   No [ ] Give Homecare.

CHILD WITH WHEEZE:

Is the child MORE THAN ONE YEAR OLD?

   Yes [ ] Refer for Assessment
           (or give salbutamol)
   No [ ] Go to next question.

Is the child BREATHING FAST?
(more than 50 times a minute?)
   Yes [ ] Refer for Admission.
   No [ ] Give Homecare.

CHILD WITH STRIDOR:

Is stridor PRESENT WHEN THE CHILD IS CALM?
   Yes [ ] Refer for Admission.
   No [ ] Go to next question.

Has child CHOKED ON FOREIGN BODY?
   Yes [ ] Refer for Amission.
   No [ ] Go to next question.

Is DIPHTHERIA COMMON IN THE AREA?
   Yes [ ] Refer for Admission.
   No [ ] Go to next question.

Is the child BREATHING FAST (more than 50 breaths per minute)?
   Yes [ ] Give Antibiotics and Homecare.
   No [ ] Give Homecare.

Figure 85-5. WHO training chart for teaching health workers to assess and manage a child with cough.

Table 85-1. Antimicrobials used for treatment of pneumococcal infections

	Outpatient Antimicrobials			Inpatient Antimicrobials		
	Procaine penicillin	Ampicillin	Cotrimoxazole	Benzyl penicillin	Chloramphenicol	Cloxacillin
Sensitivities:						
H. influenzae	Good (but 0–25% resistance)	Good (but 0–25% resistance)	Very good	Good (but 0–25% resistance)	Very good	Poor
S. pneumoniae	Very good (mild resistance in some countries)	Very good (mild resistance in some countries)	Very good (mild resistance in some countries)	Very good (mild resistance in some countries)	Good	Fair
S. aureus	Poor	Poor	Good	Poor	Fairly good	Good
Group A streptococcus	Very good	Very good	Poor	Very good	Good	Good
Chlamydia, pneumocystis	Nil	Nil	Good	Nil	Very poor	Nil
Toxicity:						
Mild, but common	0.2% acute but self-limiting psychosis or collapse	Diarrhea, rash	Rash	Rash	Nil	Rash
Severe, but rare	Fatal anaphylaxis 1 in 250,000	Fatal anaphylaxis less than 1 in 250,000	Dose-related megaloblastic anemia; bone marrow aplasia (may be fatal); Stevens-Johnson syndrome (may be fatal)	Fatal anaphylaxis 1 in 250,000	Reversible: gray syndrome, dose-dependent marrow aplasia Not reversible: fatal marrow aplasia 1 in 20,000	Fatal anaphylaxis ?1 in 250,000
Administration:						
Route	IM	PO	PO	IM (or IV)	IM (or IV), then PO	IM (or IV), then PO
Dose	50,000 U/kg once a day	25 mg/kg q 6 h	TMP 4 mg/kg q 12 h	50,000 µ/kg q 6 h	25 mg/kg q h	50 mg/kg q 6 h
Cost, 5 days, 10-kg child	U.S. $0.20	U.S. $0.40	U.S. $0.08	U.S. $0.18	U.S. $1.00	U.S. $6.00
Comments	Usually effective, long-acting; side effects rare: narrow spectrum (less risk of R factor resistance); *But* IM administration not always possible.	Usually effective, serious toxicity very rare; *but* short-acting, mild side effects common, and moderate spectrum increases risk of R factor resistance; *amoxicillin* preferable if cost is similar (with dose 15 mg/kg q 8 h).	Effective, cheap, and fairly long acting; *but* serious toxicity occurs (rare) and broad spectrum increases risk of R factor resistance.	Usually effective, side effects rare, cheap.	Effective. Side effects are rare *but* 1 in 20,000 fatal, so should only be used for severe sepsis. Fairly cheap.	Expensive. Only indicated for staphylococcal pneumonia.

100 percent of infants and preschool children will be found to harbor a pneumococcus at these sites. By adolescence and early adulthood the carriage rate has dropped sharply. One or more serotypes may be found in the nose at one time. The factors which lead to termination of nasopharyngeal carriage are inadequately understood, but it is known that in young children nasopharyngeal acquisition is often followed by elevation of homotypic serum antibody [22].

Although pneumococcal carriage is likely to be the usual precursor to pneumococcal disease, the types most frequently carried are not necessarily the types that most commonly cause disease. In fact, type 1, one of the most highly invasive types, is infrequently grown from healthy carriers. Some types, e.g., types 3, 6, and 19, are commonly carried and often cause disease, whereas other types, e.g., types 15, 16, and 17, are relatively commonly carried but do not so often cause disease.

EPIDEMIOLOGY

Central to the epidemiology of pneumococcal disease is the carriage of this organism in the upper respiratory tract by significant numbers of healthy individuals [23]. Rates of disease seem to depend on the frequency with which invasive serotypes are carried in the nasopharynx of healthy members of the population. The likelihood of transmission of pneumococci from a carrier to another individual is thought to be directly proportional to the frequency and intimacy of their contact. Carrier rates among adults are highest in barracks and in open dormitories. Spread of pneumococci within families has been well documented. This spread often occurs in conjunction with viral infection of the upper respiratory tract. Carriage rates are highest in children of preschool age and tend to decrease with increasing age. Longitudinal studies of pneumococcal carriers have shown that sometimes a serotype will be carried in the nasopharynx for up to 6 months. Reacquisition of a serotype which had been previously carried and then discontinued is common, implying that carriage of a particular serotype does not always induce a level of local immunity sufficient to prevent reacquisition.

Studies in a military population where pneumococcal disease was epidemic revealed that for each pneumococcal serotype the occurrence of pneumococcal pneumonia could be expressed with reasonable accuracy by the formula:

Rate of pneumonia = pneumococcus carrier rate
$$\times \text{ nonbacterial respiratory disease rate} \times K$$

where K varied with (1) the infectivity of the serotype of pneumococcus involved, (2) the type-specific resistance to pneumococcal infection of individuals in the population, and (3) the nature of the nonbacterial respiratory disease involved [24]. In that study, the infectivity factor for type 1 pneumococcus was 20 times higher than that for type 9.

This formula would lead us to expect epidemics of pneumococcal pneumonia in communities where rates of carriage of invasive serotypes are high and where a stream of susceptible recruits continuously enters the population. These circumstances apply in the South African gold mines, and a similar combination of circumstances probably underlies the high incidence of pneumococcal pneumonia among young adults living in the squatter settlements of the rapidly growing cities of many developing countries. A continuous stream of immigrants from the remote rural areas ensures a constant pool of susceptible new recruits who may not have previously encountered or developed immunity to the invasive serotypes prevailing in the cities. After 6 months in the gold-mining community, the risk to a new recruit of developing pneumonia falls dramatically. It seems most likely that temporary carriage of an invasive serotype by susceptible individuals induces immunity at the level of the serum or the mucosa or both. The possibility that the two levels of immunity may not depend on the same factors is suggested by the observation that parenteral immunization with capsular material is more effective for preventing serious disease than for inhibiting colonization of the respiratory tract by vaccine type organisms [25].

With the growing interest in pneumococcal vaccines there has been a resurgence of interest in the relative importance of pneumococcal serotypes. Since the 1930s, there have been secular changes in the relative incidence of disease caused by serotypes 1 and 2 which have diminished in some countries as a cause of bacteremic infection. Whereas type 46 has been shown to be a particularly common cause of bacteremia in Papua New Guinea and type 25 in South Africa, neither of these serotypes is commonly grown from blood cultures of American patients.

As well as international and secular trends in the prevalence of individual pneumococcal serotype, there are differences with age. Types 6, 14, 18, 19, and 23 are repeatedly grown from carriers and children with pneumococcal disease in childhood, whereas these types tend to be less common in published series which consist only of adults.

It follows that with variations in the invasiveness of different pneumococcal serotypes, the relative distribution of serotypes grown from carriers may be quite different from that grown from patients with disease. Vaccines against pneumococcus are formulated on the basis of surveillance carried out by the World Health Organization of serotypes recovered from blood, cerebrospinal fluid, and other body fluids of patients with disease.

PREVENTION WITH VACCINES

Adult immunization

Purified capsular polysaccharide material is highly immunogenic in young adult volunteers, and a single injection is, in most instances, followed by sustained elevation (from 3 to 8 years) of anticapsular antibody to the types included in the vaccine. A single 25-μg dose of polysaccharide stimulates what is apparently a maximal response.

A study in 1945 [25] convincingly demonstrated the efficacy of a tetravalent polysaccharide vaccine in preventing homotypic pneumococcal pneumonia among military recruits, but the vaccine became available at about the same time as penicillin, and it was little used by the medical profession. In the early 1960s it was shown that mortality from pneumococcal bacteremia was still very high [13], and that therapy with antibiotics could not reverse the toxic changes that were already present in some patients when they presented for medical care. Furthermore, the high mortality experienced by patients after splenectomy, by those with sickle cell disease, renal and liver disease, or congestive cardiac failure and by alcoholics and the elderly, led to the proposition that an effective vaccine targeted toward some of these high-risk groups would be both cost-effective and lifesaving.

A polyvalent pneumococcal vaccine is, in reality, a collection of capsular polysaccharide vaccines which must be considered independently. All components of the vaccine must meet stringent chemical requirements and be shown to be safe and immunogenic when tested in adults. The first tetradecavalent vaccine consisted of the capsular polysaccharides of pneumococcal types 1, 2, 3, 4, 6A, 7F, 8, 9N, 12F, 14, 18C, 19F, 23F, and 25. It was licensed in 1977 on the basis of a series of immunogenicity and efficacy studies carried out among recruits to the labor force in the Johannesburg gold mines. These trials demonstrated the ability of pneumococcal vaccine to reduce by 80 to 85 percent pneumococcal pneumonia associated with pneumococcal types the antigens of which were in the vaccine [26]. Over a 2-year period of observation there was no replacement of pneumonic illness associated with pneumococcal types in the vaccine by that associated with other pneumococcal types or with other bacterial or viral pathogens. Furthermore, there was an 85 percent reduction in bacteremic infection caused by pneumococcal types included in the vaccine.

Trials of polyvalent pneumococcal vaccines in various American populations, where attack rates were considerably lower than those observed in South Africa, have been much less convincing. In a study involving 13,600 persons 45 years of age or older at the Kaiser Permanente Medical Center in San Francisco, there was no reduction in the total incidence of radiologically confirmed pneumonia in the vaccinees as contrasted with control subjects. Bacteriological and serological evidence, however, suggests that pneumococcal pneumonia caused a very small part of the total burden of pneumonic illnesses while the study was in progress. A second American study involved 1300 patients resident for more than 3 months at the Dorothea Dix Hospital in North Carolina. Again, there was no reduction in total pneumonic illness demonstrated among the vaccinees, in whom the attack rate of radiologically confirmed pneumonia was higher than in the control subjects— perhaps the result, in part, of a high rate of recurring illness in a number of vaccinees with chronic respiratory disease. A

further series of recent studies of the use of vaccine in high-risk elderly North American populations has proved equally disappointing in changing the incidence of disease, and most of these studies have been too small to test whether mortality is changed in such populations by use of the vaccine. There is therefore growing uncertainty about the general benefits that will be gained from mass immunization of elderly high-risk populations, though it is still true to say that the potential benefits from use of this very safe vaccine make its routine use in such patients fully justifiable [27]. There are growing doubts, however, about the cost-benefit balance of mass use of the vaccine, particularly in those with chronic lung disease, for which the vaccine to this point has been particularly unimpressive [28].

Reactivity to the vaccine has not been a significant problem. About 40 percent of recipients experience some redness or local pain, and induration at the vaccine site and mild temperature elevation is occasionally observed. There have been no deaths reported from the several million doses now administered in the United States and only an occasional anaphylactoid reaction, which responded rapidly to conservative measures. Currently available vaccines contain the 23 serotypes which surveillance studies suggest to be the most important causes of severe pneumococcal infections including types 1, 2, 3, 4, 5, 6B, 7F, 8, 9N, 9V, 10A, 11A, 12F, 14, 15B, 17F, 18C, 19A, 19F, 20, 22F, 23F, and 33F.

Pneumococcal disease remains a major public health problem in many developing countries, including Papua New Guinea, where a controlled trial of tetradecavalent vaccine vs. saline placebo involving 12,000 adults living in a remote rural area was associated with a 44 percent reduction in mortality from pneumonia in the immunized group [29]. The protective effects were still evident during an influenza epidemic 3 years after immunization. There were 29 percent fewer cases of pneumonia in the immunized population than in the control population, and the number of cases of proven pneumococcal infection (i.e., cases in which blood cultures or lung punctures grew pneumococci) was 85 percent lower. The total reduction in pneumococcal pneumonia was less impressive than the reduction in serious cases of lobar pneumonia, bacteremic pneumonia, and death. The impact of the vaccine on adult mortality was greatest among younger individuals and among those whose pneumonia was not a complication of chronic lung disease.

Immunization of children

Although children are capable of responding with a good humoral antibody response to type 3 pneumococcal polysaccharide at the early age of 3 months, responsiveness to types 6, 14, 19, and 23, which are the very types that most commonly cause disease in early childhood, has been repeatedly shown to be poor in the early years of life [30]. For some of these serotypes, the antibody response remains relatively poor until late childhood [*31*]. A series of trials involving children who ranged in age at entry from 6 months to 6 years, have been carried out in Scandinavia, the United States, and Australia [*32–36*] in an effort to reduce the incidence of pneumococcal otitis media and other childhood pneumococcal infections by use of vaccine. The results of these trials have not been uniformly negative, but taken together, they do not indicate a sustained or consistent benefit in the prevention of morbidity in developed countries to a degree that would justify routine use of the current vaccine in childhood in these countries [*36*]. However, three double-blind placebo-controlled trials carried out in Papua New Guinea have recently been reported [*37*], and these provide evidence that in an area where severe pneumococcal disease is very common in childhood, the vaccine was effective in preventing death from pneumococcal disease even in children who were vaccinated before the age of 2 years (which is the time when antibody responses to a number of important pediatric serotypes begin to mature). These New Guinea data raise the possibility that early childhood immunization, while suboptimal in its capacity to elevate antibody, may provide the marginal improvement in humoral defense that can make a difference in outcome between survival and death in serious pneumococcal infections. Further exploration of this possibility is urgently needed before advocating widespread use of existing pneumococcal vaccines among children in developing countries, where mortality from severe pneumococcal infections continues to be enormous.

Meanwhile, other approaches to childhood immunization are being explored. Polysaccharide antigens that are poorly immunogenic in newborn mice can have their immunogenicity enhanced by conjugating them to protein antigens which are known to be immunogenic at this age. Conjugates of pneumococcal polysaccharides with various immunogenic proteins are under active development following the successful application of this approach to a similar problem which exists with vaccines of *Haemophilus influenzae* type b [*38*]. It is hoped that conjugated pneumococcal vaccines will be available for trial in childhood shortly.

CONTROL

It will be apparent from this review that the place of pneumococcal immunization in routine prophylaxis still awaits clarification. Results have been more impressive where attack rates and mortality are high. Patients with dysfunctional and absent spleens appear to have a particular need for routine vaccination. Where attack rates are low, where the responsiveness to some types in the vaccine is inadequate or ill-sustained, or where the recipients of vaccine are in chronic poor health and have other defects in their natural defenses, the results, especially in terms of morbidity effects, are less convincing. The possibility that the current generation of vaccines could con-

tribute to reduction in pneumococcal mortality in developing countries deserves further evaluation.

It is manifestly impossible to eradicate the pneumococcus, and even if therapeutic services could be optimally developed in poorer countries, they alone are unlikely to be an adequate answer to the problem of pneumococcal disease. A vaccine approach has major theoretical advantages and will continue to be sought as an adjunct to strengthening of therapeutic management of established infections.

At present, international efforts in the control of mortality from acute respiratory infections depend primarily on education of parents in the recognition of serious disease and strengthening of primary care management through the introduction of standard clinical management "packages" [*39*].

Cost-benefit considerations

The decision to embark on a mass vaccination program using the presently available polyvalent preparations requires a consideration of cost-effectiveness. This, in turn, requires information about the attack rates of pneumococcal disease in the target population, case fatality rates, hospitalization rates, and the costs of treating patients as outpatients and of delivery of vaccine to the susceptible population. In computing the costs and benefits of a vaccine program, it is important to recognize that even where pneumococcal disease is very prevalent, not all disease will be caused by types included in the vaccine and that, for a variety of reasons, the vaccine is unlikely to be more than 85 percent effective. Models for computation of cost-benefit ratios are available and have been used in estimating the benefits of routine immunization of elderly American populations [*40*].

REFERENCES

1 Austrian R: Some observations on the pneumococcus and the current status of pneumococcal disease and its prevention. Rev Infect Dis 3:S1–17, 1981

2 Tomaz A: Surface components of *Streptococcus pneumoniae*. Rev Infect Dis 3:190–211, 1981

3 Paton JC, Berry AM, Lock RA, et al: Cloning and expression of 12 *Escherichia coli* of the *Streptococcus pneumoniae* gene encoding pneumolysin. Infect Immun 3:324–352, 1981

4 Giebink GS: The pathogenesis of pneumococcal otitis media in chinchillas and the efficacy of vaccination in prophylaxis. Rev Infect Dis 3:342–352, 1981

5 Barrett DJ, Ayoub EM: IgG2 subclass restriction of antibody to pneumococcal polysaccharides. Clin Exp Immunol 63:127–134, 1986

6 Barrett DJ, Lee CG, Amman AJ, et al: IgG and IgM pneumococcal antibody responses in infants. Pediatr Res 18:1967–1971, 1984.

7 Wara DW: Host defenses against *Streptococcus pneumoniae*: The role of the spleen. Rev Infect Dis 3:299–309, 1981

8 Winkelstein JA: The role of complement in the host's defense against *Streptococcus pneumoniae*. Rev Infect Dis 3:289–298, 1981

9 Johnston RB: The host response to invasion by *Streptococcus pneumoniae*: Protection and pathogenesis of tissue damage. Rev Infect Dis 3:282–288, 1981

10 Heffron R: *Pneumonia, With Special Reference to Pneumococcus Lobar Pneumonia*. New York, The Commonwealth Fund, 1939

11 Moxon ER: Experimental infections of animals in the study of *Streptococcus pneumoniae*. Rev Infect Dis 3:354–357, 1981

12 Douglas RM, Devitt L, Macartney B: Evaluation of serum bilirubin and blood urea in pneumonia. Aust NZ J Med 4:346–351, 1974

13 Austrian R, Gold J: Pneumococcal bacteremia with especial reference to bacteremic pneumococcal pneumonia. Ann Intern Med 60:759–776, 1964

14 WHO Geneva: Respiratory infections in children: Management at small hospitals. Background notes and a manual for doctors. WHO/RSD/86.26, 1986

15 Rytel MW, Preheim LC: Antigen detection in the diagnosis and in the prognostic assessment of bacterial pneumonias. Diagn Microbiol Infect Dis 4(3) (Suppl):35S–46S, 1986

16 Schiffman G, Douglas RM, Bonner MJ, et al: A radioimmunoassay for immunologic phenomena in pneumococcal disease and for the antibody response to pneumococcal vaccines. 1. Method for the radioimmunoassay of anticapsular antibodies and comparison with other techniques. J Immunol Methods 33:133–144, 1980

17 Katz MA, Schiffman G: Comparison of an enzyme-linked immunosorbent assay with radioimmunoassay for the measurement of pneumococcal capsular polysaccharide antibodies. Mol Immunol 22:313–319, 1985

18 Ward J: Antibiotic-resistant *Streptococcus pneumoniae*: Clinical and epidemiologic aspects. Rev Infect Dis 3:254–266, 1981

19 Zighalboim S, Tomasz A: Multiple antibiotic resistance in South African strains of *Streptococcus pneumoniae*. Mechanism of resistance to β-lactam antibiotics. Rev Infect Dis 3:267–276, 1981

20 Oppenheim B, Koornhof HJ, Austrian R: Antibiotic resistant pneumococcal disease in children at Baragwanath Hospital, Johannesburg. Paediatr Infect Dis 5:520–524, 1986

21 Gratten M, Gratten H, Poli A, et al: Colonization of *Haemophilus influenzae* and *Streptococcus pneumoniae* in the upper respiratory tract of neonates in Papua New Guinea: Primary acquisition, duration of carriage, and relationship to carriage in mothers. Biol Neonate 50:114–120, 1986

22 Gwaltney JM, Sande MA, Austrian R, et al: Spread of *Streptococcus pneumoniae* in families. II. Relation of transfer of *S. pneumoniae* to incidence of colds and serum antibody. J Infect Dis 132:62–68, 1975

23 Riley ID, Douglas RM: An epidemiologic approach to pneumococcal disease. Rev Infect Dis 3:223–245, 1981

24 Hodges RG, MacLeod CM: Epidemic pneumococcal pneumonia. V. Final consideration of the factors underlying the epidemic. Am J Hyg 44:237–243, 1946

25 MacLeod CM, Hodges RG, Heidelberger M, et al: Prevention of pneumococcal pneumonia by immunization with specific capsular polysaccharides. J Exp Med 82:445–465, 1945

26 Austrian R, Douglas RM, Schiffman G, et al: Prevention of pneumococcal pneumonia by vaccination. Trans Assoc Am Physicians 89:184–195, 1976

27 Austrian R: A reassessment of pneumococcal vaccine. N Engl J Med 310:651–653, 1984

28 Leech JA, Jervais A, Ruben FL: Efficacy of pneumococcal vaccine in severe chronic obstructive pulmonary disease. Can Med Assoc J 136:361–365, 1987

29 Riley ID, Andrews M, Howard R, et al: Immunization with a polyvalent pneumococcal vaccine. Lancet i:1338–1340, 1977

30 Douglas RM, Paton JC, Duncan SJ, et al: Poor antibody response to pneumococcal vaccination in children under 5 years. J Infect Dis 148:131–137, 1983

31 Paton JC, Toogood TR, Cockington RA, et al: Antibody responses to pneumococcal vaccine in children aged 5–15 years. Am J Dis Child 140:135–138, 1986

32 Makela OH, Leinonen M, Pukander J, et al: A study of the pneumococcal vaccine in prevention of clinically acute attacks of recurrent otitis media. Rev Infect Dis 3(suppl):S124–S130, 1981

33 Douglas RM, Miles HB: Vaccination against *Streptococcus pneumoniae* in childhood: Lack of demonstrable benefit in young Australian children. J Infect Dis 149:861–869, 1984

34 Karma P, Pukander J, Sipilla M, et al: Prevention of otitis media in children by pneumococcal vaccination. Am J Otolaryngol 6:173–184, 1985

35 Rosen C, Christensen P, Hovelius B, et al: Effect of pneumococcal vaccination on upper respiratory tract infections in children. Design of a follow-up study. Scand J Infect Dis (suppl)39:39–44, 1983

36 Brunell PA, Bass JW, Daum RS, et al: American Academy of Pediatrics, Committee on Infectious Diseases: Recommendations for using pneumococcal vaccine in children. Pediatrics 75:1153–1158, 1985

37 Riley ID, Lehmann D, Alpers MP, et al: Pneumococcal vaccine prevents death from acute lower respiratory tract infections in Papua New Guinean children. Lancet ii:877–881, 1986

38 Schneerson R, Robbins JB, Parke JC Jr, et al: Quantitative and qualitative analyses of serum antibodies elicited in adults by *Haemophilus influenzae* type b and pneumococcus type 6A capsular polysaccharide–tetanus toxoid conjugates. Infect Immun 52:519–528, 1986

39 Berman S, McIntosh K: Selective primary health care: Strategies for control of disease in the developing world. XXI. Acute respiratory infections. Rev Infect Dis 7:674–691, 1985

40 Sisk JE, Riegelman RK: Cost effectiveness of vaccination against pneumococcal pneumonia: An update. Ann Intern Med 104:79–86, 1986

Streptococcal Diseases · Edward L. Kaplan*

Streptococci are ubiquitous, causing infections throughout the world. The importance of streptococci as disease-producing agents in tropical and subtropical countries, however, has not been fully recognized until recent years. The potential to reduce rheumatic heart disease in developing countries by controlling streptococcal infections is enormous [1–3].

PARASITE

The primary differentiation of pathogenic streptococci is based on their reaction when grown on blood agar. The green (α-hemolytic) or nonhemolytic (λ) streptococci normally inhabit the oral cavity and cause bacterial endocarditis, dental caries, and abscesses of the jaw. Recently, the α-hemolytic streptococci have also been shown to cause serious and life-threatening infections in immunocompromised patients. Most pyogenic infections in humans are caused by streptococcal strains that produce clear hemolysis (β-hemolysis) on blood agar.

β-Hemolytic streptococci are most reliably identified by examining well-isolated colonies grown on nutrient agar plates containing sheep or horse blood. Anaerobic cultivation is preferred; alternatively, if cultures are to be incubated aerobically, stabs made into the agar at the time of inoculation will usually facilitate the identification of strains that do not produce clear hemolysis around surface colonies.

Most β-hemolytic streptococci producing infections in humans belong to serological group A (*Streptococcus pyogenes*). More importantly, infections with strains of other serological groups do not have the capability of producing acute rheumatic fever and, with one possible exception (an outbreak of scarlet fever due to group C streptococci), have not been associated with acute glomerulonephritis. Group A streptococci can be fairly accurately differentiated from non-group A strains by inhibition of growth on subculture around specially prepared bacitracin disks, but serological confirmation is recommended. Recently, rapid antigen detection techniques have been adapted for identification of group A streptococci [4].

Group B streptococci are responsible for most streptococcal infections in human neonates. Groups C and G streptococci can produce disease in humans, and in tropical and subtropical countries appear to be commonly associated with infection as well as with carriage in the upper respiratory tract [5,6]. Groups C and G β-hemolytic streptococci have been more frequently isolated from cases of sepsis and endocarditis in recent years. Group D streptococci may be found in abdominal abscesses and in endocarditis. In contrast to other serologically groupable streptococci, group D streptococci are often nonhemolytic and resistant to penicillin. Other serological groups of streptococci are only rarely associated with human disease. One example of this is group R streptococci (*S. suis*), which have been frequently associated with infection of the central nervous system in humans who work in abattoirs [7].

More than 80 different M types of group A streptococci have been identified. The M proteins are a serologically diverse but functionally homogeneous family of proteins. Immunity to streptococcal infections is type-specific for M proteins. Other antigenic markers (the T, R, and serum-opacity proteins) are useful in identification of certain strains of group A streptococci, especially those that are difficult to M-type. Characterizing group A streptococci by opacity factor has proved very useful for the approximately 27 serotypes which are opacity-factor-positive [8]. These markers are less specific, and their biological functions are unknown. Classification according to T types often gives complex patterns corresponding only in a general way with M types.

Type-specific M proteins are surface components of group A streptococci, located on the hairlike fimbriae projecting from the streptococcal cell. In the absence of type-specific host antibody, M-positive strains resist phagocytosis and are therefore virulent. M-negative strains are readily phagocytized and avirulent. The M proteins are α-helical molecules that have a structural and chemical resemblance to tropomyosin, a mammalian muscle protein with seven residue periodicity [9].

The hairlike fimbriae on the surface of group A streptococcal cells enable adherence to epithelial cells, a first step in establishing infection. In addition to M protein, the fimbriae contain lipoteichoic acid, the specific component that appears to be responsible for attachment [10].

The group A streptococcal cell is surrounded by a watery gel or "capsule" of hyaluronic acid. Encapsulated strains, often referred to as "mucoid," have recently been associated with the resurgence of acute rheumatic fever seen in the mid-1980s in the United States [11]. The rigid cell wall results from a peptidoglycan polymer, to which the group-specific (group A) carbohydrate is bound [12a]. This peptidoglycan infrastructure, though chemically quite different from endotoxin, has many of its biological properties. Beneath the cell wall is the osmotically fragile cell membrane; a lipoprotein-containing structure which forms the outermost boundary of streptococcal protoplasts and L forms.

Toxic substances that may be released by group A streptococci into the growth medium include two cytolytic exotoxins, streptolysins S and O, which lyse a broad range of mammalian cells and cell components and the three (A, B, and C) ery-

*This is an updated version of the chapter by Lewis W. Wannamaker in the first edition of this book.

throgenic toxins (pyrogenic exotoxins), which have diverse pathological properties similar to those of gram-negative endotoxins. The streptolysins are best known for their ability to hemolyze red blood cells.

A number of other biologically active substances can be found in the extracellular fluid surrounding group A streptococci. Most of these are antigenic and blastogenic, and some have potent mitogenic properties (e.g., blastogen A). Those with specific enzymatic activity (or that trigger enzyme systems) include hyaluronidase, the two streptokinases, proteinase, nicotinamide adenine dinucleotidase (NADase), and four nucleases. Two nucleases (B and D) have both DNase and RNase activity, and two (A and C) have only DNase activity.

PATIENT

STREPTOCOCCAL SORE THROAT AND SCARLET FEVER

Streptococcal pharyngitis or tonsillitis is one of the most common infections of childhood. In Egypt, a subtropical country, prospective family studies have revealed a surprisingly high incidence of group A streptococcal infections of the throat, confirmed by a rise in antistreptolysin O titer. Infection rates of 8 in 1000 per week were found in preschool children and 6 in 1000 per week in school children [6]. These rates approach the 10/1000 per week of military recruit populations experiencing epidemic streptococcal disease. Acquisition rates for group A streptococci were remarkably high in Egyptian infants, 1.83 per infant per year as compared with 1.98 per person per year in the overall population of families. These findings are in contrast to those in the United States where streptococcal sore throat is a disease that occurs predominantly in school-age children and is rare in infants.

In tropical and subtropical countries there appears to be less seasonal fluctuation in the incidence of streptococcal sore throat than has been observed in temperate climates. Some reports from countries with distinct rainy-dry seasons indicate an increased incidence of streptococcal disease during the rainy season.

Spread of streptococcal infections of the upper respiratory tract occurs by close contact with a person currently or recently infected (and still harboring) group A streptococci [13]. Crowded living conditions, particularly in sleeping quarters, are a major determinant of spread. Environmental contamination, on the other hand, does not enhance the risk of acquiring streptococcal sore throat. Individuals with positive nose cultures and young children are especially likely to transmit infection.

Epidemics due to ingestion of milk or other foods, notably egg-containing salads, are occasionally recognized and may affect large numbers of individuals with marked toxicity [14,15]. When families or other smaller groups are exposed by this route, the hallmarks of a common-source outbreak (e.g., simultaneous onsets) may be less obvious. In tropical and/or developing countries, the use of unpasteurized milk is often widespread and the potential for transmission by ingestion may be increased, because of both the difficulties in food refrigeration and the high ambient temperatures, which may speed the multiplication of streptococci in foods.

The epidemiology of *scarlet fever* is similar to that of streptococcal sore throat. Virtually all strains of group A streptococci produce one or more erythrogenic toxins (pyrogenic exotoxins), but their production or release appears to require lysogenization (latent infection) of the strain with certain temperate bacteriophages.

The intensity of the symptoms of streptococcal sore throat is quite variable. In temperate climates, about 40 percent of streptococcal infections of the upper respiratory tract are subclinical or unrecognized. The frequency of mild or subclinical infections may be even higher in tropical or subtropical countries. Reports from the tropics indicate that the clinical manifestations of severe streptococcal sore throat (high fever, sudden onset, pharyngeal and/or tonsillar exudate) are often missing [6].

Scarlet fever is also rare in the tropics, for reasons that are not clear [16]. A scarlatinal rash is virtually pathognomonic of streptococcal infection but may occur with staphylococcal infection. Although the rash is more difficult to recognize in individuals with dark skin, it can be detected in the acute stage by the feel of the elevated cutaneous papules and retrospectively by the characteristic convalescent desquamation, which may be most obvious in the spaces between the fingers and toes.

In the absence of a scarlatinal rash, the clinical differentiation of streptococcal from other infections of the upper respiratory tract may be difficult [17]. Tender anterior cervical lymph nodes, which may occur in the absence as well as in the presence of frank pharyngitis, are one of the most reliable clinical indications of streptococcal infection. The presence of conjunctivitis, hoarseness, or cough (in the absence of frank pneumonia) should suggest other etiological agents.

Pharyngeal exudate, which may not appear until the second or third day of symptoms, occurs in viral as well as streptococcal infections. Clinical observations in temperate climates have revealed that pharyngeal exudate in infants is rarely indicative of streptococcal infection. Perhaps due to the absence of previous sensitization, infants with streptococcal infection of the upper respiratory tract are less likely to manifest acute localized inflammation of the pharynx and may present with chronic low-grade fever, nasal congestion or discharge, and generalized lymphadenopathy, known as streptococcal fever or (incorrectly) streptococcosis. In infants and young children, excoriation around the external nares is a highly suggestive sign of group A streptococcal infection. Not infrequently, the organism may be cultured from the anterior nares, but not from the throat in these infants.

Current or recent streptococcal infection in a close contact (e.g., family member or classmate) or the appearance of a nonsuppurative sequela, provides epidemiological support for the possibility of streptococcal infection.

In tropical as well as temperate climates, most patients with clinical symptoms and signs of acute pharyngitis do not have bacterial or serological evidence of streptococcal infection [17,18]. Therefore, the search for rapid and more precise methods of clinical and laboratory differentiation continues.

In adults, an elevated white blood cell count, with a shift to the left, is generally helpful in separating bacterial from viral infections, but it is not a reliable differentiation in children. The nitroblue tetrazolium (NBT) test does not distinguish streptococcal from nonstreptococcal sore throat.

When carefully taken and expertly processed, throat cultures of patients with active streptococcal infection usually show numerous colonies of β-hemolytic streptocci, and it is rare that a group A streptococcus is missed. On the other hand, cultures of streptococcal carriers (including those clinically ill with nonstreptococcal pharyngitis) may exhibit large numbers of group A streptococci. This makes differentiation of acute streptococcal infection from the carrier state impossible on the basis of culture results alone. In fact, throat cultures are more precise in excluding active streptococcal pharyngitis than in confirming its presence. Nevertheless, when used in conjunction with the clinical and epidemiological evidence, throat cultures are valuable. Even if they cannot be obtained on all patients, cultures on occasional patients are useful in sharpening diagnostic skills and in supporting the clinical impression of current prevalence of streptococcal infection in the community.

Physicians who obtain throat cultures in remote areas may need a method of transport to a central laboratory. Several simple methods are available, including a dry swab or filter-paper strip which can be easily sent through the mails [19]. During the rainy season the strips should be kept and shipped in a bottle containing desiccant (e.g., silica gel).

The need for rapid and simple means of identification of group A streptococci in the upper respiratory tract has resulted in numerous techniques for antigen detection of group A streptococci. These tests most frequently are designed to identify the group-specific carbohydrate of the group A streptococcal cell wall. The techniques which have been introduced include agglutination, coagglutination, and enzyme-linked immunosorbent assay (ELISA). While the specificity of these tests is quite good (usually approaching 95 percent), their sensitivity may be much lower [4]. The reduced sensitivity appears to be related directly to the decreased amount of antigen present on the throat swab. Because of the decreased sensitivity, many have suggested that rapid tests may not be appropriate in all clinical situations. When streptococcal pharyngitis is suspected, in the face of a negative rapid antigen detection system, a simultaneous throat culture is advisable. Two other disadvantages of these rapid antigen detection systems are also ev-

ident: They fail to identify other groups of hemolytic streptococci causing pharyngitis, and they are usually more expensive than throat cultures. Both of these latter aspects are important in tropical and developing countries.

Since an increase of streptococcal antibodies does not occur for several weeks, antibody titers are of no immediate help in making a diagnosis of acute streptococcal infection. An elevated titer at the time of presentation with a positive throat culture suggests a convalescent carrier state rather than active streptococcal infection. The antistreptolysin O test remains the most widely used streptococcal antibody test. The antideoxyribonuclease B (anti-DNase B) is also widely used, as it is now commercially available. An agglutination test for determination of multiple streptococcal extracellular antibodies is commercially available, but, generally speaking, the use of this test cannot be recommended because of technical difficulties [20].

Group C and G streptococci are sometimes isolated in patients with clinical pharyngitis. Evidence of true infection is supported by the development of an antistreptolysin O response. These group C and G infections appear to be relatively common in tropical and subtropical countries [6,18]. Hemolytic streptococci of other serological groups are occasionally found in association with pharyngitis but are rarely if ever responsible for the clinical illness.

Streptococcal carriers

In tropical and subtropical as well as temperate climates, throat carriers of hemolytic streptococci are common and may persist for many months [5,6,13]. Throat carriage of group A streptococci persists as long in warm as in colder climates, but the duration of nasal carriage appears to be shorter in warm climates and the carrier strain may lose its M protein faster. These latter two factors should lessen the risk of transmission of infection [13,21]. There is an increased prevalence of group C and G streptococci in throat-culture surveys from tropical and subtropical countries.

Streptococcal carrier rates are a poor indicator of the presence or absence of active streptococcal infection within a population group. Carrier rates may be low at the beginning of an outbreak and high when the incidence of infection is declining.

OTHER INFECTIONS RELATED TO THE RESPIRATORY TRACT

Infections of other anatomical sites related to the respiratory tract generally present as suppurative complications of streptococcal sore throat but may occur independently. Group A streptococci are a frequent cause of *acute cervical adenitis* in children. In those without clinical or bacteriological evidence of throat infection, the diagnosis can be made by aspiration and culture of an inflamed lymph node or (in retrospect) by a rise in streptococcal antibody titers. Though now a rare cause of *otitis media* in developed countries, the frequency of acquisition of group A streptococci in infants and preschool children in developing subtropical countries suggests that they may be important. Patients who acquire streptococcal *sinusitis,* with or without a recognized preceding pharyngitis, are important spreaders of infection since they often disseminate large numbers of group A streptococci for long periods. *Peritonsillar abscess* may appear in patients with streptococcal pharyngitis and may require drainage by surgical incision. Anaerobes of various kinds can often be cultured from the pus obtained at surgery and may be of etiological importance. Patients with influenza or measles may develop an *interstitial* or *bronchopneumonia* of streptococcal etiology, often complicated by empyema.

ACUTE RHEUMATIC FEVER AND RHEUMATIC HEART DISEASE

Acute rheumatic fever is poorly named since it may affect many organ systems other than the joints, most importantly the heart, where it can produce permanent crippling. A curious reversal in geographical incidence and prevalence has mysteriously transferred rheumatic fever and rheumatic heart disease from the nontropical to the tropical disease category, although the recent resurgence of acute rheumatic fever in the United States has indicated the continuing possibility for the occurrence of this disease in temperate climates [22].

Traditionally rheumatic fever and rheumatic heart disease have been recognized as important medical problems of temperate climates, with little basis for inclusion in a textbook of tropical medicine. Within the past several decades, however, rheumatic heart disease and to a lesser extent acute rheumatic fever have been diagnosed with increasing frequency in semitropical and tropical countries and with generally less frequency in countries with colder climates [23,24].

The reasons for these remarkable shifts in time and location are not clear. The lessening of the problem in temperate climates cannot be fully attributed to the more frequent or more judicious employment of antimicrobial agents, since the trend began before their introduction or widespread use. A generally improved standard of living, resulting in less-crowded housing conditions and less opportunity for spread of streptococcal infection is probably an important factor. However, it is difficult to rule out other aspects of changing socioeconomic conditions and to reconcile this decline with the continuing prevalence of group A streptococci and of streptococcal pharyngitis in temperate countries. The role of socioeconomic conditions in the epidemiology of acute rheumatic fever must be carefully reexamined, especially in view of the mid-1980s resurgence of acute rheumatic fever in the United States. In several documented geographical areas, the outbreak has occurred primarily among middle class families and not among socially and economically disadvantaged populations. The reasons for this remain unclear.

Clinical reports and autopsy surveys support the view that rheumatic fever and rheumatic heart disease were in fact rare (not merely unrecognized or unconsidered) in tropical and subtropical countries in the early decades of this century [24,26]. The factors responsible for the increased prevalence of rheumatic heart disease noted in more recent years by both clinicians and pathologists in many developing tropical countries [1,2,6,23–29] are uncertain. Recently available data from some developing countries have suggested prevalence rates of rheumatic heart disease among schoolchildren of more than 5 percent [3]. The increase may be due to urbanization and industrialization associated with the movement of rural populations into crowded city slums [24,26], as occurred with immigrant and migrant populations in the northern cities of the United States early in this century. Migration may also result in overcrowded schools and in exposure to new serotypes of group A streptococci. In developing countries, the expanding population and growing number of infants and children who survive to the age of most susceptibility for rheumatic fever are factors that may ensure continuation and perhaps further increase of the rheumatic problem in the years to come [24,30].

Reports from many developing tropical or subtropical countries have stressed the severity of the rheumatic heart disease, its frequent occurrence in young children, and the appearance in rheumatic fever victims less than 20 years old of "juvenile mitral stenosis," often with no other valvular involvement and sometimes as soon as 2 to 3 years after onset of rheumatic fever [26,31–37]. In the United States and Europe mitral stenosis has usually taken 5 to 10 years to develop, and severe isolated mitral stenosis at such a young age has always been rare, even when rheumatic fever was rampant [38]. The frequent acquisition of group A streptococci during infancy and early childhood, which has been documented in some developing countries [6], may be an important determinant in the pathogenesis of rheumatic fever [39] and may contribute to the young age of onset and rapid progression of rheumatic heart disease.

Studies in temperate climates indicate that the epidemiology of rheumatic fever follows closely the epidemiology of streptococcal infections of the upper respiratory tract [13]. This relationship may be obscured in tropical countries where scarlet fever is apparently uncommon and patients with streptococcal pharyngitis rarely exhibit the full-blown classical signs associated with this infection [6,16].

Attack rates for acute rheumatic fever after streptococcal sore throat range from less than 1 percent (in children, under endemic circumstances) to 3 percent (in young military personnel, under epidemic circumstances). This difference in attack rate is probably due (at least in part) to difficulties in distinguishing true infection from the carrier state in situations where nonstreptococcal pharyngitis is common. Variations in virulence of infecting strains or in host reactions may also be contributory. The existence of "rheumatogenic" strains has been postulated [40] and requires further critical examination. The issue of possible "rheumatogenicity" has emerged in connection with the mid-1980s outbreak of acute rheumatic fever in the United States. Of importance in this regard is the fact that no "rheumatogenic factor" has ever been isolated from a group A *Streptococcus,* making this still only a hypothesis. Furthermore, data from the United States have suggested that if rheumatogenicity exists, it may not be common to all strains of a single serotype but rather only certain individual strains [11].

In patients who have had one or more previous attacks of rheumatic fever, the risk of recurrence after acquisition of a new streptococcal infection is perilously high, ranging from 15 to 50 percent. The greatest risk is in the first few years after an attack.

The latent period between the initiating streptococcal infection and the onset of rheumatic fever ranges from 1 to 5 weeks, with an average of 18 days. In Sydenham's chorea, the latent period is generally longer, 2 to 6 months.

Pathogenesis

The well-established requisites for the development of rheumatic fever include a group A streptococcus, antibody evidence of active infection, location of the infection in the upper respiratory tract, and persistence of the infecting strain for more than a few days [41].

Many hypotheses about the pathogenesis of rheumatic fever have been entertained [12b,42]. All fall short of definitive proof, which, in the absence of a well-accepted animal model, can only be obtained in humans. The existence of a latent period before the onset of rheumatic fever does not necessarily exclude the possibility of a direct effect of one of the streptococcal toxins (e.g., streptolysin O) [41], since diphtheritic carditis and neuritis may also appear days or weeks after the acquisition of infection.

Most currently popular theories propose an aberration of the immune response. Patients who develop rheumatic fever after streptococcal infection exhibit an exaggerated humoral antibody response to streptococcal antigens. Enhancement of cellular immune responses to streptococcal cell membranes has been demonstrated in patients with acute rheumatic fever [43], whereas patients with chronic rheumatic heart disease generally exhibit suppression of cellular immune responses to several extracellular products [44]. Patients with acute rheumatic fever develop a series of cross-reacting antibodies that bind to various specific mammalian tissues and to various specific components of the streptococcal cell [12c]. The possibility of a genetically determined deviation in the immune response is enhanced by the recent demonstration of a novel B-cell alloantigen frequently found in rheumatic fever patients [45].

The current consensus is that the pathogenetic mechanism(s) responsible for the development of acute rheumatic fever is the result of a complex interaction between the human host and the bacteria. Although "rheumatogenicity" has not been documented, there is epidemiological evidence to suggest that certain serotypes are more frequently isolated from patients with rheumatic fever than are others. This is especially true, for example, with serotypes which commonly cause skin infection; these serotypes rarely are isolated from or associated with patients with rheumatic fever.

The role of the human host in rheumatic fever susceptibility remains a puzzle. A number of possible factors have been described. For example, data have been presented suggesting that B-cell alloantigens present on lymphocytes may be a marker indicating rheumatic susceptibility [45]. It has been suggested that these markers may indicate the fact that these lymphocytes process streptococcal antigens in an abnormal fashion. Although patients with rheumatic fever and/or rheumatic heart disease appear to have this B-cell alloantigen present more frequently than do nonrheumatics, this remains an hypothesis and requires further and more specific confirmation [46].

Most likely, there is a relationship between certain strains of streptococci and certain individuals which requires both factors to be present in order to cause rheumatic fever. The absence of an animal model makes precise definition of the importance of these various factors impossible except in studies of the human host.

Diagnosis of acute rheumatic fever

Difficulties in definition and diagnosis are inescapable in a polymorphic disease without a confirmatory laboratory test. For almost 40 years the Jones criteria have been helpful in alleviating but not solving these problems. The importance of a careful physical examination is emphasized by the fact that all of the major criteria (polyarthritis, carditis, chorea, erythema marginatum, and subcutaneous nodules) depend upon critical documentation of physical findings. The validity of the minor criteria is mostly dependent upon the reliability of the history (previous rheumatic fever or rheumatic heart disease, arthralgia, fever) and upon the dependability and the interpretation of laboratory tests (evidence of an active inflammatory process by an increased erythrocyte sedimentation rate, the presence of C-reactive protein or leukocytosis, prolonged PR interval). A diagnosis based on two major criteria is stronger than a diagnosis based on one major and two minor criteria. Polyarthritis as the sole major criterion is especially suspect since it can occur in a wide variety of diseases.

In developing countries with tropical or subtropical climates, the frequency of severe carditis and the infrequency of well-documented polyarthritis and other major criteria has led some observers to question the validity of the Jones criteria. Some of these reported differences in the spectrum of manifestations seem to be due to factors in patient selection, difficulties in retrospective documentation of findings, and failure to separate recurrent from first attacks [47]. Studies in Egypt have indicated that the Jones criteria are a reliable approach to the diagnosis of rheumatic fever in that country [6].

The revised Jones criteria [48a,b] have added a new requirement for diagnosis of rheumatic fever: evidence of a recent streptococcal infection (scarlet fever, elevated antistreptolysin O or other streptococcal antibodies, positive throat culture for group A streptococci). This requirement decreases the possibility of including patients with illnesses that mimic rheumatic fever. However, the Egyptian studies suggest that when streptococcal antibodies are not available, a reasonably reliable differentiation can still be made by strict adherence to the other criteria [6]. Due to the long latent period, it is more difficult to demonstrate an elevated streptococcal antibody test in patients with Sydenham's chorea, but this can often be achieved by performing antibody tests for several different streptococcal antigens.

Frequently it is difficult to make a diagnosis of acute rheumatic fever in tropical countries because of the many other conditions which may be confused with rheumatic fever. A Study Group of the World Health Organization has recently recommended modifications in the Jones criteria. In three categories, diagnosis of rheumatic fever can be accepted in the absence of two major or one major and two minor manifestations of the Jones criteria. These are chorea, insidious or late-onset carditis, and rheumatic occurrence in a well-established patient with rheumatic heart disease [3].

Among the available streptococcal antibody tests [19], the antistreptolysin O (ASO) and the antideoxyribonuclease B (anti-DNase B) are the most useful and most reproducible. An elevated single titer, or more assuredly a rise of at least two dilution increments in serial sera examined simultaneously, provides serological support of streptococcal infection. For reliable interpretation, the distribution of titers by age in the local population must be known and taken into consideration. The streptozyme test, though simple to perform, has problems in interpretation and in comparability of different lots of the complex reagent [49].

Prognosis of acute rheumatic fever

Few patients die during the first attack of rheumatic fever. Evidence of cardiac involvement may disappear during the acute attack or over a period of 5 to 10 years, especially if compliance for secondary prophylaxis is excellent [50]. The long-term prognosis is greatly enhanced by continuous antimicrobial prophylaxis against recurrent attacks [48b, see below also] and by appropriate antibiotic protection against endocarditis at the time of dental procedures or surgery of infected or contaminated tissues [48c].

STREPTOCOCCAL SKIN INFECTIONS

Erysipelas is a superficial, rapidly spreading skin lesion with a raised erythematous border. It is usually associated with group A streptococci, although other bacteria (e.g., pneumococci, staphylococci) occasionally produce erysipelas-like lesions. The disease occurs in tropical as well as temperate climates [16].

Staphylococci and streptococci are the bacterial agents commonly found in *pyoderma* and *impetigo* [51]. Bullous impetigo, caused by phage group II staphylococci, produces a thin varnishlike crust upon rupture and can be differentiated on clinical grounds from impetigo in which hemolytic streptococci are the primary agent.

Streptococcal impetigo (usually group A but occasionally C or G) is an infection of the epidermis which is vesicular or pustular in its early stages but rapidly becomes thickly crusted. Within a few days staphylococci frequently appear as secondary invaders, and they may overgrow group A steptococci in nonselective culture media. For some days or weeks before impetiginous lesions develop, group A streptococci can frequently be found on the normal skin (but not in the upper respiratory tract). Some days or weeks after the appearance of skin lesions the pyodermal strain often migrates to the upper respiratory tract but rarely produces clinical pharyngitis at this secondary site [51,52].

The serological classification (M type or T pattern) of pyoderma- or impetigo-associated group A streptococci is generally different from that of strains producing infection of the upper respiratory tract [51,53]. A few of the pyodermal types appear to be able to produce infection of the upper respiratory tract without evidence of skin infection.

A number of other striking differences between streptococcal infections of the throat and skin have been noted [51]. The antistreptolysin O response is generally muted in patients with streptococcal impetigo or pyoderma, apparently due to a natural inhibitor (free cholesterol) in the epidermis [54], whereas responses of other streptococcal antibodies (anti-DNase B and antihyaluronidase) are similar to those occurring after streptococcal pharyngitis.

Skin and wound infections have long been recognized as a common problem in tropical countries, but the frequency of group A streptococci as the initiating bacterial pathogen has not been fully appreciated until recent years [5,6,55,56]. Hot humid weather and poor hygiene appear to be important determinants of infection [57,58]. In addition to more superficial lesions, deep-seated ulcers (ecthyma or ''jungle sores''), usually on the lower extremities, may occur in wet tropical environments. These commonly yield group A streptococci as well as staphylococci on culture [59]. Recent studies have suggested that the rapid antigen detection kits for group A streptococci may have a higher sensitivity when used in the diagnosis of streptococcal pyoderma than when used for the detection of group A streptococci in the upper respiratory tract.

This may be due to larger amounts of group A streptococcal antigen present in the skin lesions.

ACUTE GLOMERULONEPHRITIS

Acute nephritis is a common problem in tropical and subtropical countries and may occur in epidemics or in epidemic waves [60,61].

Acute glomerulonephritis develops with approximately equal frequency (10 to 15 percent) after infection with a nephritogenic strain, regardless of whether the streptococcal infection occurs in the skin or in the upper respiratory tract [51]. The epidemiology of the renal complication is determined to a large extent by the epidemiology of the initiating infection.

Strains of group A streptococci associated with acute nephritis (nephritogenic strains) are limited to certain serological types which differ according to the site of infection (Table 86-1) [51,53,61]. The latent period for pyoderma-associated nephritis is much longer (generally 3 weeks) than the latent period for pharyngitis-associated nephritis (about 10 days). The increased proportion of males with acute nephritis appears to be greater in patients with pharyngitis-associated than in those with pyoderma-associated renal disease.

The pathogenic mechanism for the development of acute poststreptococcal glomerulonephritis is not known [12d]. The demonstration that immune complexes occur with equal frequency in patients with acute rheumatic fever and in those with acute nephritis have raised questions about the role of these complexes in the pathogenesis of acute nephritis [62]. A unique extracellular product of nephritogenic strains may be involved in the pathogenesis of acute nephritis [63].

Edema and hematuria are classical presenting complaints of patients with acute glomerulonephritis. Headache is common, and some patients present with or develop convulsions. Hypertension is often present, and signs of heart failure are occasionally found.

The urine of patients with acute nephritis is usually brown rather than bright red in color. Red cells and red cell casts can be identified most often in fresh specimens. Leukocytes and epithelial cells may also be present, but clean-catch quantitative urine cultures should show insignificant bacterial colony counts. The urine volume is reduced, and some patients may become anuric before diuresis begins.

Serum complement levels are typically decreased, but the low level may be missed depending on the timing of the specimen. Anemia is due to increased blood volume; transfusion to correct anemia is contraindicated since it may precipitate heart failure. Blood urea nitrogen is often elevated. Chest films may show cardiac enlargement, with or without congestive pulmonary changes.

Streptococcal antibodies furnish evidence of a recent streptococcal infection. The anti-DNase B or the antihyaluronidase titer may be a better indicator than the antistreptolysin O titer in patients with pyoderma-associated nephritis [51,53]. Group

Table 86-1. Nephritogenic M types of group A streptococci

	Pharyngitis-associated	Pyoderma-associated
Classical	12*	49
Other definite	2,3,4,25,49	2,55,57,60
Possible	6	31,52,56,59,61

* Numbers refer to M types.

Source: From [51,53,61].

A streptococci of known nephritogenic types may be isolated from the patient or from close contacts.

The prognosis is good, especially in young children who often show abnormalities in Addis counts for months but rarely develop chronic renal disease. The outlook for adults is controversial. A significant percent do develop chronic nephritis, notably after an apparent episode of endemic rather than epidemic nephritis, but it is generally difficult to rule out the possibility of preexisting renal disease.

OTHER STREPTOCOCCAL INFECTIONS

The range of infections which may be caused by streptococci is so extraordinarily broad that the clinician must constantly keep these organisms in mind (Table 86-2). For example, in tropical countries chronic streptococcal infection of lymphatic channels is frequently associated with *Filariasis (elephantiasis)* [64], see also Chap. 48.

Table 86-2. Unexpected places and guises in which streptococci may be found

Fulminating septicemia	Purpura fulminans
Newborn infants (also meningitis)	Nosocomial infections
Postpartum women (puerperal sepsis)	Foodborne epidemics
Leukemias	Perianal carriers
Solid tumors	Perianal cellulitis
Collagen diseases	Vaginitis (especially children)
Immunologically depressed patients	Omphalitis (newborn infants)
Burns	Varicella (septic complications)
Operative wounds	Streptococcal fever ("streptococcosis")
Gangrene (often fatal)	
Complications of infections of thumb	Osteomyelitis (especially infants)
Subpectoral abscesses	Hand-foot syndrome
Pleural effusion	Blistering distal dactylitis
Disseminated intravascular coagulopathy	

Source: Modified from L.W. Wannamaker, P. Ferrieri, *Streptococcal Infections—Updated. Disease-a-Month,* Chicago, Year Book Medical Publishers, October 1975, pp. 1–40. Used by permission.

Puerperal fever, a serious infection usually caused by group A streptococci, has declined in frequency but may still be a relatively common problem in developing countries. *Infections of burns* and *postsurgical wound infections* due to group A streptococci are a hazard throughout the world and may be transmitted nosocomially by medical personnel, including *anal carriers.* Outbreaks of group A streptococcal sepsis in *hospital nurseries* are infrequent but life-threatening when they occur.

Group B streptococcal infections have emerged as a major cause of neonatal sepsis and meningitis, notably in certain parts of the United States [65]. Apparently with few exceptions [66], they have not been identified as a major problem in developing or tropical countries.

Groups C and G streptococci have been seen more frequently as a cause of septicemia and other serious life-threatening infections. This is true both in temperate as well as in tropical countries. As mentioned previously, other streptococci (e.g., *S. suis*) have also proved to be important causes of serious and life-threatening infections in humans [7].

TREATMENT

Penicillin is the drug of choice for treatment of group A streptococcal infections. No strains resistant to penicillin by in vitro testing have been identified. Occasional strains of group B streptococci are moderately resistant to penicillin. Rare patients with neonatal meningitis who are responding poorly or slowly to penicillin have apparently improved after the addition of an aminoglycoside such as gentamicin. Group D streptococci are usually resistant to penicillin and require treatment with ampicillin or with penicillin plus an aminoglycoside such as gentamicin.

In patients with streptococcal sore throat or other infections of the upper respiratory tract, the goal should be to eradicate the infecting strain, which is required for the prevention of acute rheumatic fever [67]. To achieve this goal, 10 days of oral penicillin V therapy (250 mg three or four times a day) or a single intramuscular injection of benzathine penicillin G (600,000 to 1,200,000 U depending upon whether the patient weighs more or less than 27 kg) has been recommended [48b]. Erythromycin [250 mg four times a day for older children and adults, 40 mg/(kg·day) in younger children] is the drug of choice in patients sensitive to penicillin. Sulfonamides and tetracyclines should not be used for treating streptococcal infections.

Bacteriological treatment failures remain important in some populations. Some studies reveal the persistence of group A streptococci in as high as 20 percent or more of patients following treatment with oral penicillin even though a group A β-hemolytic *Streptococcus* resistant to penicillin has never been described. Several possible explanations for treatment failures have been proposed. These include antibiotic tolerance, the presence of β-lactamase–producing organisms in normal upper respiratory tract flora, and the group A streptococcal

carrier state [68–70]. It must be emphasized, though, that at the present time, penicillin remains the treatment of choice for streptococcal infections because it is widely available and inexpensive. Multiple attempts to eradicate the carrier state are not always warranted, except in high-risk individuals (e.g., from rheumatic families).

Impetigo that is limited to a few lesions can often be treated by removal of crusts and by use of soaps and antibiotic ointments. More extensive lesions may require oral or systemic antibiotics. A single intramuscular injection of benzathine penicillin G has been advocated and may provide protection against recurrence for several weeks [71]. Improvement in skin and environmental hygiene is important in reducing the possibility of recurrence. There is no evidence that antimicrobial treatment lowers the risk of nephritis in patients with established pyoderma or impetigo, and it often is initiated too late to prevent this complication in family contacts.

Acute rheumatic fever without carditis can usually be managed quite well with aspirin. However, individuals with Sydenham's chorea may require other forms of medication and careful neurological follow-up. Steroids are generally used in patients with significant carditis, although the ability of these drugs to prevent the development of rheumatic heart disease has never been fully established.

PREVENTION

Continuous penicillin or sulfonamide prophylaxis is an important aspect of management of patients who have had rheumatic fever or who present with rheumatic heart disease. The most effective protection is achieved with intramuscular benzathine penicillin G (1.2 MU) injected monthly [48b]. In compliant patients, oral prophylaxis may be used (sulfadiazine, 0.5 g once daily for patients under 60 lb (27 kg) and 1 g daily in patients over 60 lb (27 kg); penicillin, 200,000 to 250,000 U twice daily).

Recent recommendations in a number of tropical countries have suggested that it is more effective if intramuscular benzathine penicillin G is given every 3 weeks rather than every 4 weeks. Recently the World Health Organization suggested the use of 4-weekly injections except in instances when the patient is at considerably higher risk [3].

Patients with rheumatic heart disease should be given appropriate antimicrobial prophylaxis at the time of dental extraction or surgical procedures. This has been shown to reduce the frequency of bacteremia and therefore probably lessens the risk of developing bacterial endocarditis [48c]. It should be emphasized that in those patients receiving penicillin, especially oral penicillin for secondary rheumatic fever prophylaxis, penicillin is inappropriate for bacterial endocarditis prophylaxis.

In patients with acute glomerulonephritis, restriction of fluids to avoid overload, control of hypertension, and treatment of heart failure are important aspects of management. There is no evidence that long-term antimicrobial prophylaxis is of benefit in patients with acute nephritis, because the number of potentially nephritogenic serotypes of group A streptococci is rather small. However, no controlled studies have been carried out which document this point.

Since it is clear that antibiotics have not been successful in eliminating the problems of group A streptococcal infections and their complications, interest continues in the development of a streptococcal vaccine. An effective and safe vaccine would have to include M antigens for at least a majority of the prevalent M types, which may change from time to time, especially under the pressures of an immune population. Attempts to define the molecular structure of the M proteins and to produce highly purified preparations may eventually result in such a vaccine, but current approaches to control of group A streptococcal infections are dependent upon the judicious use of antimicrobial agents.

Recent research has shown more precisely the epitopes of the M protein which may be protective against subsequent streptococcal infections and therefore provide an important basis for future development of a vaccine. However, the issue of whether or not all strains are rheumatogenic must first be determined and settled, as there are more than 80 serotypes of group A streptococci and making such a vaccine may prove a formidable task.

In some tropical and developing countries, one other approach which has been proposed but never tested is a "sledgehammer" approach. Using this technique, patients with pharyngitis would be treated with penicillin whether or not a throat culture or rapid test was done. Others have suggested that the prevalence of streptococci in a pediatric population can be reduced by treating all patients at the beginning of that season of the year when streptococcal infections are more prevalent. The efficacy of these methods in preventing rheumatic fever has never been documented.

REFERENCES

1 Agarwal BL: Rheumatic heart disease unabated in developing countries. Lancet ii:910–911, 1981

*2 Anonymous: Community control of rheumatic heart disease in developing countries: I. A major public health problem. WHO Chron 34:336–345, 1980

3 World Health Organization: Rheumatic Fever and Rheumatic Heart Disease. Tech Rep Ser 764. Geneva, World Health Organization, 1988

4 Kaplan EL: The rapid identification of group A beta hemolytic streptococci in the upper respiratory tract. Ped Clin North Am 35: 535–542, 1988

5 Ogunbi O, Fadahunsi HO, Ahmed I, et al: An epidemiological study of rheumatic fever and rheumatic heart disease in Lagos. J Epid Commun Health 32:68–71, 1978

*These articles or symposia are a review of the literature.

6 El Kholy AM: Streptococcal infections and rheumatic fever in Egypt, in Read SE and Zabriskie JB (eds): *Streptococcal Diseases and the Immune Response.* pp 811–822, 1980

7 Chau PY, Huang CY, Kay R: *Streptococcus suis* meningitis: An important underdiagnosed disease in Hong Kong. Med J Aust 1:414–417, 1983

8 Johnson DR, Kaplan EL: A micro-technique for serum opacity factor characterization of group A streptococci adaptable to the use of human sera. J Clin Micro 26:2025–2030, 1988

9 Manjula BN, Fischetti VA: Tropomyosin-like seven residue periodicity in three immunologically distinct streptococcal M proteins and its implications for the antiphagocytic property of the molecule. J Exp Med 151:695–708, 1980

10 Beachey EH, Ofek I: Epithelial cell binding of group A streptococci by lipoteichoic acid on fimbriae denuded of M protein. J Exp Med 143:759–771, 1976

11 Kaplan EL, Johnson DR, Cleary PP: Group A streptococcal serotypes isolated from patients and sibling contacts during the mid-1980s resurgence of rheumatic fever in the United States. J Infect Dis 159:101–103, 1989

12 Wannamaker LW, Matsen JM (eds): *Streptococci and Streptococcal Diseases.* New York, Academic, 1972

12a Krause RM: The streptococcal cell: Relationship of structure to function and pathogenesis, pp 3–18

12b McCarty M: Theories of pathogenesis of streptococcal complications, pp 517–526

12c Ayoub EM: Cross-reacting antibodies in the pathogenesis of rheumatic myocardial and valvular disease, pp 451–464

12d Michael AF, Hoyer JR, Westberg NG, et al: Experimental models for the pathogenesis of acute poststreptococcal glomerulonephritis, pp 481–500

13 Rammelkamp CH Jr: Epidemiology of streptococcal infections. Harvey Lecture Series, Series LI, pp 113–142, 1957

14 Taylor PJ, McDonald MA: Milkborne streptococcal sore throat. A study of 835 cases. Lancet i:330–333, 1959

15 McCormick JB, Kay D, Hayes P, et al: Epidemic streptococcal sore throat following a community picnic. JAMA 236:1039–1041, 1976

16 Stransky E, Felix NS: Does scarlet fever exist in the tropics? Ann Paediatrici 177:15–20, 1951

17 Wannamaker LW: Perplexity and precision in the diagnosis of streptococcal pharyngitis. Am J Dis Child 124:352–358, 1972

18 Koshi G, Jadhav M, Myers RM: Streptococcal pharyngitis in children. Indian J Med Res 58:161–167, 1970

19 Rotta J, Facklam RR: Manual of microbiological diagnostic methods for streptococcal infections and their sequelae. World Health Organization publication, WHO/BAC/80. 1, pp 1–70

20 Editorial: Evaluation of the streptozyme test for streptococcal antibodies. Bull WHO 64:504–505, 1986

21 Krause RM, Rammelkamp CH Jr, Denny FW Jr, et al: Studies of the carrier state following infection with group A streptococci. I. Effect of climate. J Clin Invest 41:568–574, 1962

22 Kaplan EL, Markowitz M: The fall and rise of rheumatic fever in the United States: A commentary. Int J Cardiol 21:3–10, 1988

23 Shaper AG: Cardiovascular disease in the tropics—I, Rheumatic heart. Br Med J 3:683–686, 1972

24 Markowitz M: Observations on the epidemiology and preventability of rheumatic fever in developing countries. *Clin Ther,* 4: 240–251, 1981

25 Clarke JT, Late MO, Perak HO: The geographic distribution of rheumatic fever. J Trop Med Hyg 33:249–258, 1930

26 Sarrouy C, Sendra L, Duboucher G: Considerations on the evolution of heart diseases in Algeria. Am Heart J 61:145–148, 1961

27 Shrestha NK, Padmavati S: Prevalence of rheumatic heart disease in Delhi school children. Indian J Med Res 69:821–833, 1979

28 Hutt MSR: Cardiac pathology in the tropics, in Pomerance A, Davies MJ (eds): *The Pathology of the Heart,* Blackwell, Oxford, 1975, chap 18, pp 551–531

29 Strasser T: Rheumatic fever and rheumatic heart disease in the 1970s. WHO Chron 32:18–25, 1978

30 Krause RM: The influence of infection on the geography of heart disease. Circulation 60:972–976, 1979

31 Roy SB, Bhatia ML, Lazaro EJ, et al: Juvenile mitral stenosis in India. Lancet ii:1193–1196, 1963

32 Abdin ZH, Eissa A: Rheumatic fever and rheumatic heart disease in children below the age of 5 years in the tropics. Ann Rheum Dis 24:389–391, 1965

33 Al-Bahrani IR, Thamer MA, Al-Omeri MM, et al: Rheumatic heart disease in the young in Iraq. Br Heart J 28:824–828, 1966

34 D'Arbela PG, Patel AK, Somers K: Juvenile rheumatic fever and rheumatic heart disease at Mulago Hospital, Kampala, Uganda. East Afr Med J 51:710–714, 1976

35 Ayutha PSN, Ratanabanangkoon K, Pongpanich B: Juvenile rheumatic fever and rheumatic heart disease at Rheumatic Hospital, Thailand. Southeast Asian J Trop Med Public Health 1:77–80, 1976

36 Smith WM: An appraisal of rheumatic valvular disease in Western Samoa. Aust NZ J Med 9:560–565, 1979

37 Robinson RD Jr, Suttana AS, Abbasi AS, et al: Acute rheumatic fever in Karachi, Pakistan. Am J Cardiol 18:548–551, 1966

38 Bland EF, White PD, Jones TD: The development of mitral stenosis in young people. Am Heart J 10:995–1004, 1935

39 Matanoski GM, Price WH, Ferencz C: Epidemiology of streptococcal infections in rheumatic and non-rheumatic families. II. The inter-relationship of streptococcal infections to age, family transmission and type of group A. Am J Epidemiol 87:190–206, 1968

40 Bisno AL: The concept of rheumatogenic and nonrheumatogenic group A streptococci, in Read SE, Zabriskie JB (eds): *Streptococcal Diseases and the Immune Response,* New York, Academic, 1980, pp 789–803

41 Wannamaker LW: The chain that links the heart to the throat. Circulation 48:9–18, 1973

42 Markowitz M, Gordis L: *Rheumatic Fever.* Philadelphia, Saunders, 1972

43 Read SE, Fischetti VA, Utermohlen V, et al: Cellular reactivity studies to streptococcal antigens. Migration inhibition studies in patients with streptococcal infections and rheumatic fever. J Clin Invest 54:439–450, 1974

44 Gray ED, Wannamaker LW, Ayoub EM, et al: Cellular immune responses to extracellular streptococcal products in rheumatic heart disease. J Clin Invest 68:665–671, 1981

45 Patarroyo ME, Winchester RJ, Vejerano A, et al: Association of a B-cell alloantigen with susceptibility to rheumatic fever. Nature 278:173–174, 1979

46 Gray ED, Regelmann WE, Abdin Z, et al: Compartmentalization of cells bearing ''rheumatic'' cell surface antigens in peripheral blood and tonsils in rheumatic heart disease. J Infect Dis 155:247–252, 1987

47 Sanyal SK, Thapar MK, Ahmed SH, et al: The initial attack of acute rheumatic fever during childhood in North India. A prospective study of the clinical profile. Circulation 49:7–12, 1974

48a American Heart Association Committee Report: Jones criteria (revised) for guidance in the diagnosis of rheumatic fever. Circulation 69:203A–208A, 1984

48b American Heart Association Report: Prevention of rheumatic fever. Circulation 78:1082–1086, 1988

48c American Heart Association Report: Prevention of endocarditis. Circulation 70:1123A–1127A, 1984

49 Kaplan EL, Kunde C: Quantitative evaluation of variation in composition of the streptozyme agglutination reagent for detection of antibodies to group A streptococcal extracellular antigens. J Clin Microbiol 14:678–680, 1981

50 Tompkins D, Boxerbaum B, Liebman J, et al: Long-term prognosis of rheumatic fever patients receiving regular intramuscular benzathine penicillin. Circulation 45:543–551, 1972

51 Wannamaker LW: Differences between streptococcal infections of the throat and of the skin. N Engl J Med 282:23–31; 78–85, 1970

52 Ferrieri P, Dajani AS, Wannamaker LW, et al: Natural history of impetigo. I. Site sequence of acquisition and familial patterns of spread of cutaneous streptococci. J Clin Invest 51:2851–2862, 1972

53 Dillon HC Jr: Post-streptococcal glomerulonephritis following pyoderma. Rev Infect Dis 1:935–943, 1979

54 Kaplan EL, Wannamaker LW: Suppression of the antistreptolysin O response by cholesterol and by lipid extracts of rabbit skin. J Exp Med 144:754–767, 1976

55 Markham NP, Stenhouse AC: A bacteriological investigation of wound infections in Rarotonga, Cook Islands. Trans R Soc Trop Med Hyg 53:404–409, 1959

56 Allen AM, Taplin D: Skin infections in Eastern Panama. Survey of two representative communities. Am J Trop Med Hyg 23:950–956, 1974

57 Taplin D, Lansdell L, Allen AM, et al: Prevalence of streptococcal pyoderma in relation to climate and hygiene. Lancet ii:501–503, 1973

58 Mehta G, Prakash K, Sharma KB: Streptococcal pyoderma and acute glomerulonephritis in children. Indian J Med Res 71:692–700, 1980

59 Allen AM, Taplin D, Twigg L: Cutaneous streptococcal infections in Vietnam. Arch Dermatol 104:271–280, 1971

60 Lasch EE, Frankel V, Vardy PA, et al: Epidemic glomerulonephritis in Israel. J Infect Dis 124:141–147, 1971

61 Potter EV, Ortiz JS, Sharrett AR, et al: Changing types of nephritogenic streptococci in Trinidad. J Clin Invest 50:1197–1205, 1971

62 Van de Rijn I, Fillit H, Brandeis WE, et al: Serial studies on circulating immune complexes in poststreptococcal sequelae. Clin Exp Immunol 34:318–325, 1978

63 Villarreal H Jr, Fischetti VA, Van de Rijn I, et al: The occurrence of a protein in the extracellular products of streptococci isolated from patients with acute glomerulonephritis. J Exp Med 149:459–472, 1979

64 Yu-K'un L, Shu-Chen H, Tze-Ying T: The role of streptococcal infections in filariasis. Chin Med J 83:17–22, 1964

65 Anthony BF, Okada DM: The emergence of group B streptococci in infections of the newborn infant. Ann Rev Med 28:355–369, 1977

66 Chow KK, Tay L, Lam C: Prospective study of group A streptococcal colonization in parturient mothers and their infants. Ann Acad Med (Singapore) 10:79–83, 1981

67 Cantanzaro FJ, Rammelkamp CH Jr, Chamovitz R; Prevention of rheumatic fever by treatment of streptococcal infections. II. Factors responsible for failures. N Engl J Med 259:51–57, 1958

68 Kaplan EL, Gastanaduy AS, Huwe BB: The role of the carrier in treatment failures after antibiotic therapy for group A streptococci in the upper respiratory tract. J Clin Med 98:326–335, 1981

69 Kims KS, Kaplan EL: The association of penicillin tolerance with failure to eradicate group A streptococci from patients with pharyngitis. J Pediatr 107:681–686, 1985

70 Brook I, Pazzaglin G, Coolbaugh JC, et al: *In vivo* protection of group A beta-hemolytic streptococci from penicillin by beta-lactamase producing *Bacteroides* species. Antimicrob Chemother 12:599–606, 1983

71 Dillon HC Jr: The treatment of streptococcal skin infections. J Pediatr 76:676–684, 1970

C H A P T E R 87 / *Tuberculosis* · Thomas M. Daniel · S. P. Tripathy

Tuberculosis is a disease which has been of major importance for humankind throughout history. Today tuberculosis has been largely controlled in North America, Europe, and other technologically advanced regions. Nevertheless, it remains a leading cause of death and disability in most of the world. Tuberculosis is caused by *Mycobacterium tuberculosis,* a slowly growing acid-fast-staining bacillus which is transmitted from person to person via the aerial route. Disease develops only in about 5 percent of those infected and may follow primary infection by many years. A chronic and wasting infection with a high mortality rate in the absence of treatment, it afflicts primarily young adults. Exquisite cellular hypersensitivity mediated by T lymphocytes follows infection with *M. tuberculosis,* and the tubercle or granuloma formation which is the central feature of this hypersensitivity is the major determinant of the pathogenesis of tuberculosis. Thus, the evolution of disease depends primarily upon the immune status of the host. The presence of tuberculin hypersensitivity is readily recognized by tuberculin skin testing.

Tuberculosis may be effectively treated with a variety of drugs, of which isoniazid and rifampin (rifampicin) are the most effective. Infected but not yet diseased persons may be protected by the prophylactic administration of isoniazid. Public health measures for the control of tuberculosis depend heavily upon identifying and treating all infectious persons. In high prevalence areas vaccination with bacillus Calmette-Guérin (BCG) may be of value.

PARASITE

Tuberculosis is caused by *M. tuberculosis,* a bacillus first identified by Robert Koch, whose name is often attached to this organism and whose elegant and pioneering study [*1*] set the standard which has persisted to this day for the proof of bacteriological etiology of any disease. There are more than 30 recognized species in the genus *Mycobacterium* [*2*]. While most do not produce disease, others are important human pathogens. Within some of the species of mycobacteria it has been possible to recognize multiple distinct serotypes [*3*]. Additionally, there are many other mycobacteria, principally soil and water organisms, which have not yet been classified. In this chapter principal attention is given to tuberculosis, but other mycobacterial diseases will also be considered briefly. Table 87-1 summarizes the principal pathogenic mycobacteria and the diseases they produce.

Members of the genus *Mycobacterium* are characterized by their resistance to decolorizing, after staining, with strong mineral acid solutions. They are aerobic organisms with simple growth requirements. Many mycobacteria, including most pathogenic species, are slowly growing, with generation times approximating 20 to 24 h. Several weeks are required for primary isolation by culture. Characteristic of the genus is the presence of complex mycolic acid–containing lipids on the cell surface. Some of these lipids may be important to the biology of mycobacteria and the pathogenesis of disease which they produce because of their ability to inhibit phagosomal lysosomal fusion, thus facilitating the intracellular survival of mycobacteria within macrophages.

Mycobacteria do not contain or secrete toxins. However, they do contain a number of substances with significant biological activity. Both cell walls and cytoplasm contain many antigens, some species specific and others widely shared among microorganisms [*4*]. Hypersensitivity to these antigens is of major importance in the pathogenesis of tuberculosis. Importantly, the mycobacterial cell wall contains major adjuvant substances which potentiate immune responses to a wide variety of antigens. Figure 87-1 illustrates the monomeric

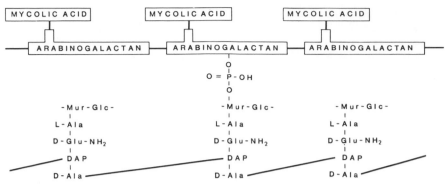

Figure 87-1. Molecular structure of the mycobacterial cell wall as proposed by Lederer [5]. Complex mycolic acid lipids are esterified to arabinogalactan, probably at an arabinose side chain. Phosphodiester linkages unite arabinogalactan to underlying muramyl peptides, such linkages probably occurring at approximately every tenth repeating arabinogalactan unit. Muramic acid-L-alanine-D-glutamic acid (MDP) is the minimal unit containing adjuvant activity. Abbreviations: Mur = muramic acid; Glc = glucosamine; Ala = alanine; Glu-NH$_2$ = glutamic acid; DAP = diaminopimelic acid. *(From T.M. Daniel, in G.P. Kubica, L.G. Wayne (eds.): The Mycobacteria—A Sourcebook, Marcel Dekker, New York, 1982.)*

structure of the mycobacterial cell wall as proposed by Lederer [5]. The arabinogalactan together with the peptide phosphodiesterified to it is a potent water-soluble adjuvant. In fact,

Table 87-1. Principal species of mycobacteria which are pathogenic for humans and the human disease syndromes produced by these organisms

Organism	Natural habitat	Principal clinical disease syndromes
M. tuberculosis	Humans	Tuberculosis
M. bovis	Cattle	Tuberculosis
M. avium	Animals, water, soil	Chronic pulmonary disease, lymphadenitis, disseminated disease in AIDS patients
M. scrofulaceum	Soil, water	Lymphadenitis in children
M. simiae	Animals	Chronic pulmonary disease
M. kansasii	Probably water	Chronic pulmonary disease, lymphadenitis in children
M. xenopi	Probably water	Chronic pulmonary disease
M. szulgai	Unknown	Chronic pulmonary disease
M. ulcerans	Unknown	Buruli (Bairnsdale) ulcer
M. marinum	Water	Swimming pool granuloma and other chronic skin granulomas
M. fortuitum-chelonei	Soil	Wound abscess
M. leprae	Humans	Leprosy

muramyl dipeptide (MDP) consisting of the *N*-acetylmuramyl-L-alanyl-D-isoglutamine moiety is by itself a potent adjuvant and is probably the minimal chemical structure with adjuvant properties. Affinity-chromatography-purified cell wall arabinogalactan has in vitro immunosuppressive properties [6], probably expressed via stimulation of suppressor monocytes.

Mycobacteria can be recognized by direct staining in sputum or other specimens. In the classical Ziehl-Neelson technique a thick smear of sputum is gently heat-fixed on a microscope slide. Alternatively, the sediment from sputum concentrated for culture may be used. Sputum may also be concentrated by digestion with household bleach followed by centrifugation, but this method renders the sample unsuitable for culture. The slide is then flooded with carbol-fuchsin stain and gently warmed to steaming with a flame for 3 min, more stain being added if necessary. The slide is then rinsed and decolorized exhaustively with a solution of 3% concentrated hydrochloric acid in 95% ethanol. Subsequently the slide is counterstained with methylene blue or brilliant green. Alternatively, Kinyoun's modification [7] uses stain containing a detergent and allows staining without heat. After staining the specimen is examined carefully using the oil immersion lens of a light microscope. Mycobacteria are stained brilliant red and may be further recognized by their characteristic appearance as thin curved rods, frequently beaded, often appearing in pairs or small clusters, sometimes linked end-to-end. The numbers of tubercle bacilli in sputum are usually small. Conscientious and prolonged search must be made before a specimen is judged to be negative.

Acid-fast staining using rhodamine-auramine fluorescent dye is also available, but a fluorescent microscope is required for reading these smears. Because of the brilliance of the fluorescence, smears thus stained may be scanned under lower magnification, thus facilitating rapid examination.

Mycobacteria may be grown on a variety of media suitable for clinical use. Most pathogenic species grow slowly, and consequently many weeks may elapse before the results of cultures are available to the clinician. The identification of individual species of mycobacteria is based on multiple cultural and cytochemical characteristics. A rapid spot test for the production of niacin is especially useful because only *M. tuberculosis, M. simiae,* and a few strains of *M. marinum* are positive. However, the niacin test cannot be performed until a sufficient growth of the cultivated organisms has taken place.

PATIENT

PATHOGENESIS

Tuberculous infection today is transmitted almost entirely by the aerial route. The control of bovine tuberculosis in many areas of the world where it once existed or where significant quantities of cow's milk are consumed has rendered this orally transmitted infection unimportant. Only a minority of patients with tuberculosis are infectious to others [8]. These persons aerosolize bacilli as droplet nuclei while coughing, speaking, singing, or otherwise forcibly expelling air from the respiratory tract. Droplets evaporate quickly, leaving desiccated bacilli which are extremely light and settle only very slowly after being suspended in the air. Although mycobacteria resist desiccation, they are rapidly killed by ultraviolet light, including open daylight, so that transmission of tuberculosis is almost always an indoor event. This is a major factor in the family clustering of tuberculosis. Tubercle bacilli in fomites, settled from the air and trapped in dust, are no longer infectious because they are not ordinarily reaerosolized as respirable particles. The premises and personal effects of infectious patients therefore, do not constitute a hazard to others [9]. Once patients are treated with effective antituberculous drug therapy, they rapidly become noninfectious, with drug killing and diminution of cough both being important factors. This, combined with the fact that most susceptible contacts have already been infected at the time of diagnosis of the index case, explains why isolation of patients does not alter the amount of tuberculosis occurring subsequently in their family contacts [10].

Probably no more than a very few bacilli reach the pulmonary air spaces to establish a primary tuberculous infection. The site of such an infection is determined primarily by the distribution of ventilation at the time of the event. At the nidus of primary infection, tubercle bacilli are rapidly ingested by macrophages and transported by these cells via lymphatics through the pulmonary parenchyma to the regional lymph nodes at the hilum of the lung. The lymphatic drainage of peripheral lung tissue is outward to the pleural surface and then across this surface to the hilum. Thus, the pleural space may be seeded during this transport. Organisms may escape beyond the regional lymph nodes and travel via the thoracic duct to

reach the circulation and be disseminated hematogenously. Unknown factors of tissue tropism appear to influence the subsequent nidation of these disseminated bacilli. Bones, meninges, and organs of the genitourinary tract appear to be particularly frequent sites for the establishment of distant foci of infection. Occasionally, dissemination is diffuse and uniform with involvement of all viscera. Dissemination via lymphatic channels may also occur, with transport to neighboring groups of lymph nodes.

During the course of the events just described, the host develops delayed hypersensitivity to mycobacterial antigens. Subsequent to this change in the host (which may be recognized clinically by the development of a positive tuberculin test) there is a profound change in the host-parasite relationship. Host macrophages become activated and develop an increased capacity to kill tubercle bacilli and probably other intracellular parasites as well. Moreover, tuberculoid granuloma formation now occurs wherever tubercle bacilli are encountered, and these granulomas entrap bacilli, limit their further dissemination, and close lymphatic routes of spread. However, despite the development of an intense delayed hypersensitivity response, mycobacteria may persist within macrophages, viable although not necessarily metabolically active and capable of producing disease at a later time. The mechanism of this persistence is not known, although failure of phagosome-lysosome fusion may be involved.

Figure 87-2 presents a schematic representation of the pathogenesis of tuberculosis. As noted in this figure, the vast majority of primary infections—probably 95 percent in the United States [11], perhaps somewhat fewer in areas of poor nutrition and general health—heal and never result in clinical disease. When reactivation occurs, it most commonly takes place in the

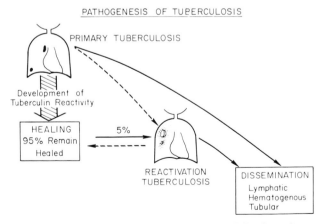

PATHOGENESIS OF TUBERCULOSIS

Figure 87-2. The pathogenesis of tuberculosis. Following primary infection, healing occurs in about 95 percent of individuals and only about 5 percent ever develop clinical disease. Dissemination via lymphatic, hematogenous, or tubular routes occurs either during primary infection or during reactivation tuberculosis, and late reactivation may occur at distant sites of dissemination.

posterior apical segments of the upper lobes of the lungs which are rarely the site of primary infection. How the organisms reach these areas and why they are sites of predilection remain unanswered questions. Endogenous reactivation may also occur at extrapulmonary sites to which dissemination has occurred. Additional dissemination may occur during reactivation disease. Similarly, the importance of exogenous reinfection in the development of clinical tuberculosis is still not well established. Prevailing thought, however, is that most clinical tuberculosis represents endogenous reactivation. Nevertheless, mycobacterial phage-typing techniques have clearly demonstrated that exogenous reinfection can occur and produce clinical disease [12].

Koch [1] observed that a guinea pig was able to contain and survive a second infection at the site of primary inoculation (the Koch phenomenon). Immunity to reinfection with *M. tuberculosis* is mediated by granuloma formation at the site of nidation and depends upon the presence of an adequate level of delayed hypersensitivity. It provides the logical basis for attempts to vaccinate against tuberculosis with attenuated strains of mycobacteria.

The formation of granulomas which protects the host is also responsible for much of the morbidity of the clinical disease. These granulomas (tuberculomas) consist of organized collections of mononuclear cells. An early infiltration of immunologically competent, predominantly T lymphocytes gives way to macrophages evoked from the circulating pool of monocytes and regulated by chemotactic factors and lymphokines produced by antigen-stimulated T lymphocytes. These macrophages undergo transformation into histiocytes, palisade, and sometimes fuse into multinucleate giant cells of the Langhans' type. During this transformation, phagocytic capacity appears to decrease. Tissue destruction results from the expansion of granulomas, and ultimately necrosis occurs in the centers of granulomas. Since neither the mononuclear cells which dominate granulomas nor tubercle bacilli contain liquefying enzymes, necrosis in tubercles does not lead to pustule formation but to the formation of cavities containing caseous material. Typically this caseum is laden with large numbers of tubercle bacilli.

The injection of soluble antigenic protein does not ordinarily lead to the development of delayed hypersensitivity. The same protein injected in the company of living or dead tubercle bacilli, however, produces typical delayed hypersensitivity. Raffel et al. [13] demonstrated that chloroform-methanol–soluble lipids from mycobacteria could substitute for the whole bacilli. More recent workers [5] have demonstrated that water-soluble fractions of the mycobacterial cell wall also have potent adjuvant properties. Some of these adjuvant moieties may be responsible for the nonspecific-immunity-producing properties attributed to mycobacteria which may protect nonspecifically against a variety of infections and tumor growth.

The tuberculin skin test is the best known but is neither the only nor the most important manifestation of delayed hypersensitivity in tuberculosis. Granuloma formation is also a manifestation of delayed hypersensitivity and probably represents the central feature of the pathogenesis of tuberculosis. The Koch phenomenon and antituberculous immunity are additional indications of tuberculin hypersensitivity. However, it should not be forgotten that it is possible to dissociate delayed tuberculin hypersensitivity from antituberculosis immunity in a number of experimental models.

Tuberculin hypersensitivity (cellular immunity) is mediated by immunologically competent cells. Delayed skin test reactivity can be transferred passively with lymphocyte-containing cellular exudates [14]. The subsequent development of methods for cell culture have made it possible to study this cellular response in vitro. Lymphocytes from a sensitive host undergo morphological dedifferentiation and incorporate thymidine in response to specific antigenic stimulation. They also produce lymphokines which regulate the activity of macrophages and other inflammatory cells. There are many complex cell-cell interactions, some involving soluble factors and some involving membrane receptors, which modulate the immune response. Specific subsets of T lymphocytes have helper and suppressor functions, and monocytes-macrophages also have suppressor functions. Aberrations of these regulatory systems may cause anergy, observed clinically in as many as 15 percent of patients with acute, bacteriologically positive tuberculosis as a paradoxically negative tuberculin skin test.

CLINICAL RESPONSE

Primary tuberculous infection rarely produces significant clinical illness. In children, enlargement of peribronchial lymph nodes may lead to bronchial compression and obstruction with collapse of a segment or lobe of lung distal to it. Pleurisy with effusion may follow closely upon primary infection when the pleural space is inoculated. However, the vast majority of primary infections are asymptomatic. Primary foci and the involved regional hilar lymph node may calcify subsequent to healing, leaving the characteristic Ghon complex usually recognized on chest radiographs of healthy persons.

Reactivated pulmonary tuberculosis is a chronic or subacute disease characterized by persistent constitutional and respiratory symptoms. Although minimally diseased persons may be completely asymptomatic, more significant disease is almost invariably accompanied by weight loss and fatigue. Low-grade fever is common, and drenching night sweats involving the upper half of the body and occurring several times weekly to once nightly are common. Cough is the commonest respiratory symptom associated with advanced or cavitary disease. Persistent cough can be used as the initial screening point in case-finding efforts. Hemoptysis is relatively common, usually minor, but sometimes major and rarely life threatening. In areas of high tuberculosis prevalence, chronic cough with hemoptysis is usually due to tuberculosis. Chest pain of mild to moderate degree is frequent, but its location correlates poorly with the location of pulmonary disease except when the pleural surface is involved. Tuberculous pleurisy is marked by an exudative effusion and a chronic course.

Disseminated tuberculosis produces symptoms related to the organs involved. Chronicity is a common feature of tuberculosis of all types. Scrofulous lymph nodes at the angle of the jaw, apparently sterile hematuria and pyuria, sharply angulated middorsal kyphosis without rotation, and chronic lymphocytic meningitis are hallmarks, respectively, of tuberculous adenitis, renal (or other urinary tract) tuberculosis, tuberculosis of the spine (Pott's disease), and tuberculous meningitis. Hematogenous dissemination produces a febrile wasting illness, sometimes characterized by twice-daily fever spikes. When hematogenously disseminated disease follows directly after primary infection, the lesions all develop at about the same rate and produce classical miliary (''millet seed'') tuberculosis lesions seen in spleen, liver, lung, and elsewhere. Patients with miliary tuberculosis characteristically present with persistent and perplexing fever, often with splenomegaly, but appear comparatively healthy with an apparently normal chest x-ray until several weeks of illness have passed. When dissemination occurs as a part of reactivation disease, the course is much more fulminant.

Untreated tuberculosis is a chronic and relapsing disease. Spontaneous remission may offer long intervals of good health only to give way to subsequent relapse. Data from the United States when sanitarium rest therapy was the only mode of treatment [15] indicate that about half of patients admitted to sanitaria ultimately died of tuberculosis, with mortality rates ranging from about 15 percent for patients admitted with minimal disease to about 70 percent for those admitted with far advanced disease. The average life expectancy of patients with tuberculosis in the high-prevalence areas of the developing world may be as short as $2\frac{1}{2}$ years after diagnosis. However, this average includes patients with a spectrum of courses ranging from fulminant to chronic disease. About 30 percent of tuberculous patients develop stable and nonprogressive disease without treatment, and only about 40 percent die [16].

Tuberculosis is a major problem in patients with the acquired immunodeficiency syndrome (AIDS). In those persons who have been infected with M. tuberculosis who develop human immunodeficiency virus-1 infections, the tuberculosis case rate is extremely high, perhaps approaching 50 percent in certain geographical areas (e.g., Haiti). Tuberculosis is often the first major infection these persons develop, preceding other manifestations of AIDS by many months. In patients with AIDS, tuberculosis is often disseminated and commonly involves lymph nodes. Pulmonary tuberculosis in patients with AIDS commonly presents as diffuse or miliary disease.

Mycobacteria other than M. tuberculosis produce a variety of clinical diseases as noted in Table 87-1 [3,17]. M. kansasii, M. avium, and M. szulgai most commonly produce chronic cavitary pulmonary disease which is similar to tuberculosis, although less prone to disseminate. All mycobacterial diseases, however, are indolent, chronic, and slowly progressive. Even in areas of low tuberculosis prevalence, disease due to other mycobacteria is much less common than tuberculosis. M. avium produces widely disseminated disease and bacteremia in patients with AIDS. Such disease is very common in these patients.

DIAGNOSIS

The diagnosis of tuberculosis rests upon the identification of M. tuberculosis in sputum or other material from the patient. When resources are limited, sputum smears should be the principal means of diagnosis. Studies from India [18] suggest that two smears of separate sputum samples are about 50 percent effective and the equal of one sputum culture in establishing the diagnosis of tuberculosis. Repeated sputum examinations increase the yield, but the maximum is reached at about five samples. There is seldom reason to obtain a greater number of samples. When expectorated sputum cannot be examined, smear and culture of early morning gastric aspirates are acceptable substitutes. Cases of minimal pulmonary tuberculosis may never have tubercle bacilli identified in the sputum despite adequate examination.

Chest x-rays are extremely helpful in evaluating the extent of pulmonary tuberculosis and following its progression and response to therapy. Although chronic infiltrative disease with cavitation located primarily in the apices is most characteristic of tuberculosis, there is no radiographic picture that is pathognomonic. Diagnoses made on the basis of chest x-ray alone should always be viewed as presumptive until confirmed by bacteriological identification of M. tuberculosis. Figure 87-3 depicts a typical chest radiograph of a patient with cavitary pulmonary tuberculosis.

Chest x-ray surveys were used in case detection in the past, but this practice has been abandoned in almost all parts of the world. In high-prevalence areas where fiscal resources are characteristically limited, x-ray surveys are not efficient because of their high cost. Emphasis is better placed on symptomatic screening and diagnosis by sputum smear. Although this approach will miss early or mild cases, it will bring the sickest and most contagious patients under treatment first. In areas of low prevalence, survey x-rays do not find significant numbers of previously unknown cases. Thus it is always most efficient to reserve x-rays for the evaluation of individuals who present with symptoms suggestive of tuberculosis, are in high-risk categories as family contacts of infectious cases, or who have a positive sputum smear. Survey chest x-rays may be appropriate for use in countries where fiscal resources are available for case detection in defined subpopulations at high risk which, for sociological or other reasons, are not readily reached by the usual health care system.

TREATMENT

In today's world it is not difficult to prescribe drug therapy which will cure the majority of patients with tuberculosis.

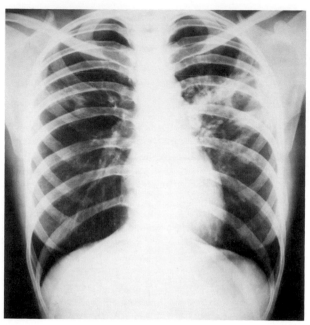

Figure 87-3. Chest radiograph of a patient with cavitary pulmonary tuberculosis. Note the typical infiltrative disease in the left upper lobe with a cavity well demonstrated. There is less extensive infiltrative disease in the right upper lobe. Lymph node calcifications are present in the left hilum.

However, if one wishes to provide maximally effective therapy, especially when large numbers of patients require treatment, then considerable thought should go into the choice of therapeutic regimens.

Drugs must be effective, with at least one bactericidal agent included in every regimen. A minimum of two agents to which the patient's bacilli are sensitive must be used. Failure to do so invites both treatment failures and the emergence of drug-resistant strains. The duration of treatment must be adequate and toxicity minimized. Hospitalization, dietary supplements, and rest are not necessary for patients given adequate chemotherapy [19]. Finally, drug regimens should have a high degree of patient acceptance. Patient noncompliance resulting in failure to complete drug therapy represents the single largest cause of treatment failure.

Although laboratory and clinical evidence is still tenuous, it is useful to think of tubercle bacilli as present in several distinct populations [20]. Patients harbor a population of rapidly growing, metabolically active, largely extracellular bacilli, a population of organisms multiplying intermittently, and a population of more slowly growing, long persisting, largely intracellular organisms. Isoniazid and streptomycin appear preferentially bactericidal for more rapidly growing organisms. Rifampin (rifampicin) is the most effective bactericidal agent for intermittently multiplying bacilli. Pyrazinamide is more bactericidal for the slowly multiplying, persisting organisms.

In addition, some organisms in every patient are dormant at any one time. These bacilli are unaffected by any drug while in this state.

Gryzbowski and Enarson [16] have reviewed the results achieved in a large number of operational treatment programs. About 30 percent of patients will achieve a satisfactory and stable clinical state without therapy. Minimally supervised mass programs have generally achieved a 60 percent favorable outcome. Individual chemotherapy under optimal circumstances has usually produced greater than 90 percent favorable treatment outcomes. There is little evidence that the choice of drug influences the potential for achieving the 90 percent success level. Low toxicity and high compliance rates become more significant when it is realized that the increment of benefit attributable to any particular drug regimen is small.

Table 87-2 lists the principal drugs available for the treatment of tuberculosis, their adult and pediatric doses, and principal toxicities. Isoniazid, first introduced in 1952, is an extraordinarily effective bactericidal agent of low cost and toxicity. Isoniazid should be used for the treatment of every patient, unless there is firm evidence of toxicity or bacterial resistance. Isoniazid toxicity includes peripheral neuropathy, which occurs primarily in the elderly, malnourished persons, and patients with other diseases predisposing to peripheral neuropathy. Peripheral neuropathy is preventable with 6 mg/day of pyridoxine and treatable with larger doses. Hepatitis occurs in some patients, the proportion rising with age from almost none in children and adolescents to approximately 2 percent in the elderly. Hepatitis occurs most frequently between 6 and 8 weeks after the initiation of therapy. It cannot be predicted by chemical monitoring of liver function because as many as one-third of patients taking isoniazid will show significant elevations of liver enzymes without progressing to hepatitis when the drug is continued.

Rifampin is a bactericidal agent whose effectiveness and safety equal that of isoniazid, but whose use in developing countries has been limited by high cost. Toxicity consists principally of hepatitis and, when used intermittently, a "flulike" hypersensitivity syndrome. The rate of hepatotoxicity of isoniazid and rifampin in combination is probably about 3 percent.

Streptomycin is used most effectively during the initial phase of treatment, and it is important not to exceed the effective daily dose, which is 0.75 g. Streptomycin must be given intramuscularly and adds significantly to the toxicity of regimens in which it is used. Major toxicities on the kidney and the auditory nerve are cumulative. Toxicity is rare in young persons with a total dose of less than 40 g. However, vestibular disturbances may occur with less than 10-g total dose in elderly persons. Most individuals who have received more than 120 g will have hearing or vestibular function loss. Dihydrostreptomycin should not be used because this agent is more toxic than streptomycin and causes deafness. Transient feelings of dizziness are common following streptomycin injection, and this symptom leads to significant patient unacceptability.

Table 87-2. Principal drugs used in the treatment of tuberculosis

| Drug | Usual daily dose | | Major toxicities |
	Adult	Pediatric	
Isoniazid	300 mg	5–10 mg/kg	Peripheral neuropathy, hepatitis
Rifampin	600 mg	10–20 mg/kg	Hepatitis, influenzalike syndrome
Streptomycin	0.75–1 g	15–20 mg/kg	Deafness, loss of vestibular function, loss of renal function
Pyrazinamide	1.5–2.0 g	30–35 mg/kg	Hepatitis, hyperuricemia
Ethambutol	15 mg/kg	15 mg/kg	Optic neuritis (extremely rare at this dose)
Thioacetazone	150 mg	2–3 mg/kg	Hepatitis, exfoliative dermatitis
Para-aminosalicylic acid	12 g	150 mg/kg	Diarrhea, hepatitis, hypersensitivity reactions

Pyrazinamide is a very effective drug which was initially seldom used because of hepatotoxicity. However, it is now apparent that it is relatively safe when used in currently recommended doses. Like streptomycin, it is probably bactericidal under at least some conditions of microbial growth. Hyperuricemia is common in patients taking pyrazinamide, and occasionally clinical gout is seen.

Ethambutol is an effective and extremely well tolerated bacteriostatic agent which has been widely accepted as a companion drug to isoniazid in two-drug regimens. Optic nerve toxicity observed during initial trials is not a problem when the daily dose is restricted to 15 mg/kg. Relatively high cost had previously limited the use of this agent in many parts of the world, but recent price reductions have made it more widely available.

Para-aminosalicylic acid is a bacteriostatic agent which has been very widely used as a second drug in two drug regimens. It is a drug of significant toxicity and low patient acceptability and has been largely replaced by other agents. Gastrointestinal symptoms are almost universal among patients taking this drug. Much of the toxicity is due to *meta*-aminophenol, a degradation product of *para*-aminosalicylic acid which is formed during storage of the drug, especially at warmer temperatures and with exposure to light.

Thioacetazone[1] is a bacteriostatic agent of very low cost and high patient acceptability. It has been in widespread use in much of the world. Significant toxicity, principally exfoliative dermatitis, hepatitis, and occasionally agranulocytosis, was a major problem when first used in high doses. At currently recommended doses, toxicity is generally low, but there appears to be a variation in the rate of toxicity which is race- or population-dependent. Thus, the general use of this drug should be preceded by carefully monitored clinical trials in each new population.

Table 87-3 lists several effective drug treatment regimens. The most effective treatment regimen of low toxicity is isoniazid and rifampin. The usual length of treatment for this regimen is 9 months, although extension to 12 months may be

warranted under conditions of slow clinical response. The major problems with this treatment regimen are its high cost and the prolonged period for which patients must be kept under surveillance. This regimen is also not satisfactory when drug resistance is suspected or known to be present. In the United States, isoniazid and rifampin have been given twice weekly after the first month of daily therapy with good results.

The least expensive drug regimen of known benefit is isoniazid and thioacetazone for 12 months. This very low cost combination is available in the form of a single tablet providing the usual adult dose of both agents. Although this regimen has been shown to produce a favorable outcome in 90 percent of patients infected with isoniazid-sensitive organisms under study conditions [21], its effectiveness is substantially lower under operating conditions. Streptomycin given during the initial 2 months of isoniazid-thioacetazone therapy has been

Table 87-3. Selected effective drug regimens for the treatment of tuberculosis

Regimen (adult drug doses)	Comment
Isoniazid (300 mg) and rifampin (600 mg) daily for 9 to 12 months.	Highly effective.
Isoniazid (300 mg) and thioacetazone (150 mg) daily for 12 to 18 months.	The least expensive effective drug regimen.
Isoniazid (300 mg) and ethambutol (15 mg/kg) daily for 18 months.	The least toxic effective regimen.
Isoniazid (300 mg), rifampin (600 mg), pyrazinamide (2 g), and streptomycin (1 g) daily for 2 months followed by isoniazid (300 mg) and thioacetazone (150 mg) daily for 6 or 7 months.	Probably the optimum short-course treatment regimen for use in developing countries.
Isoniazid (300 mg) and rifampin (600 mg) daily for 1 month followed by isoniazid (900 mg) and rifampin (600 mg) twice weekly for 8 months.	Effectiveness demonstrated in ambulatory program in the United States [26].

[1]Thioacetazone has not been approved by the United States Food and Drug Administration at the time of publication.

shown to increase efficacy, but it doubles drug cost, increases toxicity, and decreases patient acceptability.

The optimal treatment program for most countries of high tuberculosis prevalence may be a short-course regimen with an initial intensive treatment phase. Such regimens have achieved rapid sputum sterilization and permitted significant shortening of the duration of treatment. Depending on local fiscal and administrative considerations, short-course chemotherapy may lead to a significant total cost reduction. Most patient default occurs early in the course of treatment [22]. Short-term therapy, therefore, will have a major impact on patient compliance only if it leads to an increase in staff time available for patient education and follow-up. Where individual treatment costs are not a major consideration, multiple bactericidal drug regimens should be considered for all sicker patients in whom the compounded toxicity risk of multiple agents is justified by the severity of disease.

A high-intensity initial treatment phase of 1- to 2-months duration has distinct advantages for use in most multiple-agent programs [23,24]. The combination of isoniazid, rifampin, pyrazinamide, and streptomycin is probably the regimen capable of achieving the most rapid sputum sterilization. The use of this combination appears rapidly to reduce the patient bacillary load to the small residual subpopulation of persisting, largely intracellular organisms. A continuation phase of treatment is necessary to eradicate these persisting organisms, but its duration can be shortened when the initial therapy has been intense. A highly satisfactory regimen consists of 2 months initial therapy with daily isoniazid, rifampin, streptomycin, and pyrazinamide followed by 6 or 7 additional months of daily isoniazid and thioacetazone [25]. The two-drug consolidation phase can be shortened to 4 to 6 months if twice-weekly rifampin and isoniazid are used. This regimen provides the best available opportunity for fully supervised treatment with patients who are considered unreliable and at high risk for default. Ethambutol can probably be substituted for streptomycin in the initial phase of short-course regimens if an entirely oral regimen is desired or in the presence of adverse reactions to streptomycin.

There is no reason to believe that disseminated or extrapulmonary tuberculosis requires more intensive or prolonged therapy than does pulmonary tuberculosis. In fact, disseminated lesions, although numerous, are usually small with little caseation, so that drug penetration to bacilli is readily achieved. Their bacterial populations are also small, with low risk of emergence of drug-resistant organisms during treatment.

Routine follow-up of patients who have been successfully treated is not cost-effective, and resources so often allocated to this effort are probably better expended in ensuring adequate therapy and patient compliance during treatment [27].

Retreatment and management of suspected drug resistance present difficult problems. Where drug-sensitivity studies of organisms are available, retreatment should be started with a multiple drug regimen which includes at least two new agents, usually with a total of four drugs. The regimen can be adjusted later on the basis of drug-sensitivity reports.

Treatment failure should be taken to imply drug resistance where sensitivity tests are not available. Relapse after completion of treatment which was taken with regularity is due to drug-sensitive organisms in about two-thirds of cases [28]. Thus retreatment with the standard regimen is the appropriate first step in these circumstances. However, if failure occurs during treatment or following an irregular prior treatment, drug resistance is likely to be present in two-thirds of patients. In this case, a regimen including two new drugs must be found, but it is reasonable also to include the previously used agents.

It has been clearly demonstrated that the administration of isoniazid to persons who have had primary infections with *M. tuberculosis* without clinical tuberculosis protects them from the subsequent development of disease [29]. The usual dose is 300 mg daily for 6 to 12 months. Limitations on this form of therapy are imposed by its acceptability and toxicity. In most areas of the developing world, it is not used because the administration of a drug to healthy children does not have wide acceptance and limited resources are probably better expended in trying to prevent further transmission of the organism by treatment of infectious patients.

In those areas where prophylactic medicine is well accepted, the decision to use isoniazid must be based on balancing the potential therapeutic benefit against the potential drug toxicity. An elegant analysis of the competing risks in tuberculin reactors in the United States indicates that it is beneficial to give isoniazid to tuberculin reactors less than 35 years of age. At older ages the expected benefit declines and the anticipated toxicity increases. However, if risk factors predispose to tuberculosis reactivation, isoniazid should be given to older individuals as well [30].

Data are available [31] which allow one to assess the benefit and risk of isoniazid prophylaxis in older individuals with previously untreated but now inactive tuberculosis. In such persons isoniazid should probably be given if there is more than 10 to 15 years of life expectancy.

POPULATION

Tuberculosis is one of humanity's most ancient plagues with well-documented cases having been found in both old world (Egyptian) and new world (Peruvian) mummies. Today, tuberculosis remains common throughout most of the world [32,33], with half of the world's population estimated to be infected with *M. tuberculosis*. There are more than 20 million persons ill with this disease in the world. Projections for the future suggest that tuberculosis case rates will decline in most of the world. Increasing populations are expected to compensate for this decline so that the number of new cases each year is expected to remain relatively constant through the end of the century.

In technologically advanced countries, tuberculosis has been declining in incidence and prevalence for at least the last 100 years. In these areas it has become largely a disease of the urban poor [34] with three-fourths of clinical cases arising in the elderly. Cohort analysis has demonstrated that these cases represent reactivations of primary infections incurred much earlier and are the legacy of prior high infection risks in a population where current infection risk is low [35]. Indeed, the tuberculosis problem in developed countries is sufficiently restricted so that it is now possible to target control measures.

The technologically undeveloped and developing countries carry an enormous share of the world's tuberculosis burden. However, the disease is not uniformly distributed. Some countries show a continuing increase in tuberculous infection rates whereas others show declining infection rates [33,36,37]. Annual infection rates can be calculated from tuberculin skin testing data [36], and this information can be extremely useful in planning for the control of tuberculosis. In developing countries, annual infection rates are typically 1 to 3 percent. As there is a trend in developing countries toward urbanization, it is reasonable to expect that tuberculosis, now widely distributed in rural areas, will increasingly concentrate in urban centers just as it has in developed countries.

The exploding pandemic of AIDS is likely to have a substantial impact on the epidemiology of tuberculosis. Recent increases in tuberculosis case rates in the United States are probably directly attributable to the susceptibility of patients with HIV infection to mycobacterial disease, and tuberculosis is a major complication of AIDS in Africa. Disease due to *M. avium* complicates the course of about half of patients with AIDS in the United States; it may be less common in other parts of the world.

The natural history of tuberculous infection is greatly influenced by the age of the infected person [38]. Overall, about 5 percent of infected individuals in the United States will develop clinical tuberculosis [11]. The figure may be somewhat higher in developing countries. In infants, disseminated disease occurs promptly with high frequency. Infections occurring in childhood tend to remain latent until adolescence, with reactivation at that time. Infections occurring in the postpubertal years and in young adulthood tend to progress rather promptly to the development of clinical illness. In areas of high tuberculosis incidence, the disease is primarily a disease of young adults. As noted above, the prominence of tuberculosis in the elderly in developed countries is an artifact of rapidly decreasing infection risk.

We have noted that age, poverty, and urban living are all epidemiological factors associated with tuberculosis prevalence. Malnutrition can also be identified as such a factor and famines have been associated with soaring tuberculosis mortality rates. It is also clear that there are genetic factors which influence susceptibility to tuberculosis. Identical twins have been shown to have a higher concordance of tuberculosis than fraternal twins [39]. Beyond these, those specific factors which

predispose to tuberculosis are difficult to establish, and the factors which initiated the decline in tuberculosis incidence in Europe and North America during the past century are not entirely clear.

While important in the clinical diagnosis of tuberculosis, the tuberculin test has made its greatest contribution in determining the epidemiology of the disease. Koch noted that tuberculous patients treated with Old Tuberculin (OT) developed reactions directed at protein constituents of OT [40]. Von Pirquet, the father of allergy skin testing, first used OT in skin testing in 1907, and the practice was in wide use shortly thereafter. Seibert prepared tuberculin purified protein derivative (PPD) in 1934 [41]. PPD is now the standard material for all tuberculin testing. Seibert prepared a single large reference batch, designated as PPD-S. The commonly used intermediate strength of PPD in North America is that dose (5 test units) which gives reaction sizes equivalent to 0.1 μg of PPD-S. In most of the world PPD RT-23, prepared in Denmark and distributed by the World Health Organization, is in use. This PPD is assigned units according to weight. Two units of PPD RT-23 are equivalent to 5 test units of PPD-S and is the preferred dose. All PPDs in use today are prepared in a buffered diluent containing small amounts of Tween 80, which stabilizes the PPD by preventing loss on glass and plastic surfaces.

A positive reaction to 5 test units of PPD means prior primary tuberculous infection [42,43]. The tuberculin test does not discriminate between those who have had asymptomatic primary infections without sequelae and those who have active tuberculosis. Although approximately 15 percent of acutely ill tuberculous patients may have negative tuberculin tests, patients with more chronic disease are essentially all positive reactors. Age-specific tuberculin reactor rates give an accurate measure of the prevalence of tuberculous infection in a population and may be used to estimate the rate of and changes in the rate of tuberculous infection [36].

Whether PPD is used for diagnostic or epidemiological purposes, the preferred method of administration is intracutaneous injection with a syringe and needle (Mantoux technique). Multiple-puncture devices deliver an uncontrolled large amount of antigen, and therefore can only be considered as screening devices. Reactions to PPD should be measured at 48 to 72 h, and the transverse diameter of discernible induration (not erythema) recorded.

When tuberculin reactions of patients with tuberculosis are plotted in a frequency distribution histogram, a normal distribution is obtained, with mean and mode at about 17 mm in diameter and with two standard deviations including all those larger than 5 mm. Thus a 5-mm reaction has long been accepted as a positive tuberculin test. In some geographical areas, often in the tropics, a normal distribution of tuberculin reaction sizes is not present. Figure 87-4, which presents data from two Bolivian villages, demonstrates a skewed frequency distribution. This phenomenon is the result of hypersensitivity to mycobacteria other than *M. tuberculosis,* most probably soil and

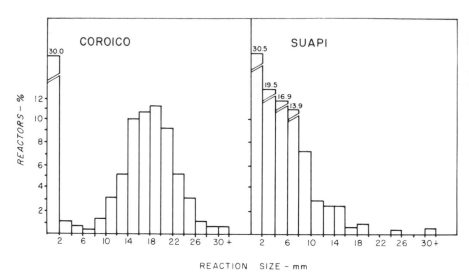

Figure 87-4. The distribution of tuberculin test reaction sizes in the Bolivian villages of Coroico and Suapi. In Coroico, the distribution is bimodal and positive reactors are clearly separated from negative reactors. In Suapi no such separation is found, and the majority of individuals have reactions which are small in size and intermediate between the size ranges identified as positive and negative in Coroico. These small, intermediate reactions probably result from cross-reactivity with antigens of nonpathogenic, environmental mycobacteria. *(From T. M. Daniel, Clinics in Chest Medicine 1:189–201, 1980.)*

water mycobacteria which do not cause disease [*42,43*]. The final skewed curve is thought to represent a summation curve, with a separate population of cross-reactors compounding the observations. When reactions to PPD are not normally distributed, then it may be advisable to consider only those reactions greater than 10 mm in diameter as positive, thus excluding most of the small cross-reactions.

CONTROL

Even in situations of extremely limited public health resources, consideration should be given to control programs for tuberculosis. Furthermore, no physician should undertake the treatment of even one tuberculous patient without also considering public health aspects of this infectious disease. Significant strides in the control and treatment of tuberculosis have been made in those communities which have assumed a measure of public responsibility both for providing treatment of affected persons and for providing control of transmission of infection. An expert committee of WHO has provided very useful guidelines for those responsible for tuberculosis control planning [*44*].

Figure 87-5 presents a simple population model of tuberculosis infection and indicates several points of attack which may help to achieve control of tuberculosis. Approximately half of the world, for the most part children, remains uninfected. This segment could be protected by an effective vaccine. Among those who are infected, recognizable by their positive tuberculin skin tests, some progress to develop tuberculosis. Of those with disease, a portion are infectious to others and are responsible for continuing to transmit infections, most commonly to the children of the same family. This transmission can be interrupted by treating the infectious patients with effective chemotherapy, and such treatment is the single most important measure available for tuberculosis control. Thus, rendering a patient noninfectious by appropriate treatment is

not solely the concern and responsibility of the patient but that of the entire community potentially at risk.

A system of reporting and registry of tuberculosis is important to every national control program that reaches the stage of trying to provide communitywide control. Contact investigation must follow reporting to have an effect on tuberculosis. The establishment of categorical registries and public health programs aimed at tuberculosis does not mean that tuberculosis

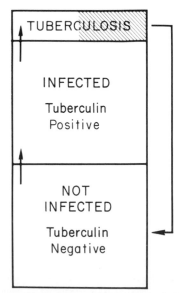

Figure 87-5. The epidemiology of tuberculosis. Uninfected persons can be recognized because their tuberculin skin tests are negative. In areas of high tuberculosis prevalence, this segment of the population is composed chiefly of children. Infected persons can be recognized by positive tuberculin skin tests. A portion of these infected persons develop tuberculosis, and some of these tuberculous individuals transmit infection to uninfected persons.

control can be divorced from the general health care system. Indeed, while categorical aspects of tuberculosis control programs are important and must be maintained, treatment must be integrated with the national health care delivery system, regardless of the nature of this system.

The general strategies employed for the control of tuberculosis must differ somewhat for high- and low-prevalence areas. In high-prevalence areas nearly all individuals are infected and hence tuberculin-positive by adulthood. Morbidity and mortality rates from dissemination during primary infections, which frequently occur during young childhood, are high. Most active disease occurs in young adults. Finally, fiscal resources are often limited. In this situation, BCG vaccination to protect uninfected children is important. Case finding among asymptomatic adults is relatively unimportant, and greatest attention should be directed at recognizing those patients who are most infectious. Thus triage by symptomatology, especially chronic cough, and diagnosis by sputum smear are appropriate.

In low-prevalence areas the major reservoir of infection is in the elderly. Young adults are generally tuberculin negative. Transmission of infection is a rare event, generally decreasing in frequency, which often occurs in microepidemics traceable to a single infectious patient. The tuberculin skin test is a useful tool for recognizing those who are infected, and isoniazid prophylaxis is appropriate for the prevention of tuberculosis in infected persons. Case finding must be targeted and vigorous follow-up of primary infections is appropriate in an attempt to recognize the source of infection. Effective chemotherapy is of great importance for preventing further transmission, and there is generally little benefit to be gained from mass BCG vaccination.

In 1908 Calmette and Guérin selected a culture of *M. bovis* and began the tedious task of attenuation by passage through cultures on artificial media and multiple animal species. By 1921 they had achieved the avirulent strain which now bears their name (bacillus Calmette-Guérin, BCG). It soon came into use in Europe. Aronson and his colleagues conducted the first controlled study of its effectiveness [45]. Native American Indian children were found to be dramatically protected by BCG, with an overall reduction in tuberculosis mortality of 82 percent during a 20-year period of follow-up. Similar effectiveness was found in England [46] and in Chicago [47], but trials in Georgia [48,49] and Puerto Rico [50] demonstrated little protection. An early trial in south India demonstrated no protection initially, but late follow-up showed protection to have reached 56 percent [51]. A good review of these studies is provided by ten Dam et al. [52].

The largest trial of BCG ever conducted was carried out in south India in the 1970s [53–55]. Among approximately 250,000 vaccinees and control subjects, no protection was observed after 7.5 years of observation. Many factors have been proposed which may contribute to the disparity between this result and those of earlier trials, but none seems totally adequate [55]. The fact that hypersensitivity to mycobacteria other than *M. tuberculosis* is common in both south India and in Georgia where BCG was also found to be ineffective suggests that the populations in these areas may have prior immunity from this hypersensitivity, thus making it difficult to demonstrate protection from BCG. It is also noteworthy that unlike most areas of similar high prevalence, age-specific tuberculosis incidence rates in south India do not peak until the fifth or sixth decade of life. Thus a prolonged period of follow-up may be necessary before it can be known if vaccination is effective in this population. This hypothesis is consonant with the earlier experience of Frimodt-Møller et al. in the same area [51]. The 15-year follow-up showed 17 percent protection against bacteriologically positive tuberculosis in subjects under 15 years of age at vaccination, and none in older subjects in the Chingleput population [56]. The low virulence and pathogenicity of the local strains of *M. tuberculosis* could have been another factor which made it difficult to demonstrate protection from BCG. Whatever the reason for the failure to demonstrate protection by BCG vaccination in south India, most experts generally agree that these results should be extrapolated to other areas only with great caution and that BCG vaccination should be continued in use throughout the world [55]. Even on the Indian subcontinent, BCG continues to be administered to infants in hopes of protecting against such more serious forms of disseminated tuberculosis as miliary tuberculosis and tuberculous meningitis, which were not studied in the vaccination trial. The greatest benefit from BCG is the protection of uninfected individuals. It is likely to have less impact than chemotherapy upon the transmission of infection because it does not change the reservoir [56,57].

Technical guidelines for the use of BCG have been published by WHO [44,58]. It is best given intradermally, and lyophilized preparations are preferred. It can be given in mass campaigns but current WHO strategy also includes BCG as one of the six childhood vaccines of the Expanded Programme on Immunization. BCG can be given indiscriminantly without prior tuberculin testing, for no adverse effects are encountered in those already infected [59]. In high-prevalence areas most adults are already infected so BCG campaigns should be targeted at those less than 15 or 20 years of age. Once mass coverage of a population is achieved, a program of vaccination of children, ideally at or close to birth, should be instituted. There is probably little value in undertaking any BCG vaccination program unless planning for this aspect is incorporated from the onset. Following BCG vaccination variable levels of tuberculin positivity are found, thus removing the tuberculin skin test from the diagnostic armamentarium. This is of no consequence in high-prevalence areas where tuberculin reactivity is nearly universal by adulthood and routine tuberculin testing is not practical.

REFERENCES

1 Koch R: Die Aetiologie der Tuberculose, a translation by Berna Pinner and Max Pinner with an introduction by Allen K. Krause. Am Rev Tuberc 25:285–323, 1932

2 Runyon EH, Wayne LG, Kubica GP: Family II. *Mycobacteriaceae,* Chester, 1897, 63, in Buchanan RE, Gibbons NE (eds): *Bergey's Manual of Determinative Bacteriology,* 8th ed. Baltimore, Williams & Wilkins, 1974, pp 681–701

3 Wolinsky E: Nontuberculous mycobacteria and associated diseases. Am Rev Respir Dis 119:107–159, 1979

4 Daniel TM, Janicki BW: Mycobacterial antigens: A review of their isolation, chemistry, and immunological properties. Microbiol Rev 42:84–113, 1978

5 Lederer E: The mycobacterial cell wall. Pure Appl Chem 25: 135–165, 1971

6 Kleinhenz ME, Ellner JJ, Spagnuolo PJ, et al: Suppression of lymphocyte responses by tuberculous plasma and mycobacterial arabinogalactan. Monocyte dependence and indomethacin reversibility. J Clin Invest 68:153–162, 1981

7 Vestal AL: Procedure for the Isolation and Identification of Mycobacteria. U.S. Department of Health, Education, and Welfare Publication No. (CDC) 77–8230, Atlanta, 1975

8 Riley RL, Mills CC, O'Grady F, et al: Infectiousness of air from a tuberculosis ward. Ultraviolet irradiation of infected air: Comparative infectiousness of different patients. Am Rev Respir Dis 85: 511–525, 1962

9 Chapman JS, Dyerly MD: Presumably infected premises with respect to conversion of the tuberculin test. Am Rev Respir Dis 89: 197–199, 1964

10 Kamat SR, Dawson JJY, Devadatta S, et al: A controlled study of the influence of segregation of tuberculous patients for one year on the attack rate of tuberculosis in a 5-year period in close family contacts in South India. Bull WHO 34:517–532, 1966

11 Comstock GW, Edwards PQ: The competing risks of tuberculosis and hepatitis for adult tuberculin reactors. Am Rev Respir Dis 111: 573–577, 1975

12 Bates JH, Stead WW, Rado TA: Phage type of tubercle bacilli isolated from patients with two or more sites of organ involvement. Am Rev Respir Dis 114:353–358, 1976

13 Raffel S, Arnaud LE, Dukes CD, et al: The role of the wax of the tubercle bacillus in establishing delayed hypersensitivity. II. Hypersensitivity to a protein antigen. J Exp Med 90:53–71, 1949

14 Chase MW: The cellular transfer of cutaneous hypersensitivity to tuberculin. Proc Soc Exp Biol Med 59:134–135, 1945

15 Alling DW, Bosworth EB: The after-history of pulmonary tuberculosis. VI. The first fifteen years following diagnosis. Am Rev Respir Dis 81:839–849, 1960

16 Grzybowski S, Enarson DA: The fate of cases of pulmonary tuberculosis under various treatment programmes. Bull Int Union Tuberc 53:70–75, 1978

17 Chapman JS: *The Atypical Mycobacteria and Human Mycobacteriosis.* New York, Plenum, 1977

18 Baily GVJ, Savic D, Gothe GE, et al: Potential yield of pulmonary tuberculosis cases by direct microscopy of sputum in a district of South India. Bull WHO 37:875–892, 1967

19 Dawson JJY, Devadatta S, Fox W, et al: A 5-year study of patients with pulmonary tuberculosis in a concurrent comparison of home and sanatorium treatment for one year with isoniazid plus PAS. Bull WHO 34:533–551, 1966

20 Grosset J: Bacteriologic basis of short-course chemotherapy for tuberculosis. Clinics in Chest Med 1:231–241, 1980

21 East African/British Medical Research Council: Isoniazid with thiacetazone (thioacetazone) in the treatment of pulmonary tuberculosis in East Africa—Fifth investigation. Tubercle 51:123–151, 1970

22 East African/British Medical Research Council: Tuberculosis in Kenya: Follow-up of the second (1974) national sampling survey and a comparison with the follow-up data from the first (1964) national sampling survey. Tubercle 60:125–149, 1979

23 Fox W, Mitchison DA: Short course chemotherapy for pulmonary tuberculosis. Am Rev Respir Dis 111:325–353, 845–848, 1975

24 Fox W: The chemotherapy of pulmonary tuberculosis: A review. Chest 76(suppl):785–796, 1979

25 East African/British Medical Research Council: Controlled clinical trial of four short-course regimens of chemotherapy for two durations in the treatment of pulmonary tuberculosis. Fifth report. Am Rev Respir Dis 118:39–48, 1978

26 Dutt AK, Jones L, Stead WW: Short-course chemotherapy for tuberculosis with largely twice-weekly isoniazid-rifampin. Chest 75: 441–447, 1979

27 Stead WW, Jurgens GH: Productivity of prolonged follow-up after chemotherapy for tuberculosis. Am Rev Respir Dis 108:314–320, 1973

28 Costello HD, Caras GJ, Snider DE Jr: Drug resistance among previously treated tuberculosis patients, a brief report. Am Rev Respir Dis 121:313–316, 1980

29 Ferebee SH: Controlled chemoprophylaxis trials in tuberculosis. A general review. Adv Tuberc Res 17:28–106, 1970

30 American Thoracic Society: Treatment of tuberculosis and tuberculous infection in adults and children. Am Rev Respir Dis 134:355–363, 1986

31 Krebs A, Farer LS, Snider WE, Thompson NJ: Five years of follow-up of the IUAT trial of isoniazid prophylaxis in fibrotic lesions. Bull Int Union Tuberc 54:65–69, 1979

32 Lowell AM: Tuberculosis in the World. U.S. Department of Health, Education, and Welfare, Public Health Service, Center of Disease Control (HEW Publication No. CDC 76-8317), Atlanta, 1976

33 Hershfield ES: Tuberculosis in the world. Chest 76(suppl):805–811, 1979

34 Center for Disease Control: Tuberculosis in the United States, 1978. HHS Publication No. (CDC) 80–8322, Atlanta, 1980

35 Frost WH: The age selection of mortality from tuberculosis in successive decades. Am J Hyg 30:91–96, 1939

36 Sutherland I, Styblo K, Sampalik M, et al: Annual risks of tuberculous infection in 14 countries derived from the results of tuberculin surveys in 1948–1952. Bull Int Union Tuberc 45:75–96, 1971

37 Bleiker MA, Styblo K: The annual tuberculosis infection rate and its trend in developing countries. Bull Int Union Tuberc 53:295–298, 1978

38 Zeidberg LD, Gass RS, Dillon A, et al: The Williamson County tuberculosis study. A twenty-four year epidemiologic study. Am Rev Respir Dis 87(suppl):1–88, 1963

39 Comstock GW: Tuberculosis in twins: A reanalysis of the Prophit survey. Am Rev Respir Dis 117:621–624, 1978

40 Long ER: *The Chemistry and Chemotherapy of Tuberculosis.* Baltimore, Williams & Wilkins, 1958, p 123

41 Seibert FB: The isolation and properties of the purified protein derivative of tuberculin. Am Rev Tuberc 30:713–720, 1934

42 Edwards PQ, Edwards LB: Story of the tuberculin test from an epidemiologic viewpoint. Am Rev Respir Dis 81(suppl):1–47, 1960

43 Comstock GW, Daniel TM, Snider DE Jr, et al: The tuberculin skin test. Am Rev Respir Dis 124:356–363, 1981

44 WHO Expert Committee on Tuberculosis: Ninth Report. WHO Tech Rep Ser 552, Geneva, 1974

45 Aronson JD, Aronson CF, Taylor RN: A twenty-year appraisal of BCG vaccination in the control of tuberculosis. Arch Intern Med 101:881–893, 1958

46 Medical Research Council: BCG and role bacillus vaccines in the prevention of tuberculosis in adolescence and early adult life. Br Med J 1:973–978, 1963

47 Rosenthal SR, Loewinsohn E, Graham ML, et al: BCG vaccination against tuberculosis in Chicago. A twenty-year study statistically analyzed. Pediatrics 28:622–641, 1961

48 Comstock GW, Palmer CE: Long-term results of BCG vaccination in the southern United States. Am Rev Respir Dis 93:171–183, 1966

49 Comstock GW, Webster RG: Tuberculosis studies in Muscogee County, Georgia. VII. A twenty-year evaluation of BCG vaccination in a school population. Am Rev Respir Dis 100:839–845, 1969

50 Comstock GW, Edwards PQ: An American view of BCG vaccination, illustrated by results of a controlled trial in Puerto Rico. Scand J Respir Dis 53:207–217, 1972

51 Frimodt-Møller J, Thomas J, Parthasarathy R: Observations on the protective effect of BCG vaccination in a south India rural population. Bull WHO 30:545–574, 1964

52 ten Dam HG, Toman K, Hitze KL, et al: Present knowledge of immunization against tuberculosis. Bull WHO 54:255–269, 1976

53 Tuberculosis Prevention Trial. Trial of BCG vaccines in south India for tuberculosis prevention: First report. Bull WHO 57:819–827, 1979

54 Tripathy SP: Fifteen-year follow-up of the Indian BCG prevention trial. Bull Int Union Tuberc 62(3):69–72, 1987

55 ICMR/WHO Scientific Group: Vaccination Against Tuberculosis. WHO Tech Rep Ser 651, Geneva, 1980

56 Styblo K, Meijer J: Impact of BCG vaccination programmes in children and young adults on the tuberculosis problem. Tubercle 57:17–43, 1976

57 Styblo K, Meijer J: Recent advances in tuberculosis epidemiology with regard to formulation or re-adjustment of control programmes. Bull Int Union Tuberc 53:283–294, 1978

58 WHO Study Group: BCG Vaccination Policies. WHO Tech Rep Ser 652, Geneva, 1980

59 Egsmose T: The effect of BCG vaccination in naturally infected tuberculin-positive individuals. Scand J Respir Dis 49:123–140, 1968

CHAPTER 88 / *Leprosy* · Richard A. Miller · Thomas M. Buchanan

Leprosy is a chronic infectious disease of humans; the causative organism is *Mycobacterium leprae*. To a great extent leprosy may be considered an immunological disease. The leprosy bacillus is virtually nontoxic, and most symptoms of the disease are due to immune reactions against antigenic constituents of *M. leprae*. The disease chiefly affects the skin, peripheral nerves, and mucous membranes, but in some forms *M. leprae* can also be found in large numbers elsewhere. Immune reactions resulting in loss of nerve function are a major cause of the chronic disability often associated with the disease. Approximately 12 million patients are estimated to suffer from leprosy throughout the world.

PARASITE

The leprosy bacillus was first seen and recognized as such by Hansen in Bergen, Norway, in 1873 [*1*]. He studied the disease in several families and found that the major hypothesis of the time, heredity, could not account for the observations made. Instead, these observations strongly indicated an infectious origin for the disease. Subsequent work resulted in the discovery of *M. leprae* in tissue from patients with leprosy.

BASIC PROPERTIES

Mycobacterium leprae is a slender acid- and alcohol-fast gram-positive rod, 6 to 8 μm long and about 0.5 μm in diameter. It is found singly or in masses of 50 or more bacilli inside macrophages, then termed *globi*.

The leprosy bacillus cannot be cultured in vitro on artificial media. Many claims to this effect have not been substantiated upon subsequent careful studies. In vivo, *M. leprae* is an obligate intracellular parasite growing mainly in macrophages, in Schwann cells of peripheral nerves, and to some extent in various other cell types, e.g., muscle cells. Its generation time in experimental in vivo models is around 12 days, longer than for other mycobacteria. This slow growth fits with the clinical evidence of a long incubation time (usually given as 1 to 7 years) and slow progression in the initial phases. The basic reason for its predilection for macrophages and Schwann cells is unknown, but its localization within the Schwann cells is of major importance for the development of nerve damage.

Classification of *M. leprae* as a mycobacterium is based on various properties which it shares with other mycobacteria. Because of lack of growth in vitro, criteria for exact species identification are few. Various staining techniques are useful for identification. Acid-fastness extractable with pyridine and oxidation of dihydroxyphenylalanine (DOPA) to quinone are considered unique properties of *M. leprae*.

Recent years have seen rapid progress in the identification and characterization of important antigens of *M. leprae*. This work, together with information obtained from analysis of the *M. leprae* genome, confirms the classification of *M. leprae* in the genus *Mycobacterium*. Among the antigens which have been well characterized are the cell wall associated with glycolipids, phenolic glycolipid 1 [2] and lipoarabinomannan [3], as well as several proteins, p70, p65, p36, p35, p28, and p12.

Murine monoclonal antibodies have been produced against all of these antigens [4–7], and the genes for most of the protein antigens have been partially or fully sequenced [8–10]. At least one *M. leprae* species-specific epitope has been found on phenolic glycolipid 1 and on the proteins of 65-, 36-, 35-, 28-, 18-, and 12-kDa mass. The lipoarabinomannan is an antigen common to all mycobacteria and *Nocardia*, and appears to be a major surface-exposed molecule. The phenolic glycolipid 1 and synthetic oligosaccharides equivalent to the terminal disaccharide or trisaccharide moieties of this molecule have been of great interest for serodiagnosis [11], and several studies have found an increased relative risk for development of leprosy in seropositive individuals. The 70- and 65-kDa proteins show considerable sequence homology with "heat-shock" or "stress" proteins common to prokaryotes and eukaryotes, and recently their potential role in autoimmunity has been under intense investigation [12].

ANIMAL MODELS

Shepard was the first to demonstrate multiplication of *M. leprae* in the footpad of the normal mouse. This growth is strictly localized with bacillary multiplication indicating a generation time of around 12 days reaching a ceiling at about 10^6 acid-fast bacilli per footpad. This model has been of tremendous importance, particularly for testing the efficiency of drug treatment, screening new drugs, and demonstrating drug resistance.

Rees introduced the early-thymectomized mouse into leprosy research. In mice with severe T-cell deficiency, the multiplication of *M. leprae* occurs with the same generation time, but is not limited by host immunity, resulting in the formation of up to 1000 times more bacilli and systemic infection. This model clearly shows the T-cell dependence of resistance. Transfer of syngeneic normal lymphoid cells to mice with systemic *M. leprae* infection leads to an immunological attack on the bacilli and a violent reaction resulting in tissue damage and clinical symptoms similar to severe reversal reactions in humans. The model has also been used to demonstrate persisting viable *M. leprae* in various tissues after prolonged drug treatment and apparent clinical cure in lepromatous leprosy in humans. The congenitally athymic nude mouse (nu/nu mouse) is also an excellent host for *M. leprae*.

In 1971, Kirchheimer and Storrs demonstrated that upon intravenous inoculation of the nine-banded armadillo, *M. leprae* established a systemic infection. After inoculation with 10^7 bacilli, about 50 percent of the animals "take" and develop a systemic infection similar to lepromatous leprosy in humans. The bacillary content is high, and large amounts of *M. leprae* may be purified from tissues of armadillos sacrificed $1\frac{1}{2}$ to 2 years after inoculation. This model created a completely new situation with regard to the availability of *M. leprae* for studies of its composition and immunological properties, and provided a basis for experiments on the development of a leprosy vaccine.

The development of systemic infection has also been observed in various nonhuman primates, including the mangabey monkey, following natural exposure to *M. leprae* or experimental inoculation with bacilli. This model most closely approximates the neurological sequelae of leprosy in humans, but availability of these animals is limited.

PATIENT

The characteristics of the clinical disease resulting from infection with *M. leprae* are determined by the complex interaction of the individual's immune response with the infecting bacilli. The host immune system plays a critical role not only in determining resistance or susceptibility to infection, but also in determining the clinical features in cases of overt disease.

It was long believed that transmission of *M. leprae* was an uncommon event, usually requiring prolonged exposure to an infectious individual(s). This belief was founded on the observations that, with the exception of a few hyperendemic areas, the prevalence of leprosy rarely exceeded 5 to 10 cases per 1000, and that the cumulative incidence of disease among household contacts of untreated patients with lepromatous leprosy was usually less than 10 percent. However, recent studies using assays for both humoral and cell-mediated immunity have found that a high percentage of the population in endemic areas shows evidence of sensitization to *M. leprae* antigens. This suggests that transmission of infection occurs much more frequently than previously thought, and that it is progression to clinically apparent disease that is the uncommon event.

The precise nature of this protective immunity is unclear, but it is probably multifactorial. Genetic determinants may be important, but environmental factors such as crowding, intensity and duration of exposure, and prior sensitization to other mycobacteria (either environmental or via BCG immunization) also seem to influence host immunity. However, regardless of how this immunity is determined, the fact remains that 85 to 95 percent of the population is resistant to the development of clinical leprosy (Fig. 88-1).

The most common initial manifestation of disease in the remainder of the population which is susceptible to *M. leprae* is a hypopigmented macule. This form of leprosy is classified as "indeterminate leprosy." These lesions are usually solitary although occasionally a small group of macules may be present. The interior of the lesion may be slightly hypesthetic, but this is not an invariant finding, particularly when the lesions

Figure 88-1. *A.* The course after infection with *Mycobacterium leprae.* *B.* Lepromatous (LL) leprosy. Multiple nodular lesions contain large amounts of bacilli. Note loss of eyebrows. *C.* Tuberculoid (TT) leprosy. The patient had a single hypopigmented lesion in the neck. (*Photographs courtesy of Armauer Hansen Research Institute, Addis Ababa, Ethiopia.*)

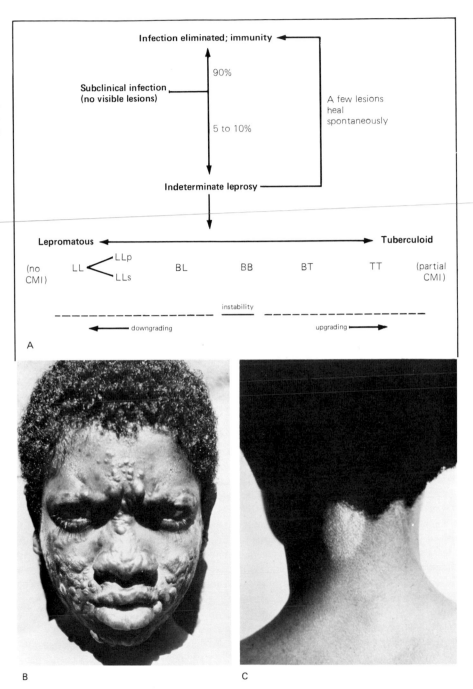

are on the face. Biopsies taken from the rim of these lesions may contain granulomas, but bacilli are uncommon.

Indeterminate leprosy is a clinically unstable entity, rarely persisting for more than 2 years. In up to 50 percent of children, the skin lesions resolve spontaneously, and all evidence of active infection disappears. This spontaneous healing also occurs in adults, but its frequency has not been determined in this age group. Those who do not spontaneously heal generally progress to overt clinical leprosy over a period of several

months to 2 years. Classification of patients with persisting disease has been a matter of prolonged discussion and dispute. They constitute a spectrum between two polar groups, those with tuberculoid leprosy (TT) with few lesions containing few bacilli, and those with lepromatous leprosy (LL) with multiple lesions in which the bacilli grow without inhibition.

Ridley and Jopling's classification of leprosy into five major groups [*13*] has been widely accepted and provides a good basis for accurate clinical diagnosis predicting the prognosis.

TT leprosy (Fig. 88-1*C*) is usually stable with few skin lesions, which show well-defined borders, central flattening, and sensory loss. Histologically there is an epithelioid granuloma with giant cells, lymphocyte infiltration, and very few bacilli. Borderline tuberculoid (BT) leprosy shows more extensive skin lesions. The nerves are commonly involved, and nerve damage may occur silently or during a reaction. There are few acid-fast bacilli in BT lesions. Mid-borderline (BB) leprosy shows many lesions, often raised with "punched out" areas. Histologically there is an epithelioid granuloma without giant cells, a clear subepidermal zone, and multiple bacilli. Borderline lepromatous (BL) leprosy shows many lesions of various forms with diffuse borders. Frequent nerve damage occurs. Histologically there is macrophage granuloma. Skin smears are strongly positive in the lesions but may be negative elsewhere. LL leprosy (Fig. 88-1*B*) has numerous symmetrical skin lesions progressing to nodular forms containing large numbers of bacilli. Classical polar lepromatous leprosy appears to arise de novo and now is denoted LLp. In other instances, borderline cases evolve toward the lepromatous end; they are termed *subpolar lepromatous leprosy* (LLs). Studies of the cell types within leprosy lesions have revealed higher T4/T8 (T-helper/T-suppressor) ratios in tuberculoid than in lepromatous lesions, and an organization pattern within tuberculoid lesions of T4 (helper) cells within the granuloma and T8 (suppressor) cells in a margin surrounding the granuloma [*14*]. In the lepromatous lesion, the helper and suppressor cells are interspersed.

In field work, which is often carried out by auxiliary personnel trained for a short period, the Ridley-Jopling classification needs simplification. The simplification, however, should not be into the three classical groups of tuberculoid, borderline, or lepromatous leprosy. In this system the "borderline" group tends to increase and will include both borderline tuberculoid and borderline lepromatous cases, which are basically different with regard to resistance, treatment, and infectiousness. It is preferable to group patients into two major categories, paucibacilliferous and multibacilliferous. Multibacillary patients are those in whom bacilli are identified in any skin biopsy or scraping. Paucibacillary patients lack demonstrable bacilli.

The host immune response after infection with *M. leprae* involves both a humoral and a cellular immune response, which need to be considered separately. An understanding of these responses is essential to understanding the pathophysiology of leprosy, as well as the potential of immunological tools for the diagnosis, treatment, or prevention of leprosy.

A humoral response to *M. leprae* antigens develops prior to the onset of clinical disease in experimentally infected animals, and can be detected in a significant percentage of healthy individuals residing in endemic areas. Individuals who remain very strongly seroreactive to phenolic glycolipid I over repeated testings during a period of 12 to 36 months appear to have an increased relative risk of developing multibacillary

leprosy, but the calculated predictive value of the test is too low to justify the enormous expenditure of money and labor necessary to repeatedly test an entire population. The currently available tests are also unable to define a cohort at increased risk for paucibacillary disease.

Antibody responses to various specific and cross-reactive mycobacterial antigens have also been studied in patients with leprosy. In general, patients with the highest number of bacilli (LL, BL, BB) have higher antibody levels than those with few organisms (BT, TT). However, since mycobacteria are easily demonstrated in skin biopsies or scrapings from multibacillary patients, a positive serological test is of little value for diagnosis. Among paucibacillary tuberculoid and indeterminate leprosy cases, where the histopathology is more difficult and less definitive, specific antibody is present only 25 to 60 percent of the time.

Resistance to *M. leprae* infection depends mainly on cellular immune reactions. Multibacillary leprosy is associated with a specific deficiency in cell-mediated immune reactivity against *M. leprae*, demonstrable both in vivo and vitro. This feature is considered directly responsible for the lack of inhibition of bacillary multiplication and is thus of the greatest significance for the progression of the disease to a multibacillary form. Resistance is correlated with cell-mediated immune reactivity demonstrable in vitro by the lymphocyte blast transformation (LBT) with various antigenic preparations from *M. leprae* or whole washed bacilli. The available evidence strongly indicates that reactivity in the LBT is more closely related to hypersensitivity than to acquired immunologically mediated resistance to *M. leprae*. Further work attempting to develop in vitro tests for the assay of true protective immunity is thus very important.

The mechanism of the lack of resistance in lepromatous leprosy is incompletely understood. Immunological tolerance has been implied, as well as excessive induction of suppressor mechanisms and genetic predisposition. The deficient cell-mediated immune reactivity in lepromatous leprosy has a pronounced specificity for *M. leprae*. Several different mechanisms may be responsible for the development of this immunodeficiency. Increased knowledge of its nature and the development of techniques for prevention or reversal after adequate chemotherapy would be of great importance.

Acute changes in the immunological balance between the host and the bacilli can be manifest clinically as "reactional states." These reactions can occur in untreated patients, but are most commonly observed during the initial 3 to 18 months of therapy. Although much has been learned of the immunological changes which occur *during* the reactional states, the underlying sequence of events which initiate the acute reactions is unknown.

Reversal reactions (also called type 1 reactions or upgrading reactions) occur in patients with BT, BB, or BL disease and appear to result from increased cellular immunity and delayed type hypersensitivity against antigens of *M. leprae*. Reversal reactions are associated with signs of neuritis and inflammation in the skin lesions. In some patients nerve symptoms predominate; in others the skin lesions are inflamed. Neuritis can lead to the loss of function in sensory and motor nerves, and, if not rapidly reversed, may lead to permanent neuropathy and the resulting claw hands, dropfoot, or cutaneous anesthesia, which in turn often results in chronic wound infections.

Erythema nodosum leprosum (ENL or type 2 reactions) presents with tender subcutaneous nodules, mainly on the arms and legs, appearing suddenly and usually disappearing after a few days. The disease is associated with general malaise and fever, and, in severe cases, there may be signs of a general immune complex disease with proteinuria, arthritis, and iridocyclitis. Both circulating and tissue-based immune complexes are detectable in most cases. Drugs which are active against T-helper lymphocytes such as cyclosporine A and thalidomide are effective in ENL, suggesting that aberrant activation of a subset of T-helper cells may be the underlying immune defect. ENL occurs in patients with lepromatous and borderline lepromatous disease.

Downgrading reactions are similar clinically to reversal reactions, although the immunological consequences are the opposite, with a general movement toward the lepromatous pole rather than toward the tuberculoid pole as is seen in reversal reactions. Downgrading reactions are seen primarily in untreated patients and during pregnancy in women on therapy.

Lucio's phenomenon is another immunologically mediated complication of leprosy. Clinically it is a necrotizing cutaneous vasculitis, and occurs almost exclusively in Mexican patients with a widely disseminated cutaneous form of lepromatous leprosy. In its most severe form it is extremely difficult to treat and is associated with a high mortality rate.

DIAGNOSIS

The diagnosis of leprosy should not be made unless there is absolute certainty. If there is the slightest doubt, the patient should be observed until further evidence confirms or excludes the disease. This will prevent psychological, social, and other damage to the patient by an incorrect diagnosis. The diagnosis is based on:

1. The presence of *M. leprae* in the skin, mucous membranes, or nerves. In practice this means the demonstration of acid-fast bacilli at one or more of these sites.
2. The presence of abnormal peripheral nerves, particularly at sites of predilection, associated with signs of nerve damage such as paralysis or sensory loss.

The following features assist in the diagnosis of the disease:

1. Skin lesions are of various kinds, and care should be taken to avoid misinterpretation due to racial differences. In dark-skinned people, the patch of tuberculoid leprosy is hypopigmented, whereas it is reddish in Caucasians. Lesions may be flat, with slightly raised borders, or nodular toward the lepromatous end of the spectrum. The lesions usually appear gradually but in some cases suddenly, do not itch, and often become anesthetic. The progression in most cases is slow, with a tendency to be prolonged over years.
2. There is often a history of paresthesia with numbness and hot and cold sensations in the extremities, especially in the area of the ulnar, median, and lateral popliteal nerves. The paresthesia may be followed by loss of cutaneous sensitivity and later by muscular weakness, paralysis, and atrophy.
3. Thickening of nerve trunks and superficial nerves occurs. During acute neuritis, nerve trunks are tender. They often become thickened and remain so for many years after the pain has subsided. Neuritis of other neurological diseases is very rarely accompanied by thickening of nerves, and on a global scale, leprosy is the most frequent cause of peripheral neuropathy.
4. Examination of skin smears for the presence of acid-fast bacilli is essential, especially in the diagnosis of lepromatous cases. The amount of bacilli in the lesions is recorded on a logarithmic scale as the bacterial index. The morphological appearance of the bacilli is recorded as the morphological index, which provides information on their viability, solid-staining bacilli being presumed viable and infectious, whereas granulated forms represent presumed dead bacilli.

Clinical examination considering the appearance of skin lesions and peripheral nerves combined with evaluation of nerve function and carefully prepared and read skin slit smears are usually sufficient for the diagnosis of leprosy and for characterization of the case as paucibacilliferous or multibacilliferous. With experience it should also be sufficient for classifying most cases within the clinical spectrum of the disease. Field personnel, even auxiliary personnel with modest training, should be able to recognize leprosy and classify cases in two broad categories, as tuberculoid or lepromatous leprosy.

Biopsies taken from the edge of active lesions are an important aid in accurate diagnosis and classification according to the full Ridley-Jopling scale.

The lepromin reaction is a skin test read at different times following intracutaneous injection of a reagent containing standardized amounts of autoclaved *M. leprae* from human lepromas or infected armadillos. The early (Fernandez) reaction is read after 48 to 72 h but is variable and of little diagnostic or prognostic importance. The late (Mitsuda) reaction is read after 1 month. A positive Mitsuda reaction consists of formation of a nodule consisting of granulomatous tissue with mononuclear cells and characteristic morphological features at the test site. A positive late lepromin reaction is *not* diagnostic for leprosy as it determines the ability of the individual to develop a cell-mediated immune reaction against *M. leprae*. The late lepromin reaction is positive in most patients with tuberculoid and borderline tuberculoid leprosy, but it is also positive in the majority of healthy individuals from leprosy-nonendemic countries. The late lepromin reaction is negative in patients with lepromatous leprosy, being an important in vivo indicator of the cellular immunodeficiency in this form of the disease.

TREATMENT

Dapsone (DDS) has been the major drug for the treatment of leprosy since its introduction in the late 1940s. The drug is cheap, easy to administer even under field conditions, and has few side effects at the regular dose of 100 mg daily. DDS is bacteriostatic, acts slowly, and needs prolonged administration. It has been extensively applied as monotherapy. The appearance of DDS resistance in leprosy patients treated with DDS alone was to be expected given the experience with monotherapy of tuberculosis. The first report of DDS-resistant leprosy appeared in 1964, but it was not until the 1970s that its widespread occurrence and serious implications were generally appreciated. Resistance which develops during DDS monotherapy is denoted *secondary resistance* and occurs after 3 to 24 years of treatment. It usually appears late due to the slow growth of *M. leprae* compared with other mycobacteria. The occurrence of secondary DDS resistance led to the introduction of combined chemotherapy, as in tuberculosis. When secondary DDS resistance became widespread, it was expected that primary DDS-resistant patients would also appear, and this was subsequently demonstrated in both tuberculoid and lepromatous leprosy. Further studies are urgently needed to determine the incidence of primary DDS resistance in various endemic countries.

Although DDS resistance is important in leprosy, it is only one of several problems faced in the treatment of multibacillary forms of leprosy. After prolonged treatment with DDS alone and the disappearance of all signs of active disease, there is still a risk of relapse upon withdrawal of chemotherapy. This is due to the presence of ''persistor'' bacilli. These are DDS-sensitive bacilli which survive in a dormant state in favored sites such as nerves. The persisting bacilli usually remain dormant while DDS is taken regularly, but when the drug is stopped, they begin to multiply and cause a relapse of the disease. Patient compliance is also a major problem in leprosy when chemotherapy lasts several years or even decades.

There is at present a marked tendency for advocating intensive chemotherapy courses, giving treatment with multiple drugs for shorter periods. Several such regimens are under clinical trial in hospital and field conditions, but there is wide agreement about certain general principles. It would be of great advantage if patients with paucibacillary leprosy could be treated with an intensive regimen for a restricted time period, which would be sufficient to ensure lack of progression or complete cure of the disease in most cases. Those patients might then be ''released from control'' to a greater extent than at present, allowing more of limited program resources to be concentrated on patients with multibacillary leprosy. Multibacillary cases need more intense and longer treatment.

The current approach to therapy of leprosy, which attempts to address several of these problems and concerns, is to use therapeutic regimens containing two or more drugs in all patients, as is done for tuberculosis. This permits more intensive chemotherapy to be administered for a shorter period of time.

Other than dapsone, the most active established agents against *M. leprae* are rifampin and clofazimine. These drugs are both more toxic and markedly more expensive than dapsone. Rifampin can cause hepatotoxicity as well as a ''flulike'' syndrome, and clofazimine is associated with gastrointestinal toxicity and skin discoloration and ichthyosis. Other agents with some activity against *M. leprae* include ethionamide, prothionamide, and some of the newer quinolones such as ofloxacin.

The following standard treatment regimens for leprosy control programs were recommended by a WHO study group in 1982:

For multibacillary patients:
Rifampin: 600 mg once monthly, supervised
Dapsone: 100 mg daily, self-administered
Clofazimine: 300 mg once monthly, supervised, together with 50 mg daily, self-administered

Where clofazimine is totally unacceptable because of skin discoloration, its replacement by 250 to 375 mg of self-administered daily doses of ethionamide or prothionamide should be considered. The optimal or essential duration of combined therapy has not been determined, but must be at least 2 years or until smear negativity.

For paucibacillary patients:
Rifampin: 600 mg once monthly, supervised
Dapsone: 100 mg daily, self-administered

The recommended duration of therapy in paucibacillary cases is 6 months unless signs of active disease persist. The preliminary results from the initial field studies with this regimen show a 3- to 5-year cumulative relapse rate of under 5 percent for paucibacillary cases.

A somewhat different approach to therapy is commonly practiced in developed countries, such as the United States, where most cases are imported, the cost of the drugs is less critical, and high-level primary dapsone resistance is uncommon. All patients are initially treated with daily rifampin and dapsone. In paucibacillary patients who show a rapid response, the rifampin is discontinued after 6 to 12 months and the dapsone after 12 to 36 months. Multibacillary cases are usually treated with just these two drugs unless there is a high likelihood of primary dapsone resistance or slow clinical response. The duration of therapy in multibacillary cases must be individualized depending on the rapidity of the clinical and histological response and the presence of any reactional states.

Reactions

During reactions the basic chemotherapy against *M. leprae* should not be discontinued. Additional drug treatment is given to reduce the inflammatory reaction. In reversal reactions with neuritis, high-dose corticosteroids are usually effective. Mild ENL symptoms are often sufficiently reduced by nonsteroidal anti-inflammatory agents. In more severe cases, high doses of glucocorticoids may be necessary to control the reaction. Thalidomide is very efficient in ENL, and severe ENL continues to be a definite indication for thalidomide treatment, provided that sufficient precautions be taken in women of childbearing age to prevent teratogenic effects. Clofazimine has anti-inflammatory activity and should be part of the regimen in patients with recurrent ENL.

The clinical diagnosis of *drug resistance* depends on demonstration of lack of improvement or the appearance of new lesions despite adequate administration of a particular drug, e.g., DDS. Resistance is confirmed by footpad testing in mice when multiplication of *M. leprae* occurs despite the addition of DDS to the food or drinking water. The significance of low-degree resistance demonstrated only by footpad testing has not been established. Various regimens are used for treatment of drug-resistant cases. The main principle is change of drugs, ensuring administration of at least two new drugs to which resistance has not been established.

Adequate medical treatment of episodes with acute neuritis is essential to reduce the risk or degree of permanent nerve damage with loss of nerve function. Deformity resulting from nerve damage is preventable in most cases. Early recognition of symptoms and early treatment is the essence of prevention, and even patients with established nerve damage can be significantly helped if they cooperate.

Health education is essential and must be adapted to the living conditions and cultural setting of the patient. Patients have to be taught how to live with their disabilities and how to avoid further damage by trauma and infection. This is particularly important for the insensitive hands and feet. Provision of protective devices such as special shoes and gloves is important. Even more so is educating the patient to recognize early damage and signs of ulcer formation so that these can be treated at an early stage, preventing the establishment of chronic secondary infection which in neglected cases is an important origin of chronic ulceration and deformity.

Surgical correction of deformity includes replacement of paralyzed muscles, tendon transplantation in limbs that are deformed but still mobile, and more extensive procedures to correct fixed deformities.

The limited resources available and the sheer volume of work imply that it is impossible to correct surgically all the deformities in leprosy patients. This fact underlines the need for early treatment and preventive care of those patients who have not yet developed serious deformities.

POPULATION

EPIDEMIOLOGY

The data on the prevalence of leprosy are unreliable in most countries, because neither case finding nor reporting is at a sufficiently high level. The number of registered patients and estimated cases is consequently too low. In 1975 WHO estimated the number of leprosy cases at 10,595,000. It is often stated that there are probably 12 million leprosy patients in the world today, mainly in Africa, India, southeast Asia, the Pacific region, and Latin America. The 1975 WHO estimate for Europe was 25,000 cases, a significant proportion being due to immigration from leprosy-endemic countries after World War II. Most cases of leprosy in the United States are attributable to immigration [*15*].

There are marked regional variations in prevalence rates. In countries with prevalence rates above 1 per 1000, leprosy constitutes a significant health problem. These variations may be due to genetic, nutritional, and socioeconomic factors, migratory patterns, and other factors which remain to be elucidated such as the roles of the environment and fomites. In most countries the occurrence of leprosy is patchy.

The incidence rate is a more accurate index of continuing transmission than the prevalence rate, but is difficult to obtain in leprosy. In practice, most leprosy control programs report prevalence and case detection rates. It would be of particular importance to compare incidence rates for infection with *M. leprae* with incidence rates of disease. Such data are unavailable and at present assayed indirectly. Over the last 15 to 20 years little variation has been recorded in overall estimates of leprosy prevalence. On a global basis, at most 50 percent of the registered cases get adequate regular treatment. For all cases this figure is probably less than 20 percent.

The problem of disability from leprosy has increased in importance and received special attention in recent years. Patients with disabilities represent significant losses of work hours, and the disabilities and deformities are among the main causes of prejudice against leprosy. A suitable criterion for the efficiency of a leprosy control program is the disability rate among newly registered cases. This rate decreases when patients are admitted for treatment at an earlier stage of the disease.

Untreated patients with multibacilliferous leprosy are highly infectious. The bacilli are mainly spread by nasal discharge, and the infection is thus transmitted as a droplet infection. *Mycobacterium leprae* is, however, of low pathogenicity. Subclinical infection is common, and clinical disease appears in only a few of the infected individuals. Among young household contacts of lepromatous cases a varying proportion (4 to 12 percent) have developed signs of leprosy within a 5-year period. Since most if not all cases have been infectious for long periods before treatment is sought, disease still occurs in household contacts despite treatment of the index case. To improve these figures, better techniques are needed for the diagnosis of subclinical infection, making it possible to start treatment at an early stage when a patient has few clinical symptoms but high infectivity.

The proportion of infected individuals who develop clinical disease may vary. In countries such as Norway, where leprosy virtually disappeared during less than 100 years, improvement in socioeconomic conditions has probably been a key factor, with infected individuals less prone to develop clinical disease and thus to transmit it to new individuals.

Leprosy control

The essence of leprosy control work is to introduce measures to decrease transmission of the infectious agent from patients to uninfected individuals. In leprosy, chemoprophylaxis in healthy individuals, environmental sanitation, and isolation of patients are inadequate means of intervention. Vaccination may become an essential factor in the future, but at present chemotherapy of known patients is the only effective tool.

The main function of a leprosy control program is thus to detect as many leprosy patients as possible at an early stage and to treat them adequately. This rapidly reduces their infectivity and helps break the chain of infection, reducing the number of new cases.

Since multibacillary cases are of the greatest importance for dissemination of the infection, work should be concentrated on early detection and treatment of such patients. To control leprosy effectively it is necessary to find and treat at least 75 percent of the multibacillary cases in a way which ensures a low incidence of relapse and renewed infectivity. This is difficult, mainly because of social and economic problems in most leprosy-endemic countries. The first step in the establishment of a leprosy control program [16] is an assessment of the baseline situation and the extent of the leprosy problem in the area. Areas with higher prevalence rates require more intensive case detection measures and considerably more work than areas of low disease prevalence where active case finding may be confined to relatively small groups of known contacts.

Diagnosis of early leprosy is based on recognition of certain clinical characteristics, which requires training of health personnel. The need for well-defined treatment regimens for various patient groups suitable for field work is to be emphasized.

When leprosy prevalence is rather low and leprosy services are reasonably well known, there is usually no need for active case finding, since a large proportion of the patients tend to report themselves spontaneously and at a sufficiently early stage. Case finding can be promoted significantly by educating the community and by good patient follow-up. When prevalence and incidence rates are high in areas where leprosy services are newly established, active case finding is important. Cost-benefit analyses should indicate areas where work should be concentrated. Mass campaigns and general surveys usually require more work per case found than does contact surveillance, particularly around households of known patients with multibacillary leprosy. Case finding is easier than case holding and continued treatment. Because of the chronic course of the disease and the need for prolonged treatment, good reporting systems are required to ensure that patients can be followed up and treatment continued even with a change of health staff or if the patient moves to another area.

Use of strict criteria for evaluation of the work is essential in leprosy because changes in patterns and incidence rates occur so slowly. The following parameters are of particular importance: extent of coverage; intensity of detection, particularly of early cases; disability rate among new cases; proportion of cases with single lesions among newly detected cases of tuberculoid leprosy; proportion of lepromatous subjects; treatment coverage rate; treatment attendance rate; and annual defaulting rate.

Patients themselves play an essential role in preventive work. They are important in detecting new patients and helping to keep them under treatment. Equally important is the fact that most of the deformities associated with leprosy are preventable, depending largely on patients' efforts to protect insensitive hands and feet. This ensures early detection of ulcers, thus preventing chronic secondary infection.

Needs and prospects

Leprosy still lags behind other important infectious diseases in the tropics with regard to knowledge, understanding of basic features, and methods for control. Predictions are difficult to make, and a multifaceted approach is recommended in leprosy research. Among the needs, the following should be stressed:

There is a great need for early and reliable detection of lepromatous leprosy, preferably in the subclinical stage. Adequate chemotherapy at this stage with a rapid decrease in infectivity of a significant proportion of these individuals is expected to have a great impact on the incidence of the disease. Antibody assays of high specificity and sufficient predictive value are needed for this purpose. Improved methods for the diagnosis of subclinical infection would also clarify the epidemiology of leprosy infection, and thus aid in defining the variables essential for the development of clinical disease.

Definition of suitable treatment regimens and the evaluation of their efficacy is a major task of the WHO Therapy of Leprosy (THELEP) program. The introduction of relatively short term, intensive treatment regimens is expected to be as valuable in leprosy as in tuberculosis, provided these regimens can be applied in the field and have an acceptable low relapse rate in multibacillary leprosy.

Improvement of program management is required to obtain better results in many leprosy control programs.

Development of a leprosy vaccine is a major priority of the WHO Immunology of Leprosy (IMMLEP) program. Current work is concentrated on the use of killed armadillo-grown *M. leprae* for this purpose. The development and application of an efficient leprosy vaccine on a sufficiently large scale is expected to be particularly valuable in reducing the incidence of the disease. The effect of BCG vaccination in protecting against tuberculosis varies considerably in different populations and in different circumstances. Testing the efficacy of a leprosy vaccine, therefore, presents great problems, particularly in view of the low incidence in many endemic countries, the long incubation period, and the slow development of the disease. The trial period would therefore need to be long. Further work is needed in animal models, especially in species closely related to humans.

Further characterization of the antigenic structure of *M. leprae* and the corresponding immune responses in leprosy patients is expected to provide much needed information on important factors involved in protective immunity and development of the disease and its complications.

Immune reactions are responsible for important clinical complications, mainly nerve damage, which cause the deformities so often associated with leprosy. Further studies of the pathogenesis of the various forms of reactions are needed as a basis for improving the treatment of these complications.

The lack of cell-mediated immune reactivity against *M. leprae* is responsible for the uninhibited growth of *M. leprae* in these individuals, leading to highly bacilliferous forms of the disease, which constitute the major infectious reservoir in the community. The nature of this immunodeficiency is poorly known and needs to be explored. Development of techniques for prevention or reversal of this immunodeficiency would have a marked impact on disease control.

Social aspects

The social consequences of leprosy are far greater than the medical consequences in many cultures. The deformities and disfiguration in advanced cases are important causes of the stigmatization of leprosy patients. Both prevention of deformity and health education of the general community are therefore important to reduce the stigma of this disease. Every effort should be made to educate the population that leprosy is a communicable disease which to a great extent can be prevented and treated. This would lessen the stigma of the disease for the individual patient and the community, thus making it possible to better control the disease.

REFERENCES

1 Harboe M: Armauer Hansen—the man and his work. Int J Lepr 41:417–424, 1973

2 Hunter SW, Fujiwara T, Brennan PJ: Structure and antigenicity of the major specific glycolipid antigen of *Mycobacterium leprae*. J Biol Chem 257:15072–15078, 1982

3 Hunter SW, Gaylord H, Brenna PJ: Structure and antigenicity of the phosphorylated lipopolysaccharide antigens from the leprosy and tubercle bacilli. J Biol Chem 26:12345–12351, 1986

4 Engers H, Abe M, Bloom BR, et al: Results of a WHO-sponsored workshop on monoclonal antibodies to *Mycobacterium leprae*. Infect Immun 48:603–605, 1985

5 Buchanan TM, Nomaguchi H, Anderson DC, et al: Characterization of antibody reactive epitopes on the 65,000 dalton protein molecule of *Mycobacterium leprae*. Mycobacterial species specificity. Infect Immun 55:1000–1003, 1987

6 Young DB, Fohn MJ, Khanolkar SR, et al: Monoclonal antibodies to a 28,000 dalton protein antigen of *Mycobacterium leprae*. Clin Exp Immunol 60:546–552, 1985

7 Young DB, Khanolkar SR, Barg LL, et al: Generation and characterization of monoclonal antibodies to the phenolic glycolipid of *Mycobacterium leprae*. Infect Immun 43:183–188, 1984

8 Young RA, Mehra V, Sweetser D, et al: Genes for the major protein antigens of *Mycobacterium leprae*. Nature 316:450–452, 1985

9 Mehra V, Sweetser D, Young RA: Efficient mapping of protein antigenic determinants. PNAS USA 83:7013–7017, 1986

10 Booth RJ, Harris DP, Love JM, et al: Antigenic proteins of *Mycobacterium leprae:* Complete sequence of the gene for the 18-kDa protein. J Immunol 140:597–601, 1988

11 Young DB, Buchanan TM: A serological test for leprosy with a glycolipid specific for *Mycobacterium leprae*. Science 221:1057–1059, 1983

12 Young DB, Lathigra R, Hendrix R, et al: Stress proteins are immune targets in leprosy and tuberculosis. Proc Natl Acad Sci USA 85:4267–4270, 1988

13 Ridley DS, Jopling WH: Classification of leprosy according to immunity. A five-group system. Int J Lepr 34:255–273, 1966

14 Modlin RL, Hofman FM, Taylor CR, et al: T lymphocyte subsets in the skin lesions of patients with leprosy. J Am Acad Dermatol 8:182, 1983

15 Neill MA, Hightower AL, Broome CV: Leprosy in the United States, 1971–1981. J Infect Dis 152:1064–1069, 1985

16 A Guide to Leprosy Control. Geneva, World Health Organization, 1980

Diphtheria · Neal A. Halsey · Margaret H. D. Smith

In 1884, Loeffler demonstrated that *Corynebacterium diphtheriae* was the etiological agent of diphtheria. During the ensuing 100-plus years, the exotoxin, which he postulated, has been discovered and its mechanism of action elaborated in exquisite detail. The subsequent development and widespread use of diphtheria toxoid in many developed countries has eliminated diphtheria as a major public health problem. However, both cutaneous and respiratory diphtheria infections remain common in most tropical countries. The mortality and morbidity associated with these infections could be prevented if appropriate resources were made available to immunization programs.

ETIOLOGICAL AGENT

MICROBIOLOGY

C. diphtheriae is a nonmotile, unencapsulated, pleomorphic bacillus with terminal swellings giving it the characteristic "club" shape [1–3]. On Loeffler's and other nutritionally deficient agar, the organisms appear to form sharp angles or "Chinese-letter" configurations. The organism is gram-positive but decolorizes easily. Methylene blue stains reveal characteristic purple-red metachromatic granules.

Gram stains of original specimens are unreliable for predicting the presence of *C. diphtheriae*. Gram stains of colonies of other *Corynebacterium* species may resemble *C. diphtheriae,* and gravis strains may not have the characteristic club shape [1–3]. Also, metachromatic granules and the Chinese-letter configurations may be seen with other *Corynebacterium* species. Therefore, cultures should always be performed with biochemical confirmation and tests for toxin production on all suspicious isolates.

C. diphtheriae grows on nutritionally enriched media used for most primary cultures of wounds and throats, but the colonies cannot be distinguished from the abundant normal throat and skin flora. Primary specimens should be inoculated onto selective media. These should include Loeffler's or Pai's agar slants and cystine-tellurite agar [3]. Blood agar should also be inoculated to detect group A β-hemolytic streptococci, which often coexist in diphtheritic infections. Some isolates of

C. diphtheriae may be completely inhibited by cystine-tellurite agar. Therefore, blood agar should be carefully examined for possible colonies in highly suspect clinical cases where characteristic colonies were not identified on selective media [3]. If these media are not readily available, culture swabs or suspect colonies from blood agar plates should be stored and transported in silica-gel packs designed for group A streptococci cultures, since *C. diphtheriae* survives drying well [4]. Tinsdale medium may be utilized instead of cystine-tellurite or Pai's agar, but its short (4 day) shelf life makes this medium impractical except in epidemics. Three colony types can be distinguished on tellurite and blood agar [2] (Table 89-1). No difference has been found in the exotoxins isolated from toxigenic strains of each type [5].

TOXIN

Diphtheria toxin is a protein with a molecular mass of 62,000 daltons [5,6]. As little as 13 μg/kg may be fatal for humans. It is produced only by strains of *C. diphtheriae* that have been lysogenized by phages containing the genetic information for toxin production. The DNA sequence responsible for insertion of the gene coding for toxin production has been identified, and hybridization techniques have allowed for epidemiological tracing of transmission of specific strains [7]. Toxin is produced at the site of local infection, absorbed through the locally inflamed tissue, and circulated throughout the body. The intact toxin molecule (which is inactive) attaches to cellular receptors by forming bonds at the fragment B portion. Exposure to trypsin results in lysis of two disulfide bridges splitting fragment A (24,000 daltons) and fragment B (39,000 daltons). Fragment A enters the cell by endocytosis and enzymatically catalyzes a reaction, resulting in the production of adenosine diphosphoribase (ADP) bound to elongation factor 2 (EF2). This EF2-ADP complex is inactive, but it binds firmly to ribosomes. Protein synthesis is stopped when a sufficient number of sites on ribosomes are occupied by inactive complexes to block the function of transfer RNA. A single molecule of fragment A introduced into a cell may result in cell death.

Toxin production can be demonstrated by two methods. The most reliable technique is the guinea pig lethality test [3]. A

Table 89-1. Characteristics of *C. diphtheriae* colony types

Colony type	Shape	Pigment on tellurite agar	Hemolysis	Fermentation Starch	Fermentation Glycogen
Mitis	Smooth, convex	Black	Weak	−	−
Gravis	Semirough, flat	Gray to black	−	+	+
Intermedius	Smooth, small	Black center	−	−	−

McFarland no. 3 standard concentration of organisms is produced from a 24-h growth on Loeffler's or Pai's medium in broth (not saline). Five milliliters of suspension is inoculated subcutaneously in the shaved skin area of each of two guinea pigs. One animal (control) has been pretreated 2 h earlier with 1000 U of diphtheria antitoxin administered intraperitoneally. Toxigenic strains will produce hemorrhagic edema at the injection site followed by local necrosis, intoxication, or death within 10 days in the test animal but not in the control animal. Nontoxigenic strains do not produce local necrosis or death. A more rapid in vitro immunodiffusion test (Ouchterlony-Elek test) is done in some laboratories [3]. A filter-paper strip dipped in 100 U/mL antitoxin is allowed to dry on Elek agar supplemented with 2% sterile rabbit serum and 0.3% potassium tellurite. A loop from a 24-h growth on Loeffler's medium is streaked up to the filter-paper strip. Toxigenic strains result in an arrow-shaped line of precipitation pointing toward the filter paper. Known toxigenic and nontoxigenic control strains should be tested simultaneously.

PATIENT

PATHOGENESIS AND PATHOLOGICAL FINDINGS

C. diphtheriae is usually acquired on mucous membranes of the upper respiratory tract or through skin disruptions such as insect bites, abrasions, or wounds. Rarely, local infection may occur on other mucous membranes, including the external ear, genitalia, and intestinal tract.

Release of exotoxin causes local tissue necrosis which provides a favorable bacterial growth medium and thereby increases toxin production [5]. An adherent, thin (1- to 3-mm) gray membrane is produced from exudative fluid, necrotic cell material, red blood cells, white blood cells, fibrinous material, and bacteria. Local and regional lymph nodes are usually enlarged, and surrounding tissues are frequently edematous.

Exotoxin is absorbed locally and circulates via the bloodstream. Although any human tissue can be affected, heart, skeletal muscle, kidneys, and peripheral neurons are most susceptible. Mild degenerative changes may be noted in other tissues including the spleen, adrenals, and liver. The changes in skeletal muscle and myocardial tissue consist of accumulation of lipids, cell necrosis, hyaline degeneration, edema, and minimal mononuclear cell infiltration [8,9]. In surviving patients, fibrosis and muscle regeneration take place.

CLINICAL MANIFESTATIONS

The pharynx is involved in at least 50 percent of patients with diphtheria of the respiratory tract. The onset of pharyngeal (respiratory) diphtheria is often insidious, with low-grade fever, listlessness, and pallor. These signs usually appear within a week after exposure. Sore throat is rarely severe, and the presenting complaints can be fatigue, headache, and vomiting.

Erythema of the pharynx appears, followed by whitish or grayish spots on one or both tonsils. These lesions coalesce to form a transparent, veillike membrane which thickens, darkens, and usually extends, often asymmetrically. The membrane is adherent and bleeds when pulled loose. It may spread to involve the uvula, soft palate, nasopharynx, larynx, trachea, bronchi, and rarely the esophagus. The characteristic red border surrounding the membrane represents the area already damaged by toxin of the advancing diphtheritic infection. The more extensive the membrane and the darker its color, the greater the toxin absorption.

Oozing of blood from the nose, mouth, or throat indicates malignant diphtheria, which has a poor prognosis [10]. Patients with malignant diphtheria characteristically have an abrupt onset of high fever and prostration. Extensive perilymphatic edema may simulate a "bull neck," with secondary pressure on the cervical veins and trachea (Fig. 89-1). In most cases, cervical and submandibular lymph nodes are enlarged but not as tender as in streptococcal infections. The lymph nodes are apt to be more edematous, even brawny, and less well delineated than in other infections. Bleeding secondary to throm-

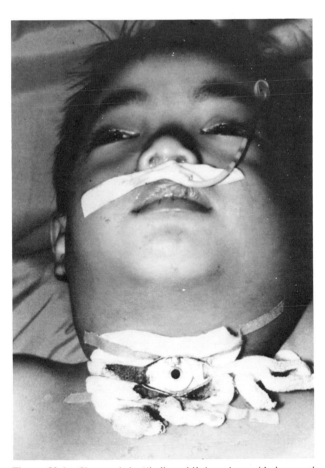

Figure 89-1. Characteristic "bull neck" in a boy with laryngeal diphtheria. A tracheostomy has been performed to relieve the obstruction. (*Courtesy of the World Health Organization Expanded Programme on Immunization.*)

bocytopenia or disseminated intravascular coagulation occurs commonly in severely affected patients [*11*].

While the pharynx is involved in most patients with diphtheria of the respiratory tract, another 25 percent suffer involvement of the larynx, either primarily or by extension from the upper airway [*10*]. Primary laryngeal diphtheria occurs most often in children under 5 years of age. These children have an abrupt onset of hoarseness, respiratory stridor, dyspnea, and steady progression to respiratory obstruction as the membrane on the vocal cords thickens. In tracheobronchial diphtheria, the membrane may form a cast of the respiratory tree, resulting in expiratory obstruction, atelectasis, and cyanosis.

Nasal diphtheria can present with thick, purulent discharge, often with marked crusting and erosion of the nostril. The discharge can be serosanguineous, which is particularly suggestive of diphtheria, especially if it is unilateral. Nasal diphtheria is apt to be chronic and toxemia minimal. These patients, however, are dangerously effective disseminators of *C. diphtheriae*.

Diphtheritic otitis media is uncommon, perhaps because the organism is highly aerobic. It develops by extension from the nasopharynx, characteristically with destruction of the tympanic membrane and secondary otitis externa.

Cutaneous diphtheria occurs most frequently in tropical and subtropical climates. High humidity, poor hygiene, and frequent skin abrasions or insect bites appear to facilitate diphtheritic infections of the skin. Cutaneous diphtheria is frequent among young children in tropical climates and probably accounts for early acquisition of immunity to diphtheria [*12,13*]. In adults, "tropical ulcers" and "desert ulcers" have been a serious problem among European and American soldiers stationed in the Mediterranean, South Pacific, and Asiatic areas [*14*].

The clinical picture is quite variable. Diphtheritic skin lesions may resemble impetigo, ecthyma, pyoderma, insect bites, dry scaly lesions, and deep punched-out lesions with or without a leathery eschar [*14–16*]. Many such lesions yield β-hemolytic streptococci and *Staphylococcus aureus* as well as toxigenic and nontoxigenic strains of *C. diphtheriae*. Although cutaneous lesions tend to be chronic, toxin absorption is rarely severe, and complications are uncommon.

Diphtheritic infection of traumatic and surgical wounds occurs particularly among young adults in the tropics. Hospital outbreaks of wound diphtheria, often disseminated by nasopharyngeal diphtheria, have been reported.

Genital diphtheria involving the penis, vulva, or vagina is not rare and must be differentiated from syphilitic chancre. Conjunctivitis due to diphtheritic infection occurs in both newborns and older individuals. It can be catarrhal or purulent in the early stages before becoming membranous and is often accompanied by enlargement of the preauricular lymph nodes and rhinitis. Corneal ulcers can occur, leading to blindness and loss of the eye. Infective endocarditis due to *C. diphtheriae* has only rarely been reported.

Complications occur in approximately 20 percent of patients hospitalized with diphtheria. The incidence depends on several factors including: (1) the biotype of *C. diphtheriae*, (2) the length of time between onset of disease and administration of antitoxin, (3) the site of infection, (4) the extent of membrane formation, and (5) the prior immune status of the patient [*10,15,17–20*]. The most common complications are respiratory obstruction, myocarditis, and paralysis.

Respiratory obstruction in diphtheria may occur in three ways [*10*]. In severe, or "malignant," tonsillar diphtheria, the edema of the tonsils, pharynx, and submandibular and cervical areas may block the upper airway necessitating tracheostomy. Attempts to remove the membrane are futile and usually result in bleeding and increased edema.

Primary localization of the membrane on the vocal cords usually occurs in infants less than 3 years of age. This produces hoarseness and inspiratory stridor with impaired oxygenation, followed by dyspnea, cyanosis, and finally fatigue, hypercapnia, and coma. Older children and adults are more likely to develop laryngeal diphtheria as an extension from the pharynx. Because of the larger size of the larynx in older individuals, complete obstruction does not occur as readily. Removal of the membrane is useless, and intubation is dangerous because it can result in downward displacement of the membrane with abrupt obstruction. Tracheostomy is far safer.

Tracheobronchial localization of the membrane can directly block the finer bronchi and bronchioles, causing atelectasis and pneumonia. Although this condition is often fatal, some patients survive with intensive supportive care, including oxygen therapy. Approximately 12 to 24 h after antitoxin administration, the membrane can loosen and cause obstruction. The tracheobronchial membrane can sometimes be withdrawn by careful bronchoscopic aspiration.

Myocarditis occurs in 20 to 80 percent of patients hospitalized for diphtheria [*9,10*]. It is far more common in pharyngeal or nasopharyngeal diphtheria than in laryngeal or cutaneous diphtheria. Myocarditis is less often associated with milder cases. This complication usually presents in the second week ("early" myocarditis) with muffled heart sounds and embryocardia, followed by depression of the T waves on electrocardiogram. The progression of myocarditis is highly variable. Early myocarditis may resolve permanently and uneventfully. However, the disease can lead to conduction disturbances (prolonged PR interval, bundle branch block, partial or complete AV block) and auricular fibrillation or flutter. Some patients have sudden onset of hypotension, pallor, and poor peripheral perfusion. Others develop marked cardiac dilatation and congestive heart failure. Occasionally in patients with marked cardiac dilatation, endocardial emboli may be dislodged, obstructing blood vessels to the brain, internal organs, or extremities. The mortality rate of early myocarditis is 10 to 50 percent. The late form of myocarditis appears during the fourth to sixth week. It is usually less severe and has a mortality rate of less than 2 percent. The survival rate is directly related to the availability and quality of supportive care.

Both forms of myocarditis may result in complete recovery, even after months of cardiac disturbances. However, sudden cardiac arrest can occur in the fourth to eighth week after onset of illness. In cutaneous diphtheria, cardiac symptoms may appear 3 to 8 weeks after the onset of skin lesions, but death is rare.

Polyneuritis occurs in at least 10 to 20 percent of patients with nasopharyngeal diphtheria [10]. Paralysis is believed to be more frequent in tropical than in temperate climates and occurs more often in older individuals than in young children. The characteristic pattern begins with palatal paralysis during the first 10 to 14 days after onset of faucial diphtheria. If the pharyngeal lesion is predominantly unilateral, palatal paralysis is more severe on, or confined to, that side. Paralysis of swallowing may occur a few days later, as well as paralysis of the muscles for accommodation and extraocular movement. These clinical signs may resolve spontaneously or be followed by symmetrical skeletal motor paralysis affecting proximal before distal muscles. Involvement of any or all muscles may occur including diaphragmatic paralysis and patchy sensory nerve loss. Even in the most extensively affected patients, the cerebral cortex is not involved.

The paralysis progresses for as long as 3 months, then recedes at the same rate and in the reverse order of its appearance. Recovery is complete by 6 months. In cutaneous diphtheria, paralysis of the cranial nerves occurs rarely, if at all. However, paresthesias are more common in cutaneous diphtheria than in faucial diphtheria. The spinal fluid in patients with neuritis shows elevated albumin content roughly proportional to the severity of paralysis, usually without pleocytosis. The presentation of diphtheritic polyneuritis may be similar to that of Guillain-Barré syndrome.

DIAGNOSIS

Bacteriological confirmation should be sought in all suspect cases of diphtheria. However, the limited availability of resources and the delay in laboratory confirmation usually necessitates initiation of therapy on the clinical findings alone. The toxic-appearing child with a bull neck and an asymmetrical, adherent, gray membrane that bleeds on removal presents no diagnostic problem. Milder illnesses, however, are often misdiagnosed.

Gram stains of membranous material are unreliable for determining the presence of *C. diphtheriae*. Cultures are obtained by inserting swabs under the membrane, if possible, or by vigorously rubbing over the surface. Nasal cultures should be taken in all suspect cases, even if no membrane is present. For cutaneous diphtheria, cultures should be obtained from more than one lesion and from nose and throat.

Negative cultures do not exclude the diagnosis of diphtheria. Poor technique in obtaining the specimens and improper media preparation could preclude the isolation of organisms.

The appearance of the membrane is the most useful char-

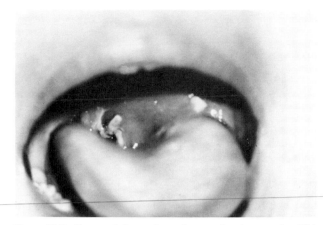

Figure 89-2. Characteristic membrane in posterior pharynx of a child with diphtheria. Note the asymmetrical pattern and the extension onto the soft palate. (*Courtesy of the World Health Organization Expanded Programme on Immunization.*)

acteristic in distinguishing diphtheria from other causes of pharyngitis (Fig. 89-2). The membrane associated with pharyngeal diphtheria is more adherent to the mucosa, sometimes darker, and often less symmetrical than that seen in membranous pharyngitis due to other agents. The diphtheritic membrane may cover only the tonsils, but frequently spreads to involve the uvula, soft palate, hard palate, nasal mucosa, or trachea.

Group A β-hemolytic streptococci cause exudative tonsillitis with petechiae and a fiery red posterior pharynx. Although streptococci are found in as many as 32 percent of patients with diphtheria, the appearance of the membrane is usually not changed. Pneumococci and other bacteria rarely cause exudative pharyngitis. Infectious mononucleosis and adenovirus infections also cause exudative pharyngitis, lymphadenopathy, and dysphagia in severe cases. The presence of an enlarged tender spleen should suggest infectious mononucleosis. Leukemia, aplastic anemia, and other blood dyscrasias can cause coalescent ulcerative lesions in the pharynx. Oral thrush (*Candida*) and coalescent herpes simplex ulcers can also produce a membranous appearance. Ingestion of paraquat, a herbicide, has been reported to cause a membrane and severe illness suggestive of diphtheria. Following tonsillectomy, some children will develop gray membranes over the surgical site. Other causes of ulcerative pharyngitis, such as Vincent's angina and tularemia, are often associated with lymphadenopathy and edema. In young children, foreign bodies in the nose are common causes of foul-smelling, purulent discharges which could resemble nasal diphtheria. Ludwig's angina caused by mixed oral flora or *H. influenzae* type b is associated with severe swelling of the neck similar to that seen in diphtheria. Peritonsillar or retropharyngeal abscesses and epiglottitis are other causes of difficulty in swallowing and respiratory tract obstruction.

TREATMENT

There are four objectives in the treatment of toxigenic diphtheria:

1. Inactivate unbound toxin as rapidly as possible.
2. Enforce bed rest and provide intensive supportive care to prevent or minimize complications.
3. Eliminate *C. diphtheriae* from the patient to prevent transmission.
4. Treat concomitant infections and complications.

Once a tentative diagnosis of diphtheria has been made, diphtheria antitoxin should be administered as quickly as possible. Mortality rates from diphtheria increase from less than 1 percent when antitoxin is administered on the first day of clinical illness to 30 percent when antitoxin is delayed beyond the sixth day [10]. As cultures take 24 to 72 h, antitoxin treatment should be given on the basis of clinical and epidemiological evidence. Diphtheria antitoxin, however, neutralizes only toxin which is circulating or which has been bound to cell surfaces for a short time.

Prior to injection of antitoxin, the patient should be tested for immediate hypersensitivity to horse serum by injecting intradermally 0.1 mL of diphtheria antitoxin, diluted 1:1000, with 0.1 mL of saline as a control. The conjuctival test, which is more sensitive and reliable, uses one drop of antitoxin diluted 1:10 in one eye, with a drop of saline in the opposite eye as a control. However, this test is useless in a crying child or an uncooperative adult. If the hypersensitivity test is negative in 20 min, the entire dose of antitoxin should be given intravenously in one dose.

Antitoxin must be diluted 1:20 in normal saline and administered at a rate not to exceed 1 mL/min. Dosage has been determined empirically and is based on the severity of clinical presentation rather than on the age or weight of the patient. Recommended doses are as follows:

Mild cases of nasal or tonsillar diphtheria, 20,000 U

Moderate cases of nasal, tonsillar, or laryngeal diphtheria, 40,000 U

Severe cases, late cases, or patients with involvement of multiple areas, 80,000 to 120,000 U

Serum sickness occurs in 5 to 10 percent of individuals who receive antitoxin, but the incidence is lower in young children. Some patients who recover from diphtheria remain Schick-positive or have recurrent disease. Therefore, immunization with diphtheria toxoid should be started during the second week of illness.

Although antibiotics do not alter the clinical course of diphtheria, all patients should be treated to eradicate *C. diphtheriae* and group A β-hemolytic streptococci, which are found frequently in both respiratory and cutaneous diphtheria infections. Either intramuscular procaine penicillin or intravenous aqueous penicillin is recommended for 10 days for all patients with toxigenic infections. Erythromycin is equally effective for penicillin-sensitive patients. [21]. Recently, several erythromycin-resistant strains of *C. diphtheriae* have been isolated from skin lesions [22]. The significance of this observation is not yet clear.

Enforced bed rest should be maintained for a minimum of 3 weeks in all patients with respiratory diphtheria. Careful physical examinations to detect changes in cardiac status and the development of paralysis should be carried out daily. Electrocardiograms should be obtained three times a week. If signs of myocarditis develop, bed rest should be extended to 4 to 6 weeks after the onset of illness. Severe cardiac failure may develop rapidly and late-onset arrhythmias may lead to sudden death. Patients with myocarditis should not be allowed to care for themselves or to get out of bed.

In patients with laryngeal diphtheria, significant local edema may compromise the airway. Equipment for suction and tracheostomy must be immediately available for these patients.

Although 50 percent or more of cutaneous diphtheria infections are caused by toxigenic strains, few result in complications [14,15,23–25]. However, both myocarditis and paralysis can occur. Antitoxin should be administered to all patients with signs of toxicity or local membrane formation. It is reasonable to treat the remaining patients with penicillin or erythromycin only and observe them closely. Topical application of penicillin has been shown effective [14] but may be associated with development of hypersensitivity. Bacitracin is a safe and effective alternative.

Digitalis administration is recommended at the earliest sign of cardiac enlargement or congestive failure, whether or not any conductive abnormality is present [26]. The majority of deaths due to diphtheria are the result of respiratory obstruction, congestive heart failure, or arrhythmias. Strict enforcement of bed rest is essential in all patients with myocarditis to minimize the cardiac workload. If signs of myocarditis develop during the first 3 weeks, then bed rest must be prolonged for 6 weeks. Digitalis levels should be monitored to avoid toxicity. Steroid therapy was not effective for prevention of myocarditis or neuritis in a randomized trial in Thailand [27].

Pharyngeal paralysis often results in difficulty in swallowing. Patients should be kept on their side and fed by nasogastric tube if necessary. The foot of the bed should be elevated to aid in removal of saliva. Paralysis of respiratory muscles requires the use of a respirator. Complete paralysis requires total nursing care, similar to that provided to quadriplegics to avoid aspiration, asphyxia, and other complications.

Persons in the same household or in close contact with a patient with diphtheria should be closely observed. Daily contact with a nurse or physician for signs or symptoms of illness should be maintained for 10 days. All close contacts should receive erythromycin, 30 to 40 mg/(kg•day) (maximum dose 1 g/day). Although slightly less effective, benzathine penicillin eradicates *C. diphtheriae* from the respiratory tract in 88 percent of individuals and should be administered if compliance is uncertain [21]. If family contacts have been inadequately immunized, they should receive two doses of the appropriate concentration of diphtheria toxoid or tetanus-diphtheria combination as listed under "Prevention and Control," below. Diphtheria antitoxin need not be given to asymptomatic individuals unless they are unimmunized, cannot be maintained under daily observation, and are at high risk of developing diphtheria.

POPULATION

EPIDEMIOLOGY

C. diphtheriae infections occur throughout the world. In tropical and semitropical climates cutaneous diphtheria infections are more common than respiratory infections. The differences in the primary site of infection result in significant changes in the patterns of immunity and the epidemiology of respiratory infections.

Humans are the only significant reservoir for *C. diphtheriae* in nature. Infection is acquired by contact with respiratory secretions or by direct contact with infected skin lesions. Cutaneous diphtheria is more contagious than respiratory diphtheria, and skin lesions are the most common source of infection in tropical countries and in crowded impoverished areas of temperate climates [15,28]. Rarely, foodborne transmission has been observed with unpasteurized milk. Since *C. diphtheriae* survives drying, transmission by fomites such as contaminated clothing and bedding is possible. However, attempts to decontaminate bedding have not been effective in decreasing the transmission of skin disease [17].

Cutaneous *C. diphtheriae* infections are infrequent causes of severe clinical illness is spite of the fact that 50 percent or more of strains isolated from skin may be toxigenic. The evidence is overwhelming that cutaneous infections result in immunity against severe respiratory diphtheria [12,13,15,18,29]. The high rates of cutaneous diphtheria infections in tropical countries, especially in coastal areas, results in immunity in most children by midchildhood. Bennett and others have noted increased rates of infection in children living near water [30]. However, these studies are confounded by the low socioeconomic status of families living over water. High rates of skin infection also occur among the native populations in northwest Canada and American Indians living in the southwest United States in semiarid conditions [28,31]. These apparently conflicting findings may be best explained by noting that poverty, crowding, poor sanitation, and increased skin trauma are the common factors correlating with a high incidence of diphtheria infections throughout the world.

In temperate zones, the frequency of respiratory and cutaneous diphtheria decreases in the warm months of the year [17]. The seasonal pattern of diphtheria in tropical climates has not been well defined. In India, respiratory diphtheria occurs most frequently during the rainy season [32]. However, Bennett did not find an association between rainfall and the frequency of skin and respiratory tract diphtherial isolates in Colombia [30].

Maternal IgG antibody to diphtheria crosses the placenta to the fetus. Thus, infants born to immune mothers are protected during the first few months of life, but the antitoxin does not prevent infants from developing an adequate response to immunization [33]. In temperate climates, the incidence of respiratory diphtheria infections and subsequent mortality is highest in young school-age children [31]. Limited data from tropical countries suggest that severe respiratory illness with subsequent death is more common in persons over 30 years of age [32]. The highest case fatality rates from diphtheria are in children less than 5 years and persons more than 40 years of age. In developing countries, cutaneous infections are most common in young children. For reasons that are unclear in the United States, the incidence of cutaneous infections increases with age [28,31].

Asymptomatic males and females have similar carriage rates of *C. diphtheriae*. However, the mortality rate is higher in males than in females. In the United States, the incidence of respiratory infections is slightly higher for males, and the incidence of cutaneous infections is eight times higher in males over 19 years of age than in females of the same age group [31].

The influence of race is difficult to differentiate from that of socioeconomic status in diphtheria infections. In the United States, the incidence of diphtheria infections among whites and blacks is similar. However, the incidence in the American Indian population is 10 to 30 times higher for both respiratory and cutaneous infections. Differences in case fatality rates by race have also been noted. The mortality rate of respiratory infections is slightly lower in the American Indians and native Canadians than in other populations [28,31]. This may be due to the high incidence of cutaneous infections observed in American Indians resulting in partial immunity and less severe respiratory infections. The incidence of diphtheria is higher in lower-socioeconomic-status populations throughout the world, probably because of limited water supply and increased transmission in crowded living conditions.

PREVENTION AND CONTROL

Immunity to *C. diphtheriae* may be acquired by natural infection or by immunization with diphtheria toxoid. Antitoxin levels of 0.01 antitoxin units per milliliter generally protect against clinical infection. However, antitoxin immunity is relative. Lower levels of antitoxin may offer some protection; high doses of toxin may produce illness despite "protective" levels of antitoxin. In areas where *C. diphtheriae* skin infections are common, most children develop antitoxin early in life. Children without detectable antitoxin may also be immune secondary to infection with nontoxigenic strains. Antibodies against somatic antigens of *C. diphtheriae* have been demonstrated in both humans and animals following infection or immunization with whole organisms. Although these individuals are Schick-positive, they may not be susceptible to *C. diphtheriae* infections [*10*]. However, there is no convenient test to determine antibacterial as opposed to antitoxic immunity. Since severe diphtheria continues to occur, all children should be immunized with diphtheria toxoid.

In 1913 Schick introduced the first practical test for immunity to diphtheria toxin. A small amount (one-fiftieth of the lethal dose for a guinea pig) of toxin is administered intradermally on the volar aspect of the forearm. Susceptible individuals develop a local inflammatory reaction that peaks in 4 to 7 days followed by desquamation or rarely by local necrosis. Persons with circulating antitoxin antibodies ($\geq$0.01 antitoxin units per milliliter) have no reaction since the toxin is neutralized. Rarely, sensitivity to other components in the toxin preparation results in a false-positive reaction, which, however, is usually maximal in 18 to 72 h rather than in 4 to 7 days. The Schick test is useful in epidemiological surveys and for evaluating the effectiveness of diphtheria immunization. However, more sensitive and specific laboratory tests for measuring antitoxin are available and should be utilized when possible. Serum antibody levels should be measured in assays standardized with international reference sera, and simplified blood collection on filter paper has proved to be satisfactory for testing small volumes of blood collected from infants [*34*].

The Moloney test is performed by injecting 0.1 mL of a 1:100 dilution of fluid toxoid intradermally. If erythema develops between 18 to 24 h, the test is positive and the individual is immune to *C. diphtheriae* and its by-products. A high percentage of Moloney-positive individuals may develop undesirable side effects if the standard pediatric diphtheria toxoid preparations are administered. Thus, this test should be useful to detect hypersensitive individuals in areas where skin infections are common.

Diphtheria toxoid induces the development of antibodies against diphtheria toxin but not against the bacterium itself. Since most symptoms and complications are due to effects of the toxin, the toxoid preparations are highly effective in preventing disease and deaths due to diphtheria.

Diphtheria toxoid is highly immunogenic. Adsorbed and alum-precipitated toxoids induce significantly higher and longer lasting antitoxin titers than plain toxoid does. Preparations designed for children usually contain 5 to 25 flocculating units (Lf) of diphtheria toxoid in addition to tetanus toxoid and pertussis vaccine (DTP or DPT). Preparations designed for adults [tetanus-diphtheria toxoid (Td)] contain only 1 to 2 Lf of diphtheria toxoid combined with tetanus toxoid without pertussis vaccine.

In susceptible individuals, a single dose of diphtheria toxoid does not induce protective levels of antitoxin. In countries where skin infections are common, children may be partially immune, and one or two doses might induce protective levels of antitoxin [*29*]. Two doses of DTP are sufficient to induce

protective levels of antibodies in 90 to 100 percent of infants [*35*]. However, to ensure immunity, three doses of DTP should be administered at 1- to 2-month intervals beginning at 6 to 8 weeks of age. A booster dose of DTP is recommended approximately 12 months after the third primary dose. In temperate climates, an additional dose is administered at 4 to 6 years of age, and Td is given every 10 years in the United States to ensure persistence of immunity. The absence of booster doses in adults has been associated with 10 to 30 percent of the population having less than protective levels of serum antibodies and outbreaks of diphtheria [*36*]. Preparations containing 6 Lf or less may be suboptimal for primary immunization of adults who did not receive routine DTP injections in childhood [*37*]. More than three doses of Td are necessary to ensure adequate immunity. The need for booster doses and the rate of hypersensitivity reactions in tropical climates where skin diphtheria is common have not been established.

Immunized individuals may become carriers of *C. diphtheriae*. In some outbreaks, no difference in carrier rates has been observed between fully immunized, partially immunized, or unimmunized individuals. However, immunized individuals harbor reduced numbers of infectious organisms, and they are less likely to transmit the infection. In highly immunized populations, a marked reduction in carrier rates of *C. diphtheriae* has been observed, and immunization may selectively decrease carriage of toxigenic strains [*38*].

REFERENCES

1 Barksdale L: *Corynebacterium diphtheriae* and its relatives. Bacteriol Rev 34:378–422, 1970

2 Wilson G: *Corynebacterium diphtheriae* and other corynebacteria organisms, in Wilson GS, Miles A (eds): *Principles of Bacteriology, Virology and Immunity,* 7th ed, vol. 12. Baltimore, Williams & Wilkins, 1983, pp. 94–113.

3 Coyle MB, Hollis DG, Groman AB: Corynebacteria, in Lennette EH, Ballows A, Hausler WJ, et al (eds): *Manual of Clinical Microbiology,* 4th ed. Washington, DC, American Society for Microbiology, 1985, pp 194–198

4 Kim-Farley RJ, Soewarso TI, Rejeki S, et al: Silica gel as transport medium for *Coyrnebacterium diphtheriae* under tropical conditions (Indonesia). J Clin Microbiol 25:964–965

5 Uchida T: Diphtheria toxin. Pharmacol Ther 19:107–122, 1983

6 Pappenheimer AM, Harper AA, Moynihan M, et al: Diphtheria toxin and related proteins: Effect of route of injection of toxicity and the determination of cytotoxicity for various cultured cells. J Infect Dis 145:94–102, 1982

7 Rappuoli R, Perugini M, Falsen E: Molecular epidemiology of the 1984–1986 outbreak of diphtheria in Sweden. N Engl J Med 318: 12–14, 1988

8 Simmons LE, Abbott JD, MaCaulay ME, et al: Diphtheria carriers in Manchester: Simultaneous infection with toxigenic and nontoxigenic mitis strains. Lancet 1:304–305, 1980

9 Boyer NH, Weinstein L: Diphtheritic myocarditis. N Engl J Med 239:913–919, 1948

10 Naiditch MJ, Bower AG: Diphtheria: A study of 1,433 cases observed during a ten-year period at the Los Angeles County Hospital. Am J Med 17:229–245, 1954

11 Wesley AG, Pather M, Chrystol V: The haemorrhagic diathesis in diphtheria with special reference to disseminated intravascular coagulation. Ann Trop Pediatrics 1:51–56, 1981

12 Tasman A, Lansberg HP: Problems concerning the prophylaxis, pathogenesis and therapy of diphtheria. Bull WHO 16:939–973, 1957

13 Kriz B, Teply V, Pecenka J, et al: Immunologic surveys of diphtheric antitoxic antibodies in some African and Asian countries. J Hyg Epidemiol Microbiol Immunol 24:42–62, 1980

14 Liebow AA, MacLean PD, Bumstead JH, et al: Tropical ulcers and cutaneous diphtheria. Arch Intern Med 78:255–295, 1946

15 Belsey MA, Sinclair M, Roder MR, et al: *Corynebacterium diphtheriae* skin infections in Alabama and Louisiana. A factor in the epidemiology of diphtheria. N Engl J Med 280:135–141, 1969

16 Funt TR: Primary cutaneous diphtheria. JAMA 176:273–275, 1961

17 Brooks GF, Bennett JV, Feldman RA: Diphtheria in the United States, 1959–1970. J Infect Dis 129:172–178, 1974

18 Griffith AH: The role of immunization in the control of diphtheria. Dev Biol Stan 43:3–13, 1979

19 Miller LW, Older JJ, Drake J, et al: Diphtheria immunization. Effect upon carriers and the control of outbreaks. Am J Dis Child 123:197–199, 1972

20 Tasman A, Minkenhof JE, Vink HH, et al: Importance of intravenous injection of diphtheria antiserum. Lancet i:1299–1304, 1958

21 McCloskey RV, Green MJ, Eller J, et al: Treatment of diphtheria carriers. Benzathine penicillin, erythromycin, and clindamycin. Ann Intern Med 81:788–791, 1974

22 Coyle MB, Minshew BH, Bland JA, et al: Erythromycin and clindamycin resistance in *Corynebacterium diphtheriae* from skin lesions. Antimicrob Agents Chemother 16:525–527, 1979

23 Bacon DF, Marples MJ: Researches in western Samoa. II. Lesions of the skin and their bacteriology. Trans R Soc Trop Med Hyg 49:76–81, 1955

24 Bezjak V, Farsey SJ: *Corynebacterium diphtheriae* in skin lesions in Ugandan children. Bull WHO 43:643–650, 1970

25 Bray JP, Burt EG, Potter EV, et al: Epidemic diphtheria and skin infections in Trinidad. J Infect Dis 126:34–40, 1972

26 Engle MA: Recovery from complete heart block in diphtheria. Pediatrics 3:222–233, 1949

27 Thisyakorn U, Wongvanich J, Kumpeng V: Failure of corticosteriod therapy to prevent diphtheritic myocarditis or neuritis. Pediatric Infect Dis 3:126–128, 1984

28 Dixon JMS: Diphtheria in North America. J Hyg Camb 93:419–431, 1984

29 Feeley JC, Curlin GT, Aziz MA, et al: Response of children in Bangladesh to adult-type tetanus-diphtheria toxoid (Td) administered during a field trial of cholera toxoid. J Biol Stand 7:249–252, 1979

30 Bennett SW: Investigation of tropical pattern of diphtheria in Buenaventura, Colombia. Proceedings of the International Symposium of Tropical Dermatoses in the Pacific Region, Tokyo, 1966, p 38

31 Diphtheria Surveillance, report no 12. Atlanta, Georgia, Centers for Disease Control, July 1978

32 Chakraborty SM: The incidence and treatment of faucial diphtheria in a rural West Bengal population. J Indian Med Assoc 55:371–375, 1970

33 Halsey NA, Galazka A: The efficacy of DPT and oral poliomyelitis immunization schedules initiated from birth to 12 weeks of age. Bull World Hlth Org 63:1151–1169, 1985

34 Shou C, Simonsen O, Heron I: Determination of tetanus and diphtheria antitoxin content in dried samples of capillary blood: A convenient method applied to infants. Scand J Infect Dis 19:445–451, 1987

35 Orenstein WA, Weisfeld JS, Halsey NA: Diphtheria and tetanus toxoids and pertussis vaccine, combined, in Halsey NA, de Quadros C (eds): *Recent Advances in Immunization*. Washington, DC, Pan American Health Organization, 1983, pp 30–51

36 Karzon DT, Edwards KM: Diphtheria outbreaks in immunized populations. N Engl J Med 318:41–43, 1988

37 Larsen Ka, Ullberg-Olsson K, Ekwall E, et al: The immunization of adults against diphtheria in Sweden. J Biol Stand 15:109–116, 1987

38 Pappenheimer AM Jr: Diphtheria: Studies on the biology of an infectious disease. Harvey Lect 76:45–73, 1982

C H A P T E R
90
/ *Pertussis* · Erik Hewlett

Whooping cough (pertussis) is a disease which continues to plague humankind around the world. In nations where pertussis vaccine was introduced 30 years ago, there was an associated decline in the incidence of disease. Subsequently, however, in some of these areas, vaccine acceptance decreased as a result of adverse publicity or changes in official immunization policy, and this resulted in marked increases in the incidence of whooping cough [1–3]. In areas of the world where pertussis vaccine has not yet become widely available, whooping cough continues to be a leading cause of childhood morbidity and mortality, resulting in an estimated 600,000 deaths worldwide annually. For these reasons, pertussis is now the object of an unprecedented research effort to develop and evaluate defined component pertussis vaccines [4,5].

PARASITE

Although infections with adenoviruses, chlamydiae, and *Haemophilus influenzae* may result in a pertussis-like illness, the focus of this chapter is on the *Bordetella* species. *Bordetella pertussis* is the most frequently identified organism in patients with whooping cough, which is therefore often referred to as "pertussis." In some areas of the world, including Mexico and eastern Europe, *B. parapertussis* has been isolated from a significant proportion (up to 30 percent) of whooping cough patients, including neonates [6,7]. Furthermore, serological surveys indicate that in many countries, including the United States, the majority of the population has antibodies against *B. parapertussis*. The disease associated with this organism is generally milder than that with *B. pertussis,* but may be life-threatening [6].

While *B. pertussis* and *B. parapertussis* appear to be natural pathogens for humans only, there is some controversy about their relationship to one another. They are sometimes isolated simultaneously from patients with clinical pertussis, and it is said that *B. parapertussis* can be converted to *B. pertussis* by phage infection and *B. pertussis* can be converted to *B. parapertussis* by mutagenesis [7]. This concept is not supported, however, by genetic analysis of multiple *Bordetella* strains [8] indicating significant diversity between *B. pertussis* and *B. parapertussis*. In contrast, *B. bronchiseptica* is an animal pathogen responsible for kennel cough in dogs and atrophic rhinitis in swine, and is only rarely implicated in human disease [9].

B. pertussis infects the respiratory tract of humans, attached to the ciliated mucosal cells. It does not penetrate the mucosa, invade the bloodstream, disseminate within the body, or survive more than a few hours in respiratory secretions. Therefore, it appears that the organism must be spread directly from infected human to susceptible individual. The organism is a small, nonmotile, non-spore-forming gram-negative coccobacillus which demonstrates homogeneous morphology on primary isolation, but may become pleomorphic with subculture, especially in a synthetic medium. Virulent strains possess fimbriae and other surface molecules which may be involved in the adherence to ciliated cells. Growth occurs in small colonies (<1 mm) that are smooth and pearly and are often likened to a drop of mercury. In clinical specimens grown on Bordet-Gengou agar, the colonies frequently are not visible until after 3 to 5 days of culture [10]. *B. pertussis* is unusual in that it does not catabolize carbohydrates, but uses amino acids (preferably glutamate and proline) as a source of energy, and most culture media are rendered alkaline by release of ammonia during growth of the organism. Growth is inhibited by fatty acids (which may be present in cotton swabs), a feature which is important to recognize when attempting clinical isolation of the organism [10]. β-Methyl-cyclodextrin has been demonstrated to enhance the growth of *B. pertussis* and the production of virulence factors in vitro; as a consequence, this component is used as an addition in some culture media [11].

B. pertussis produces a number of factors that are postulated to contribute to the virulence of the organism [12]. The role of these bacterial components can be considered in the context of the sequence of events involved in the establishment of clinical disease, namely, attachment, local damage, evasion of host defenses, and systemic disease. Filamentous hemagglutinin (FHA), pertussis toxin (PT), and perhaps fimbriae are thought to participate in the interaction of *B. pertussis* with host cells [13,14]. Tracheal cytotoxin, an oligopeptide derived from the peptidoglycan of the organism, is a leading candidate for the localized desquamation occurring in the infected respiratory tract [15]. Adenylate cyclase toxin, a bacterial enzyme which enters host cells to produce cyclic AMP from endogenous ATP, is also likely to damage the respiratory mucosa as well as facilitating evasion of host defenses such as phagocytic cells [16,17]. Dermonecrotic toxin (mouse-lethal toxin, heat-labile toxin) causes necrotic lesions in suckling mouse skin apparently by eliciting vasoconstriction [18], but its contribution to clinical pertussis is unknown.

Because of striking biological effects in experimental animals, pertussis toxin (lymphocytosis-promoting factor, histamine-sensitizing factor, islet-activating protein, pertussigen) has been hypothesized to be responsible for the systemic manifestations of clinical pertussis [19]. While this concept is accepted by many, considerable data do not support it. Pertussis toxin is a member of the family of bacterial toxins which possess ADP-ribosyl transferase activity [20]. The target molecules in host cells are guanine nucleotide binding (G) proteins involved in signal transduction by modulating adenylate cyclase, phospholipases, or ion channels. The covalent modification by pertussis toxin blocks their regulatory function. That the disease of pertussis is not solely the result of pertussis toxin action, however, is illustrated by the fact that *B. parapertussis* causes illness without producing pertussis toxin [6,21]. Furthermore, studies with *B. pertussis* mutants defective in specific virulence factors indicate that pertussis toxin mutants demonstrate only a slightly reduced LD_{50} (5×10^6 compared to 2×10^3 for wild type) [22]. In contrast, adenylate cyclase toxin–hemolysin mutants are avirulent ($LD_{50} > 3 \times 10^7$) in the suckling mouse model. Finally, Toyota et al. have injected large quantities (1 μg/kg) of pertussis toxin into volunteers, who suffered no significant adverse effects [23]. The data demonstrate clearly that pertussis is a complicated, multifactorial disease process unlike single-toxin diseases such as tetanus and diphtheria.

The classical serogrouping of *Bordetella* species has been by antisera to a series of agglutinogens (designated 1 to 6). Antibodies to these surface antigens result in agglutination of the organisms. Several of the agglutinogens have been identified and characterized biochemically. Agglutinogens 2 and 3 are fimbrial and may contribute to the protection elicited by whole-cell vaccine [24]. Agglutinogen 1 is a lipooligosaccharide molecule.

Intracerebral inoculation of mice with *B. pertussis* has served as the standard method for evaluating vaccine efficacy and potency. In a classical British Medical Research Council study, vaccine efficacy in protecting children against pertussis was shown to correlate with efficacy in the mouse potency test [25]. Although the organisms have been shown to adhere to ciliated ependymal cells in the central nervous system (CNS), the pathogenetic mechanisms involved in host susceptibility to this unnatural route of challenge are unclear, and its extrapolation to clinical pertussis is clearly limited. More recently, direct intranasal administration or exposure to an aerosol has been used to model the natural infection more closely. With respiratory inoculation, mice manifest the biological effects of pertussis toxin and ultimately either clear the infection or die [19]. These systems have been useful in evaluating the efficacy of components being considered for inclusion in an acellular vaccine.

PATIENT

Pertussis becomes clinically apparent after an incubation period of as little as 5 to as long as 21 days [26]. The first or catarrhal phase of the disease is characterized by nonspecific features such as coryza, lacrimation, mild conjunctivitis, rhinorrhea, and, occasionally, low-grade fever. Although it is virtually impossible to diagnose pertussis clinically at this point except in the setting of known contact with another case, patients are highly infectious. The catarrhal phase generally lasts 7 to 14 days and is associated with a dry cough. The evolution of the cough marks the transition to the paroxysmal phase, in which the characteristic whoop is first noted. Cough paroxysms occur spontaneously, but may be provoked by external stimuli without sufficient warning for the patient to catch a breath. After the cough spasm, the patient (especially children, but occasionally adults) gasps for breath, resulting in the characteristic whoop. Frequently, there is accompanying cyanosis and vomiting. Patients are generally afebrile during this period, which can last as little as a few days in partially immunized patients and more than a month in others. The presence of a fever during this phase of the disease suggests the possibility of an intervening suprainfection.

With decrease in the frequency and intensity of cough paroxysms, the patient enters the convalescent phase. Residua of the disease can persist for several months, and intercurrent infections or other stimuli can precipitate a return of the paroxysmal cough, sometimes interpreted incorrectly as a reinfection with *B. pertussis*.

In adults, pertussis frequently begins as a mild upper respiratory infection with cough. Although the illness is generally not of the severity seen in children, it can be extremely incapacitating, with paroxysmal cough sometimes accompanied by whoop, vomiting, and secondary infection [27]. Adults are frequently the unrecognized link between sporadic cases or major contributors to pertussis epidemics, especially in the hospital setting [27,28].

A large part of the morbidity and mortality from pertussis is caused by complications, both infectious and noninfectious. Secondary infections, such as pneumonia, are not uncommon and are often responsible for fatalities. The paroxysmal cough accounts for many sequelae including conjunctival hemorrhages, epistaxis, petechiae, hernias, rectal prolapse, and ulceration of the frenulum of the tongue. Development of subcutaneous emphysema and pneumothorax have been observed. Neurological dysfunctions, including convulsions and coma, have similarly been attributed to the severe cough and associated hypoxia resulting in focal hemorrhages in the CNS. While it has been hypothesized that pertussis toxin may be responsible for the development of encephalopathy complicating clinical disease, the available information about the toxin does not support that concept. Especially in patients who have a compromised nutritional status before the illness, the cough and subsequent vomiting can result in weight loss and life-threatening malnutrition.

DIAGNOSIS

Because other infectious agents are capable of causing a whooping cough–like illness, it is necessary to employ specific diagnostic methods to establish the presence of *B. pertussis* [10]. Current diagnostic tests are, however, relatively insensitive or nonspecific [29]. Culture is the most specific method, but is slow and time-consuming. When plates are streaked at the bedside with calcium alginate nasopharyngeal swabs rather than being held in transport medium, it is possible to recover the organism from 20 to 80 percent of patients depending upon the duration of illness [29,30]. Treatment of patients with erythromycin, trimethoprim-sulfamethoxazole, or tetracycline decreases recovery of the organism, while penicillin enhances it slightly [30]. Several media appear to be superior to the classical Bordet-Gengou medium, including charcoal agar and synthetic (blood-free) medium [11] containing cephalexin to inhibit growth of non-*Bordetella* organisms. Direct fluorescent antibody evaluation of nasopharyngeal smears can be more sensitive than culture, but there is a significant rate of false positivity, especially when read by inexperienced personnel [29].

Serological detection of agglutinating antibodies has provided a method for diagnosing pertussis retrospectively [31]. New enzyme-linked immunosorbent assays (ELISA) are being used to identify antibodies to *B. pertussis* or specific bacterial components such as filamentous hemagglutinin [32], but their sensitivity in the setting of acute illness remains to be determined [29]. The use of ELISA for detection of secretory IgA in nasal washes is specific and relatively sensitive in later stages of disease [29,33]. The need for more rapid and accurate diagnostic methods has led to the development of DNA probes for identification of B. pertussis [34] and of an enzyme assay for detection of B. pertussis based upon the activity of the extracytoplasmic adenylate cyclase [35].

TREATMENT

Although it is commonly held that antibiotics do not affect the clinical course of pertussis unless given early in the disease (before the paroxysmal phase), recent data indicate that these drugs may decrease severity of disease even later in the course [36]. Erythromycin is the mainstay of therapy, but chloramphenicol and tetracycline (with relative contraindications in children) are also effective [36]. Persistent culture positivity has been noted during treatment with erythromycin or trimethoprim-sulfamethoxasole, even though the organisms were sensitive to the drugs in vitro. The β-adrenergic agonist salbutamol has been suggested as an agent for symptomatic relief in pertussis, but controlled trials have not supported this proposal [37]. Thus, supportive care remains a mainstay of management for patients with pertussis. Close observation with discriminating use of suctioning to maintain airway patency, oxygen therapy, and parenteral nutritional supplementation are critical in reducing the threat of serious sequelae. Minimizing external stimuli may decrease the number of cough paroxysms, but patients should not be so isolated as to prevent careful observation. Hospitalization is generally indicated for children less than 1 year of age. Because many of the symptoms occur after bacteriological clearance, corticosteroids have been suggested for use in pertussis, and studies have demonstrated potential benefit [38].

POPULATION

Because whooping cough has become less common in industrialized countries since the introduction of pertussis vaccine, the current epidemiology of the disease is inadequately defined. It is presumed that this respiratory infection is transmitted by aerosol droplets, but direct contact cannot be ruled out. Whooping cough is a highly contagious illness, with attack rates reaching more than 90 percent in susceptible populations [39]. Even immunized individuals become susceptible again when the interval since last immunization is greater than 12 years [39]. It has been suggested that this population of previously "immune" adults develops mild, atypical disease after exposure to a patient with whooping cough and is unknowingly the source of infection for apparently spontaneous cases in very young infants [27,28,39]. Immune family contacts in an outbreak have been demonstrated to have a single positive culture for B. pertussis without subsequent clinical disease [27,39,40]. It is unknown whether such individuals are capable of transmitting the organism and are of epidemiological significance. There is no evidence, however, for the prolonged carriage of B. pertussis by asymptomatic persons [41].

PREVENTION

Quarantine was the first public health measure employed in the prevention and control of whooping cough. Because of high communicability during the nonspecific catarrhal phase before the disease could be diagnosed, this approach was generally unsuccessful. Next, whole serum from immune individuals was tested and found to be partially protective in preventing pertussis when given during the incubation period of the disease. Commercially available immune globulin has no proven efficacy, however, and, although widely available, it cannot be recommended. Erythromycin prophylaxis of exposed individuals, while incomplete in its effectiveness, has been shown to be beneficial in an institutional outbreak [42].

There have been several vaccines used against B. pertussis, including cell-free extracts and acellular vaccines prepared from components in culture supernate. The pertussis vaccine recommended by the WHO and in predominant use worldwide, however, is the killed, whole-cell preparation containing either alum or aluminum phosphate as adjuvant. This formulation is generally combined with diphtheria and tetanus toxoids to form the standard DTP (diphtheria-tetanus-pertussis) vaccine and given as a primary series at 2-month intervals beginning at 6 to 8 weeks of age. While it appears that infants immunized at birth may have lower antibody titers [43], overall protection may be improved by initiating immunization at 1 month of age [44]. When possible, boosters are given at 18 to 24 months and 4 to 6 years. The whole-cell vaccine has been demonstrated repeatedly to be highly efficacious, both by its evaluation in efficacy studies [45] and by the resurgence of disease associated with reduction or elimination of vaccine use [1–3]. Furthermore, immunized individuals who do get pertussis experience significantly milder disease.

The major limitation to the use of whole-cell pertussis vaccine has been its ability to produce local reactions and fever [46] and its implication in the development of neurological abnormalities such as encephalopathy [47]. Despite extensive speculation and litigation over this latter issue, however, there is not compelling evidence that the vaccine does, in fact, cause neurological damage with permanent sequelae, and assessment of the benefits and risks has repeatedly indicated that immunization with whole-cell vaccine should be continued. Nevertheless, these problems have led to the development of an acellular pertussis vaccine by Sato and coworkers [48]. This form of vaccine (which may be made differently by different manufacturers) has been in use in Japan for immunization of children ≥24 months of age since 1981 [48,49]. The vaccine, which consists primarily of formalin-inactivated pertussis toxin, filamentous hemagglutinin (FHA), some agglutinogens, and perhaps other components [48], appears to be efficacious as used in Japan [49]. In consideration for use in infants, two acellular vaccines different than those in general use in Japan (pertussis toxoid alone or pertussis toxoid plus FHA) have been tested in a double-blind placebo trial of children starting at 6 months of age in Sweden [50]. Although both preparations protected 79 to 80 percent against severe disease (positive culture with cough ≥ 30 days), neither produced 70 percent protection against culture-positive disease of any duration. Both acellular vaccines were, however, clearly associated with fewer adverse reactions than are attributed to the whole-cell vaccines. These data indicate the need for additional evaluation of multicomponent acellular vaccines which will be more likely to elicit protection equivalent to that of the whole-cell vaccine in infants.

The transition to acellular pertussis vaccines over the next decade will provide the opportunity for reevaluation of the current strategy for pertussis immunization. Since adults may be responsible for unrecognized transmission to susceptible infants, booster doses of pertussis vaccine to that population will greatly enhance control of this disease. Because of the epidemiological features of pertussis (no known carrier state, direct person-to-person transmission, no natural or animal reservoir) serious consideration of eradication will be possible.

REFERENCES

1 Cherry JD: The epidemiology of pertussis and pertussis immunization in the United Kingdom and the United States: A comparative study. Curr Probl Pediatr 14:1–78, 1984

2 Kanai K: Japan's experience in pertussis epidemiology and vaccination in the past thirty years. Japan J Med Sci Biol 33:107–143, 1980

3 Romanus V, Jonsell R, Bergquist S-O: Pertussis in Sweden after the cessation of general immunization in 1979. Pediatr Infect Dis J 6:364–371, 1987

4 Manclark CR, Burns DL: Prospects for a new acellular pertussis vaccine. Ann Inst Pasteur/Microbiol 136B:323–329, 1985

5 Robinson A, Irons LI, Ashworth LAE: Pertussis vaccine: Present status and future prospects. Vaccine 3:11–22, 1985

6 Linnemann CC, Perry EB: Bordetella parapertussis: Recent experience and a review of the literature. Am J Dis Child 131:560–563, 1977

7 Granstrom M, Askelof P: Parapertussis: An abortive pertussis infection? Lancet ii:1249–1250, 1982

8 Musser JM, Hewlett EL, Peppler MS, et al: Genetic diversity and relationships in populations of Bordetella spp. J Bacteriol 166:230–237, 1986

9 Ghosh HK, Tranter J: Bordetella bronchicanis (bronchiseptica) infection in man: Review and a case report. J Clin Pathol 32:546–548, 1979

10 Parker CD, Payne BJ: Bordetella, in Lennette EH, Balows A, Hausler WJ, et al (eds): Manual of Clinical Microbiology, 4th ed. Washington, DC, American Society for Microbiology, 1985, pp 394–399

11 Aoyama T, Murase Y, Iwata T, et al: Comparison of blood-free medium (cyclodextrin solid medium) with Bordet-Gengou medium for clinical isolation of Bordetella pertussis. J Clin Microbiol 23:1046–1048, 1986

12 Weiss AA, Hewlett EL: Virulence factors of Bordetella pertussis. Ann Rev Microbiol 40:661–686, 1986

13 Gorringe AR, Ashworth LAE, Irons LI, et al: Effect of monoclonal

14 Urisu A, Cowell JL, Manclark CR: Involvement of the filamentous hemagglutinin in the adherence of Bordetella pertussis to human WiDr cultures. Dev Biol Stand 61:205–214, 1984

15 Rosenthal RS, Nogami W, Cookson BT, et al: Major fragment of soluble peptidoglycan released from growing Bordetella pertussis is tracheal cytotoxin. Infect Immun 55:2117–2120, 1987

16 Confer DL, Slungaard AS, Graf E, et al: Bordetella adenylate cyclase toxin: Entry of bacterial adenylate cyclase into mammalian cells. Adv Cyc Nucl Prot Phosph Res 17:183–187, 1984

17 Hewlett EL, Gordon VM: Adenylate cyclase toxin of Bordetella pertussis, in Wardlaw AC, Parton R (eds): Pathogenesis and Immunity in Pertussis. Chicester, Wiley, 1988, pp 193–209

18 Endoh M, Nagai M, Nakase Y: Effect of Bordetella heat-labile toxin on perfused lung preparations. Microbiol Immunol 30:1239–1246, 1986

19 Pittman M, Furman BL, Wardlaw AC: Bordetella pertussis respiratory tract infection in the mouse: Pathophysiological responses. J Infect Dis 142:56–66, 1980

20 Gilman AG: Receptor regulated G proteins. Trends Neurosci 9:460–463, 1986

21 Arico B, Rappuoli R: Bordetella parapertussis and Bordetella bronchiseptica contain transcriptionally silent pertussis toxin genes. J Bacteriol 169:2847–2853, 1987

22 Weiss AA, Hewlett EL, Myers GA, et al: Pertussis toxin and extracytoplasmic adenylate cyclase as virulence factors in Bordetella pertussis. J Infect Dis 150:219–222, 1984

23 Toyota T, Kai Y, Kakizaki M, et al: Effects of islet-activating protein (IAP) on blood glucose and plasma insulin in healthy volunteers (phase I studies). Tohoku J Exp Med 130:105–116, 1980

24 Zhang JM, Cowell JL, Steven AC, et al: Purification of serotype 2 fimbriae of Bordetella pertussis and their identification as a mouse protective antigen. Dev Biol Stand 61:173–185, 1985

25 Medical Research Council: Vaccination against whooping cough: Relation between protection in children and results of laboratory tests. Br Med J 2:454–462, 1956

26 Lapin JH: Clinical manifestations, in Whooping Cough. Springfield, Charles C Thomas, 1942, chap VIII, pp 112–122

27 Linnemann CC Jr, Nasenbeny J: Pertussis in the adult. Ann Rev Med 28:177–185, 1977

28 Valenti WM, Pincus PH, Messner MK: Nosocomial pertussis: Possible spread by a hospital visitor. Am J Dis Child 134:520–521, 1980

29 Onorato IM, Wassilak SGF: Laboratory diagnosis of pertussis: The state of the art. Pediatr Infect Dis J 6:145–151, 1987

30 Kwantes W, Joynson DHM, Williams WO: Bordetella pertussis isolation in general practice: 1977–79 whooping cough epidemic in West Glamorgan. J Hyg (Cambridge) 90:149–158, 1983

31 Manclark CR, Meade BD, Burstyn DG: Serological response to Bordetella pertussis, in Manual of Clinical Immunology. American Society for Microbiology, Washington, DC, 1986, chap 61, pp 388–394

32 Granstrom M, Granstrom G, Lindfors A, et al: Serological diagnosis of whooping cough by an enzyme-linked immunosorbent assay using fimbrial hemagglutinin as antigen. J Infect Dis 146:741–745, 1982

33 Goodman YE, Wort AJ, Jackson RL: Enzyme-linked immunosorbent assay for detection of pertussis immunoglobulin A in naso-

antibodies on the adherence of Bordetella pertussis to Vero cells. FEMS Microbiol Lett 26:5–9, 1985 pharyngeal secretions as an indicator of recent infection. J Clin Microbiol 13:286–292, 1981

34 McLafferty MA, Bromberg K, Harcus DR, et al: Characterization of a DNA probe for identification of *Bordetella pertussis* in clinical specimens. American Society for Microbiology, Abstracts of the Annual Meeting, C-322, 1987

35 Confer DL, Eaton JW: *Bordetella* adenylate cyclase: Host toxicity and diagnostic utility. Dev Biol Stand 61:3–10, 1985

36 Bass JW: Pertussis: Current status of prevention and treatment. Pediatr Infect Dis 4:614–619, 1985

37 Mertsola J, Viljanen MK, Ruuskanen O: Salbutamol in the treatment of whooping cough. Scand J Infect Dis 18:593–594, 1986

38 Zoomboulakis D, Anagnostakis D, Albanis V, et al: Steriods in treatment of pertussis: A controlled clinical trial. Arch Dis Child 48:51, 1973

39 Lambert HJ: Epidemiology of a small pertussis outbreak in Kent County, Michigan. Pub Health Rep 80:365–369, 1965

40 Broome CV, Preblud SR, Bruner B, et al: Epidemiology of pertussis, Atlanta, 1977. J Pediatr 98:362–367, 1981

41 Linnemann CC Jr, Bass JW, Smith MHD: The carrier state in pertussis. Am J Epidemiol 83:422–426, 1968

42 Steketee RW, Wassilak SGF, Adkins WN, et al: Evidence for a high attack rate and efficacy of erythromycin prophylaxis in a pertussis outbreak in a facility for the developmentally disabled. J Infect Dis 157:434–440, 1988

43 Committee on Infectious Diseases, American Academy of Pediatrics: *Report of the Committee on Infectious Diseases*, 20th ed. Elk Grove Village, Ill, American Academy of Pediatrics, 1986

44 Abayomi I, et al: Whooping cough vaccine at birth. J Trop Pediatr 19:3–4, 1973

45 Fine PEM, Clarkson JA: Reflections on the efficacy of pertussis vaccines. Rev Infect Dis 9:866–883, 1987

46 Cody CL, Baraff LJ, Cherry JD, et al: Nature and rates of adverse reactions associated with DTP and DT immunizations in infants and children. Pediatrics 68:650–660, 1981

47 Miller D, Wadsworth J, Diamond J, et al: Pertussis vaccine and whooping cough as risk factors in acute neurological illness and death in young children. Dev Biol Stand 61:389–394, 1985

48 Sato Y, Kimura M, Fukumi H: Development of a pertussis component vaccine in Japan. Lancet i:122–126, 1984

49 Noble GR, Bernier RH, Esber EC, et al: Acellular and whole-cell pertussis vaccines in Japan. JAMA 257:1351–1356, 1987

50 Ad Hoc Group for the Study of Pertussis Vaccines: Placebo-controlled trial of two acellular pertussis vaccines in Sweden—Protective efficacy and adverse events. Lancet i:955–960, 1988

C H A P T E R
91

Tetanus · Sherwood L. Gorbach

Tetanus is a tragic disease, not only because of its severity, but because it can be completely prevented by appropriate immunizations. Indeed, prevention of tetanus by active immunization has been one of the triumphs of modern bacteriology. Experience with tetanus in the two world wars of this century demonstrated beyond peradventure the benefits of the tetanus toxoid vaccine. Universal immunization of the American forces in World War II virtually eliminated this disease as a complication of traumatic injuries in soldiers. In developing countries where immunization is not widely practiced, tetanus remains a serious public health problem.

PATHOGEN

MORPHOLOGY, LABORATORY CHARACTERISTICS

Clostridium tetani is a ubiquitous, gram-positive, anaerobic, spore-forming rod. In culture, the organism is motile and forms terminal spores which have been described as "drumsticks" or "tennis rackets." The spores, formed in reaction to adverse environmental conditions, are highly resistant to physical and chemical disinfection; they can survive exposure to simple boiling, brief autoclaving (less than 10 min), and direct exposure to quaternary ammonium compounds, mercurochrome,

alcohol, and phenol. They are, however, killed by extensive autoclaving (longer than 15 min) and exposure to ethylene oxide. The organism is widely distributed in the gastrointestinal tract of human and animals, especially cows and horses, and in soil samples. Because of their virtual indestructibility these spores achieve a form of microbial immortality, posing a threat to hapless victims of trauma.

The organism can only be grown in strict anaerobic conditions. Since *C. tetani* is usually associated with traumatic wounds, multiple other organisms, both aerobic and anaerobic, coexist at the site, making it difficult to isolate in culture. Whether due to this factor, or the relatively fastidious nature of the organism itself, *C. tetani* can be cultured from only one-third of incriminated wounds in patients with clinical tetanus.

TOXINS

Structure and pharmacology

Two toxins are produced by this organism, *tetanolysin* and *tetanospasmin* [1]. Tetanolysin has minor importance in the disease, appearing to be responsible for only local tissue damage. The potent toxin tetanospasmin accounts for all the manifestations associated with clinical tetanus. It is produced intracellularly as a 150-kDa protein molecule, which is nicked by intracellular proteases to a heavy chain (100 kDa) and a light chain (50 kDa), which are held together by a disulfide bridge. Like other α-β dichain toxins, the individual heavy and light chains are nontoxic.

Mechanism of action

The toxin initially binds to α motor neurons followed by internalization and retrograde axonal transport to the cell body. On a molecular level, the toxin proceeds through three steps, extracellular binding, membrane penetration, and internal nerve poisoning [2]. The toxin migrates from postsynaptic dendrites to presynaptic nerve terminals.

The toxin is spread from a peripheral wound to cranial nerve nuclei by two major mechanisms, intraspinal transmission among involved motor neurons and bloodstream delivery of toxin to other neuromuscular junctions.

The major action of tetanospasmin is to inhibit transmitter release and normal inhibitory input, thereby causing the lower motor neuron to increase resting tone and produce the characteristic reflex spasms. It also blocks GABA release, further preventing inhibition of the lower motor neuron by the brainstem.

PATIENT

Tetanus is a severe disease which can last for weeks or even months, taxing the patient's stamina in terms of physiological and psychological reserves, and the physician's therapeutic skills. Patients with tetanus succumb, as a rule, to complications caused by spasms and paralysis, and supportive therapy can produce a favorable result in all but the worst cases.

PATHOGENESIS

Most cases of tetanus occur after puncture wounds, lacerations, crush injuries, or burns. The spores of *C. tetani* are introduced from environmental sources or, occasionally, have been present in an old wound site for some time and are reactivated by new injury. Spores germinate to produce the toxins in a receptive environment, which includes tissue necrosis, anoxia, and other bacterial contaminants in the wound.

CLINICAL MANIFESTATIONS

The incubation period is variable, from a few days to several weeks. In general, long latency is associated with more distal injuries and has a better prognosis. The period of onset is measured from the first symptom of tetanus to the first reflex spasm; a long period before spasm, or no spasms at all, carry a better prognosis. Three clinical forms of tetanus are recognized: local, cephalic, and generalized tetanus [3].

Local tetanus is restricted to the muscles in an area of injury. The local muscle groups are set in persistent and unyielding rigidity which may last for weeks to months, but there is no progression to other muscle groups. At the spinal cord level, the dysfunction is limited to interneurons, without transmission to other central nervous system sites.

Cephalic tetanus is a rather rare form which occurs with otitis media or traumatic injuries to the head. There is usually cranial nerve involvement, especially of the VIIth nerve. Because of its proximity to the central nervous system, this condition has a poor prognosis.

Generalized tetanus, responsible for about 80 percent of cases, usually begins with trismus or "lockjaw," which is caused by tetanic spasm of the masseter muscles, preventing opening of the mouth. The spasm can spread to other facial muscles, causing a grotesque grimace, known as *risus sardonicus* (Fig. 91-1). The disease typically *descends,* initially involving the neck and back muscles, progressing to produce boardlike rigidity of the abdominal musculature, eventually causing stiffness of the extremities. Individual muscle groups go into spasm, leading to a generalized spasm, which is characterized by a toxic seizure, adduction of the arms, arching of the neck and back (known as opisthotonos), extension of the legs and clenching of the fists. The spasm may last a few

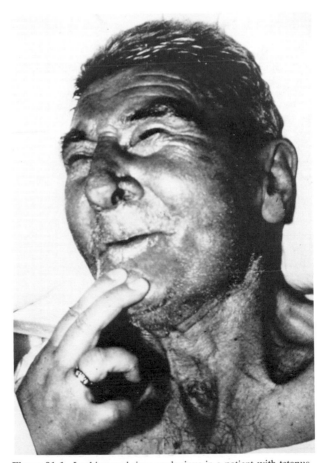

Figure 91-1. Lockjaw and risus sardonicus in a patient with tetanus.

seconds or several minutes. They can be initiated by sudden noise, such as slamming a door, touching the patient, or turning on the light, or a spasm can occur spontaneously without any stimulus.

The clinical features of tetanus have also been divided into mild, moderately severe, and severe forms. The milder cases have an incubation period greater than 10 days and a slow evolution of classical signs. While trismus and abdominal stiffness may be present, generalized spasms are absent. Moderately severe cases have an incubation period less than 10 days with progressive development of symptoms over 3 to 6 days. Generalized spasms are late in onset, occur infrequently, and are not associated with respiratory difficulty. Severe cases of tetanus have a short incubation period, often less than 7 days, with rapid evolution of signs and symptoms within 3 days of onset. The full range of clinical manifestations is present, including trismus and opisthotonos, as well as severe and frequent generalized spasms.

Autonomic dysfunction is a frequent, and often unrecognized, problem in severe forms of generalized tetanus. Clinically, there is unstable blood pressure, with swings of hypertension and hypotension, paroxysmal tachycardia and other cardiac arrhythmias, profuse sweating, and hyperpyrexia. Catecholamine concentrations are elevated in urine and plasma.

DIAGNOSIS

Tetanus is a clinical diagnosis based on the physical findings. The organism can be seen in Gram's stain of infected material, but it is often confused with other gram-positive rods, and it may be difficult to identify in the mixed flora of a grossly contaminated wound. Culturing the organism also is problematical; even an experienced microbiologist has problems with isolating this strict, fastidious anaerobe from mixed cultures. In addition, up to 20 percent of tetanus cases in some series have no apparent wound or portal of entry. For all of these reasons, the organism is isolated in less than one-third of clinical cases of tetanus.

Prior immunization with tetanus toxoid produces serum antitoxin antibodies, measured by hemagglutination or mouse-neutralizing tests. A serum antitoxin level of 0.01 IU is usually protective. Since antitoxin immunity lasts for many years after an adequate immunization, the diagnosis of tetanus should be made reluctantly in a previously immunized individual.

Differential diagnosis

Tetanus most closely resembles strychnine poisoning, since the physiological effects of the toxin and the poison are the same. Yet, strychnine poisoning comes on suddenly and lasts for a shorter period of time; there is no apparent wound or injury; and there are often criminal circumstances surrounding the situation. Many other diseases are confused with tetanus, or at least certain of the manifestations, such as trismus and opis-

Table 91-1. Differential diagnosis of tetanus

Generalized tetanus	Trismus	Opisthotonos
Strychnine poisoning	Dental abscess	Rabies
Phenothiazine reaction	Mandibular	Perforated
Bacterial meningitis	fracture	peptic ulcer
Hypocalcemic tetany	Tonsillitis	Peritonitis
Retroperitoneal	Diphtheria	Vertebral
hemorrhage	Mumps	osteomyelitis
Epilepsy		
Decerebrate posturing		
Narcotic withdrawal		
Hysteria		

thotonos (Table 91-1). Before making the diagnosis of tetanus these conditions should be considered.

THERAPY

The treatment of tetanus is mainly a physiological exercise in preventing complications [4]. Any toxin that has been elaborated and already fixed to nerve cells is in an irreversible state, so the disease cannot be interrupted once it has started. Indeed, the spasms and muscle contractions can continue for several weeks after the organism has been eradicated. The initial phases of treatment involve elimination of the organism by surgical debridement and antibiotics, and administration of antitoxin in order to neutralize circulating toxin that has not yet been fixed. The other modalities of therapy are directed at physiological stabilization and nutrition.

Surgical debridement of any obvious wound should be undertaken in order to remove necrotic tissue and anaerobic dead spaces. In some patients with tetanus the wound may be very subtle or cannot even be located. A careful search for puncture wounds, insect bites, and otitis media should be done when there is a cryptic focus.

Antibiotic therapy should be directed at the organism, and penicillin G is the treatment of choice (2 to 3 million units IV q 4 h). In the setting of a grossly contaminated wound additional antibiotics should be used according to the coexistent pathogens. The length of treatment is dictated by the extent of the traumatic injury, although in general short courses of therapy, over several days, should be sufficient.

Antitoxin, in the form of tetanal immune globulin (TIG) of human origin, should be administered in an attempt to fix any circulating toxin [5]. While the exact dose has not been determined, it is generally recommended that 3000 U be given intramuscularly as equal portions in different sites. Since the half-life is approximately 25 days, it is not necessary to give additional doses of TIG. At the same time, a full immunizing schedule of toxoid should be provided in order to prevent a second attack. Intrathecal TIG (250 U) has been given to some cases of severe tetanus with encouraging results, but this method has not been universally accepted.

Prevention of muscle contractions and spasms should be undertaken as soon as the diagnosis of tetanus is made. The most effective drugs are centrally acting inhibitory agents, particularly benzodiazepines which produce not only sedation but presynaptic inhibition of spinal reflexes. The most commonly used agent is diazepam at a usual dose of 500 mg/day or more for severe tetanus. At the higher dose mechanical ventilation is usually required. Barbiturates have been used traditionally, but they lack the specific actions of the benzodiazepines.

Respiratory therapy is a major aspect of treatment. Administration of oxygen, suction of secretions, which are abundant, and tracheostomy, after the onset of the first spasm, should be instituted. Severe cases will require neuromuscular blockade for adequate ventilation. Curare-like drugs are generally recommended, along with sedation provided by benzodiazepines or barbiturates. Severe autonomic dysfunction can be controlled by intravenous morphine therapy.

Generalized support measures are vital to a favorable outlook. The patient must be turned frequently in order to avoid bedsores and to improve respiration. Environmental stimuli should be reduced to a minimum by placing the patient in a quiet, darkened room. Loud talking and slamming of doors must be prevented, since such stimuli can initiate a series of muscular contractions and seizures.

Nutrition must be paid careful attention since these patients cannot eat for several weeks. It is best to provide these supplements by parenteral alimentation through a central venous line or enteral nutrition through a gastrostomy or small bowel tube. A thin, soft, nasogastric tube is used in some units, although it must be managed with care in order to avoid aspiration pneumonia.

COMPLICATIONS

A frequent complication and a major cause of death is pulmonary infection due to aspiration and stasis. Tension pneumothorax can also occur. Other complications are associated with prolonged bed rest in severely ill patients: pulmonary embolism, urinary catheter–associated infections, decubitus ulcers, and bacteremia from intravenous lines. The muscle spasms and seizures can lead to fractures of the spine and long bones. Muscle ruptures and hematomas are also seen.

PROGNOSIS

The average case fatality rate is 60 percent, but this figure varies greatly according to the following factors:

1. Age of the patient. The worst outlooks are at the extremes of ages, especially in neonates and persons over 50 years.
2. Incubation and period of onset. Incubations less than 10 days, and particularly less than 7 days, have a poor outlook. When the onset of generalized spasm is less than 48 h from the initial presentation of the disease, there is also a grim prognosis.
3. Severity of disease. Generalized disease carries a worse outlook than localized disease, unless the localization is in the facial muscles, in which case the outcome is guarded. Rapid evolution of symptoms and signs is associated with poor outlook. Initial presentations with generalized spasm or high fever and tachycardia have a poor outlook.
4. Respiratory complications. Pneumonia and pneumothorax presage a poor outcome.
5. Portal of entry. When entry site is close to the central nervous system, as in the scalp or middle ear, the outlook is poor.
6. Treatment facility. Specialized centers, with facilities for respiratory care, report the most favorable survival figures.

POPULATION

EPIDEMIOLOGY

There are significant differences in the epidemiology of tetanus in industrialized and developing countries [6]. Using the United States experience for the former group, there have been less than 100 cases per year for the decade 1977–1986 (Fig. 91-2) [7]. Seventy percent of these cases occur in people over 50 years of age, and approximately 2 percent in the younger-than-1-year age group. Neonatal tetanus has become an extremely rare disease. While actual incidence figures are not available for most developing countries, reports from individual hospitals show striking differences from the United States experience. Tetanus is an extremely common disease in developing countries, and entire wards of large hospitals are devoted to tetanus cases. Approximately 60 percent of the patients are less than 10 years of age, and 20 percent are in the neonatal group. On the other hand tetanus in the over-50 age group is much less common. The majority of neonatal cases come from rural settings where obstetrical practice is rudimentary. Overall mortality in the neonatal cases is over 80 percent, and death is nearly universal in those who develop the disease within 1 week of birth [8].

Another important difference is the portal of entry. In the United States, traumatic wounds cause approximately two-thirds of cases, and smaller numbers are associated with burn wounds or heroin injections. While trauma is an important cause in developing countries as well, there are many cases related to untreated otitis media, induced abortion, puerperal sepsis, neonatal practices, and injections of medications.

PREVENTION

Passive immunization

Administration of TIG of human origin offers substantial, but not complete, protection for patients with traumatic injuries. A ''tetanus-prone'' wound is characterized by tissue necrosis associated with gross contamination from the environment. Such wounds are at greatest risk of producing tetanus, but it must be emphasized that even minor puncture wounds or

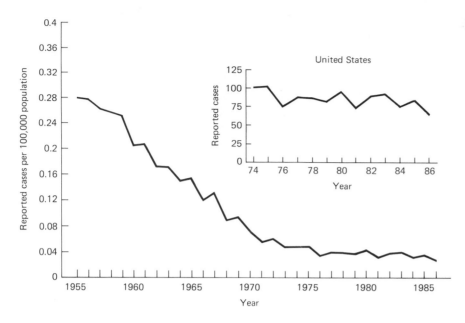

Figure 91-2. Tetanus cases, by year, in the United States, 1955–1986. (*From* [7].)

needle sticks have been the precursor to severe disease. While it is a matter of judgment who should receive preventive measures, it is best to err on the side of conservation, especially in unimmunized individuals. Table 91-2 indicates the current recommendations. With regard to the use of toxoid and TIG the following points should be made:

1. TIG is human globulin; the older preparations of horse serum should not be employed unless TIG is unavailable. When treating adults, the toxoid should be the combined tetanus-diphtheria toxoid (Td, adult type) in the form of adsorbed toxoid (with aluminum adjuvant).
2. The usual dose of TIG is 250 U, unless there is a severe injury, in which case 500 U can be employed. The TIG should be given in a different syringe and at a different site than the Td. In the event that this dose of Td constitutes a

Table 91-2. Tetanus immunization

Immunization record	Wound	Recommendation
None	Low risk	Toxoid-complete immunization
Incomplete		Toxoid-complete immunization
Unknown	High risk	Toxoid + TIG
No booster in the past	Low risk	Toxoid
10 years	High risk	Toxoid + TIG
Booster in the past	Low risk	None
10 years	High risk	Toxoid if no booster in the past 5 years

Note: Toxoid = tetanus-diphtheria toxoid, adult type, 0.5 mL IM; TIG = tetanal immune globulin, human, 250 U IM; high risk = severe, neglected for 24 h.

primary immunization, the patient should be instructed to return 28 days later to receive the second dose.

3. Antibiotic treatment and surgical debridement do not give adequate protection against tetanus. Thus, the immunization status of all patients with contaminated wounds must be ascertained and appropriate treatment initiated, as indicated in Table 91-2.

Active immunization

The standard course for active immunization of tetanus is a combined vaccine of tetanus, diphtheria, and pertussis (DPT), starting at 1 to 3 months of age, for three doses, followed by subsequent boosters at ages 1 and 4. In general, a booster injection of adsorbed toxoid, following an adequate primary vaccination series, should provide protective antibody for 10 years, during which time booster doses are not required. This interval should be shortened to 5 years in the setting of a severe injury. Multiple injections of toxoid, prompted by frequent injuries, can lead paradoxically to lower levels of circulating antibody, so this practice is discouraged. Based on the experience in World War II, the failure rate of primary tetanus immunization is less than 4 per 100 million. Neonatal tetanus should not occur when mothers are adequately immunized, since the antibody passes the placental barrier to the infant. Prevention of neonatal tetanus in developing countries can be achieved by administering at least two doses of tetanal toxoid to pregnant women, along with educational programs directed at midwives.

Control of tetanus in developing countries must proceed on several fronts. To the extent possible, tetanal toxoid should be given to all infants and children, as well as to previously unimmunized pregnant women. Carefully directed improvements in the health care delivery system and professional education programs could reduce the cases of tetanus in children, particularly neonates and those with traumatic injuries and otitis media. Tetanal toxoid is remarkably effective and extremely safe. Wider use of this vaccine could make a substantial improvement in the lives of millions of poor people in these developing countries.

REFERENCES

1 Middlebrook JL, Dorland R: Bacterial toxins: cellular mechanism of action. Microbiol Rev 48:199–221, 1984

2 Simpson LL: Molecular pharmacology of botulinum toxin and tetanus toxin. Ann Rev Pharmacol Toxicol 26:427–453, 1986

3 Weinstein L: Tetanus. N Engl J Med 289:1293–1296, 1973

4 Bleck TP: Pharmacology of tetanus. Clin Neurol 9:103–120, 1986

5 Young LS, LaForce FM, Bennett JV: An evaluation of serologic and antimicrobial therapy in the treatment of tetanus in the United States. J Infect Dis 120:153–159, 1969

6 Dowell VR Jr: Selected epidemiologic and microbiologic aspects. Rev Infect Dis 6:1, 1984

7 Summary of Notifiable Diseases, United States 1986. U.S. Department of Health and Human Services, Centers for Disease Control, Atlanta, Georgia, 1986

8 Stanfield JP, Galazka A: Neonatal tetanus in the world today. Bull WHO 62(4):647–669, 1984

CHAPTER 92 / *Anthrax* · *Philip S. Brachman*

Anthrax, a zoonotic disease, has an interesting history dating from biblical times. Although not currently a major public health problem, it has been associated with focal, devastating epidemics; it has played a significant role in developmental microbiology; and was the first disease associated with its etiological agent. Development of specific and nonspecific preventive measures has resulted in a decline in incidence so that today anthrax occurs sporadically except for an occasional report of an epidemic and in a few countries where it remains endemic. The human disease appears in three forms. In the United States, approximately 95 percent of the cases are cutaneous anthrax and the remainder are inhalation anthrax; gastrointestinal anthrax cases are reported from other countries, in some more commonly than inhalation cases. Synonyms for anthrax include charbon, malignant pustule, Siberian ulcer, malignant edema, splenic fever, milzbrand, wool-sorter's disease, and ragpicker's disease.

PARASITE

Bacillus anthracis is a gram-positive, spore-forming, nonmotile bacillus (1 to 1.3 μm by 3 to 10 μm) that grows at 37°C on ordinary laboratory media [*1*]. Growth may be noted after 8 to 12 h and becomes characteristic after 18 to 36 h of incubation, revealing round, convex, grayish-white colonies 2 to 5 mm in diameter, which may show comma-shaped outshootings. Colonial tenacity, which is typical of *B. anthracis,* may be demonstrated by drawing the inoculating loop through the colony; the disturbed part should stand perpendicular to the surface of the agar and resemble beaten egg whites. Gram-stain preparation of artificial media growth reveals gram-positive, square-ended rods in long, parallel chains. Spore stains demonstrate central or paracentral spores that do not protrude beyond the outline of the bacillus. Direct fluorescent-antibody staining of organisms grown on bicarbonate agar in a 5% CO_2 atmosphere [*2*] and bacteriophage testing may be used to confirm the identification [*3*]. Agar-grown cells suspended in saline inoculated subcutaneously or intraperitoneally into guinea pigs, mice, or rabbits will cause death of the animal in from 24 to 72 h. Autopsy reveals evidence of general toxicity and hemorrhages in multiple organs. Animals inoculated subcutaneously will demonstrate subcutaneous gelatinous hemorrhagic edema at the inoculation site in addition to general toxemia. If broth cultures are used to produce the inoculum, in order to avoid nonspecific deaths, the organisms must be centrifuged, washed, and resuspended in saline before being inoculated into animals.

Gram-stained smears of material taken directly from cutaneous lesions or from tissues have nonparallel, single-cell to short chain, gram-positive bacilli with slightly rounded ends. Spores are not seen in fresh clinical material.

Serum specimens collected during the acute phase and convalescent phase of illness (obtained at least 2 weeks apart) should demonstrate a rise in indirect hemagglutinating antibodies. A fourfold rise represents either active infection or vaccination. A single titer of 1:8 represents either current or recent infection or immunity as a result of either past infection or vaccination. A more sensitive test is the ELISA test, where a fourfold rise in titer or a single titer of 1:32 or greater is indicative of current or recent infections or immunity.

PATIENT

PATHOGENESIS

Cutaneous anthrax

Organisms, usually spores, enter the skin either through an existing wound or on a foreign body, such as a hair fiber, and are deposited in subcutaneous tissues where they germinate, multiply, and produce toxin that causes local necrosis and development of the typical anthrax lesion. Vegetative cells and toxin may be hematogenously distributed regionally or throughout the body, resulting in bacteremia and generalized toxemia. Infection may also spread locally via the lymphatics with development of regional lymphadenopathy and, rarely, lymphangitis. Once the local lesion has healed, a scar due to tissue necrosis usually remains.

Inhalation anthrax

With this form of disease, particles bearing *B. anthracis* are inhaled, and those smaller than 5 μm are transported to the terminal pulmonary alveoli, where they are ingested by macrophages and passively transported to the mediastinal lymph nodes [4]. The spores germinate, multiply, and produce toxin that causes hemorrhagic necrosis of the mediastinal nodes with associated edema and hemorrhage in the mediastinum. Hematogenous dissemination leads to septicemia and secondary manifestations such as meningitis and pneumonia. In the septicemia phase, the toxin has a direct effect upon pulmonary capillary endothelium, causing pulmonary capillary thrombosis [5]. Terminal and respiratory failure may result from the pulmonary capillary thrombosis and a poorly defined toxic effect on the respiratory center of the central nervous system.

Gastrointestinal anthrax

Ingestion of *B. anthracis*–contaminated food may result in either gastrointestinal or oropharyngeal anthrax. In gastrointestinal anthrax, there may be a primary lesion similar to that of cutaneous anthrax, located in the mucosal surface of the gut (frequently the ileum or cecum). The steps leading to development of the primary lesion have not been defined. Hemorrhagic mesenteric lymphadenitis is almost invariably present early in the course, suggesting that the initial spreading of infection is via the lymphatics. Subsequent hematogenous spread results in septicemia and secondary foci of infection at distal points.

In the oropharyngeal form, the initial lesion may be in the oropharynx or the organisms may be transported through the oral mucosa to the tonsillar or cervical lymph nodes, where they germinate, multiply, and produce toxin. The resultant lymphadenitis and associated edema may be so massive as to compress the respiratory passages.

Meningitis

Meningitis may be secondary to any of the above forms of anthrax infection. It results from hematogenous spread of bacilli from a primary focus. Rarely, a primary focus cannot be identified.

Toxin

Virulence of *Bacillus anthracis* is determined by a toxin and by capsular material, each coded by a different plasmid. The toxin consists of three components: edema factor, lethal factor, and protective antigen [6]. In human disease, sterilization of tissues with antibiotics may reduce the severity of the illness but the clinical course will continue until the toxin in the body has been metabolized or otherwise inactivated.

CLINICAL DISEASE

Cutaneous anthrax

Cutaneous anthrax usually occurs on exposed parts of the body, such as the face, neck, or arms. After an incubation period of 1 to 10 days (commonly 2 to 5 days), a round, small, pruritic, painless papule, approximately 1.0 cm in diameter, is seen at the site of inoculation. Within several days a small vesicle, or a ring of vesicles, develops, surrounded by a small ring of erythema and slight, nonpitting edema. If multiple vesicles are present, they coalesce to form a single large vesicle. There may be lymphangitis and regional lymphadenopathy. Shortly thereafter, hemorrhage occurs at the base of the vesicle. The vesicle ruptures, discharging clear to slightly yellow serous fluid containing *B. anthracis* organisms. Beneath the vesicle is a well-demarcated, depressed ulcer crater, the base of which is covered with a developing black eschar. Over the next week as the eschar dries, it slowly separates from the surrounding tissue. The ulcer slowly granulates, leaving a small scar.

Small lesions are usually round whereas larger lesions tend to be more irregularly shaped. If the lesion is located in an area of loose subcutaneous tissue, there may be extensive edematous involvement of the surrounding tissue. For example, edema resulting from a lesion beneath the eye can extend from the scalp to the upper thorax. Rarely, an individual has multiple co-primary lesions resulting from simultaneous inoculations.

Malignant edema is only rarely seen in association with cutaneous lesions and refers to development of extensive edema, induration, bulla formation, fever, and severe toxemia.

The treatment of choice is penicillin. In mild cutaneous anthrax, oral potassium penicillin 2 g/day for 5 to 7 days is recommended. Extensive lesions or those with significant symptoms should be treated with intramuscular procaine penicillin 4 to 6 million units per day for 5 to 7 days. Tetracycline or erythromycin may also be used in oral doses of 2 g/day for 5 to 7 days. In malignant edema, additional therapy with intravenous hydrocortisone 100 to 200 mg/day has been reported to be effective.

Local treatment of the lesion other than covering it with a clean dressing has not been shown to be effective; the lesion should not be excised since this has been reported to increase the severity of symptoms. Mortality for cutaneous anthrax was approximately 20 percent before antibiotic therapy. With appropriate antibiotic therapy, mortality should be less than 5 percent.

Inhalation anthrax

Inhalation anthrax, with an incubation period of 1 to 5 days (commonly 3 to 4 days), is biphasic, with the initial phase resembling a nondescript respiratory tract infection with mild fever, fatigue, malaise, myalgia, at times a nonproductive cough, and occasionally a sensation of precordial oppression [7]. Physical examination may reveal rhonchi on auscultation of the chest. Within several days there may be some clinical improvement but soon thereafter the acute phase begins with the rapid development of respiratory distress, high fever, dyspnea, cyanosis, respiratory stridor, and profuse diaphoresis. Subcutaneous edema of the neck and upper thorax may develop. The above signs progress, and physical examination reveals crepitant rales over the lungs. Radiographic examination of the chest typically reveals mediastinal widening and possibly pleural effusion. The patient usually dies within 24 h.

Therapy of inhalation anthrax is based upon empirical knowledge and data extrapolated from animal studies. Penicillin G administered intravenously in doses of 18 to 24 million units per day is the recommended treatment. Animal experimental work suggests that this therapy may be supplemented by the addition of intravenous streptomycin, 1 to 2 g/day. Supportive therapy, including the use of volume expanders and vasopressor agents, should be used as necessary. If edema becomes oppressive, a tracheostomy may be necessary. Inhalation anthrax is almost always fatal.

Gastrointestinal anthrax

Gastrointestinal anthrax has an incubation period of 2 to 5 days. The initial symptoms of the abdominal form are nausea, vomiting, anorexia, and fever. As the disease progresses, significant abdominal pain develops and hematemesis and bloody diarrhea may occur. In some cases symptoms are severe and the patient appears to have an acute surgical abdomen. Ascites may be demonstrated on physical examination. Progression of the disease leads to toxemia, cyanosis, shock, and death, which may occur 2 to 5 days after the onset of the clinical disease. There has been a report of deaths occurring in less than 2 days after onset of the first symptoms (personal communication).

In oropharyngeal anthrax, the patient develops fever, anorexia, submandibular edema, and cervical lymphadenopathy [8]. In some reports acute inflammatory lesions resembling cutaneous lesions are described in the oral cavity involving the posterior pharyngeal wall, the hard palate, or tonsils. The edema of the cervical area may become so extensive that there may be encroachment of the oral passageways causing difficulty in breathing.

Therapy of gastrointestinal anthrax is the same as for inhalation anthrax. Additionally, tetracycline 1 g/day intravenously has also been reported to be effective. The fatality rate for gastrointestinal anthrax varies from 25 to 75 percent.

Meningitis

Anthrax meningitis symptomatically resembles other forms of acute bacterial meningitis. Therapy should be the same as for inhalation anthrax.

Immunity

Serological studies suggest that immunity develops after clinical disease and persists for a number of years. Reinfections have not been confirmed. There is some evidence to support the development of subclinical infections [9].

LABORATORY DIAGNOSIS

Laboratory diagnosis of cutaneous anthrax is made by culturing the vesicular fluid on ordinary laboratory media. In inhalation anthrax, sputum may be cultured; however, unless there is secondary anthrax pneumonia, cultures are negative. In gastrointestinal anthrax, vomitus or fecal material should be cultured; in anthrax meningitis, cerebrospinal fluid should be examined. In all forms of the disease, blood cultures may be positive. Fluorescent antibody staining and/or bacteriophage testing may be used to confirm the identification of *B. anthracis*. Serology can be used to demonstrate exposure to *B. anthracis*. The indirect hemagglutination test has been used but a more sensitive test is the ELISA test [10,11]. A recent development is an electrophoretic-immunotransblots method [11].

DIFFERENTIAL DIAGNOSIS

The differential diagnosis of cutaneous anthrax includes staphylococcal skin infections, tularemia, plague, contagious pustular dermatitis (ecthyma contagiosum or orf) and milker's nodule. Inhalation anthrax must be differentiated from other diseases that cause acute respiratory insufficiency. Gastrointestinal anthrax is most easily confused with other causes of gastroenteritis such as salmonellosis, shigellosis, and *Yersinia* infection. Additionally, it can resemble acute appendicitis. The oropharyngeal form of anthrax resembles any acute infection of the cervical or tonsillar region.

POPULATION

OCCURRENCE

Whereas 35 years ago the number of cases of anthrax reported from throughout the world was estimated to be 20,000 to 200,000 [12], in 1981 the World Health Organization reported approximately 3200 cases from 43 countries, though this is an underestimation because of the lack of reporting from some countries [13]. Animal anthrax remains a significant problem in certain Asiatic, African, South American, and Caribbean countries.

In the United States, the incidence has gradually decreased. The number of annually reported cases of anthrax for the 10 years 1916 through 1925 was 127 cases, whereas the annual yearly average from 1948 to 1957 was 44; 1958 to 1967, 9.6; 1968 to 1977, 2.4; and 1978 to 1987, 1 case. From 1955 through 1987, 234 cases of anthrax were reported in the United States: 223 cases were cutaneous and 11 were inhalation anthrax.

Animal cases have also decreased in occurrence. Today, only sporadic cases are reported in the United States, frequently involving grazing areas known as ''anthrax districts'' because of the occasional cases that continue to occur there.

EPIDEMIOLOGY

Anthrax cases are classified as either industrial or agriculturally acquired [14]. In the United States, industrial anthrax accounts for approximately 80 percent of the cases. In other countries, agricultural anthrax is usually more common. An occasional case has been reported in which the source of infection is not discernible.

In the United States, the involved industries process imported goat hair, wool, skins and hides, bones, and bonemeal. Occasionally, the source of infections may be a commercial product such as animal yarn or novelties made from skins, hides, or animal hair that have not been properly disinfected. Cases sometimes occur among laboratory personnel.

Agricultural cases result from contact with carcasses of animals that have died of anthrax. Inadvertent inoculation of animal vaccine has been reported (but not documented) to cause cutaneous anthrax.

The route of transmission of cutaneous anthrax is primarily by direct contact, though occasionally indirect contact may be involved. Inhalation anthrax results from airborne transmission of organisms released into the air from equipment used to process the animal products, primarily goat hair or wool. Gastrointestinal anthrax results from eating inadequately cooked contaminated food, most often, meat.

The majority of cases are sporadic though occasional epidemics occur. In the United States the last epidemic occurred in 1957 and involved nine employees in a goat-hair processing mill; four were inhalation and five cutaneous cases [15]. All were traced to contact with a single batch of imported goat hair that appeared to be more heavily contaminated with *B. anthracis* than normal. During recent years, occasional epidemics have been reported in other countries, usually related to outbreaks of animal anthrax. An extensive epidemic occurred in Zimbabwe, which began in 1979 and by 1985 had abated; however, cases continue to occur, which may reflect the endemic occurrence. It is estimated that more than 10,000 cases, primarily cutaneous anthrax, have appeared in Zimbabwe [16].

Agriculturally related human cases parallel the existence of anthrax in the animal population. *Bacillus anthracis* spores are known for their resistance to chemical, physical, and environmental factors. They are reported to persist in nature for years, though this has not been proven under natural conditions. Anthrax districts may represent areas in which contamination persists for many years or areas that are reinfected at regular intervals by animals or other sources. These anthrax districts frequently contain alluvial soil with a pH of greater than 6.0.

Human-to-human or insect transmission has not been proven.

PREVENTION

Primary prevention of anthrax in humans involves controlling the disease in animals and preventing contamination of their products. This can be accomplished by practicing good animal husbandry, including immunization of animals at regular intervals using the Sterne strain vaccine and properly disposing of contaminated carcasses by means of deep burial or complete incineration. Animal products that are shown to be contaminated should be decontaminated with formaldehyde, ethylene oxide, pressurized steam, or gamma irradiation; they may also be discarded by burial or by incineration in a manner that does not result in contamination of the environment.

The occurrence of industrial cases can be reduced by practicing good hygiene, which primarily includes educating employees, wearing protective clothing, controlling environmental contamination, and providing medical care so that suspect lesions can be properly examined, cultured, and treated. Individuals who have regular contact with potentially contaminated animal materials should be vaccinated [17]. The human vaccine is available commercially from the Michigan Department of Public Health, Bureau of Disease Control and Laboratory Services, 3500 North Logan Street, P.O. Box 30035, Lansing, Michigan 48909.

Quarantine or embargo of potentially contaminated raw or processed materials has been an effective means of preventing the importation of contaminated materials. This has been successful in the United States in preventing the importation of contaminated drums, carpets, etc., by tourists from the Caribbean. Within a developing country, the domestic regulations concerning the sale of infected hides or carcasses are only as effective as they are enforced. Even in the United States, with a relatively high level of animal husbandry, carcasses or hides contaminated with *B. anthracis* spores occasionally do get into a processing plant and may not come to the attention of health authorities until a cutaneous case occurs. There is a direct relationship between the practice of the recommended public health practices and the occurrence of human disease.

REFERENCES

1 Doyle PJ, Keller KF, Ezell JW: *Bacillus anthracis* in Lennette EH, Balows A, Hausler W Jr, et al (eds): *Manual of Clinical Microbiology,* 4th ed. Washington, DC, American Society for Microbiology, 1985, pp 211–215

2 Cherry WB, Freeman EM: Staining bacterial smears with fluorescent antibody. V. The rapid identification of *Bacillus anthracis* in culture and in human and murine tissues. Zentralbl Bakteriol Abt 1(Orig)175:582–597, 1959

3 Brown ER, Cherry WB: Specific identification of *Bacillus anthracis* by means of a variant bacteriophage. J Infect Dis 96:36–39, 1955

4 Albrink WS, Brooks SM, Biron RE, et al: Human inhalation anthrax, a report of three fatal cases. Am J Pathol 36:457–472, 1960

5 Dalldorf FG, Beall F: Capillary thrombosis as a cause of death in experimental anthrax. Arch Pathol 83:154, 1967

6 Beall FA, Taylor MJ, Thorne CE: Rapid lethal effect in rats of a third component found upon fractionating the toxin of *Bacillus anthracis*. J Bacteriol 83:1274–1280, 1962

7 Plotkin SA, Brachman PS, Utell M, et al: An epidemic of inhalation anthrax: The first in the twentieth century. I. Clinical features. Am J Med 29:992–1001, 1960

8 Sirisantha T, Navacharoen N, Tharavichitkul P, et al: Outbreak of oral-oropharyngeal anthrax: An unusual manifestation of human infection with *Bacillus anthracis*. Am J Trop Med Hyg 33:144–150, 1984

9 Norman PS, Ray JG, Brachman PS, et al: Serological testings for anthrax antibodies in workers in a goat hair processing mill. Am J Hyg 72:32–37, 1960

10 Ezzell JW, Abshire TG: Immunological analysis of cell-associated antigens of *Bacillus anthracis*. Infect Immun 56:349–356, 1988

11 Little SF, Knudson GB: Comparative efficacy of *Bacillus anthracis* live spore vaccine and protective antigen vaccine against anthrax in the guinea pig. Infect Immun 52:509–512, 1986

12 Glassman HN: World incidence of anthrax in man. Public Health Rep 73:22, 1958

13 World Health Statistics Annual, 1980–1981, Infectious Diseases. Geneva, World Health Organization, 1981

14 Brachman PS, Fekety FR: Industrial anthrax. Ann NY Acad Sci 70:574–584, 1958

15 Brachman PS, Plotkin SA, Bumford FH, et al: An epidemic of inhalation anthrax. II. Epidemiologic investigations. Am J Hyg 72:6–23, 1960

16 Davies JCA: A major epidemic of anthrax in Zimbabwe. Centr Afr J Med Part 1: 28:291–298, 1982; Part 2: 29:8–12, 1983; Part 3: 31:176–180, 1985

17 Wright JG, Green TW, Kanode RG Jr: Studies on immunity and anthrax. V. Immunizing activity of alum-precipitated protective antigen. J Immunol 73:387, 1954

CHAPTER 93 / *Brucellosis* · A. Barnett Christie

Brucellosis is an important disease from the standpoints of economics and public health. It is primarily a disease of animals, especially farm animals, in which it can lead to poor general condition, loss of milk and wool yield, and low rate of reproduction. It spreads to humans in milk or by direct animal contact and is a serious cause of acute and chronic illness.

PARASITE

The genus *Brucella* takes its name from Dr. D. Bruce who isolated the organism from the spleen of four patients in Malta who died in 1877 from what was then called Mediterranean fever. This was *Brucella melitensis*. *Brucella abortus* was first isolated from the uterus of an aborting cow in 1895 in Copenhagen, and *Brucella suis* from the organs of a premature pig in 1914 in Indiana, U.S.A. These organisms are still the only members of the genus which commonly cause infection in animals and humans. *Brucella canis* has caused outbreaks in dogs but has only once been reported in humans [1]. *Brucella ovis* causes ram epididymitis in Australasia, but rarely infection in sheep. *Brucella neotomae* and *B. rangiferae tarandi* seem to be infections only of animals in the wild.

Growth of brucellae on agar is slow, but is speeded by the addition of animal protein, and especially by erythritol, a substance found in some animal placentas and seminal vesicles. Erythritol may play a part in the localization of brucellae in animal tissues [2]. Various other useful media are serum dextrose agar, serum potato infusion agar, and blood agar containing 5% sheep blood. *Brucella* species grow in the range of 20°C to 40°C, and best at 37°C.

Brucellae require oxygen for growth. *B. abortus* and *B. melitensis* grow best when there is also 10% CO_2 in the medium, but *B. suis* does not require this. The three organisms vary in their sensitivity to the dyes thionin, basic fuchsin, methyl violet, and pyronin and in their tendency to produce H_2S, especially when grown on liver agar, but these are not constant characteristics. The different rates of oxygen uptake by cultures of the three *Brucella* species on special media are more reliable. Strains of *B. abortus* which share this metabolic pattern are all lysed by one stable phage for *B. abortus*.

Brucellae have two main antigens, A and M, which are shared by all brucellae, but in different amounts. *B. abortus* and *B. suis* have more A than M, *B. melitensis* more M than A. This can be shown by quantitative agglutinin absorption tests, but even when monospecific sera are used there are many apparent anomalies. No one test is reliable by itself in identifying strains. When all are used nine biotypes of *B. abortus* can be distinguished, three of *B. melitensis,* and four of *B. suis* [3].

Animal inoculation is not usually necessary except when the material to be cultured is likely to be contaminated with other organisms, for example, milk.

PERSISTENCE

Brucellae survive in natural conditions for long periods. Sunlight kills them quickly, but in dry soil they may live for 6 weeks and in damp soil even longer. In animal feces in the open they have survived for over 100 days [4]. From walls and floors of cowsheds they have been isolated live for at least 4 months and from contaminated ground outside for up to 5 weeks.

Pasteurized milk is safe but raw milk is dangerous, whether from cows, goats, sheep, or camels [5]. In fresh milk brucellae survive for several days until the milk turns sour and the acidity kills them. Brucellae survive and multiply in cheese made from fresh goat or sheep milk. In one investigation they were isolated from soft cheese after 2 months' maturation [4]. Cheese and butter made from pasteurized milk are safe.

The organisms can survive in tap water for more than a month at 8°C and more than a week at 25°C. In lake water, animal urine, feces, and soil they have been isolated after more than 2 years at 25°C, but at 37°C for less than a quarter of that time. For all practical purposes, especially the control of spread, one must accept that brucellae are persistent organisms.

PATIENT

PATHOLOGY AND PATHOGENESIS

Brucellae may be implanted on the skin or the conjunctiva, be inhaled, or ingested in milk. In all cases the organisms are first conveyed to the regional lymph nodes where they may be destroyed, or, if sufficiently virulent, may overcome the defenses of the lymphoid tissue and escape into the bloodstream [3]. They then localize mainly in the cells of the reticuloendothelial system (e.g., in liver, spleen, bone marrow, lymph nodes, and kidney). The infected cells form nodules, with giant cells inside them and infiltrating lymphocytes around them.

They are like tubercles except that there is no caseation.

As intracellular parasites, brucellae are to some extent protected from antibodies and antibiotics. This may explain in part why the disease, both in animals and in humans, is sometimes so chronic. L forms may develop and be even more difficult to isolate in culture than normal forms [6]. The organisms may disintegrate inside host cells and release endotoxin [3], which may also pass into the circulation and cause symptoms. The granuloma may be the only host reaction in many patients, but in others sensitivity develops. These patients may react with a bout of fever each time endotoxin is released into the bloodstream.

CLINICAL MANIFESTATIONS

The onset of acute brucellosis may be sudden, with chills and rigors, or more gradual. The patient's temperature swings between 37.7°C and 39.4°C (100°F to 103°F) but may shoot up to 40.5°C or 41°C (105°F to 106°F) during a rigor. The patient has generalized aches and pains, especially in the back, drenching sweats, weakness, anxiety, depression, and anorexia. The patient is obviously very ill, yet little is found on examination. The spleen may be enlarged and the liver a little tender, or there may be some enlarged lymph nodes and tenderness over the lumbar spine. There are no abnormal signs in the chest although the patient may have a cough. The blood count shows leukopenia.

The acute attack usually subsides in a few weeks, with or without treatment, especially in *B. abortus* cases. But the fever tends to recur, even in patients treated with antibiotics, and the patient passes into the subacute (progressive) stage. This stage often develops slowly and insidiously with fatigue, which the patient cannot explain, as the main symptom. He or she feels well in the morning, but after an hour or two at work is tired and exhausted. A rest does no good, and by evening the patient is worn out and depressed. There may be backache and pain in the thighs, and the patient may put his or her tiredness down to "rheumatics." As in acute disease there may be fever, a palpable spleen, a few enlarged lymph nodes, but otherwise nothing to explain the symptoms. Unless specific laboratory tests are done the condition is unlikely to be diagnosed. Fortunately, the disease usually burns itself out within a year of onset and the patient regains his or her former health. In perhaps 20 percent of subacute cases the disease progresses to a chronic stage. Complications tend to occur in the subacute stage and are due to the presence of brucellae at the affected site. Brucellae have been isolated from joint fluid, liver biopsy material, and cerebrospinal fluid.

Large bones and joints are often affected. In the spine the disc and parts of the bodies of adjacent vertebrae are eroded. This may lead to collapse of vertebrae with wedging and tilting or crushing; sometimes an abscess forms, which tracks into the psoas muscle. The condition looks very much like tuberculosis of the spine. Sciatica is a common symptom. Depression, anxiety, apathy, or, during fever, delirium, are all evidence of central nervous system involvement. Deafness from effects on the eighth nerve affection is common. Occasionally meningoencephalitis or meningitis occurs. Epididymoorchitis is also common, but as in mumps the risk of sterility is slight. Damage from myocarditis is not frequent, but a few cases have been reported of endocarditis with isolation of brucellae from heart valves. Granulomatous changes in vessel walls can cause thrombosis of deep veins and pulmonary embolism may follow. Pregnancy may increase the severity of the illness, but this is a feature brucellosis shares with other diseases. In spite of the name *B. abortus,* abortion or menstrual disturbance in women is not more frequent than in any other acute septicemic illness. Brucellae are shed freely in the urine, and sometimes this may result in granulomatous lesions of the kidney, ureter, or bladder, which may closely resemble renal tuberculosis.

Pulmonary complications are rare. The liver is probably always affected, but jaundice is uncommon. The spleen is usually enlarged in the acute stage but complications caused by hypersplenism are rare. Various ocular affections have been reported. Skin rashes are uncommon except in veterinarians in whom an intensely itchy rash may occur on the arms, especially after obstetric operations on animals.

Some patients suffer for a long time with well-recognized complications, especially spinal or renal trouble. In them the diagnosis of chronic brucellosis is obvious from their history and previous laboratory tests for subacute brucellosis. Another group of patients may have only vague but disabling symptoms—lack of energy, depression, and worry. These symptoms may, of course, be psychogenic in origin, but may also be due to neurophysiological processes caused by continuing brucellar activity. The distinction can be made only by thorough physical and laboratory investigation and is never easy. One must try to avoid labeling as neurasthenic a patient suffering from a bacterial infection.

DIAGNOSIS

The only certain method of diagnosis is to isolate *Brucella* in culture from blood, urine, pus, or other material. There are several serological tests including agglutination, complement fixation, anti-human globulin, the rose Bengal plate test (useful for screening), and radioimmunoassay, which is sensitive but not readily available. The clinician and the microbiologist must work together to reach a firm diagnosis [7]. In the tropics, the physician may have to depend on clinical history and the probability of exposure to infection to make a diagnosis.

TREATMENT

In addition to full supportive nursing treatment, the patient with acute or subacute brucellosis should be treated with an antibiotic. Tetracycline in a dose of 2 to 3 g/day for 21 days is usually satisfactory. Some physicians recommend that 1 g of streptomycin be given intramuscularly daily for the same period, but this is probably unnecessary. Trimethoprim-sulfamethoxazole, 2 or 3 tablets daily, is also effective. Rifampicin has been given along with other antibiotics, but with doubtful effect [7]. The patient's temperature usually falls and his or her condition improves during the course of treatment, but intracellular brucellae may be protected against the action of the antibiotics. The resulting relapses must be treated in the same way. In chronic brucellosis it is essential to establish the diagnosis and thereafter to treat the patient during febrile episodes in the hope of eradicating the infection. For all complications it is best first to treat the patient with full courses of antibiotics before considering surgery.

POPULATION

PREVENTION

All milk should be pasteurized. All farm animals should be tested and positive reactors removed from the herd and slaughtered so that only brucellosis-free herds remain. This is ideal practice and has been achieved in many developed countries, leading to the elimination of brucellosis. Elsewhere there are immense difficulties and compromise is necessary. A human vaccine has been used and apparently protects humans but does nothing to eradicate the disease in animals. Animal vaccines are available for cattle, sheep, and goats, and one for pigs may soon be available [8,9]. A vaccine will protect an animal against future infection with brucellae, but it does nothing against infection already present.

There is no mystery about the epidemiology of brucellosis in animals or in humans. Everything needed for the elimination of the disease is known [7], but applying that knowledge throughout the world is an immense challenge.

REFERENCES

1 Swenson RM, Carmichael LE, Cundy KR: Human infection with *Brucella canis*. Ann Intern Med 76:435, 1972

2 Keppie J, Williams AE, Witt K, et al: The role of erythritol in the tissue localisation of the brucellae. Br J Exp Pathol 46:104, 1965

3 McCullough NB: Microbial and host factors in the pathogenesis of brucellosis, in Mudd S (ed): *Infectious Agents and Host Reactions.* Philadelphia, Saunders, 1970, p 324

4 King NB: The survival of *Brucella abortus* (USDA strain 2308) in manure. J Am Vet Med Assoc 111:349, 1957

5 Al-Kanderi S, Al-Enizi A, Christie AB: Brucellosis, a continuing problem. Epidemiology. Postgrad Doctor, Africa 9:316, 1987

6 Hatten BA, Sulkin SE: Intracellular production of *Brucella* forms. II. Induction and survival of *Brucella abortus* L forms in tissue culture. J Bacteriol 91:14, 1966

7 Christie AB: Brucellosis. Undulant fever. Malta or Mediterranean fever, in Christie AB: *Infectious Diseases: Epidemiology and Clinical Practice.* Edinburgh, Churchill Livingstone, 1987, pp 1130–1158

8 Joint FAO/WHO expert committee on brucellosis, 5th report. WHO Tech Rep Ser 464. Geneva, World Health Organization, 1970

9 Roux J: Les vaccinations dans les brucelloses humaines et animales. Bull Inst Pasteur 70:145, 1972

Plague · Thomas Butler

Plague is a bacterial infection of animals and humans caused by *Yersinia pestis*. The most common clinical form is acute regional lymphadenitis, called bubonic plague. Less common clinical forms include septicemic, pneumonic, and meningeal plague. The rate of mortality is high in untreated cases, but antibiotic treatment administered early in the course of the disease markedly reduces fatalities. Plague has a widespread distribution in the world with significant focuses in the Americas, Africa, and Asia. The natural reservoirs of *Y. pestis* are predominantly urban and sylvatic rodents. Plague is transmitted among animals and occasionally to humans by bites of infected fleas.

PARASITE

Y. pestis, which belongs to the family Enterobacteriaceae, is an aerobic gram-negative bacillus which is readily cultured in broth or agar media with an optimal growth rate at 28°C. It is well-adapted to a variety of mammalian hosts, especially rats, in which it maintains itself by flea transmission.

A 45-MDa plasmid, which is essential for virulence, encodes for the VW antigen, dependency on calcium for growth at 37°C, and certain outer-membrane proteins [1]. A number of other antigens and toxins may also have important roles in its virulence and pathogenicity. In the capsular envelope that surrounds the organism there is a protein called fraction I antigen, which confers antiphagocytic activity and can activate complement proteins of the host. Fraction I is readily produced at 37°C but not at 28°C, indicating that this virulence factor develops while bacteria are in their mammalian hosts but is absent in fleas. The cell walls of *Y. pestis* contain a potent lipopolysaccharide endotoxin which produces fever, leukopenia followed by leukocytosis, disseminated intravascular coagulation, complement activation, and tissue damage. In experimental systems, this plague endotoxin causes local and generalized Shwartzman reactions, is mitogenic for B lymphocytes, and stimulates gelation of limulus lysate. Additionally, *Y. pestis* elaborates exotoxins, which may play pathogenic roles. One of these is a protein called the murine toxin, which is cardiotoxic and produces β-adrenergic blockade in animals but whose role in human disease is unclear.

Another important protein secreted by *Y. pestis* is a coagulase enzyme which causes blood ingested by the flea to clot in the proventriculus, thus blocking the transit of the next blood meal into the stomach of the flea. These "blocked" fleas are efficient vectors for plague infection because they regurgitate *Y. pestis* into the bite wound while attempting to feed. The coagulase of *Y. pestis* is active at 28°C and below but is in-

active at higher temperatures such as 35°C, thus explaining the cessation of plague transmission during very hot weather.

PATIENT

Although human plague infection can assume many and protean clinical forms, the most common presentation is bubonic plague (Fig. 94-1). During an incubation period of 2 to 8 days bacteria proliferate in the regional lymph nodes. Patients are typically affected by the sudden onset of fever, chills, weakness, and headache. At about the same time, patients notice the bubo, which is accompanied by intense pain in the affected lymphatic region. The common sites of the bubo are the groin, axilla, and neck. The swelling is so tender that patients typically avoid any motion that would provoke discomfort [2,3].

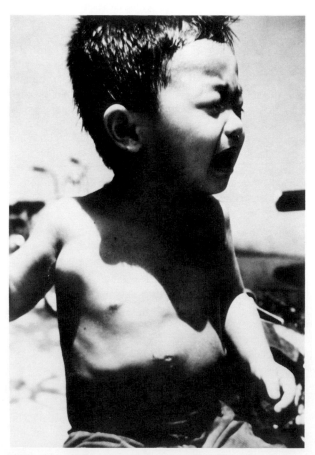

Figure 94-1. Right axillary bubo in a child with ulcerated pustule at right lower rib margin, the presumed site of fleabite inoculation.

Plague buboes are oval swellings varying from about 1 to 10 cm in length and elevate the overlying skin, which may appear stretched or erythematous. They may appear either as a smooth, uniform egg-shaped mass or in an irregular cluster of several nodes with intervening and surrounding edema. Palpation typically elicits extreme tenderness. There is warmth of the overlying skin; an underlying firm, nonfluctuant mass; and considerable gelatinous or pitting edema around the affected nodes. The acute lymphadenitis of plague is virtually unique in the sudden onset of the fever and bubo, the rapid development of intense inflammation, and the fulminant clinical course with death as soon as 2 to 4 days after the onset of symptoms. Plague is also distinctive in the absence of a detectable inoculation site and ascending lymphangitis in the anatomical region of the bubo.

In bubonic plague, patients are typically prostrate and lethargic but may exhibit restlessness or agitation [4]. Occasionally they are delirious with high fever; seizures are common in children. Temperatures are usually elevated in the range 38.5 to 40.0°C and the pulse rates are increased to 110 to 140 per minute. Blood pressures are characteristically low, in the range of 100/60 mmHg due to extreme vasodilation. The liver and spleen are often palpable and tender.

The pathology of bubonic plague is characterized by hemorrhage and necrosis. The lymph node capsule is obliterated by the destructive inflammatory process that involves the periglandular tissues as well as the lymph nodes themselves. The medulla is necrotic and contains phagocytic cells, polymorphonuclear leukocytes, red cells, and a granular material that is a pure culture of plague bacilli.

Occasionally, skin lesions at the site of the presumed flea bite appear as pustules, eschars, or papules (Fig. 94-2). The purpura of plague results from systemic disease, and with necrosis, in gangrene of distal extremities, the probable basis of the epithet "black death." These purpuric lesions contain blood vessels affected by vasculitis and occlusion by fibrin thrombi resulting in hemorrhage and necrosis.

A distinctive feature of plague is the propensity of the disease to overwhelm patients and produce systemic dissemination. In the early acute stages of bubonic plague, all patients probably have intermittent bacteremia. A hallmark of moribund patients with plague is high-density bacteremia, so that a blood smear revealing characteristic bacilli has been used as a prognostic indicator in this disease. Occasionally, bacteria are inoculated and proliferate in the body without producing a bubo. Patients may become ill with fever and actually die without detectable lymphadenitis [4–6]. This syndrome has been termed *septicemic plague* to denote plague without a bubo (Fig. 94-3).

The most feared complication of bubonic plague is secondary pneumonia. The infection reaches the lungs by hematogenous spread of bacteria from the bubo. In addition to the high mortality rate, plague pneumonia is highly contagious by airborne transmission. In the setting of fever and lymphadenop-

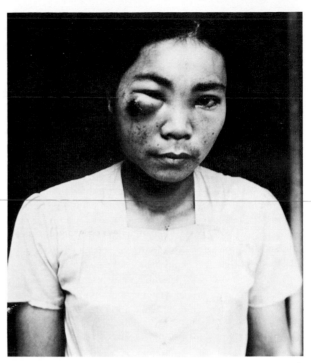

Figure 94-2. Eschar over cutaneous abscess under right eye at the presumed fleabite inoculation site. There was a right submandibular bubo.

athy it presents as cough, chest pain, and often hemoptysis [7]. Radiographically, there is patchy bronchopneumonia or confluent consolidation. The sputum is usually purulent and contains plague bacilli. Primary inhalation pneumonia is rare now but is a potential threat following exposure to a patient with plague who has a cough. It can be so rapidly fatal that persons reportedly have been exposed, become ill, and died on the same day.

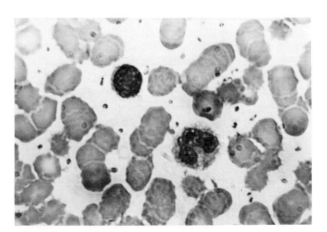

Figure 94-3. Blood smear of septicemic plague showing bipolar and pleomorphic bacilli.

Plague meningitis is a rarer complication and typically occurs more than a week following inadequately treated bubonic plague. It carries a high mortality rate when compared with uncomplicated bubonic plague. There appears to be an association between buboes located in the axilla and the development of meningitis. Rarely, plague meningitis presents as a primary infection of the meninges. Bacteria are frequently demonstrable in a Gram stain of spinal fluid sediment, and endotoxin has been demonstrated with the limulus test in spinal fluid.

Plague can produce pharyngitis that may resemble acute tonsillitis. The anterior cervical lymph nodes are usually inflamed, and *Y. pestis* may be recovered from a throat culture or by aspiration of a cervical bubo. This rare clinical form, presumed to follow the inhalation or ingestion of plague bacilli, has been related to the practice in some cultures of grooming another's hair and killing fleas by crushing them between the teeth.

The white blood cell count is typically elevated in the range of 10,000 to 20,000 cells per cubic millimeter, with a predominance of immature and mature neutrophils. Severely ill patients tend to have higher white blood cell counts. Occasionally, some patients, especially children, may develop myelocytic leukemoid reactions with white cell counts as high as 100,000 cells per cubic millimeter. Examination of the white blood cells typically reveals the so-called toxic changes characteristic of acute bacterial infections. Although patients with plague rarely develop a generalized bleeding tendency from profound thrombocytopenia, disseminated intravascular coagulation (DIC) is common.

Plague should be suspected in febrile patients who have been exposed to rodents or other mammals in the known endemic areas of the world. A bacteriological diagnosis is readily made in most patients by smear and culture of a bubo aspirate. The aspirate is obtained by inserting a 20-gauge needle on a 10-mL syringe containing 1 mL of sterile saline into the bubo and withdrawing several times until the saline becomes blood-tinged. Because the bubo does not contain liquid pus, it may be necessary to inject some of the saline and immediately reaspirate it. Drops of the aspirate should be placed onto microscope slides and air-dried for both Gram's and Wayson's stains. The Gram stain will reveal polymorphonuclear leukocytes and gram-negative coccobacilli and bacilli ranging from 1 to 2 μm in length. With Wayson's stain, *Y. pestis* appears as light-blue bacilli with dark-blue polar bodies; the remainder of the slide has a contrasting pink counterstain. Smears of blood, sputum, or spinal fluid can be handled similarly.

The aspirate, blood, and other appropriate fluids should be inoculated onto blood and MacConkey's agar plates and into infusion broth. The organism is identified in triple sugar iron agar by an alkaline slant and acid butt without gas or H_2S, by negative urease and indole reactions, failure to utilize citrate, and nonmotility. A serological test, the passive hemagglutination test utilizing fraction I of *Y. pestis,* can be performed on acute- and convalescent-phase serum. In patients with negative cultures, a fourfold or greater increase in titer or a single titer of 1:16 or more is presumptive evidence for plague infection.

TREATMENT

Untreated plague has an estimated mortality rate of greater than 50 percent and can evolve into a fulminant illness complicated by septic shock. Therefore, the early institution of effective antibiotic therapy is mandatory following appropriate cultures. In 1948, streptomycin was identified as the drug of choice for the treatment of plague by reducing the mortality rate to less than 5 percent. No other drug has been demonstrated more efficacious or less toxic. Streptomycin should be administered intramuscularly in two divided doses daily totaling 30 mg per kilogram of body weight per day for 10 days. Most patients improve rapidly and become afebrile in about 3 days. A full 10-day course is recommended to prevent relapses. The risk of vestibular damage and hearing loss caused by streptomycin is minimal. This antibiotic should be used cautiously, however, during pregnancy, in older patients who would have trouble adapting to vestibular damage, and in patients with previous hearing difficulty. Renal injury as a result of streptomycin therapy is rare with this regimen, but renal function should be monitored. If the serum creatinine level rises significantly, the dose of streptomycin should be reduced. In mild renal failure the recommended dose is about 20 mg/(kg·day) and in advanced renal failure 8 mg/kg every 3 days. Preparations of streptomycin available in the United States can be administered only intramuscularly.

For patients allergic to streptomycin or in whom an oral drug is strongly preferred, tetracycline is a satisfactory alternative. It is administered orally in a dose of 2 to 4 g/day in four divided doses for 10 days. Tetracycline is contraindicated in children younger than 7 years of age, in pregnant women, and in renal failure.

For patients with meningitis or profound hypotension, chloramphenicol should be administered intravenously. This is given as a loading dose of 25 mg per kilogram of body weight, followed by 60 mg/(kg·day) in four divided doses. After clinical improvement, chloramphenicol should be continued orally to complete a total course of 10 days. The bone marrow aplasia associated with chloramphenicol is so rare that chloramphenicol should not be withheld from patients seriously ill with plague.

Other antimicrobial drugs have been used in plague with varying success. These include sulfonamides, trimethoprim-sulfamethoxazole, kanamycin, and ampicillin. These drugs all appear to be either less effective or more toxic than streptomycin.

Antibiotic resistance to streptomycin, tetracycline, and chloramphenicol in human isolates of *Y. pestis* has never been reported nor has resistance emerged during antibiotic therapy. There is no rationale for using multiple antibiotics to treat plague.

Most plague patients are febrile with constitutional symptoms, hypotension, and dehydration. Therefore, intravenous 0.9% saline solution should be given to most patients for the first few days of the illness or until improvement occurs. Patients in shock will require additional quantities of fluid with hemodynamic monitoring. There is no evidence that corticosteroids are beneficial. Although DIC and purpura occasionally develop in severely ill patients, heparin therapy has no proven benefit.

Buboes usually recede without need of local therapy. Occasionally, however, they may enlarge or become fluctuant during the first week of treatment, requiring incision and drainage. The aspirated fluid should be cultured for evidence of superinfection with other bacteria, but this material is usually sterile.

POPULATION

EPIDEMIOLOGY

Y. pestis has caused devastating pandemics throughout history with high mortality rates. We are presently experiencing the fourth great pandemic in the world. The first pandemic originated in Egypt in 542 A.D. and spread to Turkey and Europe; the second started in the fourteenth century in Asia Minor and Africa and spread to Europe where it killed about a fourth of the population. The third occurred again in Europe during the fifteenth to eighteenth centuries. The present pandemic began around 1860 in the Chinese province of Yunnan. Subsequently plague was carried by ship to other Asian countries, India, Brazil, and California.

The plague bacillus is named after Alexandre Yersin who spent most of his life in Indochina working on bacterial diseases and the production of antisera and vaccines. During an epidemic of plague in Hong Kong in 1894, he identified bacteria in the tissues of autopsied plague victims and successfully obtained pure cultures of the organisms, which were lethal in experimental animals.

In the first half of the twentieth century, India was burdened with the largest share of reported plague in the world, with an estimated total of 10 million deaths. While plague ceased to occur in India in the 1950s, Vietnam experienced a resurgence of plague in the 1960s with as many as 10,000 deaths a year. During the 1970s Burma, Brazil, Kenya, Sudan, and Vietnam experienced more than 100 cases per year.

Plague is currently endemic in several countries of Africa, the Americas, and Asia (Fig. 94-4). The total number of human cases reported to WHO during the period 1980–1986 was 4522 with 421 deaths. Over these 7 years, Tanzania reported 927 cases, Vietnam 895, Brazil 649, Peru 512, Uganda 493, Burma 335, Madagascar 270, Bolivia 175, and the United States 148 [8].

Plague is primarily a zoonotic infection transmitted predominantly among urban and sylvatic rodents by flea bites or ingestion of contaminated animal tissues. A schematic depiction of

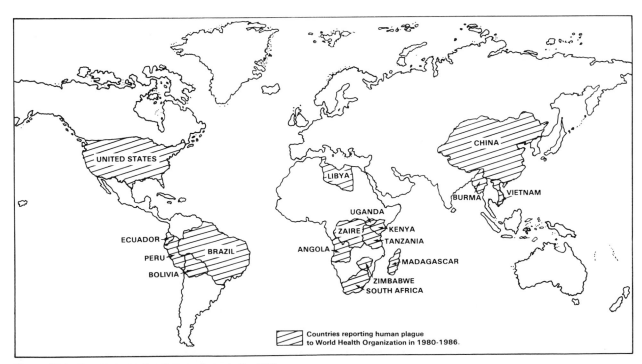

Figure 94-4. Countries reporting human plague in the 1980s.

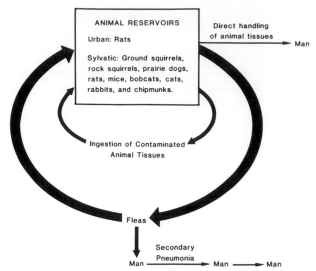

Figure 94-5. The cycle of infection of plague.

the cycle of infection is shown in Fig. 94-5. Throughout the world the urban and domestic rats, *Rattus rattus* and *R. norvegicus,* are the most important reservoirs of the plague bacillus. In sylvatic focuses of plague, however, such as in the United States, the important reservoirs are the ground squirrel, rock squirrel, and prairie dog. Human beings are accidental hosts in the natural cycle of plague when they are bitten by an infected rodent flea, and humans·appear to play no role in the maintenance of plague in nature. During the rare epidemics of pneumonic plague the infection is passed directly from person to person. On occasion humans have developed infection by handling contaminated animal tissues.

In the classic explanation of the dynamics of plague transmission, one or more relatively resistant small-animal species serve as the enzootic reservoir and one or more relatively susceptible species serve as epizootic hosts. The susceptible species may be involved in the so-called rat die-offs or ratfalls. In urban plague the same species of rat can be both the enzootic and epizootic species, whereas in rural or sylvatic plague there are usually two or more species. Some of the fluctuations in plague occurrence have been related to changing populations of the rodent reservoirs from resistant to sensitive and the reverse.

The incidence of plague in humans for any particular locality is a function of both the frequency of infection in local rodent populations and the intimacy with which the people live with the infected rodents and their fleas. All age groups and both sexes are equally susceptible to infection. Children comprise large portions of reported cases, perhaps because they spend more time in indiscriminate playing around rat-infested housing. Although humans develop acquired immunity after plague infection, the role of immunity in determining susceptibility of individuals to infection appears small.

Two other striking epidemiological features of plague infection are its focal nature and seasonality. Focuses of active plague infection are typically limited to single villages and even to single city blocks, with the adjacent villages and blocks being spared. This phenomenon is related to the parochial behavior of rats in staying near one food supply for extended periods. Only during the transport of rodents, usually on ships or trains, are epidemics of plague likely to spread to distant geographical areas.

Plague occurs predominantly in warm tropical climates. Epizootics tend to occur during humid, warm seasons and are sharply curtailed during very hot seasons when average daily temperatures exceed 30°C, and during very dry seasons. These seasonal fluctuations have been related to flea behavior and physiology. Humid conditions permit fleas longer periods between blood meals and more extended survival off their rodent hosts. On the other hand, during temperatures of 28°C and below, the coagulase enzyme of *Y. pestis* is active and blocks the digestive tract of fleas and enables them to be more efficient vectors. During these warm seasons fleas also proliferate, and when the flea index (ratio of fleas to rodents) exceeds 1, the conditions are usually optimal for a plague epidemic.

Prevention and control

Plague is one of the internationally quarantinable diseases. Accordingly, all patients with suspected plague should be reported to health department and to WHO. Patients with uncomplicated infections who are treated promptly present no health hazards to other persons. Those with cough or other signs of pneumonia must be placed in strict respiratory isolation for at least 48 h after the onset of antibiotic therapy or until the sputum culture is negative. The bubo aspirate and blood must be handled with gloves and with care to avoid aerosolization of these infected fluids. Laboratory workers who process the cultures should be alerted to exercise precautions; however, standard bacteriological techniques that safeguard against skin contact with and aerosolization of cultures should be adequate.

A formalin-killed vaccine, Plague Vaccine U.S.P. (Cutter Laboratories, Berkeley, California 94710) is available for travelers to epidemic or hyperendemic areas, for individuals who must live and work in close contact with rodents, and for laboratory workers who must handle live *Y. pestis* cultures. A primary series of two injections is recommended with a 1- to 3-month interval between them. Booster injections are given every 6 months for as long as exposure continues. In addition to vaccination, persons living in endemic areas should provide themselves with as much personal protection against rodents and fleas as possible, including living in ratproof houses, wearing shoes and garments to cover the legs, and applying insecticide dusts to houses.

The control of plague by health departments requires knowledge of the epidemiology of infected animals, vectors, and the contact of humans with these animals in any particular area.

In the United States the Plague Branch of the Centers for Disease Control in Fort Collins, Colorado has a field team of entomologists, mammalogists, and epidemiologists to investigate cases of plague. A specific approach to each case should be chosen and usually consists of insecticide use around homes, trapping of animals, and educating people to avoid contact with certain animals. Urban plague has been successfully controlled in many cities around the world by quarantine, rat control, and the use of insecticides. On the other hand, sylvatic plague defies most control measures because the wild rodent reservoirs are so widespread and diverse.

REFERENCES

1 Straley SC: The plasmid-encoded outer-membrane proteins of *Yersinia pestis*. Rev Infect Dis 10:S323, 1988

2 Butler T: *Plague and Other Yersinia Infections*. New York, Plenum Medical, 1983
3 Welty TK, Grabman J, Kompare E, et al: Nineteen cases of plague in Arizona. West J Med 142:641, 1985
4 Hull HF, Montes JM, Mann JM: Plague masquerading as gastrointestinal illness. West J Med 145:485, 1986
5 Hull HF, Montes JM, Mann JM: Septicemic plague in New Mexico. J Infect Dis 155:113, 1987
6 Leopold JC: Septicemic plague in a 14-month-old child. Pediatr Infect Dis 5:108, 1986
7 Florman AL, Spencer RR, Sheward S: Multiple lung cavities in a 12-year-old girl with bubonic plague, sepsis, and secondary pneumonia. Am J Med 80:1191, 1986
8 Human plague in 1986. Weekly Epidemiological Record, Geneva, World Health Organization, 40:299, 1987

CHAPTER 95 / *Leptospirosis* · Russell C. Johnson

Serovars of *Leptospira interrogans* are responsible for leptospirosis, a zoonosis of worldwide dimensions. Human leptospirosis can be caused by any one of a large number of serovars that infect a variety of wild and domestic animals. The majority of human cases result from contact with water and soil contaminated with the urine of leptospiruric animals. Leptospires enter through broken skin and mucosal surfaces causing an acute systemic disease characterized by an abrupt onset of fever, chills, myalgia, severe headache, and conjunctival suffusion. Since the clinical manifestations of the disease are not pathognomonic, leptospirosis is a frequently misdiagnosed disease. The majority of human infections are mild and anicteric. However 5 to 30 percent of severe icteric cases may be fatal, largely due to renal failure. The pathology associated with leptospirosis is the consequence of damage to small blood vessels. Antibiotic therapy is most efficacious if initiated during the first few days of the disease. Vaccination and rodent control are important methods of disease prevention.

PARASITE

The genus *Leptospira* is in the family Leptospiraceae of the order Spirochaetales. Although DNA-DNA annealing tests indicate at least seven distinct genetic groups exist within the genus, only two species are presently recognized. This is due to a paucity of differential phenotypic characteristics. The *Leptospira* fall into two phenotypic clusters represented by the species *L. interrogans* and *L. biflexa*. Members of each species are differentiated into serovars, the basic taxon, on the basis of antigenic composition. Serovars of *L. interrogans* are pathogenic for humans and animals and approximately 200 serovars have been isolated. For diagnostic convenience serovars of similar antigenic composition have been arranged into serogroups. The term serogroup has no taxonomic significance. The normal habitat for *L. interrogans* is the proximal convoluted tubules of the mammalian kidney.

Leptospira biflexa are free-living spirochetes that occur widely in fresh surface waters and associated soil. Several strains have been isolated from marine environments. None of the 65 serovars of *L. biflexa* are known to be infectious for experimental animals. The ubiquitous distribution of *L. biflexa* in water, combined with their ability to pass through sterilizing filters, has resulted in contamination of tissue culture and other filter-sterilized media.

Although the free-living *L. biflexa* and the parasitic *L. interrogans* are indistinguishable morphologically, several tests are available for differentiating between them. Serovars of *L. interrogans* are rapidly converted to spherical forms in hypertonic environments, whereas *L. biflexa* is relatively resistant to this morphological alteration. *L. interrogans* does not grow at 13°C or in the presence of 225 μg/mL 8-azaguanine, while *L. biflexa* does [1–3].

Leptospires are flexible, helically shaped gram-negative bacteria with dimensions of 0.1 by 6 to 20 μm that stain poorly to faintly with aniline dyes and the Giemsa stain. Unstained organisms cannot be seen with the bright-field microscope but are readily visualized with dark-field or phase microscopy.

These tightly coiled (18 coils per cell), hooked spirochetes are characterized by a very active flexuous motility. When translational motility is occurring in free liquid, one cell end is straight and the other is hooked, with movement in the direction of the straight end. Leptospires in semisolid medium display a serpentine type of movement. In contrast to bacteria with external flagella, the translational movement of *Leptospira* is enhanced as the viscosity of the milieu increases. Because of their narrow diameter, flexibility, and unique motility, leptospires can pass through sterilizing (0.22-μm pore size) filters [*1–3*].

Electron-microscopic studies of leptospires have revealed the following ultrastructural features: (1) the peripheral structure is a multilayered outer envelope or membrane; (2) enclosed by this outer envelope is the helical protoplasmic cylinder which consists of the peptidoglycan layer, cytoplasmic membrane, and the cytoplasmic contents of the cell; (3) the two periplasmic flagella (axial fibrils) lie between the outer envelope and the protoplasmic cylinder and are attached to the latter at subterminal positions. The free ends of the periplasmic flagella extend toward the cell center but rarely overlap. The helical conformation of *Leptospira* is right-handed (clockwise-coiling) [*1–3*].

Leptospira are obligate aerobes that produce oxidase, catalase, and/or peroxidase. Most serovars are easily cultivated in artificial media enriched with 10% rabbit serum or 1% bovine serum albumin–Tween 80. Their average generation time is about 12 h when cultivated in media with a pH of 7.4 and at 30°C. Diffuse to discrete nonpigmented subsurface colonies are usually formed in 1% agar medium. Colonial morphology is not a useful differentiating characteristic [*1–3*].

Nutritional requirements of leptospires are relatively simple with the only organic compounds required for growth being long-chain fatty acids in a detoxified form and vitamins B_1 and B_{12}. Fatty acids are the major carbon and energy source and also serve as a source of cellular lipids, since leptospires cannot synthesize fatty acids de novo. Ammonium salts, but not amino acids, provide a satisfactory source of nitrogen. Neither carbohydrates nor amino acids are important as carbon and energy sources. Initiation of growth of parasitic leptospires such as *hardjo* is enhanced by pyruvate, a nonessential nutrient. As a result of purines, but not pyrimidines, being metabolized by leptospires, they are resistant to the bactericidal properties of the pyrimidine analogue, 5′-fluorouracil. This compound is used as a selective agent in isolation media. Cells of leptospires are rich in lipids (20 percent) and the major phospholipid is phosphatidylethanolamine. Their peptidoglycan contains the diamino acid α,ε-diaminopimelic acid. Endotoxin is absent [*1–3*].

Serovars of *L. interrogans* have a wide host range, infecting as many as 160 different mammalian species [*4*]. The reservoir or maintenance host varies to some extent with the infecting serovar and geographical location. The primary laboratory animals used as models for leptospirosis are hamsters and guinea pigs.

PATIENT

PATHOGENESIS

Leptospirosis is most commonly acquired by direct or indirect contact with urine of leptospiruric animals. Mucosa, conjunctiva, and broken skin serve as sites of entry. A generalized infection ensues and when a critical concentration of spirochetes is reached, lesions occur. There is a marked disparity between the degree of functional impairment and the scarcity of histological lesions, suggesting damage at the subcellular level. Leptospiral toxin(s) responsible for the pathology associated with the disease have not been identified. Lesions appear to be the result of damage to the endothelial lining of capillaries. Hemorrhagic diathesis and progressive impairment of hepatic and renal function are the most notable features of severe leptospirosis. Although jaundice is due to liver dysfunction, significant hepatocellular destruction is not observed. Histological modifications seen include disorganization of hepatic cords, increased numbers of multinucleated cells, proliferation of Kupffer cells, mitochondrial damage, and cholestasis. Fatal leptospirosis is usually associated with renal failure. As was observed with hepatic dysfunction, alterations in renal function are marked and are not reflected in corresponding histological changes. The most prominent renal lesion is tubular. Survivors of severe leptospirosis have a complete recovery of hepatic and renal function reflecting the absence of significant cell destruction [*5–7*].

Pulmonary lesions which may be present in leptospirosis are due to hemorrhagic diathesis rather than inflammation. Hemorrhages may occur throughout the lungs and pleura with acute hemorrhagic lobar pneumonia being reported in some fatal cases. Myalgias often occur as an early clinical feature of this disease. In severe cases degenerative changes in striated muscle may be due to direct invasion of muscle cells but are of a transient nature.

Meningitis is the most common neurological finding in leptospirosis and may be related to the ease with which leptospires enter the cerebrospinal fluid during the leptospiremic phase of the disease. However, meningeal irritation is most frequently observed after the leptospiremic phase when antibodies are present and few if any leptospires are in the spinal fluid. Pathological changes in the meninges are minimal and may be the consequence of an immune complex reaction. Cerebrospinal fluid glucose level is normal but there may be a moderate lymphocytic pleocytosis and an elevated protein level.

Leptospires may enter the anterior chamber of the eye during the leptospiremic phase of the disease and persist for months despite high serum antibody titers. One of the sequelae of leptospirosis may be uveitis which occurs weeks to months after onset of the disease and is associated with the presence of leptospires in the anterior chamber.

As the antibody response to the infecting serovar develops, leptospires are eliminated from the host with the exception of the eye and kidney where they persist for varying periods of time. Leptospires also persist in the brains of naturally infected animals and may also do so in humans. Leptospires multiply within the renal convoluted tubules and are shed in the urine, reaching densities of 10^7 per milliliter in some animals [5–7].

HOST

The clinical manifestations of leptospirosis are not sufficiently characteristic to be pathognomonic and it is often initially misdiagnosed as meningitis, hepatic disease, fever of unknown origin, or influenza. Infections range from asymptomatic to the fulminant form. The three organ systems most frequently involved are the central nervous system, kidney, and liver. The severity of the disease is largely determined by the virulence, infecting dose of the organism, and portal of entry. Virulent strains of *L. interrogans* are relatively resistant to the bactericidal action of antibody and complement as compared to avirulent strains. The severe icteric form of leptospirosis, often referred to as Weil's disease, is frequently associated with *icterohaemorrhagiae* but can be caused by a variety of serovars. Conversely, infections with *icterohaemorrhagiae* may be anicteric or even asymptomatic. Greater than 90 percent of leptospirosis cases are the milder, anicteric type [5–7].

Although patient response to leptospirosis varies, it is typically a biphasic disease, consisting of the leptospiremic or acute phase and the leptospiruric or immune phase. After an incubation period of 1 to 2 weeks (range 2 to 20 days) there is a sudden onset of nonspecific symptoms such as fever, chills, severe headache, myalgia, malaise, and conjunctival suffusion. The leptospiremic phase generally lasts 4 to 8 days, during which time leptospires are also present in the spinal fluid. Fever is usually 39 to 40°C (102 to 104°F), sometimes increasing to 41.1°C (106°F). Headache is intense and unrelenting with tenderness of muscles of the calf, back, and abdomen frequently experienced. Anorexia, nausea, and vomiting are also commonly observed. Inflammatory exudates are not associated with the conjunctival suffusion of leptospirosis. Jaundice appears during the first week of more severe cases of leptospirosis, attaining maximal intensity 7 days after onset.

During the second week of the disease, the increasing titer of antibodies ushers in the leptospiruric or immune phase of the disease. Leptospires are eliminated from the host with the exception of the kidney, eye, and possibly the brain. The symptoms are variable but usually short febrile relapses often associated with signs of meningeal irritation are observed. Leptospiruria is present but is not associated with impaired renal function. Uveitis, which may occur in up to 10 percent of cases, is usually transient and self-limited. The biphasic nature

of leptospirosis may not be manifested in mild cases where the appearance of antibodies results in the alleviation of signs and symptoms or in patients with severe icteric illness.

Generally, the intensity of jaundice is directly related to the degree of hepatic dysfunction, hemorrhagic complications, and renal dysfunction. Mortality rates of 5 to 30 percent are reported for untreated cases of leptospirosis and are primarily due to renal failure occurring during the second and third week of the disease. Delirium, disorientation, and psychosis have resulted from infection with *pomona* and *hardjo* [5–7].

Diagnosis

Leptospirosis was the initial diagnosis in only 17 to 25 percent of the cases reported to the Centers for Disease Control since 1949 [8,9]. Meningitis was the most common initial clinical impression. Because the clinical manifestations of leptospirosis are not pathognomonic, it should be considered in the diagnosis of any febrile disease characterized by abrupt onset, chills, myalgia, and severe headache with nausea and vomiting. In particular it should be suspected in patients with febrile illness who could have been exposed directly or indirectly to the urine of leptospiruric animals.

The total and differential white cell count may be normal in mild cases but is usually elevated with a neutrophilia in patients with icteric disease. In contrast to acute viral hepatitis, individuals with icteric leptospirosis have elevated serum bilirubin levels with only minimal increases of serum glutamic oxaloacetic transaminase (SGOT) and serum glutamic pyruvic transaminase (SGPT) levels. Liver function tests are generally normal in anicteric leptospirosis. Renal involvement during the leptospiremic phase occurs in 70 to 80 percent of cases with proteinuria being the most frequent abnormality. Red and white cells and hyaline or granular casts are often observed in the urine sediment in both phases of the disease and do not necessarily reflect the extent of renal involvement. Severe renal dysfunction results in azotemia, oliguria, or anuria which usually occur during the second week of icteric leptospirosis [5–8].

A definitive diagnosis of leptospirosis requires either the demonstration of *L. interrogans* in clinical specimens, seroconversion, or a fourfold or greater rise in titer of agglutinating antibodies. Leptospires can be isolated from the blood and spinal fluid during the first week of the disease. After this, the leptospiruric phase ensues and leptospires are no longer present in the blood but can be isolated from the urine. Leptospires may be present in the kidneys and to a lesser extent in the liver in fatal cases of leptospirosis [1,2,10].

The isolation of leptospires does not require specialized techniques since they are readily cultivated in the laboratory. The two types of commercially available media commonly used are enriched with rabbit serum or bovine serum albumin (BSA)–Tween 80. The BSA–Tween 80 medium is the medium of choice for the isolation and cultivation of leptospires [*11,12*]. Semisolid media (0.2% agar) are recommended for the isolation of leptospires and should contain 100 to 200 μg/mL of the selective agent, 5′-fluorouracil, when potentially contaminated specimens such as urine are to be cultured [*13*]. Specimens are diluted 1:10 and 1:100 to decrease or eliminate the effect of inhibitory substances that are usually present. Growth of leptospires is usually detectable after 7 to 14 days incubation at 30°C but may require 6 weeks or longer. Direct microscopic examination of specimens is not recommended since the numbers of leptospires are frequently low and they are easily confused with fibrils or extrusions from tissue cells. Contaminated specimens can be injected intraperitoneally into weanling hamsters or young guinea pigs and isolated from the blood of moribund animals or from the kidneys of surviving animals 14 days after infection [*2,10*].

Blood is cultured during the leptospiremic phase of the disease. Leptospires are most frequently recovered during the first week of illness but may persist for 2 to 3 weeks. Blood is collected prior to antimicrobial therapy and 1 to 2 drops is inoculated per 5 mL media. Spinal fluid may be processed in the same manner as blood during this phase of the disease. Leptospires can be isolated from the urine, most frequently during the second week of illness, but may persist for 1 month or longer. Clean-voided, midstream, or bladder urine is diluted 1:10 and 1:100 in media containing 5′-fluorouracil as soon after collection as possible (within 1 h). Several isolation attempts on different days should be made since the shedding of leptospires is often intermittent. At necropsy the urine, kidney, and liver are cultured as soon as possible. The supernatant of a 10% tissue suspension is processed in the same manner as urine. Tissues that cannot be processed immediately should be frozen and cultured at a later date [*2,10*].

The standard serological procedure used is the microscopic agglutination (MA) test with live or formalin-fixed antigens. The serovar specificity of this test necessitates the use of a few to 15 antigens depending on the serovars present in a geographical area. The commercially available macroscopic agglutination tests lack the sensitivity of the MA test. Genus-''specific'' complement-fixation, sensitized erythrocyte lysis, and hemagglutination tests have been useful, especially in areas where a variety of different serovars exist. These ''genus-specific'' tests cannot be used for epidemological surveys since they only detect antibodies produced early in the disease. Antibodies usually reach titers of 100 to 1000 by the sixth to tenth day of illness, rising to maximal titers of 25,000 or greater by the third or fourth week of the disease. Agglutination reactions that are stronger with heterologous serovars than with the infecting serovar are frequent. Because of these paradoxical serological reactions it is important to isolate the infecting leptospires to obtain a correct identification [*14*].

Definitive typing of isolates and serological testing are available at leptospirosis reference laboratories such as the FAO/WHO Collaborating Center for the Epidemiology of Lepto-

spirosis, Bacteriology Division, Centers for Disease Control, Atlanta, Georgia 30333 USA.

Therapy

Although leptospires are susceptible to most commonly used antibiotics in vitro, the therapeutic efficacy of these drugs has not been elucidated. If treatment is initiated during the first 2 to 4 days of illness before vascular damage has occurred, antibiotic therapy appears to be effective. Controlled studies in military personnel demonstrated that doxycycline was effective when used prophylactically (200 mg/week) [*15*] and also possessed therapeutic value (100 mg twice daily for 7 days) for early leptospirosis [*16*]. After this time the effectiveness of antibiotics is controversial. Recently, high doses of intravenously administered penicillin G were found to be an effective therapy after 4 days of illness. Symptomatic and supportive care seem to be of primary importance. High doses of parenteral aqueous penicillin G [50 to 70 mg or 80,000 to 110,000 U/(kg·day) as four equal portions every 6 h for 7 to 10 days] or tetracycline [30 mg/(kg·day) perorally as four equal portions every 6 h for 7 to 10 days] are most frequently recommended. Control of hydration, electrolyte balance, and kidney and liver function is of particular importance for severe cases. Peritoneal dialysis or hemodialysis should be considered in patients with azotemia. Fortunately most cases of leptospirosis are anicteric and self-limited with an uneventful recovery in 2 to 3 weeks. Convalescence may be extended for several months with the more severe cases. Untreated, jaundiced patients have a mortality rate of 5 to 30 percent, usually due to renal failure [*5–8*].

POPULATION

Leptospirosis is a zoonosis of worldwide dimensions responsible for an acute febrile illness of humans, and its incidence is related to occupation and geographical location. Over 200 serovars of *L. interrogans* have been isolated from approximately 160 mammalian species. The number and types of serovars present vary with the geographical area. Infections in the temperate zone are often occupational and a relatively small number of serovars are involved. In tropical countries the disease is more widespread in the population and the infectious agent may be one of many serovars carried by a large variety of different hosts. Infections in maintenance hosts are generally mild to inapparent and leptospiruria persists for extended periods. Serovars are frequently associated with certain animals but can infect many different animals. Serovar *pomona* is usually associated with swine and cattle, *canicola* with dogs, and *icterohaemorrhagiae* with rats. Leptospirosis is the cause of serious economic loss in the livestock industry due to abortion and infertility. Infected domestic animals also serve as an important source of human leptospirosis. Leptospires multiply in mammalian renal tubules and are shed in the urine for varying periods of time. Maintenance hosts, such as rodents, may be leptospiruric throughout their lifetimes and carrier rates of 50 percent and higher have been reported. Domestic animals usually shed leptospires for several months to a year with decreasing intensity. Humans ordinarily do not shed leptospires for more than several weeks. Generally, rodents associated with human habitation along with domestic animals comprise the most important reservoirs and sources of human leptospirosis [8,9].

Humans acquire leptospirosis through direct or indirect contact with the urine of leptospiruric animals. Contaminated moist soil remains infective for at least 14 days and leptospires survive in natural surface waters for several months. Indirect exposure appears to be the most common mode of transmission. Direct exposure to leptospiruric urine occurs most frequently for pet owners, farm workers, and veterinarians. Rarely does human-to-human transmission occur [8,9]. Leptospirosis is an important public health problem influenced by agricultural practices and level of sanitation in many countries. Leptospirosis has been detected in practically all countries where adequate investigations were conducted.

PREVENTION

The major control measure for leptospirosis is animal vaccination. Sources of leptospirosis in livestock and dogs can be reduced through vaccination with chemically inactivated cells. The vaccine must contain sufficient immunogenic material to prevent infection as well as other manifestations of the disease. It should also contain the serovars present in the area since the immunity induced by vaccination is serovar-specific. Management of rodent populations can be another important control measure, whereas control of leptospirosis in the wildlife reservoir is not practical. Human vaccination is used in "high-risk" groups in some European and Asian countries. Through the use of recently developed protein-free media and leptospiral outer envelope preparations, human vaccines may be improved [12,17].

REFERENCES

1 Johnson RC, Faine S: *Leptospira,* in Krieg NR (ed): *Bergey's Manual of Systematic Bacteriology,* Baltimore, Williams & Wilkins, 1983, vol I

2 Johnson RC: Aerobic spirochetes: The genus *Leptospira,* in Starr PP, Stolp H, Truper HG, et al (eds): *The Prokaryotes, a Handbook on Habitats, Isolation, and Identification of Bacteria.* New York, Springer-Verlag, 1981, pp 582–592

3 Johnson RC: The spirochetes. Ann Rev Microbiol 31:89–106, 1977

4 Leptospiral serotype distribution lists according to host and geographic area. Centers for Disease Control, Atlanta, US Dept Health Education and Welfare, 1966 (Supplement 1975)

5 Feigen RD, Anderson DC: Human leptospirosis. CRC Crit Rev Clin Lab Sci 5:413–467, 1975

6 Diaz-Rivera RS, Hall HE, Ramos-Morales KY, et al: Leptospirosis in Puerto Rico. Clinical aspects of human infection. Zoonosis Res 2:159–177, 1963

7 Berman SJ, Tsar CC, Homes K, et al: Sporadic anicteric leptospirosis in South Vietnam. A study in 150 patients. Ann Intern Med 79:167–173, 1973

8 Heath, CW Jr, Alexander AD, Galton MM: Leptospirosis in the United States, analysis of 483 cases in man, 1949–1961. N Engl J Med 273:857–864; 915–922, 1965

9 Kaufmann AF: Epidemiological trends of leptospirosis in the United States, 1965–1974, in Johnson RC (ed): *The Biology of Parasitic Spirochetes.* New York, Academic, 1976, pp 177–189

10 Alexander AD: *Leptospira,* in Lennette EH, Balows A, Hausler WH, et al (eds): *Manual of Clinical Microbiology,* 3d ed. Washington, DC, American Society for Microbiology, 1980, pp 376–382

11 Johnson RC, Harris VG: Differentiation of pathogenic and saprophytic leptospires. I. Growth at low temperatures. J Bacteriol 94:27–31, 1976

12 Bey RF, Johnson RC: A protein-free medium and a low-protein medium for the cultivation of *Leptospira.* Infect Immun 19:562–569, 1978

13 Johnson RC, Rogers P: 5-Fluorouracil as a selective agent for the growth of leptospirae. J Bacteriol 87:422–426, 1964

14 Alexander AD: Serological diagnosis of leptospirosis, in Rose NR, Friedman H (eds): *Manual of Clinical Immunology,* 2d ed. Washington, DC, American Society for Microbiology, 1980, pp 542–546

15 Takafuji ET, Kirkpatrick JW, Miller RN, et al: An efficacy trial of doxycycline chemoprophylaxis against leptospirosis. N Engl J Med 310:497–500, 1984

16 Mclain JBL, Ballou WR, Harrison SM, et al: Doxycycline therapy for leptospirosis. Ann Intern Med 100:696–698, 1984

17 Bey RF, Auran NE, Johnson RC: Immunogenicity of whole cell and outer envelope leptospiral vaccines in hamsters. Infect Immun 10:1051–1056, 1974

Sexually Transmitted Diseases · Peter Piot · King K. Holmes

A better appreciation of the clinical spectrum of sexually transmitted diseases (STDs) has been made possible by improved laboratory techniques. Table 96-1 presents a list of common sexually transmitted agents and the diseases they cause. The newest STD, AIDS, is currently spreading at epidemic rates throughout the world, forcing societies to face the fact that far too little is known about sexual behavior, especially in developing countries. The contributions of previous sociological.

Table 96-1. The most important sexually transmitted pathogens and the diseases they cause

Pathogens	Disease or Syndrome
Bacterial agents:	
Neisseria gonorrhoeae	Urethritis, epididymitis, proctitis, Bartholinitis, cervicitis, endometritis, salpingitis and related sequelae (infertility, ectopic pregnancy), perihepatitis; complications of pregnancy (e.g., chorioamnionitis, premature rupture of membranes, premature delivery, postpartum endometritis); conjunctivitis; disseminated gonococcal infection (DGI)
Chlamydia trachomatis	Same as *N. gonorrhoeae,* except for DGI. Also trachoma, lymphogranuloma venereum, Reiter's syndrome, infant pneumonia
Treponema pallidum	Syphilis
Haemophilus ducreyi	Chancroid
Mycoplasma hominis	Postpartum fever, salpingitis
Ureaplasma urealyticum	Urethritis, ?low birth weight, ?chorioamnionitis
Gardnerella vaginalis, etc.*	Bacterial vaginosis
Calymmatobacterium granulomatis	Donovanosis
Shigella species, *Campylobacter* spp.	Shigellosis, campylobacteriosis (sexually transmitted among homosexual men)
?Group B β-hemolytic streptococcus	Neonatal sepsis, neonatal meningitis
Viral agents:	
Herpes simplex virus	Primary and recurrent genital herpes, aseptic meningitis, neonatal herpes with associated mortality or neurological sequelae. Spontaneous abortion and premature delivery
Hepatitis A virus	Acute hepatitis A (sexually transmitted among homosexual men)
Hepatitis B virus	Acute, chronic, and fulminant hepatitis B, with associated immune complex phenomena and sequelae including cirrhosis and hepatocellular carcinoma
Cytomegalovirus	Congenital infection: gross birth defects and infant mortality, cognitive impairment (e.g., mental retardation, sensorineural deafness), heterophile-negative infectious mononucleosis, protean manifestations in the immunosuppressed host
Human papilloma virus	Condyloma acuminata, laryngeal papilloma in infants, squamous epithelial neoplasias of the cervix, anus, vagina, vulva, and penis
Molluscum contagiosum virus	Genital molluscum contagiosum
Human immunodeficiency virus	AIDS and related conditions
HTLV-1	T-cell leukemia/lymphoma, tropical spastic paraparesis
Protozoan agents:	
Trichomonas vaginalis	Vaginitis, ?urethritis, ?balanitis
Entamoeba histolytica	Amebiasis (sexually transmitted especially among homosexual men)
Giardia lamblia	Giardiasis (sexually transmitted especially among homosexual men)
Fungal agents:	
Candida albicans	Vulvovaginitis, balanitis, and balanoposthitis
Ectoparasites:	
Phthirus pubis	Pubic lice infestation
Sarcoptis scabies	Scabies

*Vaginal bacteria associated with bacterial vaginosis include *G. vaginalis, Mobiluncus* spp. (*M. curtisii, M. mulieris*), *Bacteroides* spp. (e.g., *B. bivius, B. disiens,* black pigmented species), *Mycoplasma hominis, Ureaplasma urealyticum.*

anthropological, and clinical research really do not offer much insight into why the patterns of transmission of HIV and other STDs differ so markedly in different areas of the world. However, there is now growing awareness of the consequences of other STDs for health and society in the tropics; for example, their impact on maternal and child health, their contribution of causation of cervical and other cancers, and the recently described role of certain STDs in facilitating transmission of HIV.

It is clear that prostitution is much more important in the epidemiology of STD in developing countries than in developed countries. It seems likely that major socioeconomic-related behavioral changes have been contributing to an epidemic increase in rates of certain STDs other than AIDS for decades in many developing countries, and that lack of effective national programs for STD control and for regulating use of antimicrobials has led to a much greater problem with antimicrobial-resistant gonorrhea and chancroid in the tropics than in the northern hemisphere. Furthermore, it is clear that developed countries can no longer safely compartmentalize and ignore the problem of epidemic or hyperendemic STDs in the tropics. The international spread of HIV-1 and of antimicrobial-resistant gonorrhea are instructive, and the clinical epidemiology of HIV and other STDs in urban centers of developing countries provides a useful paradigm now being paralleled in many ways in inner-city minority populations of North America.

A discussion of the biology and clinical manifestations of all known STDs is beyond the scope of this chapter. The subject of this chapter is gonorrhea and syphilis, as well as those STDs occurring predominantly in the tropics: chancroid, lymphogranuloma venereum (LGV), and donovanosis. The sexually transmitted retroviruses are not discussed. The unique aspects of other STDs in the tropics and the differences between industrialized and developing areas will be emphasized. The interested reader is referred to textbooks on STD for in-depth information [1,2].

EPIDEMIOLOGY OF SEXUALLY TRANSMITTED DISEASES IN THE TROPICS

STDs are hyperendemic today in many areas of the developing world, including rural areas. They account for 2.5 to 15 percent of all adult outpatient diagnoses in Africa [3,4]. Reliable incidence figures do not exist for most countries in the world. Official incidence rates in Latin American countries vary between 100 and 300 cases per 100,000 population for gonorrhea, and between 10 and 300 cases per 100,000 population for syphilis. The annual incidence of gonorrhea in Africa is estimated at 3000 to 10,000 per 100,000 general population [5]. Prevalence rates of gonorrhea and serologically positive syphilis in selected groups of women are presented in Table 96-2.

STD in the tropics is also characterized by a higher incidence of complications, which include urethral strictures, congenital syphilis, pelvic inflammatory disease (PID), ectopic pregnancy, infertility, pregnancy wastage, perinatal morbidity, and certain cancers (e.g., cervical cancer) which are unusually common in the tropics. Up to 44 percent of admissions in gynecological services in Africa and Asia are for PID [19]. The highest rates of infertility are found in areas with a high prevalence of STD [19–21], and laparoscopic investigation of infertile women in developing countries shows evidence of tubal occlusion and/or past PID in the majority of cases, particularly in Africa [19,22]. Congenital syphilis was the fifth and fourth leading cause of perinatal mortality in series from Addis Ababa and Durban, respectively [23]. Gonococcal ophthalmia neonatorum occurs in up to 3.6 percent of all live births in Africa [10,24], where gonorrhea is an important cause of blindness. Sexually transmitted agents were also the leading causes of postpartum upper genital tract infections in Nairobi, Kenya, where 20 percent of puerperal women suffer from this condition [25]. Control of STDs is the most reasonable and cheapest approach to reducing the incidence of these complications.

Table 96-2. Prevalence of gonorrhea, genital chlamydial infection, and a positive serological test for syphilis in pregnant women

Country	Year	Reference	Percentage with positive culture for		VDRL or RPR	TPHA or FTA-ABS
			N. gonorrhoeae	*C. trachomatis*		
Ethiopia	1977	6	NT*	NT	12.7	10.9
Swaziland	1980	11	3.9	NT	10.0	33.3
Gambia	1984	7,8	6.7	6.7	17.5	7.2
Ghana	1985	9	3.4	7.7	NT	NT
Zambia	1985	12,13	11.2	NT	14.3	12.5
Kenya	1986	10	6.5	19.7	4	11
Thailand	1985,1986	14,15	11.9	NT	8.9	NT
Jamaica	1974	16	11.0	NT	NT	NT
Chile	1975	17	NT	NT	3.5	NT
Brazil	1980	18	NT	NT	15.7	5.0

*NT = not tested.

Management of STDs in the tropics is often poor and difficult, not only because of irreversible tissue damage from complications but frequently because of a lack of diagnostic facilities. Antimicrobial drug resistance has further complicated treatment of gonorrhea and chancroid.

The spectrum of STD is different in the developing world. Diseases such as chancroid, LGV, and donovanosis are primarily limited to the tropics and subtropics. In general, urethritis is most often due to gonorrhea in developing countries and is more often nongonococcal in the industrialized countries. Genital ulcer disease is much more frequent than in the industrialized world, but herpes simplex virus is a relatively less common cause of genital ulcers.

Growing urbanization with disruption of traditional social structures, increased mobility for economic and political reasons—especially in young men—insufficient medical facilities, a large proportion of the population composed of teenagers and young adults, who have the highest rates of STD, and high unemployment rates, are all contributing to this high incidence of STDs and their complications in developing countries. Although data on trends in incidence rates over time are lacking, as are quantitative data on trends in sexual behavior, it is very likely that progressive increases in all of the above influences have led to progressive increases in the incidence of many STDs in developing countries, particularly in urban centers. Prostitutes are named by up to 80 percent of male patients as the source of infection in Africa and Asia compared to less than 20 percent in Europe and North America [26,27]. These prostitutes are highly mobile and contribute to the interregional and international spread of STDs. Although the definition of a prostitute is difficult and depends on social attitudes, prostitutes constitute a relatively small group of promiscuous women who infect larger numbers of promiscuous men, who in their turn infect nonpromiscuous secondary contacts, usually their spouses. This pattern of sexual activity with prostitutes may be a major reason for the persistence of the ''tropical STDs''—chancroid, LGV, and donovanosis—which have largely disappeared in countries where prostitution has declined. Furthermore, self-medication among prostitutes is more common than among other STD patients and favors the emergence and spread of resistant bacterial pathogens.

Ethnic differences in circumcision practices may contribute to ethnic differences in patterns of STD infection. Lack of circumcision has recently been implicated in Nairobi as a possible risk factor for acquisition of HIV infection, and as discussed below, as a risk factor for chancroid. The possible relationship of circumcision to reduced risk of these and other STDs requires further study.

SPECIFIC AGENTS AND THE DISEASES THEY CAUSE

NEISSERIA GONORRHOEAE

N. gonorrhoeae is a fastidious aerobic gram-negative diplococcus requiring an increased CO_2 tension for isolation. Hu-

mans are the only reservoir and are infected through intimate mucosa-to-mucosa contact. Several gonococcal surface components have been very well characterized, including pili, lipopolysaccharides, and outer-membrane proteins, which play a role in the pathogenesis of gonorrhea and can be used for typing of isolates. Strains of *N. gonorrhoeae* can be further classified by antimicrobial susceptibility, β-lactamase production, nutritional requirements (auxotype), and plasmid content.

Epidemiology and clinical syndromes

Published prevalence rates of gonorrhea among women attending gynecological and family planning clinics in Africa range from 3 percent to as high as 23 percent [4,9,11,28]. Table 96-2 shows some disturbingly high isolation rates for *N. gonorrhoeae* from pregnant women in different geographical areas. However, extrapolation to the general population may not be justified, as only highly selected groups may have been examined. Large-scale random population surveys in two rural areas in Uganda [29] and in an urban center in Senegal [30] found point prevalences of gonococcal infection of 3 to 18.3 percent in women and of 4.2 to 8.9 percent in men, based on a single culture. Prevalence rates in prostitutes are generally much higher than in the general population. The prevalence of gonorrhea has usually been found to be substantially higher among unregulated street prostitutes than among those who participate in supervised programs of regular culture, diagnostic testing, and treatment. The data indicate that gonorrhea is widespread among prostitutes as well as among nonprostitutes.

In contrast to North America and western Europe, gonorrhea is the main cause of urethritis among clinic attenders in the tropics [4,31]. The lower relative frequency of nongonococcal urethritis (NGU) in developing countries probably reflects the extraordinarily high incidence of gonorrhea, as well as differences in patterns of health-care-seeking behavior and disease tolerance. Manifestations of NGU are milder than those of gonococcal urethritis, and NGU may less often lead to medical consultation in developing countries. Prevalence rates of genital infection with *C. trachomatis* are at least as high in Africa as in North America.

Stricture of the posterior urethra presumably is the most severe complication of gonococcal urethritis in males and comprises up to 80 percent of the practice of a urologist in certain parts of Africa [32]. Proper surgical treatment is rarely available, and the most common management is regular bougienage for life. Urethral strictures are seen even in young men. The time between onset of urethritis and acute urinary retention ranges between a few days and several years [33]. In population surveys in central Africa and Uganda, acute or chronic epididymitis was found in 1.5 to 27.9 percent of all men [29]. Although acute epididymitis in young men is almost always unilateral, 1 to 3 percent of men with five or more episodes of gonorrhea have experienced bilateral epididymitis [34].

Contrary to common belief, women with gonorrhea mostly do have signs or symptoms, although these may be nonspecific, such as lower abdominal pain or vaginal discharge [35]. *N. gonorrhoeae* has been recovered from the cervix of 19 to 46 percent of women with PID in Africa [25,36–38]. However, the isolation rate was much lower in one study from Asia [39]. The onset of a substantial proportion of PID cases occurs following abortion, the insertion of an intrauterine contraceptive device, or delivery [25,39–41]. Cohort studies in Sweden have shown that the risk of involuntary infertility is about 15 percent after one episode of salpingitis, 30 percent after two episodes, and over 50 percent after three or more episodes [42]. Among various Ugandan districts, there is an inverse correlation between the fertility rate and the prevalence of gonorrhea [43]. The proportion of infertility cases due to *N. gonorrhoeae* is not known.

In infants seen at clinics for severe ophthalmia neonatorum in Africa, the usual cause is *N. gonorrhoeae,* but *C. trachomatis* was the most common cause identified in a prospective cohort study in which milder cases were also recognized. Gonococcal ophthalmia is associated with keratitis in 10 to 20 percent of cases ([10,44]; Table 96-3). The risk of transmission of *N. gonorrhoeae* from an infected mother to her infant is 30 to 40 percent if ophthalmic prophylaxis is not used [10,23]. Both silver nitrate and tetracycline eye prophylaxis at birth reduce the risk of gonococcal ophthalmia neonatorum to less than 6 percent among exposed newborns [45]. *N. gonorrhoeae* is also an important cause of keratoconjunctivitis in adults in the tropics [46]. Conditions associated with neonatal gonococcal infection such as chorioamnionitis, prolonged rupture of membranes, and maternal peripartum fever [47] are common in the tropics, but their relation to genital infections has not been investigated. In one recent case control study in Kenya, maternal gonococcal infection was an independent risk factor for premature delivery [48].

Gonorrhea was the most common cause of vaginitis in girls under the age of 10 in one study from Nigeria [49]. Contaminated bed clothing, sharing of underwear and towels with older household members, and digitogenital contamination from infected adults were believed to be the most important ways of transmission, rather than sexual intercourse. However, the precise mode of infection remains unresolved.

Gonococci are generally less susceptible to antimicrobial agents in the tropics than in the industrialized world. Approximately half of the isolates in most parts of Africa and southeast Asia are now penicillinase-producing (PPNG), and a significant proportion of non-PPNG strains show high-level chromosomal resistance to penicillin as well. However, this problem so far appears to be less common in South America [50]. Penicillinase production in *N. gonorrhoeae* is encoded by a 3.2-MDa plasmid ("African" type) or a 4.2-MDa plasmid ("Asian" type), and rarely by a 2.9-MDa plasmid [51,52]. The so-called Asian type of PPNG is now also endemic in Africa [53–55].

Diagnosis

Microscopy after Gram stain of a urethral smear has a very high sensitivity and specificity for the diagnosis of gonococcal urethritis in men, and also for the diagnosis of gonococcal conjunctivitis [44]. In experienced hands the sensitivity and specificity of a Gram-stained cervical smear for the diagnosis of gonococcal infection in the female may be no more than 60 percent and 80 to 90 percent, respectively. The predictive value of a microscopic examination under suboptimal working conditions in the tropics has repeatedly been shown to be much lower. Therefore, this examination is not sufficient by itself for the diagnosis of gonorrhea in women.

Thayer-Martin chocolate agar medium is useful for culturing smears from the endocervix, anal canal, and pharynx. CO_2 is required for the isolation of gonococci and may be supplied by a candle jar. A single culture from the endocervix detects at least 80 percent of all cases in women and is the method of choice for diagnosis in women. However, routine culture facilities are expensive and rarely available, even in major centers in the tropics. Isolates should be tested for β-lactamase production with a rapid test. Serological tests for gonococcal infection are neither sufficiently sensitive nor sufficiently specific for routine use.

Treatment

The emergence of PPNG in 1976 in southeast Asia and west Africa, and the further development of high-level chromosomally mediated resistance to multiple antimicrobials, have

Table 96-3. Incidence and etiology of ophthalmia neonatorum in Nairobi, Kenya

| Etiology | Cohort study N = 1019 | | Clinic-based cross-sectional study |
	Incidence per 100 live births	Percentage of all cases N = 181	Percentage of all cases N = 149
Gonococcal	2.8	12	43
Chlamydial	7.3	32	13
Both	0.8	3	4
Neither	12.3	53	40
Total	23.2		

Source: [10] and [44].

Table 96-4. Uncomplicated urogenital gonococcal infection: recommended treatment regimens

1. In areas where less than 5 percent of strains of *N. gonorrhoeae* are penicillinase-producing or have chromosomally mediated resistance to penicillins or tetracyclines:

   Ampicillin: 3.5 g *or* amoxicillin 3.0 g, either with 1 g probenecid by mouth

   Aqueous procaine penicillin G: 3.8 million U IM at two sites, with 1 g of probenecid by mouth*

   Tetracycline hydrochloride: 0.5 g by mouth four times a day for 5 days (*Note:* Relative resistance of gonococci to tetracycline in many areas of the world, including the United States and most of the tropics, is quite high, and tetracycline is unreliable for gonorrhea in such areas.)

2. In areas where 5 percent or more of strains of *N. gonorrhoeae* are penicillinase-producing or have chromosomally mediated resistance to penicillins or tetracyclines:

   Spectinomycin hydrochloride: 2 g IM

   Ceftriaxone: 250 mg IM

   Cefotaxime: 1.0 g IM

   Cefoxitin: 2 g IM with probenecid 1 g by mouth

   Cefuroxime: 1.5 g IM with probenecid 1 g by mouth

   Trimethoprim-sulfamethoxazole: nine tablets (80 mg trimethoprim and 400 mg sulfamethoxazole) in a single dose daily for 3 days

   Norfloxacin: 800 mg by mouth

   Ciprofloxacin

*Addition of amoxicillin 250 mg plus clavulanic acid 125 mg to this regimen may be effective against infection with PPNG.

Source: Modified from [56] and [57].

dramatically changed first-line treatment of gonococcal infections in several areas when the cheapest therapy, penicillin, has become ineffective. Table 96-4 gives recommended treatment regimens for uncomplicated gonorrhea for areas with a low prevalence of PPNG and/or chromosomal resistance to penicillin, and separate recommendations for areas where such penicillin resistance is found in more than 5 percent of gonococcal strains. Tropical areas with a high prevalence of PPNG include southeast Asia and Africa. Spectinomycin-resistant strains have been isolated in the Far East [58].

CHLAMYDIA TRACHOMATIS

The biology of *C. trachomatis* is extensively discussed in Chap. 70. LGV is caused by serotypes L1, L2, and L3, which have distinct biological features such as enhanced infectivity for cells in vitro, and resistance to killing by mononuclear phagocytes.

Epidemiology

The epidemiology of genital chlamydia infections other than LGV in the tropics is still poorly documented, although it is increasingly clear that infection with *C. trachomatis* is at least as frequent as gonococcal infection (Table 96-2), and that chla-

mydial infections are associated with the same complications and sequelae as elsewhere. Among pregnant women in several studies in Africa, *C. trachomatis* was isolated from 7 to 20 percent [7,9,10]. The agent has been found in 15 to 20 percent of women with acute salpingitis in Africa [25,38], and in a case control study in Zimbabwe, there was serological evidence for a role of *C. trachomatis* in ectopic pregnancy and infertility, particularly in women with evidence of tubal disease [58].

C. trachomatis is a major cause of maternal and infant morbidity, but this has not been extensively studied in the tropics. In a trachoma-endemic area in Egypt, chlamydiae were isolated from the conjunctiva, pharynx, or rectum of 43 of 128 children [59]. A cohort study in Kenya showed that the majority of cases of ophthalmia neonatorum are due to *C. trachomatis*, and that the rate of transmission from the maternal cervix to the neonate eye is approximately 30 percent ([10], Table 96-3). Whereas both silver nitrate and tetracycline eye prophylaxis at birth initially reduced the incidence of chlamydial conjunctivitis, this practice ultimately did not influence the overall infection rate in infants exposed to maternal chlamydial infection [59]. In the same study, chlamydial infection in the neonate was associated with considerable morbidity, including conjunctivitis and pneumonia [59].

LGV is endemic in the tropics, where it may be a common cause of genital ulcer disease in certain areas (Table 96-5). In studies in southern Africa, the majority of patients with LGV were infected in the eastern subtropical areas, suggesting that there may be defined geographical foci [66]. Supposedly, LGV is not very infectious, but the exact mode of transmission and the reservoir are not known.

Clinical manifestations

Syndromes caused by *C. trachomatis* are listed in Table 96-1. For some of these conditions, the proportion actually caused by chlamydiae is not well defined, particularly in the tropics.

LGV has an incubation period of 3 to 30 days before the appearance of a primary lesion, usually a genital vesicle, papule, or ulcer. This ulcer is most often transient, painless, and small, although more extended lesions may occur. Intraurethral or cervical primary lesions probably also occur and may cause urethritis or cervicitis, but this is not well studied. In most cases the primary lesion heals spontaneously and is found in only a minority of patients at the time of presentation in a clinic.

Most heterosexual male patients with LGV seek medical care because of acute inguinal lymphadenopathy which appears a few days to several months after the primary lesion. In one-third of the cases lymphadenopathy is bilateral. Several lymph nodes are involved and initially the adenopathy is firm and not painful. Fluctuation develops in up to 75 percent of cases, starting within 1 to 2 weeks, and is often painful. A discoloration and shiny appearance of the skin anticipates rupture of the bubo, which also may regress spontaneously. Buboes are

Table 96-5. Etiology of genital ulcer disease in consecutive patients in several series (number of patients with each type of etiology)

Diagnosis	Gambia N = 104	Swaziland N = 149	Rwanda N = 109	Nairobi N = 97	Bangkok N = 120	Papua, New Guinea N = 174
Chancroid	52	42	18	62	36	0
Syphilis	22	17	16	9	1	14
Genital herpes	6	11	15	4	10	0
Lymphogranuloma venereum	4	12	7	NT*	0	9
Donovanosis	0	1	0	0	0	22
Mixed etiology	14	4	8	2	2	37
Other and unknown	27	13	36	13	51	18

*NT = not tested.

Source: From [60–65].

multiloculated abscesses which contain yellow or blood-stained viscous pus, and typically rupture at multiple points. Aspiration through normal skin reduces the risk of rupture. Inguinal scars of healed buboes are characteristic of the disease. When inguinal and femoral lymph nodes are involved, they may be divided by the inguinal ligament, giving the ''groove sign'' which is considered pathognomonic of LGV (Fig. 96-1). A penile lesion in the male and external vulvar or perineal lesions in the female are drained by inguinal lymph nodes, whereas cervical or rectal primary lesions are drained mainly by retroperitoneal lymph nodes. Anal lesions also can drain to the inguinal nodes.

Systemic manifestations such as fever, headache, malaise, anorexia, arthralgia, and myalgia generally accompany the lymphadenopathy. Leukocytosis, elevated sedimentation rate, cryoglobulinemia, and elevated IgG levels are common findings. Inclusion conjunctivitis was found in 2 of 18 patients in Ethiopia and hemorrhagic proctitis in 1 of 18 [67].

The genitoanorectal syndrome covers a wide variety of late complications that may occur sometimes without preceding primary genital lesions or secondary inguinal adenopathy. Swellings of the vulva, anus, and rectal mucosa may develop. Elephantiasis and hypertrophic ulceration of the external genitalia predominantly affects females and is termed *esthiomene* (Fig. 96-2). Lymphatic obstruction and edema of the penis and scrotum, proctitis, rectal strictures, and rectal fistulas are infrequent but severe complications. In homosexual men, LGV

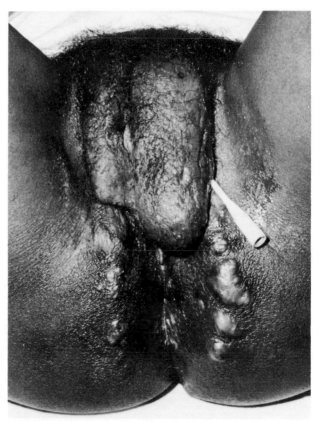

Figure 96-2. Esthiomine caused by LGV, with vulval edema and multiple perineal abscesses and fistulas. Microimmunofluorescent antibody titer to *C. trachomatis* L2 serovar was 1:1024.

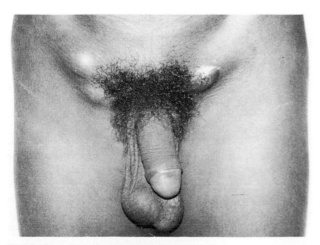

Figure 96-1. Groove sign in lymphogranulum venereum, caused by inguinal lymphadenopathy above and below the inguinal ligament.

frequently presents as an acute, severe ulcerative proctocolitis. Histopathological changes in such cases, including granulomatous inflammation of the rectum, may mimic Crohn's disease [68].

Diagnosis

The differential diagnosis of LGV includes other causes of genital ulceration listed in Table 96-5, as well as tuberculosis, actinomycosis, filariasis, lymphoma, and inguinal hernia. The intradermal Frei test has been extensively used in the past, but the antigen is no longer available. The test is negative in one-third of LGV patients and may be positive in other chlamydial infections. It remains positive for several years or for life [69]. The complement-fixation test is still the most commonly used test for the diagnosis of LGV. It becomes positive within 1 to 3 weeks following infection and titers of 1:64 are found in approximately 50 percent of the patients [67,69]. Nearly all LGV patients have a complement-fixation titer of 1:16, but this is also found in 15 to 40 percent of patients with other genital chlamydial infections such as PID. Rising titers of antibodies are seldom observed owing to late presentation of patients. The titers in the microimmunofluorescent test are usually 1:512 in a pattern showing broad reactivity with LGV and non-LGV serovars of *C. trachomitis* [66,67,70]. Micro-IF IgM antibodies are often not detected in LGV [66].

Isolation of *C. trachomatis* LGV serotypes (L1, L2, or L3) provides the most definite proof of a diagnosis of LGV. Serotype L2 is the most common of these three types. Methods for chlamydia isolation are discussed in Chap. 70. Bubo aspirate is the most rewarding material for culture, but at times the organism can be isolated from the genital ulcer base [66] and can often be isolated from rectal lesions in homosexual men with proctitis.

Management

No controlled double-blind treatment trials have been published in LGV, a disease which may show remissions and exacerbations. It was shown that the duration of buboes in patients receiving tetracycline, sulfadiazine, or chloramphenicol was significantly shorter than in symptomatically treated patients (31 days versus 69 days) [71]. LGV proctitis usually improves promptly with therapy. Early antimicrobial treatment undoubtedly is important to prevent the chronic phase of the disease. Oral tetracycline, 500 mg four times daily; or sulfamethoxazole, 1.0 g orally twice daily for at least 3 weeks; or trimethoprim-sulfamethoxazole, 80 mg trimethoprim and 400 mg sulfamethoxazole twice daily for 3 weeks, is effective. Oral sulfisoxazole for at least 3 weeks can also be recommended but may be somewhat less effective. More than one course of therapy may be necessary. Response to antimicrobial treatment in the chronic stage is uncertain. There is no relation between complement-fixation titers and response to therapy. Fluctuant

buboes should be aspirated as needed through healthy adjacent normal skin, but surgical incision is contraindicated.

SYPHILIS

The biology of the treponemes pathogenic for humans, including *Treponema pallidum*, will be discussed in Chap. 97.

Epidemiology

Syphilis is thought to be widespread in the tropics, particularly in large towns. However, accurate figures are rarely available, and interpretation of serological tests is often difficult in areas where other treponematoses have been endemic or are still occurring. The control of endemic treponematoses in the 1950s is thought to have reduced protective immunity against syphilis. Table 96-2 presents positive serology rates for selected groups in the tropics. Annual incidence rates as high as 1400 per 100,000 population have been reported in Africa [72]. Syphilis in pregnancy was responsible for 3 to 5 percent of perinatal deaths in African cities [23], and congenital syphilis is still a problem in many parts of the world. Congenital syphilis is a major cause of stillbirth in countries such as Ethiopia and Zambia, and is a significant risk factor for premature birth [71–76]. Despite the high prevalence of syphilis in the tropics, classical tertiary syphilis appears to be uncommon and the incidence of both cardiovascular and neurological syphilis would appear to be decreasing in Africa, possibly because of the widespread use of penicillins [6,77].

Manifestations

The hallmark of *primary syphilis* is a primary genital or anal chancre which is classically single, painless, indurated, with a clear base and well-defined edges. However, up to 75 percent of syphilitic ulcers may be multiple, painful, nonindurated, or have a purulent base. Moreover, mixed infections, especially with chancroid, are frequent. Thus, a clinical diagnosis of primary syphilis is often impossible. A week after the onset of the primary lesion a discrete, firm, painless, inguinal lymphadenopathy appears. The primary lesion usually heals within 6 weeks, usually without leaving a scar. The differential diagnosis in the tropics includes other causes of genital ulcer disease (Table 96-5), secondary syphilis, genital trauma, scabies, erosive spirochetal balanitis, and carcinoma of the penis.

The lesions of *secondary syphilis* are variable and appear 1 to 6 months after the onset of the primary chancre. Nonspecific systemic symptoms such as headache, malaise and fever, and lymphadenopathy may accompany or precede the mucocutaneous manifestations. The polymorphous skin rash of secondary syphilis is generalized, symmetrical, nonitching, and often maculopapular or papular. Characteristic palmar and plantar syphilis give a clue to the diagnosis. Condylomata lata are highly infectious hypertrophic papules which commonly occur on the perianal area, vulva, scrotum, or other intertriginous areas. However, the skin manifestations of secondary syphilis may yield any appearance, particularly in areas with numerous other skin diseases such as mycoses. Mucous patches inside the mouth may fuse to form "snail-track" ulcers. Iritis and patchy hair loss occur in some cases. Virtually any organ system, including the central nervous system, may be involved in secondary syphilis. Tropical aspects of the differential diagnosis of secondary syphilis include [2]: leprosy, rose spots of typhoid fever, ringworm, secondary yaws, tinea capitis, vitiligo, and onchocerciasis. Any generalized eruption is suspect of syphilis.

Latent syphilis is characterized by a positive serological test for syphilis in the absence of signs and symptoms, including a normal cerebrospinal fluid examination. Early latent syphilis (under 2 years' duration) is potentially infectious. Late latent syphilis is not infectious with the exception of pregnant women with late latent syphilis who may transmit infection to the fetus.

Benign late syphilis occurs 3 to 7 years after infection and presents as nodular, ulcerative, or noduloulcerative gummatous lesions. Gummas resemble earlier syphilis, but the lesions are more destructive and are essentially not infectious because they contain very few treponemes. They have a tendency to necrosis and are probably caused by a hypersensitivity reaction to treponemal antigens.

Cardiovascular syphilis and neurosyphilis each develop in 10 to 15 percent of untreated cases. Manifestations of *cardiovascular syphilis* include aortitis, aortic incompetence, aortic aneurysm, coronary ostitis, and angina pectoris. Histologically there is periarteritis and endarteritis with a loss of elastic tissue. Prognosis for improvement of cardiovascular syphilis after treatment is poor, because of irreversible tissue damage. The classic forms of neurosyphilis—tabes dorsalis, general paralysis of the insane, and meningovascular syphilis—have become infrequent and the diagnosis of neurosyphilis is now most often considered in atypical clinical settings [1,2].

Congenital syphilis is acquired from the mother via a placental infection. Women with untreated syphilis of under 2 years' duration are infectious to their fetus in almost all cases. The proportion of affected fetuses decreases with syphilis of longer than 2 years' duration. Approximately half of the pregnancies in mothers with primary or secondary syphilis result in abortion, stillbirth, perinatal death, or premature delivery. Most children with congenital syphilis are apparently normal at birth. Clinical features usually appear between 2 and 8 weeks, and may be quite variable, depending on the age of the infant [13,78]. In general, the features of clinical congenital syphilis are those of secondary and tertiary syphilis. The major clinical features of congenital syphilis as observed in a large series in Zambia are given in Table 96-6 [78]. Hepatosplenomegaly, skin rash, anemia, snuffles, epiphysitis and osteitis were the most common clinical abnormalities [13,78]. However, in other series swelling of the extremities, pseudoparalysis, and periostitis were present in all cases [79]. This may be due to use of different diagnostic criteria for congenital

Table 96-6. Clinical features in 202 infants with early congenital syphilis

Features	Percentage with feature	
	Neonates N = 74	Postneonatal N = 128
Hepatosplenomegaly	91	87
Joint swelling and pseudoparesis	3	34
Skin rash	31	55
Anemia	64	89
Jaundice	48	7
Snuffles	12	50
Radiological changes		
Metaphyseal dystrophy	95	91
Osteitis-like changes	29	40
Periosteal reaction	38	79
Cerebrospinal fluid changes	44	37
Mortality	54	8

Source: From [78].

syphilis. Marasmus, dactylitis, and condylomata may occur. Mucocutaneous lesions contain *T. pallidum*. Criteria for the diagnosis of congenital syphilis are given in Table 96-7.

Late congenital syphilis and stigmata of congenital syphilis are rarely seen in the tropics [2,6]. Signs include gummas, periostitis, saddle nose, Hutchinson's teeth, Clutton's joints (hydrarthrosis of both knee joints), deafness, interstitial keratitis, and neurosyphilis.

Diagnosis

Dark-field microscopy is the basis of diagnosis of infectious syphilis, i.e., primary, secondary, infectious relapsing, and early congenital syphilis. Dark-field examination requires considerable experience and a suitable microscope, which is not available in most tropical health centers or even many STD clinics. Accurate diagnosis depends on recognition of typical morphology and motility characteristic of *T. pallidum*. It is often difficult, if not impossible, to differentiate saprophytic spirochetes of the mouth from *T. pallidum*. Spirochete-associated erosive balanoposthitis is common in the tropics and may also make interpretation of dark-field examination difficult to the inexperienced observer.

Serological tests for syphilis can be subdivided into nonspecific nontreponemal reagin tests and specific treponemal tests. The quantitative or qualitative rapid plasma reagin (RPR) test is an easy test which can be performed without sophisticated laboratory equipment. It is commonly used for screening. The VDRL reaction has a comparable sensitivity and specificity. The predictive value of a positive RPR or VDRL test is low in populations which have a low prevalence of the disease. Biological false-positive reactions may occur in pregnancy and in any condition accompanied by a strong immunological response, as occurs in many chronic bacterial and parasitic diseases common in the tropics. Even positive treponemal tests

Table 96-7. Criteria for the diagnosis of early congenital syphilis

Definite criterion

1. Specimens from lesions, autopsy material, placenta or umbilical cord demonstrate *T. pallidum* by dark-field microscopy, or by histological examination.

Major criteria

2. Swelling of joints with pseudoparesis
3. Skin rash including palmar/plantar bullous lesions
4. Snuffles

Minor clinical criteria

5. Hepatosplenomegaly
6. Jaundice
7. Anemia
8. Radiological changes in bones and joints
9. Elevated cell count and/or protein and/or reactive test for reagin antibody (e.g., RPR test or VDRL) in cerebrospinal fluid

Serological criteria—mother

10. Reactive serological tests for syphilis (STS)*

Serological criteria—infant

11. Reactive STS
12. Nonreactive STS
13. Reactive STS not reverting to negativity within 4 months after birth
14. Rising RPR test antibody titer over 3 months

Maternal history

15. Documented history of adequately treated syphilis during pregnancy

Diagnosis	Criteria present
Definite	1
Probable	13, 14 or any combination of 2–9 with 10 and 11
Possible	Any of 2–9 with 10 and 11 or 12
Unlikely	10 and 15 with 11 or 12

*Reactive STS = positive RPR/VDRL and/or MHA-TP and/or FTA-ABS.
Source: Based on [78] and [80].

(described below) are difficult to interpret in areas with non-venereal treponematoses, which yield a complete serological cross-reactivity with *T. pallidum*. The quantitative VDRL or RPR tests are used to evaluate the effect of treatment, which should produce a decline in titer in patients treated for early syphilis. Older tests such as the Wasserman, Kline, and Kahn reactions are obsolete and should not be used.

Specific treponemal tests such as the FTA-ABS (fluorescent treponemal-antibody absorption) and MHA-TP (microhemagglutination antibody) use *T. pallidum* as the antigen and therefore are more specific than the RPR or VDRL. However, they are at least twice as expensive and are technically more difficult to perform. Further inconvenience in the tropics is caused by the frequently prolonged persistence of positivity of the FTA-ABS and MHA-TP. Thus, because of the extremely high in-

cidence of the disease, many individuals with previously treated syphilis will yield a positive treponemal test, with a negative RPR or VDRL. In Swaziland nearly 25 percent of the healthy adult population not attending an STD clinic showed this pattern [72]. This is very similar to the pattern found in homosexually active men in developed countries. Treponemal tests are rarely available in developing areas and, because of their cost, should be reserved for confirmation of a positive reagin test.

Management

Penicillin remains the drug of choice for the treatment of syphilis. The 1988 recommendations of the Centers for Disease Control [80] for management of syphilis can be summarized as follows.

Early Syphilis (Primary, Secondary, Latent Syphilis of Less Than 1 Year's Duration). Early syphilis should be treated with benzathine penicillin G—2.4 million U total by intramuscular injection at a single session. Patients who are allergic to penicillin should be treated with tetracycline HCl—500 mg four times a day by mouth for 15 days. Tetracycline appears to be effective but has been evaluated less extensively than penicillin. Patient compliance with this regimen may be difficult so care should be taken to encourage optimal compliance. Penicillin-allergic patients who cannot tolerate tetracycline should have their allergy confirmed. For these patients there are two options: (1) if compliance and serological follow-up can be assured, administer erythromycin 500 mg by mouth four times a day for 15 days; (2) if compliance and serological follow-up cannot be assured, the patient should be hospitalized, desensitized to penicillin, and treated with penicillin.

Syphilis of More Than 1 Year's Duration Except Neurosyphilis. Syphilis of more than 1 year's duration, except neurosyphilis (latent syphilis of indeterminate or more than 1 year's duration, cardiovascular, or late benign syphilis) should be treated with benzathine penicillin G—7.2 million U total, 2.4 million U by intramuscular injection weekly for three successive weeks. There are no published clinical data which adequately document the efficacy of drugs other than penicillin for syphilis of more than 1 year's duration.

Cerebrospinal fluid (CSF) examination should be performed to exclude neurosyphilis before therapy with these regimens: Patients who are allergic to penicillin should be given tetracycline HCl—500 mg by mouth four times a day for 30 days. Patient compliance with this regimen may be difficult so care should be taken to encourage optimal compliance. Penicillin-allergic patients who cannot tolerate tetracycline should have their allergy confirmed. The great majority of individuals with a history of penicillin allergy have negative skin tests for penicillin allergy, and can be treated safely with penicillin. For allergic patients there are two options: (1) if compliance and serological follow-up can be assured, administer erythromycin

500 mg by mouth four times a day for 30 days; (2) if compliance and serological follow-up cannot be assured, the patient should be hospitalized and managed in consultation with an expert.

Neurosyphilis. CSF examination should be performed in patients with clinical symptoms or signs consistent with neurosyphilis. This examination is also desirable in other patients with syphilis of greater than 1 year's duration to exclude asymptomatic neurosyphilis.

Potentially effective regimens, none of which have been adequately studied, include: aqueous penicillin G, 12 to 24 million U IV per day (2.4 million U every 4 h) for 10 days, followed by benzathine penicillin G, 2.4 million U IM weekly for three doses; aqueous procaine penicillin G, 2.4 million U IM daily plus probenecid 500 mg by mouth four times a day, both for 10 days, followed by benzathine penicillin G, 2.4 million U IM weekly for three doses; and benzathine penicillin G, 2.4 U IM weekly for 3 doses. Patients with histories of allergy to penicillin should have their allergy confirmed and managed in consultation with an expert.

Syphilis in Pregnancy. All pregnant women should have a nontreponemal serological test for syphilis, such as VDRL or RPR test, at the time of the first prenatal visit. In women suspected of being at high risk for syphilis, a second nontreponemal test should be performed during the third trimester and the cord blood should be tested for syphilis antibody. Seroactive patients should be expeditiously evaluated. This evaluation should include a history and physical examination as well as a quantitative nontreponemal test and a confirmatory treponemal test. If the FTA-ABS test is nonreactive and there is no clinical evidence of syphilis, treatment may be withheld. Both the quantitative nontreponemal test and the confirmatory test should be repeated within 4 weeks. If there is clinical or serological evidence of syphilis or if the diagnosis of syphilis cannot be excluded with reasonable certainty, the patient should be treated as outlined below.

Patients for whom there is documentation of adequate treatment for syphilis in the past need not be retreated unless there is clinical or serological evidence of reinfection such as dark-field-positive lesions or a fourfold titer rise of a quantitative nontreponemal test. For patients at all stages of pregnancy who are not allergic to penicillin, treatment consists of penicillin in dosage schedules appropriate for the stage of syphilis as recommended for the treatment of nonpregnant patients. For patients of all stages of pregnancy who have documented allergy to penicillin: (1) if compliance and serological follow-up cannot be assured, the patient should be hospitalized and managed in consultation with an expert; (2) because of several well-documented cases of congenital syphilis following erythromycin treatment of the pregnant woman, erythromycin probably should not be used to treat syphilis in pregnant women. Those with confirmed penicillin allergy could be hospitalized,

desensitized, and treated with penicillin under close observation. Although certain new cephalosporins are active against *T. pallidum,* they have not been sufficiently evaluated in pregnant women. Tetracycline is not recommended in pregnant women because of potential adverse effects on the fetus. Pregnant women who have been treated for syphilis should have monthly quantitative nontreponemal serological tests for the remainder of the current pregnancy. Women who show a fourfold rise in titer should be retreated. After delivery, follow-up is as outlined for nonpregnant patients.

Congenital Syphilis. If the mother has received adequate penicillin treatment during pregnancy, the risk to the infant is minimal. However, all infants should be examined carefully at birth and at frequent intervals thereafter until nontreponemal serological tests are negative. Infected infants are frequently asymptomatic at birth and may be seronegative if the maternal infection occurred late in gestation. Infants should be treated at birth if maternal treatment was inadequate, unknown, or with drugs other than penicillin, or if adequate follow-up of the infant cannot be ensured. Infants with congenital syphilis should have a CSF examination before treatment. Symptomatic infants or asymptomatic infants with abnormal CSF should be treated with aqueous crystalline penicillin G, 50,000 U/kg IM or IV daily in two divided doses for a minimum of 10 days; or with aqueous procaine penicillin G, 50,000 U/kg IM daily for a minimum of 10 days. Asymptomatic infants with normal CSF should receive benzathine penicillin G, 50,000 U/kg IM in a single dose.

Although benzathine penicillin has been previously recommended and widely used, published clinical data on its efficacy in congenital neurosyphilis are lacking. If neurosyphilis cannot be excluded, the aqueous or procaine penicillin regimens are recommended. Only penicillin regimens are recommended for neonatal congenital syphilis. Penicillin therapy for congenital syphilis after the neonatal period should be with the same dosage used for neonatal congenital syphilis. For larger children, the total dose of penicillin need not exceed the dosage used in adult syphilis of more than 1 year's duration. After 8 years of age, the dosage of tetracycline for congenital syphilis in older children who are allergic to penicillin should be individualized but need not exceed dosages used in adult syphilis of more than 1 year's duration. Tetracycline should not be given to children less than 8 years of age.

Follow-up After Treatment and Retreatment. All patients with early syphilis and congenital syphilis should be encouraged to return for repeat quantitative nontreponemal tests at least 3, 6, and 12 months after treatment. In these patients, quantitative nontreponemal test titers will decline to nonreactive or low-titer reactive within a year following successful treatment with benzathine penicillin G. Serological test results decline more slowly in patients treated for disease of longer duration. Patients with syphilis of more than 1 year's duration should also have a repeat serological test 24 months after treatment. Careful follow-up serological testing is particularly important in patients treated with antibiotics other than penicillin. Examination of CSF should be planned as part of the last follow-up visit after treatment with alternative antibiotics.

All patients with neurosyphilis must be carefully followed with periodic serological testing, clinical evaluation at 6-month intervals, and repeat CSF examinations for at least 3 years. The possibility of reinfection should always be considered when retreating patients with early syphilis. A CSF examination should be performed before retreatment unless reinfection and a diagnosis of early syphilis can be established. Retreatment should be considered when (1) clinical signs or symptoms of syphilis persist or recur, (2) there is a fourfold increase in the titer of a nontreponemal test, (3) an initially high-titer nontreponemal test fails to decrease fourfold within a year. Patients should be retreated with the schedules recommended for syphilis of more than 1 year's duration. In general, only one retreatment course is indicated because patients may maintain stable, low titers of nontreponemal tests or have irreversible anatomical damage.

Epidemiological Treatment. Patients who have been exposed to infectious syphilis within the preceding 3 months and other patients who on epidemiological grounds are at high risk for early syphilis should be treated as for early syphilis. Every effort should be made to establish a diagnosis in these cases.

DONOVANOSIS (GRANULOMA INGUINALE)

Etiology

The presumptive causal agent of donovanosis is *Calymmatobacterium granulomatis*. A gram-negative bacillus has been cultured from donovanosis lesions in the yolk sac of embryonated eggs [*81*]. This organism has a large capsule and no flagella and shares antigens with *Klebsiella rhinoscleromatis, Klebsiella pneumoniae,* and *Escherichia coli*. It is otherwise very poorly characterized, is not pathogenic for currently used laboratory animals, and its relationship to donovanosis is uncertain.

Epidemiology

The epidemiology of donovanosis is equally obscure. The disease is endemic in southeast Asia, southern India, and the Caribbean, parts of Africa and South America, and New Guinea, where it is the most common cause of genital ulcer disease [*65*]. It occurs predominantly in the lower socioeconomic classes. Sexual contact is probably the most common mode of transmission, but the exact mechanism and reservoir are unknown [*82*].

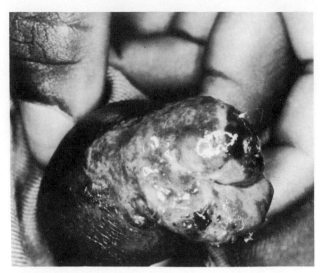

Figure 96-3. Donovanosis of the penis.

Manifestations

The incubation period in volunteers varies from 17 to 50 days and can be several months. The onset of disease is insidious with a small papule that eventually erodes and progresses into an enlarging granulomatous velvety ulcer that is indurated and beefy red (Fig. 96-3). The lesions bleed easily with trauma and are usually painless. The edges are well defined. Lesions occur most frequently on the genitals but in half of the cases they extend to the inguinal area or involve the perianal region. Lesions of the inguinal region, "pseudobuboes," usually only involve the skin and subcutaneous tissue, but not lymph nodes (Fig. 96-4). Oral lesions and systemic dissemination have been reported. Complications include stenosis of urethral, vaginal, and anal orifices, deformations of genitalia, and pseudoelephantiasis of the labia. Healing is not spontaneous and is accompanied by extensive scarring [*82*].

Diagnosis and management

Diagnosis of donovanosis is based on the demonstration of intracytoplasmic, encapsulated Donovan bodies in macrophages on stained tissue smears and section (Fig. 96-5). A small piece of tissue is obtained by curettage or biopsy and crushed between two glass slides to prepare an impression smear which is stained with Giemsa, Wright's, or Leishman's stain. Biopsy is also essential for ruling out other chronic, ulcerating conditions, such as squamous cell carcinoma. Biopsy-negative cases otherwise resembling donovanosis which have been seen in the United States have been almost uniformly culture-positive for *Haemophilus ducreyi* [*83*]. No controlled treatment trials have been reported. The treatment of choice is trimethoprim-sulfamethoxazole for at least 2 weeks [*84*].

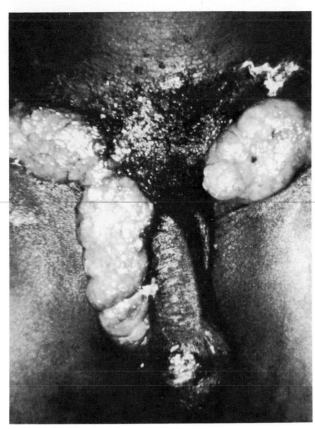

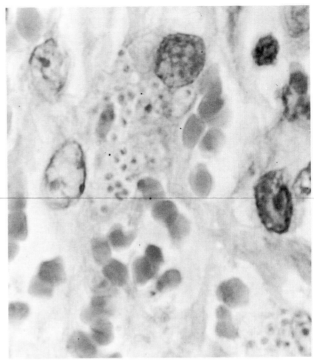

Figure 96-5. Donovan bodies seen in macrophages in tissue section from a biopsy of a genital ulcer. Hematoxylin and eosin stain.

Figure 96-4. Donovanosis extending from the penis and scrotum to both inguinal areas, producing ''pseudobuboes.''

Chloramphenicol, tetracycline, and streptomycin have been reported to be effective. Local application of an astringent lotion has been recommended but not evaluated.

HAEMOPHILUS DUCREYI (CHANCROID)

Biology

H. ducreyi is a small gram-negative facultative rod that requires hemin for growth and reduces nitrate to nitrite. Most strains are biochemically inert in standard laboratory tests except for a positive Voges-Proskauer test and alkaline phosphatase.

There is antigenic cross-reactivity of *H. ducreyi* antisera against extracts of other *Haemophilus* species. Strains can be divided into different types using electrophoresis of whole cell and outer-membrane proteins [85,86], immunofluorescence [87], and enzyme profile [88]. Major geographical variations have been found using all these methods. The organism autoagglutinates in saline. Antibodies have been detected in the serum of patients with chancroid and in experimental animals by enzyme immune assays, complement-fixation, precipitation, and indirect immunofluorescent tests [89,90].

Most recent isolates of *H. ducreyi* have been shown to produce a TEM-1 type of β-lactamase encoded by plasmids of variable size containing a Tn-2-like ampicillin-resistance transposon [91]. These plasmids are very closely related to the β-lactamase-encoding plasmids of *N. gonorrhoeae*.

Epidemiology

Chancroid is endemic in the tropics, where it is the most common cause of genital ulcer disease (Table 96-5). In sub-Saharan Africa and southeast Asia, *H. ducreyi* can be isolated from 20 to 60 percent of patients with genital ulcerations. In most countries, patients with chancroid belong to lower socioeconomic strata, and often indicate a prostitute as a source of infection [92,93]. Prostitutes seem to be a major reservoir of chancroid in several parts of the world [26]. Transmission from an infected individual to a sex partner has been well documented. Thus, in one study in Kenya, 59 percent of secondary female contacts of males with chancroid had also developed *H. ducreyi*–positive ulcers, while one contact (3 percent) who had no ulcer carried the organism in the cervix [92]. Chancroid is more common in uncircumcised men although lesions do occur in circumcised men [63,93].

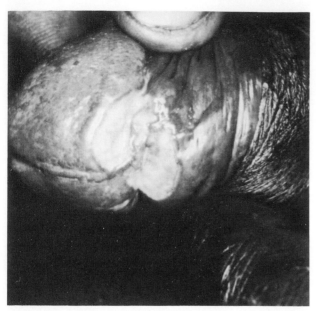

Figure 96-6. Chancroid ulcers on approximating surfaces of skin. Note purulent ulcer base.

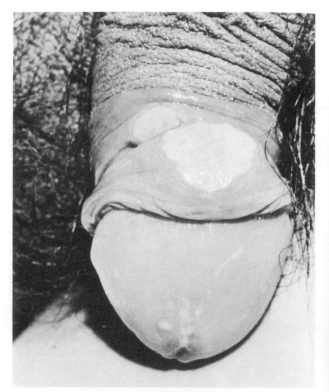

Figure 96-7. Chancroid ulcers on approximating surfaces of skin. Note suppurative ulcer base, irregular border.

Several cross-sectional and prospective studies in Africa have demonstrated not only that genital ulcers, most commonly chancroid, enhance the susceptibility to HIV infection through sexual intercourse, but that the infectiousness of HIV is also increased in individuals with a genital ulcer. This may partly explain why there is apparently much more heterosexual spread of HIV in Africa than in North America or Europe [*94–96*].

Clinical manifestations

The incubation period of chancroid is between 3 and 10 days (similar to genital herpes), when a tender papule appears on the genitals. In males, most lesions are found on the prepuce, near the frenulum or in the coronal sulcus. In females, most lesions are at the entrance to the vagina, particularly on the fourchette. Perianal lesions are not uncommon. The papules ulcerate within 1 to 2 days, when the typical chancroid lesion appears. The ulcers are painful, variably and minimally indurated, and have undermined ragged edges. The base is covered with a purulent exudate and bleeds easily during sampling. Two-thirds of the patients present with multiple ulcers, frequently due to autoinoculation (''kissing ulcers'') [*63,64,97*] (Figs. 96-6 and 96-7). Several ulcers may coalesce to form serpiginous lesions (Fig. 96-8). Pustular lesions may occur and resemble folliculitis or pyogenic infection. Edema of the prepuce and paraphimosis are common in the male.

In over half of the cases a painful inguinal lymphadenopathy appears within a week after the initial lesion. Lymphadenopathy is usually unilateral and may become fluctuant. These buboes require drainage by needle aspiration through normal skin to avoid spontaneous rupture which may result in exten-

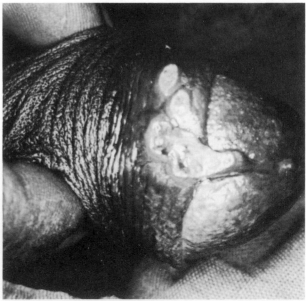

Figure 96-8. Coalescing chancroid ulcers, forming a serpiginous pattern.

sive ulceration of surrounding tissue. Bubo pus is viscous and purulent or blood-stained.

Complications include phimosis and destructive or phagedenic ulceration when there is secondary infection with anaerobes. Part or the whole of the glans penis may be lost.

The natural history of chancroid was studied before the introduction of antimicrobial chemotherapy. The mean duration of lesions was approximately 60 days. Epithelization of the ulcer is slow, and recurrence was common (but differentiation from genital herpes was not reliable at that time).

Histologically there is a superficial layer consisting of necrotic tissue, fibrin, neutrophils, and gram-negative bacilli. In the middle zone there is edema and newly formed blood vessels associated with neutrophils. The deep layer shows a dense infiltrate of neutrophils, plasma cells, and leukocytes with fibroblastic proliferation.

Diagnosis

A Gram-stained smear of material from the ulcer base is not considered reliable because of a lack of accuracy caused by the presence of numerous other bacteria in most ulcers. Smears of bubo aspirate rarely show typical gram-negative coccobacilli.

Whenever possible, diagnosis of chancroid should be supported by isolation of *H. ducreyi* from a lesion. Primary isolation should be attempted on GC agar base (BBL) enriched with 1% IsoVitalex (BBL), hemoglobin, bovine serum, and 3 mg/L vancomycin; or Mueller-Hinton agar base (BBL) with 5% horse blood heated to 75°C, 1% IsoVitalex, and 3 mg/L vancomycin [98]. The use of fresh medium (less than 1 week old) is important, and batch-to-batch variations of the agar base may influence the isolation rate. Plates should be incubated in a water-saturated 10% CO_2 atmosphere at 33 to 35°C. After 2 to 4 days of incubation, gray, small, semiopaque to translucent colonies of variable size (2 to 5 mm) appear. They can be pushed intact across the agar surface. Presumptive identification is based on the demonstration of gram-negative coccobacilli with occasional streptobacillary chaining, together with the inability of isolates to produce porphyrin from δ-amino levulinic acid.

Serological tests have been developed, but require further evaluation [85,86]. A positive serological test for syphilis does not exclude the diagnosis of chancroid, as many mixed infections occur. Thus, 37 percent of patients with proven chancroid in Johannesburg also had evidence of present or past infection with syphilis [99].

Management

In contrast to LGV and donovanosis, double-blind controlled treatment trials have been reported for chancroid. There seems to be considerable geographical variation in the antimicrobial susceptibility of *H. ducreyi* and in the effectiveness of different antimicrobial regimens. Thus, whereas trimethoprim-sulfamethoxazole is the recommended treatment in Africa [100], it cured only 55 to 87 percent of men with chancroid in Thailand [101]. Therefore, it is critical that treatment recommendations be based on local in vitro and clinical data. Whatever antimicrobial regimen is used, fluctuating buboes should be aspirated through normal adjacent skin. Because of better patient compliance, reduced toxicity, and lower price, single-dose treatment regimens are particularly interesting for the control of chancroid. Effective single-dose regimens include trimethoprim-sulfamethoxazole or trimethoprim-sulfametrole, 640 mg trimethoprim and 3200 mg sulfamethoxazole or sulfametrole by mouth [100]; ceftriaxone, 250 mg intramuscularly [101]; spectinomycin, 2 g IM [102]; and ciprofloxacin, 500 mg by mouth [103]. Erythromycin as a 10-day course is also an effective treatment [104]. The sulfonamides or tetracyclines are not recommended for the treatment of chancroid because of wide spread of resistance to these agents [104]. Recently, it was found that single-dose quinolone treatment for chancroid was significantly more likely to fail in HIV-seropositive individuals than in HIV-seronegatives. The efficacy of other regimens, therefore, should be revalidated in HIV-seropositive individuals, particularly in those who are immunosuppressed.

PREVENTION AND CONTROL OF STD

A recent WHO report [56] provides useful guidelines for prevention and control of STD, equally applicable to developing and industrialized countries. The report emphasizes essential components of a national program, training, and use of appropriate technology. Of critical importance today is more meaningful integration of programs for STD control, AIDS control, family planning, and maternal and child health. Mere lip service to integrated programs is all too common. Examples of essential steps in development of integrated programs include

1. Regular, frequent, joint program planning by leaders in each of these areas at the international, national, and where appropriate, the local level.
2. Integrated teaching of these subjects—for example in a course on reproductive health—in health science professional schools.
3. Programs to achieve 100 percent use of condoms by prostitutes with all sex partners.
4. Use of the existing family planning, maternal and child health, and public STD clinic infrastructures, which serve high-risk sexually active teenagers and young adults, to accomplish STD/AIDS control by health education, counseling, diagnostic testing for HIV and other STDs, and treatment of STDs.
5. Emphasis on improved control of STDs (e.g., genital ulcer disease) as a major strategy to reduce sexual transmission of HIV and prevent maternal and child morbidity (e.g., from congenital syphilis).

REFERENCES

1 Holmes KK, Mardh P-A, Sparling PF, et al (eds): *Sexually Transmitted Diseases,* 2d ed. New York, McGraw-Hill, 1988

2 Arya OP, Osoba AO, Bennett FJ: *Tropical Venereology,* 2d ed. Edinburgh, Churchill Livingstone, 1988

3 Piot P, Meheus A: Epidémiologie des maladies sexuellement transmissibles dans les pays en développement. Ann Soc Belge Med Trop 63:87, 1983

4 Antal G: The epidemiology of sexually transmitted diseases in the tropics, in Osoba AO (ed): *Sexually Transmitted Diseases in the Tropics.* Baillière's Clinical and Tropical Medicine and Communicable Diseases 2:1, 1987

5 Arya OP, Lawson JB: Sexually transmitted diseases in the tropics. Trop Doct 6:51, 1977

6 Friedman PS, Wright DJM: Observations on syphilis in Addis Ababa. 2. Prevalence and natural history. Br J Vener Dis 53:276, 1977

7 Mabey DC, Lloyd-Evans NE, Conteh S, et al: Sexually transmitted diseases among randomly selected attenders at an antenatal clinic in the Gambia. Br J Vener Dis 60:331, 1984

8 Mabey DCW: Syphilis in sub-Saharan Africa. Afr J Sex Transm Dis 3:61, 1986

9 Bentsi C, Klufio CA, Perine PL, et al: Genital infections with *Chlamydia trachomatis* and *Neisseria gonorrhoeae* in Ghanaian women. Genitourin Med 61:48, 1985

10 Laga M, Plummer FA, Nsanze H, et al: Epidemiology of ophthalmia neonatorum in Kenya. Lancet 2:1145, 1986

11 Meheus A, Friedman F, Van Dyck E, et al: Genital infections in prenatal and family planning attendants in Swaziland. East Afr Med J 57:212, 1980

12 Ratnam AV, Chattergee TK, Mulenga RC: Sexually transmitted diseases in pregnant women in Lusaka. Med J Zambia 14:75, 1980

13 Hira SK, Bhat GJ, Patel JB, et al: Early congenital syphilis: Clinicocardiologic features in 202 patients. Sex Transm Dis 12:177, 1985

14 Thanasoporn Y: Congenital syphilis. Asian J Infect Dis 1:75, 1977

15 Stutz DR, Spence MR, Duangmani C: Oropharyngeal gonorrhea during pregnancy. J Am Vener Dis Assoc 3:65, 1976

16 George WF: An approach to VD control based on a study in Kingston, Jamaica. Br J Vener Dis 50:222, 1974

17 Borgono JM, Falaha F, Grinspun M, et al: Pesquisa serologica de lues en embarazadar. Bol Of Sanit Panam 78:221, 1975

18 Da Silva AS, Zisman M, Ferreira OS: Incidencia de sifilis congenita em recemnascidos pre-termo e a termo. Rev Bras Resquisas Med Biol 13:105, 1980

19 Muir DG, Belsey MA: Pelvic inflammatory disease and its consequences in the developing world. Am J Obstet Gynecol 138:913, 1980

20 Romaniuk A: Infertility in tropical Africa, in Caldwell JC, Okonjo C (eds): *The Population of Tropical Africa.* London, Longmans, 1969, p 214

21 Retel-Laurentin A: *Infecondite en Afrique noire.* Paris, Masson, 1974, p 188

22 Cates W, Farley TMM, Rowe PJ: Worldwide patterns of infertility: Is Africa different? Lancet 2:596, 1985

23 Naeye RL, Kissane JM: Perinatal diseases, a neglected area of the medical sciences, in Naeye RL, Kissane JM, Kaufman N (eds): *Perinatal Diseases.* Baltimore, Williams & Wilkins, 1978, p 1

24 Galega FP, Heyman DL, Nasah BT: Gonococcal ophthalmia neonatorum: The case of prophylaxis in tropical Africa. Bull WHO 61:85, 1984

25 Plummer FA, Laga M, Brunham RC, et al: Postpartum upper genital tract infections in Nairobi, Kenya: Epidemiology, etiology and risk factors. J Infect Dis 156:92, 1987

26 D'Costa LJ, Plummer FA, Bowmer I, et al: Prostitutes are a major reservoir of sexually transmitted diseases in Nairobi, Kenya. Sex Transm Dis 12:64, 1985

27 Rajan VS: Sexually transmitted diseases on a tropical island. Br J Vener Dis 54:141, 1978

28 Mandara NA, Takulia S, Kanyawana J, et al: Asymptomatic gonorrhoea in women attending family planning clinics in Dar es Salaam, Tanzania. Trop Geogr Med 32:329, 1980

29 Arya OP, Nsanzumuhire H, Taber SR: Clinical, cultural and demographic aspects of gonorrhoea in a rural community in Uganda. Bull WHO 49:587, 1973

30 Van de Velden L, Jancloes M, M'boup S: Prevalence des gonococcies de la femme dans la zone urbaine de Pikine (Senegal) et sensibilité aux antibiotiques. Ann Microbiol (Paris) 13A:89, 1980

31 Meheus A, Ballard R, Dlamini M, et al: Epidemiology and aetiology of urethritis in Swaziland. Int J Epidemiol 9:239, 1980

32 Bewes PC: Urethral stricture. Trop Doct 3:77, 1973

33 Osegbe DN, Amaku EO: Gonococcal strictures in young patients. Urology 18:37, 1981

34 *Neisseria gonorrhoeae* and gonococcal infections. WHO Tech Rep Ser 616. Geneva, World Health Organization, 1978

35 McCormack WM, Stumacher RJ, Johnson K, et al: Clinical spectrum of gonococcal infection in women. Lancet 1:1182, 1977

36 Perine PL, Duncan MA, Krause DW, et al: Pelvic inflammatory disease and puerperal sepsis in Ethiopia. 1. Etiology. Am J Obstet Gynecol 138:969, 1980

37 Ratnam AV, Din SN, Catterjee TK: Gonococcal infection in women with pelvic inflammatory disease in Lusaka, Zambia. Am J Obstet Gynecol 138:965, 1980

38 Maheus A, Reniers J, Collet M, et al: *Chlamydia trachomatis* in women with acute salpingitis and infertility in Central Africa, p 241 in Oriel D, Ridgway G, Schachter J, et al (eds): *Chlamydial Infections.* Cambridge, Cambridge University Press, 1986

39 Shah HM, Patel S, Nagpal S: Pelvic inflammation: A study of 800 cases. J Obstet Gynaecol India 28:429, 1978

40 Kochhar M: Etiology of pelvic infections treated by the gynecologic service of the Kasturba Hospital, Delhi, India. Am J Obstet Gynecol 138:873, 1980

41 Sinnathuray TA, Yusof K, Palan VT, et al: Pattern of acute pelvic inflammatory disease in abortion-related admissions. Am J Obstet Gynecol 138:868, 1980

42 Westrom L: Incidence, prevalence, and trends of acute pelvic inflammatory disease and its consequences in industrialized countries. Am J Obstet Gynecol 138:880, 1980

43 Arya OP, Taber SR, Nsanze H: Gonorrhea and female infertility in rural Uganda. Am J Obstet Gynecol 138:929, 1980

44 Fransen L, Nsanze H, Klauss V, et al: Ophthalmia neonatorum in Nairobi, Kenya: the roles of *Neisseria gonorrhoeae* and *Chlamydia trachomatis.* J Infect Dis 153:862, 1986

45 Laga M, Plummer FA, Piot P, et al: Prophylaxis of ophthalmia neonatorum: Silver nitrate versus tetracycline. N Engl J Med 318:653, 1988

46 Kesteleyn P, Bogaerts J, Meheus A: Gonorrheal keratoconjunctivitis in African adults. Sex Transm Dis 14:191, 1987

47 Brunham R, Plummer F, Embree J, et al: STD in pregnancy, in Holmes KK et al (eds): *Sexually Transmitted Diseases,* 2d ed. New York, McGraw Hill, 1989

48 Elliot B, Brunham RC, Ndinya-Achola JO, et al: The association of maternal gonorrhea with preterm birth in Nairobi, Kenya. Submitted

49 Osoba AO, Alausa KO: Vulvovaginitis in Nigerian children. Nig J Pediatr 1:26, 1974

50 Moreno JG, Dillon JR, Assoyave R, et al: Identification of penicillinase producing *Neisseria gonorrhoeae* in Chile during clinical and microbiological study of gonococcal susceptibility to antimicrobial agents. Genitourin Med 63:6, 1987

51 Perine PL, Thornsberry C, Schalla W, et al: Evidence for two distinct types of penicillinase-producing *Neisseria gonorrhoeae*. Lancet 2:993, 1977

52 Van Embden JDA, Dessens-Kroon M, van Klingeren B: A new beta-lactamase plasmid in *Neisseria gonorrhoeae*. J Antimicrob Chemother 15:247–250, 1985

53 Bogaerts J, Vandepitte J, Van Dyck E, et al: In vitro antimicrobial sensitivity of *N. gonorrhoeae* in Rwanda. Genitourin Med 62:217, 1986

54 Plummer FA, D'Costa L, Nsanze H, et al: Development of endemic penicillinase-producing *Neisseria gonorrhoeae* in Kenya, p 101 in Schoolnik GK (ed): *The Pathogenic Neisseriae*. Washington, DC, American Society for Microbiology, 1985

55 Osoba AO, Johnston NA, Ogunbanjo BO, et al: Plasmid profile of *Neisseria gonorrhoeae* in Nigeria and efficacy of spectinomycin in treating gonorrhoea. Genitourin Med 63:1, 1987

56 World Health Organization. WHO Expert Committee on Venereal Diseases and Treponematoses. WHO Tech Rep Ser 736, Geneva, 1986

57 Bogaerts J, Tello WM, Verbist L, et al: Norfloxacin versus thiamphenicol for treatment of uncomplicated gonorrhea in Rwanda. Antimicrob Agents Chemother 31:434, 1987

58 Demuylder X, Laga M, Tennstedt C, et al: Role of *Chlamydia trachomatis* and *Neisseria gonorrhoeae* in salpingitis and its sequellae in Zimbabwe. Submitted

59 Datta P, Laga M, Plummer FA, et al: Infection and disease after perinatal exposure to *Chlamydia trachomatis* in Nairobi, Kenya. J Infect Dis 158:524, 1988

60 Mabey D: Aetiology of genital ulceration in the Gambia. Genitourin Med 63:312, 1987

61 Meheus AZ, Van Dyck E, Ursi JP, et al: Etiology of genital ulcerations in Swaziland. Sex Transm Dis 10:33, 1983

62 Bogaerts J, Ricart CA, Van Dyck E, et al: The etiology of genital ulceration in Rwanda. Sex Transm Dis, in press

63 Nsanze H, Fast M, D'Costa LJ, et al: Genital ulcer in Kenya: A clinic and laboratory study of 100 patients. Br J Vener Dis 57:378, 1981

64 Taylor DN, Duangmani C, Suvongse C, et al: The role of *Haemophilus ducreyi* in penile ulcerations in Bangkok, Thailand. Sex Transm Dis 11:148, 1984

65 Vacca A, MacMillan LL: Anogenital lesions in women in Papua New Guinea. Papua N Guinea Med J 23:70, 1980

66 Piot P, Ballard RC, Fehler HG, et al: Isolation of *Chlamydia trachomatis* from genital ulcerations in Southern Africa, in Mardh PA, Holmes KK, Oriel JD, et al: *Chlamydial Infection*. Amsterdam, Elsevier/North Holland, 1982, p 115

67 Perine PL, Andersen AJ, Krause DW, et al: Diagnosis and treatment of lymphogranuloma venereum in Ethiopia, in *Current Chemotherapy and Infectious Disease,* Washington, DC, American Society for Microbiology, 1980, p 1280

68 Quinn TC, Goodell SE, Mkrtichian E, et al: *Chlamydia trachomatis* proctitis. N Engl J Med 305:195, 1981

69 Schachter J, Smith DE, Dawson CR, et al: Lymphogranuloma venereum. I. Comparison of the Frei test, complement fixation test, and isolation of the agent. J Infect Dis 120:382, 1969

70 Philip RN, Casper EA, Gordon FB, et al: Fluorescent antibody responses to chlamydial infection in patients with lymphogranuloma venereum and urethritis. J Immunol 112:2126, 1974

71 Greaves AB, Hilleman MR, Taggart SR, et al: Chemotherapy in bubonic lymphogranuloma venereum. A clinical and serological evaluation. Bull WHO 16:277, 1957

72 Ursi JP, Van Dyck E, Van Houtte C, et al: Syphilis in Swaziland. A serological survey. J Vener Dis 57:95, 1981

73 Larsson Y, Larsson U: Congenital syphilis in Addis Ababa. Ethiop Med J 8:163, 1970

74 Ratnam AV, Din SN, Hira SK, et al: Syphilis in pregnant women in Zambia. Br J Vener Dis 58:355, 1982

75 Hira SK, Bhat GJ, Ratnam AV, et al: Congenital syphilis in Lusaka. II. Incidence at birth and potential risk among hospital deliveries. East Afr Med J 59:306, 1982

76 Hira SK, Ratnam AV, Bhat GJ, et al: Congenital syphilis in Lusaka. I. Incidence in a general nursery ward. East Afr Med J 59:241, 1982

77 Gelfand M, Warton CR, Loewenson R: Neurosyphilis—Its incidence and types, as found in the African of Zimbabwe. Cent Afr J Med 26:153, 1980

78 Hira SK, Hira RS: Congenital syphilis, in Osoba AO (ed): *Sexually Transmitted Diseases in the Tropics*. Baillière's Clinical Tropical Medicine and Communicable Diseases 2:113, 1987

79 Bwibo NO: Congenital syphilis. East Afr Med J 48:185, 1971

80 Centers for Disease Control: Guidelines for the prevention and control of congenital syphilis. Morb Mortal Weekly Rep 37:S1, 1988

81 Kuberski T: Granuloma inguinale (Donovanosis). Sex Transm Dis 7:29, 1980

82 Hart G: Chancroid, Donovanosis and Lymphogranuloma Venereum. U.S. Dept. of Health, Education, and Welfare, publication (CDC) 75-88302, Atlanta, GA, Public Health Service Center for Disease Control, 1968

83 Kraus SJ, Werman BX, Biddle JW, et al: Pseudogranuloma inguinale caused by *Haemophilus ducreyi*. Arch Derm 118:494, 1982

84 Lal S, Garg BR: Further evidence of the efficiency of cotrimoxazole in granuloma inguinale. Br J Vener Dis 56:412, 1980

85 Odumeru JA, Ronald AR, Albritton WL: Characterization of cell proteins of *Haemophilus ducreyi* by polyacrylamide gel electrophoresis. J Infect Dis 148:710, 1983

86 Taylor D, Echeverria P, Hanchalay S, et al: Antimicrobial susceptibility and characterization of outer membrane proteins of *Haemophilus ducreyi* isolated in Thailand. J Clin Microbiol 21:442, 1985

87 Slootmans L, Van den Berghe D, Piot P: Typing *Haemophilus ducreyi* using the indirect immunofluorescence assay. Genitourin Med 61:123, 1985

88 Van Dyck E, Piot P: Enzyme profile of *Haemophilus ducreyi* strains isolated on different continents. Eur J Clin Microbiol 6:40, 1987

89 Schalla WO, Sanders LL, Schmid GP, et al: Investigation of clinically suspected cases of chancroid using a dot-immunobinding assay and immunofluorescence. J Infect Dis 153:879, 1986

90 Museyi K, Van Dyck E, Vervoort T, et al: Detection of serum IgG antibodies to *Haemophilus ducreyi* in an enzyme immune assay. J Infect Dis, 157:314, 1988

91 Maclean IW, Bowden GHW, Albritton WL: TEM-type 1-lactamase production in *Haemophilus ducreyi*. Antimicrob Agents Chemother 17:897, 1980

92 Plummer FA, D'Costa LJ, Nsanze H, et al: Epidemiology of chancroid and *Haemophilus ducreyi* in Nairobi, Kenya. Lancet 2:1293, 1983

93 Hart G: Venereal disease in a war environment: Incidence and management. Med J Aust 1:808, 1975

94 Greenblatt RM, Lukehart SA, Plummer PA, et al: Genital ulceration as a risk factor for human immunodeficiency virus infection. AIDS 2:47, 1988

95 Cameron DW, D'Costa LJ, Ndinya-Achola JO, et al: Incidence and risk factors for female to male transmission of HIV. Abstract, 4th International Conference on AIDS, Stockholm, 12–16 June 1988

96 Piot P, Plummer FA, Mhalu FS, et al: AIDS: An international perspective. Science 239:573, 1988

97 Tan T, Rayan VS, Koe SL, et al: Chancroid: A study of 500 cases. Asian J Infect Dis 1:27, 1977

98 Nsanze H, Plummer FA, Maggwa AB: Comparison of media for the isolation of *Haemophilus ducreyi*. Sex Transm Dis 11:6, 1984

99 Duncan MO, Bilgen YR, Fehler HB, et al: The diagnosis of sexually acquired genital ulcerations in black patients in Johannesburg. South Afr J Sex Transm 1:20, 1981

100 Plummer FA, Nsanze H, D'Costa LJ, et al: Single-dose therapy of chancroid with trimethoprim-sulfametrole. N Engl J Med 309:67, 1983

101 Taylor DN, Pitarangsi C, Echeverria P, et al: Comparative study of ceftriaxone and trimethoprim-sulfamethoxazole for the treatment of chancroid in Thailand. J Infect Dis 152:1002, 1985

102 Fransen L, Nsanze H, Ndinya-Achola JO, et al: A comparison of single-dose spectinomycin with five days of trimethoprim-sulfamethoxazole for the treatment of chancroid. Sex Transm Dis 14:98, 1987

103 Naamara W, Plummer FA, Greenblatt RM, et al: Treatment of chancroid with ciprofloxacin. Am J Med 82:317, 1987

104 Schmid GP: The treatment of chancroid. JAMA 255:1757, 1986

CHAPTER 97 / *Yaws, Nonvenereal Treponematoses*
· Donald R. Hopkins · Peter L. Perine

Yaws, endemic syphilis, and pinta—the endemic or nonvenereal treponematoses—are chronic infections which affect skin, bones, and cartilage (yaws and endemic syphilis) or only the skin (pinta). Usually acquired by skin-to-skin contact during childhood, the three diseases are caused by closely related spirochetes belonging to the genus *Treponema*. Although they are not transmitted venereally, the endemic treponematoses are very closely related to *Treponema pallidum* which causes syphilis, a much more serious disease. Apart from the morbidity they cause, the nonvenereal treponematoses are also significant to the clinician because of the immune responses they induce. The spirochetes which produce nonvenereal treponematoses cause serological reactions indistinguishable from those of venereal syphilis by every test now known. Yaws is the most common of the nonvenereal treponematoses; it occurs in warm tropical regions of Africa, Latin America, and Asia. Endemic syphilis (bejel) is prevalent in some arid regions of the Middle East and Africa, while pinta is found only in the American tropics.

PARASITE

The treponemes which cause yaws, endemic syphilis, pinta, and venereal syphilis are believed to have evolved from a common ancestor spirochete which may have caused a disease similar to pinta. Yaws and endemic syphilis might have arisen as a result of changing environmental conditions as infected persons migrated to different areas. Some historians believe a mutation of the endemic syphilis treponeme, which was already endemic in the Mediterranean basin when Columbus sailed to the New World, gave rise to the first recognized epidemic of venereal syphilis which began in Italy in 1494. The origin of the treponematoses and their relationship to each other are still quite controversial, however [1]. Our own opinion is that for all their similarities [2], the consistent *typical* clinical and epidemiological features of yaws, endemic syphilis, and pinta are sufficiently distinct that the causative organisms must be different from each other and from the agent of venereal syphilis.

According to current nomenclature, *Treponema pertenue* causes yaws and *T. carateum* pinta. The treponeme which causes endemic syphilis is called *T. pallidum,* the same species name used to designate the organism causing venereal syphilis. In addition, *T. fribourg-blanc* is a closely related organism isolated from a few wild African monkeys and baboons. Although one or more of the primates from which this last organism was isolated had yawslike lesions and positive serological reactions, a nonhuman reservoir of yaws in Africa has not been documented. *Treponema cuniculi* causes a naturally occurring, venereal treponematosis in rabbits, but is not pathogenic for humans.

All the pathogenic treponemes are thin, cylindrical organisms which have a characteristic shape, like a corkscrew. They measure about 0.3 μm in diameter and range in length from 7 to 20 μm. *Treponema pertenue* exhibits ultrastructural features identical to those seen in electron microscopic examination of *T. pallidum* from patients with venereal syphilis.

Like *T. pallidum,* the other pathogenic treponemes appear to contain muramic acid, and manufacture a protective outer envelope of acid mucopolysaccharides. They multiply by transverse fission, with a relatively slow generation time of about 30 h. None of the pathogenic treponemes has yet been grown in artificial media or by cell culture. Usually the organisms are isolated or maintained by growing them in rabbit testicles (they can also be preserved for years by freezing at −70°C). Most laboratory studies have been done with *T. pallidum* and to a lesser extent with *T. pertenue.* The treponemes differ somewhat in the types of experimental animals they infect and the pathology which results [*3,4*].

PATIENT

PATHOGENESIS

Pathogenic treponemes usually enter the body through small abrasions or lacerations in the skin, although *T. pallidum* can penetrate intact mucous membranes [*3*]. Most cells have receptors for pathogenic treponemes on their membranes. Pathogenic treponemes can attach to the surface of living human cells and invade them without causing damage, whereas avirulent treponemes cannot. Mucopolysaccharidases produced by the pathogenic treponemes may help them pass between superficial cells to gain access to subcutaneous tissues.

Once the skin or mucous membrane barrier is breached, *T. pallidum* and *T. pertenue* multiply locally at the site of initial infection (inoculation), then spread systemically via the bloodstream. Although most tissues are exposed during the bacteremia, only the skin and osseous tissues are affected in yaws and endemic syphilis. *Treponema carateum* produces lesions only in the epithelium.

Each of the endemic treponematoses tends to progress from an initial cutaneous, or primary lesion, to a disseminated secondary stage characterized by many cutaneous lesions, followed after several years by a late, or tertiary stage. Each stage may be separated by periods of latency when no clinical signs or symptoms of infection are present, and when the only evidence of infection may be a positive serological test. Whereas early lesions in yaws and endemic syphilis are usually infectious but heal without scarring unless they become secondarily infected, the tertiary lesions are highly destructive, but not infectious.

Infection with the nonvenereal treponemes, especially yaws and endemic syphilis, elicits an immune response early in the disease. Antibodies produced in response to one treponeme invariably cross-react to varying degrees with other pathogenic treponemes. Experimental animals and patients exhibit partial resistance to reinfection after 1 year or more. This resistance is strongest against the homologous organism but substantial cross-resistance to infection with other pathogenic treponemes has been documented [*3*]. Although humoral immunity may account for the healing of the initial lesion(s), its presence does not prevent the onset of disseminated yaws or endemic syphilis, or relapses of disseminated disease. In disseminated disease infectious treponemes are plentiful in the skin lesions, despite high titers of circulating antibody. Possible explanations for this paradox are protection by the mucopolysaccharide "slime layer" which covers the surface of treponemes, incorporation of host lipid antigens by the treponemes on their surface to avoid recognition by the host's defenses, and temporary suppression of host cell-mediated immune response by pathogenic treponemes [*5,6*]. After several months of infection the host becomes partially immune to reinfection, and the mass of treponemes present in the tissues is reduced or eliminated.

Only 10 to 20 percent of patients with primary yaws or endemic syphilis patients develop late complications if left untreated [*7*]. The late destructive lesions of yaws and endemic syphilis have the same histology as the gumma of venereal syphilis. These proliferative granulomas can occur anywhere in the skin, nasopharynx, or bone. The stimulus for their formation is probably a delayed hypersensitivity response to treponemal antigens. These lesions heal by fibrosis and some degree of irreversible disfigurement or disability is common.

CLINICAL MANIFESTATIONS

Yaws

The initial lesion of yaws is a small, raised, nonindurated papule. It usually appears on the skin of the lower extremities after an incubation period of 3 to 5 weeks. The papule soon enlarges to form an elevated, superficially ulcerated, raspberrylike lesion called a papilloma or frambesioma. The papilloma may reach several centimeters in diameter and ooze a highly infectious serous exudate rich in *T. pertenue.* Unless it becomes secondarily infected by other bacteria, the papilloma is not painful. The lymph nodes draining the papilloma may become enlarged, but fever and other constitutional symptoms are rare.

Secondary lesions often appear before the initial yaws papilloma heals. They may appear anywhere on the skin or mucocutaneous junctions. The moist areas of the body such as the axilla and anal cleft are commonly involved. The morphology of disseminated cutaneous lesions varies with such factors as climate and the presence of secondary bacterial infection. Papillomata may be more numerous and larger during rainy seasons while macular, papulosquamous lesions or latency may be more prevalent in dry weather. Lesions on the soles of the feet may be accompanied by a painful hyperkeratosis. These lesions cause the patient to walk on the sides of the feet, creating a crablike gait ("crab" yaws).

Long bones of the extremities, especially the tibia, may be affected with osteoperiostitis early in yaws. Nocturnal pain in the lower legs may be the first symptom. While this osteoperiostitis usually resolves without causing permanent bone or joint disability, the tibia may become bowed anteriorly (saber tibia). Polydactylitis affecting the small joints of the hand or foot is also common in early yaws. Hypertrophic osteitis of the nasal processes of the maxilla (goundou) is much less common [8].

Disseminated yaws lesions usually heal spontaneously within the first 6 months of infection. Relapses may occur in the ensuing latent period. Late yaws lesions usually develop 5 or more years after infection. These lesions contain few treponemes, are not infectious, and are identical in clinical appearance to the gummas of late venereal syphilis, except that the gummas of yaws and endemic syphilis affect only skin and bone. The palate may be perforated and the nasal cartilage destroyed, creating a mutilation called gangosa. Healing of late cutaneous ulcers is accompanied by extensive scarring. Monodactylitis, gummatous osteoperiostitis of the skull, and juxtaarticular nodules are other manifestations of late yaws.

Endemic syphilis

Primary lesions are rarely seen in endemic syphilis. The first manifestation of infection is usually the appearance of indurated mucous patches on the mucosa of the oropharynx, tongue, and buccal mucosa, or mucocutaneous papillomata at the corners of the mouth.

As in yaws, disseminated papillomata may appear anywhere on the body, but the preferential sites are moist areas such as the axilla, nasolabial folds, and anal cleft. Painful osteoperiostitis of long bones also occurs. Generalized lymphadenopathy may appear early in infection, but constitutional symptoms are rare [9].

The late complications of endemic syphilis are identical to those of yaws. Gangosa occurs with greater frequency in endemic syphilis than in yaws. Neurological and cardiovascular complications, and gummas of the viscera have not been well documented in endemic syphilis patients because of difficulty in excluding venereal syphilis.

Pinta

The initial lesion of pinta is usually an asymptomatic erythematous papule on the skin of the legs or arms. The "pintid" slowly enlarges over several weeks or months to form a slightly elevated, psoriaform lesion that may reach several centimeters in diameter. Satellite pintids appear at the margin of the initial lesion, and are slowly incorporated into it. The color of the lesion changes slowly and irregularly to a blue or violaceous hue. Multiple lesions may occur over different parts of the body. Dyschromia may take place over several years, with the color changing to lighter shades of gray. Ultimately, lesions of pinta become achromic and the affected skin atrophic [10].

DIAGNOSIS

Dark-field examination of exudate from lesions is the diagnostic method of choice. Treponemes are usually numerous in exudate from early lesions. Exudate should be examined soon after its collection in order to observe the characteristic rapid rotational movement of pathogenic treponemes. The serodiagnostic tests used for the endemic treponematoses are the same as those used for venereal syphilis (see Chap. 96). The nontreponemal tests (VDRL, RPR, etc.) are positive in almost all yaws and endemic syphilis patients shortly after the initial lesions appear. Only about 60 percent of patients with pinta ever become reactive to nontreponemal antigen tests. The treponemal tests (FTA-ABS, TPHA) are also reactive early in infection and persist indefinitely, but do not differentiate one treponemal disease from another.

The most difficult diagnostic problems are presented by adults with positive serological reactions who may have had an endemic treponematosis in childhood. A careful clinical and epidemiological history will help in the differential diagnosis. Unfortunately, immunity produced by the endemic treponemes provides only partial protection against infection by *T. pallidum*, and venereal syphilis does occur in patients who had yaws, pinta, or endemic syphilis during childhood.

TREATMENT

Long-acting parenteral penicillin G is the treatment of choice for the endemic treponematoses [11]. All patients and contacts under 10 years of age should receive 600,000 units of benzathine penicillin G by intramuscular injection. Patients and contacts over 10 years of age should be given 1,200,000 units intramuscularly. Penicillin-allergic patients above 10 years of age should receive tetracycline hydrochloride, 500 mg orally four times a day for 10 days. To avoid staining of teeth children under 10 years of age who are allergic to penicillin can be given erythromycin, 250 mg orally four times a day for 10 days.

POPULATION

EPIDEMIOLOGY

Yaws and endemic syphilis are usually acquired between the ages of 5 and 15 years. Transmission is facilitated by crowding and poor hygiene. Minor skin trauma, including the commissural cheilitis of vitamin B deficiency, provides ideal portals of entry for *T. pallidum* and *T. pertenue*. Whereas yaws is transmitted by skin-to-skin contact with a patient who has infectious lesions, endemic syphilis is apparently more commonly transmitted by contaminated utensils. The mode of transmission of pinta is unknown, but is thought to be direct contact. *Treponema carateum* is not highly contagious, and several years of intimate family contact may be necessary for transmission. For each overt, active clinical case of endemic treponematosis in a village, there may be two or more latent cases.

PREVENTION AND CONTROL

Treatment of only active cases will not control these diseases because incubating cases and latent cases with recrudescent potential pose a constant threat [12]. Benzathine penicillin G will usually kill all the treponemes in the host and provide protection against reinfection for about 4 weeks. Thus, the rationale for controlling yaws, endemic syphilis, and pinta is to treat all patients and their contacts who are likely to be incubating the disease or to have latent infections. When the prevalence of clinically active disease is over 10 percent, the entire population should be treated (total mass treatment); for prevalences between 5 and 10 percent, all children under 15 years and obvious contacts of infectious patients should be treated (juvenile mass treatment); and when the prevalence is under 5 percent, only active cases, the household and other obvious contacts are treated (selective mass treatment).

The mass treatment campaigns organized by WHO and UNICEF in the 1950s and 1960s employed this concept with a great degree of success. About 160 million people living in endemic areas were examined for yaws and endemic syphilis, and about 60 million cases and contacts received penicillin. Although the prevalence of these diseases decreased dramatically, none of the endemic treponematoses has been eradicated. Yaws and pinta have continued to decline greatly in the Americas, but there was a substantial resurgence of yaws and endemic syphilis in west Africa in the 1970s. Yaws still appears to be declining in Asia [13].

The resurgence of yaws and endemic syphilis in Africa and the persistence of endemic foci for these diseases in other parts of the world may require new strategies for control [14,15]. Yaws surveillance and treatment should be made a component of primary health care wherever possible. All contacts should be treated as well when an infectious case of yaws, endemic syphilis, or pinta is diagnosed. The most cost-effective control method may be to create a system to detect active yaws or endemic syphilis cases, and to conduct epidemiological surveillance and treatment around these cases as was done in the smallpox eradication program. Specific control measures can never be safely discarded until the disease has been eliminated from a defined population.

REFERENCES

1 Hudson EH: Treponematosis and man's social evolution. Am Anthropol 67:885–901, 1965
2 Miao RM, Fieldsteel AH: Genetic relationship between *Treponema pallidum* and *Treponema pertenue,* two non-cultivable human pathogens. J Bacteriol 141:427–429, 1980
3 Turner TB, Hollander DH: *Biology of the Treponematoses.* WHO Monogr Ser 35, Geneva, 1957
4 Johnson RC: *The Biology of Parasitic Spirochetes.* Academic, New York, 1976
5 Fitzgerald TJ: Pathogenesis and immunology of *Treponema pallidum.* Annu Rev Microbiol 35:29–54, 1981
6 Musher DM, Schell RF: The immunology of syphilis. Hosp Prac 10:45–50, 1975
7 Guthe T, Luger A: The control of endemic syphilis of childhood. Dermatologia Internat 5:179–199, 1966
8 Perine PL, Hopkins DR, Niemal PLA, et al: *A Handbook for the Endemic Treponematoses: Yaws, Endemic Syphilis, and Pinta.* Geneva, World Health Organization, 1984
9 Murray JF, et al: Endemic syphilis in the Bakwena Reserve of the Bechuanaland Protectorate. Bull WHO 15:975–1039, 1956
10 Medina R: Pinta: Una treponematosis endemica de las Americas. Bol Sanit Panam 86:242–255, 1979
11 World Health Organization: *Treponemal Infections—Report of a WHO Scientific Group.* Geneva, World Health Organization, 1982, pp 50–51
12 Hackett CJ, Guthe T: Some important aspects of yaws eradication. Bull WHO 23:739–761, 1960
13 World Health Organization: Endemic Treponematoses. Weekly Epidemiologic Record, 61:198–202, 1986
14 Hopkins DR: After smallpox eradication: Yaws? Am J Trop Med Hyg 25:860–865, 1976
15 The international symposium on yaws and other endemic treponematoses. Rev Infect Dis 7(suppl 2):S217–S351, 1985

Relapsing Fever · Thomas Butler

Relapsing fever is an acute febrile illness of humans caused by spirochetes belonging to *Borrelia* species. The two major kinds of relapsing fever are louseborne relapsing fever, for which humans are the reservoir and the body louse is the vector, and tickborne relapsing fever, for which rodents and other animals are the predominant reservoirs and ticks the vectors. The relapsing fevers are distributed worldwide in both tropical and temperate climates.

PARASITE

The etiological agent of relapsing fever was first established in Berlin in 1873 by Obermeier, who used a microscope to observe spirochetes in the blood of patients. The transmission of *Borrelia* spirochetes by arthropod vectors was suggested in 1891 by Flugge, who postulated the body louse as a vector. In 1905 Dutton and Todd demonstrated the infection in the *Ornithodorus* ticks of Africa. The genus name *Borrelia* was proposed in 1907 in honor of the French bacteriologist Borrel.

Borrelia spirochetes are spiral organisms that measure 5 to 40 μm in length and about 0.5 μm in diameter. They are too thin to be seen reliably by light microscopy of wet prepara-

tions, but they are easily visible when viewed by dark-field or phase-contrast microscopy. They are visible with aniline dyes, such as Wright's or Giemsa stains, and stain well in tissue with silver stains, such as the Dieterle's or Warthin-Starry stains (Fig. 98-1). Like other bacteria, these spirochetes possess an outer cell wall (outer envelope) and an inner cytoplasmic membrane which contains muramic acid. Between the cell wall and cytoplasmic membrane there are 15 to 20 flagella which are anchored to the ends of the spirochete and wrap around its body until they meet at the middle region. In three dimensions the spirochetes have a helical configuration consisting of about 4 to 10 coils with amplitudes of about 1 to 4 μm. Under dark-field or phase-contrast microscopy, *Borrelia* spirochetes display an active corkscrewlike motility. Inside the cytoplasmic membrane, there are ribosomes, DNA, and RNA. These prokaryotic organisms divide by transverse binary fission.

Borrelia are microaerophilic and fermentative in their growth characteristics. Like other pathogenic spirochetes, they require long-chain fatty acids for growth. They are cultivatable in Kelly's medium, which is a complex broth containing proteose peptone, tryptone, bovine serum albumin, rabbit serum, *N*-acetylglucosamine, citric acid, and pyruvate in addition to

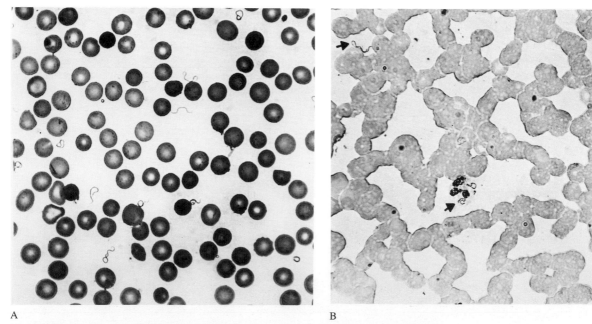

A   B

Figure 98-1. Blood smears of patient with louseborne relapsing fever. *A.* Blood smear stained with Wright's stain shows numerous plasma spirochetes. *B.* One hour after treatment with erythromycin, blood smear stained with the Dieterle's silver stain reveals both spirochetes that are extracellular and spirochetes within polymorphonuclear leukocytes (arrows).

glucose and salts. *B. recurrentis,* the agent of louseborne re-lapsing fever, is more fastidious than the tickborne *Borrelia* and requires the further addition of asparagine and choline to Kelly's medium. The *Borrelia* grow slowly in Kelly's medium with doubling times of 18 to 26 h.

Borrelia spirochetes do not possess any known endo- or exotoxins. In general, *Borrelia* spirochetes do not elicit acute inflammation, do not produce abscesses, and are confined pre-dominantly to the plasma space of their mammalian hosts. Fever is caused by a nonendotoxic pyrogen in the spirochete that elicits interleukin 1 production by mononuclear phago-cytes. The relapsing feature of *Borrelia* infections has been attributed to antigenic variation in the infecting population of spirochetes. In experimental infections of rats with *B. hermsii* separate serotypes emerge sequentially during relapses with the appearance of specific antibody response to each of the anti-genic variants. Each of the 25 serotypes of *B. hermsii* expresses different variable major proteins that are encoded by genes located on linear plasmids in the spirochete [1].

The species names of the tickborne *Borrelia* are derived from the species names of *Ornithodorus* tick vectors which carry them rather than from biochemical or antigenic charac-teristics. The more common ones in North America are *B. turicatae, B. hermsii,* and *B. parkeri;* and in Africa, *B. duttoni.*

PATIENT

After exposure to an infected louse or tick, spirochetes enter the skin and gain access to the blood and lymphatic circula-tions. The incubation period lasts from 4 to 18 days after ex-posure, during which the spirochetes divide in the blood plasma. After concentration has built up to 10^6 to 10^8 spiro-chetes per milliliter of blood, the illness begins abruptly with shaking chills, fever, headache, and fatigue [2,3]. Most pa-tients have these symptoms almost continuously throughout the day, whereas some report the intermittent appearance of these symptoms several times a day. Patients complain frequently of myalgia, arthralgia, anorexia, dry cough, and abdominal pains. These symptoms are usually mild on the first day of illness and increase in intensity over a few days, leading to prostra-tion. The nonspecific nature of these symptoms leads patients or their physicians to believe they have a "flulike" illness.

The temperature is elevated in the range of 38.5 to 40°C, and the pulse rate is increased to about 115 per minute. The blood pressure is lowered to about 105/70 mmHg. Patients appear lethargic or may be delirious. Physical signs that are common but not necessarily present include conjunctival in-jection, petechial skin rash that is usually truncal in distribu-tion, and hepatosplenomegaly with occasional jaundice [4]. Disseminated intravascular coagulation also contributes to a decrease in platelets as well as producing prolonged prothrom-bin and partial thromboplastin times and elevated titers of fibrinogen-fibrin degradation products. During acute relapsing

fever, there is evidence that activation of certain plasma pro-teins contributes to the pathogenesis of disseminated intravas-cular coagulation (DIC) and other features such as hypo-tension [5].

The diagnosis of relapsing fever depends on the demonstra-tion of spirochetemia. In most patients, this is readily accom-plished by obtaining peripheral blood by either fingerstick or venipuncture and preparing a thin film on a microscope slide. A routine blood smear stained with Wright's or Giemsa stain is adequate, but blood smears prepared for examination for malaria parasites are also satisfactory. Patients who are in the interval between relapses will have negative smears and should be reexamined when the fever reappears.

Spirochetemia may be detected, alternatively, by dark-field or phase-contrast microscopy. A drop of fresh blood is diluted with another drop of 0.9% NaCl and overlaid with a coverslip. Spirochetes are readily identified by their characteristic rota-tional motility.

Borrelia can be cultivated in Kelly's broth medium or ino-culated intraperitoneally into laboratory mice or rats, and blood of these animals examined daily for 14 days for spirochetemia. Tickborne *Borrelia* are more readily cultivated and recovered from laboratory animals than is the louseborne *B. recurrentis.* Louseborne and tickborne relapsing fever are usually differ-entiated on epidemiological grounds. If vectors can be col-lected from the patient or his or her household, they can be dissected and the hemolymph or coxal fluid examined micro-scopically for the presence of spirochetes.

Serological testing by agglutination, complement fixation, and immobilization of living spirochetes has been employed in endemic areas for purposes of seroepidemiology and examin-ing convalescent patients. None of these tests, however, is standardized or available for general use.

The majority of patients with relapsing fever recover from their illness with or without antibiotic treatment. Patients de-velop antiborrelial antibodies, which can agglutinate, kill, or opsonize the spirochetes. In the presence of opsonizing anti-body, spirochetes are rapidly phagocytized and digested by polymorphonuclear leukocytes [6]. These antibodies partici-pate also in rendering patients immune to future infection with the same serotype of *Borrelia.*

Fatal cases of relapsing fever show high blood counts in the range of 10^8 spirochetes per milliliter. Consequently, all blood-containing tissues will reveal large numbers of spirochetes in vessels when silver stains are employed. Autopsies performed in Ethiopia and Sudan in patients with louseborne relapsing fever showed that the immediate causes of death vary. The spleen is enlarged to as much as 900 g, and the cut surface shows white microabscesses which consist of necrosis and hemorrhage in the white pulp. The liver is also enlarged, and the midzonal regions show scattered necrosis and hemorrhage. The heart is normal in size but frequently shows myocarditis consisting of interstitial edema and a cellular infiltrate of lym-phocytes and plasma cells. The brain usually shows cerebral edema, and in some cases there is hemorrhage into the subarachnoid space or cerebrum [7].

TREATMENT

The relapsing fevers respond to tetracycline and erythromycin. Tetracycline is the treatment of choice except in children less than 7 years old and in pregnant women. Recent studies in Ethiopia indicate that a single oral dose of tetracycline, 500 mg, is as effective in clearing spirochetemia and preventing relapse as longer courses. Erythromycin, 500 mg given orally as a single dose, is a satisfactory alternative to tetracycline [8]. For patients unable to take oral medication, intravenous injection of 250 mg of tetracycline or erythromycin is curative. For children smaller than 30 kg, the dosage of tetracycline or erythromycin should be reduced to approximately 10 mg/kg. Penicillin G therapy results in slow clearance of spirochetes and frequent relapses [9].

In most patients with louseborne relapsing fever and in some with tickborne relapsing fever, antibiotic treatment provokes a distressing Jarisch-Herxheimer reaction. Patients are at greatest risk of dying during the reaction. Some patients undergo a similar spontaneous crisis without antibiotics. Figure 98-2 summarizes the experience of 32 Ethiopian patients with louseborne relapsing fever treated with erythromycin. A rigor occurred 2 to 3 h after treatment in 28 patients. Subsequently,

temperatures rose sharply and blood pressures declined while spirochetes were cleared from the blood [8]. Patients are extremely uncomfortable during the reaction, feeling very cold with severe headache and myalgia. They often express a sense of impending doom. Patients may require intravenous infusions of 0.9% NaCl to maintain adequate blood pressure. Over several hours, the temperature declines and patients feel improved. Attempts to ameliorate the severity of the reaction by giving antipyretic or antiinflammatory drugs have not been successful. The best approach is to anticipate the reaction and to provide intensive nursing care and the intravenous fluid support during the first day of treatment.

Complete recovery occurs in 95 percent or more of adequately treated cases of relapsing fever. The prognosis of untreated disease is grave, particularly with louseborne relapsing fever in which mortality rates of 40 percent have been reported during recent epidemics. The illness is usually fatal in neonatal infections [10].

Untreated cases will also experience relapses. In louseborne relapsing fever, the first attack lasts about 6 days and is followed by an afebrile period of about 9 days. There usually is only one relapse which characteristically lasts only 2 days. In tickborne relapsing fever, the first attack lasts about 3 days and is followed by an interval of about 7 days, after which an average of three relapses occurs, each lasting about 2 days. Relapses are usually milder in intensity than the first attacks.

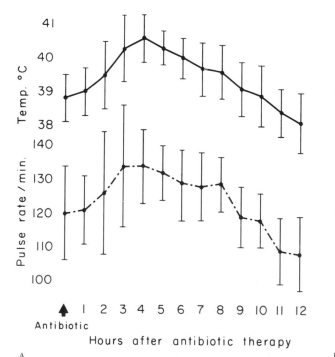

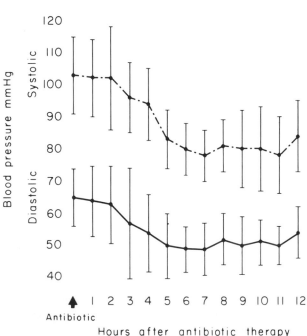

A   B

Figure 98-2. The Jarisch-Herxheimer reaction after antibiotic treatment. After a single oral dose of 500 mg erythromycin stearate, patients underwent a rigor followed by rises in temperature and pulse (**A**) and a fall in blood pressure (**B**).

POPULATION

Relapsing fever is a disease known in antiquity for its epidemic potential, particularly in times of war, migrations, and other conditions that favor human crowding and poor hygiene. Between 1910 and 1945 epidemics of louseborne relapsing fever occurred in North Africa, Sudan, Ethiopia, west Africa, central Africa, eastern Europe, and Russia. In these epidemics there were an estimated 15 million cases, over 5 million deaths, and case fatality rates as high as 73 percent.

The geographical distribution of the relapsing fevers remains widespread with occurrence in most areas of the world [11]. The only areas believed to be entirely free of the relapsing fevers are Australia, New Zealand, and Oceania. Louseborne relapsing fever has disappeared from the United States but still occurs in parts of Latin America, such as the Guatemalan and Andean highlands. During 1960 to 1979 louseborne relapsing fever was documented in Ethiopia and Sudan [11]. Although accurate statistics on the incidence of this disease are not available, Ethiopia appears to be the country with the highest incidence, estimated at approximately 10,000 or more cases a year.

Tickborne relapsing fever occurs in endemic focuses in southern British Columbia, the western United States, the plateau regions of Mexico, and in Central and South America [12]. This disease is present in all areas of Africa except for the Sahara Desert and the rain-forest belt. It occurs also in Spain and Portugal. In Asia, tickborne relapsing fever has been reported in Cyprus, Israel, Syria, Turkey, Iraq, Iran, southern Russia, China, Afghanistan, and India. Accurate statistics on tickborne relapsing fever are not available, but the small numbers of established diagnoses suggests that this form of relapsing fever occurs less frequently in humans than louseborne relapsing fever.

Louseborne and tickborne relapsing fever differ so much in their epidemiology that they must be considered separately. *Epidemic relapsing fever* refers to the louseborne kind and *endemic* or *sporadic relapsing fever* to the tickborne variety.

The only species of *Borrelia* that causes louseborne relapsing fever is *B. recurrentis.* Its vector is the human body louse, *Pediculus humanus humanus,* and the only known natural reservoir is humans. Thus, the cycle of infection is simply from person to person via the louse. Body lice acquire the infection by feeding on a spirochetemic person, and they remain infected for their entire lifespan, which is 10 to 61 days under laboratory conditions [12]. The ingested spirochetes pass through the esophagus to the midgut, where they penetrate the gut epithelium to reach the hemolymph in which they will multiply. Spirochetes do not reach the salivary glands or ovaries of the lice. Therefore, infection is not transmitted to humans by bites of lice and infection cannot be transmitted transovarially to offspring of infected lice. Infection is believed to be transmitted to humans following the crushing of lice on the skin, which allows liberated spirochetes to penetrate through a bite site or

through intact skin. Body lice prefer the normal human body temperature of 37°C to higher temperatures. Thus, lice are likely to leave the skin of a febrile patient to go to another person. This may explain, in part, the rapid transmission of infection during epidemics.

The persons at greatest risk for acquiring louseborne relapsing fever are those living under crowded, unhygienic conditions that favor infestation with body lice. Migrant workers and soldiers in war are particularly prone to develop this infection. Males are at much greater risk than females, presumably because their lives more commonly expose them to infected lice. A strain-specific and short-lived acquired immunity develops following infection. This immunity helps to explain why migrant workers coming into an endemic area are more susceptible to infection than are the permanent inhabitants. In some endemic areas, such as Addis Ababa, Ethiopia, there is an increase in incidence during the cool winter season when people wear heavier clothing that becomes louse-infested.

The vectors of tickborne relapsing fever are argasid ticks of the genus *Ornithodorus.* The major reservoirs of the tickborne relapsing fevers are wild rodents, and occasionally, lizards, toads, turtles, and owls. The infection is passed between the reservoir animals by tick bites and humans are accidental hosts when they come into contact with infected animal ticks. The exception to the animal reservoirs may be *B. duttoni* in east Africa, which is carried by the domestic tick *Ornithodorus moubata,* for which humans appear to be the reservoir. Neonates have acquired infection from their mothers' blood by either transplacental infection or exchange of blood at the time of birth.

Ticks acquire the infection by biting and sucking blood from a spirochetemic animal. The spirochetes, after entering the hemocoele, invade other tissues of the tick, including the salivary glands, coxal glands on the legs, and the ovaries. Transmission of the infection to animals or humans follows injection of infected saliva or coxal fluid through the bite site or intact skin. Ticks are more durable vectors than body lice, being able to survive as long as 15 years between blood meals and to harbor viable spirochetes for years. Additionally, female ticks can pass *Borrelia* spirochetes transovarially to their offspring, thus permitting ticks to be infective without having previously bitten an infected host [12].

Persons at greatest risk of infection are people who come into contact with infected ticks from wild rodents. In the United States the largest outbreak of tickborne relapsing fever occurred in 62 campers and employees in the national park at the northern rim of the Grand Canyon, Arizona, in 1973. Another outbreak in Washington State affected 42 boy scouts who also camped out in a log cabin. In tropical countries, people who live in dwellings that are not rodentproof are prone to infection. In east Africa, where ticks have become domesticated and humans have become a reservoir of tickborne relapsing fever, people living in endemic areas develop immunity to the disease.

PREVENTION AND CONTROL

Available approaches for control of the relapsing fevers include the detection and treatment of human cases, vector control, rodent control, and public health education [7]. Vaccines are not available.

For louseborne relapsing fever, the detection and treatment of cases has the effect of reducing the reservoir of infection and, consequently, reducing transmission. More important is the control of louse infestation. Instructing people to bathe and wash their clothes is the rational approach, but compliance is likely to be low. Delousing of clothing and bodies with insecticides, such as DDT, can be employed, as can the application of insect repellents. In known epidemic situations, prophylactic antibiotics are a temporary measure to contain spread of infection to persons at high risk. The eventual control of this disease requires improvements in personal hygiene and housing conditions.

For tickborne relapsing fever, the treatment of human cases has no impact on the animal reservoirs. It is not possible to control this infection in wild rodents. Campers and hikers going into endemic areas should be advised to avoid staying in cabins that are inhabited by rodents and their ticks, and to apply topical tick repellents to their skin. In endemic areas of Africa, people need to be assisted in building rodentproof houses.

REFERENCES

1 Barbour AG, Hayes SF: Biology of *Borrelia* species. Microbiol Rev 50:381–400, 1986

2 Southern PM, Sanford JP: Relapsing fever. A clinical and microbiological review. Medicine 48:129–149, 1969

3 Horton JM, Blaser MJ: The spectrum of relapsing fever in the Rocky Mountains. Arch Intern Med 145:871–875, 1985

4 Butler T, Hazen P, Wallace CK, Awoke S: *Borrelia recurrentis* infection: Pathogenesis of fever and petechiae. J Infect Dis 140:665–675, 1979

5 Galloway RE, Levin J, Butler T, et al: Activation of protein mediators of inflammation and evidence for endotoxemia in *Borrelia recurrentis* infection. Am J Med 63:933–938, 1977

6 Butler T, Aikawa M, Habte-Michael A, Wallace CK: Phagocytosis of *Borrelia recurrentis* by polymorphonuclear leukocytes is enhanced by antibiotic treatment. Infect Immun 28:1009–1013, 1980

7 Judge DM, Samuel I, Perine PL, et al: Louse-borne relapsing fever in man. Arch Pathol 97:136–140, 1974

8 Butler T, Jones PK, Wallace CK: *Borrelia recurrentis* infection: Single dose antibiotic regimens and management of Jarisch-Herxheimer reaction. J Infect Dis 137:573–577, 1978

9 Warrell DA, Perine PL, Krause DW, et al: Pathophysiology and immunology of the Jarisch-Herxheimer-like reaction in louse-borne relapsing fever: Comparison of tetracycline and slow-release penicillin. J Infect Dis 147:898–909, 1983

10 Yagupsky P, Moses S: Neonatal *Borrelia* species infection (relapsing fever). Am J Dis Child 139:74–76, 1985

11 Ahmed MAM, Abdel Wahab SM, Abdel Malik MD, et al: Louse-borne relapsing fever in the Sudan. A historical review and a clinicopathological study. Trop Geogr Med 32:106–111, 1980

12 Burgdorfer W: The epidemiology of the relapsing fevers, in Johnson RC (ed): *The Biology of Parasitic Spirochetes*. New York, Academic, 1976, pp 191–200

CHAPTER 99 / *Rickettsial Diseases* · Theodore E. Woodward · Joseph V. Osterman

The rickettsial diseases are acute specific febrile illnesses caused by rickettsiae, small bacterialike microorganisms transmitted to humans by arthropod vectors such as ticks, lice, mites, and fleas. Onset of illness is usually sudden with manifestations such as chills, headache, malaise, fever lasting about 2 weeks, and characteristic rashes appearing on about the third to sixth day of illness. Q fever is unassociated with a rash. Anatomical manifestations, including the rash, stem from diffuse scattered focal areas of endangiitis. In severely ill patients, there are encephalitic signs, shock, and renal failure. Serological responses include *Proteus* OX-19 agglutinins and specific antibodies of the complement fixation (CF), macroscopic agglutination (MA), and immune fluorescence antibody (IFA) types in the patient's serum during the second to third weeks of illness. Therapeutic response is prompt using chloramphenicol or tetracycline antibiotics.

Rickettsial diseases occur in all countries although their prevalence and clinical significance varies. They may be either sporadic or epidemic, dependent upon ecological or epidemiological factors. Because causative rickettsiae are well and permanently established in their natural habitat, physicians must remain alert in their recognition of these disorders in order to apply appropriate treatment and effective control.

The important global rickettsioses are Rocky Mountain spotted fever, other tickborne rickettsial diseases, epidemic typhus, murine typhus, scrub typhus, Q fever, and trench fever. Rick-

Table 99-1. The rickettsial diseases, their geographical distribution, vectors, known reservoirs, and modes of transmission*

Disease	Agent	Geographical distribution	Arthropod	Mammal	Principal means of transmission to humans
Spotted fever group					
Rocky Mountain spotted fever	*R. rickettsii*	Western Hemisphere	Ticks	Wild rodents, dogs	Tick bite
Boutonneuse fever	*R. conorii*	Africa, Europe, Middle East, India	Ticks		Tick bite
Queensland tick typhus	*R. australis*	Australia	Ticks	Marsupials, wild rodents	Tick bite
North Asian tickborne rickettsioses	*R. siberica*	Siberia, Mongolia	Ticks	Wild rodents	Tick bite
Rickettsialpox	*R. akari*	United States, Russia, Africa	Mites	House mouse, other rodents	Mite bite
Typhus fever group					
Endemic (murine)	*R. mooseri*	Worldwide	Fleas	Small rodents	Infected flea feces into broken skin
Epidemic	*R. prowazekii* *R. canada*	Worldwide North America	Body lice Ticks	Humans, flying squirrels	Infected louse feces into broken skin
Brill-Zinsser disease	*R. prowazekii*	Worldwide	Recrudescence years after original attack of epidemic typhus		
Scrub	*R. tsutsugamushi*	Asia, Australia, Pacific Islands	Trombiculid mites	Wild rodents	Mite bite
Other rickettsial diseases					
Q fever	*C. burnetii*	Worldwide	Ticks	Small mammals, cattle, sheep, goats	Inhalation of dried infected material

*Reprinted from *Harrison's Principles of Internal Medicine,* 9th ed., McGraw-Hill Book Co., 1980.

ettsialpox and Brill-Zinsser disease (recurrent typhus) occur sporadically in certain areas. Table 99-1 is a compendium of information on the rickettsial diseases.

HISTORY

Ricketts, from 1906 to 1909, first clarified the tick transmission of Rocky Mountain spotted fever (RMSF) in the Bitterroot Valley of Montana and identified the causative organisms by successfully infecting animals using blood from patients and infected ticks [1].

In 1930 RMSF was specifically identified in the eastern coastal states and in Central and South America, particularly Brazil (São Paulo typhus).

Classic louseborne typhus is the epidemic disease which accompanies wars, famine, drought, and conditions of human misery fostering louse infestation. Nicolle, working in Tunisia in 1909, incriminated the louse as vector; da Rocha Lima and Von Prowazek identified rickettsiae in louse tissues (1914). In 1915, Weil and Felix [2] reported the *Proteus* OX-19 reaction following their demonstration that blood serum from convalescent typhus patients agglutinated *Proteus* bacilli. Brill, 1910, reported a series of 211 patients observed by him from 1898 to 1910 having what resembled mild typhus fever [3].

Much later Zinsser documented that Brill's cases were recrudescent typhus which recurred years after the initial illness. This phenomenon is now called Brill-Zinsser disease [4].

In 1926, Maxcy astutely observed that mild cases of endemic typhus, often erroneously called "Brill's disease" in the southeastern United States, occurred in persons in close proximity to food depots or granaries. Maxcy proposed and Dyer subsequently confirmed that rodents such as rats or mice might serve as the reservoir and that fleas or ticks were the vectors [5]. Murine or rat-flea typhus occurs sporadically throughout the world [6].

Q fever was not recognized as a specific illness until Derrick described Australian patients whose manifestations included fever, headache, respiratory signs, and occasional hepatic involvement without rash. Burnet and Cox simultaneously reported the isolation of an organism from ticks, now called *Coxiella burnetii* [7,8]. Q fever occurred in epidemic numbers in the Balkan states and in Italy during World War II.

The vector and rodent reservoir of scrub typhus were first identified by Japanese investigators [9–11]. Investigations in Malaysia distinguished between typhus (murine typhus) and rural typhus (scrub typhus) through case identification, evaluation of the rickettsiae in animals, and the differing serological responses to *Proteus* OX-19 and *Proteus* OX-K.

PARASITE

Rickettsiae are small gram-negative bacilli that are distinct from other bacteria because of their obligate intracellular parasitism. They typically range in size from 1.0 to 2.0 μm by 0.3 μm, but pleomorphism is common. Rickettsiae multiply by transverse binary fission, and it has been shown [12] that the morphology of *Rickettsia prowazekii* is influenced by the state of its intracellular growth. Organisms in the logarithmic phase of growth evidence the classic bacillary form while those in the stationary phase become aberrant and frequently exhibit either a filamentous or coccoid form.

Coxiella burnetii is a small, extremely pleomorphic gram-variable organism with forms which vary from 0.1 to 0.3 μm by 0.1 to 2.0 μm. Electron microscope studies show that the organism has a plasma membrane and cell wall which are similar in thickness and trilaminar in structure. The extreme pleomorphism of *C. burnetii* suggested that a complex developmental cycle could be operative. Recently, definitive evidence has been presented to suggest that large cell variants (LCV) and small cell variants (SCV) exist, with the SCV originating in the periplasmic space of the LCV. Although both variants are capable of binary cell division, the SCV apparently can enlarge to form the LCV.

The basis for the obligate intracellular parasitism of rickettsiae is unknown. They are capable of some independent metabolic activities and produce energy by the catabolism of glutamate to ammonia and carbon dioxide. Rickettsiae appear to have a tricarboxylic acid cycle, but not a complete glycolytic or hexose monophosphate pathway [13]. An electron transport system is functional, and oxidative energy can be utilized to form adenosine triphosphate (ATP). In addition, typhus rickettsiae can acquire ATP from the host cell cytoplasmic milieu by a carrier-mediated ATP-ADP exchange system, presumably located in the rickettsial cytoplasmic membrane [14]. Proteins are synthesized in small quantities by rickettsiae, and formation of these macromolecules is inhibited by chloramphenicol and tetracycline. An active transport system for lysine has been described in *R. prowazekii*.

The entry of typhus rickettsiae into eukaryotic cells is an active process that requires expenditure of energy by the rickettsiae and the host cell [15]. The typhus, scrub typhus, and spotted fever group organisms all grow in the cytoplasm of infected cells, but spotted fever group rickettsiae are distinguished by their ability to grow also in the cell nucleus. Typhus and spotted fever group organisms can be differentiated by the manner in which they exit infected cells. *R. prowazekii* grows luxuriantly in the cytoplasm until the cell undergoes lysis and rickettsiae are released in a burst of viable organisms. Spotted fever group rickettsiae, on the other hand, apparently leave the cell over the entire replicative period, with minimal damage to the host cell plasma membrane [12,16].

C. burnetii shares many of the biochemical activities described for organisms in the genus *Rickettsia*, but it is set apart from them by the presence of enzymes important in the glycolytic and hexose monophosphate pathways. The in vitro metabolism of glucose by whole cells of *C. burnetii* has been found to be enhanced by low pH. The transport, catabolism, and incorporation of both glucose and glutamate were found to be highly stimulated by acidic conditions at pH 4.5 [17].

C. burnetii enters cells primarily by phagocytosis and remains within the phagocytic vacuole. Subsequent fusion of phagosomes with lysosomes results in a lowering of the pH within the phagolysosome to a point where the metabolic activities of *C. burnetii* are stimulated. This rickettsia, therefore, has evolved a possibly unique parasitic mechanism based on the regulation of microbial metabolism by hydrogen ion concentration–dependent stimulation of rickettsial function.

Genomic components of both *R. prowazekii* and *C. burnetii* have been cloned in *Escherichia coli* [18,19]. The gene for citrate synthetase in these organisms was localized to a 1.2- to 2.0-kilobase chromosomal fragment, and the translational product had a molecular weight of 46,000 to 49,000 Da.

The animals of choice for laboratory experimentation with rickettsiae are the adult male guinea pig and the adult mouse. Typhus and spotted fever organisms, as well as *C. burnetii*, are pathogenic for the guinea pig. Intraperitoneal inoculation results in a febrile response (40°C or higher), but the infections are generally self-limiting and the animals recover without sequelae. Infection with *Rickettsia typhi* and some members of the spotted fever group also results in inflammation and swelling of the scrotum. *Rickettsia rickettsii* is the most virulent species of the spotted fever group for guinea pigs. Some strains produce fever, a severe scrotal reaction with necrosis, and are lethal for the animals.

Scrub typhus rickettsiae, and one species of the spotted fever group (*Rickettsia akari*) are pathogenic for mice. The response of inbred mice to infection with *R. tsutsugamushi* is influenced markedly by the strain of rickettsiae (Karp, Gilliam, or Kato) and the genetic background of the mice. Certain strains of inbred mice are genetically resistant to lethal intraperitoneal infection with the Gilliam strain [20] and this natural resistance is controlled by a single, autosomal dominant gene not linked to the H-2 complex [21]. The other two prototype strains, Karp and Kato, appear to be lethal for all inbred strains of mice. Infection of mice with *R. akari* is also influenced both by the strain of rickettsiae (Kaplan, Hartford) and the genetic background of the mice [22]. Only C3H/HeJ mice are killed by less than 100 Kaplan.

PATHOGENESIS

Recent investigations in laboratory animals have resulted in emerging recognition of the role of cellular immune events in modulating rickettsial disease. Resistance to scrub typhus rickettsiae can be transferred passively to naive mice using either unfractionated immune spleen cells or immune thymus-derived lymphocytes (T cells) [23]. Normal macrophages can be activated in vitro by soluble products of T cells (lymphokines) to become rickettsicidal [24]. These results suggest that in vivo mechanisms of immunity to *R. tsutsugamushi* may involve the interaction of specifically sensitized T cells with rickettsial antigens for the production of lymphokines which activate macrophages to become effector cells.

Delayed-type hypersensitivity (DTH) has been demonstrated in mice infected with *R. tsutsugamushi* [25]. Temporal development of this response was similar to that for protective immunity, and DTH reactivity could be transferred from immune to normal syngeneic mice by T lymphocytes.

The immune response of the host to rickettsial infection is likely to be a surface-surface interaction, with primary recognition of rickettsial peripheral cell wall components. Six major proteins of *R. prowazekii,* ranging in molecular weight from 13,000 to 87,000 Da [26] have been identified in purified cell wall preparations. The topographical relationship of these proteins suggests that two (87,000 and 27,000 daltons) are the most peripheral and likely to be significant in immune recognition [27]. Subsequent studies established that the 87,000-Da protein is a species-specific antigen which is readily extracted from typhus rickettsiae [28] and capable of eliciting a protective response in guinea pigs against both local and systemic dissemination of rickettsiae [29]. Similar analyses have been performed on the three prototype strains of *R. tsutsugamushi* [30].

In addition to the direct interaction of rickettsiae with the immune system, it appears that T cells from immune animals are able to recognize rickettsial antigens on the cell membrane of infected cells. Mouse lymphocytes are able to specifically lyse tissue culture target cells infected with homologous rickettsiae [31]. This T-cell-mediated cytotoxic immune mechanism also exhibits H-2 restriction when lymphocytes are tested on infected target cells of a different genetic background.

Cellular immunity to *C. burnetii* has been demonstrated in human subjects with various past histories of exposure to the organism by using the lymphocyte transformation (LT) assay. Individuals with histories of exposure to Q fever organisms up to 8 years earlier demonstrated marked lymphocyte transformation in vitro to whole cell antigens. In vitro studies with guinea pig macrophages indicated that specific antiserum reacted with *C. burnetii* failed to control rickettsial intracellular replication [32], but macrophages activated by lymphokines did. Thus, it appears that protective immunity to Q fever infection depends on the development of activated macrophages produced only when T lymphocytes react with rickettsial antigen and elaborate appropriate lymphokines.

C. burnetii undergoes an apparent host-controlled modification in the chemistry of its peripheral cell wall. The organism is found in phase I in nature, but multiple passages in eggs result in the emergence of phase II rickettsiae. Phase I antigen extracted with trichloroacetic acid (TCA) causes a potent LT response in cells from immune donors. Phase II organisms are believed to be a rough variant of the rickettsiae and devoid of the capsularlike phase I antigen [33].

Rickettsial-laden feces of the tick, louse, flea, or mite which causes RMSF, epidemic, murine, and scrub typhus, respectively, are deposited in the skin when feeding at the site of arthropod attachment. Rickettsiae may also gain access via the mucous membranes and the respiratory tract. After arthropod attachment for several hours, infection is acquired through minute skin abrasions contaminated by infected feces or juices. Rickettsiae multiply initially at the site of arthropod attachment, and local lesions (eschars) develop with considerable rapidity in scrub typhus, the tickborne rickettsioses of the eastern hemisphere, rickettsialpox, and occasionally in RMSF. Figure 99-1 shows several types of primary lesions.

Q fever generally results from inhalation of rickettsial-laden aerosols derived from infected animal or tick excretions or the drinking of contaminated milk. All rickettsiae, including *C. burnetii,* are particularly hardy and maintain viability in infected hides or when dried for long periods.

Rickettsiae enter the blood from the initial site, i.e., skin, membranes, and undoubtedly circulate and penetrate endothelial cells, although the mechanism of entry is unknown. Vascular lesions develop at these randomly distributed sites of endothelial penetration and probably account for pathological abnormalities including the rash. Rickettsiae of RMSF and Q fever have been transmitted to humans from donors whose blood was taken inadvertently during the incubation of their illnesses [34].

Illness occurs after incubation periods ranging from 3 to 20 days; there is variation for each rickettsial disease. Short incubations in RMSF and epidemic typhus fever usually indicate more serious infections. Studies in volunteers ill with Q fever, murine typhus, and RMSF showed rickettsemia late in the incubation period prior to febrile onset [35]. Little is known of the pathogenesis during mid-incubation. Volunteers infected with rickettsiae of murine typhus, RMSF, and Q fever show febrile rises just prior to onset when low-grade rickettsemia is present. Conceivably this indicates release of rickettsiae into the circulation from the initial sites of multiplication with further diffuse rickettsial seeding throughout the vascular system [27,36]. It is unknown whether the capillary permeability and endovasculitis which typifies the rickettsial infections results from direct action of the rickettsiae, their toxic reactions or their immunopathological or cellular (hypersensitivity) reactions.

Endothelial cells of small blood vessels are the usual sites of rickettsial involvement with endothelial cell swelling, cellular degeneration, local thrombus formation, and complete or partial occlusion of capillaries and arterioles. Arteriolar muscle cells undergo degenerative changes such as swelling, fibrinoid infiltration, and mononuclear leukocyte invasion of the adventitia by lymphocytes and plasma cells. Vasculitis in severely ill patients with RMSF is usually randomly distributed, but diffuse, involving localized areas of arterioles, veins, and cap-

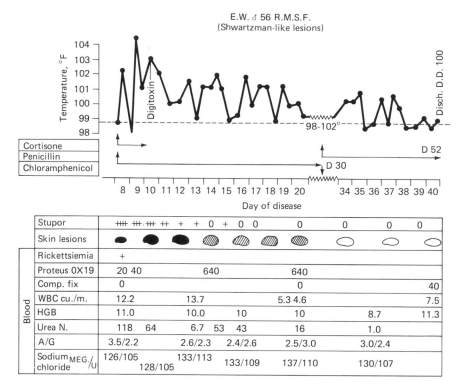

E.W. ♂ 56 R.M.S.F.
(Shwartzman-like lesions)

		Stupor	+++	+++	+++	++	+	+	0	+	0	0		0		0		0		0				
		Skin lesions																						
		Rickettsiemia	+																						
		Proteus 0X19	20 40				640				640														
		Comp. fix	0							0									40						
	Blood	WBC cu./m.	12.2				13.7				5.3 4.6									7.5					
		HGB	11.0				10.0		10			10					8.7		11.3						
		Urea N.	118	64			6.7	53		43		16				1.0									
		A/G	3.5/2.2				2.6/2.3		2.4/2.6			2.5/3.0			3.0/2.4										
		Sodium chloride MEG./U	126/105	128/105		133/113			133/109			137/110			130/107										

Figure 99-1. Shown is the graphic record of a 56-year-old man who was severely ill with Rocky Mountain spotted fever. On the eighth day of illness, when the patient was first hospitalized, he was treated immediately with chloramphenicol and corticosteroids. Patient was semidelirious with a diffuse ecchymotic rash. Careful supportive care and antibiotic treatment led to full recovery after a protracted clinical course. Rickettsemia was demonstrated, and positive Weil-Felix tests and complement-fixation reactions were confirmatory. On admission, the blood urea nitrogen determination was 118 mg/100 mL.

illaries with normal vascular architecture preserved elsewhere [37–39].

Localized and minute parenchymatous abnormalities appear diffusely adjacent to the vascular lesions. The most conspicuous of these are in the brain, cardiac and skeletal muscle, lung, and kidneys. Mental confusion and coma undoubtedly result from cerebral glial nodules which are a cellular reaction adjacent to a capillary or arteriole in patients with RMSF, epidemic, murine, and scrub typhus (see Fig. 99-2). Minute cellular infarcts result from the anemic necrosis caused by the intimal reaction and thrombotic occlusion which may occur in all tissues. Pneumonitis occurs in patients with RMSF and typhus fever and is more characteristic in patients with Q fever [35]. The alterations are primarily interstitial, resembling the pneumonic infiltrations caused by *Mucoplasma, Legionella* [40], and influenza virus. With specific fixation and staining techniques, including immunofluorescence (IF), rickettsiae (and *Legionella,* which are similar morphologically) are visualized in endothelial cells of skin, lung, muscle, brain, and other tissues by biopsy or at postmortem.

Wolbach carefully described the histological lesions of RMSF and epidemic typhus in classic monographs [37,42]. Subsequent studies attribute the character and evolution of the rash, skin necrosis, and gangrene to localized rickettsiae and the resulting angiitis [39] (see Fig. 99-3).

Following intravenous injection of a toxic fraction derived from rickettsiae [41], a specific toxin action produces vaso-

constriction, plasma leakage, and hemoconcentration in animal capillaries. This toxic effect is not potentiated by epinephrine, which distinguishes this reaction from endotoxin. Capillary leakage, tissue edema, and hemorrhage may also result from toxic action but the mechanism is not known.

Aspects of vasculitis such as diffuse skin hemorrhage and necroses late in rickettsial illness can be explained by abnormal

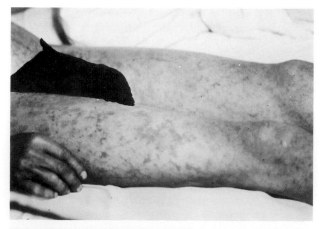

Figure 99-2. Rocky Mountain spotted fever. Extensive purpuric rash in the severely ill patient described in Fig. 99-1. These lesions are compatible with those found in those patients who manifest disseminated intravascular coagulopathy.

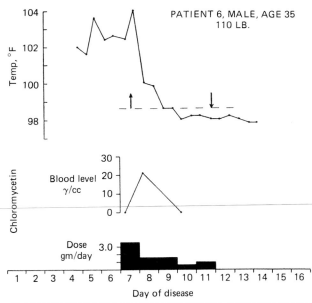

PATIENT 6, MALE, AGE 35
110 LB.

WF OX-19		128	512
WF OX-K		40	40
Rick	Murine	160	640
Aggln	Epidemic	0	80

Figure 99-3. Murine typhus fever. Shown is the graphic record of a murine typhus fever patient first treated with Chloromycetin (chloramphenicol) on the seventh febrile day. Headache and systemic manifestations abated promptly, and defervescence occurred in $2\frac{1}{2}$ days. Full recovery occurred. Clinical diagnosis was confirmed by positive *Proteus* OX-19 and rickettsial agglutination reactions. This is the characteristic type of clinical response to antibiotic treatment in rickettsial disease patients treated sufficiently early in their illness. (*Courtesy U.S. Army Scrub Typhus Team, Maylaya.*)

antigen-antibody (immune complex) reactions. These diffuse dermal and tissue changes tend to occur when measurable antibody titers are present and rickettsemia persists. Administration of hyperimmune convalescent serum at this time causes capillary leakage and tissue edema [38]. In RMSF patients studied early in their illness, however, no interactions of complement activity were found [43].

Cell-mediated immunity may be an important mechanism useful for inhibition and eradication of rickettsiae in tissues. Patients convalescent from various rickettsioses exhibit delayed hypersensitivity reactions to injected rickettsial antigens [44] and these hypersensitivity reactions could contribute to the vasculitis.

In RMSF, scrub typhus, and louseborne typhus fever, which are the life-threatening rickettsioses, there are abnormal physiological and chemical changes which require attention. Generally these changes do not occur in the first week or in mild to moderately ill patients. As a sequel to the vasculitis and resultant capillary injury, there is leakage of fluid, electrolytes,

and albumin into the tissues from the plasma [36,38] to produce an expanded extravascular space and tissue edema (see Fig. 99-4). Skin hemorrhages produce leakage of blood, first as petechiae, and later as ecchymoses. In such severely ill patients there is decreased blood volume, hypotension, hyponatremia, hypochloremia, and hypoalbuminuria, usually by the middle of the second week. Oliguria and azotemia develop in association with the hypovolemia and widespread breakdown of microinfarcted tissues. All of these findings, including mild anemia, are consequent to the vascular and tissue changes and renal decompensation. Their correction must be planned and based on clinical judgment and the pertinent pathophysiological abnormalities. Overloading of the circulation with excessive intravenous fluids must be avoided.

The clinical signs and symptoms of rickettsioses are similar and so they are described together with the significant exceptions noted.

A history of a tick bite in a wooded area (Rocky Mountain spotted fever and other tickborne rickettsioses), louse infestation in a known endemic area of epidemic typhus, flea bites in a rat-infested population (murine typhus), or exposure to mites in jungle or rural tropical settings (scrub typhus) offer important epidemiological clues. Sheep herders and abattoir workers are often exposed to the agent of Q fever.

After infection, the incubation periods are variable. Generally, shorter incubation periods result from heavier exposure to the infectious agent and are attended with more severe illnesses. The incubation period of Q fever is longer, averaging about 19 days. Before the actual onset of most rickettsioses, there are prodromata of malaise, headache, and feverish and chilly reactions. At this time, rickettsiae are probably circulating freely in the vascular system.

Prodromal symptoms increase in severity with an accompanying general ill feeling, chills or prostration, myalgia, arthralgia, and headache. Temperature may reach 104°F on the first day or two and is sustained. There may also be nausea and vomiting. Myalgia involves large muscle groups, particularly the legs, thighs, and abdominal muscles with tenderness on palpation. RMSF, epidemic, scrub, and murine typhus commonly have a sudden onset, often obvious within an hour. At other times the onset may be slower or vague with irritability, anorexia, insomnia, headache, and low-grade fever. Cough and other pulmonary manifestations may be latent and delayed. A high sustained febrile curve is maintained with slight morning remissions of only a degree or two in RMSF, epidemic, scrub, and murine typhus fevers. After about 12 to 14 days, the fever pattern becomes remittent with defervescence occurring by slow lysis during several days. Fall of temperature by crisis is uncommon. In murine typhus, Q fever, and other tickborne rickettsioses, the duration of fever is also continuous but usually shorter.

Recurrence of fever or relapse is uncommon except when effective antibiotics are given before the fifth day in scrub typhus or with secondary pyogenic infections. When fever re-

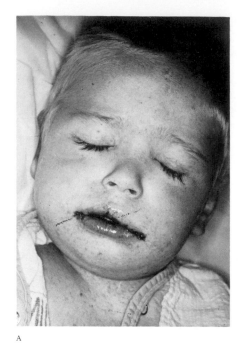

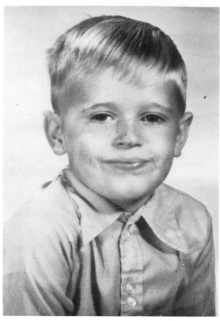

A   B

Figure 99-4. *A.* Rocky Mountain spotted fever. Facial edema of boy, aged 4, on about ninth febrile day. Note petechial rash of chin and upper trunk. Patient in coma with encephalitis. *B.* Same patient showing full recovery after about 6 weeks' convalescence. Full recovery.

curs, particularly in scrub typhus, it responds to a second course of therapy. Fortunately, rickettsiae have not developed antibiotic resistance.

Most patients ill with the major rickettsioses develop distinctive rashes by the fourth febrile day (range 2 to 6 days). In RMSF, epidemic, scrub, and murine typhus, the first lesions are flat, delicate, pink, and measure 2 to 6 mm in diameter (see Fig. 99-5). In RMSF, the lesions are initially on the palms, soles, and forearms; in epidemic and scrub typhus, they begin on the trunk and the axillae with later involvement of the buttocks, thighs, and mid-forearms but spare the periphery. In murine typhus and Brill-Zinsser disease, the rash is less prominent. The rash of tickborne typhus (*R. conorii*) is maculopapular and is diffusely distributed. Q fever is unassociated with a rash.

Primary lesions with local adenitis are noted in scrub typhus (mite), tickborne rickettsioses of the eastern hemisphere (tick), and occasionally in RMSF (tick). Rickettsialpox is typified by a primary eschar at the site of the infected mite attachment and there is a sparse vesicular rash. In seriously ill patients with unabated progress of RMSF, the skin lesions subsequently become petechial and fixed (do not fade on pressure). In such patients, purplish ecchymoses result in dermal necroses with gangrene, particularly over pressure points, the digits, and scrotum.

Headache occurs in practically all the rickettsioses. In RMSF and the typhus fevers, it is severe and often frontal. Patients are restless, irritable, unable to sleep, and complain of muscle pain, often with muscle rigidity and stiffness of the neck and back muscles. In louseborne typhus and RMSF, very ill patients look toxic, develop purposeless movements, mutter, lapse into coma, and may develop seizures. These signs are indicative of diffuse encephalitis. The cerebrospinal fluid is usually clear (not more than 15 to 20 mononuclear cells/μL) with increased pressure and normal chemical values. Deafness may occur in severely ill patients. Recovery is usually complete with adequate treatment.

In some patients with typhus fever and RMSF, a nonproductive, harassing cough occurs which is indicative of bronchiolitis. Pneumonia with consolidation is uncommon although pulmonary edema occurs with too-free use of intravenous fluids in patients with RMSF and epidemic typhus. In Q fever, lung involvement is common and roentgenographic findings simulate those of "atypical pneumonia." Lung manifestations persist beyond the febrile period.

During the first week, the pulse is regular and accelerates with the temperature rise. In severely ill patients with RMSF and epidemic typhus, the pulse weakens in the second week and hypotension develops. With sustained vascular abnormalities, there is anoxia, cyanosis, agitation, and mental confusion. At this stage, the patient becomes livid with numerous ecchymoses and beginning gangrene of the fingers, buttocks, scrotum, and occasionally the earlobes or nose. Congestive heart failure is uncommon. Electrocardiographic changes usually show transient, nonspecific myocardial changes. Rarely, myocarditis may trigger fatal cardiac arrhythmias or cardiac arrest. In Q fever, endocarditis is a late manifestation of the illness [45,46]. The aortic valve is most commonly involved

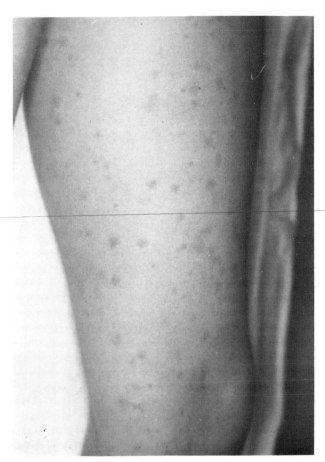

Figure 99-5. Rocky Mountain spotted fever. Characteristic pink macular rash on about the fourth febrile day. Full, rapid recovery.

and often this rickettsial infection develops on previously damaged valves [46,47]. Blood cultures are negative and diagnosis is made on suspicion and the presence of antibodies to phase I antigens of *C. burnetii*.

Oliguria, anuria, albuminuria, and azotemia occur in severely ill patients with RMSF, epidemic, murine, and scrub typhus. Oliguria and anuria result from the vascular decompensation and hypotension. Azotemia results from these vascular abnormalities plus tissue breakdown of the necroses and vascular lesions of the skin and organs and is a poor prognostic sign.

Hepatomegaly occurs in the major rickettsioses. Jaundice is uncommon and when present, there is elevation of the liver enzymes and alkaline phosphatase. In Q fever, approximately one-third of patients develop acute or chronic protracted hepatitis [47]. Biopsy specimens show diffuse granulomatous changes with multinucleated giant cells, scattered infiltrations of polymorphonuclear leukocytes, lymphocytes, and macrophages without caseation. *C. burnetii* is readily identifiable by

IF techniques. A chronic, low-grade form of hepatitis occurs in some patients.

Often in typhus and RMSF there is dehydration, conjunctivitis, and photophobia, with petechiae and/or hemorrhages occurring in the bulbar or palpebral conjunctivae. Most patients are constipated but abdominal distension without localized tenderness is indicative of ileus. Complications in the severely ill include otitis media, parotitis, bronchopneumonia, gangrene of the digits or other tissues, and indolent skin ulcerations which develop at the sites of ecchymoses and necrotic tissue. Disseminated intravascular coagulopathy (DIC) occurs in all the severe rickettsioses with thrombocytopenia, altered values of prothrombin time, thromboplastin time, and low values of fibrinogen [48].

LABORATORY DIAGNOSIS

Routine laboratory values are not diagnostic in the rickettsioses and merely reflect abnormalities in tissues. Severely ill patients may show mild microcytic anemia, and normal or only slightly elevated leukocyte counts; leukopenia occurs occasionally. Moderate leukocytosis occurs when there are hemorrhagic necroses or pyogenic complications such as parotitis or pneumonia. Severely ill patients with RMSF or epidemic typhus show hypochloremia, hyponatremia, azotemia, and hypoalbuminemia. When DIC is present, the anticipated abnormalities in coagulation occur. The sedimentation rate is elevated.

Causative rickettsiae may be isolated from the patient's blood during the first week of illness or from postmortem tissues by inoculation of laboratory animals and subsequent subculturing in hens' eggs or tissue culture systems. Isolation procedures are not recommended for routine use because of the expense, time, and hazard to laboratory personnel.

In clinical practice, the available serological tests are accurate provided the physician collects early (acute) and late (convalescent) serum specimens for submission. The *Proteus* OX-19 (Weil-Felix) agglutination reaction is positive in patients with RMSF, epidemic, murine, and tickborne rickettsioses. The *Proteus* OX-K reaction is positive in about one-half of patients with scrub typhus. The W-F reaction is negative or too low to be helpful in patients with Q fever, rickettsialpox or Brill-Zinsser disease. This test is not specific but only suggests the presence of a rickettsial infection. A titer of 1:160 is said to be diagnostic but it is more reliable to demonstrate a rise in titer.

The complement-fixation (CF) reaction using specific rickettsial antigens formerly was the most reliable confirmatory test. It has been replaced by IFA and MA tests which are now standard for most reference laboratories. It is necessary to show a rise in antibiotic titers to be specifically helpful [49].

It is possible to visualize rickettsiae by IFA techniques in specimens of skin obtained by biopsy [50] or tissue specimens such as liver or lung using either fresh specimens or after fixation in paraffin [51].

TREATMENT

In severely ill patients with RMSF or the typhus group, supportive therapeutic regimens are based on the correction of oliguria, hypotension, hypochloremia, hyponatremia, hypoalbuminemia, azotemia, edema, and coma. Careful use of serum albumin given intravenously will help support the circulation. Although it seems tempting to give intravenous fluids freely, such should be avoided in the presence of oliguria, edema, hypotension, and other circulatory changes. Dialysis may benefit some patients with renal shutdown.

Proper mouth care is needed. Frequent turning of the patient will help prevent aspiration pneumonia and pressure necroses of involved skin areas. When azotemia is minimal, nutritional support should include 2 to 3 g protein/kg. In confused or comatose patients without ileus or abdominal distension, tube feedings are helpful.

Chloramphenicol and the tetracyclines are specifically effective for the rickettsioses. These antibiotics, in spite of being only rickettsiostatic, lead to abatement of toxic and other clinical signs in 24 to 36 h and defervescence in 2 to 3 days. In scrub typhus, the response is more dramatic, whereas in Q fever clinical improvement may be less rapid. When therapy is delayed until the stage of diffuse hemorrhagic lesions with ecchymoses and skin necroses, the response is less dramatic but recovery will occur with proper management.

Generally the dosages of antibiotics are: chloramphenicol—an initial dose of 50 mg per kilogram of body weight and subsequent daily doses calculated on the same basis with treatment intervals of 6 to 8 h. For the tetracyclines, the same schedule is followed based on 25 mg per kilogram of body weight. Antibiotic treatment is given until improvement is obvious and the patient has been afebrile for about 1 day (defervescence usually occurs in moderately ill patients in 2 to 3 days). Intravenous doses of either antibiotic are given when the patient is too ill to take oral medications [52–55]. As soon as possible, the oral route should be used. Under special conditions, a single large oral dose of chloramphenicol has been effective in scrub typhus and RMSF. Under primitive conditions, a single oral dose of 200 mg doxycycline was effective in epidemic typhus fever [56].

Critically ill patients may be helped by large doses of corticosteroids given for several days in conjunction with specific antibiotics and supportive care. They are not recommended or necessary for routine use in mild or moderately ill patients. Heparin has not been effective in correcting DIC phenomena.

POPULATION

ROCKY MOUNTAIN SPOTTED FEVER

Humans are accidentally infected when ticks transmit *R. rickettsii* either through tick attachment or through contamination of conjunctivas or abrasions of skin contaminated by infected tick feces or tissue juices. Four species of ixodid ticks are natural carriers of *R. rickettsii*—*Dermacentor andersoni* (Rocky Mountain wood tick), *Dermacentor variabilis* (the American dog tick), *Amblyomma americanum* (lone-star tick), and *Haemaphysalis leporus-palustris* (rabbit tick). *D. andersoni* and *D. variabilis* are the major vectors in the western and eastern United States, respectively. *Amblyomma americanum* infestation occurs in the south central and southeastern United States [57]. The rabbit tick rarely bites humans but it transmits spotted fever to other rabbits and helps maintain rickettsiae in human-infesting species of ticks. In Brazil and Colombia, the vector tick is *Amblyomma caijenneuse*.

The tick is a natural vector and reservoir since it survives the infection and transmits the agent readily to its offspring. Ticks remain infected for life. Infected small animals infect other ticks which feed on them.

Early in the season, ticks must usually remain attached for several hours before they cause infection. During warm months, the time of feeding and transmission is shorter. This phenomenon is called *reactivation* and represents a change from a nonvirulent resting phase (after overwintering and hibernation) to a virulent phase brought about by the ingestion of fresh blood, which changes the microbes' metabolism. Spotted fever occurs in the late spring and summer months because of hibernation of ticks during winter. Rickettsialpox which is antigenically related to RMSF occurs sporadically in the eastern United States and the U.S.S.R.

EPIDEMIC TYPHUS FEVER

Epidemic typhus is transmitted to humans by the body louse, which accounts for its epidemic tendencies given conditions of poverty and low health standards. Poor sanitary conditions favor lousiness during cold months. Persons of all ages are susceptible. Usually the illness is milder in children; higher mortality rates occur in adults and the elderly.

Lice, when they feed, drop infected feces onto the skin; infection occurs through minute abrasions or through contamination of conjunctivas and mucous membranes. *R. prowazekii* is quite resistant when dried and can be infectious for months. The human body louse dies of its infection; infected females do not transmit the agent to their offspring. Usually, outbreaks of typhus cease during warm months because of better bathing practices and decreased louse infestation.

Recently, flying squirrels in many eastern states have been implicated as infected hosts of *R. prowazekii* [58]; several dozen cases have been reported in humans who were in contact with such squirrels and their ectoparasites. The entire cycle of squirrel-vector-human infestation has not been fully elucidated but these findings presumably establish that humans are not the sole reservoir of *R. prowazekii* as originally surmised [59,60]. Person-to-person transmission through contact with saliva, sputum, urine, or human feces has not been shown.

Epidemic louseborne typhus exists now in the cold environments of Europe, Africa, Asia, and Latin and South America. Although it is largely controlled and of sporadic incidence, louseborne typhus remains an important cause of morbidity and mortality when socioeconomic and environmental conditions allow proper interplay between the microbe, vectors, and susceptible populations. The principal focuses are the highlands of central Africa, including Ethiopia, Burundi, Rwanda, southern Uganda, Nigeria, and Algeria; and Bolivia, Ecuador, and Peru in South America.

MURINE TYPHUS FEVER

The rat, *Rattus rattus* and *Rattus norvegicus,* is the natural reservoir of *Rickettsia mooseri;* mice are also susceptible. Infection in rodents is nonfatal and viable rickettsiae may persist in their brains for variable periods. The rat flea, *Xenopsylla cheopis,* is infected by feeding on rats during the acute stage of their infection. Once infected, fleas discharge pathogenic rickettsiae in their feces throughout their normal life cycle. Dried flea feces may infect humans via the conjunctivas or respiratory tract. *Pulex irritans* and human body lice are susceptible to experimentally induced murine typhus infection. Guinea pigs are readily susceptible to intraperitoneal inoculation of infected tissues or blood from patients during the active stages of illness. Humans are at risk when their activities bring them in contact with infected rats and their fleas near granaries and food depots or in congested, infested areas such as harbors.

Murine typhus occurs commonly in port cities and in densely crowded populations where rats and fleas are prevalent. Epidemic louseborne typhus fever, a clinically much more severe first cousin of murine typhus, has ravaged human populations during wars, famine, and poverty, or during periods of privation.

SCRUB TYPHUS FEVER

Scrub typhus infection is well established in nature as "typhus islands" in cycles involving mites and small rodents. Presumably there is transovarial transmission of the agent in mites, although with initial infection at the larval stages, this has not been conclusively elucidated. Humans invade these infected habitats, which may vary from semidesert, disturbed rain forests to river banks, seashores, and terrain undergoing secondary vegetative growth. The secondary hosts are rats, field mice, shrews, and voles. Larvae of several species of mites, especially *Leptotrombidium* (*Trombicula*) *akamushi* and *Leptotrombidium diliensis*, infect themselves by attaching to the skin of wild rodents and ultimately to humans as an accidental host [60]. Multiple serotypes of *R. tsutsugamushi* cause illness and produce effective homologous immunity but transient cross-protection. This unfortunate fact has precluded development of an effective vaccine.

Scrub typhus fever (tsutsugamushi disease) occurs in Japan, China, Australia, the Philippines, the South Pacific islands, Malaya, Burma, Thailand, Indonesia, and in the Asian subcontinent.

Q FEVER

Humans contract Q fever by inhaling infected dusts, by handling infected animal tissues, or by drinking milk contaminated with *C. burnetii*. The rickettsiae are widely distributed in nature in ticks, small wild animals, cattle, sheep, goat herds, and humans. Infection is transmitted in nature by ticks which may infect cattle. The animal-tick-animal cycle is a basic mechanism for perpetuation of this rickettsia in nature. Cattle hides contaminated with tick feces have caused aerosol infection in humans.

Species of ticks naturally infected are *D. andersoni* and *A. americanum*. Sheep and goats are naturally infected; *C. burnetii* has been recovered from the milk of these animals. Infected cows, sheep, and goats excrete *C. burnetii* during parturition since placental and birth fluids are grossly infected. Sheep herders, veterinarians, and others who are exposed to such infected aerosols are at risk, as are stockyard workers, wool processors, and laboratory investigators who are engaged in study of the agent. There is no evidence of direct transmission from person to person.

Q fever is globally distributed with the highest incidence of reported cases in Australia, New Zealand, England, Italy and other Mediterranean countries, the United States, and South Africa.

OTHER TICKBORNE RICKETTSIOSES

The agents which cause these mild illnesses are called by various names depending on their geographical localization— *Rickettsia conorii* (fièvre boutonneuse), *Rickettsia siberica* (North Asian tickborne rickettsioses), and *Rickettsia australis* (Queensland tick typhus). Other types are South African tick typhus, Kenya tick typhus, and Indian tick typhus.

R. conorii is the prototype for the group. Ixodid ticks, small wild animals, and dogs maintain the rickettsiae in nature. Humans accidentally invade this cycle and contribute nothing to its continuity. *Rhipicephalus sanguineus,* the brown dog tick, is the dominant vector in the Medterranean countries and South Africa. In Thailand, Malaysia, Europe, Israel, India, and Pakistan, there is serological evidence of spotted fever group rickettsiae.

PREVENTION AND CONTROL

Attempts to develop effective vaccines for the major rickettsioses have been partially successful. Epidemic typhus vaccines consisting of inactivated *R. prowazekii* prepared by the chick embryo technique protected humans against mortality and severe illness. Unfortunately, such vaccines are not generally available because of diminished demand and technical difficulties in preparation. A viable attenuated strain of *R.*

prowazekii (strain E, Madrid) protects against epidemic typhus [*61*]; but it produces mild local and systemic reactions. It is not licensed but is currently available for experimental purposes.

Inactivated vaccines of *R. rickettsii* have shown limited effectiveness for RMSF. A vaccine developed in the 1970s which consists of tissue culture–derived rickettsiae was somewhat effective in volunteers. Illness in vaccinees was milder with longer incubation periods noted after exposure to pathogenic *R. rickettsii* when compared with controls [*62–64*].

The most effective rickettsial vaccine, which is also not commercially available, is an inactivated preparation of phase I *C. burnetii*, which provides good protection against Q fever. After repeated immunizing doses, a local reaction occurs at the inoculating site which has caused some difficulty.

There is no vaccine for scrub typhus. Chemoprophylactic studies in volunteers showed that exposed persons given an effective antibiotic (chloramphenicol or doxycycline) intermittently once weekly for seven doses remained well in spite of inapparent infection. Under certain conditions, with known exposure in endemic areas, this type of chemoprophylaxis is recommended [*65,66*].

Vaccines for murine typhus, the tickborne rickettsioses (*R. conorii*) and rickettsialpox have not been developed.

When persons are exposed to ticks in endemic areas of RMSF and other tickborne rickettsioses, care should be taken to avoid tick infestation. Boots and one-piece outer garments, preferably impregnated with repellent, are helpful. After exposure, a search should be made for attached ticks, particularly in children. After applying alcohol to the site ticks may be removed by forceps with careful removal of the head part. The skin site should be disinfected with soap and water or alcohol. The engorged tick should not be squeezed between the fingers. Contamination of the eyes and minor abrasions should be avoided. Although there are environmental objections to the use of residual insecticides, under certain circumstances, spraying the ground with chlordane or dieldrin helps control ticks.

Louse infestation is avoided by frequent changing of clothes and bathing. Antilousicides such as DDT had lasting effects and provided freedom from infestation for periods up to 3 weeks. At present, malathion or lindane may be used for personal louse control. Tick and louse feces contain the causative rickettsiae when excreted from infected arthropods; hence, contamination of the eyes and mucous membranes by dried feces should be avoided.

Prevention of murine typhus was attained by reducing the natural reservoir (rat) and vector (flea) through measures to eliminate rodents and use of DDT or other insecticides in rat-infested areas to control fleas.

Scrub typhus is difficult to control. In addition to protective and impregnated clothing, application of repellents such as diethyltoluamide or dimethylphthalate to clothing and exposed parts of the body prevents mite attachment. Burning of grasses and application of insecticides in infested areas of scrub typhus was necessary for control in the Pacific Islands during World War II.

REFERENCES

1 Aikawa JK: *Rocky Mountain Spotted Fever*. Springfield, Ill., Charles C Thomas, 1966

2 Weil E. Felix A: Zur serologischen diagnose des fleckfiebers. Wein Klin Wochenschr 29:33–35, 1916

3 Brill NE: An acute febrile illness of unknown origin. Am J Med Sci 139:484–502, 1910

4 Zinsser H, Castaneda MR: On the isolation from a case of Brill's disease of a typhus strain resembling the European type. N Engl J Med 209:815–819, 1933

5 Maxcy KF: Typhus fever in the United States. Public Health Rep 44:1735–1742, 1929

6 Dyer R, Rumreich A, Badger LF: A virus of the typhus type derived from fleas collected from wild rats. Public Health Rep 46: 334 (Feb. 13) 1931

7 Burnet M: Derrick and the story of Q fever. Med J Aust 2: 1067–1077, 1967

8 Cox HR: Studies of a filter-passing infectious agent isolated from ticks. V. Further attempts to cultivate in cell-free media. Public Health Rep 54:1822–1827, 1939

9 Kawamura R: Studies on tsutsugamushi disease (Japanese flood fever). Bull Coll Med Univ Cincinnati 4, spec nos 1 and 2, 1–229, 1926

10 Sasa M: Comparative epidemiology of tsutsugamushi disease in Japan (studies on tsutsugamushi, part 6). Jpn J Exp Med 24:335–361, 1954

11 Tamiya T: *Recent Advances in Studies of Tsutsugamushi Disease in Japan*. Tokyo, Medical Culture, Inc., 1962

12 Wisseman CL Jr, Waddell AD: In vitro studies on rickettsia-host cell interactions: Intracellular growth cycle of virulent and attenuated *Rickettsia prowazekii* in chicken embryo cells in slide chamber cultures. Infect Immun 11:1391–1401, 1975

13 Coolbaugh JC, Progar JJ, Weiss E: Enzymatic activities of cell-free extracts of *Rickettsia typhi*. Infect Immun 14:298–305, 1976

14 Winkler HH: Rickettsial permeability: An ADP-ATP transport system. J Biol Chem 251:389–396, 1976

15 Walker TS, Winkler HH: Penetration of cultured mouse fibroblasts (L cells) by *Rickettsia prowazekii*. Infect Immun 22:200–208, 1978

16 Wisseman CL Jr, Edlinger EA, Waddell AD, et al: Infection cycle of *Rickettsia rickettsii* in chicken embryo and L-929 cells in culture. Infect Immun 14:1052–1064, 1976

17 Hackstadt T, Williams JC: Biochemical strategem for obligate parasitism of eukaryotic cells by *Coxiella burnetii*. Proc Natl Acad Sci USA 78:3240–3244, 1981

18 Wood DO, Williamson LR, Winkler HH, et al: Nucleotide sequence of the *Rickettsia prowazekii* citrate synthase gene. J Bacteriol 169:3564–3572, 1987

19 Heinzen RA, Mallavia LP: Cloning and functional expression of the *Coxiella burnetii* citrate synthase gene in *Escherichia coli*. Infect Immun 55:848–855, 1987

20 Groves MG, Osterman JV: Host defenses in experimental scrub typhus: Genetics of natural resistance to infection. Infect Immun 19:583–588, 1978

21 Groves MG, Rosenstreich DL, Taylor BA, et al: Host defenses in

experimental scrub typhus: Mapping the gene that controls natural resistance in mice. J Immunol 125:1395–1399, 1980

22 Anderson GW Jr, Osterman JV: Host defenses in rickettsialpox: Genetics of natural resistance to infection. Infect Immun 28:132–136, 1980

23 Shirai A, Catanzaro PJ, Phillips SM, et al: Host defenses in experimental scrub typhus: Role of cellular immunity in heterologous protection: Infect Immun 14:39–46, 1976

24 Nacy CA, Osterman JV: Host defenses in experimental scrub typhus: Role of normal and activated macrophages. Infect Immun 26:744–750, 1979

25 Jerrells TR, Osterman JV: Host defenses in experimental scrub typhus: Delayed-type hypersensitivity responses of inbred mice. Infect Immun 35:117–123, 1982

26 Eisemann CS, Osterman JV: Proteins of typhus and spotted fever group rickettsiae. Infect Immun 14:155–162, 1976

27 Osterman JV, Eisemann CS: Surface proteins of typhus and spotted fever group rickettsiae. Infect Immun 21:866–873, 1978

28 Dasch GA: Isolation of species-specific protein antigens of *Rickettsia typhi* and *Rickettsia prowazekii* for immunodiagnosis and immunoprophylaxis. J Clin Microbiol 14:333–341, 1981

29 Bourgeois AL, Dasch GA: The species-specific surface protein antigen of *Rickettsia typhi:* Immunogenicity and protective efficacy in guinea pigs, in Burgdorfer W, Anacker RL (eds): *Rickettsiae and Rickettsial Diseases*. New York, Academic, 1981, pp 71–80

30 Eisemann CS, Osterman JV: Antigens of scrub typhus rickettsiae: Separation by polyacrylamide gel electrophoresis and identification by enzyme-linked immunosorbent assay. Infect Immun 32:525–533, 1981

31 Rollwagen FM, Dasch GA, Jerrells TR: Mechanisms of immunity to rickettsial infection: Characterization of a cytotoxic effector cell. J Immunol 136:1418–1421, 1986

32 Hinrichs DJ, Jerrells TR: In vitro evaluation of immunity to *Coxiella burnetii*. J Immunol 117:996–1003, 1976

33 Fiset P: Phase variation of *Rickettsia (Coxiella) burnetii*. Can J Microbiol 3:434–445, 1957

34 Wells GM, Woodward TE, Fiset P, et al: Rocky Mountain spotted fever caused by blood transfusion. JAMA 239:2763–2765, 1978

35 Woodward TE: A historical account of the rickettsial diseases with a discussion of unsolved problems. J Infect Dis 127:538–594, 1973

36 Woodward TE: Rickettsial diseases in the United States. Med Clin North Am 43:1507–1535, 1959

37 Wolbach SR: Studies on Rocky Mountain spotted fever. J Med Res XLI:1–197 (Nov.) 1919, Boston, Mass.

38 Harrell GT: Rocky Mountain spotted fever. Medicine 28:333–370, 1949

39 Walker DH, Cain BG: Pathogenesis of Rocky Mountain spotted fever. The evidence for local injury of parasitized cells, in Burgdorfer W, Anacker RL (eds.): *Rickettsiae and Rickettsial Diseases*. New York, Academic, 1981

40 Urso FP: Deceived but described Legionellosis masquerading as rickettsia pneumonia. Am J Clin Pathol 74:364–366, 1980

41 Greisman SE, Wisseman CL Jr: Studies of rickettsial toxins. Cardiovascular functional abnormalities induced by *Rickettsia mooseri* in white rats. J Immunol 81:345, 1958

42 Wolbach SB, Todd JL, Palfrey FW: *The Etiology and Pathology of Typhus*. Cambridge, Mass., League of Red Cross Societies at the Harvard University Press, 1922

43 Fine D, Mosher D, Yamada T, et al: Coagulation and complement studies in Rocky Mountain spotted fever. Arch Intern Med 138:735–738, 1978

44 Wisseman CL Jr, Batawi Y, Wood WH, et al: Gross and microscopic skin reactions to killed typhus rickettsia in human beings. J Immunol 98:194–209, 1967

45 Kristinsson A, Bentall HH: Medical and surgical treatment of Q fever endocarditis. Lancet, i:693–697, 1967

46 Kimbrough RC, Ormsbee RA, Peacock M, et al: Q fever endocarditis in the United States. Ann Intern Med 91:400–402, 1979

47 Turck WPG, Howitt G, Turnberg LA, et al: Chronic Q fever. Q J Med new series XLV:193–217, 1976

48 Yamada T, Harber P, Pettit GW, et al: Activation of the Kallikrein-Kinin system in Rocky Mountain spotted fever. Ann Intern Med 88:764–768, 1978

49 Philip RN, Casper EA, MacCormack JN, et al: A comparison of serologic methods for diagnosis of Rocky Mountain spotted fever. Am J Immunol 105:56, 1977

50 Woodward TE, Pedersen CE Jr, Oster CM, et al: Prompt confirmation of Rocky Mountain spotted fever. Identification of rickettsiae in skin tissues. J Infect Dis 134:293–301, 1976

51 Walker DH, Cain BG: A method for specific diagnosis of Rocky Mountain spotted fever on fixed, paraffin-embedded tissue by immunofluorescence. J Infect Dis 137:206–209, 1978

52 Smadel JE, Woodward TE, Ley HL Jr, et al: Chloramphenicol (Chloromycetin) in the treatment of tsutsugamushi disease (scrub typhus). J Clin Invest 28:1196–1215, 1949

53 Pincoffs MC, Guy EG, Lister LM, et al: The treatment of Rocky Mountain spotted fever with Chloromycetin. Ann Intern Med 29:656, 1948

54 Ley HL Jr, Woodward TE, Smadel JE Chloramphenicol (Chloromycetin) in the treatment of murine typhus. JAMA 143:217, 1950

55 Woodward TE: Chloromycetin and Aureomycin. Therapeutic results. Ann Intern Med 31:53, 1949

56 Wisseman CL Jr.: Personal communication

57 Burgdorfer W: Tick-borne diseases in the United States: Rocky Mountain spotted fever and Colorado tick fever. Acta Trop (Basel) 34:103–126, 1977

58 Bozeman FM, Masiello SA, Williams, MS, et al: Epidemic typhus rickettsiae isolated from flying squirrels. Nature 255:545–547, 1975

59 McDade JE, Shepard CC, Redus MA, et al: Evidence of *Rickettsia prowazekii* infections in the United States. Am J Trop Med Hyg 29(2):277–284, 1980

60 Smadel JE, Elisberg BL: Scrub typhus rickettsia, in Horsfall FL Jr, Tamm I (eds): *Viral and Rickettsial Diseases of Man*. Philadelphia, Lippincott, 1965, chap 51

61 Wisseman CL Jr: Concepts of louse-borne typhus control in developing countries. The use of living, attenuated E. strain typhus vaccine in epidemic and endemic situations, in Kohn A, Klingberg MA (eds): *Immunity in Viral and Rickettsial Diseases*. New York, Plenum, 1972, pp 97–130

62 Ascher MS, Oster CN, Harber PI, et al: Initial clinical evaluation of a new Rocky Mountain spotted fever vaccine of tissue culture origin. J Infect Dis 138:217, 1978

63 DuPont HL, Hornick RB, Dawkins AT, et al: Rocky Mountain spotted fever: A comparative study of active immunity induced by inactivated and viable pathogenic *Rickettsia rickettsii*. J Infect Dis 128:340–344, 1973

64 Clements ML, Fiset P, McNamee T, et al: Safety, immunogenicity and efficacy of chick embryo cell (CEC) derived vaccine for Rocky Mountain spotted fever (RMSF). Abstract 22 Interscience Conference on Antimicrobial Agents and Chemotherapy, Miami, October 1982

65 Smadel JE, Ley HL Jr, Diercks FH, et al: Immunization against scrub typhus: Duration of immunity in volunteers following combined living vaccine and chemoprophylaxis. Am J Trop Med Hyg 1:87–99, 1952

66 Olson JG, Bourgeois AL, Fang JC, et al: Prevention of scrub typhus. Prophylactic administration of doxycycline in a randomized double blind trial. Am J Trop Med Hyg 29:989–997, 1980

PART VI / Fungal Diseases

CHAPTER 100

Introduction · John E. Bennett

Fungal infections remain an infrequent problem in most areas of the world. Although no satisfactory prevalence figures are available, ringworm and candidiasis of the mucous membranes are probably the most common mycoses. Ringworm can be extremely prevalent in infantry units operating in wet lowland terrain. Among U.S. forces in Vietnam, 53 percent of 486 infantry soldiers surveyed had ringworm [1]. Although ringworm rarely reaches this prevalence in a general population, intertriginous lesions caused by fungi assume additional importance when they lead to bacterial cellulitis. Mycetoma, a disease caused by fungi or aerobic actinomycetes, is common in many underdeveloped areas such as sub-Saharan Africa. Mycetoma of the foot gradually impairs the patient's ability to walk. In a subsistence economy, inability to hunt or gather food makes pedal mycetoma (madura foot) a serious problem. The magnitude of the problem can be estimated from Abbott's report that 1231 cases of mycetoma were hospitalized in Sudan over a $2\frac{1}{2}$-year period [2].

The impact of the acquired immune deficiency syndrome (AIDS) on the incidence of mycoses is difficult to predict but is likely to be substantial. Retrospective studies in Africa and the USA have indicated that 58 to 81 percent of patients with AIDS develop a mycosis [3]. The most common is oral candidiasis, which can begin during the AIDS-related complex (ARC) or later. Cryptococcosis is a potentially lethal infection which has occurred in roughly 6 to 8 percent of AIDS patients in the United States [4]. If this prevalence is correct, the incidence of this mycosis should at least double in the United States, compared to the decade prior to AIDS. While histoplasmosis and coccidioidomycosis are much more severe in AIDS patients, it is as yet unclear whether the prevalence of clinically manifest infection will rise in areas endemic for these mycoses as a result of AIDS.

Although mycoses exhibit an extraordinary heterogeneity, they have certain features in common. Infection is usually acquired from nature, not from infected humans or animals. Certain types of ringworm and candidiasis are notable exceptions to this rule. Inhalation of spores into the lung is the major portal for systemic mycoses. Subcutaneous mycoses usually arise from the accidental inoculation of soil or vegetation into the skin by minor trauma. Mycoses of the keratinized layers of the skin and of the hair and nails are acquired by contact. Strong regional differences in the mycoses arise because the ecology favors certain fungi, populations differ in their use of protective clothing, and medical practice varies in the use of immunosuppressive agents. Diagnosis of mycoses is most accurately done by demonstrating the fungus in both smear and culture. Histopathological diagnosis requires special stains and expertise. However, biopsy may provide a presumptive histopathological diagnosis that permits prompt initiation of therapy. Diagnosis by culture alone is time-consuming and requires knowledge of whether or not the fungus can exist in that site as a saprophyte. Serological diagnosis is valuable only in special situations. Skin testing rarely has any diagnostic value.

REFERENCES

1 Allen AM, Taplin D, Lowy JA, et al: Skin infections in Vietnam. Milit Med 137:295–301, 1972
2 Abbott PH: Mycetoma in the Sudan. Trans R Soc Trop Med Hyg 50:11–24, 1956
3 Holmberg K, Meyer R: Fungal infections in patients with AIDS and AIDS-related complex. Scand J Infect Dis 18:179–192, 1986
4 Zuger A, Louie E, Holzman RS, et al: Cryptococcal disease in patients with the acquired immunodeficiency syndrome. Ann Intern Med 104:234–240, 1986

CHAPTER 101

Aspergillosis · Lowell S. Young

Members of the genus *Aspergillus* are one of the most commonly encountered groups of fungi in the environment and more than 300 species have been isolated from soil, water, and decaying vegetation [1]. Symptomatic human disease usually results when host defenses are bridged, as in the immunocompromised host, or when an individual develops hypersensitivity to *Aspergillus* antigens. Hypersensitivity to inhaled organisms in the upper and lower respiratory passages probably accounts for most of the symptomatic disease due to *Aspergillus* species throughout the world. Although relatively fewer cases of invasive disease occur, these are associated with high mortality and antemortem diagnosis is difficult.

The interest in *Aspergillus* among workers in the tropical disease field relates mainly to one group of syndromes, namely sinus and parasinus infections. This group of infections has been observed in warm, humid climates such as the Sudan, although symptomatic patients have been observed in a wide variety of geographical settings. Since aspergilli are ubiquitous in the environment and respiratory symptoms are often puzzling, linking the isolation of the fungus to the cause of disease often poses a major clinical challenge.

Human disease associated with *Aspergillus* colonization or infection may be on the increase because of our ability to recognize certain clinical patterns. Many unanswered questions remain, however, relating to pathogenesis of invasive disease and the mechanism for the hypersensitivity reactions which lead to bronchopulmonary symptomatology.

PARASITE

TAXONOMY AND MICROBIAL PROPERTIES

The term *Aspergillus* dates back to early microscopic descriptions of the stalks and spore-bearing heads of the basic fungal structure. The name comes from the Latin *aspergere,* "to scatter," referring to the chains of sporelike structures (conidia) radiating from the central conidial apparatus. The essential structural characteristic of the genus is the conidiophore, an elongated stalk with a globelike or vesicular ending bearing rows of short tubes or sterigmata, from which radiate chains of spherical unicellular conidia. Conidiophores and conidia are occasionally found in lung or paranasal sinus specimens, but the usual invasive form is mycelial with characteristically branching, septate hyphae. The species are identified by color and shape of conidial heads, the presence of one or two rows of sterigmata, and the morphology of the conidia. Early growth on common fungal media like Sabouraud's agar shows colonies of aspergillae to be flat, light, and velvety; these later develop the appearance of a typical mold. These colonies are usually gray-green in appearance but can be tan-yellow, and in the case of *Aspergillus niger,* are dark brown or black. The characteristic branching mycelium forms in tissue may appear as very compact entangled filaments, presenting almost as granules in "fungus ball" lesions. Aspergilli are most easily seen in tissue, sputum, or secretions using a wet mount preparation, but routinely performed stains with silver (Gomori stain) or the periodic acid Schiff (PAS) stain readily identify the branching septate structures.

The most commonly encountered *Aspergillus* species causing infection is *A. fumigatus* followed by *A. flavus.* Other encountered pathogenic species include *niger, nidulans, terreus,* and *ochraceus.* These grow on a wide variety of different substrates and under different environmental conditions. They often colonize living and dead tissues and invasive involvement of almost every organ has been reported. Most pathogenic species appear to produce exocellular substances and endotoxinlike material [4]. More than a dozen metabolites have been isolated from *Aspergillus* species and these may be virulence factors [1]. Extracts of *Aspergillus* species have been shown to cause mortality in experimental infections and are associated with infarcts and hemorrhages seen in the organs of infected animals [5].

Cell wall products of *A. fumigatus,* the most commonly studied species, appear to activate both the classic and alternative complement pathways [6,7]. Most of the investigations of virulence factors from aspergilli have focused on so-called aflatoxins [8]. This term refers to toxic metabolites of *A. fumigatus* which have been associated with cell damage and even neoplastic changes [9].

HOST DEFENSE MECHANISMS AGAINST *ASPERGILLUS* INFECTIONS

There is little question that the major site of entry of *Aspergillus* into humans is via the respiratory tract. Specific mechanisms of host resistance and the relative protective roles of different phagocytic cells (macrophages and neutrophils), delayed hypersensitivity reactions, and humoral immunity have all been investigated, but it has been difficult to assess the relative importance of these components [10–17].

The initial importance of mechanical factors should not be overlooked. *Aspergillus* conidia (spores) are small enough to reach alveoli. Ciliated epithelial cells from the trachea to the terminal bronchioles serve to clear organisms even before they reach the deeper air passageways. The majority of inhaled particles with diameters of 0.5 to 3.0 μm will be deposited on the nonciliated epithelial surface of the lower respiratory tract distal to the terminal bronchioles. Thus, phagocytic defenses must contain the latter inhaled organisms as *Aspergillus* spore size usually varies from 2 to 6 μm in diameter.

The primary phagocytes in the end-bronchial alveolar spaces of the lower respiratory tract are alveolar macrophages and neutrophils. Some studies indicate that alveolar macrophages of mice given an inhalation challenge of *Aspergillus* spores ingest virtually all spores and can inhibit their germination [10]. Nonetheless, after prolonged periods of incubation no apparent killing has been observed. The alveolar macrophages may have to be "activated" before their function is optimal. In contrast, peritoneal macrophages kill spores and prevent germination even in neutropenic and athymic mice, suggesting a less important role for T lymphocytes in host defenses.

Polymorphonuclear cells appear to have an important role against host invasion by *Aspergillus* as evidenced by the occurrence of invasive disease in patients with acute leukemia and chronic granulomatous disease [17]. While these neutrophils do not kill ingested spores [14], they have the capacity to kill mycelia in vitro and eradicate mycelia in experimental infections [11]. Additionally, there is evidence that polymorphonuclear leukocytes and monocytes can damage hyphae without ingesting them [15,17]. The available evidence suggests that both mononuclear and polymorphonuclear phagocytes are important in host defense. Interestingly, *Aspergillus* infections are relatively uncommon in patients with the acquired immune deficiency syndrome (AIDS), suggesting that T-helper lymphocyte function is not critical in host defense. Corticosteroids, whose usage in high dosage can predispose to invasive aspergillosis, inhibit the conidiacidal activity of mononuclear phagocytes and can also impair the mobilization of polymorphonuclear leukocytes. Sensitive radioimmunoassay (RIA) procedures have indicated that most normal individuals have serum antibodies against *Aspergillus* and this is associated with IgG and IgM classes of immunoglobulin [1]. Nonetheless, there is no evidence that these humoral antibodies are important in limiting the invasion of *Aspergillus* organisms [16].

EPIDEMIOLOGICAL CONSIDERATIONS

Aspergillus spores have been recovered from a wide variety of environmental sources but the greatest number have usually been found in moldy hay, straw, grasses, and leaves. Millions of spores have been found to be released per gram of hay and there is a wide prevalence (averaging approximately 50 percent) of *Aspergillus* precipitins in the sera of cattle and horses [1]. Since the apparent route of acquisition of *Aspergillus* is via the respiratory tract, a number of environmental sampling studies have been carried out in hospital settings [19]. Contamination of air conditioning ducts [1], ceiling tiles, and fireproofing materials [20] has been well documented in association with cases of invasive disease in immunosuppressed patients. It is also clear, however, that recovery of fungi from

respiratory secretions and nasal passageways does not always correlate with invasive disease. The comprehensive study of the occurrence of *Aspergillus* species in the respiratory tract of 812 patients with chronic pulmonary disease in Delhi indicated that 61 percent of patients were culture-positive, yielding a total of 29 different species of *Aspergillus* [21]. However, recovery of *Aspergillus* species did not correlate well with underlying pulmonary disease processes, suggesting that they represented saprophytes rather than true pathogens in the majority of instances. In addition to airborne contamination, medical or nonmedical products including food, medical devices, surgical dressings, and plants have been the source of infection in high-risk patients [1]. The organism has also been isolated from cannabis. Finally, it should be acknowledged that a pathway for infection not widely appreciated is the gastrointestinal tract. This has been suggested by animal studies where culture of mesenteric lymph nodes has revealed various *Aspergillus* species [22]. It has been suspected that the GI source could be an important portal of entry in immunocompromised patients [23].

PATIENT

PULMONARY DISEASE

In assessing respiratory symptoms the major clinical challenge is to distinguish apparently harmless, saprophytic colonization of respiratory passageways from invasive disease. Many variations of intermediate states exist, such as the static "fungus ball" that develops in preexisting pulmonary cavities, hypersensitivity reactions triggered by the presence of the fungus, and limited mucosal invasion in a small proportion of patients who have an essentially allergic syndrome. These states are clearly different from the frank tissue invasion leading to fatal disease involving deep organs and the central nervous system or endocarditis. Table 101-1 is an attempt to classify some of the clinical manifestations of aspergillosis in the respiratory tract. Colonization, a variant of bronchopulmonary aspergillosis, refers to that condition in which *Aspergillus* or other

Table 101-1. Pulmonary aspergillosis syndromes*

1. Saprophytic bronchopulmonary aspergillosis
2. Aspergilloma
3. Hypersensitivity syndromes
   a. Allergic bronchopulmonary aspergillosis
   b. Eosinophilic pneumonitis
   c. Granulomatous pneumonitis (extrinsic allergic alveolitis)
   d. Mucoid impaction syndrome
4. Invasive aspergillosis
   a. Necrotizing bronchopneumonia
   b. Pulmonary infarction
   c. Single or multiple abscesses of varying size

*After Bardana [24].

species may grow and multiply in lung tissue without evidence of direct tissue damage. As a result patients may develop high levels of circulating antibodies. Chronic pulmonary disease and the use of broad-spectrum antibacterial agents appear to predispose to *Aspergillus* colonization of the respiratory tract. Corticosteroids, which are often utilized in asthmatic patients, may enhance this risk. Thirty to sixty percent of sera from patients with cystic fibrosis have demonstrable precipitins to *Aspergillus* components, yet these patients do not appear to be at risk for developing significant disease related to this pathogen [25,26]. A high proportion of these patients may have so-called immediate or type I hypersensitivity reactions to *Aspergillus* antigens.

Aspergilloma or *fungus ball* is the term applied to the matted, saprophytic growth of aspergilli in a preexisting space in a patient with chronic lung disease [27–29]. The space is usually a poorly drained cavity secondary to tuberculosis, histoplasmosis, sarcoidosis, coccidioidomycosis, or even a bulla [29]. Occasionally, development of aspergilloma without apparent preexisting disease has been noted, and some patients with aspergillomas develop allergic symptoms. Aspergillomas are usually present in the nondependent or apical regions of the lung. Fungus-ball lesions can grow to very large sizes (10 cm) but the growth is usually localized and invasion is rare. It is possible that some enlargement of a lesion may be secondary to release of mycotoxins, but these lesions may also shrink due to fibrotic scarring of preexisting cavities. Calcification can occur but aspergillomas may also degenerate, with resolution or regression of the cavitary lesions.

Spontaneous disappearance has been documented in a number of cases, and is possibly related to vigorous coughing. Generally, an aspergilloma has no adverse effects in a patient without allergic tendencies [30]. Common manifestations of aspergilloma include hemoptysis, cough, sputum production, and clubbing of fingers as well as occasional fever, malaise, and weight loss [24]. The principal danger is hemoptysis. It may range from mild episodes to severe and life-threatening exsanguination requiring emergency surgery.

HYPERSENSITIVITY-INDUCED ASPERGILLOSIS

Major attention has been focused on the syndrome of allergic bronchopulmonary aspergillosis, a syndrome popularized by Pepys and collaborators [31–33]. The cardinal features of this syndrome are (1) chronic asthma, (2) transient or migratory segmental pulmonary infiltrates (usually in upper lobes), (3) type I dermal hypersensitivity reactions and demonstrable bronchial reactivity, and (4) precipitating antibodies to *A. fumigatus* antigens. Sputum usually contains eosinophils and Curschmann's spirals, and the blood eosinophil count exceeds 500 eosinophils per microliter when lung infiltrates are present. For definition of this clinical entity many investigators also require positive sputum cultures for *Aspergillus,* a history of

recurrent atelectasis, detection of visible ''plugs'' in the sputum, and radiologically demonstrable bronchiectasis [34,35].

In regard to specific humoral immunity the majority of patients with allergic bronchopulmonary aspergillosis have elevated total levels of antibodies belonging to the IgG and IgM immunoglobulin classes [36]. There have been reports of elevations of antigen-specific IgG and IgE. Such tests, however, have been difficult to standardize, and abnormalities of cell-mediated immune function have also been reported. Histologically, bronchi are characteristically dilated and filled with inspissated sputum that usually contains noninvasive fungal hyphae. Focal areas of eosinophilic pneumonia have also been observed.

A number of variants of the *Aspergillus*-associated hypersensitivity syndromes have been described by various workers and there appears to be a wide spectrum of the disease. Some individuals have mucoid impaction of bronchi with obstruction by inspissated mucous exudate containing fungal elements [37], others eosinophilic pneumonitis with severe asthma [38], and others shifting lung infiltrates involving different portions of the lungs at different times [24]. Other patients may demonstrate extrinsic allergic alveolitis. This term refers to a group of hypersensitivity lung reactions of which farmer's lung is a prototype [39]. In the granulomatous syndromes the most striking histological feature is the organizing endobronchial nodules with collections of eosinophils and minute noncaseating granulomas which develop secondary to exposure to *A. fumigatus.* Moderate blood eosinophila has also been present. Most of the patients whose lung biopsies show a more pronounced granulomatous response have a very strong history of asthma.

INVASIVE ASPERGILLOSIS

Invasive aspergillosis is diagnosed by histopathological demonstration of invasion of fungal elements, usually hyphal forms, in tissue. Culture confirmation is supportive of the diagnosis and identifies the invading species, but is not an essential requirement. The most commonly involved organ is the lung, from which dissemination occurs to deep and superficial sites. A few patients with invasive disease have not been immunocompromised [40]. However, almost all patients have some severe underlying disease such as a malignancy of the hematopoietic or lymphatic system and/or are receiving immunosuppressive therapy, such as corticosteroids or antithymocyte globulin. Granulocyte function appears to be an important host factor, as underscored by the high incidence of *Aspergillus* infections in chronic granulomatous disease [17] and acute leukemia [23,41].

It has been more difficult to precisely assess the role of antimicrobial agents. They may suppress the normal flora in immunosuppressed individuals, thereby predisposing the patient to *Aspergillus* superinfection. Indeed, over half of patients with invasive aspergillosis often have some other concurrent bacterial or viral infection and the initial therapy for a bacterial process may then predispose to fungal superinfection [23,24,41].

INVASIVE PULMONARY ASPERGILLOSIS

The lung is the most common site of invasive disease, with the route of infection being clearly airborne [42]. The initial event is colonization of the tracheobronchial tree by airborne fungi followed by superficial erosion and ulceration of bronchial mucosa. This is followed by transbronchial invasion and direct involvement of lung parenchyma. The basic process occurring in the lung, as well as in other organs that are invaded, is invasion of small- and medium-size arteries with subsequent thrombosis and infarction of tissue [43,44]. Since the major component of *Aspergillus* infection in the lung involves invasion of blood vessels, the spread of intrapulmonary disease may be both hematogenous and via endobronchial routes. Thus, a diffuse pneumonitis with an interstitial or alveolar pattern can result, mimicking cytomegalovirus or *Pneumocystis* infection [23,41].

Consolidation of the lung is usually the result of intrapulmonary hemorrhage rather than the inflammatory response of the host, which in the immunosuppressed patient is considerably blunted. The most dramatic manifestation of the necrotizing process due to *Aspergillus* infection of the lung is the development of an acute cavitating lesion in an area which was previously consolidated on the basis of hemorrhagic infarction. The necrotic or infarcted tissue may be partially expectorated thereby giving the appearance of a classic fungus ball. However, it is important to distinguish this type of acute fungus ball lesion due to infarcted tissue, which provides an excellent culture medium for the proliferation of the fungus, from the classic aspergilloma, which results from colonization of a preexisting cavity by saprophytic fungal organisms.

Miliary microabscesses due to diffuse disseminated disease without gross areas of infarction and cavitation complete the varied spectrum of pulmonary disease seen in immunosuppressed host with invasive aspergillosis [24].

Thus, a wide variety of radiological findings have been observed in invasive pulmonary aspergillosis. The most typical are focal pneumonitis reflected by a pattern of lobar consolidation or gross hemorrhagic infarction followed by necrosis and cavitation within the infarcted area.

Symptoms include fever, dyspnea, and cough with or without hemoptysis. Some of the salient clinical clues may be the development of pleuritic chest pain and/or a loud friction rub, both signs of hemorrhagic infarction which may be mistaken for evidence of a pulmonary embolus. Patients with histologically documented invasive aspergillosis may not have *Aspergillus* organisms isolated from bronchial secretions or sputum. Other studies have demonstrated a correlation between invasive pulmonic disease and the recovery of *Aspergillus* organism

from nasal swab cultures [44]. (See below for further comments on diagnosis.)

NASAL AND PERINASAL SINUS INVOLVEMENT

In view of the abundant sources of *Aspergillus* in the environment, it is not surprising that *Aspergillus* is one of the most common if not the most common fungal infection of the nose and perinasal sinuses [45]. An extensive literature documents endemic disease in the Sudan, where *A. flavus* is the most common agent isolated from sinus infection [2,3]. Sinusitis may occur in immunosuppressed patients and may be the harbinger of pulmonary and invasive disease [46], but more frequently sinusitis affects individuals without any host defect. Aspergillomas may actually be found in the sinuses and are occasionally associated with lung infection. Furthermore, even among these apparently normal individuals some may proceed to develop cranial involvement and die. The paranasal sinuses have been the most common site of involvement, followed by the sphenoid and ethmoid sinuses. Concomitant obstruction due to nasal polyps and chronic bacterial infection may predispose to or enhance fungal invasiveness. In some cases the sinus involvement is altogether benign without destruction of bone or adjacent tissue. The symptoms are primarily allergic, including rhinorrhea, congestive rhinitis, and opacification of the sinuses. The more invasive form involves bone and occasionally the orbital tissues. Ocular involvement is underscored by visual impairment and muscle palsies. The ultimate extension is intracerebral involvement, with abscesses and cavernous sinus thrombosis.

CUTANEOUS ASPERGILLOSIS

Aspergillus infection of the skin or subcutaneous tissue may result from primary infection secondary to direct trauma or burns [24]. Several cases of cutaneous lesions have been reported where the pathogenesis appears to be direct contact with materials such as adhesive tape or infusion apparatus contaminated by the organism. Indwelling vascular catheters have been associated with localized cutaneous *Aspergillus* infection [47]. Disseminated involvement leading to skin manifestations appears in immunosuppressed patients as part of the spectrum of dissemination via the hematogenous route [23]. Disseminated cutaneous involvement may result in maculopapular skinlike lesions that are violaceous, indurated, and plaquelike. These may progress to necrotizing ulcerations which may resemble the vasculitis observed in systemic gram-negative bacillary infections.

Aspergillus may also be a secondary invader complicating burns. In the latter condition diagnosis is best established by burn wound biopsy as airborne wound contamination may be mistaken for wound infection.

EXTERNAL OTITIS

Otomycotic infection is a common benign disorder caused by *A. fumigatus* or *A. niger* [24]. In this situation the fungal organisms thrive on cerumen and debris in the external auditory canal but they rarely cause damage to the crucial parts of the tympanic membrane. Further complications may include bacterial superinfection. Rarely, the disease may become invasive and involve the mastoid and temporal bone.

BONE INFECTION

Osteomyelitis caused by *Aspergillus* species is relatively uncommon [48]. Bone infection either results from direct extension from a preexisting focus or via dissemination from a pulmonary source. These patients are often immunosuppressed. Initial symptomatology includes pain, soft tissue swelling, and a palpable adjacent abscess. Lytic bone lesions are usually irregular in configuration with occasional subperiosteal new bone formation.

ENDOCARDITIS AND CARDIAC INVOLVEMENT

Although generally rare, this complication is usually associated with intravenous drug abuse, hyperalimentation, cardiac surgery [49], and bone marrow transplantation [50]. A history of valvular disease is usually present and approximately half of the cases of endocarditis have occurred on either prosthetic valves or homographs. In prosthetic valve endocarditis, obstruction of the outflow tract by the vegetative fungal growth can resemble a thrombus both grossly, radiologically, and by sonographic studies. Some theorize that an antecedent thrombus predisposes to *Aspergillus* colonization and infection. Some of these cases have occurred in temporal proximity to recent cardiac surgery and thus probably result from airborne contamination of the operative field. Secondary to endocarditis there may be metastatic myocardial abscesses or invasion of the myocardium adjacent to the focus of *Aspergillus* infection. Often, embolization to major systemic or pulmonary arteries is the presenting clinical sign. Emergency embolectomies have been performed on some patients only to find characteristic branching hyphae in microscopic sections of extirpated clots. It is only then that attention is focused on the valvular source of the infected emboli.

Mechanical valve failure, appearance of new murmurs, onset of cardiac failure, and fever are clues to endocarditis in a patient with prosthetic valves. Paradoxically, fewer than 10 percent of antemortem blood cultures have been positive and the yield has been actually greater from cultures obtained at thrombectomy. Thus, in a patient not receiving antibacterial agents who has a prosthetic valve and develops fever and evidence of mechanical valve failure wiith multiple negative blood cultures, fungal endocarditis should be strongly suspected.

CENTRAL NERVOUS SYSTEM INFECTION

Aspergilli reach the central nervous system by two main routes [23,51]. First, hematogenous spread occurs usually from a respiratory source but occasionally from the gastrointestinal tract. Second, direct extension occurs from adjacent infected tissues such as the sinuses or ear. In the brain parenchyma the same pattern of arterial invasion resulting in thrombosis and infarction of cerebral tissue followed by secondary invasion of infarcted areas occurs as has been noted for the lung. Occasionally, aneurysms of medium-sized and larger arteries have been documented. *Aspergillus* granulomas of the brain may mimic a process such as neoplasm, tuberculoma, or brain abscess. *Aspergillus* infections of the central nervous system may be a complication following neurosurgery and an occasional report documents this complication as a result of lumbar puncture. Detection of central nervous system infection is usually dependent upon tissue biopsy or aspiration. The cerebral spinal fluid is rarely culture-positive.

EYE

Primary aspergillosis of the eye is rare but keratitis is one manifestation. In compromised patients dissemination with endophthalmitis may occur. The orbit may be involved secondarily by extension of a sinus infection.

OTHER SITES INVOLVED IN DISSEMINATED DISEASE

Disseminated disease is defined as the involvement of two or more noncontiguous organs. This is clearly the most severe form of *Aspergillus* infection, can be fulminating, and is usually fatal. This occurs primarily in patients who are severely debilitated. The source is usually respiratory, but in some cases infection may originate from the GI tract. The GI tract is most commonly involved after the lung, followed by the central nervous system, liver, spleen, kidney, and thyroid gland. Aspergilli can cause erosive esophagitis in much the same manner as *Candida* species. Intestinal lesions containing aspergilli are often associated with gastrointestinal bleeding [23]. Renal involvement is almost always hematogenous but hematuria and pyuria are rather infrequent. One of the more interesting clinical manifestations is onset of the Budd-Chiari syndrome secondary to *Aspergillus*-induced thrombosis of the portal vein. In a patient with a neoplasm this is impossible to distinguish clinically from spread of underlying disease.

DIAGNOSIS

Aspergillus as a trigger mechanism in the etiology of allergic and asthmatic symptoms should be suspected if symptoms are chronic and there is a substantial yield of the fungus from sputum samples. Eosinophilia, elevated serum levels of IgE, detection of serum *Aspergillus* precipitins, and response to corticosteroids are all suggestive of the syndromes of allergic bronchopulmonary aspergillosis [52].

For the diagnosis of localized (e.g., sinusitis) or invasive disease, histopathological evidence of infection is usually required unless growth is from blood cultures or a normally sterile body fluid such as CSF. Culture isolation of fungus from blood or body fluid, even in the face of invasive disease, is variable, although the major *Aspergillus* species grow well on conventional enriched bacteriological media and Sabouraud's media. The recovery of aspergilli from mucous membranes or expectorated sputum may reflect a merely saprophytic state, although invasive disease should be strongly suspected in febrile immunosuppressed patients with lung infiltrates and positive sputum cultures for *Aspergillus* [53,54]. In suspected respiratory diseases there is increasing evidence that invasive techniques short of open lung biopsy, such as fiberoptic bronchoscopy or bronchoalveolar lavage, are valuable diagnostic procedures [55,56]. Computed tomography of the lung may be useful in evaluating acute cavitary lesions [57].

The differential diagnosis of *Aspergillus* infection in the immunosuppressed host is challenging because a wide variety of processes can mimic localized pulmonary involvement or disseminated infection. Other causes of necrotizing pneumonia must be considered, such as those due to anaerobes, gram-positive cocci (particularly *Staphylococcus aureus*), and gram-negative rods. However, the rapid onset of acute lung consolidation or cavitation, or development of diffuse pulmonary infiltrates in immunosuppressed patients already receiving broad-spectrum antibiotics is much more likely to be due to an opportunistic fungal infection rather than to a process caused by anaerobic or aerobic bacteria. *Aspergillus* infection of the lung may be indistinguishable from that observed with the zygomycoses or *Petriellidium boydii*, all of which can produce acute cavitary pneumonitis. Parenchymal involvement with evidence of infarction (e.g., a friction rub) could be due to a pulmonary embolus but in the impaired host intravascular spread of fungi should be strongly suspected.

Much attention has been focused upon noninvasive methods for the diagnosis of *Aspergillus* infections. Since so many individuals with life-threatening *Aspergillus* infections are severely debilitated, an approach which does not require direct sampling of tissue would be highly desirable. Controversy, however, surrounds the validity of interpretation of serological tests for diagnosis of invasive disease (antibody detection tests are usually positive in allergic aspergillosis and aspergilloma).

Earlier studies of crude antibodiy measurements such as agglutination, precipitation, and immunodiffusion gave conflicting results. Perhaps it would be fair to say that the timing of such studies is of crucial importance because immunosuppressed individuals dying of acute fulminating disease probably would not be expected to muster a serum antibody response to *Aspergillus* antigens.

Some studies indicate that detection of antibodies by radioimmunoassay [58] or other sensitive immunological methods, if positive, can be a valuable clue to diagnosis. On the other hand, negative serological studies do not rule out the possibility of an underlying *Aspergillus* infection [59]. More recently the opposite approach, aimed at detecting circulating *Aspergillus* antigenemia, has been attempted. Experimental studies of *Aspergillus* infection and a few scattered reports of human cases suggest that detection of circulation antigens of *Aspergillus* may be a basis for diagnosing disseminated disease [60–62]. These serological methods are not widely available and the positive predictive value of results requires confirmation from larger, multicenter, prospective studies.

TREATMENT OF ASPERGILLOSIS

Only one agent, amphotericin B, is reliably active against *Aspergillus* species, yet the results of treating invasive disease are disappointing. This is probably related to unremitting host disease rather than true drug failure. Full doses of amphotericin B in doses of up to 1 mg/(kg·day) are recommended for treating invasive aspergillosis. Although a targeted total dose of 2 g is often quoted in the literature, such a dose may be inadequate in the immunocompromised patient whose basic disease fails to improve. Conversely, an individual with disseminated infection even involving the lung may respond to far lower doses, providing the underlying disease, such as a leukemia, remits. Indeed, in the neutropenic patient the strategy of antifungal therapy is not to reach some hypothetical "curative" dose but to contain the spread of infection while other treatment hopefully improves the basic disease. Early aggressive diagnosis and initiation of treatment with amphotericin B may enhance the chance for ultimate recovery [63,64]. The efficacy of single-agent therapy of invasive aspergillosis with imidazoles such as ketoconazole or miconazole is unproven. An experimental imidazole, itraconazole, appears more active against aspergillus species but treatment studies in invasive disease are limited. Combination therapy with amphotericin B plus either flucytosine or rifampin has been suggested by in vitro or experimental studies [65,66], but there are no human studies demonstrating the superiority of these combinations over amphotericin B alone. Granulocyte transfusions have been used to treat some cases but these anecdotal reports are difficult to assess.

In the allergic bronchopulmonary aspergillosis syndromes, use of bronchodilators and iodides has been reported to ameliorate symptoms. Symptomatic relief seems to be conferred by low doses (up to 25 mg) of prednisone without serious hazard of converting localized disease into an invasive form.

The role of surgery in treating some forms of pulmonary aspergillosis is controversial. Since hemoptysis is a fair risk with aspergilloma, resection of large lesions has been advocated and is probably justified in some cases. On the other hand, some patients may spontaneously expectorate an aspergilloma and symptoms will subside. One of the critical management problems in individuals with lung lesions in invasive disease relates to the onset of uncontrolled hemoptysis. Successful resection of such lesions has been reported, but clearly these patients are high operative risks. There probably is understandable reluctance to operate on individuals who are granulocytopenic and have hemoptysis but it may be absolutely necessary in order to terminate an uncontrolled bleeding situation.

PROGNOSIS

The prognosis in allergic pulmonary and bronchopulmonary disease is fairly good, providing a low dose of steroids is all that is necessary to control asthmatic symptoms. In invasive aspergillosis the prognosis is extremely poor unless some improvement of the underlying disease is possible. Indeed, well-documented invasive pulmonary disease has responded to no specific antifungal therapy if remission in leukemia or lymphoma has been achieved. [*41*].

REFERENCES

1 Bardana EJ: The clinical spectrum of aspergillosis. I. Epidemiology, pathogenicity, infection in animals and immunology of aspergillus. CRC Crit Rev Clin Lab Sci 12:21–63, 1980

2 Milosev B, Mahgoub ES, Abdelaal O, et al: Primary aspergilloma of paranasal sinuses in the Sudan. Br J Surg 56:132, 1969

3 Veress B, Malik OA, ElTayeb AA, et al: Further observations on the primary paranasal aspergillus granuloma in the Sudan. A morphological study of 56 cases. Am J Trop Med Hyg 22:765, 1973

4 Tilden EB, Hatten EH, Freeman S, et al: Preparation and properties of the endotoxins of *Aspergillus fumigatus* and *A. flavus*. Mycopathologica 14:325, 1961

5 Wogan GN: Mycotoxins. Rev Pharmacol 15:437, 1975

6 deBracco MM, Budzko DB, Negroni R: Mechanisms of activation of complement by extracts of *A. fumigatus*. Clin Immunol Immunopathol 5:333, 1976

7 Marx JJ and Flaherty DK: Activation of the complement sequence by extracts of bacteria and fungi associated with hypersensitivity pneumonitis. J Allergy Clin Immunol 57:328, 1976

8 Detroy RW, Lillehoy EB, Cregler A: Aflatoxin and related compounds, in Cregler A, Kadis S, Aji SJ (eds): *Microbial Toxins*. 6. New York, Academic, 1971, p 1

9 Dvorackova I: Aflatoxin inhalation and alveolar cell carcinoma. Br Med J 1:691, 1976

10 Merkow LL, Epstein SM, Sidransky H, et al: Pathogenesis of experimental pulmonary aspergillosis. Am J Pathol 62:57–66, 1970

11 Shaffner A, Douglas H, Braude A: Selective protection against conidia by mononuclear and against mycelia by polymorphonuclear phagocytes in resistance to aspergillus. J Clin Invest 69:617–631, 1982

12 Turner KJ, Hackshaw J, Papadimitriou JD, et al: Experimental aspergillosis in rats infected via intraperitoneal and subcutaneous routes. Immunology 29:55–66, 1975

13 Sideransky HS, Epstein SM, Verney E, et al: Experimental visceral aspergillosis. Am J Pathol 69:55–67, 1972

14 Lehrer RI, Jan RG: Interaction of *Aspergillus fumigatus* spores with human leukocytes and serum. Infect Immun 1:345–350, 1970

15 Diamond RD, Krzesicki R, Epstein B, et al: Damage to hyphal forms of fungi by human leukocytes in vitro. Am J Pathol 91:313–328, 1978

16 Kong YM, Levine HB: Experimentally induced immunity in the mycoses. Bacteriol Rev 31:35–53, 1967

17 Lazarus GM, Neu HC: Agents responsible for infection in chronic granulomatous disease of childhood. J Pediatr 86:415–417, 1975

18 Diamond RD, Huber E, Haudenschild CC: Mechanisms of destruction of *Aspergillus fumigatus* hyphae medicated by human monocytes. J Infect Dis 147:474–483, 1983

19 Rose HS: Mechanical control of hospital ventilation and aspergillus infection. Am Rev Respir Dis 105:306–307, 1972

20 Aisner J, Schimpff SC, Bennett JE, et al: Aspergillus infections in cancer patients. Association with fireproofing materials in a new hospital. JAMA 235:411, 1976

21 Sandhu DK, Sandhu RS: Survey of *Aspergillus* species associated with human respiratory tract. Mycopathol Mycol Appl 49:77, 1973

22 Angus KW, Gilmour NJL, Dawson CO: Alimentary mycotic lesions in cattle: A histological and cultural study. J Med Microbiol 6:307, 1973

23 Young RC, Bennett JE, Vogel CL, et al: Aspergillosis: The spectrum of the disease in 98 patients. Medicine 19:147, 1970

24 Bardana EJ Jr: The clinical spectrum of Aspergillosis. II. Classification and description of saprophytic, allergic, and invasive variants of human disease. CRC Crit Rev Clin Lab Sci 12:85–159, 1980

25 Bardana EJ, Sobti SI, Cianciulli FD, et al: Aspergillus antibody in patients with cystic fibrosis. Am J Dis Child 129:1164, 1975

26 Galant SP, Rucker RW, Groncy CE, et al: Incidence of serum antibodies to several *Aspergillus* species and to *Candida albicans* in cystic fibrosis. Am Rev Respir Dis 114:325, 1976

27 Aslam PA, Eastridge CE, Hughes FA: Aspergillosis of the lung—an 18 year experience. Chest 59:28, 1971

28 Villar TG, Pimental C, Costa MO: The tumor-like forms of aspergillosis of the lung (aspergilloma). Thorax 17:22, 1962

29 Davis D (ed): British thoracic and tuberculosis association report. Aspergilloma and residual tuberculous cavities. Tubercle 51:227, 1970

30 Varkey B, Rose HD: Pulmonary aspergilloma. A rational approach to treatment. Am J Med 61:626, 1976

31 Longbottom JL, Pepys J: Pulmonary aspergillosis: Diagnostic and Immunological significance of antigens and C. substances in *Aspergillus fumigatus*. J Pathol Bacteriol 88:141, 1964

32 Saferstein B, D'Souza M, Simon G, et al: Five year follow up of allergic bronchopulmonary aspergillosis. Am Rev Respir Dis 108:450, 1973

33 Pepys J: *Hypersensitivity Diseases of the Lungs Due to Fungi and Organic Dusts*. Basel, Karger, 1969, 324 pp

34 Henderson AH: Allergic aspergillosis. Review of 32 cases. Thorax 23:501, 1968

35 McCarthy DS, Simon G, Hargreave FE: The radiological appearances in allergic bronchopulmonary aspergillosis. Clin Radiol 21:366, 1970

36 Wang JLF, Patterson R, Rosenberg M: Serum IgE and IgG antibody activity against *Aspergillus fumigatus* as a diagnostic aid in allergic bronchopulmonary aspergillosis. Am Rev Respir Dis 117:917, 1978

37 Urschel H, Parkson D, Shaw R: Mucoid impaction of the bronchi. Ann Thorac Surg 2:1, 1966

38 Middleton WG, Paterson IG, Grant IWB, Douglas AC: Asthmatic pulmonary eosinophilia: A review of 65 cases. Br J Dis Chest 71: 115, 1971

39 Katzenstein AL, Liebow AA, Friedman PJ: Bronchocentric granulomatosis, mucoid impaction, and hypersensitivity reactions to fungi. Ann Rev Respir Dis 111:497, 1975

40 Karam GH, Griffin FM Jr: Invasive pulmonary aspergillosis in nonimmunocompromised, nonneutropenic hosts. Rev Infect Dis 8:357–363, 1986

41 Meyer RD, Young LS, Armstrong D, Yu B: Aspergillosis complicating neoplastic disease. Am J Med 54:6–15, 1973

42 Levitz SM, Diamond RD: Changing patterns of aspergillosis infections. Adv Intern Med 30:153–174, 1984

43 Orr DP, Myerowitz RI, Dubois PJ: Pathoradiologic correlation of invasive pulmonary aspergillosis in the compromised host. Cancer 41:2028, 1978

44 Aisner J, Murillo J, Schimpff SC, et al: Invasive aspergillosis in acute leukemia: Correlation with nose cultures and antibiotic use. Ann Intern Med 90:4, 1979

45 Jahrsdoerfer RA, Ejerato VS, Johns MME: Aspergillosis of nose and paranasal sinuses. Am J Otolaryngol 1:6, 1979

46 Viollier AF, Peterson DE, DeJongh Ca, et al: Aspergillus sinusitis in cancer patients. Cancer 58:366–371, 1986

47 Allo MD, Miller J, Townsend T, Tan C: Primary cutaneous aspergillosis associated with Hickman intravenous catheters. N Engl J Med 317:1105–1108, 1987

48 Simpson MB, Merz WG, Kurlinski JP, et al: Opportunistic mycotic osteomyelitis: Bone infections due to *Aspergillus* and *Candida* species. Medicine 56:475, 1977

49 Rubinstein E, Noriega ER, Simberkoff MS, et al: Fungal endocarditis: Analysis of 24 cases and review of the literature. Medicine 54:331, 1975

50 Johnson RB, Wing EJ, Miller TR, Rosenfeld CS: Isolated cardiac aspergillosis after bone marrow transplantation. Arch Intern Med 147:1942–1943, 1987

51 Mukuyama M, Gimple K, Poser CM: Aspergillosis of the central nervous system: A review of the literature. Neurology 19:967, 1969

52 Greenberger PA, Patterson R: Diagnosis and management of allergic bronchopulmonary aspergillosis. Ann Allergy 56:444–448, 1986

53 Treger TR, Visscher DW, Bartlett MS, Smith JW: Diagnosis of pulmonary infection caused by aspergillus: Usefulness of respiratory cultures. J Infect Dis 152:572–576, 1985

54 Yu VL, Muder RR, Poorsattar A: Significance of isolation of aspergillus from the respiratory tract in diagnosis of invasive pulmonary aspergillosis. Am J Med 81:249–254, 1986

55 Albelda SM, Talbot GH, Gerson SL, et al: Role of fiberoptic bronchoscopy in the diagnosis of invasive pulmonary aspergillosis in patients with acute leukemia. Am J Med 76:1027–1034, 1984

56 Kahn FW, Jones JM, England DM: The role of bronchoalveolar lavage in the diagnosis of invasive pulmonary aspergillosis. ACJP 86:518–523, 1986

57 Kuhlman JE, Fishman EK, Burch PA, et al: Invasive pulmonary aspergillosis in acute leukemia. The contribution of CT to early diagnosis and aggressive management. Chest 92:95–99, 1987

58 Bardana EJ, Gerber JD, Craig S, Cianculli FD: The general and specific humoral immune response to pulmonary aspergillosis. Am Rev Respir Dis 112:799, 1975

59 Young RC, Bennett JE: Invasive aspergillosis: Absence of a detectable antibody response. Am Rev Respir Dis 104:710, 1971

60 Weiner MH: Antigenemia detected by radioimmunoassay in systemic aspergillosis. Ann Intern Med 92:793–796, 1980

61 Shaffer PJ, Kobayashi GS, Medoff G: Demonstration of antigenemia in patients with invasive aspergillosis by solid phase radioimmunoassay. Am J Med 67:627–630, 1979

62 Bennett JE: Rapid diagnosis of candidiasis and aspergillosis. Rev Infect Dis 9:398–402, 1987

63 Pennington JE: Successful treatment of *Aspergillus* pneumonia in hematologic neoplasia. N Engl J Med 295:426, 1976

64 Aisner J, Schimpff SC, Wiernik PH: Treatment of invasive aspergillosis. Relation of early diagnosis and treatment to response. Ann Intern Med 86:539, 1977

65 Kitahara M, Seth VK, Medoff G, et al: Activity of amphotericin B, 5-flurocytosine, and rifampin against 6 clinical isolates of *Aspergillus*. Antimicrob Agents Chemother 9:915, 1976

66 Arroyo J, Medoff G, Kobayashi GS: Therapy of murine aspergillosis with amphotericin B in combination with rifampin or 5-flurocytosine. Antimicrob Agents Chemother 11:21, 1977

CHAPTER 102

Blastomycosis · Robert W. Bradsher

Blastomyces dermatitidis causes the systemic fungal infection called *blastomycosis*. The disease ranges from mild or asymptomatic infections to focal destructive lesions in the lung, skin, or various other organs which may lead to progressive, fulminant infection.

Diagnosis is made by visualization of the organism in tissue, sputum, or exudate, or by culture, because routine serological methods are not reliable for this pathogen. This chapter describes the organism and its effects in humans, the treatment for the infection, and the types of persons who typically develop blastomycosis.

PARASITE

ORGANISM

B. dermatitidis is a *dimorphic fungus,* which means that mycelial forms are present in nature with conversion to yeast forms in tissue [1]. In contrast to some organisms, the relatively easy visualization of the thick-walled budding yeast cell in clinical specimens allows a sure diagnosis of blastomycosis. The fungus varies in size from 5 to 15 μm as well as in the number of organisms found in tissue [2]. Methenamine silver or periodic acid Schiff (PAS) stain is helpful although the organism may be detected on routine histology without these special stains. Atypical forms may be noted, but most organisms are round with a double wall and a broad-based daughter bud [2].

Examinations of sputum or other clinical specimens by wet preparations with potassium hydroxide are often the means of diagnosis [3]. Visualization of the fungus after Papanicolaou staining for cytology may give the diagnosis since the clinical picture of chronic pneumonia due to blastomycosis may closely resemble carcinoma of the lung, prompting cytological examinations of sputum.

CULTURE

Colonization or contamination does not occur with *Blastomyces* as it does with *Candida* or *Aspergillus*. Cultures are routinely positive in blastomycosis cases when smears show the organism. *B. dermatitidis* displays *thermal dimorphism,* which is the transition from mycelial forms in nature to yeast in tissue. This also means that growth in cultures occurs as mycelia at 25°C and as yeast at 37°C. The mycelial or conidial stage is how the fungus is grown to confirm the diagnosis in most clinical laboratories. Growth appears as a fluffy, white mold on media at room temperature, but can also be identified from the brown, wrinkled, folded colonies of yeast if cultures are incubated at 37°C. Exoantigen testing can aid diagnosis by detecting species-specific antigen in broth cultures [4]. This is particularly helpful in poorly sporulating cultures.

SEROLOGY

Diagnostic techniques other than direct smear or culture are not as reliable for blastomycosis as for other infections [3]. Serological tests include complement-fixation (CF) antibodies, enzyme-linked immunoassay (EIA) antibodies, and immunodiffusion (ID) precipitin bands. Delayed hypersensitivity skin testing with blastomycin has also been used in past years. These assays have been useful as tools for epidemiological assessments [1,5–7] but not for clinical diagnosis. Cross-reactivity to antigens of other fungi, particularly *H. capsulatum,* is a major limiting factor. For example, a person with culture-proven blastomycosis is just as likely to demonstrate CF antibodies against histoplasmin as against blastomycin [1,3]. None of a group of patients from Arkansas had titers of CF blastomycin antibodies greater than a 1:8 dilution [8]. Immunodiffusion testing for blastomycosis has been reported to result in higher sensitivity rates of 80 percent, but there is a general lack of clinical availability for this test. Klein et al. [6] reported better results with EIA techniques using a yeast-phase antigen than with immunodiffusion tests in sera of patients with localized blastomycosis, but the same problem of lack of availability exists. In the largest outbreak of blastomycosis reported, Klein et al. [7,9] described antibody detection by EIA, ID, and CF techniques in 77 percent, 28 percent, and 9 percent, respectively. Therefore, serodiagnosis of blastomycosis is difficult because of low sensitivity and low specificity rates for available tests as noted by Davies and Sarosi [3]. Skin testing with blastomycin is no better diagnostically. Sufficient specificity and sensitivity is not provided by this mycelial-phase antigen for reliable patient assessment. In two series of blastomycosis, 59 percent and 100 percent of those with infection had negative skin tests [10,11]. Blastomycin skin test reactions also rapidly diminish in size of induration and become negative upon repeated testing so that usefulness of this intradermal test is limited even for epidemiological investigations [1]. None of the screening tests are totally reliable in the diagnosis of blastomycosis. The diagnosis of blastomycosis depends on visualization of the fungus on smear, in tissue, or in culture of infected material.

PATHOPHYSIOLOGY

Infection begins with inhalation of conidia into the lung. At body temperature, the fungus undergoes transition to yeast cells with subsequent growth in the parenchyma of the lung and in metastatic foci spread to various organs by the bloodstream and lymphatics [1]. With the development of immunity, inflammatory reactions form at the initial and distant sites of infection. The pathological reaction to the fungus is both suppurative and granulomatous showing polymorphonuclear cells, and monocytes and macrophages [2]. Pathology of the skin and laryngeal lesions of this infection may show pseudoepitheliomatous hyperplasia, prompting an erroneous diagnosis of squamous carcinoma. Endogenous reactivation may occur at either pulmonary or extrapulmonary sites whether previous therapy has been given or not.

IMMUNOLOGY

Cellular immunity is considered to be the primary host defense in blastomycosis [12]. Experimental animal models have demonstrated that this arm of immunity rather than humoral immunity is the critical host defense in preventing progressive disease. Delayed hypersensitivity to *Blastomyces* antigens was shown to be transferable by lymphocyte, but not serum, with the additional finding that immunization protected animals on subsequent challenge with live organisms [13]. Cox and others developed a yeast-phase antigen of *B. dermatitidis* which identified *Blastomyces*-sensitized animals as compared to *Histoplasma*-sensitized animals [14,15] by lymphocyte transformation assays and skin tests. Although Cox demonstrated cross-reactivity in lymphocyte reactivity assays of persons without infections using various fungal antigens of *C. immitis, H. capsulatum,* and *B. dermatitidis* [16], the antigen that Cox had prepared was used to differentiate patients with treated blastomycosis from those with histoplasmosis [17]. In additional studies, pulmonary blastomycosis patients were shown to have no evidence of immunity with this antigen at the outset of therapy, but this marker of specific *Blastomyces* cellular immunity developed over a 4-week period [17].

In human infection with *B. dermatitidis,* histology frequently shows the fungus inside or attached to macrophages or giant cells. Schwarz and Salfelder [2] routinely found one or more yeast cells located in the cytoplasm of giant cells from pathology sections from 152 cases. Enhanced phagocytosis as well as intracellular inhibition of growth of the fungus was found with macrophages from *Blastomyces*-immune mice, but not the control animals in coculture experiments of *B. dermatitidis* and macrophages [13]. Similar experiments using macrophages from humans with treated blastomycosis showed greater efficiency of phagocytosis of live *Blastomyces* than cells from normal persons [12]. In addition, a decreased proliferation of intracellular yeast *in vitro* in macrophage cultures from infected patients was noted when compared with the growth rate of the fungus in cells from controls [12]. No differences were noted between alveolar and peripheral macrophages from the same donor. The demonstration of activated macrophage function is evidence of defense by cellular immunity. Brummer et al. have shown that recombinant murine γ-interferon had an immunoregulatory effect on the murine macrophage defense system against *B. dermatitidis* [18].

The effect of other leukocytes in the defense against blastomycosis has been less clear even though these cells are almost universally present in histological sections from a site of infection. Brummer and Stevens suggested an actual enhancement of the replication of the fungus by polymorphonuclear leukocytes [19], but others have shown the opposite effect. Drutz and Frey [20] reported in vitro studies showing extensive damage to mycelia by polymorphonuclear leukocytes, but that the yeast forms of *B. dermatitidis* were more difficult for the cells to destroy. These studies indicated that these leukocytes may have a role in early host defense against *B. dermatitidis*. If only a few spores have been inhaled, this limited defense by leukocytes may be successful. This could account for patients with subclinical or asymptomatic blastomycosis who display specific immune markers.

PATIENT

GENERAL CLINICAL FEATURES

Blastomycosis can cause unusual manifestations of infection leading to difficulty in diagnosis. Even the more common features of skin lesions or pneumonia may not be quickly diagnosed because of the rarity of this infection in most geographical areas. Weight loss, fever, malaise, fatigue, and other nonspecific complaints are usually present but offer little diagnostic help. In an epidemic of infection, a person of any age or sex may develop blastomycosis, but in endemic areas, the typical patient is an adult male. The male-female ratios in large series have been reported with a range of 4:1 to 15:1 [10,11,21,1]; this most likely represents greater occupational or recreational exposures to outdoor areas with greater potential for infection [1,22].

PULMONARY FEATURES

The most common finding in patients with blastomycosis is a pulmonary infiltrate. The majority of patients have either an alveolar or masslike infiltrate, although a reticulonodular or miliary pattern may be found. Upper-lobe localization has been more commonly reported, but the lobar location of the infiltrate of blastomycosis is not actually helpful diagnostically [1]. Cavitary disease may occur, but this pattern is not found as commonly as in chronic pulmonary histoplasmosis or tuberculosis. Based on radiographic appearance, many blastomycosis patients are initially thought to have pulmonary neoplastic diseases. Pleural disease is considered by some to be common, and by others to be distinctly unusual in this manifestation. In summary, none of the radiographic patterns are diagnostic.

Patients with acute blastomycotic pneumonia present similarly to those with bacterial disease with fever, chills, and a productive cough with purulent sputum and perhaps hemoptysis. Antibacterial antibiotics are not effective, but some patients with either epidemic or endemic disease have been reported to have spontaneous resolution of their acute pneumonia [6,7,12,17]. This may erroneously suggest a response to routine antibiotics.

Chronic pneumonia due to blastomycosis usually causes symptoms for 2 to 6 months, including weight loss, night sweats, fever, cough with sputum production, and chest pain. These patients would likely be considered to have a malignancy or tuberculosis. Blastomycosis patients with pulmonary infiltrates may have no pulmonary symptoms and may be discovered via routine radiographs or routine examinations performed for other reasons.

EXTRAPULMONARY FINDINGS

The skin lesions seen in blastomycosis have been of two major types: *verrucous* and *ulcerative* [11]. The verrucous form has an irregular elevated border with obvious crusting above the abscess in the subcutaneous tissue (Fig. 102-1). Histologically, these lesions may show papillomatosis, downward proliferation of the epidermis with abscesses, with specific histological stains showing the organisms [2]. The ulcerative form of blastomycosis has similar histology (Fig. 102-2). The borders are elevated, and the base of the ulcer usually has exudate present. The majority originate from subcutaneous pustules which subsequently drain.

Osteomyelitis due to *B. dermatitidis* is reported in 25 to 50 percent of cases [11]. The vertebrae, pelvis, sacrum, skull, ribs, or long bones are more commonly reported, but any bone may be involved [1,11]. The radiographic appearance of involvement is not distinguishable from that of other fungal, bacterial, or neoplastic disease.

The next most common site of involvement is the genitourinary system; prostatitis and epididymoorchitis have frequently been reported [1,11]. The detection of genitourinary involve-

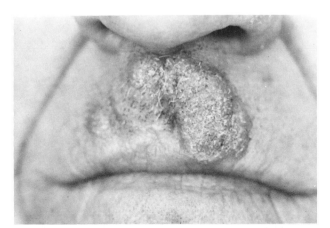

Figure 102-1. Facial lesion due to blastomycosis. The fungating, irregularly elevated lesion is typical of the nodular verrucous form of cutaneous blastomycosis.

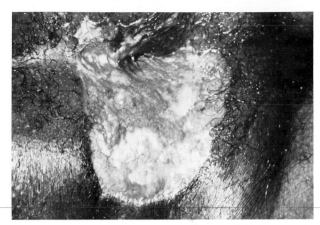

Figure 102-2. Ulcerative form of blastomycosis. This lesion on the buttocks shows the mounded margins of the ulcer. Exudate containing the organisms covers the base of the ulcer.

ment will be improved if urine cultures are collected after prostatic massage. As is the case with skin or bone infection, the organism will usually be present in the lung as well as the prostate or epididymis.

Blastomycosis involves the nervous system in a small number of cases of disseminated disease [1,11] with meningitis or with epidural or cranial abscesses. Meningitis may be more difficult to diagnose than abscesses which are localized by radiographic studies. Evaluation of spinal fluid may not be diagnostic, requiring culture of ventricular fluid. In a review of cases, lumbar puncture gave the diagnosis in only 2 of 22 cases, while ventricular fluid specimens were positive in 6 of 7 cases [23].

Abscesses are most common in the subcutaneous tissue, but, as already noted, they may be found in virtually any organ. This includes lesions in the myocardium, pericardium, orbit, sinuses, pituitary, adrenal glands, liver, or other organs as reviewed by Witorch and Utz [11]. Of particular note is laryngeal involvement in this infection. The hyperplasia and acanthosis histologically, and the fungating appearance of the lesion on the larynx has led to the erroneous diagnosis of neoplasm rather than blastomycosis. Widely disseminated or miliary blastomycosis may occur with an acute presentation or one which is overwhelming. Patients with overwhelming disease may present with adult respiratory distress syndrome [24]. Almost all of these patients with diffuse infiltrates, noncardiac pulmonary edema, and refractory hypoxemia die very quickly following presentation.

TREATMENT

The first consideration for the patient with blastomycosis is whether or not to treat with an antifungal agent. If the patient is not very ill, observation of pneumonia for one to two weeks may show resolution of the infection. Observation alone may also be indicated in the patient with acute pneumonia that resolves before the organism is identified by culture. Observation following surgical resection of a solitary pulmonary lesion if no other disease is present has been recommended by some rather than treating with systemic antifungal drugs. The presence of pleural disease or any extrapulmonary infection during the course of illness requires antifungal treatment. All other forms of blastomycosis should be treated.

Amphotericin B has been shown to be effective in the treatment of blastomycosis. A dose of 2.0 g has been associated with cure rates up to 97 percent but with toxicities of renal dysfunction, anemia, fever, hypokalemia, and thrombophlebitis [21]. Relapse after amphotericin B is rare. The main reason for considering not giving or postponing treatment of pulmonary blastomycosis has been the toxicity of amphotericin B, which was the only therapy until recent years.

Ketoconazole is an imidazole antifungal agent which has in vitro activity against *B. dermatitidis* comparable with that of amphotericin B [25,26]. The major advantage of the drug is that it is given orally and is generally not very toxic as compared to amphotericin B. Adverse reactions include rare episodes of hepatitis and dose-related endocrinologic abnormalities. Two large trials of ketoconazole in the treatment of blastomycosis resulted in cure rates of greater than 85 percent in those who were compliant with therapy [8,26]. With the lower potential for toxicity and the cost savings of outpatient therapy, ketoconazole is considered to be the drug of choice for less than life-threatening infection. Newer imidazole and triazole antifungal agents, such as itraconazole, are being developed which appear promising for use in blastomycosis. For the very ill patient, amphotericin B remains the treatment of choice, with a switch to ketoconazole following improvement.

POPULATION

EPIDEMIOLOGY

Endemic or sporadic cases account for the majority of cases of blastomycosis, but a few epidemics of infection from point sources have also been described. Unfortunately, *B. dermatitidis* has been very difficult to isolate from the soil—in contrast to the ease of growing other fungi from soil, such as *Histoplasma capsulatum*. Klein and coworkers [6,7] reported the isolation of *B. dermatitidis* from soil for the first time in association with epidemics of infection. Both isolations were from moist soil with high organic content, thus providing evidence that the fungus exists in microfoci in soil. In both epidemics, the isolation of the fungus from soil was noted to be associated with either animals or bodies of water [7,22]. Whether these associations are the primary factor or simply represent a greater exposure opportunity to humans because of increased recreational activities in areas with wildlife or water remains to be determined.

The geographical distribution of blastomycosis is primarily in the Americas and Africa. The finding of this infection in Africa is the reason for abandoning the term North American blastomycosis. Within the Americas, blastomycosis extends from Canada southward to Central America. Cases in South America have been rare. African cases have been rare but widely distributed over the continent with most cases occurring in Zimbabwe. Cases have been recently reported from the Middle East (Lebanon, Israel, Saudi Arabia), India, and Poland [27].

REFERENCES

1 Sarosi GA, Davies SF: Blastomycosis. State of the art. Am Rev Respir Dis 120:911–938, 1979
2 Schwarz J, Salfelder K: Blastomycosis: A review of 152 cases. Curr Top Pathol 65:165–200, 1977
3 Davies SF, Sarcosi GA: Serodiagnosis of hystoplasmosis and blastomycosis. Am Rev Respir Dis 136:254–255, 1987
4 Kaufman L, Standard P, Padhye AA: Exoantigen tests for the immunoidentification of fungal cultures. Mycopathologia 82:3–12, 1983
5 Furcolow ML, Chick EW, Busey JF, et al: Prevalence and incidence studies of human and canine blastomycosis. I. Cases in the United States 1885–1968. Am Rev Respir Dis 102:60–67, 1970
6 Klein BS, Vergeront JM, DiSalvo AF, et al: Two outbreaks of blastomycosis along rivers in Wisconsin: isolation of *Blastomyces dermatitidis* from riverbank soil and evidence of its transmission along waterways. Am Rev Respir Dis 136:1333–1338, 1988
7 Klein B, Vegeront JM, Weeks RJ, et al: Isolation of *Blastomyces dermatitides* in soil associated with a large outbreak of blastomycosis in Wisconsin. N Engl J Med 314:529–534, 1986
8 Bradsher RW, Rice DC, Abernathy RS: Ketoconazole therapy of endemic blastomycosis. Ann Intern Med 103:872–879, 1985
9 Klein B, Vergeront JM, Kaufman L, et al: Serological tests for blastomycosis: Assessments during a large point-source outbreak in Wisconsin. J Infect Dis 155:262–268, 1987
10 Busey JF: Blastomycosis: A review of 198 collected cases in VA hospitals. Am Rev Respir Dis 89:659–672, 1964
11 Witorch P, Utz JP: North American blastomycosis: A study of 40 patients. Medicine 47:169–200, 1968
12 Bradsher RW, Balk RA, Jacobs RF: Growth inhibition of *Blastomyces dermatitidis* in alveolar and peripheral macrophages from patients with blastomycosis. Am Rev Respir Dis 135:412–417, 1987
13 McDaniel LS, Cozad GC: Immunomodulation of *Blastomyces dermatitidis:* Functional activity of murine peritoneal macrophages. Infect Immun 40:733–740, 1983
14 Cox RA, Larsh HW: Isolation of skin test-active preparations from yeast-phase cells of *Blastomyces dermatitidis*. Infect Immun 10:42–47, 1974
15 Deighton F, Cox RA, Hall NJ, et al: *In vivo* and in vitro cell-mediated immune responses to a cell wall antigen of *Blastomyces dermatitidis*. Infect Immun 15:429–435, 1977
16 Cox RA: Cross-reactivity between antigens of *Coccidioides immitis, Histoplasma capsulatum,* and *Blastomyces dermatitidis* in lymphocyte transformation assays. Infect Immun 25:932–938, 1979
17 Bradsher RW: Development of specific immunity in patients with pulmonary or extrapulmonary blastomycosis. Am Rev Respir Dis 129:430–434, 1984

18 Brummer E, Morrison CJ, Stevens DA: Recombinant and natural gamma-interferon activation of macrophages *in vitro:* Different dose requirements for induction of killing activity against phagocytizable and nonphagocytizable fungi. Infect Immun 49:724–730, 1985

19 Brummer E, Stevens DA: Opposite effects of human monocytes, macrophages, and polymorphonuclear neutrophils on replication of *Blastomyces dermatitidis in vitro.* Infect Immun 36:297–303, 1982

20 Drutz DJ, Frey CL: Intracellular and extracellular defenses of human phagocytes against *Blastomyces dermatitidis,* conidia and yeasts. J Lab Clin Med 105:737–750, 1985

21 Abernathy RS: Amphotericin therapy of North American blastomycosis. Antimicrob Agents Chemother 3:208–211, 1967

22 Bradsher RW: Water and blastomycosis: Don't blame beaver. Am Rev Respir Dis 136:1324–1326, 1987

23 Kravitz GR, Davies SF, Eckman MR, et al: Chronic blastomycotic meningitis. Am J Med 71:501–505, 1981

24 Evans ME, Haynes JB, Atkinson JB, et al: *Blastomyces dermatitidis* and the adult respiratory distress syndrome. Am Rev Respir Dis 126:1099–1102, 1982

25 Dismukes WE, Stamm AM, Graybill JR, et al: Treatment of systemic mycoses with ketoconazole: Emphasis on toxicity and clinical response in 52 patients. Ann Intern Med 98:13–20, 1983

26 National Institutes of Allergy and Infectious Disease, Mycosis Study Group: Treatment of blastomycosis and histoplasmosis with ketoconazole: Results of a prospective, randomized clinical trial. Ann Intern Med 103:861–872, 1985

27 Anon. Blastomycosis—one disease or two? Lancet 1:25–26, 1989

CHAPTER 103 / *Candidiasis* · Jeffrey M. Jones

Oral thrush, characterized by reddening and white flocculent stippling of the oral mucosa, was first described in the fourth century B.C. by Hippocrates in a patient debilitated by an enteric fever; however, *Candida albicans,* the microorganism causing thrush, was not described until 1839 [*1*]. In ensuing years it became clear that this fungus can infect virtually every tissue of the body. Severe *Candida* infections have been observed with increasing frequency in immunocompromised patients during the past decade and literature dealing with *Candida* infections has increased accordingly.

PARASITE

NOMENCLATURE AND ECOLOGY

The term *candidiasis* is applied to infections produced by members of the genus *Candida. C. albicans* and *C. tropicalis* are the species most frequently causing human candidiasis. *C. stellatoidea, C. krusei, C. pseudotropicalis, C. guilliermondii, C. parapsilosis,* and the closely related yeast *Torulopsis glabrata* are also medically important. Moniliasis, an older name for *Candida* infection, arose because these yeasts were classified at one time in the genus *Monilia,* yeastlike fungi commonly inhabiting decaying vegetation [*2*]. In contrast to other yeasts, which are ubiquitous in terrestrial and aquatic habitats, *Candida* species have been isolated primarily from humans and other warm-blooded animals. Some authors consider *C. albicans, C. stellatoidea,* and *T. glabrata* obligatory animal saprophytes [*2*]. Transfer of *C. albicans* from maternal mucous membranes to those of the newborn infant occurs during birth or soon thereafter and colonization of mouth, intes-

tines, and skin of intertriginous zones is completed soon after birth. Thus, in humans it is the breakdown of normal barriers to infection or overgrowth of the endogenous yeast flora which results in candidiasis.

MORPHOLOGY AND ULTRASTRUCTURE

Figure 103-1 demonstrates the large size of *Candida* relative to bacteria. All *Candida* species can reproduce as oval budding structures, called blastospores, measuring about 2.5×5 μm. The blastospore is endowed with a thick cell wall (Fig. 103-2) and up to five layers are recognizable in the cell wall [*3*] by transmission electron microscopy. Host tissues have a lower oxygen tension than that of the atmosphere. This lower oxygen tension, and the presence of serum and other substances, stimulate the growth of cylindrical structures, called germ tubes, from blastospores of *C. albicans* and many isolates of *C. stellatoidea* [*2*]. A germ tube forms no constriction at its point of origin and only one germ tube is produced by each blastospore. Elongation of the germ tube may continue with septa forming behind its extending apical end and blastospores budding from the resultant cylindrical septate hypha. *Candida albicans* and other *Candida* species undergo a budding process in which elongated elements are formed that remain attached to each other to produce pseudohyphae. *T. glabrata* reproduces exclusively as a budding blastospore. In all other species, blastospores will bud from each other and from the pseudohyphae near their constriction points. Only *C. albicans* can produce thick-walled chlamydospores at the ends of pseudohyphae; however, these chlamydospores are readily produced on certain culture media but are rarely seen in infected tissue.

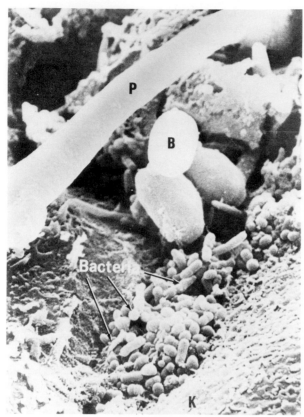

Figure 103-1. Scanning electron micrograph showing long pseudohypha (P) and blastospores (B) of *C. albicans* as well as numerous bacteria on the surface of keratinized cells (K) in oral candidiasis (original magnification, × 6700). Note difference in size between yeast and bacteria. (*From* [*33*].)

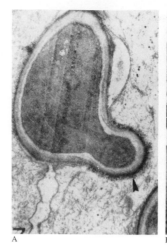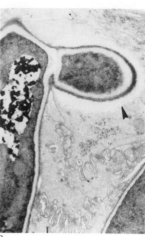

Figure 103-2. Transmission electron micrographs showing *C. albicans* penetrating epithelial cells. *A.* Original magnification, × 15,000; the outer layer of cell wall is inconspicuous where the fungus is in close association with the cell membrane but is evident where penetration of the epithelial cell has occurred (arrow). *B.* Original magnification, × 10,000; dissolution of epithelial cell membrane is limited and loss of cytoplasmic material around the fungal profile (arrow) is seen infrequently. (*From* [*3*].)

BIOCHEMISTRY, PHYSIOLOGY, AND IN VITRO CULTURE

Candida is an aerobic eukaryote with a cytoplasm containing vacuoles, ribosomes, and mitochondria. The organism's cell membrane, which maintains its osmotic integrity, is rich in ergosterol. The imidazole antimicrobials, miconazole and ketoconazole, inhibit ergosterol synthesis and the polyene antimicrobials, nystatin and amphotericin B, bind to ergosterol. Therefore, all these antifungal agents produce leakage of the cell membrane that results ultimately in death of the organism. Biotyping of isolates by observing growth on various media has been described and typing of isolates by use of nuclear or mitochondrial DNA polymorphism is under investigation [*4*].

To maintain viability of *Candida* after their recovery from the host, swabs or tissues bearing the organism may be placed in any transport medium that will prevent desiccation, including sterile water. *Candida* species will grow on a variety of common culture media including blood and chocolate agar. They grow poorly on eosin-methylene blue agar. Sabouraud's dextrose agar is the medium of choice for isolation and if *Candida* is to be recovered from specimens heavily contaminated with bacteria, culture should be done at 22 to 30°C on this medium to which chloramphenicol has been added. Isolation of *Candida* should not be attempted on media supplemented with cycloheximide. This reagent, which is added to media to inhibit growth of saprophytic molds, may prevent growth of *Candida* [*5*].

Recovery of *Candida* from the blood is difficult. Experimental studies in rats and rabbits support the view that *Candida* are cleared much more rapidly from the blood than bacteria because their larger size results in their being caught in capillaries or engulfed by reticuloendothelial cells [*6*]. Therefore, multiple blood cultures must be taken when *Candida* fungemia is suspected and measures must be taken to enhance growth of the fungus from the blood specimens.

Since *Candida* grow best aerobically, it is essential that "aerobic" culture bottles be used. Lysis of blood followed by centrifugation and culture of concentrate on solid medium enhances recovery of *Candida*. A commercially available lysis-centrifugation system (Isolator Microbial Tubes, DuPont and Co., Wilmington, DE) is available. Although this system yields more positive cultures for yeasts than another widely used broth system (Bactec, Johnston Laboratories, Towson, MD), bacterial contaminants are more common using the lysis-centrifugation system [*7*].

When *Candida* is to be isolated from a specimen containing a mixture of microorganisms, culturing on differential solid media containing bismuth sulfite (Nickerson medium) or a tetrazolium dye and neomycin (Pagano-Levin medium) may be useful.

After initial isolation of *Candida*, subculture on bromocresol green agar containing neomycin may be done to ensure that a pure culture will be obtained for speciation. The first step in speciation is inoculation into serum and incubation at 35°C for 0.5 to 3 h. Over 95 percent of *C. albicans* isolates and some *C. stellatoidea* isolates will produce germ tubes under these conditions. If this germ tube test is negative, the organism is inoculated onto glucose-free corn meal agar containing 0.3% Tween 80 [5]. A coverslip is placed on the agar surface and the covered area is examined under the microscope after incubation at 22 to 26°C for 18 to 24 h. *Candida albicans* will produce well-developed pseudohyphae with terminal chlamydospores on this medium, *T. glabrata* will show only blastospores, and all other species will produce pseudohyphae but no chlamydospores. Final speciation is accomplished by carbon assimilation tests [5]. Kits such as the API-20C strip (Analytab Products, Inc., Plainview, NY) and Uni-Yeast-Tek plate (Flow Laboratories, Inc., Roslyn, NY) are available for this purpose.

ANIMAL MODELS

Experimental models for cutaneous infection by *C. albicans* have been described for the mouse and rat [8], guinea pig [9],

and humans [10]. Oral thrush has been produced experimentally in rats and rabbits, and mechanisms of resistance to disseminated candidiasis have been studied in mice and rats [11], guinea pigs, rabbits [6], and dogs. Hypovitaminosis A, B_1, B_2, and B_6 increases the susceptibility of the rat to *Candida* infection and presumably the same is true for humans [2].

PATIENT

HOST-PARASITE INTERFACE

There are a variety of materials in the cell wall and cytoplasm of *C. albicans*, some of which are released into the environment surrounding the microorganism to interact with the host (Table 103-1). Most of our knowledge about all these substances has developed during the past decade and one can anticipate that our knowledge about interaction of *C. albicans* with the host will expand even more rapidly during the next decade.

It is now clear that the microenvironment at host surfaces or in host tissue influences the morphology of *Candida*, the chemistry of its surface structures, its metabolism, and ultimately its interaction with the host. For example, human saliva has been shown to promote germination of *C. albicans*. Surfaces of germ tubes posses proteins that bind to epithelial or fibrin-platelet matrices (Table 103-1). This may explain the

Table 103-1. Important components of *Candida albicans*

Component	Location in *Candida*	Importance to *Candida*	Interactions with host	Relevance to diagnosis
Glucan	Cell wall	Polysaccharide, provides rigid structure of cell wall [4]	Induces granuloma formation [12]	Organism is gram-positive and stains with silver methenamine or periodic acid Schiff reagent
Mannan	Cell wall	Polysaccharide, abundant in innermost and outermost layers of cell wall [4]	Induces antibody production, activates alternate complement pathway, possible role in attachment [13,16]	Elevation of antimannan antibody levels and detection of mannan in sera of patients with deep organ infection [14,15]
Cell wall proteins and glycoproteins	Cell wall	Attachment to epithelial cells or to fibrin-platelet matrix; germ tube antigen described [16,17]	Attachment sites for neutrophils	Under investigation
Numerous other proteins	Cytoplasm and cell membrane	Numerous enzymatic and structural functions	Released from dead organisms, induce antibody and delayed hypersensitivity responses [14,18]	Antibody detectable in patients with deep organ infection; antigen detection under study
Proteolytic enzymes and phospholipase	Secreted	Possible role in penetration of keratinized cells	Very limited destruction of cell membrane and cytoplasm of host cells (Fig. 103-2)	None
D-arabinitol	Secreted metabolite	Used as energy source when glucose depleted	Released into tissue fluids at site of infection	Elevation of levels in sera of patients with deep organ involvement [19]

tendency of *C. albicans* to colonize epithelial surfaces and to adhere in large numbers to ulcerations of mucous membranes. While some features of host surfaces favor attachment of the fungus, other characteristics of the microenvironment may favor colonization of the host by the microorganism by stimulating its proliferation. For example, treating a woman with a tetracycline orally is known to increase vaginal *Candida* carriage [2] and can precipitate symptomatic *Candida* vaginitis. The antibacterial removes flora from the vaginal surface that normally compete with *Candida* for nutrients, leading to proliferation of the *Candida*. Just prior to menses and particularly during the third trimester of pregnancy, epithelial glycogen increases. Action of Döderlein bacilli on this glycogen results in a low vaginal pH, which is unfavorable to growth of many bacteria but favors growth of *Candida*. Proliferation of the yeast in this situation leads to extensive colonization of the vaginal surface and may lead to symptomatic candidiasis.

Invasion of epithelial surfaces

Epithelial cells of skin and mucous membranes are the major barriers to penetration of the host by *Candida* species. Only *C. albicans* and *C. stellatoidea* can invade cornified epithelium of rodents [8]. Although *C. albicans* produces small amounts of hydrolytic enzymes, the mechanical support offered by the close attachment of the microorganism to the epithelial cells along with linear growth of filamentous structures produced by the microorganism appear more important than enzymatic activity in penetration of epithelial cells [3] (Fig. 103-2).

Host responses

Complement, specific antibodies, neutrophils, and thymus-dependent lymphocytes are all important in attacking *Candida* that have penetrated the epithelial barrier of the host. Patients with chronic mucocutaneous candidiasis, the clinical features of which will be discussed in detail later, have defects of the thymus-dependent lymphocyte system. Skin biopsies of infected skin from these patients show massive infiltrations of the dermis and epidermis by monocytes, lymphocytes, and neutrophils. Some patients with this disorder will present with so-called *Candida* granulomas of the skin. Microscopic examination of a biopsy of such a lesion reveals gross hyperkeratosis, parakeratosis, and acanthosis. Epithelioid cells and giant cells are present at the border between the lesion and surrounding normal tissue. These histological observations and in vitro studies of lymphocytes and monocytes from patients with chronic mucocutaneous candidiasis have shown that they can bring phagocytic cells to sites of *C. albicans* invasion but that either their thymus-dependent lymphocytes fail to produce lymphokines needed to activate these phagocytes to kill the *Candida* or their phagocytic cells are not activated appropriately by these mediators [20].

Anti-*Candida* IgA is accepted by the vaginal mucosa and presumably by other mucous membranes [35]; however, the role of such antibody in preventing attachment of *Candida* to mucous membranes is unknown. IgG antibody against the cell wall mannan of *Candida* is present in serum from virtually all immunocompetent humans [14]. Attachment of this antibody to *C. albicans* blastospores enhances their phagocytosis by neutrophils. *Candida* cell walls can activate the alternative complement pathway. The presence of the C3 component of complement on the ingested microorganism mediates ingestion and killing of the microbe by neutrophils [13].

Although both neutrophils and macrophages can ingest and kill *Candida* blastospores, neutrophils appear to be the most important single defense for eliminating *Candida* which have penetrated through the skin and mucous membranes into deeper tissues. Patients who are granulocytopenic are more prone to develop *Candida* fungemia and disseminated candidiasis than any other patient population [21]. Trapping and ingestion of *Candida* by macrophages of the reticuloendothelial system is of major importance in clearing the microbe from the blood [12].

PATHOGENESIS, PATHOPHYSIOLOGY, AND PATHOLOGY

The pustular dermatitis typically produced by *C. albicans* (Fig. 103-3) can be produced experimentally in normal human volunteers by placing occlusive tape for several hours over a site where *C. albicans* has been applied [10]. The likelihood pustules will form increases as one increases either the time of occlusion or the number of organisms applied. Thus, occlusion of the skin and circumstances favoring the growth of the fungus are the chief factors promoting development of dermatitis. Experiments have also shown that penetration of normal human

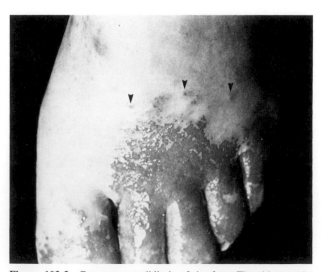

Figure 103-3. Cutaneous candidiasis of the foot. The shiny, moist erythematous area over the toes indicates where cornified epithelium has been shed. Subcorneal pustules, which have not become confluent, appear as "satellite lesions" (arrows).

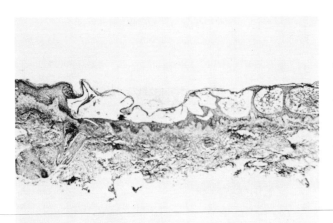

Figure 103-4. Histological appearance (hematoxylin and eosin stain, original magnification, × 32) of *Candida* dermatitis lesion. Note fusion of pustules to produce a large subcorneal suppurative lake occupying the entire upper epidermis. The horny roof easily ruptures and is rapidly lost. (*From [10].*)

epithelium by *C. albicans* is limited to stratum corneum and the Malpighian layers of epidermis. Mannan and other materials released from *C. albicans* trigger an outpouring of inflammatory cells into the deep epithelium of the skin, resulting in development of subcorneal pustules (Fig. 103-4). This chemotaxis of inflammatory cells is mediated by complement and specific antibodies and thymus-dependent lymphocytes [8,13,18]. Sheets of cornified epithelial cells are shed as subcorneal pustules coalesce. Therefore, a fully developed *Candida* dermatitis presents with a central, moist, hyperemic area corresponding to the location where the upper layer of the epithelium has sloughed. "Satellite lesions," red papules which represent newly formed subcorneal abscesses, are present on skin surrounding the erythematous, moist patch (Fig. 103-3). It should be noted that by shedding the infected cornified epithelium, the host actually rids itself of the bulk of the invading microorganisms.

Reproducible experimental human models for infection of buccal mucosa have not been obtained. This may mean that abnormalities of the mucous membranes such as atrophy or ulceration must be present before *Candida* infection can occur. Such mucosal defects occur in patients wearing dentures and patients receiving cytotoxic chemotherapy or steroids.

Patients with severe burns, penetrating wounds of the bowel, or surgical anastomoses of the bowel have serious defects in barriers to *Candida* penetration and may develop disseminated candidiasis [34,42]. *C. albicans* and less commonly *C. parapsilosis, C. tropicalis,* or other *Candida* species may be directly inoculated into the bloodstream by intravenous devices or fluids. This occurs most commonly in patients receiving parenteral hyperalimentation or in heroin addicts [34]. The pattern of disease produced by bloodborne dissemination de-

pends upon the portal of entry of the yeast, and the organs in which greatest infection occurs.

CLINICAL MANIFESTATIONS

Since *C. albicans* is commonly inoculated into the mouth of the infant during passage through the birth canal, it is not surprising that oral candidiasis or thrush may occur shortly after birth. Thrush begins as soft white patches on tonsils, cheeks, gingivae, or tongue (Fig. 103-5). These patches, which are composed of cellular debris, inflammatory exudate, and *Candida,* are readily removed by a swab to expose an erythematous mucosal surface. In time, reddening of the entire oral mucosa can occur. Breast-feeding an infant with thrush will frequently result in localized candidiasis of the mother's nipple. Thus, the fungus can be continually passed between mother and infant. The same cycle can occur when nipples used in bottle-feeding are not adequately disinfected. Oral thrush is usually self-limited in infants but topical treatment may be needed when symptoms are severe. Some babies will fail to thrive when they develop painful ulcerations of the oral mucosa or have extension of candidiasis onto skin around the lips or into the upper esophagus. In childhood and adulthood, vitamin deficiencies and iron deficiency may lead to *Candida* glossitis. *Candida albicans* may contribute to stomatitis of dentures, angular cheilitis, and folliculitis of the beard.

Colonization of the intestinal mucosa by *Candida* occurs within the first weeks of life. Thereafter, skin of the infant's perineum will be inoculated with yeast shed in the feces and occlusion of this area by diapers will lead to cutaneous candidiasis that will be recognized as a diaper rash.

In adults, cutaneous candidiasis can occur in any area of skin that is colonized with *Candida* and becomes occluded for prolonged periods of time (Fig. 103-3); however, intertrigo of the groins, perineum, secondary folds of obesity, submammary folds, or axillae is the most common presentation of cutaneous

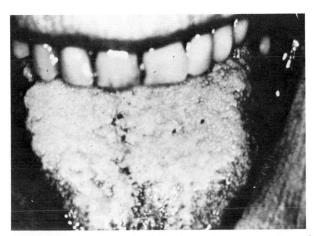

Figure 103-5. Oral thrush. A thick white exudate covers portions of the tongue and oral mucosa.

candidiasis in older patients. In all cases, the infection presents as a shiny, reddened area moistened with an inflammatory exudate where cornified epithelium has been lost. The edge of this area will be slightly elevated by a readily detachable epithelial fringe. Punctiform "satellite lesions" will be present beyond this edge. The patient will complain of burning and itching, and lichenification of surrounding skin may be present.

Candida vaginitis has an appearance similar to oral thrush and may be accompanied by cutaneous candidiasis of the vulva. The infection most commonly occurs during late pregnancy, and in women with diabetes mellitus or who are using oral contraceptives. Vaginal or vulvar itching, or burning on urination, simulating a urinary tract infection, may be noted.

Candida balanitis presents as pustular or vesicular lesions on a reddened glans penis. Burning is the most common symptom. The infection occurs in diabetics and in men whose sexual partners have high vaginal carriage of *Candida*.

Erosio interdigitalis blastomycetica and *Candida* paronychia are two infections of the skin of the hand which are clearly initiated by *C. albicans*. The former is an erosive dermatitis of the third finger web and the latter is a warm, tense area of inflammation adjacent to the nail. Both lesions are associated with frequent immersion of the hands in water and are probably sustained by bacterial superinfection [*23*].

Although *C. albicans* frequently can be isolated from loci of esophagitis present in patients known to have reflux of gastric contents or retention of esophageal contents due to abnormal esophageal motility, chemical or physical damage to the esophageal mucosa is probably more important than *Candida* in sustaining esophagitis in either of these settings.

The histopathology and pathogenesis of chronic mucocutaneous candidiasis have been discussed previously. Patients with this syndrome can present with a variety of findings such as chronic paronychia, chronic oral thrush with or without esophagitis, or exuberant keratotic skin plaques called *Candida* granulomas. Chronic *Candida* esophagitis may result in esophageal stricture formation. The vast majority of cases begin in infancy, are clearly familial, and are associated with endocrinopathies such as hypothyroidism, diabetes mellitus, hypoparathyroidism, and Addison's disease [*20*]. The syndrome may also begin after infancy in the first two decades of life by genetically determined or unknown factors.

Rarely, *Candida* can colonize the bronchial tree and elicit allergic reactions that lead to episodes of pulmonary infiltrates, asthma, and eosinophilia [*24*].

With the exception of *Candida* endocarditis in heroin addicts, deep organ involvement is seen in abnormal hosts, many of whom will have had major medical or surgical interventions. In such patients, severe localized infections such as necrotizing candidiasis of the esophagus and intestines, peritonitis, pneumonitis, and pyelonephritis can occur. A variety of disease manifestations related to bloodborne dissemination have been described including endophthalmitis, septic arthritis or osteomyelitis (Fig. 103-6), meningitis, embolic skin lesions, en-

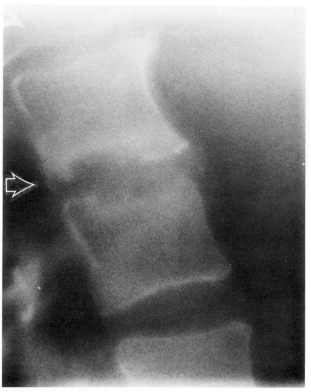

Figure 103-6. *Candida* osteomyelitis of the lumbar spine demonstrated as bony defects in a lateral view x-ray of the spine. The patient, who had acute leukemia and was neutropenic, had numerous negative blood cultures. He developed back pain and fever. Diagnosis was confirmed by needle aspiration of the vertebra indicated by arrow.

docarditis, hepatitis, renal infection, and possibly pneumonitis [*21,34,46*]. Most reported cases of *Candida* meningitis have occurred in infancy, chiefly in premature infants.

DIAGNOSIS

The diagnosis of cutaneous or mucous membrane candidiasis will frequently be based largely on the appearance of the lesions present. Blastospores and pseudohyphae can be demonstrated in potassium hydroxide preparations of scrapings taken from the edges of skin lesions and in wet mounts or Gram stains of swabs of white patches from mucous membranes (Fig. 103-7). Scaping or swabs can be cultured on Sabouraud's agar if speciation of the *Candida* is desired.

A quantitative culture of a clean-catch urine specimen showing ≥100,000 bacteria per mL is frequently used as a criterion for significant bacteriuria. By contrast, it appears that ≥20,000 colony-forming units of *Candida* per mL clean-catch urine suggests the presence of a *Candida* urinary tract infection [*26*]. This difference is thought to be due to the fact that *Candida* divide more slowly in urine than bacteria. It should be emphasized that urine containing over 100,000 *Candida* per mL

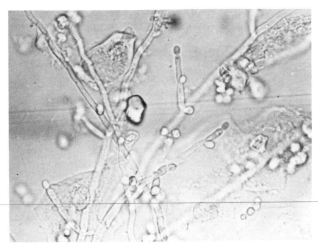

Figure 103-7. Wet mount of exudates scraped from the vagina of a patient with vulvovaginal candidiasis (original magnification, × 420). Multiple mycelial elements with attached blastospores are seen. (*Courtesy of Dr. Jack Sobel.*)

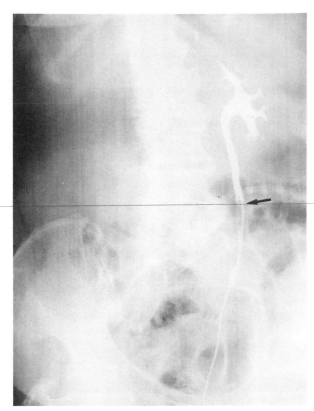

Figure 103-8. Retrograde pyelogram of an elderly woman who presented with rigors, temperature of 39°C orally, and flank tenderness. Urinalysis showed numerous yeasts and pseudomycelia, and blood cultures grew *C. albicans*. She had a past history of recurrent bacterial urinary tract infections and *Candida* vaginitis. *Candida,* which had refluxed into the ureter, produced a "fungus ball," which partially occluded the ureter (arrow). Acute pyelonephritis and septicemia resulted.

may be obtained from a patient whose urinary tract has been inoculated with the fungus through an indwelling urinary catheter. Such catheterized patients will rarely develop a significant *Candida* urinary tract infection providing drainage is adequate. If an uncatheterized patient has symptoms of cystitis, a urine sediment consistent with a urinary tract infection, and ≥20,000 colonies of *Candida* per mL clean-catch urine, another urine specimen should be taken for culture and antifungal therapy may be begun [27]. In general, the asymptomatic patient with *Candida* in the urine will require no therapy since the infection will usually clear spontaneously with time. Pyelonephritis due to *Candida* rarely occurs without obstruction of the upper urinary tract [28]. Therefore, a patient with flank pain and ≥20,000 *Candida* per mL clean-catch urine should be investigated for the presence of an obstruction of the upper urinary tract by echography, intravenous pyelography, or cystoscopy, depending upon the clinical situation. Occasionally, a patient who has had *Candida* present in the urine for some time will develop a "fungus ball" that will occlude the ureter and lead to *Candida* pyelonephritis (Fig. 103-8) [46].

Generally, the diagnosis of visceral candidiasis will be considered only in patients who are severely compromised hosts. Necrotizing *Candida* esophagitis is diagnosed by barium esophagram and endoscopy (Fig. 103-9). A careful fundoscopic examination searching for endophthalmitis should be done in patients suspected of having disseminated candidiasis [20] (Fig. 103-10). Erythematous papular skin lesions can be biopsied, sectioned, and stained with Gomori methenamine silver stain to look for *Candida* if bloodborne dissemination is suspected [20]. In a patient who has received cytotoxic drugs and has granulocytopenia, strikingly elevated serum alkaline phosphatase level, and unexplained fever, examination of a silver-

stained liver biopsy section may demonstrate granulomatous lesions containing *Candida* [25] (Fig. 103-11). The usefulness of quantitation of anti-*Candida* antibodies in the diagnosis of severe candidiasis is under investigation and there is evidence that it may be feasible to detect antigens or metabolites of *Candida* in sera from patients with severe candidiasis [14,15].

MANAGEMENT

Successful treatment of cutaneous candidiasis requires application of topical antifungal agents and removal of factors that initiated the infection. Creams or lotions containing nystatin, miconazole nitrate, or clotrimazole should be applied two to three times daily and be continued for several days after resolution of the lesions. Since all these preparations work well, cost will determine which preparation is selected. Although Castellani's paint (0.3% basic fuchsin, 4.5% phenol, 5% acetone, 10% resorcinol, 10% ethanol) and 0.1 to 1.0% gentian violet are inexpensive, possess excellent antifungal activity,

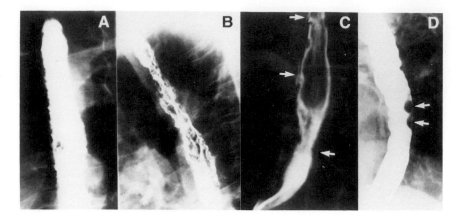

Figure 103-9. *Candida* esophagitis demonstrated by barium esophagrams. *A* and *B.* "Cobblestone" pattern of the mucosa, which correlates with edema of the mucosa at sites invaded by the organism. *C.* "Tram-track" pattern, which correlates with deep, undermining ulceration of the esophageal wall. *D. Candida* granulomas of the esophageal mucosa mimicking an esophageal neoplasm. Patients shown in *A, B,* and *C* had received immunosuppressive drugs while the patient in *D* was an elderly man who presented with dysphagia. His swallow also demonstrated presbyesophagus. (*From* [*34*]).

and are good drying agents, their use raises cosmetic problems, and they may be painful to apply to large areas of infection. Castellani's paint has been used primarily for treating skin web infections of the feet and *Candida* paronychias.

Because topical agents penetrate paronychias poorly, it may be necessary to give an orally absorbed oral antifungal such as ketoconazole or flucytosine to effectively treat paronychias. Burow's solution has weak antifungal activity and, when applied to the inflamed, moist areas of cutaneous candidiasis on wet to dry dressings, it will reduce itching and dry the lesions. For relief of burning and itching, 0.025% triamcinolone acetonide or 0.5% hydrocortisone cream can also be used. How-

ever, it should be emphasized that unless a topical antifungal is given, topical steroids should not be used. For intertrigo of the groins or perineum, where areas denuded of epithelium may be uncomfortable and readily infected with bacteria, it is logical to use commercially available creams or lotions such as Mycolog (Squibb and Sons, Inc.) which contain nystatin, an antibacterial, and triamcinolone.

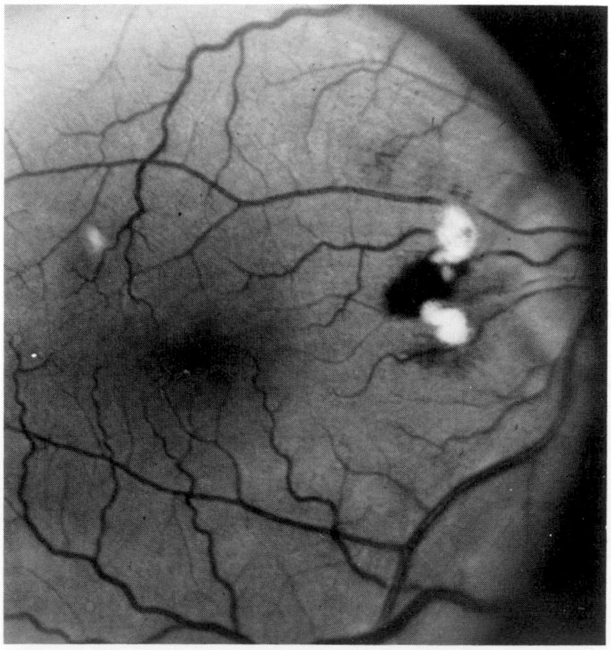

Patients with cutaneous candidiasis should be instructed to wear absorbent, nonocclusive garments over infected areas. Patients with *Candida* paronychias must avoid immersing their affected extremity repeatedly in water. Successful treatment of *Candida* balanitis may require treatment of vaginal candidiasis in the patient's sexual partner. Urinalysis and fasting blood sugar should be obtained from any patient with recurrent cutaneous or mucous membrane candidiasis.

Chronic mucocutaneous candidiasis is very difficult to treat. Topical agents will not penetrate thickly keratinized lesions of these patients and infection will recur after treatment with systemically absorbed antifungal agents is stopped. Recent work indicates that it may be possible to give oral ketoconazole [6.7 mg/(kg·day) up to 200 mg daily] for months with resolution of the lesions and no serious untoward effects [*29*].

Oral thrush can be treated with oral nystatin suspension, giving 200,000 U four times daily to infants and 400,000 to 600,000 U four times daily to adults. Treatment should be continued for 48 h after clinical resolution of the infection. The infection may recur in infants unless candidiasis of the mother's nipple is treated or rubber nipples used in feeding are adequately disinfected.

For vaginal candidiasis, topical nystatin, miconazole, or clotrimazole cream or troches are given daily for 7 days. Recently, ketoconazole (200 mg orally twice or three times daily for 2 to 3 days) has been found to be effective for treating *Candida* vaginitis [*30*]. Presently, oral ketoconazole cannot be recommended for treatment of vaginitis during pregnancy. Women with frequently recurrent *Candida* vaginitis pose particular problems. These women can be treated for 2 weeks with ketoconazole (400 mg daily). This is followed by prophylactic

Figure 103-10. *Candida* endophthalmitis. Fluffy white lesions are characteristic.

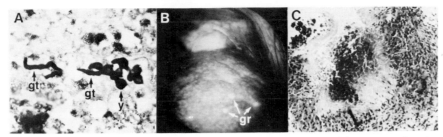

Figure 103-11. *Candida* hepatitis. *A. Candida* yeasts (y) and germ tubes (gt) present at the edge of a suppurative granuloma found in a liver biopsy from a patient with acute leukemia (Gomori methenamine silver; original magnification, × 800). *B.* Photograph of liver surface of another patient taken through a laparoscope just before biopsy. Granulomas (gr) can be seen beneath the capsule of the liver and the right hemidiaphragm is seen arching over the surface of the liver. *C.* Caseating granuloma seen in a biopsy of one of the lesions shown in *B* (hematoxylin and eosin; original magnification, × 125). *(From [25]).*

treatment consisting of either ketoconazole (400 mg daily for 5 days beginning with the onset of each menses or 100 mg daily). In women treated for 6 months with such prophylaxis, recurrences of vaginitis were nearly eliminated. Although the vaginitis often recurred after stopping the prophylaxis, recurrences were still less frequent than before prophylaxis was given [31].

Treatment of visceral candidiasis requires use of systemically absorbed antifungal agents. Because amphotericin B was the first effective intravenous antifungal introduced, most published accounts of treatment of visceral candidiasis have described use of this agent. Therapy with amphotericin B is begun with infusion of 0.15 to 0.25 mg/kg given over 2 to 6 h; infusions are repeated daily with the dose gradually being increased to 0.5 mg/(kg·day). Infusions are then given daily or on alternate days for 2 to 6 weeks, depending upon the clinical situation.

Because of the acute side effects of amphotericin B and its nephrotoxicity, alternative systemically absorbed drugs have been developed. For example, miconazole, which lacks nephrotoxicity, has been given intravenously at a dose of 600 mg every 8 h to treat severe candidiasis [51] but the efficacy of this regimen remains controversial. Flucytosine is distributed throughout the entire body and is excreted in high concentrations in the urine. It is given orally at a dose of 100 to 150 mg/(kg·day) at 6-h intervals. A parenteral preparation can be obtained from the manufacturer and is given intravenously at the same dose. Dosage must be adjusted downward in renal failure. Depending on the method of testing, 5 to 40 percent of pretreatment *Candida* isolates will be resistant to this drug and resistance to the drug may emerge during treatment. Therefore, flucytosine should not be given alone for initial treatment of severe candidiasis and even when the initial isolate is sensitive to the drug, it should not be given alone for prolonged therapy of serious *Candida* infections. A urinary tract infection due to susceptible *Candida* will respond quickly to this drug. Because it reaches therapeutic levels in cerebrospinal fluid,

flucytosine can be paired with amphotericin B or miconazole to treat *Candida* meningitis. Similarly, because it reaches high levels in the serum it can be paired with another antifungal to treat *Candida* endocarditis. It should be noted that *Candida* endocarditis is difficult to treat. Even when the infected heart valve is removed and replaced with a prosthetic valve, *Candida* infection may recur along the suture site of the prosthetic valve. Although ketoconazole, given at a dosage of 200 to 400 mg/day orally, has been effective in treating severe mucocutaneous candidiasis, there is not sufficient data to recommend its use in treatment of disseminated candidiasis.

REFERENCES

1 Winner HI, Hurley R: *Candida albicans*. London, Churchill, 1964, pp 1–175

2 Odds FC: Candida *and Candidosis*. Baltimore, University Park Press, 1979, pp 1–228

3 Howlett JA, Squier CA: *Candida albicans* ultrastructure: Colonization and invasion of oral epithelium. Infect Immun 29:252–260, 1980

4 Olivo PD, McManus EJ, Riggsby WS, et al: Mitochondrial DNA polymorphism in *Candida albicans*. J Infect Dis 156:214–215, 1987

5 Cooper BH, Silva-Hunter M: Yeasts of medical importance, in Lennette EH et al (eds): *Manual of Clinical Microbiology,* 4th ed. Washington, D.C., American Society for Microbiology, 1985, pp 528–533

6 Baine WB, Koenig MG, Goodman JS: Clearance of *Candida albicans* from the bloodstream of rabbits. Infect Immun 10:1420–1425, 1974

7 Brannon P, Kiehn TE: Large-scale clinical comparison of the lysis-centrifugation and radiometric systems for blood culture. J Clin Microbiol 22:951–954, 1985

8 Ray TL, Wuepper KD: Experimental cutaneous candidiasis in rodents. II. Role of the stratum corneum barrier and serum complement as a mediator of a protective inflammatory response. Arch Dermatol 114:539–543, 1978

9 Van Cutsem J, Thienpont D: Experimental cutaneous *Candida albicans* in guinea pigs. Sabouraudia 9:17–20, 1971

10 Mailbach HI, Kligman AM: The biology of experimental human cutaneous moniliasis (*Candida albicans*). Arch Dermatol 85:233–254, 1962

11 Rogers TJ, Balish E: Immunity to *Candida albicans*. Microbiol Rev 44:660–682, 1980

12 Meister H, Heymer B, Schafer H, et al: Role of *Candida albicans* in granulomatous tissue reactions. II. In vivo degradation of *C. albicans* in hepatic macrophages of mice. J Infect Dis 135:235–242, 1977

13 Kozel TR, Brown RR, Pfommer GST: Activation and binding of C3 by *Candida albicans*. Infect Immun 55:1890–1894, 1987

14 Jones JM: Kinetics of antibody responses to cell wall mannan and a major cytoplasmic antigen of *Candida albicans* in rabbits and humans. J Lab Clin Med 96:845–860, 1980

15 Kahn FW, Jones JM: Latex agglutination tests for detection of *Candida* antigens in sera of patients with invasive candidiasis. J Infect Dis 153:579–585, 1986

16 Rotrosen D, Calderone RA, Edwards JE: Adherence of *Candida* species to host tissues and plastic surfaces. Rev Infect Dis 8:73–85, 1986

17 Ponton J, Jones JM: Identification of two germ tube specific cell wall antigens of *Candida albicans*. Infect Immun 54:864–868, 1986

18 Ellsworth JH, Reiss E, Bradley RL, et al: Comparative serological and cutaneous reactivity of *Candida* cytoplasmic proteins and mannan separated by affinity for concanavalin A. J Clin Microbiol 5:91–99, 1977

19 Kiehn TE, Bernard EM, Gold JWM, et al: Candidiasis: Detection by gas-liquid chromatography of D-arabinitol, a fungal metabolite, in human serum. Science 206:577–580, 1979

20 Edwards JE, Lehrer RI, Stiehm ER, et al: Severe candidal infections—Clinical perspective, immune defense mechanisms, and current concepts of therapy. Ann Intern Med 89:91–106, 1978

21 Muenier-Carpentier F, Kiehn TE, Armstrong D: Fungemia in the immunocompromised host. Changing patterns, antigenemia, high mortality. Am J Med 71:363–370, 1981

22 Solomkin JS, Flohr AB, Quie PG, et al: The role of *Candida* in intraperitoneal infections. Surgery 88:524–530, 1980

23 Rebora A, Marples RR, Kligman AM: Erosio interdigitalis blastomycetica. Arch Dermatol 108:66–68, 1973

24 Pepys J, Faux JA, McCarthy DS, et al: *Candida albicans* precipitins in respiratory disease in man. J Allergy 41:305–318, 1968

25 Jones JM: Granulomatous hepatitis due to *Candida albicans* in patients with acute leukemia. Ann Intern Med 94:475–477, 1981

26 Wise GJ, Goldberg P, Kozinn PJ: Genitourinary candidiasis: Diagnosis and treatment. J Urol 116:778–780, 1976

27 Rohrer TJ, Tuliszewski RM: Fungal cystitis: Awareness, diagnosis and treatment. J Urol 124:142–144, 1979

28 Robbins JS, Mittemeyer BT, Borski AA: Primary renal candidiasis masking transitional-cell carcinoma. Urology 4:332–333, 1974

29 Petersen EA, Alling DA, Kirkpatrick CH: Treatment of chronic mucocutaneous candidiasis with ketoconazole. A controlled clinical trial. Ann Intern Med 93:791–795, 1980

30 Fregoso-Duenas F: Ketoconazole in vulvovaginal candidosis. Rev Infect Dis 2:620–624, 1980

31 Sobel JD: Recurrent vulvovaginal candidiasis: A prospective study of the efficacy of maintenance ketoconazole therapy. New Engl J Med 315:1455–1458, 1986

32 Jordan WM, Bodey GP, Rodriguez V, et al: Miconazole therapy for treatment of fungal infections in cancer patients. Antimicrob Agents Chemother 16:792–797, 1979

33 Wilborn WH, Montes LF: Scanning electron microscopy of oral lesions in chronic mucocutaneous candidiasis. JAMA 244:2294–2297, 1980

34 Jones JM: The recognition and management of *Candida* esophagitis. Hosp Pract 16:64A–64V, 1981

CHAPTER 104 / *Chromoblastomycosis* · Michael McGinnis

The clinical entity of chromoblastomycosis is caused by five species of dematiaceous fungi: *Fonsecaea pedrosoi, Phialophora verrucosa, Cladosporium carrionii, F. compacta,* and *Rhinocladiella aquaspersa.* Dematiaceous fungi have either hyphae, conidia, or both that are brown to black in color. The etiological agents of this mycosis have been recovered from wood, vegetable debris, soil, and similar substrates.

Chromoblastomycosis (Fig. 104-1) occurs following the traumatic implantation of one of the etiological agents. The primary lesions are small, pink, scaly papules that gradually increase in size to form a superficial verrucous nodule. They occur most frequently on the feet and legs. Carrión characterized five different types of lesions: nodular, tumorous, verrucous, plaque, and cicatricial [1]. Satellite lesions occur via either autoinoculation or by spread through the superficial lymphatics. Rare hematogenous dissemination to the central nervous system has been reported for *F. pedrosoi.* Early lesions can be managed with wide and deep excision followed by grafting. Locally applied heat and cryosurgery have been curative, too. 5-Fluorocytosine or 5-fluorocytosine combined with amphotericin B are the choices for chemotherapy. Ketoconazole has been used with occasional success. Resistance, partial cure, and relapse are common.

The lesions of chromoblastomycosis show hyperkeratotic pseudoepitheliomatous hyperplasia, dermal granulomata, fibrosis, and keratolytic microabscess formation in the epidermis [2]. The lesions contain dematiaceous muriform cells, which have vertical and horizontal septa. In vitro, muriform

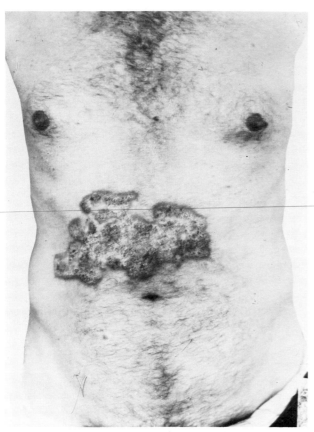

Figure 104-1. Chromoblastomycosis caused by *F. pedrosoi*. (*Courtesy of Dr. Carlos da Silva Lacaz.*)

cells result from the inhibition of bud emergence by yeastlike cells without the inhibition of growth, nuclear division, and cytokinesis. They apparently represent an intermediate vegetative form that is phenotypically arrested between a yeast and hyphal morphology. Muriform cells and the contents of the inflammatory response may occur on the lesion as "black dots," which are the result of a transepithelial elimination process.

This mycosis has been reported from Africa, the Americas, Asia, Australia, Europe, and Oceania. The majority of patients live in tropical or subtropical regions and are engaged in farming or some similar form of manual labor. All ages appear to be susceptible, but most patients are between 30 to 50 years of age. Most patients are Caucasians, whereas blacks are the second most frequently infected group.

LOBOMYCOSIS

The etiological agent of lobomycosis, *Loboa loboi,* has not been cultivated in vitro. Therefore, nothing is known of its growth requirements. Material obtained from human infections has been used to initiate lobomycosis in other humans, a six-banded armadillo, and in the cheek pouches of hamsters. Tissue containing *L. loboi* obtained from a dolphin has been passed through mouse foot pads for three generations [2]. In two human infections, one experimental and the other accidental, the incubation period was estimated to be 12 to 24 months.

Lobomycosis develops following trauma to the skin. As the disease progresses, the initial lesions are nodular and keloidal in appearance. The nodules are free-moving and sharply delimited from the surrounding normal skin. The lesions spread peripherally to form large verrucose, nodular plaques. Satellite lesions may occur, which are apparently the result of autoinoculation. Silva [3] differentiated five clinical forms of lobomycosis: infiltrative, keloidiform, gummatous, ulcerated, and verrucoid. There is little discomfort to patients having lobomycosis. The lesions of lobomycosis do not heal spontaneously.

The diagnosis of lobomycosis is made by observing the characteristic yeast cells in the direct examination of clinical specimens, or by the characteristic histopathology. The yeast cells are round to oval, 6 to 13.5 × 5 to 11 μm, hyaline, and occur in simple or branched chains consisting of two to eight cells. Between the yeast cells, short bridges occur.

Histopathologically [2], the dermis is replaced by a granulomatous inflammatory reaction consisting of packed histiocytes and Langhans' and foreign body types of giant cells. Langhans' giant cells most frequently contain abundant numbers of yeast cells. Areas of tissue necrosis and other kinds of inflammatory cells are infrequent. Lobomycosis is treated by surgical excision.

The majority of cases, which are predominately in males, have occurred in Brazil, especially in the Amazon region. An extremely high prevalence of lobomycosis is found in the Caiabi Indians. Other human cases have been reported from Mexico to central Brazil. Lobomycosis occurs in whites, blacks, and Indians in the Americas. Most patients are involved in farming, trapping, or prospecting for minerals in tropical areas having high temperatures and humidity.

PHAEOHYPHOMYCOSIS

A large number of dematiaceous fungi have been reported as etiological agents of phaeohyphomycosis (Table 104-1). The principal fungi include *Exophiala jeanselmei, Wangiella dermatitidis,* and *Xylohypha bantiana* (syn. *Cladosporium bantianum* and *C. trichoides*). These fungi have been recovered from soil, wood, and other plant materials. The various agents of phaeohyphomycosis are cosmopolitan fungi seen throughout the world.

Phaeohyphomycosis can be classified into four clinical forms [6]. In each of these, the dematiaceous etiological agents occur in tissue as either yeastlike cells, pseudohyphaelike elements, hyphae, or in any combination. In some instances, the dematiaceous nature of the fungal forms in tissue may not be

Table 104-1. Agents of phaeohyphomycosis

Superficial infections
  Phaeoannellomyces werneckii (syn. *Exophiala werneckii,*
    Cladosporium werneckii)
  Piedraia hortae
  Stenella araguata
Cutaneous and corneal infections
  Alternaria sp.
  Botryodiplodia theobromae (syn. *Lasiodiplodia theobromae*)
  Curvularia geniculata
  C. lunata
  C. senegalensis
  Exophiala jeanselmei
  Exserohilum rostratum (syn. *Drechslera rostrata*)
  Phyllosticta sp.
  Rhizoctonia sp.
  Scytalidium synanamorph of *Hendersonula toruloidea*
  Taeniolella stilbospora
  Tetraploa sp.
Subcutaneous infections
  Alternaria alternata
  Bipolaris spicifera (syn. *Drechslera spicifera*)
  Exophiala jeanselmei
  E. moniliae
  E. spinifera
  Phialophora bubakii
  P. parasitica
  P. repens
  P. richardsiae
  P. verrucosa
  Phoma sp.
  P. hibernica
  Scytalidium lignicola
  Wangiella dermatitidis (syn. *Exophiala dermatitidis*)
  Xylohypha bantiana (syn. *Cladosporium bantianum,*
    C. trichoides)
Systemic infections
  Bipolaris hawaiiensis (syn. *Drechslera hawaiiensis*)
  B. spicifera
  Cladosporium cladosporioides
  Curvularia geniculata
  C. pallescens
  Exophiala jeanselmei
  Exserohilum rostratum
  Mycelia Sterilia
  Mycocentrospora acerina (syn. *Cercospora apii* sensu Emmons)
  Wangiella dermatitidis
  Xylohypha bantiana

apparent. In these cases, the dematiaceous character of the fungus is readily evident in the colonies growing on laboratory media. Sclerotic bodies are not produced in tissue by the etiological agents of phaeohyphomycosis.

Superficial phaeohyphomycosis includes infections that involve the stratum corneum with little or no tissue response, such as in the case of tinea nigra. If hair is involved, as in black piedra, the fungi grow superficially around the hair shaft.

Cutaneous and corneal phaeohyphomycosis involves the keratinized tissues, in which there is frequently extensive tissue destruction and often an immunological response. Subcutaneous phaeohyphomycosis typically results from the traumatic implantation of the etiological agent. The disease process usually results in an abscess. The most commonly encountered etiological agent of subcutaneous phaeohyphomycosis is *E. jeanselmei*. Systemic phaeohyphomycosis involves deep organs such as the brain and may have a grave prognosis, especially infections involving the central nervous system. The most common agent of cerebral phaeohyphomycosis is *X. bantiana*. Patients with this form of phaeohyphomycosis typically exhibit headache, convulsions, nuchal rigidity, papilledema, hemiplegia, diplopia, confusion, coma, fever, nausea, vertigo, and hemiparesis as principal symptoms. The diagnosis of phaeohyphomycosis is made by the demonstration of dematiaceous fungal elements in tissue.

Subcutaneous infections are treated by surgical excision of the cyst, and the concurrent use of drugs appears to be unnecessary. Cerebral infections are treated surgically because antifungal agents seem to have little effect upon the disease process. If intravenous amphotericin B is to be used, 5-fluorocytosine should be considered in addition because of its good penetration into the brain. The prognosis for cerebral infections is poor.

It is impossible to draw accurate conclusions regarding the epidemiology and human population infected. There are a large number of different etiological agents of phaeohyphomycosis. In many instances, these fungi have been documented as the etiological agent of an infection in only one or two case reports.

PROTOTHECOSIS

Species of *Prototheca* are achlorophyllous microorganisms that are morphologically similar to the green algae and fungi. *Prototheca wickerhamii* and *P. zopfii* are the only species known to cause infections in humans and lower animals. Members of the genus *Prototheca* have been isolated from the slime flux of trees, streams, ponds, soil, animal feces, sludge in waste stabilization ponds, and similar environments throughout the world.

Prototheca species occur in vivo and in vitro as hyaline sporangia that are 8 to 20 μm in diameter when mature. The sporangia divide internally by progressive cleavage to form two to 20 or more sporangiospores. The sporangia often have a centrally positioned sporangiospore with the other spores surrounding it. Following the rupture of the sporangial wall, and subsequent release of the sporangiospores, the spores mature and repeat the cycle. Budding cells, pseudohyphae, and hyphae are not produced by species of *Prototheca*.

The pathogenesis of *Prototheca* infections is not well understood. The majority of reported infections involve cutaneous-subcutaneous tissues. In these infections, the tissue reaction [2] consists of varying degrees of hyperkeratosis, parakeratosis, and acanthosis. Intraepidermal abscesses may be present. If the dermal reaction is chronic granulomatous, there is often seen pseudoepitheliomatous hyperplasia of the overlying epidermis. There is typically a mixed inflammatory reaction in the dermis. *Prototheca* organisms can be found in either the epidermis, dermis, subcutaneous tissue, or any combination of these. Clinically, the lesions are single or multiple, slow-developing, localized, papulonodular lesions, nodules, crusted papules with ulceration, or rarely granulomatous eruptions that do not heal spontaneously.

Olecranon bursitis is the second type of infection caused by *Prototheca* spp. The lesions of the bursal lining contain a central zone of caseous necrosis that is surrounded by a layer of palisading epithelioid cells, foreign body, and Langhans' giant cells, this being surrounded by dense fibrous tissue or granulation tissue [2]. The caseous material, as well as the interface of the necrotic and intact tissues contain the *Prototheca* cells. Patients show symptoms of chronic, persistent olecranon bursitis, with pain and marked swelling often being present. In several patients, a nonpenetrating injury to the elbow can be recalled. In one patient, systemic protothecosis has been reported.

The diagnosis of protothecosis is made by demonstrating the presence of *Prototheca* in tissue. The fluorescent antibody (FA) technique can be used to stain *Prototheca* cells in tissue sections, even those that have been previously stained by the hematoxylin and eosin and Giemsa procedures. Concurrently, *Prototheca* can be easily recovered in the laboratory on routine microbiological media.

Protothecosis is an exogenous infection that is relatively uncommon, even though it is worldwide in distribution. A number of patients having the cutaneous-subcutaneous form of protothecosis have had preexisting problems such as metastatic carcinoma, diabetes, previous surgery at the site of the infection, and immunosuppressive chemotherapy. The patient who had the systemic infection had a defective cell-mediated immunity. Surgical excision of the lesions is the therapy of choice in protothecosis. Chemotherapy is generally unsuccessful, except in three cases that have been successfully treated with amphotericin B [7].

REFERENCES

1 Carrión AL: Chromoblastomycosis. Ann NY Acad Sci 50:1255–1282, 1950

2 Chandler FW, Kaplan W, Ajello L: *A Colour Atlas and Textbook of the Histopathology of Mycotic Diseases*. London, Wolfe Medical Publications, 1980

3 Silva D: Micose de lobo. Rev Soc Brasil Med Trop 6:86–89, 1972

4 Silva ME, Kaplan W, Miranda JL: Antigenic relationships between *Paracoccidioides loboi* and other pathogenic fungi determined by immunofluorescence. Mycopathol Mycol Appl 36:97–106, 1968

5 McGinnis MR: *Laboratory Handbook of Medical Mycology*. New York, Academic, 1980

6 McGinnis MR: Chromoblastomycosis and phaeohyphomycosis: New concepts, diagnosis, and mycology. J Am Acad Dermatol 8:1–16, 1983

7 Venezio FR, Lavoo E, Williams JE et al: Progressive cutaneous protothecosis. Am J Clin Pathol 77:485–493, 1982

CHAPTER
105

Coccidioidomycosis · John N. Galgiani

Coccidioidomycosis is a pulmonary infection caused by the dimorphic fungus *Coccidioides immitis*. The infection is limited to certain desert areas of the new world. The major endemic areas include the southwest United States and northern Mexico. Other foci are located in Central and South America. In these regions, infection is common and often subclinical. Symptomatic illness usually is expressed as a subacute pneumonia. Only a minority of patients develop persistent pulmonary difficulties or destructive coccidioidal lesions elsewhere in the body. The horizontal spectrum of disease is mainly influenced by host factors. Immunocompromised patients are particularly susceptible to disseminated disease. Although most patients are able to limit their infection without therapy, the few who cannot frequently pose formidable therapeutic problems. Despite efforts to reduce the risk of acquiring coccidioidomycosis through attempts at vaccination and environmen-

tal control, coccidioidomycosis is likely to remain a serious public health problem in the foreseeable future.

PARASITE

LIFE CYCLE AND MORPHOLOGY

C. immitis is classified as a deuteromycete since no sexual state of reproduction has been described. It exhibits dimorphic growth depending on its environment. In desert soil and on culture media, *C. immitis* develops as mycelia whereas its parasitic form grows as a unique spherical structure in tissue and on specialized media. The mycelial growth results from apical elongation into branching, septated hyphae [1]. With maturity, alternating compartments lose their cytoplasm. The walls of these degenerating cells are easily fractured so the infectious spore, the arthroconidium, can be released. Once the arthroconidium is inhaled, as in naturally acquired infection, or inoculated into special synthetic media, it becomes spherical. The spherule enlarges and within days undergoes internal septation to form scores of subcompartments, each of which contains an endospore. By rupturing its outer wall, the endospores are released, each of which perpetuates the spherule cycle in the infection. Alternatively, if removed to the external environment, spherules revert to mycelial growth. Wall structure of the various forms of growth is not uniform. Spherule walls appear to have two layers of different compositions which vary in organization with stages of maturity [2]. Chitin appears to be an important structural element in the spherule, whereas this function of chitin is less apparent in mycelia.

ECOLOGY

The natural habitat of the fungus is the deserts of the western hemisphere, roughly following the lower Sonoran lifezone. The weather in these areas is characterized by high temperatures, low humidity, but predictable slight seasonal precipitation. *C. immitis* grows in the upper few inches of the desert soil where conditions are too hostile for most competing microorganisms. The distribution within the desert areas, however, is not uniform. In areas where new irrigation has started, the fungus has trouble surviving. Influencing soil ecology has been applied to the control of the disease but in most instances this is not a practical or permanent solution.

ANIMAL MODELS

C. immitis is virulent for many of the animals living in the desert areas such as rodents, dogs, and livestock. In addition, several laboratory animal models for coccidioidomycosis exist. The murine model is the best-developed. The murine disease is normally disseminated and there are marked inoculum and fungal strain effects. The major histocompatibility complex has no effect on type of disease seen. Immunity to infection is T-lymphocyte-mediated [3].

PATIENT

PATHOGENESIS

Usual infection

Essentially all naturally acquired infections with *C. immitis* enter via the respiratory route. Direct cutaneous inoculation can occur but is convincingly documented only as a result of laboratory accidents. Low inoculum, perhaps approaching a single arthroconidium, is probably sufficient to cause infection in humans. When exposure is highly concentrated, such as during archeological excavations, symptomatic disease is more frequent, suggesting that inoculum effect can be important.

The immunology of coccidioidomycosis is incompletely understood. The data obtained from in vitro studies and in vivo animal experiments suggest that the following parasite-host interactions take place. After an arthroconidium has been inhaled and a pulmonary focus has been established, inflammation ensues [4]. The mycelial form of *C. immitis* activates complement with the formation of chemotactic active fragments such as C5a. Leukocytes are then recruited and influence the mycelia to become spherules [5]. Whether human leukocytes during this initial contact with arthroconidia are fungicidal is unknown. However, murine phagocytic cells alone do not appear to kill the fungus [6]. The monocytes recruited to the area of inflammation process fungal antigens. This is followed by clonal expansion of T lymphocytes bearing receptors for coccidioidal antigens. This development of a specific cell-mediated immune response is essential for resistance to reinfection [3] and may be required for successful control of the primary infection. Which cell or cells are ultimately responsible for inhibition or destruction of the parasitic fungus has not been established.

Aberrant infection

The initial infection is not always contained. Progressive disease or dissemination occurs when the initial parasite-host interaction favors the former. Such conditions include large fungal inoculum and an immunosuppressive state of the patient. Diseases or treatment that affect expression of cell-mediated immunity particularly predispose to dissemination. However, certain persons who develop progressive infection have had no immunological deficiency identified. The immune response in these instances is predominantly at the B-cell level with production of high amounts of specific complement-fixing (IgG) coccidioidal antibodies. Circulating immune complexes can also be demonstrated [7]. In contrast, delayed-type hypersensitivity skin test reaction is absent. These findings are very similar to those seen in both leprosy and leishmaniasis. It is, therefore, likely that T suppressor cells and/or macrophage suppressors play a role in the fungal-specific immune suppression that is seen in the more severe forms of coccidioidal disease.

Pathology

The pathology from an infection is usually characterized by granulomatous inflammation [8]. However, the histology is frequently variable with acute and chronic inflammation often seen in adjacent areas. Chronic inflammation is most often associated with mature, intact spherules whereas acute inflammation is associated with rupturing spherules and endospores. Tissue destruction due to fungal substances has not been demonstrated and more likely results from the inflammatory response of the host.

CLINICAL MANIFESTATIONS

Pulmonary

Usual Infection. It is estimated that two-thirds of primary infections result in no symptoms or respiratory illness so mild that the patients do not seek medical attention [9]. Those with symptoms usually manifest findings of subacute pneumonia: dry cough, pleuritic chest pain, fatigue, low-grade fever, and night sweats. Hypersensitivity phenomena associated with the primary infection are frequent and include a diffuse maculopapular skin rash, erythema nodosum, erythema multiforme, phlyctenular conjunctivitis, and a polyarthritis for which the illness has become known as "desert rheumatism." Although these lesions may be discomforting and persist for several weeks, they eventually resolve and do not represent sites of infection. Laboratory findings include leukocytosis of which eosinophilia is often a prominent feature. The erythrocyte sedimentation rate is often increased. A characteristic chest x-ray finding is perihilar adenopathy with or without evidence of pneumonitis. Peripneumonic effusions may be present. Ninety-five percent of clinically recognized primary pulmonary coccidioidomycosis is self-limited. However, fatigue that is disproportionate to the physical and laboratory findings may last weeks or months. Diabetes mellitus may contribute to slow resolution. Except in immunocompromised patients, reactivation or second infections later in life rarely occur [10].

Common Sequelae. The most frequent residual lesions are pulmonary nodules or cavities which are evident in approximately 5 percent of patients [11]. This may follow a subclinical infection. In this setting, a coccidioidal nodule may pose a significant diagnostic problem and may lead to surgical resection since the appearance may be indistinguishable from cancer. Otherwise, the nodules are unlikely to cause further problems for the patient, despite the fact that these foci frequently contain viable spherules.

On the other hand, coccidioidal cavities are often a cause of concern. Typically, they are thin-walled and located in the peripheral lung field. If left alone long enough, over 85 percent of cavities will resolve spontaneously. However, cavities may be associated with pleuritic pain and hemoptysis, which are disturbing symptoms even though usually not of dramatic proportions. Like any cavity, superinfection or mycetomas with other fungi may develop. Because of their peripheral nature, coccidioidal cavities may rupture into the pleural space. This uncommon event can usually be distinguished from the simpler peripneumonic effusion seen with primary coccidioidomycosis by the presence of an air-fluid level on radiographs caused by the continuity of the cavity with the bronchus. Thus, despite the usual benign course of these lesions, treatment is often aggressive to avoid future problems.

Progressive Pneumonias. A very small percentage of patients do not resolve a primary illness and the infection continues to involve other parts of the lung. Their course is commonly protracted over a period of years with progressive development of pulmonary fibrosis and may eventually lead to respiratory insufficiency [12]. Despite continued activity of their pulmonary infection, these patients rarely develop destructive lesions elsewhere. Miliary pneumonia is another progressive form of

pulmonary coccidioidomycosis [13]. It is most often seen in immunocompromised patients, especially those with the acquired immune deficiency syndrome (AIDS). As with tuberculosis, this appears to be a hematogenous event, occurring either during the primary infection or later as reactivation disease and is frequently associated with lesions in other organs [14].

Extrapulmonary infection

Nonmeningeal Dissemination. Subclinical spread of *C. immitis* from the lungs may not be uncommon [15]. However, extrathoracic destructive lesions occur in less than 1 percent of patients. The most common sites for dissemination are skin and subcutaneous tissue, bone, and meninges. Autopsy findings indicate that nearly any part of the body can be involved. The only organs routinely spared are the gastrointestinal tract and the urinary bladder. The symptoms from dissemination depend on the organ affected. When the skin or soft tissues are involved, chronic abscess formation is the rule. Involvement of bone and joint gives rise to chronic osteomyelitis and joint infection. The disease presentation mimics tuberculosis and can be clinically and radiographically indistinguishable from this entity.

Several factors have been associated with dissemination and include male sex, dark-skinned race [16], pregnancy [17], immunocompromised state [10], and B-antigen blood group. Very few studies have had defined populations from which these associations have been derived, and their validity may be suspect because of the possibility of sampling bias.

Meningeal Dissemination. Coccidioidal meningitis is most often devastating [18]. In as many as one-third of patients whose disease disseminates, it does so to the meninges. This can be the only clinical manifestation of coccidioidal disease. The meningitis is characteristically chronic and develops over weeks to months. The infection involves many areas of the meninges but is most prominent at the base of the brain. Early symptoms include headache. Later symptoms result from increased infection activity around the aqueduct of Sylvius with subsequent partial or total hydrocephalus. CSF abnormalities include increased white blood cell count often with eosinophils and basophils present, and increased protein and decreased glucose levels. Untreated meningitis results in death within 2 years.

DIAGNOSIS

Isolation of organism

The definitive diagnosis of coccidioidomycosis is made by the isolation of *C. immitis* or the demonstration of typical coccidioidal spherules in body fluids or tissue. The diagnosis of acute or chronic pulmonary coccidioidomycosis is often made by isolating the fungus from pulmonary secretions. Even lightly productive sputa are frequently culture positive. When extrathoracic destructive lesions are present, biopsy material will help identify the organism. Hematoxylin-eosin stain is usually sufficient to see the parasitic spherule; however, on occasion specific fungal stains are required. Cultures of concentrated first-morning voided urine specimens may also yield a few colonies of the fungus [15]. In the laboratory, the culture of *C. immitis* requires special precautions. The fungus grows rapidly as a nonpigmented mold on most simple media. Within 1 to 2 weeks, arthroconidia appear. Such cultures are extremely infectious and should only be grown in sealed containers and handled in biohazard hoods.

Serology

Without culture evidence of coccidioidomycosis, positive coccidioidal serology is presumptive evidence of infection. Two types of serological tests are available, one which identifies IgM and another which identifies IgG antibody. The IgM antibody appears early and disappears first in the infection and is measured by either a latex agglutination or an IgM immunodiffusion test. The original tube precipitin antibody test is now rarely used. The IgG response appears later in the infection. The standard method for identifying IgG is by a complement-fixation assay (CF). CF can also be quantitated, and this is very helpful in certain clinical settings. Thus, CF titers greater than 1:32 are frequently associated with extrathoracic involvement. IgG can also be detected by an immune diffusion technique. Radioimmunoassay and enzyme-linked immunosorbent assay (ELISA) techniques for both antibody and antigen detection are at the present only used in research laboratories.

These serological tests are of paramount importance in some clinical situations. Any positive serological test in a patient without a history of coccidioidomycosis suggests a recent infection, since the antibodies usually become undetectable within months of a self-limited infection. Serology is also a very important means of diagnosing meningeal coccidioidomycosis, since spinal-fluid cultures are positive in less than 40 percent of such patients. Thus CF antibody in spinal-fluid samples suggest coccidioidal meningitis.

Skin tests

Two different skin test preparations are available. Coccidioidin is prepared from the mycelial form of the fungus and spherulin is prepared from the parasitic form of the fungus. The use of skin testing has two major applications. It is very helpful in obtaining epidemiological data on the prevalence of acquired coccidioidomycosis in an area. The development of delayed hypersensitivity to coccidioidal antigen is also a good prognostic indicator suggesting that a particular patient is more likely to control his or her disease successfully. Skin testing, however, has very little value in the diagnosis of acute coccidioidal disease unless it can be documented that a patient just recently has converted to a positive.

MANAGEMENT

Most patients need only supportive measures. Only a few require therapy to resolve their illness. Although pulmonary infections which persist for many weeks may lead to treatment, it is unknown whether this intervention shortens their course. Similarly, medical therapy of patients with symptomatic cavities is of undocumented benefit. A ruptured coccidioidal cavity is treated surgically, and resection of the cavity should be part of the procedure. Although dissemination has a variable course, any extrathoracic destructive lesion identifies a patient as having a disease more severe than 99 percent of those infected. The consensus is that such patients normally should be treated with systemic antifungal agents, surgery, or both, depending on the lesion. Coccidioidal meningitis represents a special therapeutic problem and always requires intrathecal administration of an antifungal agent.

A more difficult decision concerns instituting therapy for "impending dissemination." Such decisions are individualized for each patient. Seventy-five percent of immunosuppressed patients disseminate, therefore all should probably be given treatment [10]. In other patients, a persistently high CF antibody titer, negative coccidioidin skin test, eosinophilia, and development of peritracheal nodes are relative indications for treatment.

Amphotericin B has until recently been the only antifungal agent with apparent efficacy. Currently, miconazole and ketoconazole are new agents also approved by the Food and Drug Administration for use in coccidioidomycosis. The dose of amphotericin is often limited by toxicity [19] and that of miconazole both by side effects and by the practical limits imposed by the prolonged hospitalization required for its use [20]. Ketoconazole, available only as an oral preparation, is usually administered as a single dose of 400 mg per day for at least 6 months [21]. Now under investigation are itraconazole, fluconazole, and other agents structurally related to ketoconazole, and it is hoped that these may have fewer side effects.

REFERENCES

1 Sun SH, Sekhah SS, Huppert M: Electron microscopic studies of saprobic and parasitic forms of *Coccidioides immitis*. Sabouraudia, 17:265–273, 1979

2 Hector RF, Pappagianis D: Enzymatic degradation of the wall of spherules of *Coccidioides immitis*. Experimental Mycology 6:136–152, 1982

3 Beaman L, Pappagianis D, Benjamini E: Significance of T cells in resistance to experimental murine coccidioidomycosis. Infect Immun 17:580–585, 1977

4 Savage DC, Madin SH: Cellular responses in lungs of immunized mice to intranasal infection with *Coccidioides immitis*. Sabouraudia 6:94–102, 1968

5 Galgiani JN, Hayden R, Payne CM: Leukocyte effects on the dimorphism of *Coccidioides immitis*. J Infect Dis 146:56–63, 1982

6 Beaman L: Fungicidal activation of murine macrophages by recombinant gamma interferon. Infect Immun 55:2951–2955, 1987

7 Yoshinoya S, Cox RA, Pope RM: Circulating immune complexes in coccidioidomycosis. J Clin Invest 66:655–663, 1980

8 Huntington RW, Waldmann WJ, Sargent JA, et al: Pathological and clinical observations in 142 cases of fatal coccidioidomycosis with necropsy, in Ajello L (ed): *Coccidioidomycosis*. Tucson, University of Arizona Press, 1967, pp 143–167

9 Smith CE, Saito MT, Simmons SA: Pattern of 39,500 serologic tests in coccidioidomycosis. JAMA 160:546–552, 1956

10 Bronnimann DA, Adam RD, Galgiani JN, et al: Coccidioidomycosis in the acquired immunodeficiency syndrome. Ann Intern Med 106:372–379, 1987

11 Drutz DJ, Catanzaro A: State of the art. Coccidioidomycosis, Part II. Am Rev Respir Dis 117:727–771, 1979

12 Sarosi GA, Parker JD, Doto IL, et al: Chronic pulmonary coccidioidomycosis. N Engl J Med 283:325–329, 1970

13 Bayer AS: Fungal pneumonias: Pulmonary coccidioidal syndrome (Part II). Chest 79:686–691, 1981

14 Ampel NM, Ryan KJ, Carry PJ, et al: Fungemia due to *Coccidioides immitis*. An analysis of 16 episodes in 15 patients and a review of the literature. Medicine (Baltimore) 65:312–321, 1986

15 DeFelice R, Wieden MA, Galgiani JN: Incidence and implications of coccidioidouria. Am Rev Respir Dis 125:49–52, 1982

16 Johnson WM: Coccidioidomycosis mortality in Arizona, in Ajello L (ed): *Coccidioidomycosis, Current Clinical and Diagnostic Status*. New York, Symposium Specialist, 1977, pp 33–44

17 Pappagianis D: Epidemiology of coccidioidomycosis, in Stevens DA (ed): *Coccidioidomycosis, A Text*. New York, Plenum, 1980, pp 63–85

18 Labadie EL, Hamilton RH: Survival improvement in coccidioidal meningitis by high-dose intrathecal amphotericin B. Arch Intern Med 146:2013–2018, 1986

19 Drutz DJ: Amphotericin B in the treatment of coccidioidomycosis. Drugs 26:337–346, 1983

20 Stevens DA: Miconazole in the treatment of coccidioidomycosis. Drugs 26:347–354, 1983

21 Galgiani JN, Stevens DA, Graybill JR, et al: Ketoconazole therapy of progressive coccidioidomycosis. Comparison of 400 and 800 mg dosages and observations at higher doses. Am J Med 84:603–610, 1988

CHAPTER
106

Cryptococcosis · John R. Graybill

Until recently, *Cryptococcus neoformans* was classified as an asexually reproducing yeast. Within the past few years, the perfect mycelial form has been identified as the basidiomycete, *Filobasidiella neoformans* [1]. Cryptococcus neoformans is found worldwide in temperate and tropical climates and has been recovered in high numbers from excreta of pigeons, and less commonly, other birds. Cryptococci are small enough to be inhaled and produce pulmonary infection in mice allowed to run on the inoculated soil. These studies support the clinical impression that most patients acquire cryptococcosis after inhaling the fungus [2,3].

PARASITE

The major feature which distinguishes *C. neoformans* from other fungi is a thick, mucoid capsule. This stains pink with mucicarmine, a helpful test for identification in tissues. *C. neoformans* is the only pathogenic encapsulated fungus, and will grow on most laboratory media, producing white, tan, or cream-colored mucoid colonies in about 48 to 72 h. In the presence of caffeic acid or other precursors of melanin, *C. neoformans* uniquely produces a tan melanin-like pigment, visible in 4 to 5 days [4]. Cryptococci also contain urease,

which forms the basis for a commonly used test to separate them from *Torulopsis* and *Candida* species.

The capsule is composed of a backbone of α-linked D-mannopyranoside residues [1,3], linked in polymeric units substituted with D-xylopyranosyl and D-glucuronopyranosyl residues [5]. It is important not only for identification of the fungus, but also for the pathogenicity in laboratory animals.

The most susceptible animals are the mouse and rat; they develop widespread disease with wasting and cerebritis after intraperitoneal or intrathecal challenge.

PATIENT

HOST-PARASITE RELATIONSHIP

Both in vitro and animal studies have suggested that host immune response to *C. neoformans* is complex and involves both humoral and cell-mediated responses. Encapsulated cryptococci are much more virulent to mice than stable nonencapsulated mutants [6–8]. This is probably because the capsule enables cryptococci to resist phagocytosis and killing by polymorphonuclear (PMN) leukocytes. Complement depletion of experimental animals is also associated with increased susceptibility [8,9].

However, mice can also be protectively immunized with cryptococcal antigens in Freund complete adjuvant. This stimulates cell-mediated immunity more than humoral immunity [10]. Treatment with corticosteroids or antithymocyte serum, procedures which depress cell-mediated immunity, accelerate the course of cryptococcosis [12]. Congenitally athymic mice, which have no functional cell-mediated immunity, are far more susceptible than normal mice. Thymus transplantation into these mice heightens their resistance to cryptococcal challenge [11].

While cryptococcosis does not appear frequently in leukopenic patients, it does occur in the setting of depressed cell-mediated immunity [13], not humoral immunity. In recent years, cryptococcosis has become the fourth most common mycosis after *Candida* mucosal infection [14,15]. The acquired immune deficiency syndrome (AIDS) is now the most common setting for cryptococcal meningitis. In non-AIDS patients, tissue infiltrates include granulomas and lymphocytes, but few PMN. This suggests that cell-mediated immunity is the major protective arm. However, in AIDS patients there is often remarkably little histopathological reaction to the fungus.

CLINICAL MANIFESTATIONS

With cryptococci, as with other pathogenic fungi, infection occurs far more commonly than disease. Inhalation of either spores or small yeast cells is the presumed route. Despite the relatively frequent inhalation of cryptococci, cryptococcosis restricted to the lungs is relatively uncommon. Chronic pulmonary histoplasmosis is manifested by cough, occasional fevers, and radiographic changes of pulmonary infiltrates or cavities. The illness is often mild, and may undergo a course of many months to eventually resolve [16]. Calcification does not occur in cryptococcal lesions, and dissemination in these patients has been considered very uncommon. However, recently it has been appreciated that some patients presenting with pulmonary disease, particularly if concurrently immune-suppressed, will undergo dissemination to other organs, including the brain [17]. The most severe form of cryptococcosis is meningitis, which may present following a completely asymptomatic pulmonary infection. Dissemination is presumably bloodborne. Quiescent pulmonary primary lesions are regularly encountered at autopsy of patients succumbing to cryptococcal meningitis. Cryptococcal meningitis presents with features common to tuberculosis or coccidioidal meningitis, and must be distinguished from these. Patients frequently have chronic headache, personality changes, and may have cranial nerve findings caused by basilar meningitis.

In AIDS patients, despite the usual widespread dissemination to many organs, the clinical symptoms reflected chronic meningitis or meningoencephalitis in 17 or 27 cases in one series (Table 106-1) [14]. In 9 patients cryptococcosis occurred as the initial clinical presentation of AIDS. However, 25 patients had opportunistic processes other than cryptococcosis

Table 106-1. Clinical findings at presentation in 27 patients with AIDS and cryptococcosis

Symptoms	Number	Signs	Number
Headache	27	Meningismus	5
Nausea, vomiting	10	Focal signs	3
Photophobia	5	Papilledema	1
Skin lesions	2	Peritonitis	1
Lung infiltrate	1		
Abdominal pain	1		
Postmortem diagnosis:	1		
Asymptomatic	2		

Source: Adapted from [14].

documented at some time during their course. This overlapping of multiple severe diseases may confound determination of the cause of death in some of these patients. Signs and symptoms of an acute meningitis, such as fever and nuchal rigidity, are frequently lacking, and the patient may be completely asymptomatic in the first weeks of cryptococcal meningitis. Critical areas such as the aqueduct of Sylvius may be involved, and ultimately produce obstructive hydrocephalus, with death from herniation.

Patients with cryptococcal meningitis commonly have underlying depressed cell-mediated immunity. This may be caused by lymphoreticular neoplasm, renal transplantation, subsequent immunosuppression or corticosteroids given for other reasons, or AIDS [13–15,17–19]. Some patients may have definite but subtle abnormalities of immune response not associated with a definite underlying disease. These may be detected only by skin tests for common recall antigens [20]. Untreated, cryptococcal meningitis usually runs a fatal course in months.

Of the other forms of extracerebral cryptococcosis, the most common is skin lesions. These may be painless ulcerative or nodular lesions appearing anywhere, either in the dermis or subdermis [21]. On biopsy, there may be many cryptococci with minimal host response, or a lymphocyte-histiocyte response with granuloma formation. Bone disease is considerably less common. Patients who are terminally ill and severely immune-suppressed may have widespread sepsis with positive blood culture for cryptococci [9].

DIAGNOSIS

Although nodular pulmonary infiltrates are said to characterize pulmonary cryptococcosis, there is no specific radiographic pattern. Similarly, routine studies of cerebrospinal fluid show a lymphocyte-predominating pleocytosis, up to several hundred cells per milliliter, modest elevation of the protein, and depressed cerebrospinal fluid glucose, the latter apparent in about half the patients at hospitalization. These findings are consistent with coccidioidal, tubercular, or carcinomatous meningitis and with other causes. However, there is an important difference in patients with AIDS. Because of the minimal host immune response, there is little inflammatory reaction in cerebrospinal fluid, despite massive numbers of organisms seen in India ink preparations, and antigen titers which range into the tens of thousands [14,15]. In one series, 11 of 17 had fewer than five leukocytes per milliliter, and 11 of 16 had cerebrospinal fluid glucose over 40 mg per 100 mL [14]. Extraordinarily high serum titers of antigen may also be seen in AIDS patients with cryptococcal meningitis. Therefore, more specific microbiological methods must be used.

Culture of cryptococci from sputum may or may not be significant [16]. Repeated cultures, associated with biopsy material showing C. neoformans, confirm a diagnosis of cryptococcal pneumonia, but a single culture may not be meaningful. On the other hand, culture of C. neoformans from skin biopsies, cerebrospinal fluid, or blood is synonymous with active disseminated disease, and indicates the need for treatment. Unfortunately, C. neoformans is not always cultivable from patients with meningitis, and a positive culture often requires several lumbar punctures and culture of a large volume of fluid. One alternative to culture is the India ink test. This suspension of particles of India ink will outline the translucent capsule of C. neoformans, with the enclosed fungus. It is positive in only two-thirds of non-AIDS patients with cryptococcal meningitis [13]. There is also available an indirect serological test, the latex cryptococcal agglutination test, or LCAT [22]. This test is subject to false-positive reactions caused by rheumatoid and other factors, which produce a nonspecific positive latex agglutination test. However, these can be neutralized by procedures which eliminate IgM antibody, and then the test is quite specific. It is also sensitive, being positive in up to 70 percent of sera of patients with cryptococcal meningitis, and 94 percent of cerebrospinal fluid of patients with meningitis. A positive cerebrospinal fluid LCAT, in any titer, is almost equivalent to a diagnosis of cryptococcal meningitis, but there are false-positive results [23]. One must be sure the spinal fluid is not contaminated by blood, which could give a positive test in nonmeningeal cryptococcosis.

MANAGEMENT

The management of cryptococcosis continues to evolve at the present time. Chemotherapy was not always recommended for pulmonary cryptococcosis. However, recent studies suggest that the casual approach is not warranted, as many patients with pulmonary disease undergo dissemination [17]. Therapy for meningitis was amphotericin B, given intravenously and sometimes intrathecally as well. More recently, with the development of flucytosine, combination therapy has been frequently used. This was based on an additive or synergistic sensitivity test in vitro. As flucytosine saw increased use, problems of gastrointestinal toxicity and bone marrow depression became apparent [24]. Initially, a dose of 2.5 g of intravenous amphotericin B was used in conjunction with flucytosine at

150 mg/(kg·day) for prolonged therapy. Recently, investigators in a collaborative study found that treatment could be shortened to 6 weeks with amphotericin B given at 0.3 mg/(kg·day) intravenously, combined with oral flucytosine [25]. This regimen was found to be just as effective as the longer 10-week regimen of amphotericin B alone. Mortality was still high at 21 percent, although relapses and clinical failures were fewer (12 percent) with the combination than with amphotericin B alone (40 percent) [25]. Therefore, this new regimen became the treatment of choice in cryptococcosis. Some patients failed this regimen, and others relapsed after completion of therapy. In those patients with persistent meningitis on intravenous amphotericin B, amphotericin B may be given intrathecally at 0.5 mg three times per week.

Because much of the mortality of cryptococcosis occurs early in treatment, a recent study was done to determine whether shortening therapy to 4 weeks would reduce the morbidity of treatment and not increase the mortality [26]. In this study of non-AIDS patients, 14 percent died in the first 4 weeks of treatment. Of the 45 randomized to 6 weeks of treatment, the relapse rate was 15 percent versus 25 percent for those randomized to 4 weeks of treatment. In a complex data analysis, the authors found that 4 weeks of treatment was sufficient for those with no neurological complications, no immunosuppressive therapy, cerebrospinal fluid leukocyte counts above 20 per milliliter, LCAT <1:32 at 4 weeks of treatment, and a negative India ink preparation.

While this regimen is appropriate for many non-AIDS patients, combined amphotericin B–flucytosine therapy is too myelotoxic for most AIDS patients [14]; also failures and relapses occur in well over two-thirds of these patients [13,14]. With such a dismal record for traditional therapy, there has been a turn to the newer triazoles for antifungal therapy [27]. With excellent gastrointestinal absorption and cerebrospinal fluid penetration, orally administered fluconazole has been the subject of intense investigation, both as treatment to suppress clinical relapses after amphotericin B, and as primary treatment [28]. Comparative trials of fluconazole versus chronic amphotericin B [1 mg/(kg·week) after initial treatment] are in progress. Itraconazole is also being explored as chronic suppressive therapy [29]. Finally, there are others who have successfully treated patients with prolonged maintenance amphotericin B at 0.7 to 1.5 mg per kilogram of body weight [30]. Successful maintenance was extended for up to 77 weeks in one patient. It is uncertain which of these approaches is optimal; what is certain is that within a few years treatment will undergo major revisions.

POPULATION

The population at risk for cryptococci is the immunosuppressed. Because the majority of patients are those severely immune-suppressed by AIDS, there is little clinical applicability for any vaccine, even though murine models suggest this may be feasible [*10*].

REFERENCES

1 Kwon-Chung KJ: A new genus, *Filobasidiella,* the perfect state of *Cryptococcus neoformans.* Mycologia 67:1197–1200, 1975

2 Neilson JB, Fromtling RA, Bulmer GS: *Cryptococcus neoformans*: Size range of infectious particles from aerosolized soil. Infect Immun 17:634–638, 1977

3 Smith CD, Ritter R, Larsh HW, et al: Infection of white mice with airborne *Cryptococcus neoformans.* J Bacteriol 87:1364–1368, 1964

4 Wang HS, Zeimis RT, Roberts GD: Evaluation of a caffeic acid-ferric citrate test for rapid identification of *Cryptococcus neoformans.* J Clin Microbiol 6:445–449, 1977

5 Bhattacharjee AK, Kwon-Chung KJ, et al: On the structure of the capsular polysaccharide from *Cryptococcus neoformans,* serotype C. Immunochemistry 15:673–679, 1978

6 Diamond RD, Root RK, Bennett JE: Factors influencing killing of *Cryptococcus neoformans* by human leukocytes in vitro. J Infect Dis 125:367–375, 1972

7 Graybill JR, Hague M, Drutz DJ: Passive immunization in murine cryptococcosis. Sabouraudia 19:237–244, 1981

8 Graybill JR, Ahrens J: Immunization and complement interaction in host defense against cryptococcosis. J Reticuloendothel Soc 30:347–357, 1981

9 Macher AM, Bennett JE, Gadek JE, et al: Complement depletion in cryptococcal sepsis. J Immunol 120:1685–1690, 1978

10 Graybill JR, Taylor RL: Host defense in cryptococcosis. I. An in vivo model for evaluating immune response. Int Arch Allergy Appl Immunol 57:101–113, 1978

11 Graybill JR, Mitchell L: Host defense in cryptococcosis. In vivo alteration of immunity. Mycopathologia 69:171–178, 1979

12 Graybill JR, Mitchell L, Drutz DJ: Host defense in cryptococcosis. III. Protection of nude mice by thymus transplantation. J Infect Dis 140:546–552, 1979

13 Diamond RD, Bennett JE: Prognostic factors in cryptococcal meningitis: A study of 111 cases. Ann Intern Med 80:176–181, 1974

14 Kovacs JA, Kovacs AA, Polis M, et al: Cryptococcosis in the acquired immunodeficiency syndrome. Ann Intern Med 103:533–538, 1985

15 Eng RHK, Bishburg E, Smith SM, et al: Cryptococcal infections in patients with acquired immune deficiency syndrome. Am J Med 81:19–23, 1986

16 Hammerman KG, Powell KE, Christianson CS, et al: Cryptococcosis: Clinical forms and treatment. Am Rev Respir Dis 108:1116–1123, 1973

17 Kerkering TM, Duma RJ, Shadomy S: The evolution of pulmonary cryptococcosis. Ann Intern Med 94:611–616, 1981

18 Schroder GPJ, Temple DR, Husberg BS, et al: Cryptococcosis after renal transplantation: Report of ten cases. Surgery 79:268–277, 1976

19 Kaplan MH, Rosen PP, Armstrong D: Cryptococcosis in a cancer hospital. Clinical and pathological correlates in forty-six patients. Cancer 39:2265–2274, 1977

20 Graybill JR, Alford RH: Cell-mediated immunity in cryptococcosis. Cell Immunol 14:12–21, 1974

21 Schupbach CW, Wheeler CF, Briggaman RA: Cutaneous manifestations of disseminated cryptococcosis. Arch Dermatol 112:1734–1740, 1976

22 Snow RM, Dismukes WD: Cryptococcal meningitis: Diagnostic value of cryptococcal antigen in cerebrospinal fluid. Arch Intern Med 135:1155–1157, 1975

23 MacKinnin S, Kane JG, Parker RH: False-positive cryptococcal antigen test and cervical paravertebral abscess. JAMA 240:1982–1983, 1978

24 Bryan CS, McFarland JA: Cryptococcal meningitis: Fatal marrow aplasia from combined therapy. JAMA 239:1068–1969, 1978

25 Bennett JE, Dismukes WE, Duma RJ, et al: A comparison of amphotericin B alone and combined with flucytosine in the treatment of cryptococcal meningitis. N Engl J Med 301:126–131, 1979

26 Dismukes WE, Cloud G, Gallis HAS, et al: Treatment of cryptococcal meningitis with combination amphotericin B and flucytosine for four as compared with six weeks. N Engl J Med 317:334–341, 1978

27 Dismukes WE: Azole antifungal drugs: Old and new. Ann Intern Med 109:177–179, 1988

28 Dismukes WE: Cryptococcal meningitis in patients with AIDS. J Infect Dis 157:624–628, 1988

29 deGans J, Schattenkerk JKM, van Ketel RJ: Itraconazole as maintenance treatment for cryptococcal meningitis in the acquired immune deficiency syndrome. Br Med J 296:339, 1988

30 Zuger, A, Schuster M, Simberkoff MS, et al: Maintenance amphotericin B for cryptococcal meningitis in the acquired immunodeficiency syndrome (AIDS). Ann Intern Med 109:592–593, 1988

Histoplasmosis · James E. Loyd
· Roger M. DesPrez · Robert A. Goodwin

Histoplasmin skin test surveys [*1*] have defined foci of histoplasmosis as being mostly scattered in the tropical zones of the world but occurring also in the temperate zones; the most heavily endemic area is the central United States. The agent is a dimorphic fungus, *Histoplasma capsulatum,* found in soil in its mycelial form. Inhaled airborne spores release a yeast form infectious for humans and other mammals. With usual inhalation exposures human infections and reinfections are generally asymptomatic; unusually heavy inhalation exposures induce an acute self-limiting illness. This organism of low pathogenicity may, however, produce uncommon but severe opportunistic infections.

PARASITE

Histoplasma capsulatum is a dimorphic fungus, native to soil in its mycelial phase and a parasite of mammalian mononuclear phagocytes in its temperature-sensitive (37°C) yeast phase.

The mycelial phase consists of septate branching hyphae about 2 μm (range 1 to 3 μm) in diameter. Spores are generally small (microconidia, averaging 1.6 μm) and smooth, but approximately 5 percent are larger (macroconidia, 8 to 14 μm) and many of these are tuberculated, their surface covered by fingerlike appendages. These tuberculated macroconidia serve to identify the fungus (Fig. 107-1*A*). All spores are readily airborne and small enough to reach small bronchi and alveoli when inhaled. Growth of *H. capsulatum* in the soil is depend-

ent on humidity, temperature, and pH, but by far the most significant factor is the presence of deposits of avian or bat feces. Bats (mammals) may have intestinal lesions with infection and deposit organisms in their excrement; but avian species are not themselves infected because of their high body temperature. The affinity of the organism for soil fertilized by avian and bat feces is not understood.

The yeast phase is an ovoid body ranging in size from 1.5 to 2.0 μm × 3.0 to 3.5 μm. Reproduction takes place by budding. Tissue fixatives cause contraction of the cytoplasm, giving an erroneous impression of a capsule when viewed with cytoplasmic stains, but not when stained with cell wall–specific stains such as methenamine silver. With rare exceptions, active infection in normal tissue is intracellular (macrophages) (Fig. 107-1*B*).

PATIENT

Histoplasmosis in humans is an accidental, nontransmittable infection resulting from inhalation of airborne spores of *H. capsulatum.* There are three distinct categories of disease: (1) *acute pulmonary histoplasmosis* (the infection in normal hosts) and its rare complications; and the uncommon opportunistic infections (2) *disseminated histoplasmosis* (immune defect) and (3) *chronic pulmonary histoplasmosis* (structural defect of the lung).

ACUTE PULMONARY HISTOPLASMOSIS

Pathogenesis, pathology, and immunology

Inhaled spores reach bronchioles and alveoli where they germinate, releasing yeast forms of the fungus. These are promptly phagocytized by mononuclear phagocytes (macrophages) where they proliferate within the cells for a period of time. In established infections, more macrophages are recruited to the site and in turn become parasitized, resulting in a focal accumulation of infected macrophages together with a few lymphocytes and plasma cells. Whether few or many such patches of pneumonitis develop depends upon the quantity of spores inhaled. Infected macrophages produce similar but larger lesions in the hilar and mediastinal lymph nodes, and to a lesser extent in the spleen and liver. Cellular immunity and tissue hypersensitivity develop in an average of 14 days, producing an intense vasculitis with central tissue necrosis at the site of all focal lesions, together with macrophage fungicidal capability. Necrotic tissue caseates, the lesions heal by fibrous encapsulation, and eventually calcification ensues. Stainable yeast forms of unknown viability are trapped in the caseum and persist, often in large numbers, even after calcification.

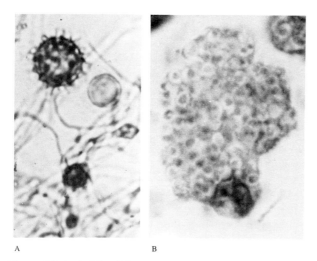

A   B

Figure 107-1. *A.* Mycelial phase of *H. capsulatum* showing spores of various sizes. Large tuberculated spore (upper left) identifies the organism. *B.* Yeast phase parasitizing macrophage in case of disseminated histoplasmosis. Hematoxylin and eosin stain. (Original magnification of both, 35 mm film × 1000.)

In the fully immune host, reinfection induces similar changes with the exception that specific immune mechanisms develop 24 to 48 h after yeast forms first appear, there is less opportunity for intracellular proliferation, consequently less antigen develops, and there is much less inflammatory reaction with little or no necrosis.

It is characteristic of histoplasmosis that acquired immunity and skin test hypersensitivity wane with time, and after several years an individual may come to respond to new infection as if he or she had never been infected. Therefore all states of immunity ranging from immunologically naive (never infected or hypersensitivity entirely waned) to fully immune (recent or repeated infection) are characteristic of populations in endemic areas [2].

Clinical manifestations

The usual inhalation exposure to airborne spores sufficient to induce or reinduce skin hypersensitivity to histoplasmin is asymptomatic and benign in the vast majority of people. Very large inhalation exposures are likely to produce highly symptomatic illness both in nonimmune and immune individuals, in all age groups. Infection in infancy and to a lesser degree in young children is more likely to become symptomatic than in older persons. In general, with mild exposure, adults (immune or nonimmune) develop asymptomatic infections, while some infants may become symptomatic. With moderate exposures the immune may develop no discernible illness or only a mild or short-lived one, whereas the nonimmune person usually develops symptoms, at times quite severe. With heavy exposures, even the fully immune person will develop symptomatic illness, although it will be less severe, of shorter duration, and will have a much shorter incubation period. The incubation period usually varies from 3 to 5 days in the fully immune, and 10 to 18 days in the nonimmune, with the partially immune falling in between. The symptoms of histoplasmosis, with one exception, are nonspecific and influenza-like, with fever, headache, and cough being most common. In two-thirds of symptomatic patients a deep substernal discomfort or pain related to mediastinal adenitis may be conspicuous and diagnostically important. Chilliness and chills are common with severe illness, myalgia may occur, and in prolonged illness weight loss is prominent. In children, nausea and vomiting and even coryza, sore throat, and some stiffness of the neck are not uncommon. Dyspnea may accompany extensive pulmonary infiltrations. Asthenia and fatigability occasionally last for weeks or even months after severe infections. With moderately heavy or heavy inhalation exposure the illness in a given individual may vary, with a low-grade fever lasting a few hours or a day or two to a high fever of 102° to 106°F, with severe constitutional symptoms lasting an average of 7 to 10 days, occasionally up to 14 days, and rarely to 3 weeks or more. Symptoms tend to be aggravated by activity and reduced by rest. There is a paucity of physical findings. Erythema nodosum or erythema multiforme occurs occasionally in both symptomatic and asymptomatic infections, most often in women. Hepatosplenomegaly is occasionally found in more severe infections, particularly in infants. If persistent or extensive, it may signal transition to disseminated histoplasmosis.

Diagnosis

A history of exposure and characteristic roentgenographic changes are often diagnostic. Diagnosis may be confirmed by the complement-fixation (CF) test, which will be positive after 3 to 4 weeks in the majority of patients with acute histoplasmosis. Three out of four usual infections show no chest roentgenographic findings or later calcifications. Twenty-five percent will show recognizable mediastinal adenopathy and possibly one or more small pulmonary infiltrates (Fig. 107-2). Unusually heavy inhalation exposures result in prominent, diffusely scattered, fairly uniform and small pulmonary infiltrates ranging in size in different individuals from 3 to 10 mm, the larger ones having a soft appearance, the smaller more nodular (Fig. 107-3). In the fully immune individual, the nodulations have the appearance of a granulomatosis, are smaller (1 to 2 mm), more uniform, and do not visibly calcify.

Histoplasmin Skin Test. The skin test, positive in 2 to 10 weeks, is rarely helpful diagnostically in endemic areas, because the high frequency (90 percent) of positives precludes any diagnostic value.

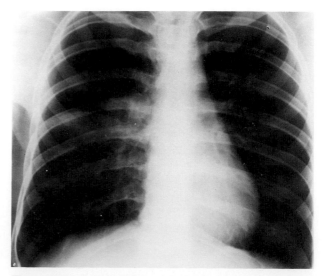

Figure 107-2. Acute histoplasmosis with hilar adenopathy. The chest roentgenogram of a young man from a nonendemic area who developed an influenza-like illness after a visit to Tennessee. There is a cluster of small infiltrates in the right 4th and 5th anterior interspaces and right hilar adenopathy. (*From* [2].)

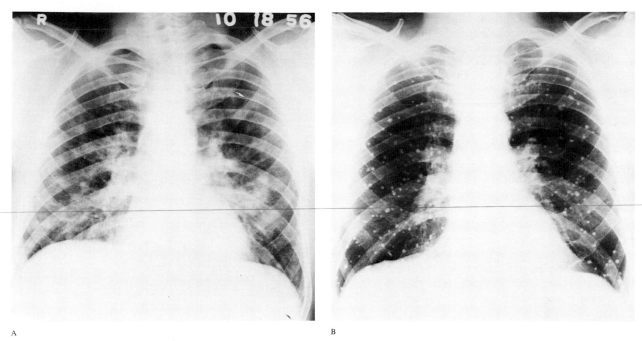

Figure 107-3. *A.* Multiple, soft, pneumonic infiltrates and hilar adenopathy characteristic of acute histoplasmosis after a heavy inhalation of organisms in a nonimmune individual. *B.* Chest radiograph of the same individual 10 years later showing typical "buckshot" calcification. (*From RA Goodwin, RM DesPrez, Am Rev Respir Dis 117:929–955, 1978.*)

Serodiagnosis. Of the many tests reported which detect serum antibody to *H. capsulatum,* the most experience is with complement fixation. The CF test for the yeast-phase antigens is more sensitive than that for the mycelial phase, which may be boosted by a prior histoplasmin skin test and is of little value. A titer of 1:32 or greater, or an appropriately timed fourfold increase in titer, is evidence of active or recent infection. Background positivity of CF titers in endemic areas may be as high as 30 percent of persons and may reach titers of 1:32. Cross-reactivity to antigens shared with other fungi (especially *Blastomyces*) is a recognized problem.

Immunodiffusion (ID) is a simple agar gel diffusion test which is more specific but less sensitive than CF. The ID test measures two bands of immunoprecipitation, the "M" band and/or the "H" band. The presence of both bands is the most specific serodiagnostic test for histoplasmosis but is uncommonly observed. A positive "M" band alone is fairly specific, more so than a positive CF; a positive "H" band alone almost never occurs.

Newer and more sensitive tests (radioimmunoassay) for the serological detection of histoplasmosis have been developed, but their higher sensitivity is associated with more false positives, because of background positives from remote histoplasmosis infection and cross-reactivity with shared antigens of other fungi. However, a negative result is strong evidence against recent or active infection. Experimental methods for detection of antigens of *H. capsulatum* in clinical specimens have been reported to be useful in some clinical syndromes (disseminated histoplasmosis).

Treatment

The great majority of cases of acute pulmonary histoplasmosis require no specific treatment. Bed rest will diminish symptomatic disease. In severe and prolonged infections (10 to 14 days) in both infants and adults, the use of short-course amphotericin B has been recommended. The dose in infants is 1 mg/(kg·day) for 3 to 4 weeks and in adults 50 mg/day for 10 days, both intravenously. Ketoconazole (400 mg/day) has not been investigated in acute histoplasmosis, but most believe it would be an appropriate alternative to amphotericin in the occasional patient with very severe or prolonged symptoms.

Complications of acute pulmonary histoplasmosis

Rarely, complications attend unusually vigorous acute mediastinal adenitis or the encapsulating fibrosis of healing.

Acute Adenitis. The hilar and mediastinal lymph nodes may rarely become markedly enlarged, causing acute tracheal obstruction or dysphagia requiring surgery, or, in the case of bronchi, obstructive pneumonia or bronchiectasis. In less critical circumstances amphotericin B may be tried. Adhesions from healing of such lesions may cause traction diverticuli of the esophagus or interfere with motility. Rarely, large caseous nodes liquefy, resulting in tracheal, esophageal, or mediastinal fistulas which require surgical excision. In the vast majority enlarged nodes subside spontaneously without complications, and require no treatment.

Acute Pericarditis. Rarely, large caseous lymph nodes contiguous to the pericardium may either rupture in the pericardium, causing an acute granulomatous pericarditis, or, more often, by means of a contiguous inflammatory reaction, induce an acute fibrinous pericarditis. In either case, the infection and inflammation will subside spontaneously. Acute tamponade must be decompressed by pericardiocentesis or anterior pericardiectomy. Short-course amphotericin B (50 mg/day for 10 to 15 days) is recommended by some physicians hoping to shorten the course and reduce the 15 percent chance [2] of constrictive pericarditis.

Mediastinal Granuloma. Rarely, a group of large caseous lymph nodes break down into a single encapsulated caseous mass up to 8 to 10 cm in diameter, usually in the right paratracheal area [2]. These lesions sometimes cause superior vena caval obstruction or dysphagia due to esophageal compression and require surgery, but more often are asymptomatic and benign.

Mediastinal Fibrosis. Rarely, the elaboration of encapsulating fibrosis about a caseous mediastinal lymph node will continue for years and the capsule will become far thicker than the usual 1 to 2 mm, resulting in a fibroma-like capsule 1 to 2 cm in thickness [2]. Since the encapsulating fibroblasts arise from contiguous normal tissue, fibrosis is laid down in these tissues, destroying them to the depth of the fibrous capsule. Bronchial stenosis (Fig. 107-4), superior vena caval stenosis, pulmonary artery or pulmonary vein stenosis, or some combination may develop, often with eventually fatal results. Surgery is hazardous and rarely of therapeutic value; amphotericin B is not likely to be helpful.

Broncholithiasis. Pulmonary calcifications and, more commonly, calcifications from bronchial lymph nodes, are occasionally expectorated as ''stones'' or gritty material [2]. The extrusion of a stone into a bronchus may cause hemoptysis and sometimes bronchial obstruction, requiring bronchoscopic removal but these occurrences are usually benign.

Histoplasmoma. The same host-specific tendency to excessive fibrotic response seen in mediastinal fibrosis may induce a slowly (1 to 2 mm a year) enlarging capsule around a small,

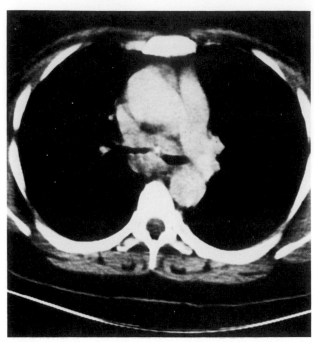

Figure 107-4. Chest computed tomographic scan of a patient with subcarinal mediastinal fibrosis causing severe obstruction of both mainstem bronchi.

healing pulmonary caseous focus following acute pulmonary histoplasmosis [2]. This enlarging fibroma-like lesion, often mistaken for malignancy, can usually be recognized roentgenologically (Fig. 107-5) by its central or concentric laminated (''bulls-eye'') calcification, and surgery may be avoided.

DISSEMINATED HISTOPLASMOSIS

Disseminated histoplasmosis is a rare but usually fatal opportunistic infection which occurs when acquired cellular immunity is inadequate to render macrophages capable of killing intracellular yeast. It occurs in the immature immune state of infants and in known immunosuppressed or immunodeficient states, but can also develop in individuals without a recognized immune defect. It usually occurs as a direct result of either asymptomatic or symptomatic recent inhalation exposure, although it can also appear after a long period of latency following a remote infection. It has been included by the Centers for Disease Control (CDC) as one of the defining infections in the acquired immune deficiency syndrome (AIDS), and in some endemic areas is the most common one. Of special importance is the fact that some reports of disseminated histoplasmosis in AIDS have originated from nonendemic areas (New York), in patients long removed from endemic areas (the Caribbean or South America). Diagnosis is usually established by culture or histological examination of bone marrow, skin, liver, or lymph

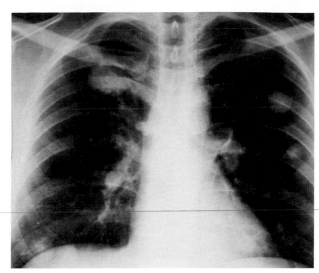

Figure 107-5. Chest radiograph of a patient with multiple pulmonary histoplasmomas.

nodes, or Wright's stain of a buffy coat smear or marrow smear.

Pathology

Parasitized macrophages are diffusely scattered throughout the entire mononuclear phagocyte system (MPS) with little or no inflammatory response [3]. The number of parasitized macrophages in the MPS varies from a few to enormous numbers. In less severe infections, focal accumulations of parasitized cells may cause destructive effects in certain organs.

Clinical manifestations

Clinical symptoms closely correlate with the degree of diffuse involvement of the MPS [3]. *Severe degrees*, most often found in infants, are associated with an acute, highly febrile illness, marked hepatosplenomegaly, severe anemia, leukopenia, and thrombocytopenia, with death occurring in 4 to 5 weeks from debility and hematological disturbances. *Moderate degrees* of MPS involvement, seen occasionally in infants but more often in children or adults, run an eventually fatal subacute course over months with moderate and often intermittent fever, moderate hepatosplenomegaly, moderate anemia, leukopenia, or thrombocytopenia. A tendency to focal organ lesions may cause intestinal ulcers (which occasionally perforate), oropharyngeal ulcers and, more uncommonly, endocarditis or perivascular lesions which result in adrenal insufficiency or meningitis.

Mild degrees of parasitization of the MPS, usually limited to adults, may run a very chronic course over years with intermittent episodes of low-grade fever or none at all, mild

fatigability, weakness and weight loss, with minimal or no hepatosplenomegaly or hematological disturbance. However, there may be a tendency to focal organ lesions (as above), most typically oropharyngeal ulcers.

Diagnosis

Wright-stained blood smears or bone marrow aspirates are usually positive in severe or moderate but are rarely so in mild disease. Liver biopsy with methenamine silver stain is more reliable but may also be negative in mild disease. Biopsy or smear of oropharyngeal ulcers is consistently diagnostic.

Treatment

If the patient lives as long as a week after treatment is started, amphotericin B in full dosage is highly effective [50 mg/day or three times weekly to a total dose of 2.0 g (4.0 g in endocarditis) in adults and 1 mg/kg for 4 to 6 weeks in children] and is the drug of choice in severe cases and for endocarditis or meningitis. Ketoconazole (400 mg/day for 6 months) is more convenient and is an effective alternative [4] in less severe cases, but should not be used alone for initial therapy in immunocompromised or AIDS patients. Most AIDS patients with disseminated histoplasmosis suffer later relapse after amphotericin B therapy, which has led to the recommendation for chronic ketoconazole therapy or once weekly amphotericin B after a full course of amphotericin B (total of 2 g).

CHRONIC PULMONARY HISTOPLASMOSIS

A chronic low-grade infection in the apical-posterior areas of the lung, which is often confused with tuberculosis but is more akin in severity to atypical mycobacterial infections, may develop in individuals (mostly middle-aged white men) with centrilobular and bullous emphysema.

Pathogenesis

After inhalation the yeast phase of *H. capsulatum* can only survive in abnormal air spaces in emphysematous lungs (or in abnormal macrophages as seen in disseminated histoplasmosis). Three types of lesions are seen. The least well known of these is *infection of one or more small centrilobular emphysematous spaces* which then become fluid-filled and appear roentgenographically as one or more coin lesions. Such lesions are intrinsically unstable and when they spill into peripheral bronchi may lead to the second, and roentgenographically almost pathognomonic, type of lesion, *the pneumonic phase* (Fig. 107-6) of pulmonary histoplasmosis. This is typically a wedge-shaped infiltrate with its base towards the pleura in the posterior apical or subapical areas of the upper lobes. The basic process is an interstitial pneumonitis leading to a fine homogeneous infiltrate often containing centrally a denser area of infarcted lung due to large-vessel vasculitis in the pneu-

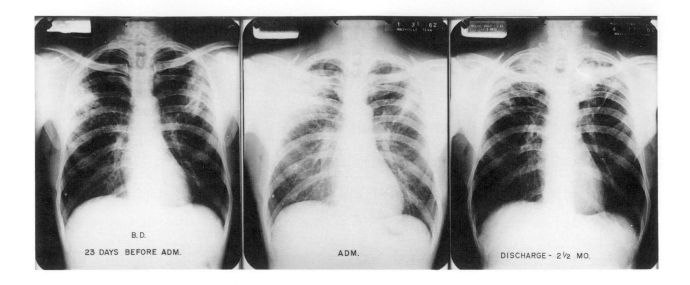

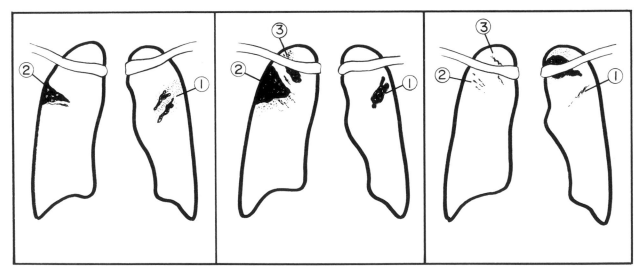

Figure 107-6. Series of chest radiographs (top panel) and corresponding drawings (bottom panel) of a patient with chronic pulmonary histoplasmosis. They depict the evolution and resolution of bilateral infiltrates during a 4-month period. During the 3 weeks between the first and second radiograph, lesion 1 contracted, lesion 2 progressed, and lesion 3 appeared. The third radiograph is after 9 more weeks, during which time lesions 1, 2, and 3 healed, but lesion 4 developed. (*From RA Goodwin et al., Am Rev Respir Dis 93:47–61, 1966.*)

monic area. Underlying emphysema may be made more visible by this process. Healing begins in a week or so, and occurs over a period of several months, typically with considerable loss of lung volume as the affected area contracts. Frequently a new lesion will appear on the contralateral side while the initial one is undergoing involution. The third typical lesion of chronic pulmonary histoplasmosis (Fig. 107-7) is the *infected apical bullous* or emphysematous space, which because of its tendency to progression is the lesion which determines the outcome of the disease. Apical bullae may be infected by direct

inhalation, but most often, when evidence is available, such spaces will be seen to have been infected in close temporal association with a pneumonic episode.

Symptoms

Pneumonic lesions and the more severe chronic cavitary infections are usually attended by nonspecific tuberculosis-like symptoms but of milder degree. Often, the symptoms are minimal or masked by the preexisting chronic bronchitis.

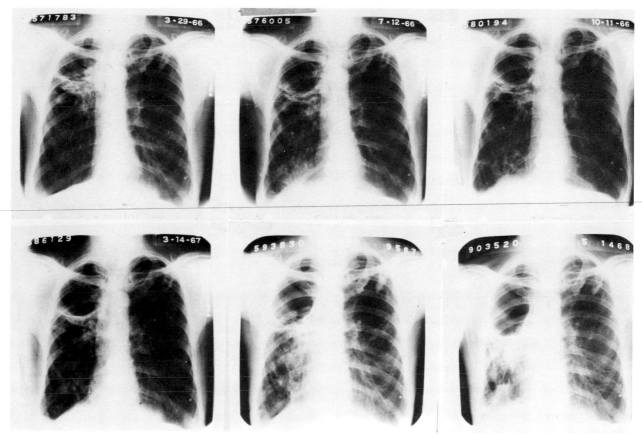

Figure 107-7. Series of chest radiographs of a thick-walled "marching cavity" showing progressive necrosis of the dependent wall of the cavity and also progressive fibrosis of the right lower lobe from the "spillover" effect. (*From RA Goodwin, RM DesPrez, Am Rev Respir Dis 117:929–955, 1978.*)

Diagnosis

The segmental interstitial pneumonitis and the contraction of the infarctlike necrosis, particularly in a setting of bullous emphysema, can usually be recognized on chest roentgenogram [5]. Positive sputum cultures are definitive but many specimens may be required for positive findings in pneumonic lesions or thin-walled infected air spaces (cavities); patients with thick-walled cavities usually will be positive. CF tests are negative in one-third, of suggestive titer only (1:8 to 1:32) in one-third, and in diagnostic titer (>1:32) in only one-third of patients [5].

Treatment

Bed rest when the patient is symptomatic and limitation of activity for 6 to 8 weeks seem to afford the best opportunity for more rapid healing of pneumonic lesions without persistent cavitation, although satisfactory healing may occur without limited activity or chemotherapy. Thin-walled cavities usually do not require antimicrobial therapy. Persistent cavitation may be treated with ketoconazole (400 mg in a single oral daily dose for 6 months). Amphotericin B in full dosage (50 mg/ day or three times weekly intravenously to a total dose of 2.0 g) may be necessary for thick-walled cavities (2 to 4 mm) or treatment failures.

HISTOPLASMOSIS DUE TO *HISTOPLASMA CAPSULATUM* VAR. *DUBOISII*

A stable variant, *Histoplasma capsulatum* var. *duboisii* [7], found in Africa, causes somewhat different disease manifestations and differs morphologically in that the yeast phase is much larger (7 to 15 μm). The lesions of the human disease entity, which is probably not yet fully described, correspond to the focal lesions seen in the milder chronic range of disseminated histoplasmosis but differ in being more reactive, displaying more parasitized multinucleated macrophages (giant cells), and having a greater tendency to break down, causing cold abscesses. The focal granulomas containing many parasitized giant cells occur mainly in the skin and bone and less often in the submucosa of the oropharynx and intestinal tract, lymph nodes, spleen, and liver.

The clinical spectrum varies from single or sparse lesions with no constitutional symptoms to many lesions usually attended by fever, anemia, weight loss, often with lymphadenopathy and hepatosplenomegaly, and, in the more severe cases, a progressive and eventually fatal course. Cutaneous [8] or subcutaneous lesions occur in almost all cases. The former are usually painless, warty, dome-shaped papules a few millimeters across, some of which heal spontaneously, while new lesions appear elsewhere and others ulcerate, displaying rolled edges. Occasionally, cutaneous lesions may be eczematoid or psoriasis-like plaques, or circinate with advancing edges and healing centers. Subcutaneous lesions are usually nodular, painless, and often felt rather than seen. Occasionally, they are larger and painful at the onset; these often break down to produce cold abscesses. Focal lesions may involve any bone but most commonly the femur, ribs, and skull; are painless at the onset, tend to erode the cortex, and present a protruding granulomatous mass or, more commonly, a cold abscess, often with sinus formation.

Diagnosis

The diagnosis may be suggested by the character of the skin lesions or of the roentgenographically demonstrated focal lesions of bone and confirmed by demonstration of typical large budding yeast forms on pus smear, biopsy, histology, or culture of either. The histoplasmin skin test is equivocal and CF testing has not been adequately studied.

Treatment

Amphotericin B intravenously in full dosage (total 2 g) is highly effective, is the drug of choice, and should always be used in severe cases. Sulfamethoxazole (800 mg)–trimethoprim (160 mg) 2 or 3 times daily for 1 year has been shown to have some success in mild and limited cases and may be used alone or following a shorter (0.5 to 1.0 g) course of amphotericin B.

Ketoconazole has activity in vitro and has been effective in individual cases, but has not been studied extensively.

POPULATION

EPIDEMIOLOGY

Significant sources of airborne spores, known as point sources, almost always are sites within endemic areas where avian or bat excrement has collected in quantity and the site has become infested with *H. capsulatum* (not all do). The number of point sources, proximity to them, wind velocity and direction, and the presence or absence of dusty circumstances determine the usual baseline of infection in various communities. Wind is likely to keep enough spores airborne near point sources sufficient to produce mild infections, but mechanical disturbances of point sources under dusty circumstances may raise enormous numbers of spores and produce clinically significant infections in those living nearby or in large populations downwind. Significant instances of mechanical disturbance of point sources have been the bulldozing of blackbird roosts, sweeping and cleaning of chicken houses, collecting and spreading of chicken manure, cleaning of belfries and other pigeon roosts, spelunking, cleaning of bat-infested attics and cellars, cutting up hollow trees, demolishing buildings that have served as bat or pigeon roosts, cleaning of bridges and, in South and Central America, collecting oilbird guano.

CONTROL

Elimination of many or most point sources has not yet proved feasible. Soaking blackbird or pigeon roosts with 3% formalin [6] is recommended if cleanup activities are planned. It is also advantageous to use histoplasmin-positive workers, to water down the site to minimize dust, and possibly to use masks. Attempts to reduce blackbird populations have been controversial and not very successful.

REFERENCES

1 Edwards PQ, Billings EL: World wide pattern of skin sensitivity to histoplasmosis. Am J Trop Med Hyg 20:288–319, 1971
2 Goodwin RA, Loyd JE, DesPrez RM: Histoplasmosis in normal hosts. Medicine 60:231–266, 1981
3 Goodwin RA, Shapiro JL, Thurman GH, Thurman SS, DesPrez RM: Disseminated histoplasmosis: Clinical and pathologic correlations. Medicine 59:1–33, 1980
4 National Institute of Allergy and Infectious Diseases Mycoses Study Group: Treatment of blastomycosis and histoplasmosis with ketoconazole; Results of a prospective randomized clinical trial. Ann Intern Med 103:861–872, 1985
5 Goodwin RA, Owens FT, Snell JD, et al: Chronic pulmonary histoplasmosis. Medicine 55:413–452, 1976
6 Tosh FE, Weeks RJ, Pfeiffer SL, et al: The use of formalin to kill *Histoplasma capsulatum* at an endemic site. Am J Epidemiol 85: 259–265, 1967
7 Cockshott WP, Lucas AO: Histoplasmosis Duboisii. Quarterly Journal of Medicine 33:223–238, 1964
8 Lucas AO: Cutaneous manifestations of African histoplasmosis. Brit J Derm 82:435–447, 1970

Mucormycosis · Richard D. Meyer

Fungi of two orders of the class Zygomycetes cause human disease. The term *mucormycosis* refers to infections caused by fungi of the order Mucorales; its families include Cunninghamellacae, Mortierellaceae, Saksenaeaceae, Syncephalastraceae, Thamnidiaceae (member *Cokeromyces recurvatus*), and the more commonly encountered Mucoraceae, with its genera *Absidia, Mucor,* and *Rhizopus.* Fungi of the other order include Entomophthorales (see Chap. 109) and *Conidiobulus coronatus,* which causes rhinoentomophthoramycosis [1–3].

PARASITE

All these fungi are saprobic in nature. Mycelia are generally found in both the parasitic and saprophytic state. They are distinguished in culture by the gross colony appearance and on microscopic examination by occurrence of, or type of, stolons, rhizoids, and sporangia. In both mucormycosis (except for *C. recurvatus*) and rhinoentomophthoramycosis broad (6 to 50 μm), nonseptate hyphae with right-angle irregular branching are found on histopathological examination. In mucormycosis (except for *C. recurvatus*) there is prominent invasion of blood vessels with subsequent hemorrhagic infarction. In rhinoentomophthoramycosis, on the other hand, granulomata, hyaline material, and eosinophils are found.

Mucoraceae are ubiquitous and grow in soil, and on fruit or bread. Thus the exposure of a predisposed patient is the most important factor. Almost all cases of mucormycosis, which is worldwide in distribution, have occurred in patients predisposed by an underlying condition [4]. Rhinoentomophthoramycosis, on the other hand, usually occurs in patients with no known underlying diseases; usually in men in Africa and the West Indies, less commonly in tropical South America and India, and uncommonly in the United States [4].

PATIENT

HOST FACTORS, PATHOGENESIS, AND PATHOLOGY

In experimental infections acidosis alone or corticosteroid administration but not hyperglycemia itself predisposes to mucormycotic infection [1]. Acidosis normally precedes rhinocerebral mucormycosis; it is usually caused by diabetes mellitus and, less commonly, by renal insufficiency or in infants by diarrhea [1,4]; deferoxamine use in hemodialysis patients has been linked to it [5]. Less frequently, mucormycosis is seen in immunosuppressed patients with tumors or in organ transplant recipients [1,4]. It occurs uncommonly in patients with well-controlled diabetes mellitus without acidosis.

The fungus invades the mucous membranes of the paranasal sinuses, nose, or the palate, and extends with hemorrhagic

thromboses in contiguous areas (e.g., paranasal sinuses, orbit, meninges, and frontal lobes of the brain) (see Fig. 108-1).

Pulmonary mucormycosis is also found in a minority of patients with rhinocerebral disease but usually occurs in patients with leukemia or lymphoma who have received corticosteroid therapy [1,4,6]. It is found less commonly in patients with diabetes mellitus, organ transplants, renal insufficiency, or burns. Spread occurs locally and at distant sites from blood vessel invasion with hemorrhagic infarction or spread through a bronchus.

Surgical or traumatic wounds and, more frequently, burn wounds may be involved with localized or disseminated dis-

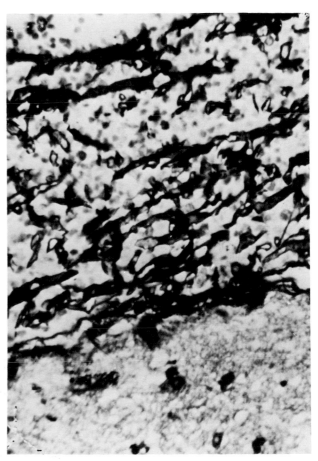

Figure 108-1. Hyphal invasion by mucormycosis of meninges and frontal lobe of cerebrum (methenamine silver stain, × 200). (*After Meyer RD, chap. 213 in Mandell GL, Douglas RG, Bennett JE (eds): Principles and Practice of Infectious Diseases. New York, Wiley, 1979. Used by permission.*)

ease [1,4,7,8]. Hospital-acquired mucormycosis has resulted from contaminated Elastoplast bandages [7]. Isolated hemorrhagic cerebral infarcts in intravenous drug abusers or in immunosuppressed patients occur rarely [4,6,9]. Intestinal mucormycosis results from ingestion of fungi by susceptible individuals, e.g., those malnourished. *C. coronatus* is introduced by incidental trauma or by insects [3]. Rarely, *C. coronatus* may be associated with intestinal infection in normal individuals [10].

Pathological examination in mucormycosis shows hemorrhagic infarcts with hyphal invasion of blood vessels, nerves, and other tissues, hemorrhagic thrombosis, and necrosis. The broad, nonseptate hyphae with right-angle branching stain better with either the Gomori methenamine silver stain or periodic acid Schiff (PAS) stain than with the hematoxylin and eosin stain. The Mucoraceae cannot be distinguished from each other by histopathological examination. *C. coronatus* is associated with a PAS-positive perifungal eosinophilic material, granulomata, microabscesses, and absence of vessel invasion [1,10].

CLINICAL MANIFESTATIONS, DIAGNOSIS, AND THERAPY

Rhinocerebral mucormycosis should be suspected early in predisposed patients with infections of the paranasal sinuses, eye, orbit, and brain; the course is usually fulminant but durations of weeks to months occur uncommonly [1,4]. Early symptoms are headache, eye irritation and swelling, lacrimation, periorbital numbness, nasal stuffiness, or epistaxis. The level of consciousness is usually depressed. Frequently, examination shows proptosis or cellulitis of the orbit or face, and black necrotic lesions on the nasal mucous membranes or hard palate. Internal and external ophthalmoplegia, corneal anesthesia, anhidrosis, and blindness are found with orbital involvement. Paralysis of the facial nerve and internal carotid artery involvement occur in about a third of patients [1,4].

Routine laboratory examination usually shows evidence of the underlying disease and acidosis. Examination of cerebrospinal fluid in patients with intracranial extension usually shows a normal or slightly increased pressure, up to 500 cells per cubic millimeter with both neutrophils and/or mononuclear cells, a few to thousands of red blood cells, and a modestly elevated protein concentration; the glucose concentration varies with control of the diabetes mellitus. Cultures are negative.

Roentgenographic findings include fluid or clouding of the paranasal sinuses and, less commonly, osteomyelitis. Brain scan may be positive in involved areas. Computed tomography may show masses, proptosis, lateral displacement of a thickened medial rectus muscle, bone destruction, or cerebritis. Angiograms of the common carotid artery may show narrowings or occlusions of the ophthalmic artery or internal carotid artery with secondary infarctions [4,11].

Pulmonary mucormycosis is manifested usually by fever and rapidly progressive pulmonary infiltrates in immunosuppressed patients; pleuritic pain and hemoptysis are uncommon but helpful clues [4,6]. Pulmonary mucormycosis in patients with diabetes mellitus or renal insufficiency usually has a more subacute course with fever and hemoptysis. Common roentgenographic findings are patchy infiltrates or bronchopneumonia; diffuse infiltrates, consolidation, cavitation, and mycetoma are less common [4,6,12,13]. Histopathological examination of tissue is usually necessary in addition to culture and direct examination of respiratory secretions. Noninvasive mycetomas may follow pyogenic lung infection [14].

Disseminated mucormycosis in immunosuppressed patients spreads from the lungs to the central nervous system and less commonly to other organs, including the skin where hemorrhagic infarcts are found rarely. In central nervous system disease, disorientation, obtundation, or coma with focal signs are commonly found; the cerebrospinal fluid usually resembles that of rhinocerebral mucormycosis. Brain biopsy is usually necessary.

Mucormycosis of the gastrointestinal tract is associated with malnutrition, kwashiorkor, uremia, or amebiasis. It is manifested by acute crampy abdominal pain and distension, vomiting, bloody diarrhea, or signs of intestinal perforation from the necrotic ulcers with thromboses. The terminal ileum and colon are affected most frequently.

Burn and wound infections may be papular lesions but indurated necrotic ulcers, eschars, or extensive cellulitis with necrosis are more common [4,7,15].

In rhinoentomophthoramycosis, systemic symptoms are rare and the course is usually chronic [3]. Lesions in the nasal mucosa may cause obstruction or spread to the paranasal sinuses and then to the skin of the nose, face, and neck where swelling and induration are noted or to the mediastinum.

Diagnosis is made most frequently by examination of scrapings, biopsies, or, unfortunately, autopsy specimens. Specimens should be cultured on Sabouraud's glucose agar although histopathological confirmation is required. Other considerations in rhinocerebral mucormycosis include cavernous sinus thrombosis or orbital syndromes caused by other fungi or by bacteria. Pulmonary involvement with mucormycosis mimics aspergillosis in immunosuppressed patients. Direct examination of tissues is frequently required.

Therapy involves several approaches. The most important aspect is the correction of the underlying predisposing condition (e.g., acidosis) in rhinocerebral disease. Tapering or discontinuation of immunosuppressive therapy should be considered unless it is required to achieve a remission in hematological malignancy. Surgical removal of infected tissue is another mainstay. Finally, amphotericin B should be given intravenously after the diagnosis has been established but it is adjunctive. Local irrigations of amphotericin B or therapy with intravenous miconazole, oral flucytosine, or ketoconazole are not effective. Early recognition and correction of the underlying condition controls the infection uncommonly but limits the need for extensive surgery in other cases [4].

In pulmonary mucormycosis control of the underlying disease with amphotericin B therapy and, sometimes, surgery is recommended. Therapy of mucormycosis in other areas generally includes the tripartite approach also.

Amphotericin B therapy should be given as outlined in Chap. 116. The total dose required is variable but usually is 30 to 40 mg per kilogram of body weight given over 2 to 3 months. Prognosis depends upon early recognition, control of the underlying disease, and institution of therapy. Amphotericin B is also the drug of choice for rhinoentomophthoramycosis but oral iodides may be useful in some cases.

PREVENTION AND CONTROL

Prevention of mucormycosis involves protection of the susceptible host since the fungi are ubiquitous; in rhinoentomophthoramycosis, control involves avoidance of incidental trauma from a contaminated site.

REFERENCES

1 Baker RD: Mucormycosis (opportunistic phycomycosis), in Baker RD (ed): *The Pathologic Anatomy of Mycoses. Human Infection with Fungi, Actinomyces and Algae.* New York, Springer-Verlag, 1971, pp 832–918

2 Ainsworth GC: Introduction and keys to higher taxa, in Ainsworth GC, Sparrow FK, Sussman AS (eds): *The Fungi IV-B—An Advanced Treatise,* New York, Academic, 1973, pp 1–7

3 Axelrod P, Kwon-Chung KJ, Frawley P, et al: Chronic cystitis due to *Cokeromyces recurvatus*: A case report. J Infect Dis 155: 1062–1064, 1987

4 Meyer RD, Armstrong D: Mucormycosis—changing status. CRC Crit Rev Clin Lab Sci 4:421–451, 1973

5 Windus DW, Stokes TJ, Julian BA, et al: Fatal Rhizopus infections in hemodialysis patients receiving deferoxamine. Ann Intern Med 107:678–680, 1987

6 Meyer RD, Rosen P, Armstrong D: Phycomycosis complicating leukemia and lymphoma. Ann Intern Med 77:871–879, 1972

7 Gartenberg G, Bottone EJ, Keusch GT, et al: Hospital-acquired mucormycosis (*Rhizopus rhizopodiformis*) of skin and subcutaneous tissue. N Engl J Med 299:1115–1118, 1978

8 Codish SC, Sheridan ID, Monaco AP: Mycotic wound infections. Arch Surg 114:831–835, 1979

9 Cuadrado LM, Guerrero A, Lopez Garcia Asenjo JA, et al: Cerebral mucormycosis in two cases of acquired immunodeficiency syndrome. Arch Neurol 45:109–111, 1988

10 Bittencourt AL, Ayala MAR, Ramos EAG: A new form of abdominal zygomycosis different from mucormycosis. Am J Trop Med Hyg 28:564–569, 1979

11 Lazo A, Wilner HI, Metes JJ: Craniofacial mucormycosis: Computed tomographic and angiographic findings in two cases. Radiology 139:623–626, 1981

12 Medoff G, Kobayashi GS: Pulmonary mucormycosis. N Engl J Med 286:86–87, 1972

13 Kiehn TE, Edwards F, Armstrong D, et al: Pneumonia caused by *Cunninghamella bertholletiae* complicating chronic lymphatic leukemia. J Clin Microbiol 10:374–379, 1979

14 Fahey PJ, Utell MJ, Hyde RW: Spontaneous lysis of mycetoma, after acute cavitating lung disease. Am Rev Respir Dis 123:336–339, 1981

15 Koren G, Polachek I, Kaplan H: Invasive mucormycosis in a nonimmunocompromised patient. J Infect 12:165–167, 1986

C H A P T E R / *Mycetoma* · *Jerrold J. Ellner* · *Anne Morrissey*
109

A *mycetoma* is a chronic, progressively destructive infection of the skin, subcutaneous tissues, fascia, muscles, and often bone, most common worldwide between 15° S and 30° N latitudes and hyperendemic in the thorny semideserts of Central and South America, Africa, and India. The characteristic appearance is that of a tumor or fungating nodules with multiple draining sinus tracts and fistulas discharging purulent material containing granules. Numerous filamentous soil-dwelling organisms are capable of causing this syndrome following trauma to the skin. The mycetoma most often involves the foot, which represents the usual site of inoculation, and for this and historical reasons the terms ''Madura foot'' and *maduramycosis* have been used to describe the clinical entity [1–9].

CAUSATIVE AGENT

Mycetoma may be caused by a wide variety of agents (Table 109-1). Determination that a mycetoma is eumycotic (caused by a true fungus) or actinomycotic (caused by filamentous bacteria) is of some importance as regards management. The relative proportion of cases due to particular agents varies with geography and climatic conditions. For example, *Madurella mycetomi* and *Streptomyces somaliensis* predominate in some arid areas, whereas *Nocardia* spp. prefer areas receiving good rainfall. The main causes of mycetoma in various regions are shown in Table 109-2 [1–9]. In Mexico, 98 percent of mycetomas are actinomycotic, whereas in India the distribution is

Table 109-1. Common etiological agents of mycetoma in humans and animals

Agent	Grain color	Occurrence*
Actinomycotic mycetoma (thin, branching, intertwined filaments)		
Actinomyces israelii	White to yellow	R
Nocardia asteroides	Grains rare—white	R
N. brasiliensis	White	C
N. caviae	White to yellow	R
N. farcinica	White to yellow†	R
Actinomadura madurae	White to yellow or pink	C
A. pelletieri	Garnet red	O
Streptomyces somaliensis	Yellow to brown	O
Eumycotic mycetoma (wide, branching, intertwined hyphae and cystlike cells)		
Pseudallescheria boydii	White	C
Madurella grisea	Black‡	R
M. mycetomatis	Black	C
Acremonium kiliense	White	R
A. falciforme	White	E
A. recifei	White	
Leptosphaeria senegalensis	Black	R
L. tompkinsii	Black	E
Exophiala jeanselmei	Black	E
Neotestudina rosatii	White	E
Pyrenochaeta romeroi	Black‡	R
Curvularia geniculata	Black§	E
C. lunata	White	E
Cochliobolus spicifer	Black§	E
Fusarium spp.	White	E
Aspergillus nidulans	White	E

*Key: C = common; O = occasional; E = extremely rare.
†Some authors believe that this organism is within the species limits of *N. asteroides*.
‡It is believed that the two species are related, if not identical.
§From animals.
    Some lesions induced by dermatophytes superficially resemble mycetoma; however, true grains and sinus tracts are lacking.

Source: Modified from JW Rippon: *Medical Mycology*. Philadelphia, Saunders, 1982.

Table 109-2. Geographic distribution of organisms causing mycetomas

Europe, United States	*Pseudoallescheria boydii* (eu)*
Mexico	*Nocardia brasiliensis* (actino)
South America	*Madurella grisea* (eu)
	N. brasiliensis (actino)
Tunisia	*Actinomadura madurae* (actino)
West Africa	*A. pelletier* (actino)
East Africa	*Streptomyces somaliensis* (actino)
India	*A. madurae* (actino)
	N. brasiliensis (actino)
	M. mycetomatis (eu)

*Eu, eumycotic; actino, actinomycotic.

about 50 percent actinomycotic and 50 percent eumycotic. Direct smear of a freshly crushed grain may show wide filaments indicating fungal origin or thinner actinomycotic forms. Grains can be difficult to localize in histological sections, requiring additional sectioning of tissues. Hematoxylin and eosin staining is usually adequate for detection of the grains. A Gram-stained preparation of tissue permits demonstration of the fine, branching structures within actinomycotic grains, and Gomori methenamine silver the larger and broader hyphae of eumycotic mycetomas. The color and appearance of the grains allows tentative identification of the causal agent. Of particular significance is the microscopic appearance and staining characteristics of the grains, including the presence of "cement" and clubs [3,6] (Figs. 109-1 and 109-2). Definitive identification requires culture. The grains should be washed in sterile saline

Figure 109-1. Grains in sections of mycotic mycetomas. *A*. *M. mycetomi,* filamentous and vesicular areas in the same grain (biopsy sample BB 2160, H and E, × 150). *B*. *L. senegalensis*: The grain is surrounded by a plasmodial reaction (biopsy sample Bi 1025, H and E, × 150). *C*. *M. grisea* (biopsy sample Y 925, H and E, × 150); the same morphology appears for *P. romeroi*. *D*. *N. rosatii* (biopsy sample Bi 2509, H and E, × 70). *F*. Same grain as in *E*, stained by Gomori Grocott (biopsy sample Bi 2509, × 260). The same morphology is observed in *P. boydii*. (*Courtesy of F. Mariat et al. [3], S. Karger AG, Basel.*)

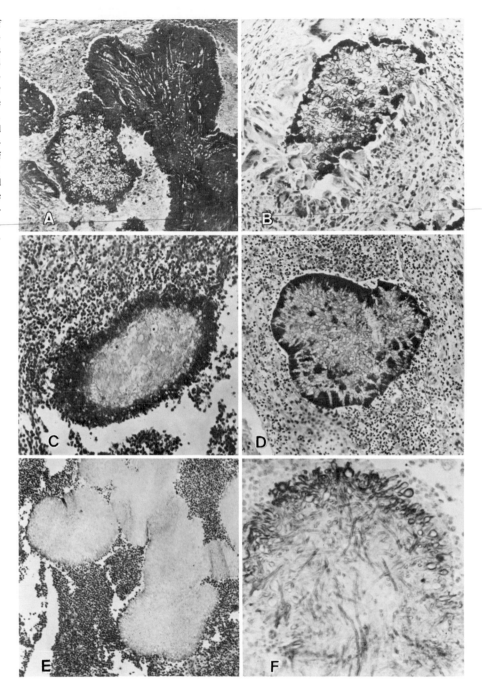

to decrease contamination [3]. Sabouraud's agar is an appropriate culture medium. Antibiotics added to the agar decrease skin contaminants, but interfere with the isolation of actinomycotic agents. Dextrone-peptone agar medium (pH 7) or Lowenstein medium also can be used to isolate actinomycetes. The appearance of colonies, the sexual and asexual forms of the fungi, and metabolic profiles allow definitive characterization of isolates.

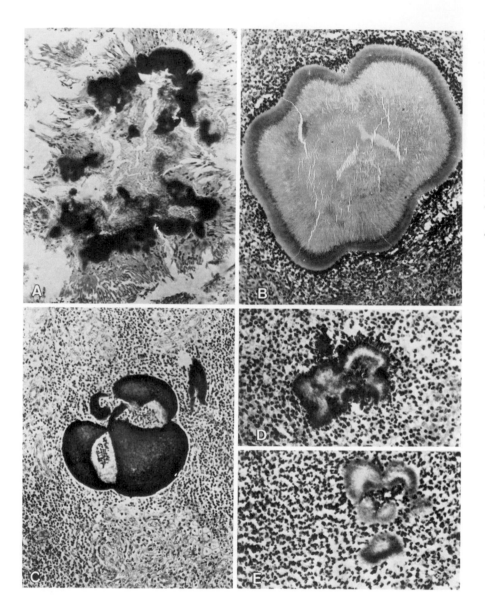

Figure 109-2. Grains in sections of actinomycotic mycetomas. *A. A. madurae,* with irregular edges and long fringes (biopsy sample BD 2661, H and E, × 150). *B. S. somaliensis,* containing a hard cement (biopsy sample BA 81, H and E, × 150). *C. A. pelletieri,* bursting of a spherical grain due to the cellular reaction (biopsy sample Bi 1640, H and E, × 150). *D. Nocardia* spp., with clubs (biopsy sample Z 108, H and E, × 260). *E. N. asteroides,* without clubs (biopsy sample 1008, H and E, × 260). (*Courtesy of F. Mariat et al.* [*3*], *S. Karger AG, Basel.*)

PATIENT

PATHOGENESIS AND CLINICAL MANIFESTATIONS

Most of the causal organisms have been isolated from soil or plants [*10*]. For example, in the Senegal valley, *L. senegalensis* and *L. tompkinsii* are found in about 50 percent of dry thorns of acacia, particularly when they are covered with mud during the rainy season. In the same valley, *N. rosatii* can be isolated from dry sand and *M. mycetomi* from soil on the surface of termitaria [*11*]. The saprophytic soil fungi enter the subcutaneous tissues after a barefooted individual sustains local trauma, frequently by stepping on a thorn. The chest wall,

back, and shoulders may be inoculated by trauma caused by carrying sacks contaminated with soil (Fig. 109-3). Head and neck mycetomas are associated with carrying bundles of wood.

Typically, males develop mycetoma between the ages of 20 and 40. It tends to be an occupational disease of farmers and others likely to be exposed to injury from thorns and splinters. The most common site of injury and consequent infection is the foot. The initial sign is an atypical wart or subcutaneous nodule. Nodules swell and discharge through sinus tracts. New nodules appear near the initial one with spread between muscular layers. Old sinuses heal and scar over, but new ones develop. A chronic necrotizing infection ensues with painless

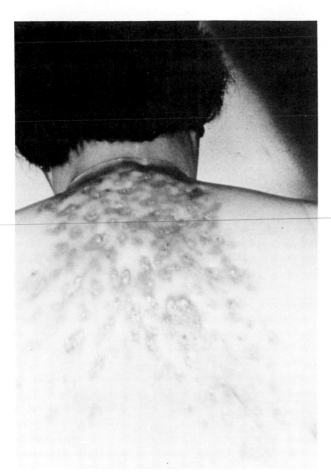

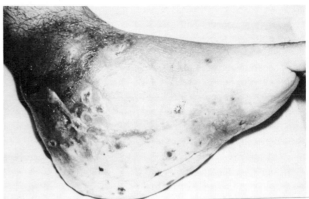

Figure 109-4. Mycetoma: foot, clinical photograph. This convex surface of a foot with advanced infection shows multiple, draining sinuses with gross deformity of the foot. Maduromycosis most often occurs on the extremities, particularly the feet. (*Reproduced from the* Atlases of Clinical Mycology: Subcutaneous Mycoses, *CT Dolan et al. © 1976 by American Society of Clinical Pathologists, Chicago. Used by permission.*)

Figure 109-3. Mycetoma: back, clinical photograph. This case of widespread mycetoma shows a plaqueform area of granulomatous inflammation with multiple draining sinuses. Keloidal scarring is present.

has emerged as an important opportunistic agent involving the skin, lungs, bones, and joints in immunosuppressed patients [*15,16*].

Radiographs of involved bony areas show osteolytic lesions and periosteal inflammation [*8*].

PATHOLOGY

A typical mycetoma consists of large granulomatous areas with a purulent center surrounded by a thick fibrous capsule. The subcutaneous region, modified by intricate necrotic lesions and

swelling, and repeated drainage of pus-containing grains of fungal particles through sinus tracts and fistulas (Fig. 109-2 through 109-5). The appearance in eumycetoma can be particularly dramatic with black grains discharging from fungating nodules. The process may extend to invade bone. Tendons usually are spared. Destruction of the tarsal bones with widespread plantar fibrosis produces a characteristic foreshortened and raised appearance to the foot known as "Madura foot" [*12,13*].

The course is slowly progressive with recurring cycles of swelling, suppuration, and scarring. Despite distortion of anatomy with marked edema and erythema, there is little pain unless bacterial superinfection supervenes. Lymphatic involvement is common, and occasionally there is inguinal lymphadenopathy [*14*]. Systemic infection is extremely rare and then mainly with *Nocardia* spp. and other actinomycetes, possibly because of the small size of the grains. *Pseudallescheria boydii*

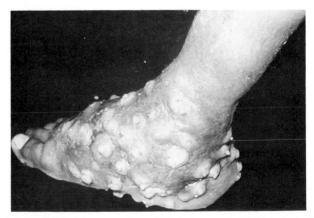

Figure 109-5. Mycetoma: foot, clinical photograph. Multiple foci of suppuration and nodulation with sinus-tract formation can be seen in the swollen, distorted foot shown in this slide. Note the large number of draining abscesses. (*Reproduced from the* Atlases of Clinical Mycology: Subcutaneous Mycoses, *CT Dolan et al. © 1976 by American Society of Clinical Pathologists, Chicago. Used by permission.*)

areas of extensive fibrosis, gives the mycetoma its typical pseudotumor aspect. The necrotic and purulent process can involve muscle with resultant degenerative myositis. The tendons generally are spared.

Bone frequently is invaded and destroyed (Fig. 109-6). Small cavities are formed in the bone with a grain in the middle, appearing as an osseous "geode," 2 to 10 mm in diameter. The medullary canal and epiphyses frequently are invaded. Destruction of bone and formation of osteophytes from periosteal reaction can produce complete remodeling of bone [17–19].

The granuloma consists of a central suppurative zone, surrounded by a ring of histiocytes, often arranged in palisades. In a third concentric zone, a subacute, nonspecific, and limiting fibrous tissue reaction is observed. Histiocytes can aggregate to form giant cells. Neutrophils and giant cells occasionally engulf, split, and destroy the grain.

The inflammatory response is not specific, only its extensive development is characteristic. Contrariwise, the morphology of the parasitic grain is helpful in the specific diagnosis of the etiological agent. The morphology in histological sections stained by hematoxylin and eosin (H and E) is described above with the characteristics of the individual agents.

DIAGNOSIS

The clinical appearance of mycetoma usually allows the diagnosis (Fig. 109-7). Results of culture are key, however, both

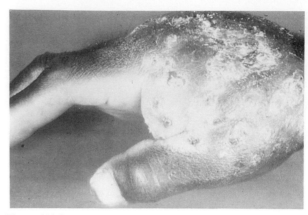

Figure 109-7. Mycetoma: hand, clinical photograph. Illustrated here is mycetoma of the hand, showing multiple draining sinuses with a large area of swelling and induration. (*Reproduced from the* Atlases of Clinical Mycology: Subcutaneous Mycoses, *CT Dolan et al.* © *1976 by American Society of Clinical Pathologists, Chicago. Used by permission.*)

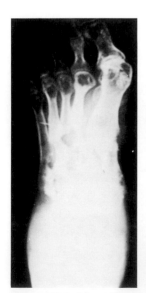
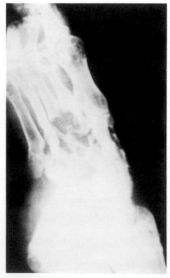

Figure 109-6. Mycetoma: foot roentgenogram. This roentgenogram of the foot reveals extensive destruction and deformity in the cuneiform and proximal part of the metatarsals. Localized lytic lesions characteristic of mycetoma are present. (*Reproduced from the* Atlases of Clinical Mycology: Subcutaneous Mycoses, *CT Dolan et al. Copyright 1976 by American Society of Clinical Pathologists, Chicago. Used by permission.*)

because of management considerations and to distinguish mycetoma from botromycosis, a clinically similar chronic bacterial infection caused by cocci (staphylococci, streptococci) or short rods (actinobacillus, gram-negative enteric bacilli) and from chronic bacterial osteomyelitis. Tuberculosis also can cause a slowly progressive destructive process involving the foot. Both serological tests and delayed-type hypersensitivity skin testing are of potential value but not of practical use in the diagnosis of mycetoma.

TREATMENT

The treatment of mycetoma is unsatisfactory. The best chance of cure is amputation with a wide margin free of infection, but this is not an acceptable alternative for most patients because of the ensuing loss of livelihood. Medical therapy has some role, particularly if combined with surgical debridement. The fungal agents causing mycetoma are resistant to amphotericin B and flucytosine. Some of these organisms are sensitive to Miconazole and ketoconazole which have produced improvement in individual cases [16,22]. The treatment options are broader for actinomycotic mycetomas. *Nocardia* spp. can be treated with trimethoprim-sulfamethoxazole combination or dapsone [23,24]. The adjunctive use of streptomycin or amikacin has had a positive effect in some instances and appears indicated in mycetomas caused by *Actinomadura* spp. or *S. somaliensis* [23–25].

Eventually, many mycetomas require amputation. If this is performed too close to the infected area, recurrence is likely. Fortunately, mycetomas remain localized in most instances so that the prognosis for survival is good. Involvement of the scalp, however, requires aggressive medical and surgical therapy to forestall intracranial extension.

REFERENCES

1 Abbott PH: Mycetomas in the Sudan. Trans R Soc Trop Med Hyg 50:11–24, 1956

2 Mahgoub ES, Murray IG: *Mycetoma*. London, Heinemann, 1973

3 Mariat F, Destombes P, Segretain G: The mycetomas: Clinical features, pathology, etiology and epidemiology. Contrib Microbiol Immunol 4:1–39, 1977

4 Rey M: Less Mycétomes dan l'ouest Africain. Medical thesis, Foulon, Paris, 1961

5 Zaias N, Taplin D, Rebell G: Mycetoma. Arch Dermatol 99:215–225, 1969

6 Develoux M, Audoin J, Treguer J, et al: Mycetomas in the Republic of Niger: Clinical features and epidemiology. Am J Trop Med Hyg 38:386–390, 1988

7 Joshi KR, Sanghvi A, Vyas MC, et al: Etiology and distribution of mycetoma in Rajasthan, India. Indian J Med Res 85:694–698, 1987

8 Bendl BJ, Mackey D, Al-Saati F, et al: Mycetoma in Saudi Arabia. J Trop Med Hyg 90:51–59, 1987

9 Tight RR, Bartlett MS: Actinomycetoma in the United States. Rev Infect Dis 3:1139, 1981

10 Basset A, Camain R, Lambert D: Rôles des épines de mimosacees dans l'inoculation des mycétomes (A propos de deux observations). Bull Soc Pathol Exot 58:22–24, 1965

11 Segretain G, Mariat F: Recherches sur la présence d'agents de mycétomes dans le sol et sur les épineux du Sénégal et de la Mauritanie. Bull Soc Pathol Exot 61:194–202, 1968

12 Bezes H: L'aspect chirurgical des mycétomes à Dakar. A propos d'une statistique personnelle de 60 observations. J Chir (Paris) 82:13–32, 1961

13 Camain R: Processus d'extension et de limitation des mycétomes africains. Bull Soc Pathol Exot 61:517–523, 1968

14 El Hassan AM, Mahgoub ES: Lymph node involvement in mycetoma. Trans R Soc Trop Med Hyg 66:165–169, 1972

15 Ansari RA, Hindson DA, Stevens DL, et al: Pseudallescheria boydii arthritis and osteomyelitis in a patient with Cushing's disease. South Med J 80:90–92, 1987

16 Willsteed E, Regan W: Treatment of Pseudallescheria boydii infection with oral ketoconazole and topical miconazole. Australas J Dermatol 28:21–23, 1987

17 Davies AGM: The bone changes of Madura foot. Observations of Uganda Africans. Radiology 70:841–847, 1958

18 Destombes P: Histopathologie des mycétomes. Ann Soc Belg Med Trop 52:261–276, 1972

19 Destombes P: Mycoses osseuses. *Encyclopédie Médico Chirurgicale,* 1972

20 Camain R, Segretain G, Nazimoff O: Etude histopathologique des mycétomes du Sénégal. Sem Hôp Paris 33:923–938, 1957

21 Destombes P, Segretain G: Les mycétomes fongiques. Caractères histologiques et culturaux. Arch Inst Pasteur, Tunis 39:273–290, 1962

22 Fernandez-Guerrero ML, Ruiz Barnes P, Ales JM: Postcraniotomy mycetoma of the scalp and osteomyelitis due to Pseudallescheria boydii (letter). J Infect Dis 156:855, 1987

23 Latapi F, y Ortiz Y: Los micetomas en Mexico: Algunos datos clinicos y epidemiologicos relativos a 197 casos. Mem 1° Congr Mex Dermat 1963, pp 126–144

24 Mahgoub ES: Medical management of mycetoma. Bull WHO 54:303, 1976

25 Welsh O, Sauceda E, Gonzalez J, et al: Amikacin alone and in combination with trimethoprim-sulfamethoxazole in the treatment of actinomycotic mycetoma. J Am Acad Dermatol 17:443–448, 1987

CHAPTER
110

Paracoccidioidomycosis · Donald L. Greer

Paracoccidioides brasiliensis is a thermal dimorphic fungus found in soil, although its precise micro-niche in soil is still unknown. Its geographical distribution is restricted to the Latin American countries, for example, Mexico, Central, and South America. The infection is exogenously acquired after inhalation of the spores. The fungus produces an acute to chronic disease, paracoccidioidomycosis (South American blastomycosis). Primary lesions of the lungs frequently disseminate to the lymph nodes, reticuloendothelial system, skin, and mucous membranes. Infection occurs in both males and females, but adult males working in agriculture or soil-related employment most frequently develop disease. Natural disease in lower animals, domestic or feral, is virtually unknown. The disease is noncommunicable. Diagnosis is readily confirmed by direct examination of clinical material or serological tests. Rapid recognition of the disease is essential to successful management. Chemotherapy is effective with sulfonamides, amphotericin B, and ketoconazole; the latter being the present drug of choice.

PARASITE

Lack of evidence of the exact source of the fungus in nature and the absence of disease in animals have hampered the studies of the ecology of this disease and its agent. All evidence suggests that the soil is the common source for *P. brasiliensis.* It has been successfully isolated from soil on two occasions [1].

Animal reservoirs

The disease is found only in humans. Data from skin test surveys in domestic animals indicate that they may acquire the infection, but overt disease does not develop [2]. Overt natural disease is unknown in feral animals. The positive histopathological finding of *P. brasiliensis* in a squirrel monkey from Bolivia and in four armadillos from Brazil are the only acceptable reports of natural nonhuman disease [3,4]. Bats are not naturally infected and play no role in the distribution of the fungus in nature.

Geographical distribution

Based on morbidity and mortality data, *P. brasiliensis* is confined to specific ecologically defined zones corresponding to the tropical and subtropical forests of Latin America, from Mexico to Argentina. These zones are well demarcated by narrow criteria of rainfall, temperature, and altitude. However, not all countries within this endemic region have reported cases nor is the disease evenly distributed within a single country. No cases have been reported from the Caribbean Islands. Authentic cases outside Latin America, i.e., in the United States, Europe, and Africa, were all reported in patients who had previously resided in the endemic area [2].

MORPHOLOGY OF AGENT

P. brasiliensis is a temperature-dependent dimorphic fungus which grows as a mold in nature at 25°C and as a yeast in tissue or at 37°C. As a mold it is seen as a slow-growing, wrinkled colony with short, white, aerial hyphae. Microscopically it produces arthroconidia and microconidia attached to thin, septate hyphae [5]. Identification of the fungus cannot be made from the mold phase. In tissue, or on Kelly's medium [6] at 37°C, the fungus grows as a wrinkled cream-colored yeast colony. Microscopically, spherical double-walled yeast cells are seen ranging in size from 10 to 30 μm. They reproduce by multiple budding. The distinctive "pilot wheel" configuration consists of a large mother cell surrounded by smaller daughter cells or buds. The definite identification is made from the yeast phase.

BIOCHEMISTRY AND PHYSIOLOGY

Both phases of *P. brasiliensis* require oxygen for growth; on occasion, primary isolation may be enhanced by microaerophilic conditions. The fungus grows best at pH 6.8 to 7.0.

The biochemical composition of the cell wall appears associated with the virulence of the agent. The antigenic component of fungus is related to the presence of galactomannan in the cell wall. Both the yeast and mold phases contain chitin and polysaccharides; however, the principal polysaccharide of the yeast form consists of α-1-3 glucan, while the mold form consists of β-1-3 glucan.

ANIMAL MODELS

Attempts to reproduce the disease in laboratory animals using the mycelial phase via the natural route of inhalation have met with little success. Experimentally, many laboratory animals have been infected by numerous routes of inoculation using the yeast phase; however, the study of pathogenesis in animals after the inhalation of the mycelial phase of *P. brasiliensis* has been reproduced only in mice [8]. Similar animal studies using the yeast phase have been accomplished in hamsters and bats [9].

PATIENT

PATHOGENESIS

Asymptomatic infection occurs in "normal" individuals of both sexes after inhalation of the arthroconidia and microconidia produced by the fungus. The intradermal skin test converts from a negative to a positive (> 5-mm induration). It is well-established that the portal of entry is the lung [10]. Clinical disease affects primarily males and may vary from primary pulmonary forms to acute or chronic disseminated cases. A comprehensive discussion of the prognosed pathogenesis and clinical forms has been reported [11].

CLINICAL MANIFESTATIONS

Paracoccidioidomycostic disease has many clinical facets [11]. Although relatively rare in children, the acute to subacute juvenile form progresses rapidly and is usually fatal. Primarily the reticuloendothelial system (RES) and lymphatics are involved (Fig. 110-1). Most commonly seen in endemic areas is the chronic progressive adult form of paracoccidioidomycosis [12]. Occasionally the disease may be localized to a single organ or system, i.e., the respiratory system (Fig. 110-2); however, most frequently the patient presents with both pulmonary and mucocutaneous pathology (Fig. 110-3). Patients who sur-

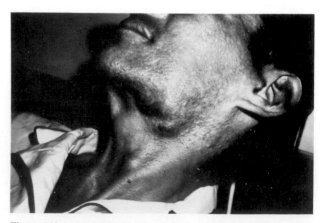

Figure 110-1. Lymphatic involvement in a young Colombian patient.

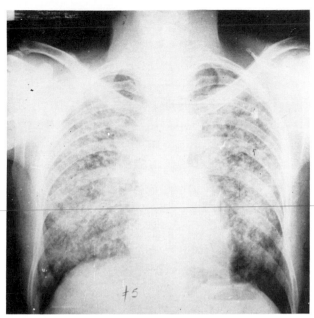

Figure 110-2. Extensive micronodular infiltration seen on x-ray from a patient with pulmonary disease.

vive the juvenile or adult forms of paracoccidioidomycosis may continue to develop sequelae such as pulmonary fibrosis or laryngeal stenosis. Frequently physical examination reveals mucocutaneous lesions, dysphagia and dyspnea accompanied by varying degrees of weight loss, malaise, and low-grade fever. Mucocutaneous lesions are ulcerated and granulomatous with an irregular surface (Fig. 110-4). Bleeding petechiae give the lesions a "mulberry" appearance.

Radiographic images of the lungs reveal chronic pulmonary disease simulating tuberculosis. Often, the x-ray findings appear more severe than the physical examination of the patient may suggest. The infiltrates are concentrated toward the central and lower lobes and consist of micro- and macronodules which may progress toward consolidation. Cavitation and calcification are not common. Differential diagnosis includes any of the respiratory mycoses, tuberculosis, or neoplasms.

The early involvement of the reticuloendothelial system (RES) after dissemination may result in hepatosplenomegaly, generalized lymphadenopathy, and impaired adrenal gland function leading to Addison's disease. The acute disseminated form often seen in juveniles shows extensive lymphadenopathy simulating Hodgkin's disease.

LABORATORY DIAGNOSIS

The laboratory diagnosis may be accomplished readily by visualizing the yeast directly in clinical material and tissue biopsy. Serological methods of immunodiffusion and/or complement fixation are both diagnostic and prognostic.

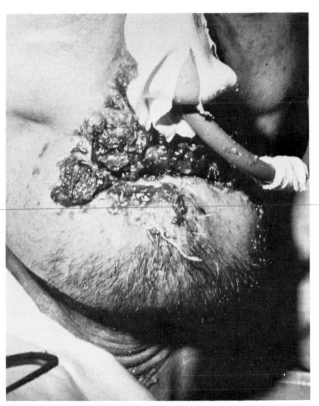

Figure 110-3. Extensive mucocutaneous lesions in a Colombian patient with chronic disseminated paracoccidioidomycosis.

DIRECT EXAMINATION

Any type of clinical specimen may be examined using the direct wet preparation with 10% KOH. Early morning sputum, exudates from oral lesions, and biopsies are preferred; positive specimens for paracoccidioidomycosis show spherical double-

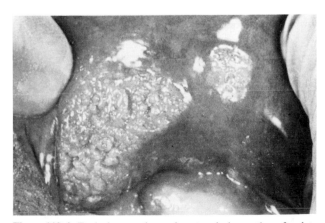

Figure 110-4. Typical mucosal granulomatous lesion on the soft palate showing "mulberry" surface characteristics.

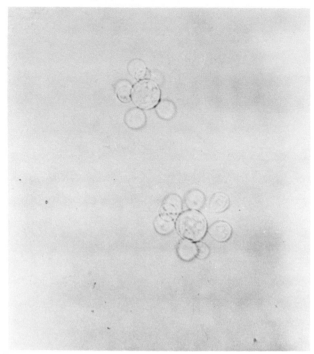

Figure 110-5. Multiple budding yeast cells from culture grown at 37°C on Kelly's medium. × 400.

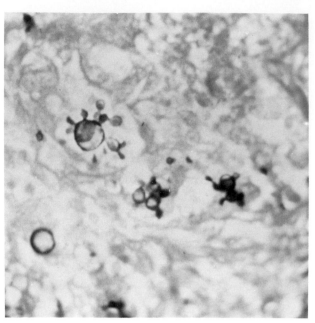

Figure 110-6. Multiple budding yeast cells or pilot-wheel configuration in tissue stained with methenamine silver. × 400.

walled multiple budding yeast cells (10 to 30 μm in diameter). The characteristic pilot-wheel formation is diagnostic of this disease.

CULTURES

Clinical material must be plated on at least two media: Sabouraud's dextrose agar with cycloheximide and chloramphenicol (Mycosel BBL); and brain-heart infusion agar with gentamicin. All cultures are incubated at 25°C. Growth is slow, requiring 3 to 4 weeks for the appearance of small, white to tan, glabrous colonies. Microscopic examination of these colonies shows sterile hyphae and rare arthroconidia and microconidia attached to narrow septate hyphae. The morphology of the conidia and/or hyphae may be confused with some saprophytic Hyphomycetes such as *Chrysosporium,* and cannot be used for final identification. Conversion of the fungus to the yeast phase is necessary for complete identification. This is accomplished in about 7 days on Kelly's agar [6] incubated at 37°C. Microscopic examination of the yeastlike growth shows the spherical multiple budding yeast cells characteristic of the fungus (Fig. 110-5).

HISTOPATHOLOGY

The primary tissue reaction seen on H&E sections is a nonspecific granuloma complete with multinucleate giant cells.

The fungal yeast cells are refractile double-walled spheres which do not stain and may be difficult to see. Tissues stained with methenamine silver (Gomori) readily reveal the characteristic fungal yeast cells (10 to 30 μm) as dark-staining bodies with multiple buds (Fig. 110-6). The presence of the pilot wheel is diagnostic. A small form of *P. brasiliensis* only 3 to 5 μm in diameter and resembling *Histoplasma capsulatum* in tissue has been reported.

SEROLOGICAL DIAGNOSIS

Two serological tests are routinely used for diagnosis and prognosis of paracoccidioidomycosis: double immunodiffusion (ID) and complement fixation (CF).

The ID test is rapid, sensitive, and selective for paracoccidioidomycosis. It is also simple and inexpensive, making it the test of choice in small diagnostic laboratories throughout Latin America. Approximately 93 to 95 percent of patients with active disease develop one to three bands. This is an indication of active disease. The use of a positive control and a line of identity between the control band and the band produced by the patient's serum makes the test specific. These bands may disappear with treatment [13].

The more quantitative CF test also can be used for both diagnosis and prognosis. Approximately 85 to 90 percent of patients with active disease will give titers of 1:16 or higher. Cross-reactions occur with antigens of the respiratory mycosis so that careful controls must be used. Upon successful treatment, the titers fall, indicating a good prognosis [13].

SKIN TESTING ANTIGENS

The intradermal skin test procedure using the polysaccharide extracted from the yeast phase of *P. brasiliensis* is reserved for epidemiological surveys. Skin tests are not diagnostic. Throughout the endemic areas some 8 to 54 percent of the "normal" population may present with a positive reaction [2] and about 40 to 60 percent of the patients have negative skin test at the time of diagnosis. As the patient recovers with treatment, a negative skin test may become positive. Likewise, the conversion of a positive to a negative skin test and a rising CF titer usually indicate a poor prognosis.

MANAGEMENT

Paracoccidioidomycosis is a treatable fungal disease. Early diagnosis is essential for ensuring a good clinical response. Underlying debilitating illness may complicate the medical treatment. The sulfonamides have been the classical drugs, giving approximately 60 to 75 percent patient response. Both slow and rapid action sulfas can be used; however, therapy must be continued for a prolonged period [14]. Amphotericin B treatment is successful in all forms of the disease and in those cases resistant to sulfonamides. Its use is similar to that prescribed for the other mycotic respiratory diseases. A combination of amphotericin B (total of 1.0 to 1.5 g) later followed by sulfonamides has been successfully used. However, relapses have been reported. The oral imidazole compound ketoconazole is now the drug of choice. A total of 200 mg/day for at least 6 months gives excellent results and is relatively nontoxic [15]. Liver enzymes should be monitored during treatment. Relapses are uncommon if treatment is continued until all clinical signs are clear and patients present with negative serology.

Regardless of the type of treatment, the outcome depends largely upon the patient's condition at the beginning of therapy. About 8 percent of the patients die of the disease regardless of therapy [15].

POPULATION

PREVALENCE AND INCIDENCE

Unlike the other respiratory mycoses, paracoccidioidomycosis occurs as isolated cases in the general population. Epidemics or even small outbreaks are unknown. Like the other mycoses, it is noncommunicable, and human to human transmission has not been reported. The disease is the most prevalent respiratory mycosis in Latin America. To date, in excess of 6000 cases have been reported in the literature. Actual figures are difficult to acquire because of underreporting and misdiagnoses of mycoses, often as tuberculosis. Over 69 percent of the published cases are reported from Brazil. Venezuela and Colombia occupy second and third place in reported cases with approximately 13 percent and 10 percent, respectively. The remaining 12 countries reporting the disease total only 8 percent of the cases; the majority of these are seen in Argentina, Ecuador, Paraguay, and Peru. Only 13 nonautochthonous cases have been documented in the United States, and 11 from Europe, Asia, and Africa. All cases were reported in individuals who had previously lived in an endemic country. No cases have been reported from Chile, Cuba, the Dominican Republic, Guyana, Haiti, Jamaica, Nicaragua, Trinidad and Tobago, or Puerto Rico [2].

AGE AND SEX DISTRIBUTION

Paracoccidioidomycosis is rare in children and uncommon in young adults under 20 years of age. It is diagnosed most frequently in adults between 30 and 60 years of age. Skin test surveys show that infection occurs equally in males and females; however, the disease is diagnosed most frequently in males in an overall ratio of 13:1. Exposure alone does not explain this discrepancy. Hormonal factors appear to give the female more resistance to disease. Most patients live in rural zones and work in agriculture, ranching, or other soil-related employment. Cases are often reported, however, from urban populations [2].

Infection and disease

Subclinical infection as demonstrated by skin test surveys within the endemic areas occurs in the normal population. The sensitivity is low when compared to other systemic mycoses. In Colombia, surveys show approximately 10 to 12 percent intradermal hypersensitivity in the normal population. There is no standard skin test antigen.

Prevention and control

Paracoccidioidomycosis is not considered an occupational disease. Control of the mycoses and identifying the occupation will not be possible in the absence of more precise knowledge of the source of infection. Fortunately, *P. brasiliensis* is not considered to be a particularly infectious fungus; it produces a low infection rate, does not cause epidemics in the normal population, and only one case of a laboratory infection has been reported—autoinoculation with infected material. It appears that prolonged and intimate contact with the fungus is necessary for infection to occur. The latent period is unknown, but can be as long as 60 years [2]. All these factors make prevention and control impractical at this time.

REFERENCES

1 Albornoz M: Isolation of *P. brasiliensis* from rural soil in Venezuela. Sabouraudia 9:248–253, 1971
2 Greer DL, Restrepo M: The epidemiology of paracoccidioidomycosis, in Al-Doory Y (ed): *The Epidemiology of Human Mycotic Disease*. Springfield, Charles C Thomas, 1975, pp 117–141

3 Johnson WD, Lang CM: Paracoccidioidomycosis (South American blastomycosis) in a squirrel monkey. Vet Pathol 19:368–371, 1977

4 Naiff RD, Ferreira CL, Barrett TV, et al: Paracoccidioidomicose enzoótica em tatus (*Dasypus novemcinctus*) no estado do Pará. Rev Inst Med Trop São Paulo 28(1):19–27, 1986

5 Restrepo A: A reappraisal of the microscopical appearance of mycelial phase of *P. brasiliensis*. Sabouraudia 8:141–144, 1970

6 Kelley WH: A study of the cell and colony variations of *B. dermatitidis*. J Ing Dis 64:293–296, 1939

7 San-Blas G, San-Blas F: Variability of cell wall composition in *Paracoccidioides brasiliensis:* A study of two strains. Sabouraudia 20:31–40, 1982

8 Restrepo A, Guzman G: Paracoccidioidomycosis experimental del raton inducida por via aerogena. Sabouraudia 14:299–311, 1976

9 Greer DL, McMurray DN: Pathogenesis and immune response to *Paracoccidioides brasiliensis* in the fructivorous bat, *Artibeus lituratus*. Sabouraudia 19:165–178, 1981

10 Gonzalez-Ochoa A: Theories regarding the portal of entry of *Paracoccidioides brasiliensis:* A brief review, in Paracoccidioidomycosis, Proceedings of the First Pan American Symposium, PAHO sci publ no 254, 1972, pp 278–283

11 Restrepo A, Robledo M, Giraldo R, et al: The gamut of paracoccidioidomycosis. Am J Med 61:33–42, 1976

12 Londero AT, Ramos CD, Lopez JOS: Progressive pulmonary paracoccidioidomycosis. A study of 34 cases observed in Rio Grande do Sul (Brazil). Mycopathol 63:53–56, 1978

13 Restrepo A, Restrepo M, Restrepo F, et al: Immune responses in paracoccidioidomycosis. A controlled study of 16 patients before and after treatment. Sabouraudia 16:151–163, 1978

14 Negroni P: Prolonged therapy for paracoccidioidomycosis. Approaches, complications and risks, in Paracoccidioidomycosis, Proceedings of the First Pan American Symposium PAHO sci publ no 254, 1972, pp 147–155

15 Marques SA, Dillon NL, Franco MF, et al: Paracoccidioidomycosis: A comparative study of the evolutionary serologic, clinical, and radiologic results for patients treated with ketoconazole or amphotericin B plus sulfonamides. Mycopathologia 89:19–23, 1985

16 Del Negro G: Ketoconazole in paracoccidioidomycosis: A long-term therapy study with prolonged follow-up. Rev Inst Med Trop Sao Paulo 24(1):27–39, 1982

CHAPTER 111 / *Pneumocystosis* · Peter D. Walzer

Pneumocystis carinii is an organism of uncertain taxonomy and worldwide distribution that resides in the lung. For many years *P. carinii* has been recognized as an important cause of pneumonia in the immunocompromised host. The emergence of the acquired immunodeficiency syndrome (AIDS) has been accompanied by a dramatic rise in the number of cases of pneumocystosis. *P. carinii* has provided important new clinical challenges in AIDS as well as opportunities to study the host-parasite relationship. Yet our knowledge of the basic immunobiology of this organism remains at a rudimentary level because of a lack of a widely available in vitro cultivation system.

PARASITE

LIFE CYCLE

The precise taxonomic status of *P. carinii* is unsettled. Most authors have favored a protozoan classification, but analysis of *P. carinii* ribosomal RNA, a technique of phylogenetic investigation that is finding increasing application, suggests a close relationship to fungi [1,2]. It therefore seemed reasonable to consider *P. carinii* among fungi in this book until its classification can be formally established. The life cycle stages of *P. carinii* have been based on terminology for protozoa, and three principal forms have been identified: the *trophic* form, or *trophozoite*, the most numerous stage; the *cyst*, which contains up to eight intracystic bodies, or *sporozoites*; and the *precyst*, an intermediate stage. Knowledge of the life cycle of *P. carinii* has mainly been obtained from studies of the organism in lung sections, although recently tissue culture has been used [3]. It is generally considered that there is an asexual cycle in which trophozoites replicate by binary fission, but definitive proof of this is lacking. A sexual cycle has been proposed for the development of trophozoites into cysts, and support for this hypothesis has come from the demonstration of synaptonemal complexes in precysts [4]. At maturity, cysts liberate the intracystic bodies, which then develop into trophozoites. The conditions that stimulate encystation or excystation are unknown.

MORPHOLOGY AND ULTRASTRUCTURE

The trophozoite is small (1 to 4 μm), pleomorphic, and is commonly found in clusters. On Giemsa stain the organism has a reddish nucleus and blue cytoplasm. Electron microscopy reveals a few organelles and tubular cytoplasmic extensions termed *filopodia*. The large (5- to 8-μm) cyst is easily identifiable by its thick cell wall and intracystic bodies (Fig. 111-1A and B). Stains such as Grocott or Gomori methenamine

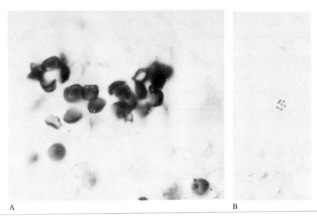

Figure 111-1. *A. Pneumocystis carinii* cysts. Methenamine silver stain, × 1000. *B. P. carinii* cyst containing intracystic bodies. Giemsa stain, × 1000.

silver, which selectively stain the cyst wall, are used to identify this stage of the organism in histopathological sections. The definition of the intermediate (4- to 6-μm) precyst stage varies among different workers.

METABOLISM AND CULTURE

The metabolic pathways of *P. carinii* are poorly understood. The organism presumably obtains nutrients from the contents of the alveolar fluid; the primitive organelle system suggests metabolism of low-molecular-weight substances, although endocytosis may also occur. The few metabolic studies that have been performed have used nonreplicating organisms [5]. The data suggest that *P. carinii* can metabolize carbohydrates, synthesize proteins, nucleic acids, and phospholipids, and utilize molecular oxygen; the use of histochemical stains has revealed the presence of several important dehydrogenase enzymes.

Modest growth (up to 10-fold) of rat, but not human, *P. carinii* has been achieved using several different cell lines [6]. Cultivation of *P. carinii* has been significantly limited by lack of reproducibility among laboratories and the lack of commonly accepted standards of organism growth; thus, no culture system has achieved widespread application. Despite these limitations, in vitro cultivation of *P. carinii* has been useful in analyzing the developmental stages of the organism, in testing susceptibility to antimicrobial drugs, and in obtaining preparations of improved purity for immunological studies.

ANIMAL MODELS

Rats administered corticosteroids for about 8 weeks spontaneously develop *P. carinii* pneumonia with histopathological features identical to the disease in humans; the mechanism involves reactivation of latent infection. This animal model system has been used extensively in studies of pathogenesis and host immune responses and in the development of new treatment modalities [7]. Pneumocystosis has also been in-

duced by corticosteroids in mice, rabbits, guinea pigs, and ferrets. The low virulence of *P. carinii* has frustrated attempts to produce pneumonia in animals with exogenous organisms. *P. carinii* can be transmitted experimentally among athymic mice but results in little overt disease. Yet, the occurrence of outbreaks of pneumocystosis in colonies of immunodeficient mice emphasizes the pathogenicity of the organism in this animal population under natural conditions.

Intermediate and reservoir hosts

P. carinii can be found in the lungs of humans and a wide variety of animals in nature. Although organisms from these hosts are morphologically indistinguishable, antigenic studies suggest that species and strain differences exist [8]. Thus, there is little evidence to support the notion that *P. carinii* infection represents a zoonosis.

PATIENT "HOST"

PREDISPOSING HOST FACTORS

P. carinii was first associated with human illness when it was found to cause interstitial plasma cell pneumonia, a disease which occurred in malnourished, premature infants in orphanages in Europe after World War II. Since interstitial plasma cell pneumonia sometimes occurred in explosive outbreaks, it has been called the "epidemic" form of pneumocystosis. Interstitial plasma cell pneumonia is now uncommon but still can be found in parts of the world where poor socioeconomic conditions exist.

The more widely recognized form of *P. carinii* pneumonia is as a complication of medical progress. Major target populations include children with primary immunodeficiency diseases (particulary severe combined immunodeficiency disease); patients receiving immunosuppressive therapy (especially corticosteroids) for organ transplantation, cancer, and other disorders; and patients with AIDS [9,10]. Pneumocystosis is the leading opportunistic infection in AIDS, occurring in greater than 60 percent of patients. Although the specific immune defects that predispose to *P. carinii* pneumonia are poorly understood, it is generally considered that impaired cellular immunity plays a major role in the development of this disease. AIDS, which has emerged as the most common underlying condition in *P. carinii* infection, is characterized principally by a reduction in the number and function of CD4 T helper cells. Patients infected with the human immunodeficiency virus (HIV) have impaired lymphocyte proliferative responses to *P. carinii* that parallel different stages of the viral infection [11]. Other important *P. carinii* predisposing factors, such as protein malnutrition and corticosteroid therapy, have broad inhibitory effects on host cell-mediated immunity.

Antibodies are produced locally and systemically in response to infection with *P. carinii*, but their role in host defenses against the organism is unclear. Perhaps the antibodies function as opsonins and enhance phagocytosis [*12*]. Once engulfed by alveolar mcrophages *P. carinii* is immediately digested, thus supporting the concept that the organism does not have an intracellular stage in its life cycle.

PATHOGENESIS AND PATHOLOGY

P. carinii interacts with a variety of factors in alveoli which may contribute to its evasion of host defenses or development of disease. Foremost among these is the tight attachment of *P. carinii* to a specific alveolar lining cell, the type 1 pneumocyte [*13*]. The nature of the organism's antigens, surface carbohydrates, and other structures, and their relationship to alveolar fluid constituents are receiving increasing attention.

The sequential changes during the development of pneumocystosis have been studied in detail in the rat model. The slow propagation of organisms within alveoli is accompanied by changes in the surface properties of lining cells, alveolar-capillary membrane permeability, respiratory mechanics, and surfactant phospholipids; the process culminates with damage to the type 1 cell. On hematoxylin and eosin stain in the rat and in humans, the alveoli are filled with a frothy honey-combed material that reveals numerous organisms when stained with silver. There may be interstitial edema with hyperplasia and hypertrophy of alveolar type 2 pneumocytes (a typical host reparative response), but other host inflammatory changes are mild and nonspecific. Only in premature infants is there a prominent interstitial plasma cell infiltrate.

CLINICAL FEATURES

Pneumocystosis presents as a respiratory illness characterized by fever, shortness of breath, and a nonproductive cough. In patients receiving immunosuppressive therapy, symptoms may begin during corticosteroid administration or after these drugs

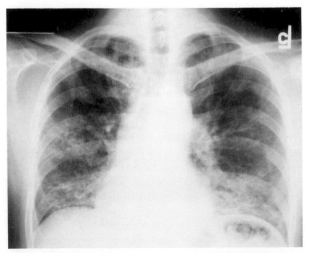

Figure 111-2. Chest radiograph of a patient with *P. carinii* pneumonia showing bilateral infiltrates.

have been tapered or discontinued. The duration of illness varies considerably among individual patients, but typically is 1 to 2 weeks. In contrast, *P. carinii* pneumonia in AIDS patients is frequently a subtle illness with symptoms continuing for weeks to months [*14*]. Findings on physical examination vary from no abnormalities to tachypnea, tachycardia, and cyanosis. Rales are present in about one-third of the patients, but other auscultatory findings are uncommon.

Pulmonary function abnormalities include hypoxemia, increased alveolar-arterial oxygen gradient, respiratory alkalosis, and impaired vital and total lung capacity. Classic findings on chest roentgenogram consist of diffuse alveolar infiltrates emanating from the perihilar region (Fig. 111-2). A variety of atypical radiological changes (e.g., nodules, abscess) have been reported. Some patients may have a normal x-ray but show increased lung uptake on gallium scan; others may have increased clearance of inhaled technetium-99m diethylene triamine penta-acetate (tc DTPA), a marker for alveolar-capillary membrane permeability. Changes in other laboratory values (e.g., white blood cell count) usually reflect the status of the underlying disease rather than activity of *P. carinii*.

DIAGNOSIS

The clinical features of *P. carinii* pneumonia can be produced by a variety of other agents, and thus specific diagnosis must be made by histopathological demonstration of the organism. Since the development of AIDS, laboratories have become considerably more proficient in detecting the organism in body tissue or fluids. Selective cell wall stains such as methenamine silver or its simpler variants (cresyl echt violet, toluidine blue 0, Gram-Weigert) have been widely used because they are easy to perform and to interpret (Fig. 111-1*A*). Limiting factors are the lack of information provided about internal cyst contents and the possible confusion of *P. carinii* with fungi in cases of light infection. Giemsa and its congener stains (Diff Quik, polychrome methylene blue) can be performed rapidly and provide information about the developmental stages of *P. carinii* (Fig. 111-1*B*); since these reagents also stain host cells, they require a greater degree of expertise for proper interpretation. Diagnosis of pneumocystosis by immunofluorescence correlates well with the use of histological stains, but attempts to detect soluble antigens of the organism have been unrewarding. Special light-microscopic techniques such as phase or Nomarski interference contrast microscopy provide excellent views of *P. carinii* in fresh body fluid specimens [*15*]; there is increasing interest in applying these techniques to studying the effects of treatment on organism viability and life cycle stages.

Collection of adequate specimens has been essential to the histological diagnosis of pneumocystosis. Traditionally, *P. carinii* has been found only rarely in sputum or tracheal aspirates, and thus an invasive procedure has been necessary to establish the diagnosis. However, among AIDS patients examination of sputum that has been induced by inhalation of a saline mist has revealed the presence of the organism in a high frequency of patients at selected institutions [16]. If this technique can gain widespread use, it will offer considerable benefits in terms of patient safety, comfort, and cost. The most widely used diagnostic procedure today is fiber-optic bronchoscopy with bronchoalveolar lavage or transbronchial biopsy [17]. This technique is well-tolerated and has a high diagnostic yield both in AIDS and non-AIDS patients. Open lung biopsy, the most invasive procedure, is performed less often than in the past; nevertheless, this technique remains a useful procedure because it can provide diagnosis when other approaches have failed.

The diagnosis of pneumocystosis should be pursued aggressively and early in the patient's course in order to limit the risk of complications of the procedures and to facilitate the initiation of specific antimicrobial therapy. This requires close cooperation with the patient's primary care physician, consulting services, and hospital laboratory. A high index of suspicion should be maintained for other opportunistic pathogens which frequently coexist with *P. carinii*.

Course and prognosis

P. carinii infection in the normal host is a subclinical illness requiring no therapy. The natural history of untreated pneumocystosis in the compromised host is usually one of progressive hypoxemia, respiratory insufficiency, and death. Prognosis may be related to such factors as the extent of *P. carinii* involvement in the lung, the status of the host's underlying disease and nutrition, prior pulmonary damage, leukocyte or lymphocyte count, and the presence of other opportunistic infections [9,18]. The outlook is especially poor if mechanical ventilation is required. Spread of *P. carinii* beyond the lungs, probably by hematogenous or lymphatic routes, is uncommon but has been reported in patients with AIDS and other compromised hosts. Follow-up studies of patients who have recovered from pneumocystosis have demonstrated residual pulmonary function abnormalities in adults but not in children.

TREATMENT

The principal drugs used in the therapy of pneumocystosis have been trimethoprim-sulfamethoxazole (TMP-SMX) and pentamidine isethionate. These agents are equally effective in persons with AIDS and other immunosuppressed patients, with an overall success rate of about 75 percent. Even greater efficacy can be achieved in mild forms of the disease when treatment is instituted early [19]. TMP-SMX and pentamidine are administered for 14 days in non-AIDS patients. It takes on average about 4 days of therapy to observe a clinical response, but this is somewhat variable among individuals; if there is no improvement with one agent after 5 to 6 days, it is prudent to consider switching to the other drug. Combination therapy of TMP-SMX and pentamidine does not improve efficacy but

does increase the risk of adverse reactions. AIDS patients with pneumocystosis respond more slowly to therapy and have a high rate of recurrence; thus, it has become customary to treat these persons for 21 days and to wait at least 7 days before declaring therapeutic failure.

TMP-SMX is administered orally or intravenously in a dose of 20 mg/(kg·day) TMP and 100 mg/(kg·day) SMX in four divided doses, but this regimen should be adjusted based on serum concentrations of the drug. Optimal levels of TMP are 3 to 5 µg/mL in children and ≥5 µg/mL in adults and of SMX are 100 to 150 µg/mL. TMP-SMX is well-tolerated by non-AIDS patients, with side effects usually limited to skin rash or gastrointestinal complaints. In contrast, over half the AIDS patients experience adverse reactions to TMP-SMX, including rash, fever, thrombocytopenia, leukopenia, and abnormalities in liver function [10]. These effects usually begin during the second week of treatment, and frequently are of such severity that the drug has to be withdrawn. These reactions, which are mainly due to the sulfonamide component, probably represent a form of drug hypersensitivity, but the mechanism is poorly understood. Rechallenge with TMP-SMX or substitution of another sulfonamide or sulfone have led to widely varying results; thus, because of the risk of serious adverse reactions, considerable caution is needed if such actions are contemplated.

Pentamidine is administered parenterally in a single dose of 4 mg/(kg·day). The intravenous route has caused no more side effects than the intramuscular route as long as the drug is diluted in 50 to 250 mL of a 5% dextrose solution and infused over a period of at least 1 h. Pentamidine is a toxic drug. Adverse reactions occur in over half of the non-AIDS or AIDS patients and can be severe [20]. Side effects include hypotension, cardiac arrhythmias, hypoglycemia, hyperglycemia, azotemia, neutropenia, abnormal liver function tests, hypocalcemia, and reactions at intramuscular injection sites. Pharmacokinetic studies have suggested that pentamidine is bound to host tissues and released slowly over time; serum concentrations of the drug are not materially altered by impaired renal function, but there may be accumulation of pentamidine with repeated dosing [21].

At the present time TMP-SMX is the preferred agent in the treatment of pneumocystosis in non-AIDS patients, but there is no clear-cut drug of choice in AIDS patients. Considerable interest has arisen in developing new forms of *P. carinii* therapy, but these agents have not yet been studied in controlled clinical trials and must be considered investigational. Trimetrexate, a lipid-soluble derivative of methotrexate and potent inhibitor of dihydrofolate reductase, has shown promising results in the treatment of pneumocystosis when used alone or in combination with a sulfonamide [22]. Dapsone has shown good anti-*P. carinii* activity and may be better tolerated than sulfonamides by AIDS patients. The administration of pentamidine via aerosol, which results in higher drug levels in the lung with less systemic absorption, has shown promising results in the treatment of mild cases of pneumocystosis [23]. α-Difluoromethylornithine (DFMO), an inhibitor of polyamine biosynthesis, has been successful in the treatment of *P. carinii* pneumonia in patients who failed with or became intolerant to TMP-SMX or pentamidine. Other compounds that have shown promising anti-*P. carinii* activity in experimental systems include diamidines (e.g., diminazene) and related cationic anti-trypanosomal drugs; 9-deazainosine, a purine nucleoside; and the combination of clindamycin and primaquine.

General supportive measures constitute an important part of *P. carinii* therapy. Careful attention should be given to maintaining adequate nutrition, oxygenation, and fluid and electrolyte balance. Controversies have arisen over the use of corticosteroids because of the feeling among some observers that the host inflammatory response may be playing a role in the clinical manifestations of pneumocystosis. Among patients receiving corticosteroids or other immunosuppressive drugs for the treatment of malignancies or other diseases, it seems prudent to lower the dose of these agents to the lowest level permitted by the underlying disorder. Recent studies have suggested that corticosteroids may be helpful as adjunctive therapy of *P. carinii* pneumonia in AIDS patients; however, because of the well-known serious side effects of these drugs, this author feels they should not be used until their benefits can be clearly shown in controlled trials.

POPULATION

Epidemiology

Seroepidemiological studies using the indirect fluorescent antibody technique or enzyme immunoassay have shown that most healthy people develop antibodies to *P. carinii* by an early age [24]. Antigens in these assays have consisted of whole organisms or crude preparations, and thus it has not been possible to distinguish persons with active pneumocystosis from healthy controls. Perhaps with improvement in knowledge of specific *P. carinii* antigens serology will become more valuable as an epidemiological or diagnostic tool.

The communicability of *P. carinii* has been clearly demonstrated under experimental conditions, and the airborne route appears to be the major mode of transmission [25]. Outbreaks of pneumocystosis have been reported in orphanages and cancer hospitals, and cases of the disease have been noted in patients who have had prolonged contact with each other. The incubation period has been estimated to be 4 to 8 weeks.

Environmental factors

P. carinii has worldwide distribution, but there are no data available concerning intermediate versus definitive hosts, vectors, or environmental sources of the organism.

Prevention and control

Recovery from pneumocystosis is not accompanied by the development of an acquired immunity, and hence the host remains at risk of recurrences of the disease as long as the immunosuppressive conditions persist. It is unclear whether these recurrent episodes of *P. carinii* pneumonia are due to relapse or reinfection. AIDS patients have the highest rate of recurrence (about 50 percent at 1 year of follow-up), probably reflecting their higher rate of organism burden or degree of immunological impairment. *P. carinii* can be found frequently on repeat bronchoscopy in AIDS patients following successful therapy, but the viability and clinical significance of these organisms are unknown. Controlled trials have shown that TMP-SMX in a dose of 5 mg/(kg·day) TMP and 25 mg/(kg·day) SMX administered daily or three times a week can prevent the development of pneumocystosis in immunosuppressed patients [26]. The drug is not lethal for *P. carinii*, and hence is effective in chemoprophylaxis for only as long as it is being given. Chronic TMP-SMX administration, though usually well-tolerated, requires careful medical follow-up, because serious adverse reactions can occur in transplant recipients or persons with impaired renal function who are taking immunosuppressive drugs.

Chemoprophylaxis with TMP-SMX is effective in AIDS patients, but the problem of side effects has significantly limited its use. Regimens involving other antifol compounds and aerosolized pentamidine also appear to be effective and are currently undergoing clinical evaluation.

Environmental measures for the prevention of pneumocystosis have not yet been developed. It seems reasonable within the hospital setting to place *P. carinii* patients in respiratory isolation or to separate them from direct contact with other immunocompromised hosts.

REFERENCES

1 Edman JC, Kovacs JA, Masur H, et al: Ribosomal sequence shows *Pneumocystis carinii* to be a member of the fungi. Nature 334:519–522, 1988

2 Stringer SL, Stringer JR, Blase MA, et al: *Pneumocystis carinii*: Sequence from ribosomal RNA implies a close relationship with fungi. Exp Parasitol 68:450–461. 1989

3 Cushion MT, Ruffolo JM, Walzer PD: Characterization of the developmental stages of *Pneumocystis* by light microscopic techniques. Lab Invest 58:324–331, 1988

4 Matsumoto Y, Yoshida Y: Sporogony in *Pneumocystis carinii*: Synaptonemal complexes and meiotic nuclear divisions observed in precysts. J Protozool 31:420–428, 1984

5 Pesanti EL: Phospholipid profile of *Pneumocystis carinii* and its interacting with alveolar type II epithelial cells. Infect Immunol 55:736–741, 1987

6 Cushion MT, Ruffolo JJ, Linke MJ, et al: *Pneumocystis carinii*: Growth variables and estimates in the A549 and WI-38 VA 13 human cell lines. Exp Parasitol 60:43–54, 1985

7 Walzer PD: Experimental models for *Pneumocystis carinii* infection, in Young LS (ed): Pneumocystis carinii *Pneumonia*. New York, Dekker, 1984, pp 7–75

8 Walzer PD, Linke MJ: A comparison of the antigenic characteristics of rat and human *Pneumocystis carinii* by immunoblotting. J Immunol 138:2257–2265, 1987

9 Walzer PD, Perl DP, Krogstad DJ, et al: *Pneumocystis carinii* pneumonia in the United States: Epidemiologic, clinical and diagnostic features. Ann Intern Med 80:83–93, 1974

10 Mills J: *Pneumocystis carinii* and *Toxoplasma gondii* infections in patients with AIDS. Rev Infect Dis 8:1001–1011, 1986

11 Hagler DW, Deepe GS, Pogue CL, et al: Blastogenic responses to *Pneumocystis carinii* among patients with human immunodeficiency virus (HIV) infection. Clin Exper Immunol 74:7–13, 1988

12 Masur H, Jones TC: The interaction in vitro of *Pneumocystis carinii* with macrophages and L cells. J Exp Med 147:157–170, 1978

13 Walzer PD; Attachment of microorganisms to host cells: Relevance of *Pneumocystis carinii*. Lab Invest 54:589–592, 1986

14 Kovacs JA, Hiemenz JW, Macher AM et al: *Pneumocystis carinii* pneumonia: A comparison between patients with the acquired immunodeficiency syndrome and patients with other immunodeficiencies. Ann Intern Med 100:663–671, 1984

15 Ruffolo JJ, Cushion MT, Walzer PD: Microscopic techniques for studying *Pneumocystis carinii* in fresh specimens. J Clin Microbiol 23:17–21, 1986

16 Kovacs JA, Ng VL, Masur H, et al: Diagnosis of *Pneumocystis carinii* pneumonia: Improved detection in sputum with use of monoclonal antibodies. N Engl J Med 318:589–593, 1988

17 Murray JF, Garay SM, Hopewell PC, et al: Pulmonary complications of the acquired immunodeficiency syndrome: An update. Am Rev Resp Dis 135:504–509, 1987

18 Brenner M, Ognibene FP, Lack E, et al: Prognostic factors and life expectancy of patients with acquired immunodeficiency syndrome and *Pneumocystis carinii* pneumonia. Am Rev Resp Dis 136:1199–1206, 1987

19 Wharton JM, Coleman DL, Wofsy CB, et al: Trimethoprim-sulfamethoxazole or pentamidine for *Pneumocystis carinii* pneumonia in the acquired immunodeficiency syndrome. Ann Intern Med 105:37–44, 1986

20 Pearson RD, Hewlett EL: Pentamidine for the treatment of *Pneumocystis carinii* pneumonia and other protozoal diseases. Ann Intern Med 103:782–786, 1985

21 Conte Jr JE, Upton RA, Lin ET: Pentamidine pharmacokinetics in patients with AIDS with impaired renal function. J Infect Dis 156:885–890, 1987

22 Allegra CJ, Chabner BA, Tuazon CU, et al: Trimetrexate for the treatment of *Pneumocystis carinii* pneumonia in patients with the acquired immunodeficiency syndrome. N Engl J Med 317:978–985, 1987

23 Montgomery AB, Debs RJ, Luce JM, et al: Aerosolised pentamidine as sole therapy for *Pneumocystis carinii* pneumonia in patients with acquired immunodeficiency syndrome. Lancet 29:480–483, 1987

24 Meuwissen JHE, Tauber I, Leeuwenberg ADEM, et al: Parasitologic and serologic observations of infection with *Pneumocystis* in humans. J Infect Dis 136:43–49, 1977

25 Hughes WT: Natural mode of acquisition for de novo infection with *Pneumocystis carinii*. J Infect Dis 145:842–848, 1982

26 Hughes WT, Rivera GK, Schell MJ, et al: Successful intermittent chemoprophylaxis for *Pneumocystis carinii* pneumonitis. N Engl J Med 316:1627–1632, 1987

CHAPTER 112 / *Rhinosporidiosis* · L. N. Mohapatra

Rhinosporidiosis is a chronic infection caused by *Rhinosporidium seeberi* which most commonly involves the nasal mucosa and produces a polypoid growth. The disease may also affect the conjunctiva, the skin, and other parts of the body [1].

EPIDEMIOLOGY

The majority of reported cases are from India and Sri Lanka. Occasional cases are reported from other countries of the world except Australia and New Zealand. The first two cases were recorded by Malbran in 1892 and by Guillermo Seeber in 1900, from Argentina. O'Kinealy reported the first case from India in 1903. In the subsequent years cases were reported from Africa, Cuba, England and Scotland, Indonesia, Iran, Italy, Malaysia, Mexico, the Philippines, Russia, South America (Argentina, Bolivia, Brazil, Ecuador, Paraguay), Thailand, Turkey, the United States, and Vietnam [2]. The infection also occurs in domestic animals, i.e., horse, cattle, buffalo, mule, and dog [3].

The disease is seen most frequently in the younger age group (20 to 30 years old) but may occur at any age. The largest number of reported cases from India and Sri Lanka is in the age group 15 to 39 years [2]. Males are infected more often than females (3:1). There is no difference in the susceptibility of different races or communities to this infection, but it is seen more often in persons of the working class who are exposed to water in tanks and pools [4]. The infection is exogenous in origin, and the etiological agent is suspected to be present in stagnant water or water vegetations [5]. The disease is not contagious and does not spread from person to person.

PARASITE

The organism is seen in the infected tissue in abundance. The sporangia vary in size and maturity: the small young ones with a well-defined wall are empty-looking. In a fully matured sporangium measuring up to 250 to 300 μm there are 15,000 to 20,000 young spores. These spores vary in size; the matured ones, measuring 8 to 9 μm in diameter, contain a number of highly refringent granules. The sporangium wall and spore wall are rich in mucopolysaccharides. The spores possess periodic acid–Schiff (PAS) reactivity. Histochemical reactions indicate the presence of protein in the spores [6]. The fungus has not been cultured in vitro, nor has the infection been transmitted to animals in vivo [7]. A recent report about cultivation in vitro and interaction with epithelial cells states that the original culture was maintained for 63 days with growth of the organism and induction of polyplike proliferation of the cells [8].

PATIENT "HOST"

CLINICAL FEATURES

The commonest site of rhinosporidiosis in humans is the nose. The nose is affected in 70 percent of cases [2], and the polypoid growth is confined most frequently to the septum, inferior turbinate, or the floor of the nose. Multiple lesions are not rare. Usually only one nostril is affected, but bilateral infection is occasionally seen. The patient has a sessile or pedunculated growth which is vascular, friable, and sometimes ulcerated (Fig. 112-1). Infections of the nasopharynx, epiglottis, uvula, palate, tonsils, larynx, and trachea are reported [9,10].

The eye lesions are mostly confined to the palpebral conjunctiva. Lesions in the conjunctiva are more conspicuous and produce lacrimation and photophobia. The lesion is usually small, and because of its location medical advice is sought

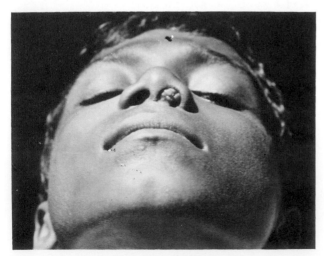

Figure 112-1. Rhinosporidiosis. A polypoid growth protrudes from the left nostril. (*Courtesy of S. Subramanian and V. Chitravel, Madras.*)

early [11]. Infection of the lacrimal sac presents as a swelling which may suppurate, and the skin over it is ulcerated. Skin lesions are also seen occasionally [12].

Lesions involving rare sites such as the oral cavity, the ear, the urethra, and the bronchus have been recorded [13–15]. The infection remains strictly localized to the site for long periods. Unless surgically removed, the growth increases in size and may ulcerate with secondary bacterial infection.

DIAGNOSIS

Examination of the surface of the polypoid growth shows small white specks which contain sporangia of varying size. The mucoid exudate on the surface of the lesion may show the presence of spores discharged from the sporangia. Examination of the stained (hematoxylin and eosin) section of the biopsy taken from the lesion readily reveals the histological diagnosis. The stroma is dense with a chronic inflammatory reaction having neutrophils, plasma cells, and lymphocytes, and occasional giant cells of the foreign body type. The epithelium (squamous or columnar) covering the polypoid growth shows considerable hyperplasia. The sporangia of varying size and age are quite conspicuous as well-circumscribed globular structures in the stroma.

No immunological test is designed for diagnosis of a case.

TREATMENT

Several chemotherapeutic agents and antibiotics (antifungal) have been tried without success. Surgical removal of the lesion is usually curative. In advanced cases extensive surgical excision may be supplemented by cauterization to prevent recurrence [16].

REFERENCES

1 Rippon JW: The pathogenic fungi and the pathogenic actinomycetes, in *Medical Mycology*. 2d ed. Philadelphia, Saunders, 1982, pp 325–334

2 Karunaratne WAE: *Rhinosporidiosis in Man*. University of London, Athlone Press, 1964, p 146

3 Ramachandra Rao PV, Jain SN: Rhinosporidiosis in animals. Indian J Otolaryngol 23:106–109, 1971

4 Jain SN: Aetiology and incidence of rhinosporidiosis. Indian J Otolaryngol 19:1–21, 1967

5 Cherian PV, Satyanarayana C: Rhinosporidiosis. Indian J Otolaryngol 1:15–19, 1949

6 Narayana Rao S: *Rhinosporidium seeberi*—a histochemical study. Indian J Exp Biol 4:10–14, 1966

7 Reddy DG, Lakshminarayana CS: Investigation into transmission, growth, and serology in rhinosporidiosis. Indian J Med Res 50:363–370, 1962

8 Levy MG, Meuten DJ, Breitschwerdt EB: Cultivation of *Rhinosporidium seeberi* in vitro: Interaction with epithelial cells. Science 234:474–476, 1987

9 Gupta OP: Unusual extranasal manifestations of rhinosporidiosis. Laryngoscope (St. Louis) 76:1842, 1966

10 Satyanarayana C: Rhinosporidiosis with a record of 255 cases. Acta Otolaryngol 51:348–366, 1960

11 Sood NN, Narayana Rao S: Rhinosporidium granuloma of the conjunctiva, Br J Ophthalmol 51:61–64, 1967

12 Acharya PV, Gupta RL, Darbari BS: Cutaneous rhinosporidiosis. Indian J Vener 39:22–25, 1973

13 Dhayagude RG: Unusual rhinosporidiosis infection in man. Indian Med Gaz 76:513–515, 1941

14 Koshal KD, Sinha SC, Tiwari RR, et al: Rhinosporidiosis of urethra. Indian J Surg 43:599–601, 1981

15 Thomas T, Gopinath N, Betts RH: Rhinosporidiosis of the bronchus. Br J Surg 44:316–319, 1956

16 Kameswaran S: Surgery in rhinosporidiosis, experience with 293 cases. Int Surg 46:602–605, 1966

CHAPTER 113 / *Ringworm and Other Superficial Mycoses* · Robert A. Salata

Ringworm, a mycotic infection of keratinized tissue, is caused by a group of filamentous fungi collectively known as *dermatophytes*. These organisms occupy a unique ecological niche through their ability to degrade and subsist in the keratinized and cornified tissues of the skin, hair, and nails. These fungi are virtually always found in the avascular, nonliving elements of the epidermis and its appendages, where they grow, causing the superficial infections called *ringworm*. These infections have been described since antiquity, and the designation *ringworm* is from Greek and Latin roots. The nature of the infection in a particular individual is a function of the dermatophyte, the tissue affected, the anatomical location, and the immunological response of the host.

The dermatophytes are commonly identified by assignment to the three genera of the Fungi Imperfecti: *Epidermophyton*, *Trichophyton*, and *Microsporum*. However, some of these imperfect organisms can be grown in the perfect state (i.e., with sexual spores), and they are then classified according to two genera, *Nannizzia* and *Arthroderma* in the class Ascomycetes (Table 113-1). Although there are 37 species of dermatophytes, most of these are rarely implicated in disease, and a mere seven species account for almost 95 percent of the clinical infections in the United States [1].

The categorization of dermatophytes by their primary reservoir predicts the epidemiology and host response. Anthropophilic dermatophytes are primarily acquired from humans and usually do not induce marked inflammation in infected individuals (Table 113-1). Zoophilic dermatophytes are acquired predominantly from animals and cause marked inflammatory reactions in infected humans. Soil is the predominant reservoir for geophilic dermatophytes which cause an inflammatory response in infected hosts.

This is a revision of the chapter by Richard S. Salzman and Henry E. Jones in the first edition of this book.

PARASITE

ECOLOGY

The dermatophytes are found throughout the world. Attempts to delineate their distribution may be made by assessing the organisms responsible for clinical infections, by soil-baiting

Table 113-1. Nomenclature of dermatophytes

Imperfect name	Perfect state
Microsporum audouini*	
Microsporum canis†	
Microsporum distortum†	
Microsporum ferrugineum*	
Microsporum fulvum‡	*Nannizzia fulva*
Microsporum gypseum‡	*Nannizzia gypsea*
	Nannizzia incurvata
	Nannizzia obtusa
Microsporum nanum†	
Trichophyton concentricum*	
Trichophyton equinum†	
Trichophyton gourvillii*	
Trichophyton megninii*	
Trichophyton mentagrophytes	
var. *interdigitale**	*Arthroderma benhamiae*
var. *mentagrophytes*†	*Arthroderma benhamiae*
Trichophyton rubrum*	
Trichophyton schoenleinii*	
Trichophyton simii†	*Arthroderma simii*
Trichophyton soudanense*	
Trichophyton tonsurans*	
Trichophyton verrucosum†	
Trichophyton violaceum*	
Trichophyton yaoundei*	
Epidermophyton floccosum*	

*Anthropophilic.
†Zoophilic.
‡Geophilic.

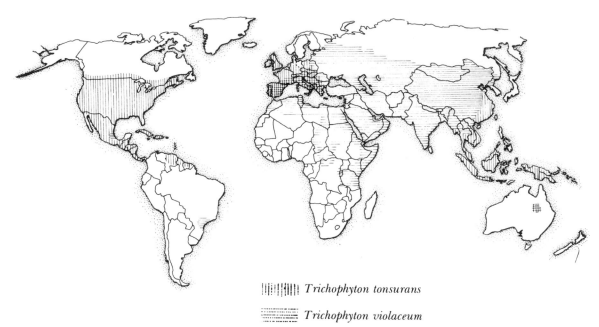

|‖|‖|‖|‖|‖| *Trichophyton tonsurans*

⸭⸭⸭⸭⸭⸭   *Trichophyton violaceum*

Figure 113-1. Distribution of *Trichophyton tonsurans* and *Trichophyton violaceum*. (*From Rippon JW: Medical Mycology: The Pathogenic Fungi and the Pathogenic Actinomycetes. Philadelphia, Saunders, 1974. Used with permission.*)

techniques, or by person-to-person epidemiological surveys. In practice, statements about distribution are generally based on surveys of patients who seek medical aid, which may be at variance with the true prevalence of the organism. It seems, however, that some dermatophytes are relatively restricted geographically, while others are found worldwide [2] (Fig. 113-1).

BIOCHEMISTRY

The dermatophytes elaborate a number of enzymes which presumably enable them to parasitize the seemingly inhospitable environment of cornified skin, hair, and nails. Elastase [3], collagenase [4], keratinase [5], and other proteases degrade tissue and supply the nutritional requirements for their growth. Dermatophyte exocellular protease production in vitro can be significantly affected by glucose and metal ions, emphasizing the need for caution in evaluating in vitro enzyme determinations [6].

Despite this array of enzymes which facilitate tissue invasion, the dermatophytes are almost always limited to the non-living keratinized tissue; hence, their historical designation as keratinophilic. One of the major barriers to dermatophyte invasion of the living tissue is probably unsaturated transferrin [7].

CULTURE

Dermatophytes are readily grown in vitro because of their minimal nutritional requirements. The initial step in culturing these fungi is collection of an adequate sample. With scalp involve-

ment, an attempt should be made to pluck a few infected hairs which can be implanted directly into the agar. If the hairs are broken at the scalp level and unobtainable, the scalp can be scraped with a scalpel blade and the scrapings implanted into the medium. Glabrous skin involvement should be scraped at the advancing edge. When the nails are infected, the most suitable material for culture is the subungual hyperkeratotic debris at the base of the nail plate.

Once the specimens have been inoculated, most dermatophytes will, within 10 to 25 days, show good evidence of growth at 30 to 35°C or at room temperature (25°C). Exceptions are *Trichophyton verrucosum* and rare strains of *Trichophyton tonsurans,* which grow better at 37°C. For convenience, cultures are usually incubated at room temperature.

The standard medium for mycological culture is Sabouraud's agar. The colonial morphology of the dermatophytes varies greatly depending on the media employed, and since traditional identification is based on their growth in Sabouraud's agar, this medium has retained its status as the standard agar. It is a mixture of beef extract (neopeptone) and dextrose. There are different formulas for Sabouraud's agar, which can affect morphology, making it important to know exactly what medium is being used.

Sabouraud's agar tends to promote mycelial growth and suppress sporulation, and, for this reason, other media are sometimes employed that are more conducive to spore formation and, hence, microscopic identification. These so-called deficient media, such as cornmeal agar and potato dextrose agar, are made from plant extracts. The dermatophyte test medium (DTM) is a relatively recent attempt to simplify dermatophyte culturing [8]. It contains antibacterials and cycloheximide, plus phenol red as a pH indicator. During the first 10 to 14 days of dermatophyte growth, the fungi release more alkaline metabolites into the medium than most nondermatophytic fungi, thus causing an increase in pH and a color change to red. This is presumptive of a dermatophyte. Subculturing on an identification agar must then be done because morphology is usually not characteristic on DTM.

Some research laboratories perform susceptibility testing of these organisms to antimycotic agents in vitro [9]. However, no standard methods are available, and clinical indications for performing the tests are unclear with the imidazoles and triazoles. Correlation between susceptibility in vitro and clinical results have been poor with many fungi, although experience with dermatophytes is limited.

ANIMAL MODELS

Although dermatophyte infections in animals are commonplace and have been experimentally induced for decades, their relevance to understanding this disease in humans is limited. There is not an adequate animal model for chronic dermatophytosis.

Guinea pigs are probably the most frequently used experimental model of acute dermatophyte infection. It is interesting that other rodents, such as mice, rats, and hamsters, are unsuitable because they differ from humans in being susceptible to these organisms only during a very limited phase of the hair cycle [10]. It has been well documented that the unsensitized guinea pig develops an acute inflammatory infection which can be divided into several phases [11]:

1. Incubation phase, 4 to 6 days
2. Spreading phase, 7 to 10 days
3. An inflammatory phase or climax reached on day 12 to 15
4. A healing or clearing phase, which takes an additional 30 to 35 days

If the animal is reinfected, the entire process is accelerated such that the incubation and spreading phases are shorter, the climax is reached at an earlier time, and complete clearing occurs at least 1 to 2 weeks sooner.

Such experimental infections have been shown to be accompanied by changes in cell-mediated immunity (CMI) [12]. As unsensitized animals undergo a primary infection, intradermal skin tests (to dermatophyte antigen) become positive at days 7 to 10 and remain positive for months. In vitro studies to determine the macrophage and lymphocyte responses to the dermatophyte infection were also performed [12]. Using specific dermatophyte antigens, it was found that both macrophage migration inhibition and lymphocyte transformation were significantly increased in the previously infected guinea pigs, revealing that systemic sensitization had occurred and that immunocompetent cells were reacting to the antigens which had yielded positive skin test results.

Table 113-2. Acute and chronic dermatophytosis

Parameter	Acute	Chronic
Signs and symptoms	Erythema, vesicles, pustules, exudation, tenderness, pruritus	Erythema, scaling, hyperkeratosis, pruritus
Extent of process	Usually limited to discrete focus on skin	May be extensive
Immunological response to trichophytin	CMI	Immediate, CMI, both, neither
Depth of fungal penetration	Stratum corneum	Stratum corneum
Histology	Few fungi, acute dermatitis	Many fungi, chronic dermatitis
Response to therapy	Excellent	Poor, relapsing

It thus seems that the abbreviated course of secondary and subsequent dermatophyte infections is associated with the accelerated and intense cutaneous inflammation produced by fungal-antigen-activated CMI mechanisms. This corresponds nicely to what we know about infections in humans and does provide a model for the study of other immune mechanisms, prophylaxis, and certain therapeutic agents.

However, the shortcomings of the guinea pig model are obvious when the bivalent nature of dermatophytosis in humans is considered. It is, of course, a gross oversimplification, but dermatophytosis in humans has two fundamental natural forms: an acute inflammatory type and a chronic noninflammatory type (Table 113-2). It is likely that the chronic, noninflammatory type of infection produces the most prevalent and most significant morbidity in humans, and the guinea pig only provides a model for acute inflammatory infection that humans expediently deal with naturally [13]. At this time, a suitable model for the chronic, noninflammatory type of infection has not been described.

PATIENT

LOCAL FACTORS

The human integument is an excellent barrier against mycotic intruders; however, various factors can alter one's susceptibility to infection. The primary local factors involved seem to be moisture and maceration, which may be promoted by occluding skin surfaces or may be a function of clothing, climate, and lifestyle. The propensity of dermatophytes to invade the toe web spaces and the inguinal region, two areas of the body particularly likely to be occluded and moist, is well known.

Experimental work in humans has demonstrated that soaking the feet in fungal solutions does not lead to infection if the feet are allowed to dry [14]. It is relatively easy, however, to produce at least transient infection if occlusion is employed for a few days [15,16]. This may be due to the increased hydration of the stratum corneum that results and is felt by some to be extremely important in microbial proliferation [17]. As English [18] has pointed out, tinea pedis is practically unknown among the unshod people of the tropics. Also, Allen and Taplin [19] found that occlusion and maceration provided by prolonged exposure to wet clothing among soldiers in the tropics led to a high prevalence of tinea corporis. Allen and King [20] hypothesized that the significant effect of occlusion is to raise the local CO_2 tension.

Abrasion of the skin has also been experimentally shown to be an important factor. Kligman [21] was able to produce tinea capitis by applying infected hairs to the scalp and rubbing them, whereas merely applying them led to no infection. This type of superficial breakdown of the skin is common in the intertriginous areas due to the close apposition of the skin surfaces. This apparently aids the dermatophytes by allowing the organisms to bypass the intact, relatively dry exterior surface of the stratum corneum and lodge in the overly hydrated layers of the stratum corneum underneath.

IMMUNE RESPONSE

Intradermal skin testing with a commercially available extract called trichophytin frequently demonstrates immediate hypersensitivity in chronic infections and delayed-type hypersensitivity (DTH) in acute, self-limited disease. Prior infection apparently increases host resistance to repeated infection. Experimental work has shown that an increased inoculum of spores is necessary to incite infection in an experienced immune host [22]. Thus, resistance is relative, not absolute.

Antigens

It has been well demonstrated that extensive cross-reactivity among antigens exists among the species and genera of dermatophytes [23]. Even "purified" antigen from E. floccosum will elicit a positive skin test in animals sensitized to T. mentagrophytes [24]. Antigens from the different genera cross-react with host antibodies to such an extent that determination of the infecting organism by this method is virtually impossible [25]. This limits the clinical use of trichophytin skin testing since positive tests only indicate past or present infection and do not identify the infecting species.

Numerous investigators, since Bloch in 1925 [26], have attempted to separate and characterize the constituents of these antigens. This literature is extensively reviewed by Grappel et al. [27]. Purification of the antigen has been exceedingly difficult. Antigens produced from the same strain of a given dermatophyte can vary in molecular weight and structure depending on substrate, surface versus suspension cultures, oxygen tension [28], and age of culture [29]; however, immunological activity remains essentially the same. It appears from fluorescent antibody staining that immunogens are often located near the growing hyphal tips and in young mycelia [29].

Ito demonstrated 22 separate antigenic fractions from T. mentagrophytes [30]. These had distinctive chemical com-positions and varying degrees of antigenicity, and most were peptide-containing polysaccharides. The other constituents, such as sugar-containing peptides, simple peptides, and simple polysaccharides, were much less active.

It has more recently been shown by Christiansen and Svejgaard [31] that the number of antigens in four common species varied from 25 to 35, and they stressed that this is a minimum number. They were able to find only two common antigens shared by T. rubrum, T. mentagrophytes, Microsporum canis, and E. floccosum.

Humoral immune response

Animal and human hosts have a weak antibody response to dermatophyte infection. Skin testing with trichophytin may lead to an immediate (15-min) anaphylactic-type hypersensitivity response. This is mediated by IgE and is exceptionally prevalent in T. rubrum infections [28]. It seems to be found most often in patients with chronic infections [32] and may play a role in preventing the host's rejection of the organism.

Antibodies of the IgG and IgM classes may also be produced in response to dermatophytes. Grappel et al. [33] showed circulating antibodies in patients with tinea capitis and tinea corporis. Both inflammatory and noninflammatory tinea capitis were associated with antibodies. Svejgaard and Christiansen [34] found circulating antibodies in all four patients with scalp kerions (all zoophilic infections), in 62 percent of patients with acute tinea pedis complicated by dermatophytids of the hands, in 16 percent of patients with chronic infections (T. rubrum), and in only 2.8 percent of patients with acute, uncomplicated dermatophytosis. They also reported that the antibodies persisted in chronic infection and disappeared by 3 months in acute disease. All the patients had only one specific antibody except those with chronic infections (who had two to four), suggesting antibodies to more than one of the antigens present. This would be consistent with an increased antigenic stimulus over a longer period of time. However, Kaaman [25] found no difference between total antidermatophyte antibody levels in chronic and acute infections, although he did report that T. rubrum seemed to elicit the greatest antibody response.

Cellular immune response

It has been demonstrated in human [15] and experimental infections [35] that DTH to trichophytin develops at approximately the time that the clinical ringworm infection becomes erythematous and inflamed, just a few days before maximal size is attained and resolution begins. As an in vitro correlate, lymphocyte transformation tests to dermatophyte antigens have been shown to accompany this DTH in both humans [36] and guinea pigs [35]. Thus, as an acute dermatophyte infection is nearing its zenith, CMI is developing, as shown by both in vivo and in vitro determinations.

An important finding in this regard is the difference in immunological responses between individuals with acute and chronic dermatophytosis. In contrast to the development of CMI and subsequent resolution in acute infections, it has been shown that patients with chronic infections less frequently develop trichophytin DTH skin test positivity [32,37–39]. Patients with chronic infections and no DTH reactions also have decreased lymphocyte responses to trichophytin in vitro [36,40]. The deficits are usually specific, as skin testing to PPD [41], Candida [36], and a battery of allergens [41] were not affected. However, one report [40] of patients with dermatophytoses of the deeper tissues (dermis, lymph nodes) indicated a more severe impairment of CMI. These patients had a marked reduction in T cells and depressed responses (in vitro and in vivo) to the whole range of antigenic stimuli.

Diseases and conditions that depress CMI have been associated with dermatophytosis. These include immunodeficiency diseases, including the acquired immunodeficiency syndrome (AIDS), Cushing's syndrome, iatrogenic immunosuppression, and lymphoma [29,42–45].

Other factors

It has been suggested that genetics may play a role in immunity, as household surveys have revealed an increased prevalence among family members but not among conjugal partners [46]. The strong association of chronic dermatophytosis and atopy [47] could be based on genetic predisposition. There is also an interesting report concerning tinea imbricata in New Guinea, suggesting an autosomal recessive inheritance pattern [48]. However, studies of HLA haplotypes among infected patients have been unrevealing [49].

It is curious that except for tinea capitis dermatophytosis occurs most commonly when the dominant sexual hormones are androgenic [28]. Men rarely develop tinea pedis or cruris before puberty, and women have a lower prevalence until they are postmenopausal. An explanation for this association is lacking.

PATHOLOGY

The histological picture of dermatophytosis is extremely variable, depending on the site of involvement and the intensity of the inflammatory response. Demonstration of the fungal organisms is enhanced with either the PAS (periodic acid-Schiff) reaction, which stains the polysaccharide-rich fungal walls red, or the methenamine silver nitrate method, which stains them black. The fungi may be present as either hyphae or arthrospores. They are generally located exclusively in the stratum corneum, the follicle walls, and in and around the hair shafts; although when a severe inflammatory reaction exists around a ruptured follicle, they may be found within the intense inflammatory infiltrate in the dermis [50].

The variability of the pathology has been extensively detailed by Graham and Barroso-Tobila [51]. The noninflammatory chronic infections of glabrous skin show hyperkeratosis, parakeratosis, mild acanthosis, and a predominantly perivascular lymphohistiocytic infiltrate. Acute, inflammatory infections have extensive spongiosis and vesiculation with the epidermis. When the follicles become involved, either in tinea capitis, tinea barbae, or tinea corporis, a folliculitis of varying intensity ensues. The infiltrate may be lymphohistiocytic and perifollicular, but in inflammatory disease, especially kerion celsi, polymorphonuclear leukocytes and giant cells are also present in and around the disrupted follicles. The giant cell granulomatous response may lead to fibrosis.

CLINICAL MANIFESTATIONS

Ringworm infections have classically been described and designated by the area of the body that is involved. Although there are organisms with a propensity to establish themselves in certain anatomical locales, most dermatophytes can infect various parts of the body.

Tinea pedis

Involvement of the feet and toes is the most common clinical presentation of dermatophytosis among shoe-wearing people, comprising 47 percent of these infections in the United States [52]. The infection may be limited to the toe web spaces, usually the third and fourth. This type of infection may be asymptomatic; fungi have been recovered from 2.5 percent to 8.9 percent of normal adult web spaces [53]. Symptomatic infection certainly occurs, and scaling, fissuring, erythema, edema, and inflammation can occur, varying in intensity from mild to severe. Diagnosis is complicated by the fact that these same signs and symptoms often result from bacterial overgrowth in overhydrated, macerated skin. Bacterial superinfection can occur [53]. Toe web tinea pedis can have a tendency to recur because therapy of the acute condition will eliminate the bacteria and clinical signs while leaving resident fungi extant to incite another episode. It is noteworthy that the ability to demonstrate organisms in KOH preparations or culture declines as the inflammation increases [53]. T. rubrum, T. mentagrophytes, and E. floccosum are the organisms usually isolated from web spaces.

Another common variety of foot infection presents with the "sandal" or "moccasin" distribution of hyperkeratosis and scaling involving the plantar aspect and sides of the foot. Among adults, this pattern of infection is more common than web space infection and is perhaps the most prevalent form of dermatophytosis today. This type is noninflammatory, chronic, and extremely difficult to eradicate. Nail involvement is also common, while the dorsal aspects of the toes and foot are spared. T. rubrum is the predominant organism, although T. mentagrophytes may be found in some patients.

Tinea pedis may also present as an acute inflammatory process with vesicles, bullae, and even pustules on the plantar aspect on the foot (Fig. 113-2). The blister top contains the pathogen. It is felt that this is often secondary to a toe web infection which has spread and elicited a greater response from

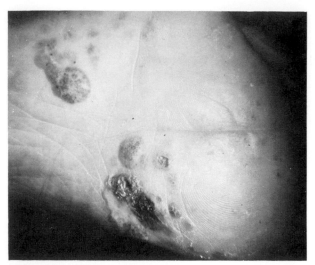

Figure 113-2. Tinea pedis with vesicles, some slightly hemorrhagic, on sole of foot. (*Courtesy of R. S. Salzman.*)

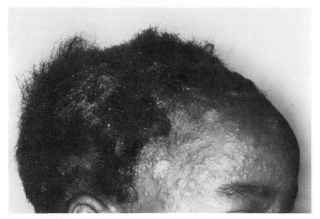

Figure 113-3. Tinea capitis showing areas of hair loss and accompanying id reaction on forehead. (*Courtesy of H. E. Jones.*)

the host. One form of vesicular infection affects mainly the skin of the lateral margins and instep of the foot. This particular pattern of infection is typically recurrent. This is puzzling as practically all other forms of inflammatory dermatophytosis are self-limited and not subject to recrudescence.

Tinea capitis

Ringworm of the scalp (Fig. 113-3) is characterized by involvement of the follicles and hair shafts, as well as the skin, and the clinical manifestations may vary considerably. The fungi which invade the follicles and hair shafts may form arthrospores on the outer surface of the hair; this is an ectothrix infection. Hairs infected in this manner tend to break off a few millimeters above the scalp surface, and the surrounding scalp is often slightly scaly. There may be several such patches, usually well-defined, randomly located on the scalp. Inflammation of the scalp may be minimal or fairly intense and has been thought to depend on the species of dermatophyte. Many isolates of both *Microsporum* and *Trichophyton* may cause ectothrix infections, although *Microsporum audouini* (noninflammatory) and *Microsporum canis* (inflammatory) are the most common.

Certain *Trichophyton* species, especially *T. tonsurans* and *T. violaceum,* form arthrospores within the hair shafts, causing endothrix infections. This process severely weakens the hairs, and they break off at the follicular orifice of the scalp. This causes the appearance of "black dots" on the scalp in a patch of baldness. Accompanying clinical findings may include scaling, folliculitis, or even frank kerions. Recently, Rasmussen and Ahmed [54] have shown that the intensity or degree of inflammation present in *T. tonsurans* tinea capitis is correlated with the presence or absence of DTH to fungal antigen. Fifteen

of 16 patients with kerions had DTH, while none of 36 patients with "black dot" infections had DTH. In light of our current understanding of fungal immunology and inflammation, this finding is highly relevant to understanding the variance seen in these clinical manifestations.

The classical favic infection caused by *Trichophyton schoenleinii* is characterized by yellowish follicular crusts known as *scutula.* These crusts may coalesce to cover large areas of the scalp. In long-standing cases, cicatricial alopecia can develop among the areas of crusts.

The most inflammatory forms of tinea capitis are collectively referred to as *kerion celsi.* In these instances, the colonized skin and hair follicles are severely damaged by an intense inflammatory process with weeping and pustulation. This leads to painful, purulent, edematous masses, either focal or spread over the scalp. Remaining hairs are loose, lymphadenopathy is common, and an accompanying bacterial superinfection must be sought. Although historically associated with zoophilic organisms, kerion formation occurs with common anthropophilic species [55] and appears to be determined by the nature of the host immune response.

Tinea corporis

Dermatophytosis of the glabrous skin generally occurs in either the acute or chronic form as discussed above (Fig. 113-4). Acute infection is often not noticed until it becomes inflammatory after a few weeks of radial spread. It then appears as an erythematous, annular lesion, often with some central clearing. A papular border with a distinct, well-defined edge is characteristic. Vesicles, and even pustules, may occur; there is slight evident scaling.

The acute process usually resolves spontaneously within 60 to 90 days, although it may, in immunologically susceptible individuals, transform into a chronic infection characterized by less erythema, less inflammation, and more scaling [37]. There

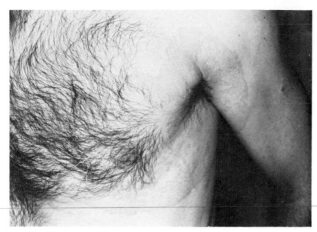

Figure 113-4. Chronic tinea corporis with a well-defined border and some central clearing. (*Courtesy of R. S. Salzman.*)

is a diminished tendency to central clearing, and there may be multiple sites of involvement or extensive coalesced areas of infected skin. The entire body skin, hair, and nails may remain infected for decades, or a lifetime.

Sometimes hair follicles become severely involved in tinea corporis. A deep dermal inflammatory reaction and abscess formation may ensue, forming a so-called Majocchi's granuloma. This process is reminiscent of the kerion celsi type of scalp infection. In this condition, segments of hyphae have been found associated with giant cells in the dermis [56] outside disrupted hair follicles.

A unique variant of tinea corporis, caused by *Trichophyton concentricum,* is known as *tinea imbricata;* it has a rather restricted geographical distribution (southeast Asia, South Pacific islands, Guatemala, southern Mexico, Brazil). Concentric rings of scaling radiate out in waves from the focus of infec-

tion, giving it a distinctive appearance. It is usually a chronic infection that can involve extensive areas of skin. Not uncommonly it begins in infancy [48].

Tinea cruris

Tinea cruris refers to infection of the groin area and is quite common in men. It begins in the intertriginous zone and spreads to the thigh with a well-defined arciform erythematous border. There can be considerable inflammation, vesiculation, and pustule formation. In contrast to the many satellite lesions seen in candidiasis, there are few or none in all types of tinea cruris. It can involve the scrotum, although the clinical findings of erythema and slight scaling are very subtle and easily missed [57]. *Epidermophyton floccosum* is a frequent isolate from this region. *T. rubrum* is commonly found also, especially in patients with chronic tinea pedis.

Tinea unguium

The nails often become infected when the adjacent skin is chronically involved, although isolated nail infection does occur. The process begins at the free nail border or lateral nail folds as the hyphae invade the nail bed and the ventral nail plate, producing an area of yellowish discoloration. This can continue until the central and medial portions of the nail plate are almost entirely consumed, and the thickened subungual debris grossly distorts the remaining dorsal nail plate (onychodystrophy). An intermediate finding consists of discoloration, subungual hyperkeratosis, onycholysis, and varying degrees of onychodystrophy (Fig. 113-5).

Although onychodystrophy is the most prominent feature of fungal involvement, it is not diagnostic of it. In one group of over 2000 nails and subungual hyperkeratosis and discoloration, only 46 percent could be demonstrated by KOH or culture to be fungal in origin [58]. Another group of 183 such nails yielded dermatophytes in only 23 percent, while bacteria, yeasts, and molds were found in the rest [59].

On occasion, the exposed portion of the dorsal nail plate is infected in a condition called superficial white onychomycosis. Clinically, one sees a well-circumscribed white patch, which can be easily scraped away, on one of the toenails. It is asymptomatic, noninflammatory, and usually caused by *T. mentagrophytes* [60].

It is interesting that in contrast to dermatophyte infections elsewhere in the integument, no form of tinea unguium is of the acute inflammatory type. This is true even when the entire nail is infected, in fact destroyed, and the infected nail bed is in contact with vascularized living skin.

Other tineas

There are numerous other types of dermatophytosis, e.g., tinea manus, tinea facei, and tinea barbae, which merely represent variations on the common themes already described.

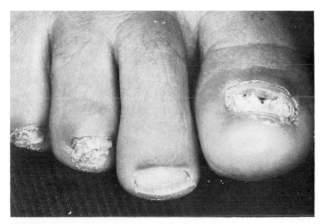

Figure 113-5. Characteristic onychodystrophy in tinea unguium. (*Courtesy of R. S. Salzman.*)

Tinea manus frequently presents an interesting picture because of its peculiar association with moccasin-type tinea pedis in the so-called "one-hand-two-foot syndrome." No adequate explanation exists for this intriguing, frequently seen clinical entity. The dorsum of the feet or hand is never infected, only the plantar-palmar surface. Yet the palmar skin of the uninfected hand remains normal despite years or decades of a stable one-hand-two-foot infection.

Tinea facei may involve any part of the face, including the beard area, and such infection is unusual in the frequency with which it may be misdiagnosed [61]. Its presentation often varies from classical ringworm, and it has been diagnosed as contact dermatitis, lupus erythematosus, and even granuloma annulare.

Tinea barbae is most commony seen in farm workers, who often contract their dermatophytosis from cattle or other animals. *Trichophyton verrucosum* and *T. mentagrophytes* (*granulare*) are frequently responsible for this acute, inflammatory infection.

Dermatophytids

These infrequent, mysterious concomitants of dermatophytosis apparently represent allergic reactions to a focus of fungal infection. The most common clinical forms of dermatophytids are: (1) follicular erythematous eruptions that may involve the trunk and extremities and are usually associated with inflammatory tinea capitis of the kerion type; and (2) vesicular eruptions on the palms and fingers, which are usually associated with tinea pedis.

The general criteria that have historically been used to diagnose id reactions include: (1) negative fungal determinations from the id, (2) proven dermatophytosis in another location, and (3) resolution of the id as the fungal infection clears [62]. Other clinical manifestations have been reported on rare occasions which meet these criteria and probably represent other forms that this "allergic" response may take. These include erythema nodosum [63], erythema annulare centrifugum [64], urticaria, and erythema multiforme [65].

Dermatophyte infection in immunocompromised hosts

Although localized invasive dermatophyte infection has been occasionally reported in normal hosts [44], in certain clinical situations, such as in immunocompromised hosts, deep local invasion, multivisceral dissemination, or even death has been reported [44]. In these cases, *T. rubrum* has been most frequently encountered.

Underlying systemic conditions such as leukemia, lymphoma, dysproteinemia, diabetes mellitus, Cushing's syndrome, graft-versus-host disease, or AIDS, as well as the administration of corticosteroids or cytotoxic agents, can predispose to atypical, extensive, or invasive *T. rubrum* infec-

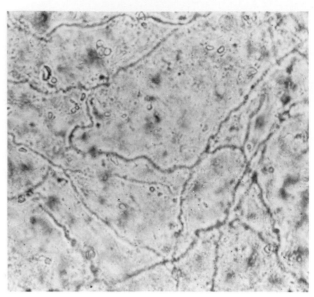

Figure 113-6. Branching hyphal elements as seen in a well-cleared KOH preparation. (*Courtesy of H. E. Jones.*)

tions [42–45]. In nearly all circumstances, chronic cutaneous *T. rubrum* infection preceded deep invasion, and tissue invasion was attributed to alterations in host resistance.

DIAGNOSIS

Clinical features

As mentioned above, the clinical manifestations of dermatophytosis are often distinctive enough to allow a diagnosis to be made on morphological grounds alone. However, it is sometimes difficult to distinguish contact dermatitis, nummular eczema, dyshidrosis, pityriasis rosea, secondary syphilis, lichen planus, trichotillomania, seborrheic dermatitis, and other entities from a fungal infection.

Wood's light

One of the traditional aids in diagnosing ringworm, especially tinea capitis, has been Wood's light. It has an ultraviolet (UV) light source and a special glass of barium silicate with approximately 9% nickel oxide which transmits UV light above 365 nm in wavelength (UVA). This causes hair infected with certain dermatophytes to fluoresce a greenish hue. Some pathogens of tinea capitis, such as *M. audouini, M. canis,* and *T. schoenleinii,* fluoresce, although the hair may have to be plucked to expose the portion with fungal involvement. *T. tonsurans*–infected hairs do not fluoresce, which is unfortunate given that today it is by far the most common cause of tinea capitis in the United States.

Direct examination

The most clinically useful diagnostic aid is direct microscopic examination of potassium hydroxide (KOH)–treated skin scales, hair, or nail debris [66]. After an appropriate sample of glabrous skin or hair has been placed on a glass slide, one or two drops of KOH solution (10%) is added and a coverslip applied. With dystrophic nails, the subungual hyperkeratotic material should be examined and when vesicles are present, the top of one should be pared off and placed on the slide. After the KOH and coverslip are in place, gentle heating (no boiling) over a flame or mild pressure on the coverslip will facilitate the clearing process. Thicker specimens, e.g., vesicle tops, may require hours to clear adequately.

The hyphae will be seen as thin (2 to 3 μm), refractile strands, often branching, transversing cellular membranes (Fig. 113-6). Arthrospores will be seen within or around involved hairs. Possible sources of confusion include fibers, which are usually larger, and mosaic artifact of intercellular lipid material between irregular polygonal cells. The hyphae of all dermatophyte species appear similar in a KOH preparation, and, in fact, dermatophyte hyphae cannot be distinguished with certainty from those of *Candida* species.

Culture

Under certain circumstances, fungal culture is warranted, although it is unusual for it to be the sole basis for the diagnosis. Frequently, culture is positive while microscopic examination is negative in dermatophyte infections. Nails should always be cultured, as *Candida* species and nonpathogenic molds have similar hyphal morphology in a KOH preparation. Culture identification is important in any clinical setting where other fungi, especially *Malassezia furfur* or *Candida* species, may confuse KOH confirmation of dermatophytosis.

THERAPY

General principles

Although the treatment of dermatophytosis may be viewed as routine and simplistic, it is important to individualize therapy based on the clinical-anatomical syndrome and the nature of the infection. It is necessary to keep in mind the acute and chronic varieties (Table 113-2) and the different responses to therapy which may be expected. Thus, at different ends of the clinical spectrum, acute inflamed sites of glabrous skin often spontaneously heal and may require minimal treatment, while chronic scaling lesions may respond only slowly to aggressive therapy and relapse when treatment is halted.

If the affected skin is denuded, severely inflamed, or near the eyes or genitalia, strong, irritating topical medication is contraindicated. Evidence of bacterial infection necessitates topical cleansing as well as possible antibiotic coverage. When the patient has a kerion celsi or a severe dermatophytid, a short course of corticosteroids and antifungal therapy can reduce the morbidity from this allergic condition.

But the mainstays of antifungal therapy are the topical and oral preparations which are available. They are fungistatic agents which, by halting proliferation of the fungi, allow the organism to be shed by the body during the normal course of epidermal turnover. Topical therapy is often all that is necessary to control minimal infections in toe web spaces, localized glabrous skin involvement, and scaly, pruritic foot infections. The latter, when extremely hyperkeratotic, may benefit from adjunctive keratolytic therapy with urea, salicylic acid, or topical retinoic acid. If the infection is extensive, fails to respond to topical therapy, or involves the hair or nails, then oral therapy is warranted, although chronic dermatophytosis is often not cured, merely temporarily interrupted, by such treatment. The acute type of infection is probably shortened by oral therapy.

Topical preparations

Over the past decade, an impressive array of topical antifungal preparations have been marketed. However, the old-time remedies of Whitfield's ointment (6% benzoic acid, 3% salicylic acid) and Castellani's paint (carbol-fuchsin) are far less costly and often equally effective [67,68]. The drawbacks of Whitfield's ointment are its acidic nature, which contraindicates use for fissured or denuded skin, and potential problems from absorption (salicylism) if applied to extensive areas. Castellani's paint works well in toe web infections, especially when coinfection with bacteria exists, but its messy color can be a nuisance. Aluminum chloride or aluminum acetate (20% solutions) are reported to be efficacious for this condition also [68].

The newer antifungal preparations include imidazole derivatives (clotrimazole, miconazole, econazole), which are generally well tolerated, nonirritating, and effective against both ringworm and candidiasis. They penetrate the epidermis well; a small amount enters the dermis and can be recovered in urine and feces [69]. Haloprogen is probably slightly less effective but also possesses anticandidal as well as antidermatophyte activity [70]. Tolnaftate, despite potency in the in vitro assays, does not seem to be as clinically effective as the others mentioned [70]. Application of these preparations for 2 to 4 weeks is usually sufficient. An exception is chronic sandal-type tinea pedis, for which long-term therapy may be needed to minimize symptomatology.

Oral medication

Griseofulvin. This, the first orally effective antifungal agent, was isolated from *Pencillium griseofulvum* in the 1930s and introduced into clinical medicine in 1958. It is only slightly soluble in water, which creates some difficulties with intestinal absorption, but solubility may be facilitated by smaller-sized particles [71]. The serum level peaks a few hours after administration, at which time the drug can be found in the stratum corneum, although levels in the skin will continue to rise for days if the drug is taken regularly [72]. Both serum and skin levels decline rapidly once oral administration has been stopped.

Griseofulvin apparently reaches the cornified tissue by two mechanisms: (1) from the circulating pool which diffuses into the newly forming cellular elements and (2) via eccrine sweat. The sweat must evaporate to concentrate and deposit the drug. However, excess sweating has been shown to lead to a decreased concentration of the drug in the stratum corneum [73], suggesting that dosages may need to be adjusted, depending on the ambient humidity and rate of sweat evaporation. Considering that the drug can reach the skin through sweating, it is interesting that topical griseofulvin, despite adequate levels in the skin, is ineffective clinically [72]. The effects of this agent on dermatophytes, as observed by electron microscopy, have been described [74], although the exact mode of action is not known. The growing hyphal tips are seen to become swollen and distorted, while the cell walls weaken with occasional collapse. However, most of the dormant mass of mycelia is unaffected. Microtubule formation or assembly is probably affected, but it is not clear if this is the relevant mechanism of action.

The general indications for administration of griseofulvin include: tinea capitis, tinea unguium, extensive infections, and infections unresponsive to topical therapy. The dosage of standard griseofulvin is 1000 mg/day for an adult, but the newer formulations of microsize and ultramicrosize griseofulvin have increased intestinal absorption and reduced the daily dose such that 250 mg/day is the recommended dose for the ultramicrosize form. Many clinicians prefer the microsized dose form, feeling that supposed equivalent doses of the ultramicrosized dose form are less effective. It may be necessary, though, to increase the dosage if the clinical response is inadequate, provided that the drug is well-tolerated by the patient.

The clinical effectiveness of griseofulvin has been reviewed [75] and demonstrates that certain types of dermatophytosis can be rather recalcitrant to therapy (Table 113-3). These figures include a second clinical trial when needed. The duration of therapy varies with the involved area and its expected turnover time.

There are many hypothetical reasons for griseofulvin failures which occur. Some patients have a natural predilection to chronic dermatophytosis. In others, their lack of response to griseofulvin has been shown to correlate with in vitro microbial resistance to the drug [76]. This resistance might be relative; i.e., higher concentrations of the drug could be effective, or absolute, with the minimal inhibitory concentration (MIC) being higher than the solubility limits of the drug in serum. The nature of the resistance to this drug is unknown but may involve demethylation and inactivation of the drug by fungal enzymes. Microbial resistance to griseofulvin is important, and in vitro testing can be a useful tool in certain circumstances.

The list of potential side effects is long and varied; however, griseofulvin is generally well-tolerated. Headaches, which may be severe enough to warrant cessation of therapy, and gastrointestinal or abdominal distress are the most frequently encountered complaints. Photosensitivity and mental confusion may also occur occasionally, while other complications are decidedly rare.

Griseofulvin may interact with phenobarbital and coumadin. It has been found that concurrent phenobarbital therapy can lower the serum griseofulvin level, probably by reducing intestinal absorption [72]. This may necessitate increasing the dose of griseofulvin. On the other hand, the anticoagulant effect of coumadin may be diminished by griseofulvin [77], necessitating an adjustment in the coumadin dosage.

Imidazoles. Ketoconazole possesses potent antifungal activity. It is a water-soluble imidazole derivative with adequate intestinal absorption leading to good serum levels. It has a much broader spectrum of activity than griseofulvin and may be used for candidiasis and some deeper fungi, as well as dermatophytes. The normal dosage is 200 mg/day, taken with meals. In some instances, 400 mg/day may be necessary. Stomach acidity enhances the bioavailability of the drug, and concurrent use of cimetidine or antacids may markedly reduce absorption. Peak serum levels of 3 to 4 μg/mL are reached 1 to 2 h after administration; relevant skin tissue levels have not been determined [78].

Its mechanism of action against the dermatophytes is not specifically known; however, it is likely that the sterol metabolism of the fungal cells is selectively impaired, resulting in defective cellular membranes. Scanning electron microscopy has shown cell wall changes in the hyphae with some internal necrosis by the ninth day of treatment [79].

Because of its relative expense, this drug will probably not replace griseofulvin as the primary oral antifungal agent. However, because of the proven resistance of some dermatophytes to griseofulvin and the problems that chronic, recalcitrant dermatophytosis can engender, there is a definite role for ketoconazole in dermatophytosis. It has been shown in double-blind studies to be more effective than griseofulvin [80] and

Table 113-3. Griseofulvin therapy

Type infection	% cure	Duration
Tinea capitis	93	2 months
Tinea corporis	100*	1 month
Tinea pedis/manus	53	2–4 months
Tinea unguium (hands)	57	4–6 months
Tinea unguium (feet)	17	6–12 months

*Excluding patients with tinea imbricata. This subgroup had a cure rate of 20%.

Source: [75]

has been shown in open studies to clear chronically infected patients who had little response to griseofulvin [81]. It should be noted, though, that relapses do occur, and in the chronically infected patients, 75 percent had clinical evidence of reinfection at 5 months [82].

Although this drug has not been extensively used over a long period of time, it appears to be well-tolerated. Dose-related nausea and abdominal pain are the most common side effects. Gynecomastia in men is related to dose and duration. Doses above 500 mg/day decrease testosterone and cortisol synthesis, but this is usually asymptomatic. Ketoconazole is contraindicated in pregnancy and during breast-feeding. The most serious complication is hepatotoxicity, which can be fatal and can occur at virtually any time during therapy, from the first week to beyond the twelfth week. While transient liver function abnormalities are common, fatal hepatotoxicity is rare. Patients receiving cyclosporine, oral anticoagulants, or phenytoin should have blood levels assessed because ketoconazole may slow metabolism of these drugs. H_2 blockers decrease ketoconazole levels dramatically; oral antacids only interfere with absorption if taken simultaneously. Food does not change absorption. Rifampin decreases ketoconazole blood levels significantly.

Itraconazole, a new antifungal drug, is lipophilic and absorbed after oral administration. Serum levels of the drug are low, but levels of drug in tissues, especially liver and skin, may exceed serum values [83]. When used for treatment of superficial fungal infections (tinea corporis, tinea cruris, and tinea pedis) itraconazole has been very effective. Most of the infections treated have been caused by *T. rubrum* [83]. More data are necessary on the efficacy of this drug against species other than *T. rubrum,* as well as in groups of patients failing other therapy and in treatment of onychomycosis or dry-type *T. rubrum* infections of the feet.

POPULATION

EPIDEMIOLOGY

Dermatophytosis is a worldwide problem. No exact data for incidence and prevalence within a given population exist, and the obstacles to compiling such information are formidable.

Most infections are probably never seen by a physician because they are acute and self-limited. These fungi can also be carried by people on clinically normal skin. Thus, estimates of incidence and prevalence tend to reflect clinically significant infections which have been brought to a physician's attention.

The magnitude of the problem can be seen by looking at such clinical data. In two of the developing countries, Egypt and Nigeria, the percentage of new patients with dermatophytosis seen in dermatology clinics has been reported to be 15 to 20 percent [84,85]. In many of the developed countries, dermatophytosis accounts for 5 to 7 percent of the dermatological visitors. The same is true in large U.S. Army hospital dermatology clinics. It has been estimated from the National Health Survey that 9 percent of the people in the United States have a cutaneous fungal infection [86].

Tremendous variability exists between population groups concerning the types of infection that are seen clinically (Table 113-4). This is due to significant differences in climate, clothing, age, socioeconomic factors, and rural-versus-urban living patterns [87–90]. The impacts of climate and clothing have been discussed above. Socioeconomic situations, e.g., crowded living conditions, can foster the spread of disease among animals and humans and increase prevalence rates.

Rural and urban ringworm often seem to have distinctive patterns [91]. Rural infections are more often of zoophilic origin, tend to be more acute, more suppurative, more likely to be accompanied by a dermatophytid, and are more likely to occur on exposed body surfaces. On the other hand, urban ringworm is more often caused by anthropophilic organisms with a greater tendency to be chronic, less inflamed, and involve covered body parts. A notable exception to this is tinea capitis caused by *M. canis*, which may become very prevalent among children in a crowded urban environment.

There are a few other generalizations which usually apply to different population groups. Tinea capitis is essentially a disease of childhood which, for unexplained reasons, is uncommon after puberty. Conversely, tinea pedis and tinea cruris become much more common after puberty. The most significant difference between the sexes is the propensity of young males to develop tinea cruris, probably because of the occlusion provided by the scrotum.

Table 113-4. Types of dermatophytosis seen in different locales

	Tinea cruris	Tinea pedis	Tinea unguium	Tinea corporis	Tinea capitis
Christchurch, New Zealand [87]	35%	20%	5%	19%	6%
Salamanca, Spain [88]	25%	18%	8%	42%	4%
Kuwait [89]	5%	4%	3%	16%	71%
San Francisco, U.S.A. [90]	19%	31%	11%	17%	10%
Nigeria [85]	17%	30%	9%	26%	14%
United States [86]	29%	53%	12%	<5%	<5%

TRANSMISSION

Dermatophytes may be spread by person-to-person, animal-to-person, and person-to-animal contact, as well as via fomites.

Person-to-person transmission is perhaps most important in tinea capitis, where it may rapidly spread among the children in the confined area of a classroom. It is not even necessary for the children to touch each other since the dust in the room where infected people have been has been shown to contain fungal elements [92], and caged guinea pigs have contracted fungal infections by airborne spread [93]. Humans working in a laboratory containing fungi became infected at sites on their body that were sprayed with an aerosol adhesive [94]. This suggests that under specific circumstances, airborne spread does occur.

A study comparing scalp carriage of dermatophytes by children in classes with and without cases of ringworm showed a substantially higher carriage rate among those who had been exposed to ringworm in their classrooms, even though the index cases were no longer present [92].

Spread from animals to humans has been reported for dozens of different animals. The most common occurrences are probably transmission of *T. verrucosum* from cattle, *M. canis* from cats, and *T. mentagrophytes (granulare)* from a variety of animals. The infective fungal elements may be present not only on the animals themselves but also in their nesting material [95] and on scratching posts and barn walls with which they have had contact [96].

As can be seen, fomites are commonly implicated in the spread of these infections. In an area of Nigeria where 64 percent of the primary school children had tinea capitis, the scissors of the traveling barber were found to harbor the causative agent [85]. Viable fungal elements have also been found on combs, brushes, the backs of theater seats, bed linens, towels, underwear, and jockstraps. It has also been shown that the floors of public baths contain dermatophyte elements [97].

It is not known how long these fungal remnants remain viable under natural conditions. When kept in dry laboratory conditions, they have been found to be infective after a year or more [95,96]. However, when some of the samples were dampened, they survived less than a week, as they were presumably overgrown by other organisms [95].

CONTROL

It can be seen that infective particles may be virtually ubiquitous in an environment where dermatophytosis is prevalent. Given the seemingly high prevalence of dermatophytosis in humans, exposure to dermatophytes can almost be taken for granted. However, control measures may properly be utilized in certain circumstances.

Tinea capitis may spread among schoolchildren. When cases are found, prompt treatment with griseofulvin, clipping of infected hair, exclusion from school, and appropriate cleaning of the environment can reduce the spread of disease, especially when anthropophilic organisms are the source. Screening children with Wood's light will pick up some infections (*M. canis, M. audouini, T. schoenleinii*), but *T. tonsurans* does not fluoresce. A more thorough approach employs a circular brush which is embedded into culture media after the child's scalp has been brushed [92]. This can facilitate treatment of all children carrying the organism, since it has been shown that they may later develop a clinical infection [98]. When *M. canis* is the pathogen, if the infected cat (or dog) can be located, it can be treated with griseofulvin; however, a certain percentage of cats are asymptomatic carriers of this fungus [99].

It is also important to realize that many common domestic animals may harbor or be infected by dermatophytes. Recognition of this condition in animals will facilitate appropriate handling and hygienic measures which may reduce the possibility of animal-to-person spread.

Tinea pedis becomes more common where enclosed footwear is fashionable. Because it may easily be transmitted at public baths, pools, etc. frequent hosing down of floors and walkways is recommended to reduce the dermatophyte count [95]. Use of topical antifungal agents in these places may also be efficacious. However, neither practice has been subjected to rigorous trials, and proof of efficacy is lacking. Control of tinea pedis, either by prevention or by merely limiting it with topical agents, can be important in reducing the spread of the infection, so that nails and other body areas, especially the groin, become involved less frequently.

Spread of both tinea pedis and tinea cruris from one person to another may be hindered by good hygienic practices concerning towels, bathmats, footwear, and clothes which may act as fomites. The value of hygienic measures, disinfectant procedures, and the discarding of fomites is not clear. During a successful course of therapy, patients with acute, and especially chronic, infections frequently ask the appropriate questions. Unfortunately, there are no definite answers available.

REFERENCES

1 Jones HE: Superficial infections of the skin, in Hoeprich PD (ed): *Infectious Diseases,* 3d ed. Hagerstown, Md, Harper & Row, 1983, pp 966–978

2 Philpot CM: Geographical distribution of the dermatophytes. A review. J Hyg (Lond) 80:301, 1978

3 Rippon JW: Elastase: Production by ringworm fungi. Science 157: 947, 1967

4 Rippon JW: Extracellular collagenase from *Trichophyton schoenleinii.* J Bacteriol 95:43–46, 1968

5 Weary PE, Canby CM: Further observations on the keratinolytic activity of *Trichophyton schoenleinii* and *Trichophyton rubrum.* J Invest Dermatol 53:58–63, 1969

6 Meevootisom V, Niederpruem DJ: Control of exocellular proteases in dermatophytes and especially *Trichophyton rubrum.* Sabouraudia 17:91–106, 1979

7 King RD, Khan HA, Foye JC, et al: Transferrin, iron and dermatophytes. I. Serum dermatophyte inhibitory component defi-

nitely identified as unsaturated transferrin. J Lab Clin Med 86:204–212, 1975

8 Taplin D, Zaias N, Rebell G, et al: Isolation and recognition of dermatophytes on a new medium (DTM). Arch Dermatol 99:203, 1969

9 Granade TC, Artis WM: Antimycotic susceptibility testing of dermatophytes in microcultures with a standardized fragmented mycelial inoculum. Antimicrob Ag Chemother 17:725–729, 1980

10 Kligman AM: Pathophysiology of ringworm infections in animals with skin cycles. J Invest Dermatol 27:171–185, 1952

11 DeLamater ED, Benham RW: Experimental studies with dermatophytes. I. Primary disease in laboratory animals. J Invest Dermatol 1:451–467, 1938

12 Hunjan BS, Cronholm LS: An animal model for cell-mediated immune responses to dermatophytes. J Allergy Clin Immunol 63:361–369, 1979

13 Jones HE: Animals models of human dermatophyte infection, in Maibach H (ed): *Animal Models in Dermatology.* New York, Churchill Livingstone, 1975

14 Baer RL, Rosenthal SA, Rogachefsky H, et al: Newer studies on the epidemiology of fungus infections of the feet. Am J Public Health 45:784, 1955

15 Jones HE, Reinhardt JH, Rinaldi MG: Acquired immunity to dermatophytes. Arch Dermatol 109:840, 1974

16 Knight AG: A review of experimental human fungus infections. J Invest Dermatol 59:354, 1972

17 Taplin D, Zaias N, Rebell G: Environmental influences on the microbiology of the skin. Arch Environ Health 11:546, 1965

18 English MP: Comment: Tinea pedis as a public health problem. Br J Dermatol 81:705, 1969

19 Allen AM, Taplin D: Epidemic *Trichophyton mentagrophytes* infections in servicemen: Source of infection, role of environment, host factors, and susceptibility. JAMA 226:864, 1973

20 Allen AM, King RD: Occlusion, carbon dioxide, and fungal skin infections. Lancet, Feb 18, 1978, p 360

21 Kligman AM: The pathogenesis of tinea capitis due to *Microsporum audouini* and *Microsporum cansi.* J Invest Dermatol 18:231, 1952

22 Jones HE, Reinhardt JH, Rinaldi MC: Model dermatophytosis in naturally infected subjects. Arch Dermatol 110:369, 1974

23 Basarab O, How MJ, Cruickshank CND: Immunological relationships between glycopeptides of *Microsporum canis, Trichophyton rubrum, Trichophyton mentagrophytes,* and other fungi. Sabouraudia 6:119, 1968

24 Kaaman T, Wasserman J: Cell-mediated cross reactivity *in vivo* and *in vitro* to purified dermatophyte antigen preparations in sensitized guinea pigs. Acta Derm Venereol (Stockh) 63:404, 1983

25 Kaaman T, von Stedingk LV, von Stedingk M, et al: ELISA-determined serological reactivity against purified trichophytin in dermatophytosis. Acta Derm Venereol (Stockh) 61:313, 1981

26 Bloch B, La bouchere A, Schaaf F: Versuche einer Chemischen Charakterisierung und Reindarstellung des Trichophytins (des aktiven, antigenen Prinzips pathogener Hautpilze). Arch Dermatol Syph 148:413, 1925

27 Grappel SF, Bishop CT, Blank F: Immunology of dermatophytes and dermatophytosis. Bacteriol Rev 38:222, 1974

28 Jones HE, Artis WM: Dermatophytosis, in Safai B, Good RA (eds): *Immunodermatology.* New York, Plenum, 1981

29 Stuka AJ, Burrell R: Factors affecting the antigenicity of *Trichophyton rubrum.* J Bacteriol 94:914, 1967

30 Ito Y: On the immunologically active substances of the dermatophyte II. J Invest Dermatol 45:285, 1965

31 Christiansen AH, Svejgaard E: Studies of the antigenic structure of *Trichophyton rubrum, Trichophyton mentagrophytes, Microsporum canis,* and *Epidermophyton floccosum* by crossed immunoelectrophoresis. Acta Pathol Microbiol Scand (C) 84:337, 1976

32 Jones HE, Reinhardt JH, Rinaldi MG: A clinical, mycological, and immunological survey for dermatophytosis. Arch Dermatol 108:61, 1973

33 Grappel SF, Blank F, Bishop CT: Circulating antibodies in dermatophytosis. Dermatologica 144:1, 1972

34 Svejgaard E, Christiansen AH: Precipitating antibodies in dermatophytosis demonstrated by crossed immunoelectrophoresis. Acta Pathol Microbiol Scand (C) 87:23, 1979

35 Kerbs S, Greenberg J, Jesrani K: Temporal correlation of lymphocyte blastogenesis, skin test responses, and erythema during dermatophyte infections. Clin Exp Immunol 27:526, 1977

36 Hanifin JM, Ray LF, Lobitz WC: Immunologic reactivity in dermatophytosis. Br J Dermatol 90:1, 1974

37 Jones HE, Reinhardt JH, Rinaldi MG: Immunologic susceptibility to chronic dermatophytosis. Arch Dermatol 110:213, 1974

38 Kaaman T: The clinical significance of cutaneous reaction to trichophytin in dermatophytosis. Acta Derm Venereol (Stockh) 58:139, 1978

39 Kaaman T: Cell-mediated reactivity in dermatophytosis: Differences in skin responses to purified trichophytin in tinea pedis and tinea cruris. In press

40 Brahmi Z, Liautaud B, Marill F: Depressed cell-mediated immunity in chronic dermatophytic infections. Ann Immunol (Inst Pasteur) 131:143, 1980

41 Sorensen G, Jones HE: Immediate and delayed hypersensitivity in chronic dermatophytosis. Arch Dermatol 112:40, 1976

42 Noppakun N, Head ES: Proximal white subungual onychomycosis in a patient with acquired immune deficiency syndrome. Int J Dermatol 25:586–587, 1986

43 Basuk PJ, Scher RK: Onychomycosis in graft versus host disease. Cutis 40:237–241, 1987

44 Novick NL, Tapia L, Bottone EJ: Invasive *Trichophyton rubrum* infection in an immunocompromised host. Am J Med 82:321–325, 1987

45 Baker RL, Para MF: Successful use of ketoconazole for invasive cutaneous *Trichophyton rubrum* infection. Arch Intern Med 144:615–616, 1984

46 Many H, Derbes VJ, Friedman L: *Trichophyton rubrum:* Exposure and infection within household groups. Arch Dermatol 82:226, 1960

47 Jones HE: The atopic-chronic-dermatophytosis syndrome. Acta Derm Venereol (Stockh) (Suppl) 92:81, 1980

48 Serjeantson S, Lawrence G: Autosomal recessive inheritance of susceptibility to tinea imbricata. Lancet i:13, 1977

49 Jones HE, Terasaki P: Unpublished data

50 Lever WF, Schaumburg-Lever G: *Histopathology of the Skin,* 5th ed. Philadelphia, Lippincott, 1975, chap 18

51 Graham JH, Barroso-Tobila C: In Baker RD (ed): *The Pathologic Anatomy of the Mycoses.* Berlin, Springer-Verlag, 1971

52 *The National Ambulatory Medical Care Survey: 1973.* National Center for Health Statistics, Department of Health, Education and Welfare, publication no HRA 76–1772, 1975

53 Leyden JJ, Kligman AM: Interdigital athlete's foot: The interaction

of dermatophytes and resident bacteria. Arch Dermatol 114:1466, 1978

54 Rasmussen JE, Ahmed R: Trichophytin reactions in children with tinea capitis. Arch Dermatol 114:371, 1978

55 Erbaken N, Nur Or A, Palali Z, et al: Factors influencing the formation of tinea capitis profundus, "kerion celsi." Mykosen 18: 35, 1975

56 Blank H, Smith JG: Widespread *Trichophyton rubrum* granulomas treated with griseofulvin. Arch Dermatol 81:779, 1960

57 LaRouche CJ: Scrotal dermatophytosis: An insufficiently documented aspect of tinea cruris. Br J Dermatol 79:339, 1967

58 Davies RR: Mycological tests and onychomycosis. J Clin Pathol 21:729, 1968

59 Zaias N, Oertel I, Elliott DF: Fungi in toenails. J Invest Dermatol 53:140, 1969

60 Zaias N: Superficial white onychomycosis. Sabouraudia, 5:99, 1966

61 Elton RF, Mehregan AH, Grekin JN: Tinea faciei: A report of 14 cases with non-specific skin lesions. Cutis 12:394, 1973

62 Peck SM: Epidermophytosis of the feet and epidermophytids of the hands: Clinical, histological, cultural, and experimental studies. Arch Derm Syph 22:40, 1930

63 Franks AG, Rosenbaum EM, Mandel EH: *Trichophyton sulfureum* causing erythema nodosum and multiple kerion formation. Arch Derm Syph 65:95, 1952

64 Jillson OF, Hoekelman RA: Further amplification of the concept of dermatophytid. 1. Erythema annulare centrifugum as a dermatophytid. Arch Dermatol 66:738, 1952

65 Weary PE, Guerrant JL: Chronic urticaria in association with dermatophytosis: Response to the administration of griseofulvin. Arch Dermatol 95:400, 1967

66 Lefler E, Haim S, Merzbach D: Evaluation of direct microscopic examination versus culture in the diagnosis of superficial fungal infections. Mykosen 24(2):102, 1981

67 Clayton YM, Connor BL: Comparison of clotrimazole cream, Whitfield's ointment, and nystatin ointment for the topical treatment of ringworm infections, pityriasis versicolor, erythema, and candidiasis. Br J Dermatol 89:297, 1973

68 Leyden JJ, Kligman AM: Aluminum chloride in the treatment of symptomatic athlete's foot. Arch Dermatol 111:1004, 1975

69 Raab W: Clinical pharmacology of modern topical broad-spectrum antimicrobials. Curr Ther Res 22:65, 1977

70 Carter VH: A controlled study of haloprogen and tolnaftate in tinea pedis. Curr Ther Res 14:307, 1972

71 Chiou WL, Riegelman S: Absorption characteristics of solid dispersed and micronized griseofulvin in man. J Pharm Sci 60:1376, 1971

72 Epstein WL, Shah V, Riegelman S: Dermatopharmacology of griseofulvin. Cutis 15:271, 1975

73 Shah VP, Epstein WK, Riegelman S: Role of sweat in accumulation of orally administered griseofulvin in skin. J Clin Invest 53: 1673, 1974

74 Blank H, Taplin D, Roth F: Electron microscopic observations of the effects of griseofulvin on dermatophytes. Arch Dermatol 81: 667, 1960

75 Anderson DW: Griseofulvin: Biology and clinical usefulness. A review. Ann Allergy 23:103, 1965

76 Artis WM, Odle BM, Jones HE: Griseofulvin-resistant dermatophytosis correlates with *in vitro* resistance. Arch Dermatol 117:16, 1981

77 Cullen SI, Catalano PM: Griseofulvin-warfarin antagonism. JAMA 199:582, 1967

78 Heel RC: Pharmacokinetic properties, in Levine HB (ed): *Ketoconazole in the Management of Fungal Disease*. New York, Adis, 1982

79 Borgers M, Van den Bossche H: The mode of action of antifungal drugs, in Levine HB (ed): *Ketoconazole in the Management of Fungal Disease*. New York, Adis, 1982

80 Heel RC: Dermatomycoses, in Levine HB (ed): *Ketoconazole in the Management of Fungal Disease*. New York, Adis, 1982

81 Jones HE, Simpson JG, Artis WM: Oral ketoconazole: An effective and safe treatment for dermatophytosis. Arch Dermatol 117:129, 1981

82 Heel RC: Toxicology and safety studies, in Levine HB (ed): *Ketoconazole in the Management of Fungal Disease*. New York, Adis, 1982

83 Sa'ul A, Borif'az A, Arias I: Itraconazole in the treatment of superficial mycoses: An open trial of 40 cases. Rev Infect Dis (Suppl) 1:S100–S103, 1987

84 Amer M, Taha M, Tosson Z, et al: The frequency of causative dermatophytes in Egypt. Int J Dermatol 20:431, 1981

85 Soyinka F: Epidemiologic study of dermatophyte infections in Nigeria (clinical survey and laboratory investigation). Mycopathologia 63:99, 1978

86 Johnson MLT: Skin conditions and related need for medical care among persons 1–74 years. US Department of Health, Education, and Welfare, series 11, no 212, publication (PHS) 79–1660, November 1978

87 Bridger RC: Superficial mycoses in a southern New Zealand district. Sabouraudia 17:107, 1979

88 Benito JAV, Martin-Pascual A, Perez AG: Epidemiologic study of dermatophytoses in Salamanca (Spain). Sabouraudia 7:113, 1979

89 Karaoui R, Selim M, Mousa A: Incidence of dermatophytosis in Kuwait. Sabouraudia 17:131, 1979

90 Aly R: Incidence of dermatophytes in the San Francisco Bay area. Dermatologica 161:97, 1980

91 Georg LK, Hand EA, Menges RA: Observation on rural and urban ringworm. J Invest Dermatol 27:335, 1956

92 Midgley G, Clayton YM: Distribution of dermatophytes and *Candida* spores in the environment. Br J Dermatol 86:69, 1972

93 Chittasobhon N, Smith JMB: The production of experimental dermatophyte lesions in guinea pigs. J Invest Dermatol 73:198–201, 1979

94 Jones HE: Unpublished data

95 English MP, Morris P: *Trichophyton mentagrophytes* var. *erinacei* in hedgehog nests. Sabouraudia 7:118, 1969

96 Walker J: Possible infection of man by indirect transmission of *Trichophyton discoides*. Br Med J 2:1430, 1955

97 Gip L: Estimation of incidence of dermatophytes on floor areas after barefoot walking with washed and unwashed feet. Acta Derm Venereol (Stockh) 47:89, 1967

98 Ive FA: The carrier stage of tinea capitis in Nigeria. Br J Dermatol 78:219, 1966

99 Woodgyer AJ: Asymptomatic carriage of dermatophytes by cats. NZ Vet J 25:67, 1977

Sporotrichosis · John E. Bennett

AGENT

Sporotrichosis is the infection caused by *Sporothrix schenckii*. This fungus grows as a budding yeast in tissue or in enriched medium at 37°C. Size and shape of the yeast form is quite variable in tissue, ranging from spherical to cigar-shaped. In vitro, ovoid or fusiform yeast cells, 2.5 to 5 by 3.5 to 6.5 μm, grow on special media at 37°C. Budding may be single or multiple. At 25°C, a white mold forms and darkens to black with age. Slide culture shows hyaline, regularly septate mycelial filaments 1 to 2 μm wide; and oval, pyriform, or elongated conidia born singly or in groups, each attached to the conidiophore by a small denticle. Identification is most secure when both the yeast and mycelial forms are examined.

PATIENT

PATHOGENESIS AND PATHOLOGY

S. schenckii has been isolated from a variety of natural sources, especially soil, plants, and dead vegetation such as wood or straw. Rodents and domestic animals, such as cats and dogs, may acquire sporotrichosis. Scratches or bites of animals occasionally lead to sporotrichosis, usually without obvious infection in the animal. More commonly, infection follows scratches or puncture wounds from plants. Workers handling sphagnum moss, roses, and hay are predisposed to infection [1]. No age or sex predisposition is apparent.

The highest incidence of sporotrichosis appears to be in southern Brazil and the highlands of Mexico. Infection is sporadic in most countries of the world, although nearly nonexistent in western Europe. The greatest epidemic occurred in the Transvaal mine of South Africa, where up to 2825 cases were reported from 1941 to 1944. Treating timbers with fungicide stopped the epidemic.

Sporotrichosis excites both a neutrophilic and granulomatous response in tissue. Fungal cells are infrequent in tissue and require special stains for visualization. Occasionally an asteroid body is seen in tissue. This is a 5- to 8-μm thick-walled fungal cell surrounded by a radiating ring of eosinophilic material 1 to 12 μm thick [2]. Rarely, *S. schenckii* in brain or eye has had a thick capsule resembling *Cryptococcus*.

CLINICAL MANIFESTATIONS

A painless red nodule forms slowly at the site of inoculation followed by the appearance after 1 week or more of similar nodules along proximal lymphatics (Fig. 114-1). Each nodule tends to wax and wane, intermittently discharges serosanguineous pus, and may persist for months. Infection remains confined to the soft tissue of the infected extremity. Systemic symptoms such as fever are absent. Plaque sporotrichosis is the name given to solitary lesions without extension.

Extracutaneous sporotrichosis probably enters by the lung, though a pulmonary focus is only seen occasionally. Infection confined to the lung forms a chronic, fibrocavitary lesion, usually single, with no predilection for apical segments. Osteoarticular infection presents as a chronic asymmetrical arthritis of the peripheral joints, particularly knee or wrist. Over months or years, draining sinuses or patchy radiolucencies of underlying bone help distinguish this entity from degenerative osteoarthritis. Other sites of hematogenous spread include skin, meninges, and kidney, but all are rare.

DIFFERENTIAL DIAGNOSIS

Skin lesions closely resembling sporotrichosis can be caused by *Nocardia brasiliensis* or leishmaniasis. Plaque sporotrichosis can resemble chromomycosis or lobomycosis. A single thin-walled cavity of pulmonary sporotrichosis can be identical on chest x-ray to coccidioidomycosis. Early manifestations of osteoarticular sporotrichosis are frequently mistaken for osteoarthritis or rheumatoid arthritis.

Diagnosis of sporotrichosis requires culture of the fungus from pus, sputum, or biopsied tissue. Pus from skin lesions is usually positive by culture and occasionally by smear. Skin biopsy for culture is also useful but finding the fungus in histopathological stain requires patience and special stains such as Gomori methenamine silver or periodic acid Schiff. Similarly, culture of joint fluid or a draining sinus is more useful than synovial biopsy. Serological diagnosis and skin testing are still research procedures, although a great deal is known of the immunochemistry of this pathogen [2].

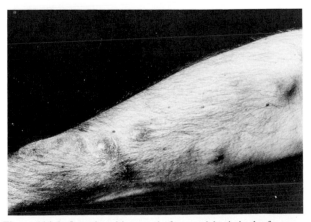

Figure 114-1. Lymphangitic spread of sporotrichosis in the forearm.

TREATMENT

Cutaneous sporotrichosis responds well to 4 or more weeks of oral iodide, given as a saturated solution of potassium iodide (SSKI). Treatment is begun as 1 drop three times daily for a small child or 5 drops three times daily in older children or adults. For ease of ingestion, the drops are put in a small amount of water or juice. The amount is increased daily as tolerated to a maximum dose of 10 drops three times a day for a small child [3] to 30 or 40 drops three times a day for an adult. Treatment continues until all induration is gone, typically 4 to 6 weeks. Relapse is uncommon and responds to retreatment with iodide. Eructation, anorexia, and nausea are common with the highest doses of this bitter medicine. An acneiform rash over the cape area of the chest can occur. Enlarged salivary and lacrymal glands may be noticed. None of these are indications for discontinuing therapy prematurely. Patients able to tolerate only a low dose of SSKI may nevertheless be cured, though improvement may be slow. Patients with a known history of allergic reactions to iodides or who develop allergic skin rashes to SSKI may respond to systemic therapy with one of the imidazoles. Ketonazole, given to adults in oral doses of 400–600 mg once daily, will cure an occasional patient. Early experience with oral itraconazole in lymphocutaneous sporotrichosis appears promising [4]. For lesions confined to the distal portions of an extremity, immersing the area in very hot water for 15 to 30 min three times a day can aid healing. Osteoarticular disease does not respond well to any available therapy, but intravenous amphotericin B is the drug of choice. Resection of localized pulmonary lesions should be considered [5].

REFERENCES

1 Powell KE, Taylor A, Phillips BJ, et al: Cutaneous sporotrichosis in forestry workers. JAMA 240:232–235, 1978
2 Bullpitt P, Weedon D: Sporotrichosis: A review of 39 cases. Pathology, 10:249–256, 1978
3 Orr ER, Riley HD: Sporotrichosis in childhood: Report of ten cases. J Pediatr 78:951–957, 1971
4 Restrepo A, Robledo J, Gomez I, Tabares MT, Gutierrez R: Itraconazole therapy in lymphangitic sporotrichosis. Arch Dermatol 122: 413–417, 1986
5 Pluss JL, Opal S: Pulmonary sporotrichosis: Review of treatment and outcome. Medicine 65:143–153, 1986

CHAPTER
115

Entomophthoramycosis Caused by Basidiobolus haptosporus

· J. W. Mugerwa

Lei Kian Joe and others reported the first two cases of subcutaneous zygomycosis from Indonesia in 1956. Both cases were in boys less than 10 years of age. Fungal hyphae were recognized in histological sections, and from one of the cases a fungus identified at that time as *Basidiobolus ranarum* was isolated [1]. In the same year Raper [2] described five cases of creeping subcutaneous granuloma with similar histology in Ugandan Africans—these were later confirmed to be due to subcutaneous phycomycosis [3]. This deep mycosis is now known to be caused by *Basidiobolus haptosporus (ranarum)* or closely related species such as *B. meritosporus* [4,5].

AGENT

B. haptosporus is found as a saprophyte in the intestinal tract of reptiles and amphibia such as lizards, chameleons, and frogs [6]. It has also been recovered from mites and insects on which the reptiles and amphibia feed. It grows on decomposing vegetables and leaves, possibly as a result of droppings on them from lizards and frogs. Kangaroos and wallabies have been reported to carry *B. haptosporus*.

PATIENT

PATHOLOGY

The characteristic lesions of *B. haptosporus* are found in the subcutaneous tissues and the dermis is usually normal or shows nonspecific inflammation. In the earlier stages of the disease there is inflammation of the areolar tissue with focal collections of eosinophils in which fungal hyphae can be seen as round or longitudinal structures with occasional septae (Fig. 115-1). The width of the hyphae is estimated to be 8 to 20 μm, and it is unusual to see protoplasm within the hyphae walls. The fungi can most easily be identified with the Grocott or periodic acid-Schiff (PAS) stain (Fig. 115-2). An eosinophilic granular material, the Splendore-Hoeppli phenomenon, surrounding the hyphae (Fig. 115-3) is from the deposition of antigen-antibody complexes there [7]. In older lesions a granulomatous reaction is seen in the subcutaneous fat with groups of macrophages and foreign body–type giant cells arranged around hyphae, many of which are distorted. Fragments of hyphae may be present in these giant cells, and there are collections of lym-

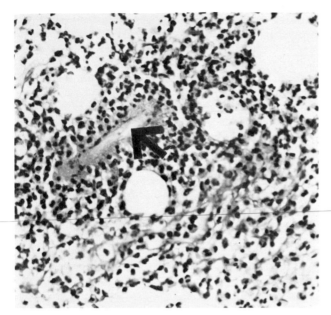

Figure 115-1. Inflammatory cells with eosinophils in subcutaneous fat. A hypha cut longitudinally (arrow) is surrounded by a granular zone. (Splendore-Hoeppli phenomenon). H&E, × 400.

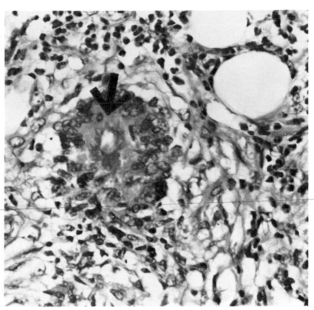

Figure 115-3. Cross section of *B. haptosporus* hypha with Splendore-Hoeppli phenomenon (arrow).

phocytes and plasma cells adjacent to the granulomas (Fig. 115-4). Concomitantly there is increasing fibrosis and a decreasing number of eosinophils; the appearances suggest the gradual development of a type IV delayed hypersensitivity reaction. On rare occasions, the fungus invades blood vessels and metastasizes by blood or lymph [8].

CLINICAL FEATURES

In two-thirds of patients the lesion is on the buttocks or the thighs and may extend from there to the external genitalia and the perineum. In about one-third of patients the lesion is on the upper limbs, legs, or trunk; rarely is the head or neck

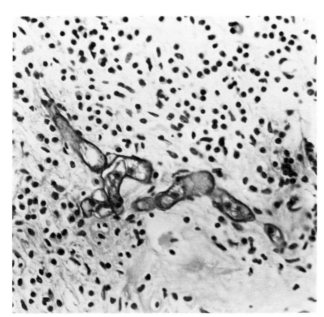

Figure 115-2. Hyphae of *B. haptosporus* in the subcutaneous tissues. Note wide hyphae and occasional septa. (Grocott, × 400.)

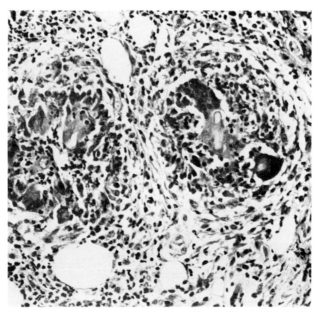

Figure 115-4. Granulomatous reaction to degenerating hyphae in the subcutaneous tissues. (H&E, × 250.)

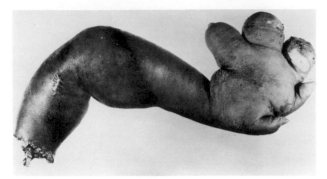

Figure 115-5. Amputated right arm of 6-year-old male Ugandan child. Subcutaneous zygomycosis.

involved. The sole of the foot and the palms of the hands are hardly ever affected, which is in marked contrast to Madura foot (mycetoma), in which the organisms are likely to be introduced by thorn pricks. The size of the lesion varies; it can be as small as a boil, or can attain grotesque dimensions, (Fig. 115-5), involving a large area of the body or a whole limb [1,8,9]. The edges of the skin lesion are usually sharply demarcated, but there may be palpable peripheral, extending nodules. The lesion is woody and hard, painless, attached to the skin, and mobile on deep structures. The overlying skin may be hyperpigmented and roughened, but it rarely ulcerates. Draining central lymph nodes may be enlarged, although not because of direct involvement by the fungus. Patients usually have no constitutional disturbances, but in a few cases ulceration, fever, and eosinophilia have been reported. Gastrointestinal lesions [10] and spread from perianal lesions into the pelvis with involvement of retroperitoneal tissues around the rectum and pelvis are occasionally seen [8].

DIAGNOSIS

The histological appearance of a chronic panniculitis with tissue eosinophilia and/or a granulomatous reaction should alert the pathologist to a diagnosis of subcutaneous zygomycosis. The histological appearance of hyphae surrounded by the eosinophilic granular material in the subcutaneous tissue is pathognomonic of *B. haptosporus,* though a similar reaction is found in cases of nasal sinus infection from a related fungus, *Conidiobolus coronatus.* In late cases with a marked granulomatous reaction, the hyphae may be fragmented and only present in giant cells, but they are still easily identified in Grocott or PAS-stained sections. In a suspected case, material from the lesion may be inoculated on Sabouraud's medium. The organism usually grows better at 37°C than at 25°C, although it is capable of growing at 40°C. Isolates from different patients may have different optimal growth temperature [6]. On Sabouraud's agar, glabrous, radially folded gray to yellowish colonies are followed by the appearance of a white bloom which is due to short aerial hyphae, sporangia, chlamydos-

pores, and zygospores. Most isolates form smooth-walled zygospores [4].

TREATMENT

The evaluation of drugs used in the treatment of subcutaneous zygomycosis is difficult because in some patients the disease may regress spontaneously. Potassium iodide in doses of 30 mg per kilogram of body weight once a day usually causes a regression of the disease but must be continued for several weeks or even months [3,11]. Treatment with seprin alone or with hydrocortisone in spreading lesions is reported to be superior to potassium iodide. Occasional successes have been reported in patients treated with trimethoprim-sulfamethoxazole or ketoconazole. The 3-year-old girl shown in Fig. 115-6 had complete regression while receiving ketoconazole 100 mg twice a day [13]. However, the place of drugs other than iodides in therapy awaits further study.

Amputation of limbs with severe deforming lesions (Fig. 115-5) or a wide excision is, in view of recent findings, unnecessary.

POPULATION

Subcutaneous zygomycosis is a tropical disease which has been reported largely from sub-Saharan tropical Africa and some Asian countries. In Africa, the largest number of cases (70) has been reported from Uganda (Fig. 115-7), where it occurs particularly in the more arid northern regions [9]. The condition also occurs quite commonly in Nigeria [12] and Kenya [8], with a few cases reported from other western, central and east African countries [12]. From Asian countries besides Indonesia [1], it has been reported from India, Burma, and Iraq. It is assumed that spore inoculation occurs through the skin as

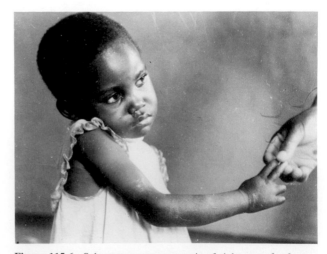

Figure 115-6. Subcutaneous zygomycosis of right arm of a 3-year-old female Ugandan before treatment.

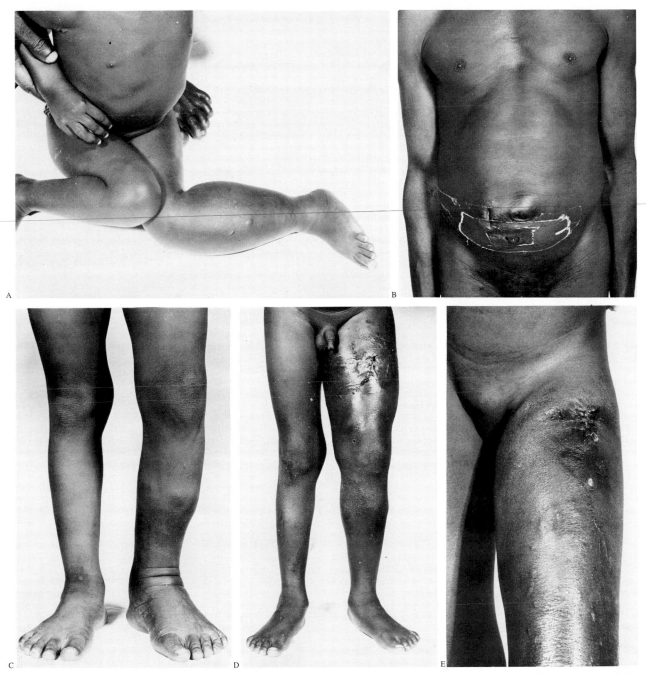

Figure 115-7. Subcutaneous zygomycosis. *A.* A 3-year-old female. Note left lower leg. *B.* Male adult Ugandan with zygomycosis of the anterior abdominal wall. *C.* An 8-year-old Ugandan male. Note left lower leg. *D.* A 10-year-old male Ugandan. Note left thigh. *E.* A 14-year-old female. Note left thigh.

a result of minor trauma, but the natural history of early infection is not established. It is possible that the fungus sometimes gains entry through the skin from leaves which are used instead of toilet paper after defecation, or when naked skin comes in contact with contaminated soil. Insect bites have also been suggested as a route of infection. The disease is usually seen in children, and over half the cases reported have been below 10 years. Although the frequency falls off with advancing age, a few cases in patients in their sixties have occurred. There is a predominance of male over female patients.

REFERENCES

1 Lei Kian Joe, et al: *Basidiobolus ranarum* as a cause of subcutaneous phycomycosis in Indonesia. Arch Derm Syph 74:378–383, 1956

2 Raper AB: Subcutaneous granuloma of unknown aetiology. East Afr Med J 33:365–366, 1956

3 Burkitt DP, Wilson AMM, Jelliffe DB: Subcutaneous phycomycosis: A review of 31 cases seen in Uganda. Br Med J 1:1669–1672, 1964

4 Greer DL, Friedman L: Studies of the genus *Basidiobolus* with reclassification of the species pathogenic to man. Sabouraudia 4:231–241, 1966

5 Yangco BG, Nettlow A, Okofor JI, et al: Comparative antigenic studies of species of *Basidiobolus* and other medically important fungi. J Clin Microbiol April 23(4), 1986, pp 679–682

6 Clark BM: The epidemiology of phycomycosis, in Wolstenholme GEW, Porter R (eds): *Systemic Mycoses*. London, Churchill, 1968, pp 179–192

7 Williams A, Lichtenberg FV, Smith JH, et al: Ultrastructure of phycomycosis. Arch Pathol 87:459–468, 1969

8 Cameroon HM, Gatei D, Bremner AD: The deep mycoses in Kenya, a histopathological study. 2. Phycomycosis. East Afr Med J 50: 396–405, 1973

9 Mugerwa JW: Subcutaneous phycomycosis in Uganda. Br Dermatol 94:539–544, 1976

10 Schmidt JH, Howard RJ, Chen JL, et al: First culture-proven gastrointestinal entermophthoramycosis in the United States: A case report and review of the literature. Mycopathologia Ang. 95:101–104, 1986

11 Kelly S, Gill N, Hutt MSR: Subcutaneous phycomycosis in Sierra Leone. Trans R Soc Trop Med Hyg 74:396–397, 1980

12 Clark BM: The epidemiology of entomophthoromycosis, in Al-Doory (ed): *The Epidemiology of Human Mycotic Diseases*. Springfield, Illinois, Charles C Thomas, 1975, pp 178–196

13 Okello DO: Personal communication, 1988

CHAPTER 116 / *Treatment of the Systemic Mycoses* · Edward C. Oldfield, III

AMPHOTERICIN B

Amphotericin B, first introduced in 1956, remains the standard therapeutic agent for the treatment of most of the deep mycoses. It has maintained this position despite its formidable and essentially unavoidable toxicity. Amphotericin B is a product of *Streptomyces nodosus,* originally isolated from a soil sample from the Orinoco River region of Venezuela, and a member of the class of antibiotics called *macrolide polyenes.* The polyene structure accounts for its unique properties and is felt to be responsible for both the therapeutic and the toxic effects of the drug.

MECHANISM OF ACTION

All cells susceptible to polyenes contain sterols in their membranes [*1*]. The major function of these sterols is maintenance of membrane integrity. Interaction of amphotericin B with membrane sterols leads to an alteration of membrane permeability with leakage of intracellular contents such as potassium. In the fungi, the primary sterol is ergosterol, while in humans it is cholesterol. The interaction with ergosterol is responsible for the therapeutic effect, while that with cholesterol is probably responsible for some of the toxicity. This sterol interaction also explains the total lack of activity against bacteria, which do not contain sterols in their cell membranes.

SENSITIVE ORGANISMS

Amphotericin B is a broad-spectrum antifungal agent. Most of the fungi responsible for systemic mycotic infections are sensitive. These include *Histoplasma capsulatum, Cryptococcus neoformans, Coccidioides immitis, Blastomyces dermatitidis, Candida* species, *Torulopsis glabrata, Aspergillus species, Sporothrix schenckii, Paracoccidioides brasiliensis,* and the causative agents of mucormycoses.

Interpretation of data on minimum inhibitory concentrations (MIC) is difficult, largely because of a lack of standardization among laboratories on important details of testing and the variance between clinical response and in vitro results. Even when laboratories with a special interest in fungal susceptibility testing used the same isolates and very similar methodology, the difference in MIC between laboratories was marked, varying 8- to 32-fold [*2*]. It would seem that there is little to be gained clinically by susceptibility testing or measurement of serum levels of amphotericin B at the present time.

Activity has also been noted against a number of protozoan pathogens, including trichomonads, *Entamoeba, Naegleria, Leishmania,* and trypanosomes [*3*].

RESISTANCE

The development of clinical resistance during therapy has not been a problem. The organisms isolated from patients who have been treated with amphotericin B and subsequently relapsed have been as sensitive as the previously isolated organisms.

Resistance remains rare among *Candida* species, but has been well reported. This is especially true for isolates from patients with extensive chemotherapy, prolonged neutropenia, and treatment with polyenes [4]. This resistance has almost always been associated with a marked loss of ergosterol from the cell membrane. *Candida lusitaniae* appears to be the most resistant, while *Candida parapsilosis* has been reported to show tolerance to amphotericin B [2]. Among the filamentous fungi, *Pseudallescheria boydii* and *Fusarium* species do not respond clinically or in vitro to amphotericin B.

Of increasing concern are reports that the combined use of ketoconazole and amphotericin B may lead to resistance to amphotericin B by ketoconazole inhibition of ergosterol synthesis in both *Candida* and *Aspergillus* [5].

SYNERGISM

Amphotericin B has been shown to be synergistic with a number of antibiotics which normally have no effect against fungi because of their inability to penetrate the cytoplasmic membranes of the organisms. Alteration of the permeability of the fungus by amphotericin B might allow an increased penetration of the second agent. This enhancement of activity has been demonstrated in animal models for rifampin, tetracycline, and minocycline against a variety of fungi [6]. However, the clinical importance of this enhancement has not been established in human studies. (See ''Flucytosine'' for clinical uses of synergism.)

PHARMACOLOGICAL PROPERTIES

Peak serum concentrations of amphotericin B with standard therapeutic doses are in the range of 0.5 to 2.0 µg/mL and are usually consistent from patient to patient [7]. Only 10 percent of an injected dose can be found in the serum immediately after termination of an infusion [7]. The fate of the drug within the body is unknown, and no metabolites have been identified [8]. Amphotericin B is 95 percent bound to serum proteins, predominantly lipoproteins. There is an initial rapid elimination with a half-life of 24 h, followed by a more prolonged terminal phase of elimination with a half-life of 15 days [8]. The drug can usually be detected in serum or urine for 4 weeks or more after completion of therapy. Renal excretion is minimal, being only 3 to 5 percent of total drug elimination [8,9]. Importantly, there is no significant increase in amphotericin B serum levels with decreased renal function or in the anephric patient, and disappearance from serum is similar to that in patients with normal renal function [7]. Therefore, no dosage reduction is necessary with renal insufficiency to avoid accumulation of the drug in serum. However, a dosage reduction may be necessary to avoid further progression of nephrotoxicity. It should be noted that this will lead to a reduction in

serum levels. Amphotericin B is not removed by hemodialysis or peritoneal dialysis [10]. Biliary excretion has been noted to be 19 percent [11], and hepatic failure has not been felt to affect serum levels or to be an indication for dosage reduction.

Amphotericin B is very poorly absorbed from the gastrointestinal tract. Doses up to 5 g have resulted in inadequate serum levels, varying from 0.04 to 0.5 µg/mL [9].

Penetration into body fluids

Cerebrospinal fluid (CSF) penetration has been poor with both inflamed and noninflamed meninges. The CSF levels are 30 to 50 times lower than concomitant serum levels [9]. The concentration of amphotericin B in pleural, peritoneal, and synovial fluid is approximately two-thirds of trough serum levels. In the inflamed eye, the concentration in aqueous humor is also about two-thirds of trough serum levels, but vitreous humor penetration is poor. Urine concentrations are similar to those of serum.

PREPARATIONS

Amphotericin B (Fungizone, Squibb) is available as a sterile lyophilized powder for intravenous use in vials containing 50 mg of amphotericin B plus 41 mg of deoxycholate to create a colloidal dispersion of the insoluble antibiotic. It is reconstituted with 10 mL of sterile water (without a bacteriostatic agent) and is added to 5% dextrose in water. It is important to note that addition of as little as 1.5 meq of sodium chloride will aggregate the colloidal drug and lead to the prompt appearance of turbidity [12]. Cloudy solutions probably give poorer serum drug levels and should not be infused. Therefore, amphotericin B should not be mixed with electrolytes, preservatives, or acid solutions. The addition of heparin or hydrocortisone in an attempt to reduce toxic reactions does not result in loss of activity over 24 h [12].

Although amphotericin B is light-sensitive, it has been shown that there is no appreciable loss of activity on exposure to fluorescent light for up to 24 h at 25°C (room temperature) [12]. Therefore, no special precautions are needed to protect the amphotericin B during infusion. More prolonged exposure to light for 3 to 15 days has been shown to cause a definite reduction in activity, but these precautions are more relevant to storage by the pharmacy or on nursing units. Because amphotericin B is a colloidal suspension, the use of in-line membrane filters of less than 1.0 µm may result in significant loss of active drug and should be avoided.

The formidable toxicity of amphotericin B has resulted in attempts to develop less toxic formulations. Amphotericin B methylester hydrochloride is a water-soluble derivative which appears to be only one-eighth to one-twenty-fifth as toxic as the parent compound in animal studies. Unfortunately, in clinical studies a high incidence of progressive neurological deterioration has been noted which appears dose-related. Pathologically, diffuse white matter degeneration was noted [13].

More promising is liposomal amphotericin B. Incorporation of amphotericin B into phospholipid-containing liposomes has markedly decreased toxicity to mammalian cells while maintaining toxicity to fungal cells. Infusions of up to 5 mg/kg over 5 to 20 min are well-tolerated, and early clinical data are encouraging [14].

Initiation of therapy

The decision to initiate therapy with amphotericin B must always include careful evaluation of the expected benefits balanced against the toxicity of the drug. Therapy is initiated with a test dose of 1 mg to evaluate the extent of the commonly encountered infusion-related reactions. This dose is given in 5% dextrose over 10 to 20 min intravenously. The vital signs should be monitored closely during the initial infusion. The rapidity of subsequent dosage increments to a full therapeutic dose of 0.3 to 1.0 mg/kg is determined by the severity of the toxic reaction balanced by the severity of the fungal infection. For chronic or indolent fungal disease, it has been traditional to increase the dose daily until the desired level is reached. For instance, the daily dose of amphotericin B is increased from 1 mg on the first day to 5-, 10-, 20-, and 30-mg doses in 500 mL of 5% dextrose on days 2, 3, 4, and 5, respectively. Duration of infusion is commonly 2 to 3 h [15], or up to 6 h. In cases where the disease is of a fulminating nature, more rapid attainment of therapeutic dosage is necessary. One method has been to place amphotericin B, 0.3 mg/kg in 500 mL of 5% dextrose in water and infuse 25 mL (1.0 mg of amphotericin B) over 10 to 15 min as a test dose. If no severe reactions are encountered, the remainder can be infused over 2 h with frequent monitoring of vital signs [15].

The rapidity of escalation to a full therapeutic dose is also determined by the severity of the toxic reactions encountered, which may include fever, violent chills, sweating, prostration, dyspnea, cyanosis, hypotension, or delirium. The severity of these reactions is variable, but reactions are more pronounced with preexisting fever, cardiac, or pulmonary disease. The addition of 25 mg hydrocortisone to the infusion bottle can be used to decrease these untoward effects. This dose has been shown to decrease the frequency but not the severity of fever and chills from 78 to 56 percent; increasing the dose of hydrocortisone to 50 mg does not result in a further reduction in reactions [16]. Oral prednisone should probably be avoided because of its long half-life. Combined oral premedication with aspirin and diphenhydramine does not further reduce reactions, but routine premedication with these agents is a common practice in many centers. If toxic reactions are not noted, the hydrocortisone should be excluded. Tolerance to the febrile reactions will often develop with time, allowing a decrease or discontinuation of hydrocortisone. It has been noted that meperidine hydrochloride in a mean dose of 45 mg is more effective in eliminating chills and fever than stopping the infu-

sion [17]. Meperidine has also been used prior to the infusion in an attempt to prevent rigors. Dantrolene has also been noted to reduce rigors. Because amphotericin B is a potent inducer of prostaglandin E_2 synthesis in peripheral blood mononuclear cells, ibuprofen at a dose of 10 mg/kg, or a maximum of 600 mg, has been used to prevent infusion-related side effects. Ibuprofen administered 30 min prior to the amphotericin B infusion reduced the incidence of chills in patients having reactions from 87 to 49 percent and of severe chills from 69 to 15 percent [18]. Although no toxicity was noted in the study, ibuprofen has multiple potential adverse effects on the kidney which could possibly enhance amphotericin B–induced nephrotoxicity. The renal effects of ibuprofen include a reduction in renal blood flow and glomerular filtration rate as well as tubular toxicity, which is enhanced in patients with preexisting renal toxicity [19]. Heparin, 500 to 1000 U, is commonly added to the infusion to decrease the incidence of phlebitis.

Maintenance of therapy

Total daily dosage recommendations are variable depending on the fungus, the use of synergistic drugs, and severity of disease. The usual recommended dose is 0.3 to 1.0 mg/(kg·day), not exceeding 50 mg/day. If the patient does not require other intravenous medications, it is best to remove the needle after each infusion to decrease the incidence of phlebitis and preserve venous access. The duration of the infusion is commonly 2 to 3 h, although others have recommended 4 to 6 h or as tolerated by the patient [15]. One study reported the use of 1-h infusions and noted a decreased incidence of nausea and chills without serious arrhythmias or any increase in renal dysfunction [20]. More rapid infusions are usually avoided because of fatal cardiac arrhythmias noted in dogs given rapid infusions.

The use of a double dose on alternate days (usually not exceeding 70 mg) has been shown to be equally efficacious. The trough concentrations have been shown to be similar, and the peak concentrations with either regimen have a tendency to plateau at doses exceeding 50 mg. There is no reduction in renal toxicity with alternate-day therapy, but patients usually feel better on the off day, and it is especially convenient for prolonged outpatient therapy.

The development of toxicity is to be expected and can be monitored by twice-weekly measurements of serum creatinine, blood urea nitrogen, serum magnesium and potassium; and hematocrit.

Duration of therapy is variable and depends on the particular fungus, anatomical site of involvement, and clinical response.

Intrathecal therapy

Intrathecal therapy may be required for fungal meningitis because of the poor CSF levels obtained with intravenous amphotericin B. All cases of coccidioidal meningitis require intrathecal therapy. Only special cases of cryptococcal meningitis require this form of therapy. Treatment is commonly begun on a thrice-weekly schedule, although some researchers have suggested that daily injections may be needed to maintain therapeutic levels [21]. An initial intrathecal dose of 0.1 mg is often used, followed by 0.1-mg increments until a total daily dose of 0.5 mg has been reached [15]. Recent experience in treating coccidioidal meningitis suggests that maintenance doses of 1.0 mg may be associated with better outcomes. Lumbar injections may be followed by a number of toxic reactions, including radicular pain, urinary retention, lower extremity monoparesis, paraparesis, paresthesias, and acute toxic delirium [15]. The etiology of these symptoms is unknown; some postulate an arachnoiditis while others suggest a vascular etiology. Hydrocortisone hemisuccinate (10 to 25 mg) may be added to the injection to decrease radicular pain. Some authors have recommended infusion with hyperbaric 10% glucose solutions in combination with a head-down position to reduce radiculitis and improve flow to the basilar meninges [22]. As therapy is continued, an arachnoiditis commonly develops making instillation increasingly difficult in the lumbar region. Cisterna magna injections have been used, but the high potential for serious complications in inexperienced hands makes this approach less satisfactory.

Some centers have utilized the implantation of siliconized rubber subcutaneous reservoirs connected by tubing to the lateral ventricle. Unfortunately, this has not proved to be a panacea because of the high incidence of untoward effects related to the reservoir. These effects have included hemiparesis, intracranial hemorrhage, bacterial meningitis, wound infections, nonfunctioning tubing, and, possibly, persistence of fungal meningitis secondary to the reservoir serving as a foreign body [23]. Nonetheless, some centers have reported a low incidence of complications associated with insertion and use of subcutaneous reservoirs [24].

Other routes of administration

Intraperitoneal administration has been recommended at a dose of 1 mg added to 1000 mL of dialysis fluid. Bladder irrigation may be accomplished with 50 mg in 1000 mL of sterile water. Intraarticular use has been reported in the treatment of coccidioidal arthritis in doses of 25 to 50 mg per injection, particularly for knee joints, while others have recommended intraarticular doses of 5 to 15 mg. The injection itself has been noted to cause acute inflammation. Ocular penetration is poor with intravenous administration, and direct intravitreous administration has led to retinal necrosis and detachment in rabbits even at very low doses. For a detailed discussion of the use of amphotericin B in ophthalmology see Ref. 25.

TOXICITY

Almost all patients treated with amphotericin B will develop some form of toxicity. Despite this formidable toxicity, with appropriate management most patients can complete a therapeutic course. In general, toxicity appears to be similar or milder in children and infants [26].

General

Generalized side effects associated with the infusion of amphotericin B have been noted in 78 to 93 percent of patients. These include fever (occasionally in excess of 40°C), chills or severe rigors, headache, anorexia, nausea, and vomiting. Idiosyncratic reactions have been noted including anaphylactoid shock, flushing, vertigo, cardiac arrhythmias, seizures, and generalized pain [30].

Renal

The most severe form of amphotericin B toxicity is renal. During an average course of therapy, it is common for the serum creatinine level to rise to the range of 2.0 to 3.0 mg/dL. In many cases, the serum creatinine level will plateau in this range, while in others it will continue to rise. In some series, more than 80 percent of patients developed significant alteration in renal function [27]. There is usually a significant correlation between the total dose of amphotericin B and the permanent rise in serum creatinine level. In patients who receive a total dose of amphotericin B of less than 4 g, the renal insufficiency is usually reversible. However, in those receiving greater than 4 or 5 g, persistent abnormalities have been noted in 44 and 88 percent, respectively [27]. One study has suggested that the combination of gentamicin with amphotericin B may enhance this already formidable nephrotoxicity. Pathologically, the most consistently observed lesions are focal calcifications, both intratubular and interstitial, associated with degenerative changes of tubules. Glomerular lesions are more variable, and in one series no specific glomerular lesions were noted on renal biopsy by light or electron microscopy [28].

The mechanism of the nephrotoxicity has been postulated to be a result of a combination of direct tubular damage, primarily distal, and renal artery constriction [28]. Studies of renal function have shown a consistent decrease in glomerular filtration rate and decreased renal blood flow [29]. There has been a consistent impairment of distal tubular function with an increased potassium clearance, and the development of renal tubular acidosis with decreased hydrogen ion secretion. A vasopressin-resistant renal concentrating defect has also been noted, manifested by polyuria in excess of 4 L/day. The urine sediment has consisted of white blood cells without red blood cells, casts, macroscopic hematuria, or significant proteinuria.

The use of mannitol has been suggested as a means of decreasing nephrotoxicity by preventing the amphotericin B–induced decrease in renal blood flow. However, a double-blind controlled study showed no protective action [29], and at present mannitol is not used with amphotericin B. Once the creatinine level rises above 3.0 mg/dL, it may be advisable to discontinue the amphotericin B infusion for a few days or to decrease the dose to prevent further decrease in glomerular filtration and the associated problems of uremia.

Renal toxicity appears to be enhanced by intravascular volume depletion whether secondary to low sodium intake, diuretics, vomiting, or cirrhosis with ascites. Correcting volume depletion by rehydration, high-salt diet, discontinuing diuretics, or volume expansion has been noted to improve renal function. Even patients who are not volume-depleted may benefit by an infusion of intravenous saline on the day they receive amphotericin B, provided they do not have conditions which contraindicate sodium loading [31].

Hematological

Anemia is another common side effect. In one study, a decrease in hematocrit of 10 U was noted in 76 percent of patients, and a drop of 15 U or greater in 33 percent [30]. The anemia is normochromic and normocytic. There is no correlation with the degree of azotemia or total dose of drug. Usually the hematocrit decreases early in therapy to between 20 and 30 U and then stabilizes; there is no reticulocytosis, and chromium-51 red cell survival studies show no shortening of survival time. The bone marrow usually reveals normal erythroid activity, but erythropoietin levels are consistently much lower than would be expected for the degree of anemia. Transfusions have not been shown to be beneficial; with transfusions, the hematocrit has gradually returned to the pretransfusion level. After therapy, the hematocrit almost always returns to pretreatment levels. Thrombocytopenia has occasionally been noted, and neutropenia occurs very rarely.

Electrolyte abnormalities

A significant decrease in serum potassium concentration requiring oral supplementation occurs in about 25 percent of patients. Hypomagnesemia has also been noted. Both occur as a result of tubular defects with resultant decrease in potassium and magnesium reabsorption.

Allergic reactions

Amphotericin B is remarkably free of allergic reactions. Because reported cases of well-documented drug eruptions are so rare, a rash appearing during therapy can usually be attributed to some other cause.

Hepatic

Alteration in hepatic function has rarely been reported.

Pregnancy

Amphotericin B has been used during pregnancy without evidence of teratogenesis or persistent toxicity in infants [32]. Treatment of a pregnant woman should not be considered an indication for termination of pregnancy.

THERAPEUTIC INDICATIONS

For specific indications, dosage, and duration of therapy refer to the chapter on the particular fungal disease.

FLUCYTOSINE (5-FLUOROCYTOSINE)

Flucytosine is a narrow-spectrum oral antifungal drug first synthesized in 1957 as an antitumor agent. It is a fluorinated pyrimidine used primarily today in combination with amphotericin B to provide an additive or synergistic effect against certain fungi.

MECHANISM OF ACTION

Flucytosine enters the fungal cell by means of cytosine permease and is then deaminated by cytosine deaminase to 5-fluorouracil, a commonly used antitumor agent. The effectiveness of flucytosine appears to be limited to cells which possess cytosine deaminase. Studies of human liver, mucosal, and bone marrow cells have failed to detect this enzyme [33]. This may explain the relatively low toxicity of this agent. 5-Fluorouracil is incorporated into fungal RNA as 5-fluorouridine triphosphate, replacing up to 50 percent of the normal uracil. Flucytosine has also been noted to block thymidylate synthetase by the formation of 5-fluorodeoxyuridine monophosphate, leading to a decrease in DNA synthesis [34]. The relative importance of these two mechanisms has not been determined at present.

SENSITIVE ORGANISMS

Flucytosine has a limited spectrum, with its most important activity directed against *Cryptococcus neoformans, Candida albicans* and some other *Candida* species, *Torulopsis glabrata,* and the causative agents of chromomycosis. Variable activity has been noted against *Aspergillus fumigatus*. In performing sensitivity tests, it should be noted that the antifungal activity of flucytosine is markedly inhibited by the presence of peptones or beef and yeast extracts. Therefore, Sabouraud's medium is inappropriate, and media such as Bacto Yeast-Nitrogen Base (Difco) with the addition of 1% glucose are appropriate [33].

Resistance

Primary resistance among *C. neoformans* and *Torulopsis* species has been rare, with respectively, 98 and more than 90 percent of initial isolates being sensitive. If resistance is defined as an MIC $\geq$ 12.5 μg/mL after 2 days of incubation, the resistance rate for *C. albicans* varies from 11.5 to 35 percent [36]. Resistance has been lower in Europe, ranging from 4.5 to 11.7 percent.

Primary resistance occurs through spontaneous mutation and may be secondary to an enzyme deficiency at any step in the metabolic pathway or to an increased synthesis of pyrimidines.

These mutants are genetically stable and do not appear to have decreased pathogenicity. Increasing data suggest the possibility that *C. albicans* isolates are diploid and that as many as 37 percent of strains may have heterozygosity for resistance and are capable of giving rise to resistant variants at high frequency by segregation [37].

Secondary resistance has been a considerable problem with flucytosine [38] and is the primary reason why it is rarely used alone. This is the most common cause of treatment failures and relapses, especially after an initial encouraging clinical response. As many as two-thirds of isolates cultured during therapy have been resistant. Secondary resistance occurs by the same mechanisms as primary resistance and is related to selection of resistant strains by the suppression of sensitive ones, rather than by drug induction [38]. When tested, all flucytosine-resistant isolates are sensitive to amphotericin B.

Synergism

The synergism of flucytosine with amphotericin B has provided the most important uses for this drug. This synergism has been noted with *C. neoformans* and with *Candida* species. An additive or synergistic effect with amphotericin B has been noted in 86 percent of *Candida* species resistant to flucytosine alone.

PHARMACOKINETICS

Absorption of flucytosine after oral administration is 76 to 89 percent. Ingestion with meals decreases the rate but not the total absorption. In the presence of renal failure, absorption remains excellent and similar to that of normal persons. The peak serum concentration ranges from 50 to 100 μg/mL with a dose of 37.5 mg/kg every 6 h. Binding to serum proteins is negligible.

Flucytosine concentrations in liver, kidney, spleen, heart, and lung tissue have been noted to be equal to or greater than serum concentrations. CSF concentrations have been reported to vary from 50 percent of simultaneous serum levels to approximately the same as serum, with an average of 75 percent [39]. Concentrations similar to those in serum have also been noted in bone, peritoneal fluid, and joint fluid. Flucytosine concentrations in urine are markedly higher than in serum, in the range of 1000 to 2000 μg/mL. Although urine levels decrease proportionally with increasing renal insufficiency, the levels have been adequate even with severely impaired renal function [40].

Excretion of flucytosine is primarily by glomerular filtration. There is very minimal metabolism (1 percent) in humans, with 98 percent of the absorbed drug excreted unchanged in the urine [41]. The half-life is 3 to 4 h with normal renal function but is prolonged even with minor degrees of renal insufficiency. The clearance is about 75 percent of that of creatinine with a positive linear correlation between serum creatinine level and the half-life of flucytosine. Hemodialysis very effectively removes flucytosine at the same rate as creatinine [10].

Peritoneal dialysis also removes significant amounts of drug. Hepatic disease does not alter drug excretion or result in accumulation in serum.

DOSAGE AND ADMINISTRATION

Flucytosine is manufactured by Hoffman-LaRoche as Ancobon in capsules of 250 and 500 mg. The standard daily dosage is 150 mg/kg divided into four doses of 37.5 mg/kg each. This dose will usually maintain serum levels above 25 μg/mL and below the toxic level of 100 to 125 μg/mL.

It is critical that the dose be adjusted in the presence of renal insufficiency, as even mild azotemia has been noted to cause significant increases in serum levels of flucytosine. In one study, with patients receiving 150 mg/(kg·day), the mean serum level with creatinine concentration less than 1.4 mg/dL was 78 mg/L, versus a serum level of 119 mg/L with a creatinine concentration between 1.4 and 1.9 mg/dL [42]. Recommendations for dosage adjustment from a large treatment trial of cryptococcal meningitis (194 patients) were for a dose of 150 mg/(kg·day) with a creatinine clearance (CrCl) above 50 mL/min, 75 mg/(kg·day) with a CrCl between 26 and 50 mL/min, and 37 mg/(kg·day) with a CrCl between 13 and 25 mL/min [43]. Because there is no metabolism of flucytosine, with rapid decreases in renal function dialysis may be required to remove the drug [44]. For patients on hemodialysis, a dose of 37.5 mg/kg after each dialysis has been recommended. Others have recommended a lower dose of 20 mg/kg after dialysis. Serum flucytosine levels should be monitored in patients with renal insufficiency.

During treatment, it is essential to monitor the platelet count, white blood cell count, creatinine and blood urea nitrogen levels, and liver function tests twice weekly. Particular caution must be used when flucytosine is used with preexisting neutropenia, renal insufficiency, or liver disease, although none of these are absolute contraindications to usage of the drug. One study has shown no increase in bone marrow toxicity with hematological malignancies or immunosuppressive therapy [43].

TOXICITY

Flucytosine has, as a rule, been well-tolerated. In one large series, 18 percent of patients experienced gastrointestinal, 7 percent hepatic, and 18 percent hematological complications [43].

The gastrointestinal toxicity is most commonly nausea, vomiting, and diarrhea. This is usually not severe, but fatal colitis with multiple perforations has been reported. Elevations of transaminases and alkaline phosphatase have been reported. These abnormalities are not usually progressive and return to normal after cessation of the drug. Preexisting liver disease has not been exacerbated by use of flucytosine.

Hematological abnormalities have included neutropenia, thrombocytopenia, or a combination of the two. This toxic effect on the bone marrow is usually reversible with decreased dosage or discontinuation of the drug, although fatal bone marrow suppression has been reported in a number of cases. Hematological toxicity has been correlated with serum levels in excess of 100 to 125 μg/mL, often in association with renal insufficiency [44]. Levels greater than 100 μg/mL should be avoided. Most authors recommend close attention to serum levels, especially with renal insufficiency which may be common during combination therapy with amphotericin B. Serum levels can be determined by bioassay and by gas-liquid chromatography.

Other reported toxicity has included eosinophilia, photosensitivity, and maculopapular rashes. Flucytosine has been teratogenic in rats and thus should be used with caution in females of childbearing age, and should be avoided in pregnancy.

The mechanism of flucytosine toxicity is unknown. In one study, 20 of 41 patients had 5-fluorouracil levels in the serum of greater than 1000 ng/mL, which is in the range noted during chemotherapy and associated with hematological toxicity [45]. The 5-fluorouracil may be derived from the metabolism of flucytosine by the intestinal microflora.

THERAPEUTIC INDICATIONS

The combined use of amphotericin B and flucytosine is the regimen of choice for cryptococcal meningitis. A prospective randomized controlled study of flucytosine plus amphotericin B versus amphotericin B alone has shown improved cure rates, fewer relapses, more rapid sterilization of the cerebrospinal fluid, and less nephrotoxicity with the two-drug regimen [42]. Flucytosine plus amphotericin B also appears indicated in disseminated cryptococcal disease and severe infections with *Candida* species, especially meningitis, and with *Torulopsis* infections [47]. The combination of amphotericin B and flucytosine allows for a decreased amphotericin B dose and, hence, a decrease in renal toxicity and a decreased duration of therapy. The presence of amphotericin B also decreases the possibility of emerging flucytosine resistance but may increase flucytosine toxicity [33]. In the treatment of the deep mycoses, there appear to be few indications for flucytosine alone. Chromomycosis may be an indication for flucytosine alone, and some have used flucytosine alone to treat urinary candidiasis, but eradication was not successful in those patients with an indwelling Foley catheter [49].

KETOCONAZOLE

Ketoconazole is a synthetic imidazole with a broad antifungal spectrum. It was first introduced for the treatment of deep mycoses in 1977 and released for general use in 1981. Ketoconazole is the most important new antifungal agent since the introduction of amphotericin B in the 1950s. Ketoconazole offers many advantages over amphotericin B including a single daily oral dose, minimal side effects, and the potential for prolonged outpatient treatment.

MECHANISM OF ACTION

Ketoconazole has been shown to be a potent inhibitor of ergosterol synthesis, the major membrane sterol of fungi [50]. This is thought to be due to inhibition of the removal of the 14-α-methyl group from lanosterol, an ergosterol precursor. Other effects include inhibition of triglyceride and phospholipid biosynthesis and suppression of peroxidase and catalase activity leading to intracellular accumulation of toxic hydrogen peroxide [51]. Ketoconazole has been found to enhance the action of neutrophils against *Candida*, presumably by preventing transformation of the yeast phase to the mycelial phase, which is much more difficult for the neutrophil to kill. A possible explanation for the minimal toxicity of ketoconazole is the 600 times higher concentration needed to inhibit sterol synthesis of mammalian cells as compared to fungal cells [51].

SENSITIVE ORGANISMS

Ketoconazole is a very broad spectrum antifungal agent, active against many of the dermatophytes, yeasts, and dimorphic fungi. *Blastomyces dermatitidis* and *Histoplasma capsulatum* are highly sensitive, with MICs ≤ 0.39 μg/mL; *Coccidioides immitis* has intermediate sensitivity, with some strains resistant to 100 μg/mL. *Cryptococcus neoformans*, *Sporothrix schenckii*, and *Aspergillus* species are less sensitive, with many resistant strains [54]. There is also some activity against gram-positive bacteria, *Leishmania*, *Trypanosoma cruzi*, and *Plasmodium falciparum*.

Interpretation of MICs is difficult and varies among different laboratories depending on many factors related to incubation duration, medium composition, and phase of the fungus. Furthermore, in some instances there appears to be a dissociation between in vitro and in vivo results [54]. The impressive in vivo effects of ketoconazole could not have been predicted with the classical in vitro test models. Using these test models, the drug would have been rejected for further study [53].

Synergism with other antifungal agents cannot usually be detected in vitro. Resistance developing during therapy, or in patients who have relapsed, has not been noted as a clinical problem. The response of a patient to ketoconazole seems to be unchanged by previous failure of other antifungal agents.

PHARMACOKINETICS

Ketoconazole is supplied as a 200-mg tablet for oral use (Nizoral, Janssen Pharmaceutica). Peak serum concentrations occur 2 to 4 h after oral administration with levels of 2 to 4, 6 to 8, and 8 to 10 μg/mL after doses of 200, 400, and 800 mg. Ketoconazole is a base which is converted in the gastric acid to a hydrochloride salt. It requires sufficient gastric acid for dissolution and complete absorption. Concomitant use of drugs that lower gastric acidity should be avoided. If their use is felt to be mandatory, administration should be 2 h after the dose of ketoconazole. In cases of achlorhydria, the manufacturer has recommended dissolving ketoconazole in 4 mL aqueous solution of 0.2 N HCl and ingesting through a straw to protect tooth enamel. Administration with meals has been noted by some authors to decrease absorption, while others have noted no effect [55,56].

Following oral administration, ketoconazole is extensively metabolized; only 2 to 4 percent of the dose is excreted unchanged in the urine [57]. The half-life is biphasic with a first phase of 1.4 to 2.2 h and a second phase of 7 to 10 h. The half-life is not prolonged in renal insufficiency; therefore, no dosage adjustment is indicated with reduced function. The need for and amount of dose reduction with abnormal liver function has not been determined. Protein binding is in excess of 90 percent, and urine concentrations are low, only about 0.4 μg/mL. Concentrations in CSF have been low, only 2 to 4 percent of serum levels, and failures have been reported in the treatment of fungal meningitis. Some data have demonstrated that ketoconazole may have a role in long-term suppression of meningeal infections at doses of 800 to 1200 mg/day [58]. Only minimal levels of ketoconazole can be detected in the peritoneal fluid of patients on chronic peritoneal dialysis, and serum levels are not altered by hemodialysis.

DRUG INTERACTIONS

The drug does not interfere with warfarin metabolism, and there is no evidence for induction of hepatic microsomal enzymes with repeated doses as occurs with clotrimazole [57]. Rifampin, by induction of hepatic microsomal enzymes, decreases ketoconazole levels. The addition of isoniazid further depresses ketoconazole serum levels. Conversely, ketoconazole decreases serum rifampin levels [59]. The combination of cyclosporin and ketoconazole in organ transplant patients has resulted in substantial elevations of serum cyclosporin levels [60]. Other drug interactions include decreased clearance of methylprednisolone by inhibition of excretion, decreased clearance of chlordiazepoxide by 38 percent, and a possible disulfiram-like reaction with alcohol.

TOXICITY

One of the most consistently impressive aspects of ketoconazole therapy, especially in comparison to other antifungal agents, has been the lack of significant toxicity. The most common side effect has been nausea and or vomiting in about 20 percent. The incidence increases as dosage is increased, but often decreases with continued therapy and when administered with meals. Pruritus and abdominal pain have been noted in 1.7 percent of patients. Other less common side effects include diarrhea, dizziness, somnolence, rash, and headache. Side effects severe enough to stop therapy have been noted in only 2 percent of patients [53].

Hepatitis is the most common serious toxicity associated with ketoconazole. The incidence of symptomatic hepatotoxicity has been estimated to be 1 in 15,000 exposed individuals [60]. The hepatitis appears to be idiosyncratic, and in many ways appears similar to hepatitis caused by isoniazid. The hepatitis is most common in women over 40 years of age and has been reported as early as at 10 days or as late as at 219 days of therapy with a mean of 49 days. It is not associated with rash or eosinophilia. The hepatitis is most commonly manifested as hepatocellular damage, but may be cholestatic or mixed. Chronic hepatitis has not been reported. Fatalities have been reported, and have occurred even when ketoconazole was stopped prior to the onset of jaundice. In addition, mild, asymptomatic, and reversible elevations of liver function tests occur in about 12 percent of patients [60]. Monitoring of liver function tests every 2 weeks for the first 2 months of therapy and then monthly or bimonthly has been recommended [60]. If biochemical abnormalities develop, closer monitoring is indicated. If there is a continued rise in transaminases to three to five times normal or the development of clinical symptoms or jaundice, ketoconazole should be discontinued immediately.

Ketoconazole has multiple interactions with the endocrine system which are dose-dependent and usually reversible. The mechanism of the endocrine effects of ketoconazole is a dose-dependent inhibition of mitochondrial cytochrome P_{450} enzymes. Multiple enzymes involved in steroid hormone synthesis are inhibited, including C_{17-20} lyase, cholesterol side chain cleavage, and 11-β and 18 hydroxylation [61].

The inhibition of testosterone synthesis has resulted in gynecomastia, decreased libido, impotence, and azoospermia. It has also resulted in the use of ketoconazole in the treatment of prostate cancer, precocious puberty, and hirsutism. Inhibition of cortisol synthesis has rarely led to adrenal insufficiency in the doses commonly used to treat fungal infections, but higher doses have been used in the treatment of Cushing's syndrome and metastatic adrenal carcinoma. Other endocrine effects include decreased serum cholesterol levels, decreased 1,25-dihydroxyvitamin D levels, and hypothyroidism.

Inhibition of testosterone synthesis has occurred at doses of 200 to 400 mg each day, while cortisol inhibition has usually occurred at higher doses (600 to 1200 mg). The inhibition of hormone synthesis persists for 8 to 16 h after a single dose and is increased by split doses. Because of this, treatment of fungal infections should usually be by single daily dose to decrease endocrine side effects.

Teratogenic and embryotoxic effects have been noted in rats, but no mutagenic effect has been detected. The drug is contraindicated in pregnancy.

THERAPEUTIC USES

Ketoconazole has proved most effective in the treatment of paracoccidioidomycosis and chronic mucocutaneous candidiasis. Excellent results have been obtained with cases of histoplasmosis and blastomycosis in immunocompetent patients with infections which were not meningeal and not life-threatening [62]. Success has also been noted with *Pseudallescheria boydii,* which is resistant to amphotericin B. There have also been reports of successful therapy of some cases of chromomycosis, mycetoma due to various fungi, and entomophthoramycosis [63]. In coccidioidomycosis, there is often a suppression of clinical symptoms, but relapses may occur after years of apparently successful therapy.

Ketoconazole has been used prophylactically in neutropenic patients and critically ill surgical patients to prevent candidal infections. There has been some concern that by inhibiting ergosterol synthesis, ketoconazole may antagonize the subsequent activity of amphotericin B [5].

For specific indications, dosage, and duration of therapy, refer to the chapter on the particular fungal disease.

TRIAZOLES

Two new oral triazoles, itraconazole and fluconazole, are currently under clinical investigation [64]. Itraconazole is highly protein bound with low levels in body fluids, but high tissue levels. Clinical activity is similar to that of ketoconazole, but in addition there appears to be improved activity against the causative agents of chromomycosis, cryptococcosis, sporotrichosis, and aspergillosis. Studies to date have failed to detect inhibition of steroid hormone synthesis, as occurs commonly with ketoconazole.

In contrast, fluconazole is water-soluble, weakly protein bound, attains high cerebrospinal fluid levels (60 to 80 percent of serum levels), and is excreted unchanged in the urine with minimal metabolism. Dosage reduction is required with renal insufficiency. Fluconazole may be especially useful in fungal meningitis and urinary tract infections.

MICONAZOLE

Miconazole is a broad-spectrum antifungal agent of the imidazole class. The drug is available in topical formulations and in an intravenous form with a carrier of polyethoxylated castor oil. The commonly used dose is 600 to 1200 mg/day in three divided doses infused in 5% dextrose over a 1-h period. Toxicity includes anemia, thrombocytopenia, hyponatremia, hyperlipemia, rouleaux formation on peripheral blood smear, nausea, vomiting, and pruritus [65]. Phlebitis has been noted in up to 70 percent of patients but can be markedly decreased by the use of central venous catheters [65].

Despite a spectrum of activity similar to ketoconazole, miconazole appears to have no primary indications. The need for hospitalization, intravenous use, and increased incidence of toxicity limit its use to treatment failures with amphotericin B or ketoconazole.

REFERENCES

1 Hamilton-Miller JMT: Chemistry and biology of the polyene macrolide antibiotics. Bacteriol Rev 37:166–196, 1973

2 Drutz DJ: In vitro antifungal susceptibility testing and measurement of levels of antifungal agents in body fluids. Rev Infect Dis 9:393–397, 1987

3 Medoff G, Brajtburg J, Kobayashi GS: Antifungal agents useful in therapy of systemic fungal infections. Ann Rev Pharmacol Toxicol 23:303–330, 1983

4 Dick JD, Merz WG, Saral R: Incidence of polyene-resistant yeasts recovered from clinical specimens. Antimicrob Agents Chemother 18:158–163, 1980

5 Schaffner A, Frick PG: The effect of ketoconazole on amphotericin B in a model of disseminated aspergillosis. J Infect Dis 151:902–910, 1985

6 Kwan CN, Medoff G, Kobayashi GS, et al: Potentiation of the antifungal effects of antibiotics by amphotericin B. Antimicrob Agents Chemother 2:61–65, 1972

7 Bindschadler DD, Bennett JE: A pharmacologic guide to the clinical use of amphotericin B. J Infect Dis 120:427–436, 1969

8 Atkinson AJ, Bennett JE: Amphotericin B pharmacokinetics in humans. Antimicrob Agents Chemother 13:271–276, 1978

9 Louria DB: Some aspects of the absorption, distribution and excretion of amphotericin B in man. Antibiot Med Clin Ther 5:295–301, 1958

10 Block ER, Bennett JE, Livoti LG, et al: Flucytosine and amphotericin B: Hemodialysis effects on plasma concentration and clearance. Ann Intern Med 808:613–617, 1974

11 Craven PC, Ludden TM, Drutz DJ, et al: Excretion pathways of amphotericin B. J Infect Dis 140:329–341, 1979

12 Block ER, Bennett JE: Stability of amphotericin B in infusion bottles. Antimicrob Agents Chemother 4:648–649, 1973

13 Ellis WG, Sobel RA, Nielsen SL: Leukoencephalopathy in patients treated with Ampotericin B Methyl ester. J Infect Dis 146:125–137, 1982

14 Lopez-Berestein G, Bodey GP, Frankel LS, et al: Treatment of hepatosplenic candidiasis with liposomal-amphotericin. Br J Clin Oncol 5:310–317, 1987

15 Bennett JE: Treatment of cryptococcal, candidal, and coccidioidal meningitis, in Remington JS, Swartz MN (eds): *Current Clinical Topics in Infectious Disease.* New York, McGraw-Hill, 1980, pp 54–67

16 Tynes BS, Utz JP, Bennett JE, et al: Reducing amphotericin B reactions: A double blind study. Am Rev Respir Dis 87:264–268, 1963

17 Burks LC, Aisner J, Fortner CL, et al: Meperidine for the treatment of shaking chills and fever. Arch Intern Med 140:483–484, 1980

18 Gigliotti F, Shenep JL, Lott LL, et al: Induction of prostaglandin synthesis as the mechanism responsible for the chills and fever produced by infusing amphotericin B. J Infect Dis 156:784–789, 1987

19 Clive DM, Stoff JS: Renal syndromes associated with nonsteroidal antiinflammatory drugs. N Engl J Med 310:563–572, 1984

20 Barreuther AD, Dodge RR, Blondeaux AM: Administration of amphotericin B. Drug Intell Clin Pharm 11:368–369, 1977

21 Atkinson AJ, Bindschadler DD: Pharmacokinetics of intrathecally administered amphotericin B. Am Rev Respir Dis 99:917–924, 1969

22 Alazraki NP, Fierer J, Halpern SE, et al: Use of a hyperbaric solution for administration of intrathecal amphotericin B. N Engl J Med 290:641–646, 1974

23 Diamond RD, Bennett JE: A subcutaneous reservoir for intrathecal therapy of fungal meningitis. N Engl J Med 288:186–188, 1973

24 Polsky B, Depman MR, Gold JWM, et al: Intraventricular therapy of cryptococcal meningitis via a subcutaneous reservoir. Am J Med 81:24–28, 1986

25 Havener WH: *Ocular Pharmacology*. St. Louis, Mosby, 1983, pp 133–137

26 Starke JR, Mason EO, Kramer WG, et al: Pharmacokinetics of amphotericin B in infants and children. J Infect Dis 155:766–774, 1987

27 Butler WT, Bennett JE, Alling DW, et al: Nephrotoxicity of amphotericin B: Early and late effects in 81 patients. Ann Intern Med 61:175–187, 1964

28 Bhathena DB, Bullock WE, Luke RG: The effects of amphotericin B therapy on the intrarenal vasculature and renal tubules in man. Clin Nephrol 9:103–110, 1978

29 Bullock WE, Luke RG, Nuttall CE, et al: Can mannitol reduce amphotericin B nephrotoxicity? Double blind study and description of a new vascular lesion in kidneys. Antimicrob Agents Chemother 10:555–563, 1976

30 McCurdy DK, Frederic M, Elkinton JR: Renal tubular acidosis due to amphotericin B. N Engl J Med 278:124–131, 1968

31 Heidemann HT, Gerkens JF, Spickard WA, et al: Amphotericin B Nephrotoxicity in humans decreased by salt repletion. Am J Med 75:476–481, 1983

32 Ismail MA, Lerner SA: Disseminated blastomycosis in a pregnant woman. Am Rev Respir Dis 126:350–353, 1982

33 Scholer HJ: Flucytosine, in Speller DCE (ed): *Antifungal Chemotherapy*. New York, Wiley, 1980, pp 35–106

34 Waldorf AR, Polak A: Mechanism of action of 5-fluorocytosine. Antimicrob Agents Chemother 23:79–85, 1983

35 Bennett JE: Flucytosine. Ann Intern Med 86:319–322, 1977

36 Stiller RL, Bennett JE, Scholer HJ, et al: Susceptibility to 5-fluorocytosine and prevalence of serotype in 402 *Candida albicans* isolates from the United States. Antimicrob Agents Chemother 22:482–487, 1982

37 Defever KS, Whelan WL, Rogers AL, et al: *Candida albicans* resistance to 5-fluorocytosine: Frequency of partially resistant strains among clinical isolates. Antimicrob Agents Chemother 22:810–815, 1982

38 Block ER, Jennings AE, Bennett JE: 5 Fluorocytosine resistance in *Cryptococcus neoformans*. Antimicrob Agents Chemother 3:649–656, 1973

39 Block ER, Bennett JE: Pharmacological studies with 5-fluorocytosine. Antimicrob Agents Chemother 1:476–482, 1972

40 Dawborn JK, Page MD, Schiavone DJ: Use of 5-fluorocytosine in patients with impaired renal function. Br Med J 4:382–384, 1973

41 Schonebeck J: Mode of action and resistance to 5-fluorocytosine, in Williams JD, Geddes AM (eds): *Chemotherapy*. New York, Plenum, 1975, vol 6, pp 127–135

42 Bennett JE, Dismukes WE, Duma RJ, et al: A comparison of amphotericin B alone and combined with flucytosine in the treatment of cryptococcal meningitis. N Engl J Med 301:126–131, 1979

43 Stamm AM, Diasio RB, Dismukes WE, et al: Toxicity of amphotericin B plus flucytosine in 194 patients with cryptococcal meningitis. Am J Med 83:236–242, 1987

44 Kauffman CA, Frame PT: Bone marrow toxicity associated with 5-fluorocytosine therapy. Antimicrob Agents Chemother 11:244–247, 1977

45 Diasio RB, Lakings DE, Bennet JE: Evidence for conversion of

5-fluorocytosine to 5-fluorouracil in humans: Possible factor in 5-fluorocystine toxicity. Antimicrob Agents Chemother 14:903–908, 1978

46 Washburn RG, Klym DM, Kroll MH, et al: Rapid enzymatic method for measurement of serum flucytosine levels. J Antimicrob Chemother 17:673–677, 1986

47 Smego RA, Perfect JR, Durack DT: Combined therapy with amphotericin B and 5-fluorocytosine for *Candida* meningitis. Rev Infect Dis 6:791–801, 1984

48 Bennett JE: Chemotherapy of systemic mycoses. N Engl J Med 290:320–322, 1974

49 Wise GJ, Kozinn PJ, Goldberg P: Flucytosine in the management of genitourinary candidiasis: 5 years of experience. J Urology 124:70–72, 1980

50 Ven Den Bossche H, Willemsens G, Cools W, et al: In vitro and in vivo effects of the antimycotic drug ketoconazole on sterol synthesis. Antimicrob Agents Chemother 17:922–928, 1980

51 Borgers M: Mechanism of action of antifungal drugs, with special reference to the imidazole derivatives. Rev Infect Dis 2:520–534, 1980

52 Levine HB (ed): *Ketoconazole in the Management of Fungal Disease*. New York, ADIS Press, 1982

53 Symoens J, Moens M, Dom J, et al: An evaluation of two years of clinical experience with ketoconazole. Rev Infect Dis 2:674–687, 1980

54 Shadomy S, White SC, Yu HP, et al: NIAID Mycoses Study Group: Treatment of systemic mycoses with ketoconazole: In vitro susceptibilities of clinical isolates of systemic and pathogenic fungi to ketoconazole. J Infect Dis 152:1249–1256, 1985

55 Mannisto PT, Mantyla R, Nykanen S, et al: Impairing effect of food on ketoconazole absorption. Antimicrob Agents Chemother 21:730–733, 1982

56 Daneshmend TK, Warnock DW, Ene MD, et al: Influence of food on the pharmacokinetics of ketoconazole. Antimicrob Agents Chemother 25:1–3, 1984

57 Graybill JR, Drutz DJ: Ketoconazole: A major innovation for treatment of fungal disease. Ann Intern Med 93:921–923, 1980

58 Craven PC, Graybill JR, Jorgensen JH, et al: High-dose ketoconazole for treatment of fungal infections of the central nervous system. Ann Intern Med 98:160–167, 1983

59 Engelhard D, Stutman HR, Marks MI: Interaction of ketoconazole with rifampin and isoniazid. N Engl J Med 311:1681–1683, 1984

60 Lewis JH, Zimmerman HJ, Benson GD, et al: Hepatic injury associated with ketoconazole therapy. Gastroenterology 83:503–513, 1984

61 Sonino N: The use of ketoconazole as an inhibitor of steroid production. N Engl J Med 317:817–818, 1987

62 NIAID Mycoses Study Group: Treatment of blastomycosis and histoplasmosis with ketoconazole. Ann Intern Med 103:861–872, 1985

63 Drouhet E, Dupont B: Laboratory and clinical assessment of ketoconazole in deep-seated mycoses. Am J Med 74 (1B):30–47, 1983

64 Saag MS, Dismukes WE: Azole antifungal agents: Emphasis on new triazoles. Antimicrob Agents Chemother 32:1–8, 1988

65 Stevens DA, Levine HB, Deresinski SC: Miconazole in coccidioidomycosis: Therapeutic and pharmacological studies in man. Am J Med 60:191–202, 1976

PART VII / Nutritional Diseases

Introduction · *Gerald T. Keusch*

Among the early triumphs of the application of biochemistry to medicine was the identification and description of specific nutrient deficiency diseases, paving the way for direct therapeutic and preventative action. As a result, many of these diseases have disappeared from regions of the world where formerly they were prevalent. At the same time the list of required specific nutrients, including vitamins, minerals, and trace elements, has enlarged and with it the number of defined clinical deficiency syndromes has increased. When one adds the number of individuals in the world affected by protein-energy malnutrition to those at risk of specific nutrient deficiency disease, the number becomes very large indeed, particularly in the developing countries of the world.

In this section, the most important of these deficiency syndromes are described in a manner that presents the relevant pathogenesis and pathophysiology, clinical manifestations, and diagnosis. Epidemiology stressing those factors of specific importance for the developing nations is included because these may be of utmost importance to the development of cost-effective public health interventions to treat or prevent the problem.

In some very specific examples, notably in hookworm disease, a single nutritional problem results from the infectious disease. However, due to the ecology of infection and malnutrition in developing nations, it is unlikely that iron deficiency due to hookworm will occur alone. Rather, other infections and other nutrient deficiencies are likely to coexist. Specific deficiency syndromes must be recognized and treated (or better still prevented), but once treatment is accomplished, the clinician practicing in the developing countries must not be satisfied that he or she has, in a single stroke, restored good health to the patient.

This section of the text has been organized in a systematic fashion by nutrient. The section must be read as a whole, however, with the perspective of nutrient interactions kept clearly in view. For example, some of the immune defects present in the individual with protein-energy malnutrition may be due to concomitant zinc deficiency, while the occurrence of an acute infection in such a patient may precipitate vitamin A deficiency, which unless treated rapidly progresses to irreversible keratomalacia and blindness. Equally tragic would be the setting in which goiter was found to be prevalent but the presence of cretinism was overlooked and nutritional interventions were not introduced.

With appropriate community nutrition information and political will of a government, most specific nutrient deficiency diseases are preventable by appropriate agricultural planning, food distribution, fortification methodology, or direct supplementation of the diet or periodic mass administration. The continued existence of these diseases is an indictment of health delivery systems and/or the setting of priorities for national action.

Protein-Energy Malnutrition
· *Benjamin Torún* · *Fernando E. Viteri*

Protein-energy malnutrition (PEM) is the most important nutritional disease in the developing countries because of its high prevalence and its relationship with child mortality rates, impaired physical growth, and inadequate social and economic development. While associated deleterious effects on mental growth and maturation have been demonstrated in experimental animals and they seem to occur in humans, it has not been possible to disassociate completely the nutritional factors from other environmental conditions, nor to ascertain the irreversibility of the nutritional mental damage [1,2].

PEM mainly affects infants, preschool-aged children, and the elderly. It occurs more frequently when infections reduce appetite and impose additional demands or induce greater losses of dietary energy, total nitrogen, and essential amino acids. The inability to satisfy the needs for these nutrients leads to PEM of varying degrees of severity. It is estimated that about 40 percent of all children under 5 years of age in the developing world had or presently have PEM [3]. Mild and moderate forms of PEM affect the physical and physiological performance of many millions of adults, especially when living conditions demand greater energy expenditure, as in heavy physical work.

PEM encompasses a wide spectrum of clinical syndromes conditioned by the relative intensity of protein or energy deficit, the severity and duration of the deficiencies, the age of the host, the etiology of the deficiency, and the association with other nutritional or infectious diseases. Its severity ranges from weight loss without other clinical manifestations to kwashiorkor or marasmus. Its origin can be *primary,* as a result of inadequate food intake, or *secondary,* as a result of other diseases that lead to low food intake, inadequate nutrient utilization, and/or increased nutritional requirements.

This chapter deals only with *primary PEM of a relatively chronic onset,* where inadequate energy and/or protein intakes lead to the nutritional disease. The metabolic alterations and clinical characteristics of specific vitamin and mineral deficiencies are described in other sections of this book.

NUTRIENTS

Primary PEM results from insufficient food intake or from the ingestion of foods with proteins of poor nutritional quality. Dietary energy and protein deficiencies usually occur together, but sometimes one predominates and, if severe enough, may lead to the distinct clinical syndromes of *kwashiorkor* (predominant protein deficiency), *marasmus* (mainly energy deficiency), or *marasmic kwashiorkor* (chronic energy deficiency with chronic or acute protein deficit). It is difficult to recognize which deficit predominates in milder forms of the disease.

ABSORPTION AND UTILIZATION

Energy

The main dietary energy sources are carbohydrates and fats, but proteins can also provide energy. In order to be absorbed, carbohydrates must be hydrolyzed to monosaccharides by the action of amylases and disaccharidases; fats must be converted into fatty acids and monoglycerides, which requires bile salts and lipases; and proteins must be hydrolyzed into amino acids by several gastrointestinal proteases and peptidases. Assuming that carbohydrates, fats, and proteins are 99, 95, and 92 percent absorbed, respectively, and that each gram of urinary nitrogen represents 1.25 kcal of protein energy that was not utilized by the human body, Atwater proposed that the "metabolizable" energy contents of those food components were 4, 9, and 4 kcal/g, respectively. It is now known that the proteins of most predominantly vegetable diets are only 65 to 85 percent absorbed and total energy absorption from mixed animal-vegetable diets is usually 90 to 95 percent [4]. Nevertheless, the Atwater factors are still practical and their use results in a relatively small error.

Protein

The utilization of dietary proteins depends on their digestibility (i.e., absorption) and their amino acid composition. A protein that is deficient in one or more essential amino acids is not used adequately for the body's protein metabolism, although the nonutilized amino acids are potential energy sources when dietary carbohydrates and fats do not provide sufficient energy. The rational combination of poor-quality proteins will combine and complement the essential amino acids that each one lacks and improve the protein quality of a diet. This quality can be expressed as a chemical or amino acid score, relative to a standard essential amino acid pattern. If the score is corrected by the protein digestibility, a good estimate of the protein's nutritional value is obtained [5]. Protein deficiency can result from the intake of insufficient amounts of digestible protein (total nitrogen deficit), from the ingestion of poor-quality protein (essential amino acid deficit), or from a combination of both. A deficient dietary energy intake will also contribute to the development of protein deficiency by reducing the efficiency of protein utilization, altering amino acid metabolism, and increasing the nutritional requirements for protein [6].

ENERGY AND PROTEIN DENSITIES OF FOODS

Some vegetable foods have proteins and energy of good nutritional quality, but they are bulky and become more so as a result of the water absorbed during cooking. Consequently, their energy and protein densities (i.e., energy and protein per gram of cooked food, ready to be eaten) are low and they must be consumed in relatively large amounts to meet the body's requirements for these nutrients. This may lead to PEM, particularly in infants and preschool children whose appetites are satisfied and whose stomachs are filled with quantities of bulky foods that do not provide sufficient amounts of proteins or energy [7].

INTERACTIONS WITH OTHER NUTRIENTS

Poor energy and protein intakes are accompanied by insufficient intakes of other essential nutrients. In severe PEM there can be deficiencies of vitamins, such as A, D, folic acid, and B_{12}; minerals such as iron and zinc; and electrolytes such as potassium and magnesium. Their clinical and metabolic significance depend on the severity of the specific micronutrient deficit relative to that of PEM. In kwashiorkor and marasmus, manifestations of energy and protein insufficiency usually predominate, and some of the other nutrient deficiencies only become clinically evident during the course of protein-energy repletion. This can be either because the derangement caused by severe PEM overshadows other symptoms or because the functional requirements for some micronutrients diminish in severely malnourished patients and increase only during the period of nutritional rehabilitation.

These "hidden" nutrient deficits are important during treatment of PEM. For example, functional anemia and hypoxia may develop if hematinics are not provided as tissue synthesis and oxygen demands increase [8]; failure to replete nearly exhausted vitamin A stores can precipitate severe ocular manifestations of hypovitaminosis A; muscular tone and other cell functions will recover very slowly unless enough potassium is provided to overcome the intracellular depletion of this electrolyte; covert zinc deficiency may retard catch-up growth.

PATIENT

PATHOPHYSIOLOGY AND ADAPTIVE RESPONSES

PEM develops gradually over many days or months. This allows a series of metabolic and behavioral adaptations which result in decreased nutrient demands and in a nutritional equilibrium compatible with a lower level of cellular nutrient availability. Patients whose PEM develops slowly—as is usually the case in marasmus—are better-adapted to their current nutritional status and maintain a less fragile metabolic equilibrium than those with more acute PEM, as in kwashiorkor of rapid onset.

Energy mobilization and expenditure

A decrease in energy intake is quickly followed by a decrease in energy expenditure, accounting for shorter periods of play and physical activity in children [9,10] and for longer rest periods and less physical work in adults [11]. When the decrease in energy expenditure cannot compensate for the insufficient intake, body fat is mobilized with a decrease in adiposity and weight loss. Lean body mass diminishes at a slower rate, mainly as consequence of muscle protein catabolism with increased efflux of amino acids, primarily alanine. As the cumulative energy deficit becomes more severe, subcutaneous fat is markedly reduced, and protein catabolism leads to muscular wasting. Visceral protein is preserved longer, especially in the marasmic patient. In marasmus, these alterations in body composition lead to increased basal oxygen consumption (i.e., basal metabolic rate) per unit body weight. In kwashiorkor, the severe dietary protein deficit leads to an earlier visceral depletion of amino acids that affects visceral cell function and reduces oxygen consumption; therefore, basal energy expenditure decreases per unit of lean or total body mass. Blood glucose concentration remains normal, mainly at the expense of fats and gluconeogenic amino acids, and it falls in very severe PEM or when complicated by serious infections or fasting.

Protein metabolism

The most striking changes are a marked recycling of amino acids and a reduction in urea synthesis and excretion. The poor availability of dietary amino acids decreases protein synthesis in viscera and muscles. This is followed by increased muscle protein catabolism, modified composition of the free amino acid pool, and increased visceral amino acid availability. In the steady state, the amount of free amino acids entering the body pool is equal to the amount leaving it. The latter is represented by the amino acids synthesized into body protein and the amount of amino acid nitrogen that is excreted. On a normal protein intake, 25 percent of the amino acids leaving the total body pool are excreted as nitrogenous compounds and 75 percent are recycled or reutilized for protein synthesis. This

latter fraction may rise to 90 to 95 percent when protein intake is reduced [12]. Therefore, the adaptive change is not so much a reduction of total nitrogen or amino acid turnover but an increase in the proportion turned over that is used for synthesis and a corresponding reduction in the proportion of nitrogen that is excreted.

The half-life of some proteins increases. The rate of albumin synthesis decreases, but after a time lag of a few days the rate of breakdown also falls. In addition to its increased half-life, a shift of albumin from the extravascular to the intravascular pool assists in maintaining adequate levels of circulating albumin in the face of reduced synthesis, until protein depletion becomes so severe that it disrupts these adaptive mechanisms. The ensuing reduction in intravascular oncotic pressure and the outflow of water into the extravascular space contribute to the development of the edema of kwashiorkor.

These adaptations lead to the sparing of body protein and the preservation of essential protein-dependent functions. The gradual and inevitable loss of body protein as a result of long-term dietary protein deficit is primarily from skeletal muscle. Some visceral protein is lost in the early development of PEM but then becomes stable until the nonessential tissue proteins are depleted; the loss of visceral protein then increases, and death may be imminent unless nutritional therapy is successfully instituted.

Endocrine changes

Hormones play an important role in the adaptive metabolic processes. Endocrine changes may not be wholly explained by the circulating levels of hormones, since cellular responses to hormonal stimulation may also be altered in PEM. Table 118-1 summarizes the main changes in hormonal activity seen in patients with severe energy or protein deficiencies [13]. The functional capacities of the hypothalamic-pituitary axis and the adrenal medulla are preserved. Consequently, patients can still show endocrine and metabolic responses to stress conditions.

Some endocrine adaptive functions in severe PEM are related to energy metabolism (Fig. 118-1); (1) The decreased food intake tends to reduce plasma concentrations of glucose and free amino acids which, in turn, *reduce insulin* secretion and *increase epinephrine* release. The low plasma amino acid levels, seen mainly in kwashiorkor, also *stimulate the secretion of human growth hormone*. (2) The *low plasma somatomedin* activity, also seen mainly in kwashiorkor, probably contributes to the high circulating levels of growth hormone, due to the absence of the feedback inhibition postulated for somatomedins. (3) The stress induced by the low food intake and further amplified by fever, water and electrolyte losses, and other manifestations of the infections that frequently accompany PEM, also *stimulates epinephrine release* and *corticosteroid secretions,* more so in marasmus than in kwashiorkor, probably because of the greater severity in energy deficit that characterizes marasmus. (4) The plasma concentrations of T_3 and T_4

Table 118-1. Some metabolic effects and hormonal changes usually seen in severe protein-energy malnutrition

Hormone	Influenced in PEM by	Hormonal Activity in		Metabolic effects of changes in PEM
		Energy deficit	Protein deficit	
Insulin	Low food intake ($\downarrow$ glucose) ($\downarrow$ amino acids)	Decreased	Decreased	$\downarrow$ muscle protein synthesis $\downarrow$ lipogenesis $\downarrow$ growth
Growth hormone	Low protein intake ($\downarrow$ amino acids) Reduced somatomedin synthesis	Normal or moderately increased	Increased	$\uparrow$ visceral protein synthesis $\downarrow$ urea synthesis $\uparrow$ lipolysis
Somatomedins	Low protein intake?	Variable	Decreased	$\downarrow$ muscle and cartilage protein synthesis $\downarrow$ collagen synthesis $\downarrow$ lipolysis $\downarrow$ growth $\uparrow$ production of growth hormone
Epinephrine	Stress of food deficiency, infections ($\downarrow$ glucose)	Normal but can increase	Normal but can increase	$\uparrow$ lipolysis $\uparrow$ glycogenolysis inhibits insulin secretion
Glucocorticoids	Stress of hunger Fever ($\downarrow$ glucose)	Increased	Normal or moderately increased	$\uparrow$ muscle protein catabolism $\uparrow$ visceral protein turnover $\uparrow$ lipolysis $\uparrow$ gluconeogenesis
Aldosterone	$\downarrow$ blood volume $\uparrow$ extracellular K? $\downarrow$ serum Na?	Normal	Increased	$\uparrow$ sodium retention and $\uparrow$ water retention contribute to appearance of edema
Thyroid hormones	?	T_4 normal or decreased; T_3 decreased	T_4 usually decreased; T_3 decreased	$\downarrow$ glucose oxidation $\downarrow$ basal energy expenditure $\uparrow$ reverse T_3
Gonadotropins	Low protein intake? Low energy intake?	Decreased	Decreased	Delayed menarche

Note: $\downarrow$ = low or reduced; $\uparrow$ = high or increased.

Source: From [*13*].

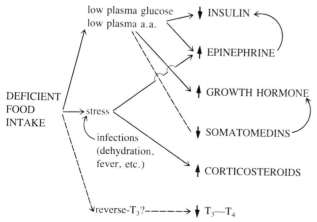

Figure 118-1. Endocrine adaptive functions in severe PEM related to energy metabolism.

decrease, by mechanisms that are not yet defined; the iodination of tyrosine may be involved, as the reduction in T_3 (3,5,3′-triiodothyronine) is accompanied by an increase in the circulating levels of the metabolically inactive reverse-T_3 (3,5,5′-triiodothyronine). All these changes contribute to the maintenance of energy homeostasis through increased glycolysis and lipolysis; increased amino acid mobilization; decreased storage of glycogen, fats, and proteins; and decreased energy metabolism. They also participate in the preservation of visceral protein through increased breakdown of muscle protein and increased availability and turnover of amino acids in viscera, particularly liver. Some investigators [*14*] have postulated that the evolution of PEM into either kwashiorkor or marasmus may be partly related to differences in adrenocortical response, whereby the better response will preserve visceral proteins more efficiently and lead to the better-adapted syndrome of marasmus.

Disruption of adaptation

Patients with severe PEM adapt to a new, but fragile, state of metabolic equilibrium. The adaptive mechanisms can be upset by large increases in the intake of energy relative to proteins, by infections, and by a sudden, large increase in energy and/or protein intake. For example, the abrupt administration of high-carbohydrate diets with poor protein intake will induce insulin secretion and reduce the release of epinephrine, growth hormone, and cortisol. Consequently, fat oxidation and gluconeogenesis decrease and the availability of muscle amino acids for liver protein synthesis diminishes. These changes may lead to the development or exacerbation of kwashiorkor.

Patients with kwashiorkor suddenly fed large amounts of proteins or given large transfusions of plasma or blood may experience a rapid increase in intravascular protein concentration and entry of extracellular fluid into the vascular compartment leading to cardiovascular insufficiency and pulmonary edema. In fact, a too early introduction of high-energy or high-protein diets to a severely malnourished patient may be fatal [15].

ASSESSMENT OF NUTRIENT STATUS

Severe PEM can be classified qualitatively to distinguish kwashiorkor, marasmus, and intermediate forms, based on clinical and biochemical criteria. The assessment and classification of mild and moderate forms of PEM is based on anthropometric measurements, since biochemical indexes usually do not show changes unless the disease is well advanced. More accurate measurements, such as assessment of body composition, are not practical or feasible in most of the settings where PEM occurs, and the so-called functional indicators are difficult to measure or are not as yet well defined or standardized.

Anthropometric measurements

The anthropometric assessment of nutritional status employs a standard reference of comparison that is not necessarily an ideal or a target. Any set of reliable anthropometric data can be used as the standard, but the interpretation of their use (i.e., the line that separates "normal" from "deficient" and further subdivisions into "mild," "moderate," and "severe" forms) is a matter of judgment. In order to allow international comparisons, it is sensible to use the same standard of reference for various populations. The value judgment comes into play when deciding whether the expected normal value for a given population should be 100 percent, 90 percent, or other proportion of the standard. Setting different cutoff points relative to a single standard is more practical than constructing local standards which, in a country with heterogeneous population groups, may pose the same problem as a "foreign," commonly used reference. The World Health Organization presently recommends the data from the U.S. National Center for Health Statistics (NCHS) [16] as reference.

The choice of anthropometric indexes will depend on the simplicity, accuracy, reproducibility, and sensitivity of the measurements, and on the availability of measuring instruments. The most widely used index for children, although not the best, is *weight for age*. This was the basis for classifying PEM into three degrees [17]: first degree = 90 to 75 percent of standard, second degree = 74 to 60 percent, third degree = less than 60 percent. The use of this index, however, does not differentiate between a truly underweight child and one who is short in stature but well-proportioned in weight. Furthermore, the information about chronological age is not always reliable.

The measurement of height or length, in addition to weight, is important. It allows the use of two indexes: *weight for height,* as an index of *current* nutritional status, and *height for age,* as an index of *past* nutritional history which, when deficient, may represent a short period of growth failure at an early age or a longer period at a later age. Waterlow [18] suggested the term *wasting* for a deficit in weight for height, and *stunting* for a deficit in height for age. Children may fall into four categories that are qualitatively different: (1) normal, (2) wasted but not stunted (suffering from acute PEM), (3) wasted and stunted (suffering from acute and chronic PEM), and (4) stunted but not wasted (past PEM with present adequate nutrition, or "nutritional dwarfs"). The severity of wasting and stunting can be graded using, respectively, weight as percentage of the expected median weight of a standard child of the same height, and height as percentage of the median standard height for age. The grading shown in Table 118-2 is suggested for most countries. It may be convenient to use different points of demarcation for some populations (e.g., normal height for age in groups that are genetically short could be less than 95 percent of the standard).

Better statistical but less practical approaches of grading use *Z values* or standard deviations apart from the NCHS/WHO median values or express weight for height and height for age as the corresponding centile of the NCHS/WHO reference tables [16].

For adults, in addition to weight deficit for a given height and age, another practical indicator is the body mass index, or BMI (weight in $kg/height^2$ in m), which is used primarily as an indicator of fatness. There are no international standards of comparison, but reference charts have been calculated for

Table 118-2. Grading of severity of current ("wasting") and past or chronic ("stunting") malnutrition

	Normal	**Mild**	**Moderate**	**Severe**
Weight for height (deficit = wasting)	90–110*	80–89	70–79	<70
Height for age (deficit = stunting)	95–105	90–94	85–89	<85

*Percentage of the median NCHS standard [16].

Source: From [18].

Table 118-3. Fifth percentile values for the body mass index of white and black adults from the United States*

Age, years	Males, kg/m²	Females, kg/m²
18–29	18–19	17–18
30–50	18–20	18–19

*Calculated from tables of C. E. Cronk and A. F. Roche [*19*].

white and black men and women [*19*] from data of a U.S. national survey [*20*]. A person with a BMI lower than the fifth percentile value shown in Table 118-3 may be malnourished. Clinical evaluation will establish whether the individual is truly malnourished or normal but extremely lean.

Other anthropometric measurements and indexes have been used, based on arm circumference, skin-fold thicknesses, or their combination with height and weight. Accurate measurements are more difficult to standardize, and no international standards of reference have been validated.

Body composition

Measurements of adiposity and lean body mass provide a better assessment of mild and moderate PEM than anthropometric measurements in adults. Since energy deficiency is usually more common than protein deficiency, the most striking change is a reduction of adiposity below the average 12 and 20 percent expected in normal, well-nourished men and women, respectively.

Fat stores are reduced in severe PEM and virtually depleted in marasmus; a notable exception are the classic cases of kwashiorkor where fat stores are preserved due to an adequate energy intake with a very poor protein intake.

Body protein decreases at a slow rate, most of it from muscle, and the greater loss of adipose tissue results in a relative increase of total body water (i.e., per unit of body mass), mainly as intracellular water. In severe protein deficiency (kwashiorkor) there is also an increase in extracellular water. The intracellular concentrations of potassium and magnesium decrease and that of sodium increases, although the serum concentrations of electrolytes do not necessarily reflect these alterations [*21*].

Functional alterations

Although spontaneous physical activity and total energy expenditure decrease with insufficient dietary energy intake [*11–13,22*], the methods to assess such changes are complex. Physical fitness is reduced in children and adults [*23*], but in individuals who engage in daily heavy physical work this may be evident only through endurance tests.

PEM reversibly reduces immune response (see Chap. 24). Severely malnourished patients are highly susceptible to gram-negative bacterial sepsis [*24,25*]. Skin test anergy and a poor febrile response due to reduced production of interleukin 1 [*26*] interfere with the diagnosis of some infectious complications.

Reductions in gastric, pancreatic, and bile secretions and in disaccharidase activities decrease digestion and absorption. Malnourished persons are prone to more prolonged episodes of diarrhea [*27*] because of these alterations and possibly also because of irregular intestinal motility and depressed immune responses that favor intestinal bacterial overgrowth.

Other functional alterations include a tendency for malnourished women to have low-birth-weight babies and for children to have shortened attention spans and to perform poorly in school.

CLINICAL MANIFESTATIONS

Mild and moderate PEM

The main clinical feature of mild and moderate PEM in children is a retardation in physical growth (Fig. 118-2). Present malnutrition results in wasting (low weight for height) and past malnutrition in stunting (low height for age). The combination of wasting and stunting suggests chronic malnutrition with present inadequate nutritional status. In adults, mild to moderate or chronic PEM results in leanness with a more or less marked reduction in subcutaneous tissue.

Children become more sedentary and spend less time in energy-demanding play and other activities. There are a series

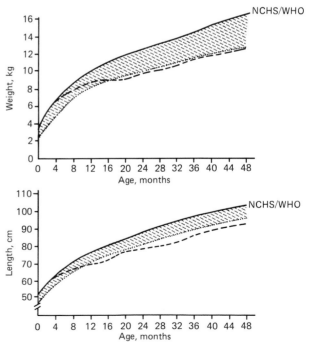

Figure 118-2. Growth retardation due to primary protein-energy malnutrition (shaded area = 2 SD below the NCHS/WHO standard of reference).

of nonspecific manifestations, which include frequent and prolonged episodes of diarrhea, apathy and lack of liveliness, and short attention spans that may interfere with school performance. Adults show a reduced capacity for prolonged, intense physical work and tend to take long naps or rest periods.

Marasmus

Severe muscular wasting and absence of subcutaneous fat give the patient a ''skin-and-bones'' appearance (Fig. 118-3). Marasmic persons frequently have 60 percent or less of the weight expected for their height, with marked retardation in longitudinal growth. The hair is sparse, thin, and dry. The skin is usually dry, thin, with little elasticity, and it wrinkles when pinched; lymph nodes are easily palpable. The patient is weak and frequently cannot stand without help. Heart rate, blood pressure, and body temperature may be low. Hypothermia of 35°C or less can occur, especially after a fasting period, and is often accompanied by hypoglycemia.

The marasmic child is apathetic but usually aware and with a look of anxiety on his or her face. These features and the sunken cheeks caused by disappearance of the Bichat fat pads, which are among the last subcutaneous adipose depots to disappear, give the marasmic child's face the appearance of a monkey's or an old person's. Some patients are anorexic while others are ravenously hungry, but they seldom tolerate large amounts of food and vomit easily.

Common complicating features are diarrhea, dehydration, respiratory infections, eye lesions due to hypovitaminosis A, and skin infections. Systemic infections can be present without an appropriate febrile response, tachycardia, or leukocytosis.

Kwashiorkor

The predominant feature is soft, pitting, painless edema, usually in the feet and legs, but extending to perineum, upper extremities, and face in severe cases (Fig. 118-4). Subcuta-

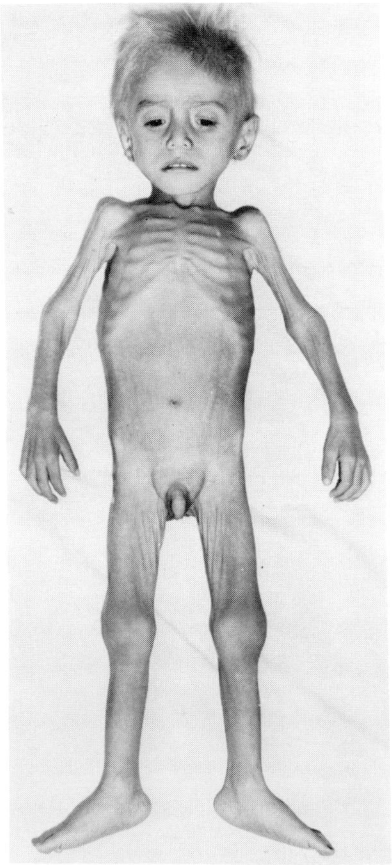

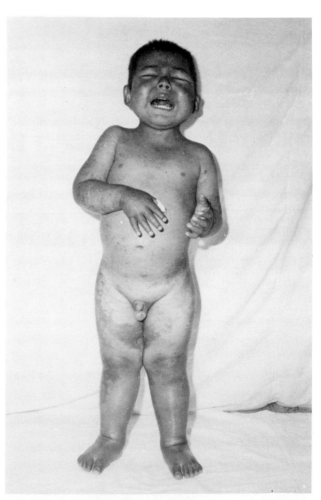

Figure 118-3. Severe wasting in marasmus. Note the dry, wrinkled skin and the sparse, often discolored, hair.

Figure 118-4. Edema and skin lesions in kwashiorkor. Note that subcutaneous fat is preserved in the trunk, arms, and face (*From* [*13*].)

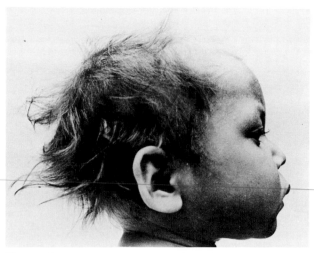

Figure 118-5. Dry, brittle hair which falls off or can be pulled out without pain. More frequently seen in kwashiorkor but may also occur in marasmus.

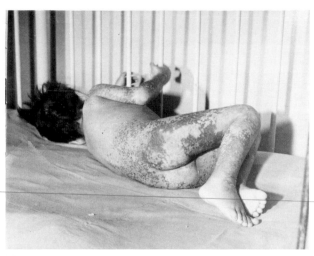

Figure 118-7. Skin lesions in edematous PEM. The epidermis peels off in large scales.

neous fat is preserved, although there may be some muscle wasting. Weight deficit, after accounting for the edema, is not as severe as in marasmus. Height is variable and may be normal or retarded, depending on the chronicity of the current episode and on past nutritional history. The hair is dry, brittle, without its normal sheen, and can be pulled out easily and without pain (Fig. 118-5). Curly hair becomes straight, and there usually are changes in pigmentation; hair becomes dull brown, reddish, or even yellowish-white. Alternating periods

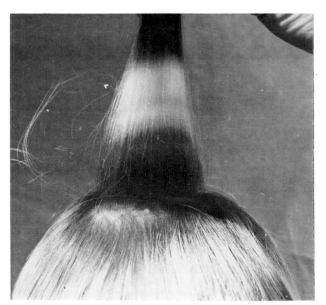

Figure 118-6. ''Flag sign'': bands of depigmented and normal hair due to alternating periods of poor and relatively good protein intake.

of poor and relatively good protein intake can produce alternating bands of depigmented and normal hair, which have been termed the ''flag sign'' (Fig. 118-6). Skin lesions, often confused with pellagra, are very characteristic of kwashiorkor (Fig. 118-7). They occur in many but not all patients, more frequently in the areas of edema, continuous pressure (e.g., buttocks and back), or frequent irritation (e.g., perineum and thighs). In those areas the skin may be erythematous; it glistens in the edematous regions and has zones of dryness, hyperkeratosis, and hyperpigmentation, which tend to become confluent. The epidermis peels off in large scales, exposing underlying tissues that are easily infected.

The patients may be pale, with cold and cyanotic extremities. Hepatomegaly with a soft, round edge, caused by severe fatty infiltration is usually present. The abdomen is frequently protruding because of distended stomach and intestinal loops. Peristalsis is irregular. Muscle tone and strength are greatly reduced and tachycardia is common. Both hypothermia and hypoglycemia can occur after short periods of fasting.

Patients are alternately apathetic and irritable and have an expression of misery and sadness. Anorexia, sometimes necessitating nasogastric tube feeding, postprandial vomiting, and diarrhea are common. These improve as nutritional recovery progresses.

Diarrhea and respiratory infections are more frequent and severe in kwashiorkor compared to marasmus. Severe, even fatal infections may occur as in marasmus, often without fever, tachycardia, respiratory distress, or leukocytosis.

Marasmic kwashiorkor

This form of edematous PEM combines clinical characteristics of kwashiorkor and marasmus. The main features are the

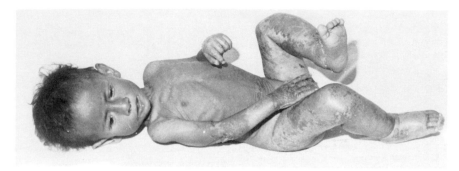

Figure 118-8. Marasmic kwashiorkor. Note the wasting of the arms and thorax, characteristic of marasmus; the edema and skin lesions, characteristic of kwashiorkor; and the sparse, discolored hair that occurs in both syndromes.

edema of kwashiorkor, with or without its skin lesions, and the muscle wasting and decreased subcutaneous fat of marasmus (Fig. 118-8). When edema disappears during early treatment, the patient's symptoms resemble those of marasmus. Biochemical features of both marasmus and kwashiorkor are seen, but the alterations of severe protein deficiency usually predominate.

DIAGNOSIS

Mild and moderate PEM

The diagnosis is based on dietary history and anthropometric measurements. Biochemical indicators are of little help, although the patients may have low urinary excretions of urea nitrogen, creatinine, hydroxyproline, and 3-methylhistidine, and a small decrease in serum concentrations of branched-chain essential amino acids, albumin, and transferrin.

Severe PEM

The diagnosis is principally based on dietary history and clinical features. The most common biochemical findings are that serum concentrations of total proteins and albumin are markedly reduced in edematous PEM, and normal or moderately low in marasmus; hemoglobin and hematocrit are usually low, more so in kwashiorkor than marasmus; the ratio of nonessential to essential amino acids in plasma is elevated in kwashiorkor and usually normal in marasmus; serum levels of free fatty acids are elevated, particularly in kwashiorkor; blood glucose level is normal or low, especially after fasting 10 to 12 h; urinary excretions of creatinine, hydroxyproline, 3-methylhistidine and urea nitrogen are low; children with kwashiorkor or marasmic kwashiorkor usually have low urinary creatinine excretions in relation to their height, leading to a low creatinine-height index [28], whereas marasmic children may have a normal or somewhat low index.

Plasma levels of other nutrients vary and tend to be moderately low. They do not necessarily reflect the body stores. For example, serum iron and retinol may be normal with almost depleted body stores, or in kwashiorkor they may be relatively low with adequate stores because of alterations in the transport proteins, transferrin and retinol-binding protein, respectively.

Many other biochemical changes have been described in severe PEM. They have little practical diagnostic importance but give an insight into the pathophysiological changes (Table 118-4).

PROGNOSIS AND RISK OF MORTALITY

Treatment usually takes longer in marasmus than kwashiorkor. Mortality rates in severe PEM can be as high as 40 percent. Immediate causes of death are usually infections. Table 118-5 lists the characteristics that generally indicate a poor prognosis.

Table 118-4. Selected biochemical changes observed in severe protein-energy malnutrition

	Marasmus	Edematous PEM
Body composition		
Total body water	High	High
Extracellular water	High	Higher
Total body potassium	Low	Lower
Total body protein	Low	Low
Serum or plasma		
Transport proteins*	Normal or low	Low
Branched-chain amino acids	Normal or low	Low
Tyrosine/phenylalanine ratio	Normal or low	Low
Enzymes (in general)†	Normal	Low
Transaminases	Normal or high	High
Liver		
Fatty infiltration	Absent	Severe
Glycogen	Normal or low	Normal or low
Urea cycle and other enzymes‡	Low	Lower
Amino acid-synthesizing enzymes	High	Not as high

*For example, transferrin, ceruloplasmin, retinol-, cortisol-, and thyroxine-binding proteins, α- and β-lipoproteins.
†For example, amylase, pseudocholinesterase, alkaline phosphatase.
‡For example, xanthine oxidase, glycolic acid oxidase, cholinesterase.

Table 118-5. Manifestations in patients with protein-energy malnutrition that generally indicate a poor prognosis

1. Age less than 6 months
2. Deficit in weight for height of greater than 30%, or in weight for age of greater than 40%
3. Extensive exfoliative or exudative cutaneous lesions or deep decubitus ulcerations
4. Dehydration and electrolyte imbalances, especially hypokalemia and severe acidosis
5. Clinical jaundice or elevated serum bilirubin concentrations, with or without elevations in the transaminases
6. Hypoglycemia or hypothermia
7. Total serum protein concentrations less than 3 g/dL
8. Severe anemia with clinical signs of hypoxia
9. Petechiae or hemorrhagic tendencies (purpura is usually a sign of septicemia or a viral infection)
10. Intercurrent infections, particularly measles and bronchopneumonia
11. Persistent tachycardia, signs of heart failure, and/or respiratory difficulty
12. Coma, stupor, or other alterations in mental status and consciousness

Source: Modified after B. Torún, F.E. Viteri, Rev. Col. Med. (Guatemala) 27:43–62, 1976.

Anthropometric characteristics are also associated with mortality rates, as in the classification of severe PEM into first, second, or third degrees, based on weight for age [*17*]. A higher mortality rate is associated with the more intense anthropometric deficits but not with mild or moderate deficiencies [*29*].

TREATMENT

Severe PEM

Whenever possible, patients with noncomplicated PEM should be treated on an outpatient basis. Hospitalization increases the risk of cross-infections, and the unfamiliar setting may increase apathy and anorexia in children, making feeding more difficult. When hospitalization is necessary, treatment strategy can be divided into three stages: (1) resolving life-threatening conditions, (2) restoring nutritional status without disrupting homeostasis, and (3) ensuring nutritional rehabilitation.

Resolving Life-threatening Conditions. Most in-hospital deaths occur in the first week of treatment. Nutritional rehabilitation can be delayed until emergencies are solved. The most frequent complications that require immediate treatment are discussed below.

1. Fluid and Electrolyte Disturbances. The assessment of dehydration is not easy in severe PEM, as classical signs of dehydration, such as sunken eyeballs and decreased skin turgor, are frequently found in well-hydrated patients, while hy-

povolemia may coexist with subcutaneous edema. Useful signs are thirst, low urinary output, weak and rapid pulse, and low blood pressure and a declining state of consciousness, which indicate impending circulatory collapse.

Whenever possible, oral or nasogastric rehydration should be used. Intravenous fluids must be used in severe dehydration with hypovolemia, impending shock, frequent vomiting, and persistent abdominal distension. The therapeutic approach differs from that in well-nourished patients because of hydroelectrolytic peculiarities of severe PEM, namely: (1) hypoosmolarity with moderate hyponatremia, frequently with intracellular sodium excess; (2) intracellular potassium depletion, usually without hypokalemia; (3) mild-to-moderate metabolic acidosis, which decreases or disappears when the patient receives dietary or parenteral energy, and electrolyte balance is reestablished; (4) high tolerance to hypocalcemia, partly because of the acidosis, which produces a relative increment in ionized Ca^{2+}, and partly because of hypoproteinemia, which makes less protein available to bind Ca^{2+}; and (5) decreased body magnesium, with or without hypomagnesemia.

The volume of fluids will depend on diuresis and the clinical signs of dehydration. Fluid repletion should allow a diuresis of at least 200 mL in 24 h in children and 500 mL in adults, or a micturition every 2 to 3 h. As a guideline, 10 to 20 mL/(kg·h) by mouth or nasogastric tube every 1 to 2 h can be given initially to be modified according to patient response.

It may be practical to use the solution of oral rehydration salts (ORS) recommended by WHO and UNICEF, especially in nonedematous patients. One liter of this solution has 3.5 g NaCl, 2.9 g trisodium citrate (*or* 2.5 g sodium bicarbonate), 1.5 g KCl, and 20 g anhydrous glucose (*or* 40 g sucrose). This corresponds to molar concentrations (in mmol/L) of Na^+, 90; K^+, 20; Cl^-, 80; citrate 10 (*or* bicarbonate 30); and glucose, 111. There is, however, some concern about the administration of so much sodium to patients with kwashiorkor, the relatively low content of potassium, and the lack of calcium. An alternative is the following treatment plan, based on extensive experience at the Institute of Nutrition of Central America and Panama (INCAP). Patients with edema who are urinating should receive about 6 meq K, 2 to 3 meq Na, 2 to 3 meq Ca, and 20 to 30 kcal/day per kilogram of body weight. This can be accomplished by dissolving in 1 L of water, 3 g KCl, 1 g table salt (NaCl), 2 g $CaCl_2 \cdot 6H_2O$ (or 4 g calcium gluconate), and 50 g glucose or cane sugar. Potassium should be withheld when there is no diuresis. Additional fluids must be given to compensate for the losses of diarrhea and vomiting, providing about 35 meq Na and 30 meq K per kilogram of excreta (i.e., 2 g table salt and 2 g KCl per liter). Dietary formula with calcium (e.g., milk formula) should be started as early as possible, if necessary alternating with the electrolyte solution. Total K intake should be raised to 8 to 10 meq/(kg·day), while for Mg 0.5 to 1 meq/(kg·day) should be given.

When intravenous infusions are necessary, osmolarity must be kept low (200 to 280 mosmol/L), K (when urinating) and

Na should not exceed 6 and 3 meq/(kg·day), respectively, and glucose must provide 15 to 30 kcal/(kg·day). During the first hour, 10 to 30 mL/kg is infused, depending on the patient's condition. Subsequent volumes are calculated at 2- to 4-h intervals. Additional losses through diarrhea and vomiting must be compensated with about 3 meq Na, 3 meq K, 6 meq Cl, and 15 kcal per 100 g (i.e., 20 mL isotonic saline, 2 mL of 10% KCl, and 78 mL of 5% dextrose per 100 g excreta). An increase in pulse and respiratory rate with weight gain after accounting for weight of excreta, pulmonary rales, and appearance or exacerbation of edema indicates overhydration. An increase in pulse and respiratory rate with weight loss, low urine output, and continuing losses from diarrhea and vomiting suggests insufficient fluid therapy.

Patients with severe hypoproteinemia (less than 3 g/dL), anuria, and signs of hypovolemia or impending circulatory collapse should be given 10 mL plasma per kilogram in 1 to 2 h, followed by 20 mL/(kg·h) of a mixture of two parts of 5% dextrose and one part of isotonic saline, for 1 or 2 h. This will increase plasma protein concentration by about 0.5 to 1 g/dL and help prevent the rapid exit of water from the intravascular compartment. If diuresis does not improve, the dose of plasma can be repeated 2 h later. Further treatment is similar to that of well-nourished patients.

Some clinicians advocate the routine use of lactate- or bicarbonate-containing solutions. However, the mild metabolic acidosis of malnutrition usually disappears with energy intake. Therefore, treatment for acidosis should be withheld unless blood pH is below 7.25, urinary pH is below 5, or there are clinical signs of severe acidosis.

Hypocalcemia may be secondary to magnesium deficiency. When there is hypomagnesemia or clinical signs similar to hypocalcemia that do not respond to calcium infusion, magnesium should be given intramuscularly as a 50% solution of magnesium sulfate in doses of 0.5, 1, and 1.5 mL, respectively, for patients who weigh less than 7, between 7 and 10, and more than 10 kg. The dose can be repeated every 12 h until there is no recurrence of the hypocalcemic symptoms and oral Mg supplementation of 0.5 to 1 meq/(kg·day) can be given as described later.

2. Infections. Malnourished patients are particularly prone to infections. While these are often severe and life-threatening, paradoxically, clinical manifestations may be mild and the classical signs of fever, tachycardia, and leukocytosis absent. Antigen-antibody reactions are often impaired and skin tests, such as tuberculin, often give falsely negative results.

Antibiotics should not be used prophylactically, but when an infection is suspected appropriate antibiotic therapy must be started immediately, even before obtaining the results of microbiological cultures. The choice of drug will vary with the suspected etiological agent, the severity of the disease, and the pattern of the drug resistance in that area. Clinicians should be aware that gastrointestinal, hepatic, and renal alterations that might accompany severe PEM could potentiate a drug's toxic effects. Where septicemia is suspected, a broad-spectrum antibiotic or a combination, such as ampicillin and gentamicin (two inexpensive antibiotics generally available in developing countries), is usually given intravenously. Other supportive treatment may also be necessary, for instance, for respiratory distress, hypothermia, and hypoglycemia.

Treatment for intestinal parasites is rarely urgent and can be deferred until nutritional rehabilitation is underway. This will decrease the risks of potential toxicity, including the possibility of absorbing drugs normally not absorbed by a healthy intestine.

3. Hemodynamic Alterations. Cardiac failure may develop during or after administration of intravenous fluids, or shortly after the introduction of high-protein and high-energy feedings, leading to pulmonary edema and secondary pulmonary infection. These alterations may be the result of impaired cardiac function, sudden expansion of the intravascular fluid volume, severe anemia, or impaired membrane function. Diuretics such as furosemide (10 mg IV or IM, repeated as necessary) should be given, as well as other supportive measures. Many clinicians advocate the use of digoxin (0.03 mg/kg IV, every 6 to 8 h). The use of diuretics merely to accelerate the disappearance of edema in kwashiorkor is contraindicated.

4. Severe Anemia. Blood transfusions should be given only in cases of severe anemia with less than 4 g hemoglobin per deciliter, or with signs of hypoxia or impending cardiac failure. In many developing countries with high prevalence of infection with human immunodeficiency virus (HIV) and few or no resources for screening the blood supply, the risk of transmission of HIV is significant and should restrict use of transfusion except in life-threatening situations. Whole blood (10 mL/kg) can be used in marasmic patients, but it is better to use packed red blood cells (6 mL/kg) in edematous PEM. The transfusion should be given slowly, over 2 to 3 h, and repeated if necessary after 12 to 24 h. The routine use of blood transfusions endangers the patient, and hemoglobin levels will improve with proper dietary treatment supplemented with hematinics.

5. Hypothermia and Hypoglycemia. Body temperature below 35.5°C and plasma glucose concentration below 60 mg/dL can be due to either impaired thermoregulatory mechanisms, reduced fuel substrate availability, or severe infection. Asymptomatic hypoglycemia can be treated (and prevented) by the frequent feeding of small volumes of glucose- or sucrose-containing diets and solutions. Severe symptomatic hypoglycemia must be treated intravenously with 10 to 20 mL of 50% glucose solution followed by oral administration of 25 to 50 mL of 5% glucose solution at 2-h intervals for 24 to 48 h.

Body temperature usually rises in the hypothermic patient with frequent feedings of glucose-containing diets or solutions. Caution and close monitoring of body temperature must be used with external heat sources and devices to reduce the loss of body heat, as these patients may rapidly become hyperthermic. It is best to keep the seminude patients in an ambient temperature of 30 to 33°C.

6. Severe Vitamin A Deficiency. Severe PEM is often associated with vitamin A deficiency. A large dose of vitamin A should be given on admission, since ocular lesions can develop as adequate protein and energy feeding begins and the metabolic demands for retinol increase. Water-miscible vitamin A should be given orally or IM on the first day, at a dose of 50,000 to 100,000 IU for infants and preschool children, or 100,000 to 200,000 IU for older children and adults, followed by 5000 IU orally each day for the duration of treatment. The initial dose should be repeated two more days in symptomatic cases. Corneal ulcerations should be treated with ophthalmic drops of 1% atropine solution and antibiotic ointments or drops until the ulceration heals.

Homeostatic Restoration of Nutritional Status. The next objective of therapy is to replace tissue deficits as rapidly and as safely as possible. It is best to begin with a liquid formula fed orally or by nasogastric tube, divided equally into 5 to 12 feedings per day, depending on the patient's age and general condition. This frequent feeding of small volumes avoids vomiting and prevents the development of hypoglycemia and hypothermia. Intravenous feeding is rarely justified in primary PEM.

The protein source must be of high biological value and easily digested. Cow's milk is frequently available, but some clinicians worry about the possibility of lactose malabsorption in severe PEM. However, cow's milk is well-tolerated and assimilated by severely malnourished children and can be safely advocated [30,31]. Goat's, ewe's, buffalo's, and cam-

el's milk can also be used. Human, mare's, and ass's milk, however, have very low protein concentrations. Eggs, meat, fish, soy, and some vegetable-protein mixtures are also sources of good protein. Most vegetable mixtures have protein digestibilities that are 10 to 20 percent lower than animal proteins, making it necessary to feed larger amounts. Their bulk may pose a problem in feeding small children, but energy density can be increased by adding sugar and/or vegetable oil. The latter will also provide the essential fatty acids needed.

Based on the premise that the patient is adapted to the malnourished state, nutritional treatment must begin slowly to avoid deleterious metabolic disruptions. Various regimens provide a diet that meets daily maintenance requirements for a few days, followed by a gradual increase in nutrient delivery. A practical therapeutic strategy is based on a basic liquid food with high protein concentration and high energy density; Table 118-6 gives several examples. Delivery of proteins and energy is gradually increased using different concentrations of the basic food, as shown in Table 118-7; the additional sugar compensates for the dilution of dietary energy. The liquid preparations must be fed at a dose of 100 mL/(kg·day). Additional water must be given to provide at least 1 mL of total fluids per kilocalorie in the diet. After day 7 the patient can be allowed larger amounts of food (ad libitum). The only difference between the treatment of kwashiorkor and marasmus is that the latter often requires larger amounts of dietary energy, which must be raised at 5-day intervals, depending on the patient's weight gain. The intervals for the dietary increments in Table 118-7 can be lengthened to 3 to 5 days in very severely malnourished children, especially those with plasma protein less than 3 g/dL or with serious metabolic disturbances.

The attitude of the person who feeds the patient and the appearance, color, and flavor of the foods influence appetite. For older children with good appetite, the liquid formula can

Table 118-6. Formulations for high-protein, high-energy liquid foods (3–4 g protein and 135–145 kcal per 100 mL)

Food used as protein source	Amount, g	Sucrose, g	Oil,* g	Water, mL
Cow's, goat's, or camel's milk, fresh	1000	100	40	——
Cow's milk, full-cream powder	140	100	40	900
Cow's milk, skimmed powder	110	100	70	900
Yogurt (cow's or goat's milk)	900	100	40	——
Buffalo's or ewe's (sheep's) milk, fresh	850	100	15	150
K-Mix 2†	140	70	70	900
ICSM‡	170	100	40	900
Incaparina§	140	100	55	900

*Amount of vegetable oil can be substituted for up to one-half with isoenergetic amounts of sugar.
†Mixture of 17% calcium caseinate, 28% skimmed milk powder, 55% sucrose, and vitamin A, distributed by UNICEF.
‡Mixture of 63% cornmeal, 24% defatted soy flour, 5% skimmed milk powder, 5% soy oil, and 3% vitamin and mineral mix, distributed by U.S. AID and CARE.
§Mixture of 58% lime-treated corn flour, 38% cottonseed flour, and 4% vitamin, mineral, and lysine mix, developed by INCAP.

Table 118-7. Example of a dietary therapeutic regimen for children based on dilutions of the basic high-energy foods shown in Table 118-6*

Days from beginning of treatment	Proportions of Basic food	+ Water	Additional sugar, g/100 mL	Additional oil, mL/100 mL	100 mL will provide Protein, g	Energy, kcal
1	1 +	2	10	——	1–1.3	85–90
3	1 +	1	10	——	1.5–2	110–115
5	3 +	1	5	——	2.3–3	120–130
7	Undiluted		——	——	3–4	135–145
Marasmus†						
12	Undiluted		——	3	3–4	160–170
17	Undiluted		——	6	3–4	185–195
22	Undiluted		——	9	3–4	210–220
etc.	Undiluted		——	†	3–4	†

*The formulas must be fed at 100 mL/(kg·day). They must be supplemented with adequate amounts of vitamins, minerals, and electrolytes. Additional water must be given to provide at least 1 mL of total fluids per kcal in the diet.

†Marasmic patients may require more dietary energy; 2 to 3 mL (half a teaspoon) of vegetable oil per 100 mL of liquid diet should be added at 5-day intervals until the rate of weight gain becomes adequate.

be partly substituted with solid foods that have high concentrations of good-quality, easily digestible nutrients.

The diet must be supplemented to provide 8 to 10 meq of potassium, 3 to 5 meq of sodium, 5 to 8 meq of calcium, and 1 to 2 meq of magnesium per kilogram of body weight per day. This can be accomplished by adding 0.3 g KCl and 0.1 g NaCl per 100 mL to milk formulas, or by adding appropriate amounts of the mineral mixture shown in Table 118-8 to most other diets. Additional supplements should include daily doses of 60 to 120 mg elemental iron, 10 mg elemental zinc, 0.3 mg folic acid, 5000 IU vitamin A, and other vitamins and trace elements in the doses provided by most commercial preparations.

Therapeutic diets for children of school age and adults must be adjusted to their age. Initial treatment should provide average energy and protein requirements, followed by a gradual increase to about 1.5 times the energy and three to four times the protein requirements by the seventh day. Dietary energy delivery to marasmic patients may have to be increased further.

The initial response to diet is either no change in weight or a decrease due to loss of edema, accompanied by large diuresis. After some time, commonly 7 to 15 days, a period of rapid weight gain or "catch up" begins. The rate of catch up usually is slower in marasmus than kwashiorkor. In children, this rate of weight gain generally is 10 to 15 times that of a normal child of the same age, and it can be as high as 20 to 25 times greater. Some patients only show a four- or fivefold increase in catch up; most times this is associated with insufficient energy intakes (formula inadequately prepared, insufficient amounts of formula given at each feeding, too few feedings per day, anorexia, or lack of patience of the person who feeds the child) or with overt or asymptomatic infections. Urinary infections and tuberculosis are among the most commonly seen asymptomatic diseases.

Ensuring Nutritional Rehabilitation. This last stage of treatment may begin in the hospital and continue on an outpatient basis, but making sure that the patient continues eating adequate amounts of protein, energy, and other nutrients, especially when traditional foods are introduced into the diet. Emotional and physical stimulation must be provided, and persistent diarrhea, intestinal parasites, and other minor complications treated. Children can be vaccinated during this period as well.

1. Introduction of Traditional Foods. Other foods, especially those available at home, are gradually introduced into the diet in combination with the high-energy, high-protein formula. This should be done when edema has disappeared, the skin lesions are notably improved, the patient becomes active and interacts with the environment, appetite is restored, and adequate rates of catch-up growth have been achieved. For children, a daily minimum intake of 3 to 4 g of protein and 120 to 150 kcal per kilogram of body weight (or more in marasmus) must be ensured. To achieve this, the energy density of solid

Table 118-8. Mineral mixture to complement liquid formulas

Salt	Amount, g	1 g mixture provides, meq	
KCl	44	K^+	8.5
NaCl	9	Na^+	3.5
Na_2HPO_4	7	Ca^{2+}	1.4
$CaCO_3$	5	Mg^{2+}	0.6
$MgSO_4,·7H_2O$	5	HPO_4^{2-}	1.4

foods must be increased with oil or fat, and protein density and quality must be high, using animal proteins, vegetable protein mixtures, or soybean protein concentrates and isolates. Local traditional foods can be used in appropriate combinations, *in addition to the liquid formula,* as in the following examples: (1) one part of a dry pulse or its flour (black beans, soybeans, kidney beans, cowpeas) and three parts of a dry cereal or flour (corn, rice, wheat); fat or oil should be added to the mashed or strained pulse during or after cooking, in amounts equal to the weight of the dry pulse or flour, and to the cereal preparations in amounts of 10 to 30 mL oil per 100 g dry cereal product, depending on the type of preparation. (2) Four parts of dry rice and two parts of fresh fish; fat or oil should be added in amounts equal to 20 to 40 percent of the dry weights. The foods can be served as separate dishes or they can be mashed or blended and fed as paps to infants and young children.

2. Emotional and Physical Stimulation. The malnourished child needs affection and tender care from the beginning of treatment. This requires patience and understanding by the hospital staff and the relatives. Involvement of parents or relatives is usually very helpful. Hospitals should be brightly colored, cheerful, with audible stimulation such as music. As soon as the child can move without assistance and is willing to interact with the staff and other children, he or she must be encouraged to explore, to play, and to participate in activities that involve body movements. These principles are rarely achieved in practice in developing countries. Relatively small increments in physical activity and energy expenditure during the course of nutritional rehabilitation result in faster longitudinal growth and accretion of lean body tissues [10].

Parents should be encouraged to stimulate and teach their children by playing and talking. Toys and play materials can often be made from discarded local articles.

3. Persistent Diarrhea and Other Health Problems. Mild diarrhea does not interfere with nutritional rehabilitation, as long as fluid and electrolyte intakes maintain satisfactory hydration, and often disappears without specific treatment as nutritional status improves. Persistent diarrhea can contribute to the development of a new episode of PEM and should be treated. This is determined by the underlying cause of diarrhea, usually intestinal infections, excessive bacterial flora in the upper gut that ferment food substrates and deconjugate bile salts, intestinal parasites (particularly giardiasis, cryptosporidiosis, and trichiuriasis), and intolerance to food components. Among the latter, lactose, milk protein, and gluten have often been held responsible. This is often founded on inadequate diagnostic procedures (e.g., intolerance to 2 g lactose per kilogram of body weight in aqueous solution, rather than to the 7 to 15 g lactose contained in a milk meal) [32]. When food intolerance is suspected, the diet should be modified, taking care to preserve its nutritional quality and nutrient density. Before brand-

ing a patient as intolerant to a given food, it should be reintroduced into the diet to confirm the diagnosis and adequate diagnostic tests should be done.

4. Criteria for Recovery. The most practical criterion is weight gain. A patient should be discharged from in-hospital or outpatient treatment when he or she has reached a body weight equal to or near the expected weight for height. A premature discharge increases the risk of a recurrence of malnutrition. If urine can be collected for 24 h in children, the creatinine-height index [28] can be used as an indicator of body protein repletion. Specific treatment of other nutritional problems (e.g., iron deficiency) may have to be prolonged beyond discharge for PEM.

When discharged, patients or their parents must be taught about the causes of PEM, emphasizing rational and nutritious use of household foods, personal and environmental hygiene, appropriate immunizations, and early treatment of diarrhea and other diseases.

Mild and moderate PEM

The less-severe forms of PEM should be treated in an ambulatory setting, supplementing the home diet with easily digested foods that contain proteins of high biological value and a high energy density. In some instances, therapy can be achieved merely by instructing the adult patient about adequate eating habits and a better use of food resources or by instructing mothers in improved child-feeding practices and in more nutritious culinary habits. It is almost always necessary, however, to provide both nutritious food supplements and instructions in their use.

The quantity of food supplements will vary depending upon the degree of malnutrition and the relative deficit of proteins and energy. As a general guideline, the goal should be to provide a total intake—including the home diet—of *at least* twice the protein and 1.5 times the energy requirements. For preschool children, this would signify a daily intake of about 2 to 2.5 g of high-quality protein and 120 to 150 kcal per kilogram of body weight, and for infants under 1 year, about 3.5 g protein and 150 kcal/(kg·day).

The ingestion of the food supplement by the malnourished person must be ensured. This is more likely to occur if it is appetizing to both the child and the mother, if it is ready-made or easy to prepare, if additional amounts are provided to feed the siblings, and if it does not have an important commercial value outside the home that would make it easy and profitable for the family to sell the item for cash. A substitution effect on the home diet (i.e., a decrease in the usual food intake) is almost unavoidable, but it can be reduced by using low-bulk supplements with high protein and energy concentrations. Special attention should be given to avoid a decrease in breast-feeding; the supplements for breast-fed infants should be paps or solid foods that will not quench the infant's thirst and thus not change the infant's demand nor the mother's attitude toward lactation.

Adequate amounts of vitamins and minerals must be ensured, although mild deficiencies can be overcome by the micronutrients in the food or using fortified vehicles such as iron-enriched bread or sugar fortified with retinol.

POPULATION

The epidemiology of PEM is discussed in Chap. 23. Certain aspects, however, should be further emphasized.

POPULATION ECOLOGY

PEM can affect all age groups but it is more frequent among children whose growth increases nutritional requirements, and especially among the very young who cannot obtain food and ensure adequate intakes by their own means. Older children usually have milder forms of PEM because they can cope better with social and food availability constraints, because infections and other precipitating factors become less severe, and because early survival may imply a natural selection of the more fit. Pregnant and lactating women can also have PEM, but the consequences of the dietary deficiencies are seen mainly in the growth, nutritional status, and survival rates of their fetuses, newborn babies, and infants. Adult men and nonpregnant, nonlactating women usually have the lowest prevalence and the mildest forms of the disease, because of greater opportunities to obtain food and social and cultural practices that protect the productive members of the family.

Poverty, low food availability, and infectious disease stress are causes of PEM (see Chaps. 22 to 24). In some families or societies, ignorance may lead to poor infant- and child-rearing practices, misconceptions about the use of certain foods, inadequate feeding practices during illnesses, and improper food distribution among the family members. Poor environmental conditions favoring infections, and social problems such as child abuse, maternal deprivation, alcoholism, and drug addiction can lead to PEM in children and adults. Other circumstances that contribute to or precipitate PEM are agricultural patterns and climatic conditions leading to cyclic or sudden food scarcities, social and cultural practices which impose food taboos, the migration from traditional rural settings to urban slums, and a decline in the practice or duration of breast-feeding.

A profile of risk factors can indicate which individuals or societies are more prone to PEM. Thus, the most likely victims are children under 2 years of age from low socioeconomic strata whose parents have a series of misconceptions concerning the use of foods, whose families are known to have a high prevalence of alcoholism and unstable marriages, who live under poor sanitary conditions in urban slums or in rural areas frequently subject to droughts or floods, and whose societal beliefs prohibit the use of many nutritious foods.

PREVENTION AND CONTROL OF PEM

Measures that will prevent the recurrence of PEM or the appearance of new cases include the availability and rational use of foods that optimize nutrient utilization, the control or reduction of infections, and health and nutrition education programs for the individual, the family, and the community.

Food availability

Inadequate food availability caused by poverty, cultural customs, cyclical climatic conditions, and natural disasters and those of human origin are the major constraints in the control of malnutrition. The solution of some conditions is dependent on social and economic changes while others, as natural disasters, are beyond human control. However, the pediatrician, nutritionist, public health worker, and educator can and *must* play an active role in ameliorating or solving other conditions.

Animal foods are the best protein sources but they tend to be expensive, not always available, or prohibited by religious practices. Under such circumstances, the staple foods can be complemented or substituted with vegetable foods combined in ways to permit a good essential amino acid complementation and improve the biological value of dietary protein. For example, corn and black bean combinations that provide proteins in a proportion of about 60:40, equivalent to about three parts of dry corn and one part of dry beans, have an excellent amino acid composition and permit adequate growth and function [33,34]. The same is true of a series of combinations of grains and/or legumes [4]. The relatively low nitrogen digestibility of these vegetable sources must be considered in recommending the amounts to be eaten. Energy density can be increased by adding fats or carbohydrates.

It will often be necessary to convince parents about the safety of using foods which, in some cultures, are fed only to adults and older children. This is especially true in the case of weaning foods. Trials at INCAP have shown that it is feasible to feed pablums based on legumes, a cereal, and vegetable oil to babies as young as 3 months without intestinal symptoms and without decreasing breast-milk intakes. Examples of such paps are shown in Table 118-9. Promotion of breast-feeding must accompany the recommendation for weaning foods.

Reduction of morbidity rates

This is a logical consequence of the interactions of nutrition with infection [35,36]. Since young children are at higher risk of malnutrition, high priority must be given to immunizations, sanitary measures to reduce fecal contamination, and early oral rehydration of children with diarrhea [37].

Education

The presence of a malnourished child in a family suggests that other members of the household might also be at risk of malnutrition. Therefore, nutritional and health education must not

Table 118-9. Paps to complement breast milk, using common foods and based on combinations of a legume, a grain, and vegetable oil

	A	B	C	D
Cooked beans*	25 g	20 g	20 g	25 g
Vegetable oil	12 g	7 g	7 g	10 g
Corn dough†	20 g	—	—	—
White bread‡	—	10 g	—	—
Boiled rice	—	—	22 g	—
Boiled potatoes	—	—	—	31 g
Protein, g/100 g§	5.6	7.1	6.1	5.5
Energy, kcal/100 g§	312	268	269	232

*Black beans (*Phaseolus vulgaris*), cooked and strained according to Guatemalan customs.
†Cooked, lime-treated corn dough.
‡Moistened with about 50 percent water.
§Protein and energy content of 100 g of pap, ready to eat.

Source: From F.E. Viteri, B. García, B. Torún, unpublished observations.

be restricted to the rehabilitation of the index case, but to prevention of nutritional deterioration of other family members, especially siblings and pregnant and lactating women. Similarly, a high prevalence of children with malnutrition or growth retardation indicates that the entire community is at some risk of impaired nutrition. Consequently, education programs must be devised for community leaders, civic action groups, and the community as a whole. Such programs must emphasize promotion of breast-feeding, appropriate use of weaning foods, nutritional alternatives using traditional foods, personal and environmental hygiene, feeding practices during illness and convalescence, and early treatment of diarrhea and other diseases. Personal and communal involvement should be pursued through commitments to apply the recommendations. Toward this aim, it is very important that all educational programs incorporate the people's own assessment of their nutritional problems and their feelings toward personal participation to contribute to the solution.

REFERENCES

1 Brozek J: Nutrition, brain and behaviour, in Harper AE, Davis GK (eds): *Nutrition in Health and Disease and International Development.* New York, Alan R Liss, 1981, pp 371–382
2 Grantham-McGregor S: The effect of childhood malnutrition on mental development, in Taylor TG, Jenkins NK (eds): *Proceeding of the XIII International Congress of Nutrition.* London, John Libbey, 1986, pp 68–74
3 UNICEF: *The State of the World's Children 1988.* Oxfordshire, P & L Adamson, 1988
4 Torún B, Young VR, Rand WM (eds): *Protein-Energy Requirements of Developing Countries: Evaluation of New Data.* Food Nutr Bull (suppl 5), 1981
5 *Energy and Protein Requirements:* Report of a joint FAO/WHO/UNU expert consultation. WHO Tech Rep Ser 724, Geneva, World Health Organization, 1985
6 Torún B: Energy-nutrient interactions, in Bodwell CE, Erdman JW (eds): *Nutrient Interactions.* New York, Dekker, 1988
7 Torún B: Proteínas y aminoácidos: Características y satisfacción de requerimientos con dietas latinoamericanas. Arch Latinoam Nutr, in press
8 Viteri FE, Alvarado J, Luthringer DG, et al: Hematological changes in protein-calorie malnutrition. Vitam Horm 26:573–615, 1968
9 Rutishauser IHE, Whitehead RG: Energy intake and expenditure in 1–3-year-old Ugandan children living in a rural environment. Br J Nutr 28:145–152, 1972
10 Viteri FE, Torún B: Nutrition, physical activity and growth. in Ritzén M et al (eds): *The Biology of Normal Human Growth.* New York, Raven, 1981, pp 265–273
11 Viteri FE, Torún B: Ingestión calórica y trabajo físico de obreros agrícolas en Guatemala: Efecto de la suplementación alimentaria y su lugar en los programas de salud. Bol Sanit Panam 78:58–74, 1975
12 Waterlow JC: Adaptation to low-protein intakes, in Olson RE (ed): *Protein-Calorie Malnutrition.* New York, Academic, 1975, pp 23–35
13 Torún B, Viteri FE: Protein-energy malnutrition, in Shils ME, Young VR (eds): *Modern Nutrition in Health and Disease,* 7th ed. Philadelphia, Lea & Febiger, 1988, pp 746–773
14 Reddy V: Protein-energy malnutrition: An overview, in Harper AE, Davis GK (eds): *Nutrition in Health and Disease and International Development.* New York, Alan R Liss, 1981, pp 227–235
15 Patrick J: Death during recovery from severe malnutrition and its possible relationship to sodium pump activity in the leucocyte. Br Med J 1:1051–1054, 1977
16 *Measuring Change in Nutritional Status.* Geneva, World Health Organization, 1983
17 Gómez F, Ramos Galván R, Frenk S, et al: Mortality in second and third degree malnutrition. J Trop Pediatr 2:77–83, 1956
18 Waterlow JC: Classification and definition of protein-energy malnutrition, in Beaton GH, Bengoa JM (eds): *Nutrition in Preventive Medicine.* Geneva, World Health Organization, 1976, pp 530–555
19 Cronk CE, Roche AF: Race- and sex-specific reference data for triceps and subscapular skinfolds and weight/stature^2. Am J Clin Nutr 35:347–354, 1982
20 National Center for Health Statistics: Plan and Operation of the HANE Survey, United States 1971–73. Department of Health, Education and Welfare publication (HSM)73–1310, 1973
21 Nichols BL, Alvarado J, Hazlewood CF, et al: Significance of muscle potassium depletion in protein-calorie malnutrition. J Pediatr 80:319–330, 1972
22 Torún B, Chew F: Spontaneous physical activity and energy expenditure of low-income preschool children. Submitted for publication
23 Spurr GB: Effects of chronic energy deficiency on stature, work capacity and productivity, in First Meeting of the International Dietary Energy Consultative Group in Guatemala. Lausanne, International Dietary Energy Consultative Group, 1987
24 Keusch GT, Torún B, Johnson RB, et al: Impairment of hemolytic complement activation by both classical and alternative pathways in serum from patients with kwashiorkor. J Pediatr 105:434–436, 1984

25 Chandra RK, Puri S: Nutritional regulation of host resistance and predictive value of immunologic tests in assessment outcome. Pediatr Clin North Am 32:499–515, 1985

26 Kauffman CA, Jones PG, Kluger MJ: Fever and malnutrition: Endogenous pyrogen/interleukin-1 in malnourished patients. Am J Clin Nutr 44:449–452, 1986

27 Black RE, Brown KH, Becker S: Malnutrition is a determining factor in diarrheal duration, but not incidence, among young children in a longitudinal study in rural Bangladesh. Am J Clin Nutr 39:87–94, 1984

28 Viteri FE, Alvarado J: The creatinine-height index: Its use in the estimation of the degree of protein depletion and repletion in PCM children. Pediatrics 46:696–706, 1970

29 Chen LC, Chowdry AKMA, Huffman SL: Anthropometric assessment of energy-protein malnutrition and subsequent risk of mortality among preschool aged children. Am J Clin Nutr 33:1838–1845, 1980

30 Solomons NW, Torún B, Caballero B, et al: The effect of dietary lactose on the early recovery from protein-energy malnutrition I: Clinical and anthropometric indices. Am J Clin Nutr 40:591–600, 1984

31 Torún B, Solomons NW, Caballero B, et al: The effect of dietary lactose on the early recovery from protein-energy malnutrition. II. Indices of nutrient absorption. Am J Clin Nutr 40:601–610, 1984

32 Torún B, Solomons NW, Viteri FE: Lactose malabsorption and lactose intolerance: Implications for general milk consumption. Arch Latinoamer Nutr 29:445–494, 1979

33 Torún B, Viteri FE: Energy requirements of preschool children and effects of varying energy intakes on protein metabolism. Food Nutr Bull supp 5:229–241, 1981

34 Viteri FE, Torún B, Arroyave G, et al: Use of corn-bean mixtures to satisfy protein and energy requirements of preschool children. Food Nutr Bull (suppl 5):202–209, 1981

35 Whitehead RG: Infection and the development of kwashiorkor and marasmus in Africa. Am J Clin Nutr 30:1281–1284, 1977

36 Mata LJ: *The Children of Santa María Cauqué: A Prospective Field Study of Health and Growth.* Cambridge, Mass, MIT Press, 1978

37 Keusch GT, Katz M (eds): Effective interventions to reduce infection in malnourished populations. Am J Clin Nutr 31:2035–2126, 2202–2356, 1978

CHAPTER 119 / *Folate and Vitamin B$_{12}$* · Joel B. Mason · Irwin H. Rosenberg

The two vitamins folate and vitamin B$_{12}$ are related in certain biochemical functions and especially in the sequela of their deficiency state: megaloblastic anemia [1]. This chapter examines the assimilation and utilization of the two nutrients by human beings, the diagnosis and consequences of their deficiency states, and the epidemiological patterns of deficiency.

THE NUTRIENTS

CHEMISTRY

The chemical structure for the family of cobalamins commonly referred to as vitamin B$_{12}$ is seen in Fig. 119-1. According to the nomenclature rules established by the International Union of Pure and Applied Chemistry (IUPAC), the term *vitamin B$_{12}$* refers only to cyanocobalamin. In practice, the other forms of cobalamin that are listed in the upper right-hand corner of Fig. 119-1 are also referred to by that name because, biologically, all are effective in the treatment of vitamin B$_{12}$ deficiency (except in those rare instances where there is a metabolic block impairing interconversion of different forms of the vitamin). Methylcobalamin, deoxyadenosylcobalamin (coenzyme B$_{12}$), and hydroxycobalamin account for nearly all the vitamin B$_{12}$ in the human. In this chapter *vitamin B$_{12}$* refers to any of the biologically active congeners of cobalamin.

The core structure of the cobalamins is a planar corrin ring system, the center of which is a cobalt atom coordinated to four nitrogen atoms. Various R groups may occupy one of the coordination positions of the cobalt atom and thus determine the particular congener of vitamin B$_{12}$. Cyanocobalamin, the pharmaceutical form of vitamin B$_{12}$, is rarely, if ever, found in nature. Naturally occurring vitamin B$_{12}$ exists in a variety of reduced forms and is usually linked to a peptide through an amide bond.

Like *vitamin B$_{12}$, folate* is a generic term: it refers to a family of structurally and functionally related compounds. Folic acid (pteroylglutamic acid) is the parent compound and is the pharmaceutical form of the vitamin. The structure of folic acid is shown in Fig. 119-2 and can be seen to be composed of three moieties: a pterin ring linked to a para-aminobenzoic acid moiety, which in turn is linked to a glutamic acid residue through an amide bond.

All naturally occurring folates are reduced: in the case of dihydrofolate, at the 7 and 8 positions of the pterin ring and in the case of tetrahydrofolate, at the 5,6,7, and 8 positions of the ring. Naturally occurring folates have two other major structural additions compared to folic acid. The first is that one-carbon moieties of varying oxidation states may be linked to the number 5 and/or number 10 nitrogen atoms, which confers its major function to folate as a one-carbon carrier. The other special feature of naturally occurring folates is that many have multiple glutamic acid residues. Each successive glutamic acid residue is linked to its proximate neighbor by a γ-amide

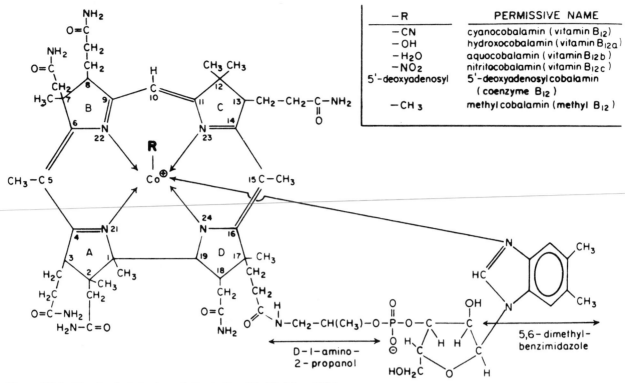

-R	PERMISSIVE NAME
-CN	cyanocobalamin (vitamin B$_{12}$)
-OH	hydroxocobalamin (vitamin B$_{12a}$)
-H$_2$O	aquocobalamin (vitamin B$_{12b}$)
-NO$_2$	nitritocobalamin (vitamin B$_{12c}$)
5'-deoxyadenosyl	5'-deoxyadenosylcobalamin (coenzyme B$_{12}$)
-CH$_3$	methylcobalamin (methyl B$_{12}$)

Figure 119-1. The chemical structure of vitamin B$_{12}$. (*Modified from* [36].)

linkage. In mammalian systems most folates have 1 to 7 residues, although other biologically derived folates have been noted to have as many as 11.

PHYSIOLOGY

Intestinal absorption

Considerable evidence suggests that the absorption of folate is most avid in the proximal one-third of the small intestine and that the vast majority of dietary folate is absorbed in this portion of the gastrointestinal tract. At the concentrations of folate usually found in the proximal small intestine virtually all of the absorption proceeds by a carrier-mediated process that is located in the brush border of the enterocyte. Absorption is markedly sensitive to the pH of the intestinal lumen: it proceeds maximally at a luminal pH of 6.0 and decreases rapidly as a neutral pH is approached. All of the various reduced and one-carbon substituted forms of folate seem to share this transport system.

Most dietary folates are polyglutamates. As such, they cannot be absorbed by the above-mentioned transport system until they have undergone hydrolysis in the lumen of the intestine to the monoglutamate form. This is accomplished by an enzyme called *folyl polyglutamate hydrolase* (or trivially, *conjugase*) that is found in the small intestine. The extent to which dietary folate is absorbed appears to be markedly influenced

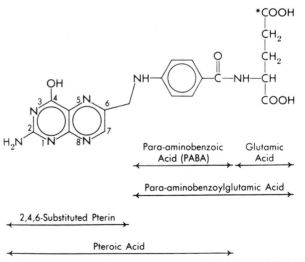

Folic Acid (Pteroylglutamic Acid)

Figure 119-2. The chemical structure of folic acid and the various components of the molecule. (*From V. Herbert in L.S. Goodman, A. Gilman (eds.): The Pharmacological Basis of Therapeutics, New York, Macmillan, 1975.*)

by the form in which it is ingested. Approximately 70 to 100 percent of a dose of purified folic acid is absorbed; the absorption of purified polyglutamyl folic acid being about 80 percent of that value. Tamura and Stokstad [2] have demonstrated that the extent of absorption of dietary folate and its subsequent availability for metabolism can be substantially less than for corresponding pure forms of the vitamin. Their data suggest that the bioavailability of food folate is 30 to 100 percent and is substantially influenced by the nature of the foodstuff containing the folate. The factors associated with foodstuffs that determine the absorption of folate are poorly defined although it is known that certain foods, such as yeast extract and a wide variety of pulses, contain conjugase inhibitors that may interfere with intestinal absorption. Some investigators have found the availability of folate from brewer's yeast to be as low as 10 percent. The impact of these foodborne conjugase inhibitors on the folate status of marginally nourished populations has yet to be defined. The concern is that if such a population ingested the majority of its calories in the form of a single pulse, as is frequently the case, then what little folate was present in the diet would not be effectively absorbed.

Intestinal absorption of vitamin B_{12} proceeds by a very different mechanism. Dietary vitamin B_{12} is released from its association with polypeptides by gastric acid and gastric and intestinal enzymes. Gastric intrinsic factor (IF, a glycoprotein produced by gastric parietal cells) and R-binders (produced by the salivary glands), both of which avidly bind free vitamin B_{12}, are available in the stomach and upper small intestine. Vitamin B_{12} binds preferentially to the R-binders. However, R-binders are subsequently destroyed by trypsin digestion in the small bowel, enabling vitamin B_{12} to bind to IF. In the ileum specific mucosal receptors recognize the complex and mediate the absorption of the vitamin. Approximately 50 percent of a 1-μg dose of crystalline cyanocobalamin is absorbed. However, dietary B_{12}, most of which is protein-bound, is absorbed with much lower efficiency: only 2.5 percent of B_{12} in such form is absorbed. Patients with hypochlorhydria may exhibit normal absorption of crystalline B_{12} but severe impairment of protein-bound B_{12} [3]. This may be due to inadequate protein digestion by the stomach, to the bacterial overgrowth associated with hypochlorhydria, or to some other, unknown factors. A Schilling test in such an individual can thus be highly misleading.

Transport, distribution, and excretion

Virtually all of the folate circulating in the portal and systemic circulation is 5-methyltetrahydrofolate (5-methyl-THF). More than one-half of this folate is bound nonspecifically to a variety of low-affinity binding proteins such as serum albumin. Less than 5 percent of circulating folate is bound specifically to a high-affinity folate-binding protein. The function of this high-affinity binding protein remains unclear. The remaining portion of circulating folate is unbound. Circulating folate is delivered to most tissues by specific active transport systems, thus enabling concentrations to be achieved in those tissues that exceed the concentration found in the blood.

Total body folate content in the adult is thought to be 5 to 10 mg. Approximately one-half of this is present in the liver. Most intracellular folates in the body exist in a polyglutamate form. Since monoglutamyl, but not polyglutamyl, folates can cross cellular membranes, the interconversion of folate between these forms is thought to play a major role in the distribution of folate among the various body compartments.

Significant excretion of folate occurs by both fecal and urinary routes. The amount lost by these two routes is thought to be approximately equal, although the total folate content of feces in considerably greater because substantial quantities of the vitamin are produced by enteric bacteria. The concentration of biologically active folates in the bile is about five times the concentration in serum. Enterohepatic circulation of this biliary folate is felt to play an important role in the body's economy of this vitamin.

Vitamin B_{12} circulates in the blood primarily as methylcobalamin. It is entirely protein-bound; the binding being distributed among three specific binding proteins: transcobalamin I, II, and III (TC I–III). Only TC II appears to be important in delivering vitamin B_{12} to receptors that recognize the vitamin-binding protein complex and mediate the uptake of B_{12} into the cell.

Total body vitamin B_{12} is thought to be between 1 and 10 mg, 50 to 90 percent of which is stored in the liver. Coenzyme B_{12} appears to be the major storage form of the vitamin. The enterohepatic circulation reclaims virtually all of the vitamin excreted through the bile. The frugal nature of this enterohepatic circulation of B_{12} is a major reason why, even in vegetarians, decades may pass before inadequate dietary intake results in a clinical deficiency state.

Metabolic utilization

Folate is a necessary coenzyme in the synthesis of thymidylate and is thus critical in the synthesis of DNA. The metabolic interdependence of folate and B_{12} stems from the fact that the 5-methyl-THF that is destined to mediate the synthesis of thymidylate from deoxyuridylate can only enter the pathway through a methylcobalamin-dependent step. The respective functions of the two vitamins in this pathway are outlined in Fig. 119-3. Cellular deficiency of methylcobalamin produces a so-called "methylfolate trap" in which the 5-methyl-THF becomes metabolically isolated and therefore useless. This also explains why the hematological sequelae of both vitamin B_{12} and folate deficiencies are so similar: the final common pathway in each instance is a deficiency of 5,10-methylene-THF. Defective DNA synthesis results and manifests as megaloblastic bone marrow, ineffective hematopoiesis, and, eventually, macrocytic anemia. Similarly, all dividing cells in the body

Figure 119-3. The metabolic interrelationship of vitamin B$_{12}$ and folate. (*From* [*36*].)

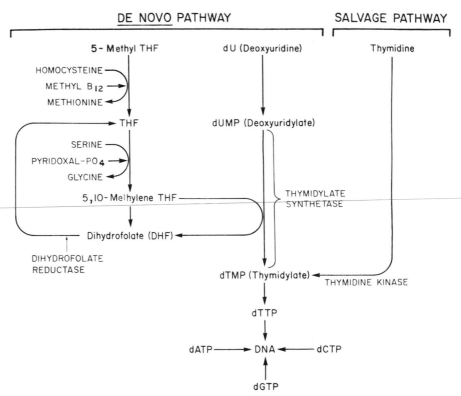

are affected, resulting in megaloblastic epithelium and functional abnormalities in locations such as the gastrointestinal tract [4].

As a coenzyme involved in the transfer of one-carbon units, folate is necessary in a number of other important metabolic pathways. The interconversion of serine and glycine as well as the metabolism of the essential amino acids histidine and methionine are folate-dependent pathways. In addition, folate is involved in the de novo synthesis of purines, in the methylation of transfer RNA, and in the metabolism of formate.

Vitamin B$_{12}$ has a number of other functions. It is somehow necessary for the synthesis of myelin, although its role in this pathway is unclear. In addition, B$_{12}$ is involved in fat and carbohydrate metabolism by virtue of its role in converting methylmalonate to succinate and in protein metabolism by mediating the synthesis of methionine from homocysteine. Finally, B$_{12}$ also appears to serve an antioxidant function by maintaining sulfhydryl groups in a reduced form: in vitamin B$_{12}$ deficiency the liver develops decreased levels of the reduced form of glutathione.

DIETARY SOURCES AND REQUIREMENTS

Folate is present in a wide variety of foodstuffs. Foods containing particularly high concentrations are leafy vegetables, some fruits, liver and other organ meats, yeast, and pulses. The latter two foodstuffs, as mentioned above, have been identified as containing folyl polyglutamate hydrolase inhibitors

which are reported to significantly reduce folate absorption. Folates are very susceptible to oxidative degradation. Consequently, protracted cooking of foodstuffs and other forms of food processing can result in substantial losses of the folate content in foods.

Considerable evidence now exists that 3.0 to 3.1 μg folate per kilogram per day (approximately 200 μg/day for adult men, 170 for adult women) is an adequate dietary goal to ensure nutritional repletion in a population of normal adults [5]. Infants up to 1 year of age should receive 3.6 μg/(kg·day), and children aged 1 to 9 years should receive 3.3 μg/(kg·day). Human and bovine milk contain sufficient folate for an infant fed entirely with milk. However, infants fed entirely on goat's milk should receive folate supplementation, since the content and availability of folate in goat milk is quite low. Pregnancy and lactation are situations that cause substantial increases in folate utilization. Folate deficiency is common enough among pregnant women that most experts agree that all pregnant women should receive folate supplementation (see below). A dietary intake of 500 μg/day is recommended for pregnant women. For lactating women, 100 μg/day above their basal goal of 3 μg/(kg·day) is probably sufficient.

In contrast to the circumstances in the case of folate, vegetables and fruits are generally poor sources of vitamin B$_{12}$. Natural vitamin B$_{12}$ is thought to be derived entirely from bacterial synthesis. Consequently the only B$_{12}$ in plants is from soil or fecal contamination or, as is the case with some legumes, by bacterial synthesis in root nodules. Fortunately, the requirement for the vitamin is so small that even these sources may be sufficient for vegetarians. Rich sources of B_{12} are organ meats and bivalve molluscs, with lesser quantities in other meats, milk, and milk products. An extensive review of the presently available literature suggests that 2 μg of vitamin B_{12} per day is sufficient dietary intake to maintain normal body stores of the vitamin in adults while 0.06 μg/(kg·day) is sufficient for preadolescent children [6]. Pregnancy and lactation do not typically predispose to B_{12} deficiency, but because of increased utilization, the recommended intake during such times is 2.5 μg/day.

PATIENT

PATHOGENESIS OF DEFICIENCY STATES

Vitamin B_{12} and folate deficiency may arise from inadequate dietary intake, intestinal malabsorption, ineffective utilization, or increased excretion. The margin of safety between average dietary intake and daily metabolic needs is considerably smaller with folate than with B_{12}. As a result, insufficient dietary intake frequently plays a role in folate deficiency whereas diet is rarely a factor in B_{12} deficiency except in strict vegetarians.

Intestinal malabsorption is another frequent cause of folate deficiency. It may arise in situations in which there is a disease involving the small bowel such as sprue or inflammatory bowel disease. The role of naturally occurring conjugase inhibitors remains unclear. Certain drugs are capable of causing folate malabsorption, the most common of these being salicylazosulfapyridine (sulfasalazine) and diphenylhydantoin.

Ineffective utilization of folate is a common cause of folate deficiency in the form of alcohol abuse. Not only do many alcoholics consume a folate-deficient diet, but the folate they do ingest appears to be sequestered into certain body compartments, such as the liver, rendering the folate unavailable for general metabolism [7]. Less commonly drugs other than alcohol are the cause of ineffective utilization of the vitamin. Methotrexate, pyrimethamine, trimethoprim, triamterene, the sulfonamides, and pentamidine are all dihydrofolate reductase inhibitors ("antifols"). Many, if not all, of these antifols are capable of precipitating functional folate deficiency or exacerbating a preexisting deficiency state. As previously mentioned, B_{12} deficiency may also impair folate utilization: first, by blocking cellular uptake or retention of methylfolate, and second, by isolating the methylfolate that is present intracellularly from folate-dependent pathways.

The most common situations in which there is an increased requirement for folate are pregnancy and lactation. Pathological states where cell turnover is very high, such as chronic hemolysis or the lymphoproliferative disorders, also predispose to folate deficiency. Increased urinary excretion of folate may play a significant role in the development of folate deficiency in alcoholics [8], although this remains a controversial issue. In developed countries, where dialysis is frequently available, increased excretion of folate through chronic peritoneal dialysis and hemodialysis are important causes of deficiency among patients with renal disease.

Malabsorption of vitamin B_{12} accounts for 95 percent of all cases of B_{12} deficiency. It may be caused by gastric disorders, such as pernicious anemia or gastrectomy; by small-intestinal disease, such as Crohn's disease, involving the ileum, or by chronic pancreatic disease where the lack of trypsin prevents degradation of R-binders and the lack of pancreatic bicarbonate interferes with the maintenance of the alkaline environment necessary for optimal B_{12} absorption. In the case of bacterial overgrowth, bacteria compete for vitamin B_{12} with the host.

DIAGNOSIS OF DEFICIENCY

Laboratory diagnosis

The development of most vitamin deficiencies, including those of B_{12} and folate, follows a common progression of events. A drop in the serum level of the vitamin occurs first and is followed by a decrease in the vitamin concentration found in peripheral blood cells. Significant functional impairment of cellular function comes next, when enzyme systems dependent on that particular vitamin begin to malfunction. This is followed by evidence of impaired physiological functioning that is evident initially only under stress but eventually even in an unstressed state. Clinical signs and symptoms of deficiency usually begin to manifest themselves at this stage. Finally irreversible tissue damage occurs, and if left unchecked, may result in death.

This general scheme is reflected in Fig. 119-4. It shows the progression of abnormalities that occurred in a healthy adult man after he had been placed on a folate-free diet. It is worthwhile noting that evidence of cellular and organ dysfunction, as manifest by increased urinary formiminoglutamic acid (FIGLU) excretion and megaloblastic bone marrow, is more closely related chronologically to red blood cell (RBC) folate than serum folate levels. Furthermore, it is clear that the serum folate is a useful screen for folate status, but RBC folate is a considerably more accurate indication of folate stores in other

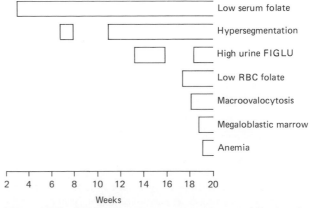

Figure 119-4. The chronological sequence of events following the elimination of folate from the diet (*From* [36].)

tissues than is the serum folate [9]. Serum levels correlate poorly with tissue levels and are really more a reflection of recent dietary intake. For this reason RBC folate is the preferable choice for assessing an individual's folate stores. A precautionary note about interpreting blood folate levels, however, is that B$_{12}$ deficiency may cause high serum levels and falsely low RBC folate levels. Serum and RBC folate levels traditionally have been assayed by a microbiological method, although suitable radioisotope binding assays have been developed over the past decade. Because the microbiological method is based on the growth of a folate-dependent bacterium, its results are susceptible to distortion by individuals whose blood contains antibiotics or other growth inhibitors.

With routinely available methods, the best way to assess vitamin B$_{12}$ status is by determining the serum B$_{12}$. Unlike serum folate, serum B$_{12}$ tends to be an accurate predictor of depleted tissue stores, although in pregnancy there is a physiological decrease in the serum B$_{12}$. After deficiency is documented, a Schilling test is frequently used to determine whether a malabsorptive disorder is responsible for the deficiency and what type of malabsorptive disorder it might be. Failure to absorb a normal quantity of radiolabeled B$_{12}$ documents malabsorption (part I); failure to correct the malabsorption with coadministration of intrinsic factor suggests a defect other than intrinsic factor deficiency (part II); and failure to correct malabsorption by previously administered antibiotics suggests something other than bacterial overgrowth (part III).

The megaloblastic anemia that develops in either vitamin B$_{12}$ or folate deficiency is characterized by macroovalocytic erythrocytes in the peripheral blood. As the anemia becomes more severe, anisocytosis and poikilocytosis become evident, as do leukopenia and thrombocytopenia. Hypersegmented polymorphonuclear neutrophils (five or more nuclear lobes) appear as an increasing proportion of the polymorph population, reaching 15 percent of the total in severe anemia. Examination of the bone marrow reveals the disassociation between nuclear and cytoplasmic maturation that is characteristic of megaloblastic tissue (see Fig. 119-5).

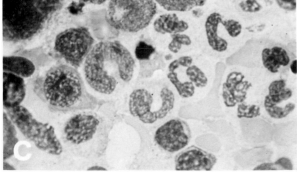
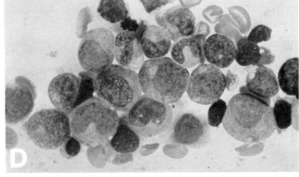
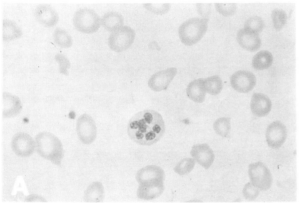
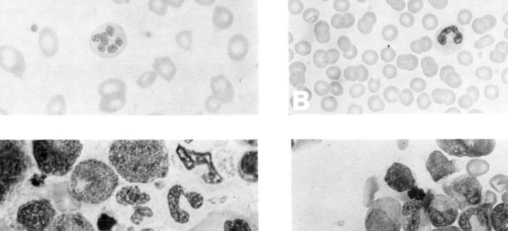

Figure 119-5. *A* and *B* are peripheral blood smears from a patient with megaloblastic anemia and from a normal individual, respectively. In addition to the macroovalocytes that are present in the abnormal smear, note the marked anisocytosis and poikilocytosis. A hypersegmented polymorphonuclear leukocyte is present in *A*. *C* and *D* are bone marrow smears from a patient with megaloblastic anemia and from a normal individual, respectively. Megaloblastic changes evident in *C* include the increased cellular size and the relative immaturity of the nucleus relative to the cytoplasm. Note the finer, more delicate pattern of chromatin in the megaloblastic nuclei. A giant band form, commonly found in megaloblastic marrow, is present left of center in *C*. Each panel × 100 with oil immersion. (*Courtesy of Pauline Cleary.*)

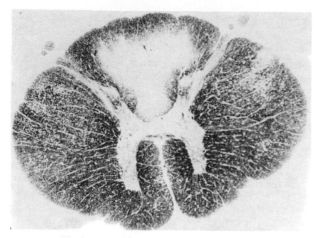

Figure 119-6. Cross section of a spinal cord from a patient with neuropathological complications of pernicious anemia. The stain for myelin indicates severe demyelination of the posterior spinal tracts. In this patient there was relatively mild demyelination of the lateral spinal tracts.

CLINICAL MANIFESTATIONS OF NEUROPATHOLOGY

Myelin synthesis is impaired in B_{12} deficiency resulting in damage to both peripheral and central myelinated nerves. A syndrome of peripheral neuropathy usually develops insidiously as the first sign of further neuropathology. Demyelination in the central nervous system is most evident in the lateral and posterior tracts of the spinal cord (see Fig. 119-6) with lesser degrees of damage in the brain. These central lesions are initially evidenced by the loss of position and vibration sense, with findings in the lower extremities usually more prominent than in the upper. Motor defects appear later, initially as ataxia and later superimposed with spasticity. Alterations in mentation are frequent and include irritability, apathy, emotional lability, intellectual deterioration, and psychosis. Optic neuropathy and central scotomas have been frequently reported. The term *subacute combined degeneration of the spine* is somewhat of a misnomer: a gradual, not subacute, onset is more common. In addition, an isolated peripheral syndrome, not necessarily combined with a central one, is common early on in the disease.

Folate deficiency does not cause demyelination. However, alterations in mood and mentation that can quickly resolve with nutritional repletion are well-documented. Other neurological lesions have been ascribed to folate deficiency but not convincingly so.

POPULATION

Nonindustrialized nations share with the industrialized world many risk factors for folate deficiency: pregnancy, lactation, low socioeconomic status, and alcoholism [10]. However, nonindustrialized and tropical nations also harbor their own distinctive ecological and demographic features that predispose segments of their populations to folate deficiency. A representative survey of folate status in an underdeveloped area is that performed by Colman et al. [11] (Fig. 119-7) on rural South African blacks. As is the case in the developed world, the segment of the population at greatest risk is clearly women of childbearing age. Parity as a risk factor for folate deficiency is particularly problematic in the underdeveloped world because of the extremely high birth rates that frequently exist. This particular survey also points to the elderly as a group at high risk of folate deficiency. Old age, as a risk factor for folate deficiency still needs to be confirmed by other surveys before it can be considered a general feature of this disease in underdeveloped nations.

The prevalence of vitamin B_{12} deficiency is considerably less than that of folate deficiency, presumably for the same reasons as in the developed world: the vanishingly small dietary requirement for the vitamin and the large storage capacity of the liver. Nevertheless, there are factors particular to the underdeveloped world that can produce vitamin B_{12} deficiency.

The following discussion highlights those factors in tropical and underdeveloped environments that predispose populations to deficiencies of these two vitamins.

PREGNANCY AND LACTATION

Pregnancy

From a global perspective pregnancy ranks among the most important of all the factors that contribute to folate deficiency. The additional metabolic requirements imposed by pregnancy put any woman with low or marginal dietary folate intake at risk. A joint Food and Agriculture Organization (FAO) and World Health Organization (WHO) group has estimated that depleted tissue folate stores are present in one-third of pregnant women worldwide [10]. This figure has been substantiated by

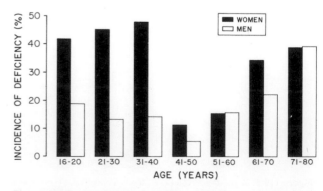

Figure 119-7. The incidence of folate deficiency in a rural South African population. Note the particularly high incidence of deficiency among women of childbearing age and among the elderly. See [11]. (*From [36].*)

a number of studies performed in the underdeveloped world as well as by studies performed in prenatal clinics serving women of low socioeconomic status in developed countries. Whether a particular pregnant woman will develop folate deficiency is largely dependent on factors such as her folate stores at the beginning of the pregnancy and the adequacy of dietary folate during the pregnancy. The presence of a twin pregnancy, a history of multiple prior pregnancies, and prolonged breast-feeding after prior pregnancies all appear to increase the risk of developing folate deficiency. What percent of pregnant women with evidence of depleted folate stores go on to develop frank megaloblastic anemia remains unclear. What is clear is that 25 to 30 percent of all pregnant women in surveys of western industrialized countries have evidence of megaloblastic changes in their bone marrow and that 0.5 to 5 percent have megaloblastic anemia [12]. Comparable figures from the underdeveloped world are less plentiful, although a survey of pregnant south Indian women, most of whom were from low and middle income families, demonstrated megaloblastic bone marrow in 54 percent and megaloblastic anemia in 20 percent [13].

The megaloblastic anemia of pregnancy usually appears during the latter portion of the third trimester and during the first month of the postpartum period. The anemia may be severe and fatal, and although the usual hematological profile is solely one of diminished red cell mass, it may present as severe pancytopenia. The degree to which the fetus is affected remains controversial: most investigators have found an increased incidence of stillbirths among women with megaloblastic anemia, although a couple of dissenting studies exist. Whether other obstetrical complications such as toxemia, prematurity, and fetal malformations are increased is even less clear, although one study from India and another from Africa suggest that in populations with a relatively high prevalence of folate deficiency, prenatal supplementation with folate substantially decreases the incidence of low-weight-for-date births and prematurity, respectively [14,15].

Although the recommended daily intake for vitamin B$_{12}$ is increased for pregnant women to compensate for increased utilization of the vitamin, epidemiological studies fail to demonstrate pregnancy as a significant risk factor for deficiency of the vitamin.

Lactation

The concentration of folate in human milk is high: it is variably reported as 50 to 150 ng/mL. Furthermore, dietary folate is preferentially incorporated into milk rather than into depleted maternal stores to such an extent that a lactating woman with depleted folate stores who receives supplementation will experience a rise in milk folate before rises are observed in her serum or RBC folate. Similarly, a lactating woman with folate deficiency is frequently able to maintain a normal level of folate in her milk. Thus, lactation serves as a factor that can

either sustain pregnancy-associated folate deficiency or predispose to the onset of postpartum folate deficiency [16]. This is a particular problem in many areas of the underdeveloped world where an extended period of breast-feeding is common.

In lactating women fed diets intentionally low in folate a supplement of 200 to 300 µg of folic acid per day is sufficient to maintain normal levels of serum folate in the mother. It remains less clear whether the same is true in populations in which there is high prevalence of folate deficiency.

As is the case with pregnancy, lactation does not seem to predispose toward B$_{12}$ deficiency.

AGE

Although there exists a single study reporting impaired absorption of folate polyglutamates in the elderly [17], there are otherwise few data to suggest significant alteration in the physiology of assimilation, utilization, and excretion of folate in the elderly. The increased prevalence of deficiency noted by Colman et al. (see Fig. 119-7) among elderly black South Africans has not yet been confirmed in other underdeveloped areas. It may be related to the edentulous state, the altered diet, and the chronic illnesses associated with old age.

INFECTION

Infectious diseases play a prominent role in human morbidity and mortality in the underdeveloped world because of, among other things, the widespread lack of adequate sanitation and the increased susceptibility to infection engendered by malnutrition. Serious bacterial infections in general are associated with folate deficiency; the mechanism of which is thought to be increased utilization and intestinal malabsorption [18]. However, a number of features associated with particular infectious illnesses can contribute to folate and B$_{12}$ deficiencies and are discussed below.

Diarrhea

Diarrhea [19] is particularly common among infants and children in the underdeveloped world and in many areas is the leading cause of death in children under the age of 3. A diarrheal illness frequently leads to a temporary compromise in both the quantity and quality of dietary intake, which in an individual with underlying marginal vitamin stores may lead to frank vitamin deficiency. In addition, it is clear that the malabsorption of macronutrients associated with some infectious diarrheas is accompanied by malabsorption of some micronutrients, including folate and B$_{12}$. In studies of patients with acute diarrhea due to a variety of organisms (the majority of which are bacterial), the prevalence of B$_{12}$ and folate malabsorption exceeds 50 percent [20,21]. Perhaps more significant is the observation that, in a minority of patients, malabsorption of these nutrients persists for days to weeks after resolution of the clinical illness. The entity of chronic diarrhea due to bacterial infection is less well understood, but its prolonged nature suggests that it might prove to be substantially more threatening to the host's vitamin status than acute diarrhea.

The mechanisms by which bacterial infections of the gastrointestinal tract produce malabsorption of folate and B_{12} remain unclear. In those instances where an overgrowth of the pathogenic organism develops in the small intestine the organism may compete with the host for uptake of ingested nutrients; this phenomenon has been well described in the case of vitamin B_{12} [22]. The other intraluminal and mucosal events associated with infectious diarrhea that result in vitamin malabsorption remain ill-defined.

Infestation with a number of intestinal parasites has been associated with deficient blood levels of folate and B_{12}. Infections with the protozoan *Giardia lamblia,* as well as with the helminths *Diphylobothrium latum, Strongyloides stercorales, Necator americanus,* and *Ancylostoma duodenale,* have been associated with low serum levels of vitamin B_{12}, and all of the above, with the exception of *D. latum,* have been associated with low levels of serum folate [23]. Whether the reports of low vitamin levels in these infections are truly due to parasite-induced malabsorption or not remains unclear, although malabsorption of folate and B_{12} has been documented in a few instances. The "tapeworm pernicious anemia" that affects about 1 to 2 percent of individuals infected with *D. latum* has been convincingly shown to be caused by malabsorption of vitamin B_{12} due to competition for the vitamin between the host and the parasite. However, *D. latum* not only is able to concentrate B_{12} in its tissues but also appears to be capable of interfering with the gastric secretion of intrinsic factor and with the subsequent binding of B_{12} to intrinsic factor.

Tropical enteropathy and tropical sprue

Whether tropical enteropathy and tropical sprue represent entities along the spectrum of a single disease or distinct pathophysiological processes is unclear and is discussed further in Chap. 3. What is clear is that tropical sprue continues to be an endemic and occasionally, an epidemic, problem in many tropical countries. An infectious etiology is presumed although not proven. Intestinal malabsorption of both folate and B_{12} is present in the majority of cases, as are deficient serum levels of the vitamins. The malabsorption of folate is thought to be due to impaired mucosal transport of monoglutamyl folate and not to impaired hydrolysis of the polyglutamyl forms of the vitamin [24]. The malabsorption of vitamin B_{12} has been ascribed to bacterial utilization in some instances and impaired function of the ileal mucosa in others. Deficiencies of B_{12} and folate are the principal factors responsible for the anemia that frequently accompanies the disease.

Folate, and probably B_{12}, deficiency is not only a consequence of tropical sprue but a factor that propagates the disease process. Deficiency of either vitamin causes megaloblastic

changes in the small-intestinal epithelium as well as blunting and other abnormalities of the villous architecture. In the case of folate deficiency these morphological changes have been clearly shown to be associated with functional abnormalities of the mucosa [24]. The hypothesis that folate and B_{12} are causative, as well as consequential, factors in the disease is supported by the repeated observation that pharmacological doses of either vitamin cause prompt resolution of all symptoms of the disease, although in practice the patient frequently receives antibiotics as well. Vitamin B_{12} should be given in conjunction with folic acid in those instances in which B_{12} levels are not available or in which B_{12} deficiency is documented. Otherwise the megaloblastic anemia may relapse after initial response to folate. Furthermore, there are rare reports of neurological damage due to B_{12} deficiency in this disease, and folate administration alone could feasibly exacerbate the problem.

Malaria

Low serum levels of folate have been inconsistently noted in patients with malaria, and low cerebrospinal fluid (CSF) levels have been noted in those with cerebral malaria [25,26]. However, it is not yet clear whether a true deficiency state with hematological sequelae is associated with the disease. Increased utilization of the vitamin due to recurrent fever and the chronic hemolytic state (see below) are thought to be contributing factors, although impaired intestinal absorption has been reported in a minority of patients [26]. Furthermore, pyrimethamine and the sulfonamides, drugs that are commonly used in the treatment of malaria, are inhibitors of dihydrofolate reductase. As such, they have the capacity to produce a metabolic block in folate-mediated biochemical pathways. Megaloblastic anemia has been sporadically reported to be exacerbated by these drugs.

Tuberculosis of the gastrointestinal tract

Infection of the gastrointestinal tract with *Mycobacterium tuberculosis* (or less frequently, *M. bovis*) is still a common problem in many tropical countries. Concurrent pulmonary involvement is only present in about one-half of the cases. The ileocecal region is the most commonly involved region, presumably a consequence of initial infection of the Peyer's patches. Malabsorption and diarrhea may develop secondary to ileal dysfunction. Anemia is common although only in rare instances is it due to B_{12} deficiency: the majority of cases are due to either blood loss or the "anemia of chronic disease."

MALNUTRITION

Protein-calorie malnutrition causes marked structural and functional abnormalities of the small-intestinal mucosa and pancreas, all of which appear to be reversible with nutritional repletion [27]. Marked blunting, or total absence, of the intestinal villi is observed and is associated with decreased levels of disaccharidases and aminopeptidases in the mucosa. Clinically, malabsorption of carbohydrates, fat, and fat-soluble vitamins has been observed; the degree of steatorrhea being proportional to the severity of protein depletion. In nonhuman primates, intestinal absorption of folate is decreased 50 percent by chronic protein malnutrition. The absorptive defect is completely reversible with nutritional repletion [28]. Folate and B$_{12}$ malabsorption almost certainly occur in the human in this setting.

MISCELLANEOUS

Sickle cell disease and trait [29]

Chronic hemolytic states are associated with folate deficiency and megaloblastic hematopoiesis because of the increased utilization required for the compensatory rise in the rate of hematopoiesis. Clinically, folate deficiency is usually manifest in these individuals by the development of an anemia that is more severe than is typical for that individual. Production of hemoglobin S seems to be affected to a greater extent than hemoglobin A by folate deficiency and thus might further exacerbate the problem. There is also evidence that individuals suffering from hemoglobin SS disease and megaloblastic anemia require greater doses of folic acid to produce a hematological response than do individuals without the hemolytic process: such individuals with SS disease have been noted to respond to 500 μg, but not to 200 μg, per day.

Individuals with the hemoglobin AS trait have not been clearly documented to suffer from a greater prevalence of megaloblastic anemia. However, they do have lower serum and RBC folate levels than hemoglobin AA individuals and thus seem to be susceptible to a clinical deficiency state [30].

Immunoproliferative disease of the small intestine [31]

Immunoproliferative disease of the small intestine [31], commonly called Mediterranean lymphoma, is a spectrum of immunoproliferative B-cell disorders that primarily affect the small-intestinal mucosa and mesenteric lymph nodes. Most cases are reported from the Middle East and north Africa, although cases from South Africa and South America are well-documented. The vast majority of afflicted individuals are from lower socioeconomic classes.

The disease typically causes severe, generalized malabsorption. Anemia is common and is often associated with decreased serum values for folate and/or B$_{12}$.

PREVENTION AND TREATMENT

Folate

Measures to prevent the development of folate deficiency should be primarily directed toward pregnant women, who clearly constitute a high-risk segment of any population. Folic acid supplementation, at a dose of 500 μg/day, should be provided to all pregnant women. However compliance with prenatal dietary supplements can be a substantial problem. The issue of compliance led Colman et al. [32,33] to investigate whether folic acid fortification of cornmeal was sufficient to prevent the development of deficiency during pregnancy in a rural South African population that has a high prevalence of folate deficiency. These investigators found that as little as 300 μg of folate in this form was sufficient to prevent folate deficiency. Approximately 55 percent (170 μg) of this 300 μg was considered to be bioavailable when compared to an equivalent dose of uncooked, crystalline folic acid. Other investigators have tried to circumvent the problem of compliance by providing weekly supplements. Unfortunately, this has not yet been shown to be effective: Nigerian women receiving 2.5 to 5.0 mg of folic acid weekly still had a substantial risk of developing folate deficiency [34].

One fresh fruit or one fresh vegetable each day is probably sufficient to prevent the development of folate deficiency in a nonpregnant population.

Treatment of established folate deficiency should involve a daily oral dose of 0.5 to 1.0 mg. There is no evidence that larger doses provide additional benefit. Parenteral therapy is usually not necessary. If taken in doses greater than 100 μg/day, folic acid can correct the megaloblastic anemia of B$_{12}$ deficiency without improving the neurological manifestations. Inappropriate treatment such as this can mask, and even exacerbate, the neurological sequelae of B$_{12}$ deficiency. In the setting of megaloblastic anemia where there is a reasonable possibility of B$_{12}$ deficiency, the serum B$_{12}$ value should be checked. Alternatively, a daily 100-μg oral dose of folic acid daily can be administered: a maximal hematological response is noted to such a therapeutic trial if the anemia is due to folate, but not B$_{12}$, deficiency [35].

Vitamin B$_{12}$

Individuals at risk of developing B$_{12}$ deficiency due to inadequate dietary intake are those who, for reasons of poverty or because of their adherence to strict vegetarianism, consume no animal products for extended periods of time. Prevention of deficiency in these individuals can be accomplished by altering the diet to include B$_{12}$ or by supplying 1 μg B$_{12}$ per day as a supplement.

Diet-induced vitamin B$_{12}$ deficiency can be treated by oral administration of 1 μg daily. A deficiency state created by malabsorption should be treated with parenteral administration of B$_{12}$: 100 μg of intramuscular cyanocobalamin is typically given on a daily basis for 1 week followed by periodic intramuscular injections such that 2000 μg is given over the first 6 weeks. This should be sufficient to replete body stores. Thereafter, a 100-μg intramuscular dose per month is sufficient maintenance therapy.

REFERENCES

1 Herbert VD, Colman N: Folic acid and vitamin B_{12}, in Shils ME, Young VR (eds): *Modern Nutrition in Health and Disease*. Philadelphia, Lea & Febiger, 1988, pp 388–416

2 Tamura T, Stokstad ELR: The availability of food folate in man. Br J Haematol 25:513–532, 1973

3 King CE, Leibach J, Toskes PP: Clinically significant vitamin B_{12} deficiency secondary to malabsorption of protein-bound vitamin B_{12}. Dig Dis Sci 24:396–402, 1979

4 Davidson GP, Townley RRW: Structural and functional abnormalities of the small intestine due to nutritional folic acid deficiency in infancy. J Pediatr 90:590–594, 1977

5 Herbert V: Recommended dietary intakes (RDI) of folate in humans. Am J Clin Nutr 45:661–670, 1987

6 Herbert V: Recommended dietary intakes (RDI) of vitamin B-12 in humans. Am J Clin Nutr 45:671–678, 1987

7 Hillman RS, Steinberg SE: The effects of alcohol on folate metabolism. Ann Rev Med 38:345–354, 1982

8 Russell RM, Rosenberg IH, Wilson PD, et al: Increased urinary excretion and prolonged turnover time of folic acid during ethanol ingestion. Am J Clin Nutr 38:64–70, 1983

9 Hoffbrand AV, Newcombe FBA, Mollin DL: Method of assay of red cell folate activity as a test for folate deficiency. J Clin Pathol 19:17–28, 1966

10 Joint FAO/WHO Expert Group: Requirements of ascorbic acid, vitamin D, vitamin B_{12}, folate and iron. Geneva, World Health Organization, WHO Tech Rep Ser 452, 1970

11 Colman N, Barker EA, Barker M, et al: Prevention of folate deficiency by food fortification. IV. Identification of target groups in addition to pregnant women in an adult population. Am J Clin Nutr 28:471–476, 1975

12 Chanarin I: *The Megaloblastic Anemias*. Oxford, Blackwell Scientific Publications, 1969, pp 786–829

13 Karthigaini S, Gnanasundaram D, Baker SJ: Megaloblastic erythropoiesis and serum vitamin B_{12} and folic acid levels in pregnancy in south Indian women. J Obstet Gynecol Br Commonw 71:115–122, 1964

14 Iyengar L, Rajalakshmi K: Effect of folic acid supplement on birth weights of infants. Am J Obstet Gynecol 122:332–336, 1975

15 Baumslag N, Edelstein T, Metz J: Reduction of incidence of prematurity by folic acid supplementation in pregnancy. Br Med J 1:16–17, 1970

16 Metz J: Folate deficiency conditioned by lactation. Am J Clin Nutr 23:843–847, 1970

17 Baker H, Jaslow HP, Frank O: Severe impairment of dietary folate utilization in the elderly. J Am Geriatr Soc 26:218–221, 1978

18 Cook GC: Impairment of folate absorption by systemic bacterial infections. Lancet ii:1416–1417, 1974

19 Rosenberg IH, Solomons NW, Schneider RE: Malabsorption associated with diarrhea and intestinal infections. Am J Clin Nutr 30:1248–1253, 1977

20 Lindenbaum J: Malabsorption during and after recovery from acute intestinal infection. Br Med J 2:326–329, 1965

21 Butler T, Middleton FG, Earnest DL, et al: Chronic and recurrent diarrhea in American servicemen in Vietnam. Arch Intern Med 132:373–377, 1973

22 Donaldson RM: Role of enteric microorganisms in malabsorption. Fed Proc 26:1426–1431, 1967

23 Brasitus TA: Parasites and malabsorption, in Sleisenger MH (ed): *Malabsorption and Nutritional Support*. Philadelphia, Saunders, 1983, pp 495–510

24 Corcino JJ, Risenauer AM, Halsted CH: Jejunal perfusion of simple and conjugated folates in tropical sprue. J Clin Invest 58:298–305, 1976

25 Arrekul S, Pinyawatana W, Charoenlarp P: Serum folate and folic acid absorption in patients with *Plasmodium falciparum* malaria. Southeast Asian J Trop Med Pub Health 5:353–358, 1974

26 Arrekul S, Cherraratna C: Cerebrospinal fluid folate activity in patients with *Plasmodium falciparum* cerebral malaria. Trop Geogr Med 37:227–230, 1985

27 Viteri FE, Schneider RE: Gastrointestinal alterations in protein-calorie malnutrition. Med Clin North Am 58:1487–1505, 1973

28 Gyr K, Wolf RH, Felsenfeld O: Intestinal absorption of D-xylose and folic acid in protein-deficient patas monkeys. Am J Clin Nutr 27:350–354, 1974

29 Chanarin I: *The Megaloblastic Anemias*. Oxford, Blackwell Scientific Publications, 1969, pp 866–889

30 Osifo BOA, Lukanmbi FA, Bolodeoku JO: Reference values for serum folate, erythrocyte folate, and serum cobalamin in Nigerian adolescents. Trop Geogr Med 38:259–264, 1986

31 Rambaud JC, Seligmann M: Alpha-chain disease. Clinics Gastroenterology 5:341–358, 1976

32 Colman N, Larse JV, Barder M, et al: Prevention of folate deficiency by food fortification. III. Effect in pregnant subjects of varying amounts of added folic acid. Am J Clin Nutr 28:465–470, 1975

33 Colman N, Barker M, Green R, et al: Prevention of folate deficiency in pregnancy by food fortification. Am J Clin Nutr 27:339–344, 1974

34 Fleming AF, Hendrickse JP, Allan NC: The prevention of megaloblastic anemia in pregnancy in Nigeria. J Obstet Gynaecol Br Commonw 75:425–432, 1968

35 Herbert V: Megaloblastic anemia. N Engl J Med 268:201–203, 368–371, 1963

36 Colman N, Herbert V: Folate and vitamin B_{12}, chap 115 in Warren KS, Mahmoud AF: *Tropical and Geographical Medicine*. New York, McGraw-Hill, 1984

Beriberi, Pellagra, and Scurvy

· *Aree Valyasevi* · *Hamish N. Munro*

In contrast to western countries, most tropical populations subsisting on a rice-based diet show a significant incidence of beriberi due to thiamine deficiency, while those consuming a corn-based diet report cases of pellagra due to lack of nicotinic acid. On the other hand, scurvy in adults due to ascorbic acid deficiency is even rarer in the tropics than in developed countries, although infantile scurvy is occasionally seen. Detailed accounts of the biochemical and metabolic background to these diseases as well as their clinical and epidemiological features can be obtained in specialized texts [1–3].

BERIBERI

Beriberi became prevalent in the early nineteenth century in rice-eating populations due to introduction of mechanical removal of the vitamin-rich rice husk. In 1897, Eijkman demonstrated a curative agent in extracts of the husks, and this was later identified as thiamine (vitamin B_1), now available by chemical synthesis.

NUTRIENT

The main dietary sources of thiamine are fish, meat, eggs, pulses (legumes), and pork. In rice-eating populations, the thiamine content of rice as grown and as eaten is critical, being affected by methods of milling and cooking. Up to 80 percent of the original thiamine in the grain can be lost in milling and washing procedures prior to cooking, and in boiling, which can further reduce thiamine content. Thiamine already present in the diet can be made unavailable by the enzyme thiaminase, which is present in some raw fish and vegetables consumed in southeast Asia [4], while in Burma an antithiamine factor has also been identified in fish [5] and tea [6]. Such antagonists can aggravate thiamine deficiency in the diet, especially in groups of pregnant and lactating women and their offspring.

Structurally, thiamine consists of a pyrimidine ring joined to a thiazole nucleus by a methylene bridge. It occurs in the tissues as the active pyrophosphate form. Following active transport across the intestinal mucosa, thiamine is phosphorylated in the liver to thiamine pyrophosphate, a form in which it is exported into the peripheral blood for use by other tissues [2]. Excess thiamine is excreted in the urine as several metabolites (pyrimidine carboxylic acid, thiazole acetic acid, and thiamine acetic acid). Deficiency impairs notably the activity of the decarboxylases of ketoacids such as pyruvate and α-ketoglutarate and in the hexose monophosphate shunt where it serves as the cofactor for transketolase. The activity of the latter enzyme in red cells provides a measure of deficiency in humans. Since thiamine pyrophosphate is especially involved as a cofactor for enzymes of carbohydrate metabolism, the amount of carbohydrate consumed can determine thiamine requirement.

PATIENT

Pathogenesis

The nervous system and the heart are most sensitive to the disordered intermediary metabolism due to lack of thiamine pyrophosphate [7]. In the peripheral nerves, loss of myelin sheath and disruption of axoplasm have been observed. In adult beriberi, dilatation and/or hypertrophy of the heart are recorded, with cloudy swelling, fatty infiltration, and fragmentation of myocardial fibers seen microscopically, as well as occasional foci of necrosis.

Clinical manifestations

The syndrome of thiamine deficiency seen clinically can range from peripheral neuropathy (dry beriberi) and cardiac beriberi (wet beriberi), through Wernicke's encephalopathy and Korsakoff's syndrome, to alcoholic polyneuropathy, partly depending on the degree of deprivation [8]. Encephalopathy and Korsakoff's syndrome result from deprivation in individuals of European origin with a genetic susceptibility to these diseases [9]. Some evidence, however, indicates that the incidence of Wernicke's encephalopathy is higher in Australia than in other countries [10].

Wernicke's encephalopathy may be of acute onset, presenting with ophthalmoplegia, ataxia, and mental confusion; about three-fourths of cases show signs of peripheral neuropathy. On the other hand, the symptoms of Korsakoff's syndrome are usually retrograde and anterograde amnesia. It is reported that 84 percent of Wernicke's encephalopathy developed Korsakoff's psychosis after recovery from the acute onset [11].

Infantile beriberi occurs during the first year of life, most frequently in infants between 2 to 4 months old who are breast-fed by thiamine-deficient mothers. The earliest symptoms may be a disinclination for the breast followed by restlessness, attacks of crying, as if with abdominal pain, and vomiting of breast milk. An observant mother will notice that less urine has been passed and that the baby seems puffy. The bowels are usually normal at this stage, although mild constipation or diarrhea may occur. However, in many instances these early signs are overlooked by the mother, and consequently the disease often appears to be fulminating in onset. A diagnosis of infantile beriberi should be entertained if (1) the nursing mother gives a history of restricted diet; (2) she reports having numbness and/or weakness, notably of both lower extremities; (3) the infant shows signs of incipient cardiac failure (dyspnea, tachycardia, cyanosis, edema, and enlargement of heart and liver); and (4) the infant is aphonic (laryngeal nerve paralysis) and subject to attacks of muscular rigidity.

Beriberi in older children and adults can be divided into dry (neurological or paralytic) and wet (cardiac) types, although mixed forms are frequently observed. The clinical manifestations of the dry type include tenderness over the calf muscles and difficulty in rising from a squatting position, and abnormalities of deep tendon reflexes which may be exaggerated at first but later become diminished or absent. Cardiovascular manifestations are observed only in wet beriberi (Fig. 120-1), often starting with palpitation, rapid heartbeat, breathlessness, and peripheral edema. Progressive dyspnea and orthopnea may appear, evidencing left-sided heart failure. Cardiac enlargement, jugular vein engorgement, bounding pulse, and gallop rhythm are commonly observed. Cardiomegaly and pulmonary congestion have been frequently observed radiologically in wet beriberi, and the electrocardiogram usually exhibits nonspecific S-T wave changes accompanying generalized low voltage.

Diagnosis and management

The diagnosis of beriberi is assisted by a dietary history revealing low thiamine intake and clinical manifestations. However, objective biochemical tests of thiamine status, particularly measurement of erythrocytes transketolase activity (ETKA) and of the thiamine pyrophosphate effect (TPPE), provide a sensitive test for thiamine deficiency [12]. TPPE is expressed as the percentage increase in ETKA obtained after addition of TPP to the erythrocyte. The biochemical diagnostic

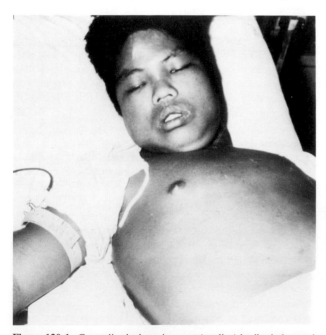

Figure 120-1. Generalized edema in a wet (cardiac) beriberi observed in a 16-year-old boy who consumed only milled rice and fish sauce.

criteria of thiamine deficiency consist of low ETKA and high TPPE (normal range 0 to 15 percent). However, since beriberi is seen in remote areas without laboratory facilities, diagnosis can and should be based on the diet history and clinical manifestations. In locations where the condition is prevalent, thiamine should be given for diagnostic and therapeutic purposes if the condition is even suspected. If the diagnosis is correct, improvement will begin within a few hours and be progressive. For infants acutely ill with cardiac failure, 25 to 50 mg of thiamine should be given intramuscularly or intravenously, often resulting within an hour in reduction of respiratory and heart rate, decreased restlessness, and disappearance of cyanosis. For children and adults with cardiac failure, 50 to 100 mg of thiamine should be given. During the acute cardiorespiratory phase, there is no contraindication to digitalization in addition to thiamine administration, and other supportive treatments. Thereafter, 25 to 50 mg of thiamine should be given orally or intramuscularly once or twice daily until symptoms have subsided, after which 10 mg daily should be maintained orally for some time and advice on proper diet should be given.

POPULATION

Epidemiology

Beriberi was once a major health problem in many Asian countries where milled rice is the main staple diet. Today, its prevalence has been greatly reduced, although it remains endemic in some southeast Asian countries such as Thailand [13] and Burma [14]. Beriberi heart disease has been recently reported in 23 young Japanese adults who consumed sweet carbonated drinks, instant noodles, and polished rice [15]. Thiamine deficiency in alcoholic populations derives from multiple causes, an important one being inadequate intake of thiamine [16]. Alcohol can also cause deficiency by decreasing conversion of thiamine to the active pyrophosphate form, reducing hepatic storage in patients with fatty infiltration, inhibiting intestinal thiamine transport, and impairing thiamine absorption secondary to other states of nutritional deficiency induced by ethanol [2]. As mentioned earlier, Wernicke's encephalopathy and Korsakoff's psychosis occur in populations with a genetic susceptibility to thiamine deficiency.

Prevention

Beriberi is entirely preventable if one consumes food containing adequate amounts of thiamine. The recommended daily allowance of the U.S. National Research Council [17] for thiamine is 0.5 mg per 1000 kcal, which applies to infants, children, and adults. The intakes for infants from 0 to 6 months and 6 to 12 months are 0.3 mg and 0.5 mg, respectively. Children 1 to 3 years and 4 to 6 years of age should have daily thiamine intakes of 0.7 and 0.9 mg, respectively. In older children and adults the intake should be 1.0 to 1.5 mg, and in pregnant and lactating women, an additional allowance of 0.4

to 0.5 mg of thiamine per day is recommended. Synthetic thiamine, which is low in cost, can also be used for the prevention of beriberi, if taken regularly.

PELLAGRA

This condition is prevalent among populations subsisting on corn (maize). In 1937, Elvejhem showed that nicotinic acid is effective in curing both experimental pellagra in dogs and also the clinical disease.

NUTRIENT

Nicotinic acid, also known as niacin, occurs as such in the diet and also is available to the body as a metabolite of tryptophan. This essential amino acid becomes a source of nicotinic acid through conversion to quinolinic acid and hence to nicotinic acid ribonucleotide. In humans, 60 mg of dietary tryptophan can form 1 mg of nicotinic acid through this pathway [17]. Indeed, Horwitt [18] emphasizes that most foods provide more nicotinic acid from tryptophan than does the preformed vitamin. Animal meats are rich sources of each of these, whereas cereals tend to be deficient in both, especially corn, which is low in tryptophan and also contains nicotinic acid in a form only made available by pretreating the cereal with alkali.

Nicotinic acid consists of a heterocyclic (pyridine) ring compound present in cells mainly in the form of its amide, nicotinamide. The latter is a structural component of the pyridine nucleotide coenzymes nicotinamide adenine dinucleotide (NAD) and nicotinamide adenine dinucleotide phosphate (NADP) that function in tissue respiration. Dietary nicotinic acid and nicotinamide are readily absorbed and converted to these pyridine nucleotides. Breakdown of nicotinic acid in the body results in urinary excretion of a series of pyridine derivatives, notably N-methylnicotinamide.

PATIENT

Pathogenesis

NAD and NADP are involved as cofactors in many oxidation-reduction reactions central to tissue respiration. Consequently, tissues with a high respiration rate, such as the central nervous system, are most extensively affected by deficiency.

Clinical manifestations

The initial clinical features of pellagra are nonspecific and include anorexia, prostration, weight loss, headache, and a burning sensation in the mouth. The fully developed syndrome, known as the "three D's," consists of dermatitis, gastrointestinal symptoms (diarrhea), and finally mental impairment (dementia). The clinical manifestations of pellagra are described below.

1. Dermatitis occurs on the exposed surfaces of the body, namely the face, neck, back of the arms and hands, lower legs and feet (Fig. 120-2A), and is exacerbated by exposure to sunlight and wind or even mechanical irritation. It may start with erythema on the exposed surfaces, these areas darkening to a purple color. Pigment then accumulates so that areas of dark, rough, crackled dermatitis occur with sharply defined margins. These skin lesions can be regarded as characteristic and almost specific to the disease.

2. Stomatitis and glossitis may occur in association with riboflavin deficiency. However, early signs of glossitis may be restricted to hyperemia of the lip and margin of the tongue, later developing into a raw, beefy tongue (Fig. 120-2B).

3. Diarrhea—attacks of loose, watery stool—is one of the most constant features of pellagra, but in addition superficial inflammation occurs to a variable degree in the whole gastroin-

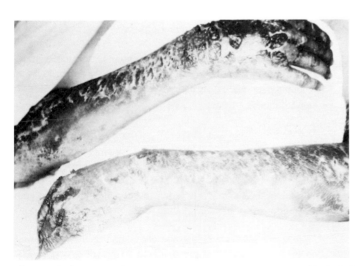
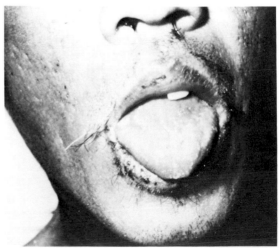

Figure 120-2. Dermatitis, glossitis, and stomatitis in a 25-year-old alcoholic man who suffered from pellagra.

testinal tract, causing a variety of signs and symptoms including dysphagia, nausea, and vomiting.

4. Dementia usually occurs after the other manifestations and may start with apathy, insomnia, and irritability, which can develop into psychosis, a feature of the chronic phase of the disease in adults. The incidence of dementia and neuropathy is higher when pellagra is associated with alcohol abuse.

Diagnosis

Although the triad of dermatitis, diarrhea, and dementia is distinctive, these symptoms do not all occur in every patient. The earliest manifestations lack dermatitis [19] and in one-third of florid cases dermatitis is the only sign [20]. In addition to the clinical signs, the socioeconomic and cultural circumstances of the patient and patterns of diet, including alcohol consumption, can all be relevant to intake of nicotinic acid. The diagnosis can be confirmed therapeutically by administering nicotinamide (100 to 200 mg to adults and 10 to 25 mg to small children) three times daily by mouth or intravenously. Cases of pellagra respond promptly to this treatment.

Measurement of urinary excretion of *N*-methylnicotinamide has been used in the diagnosis of pellagra, since decreased excretion coincides with the onset of clinical symptoms. An excretion rate per gram of urinary creatinine in random samples of fasting urine that exceeds 1.6 mg for adults and 2.5 mg for pregnant women in the third trimester has been thought to indicate adequate niacin nutritional status. Unfortunately, this test is neither simple nor readily available, and the results do not unequivocally identify deficiency.

Management

Pellagra will respond promptly to treatment with nicotinamide, which is preferred to nicotinic acid, since it has less side effects. The vitamin should be given three times daily at the levels recommended above for therapeutic diagnosis until the symptoms subside. Diarrhea will usually stop within 1 or 2 days, while dementia and dermatitis will significantly improve within the first week after the start of therapy. In addition the consumption of protein of high biological value should be encouraged as a source of tryptophan. If a satisfactory response does not occur, administration of other members of the vitamin B complex should be considered, since multiple deficiencies may prevent a response to nicotinic acid therapy alone.

POPULATION

Epidemiology

Pellagra occurs among adults whose niacin intakes are deficient, but it is rare in childhood. Endemic pellagra is characteristically reported in populations which derive a large proportion of their energy intakes from corn, because of its rather small content of nicotinic acid and tryptophan. Although pellagra still occurs in some parts of Africa and the Middle East

where corn is the main staple, it is seldom seen in Central America and Mexico, where corn provides up to 80 percent of the energy intake, since treatment of corn with lime for the preparation of tortillas makes more nicotinic acid available. Pellagra is also observed in Central India, where the staple food is sorghum [21].

An excessive intake of alcohol is another important factor inducing pellagra in adults. Alcohol contributes to the development of pellagra by replacing a more nutritionally balanced caloric intake, but this will be significant only when the diet is marginal. Other less frequent causal factors include malabsorption leading to impairment in assimilation of nutrients, alterations in tryptophan metabolism, such as Hartnup disease (intestinal malabsorption and urinary loss of a number of amino acids including tryptophan), and carcinoid tumors diverting significant amounts of tryptophan to the synthesis of serotonin. Isoniazid therapy can also serve to exacerbate a latent deficiency of niacin since it is a pyridoxine antagonist which interferes with the conversion of tryptophan to niacin.

Prevention

The recommended allowances [17] range from 13 to 15 mg nicotinic acid equivalent daily for women and 16 to 19 mg for men. During pregnancy and lactation 2 and 5 mg nicotinic acid, respectively, should be added. For infants and children, 6 and 11 mg daily are recommended, respectively.

SCURVY

Scurvy has been recognized clinically since the Middle Ages when it was endemic among populations in northern Europe until the introduction of the potato in the seventeenth century. In the sixteenth, seventeenth, and eighteenth centuries, scurvy was a major cause of death on long sea voyages of exploration because of the lack of fresh fruits and vegetables. The active factor, ascorbic acid, was isolated by Szent-Györgyi in 1928 and is now available in synthetic form. Nowadays, scurvy is occasionally seen in western countries in adults and infants on inadequate intakes. In tropical populations, rare cases of infantile scurvy have been recorded, and scurvy has been noted in adult populations on high iron intakes, notably South African Bantus.

NUTRIENT

Ascorbic acid is most abundant in growing vegetables and fruits, notably citrus fruits, whereas grains contain little of the vitamin. Much of the ascorbic acid of vegetables can be lost in cooking because of extraction in the water and by its ready oxidation, especially in alkaline water and in the presence of copper.

Ascorbic acid is a six-carbon compound related structurally to glucose. It is reversibly oxidized to dehydroascorbic acid, and by further irreversible degradation to breakdown products including oxalic acid. Ascorbic acid is readily absorbed in the small intestine. Its functions in the tissues include acting as a cofactor in a variety of hydroxylations, such as formation of hydroxyproline in collagen synthesis, 5-OH-tryptophan in serotoninergic neurones, hydroxylation of lysine in carnitine production, and hydroxylation of adrenal steroid hormones, and also in the metabolism of tyrosine [1]. Being a powerful antioxidant, it is thought to protect fat-soluble nutrients such as vitamins A and E and essential fatty acids against oxidation. It also facilitates absorption of nonheme iron taken in the same meal [22].

PATIENT

Pathogenesis

Synthesis of intercellular substances such as collagen, tooth, and bone matrix are impaired in ascorbic acid deficiency. It is also suggested that formation of the intercellular cement of capillary endothelium requires adequate supplies of ascorbic acid. Scurvy is thus associated with failure of wounds to heal because of absence of new collagen, defects in tooth formation, and weakening of capillary walls, the latter accounting for the subcutaneous petechiae and sheets of ecchymoses characteristic of florid scurvy. Subcutaneous capillary hemorrhages may alternatively be due to reduced support of pericapillary collagen. A specific need for ascorbic acid in hemoglobin formation appears to account for the anemia of scurvy.

Clinical manifestations

Scurvy can occur in adults and in infants up to 2 years of age receiving diets lacking ascorbic acid. The infant fails to thrive and is irritable, resenting being touched because of painful hematomas under the periosteum of the long bones. These can be seen by x-ray of the bones (Fig. 120-3), which can also reveal delayed ossification. Hemorrhages also occur elsewhere, notably subcutaneously, and the infant may exhibit hematuria and bloody diarrhea.

Adult scurvy is occasionally seen in western countries among the elderly living alone on inadequate diets [23], and in alcoholics and drug addicts. Usually there is a long history of consuming diets lacking fruits, vegetables, and potatoes. Scurvy also occurs among the Bantu of South Africa, where an iron overload due to enormous intakes of iron leads to destruction of ascorbic acid within the tissues [24]. Typically, cases of frank scurvy show subcutaneous hemorrhages on the legs and less frequently on the arms, either as discrete petechiae but more often occurring as sheets of ecchymoses. Gingival hemorrhages occur around the teeth (Fig. 120-4), and some cases show perifollicular hyperkeratosis around the hair follicles. There is also a mild hypochromic anemia.

Diagnosis and management

Given the dietary history and the characteristic sheets of subcutaneous hemorrhage, diagnosis is usually obvious. Plasma

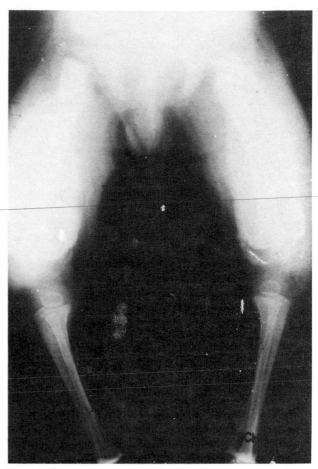

Figure 120-3. Infantile scurvy. Note subperiosteal hemorrhage of both femurs.

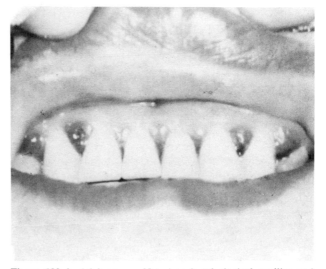

Figure 120-4. Adult scurvy. Note interdental gingival swelling and hemorrhage.

ascorbic acid levels below 0.2 mg/dL confirm the diagnosis. Tests for capillary weakness, once popular, are no longer in use since not all cases of scurvy show a positive response, and some who display weakness continue to respond positively after cure [23], suggesting a constitutional capillary defect that may be a precipitating factor in the onset of scurvy. The treatment of frank scurvy is to give 1 g ascorbic acid daily until the signs disappear, which also constitutes therapeutic confirmation of the diagnosis. Thereafter, a diet containing adequate sources of ascorbic acid should be instituted.

POPULATION

Epidemiology

Scurvy is seen sporadically in adults on diets providing little vitamin C, usually elderly impoverished men without access to fresh fruits and vegetables, and also in alcoholics and drug addicts. A substantially impaired vitamin C status was reported in cigarette smokers as compared to nonsmokers with comparable vitamin C intakes, suggesting an increased risk of marginal vitamin C deficiency among smokers [25]. Vitamin C deficiency also occurs in the Bantu of South Africa, who consume Kaffir beer made in iron pots, which provides up to 100 mg of iron daily to the Bantu diet. The resulting iron overload causes excessive oxidation of ascorbic acid, so that blood levels of ascorbic acid normally achieved by adults consuming 60 mg ascorbic acid daily can require an intake of 200 mg daily by the Bantu, in whom frank scurvy has been seen [24]. Iron overload resulting from repeated blood transfusions for β-thalassemia has a similar oxidative effect on ascorbic acid, and frank scurvy has also been recorded in such patients [26].

Prevention

Prevention consists in providing adequate sources of dietary ascorbic acid [17]. Breast milk normally contains 35 to 55 mg of ascorbic acid per liter [27], so that the average breast-fed infant receives about 35 mg daily. Premature infants require more (up to 100 mg) to prevent accumulation of tyrosine. The growing child should have an allowance of 45 to 60 mg daily, and the adult should receive 60 mg.

REFERENCES

1 Danford DE, Munro HN: Water-soluble vitamins. The vitamin B complex and ascorbic acid, in Gilman AG, Goodman LS, Gilman A (eds): *The Pharmacological Basis of Therapeutics,* 6th ed. New York, Macmillan, 1980, pp 1560–1582

2 Danford DE, Munro HN: The liver in relation to the B-vitamins, in Arias IM, et al (eds): *The Liver: Biology and Pathobiology.* New York, Raven, 1982, pp 367–384

3 Goodhart RS, Shils ME (eds): *Modern Nutrition in Health and Disease,* 6th ed. Philadelphia, Lea & Febiger, 1980

4 Shimazono N, Katsura E: *Review of Japanese Literature on Beri-Beri and Thiamine.* Vitamin B Research Committee of Japan, 1965

5 Kin-Maung-Naing, Tin-Tin-Oo, Kywe-Thein: Antithiamine activity in Burmese fish. Union Burma J Life Sci 2:63–66, 1969

6 Vimokesant SL, Nakornchai S, Dhanamitta S, et al: Nutr Rept Int 9:371, 1974

7 Follis RH Jr: Effect of tea consumption on thiamin status in man. Fed Proc 17:20, 1958

8 McLaren D: Metabolic disorders, in Conn HF (ed): *Current Therapy.* Philadelphia, Saunders, 1978, pp 409–410

9 Blass JP, Gibson GE: Abnormality of a thiamine-requiring enzyme in patients with Wernicke-Korsakoff syndrome. N Engl J Med 297: 1367–1370, 1977

10 Wood B, Breen KJ: Clinical thiamine deficiency in Australia. The size of the problem and approaches to prevention. Med J Aust 1:461–464, 1980

11 Tanphaichitr V, Wood B: Thiamine, in Olson RE (ed): *Nutrition Review's Present Knowledge in Nutrition,* 5th ed. Washington DC, The Nutrition Foundation, Inc. 1984, pp 273–281

12 Tanphaichitr V: Beri-beri. Clin Nutr 3:9–14, 1987

13 Valyasevi A, et al: *Nutritional Diseases in Thailand.* Bangkok, Thailand, Ramathibodi Publications, 1977, p 30

14 Kywe-Thein, Tin-Tin-Oo, Khin-Mauang-Naing: Thiamin nutriture of the Burmese. Burma J Life Sci 3:151, 1970

15 Kawai C, Wakabayashi A, Matsummura T, et al: Reappearance of beriberi heart disease in Japan: A study of 23 cases. Am J Med 69: 383, 1980

16 Hoyumpa AM: Mechanisms of thiamine deficiency in chronic alcoholism. Am J Clin Nutr 33:2750, 1980

17 National Research Council: Recommended Dietary Allowances, 9th ed. Washington, DC, National Academy of Sciences, 1980

18 Horwitt MK: Niacin, in RS Goodhard, ME Shils (eds): *Modern Nutrition in Health and Disease,* 6th ed. Philadelphia, Lea & Febiger, 1980, pp 203–208

19 Goldsmith GA, et al: Studies of niacin requirement in man. I. Experimental pellagra in subjects on corn diet low in niacin and tryptophan. J Clin Invest 31:533, 1952

20 Spivak J, Jackson DL: Pellagra, an analysis of 19 patients and a review of the literature. John Hopkins Med J 140:295, 1977

21 Gopalan C, Faya Ras KS: Pellagra and amino acid imbalance. Vitam Horm 33:505, 1975

22 Monsen ER, et al: Estimation of available dietary iron. Am J Clin Nutr 31:134–141, 1978

23 Lazarus S, Munro HN, Bell GH: Capillary strength test in scurvy and their reactions to vitamin C and vitamin P therapy. Clin Sci 7:175–184, 1948

24 Nienhuis AW: Vitamin C and iron. N Engl J Med 304:170–171, 1981

25 Hornig D, Glatthar B: Vitamin C and smoking. Intern Med 1:244–248, 1985

26 Cohen A, Cohen IJ, Schwartz E: Scurvy and altered iron stores in thalassemia major. N Engl J Med 304:158–160, 1981

27 Irwin MI, Hutchins BK: A conspectus of research on vitamin C requirements of man. J Nutr 106:823–879, 1976

CHAPTER 121

Vitamin A · Elizabeth A. Phelan · Robert M. Russell

Vitamin A refers to all compounds with the biological activity of retinol. Vitamin A is an essential nutrient which occurs in foods in two forms: as preformed vitamin A (found in animal foods such as liver, kidney, egg yolk, and milk) and as provitamin A carotenoids (found mainly in plant foods, especially green, leafy and yellow-red vegetables). Carotenoids are substances structurally related to vitamin A and converted in part in vivo to the vitamin. The typical American and European diet provides about half of the total vitamin A as preformed and half as carotenoid–vitamin A precursors. Diets in less-developed countries supply the majority of vitamin A as carotenoid vitamin A precursors, although rich sources of provitamin A are, for a variety of reasons, often not consumed.

NUTRIENT

The structure of retinol is shown below:

Three important features of the vitamin A molecule are (1) a hydrophobic head: the β-ionone ring; (2) a conjugated isoprenoid side chain that lends itself to isomerization (by enzyme or light); (3) a polar terminal group that can be modified to the ester, aldehyde, or carboxylic acid derivatives [1]. Vitamin A exists in cis and trans isomeric forms; the major naturally occurring form is the all-trans alcohol isomer.

Among the carotenoids, β-carotene is the most biologically active provitamin A compound. It is a symmetrical molecule with two β-ionone rings connected by a conjugated chain, as shown below:

Both preformed vitamin A and the carotenoids are unstable in oxygen due to their conjugated double bond structure. Their destruction by oxygen is accelerated by exposure to light. Light also catalyzes isomerization. Thus, retinol and β-carotene are highly sensitive compounds. Their stability is enhanced in the presence of inert gases and antioxidants (e.g., vitamin E) and in the absence of direct light.

REQUIREMENTS

Vitamin A activity is expressed in retinol equivalents (RE), defined as 1 μg or its equivalent of all-trans retinol. In humans, 1 μg retinol is thought to be equivalent to 6 μg carotene or 12 μg of other provitamin A carotenoids. In 1986, WHO recommended that women 18 years and older, excepting those either pregnant or lactating, should consume 500 RE per day; for men 18 years and older, the figure is 600 RE/day [2]. For pregnant women, 600 RE/day is considered appropriate; higher levels may increase the risk of birth defects. For lactating females, 850 RE/day is recommended.

Allowances increase during childhood but level off at adolescence. For children aged 1 to 10 years, the amount recommended is 400 RE; between the ages of 10 and 12, 500 RE is recommended. For males between 12 and 18 years and for females aged 12 to 15, 600 RE is recommended, while 500 RE is recommended for females aged 15 to 18 years. Newborns have a relatively small vitamin A reserve due to rapid growth during the last trimester. A recommended daily intake of 350 RE for infants is advised to meet the continued demands for growth as well as to augment the body's reserves. It should be stressed that a precise optimal intake does not exist; recommended levels are approximations of optimal intakes which take into account factors such as age and physiological status.

Vitamin A–nutrient interactions (Table 121-1)

Changes in the efficiency of digestion and absorption of vitamin A occur in the presence of protein-energy malnutrition (PEM). For example, decreased synthesis and release of proteolytic and lipolytic enzymes of the intestine and pancreas as a result of PEM impair the hydrolysis of retinyl ester and the formation of retinol- or carotene-containing micelles. In addition, synthesis of plasma vitamin A transport proteins [i.e.,

Table 121-1. Effects of different nutrients on vitamin A levels

Nutrient	Interaction
↓ Protein	Decreases vitamin A absorption
	Decreases retinol-binding protein
↓ Fat in diet	Decreases retinol absorption
	Impairs vitamin A transport
↓ Zinc	Decreases vitamin A mobilization
	Decreases enzyme activity
Vitamin E	Protects vitamin A from oxidation
Ethanol	Decreases liver storage of vitamin A

retinol-binding protein (pRBP), and transthyretin (TTR)] by the liver and intestinal synthesis of retinol from β-carotene are diminished.

Dietary fat has a marked stimulatory effect on vitamin A absorption, particularly of carotenoids. Where diets are unusually low in fat, inefficient absorption of dietary carotenoids has been implicated in the development of xerophthalmia. Ingested fat stimulates pancreatic lipase and cholecystokinin secretion, gallbladder contraction, and bile salt secretion which is essential for hydrolysis of both retinyl esters and carotenoids and for the formation of micelles within the intestinal lumen.

Vitamin A mobilization is impaired in zinc deficiency, probably through an indirect action on protein (and thus pRBP) synthesis [3]. Retinol dehydrogenase activity is also significantly depressed (resulting in night blindness), since this enzyme requires zinc for activity. While a vitamin A–vitamin E interrelationship exists, there is conflicting evidence as to the nature of vitamin E's effect on serum levels of vitamin A. Nevertheless, high vitamin E levels in the diet spare vitamin A, leading to an increase of liver stores of vitamin A. This effect may be due to decreased utilization of vitamin A by peripheral tissues, increased uptake of vitamin A by the liver, and/or decreased mobilization of vitamin A from the liver. Moreover, as an antioxidant, vitamin E may protect vitamin A and carotenoids from oxidation within the intestinal lumen.

Chronic alcohol ingestion associated with alcoholic liver disease results in lowered liver storage as well as lower plasma levels of vitamin A. Ethanol may interfere with the absorption of fat-soluble vitamins like vitamin A and alter their metabolism in the liver. One possible explanation is that alcoholics may not have adequate nutrient intakes. A second explanation is that alcohol induces an increase in hepatic microsomal cytochrome P-$_{450}$ enzyme activity, a metabolic pathway that catabolizes retinol.

Significant positive associations exist between serum vitamin A and hemoglobin and other biochemical indicators of iron nutriture. In the vitamin A–deficient state, hemoglobin and serum iron values decrease despite adequate iron intake [4] and, furthermore, liver iron stores become elevated [5]. These observations suggest that vitamin A is involved in the release of iron from the liver and in iron transport throughout the body. Vitamin A fortification seems to improve iron status. Through this relationship, vitamin A deficiency may be a contributing factor in the occurrence of anemia.

METABOLISM

Vitamin A metabolism involves (1) ingestion and absorption, (2) transport to and uptake and storage by the liver, (3) release from the liver and transport in the plasma to target tissues, and finally, (4) hemostatic control and excretion (Fig. 121-1).

Vitamin A is ingested either as retinyl ester from foods of animal origin or as carotene from vegetable sources. Pepsin, chymotrypsin, and trypsin effect the dissociation of preformed vitamin A and carotene from dietary proteins; once liberated, vitamin A is dissolved in fatty globules which move to the small intestine. Uptake of both retinol and carotene by the intestine requires the presence of bile salts and adequate dietary products of fat digestion to form micelles. Retinyl esters are hydrolyzed to retinol in the intestinal lumen by pancreatic esterases and hydrolases associated with the brush border.

How β-carotene is converted to retinol within the intestinal epithelial cell after absorption is less certain. The cleavage of β-carotene to β-apocarotenals by β-carotene dioxygenase may occur in a random or sequential manner or possibly both. Cellular retinol-binding protein type II (cRBP II), a retinol-binding protein found in the absorptive cells of the small intestine, may, in addition to binding retinol, also serve as the acceptor for the retinaldehyde generated by oxidative cleavage of β-carotene in the gut. Retinol dehydrogenase then reduces retinaldehyde to retinol. Theoretically, two molecules of retinol are formed from each molecule of carotene. However, the actual yield under optimal conditions of feeding a physiological, pure β-carotene dose in oil to rats approaches just 50 percent. The absorption of β-carotene in human beings is much less efficient than that of vitamin A and varies depending on the dose administered and the food with which it is eaten.

Retinol, either newly absorbed or synthesized from carotene, is reesterified in the mucosal cell by a mechanism involving its reaction with a fatty acyl-CoA ester (mostly palmitate) and catalyzed by an acyltransferase. Cellular RBP II probably functions in presenting retinol to the esterifying enzyme. Retinyl ester, associated with chylomicrons, is then released and carried via the lymphatics into the general circulation.

With the removal of the chylomicron's triglyceride a chylomicron remnant is formed containing the retinyl ester originally present in the chylomicron along with cholesterol and other lipids. This is taken up by the liver via receptor-mediated endocytosis; the retinyl esters are hydrolyzed to retinol, which is taken up by the hepatic parenchymal cells. Retinol is then reesterified (mostly to retinyl palmitate), secreted in association with plasma RBP (pRBP), and taken up by hepatic nonparenchymal (stellate) cells via pRBP receptors and stored. About 80 percent of total liver vitamin A is stored in stellate cells; however, in hypervitaminosis A, these cells may contain still more. Moreover, pRBP is synthesized not only in parenchymal cells but also by extrahepatic tissues (e.g., lungs, spleen, brain, stomach, skeletal muscle, heart) in small amounts, a fact which, considered with some extrahepatic storage of retinol, suggests a recylcing of retinol between various tissues.

Retinol mobilization and delivery are highly regulated processes, controlled by the rate of synthesis and secretion of plasma retinol-binding protein (apo-pRBP) produced by hepatic parenchymal cells. Retinol binds to apo-pRBP in a 1:1 molar complex before being secreted; the holo-pRBP thus formed combines with transthyretin (TTR) in the plasma before moving to target tissues. Specific cell membrane receptors recognize pRBP; whereas retinol is internalized by the target cell,

VITAMIN A ABSORPTION

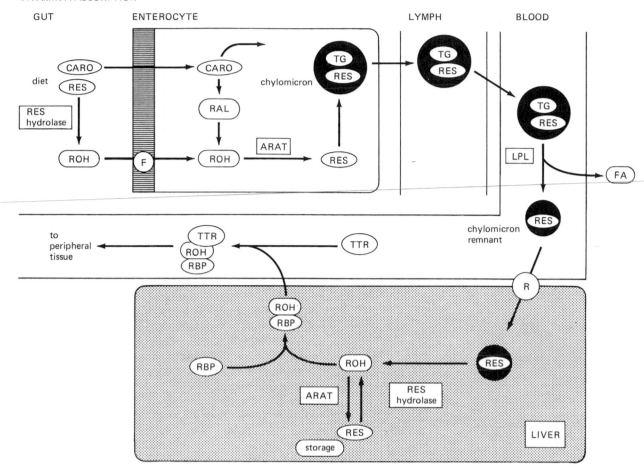

Figure 121-1. Pathways of vitamin A absorption. CARO, β-carotene; RES, retinyl esters; ROH, retinol; RAL, retinaldehyde; RBP, retinol-binding protein; FA, fatty acids; TTR, transthyretin (prealbumin); ARAT, acylCoA:retinol acyltransferase; F, facilitated uptake; R, re-ceptor-mediated uptake. (*From S.A. Krainski: Vitamin A nutritional status and metabolism among older human subjects: A relationship to postprandial plasma vitamin A transport (thesis), p. 8.*)

apo-RBP is not transported across the cell membrane. The liver and kidney both participate in the tissue catabolism of pRBP.

Within all cells, retinol is not free in solution but is associated with either cellular proteins, enzymes, or lipid-rich aggregates. Retinol may be esterified or oxidized to polar metabolites (retinaldehyde, retinoic acid, retinyl taurine, glucuronide), or it may be phosphorylated to retinyl phosphate, which can then participate in glycoprotein synthesis. In certain tissues (liver, eye, gut) retinol interconverts between the trans and various cis forms.

In the rat, about 20 percent of an ingested vitamin A dose is rapidly excreted in the feces; 20 to 50 percent is absorbed but excreted within several days; the remainder (30 to 60 percent) is stored in the liver [6]. Extensive recycling of retinol occurs between plasma, liver, and kidney, allowing for rapid modification of vitamin A distribution relative to nutritional or metabolic changes. The concentration of retinol in plasma re-mains fairly constant (~ 30 to 70 μg/100 mL) despite large variations in intake. Unlike plasma retinol, plasma carotenoid levels directly reflect the amount of carotenoid ingested in the diet. Due to its large storage capacity and its ability to release vitamin A when needed, the liver plays an important role in maintaining a relatively stable state of vitamin A throughout the body. Since the biliary excretion mechanism is also sensitive to the total body pool of vitamin A, the liver serves as a buffer to conserve vitamin A when stores are low and to eliminate vitamin A when stores or intake are high.

PHYSIOLOGICAL ROLES OF VITAMIN A

Maintenance of epithelial tissue integrity

Vitamin A promotes differentiation of epithelial cells through its control of synthesis of messenger RNA for keratin. In vita-min A deficiency, mucus-secreting cells are either replaced by keratinizing cells (as in olfactory glands, taste buds, prostate gland, etc.) or decreased in number (as in the intestine).

Molecular role in glycoprotein synthesis

Retinoids influence the biosynthesis of glycoproteins. Epithelial tissues phosphorylate retinol, and the retinyl phosphate thus formed functions as an acceptor and donor of specific sugar moieties to glycoconjugates. Incorporation of radiolabeled sugars into glycoconjugates is significantly reduced in vitamin A deficiency and restored following retinoid repletion.

Vision

Vitamin A is necessary to maintain the visual process. Retinol is the precursor for the 11-*cis*-retinaldehyde prosthetic group of opsin, a transmembrane glycoprotein contained in the photoreceptor cells of the retina. Thus, retinol must be supplied to the eye from the circulation, stored in eye tissue (retinal pigment epithelial cells), and transported between cells of the retinal pigment epithelium and the photoreceptor cells. All-trans retinol is the form taken up by the pigment epithelium. It is so stored until isomerized to the 11-*cis* form to be delivered to the photoreceptors. Interstitial retinol-binding protein (iRBP), a high-molecular-weight glycoprotein, transfers endogenous retinol from the retinal pigment epithelium to the photoreceptors in the presence of light and back after illumination (Fig. 121-2).

Reproduction, development, and growth

Adequate supplies of retinol are necessary for spermatogenesis, maintenance of the testicular and the vaginal epithelia, and for the proper development of the fetus. The placenta regulates transfer of vitamin A from the mother to the developing child via a retinol-RBP complex. Maternal holo-RBP is the likely form of transfer of vitamin A until midgestation; fetal RBP may sequester retinol from the placental circulation in the latter part of gestation. Since the fetus is more sensitive to extremely low levels of dietary vitamin A than is maternal tissue [7], insufficient maternal intake of the vitamin may result in fetal death, congenital defects, or signs of vitamin A deficiency. Fetal abnormalities also arise as a result of excessively high vitamin A intakes, which alter cell differentiation and growth. Vitamin A participates in the maintenance of mesenchymal structures such as bone and cartilage. In a vitamin A–deficient state, bones become shorter and thicker and osteoblast distribution is abnormal.

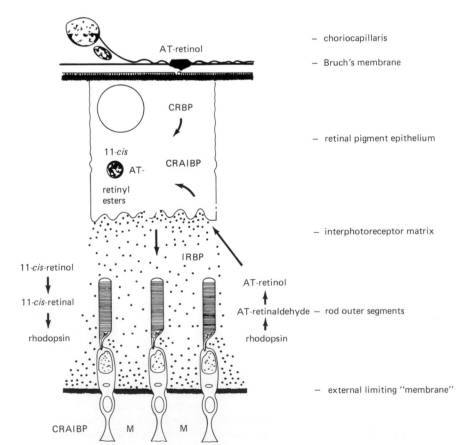

Figure 121-2. Visual cycle retinoids and location of retinoid-binding proteins in the pigment epithelium, interphotoreceptor matrix, and distal retina. AT, all-trans configuration; M, Müller cell, a glial cell that spans the retina from the vitreous surface to the external limiting "membrane." This membrane is formed by the Müller cell ciliary processes that project into the space filled with interphotoreceptor matrix (*dotted area*). (*From C.D.B. Bridges: Retinoids in photosensitive systems, in The Retinoids, vol. 2, New York, Academic, 1984, p. 137.*)

Immune function

Vitamin A has frequently been termed an ''anti-infective'' agent, because animals maintained on vitamin A–deficient diets exhibit increased susceptibility to a wide variety of infections. The frequency and severity of infections also increase. Changes in surface epithelium resulting from deficiency may disrupt the epithelium's normal barrier function, with keratinization of upper intestinal mucosal cells and consequent reduction in mucus secretion facilitating the entry of bacteria into the bloodstream. The immune response in the vitamin A–deficient state has also been shown to be impaired. High doses of vitamin A administered to normal animals produce an increased resistance to infection.

Skin

In addition to keratinization, 11-*cis*-retinoic acid, by an unknown mechanism, inhibits sebum production and so is frequently prescribed for the treatment of cystic acne.

PATIENT

HYPOVITAMINOSIS A

In developed countries, severe vitamin A deficiency is uncommon except in some subgroups of the population—alcoholics, patients with gastrointestinal disease, and Mexican-Americans. Seventy-three less-developed countries and territories are considered to have a potentially serious vitamin A deficiency problem, with Africa, the Middle East, the Caribbean, and southeast Asia most affected. [*13*].

The bioavailability of stored vitamin A depends on general nutritional status. Severe hypovitaminosis A seldom occurs in isolation; it is usually found in combination with PEM. When pRBP is synthesized at a decreased rate, serum retinol levels may drop while hepatic retinol stores remain adequate. Diseases which affect fat absorption (e.g., pancreatic insufficiency, diarrhea, parasitic disease) also increase the risk of developing vitamin A deficiency, since as liver vitamin A stores become depleted, serum retinol levels drop. Infection induces changes in vitamin A metabolism which result in a drop in circulating retinol levels not necessarily related to a depletion of hepatic vitamin A stores. Low serum retinol levels may be due to increased pRBP turnover, to impaired release of retinol from the liver, or increased excretion of vitamin A. Impaired absorption as seen in gastrointestinal diseases and diarrhea may also contribute to depressed serum retinol levels. The depression in serum retinol levels associated with infectious diseases—diarrhea, pneumonia, chickenpox, measles, rheumatic fever, and respiratory infection—may result in the development of acute vitamin A deficiency syndromes.

Any vitamin A deficiency which results from the inability to metabolize or transport the vitamin is termed a *functional deficiency*, as opposed to a true deficiency, wherein stores of the vitamin are themselves inadequate. For example, in zinc deficiency retinol cannot be converted to retinaldehyde without the zinc metalloenzyme retinol dehydrogenase.

Xerophthalmia

The most debilitating manifestation of severe vitamin A deficiency is the irreversible loss of eyesight. Vitamin A deficiency is the most common cause of blindness in children in rural communities of less-developed countries and one of the most prevalent and serious of all nutritional deficiency diseases. The eye is affected by vitamin A deficiency in two principal ways: (1) by reduction of rhodopsin in the retina, leading to abnormal dark adaptation (i.e., impaired night vision, or night blindness) and (2) by keratinization of epithelial layers of the cornea and conjunctiva, which can lead to corneal ulceration and can progress, if untreated, to permanent, irreversible blindness. Xerophthalmia is the general term for all ocular manifestations of impaired vitamin A metabolism. The duration of inadequate vitamin A intake required for xerophthalmia to occur depends on (1) the amount of vitamin A ingested, (2) the extent of preexisting liver stores, and (3) the rate at which vitamin A is utilized by the body [*8*].

Severe xerophthalmia with extensive corneal involvement, resulting from a gradual depletion of vitamin A stores, is less prevalent than mild xerophthalmia, which is characterized by night blindness, conjunctival dryness, or both. While 5 million Asian children may show signs of mild xerophthalmia every year, 0.5 million develop corneal disease [*9*]. The extent to which the cornea has been destroyed (as opposed to the appearance of corneal involvement) is used as the index of severity of the vitamin A deficiency in individual cases [*8*]. The major signs and symptoms of xerophthalmia have been classified [*10*] as seen in Table 121-2.

Assessment of deficiency

Dietary surveys remain inadequate for use in the assessment of hypovitaminosis A in individuals, as it is difficult to obtain quantitatively precise records of vitamin A intake. Food composition tables used in conjunction with surveys frequently assess vitamin A content of foods having made unwarranted assumptions about carotenoid content. Furthermore, the reliability of extrapolating short-term food intake histories to provide an estimation of vitamin A status is limited. However, such dietary surveys are useful as indicators, allowing estimations of the adequacy of a population's diet and thereby permitting predictions of deficiency risk for any given population.

Evidence has been provided that thorough questioning in regard to night blindness can be a simple and reliable screening test for xerophthalmia in a given community. Examination of the eye in search of ocular changes is also a good means by which to make an initial assessment of a population while at the same time serving to identify active cases of vitamin A deficiency. Blood levels of vitamin A give limited information

Table 121-2. Classification of xerophthalmic condition

Condition (classification)	Characteristics	
Night blindness (XN)	Rhodopsin production compromised; rod function impaired	
Conjunctival xerosis (X1A)	Conjunctival epithelium becomes stratified squamous cell layer; loss of goblet cells; formation of granular cell layer; keratinization of surface; eyes dry; fine droplets or bubbles on surface rather than smooth, glistening appearance	**Fig. 121-3**
Bitot's spot (X1B)	Dry, rough, oval, or triangular grayish-white patch in temporal quadrant; surface rippled; foamy, cheesy appearance to white of eye indicative of presence of *Corynebacterium xerosis* (Fig. 121-3)	
Corneal xerosis (X2)	Inferior and/or superior quadrants affected; dry, skinlike, corrugated conjunctiva overlying hazy, lustreless cornea (Fig. 121-4)	**Fig. 121-4**
Corneal ulceration— keratomalcia $< \frac{1}{3}$ corneal surface (X3A) $\geq \frac{1}{3}$ corneal surface (X3B)	Permanent destruction of part or all of corneal stroma (Figs. 121-5 and 121-6); "punched-out" oval ulcers; opaque, gray, or yellow mounds, cental pupillary zone involved; perforation, extrusion of intraocular contents; loss of globe	**Fig. 121-5** **Fig. 121-6**
Xerophthalmic fundus (XF)	Small white retinal lesions in midperipheral region	

Source: Figures are from A. Sommer, Field Guide to the Detection and Control of Xerophthalmia. Geneva, WHO, 1982.

in individual cases, since serum retinol levels are controlled by regulatory mechanisms that maintain circulating levels relatively constant as long as vitamin A stores stay in the normal range (i.e., 20 to 300 μg per gram of liver); thus, marginal stores would not be detected. Blood levels are more predictive for cases of extreme deficiency. However, a high prevalence of low total serum vitamin A levels can serve as a marker of compromised vitamin A status for a given population.

Diagnosis

Liver stores serve as the best indicator of vitamin A status in individuals, but this is difficult to assay in humans. A guideline for hepatic reserves of 20 μg per gram of liver is the minimum acceptable level, since above such a concentration, humans have steady state levels of serum retinol. Newborns tend to have liver reserves of 20 μg/g or lower; however, these reserves increase over time provided the dietary intake of vitamin A remains adequate. A liver reserve of 20 μg/g would provide an adult with over 100 days of protection on a vitamin A–free diet, given that the half-life of retinol in adults is greater than 100 days.

Along with clinical observations and biochemical assessment, functional tests are useful in evaluating vitamin A status in individual cases. Quantitative dark-adaptation tests, of approximately 30 to 45 min in length, are useful tools for identifying subclinical vitamin A deficiency, as impairment of dark adaptation is an early symptom of vitamin A depletion (Fig. 121-7). However, the equipment used is cumbersome, and the test is time-consuming. Rapid dark-adaptation tests (6 to 15 min) have been described but have not been validated in the field.

The electroretinogram (ERG) gives a measure of the change in electrical potential across the retina caused by a light stimulus. However, since the ERG apparatus is large and expensive, and since the procedure is invasive, necessitating contact of the electrode with the eye surface, this method is unsuitable for field use. A drawback of all retinal function tests is that protein-energy malnutrition, zinc deficiency, and eye disease may produce ERG or electrooculogram abnormalities independent of vitamin A status.

A promising approach to assessing vitamin A nutriture in the individual is the examination of a relative response to an oral dose of vitamin A. During vitamin A deficiency, apo-RBP

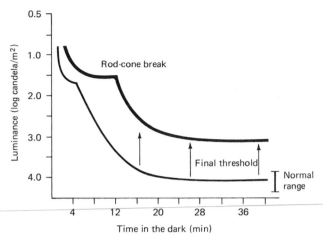

Figure 121-7. Classical dark adaptation curve as measured by a Goldmann-Weekers adaptometer showing a normal curve (*lower*) and that seen in vitamin A deficiency (*upper*). When the logarithm of the light perception threshold is plotted as a function of time in darkness, the change in threshold follows a characteristic course. There is an initial rapid fall in threshold attributed to cone adaptation, followed by the curve plateau. At the rod-cone break, a slower descent begins, attributed to the rods. The final dark-adapted threshold is reached in 35 to 40 min. (*From N.E. Vinton, R.M. Russell: Evaluation of a rapid test of dark adaptation, Am J Clin Nutr 9:1925–1934, 1981.*)

increases in concentration in liver cells, while hepatic vitamin A levels are very low. Upon administration of a small dose of vitamin A to such an individual, the apo-RBP is quickly mobilized and secreted as holo-RBP when joined to retinol. Thus, plasma retinol levels rise in serum under vitamin A–deficient conditions. In cases of sufficiency, newly ingested vitamin A enters the hepatocyte to become part of the hepatic vitamin A ester storage pool rather than becoming immediately bound to pRBP for secretion. Thus, a lesser rise in serum retinol is observed in sufficient states. A relative dose reponse (RDR; i.e., the calculated difference between the 5-h and fasting plasma retinol level divided by the absolute value at 5 h) of > 20 percent indicates marginal vitamin A stores in the liver. This test may not be a reliable indicator of vitamin A status for individuals suffering from gastrointestinal disease, liver dysfunction, or severe protein deficiency, since test results depend on the absorption and liver uptake of a dose of vitamin A, adequate pRBP synthesis, and mobilization of vitamin A by the liver, all of which are adversely affected by the disorders mentioned.

Treatment

To meet an acute need, a massive dose (e.g., 60,000 RE retinyl palmitate) is given upon diagnosis and again the following day. Infants less than 1-year-old and very low weight children are given approximately one-half of this dose on the same schedule. An additional dose should be given 1 to 2 weeks later to boost liver stores and at least two times a year thereafter, and preferably every 3 to 4 months. If the individual is severely protein-deficient, it is recommended that dosing continue biweekly until protein status improves [*11*]. An oral preparation is safe and inexpensive. When not available, treatment should be initiated by feeding food rich in vitamin A (e.g., liver, fish liver oils, egg yolk, milk) or β-carotene (red palm oil, carrots, tomatoes, mangoes, papayas, yellow sweet potatoes, dark-green, leafy vegetables) along with small amounts of oil to enhance absorption. Xerophthalmic conditions in their early stages of development respond rapidly to vitamin A therapy. In addition, vitamin A supplementation reduces the incidence of mortality in severely deficient individuals. Thus, prompt and appropriate treatment can preserve both sight and life.

HYPERVITAMINOSIS A

Excessive intakes of vitamin A—that is, intakes greater than an individual can metabolize, either a single, acute dose or very high intakes over a period of time—have deleterious effects. Variation in sensitivity to vitamin A may cause some individuals, though not others, to experience hypervitaminotic symptoms (e.g., headache, nausea). *Hypervitaminosis A* is the set of biochemical and clinical abnormalities resulting from misuse or overconsumption of excessive amounts of vitamin A. While hypovitaminosis A in less-developed countries poses a far graver health problem, hypervitaminosis A and its resultant effects continue to occur in developed nations.

In most cases of reported hypervitaminosis A, vitamin A intakes are reported by the individual; hence, the intake value should be treated as an alleged one, as the self-medicating individual is often reticent about admitting actual intakes. Depending on the origin of the dose—oil or water—rates of absorption, and thus the appearance of toxic effects, vary. Oil solutions are generally tolerated better than aqueous dispersions, since aqueous dispersions are absorbed more rapidly.

Hypervitaminosis A develops when the body's intake of vitamin A exceeds the liver's capacity to remove it from circulation and store it at a sufficient rate. Although the liver's ability to take up, store, and secrete retinol bound to its carrier protein (pRBP) is extensive, when the liver becomes saturated with vitamin A, increasing amounts of retinyl esters circulate in association with serum lipoproteins and not bound to pRBP. Clinical toxicity is associated with elevated fasting serum concentrations of total vitamin A (>100 μg/dL) and more specifically, with dramatically increased levels of retinyl esters. By contrast, concentrations of plasma holo-pRBP may be normal in individuals with symptoms of vitamin A toxicity. In assessing vitamin A status, the ratio of total vitamin A to pRBP is useful. Since pRBP binds only one molecule of retinol, the normal ratio would be 1:1; however, vitamin A toxicity is characterized by a large molar excess of total vitamin A.

The appearance of clinical manifestations of hypervitaminosis A coincides with the observation of elevated retinyl ester levels. Symptoms observed in cases of hypervitaminosis A can be explained as effects of the nonspecific delivery of free retinol to somatic cell membranes following hydrolysis of retinyl ester by lipoprotein lipase. Free retinol causes cell membrane damage which is evidenced clinically in bodily detriment. Normally, pRBP protects body tissues against surface-active properties of retinol.

Hypervitaminosis A can be classified as either acute (a single oral dose) or chronic (intake over a period of one month or longer). Acute hypervitaminosis A in humans occurs primarily from the consumption of cooked liver from various mammalian sources (polar bear, seal, walrus) or from fish (halibut, shark) with high vitamin A content. Symptoms of hypervitaminosis A have been observed in children aged 9 months to 6 years following single oral doses of 1.7 to 5 million RE of preformed vitamin A [11]. In adults, acute vitamin A toxicity has been observed following ingestion of 1.1 to 16.5 million RE of preformed vitamin A [11]. Physical manifestations from the ingestion of a very high dose appear in hours and include reddening, itchiness and scaliness of the skin, headaches, dizziness, nausea, and vomiting.

Chronic toxicity arises primarily as a result of overdosing by either the individual or parents, whether due to carelessness, ignorance, or the misconception that continued high intakes are beneficial. Toxic manifestations develop at a rate proportional to the level of vitamin A consumed. Symptoms of chronic toxicity include joint and bone pain, pigmentation of the skin, fatigue, insomnia and malaise, pruritus, alopecia, hepatomegaly, hyperostosis, and weight loss. Symptoms have been observed in as short a time as 2 months, with vitamin A at levels of 6000 to 90,000 RE in children and 60,000 to 150,000 RE in adults, but also over longer periods at much lower intakes [11]. For example, one case of reported toxicity occurred at intakes of 13,800 RE over a period of 7 to 10 years. Serum vitamin A levels fall more rapidly in cases of acute (as opposed to chronic) intoxication, since liver stores in acute intoxication are not as great.

Certain conditions may predispose an individual to the development of hypervitaminosis A: alcoholism, hepatitis, hyperlipidemia, and renal disease. The elderly population may be more susceptible to developing vitamin A toxicity as a result of enhanced absorption and/or delayed clearance of vitamin A, which has been demonstrated in this age group.

HYPERCAROTENURIA

Excessive intake of carotenoids does not result in elevated vitamin A levels in body tissue and has not been reported to cause hypervitaminosis A. This situation is due to the slow rate of conversion of carotenoids to vitamin A in the body, their inefficient absorption by the intestine, and their markedly reduced absorption efficiency at high doses. The only clinical manifestation of high levels of intake of carotenoids is a yellow or orange pigmentation of the epidermis which is reversible

upon discontinuing intake of carotenoids. High carotenoid levels in the blood (>200 μg/dL) drop over several months following elimination of the carotenoid source from the diet.

POPULATION

Whether too little or too much vitamin A is consumed, health is always compromised by inappropriate vitamin A nutriture. Although it is difficult to separate the effects of less than optimal vitamin A nutriture from effects of unsuitable nutriture in regard to other nutrients, it can be assumed that the most desirable state of health is attained by maintaining body reserves (and thus, serum retinol levels) through adequate dietary intake of vitamin A.

Age-specific prevalence patterns and morbidity patterns of xerophthalmia are best understood in the context of early childhood feeding practices. Xerophthalmia is rare among breastfed infants and among children who continue to be breast-fed into the second year of life, provided the mother has adequate concentrations of vitamin A in her milk. Since infants have limited vitamin A stores, their ability to maintain and improve their vitamin A status depends on the maternal milk supply. Two patterns observed among the underprivileged in less-developed countries—early weaning to diets inadequate in vitamin A and the rarity of complementary feeding of vitamin A–rich foods along with breast milk—lead to a lack of accumulation of body reserves in early life and a high prevalence of severe deficiency states in preschool populations. Where children are undernourished with respect to vitamin A, intakes of calories, protein, and other micronutrients are often found to be low as well. If undernutrition is not severe, unusual vulnerability to infection may not be in evidence. However, when challenged by a variety of pathogens and subjected to unsanitary environments, these children frequently suffer more severe and more persistent morbid episodes. Infectious morbidity decreases appetite and impairs nutrient metabolism, leading to severe PEM and thus contributing to the development of xerophthalmia [12].

A decrease in the prevalence of xerophthalmia has been noted in instances where impoverished women experience improved economic and social status. Women, more than men, tend to use additional income to improve the quality of their children's diet. Furthermore, added income usually is linked with improved environmental conditions and thus could contribute to decreased morbidity among children. Greater wealth, however, does not reduce morbidity if mothers remain illiterate [13]. Thus, upgrading the social status of women is crucial to alleviating childhood vitamin A deficiency. Recent data strongly suggest that increased morbidity and mortality are related to vitamin A deficiency in humans [14]. In a randomized, controlled community trial in vitamin A–deficient Indonesian children, mortality decreased significantly with vitamin A supplementation [15]. Epidemiological investigations also suggest that marginal or deficient vitamin A levels are associated with increased risk of cancer in a variety of organs (e.g., lung, bladder, oral cavity). High doses of vitamin A compounds have been shown to suppress induction and development of tumors in animal models. Epidemiological studies implicate β-carotene more than retinol in the prevention of cancer; animal studies indicate that dietary carotenoid supplementation can inhibit the process of cancer induction. However, at least one human study demonstrates a negative association between β-carotene intake and risk of esophageal cancer [16]. Thus, existing data do not definitively suggest a protective effect conferred by dietary β-carotene.

PREVENTION

Only by ensuring the adequate intake of vitamin A among those at risk of becoming or those already vitamin A–deficient will the underlying cause of hypovitaminosis A be eliminated. A solution must take into account such complicating factors as reduced absorption, decreased vitamin A stores, and increased requirements in cases of gastroenteritis, parasitism, measles, and other infectious diseases. The ultimate goal of a prevention program must thus be the regular, adequate, dietary intake of vitamin A. Intervention programs to treat hypovitaminosis A either increase the intake of the vitamin directly or increase the efficiency of utilization by minimizing factors that elevate vitamin A requirements (e.g., reduced absorption, decreased stores, intestinal and infectious diseases). Most often, a combination of short- and long-term methods is employed. Measures currently being implemented which will lead to the realization of this goal include: (1) periodic administration of large vitamin A doses to the most highly vulnerable segment of the population—preschoolers; (2) fortification of foods frequently consumed; and (3) increasing the amount of vitamin A–rich foods in the diet.

Periodic dosing is effective as a short-term interventive measure. Since large quantities of vitamin A are stored in the liver for future use, oral administration of 110 mg retinyl palmitate or 66 mg retinyl acetate (one half this dose for children less than 1 year) every 6 months protects recipients from xerophthalmia [8]. The provision of a standard high-dose capsule by UNICEF has facilitated this approach. The major difficulty in terms of both cost and efficacy is distribution. Since vitamin A deficiency and xerophthalmia cluster, distribution of capsules should be targeted to areas where xerophthalmia is particularly prevalent. Another approach is to dose newborns (15,125 RE) and their mothers (90,750 RE) with retinyl palmitate [8]. Pregnant women in high-risk communities may receive frequent, low-dose (1512 RE/day or 6050 RE/week) supplementation of retinyl palmitate, which avoids the potential risk of teratogenicity from a larger dose.

Fortification of inexpensive, commonly consumed foods (such as bread, salt, sugar, monosodium glutamate) with vitamin A is another effective means by which to improve the vitamin A status of a population. Although theoretically for-

tification should be a low-cost, easily controllable long-term solution, numerous economic and political restraints—the cost of imported synthetic vitamin A, for example—have arisen. It remains technically feasible as an approach, however, and does have the potential to improve vitamin A status of groups at risk.

The most reasonable and least expensive long-range solution to improving vitamin A status lies in altering the inappropriate dietary practices of those at risk. This approach should have two aims: in the first place, to increase the availability of food sources of vitamin A through promotion of home gardening or other horticultural programs; and secondly, to heighten family awareness through the institution of health education programs of the importance of prolonging breast-feeding and of consuming vitamin A–rich foods.

Unlike hypovitaminosis A, hypervitaminosis is not a problem of public health magnitude for any population of the world [12]. This is due in large part to the fact that most symptoms and signs of toxicity revert to normal following removal of the vitamin from the diet, with liver damage and growth stunting in children being the exceptions. However, concern is mounting in regard to the anticipated increase in prevalence of chronic hypervitaminosis A in developed countries in the future. The common practice of parental administration of concentrated vitamin supplements to young children who also consume foods fortified with vitamin A may result in an increase in the numbers of individuals with reserves at toxic levels. In addition, reported associations between retinoids and cancer prevention may lead the uninformed public to increase their consumption of vitamin A.

REFERENCES

1 Zile M, Cullum M: The function of vitamin A: Current concepts. Proc Soc Exp Biol Med 172:139–152, 1983

2 World Health Organization: Requirements of vitamin A, folate, and B_{12}. Geneva, FAO/WHO Joint Expert Presentation, March 1985

3 Bauernfeind JC: *Vitamin A Deficiency and Its Control.* New York, Academic, 1986

4 Hodges RE, Sauberlich HE, Canham JE, et al: Hematopoietic studies in vitamin A deficiency. Am J Clin Nutr 31:876–885, 1978

5 Mejia LA, Hodges RE, Rucher RB: Role of vitamin A in the absorption, retention and distribution of iron in the rat. J Nutr 109:129–137, 1979

6 Deluca LM, Gover J, Heller J, et al: Guidelines for the eradication of vitamin A deficiency and xerophthalmia. Recent advances in the metabolism and function of vitamin A and their relationship to applied nutrition. A report of the International Vitamin A Consultative Group. Washington, DC, The Nutrition Foundation, 1977

7 Wallingford J, Underwood B: Vitamin A status needed to maintain vitamin A concentrations in nonhepatic tissues of the pregnant rat. J Nutr 117:1410–1415, 1987

8 Sommer A: *Field Guide to the Detection and Control of Xerophthalmia.* Geneva, World Health Organization, 1982

9 Sommer A, Tarwotjo I, Hussaini G, et al: Incidence, prevalence, and scale of blinding malnutrition. Lancet i:1407–1408, 1981

10 World Health Organization: Report of a joint WHO/USAID/UNICEF/HKI/IVACG Meeting. WHO Tech Rep Ser 672, Geneva, World Health Organization, 1982

11 Bauernfeind J: The safe use of vitamin A. A report of the International Vitamin A Consultative Group. Washington, DC, The Nutrition Foundation, 1980

12 Underwood B: Vitamin A in animal and human nutrition, in *The Retinoids.* New York, Academic, 1984, vol 1, pp 282–377

13 Mamarbachi D, Pellett PLL, Basha HM, et al: Observations on nutritional marasmus in a newly rich nation. Ecol Food Nutr 9:43–53, 1980

14 Sommer A, Tarwotjo I, Hussaini G, et al: Increased mortality in mild vitamin A deficiency. Lancet ii:585–588, 1983

15 Sommer A, Tarwotjo I, Djunaedi E, et al: Impact of vitamin A supplementation on childhood mortality. Lancet i:1169–72, 1986

16 Decarli A, Liati P, Negri E, et al: Vitamin A and other dietary factors in the etiology of esophageal cancer. Nutr Cancer 10:29–37, 1987

CHAPTER 122 / *Vitamin D* · Michael D. Sitrin

NUTRIENT

The term *vitamin D* denotes a group of secosteroids which cause healing of rickets and osteomalacia in humans and experimental animals. The two forms of vitamin D of most nutritional importance are *cholecalciferol, vitamin D₃*, produced in animal skin by the action of ultraviolet light on precursor 7-dehydrocholesterol; and *ergocalciferol, vitamin D₂*, which is widely used in food fortification and dietary supplements and is produced by ultraviolet radiation of the plant sterol ergosterol [1]. In mammals, these secosteroids have a nearly identical metabolism and action and will therefore be considered together as vitamin D. Vitamin D is not itself biologically active at physiological concentrations, but it is extensively metabolized to other compounds that stimulate intestinal calcium and phosphate absorption, and participate in the maintenance of a normal serum calcium, thereby causing bone mineralization. Vitamin D is, therefore, not a vitamin in the classical sense, but is part of a complex endocrine system for regulating mineral and bone metabolism [1].

CUTANEOUS PHOTOSYNTHESIS OF VITAMIN D

It is now established that cutaneous photosynthesis of vitamin D₃, cholecalciferol, provides from 40 to 80 percent of the circulating vitamin in individuals eating typical western diets. Photosynthesis of vitamin D causes the observed seasonal variation in serum vitamin levels, which peak in late summer when sun exposure and ultraviolet radiation are maximal and are lowest in late winter [2]. Ultraviolet B radiation, 290 to 320 nm, converts skin 7-dehydrocholesterol to previtamin D₃, which subsequently undergoes a temperature-dependent thermal isomerization to vitamin D₃ over several days [3]. Vitamin D₃ is carried from the skin into the circulation bound to the plasma vitamin D–binding protein. With prolonged ultraviolet B exposure, previtamin D photoisomerizes to the inactive products lumisterol and tachysterol, so that the maximum amount of previtamin D produced is about 15 percent of the original 7-dehydrocholesterol concentration. These reactions provide an explanation for the observation that vitamin D toxicity has not been reported from protracted sun exposure [3]. Darker skin pigmentation increases the exposure time to ultraviolet B radiation that is required to maximize previtamin D synthesis; melanin competes with 7-dehydrocholesterol for ultraviolet B photons [4]. The required exposure time for maximum previtamin D synthesis lengthens with increasing latitude from the equator, reflecting decreased ultraviolet radiation with increased zenith angle of the sun [3]. Window glass and industrial pollution filter out much of the ultraviolet B radiation.

DIETARY SOURCES OF VITAMIN D

Most natural diets contain little vitamin D, with certain fatty fish being the only common foods which provide substantial amounts. Cod liver oil has long been appreciated as a cure for rickets. Liver, eggs, butter, and cheese contain small amounts of the vitamin [5]. Human breast milk also is relatively poor in vitamin D, providing only about 40 IU/L [6]. In the United States, most of the vitamin D in the diet is provided by fortification of dairy products, with vitamin D being added to most milk to provide a concentration of 10 μg/quart (400 IU/quart).

REQUIREMENT

The U.S. Recommended Dietary Allowance and the WHO recommended intake for vitamin D is 400 IU/day for infants, children, and adolescents, although a lesser amount, 100 IU, is sufficient for preventing rickets [7]. For individuals aged 19 to 22 years, the recommended dietary allowance is reduced to 300 IU, and it is further reduced to 200 IU after age 22. An additional 200 IU is recommended during pregnancy and lactation.

VITAMIN D ABSORPTION AND METABOLISM

Vitamin D is a fat-soluble vitamin, absorbed mainly in the duodenum and jejunum [8]. Bile salts in the intestinal lumen facilitate absorption by solubilizing the vitamin in mixed micelles. The bile salt requirement may be influenced by the amount of other dietary fats in the intestinal lumen [9]. Vitamin D enters the enterocyte from the mixed micelle by passive diffusion; much of the vitamin is packaged into chylomicron particles and released with triglyceride into mesenteric lymph, although some goes directly into portal blood [9].

Vitamin D derived from the diet or photocutaneous synthesis is inactive at physiological concentration. The first step in bioactivation occurs in the liver with formation of 25-(OH) vitamin D, the major metabolite of vitamin D circulating in the plasma, where it is bound to a specific vitamin D–binding protein in the α-globulin fraction. The control of hepatic 25-hydroxylase activity is poorly understood; hydroxylation is enhanced in vitamin D deficiency. At physiological concentrations, 25-(OH) vitamin D does not significantly stimulate intestinal calcium absorption. In the kidney, 25-(OH) vitamin D is further hydroxylated, forming 1,25-(OH)$_2$ vitamin D, the vitamin metabolite which stimulates intestinal calcium and phosphate absorption. Renal 1-hydroxylation is enhanced by parathyroid hormone and by hypophosphatemia and hypocalcemia. If serum levels of calcium or phosphate fall, production of 1,25-(OH)$_2$ vitamin D is stimulated, resulting in enhanced calcium and phosphate absorption [10]. In the absence of parathyroid hormone or hypophosphatemia, the kidney produces another vitamin D metabolite, 24,25-(OH)$_2$ vitamin D. Some evidence suggests that 24,25-(OH)$_2$ vitamin D may play a role in mineralization of cartilage and bone [11], but other data indicate that this is an inactivation pathway. Other vitamin D metabolites, including di- and trihydroxy derivatives, lactones, and acids, have been identified in serum and tissue, but their physiological function remains uncertain.

1,25-(OH)$_2$ vitamin D acts in the intestine and other tissues by a mechanism analogous to that of classical steroid hormones [12]. 1,25-(OH)$_2$ vitamin D interacts with a specific receptor protein, and the hormone-receptor complex associates with nuclear chromatin altering gene expression. Although the exact mechanism by which 1,25-(OH)$_2$ vitamin D causes active calcium transport remains uncertain, 1,25-(OH)$_2$ vitamin D does stimulate production of a calcium-binding protein and other proteins which may play a role in calcium absorption [13]. Additional nongenomic effects of 1,25-(OH)$_2$ vitamin D on intestinal membranes may also participate in the stimulation of calcium absorption [14]. Active intestinal phosphate transport is also enhanced by 1,25-(OH)$_2$ vitamin D. In bone, 1,25-(OH)$_2$ vitamin D, along with parathyroid hormone, causes mobilization of calcium, increasing the serum calcium. In the kidney, 1,25-(OH)$_2$ vitamin D increases tubular calcium and phosphate reabsorption.

Receptors for 1,25-(OH)$_2$ vitamin D are found in many cell types other than the classical target tissues for vitamin D. 1,25-(OH)$_2$ vitamin D has been demonstrated to have potent effects on cell proliferation and differentiation, immune function, and other cellular events [15,16].

ASSESSMENT OF VITAMIN D STATUS— ASSAYS FOR VITAMIN D METABOLITES

Methods are currently available for measurement of the serum concentration of the major vitamin D metabolites. The most useful indicator of vitamin D nutritional status is the 25-(OH) vitamin D concentration, most commonly measured by a competitive protein-binding assay [17]. Serum 25-(OH) vitamin D levels must be compared with appropriately timed controls because there is a seasonal variation in serum 25-(OH) vitamin D concentration. Measurements of serum levels of other vitamin D secosteroids are more difficult since they are present in much lower concentrations and require extensive separation by column and high-pressure liquid chromatography before assay. Serum 1,25-(OH)$_2$ vitamin D concentration has not been a consistently reliable measure of vitamin D status [18]. Since the half-life of this secosteroid is rather short, serum concentration may not accurately reflect the rate of synthesis or the concentration in target tissues.

PATIENT

CLINICAL MANIFESTATIONS OF VITAMIN D DEFICIENCY

The skeletal manifestations of vitamin D deficiency will vary greatly depending upon the stage of skeletal growth [19]. With congenital or infantile rickets, the most common abnormality is craniotabes, softening of the bones of the skull. In children, vitamin D deficiency predominantly affects the cartilaginous growth plate and primary spongiosa of bone causing the characteristic abnormality called rickets. In the first year, rapid growth of arms and ribs leads to enlargement of the costochondral junctions (the rachitic rosary) and thickening at the wrist. As the child begins to walk, deformities in the lower extremities, including bow legs or knock knees, are more commonly observed; growth may be impaired. "Late rickets" represents a form of mild chronic rickets which may become clinically apparent during the pubertal growth spurt. These adolescents complain of pain in the back or limbs and weakness, and may have only mild deformities such as knock knees.

In the adult, vitamin D deficiency produces the clinical syndrome of osteomalacia [20]. Bone pain, particularly in the spine, pelvis, legs and ribs, is commonly seen and may be worsened by weight bearing, activity, or pressure over the bone. These symptoms may be vague and nonspecific leading to incorrect diagnoses such as arthritis, rheumatism, or psychosomatic disease. With advanced osteomalacia, deformities such as bowing of the legs, gibbus, pigeon chest, kyphoscoliosis, or loss of trunk height ensue. Patients who have associated osteoporosis may develop vertebral compression fractures.

Proximal muscle weakness is often a prominent feature of vitamin D deficiency and may lead to a waddling gait or lordotic stance. Muscle strength improves rapidly with treatment with vitamin D, long before bone healing is complete. Most patients with vitamin D deficiency have normal or low normal serum calcium, but occasionally vitamin D deficiency results in severe enough hypocalcemia to produce paresthesias, muscle cramps, or tetany. Hypocalcemic convulsions may occur with neonatal vitamin D deficiency.

DIAGNOSIS AND DETECTION OF VITAMIN D DEFICIENCY

Biochemical indices

The most sensitive and reliable biochemical test of depletion of vitamin D is the circulating 25-(OH) vitamin D concentration. In the earliest stages of deficiency the low 25-(OH) vitamin D level may be the sole abnormality. Serum calcium and phosphate levels may be reduced and serum alkaline phosphatase activity elevated in patients with vitamin D deficiency, but will be normal in significant numbers of deficient patients.

Radiological signs

In rickets, the growth plates of rapidly growing metaphyses are widened due to hypertrophy of cartilage cells whose matrix is not being calcified and transformed into bone. The metaphyses develop an irregular appearance as the recently calcified cartilage is invaded by the adjacent bone. With more severe rickets, the subperiosteal bone is also undercalcified, leading to a fuzzy outer margin of the shafts. Radiological evidence of secondary hyperparathyroidism with erosion of subperiosteal bone is also found. With osteomalacia, the bones will often be relatively radiolucent, although many patients will have radiologically normal bone. A more specific sign is the finding of Looser's zones or Milkman's fractures. These are "ribbon-like zones of rarefaction" seen in the shafts of long bones and certain flat bones such as the scapula. Such areas reflect sites of recurrent stress microfractures which fail to calcify properly during healing. With long-standing osteomalacia, bone deformities such as biconcave vertebrae and narrowing of the pelvis also occur [21].

Histology

The most sensitive and accurate technique for the diagnosis of rickets and osteomalacia is bone biopsy, generally performed at the anterior iliac crest. Much vitamin D deficiency bone disease is subclinical, producing no clinical, radiological, or biochemical abnormalities, and will only be found by histological examination of bone. Thin, undercalcified sections of bone are stained to demonstrate the extent and width of unmineralized bone matrix, termed *osteoid*, covering trabecular and cortical bone surfaces. In vitamin D deficiency, wide osteoid seams cover more of the bone surface than in normal age- and sex-matched controls [22]. The calcification front can be labeled by administering tetracycline to the patient prior to biopsy, allowing measurement of the extent of mineralizing surface and the mineral appositional rate, which are both reduced in rickets and osteomalacia [23].

POPULATION

VITAMIN D DEFICIENCY IN TROPICAL COUNTRIES

Vitamin D deficiency has traditionally been viewed as a nutritional problem of industrial northern Europe. With the growth of industrial cities, rickets became very prevalent in the lower socioeconomic classes who lived in overcrowded conditions limiting sun exposure and who ate a poor diet. It is somewhat surprising that rickets and osteomalacia are regularly observed in tropical and subtropical countries where solar irradiation is high. Several reports from India indicate a 2 to 5 percent prevalence of rickets in young children and a high prevalence of osteomalacia in adult women [24]. In the Middle East, rickets and osteomalacia have been reported as significant problems in Iran, Iraq, Saudi Arabia, and among the bedouin population of Israel [25–28]. Three to eighteen percent of children under age 5 in Algeria, Libya, Morocco, and Tunisia who were examined in 1965 by a WHO consultant had clinical signs of severe rickets [29]. In Algeria, 5.7 percent of pregnant women admitted for delivery had clinically apparent osteomalacia [30]. In South Africa, vitamin D deficiency, rickets, and osteomalacia are seen mainly in the black and mulatto population [31,32]. A report of nine Jamaican children with vitamin D deficiency rickets suggests that this problem may be more common in the Caribbean than previously thought [33]. Even in Greece, 15 percent of 327 infants had elevated serum alkaline phosphatase levels which returned to normal with vitamin D treatment [34]. Fifty-eight percent of these infants had radiological evidence of rickets in the wrist, while clinical signs of rickets were found in 94 of the 327 children.

The pathogenesis of vitamin D deficiency in tropical countries characteristically involves several factors which limit dietary vitamin D intake and cutaneous vitamin D synthesis [5]. In the Middle East, many people live in high-walled, relatively sunless houses, and industrial pollution in some cities filters out much ultraviolet irradiation. Avoidance of sun exposure and practices of purdah (seclusion of females and children), wearing full-length veils, and swaddling of infants in Moslem countries markedly reduce cutaneous vitamin D synthesis. Dark skin pigmentation increases the exposure time necessary for maximum conversion of previtamin D [4]. In less-developed countries, dietary sources of vitamin D are sparse, and foods rich in vitamin D such as fish and fortified dairy products are expensive.

In tropical countires, vitamin D deficiency during pregnancy is a particularly serious problem, presenting major health hazards for both the mother and newborn. Osteomalacia may lead to narrowing of the pelvic outlet, making vaginal delivery extremely difficult. Both mother and child may die after protracted difficult labor. Osteomalacia is often more severe in women who have had multiple pregnancies with prolonged lactation. Reduced dietary intake of vitamin D and decreased sun exposure during pregnancy and lactation contribute to the development of vitamin D deficiency.

Infants of Vitamin D–depleted mothers are at high risk for vitamin D deficiency, neonatal rickets, hypocalcemic seizures, and abnormalities of dental enamel [35]. There is a strong correlation between maternal vitamin D status and cord blood vitamin D activity, reflecting significant transplacental transfer of vitamin D and its metabolites [36]. Maternal vitamin D status also influences the vitamin D content of her milk, and dietary supplementation or increased sun exposure will increase breast milk vitamin D activity [37]. Prolonged breast-feeding without addition of vitamin D–rich foods or supplements to the baby's diet may contribute to the development of rickets. In some populations, however, breast-feeding reflects a higher standard of infant care, with increased sun exposure compensating for the relatively poor vitamin D content of human milk.

VITAMIN D DEFICIENCY, RICKETS, AND OSTEOMALACIA IN WESTERN COUNTRIES

Despite the availability of cod liver oil as a vitamin D supplement in the 1920s, rickets continued to be observed in 2 to 8 percent of infants in Great Britain until World War II. With the outbreak of World War II, measures were taken by the English government to safeguard health, including fortification with vitamin D of margarine, milk, and infant milks and cereals [5]. Vitamin D supplements were also provided for pregnant women. With these steps and improved socioeconomic conditions, the incidence of rickets in England dropped dramatically after World War II. In the 1950s, hypercalcemia was observed in some infants and young children, and was presumed related to excessive intake of vitamin D–fortified foods [38]. The amount of vitamin D in milk, cereals, and cod liver oil was reduced, but rickets has not reappeared as a major problem in the native white English population.

Beginning in the 1960s and 1970s, rickets and osteomalacia were appreciated as common diseases in the growing Asian immigrant population in Great Britain [39,40]. The factors responsible for rickets and osteomalacia in immigrant Asians are complex [41]. Dietary vitamin D intake is lower in this population than in the native white population, and serum 25-(OH) vitamin D levels correlate with dietary vitamin D intake. Limited sun exposure among the Asian population has been reported as an important pathogenetic mechanism. Skin pigmentation does not appear to be a major factor, since vitamin D deficiency is more common among light-skinned Asians than the darker-skinned immigrants from the West Indies [5].

Ingestion of chappatis, bread made without yeast and therefore high in phytate, has been suggested as a contributing cause of rickets and osteomalacia, but this is disputed [41,42]. Calcium deficiency, which can occur with high-fiber diets, has been reported to accelerate 25-(OH) vitamin D turnover and contribute to vitamin D depletion [43].

Vitamin D deficiency rickets is rarely seen in the United States, except in certain susceptible groups. Several reports emphasize that black inner-city children may develop rickets, particularly if they breast-feed for a prolonged time and their mothers have a poor vitamin D nutritional status. Many of these children belong to Muslim sects, wear clothing which covers all but their eyes and forehead, and are weaned to vegetarian diets [44]. Serum 25-(OH) vitamin D levels are often low in breast-fed infants from northern Europe who have little UV-B exposure in winter, although clinical rickets is unusual [45]. Premature infants often require vitamin D deficiency supplementation.

Currently, vitamin D deficiency is unusual in adult caucasians in western countries. Elderly individuals are at increased risk for vitamin D deficiency and bone disease, particularly if they are housebound or require institutional care [46]. Dietary vitamin D intake is often low in the elderly, typically less than 100 IU/day, and exposure to sunlight is often limited. Some studies in animals and humans suggest that intestinal absorption of vitamin D decreases with advancing age [47]. Metabolism of vitamin D, particularly renal 1-hydroxylation, may also decrease with aging. Exposure to ultraviolet light produces similar increases in serum 25-(OH) vitamin D concentration in both young and elderly subjects. Some studies have indicated that vitamin D deficiency is common in patients with hip fractures [48]. Osteomalacia and secondary hyperparathyroidism could contribute to bone loss, and vitamin D deficiency myopathy may predispose to frequent falls.

CONDITIONED DEFICIENCY

In western countries, rickets and osteomalacia are most commonly caused by diseases which interfere with the normal absorption, metabolism, or action of vitamin D (Table 122-1). Patients with gastrointestinal diseases, such as postgastrectomy syndromes, celiac sprue, Crohn's disease, the short-bowel syndrome, and exocrine pancreatic insufficiency, are at increased risk of vitamin D deficiency and metabolic bone disease [49]. These patients are often on fat-restricted diets or are lactose-intolerant and may therefore have low vitamin D intakes. Malabsorption of both vitamin D and calcium also contributes to the development of bone disease. Patients with liver disease, particularly chronic cholestatic liver diseases such as primary biliary cirrhosis, often have severe metabolic bone disease. Malabsorption of dietary vitamin D, impaired hepatic 25-hydroxylation, and increased urinary losses of vitamin D metabolites all contribute to vitamin D deficiency. Chronic renal failure commonly causes metabolic bone disease which is a

Table 122-1. Examples of conditioned vitamin D deficiency

Mechanism	Disease
Vitamin D malabsorption	Postgastrectomy; small-intestinal diseases, e.g., sprue; pancreatic insufficiency
Impaired hepatic 25-hydroxylation	Cirrhosis
Increased hepatic metabolism or excretion	Anticonvulsants
Increased renal excretion	Cholestatic liver disease; nephrotic syndrome
Impaired renal 1-hydroxylation	Chronic renal failure; hypoparathyroidism; vitamin D–dependent rickets—type 1
Target organ resistance to 1,25-$(OH)_2$ vitamin D	Vitamin D–dependent rickets—type 2

combination of hyperparathyroidism and osteomalacia [*50*]. With phosphate retention and decreased functional renal mass, production of 1,25-$(OH)_2$ vitamin D diminishes and intestinal calcium absorption is reduced. Children with vitamin D–dependent rickets have genetic defects in either the renal production of 1,25-$(OH)_2$ vitamin D or its action on target tissues [*51,52*]. Drugs may also interfere with vitamin D absorption or metabolism. The anion exchange resin cholestyramine binds vitamin D and may result in osteomalacia. Inducers of hepatic microsomal activity, such as the anticonvulsant diphenylhydantoin, accelerate the metabolism of vitamin D to inactive compounds and may cause rickets or osteomalacia.

PREVENTION AND TREATMENT OF VITAMIN D DEFICIENCY

As a public health measure, fortification of foods such as infant formulas, cereals, and dairy products with vitamin D has been effective in dramatically decreasing the incidence of vitamin D deficiency rickets in the United States and western Europe. In the United States, a daily intake of 400 IU is recommended for infants and children. Concern has been raised, however, about toxicity from routine fortification of foods with vitamin D. In the mid-1950s, workers in England and Switzerland reported hypercalcemia in infants, which responded to removing vitamin D and calcium from the diet [*38*]. Because the extent of food fortification was poorly regulated, many of these children were ingesting more than 4000 IU/day of vitamin D; some children developed hypercalcemia wth lower vitamin D intakes. The amount of vitamin D added to various foods was reduced, and the incidence of hypercalcemia in infancy declined. In the United States, a more controlled fortification of infant foods and dairy products with vitamin D has been employed, and hypercalcemia in infants is rarely reported. A more directed approach to fortification is the addition of vitamin D to foods used only by the population groups at higher risk for deficiency. For example, fortification of the chappati flour used

by the immigrant Asians in England has been effective in preventing vitamin D deficiency in that group.

Daily vitamin D supplements providing about 400 IU/day are often used to prevent vitamin D deficiency. The supplements are typically provided in clinics caring for children and pregnant women, but poor compliance often limits their effectiveness. In situations where compliance is poor and medical supervision is limited, large oral or intramuscular doses of vitamin D have been periodically given (e.g., 200,000 to 600,000 IU every 6 months), although the risk of toxicity is somewhat higher with this regimen.

Patients with clinically apparent rickets or osteomalacia are treated with approximately 5000 IU/day of vitamin D for several weeks, followed by prolonged supplementation with lower doses. Patients with malabsorption may require higher doses of vitamin D, 4000 to 20,000 IU/day, and should optimally be followed by monitoring serum 25-(OH) vitamin D levels as dosage adjustments are made. In less-developed countries, large oral or intramuscular doses are given every few months as treatment for vitamin D deficiency. The hydroxy vitamin D metabolites, 25-(OH) vitamin D_3 and 1,25-$(OH)_2$ vitamin D_3 are now available for oral therapy. Patients with chronic cholestatic liver disease, where absorption and hepatic hydroxylation may be impaired, may respond to oral doses of 50 to 100 μg of 25-(OH) vitamin D when therapy with vitamin D is ineffective. Renal osteodystrophy will respond either to 25-(OH) vitamin D or 1 to 3 μg of 1,25-$(OH)_2$ vitamin D [*53*]. Similar doses of 1,25-$(OH)_2$ vitamin D can correct disordered calcium metabolism and heal bone disease in hypoparathyroidism, pseudohypoparathyroidism, and vitamin D–dependent rickets.

Vitamin D toxicity presents as hypercalcemia resulting from increased intestinal calcium absorption and mobilization of calcium from bone. Manifestations include neurological symptoms such as coma or hypotonia, constipation, polyuria and polydipsia due to decreased renal concentrating ability, cardiac rhythm disturbances, renal stones, nephrocalcinosis which may lead to renal failure, and ectopic calcification in various organs. Appropriate monitoring of 25-(OH) vitamin D levels or serum and urinary calcium can guide the safe and effective use of vitamin D or metabolites of the vitamin.

REFERENCES

1 Haussler MR, McCain TA: Vitamin D metabolism and action. N Engl J Med 297:974–1041, 1977

2 Poskitt EME, Cole TJ, Lawson DEM: Diet, sunlight, and 25-hydroxyvitamin D in healthy children and adults. Br Med J 1:221–223, 1979

3 Holick MF: The cutaneous photosynthesis of previtamin D_3: A unique photoendocrine system. J Invest Dermatol 76:51–58, 1982

4 Clemens TL, Adams JS, Henderson SL, et al: Increased skin pigment reduces the capacity of skin to synthesize vitamin D_3. Lancet 1:74–76, 1982

5 Rickets and Osteomalacia, Report on Health and Social Subjects, Department of Health and Social Security, London 1980

6 Hollis BW, Pittard WB, Reinhardt TA: Relationships among vitamin D, 25-hydroxyvitamin D, and vitamin D-binding protein concentrations in the plasma and milk of human subjects. J Clin Endocrinol Metab 62:41–44, 1986

7 Recommended Dietary Allowances, National Academy of Sciences, Washington, DC, 1980

8 Schachter D, Finkelstein JD, Kowarski S: Metabolism of vitamin D. I. Preparation of radioactive vitamin D and its intestinal absorption in the rat. J Clin Invest 43:787–796, 1964

9 Sitrin MD, Pollack KL, Bolt MJG, et al: Comparison of vitamin D and 25-hydroxyvitamin D absorption in the rat. Am J Physiol 5:G326–G332, 1982

10 Tanaka Y, DeLuca HF: The control of 25-hydroxyvitamin D metabolism by inorganic phosphorus. Arch Biochem Biophys 154:566–574, 1973

11 Kanis JA, Cundy T, Bartlett M, et al: Is 24-25 dihydroxycholecalciferol a calcium-regulating hormone in man? Br Med J 1:1382–1386, 1978

12 Norman AW, Roth J, Orci L: The vitamin D endocrine system: Steroid metabolism, hormone receptors, and biological response (calcium binding proteins). Endocr Rev 3:331–366, 1982

13 Wasserman RH, Corradino RA, Fullmer CS, et al: Some aspects of vitamin D action: calcium absorption and vitamin D-dependent calcium-binding protein. Vitam Horm 32:299–324, 1974

14 Brasitus TA, Dudeja PK, Lau K: Correction by 1-25-dihydroxy cholecalciferol of the abnormal fluidity and lipid composition of enterocyte brush border membranes in vitamin D-deprived rats. J Biol Chem 261:16,404–16,409, 1986

15 Manolagas SC: Vitamin D and its relevance to cancer. Anticancer Res 7:625–638, 1987

16 Gray TK, Cohen MS: Vitamin D, phagocyte differentiation and immune function. Surv Immunol Res 4:200–212, 1985

17 Haddad JG, Chyu KJ: Competitive protein-binding radioassay for 25-hydroxycalciferol. J Clin Endocrinol Metab 3:992–995, 1971

18 Eastwood JB, Wardener HE: Normal plasma 1,25-$(OH)_2$-vitamin D concentrations in nutritional osteomalacia. Lancet i:1377–1378, 1979

19 Loveinger RD: Rickets. Pediatrics 66:359–365, 1980

20 Frame B, Parfitt AM: Osteomalacia: Current concepts. Ann Intern Med 89:966–982, 1978

21 Dent CE, Stamp TCG: Vitamin D, rickets, and osteomalacia, in Avioli LV, Krane SM (eds): *Metabolic Bone Disease*. New York, Academic, 1977, pp 184–231

22 Arnestein AR, Frame B, Frost HM: Recent progress in osteomalacia and rickets. Ann Intern Med 67:1296–1330, 1967

23 Frost HM: Tetracycline-based histological analysis of bone remodeling. Calcif Tissue Res 3:211–217, 1969

24 Chaudhuri MK: Nutritional profiles of Calcutta pre-school children. II. Clinical observations. Indian J Med Res 63:189–195, 1976

25 Salimpour R: Rickets in Tehran: Study of 200 cases. Arch Dis Child 50:62–66, 1975

26 Nagi NA: Vitamin D deficiency rickets in malnourished children. J Trop Med Hyg 75:251–254, 1972

27 Sedrani SH: Vitamin D status of Saudi men. Trop Geogr Med 36:181–187, 1984

28 Groen JJ, Echchar J, Ben-Ishay D, et al: Osteomalacia in Negev bedouin. Arch Intern Med 116:195, 1965

29 Food and Agriculture Organization of the United Nations/World Health Organization: Rickets, in Joint FAO/WHO Expert Committee on Nutrition, 7th Report. Rome, Food and Agriculture Organization of the United Nations, 1967, pp 31–34

30 Castodot RG: Osteomalacia in Algeria. Am J Obstet Gynecol 102:749–751, 1968

31 Sochett EB, Pettitor JM, Moodley G, et al: Vitamin D status in hospitalized black children under 2 years of age. S Afr Med J 87:1041–1044, 1985

32 Robertson I: Survey of clinical rickets in the infant population in Cape Town. S Afr Med J 43:1072–1076, 1969

33 Miller CG, Chutkan W: Vitamin D deficiency rickets in Jamaican children. Arch Dis Child 51:214–218, 1976

34 Lapatsanis P, Deliganni V, Doxiadis S: Vitamin D deficiency rickets in Greece. J Pediatr 73:195, 1968

35 Elidrissy ATH, Sedrani SH, Lawson DEM: Vitamin D deficiency in mothers of rachitic infants. Calcif Tissue Int 36:266–268, 1984

36 Markestad T, Elzouki A, Legnain M, et al: Serum concentrations of vitamin D metabolites in maternal and umbilical cord blood of Libyan and Norwegian women. Hum Nutr Clin Nutr 38C:55–62, 1984

37 Specker BL, Tsang RG: Vitamin D in infancy and childhood: Factors determining vitamin D status. Adv Pediatr 33:1–22, 1986

38 Lightwood RC: Idiopathic hypercalcemia in infants with failure to thrive. Arch Dis Child 27:302, 1952

39 Holmes AM, Enoch BA, Taylor JL, et al: Occult rickets and osteomalacia amongst the Asian immigrant population. Q J Med XLII:125–149, 1973

40 Shaunak S, Colston K, Ang L, et al: Vitamin D deficiency in adult British Hindu Asians: A family disorder. Br Med J 291:1166–1168, 1985

41 Henderson JB, Dunnigan MG, McIntosh WB, et al: The importance of limited exposure to ultraviolet radiation and dietary factors in the aetiology of Asian rickets: A risk factor model. Q J Med 63:413–425, 1987

42 Dent CE, Rowe DJF, Round JM, et al: Effect of Chappatis and ultraviolet irradiation on nutritional rickets in an Indian immigrant. Lancet i:1282, 1973

43 Clements MR, Johnson L, Fraser DR: A new mechanism for induced vitamin D deficiency in calcium deprivation. Nature 325:62–75, 1987

44 Bachrach S, Fisher J, Parks JS: An outbreak of vitamin D deficiency rickets in a susceptible population. Pediatrics 64:871–877, 1979

45 Markestad T: Effect of season and vitamin D supplementation on plasma concentrations of 25-hydroxyvitamin D in Norwegian infants. Acta Paediatr Scand 72:817–821, 1983

46 Parfitt AM, Gallagher JC, Heaney RP, et al: Vitamin D and bone health in the elderly. Am J Clin Nutr 36:1014–1031, 1982

47 Barragry JM, France MW, Corless D, et al: Intestinal cholecalciferol absorption in the elderly and in younger adults. Clin Sci Molec Med 55:213–220, 1978

48 Harju E, Sotaniemi E, Puranen J, et al: High incidence of low serum vitamin concentration in patients with hip fracture. Arch Orthop Trauma Surg 103:408–416, 1985

49 Sitrin M, Meredith S, Rosenberg IH: Vitamin D deficiency and

bone disease in gastrointestinal disorders. Arch Intern Med 138: 886–888, 1978

50 Recker R, et al: The efficacy of calcifediol in renal osteodystrophy. Arch Intern Med 138:857, 1978

51 Scriver CR, Reade T, DeLuca HF, et al: Serum 1,25-dihydroxy-vitamin D levels in normal subjects and in patients with hereditary rickets or bone disease. N Engl J Med 299:976–979, 1978

52 Marx SJ, Spiegel AM, Brown EM, et al: A familial syndrome of decrease in sensitivity to 1,25-dihydroxyvitamin D. J Clin Endocrinol Metab 47:1303–1310, 1978

53 Pierides AM, Aljama P, Kerr DNS, et al: Effect of 1-OHD$_3$, 1,25(OH)$_2$D$_3$, 3-deoxy-1 OHD$_3$, 24R 25(OH)$_2$D$_3$ and successful renal transplantation on calcium absorption in hemodialysis patients. Nephron 20:203–211, 1978

CHAPTER 123 / *Vitamins E and K* · *Coy D. Fitch*

Vitamin E is generally accepted as an essential nutrient for humans, although its usefulness as a therapeutic agent remains controversial. In experimental animals, vitamin E deficiency causes sterility [1], myopathy [2], axonopathy [3], anemia [4], and a variety of other syndromes depending on the species and the type of stress imposed by the experimental design. Vitamin K deficiency causes hemorrhagic disease in humans as well as in experimental animals [5]; and, in contrast to vitamin E, the therapeutic usefulness of vitamin K is well established. Clinically significant disease from isolated deficiencies of vitamins E and K would be expected to occur rarely if at all in any human population. Nevertheless, deficiencies of these two vitamins may cause significant morbidity in association with the stress of certain diseases and therapeutic interventions.

VITAMIN E

NUTRIENT

There are several natural fat-soluble antioxidants that exhibit vitamin E activity in experimental animals. [6]. The natural product with the greatest activity in vivo is D-α-tocopherol. It has a chroman ring system with an alcohol group that contributes to its antioxidant properties—these properties constituting the only well-substantiated biochemical function of vitamin E—and a saturated isoprenoid side chain that contributes to lipid solubility. There also are methyl groups on the ring system that are important for biological activity. Other closely related natural products with vitamin E activity differ from D-α-tocopherol in the number and position of the methyl groups, or by having an unsaturated side chain, or both. The best sources of these compounds are vegetable oils. Usually, compounds with vitamin E activity are present in greater concentrations in the more unsaturated oils.

The commercially available synthetic preparation of vitamin E is commonly designated DL-α-tocopherol, although it is actually a mixture of eight steroisomers which probably vary widely in biological activity. Further evaluation of the activity of synthetic α-tocopherol in humans is needed, for it may have

as little as 50 percent of the potency of the natural D-α-tocopherol [7]. Despite lower potency in vivo, synthetic α-tocopherol is a good lipid antioxidant, and it apparently serves all the functions of vitamin E in experimental animals and humans.

The daily dietary allowance of vitamin E currently recommended by the Food and Nutrition Board of the United States varies from 3 mg of D-α-tocopherol equivalent (4.5 IU) for infants to 10 mg of D-α-tocopherol equivalent (15 IU) for adults [8]. These amounts ordinarily are supplied by balanced diets. It must be remembered, however, that vitamin E is vulnerable to destruction by oxidation, so the vitamin E content of a food may be reduced significantly by storage, heat, processing, or exposure to oxidants. Thus, the potential exists for unwittingly producing a vitamin E–deficient diet for human consumption. Furthermore, the vitamin E requirement may increase if the individual is subjected to increased oxidant stress as can be done simply by increasing the unsaturated fatty acid content of the diet.

Vitamin E is widely distributed throughout the body with relatively large amounts being stored in liver and adipose tissue. These stores may be sufficient to protect an individual from developing a deficiency syndrome for many months. With vitamin E deprivation, the plasma vitamin E concentration falls rapidly for the first few weeks and then more slowly. In rhesus monkeys, the plasma vitamin E concentration may be measurable for a year or more after starting a vitamin E–deficient diet. Then another year or more may elapse before the monkeys develop the clinical syndromes of vitamin E deficiency [9]. There is evidence that adult humans require even longer periods of time to develop clinical evidence of vitamin E deficiency [10]. Younger individuals, particularly infants, are more susceptible to vitamin E deficiency, in part because they have smaller tissue stores of the vitamin. Apparently vitamin E crosses the placenta poorly, if at all, and the ability of infants to absorb vitamin E from the gastrointestinal tract may be suboptimal.

The absorption of vitamin E from the gastrointestinal tract

occurs along with other lipids in chylomicrons [*11*]. As the chylomicrons are removed from the circulation, the concentration of vitamin E in the blood decreases to a plateau, which is a function of the amount of lipid in lipoprotein. Consequently, when the plasma lipid concentration is low, the plasma vitamin E concentration also will be low. Indeed, it is not advisable to use the plasma vitamin E concentration to assess the vitamin E status of an individual without knowledge of the plasma lipid concentration [*6*]. When lipid concentrations are normal, the normal range of plasma vitamin E (measured as total tocopherols) is 0.5 to 1.2 mg/dL. Concentrations of vitamin E of less than 0.5 mg/dL are common, but symptoms of vitamin E deficiency are not. At present, a positive response to a therapeutic trial of vitamin E is the only acceptable evidence that a disease in humans may be the result of a relative or absolute deficiency of vitamin E.

PATIENT

From the long list of syndromes described in experimental animals, myopathy, axonopathy, and anemia merit discussion as potential manifestations of vitamin E deficiency in humans. Each of these syndromes occurs in vitamin E–deficient non-human primates, and there is reason to suspect that each may occur in humans. In rhesus monkeys, the myopathy usually is rapidly progressive. It is characterized by necrosis of skeletal muscle fibers, infiltration of the muscle with macrophages and inflammatory cells, and creatinuria. All these abnormalities are corrected by treatment with vitamin E [*9*]. Histopathological evidence of a similar myopathy has been observed in patients who demonstrate a chronic malabsorption of vitamin E [*12*]. Creatinuria also may occur in these patients, and it can be corrected by treatment with vitamin E [*13*].

Patients with chronic vitamin E malabsorption also may develop an axonopathy [*14,15*] that resembles the axonopathy in vitamin E–deficient rhesus monkeys [*3*]. The monkeys exhibit a progressive loss of sensory axons in the peripheral nerves, sensory roots, and posterior columns of the spinal cord. Large-caliber myelinated fibers are selectively involved. Remarkably similar neuropathological lesions have been found in patients with cystic fibrosis or biliary atresia, and they may occur in patients with abetalipoproteinemia [*3*], who regularly have very low serum vitamin E concentrations [*16*]. Vitamin E presently is being used by some physicians in an effort to prevent the neuropathology associated with abetalipoproteinemia and with severe vitamin E malabsorption [*14,15,17*]. The efficacy of this treatment requires further evaluation.

There is a dispute about the need for vitamin E for erythropoiesis [*4*], but there is unambiguous evidence that oxidant stress increases the requirement for vitamin E to protect the erythrocyte and other oxidant-sensitive tissues. This evidence has been obtained primarily in low birth weight infants who normally have minimal tissue stores of vitamin E. When these infants are stressed by the administration of large amounts of iron, they may develop a vitamin E–responsive, hemolytic anemia [*18*]. Low birth weight infants also may develop retrolental fibroplasia when exposed to high concentrations of oxygen, and vitamin E treatment may partially protect against this toxicity [*19*]. A recent review describing the results of therapeutic trials of vitamin E for various other clinical syndromes is available [*20*].

Therapeutic use

All therapeutic uses of vitamin E at the present time should be considered to be experimental. This statement is not made to discourage the use of vitamin E, but only to emphasize the need for carefully controlled studies when it is used. Vitamin E is available as the free alcohol, as an acetate ester, and as a water-solubilized preparation. The acetate ester is preferred over the free alcohol for oral therapy because it is less susceptible to oxidation during storage, and it is hydrolyzed to the free alcohol in the intestine. The correct amount of vitamin E to use in therapeutic trials is unknown, but most investigators use very large doses, on the order of 300 mg (400 IU) of D-α-tocopherol acetate once or twice daily for adults. Concern is expressed from time to time about the possibility of toxicity from large doses of vitamin E [*21*], but there is little objective evidence that the doses commonly used are toxic. Vitamin E has been well tolerated by adults in doses of 800 IU per day for years [*12*].

VITAMIN K

NUTRIENT

The vitamin K produced by plants is phylloquinone (2-methyl-3-phytyl-1,4-naphthoquinone) [*22*] which was formerly known as vitamin K_1. Other compounds with vitamin K activity, menaquinones (formerly vitamin K_2), are found in animal tissues. These compounds have unsaturated side chains and are synthesized primarily by the intestinal microflora, but animals can synthesize a menaquinone with 4 isoprene units in the side chain (menaquinone-4) if they are provided with menadione [*23*].

Green, leafy vegetables are the best dietary sources of vitamin K. Animal products, particularly milk, are relatively poor sources. As expected for a lipid-soluble factor, dietary vitamin K is absorbed in chylomicrons for distribution to the liver and other tissues. Vitamin K produced by the intestinal microflora probably is absorbed from the distal ileum [*24*]. Although the human requirement for vitamin K remains to be established, it probably is on the order of 30 μg/day. A normal mixed diet in the United States will contain approximately 300 μg/day of vitamin K [*24*].

The biosynthesis of prothrombin and blood clotting factors VII, IX, and X in the liver requires vitamin K. Because of this requirement, it is common practice to monitor the vitamin K status of experimental animals and humans by measuring prothrombin activity [*5*]. The finding of low prothrombin activity, which increases after a therapeutic trial of vitamin K, is indicative of vitamin K deficiency. A low prothrombin activity which does not increase with vitamin K treatment can occur with serious liver disease.

Vitamin K catalyzes the carboxylation of glutamic acid residues in precursors of prothrombin and other vitamin K–dependent proteins [25], converting them from inactive to active forms. Vitamin K also catalyzes the carboxylation of proteins other than clotting factors, raising the possibility that it may be important for physiological processes other than blood clotting [25].

PATIENT

The only known vitamin K deficiency syndrome in humans is hemorrhagic disease secondary to reduced concentrations of prothrombin and other vitamin K–dependent clotting factors. A natural deficiency of vitamin K is unusual in humans but can occur in newborn infants who are born with low body stores of the vitamin [24]. A deficiency may also develop in association with fat malabsorption or with the use of antibiotics that reduce vitamin K production by the intestinal microflora [24]. In addition, coumarin and phenindione derivatives, which function as vitamin K antagonists, are commonly used therapeutically as anticoagulants. An undesirable side effect of these drugs is hemorrhagic disease, which is reversible with vitamin K treatment.

Therapeutic use

Although the daily requirement for vitamin K is in the microgram range, it is common practice to use milligram amounts in therapeutic trials. For example, as much as a milligram parenterally may be used as treatment or prophylaxis of hemorrhagic disease of the newborn [26]. Occasionally, very large doses (10 mg or more) may be required to reverse the effect of anticoagulant drugs. Phylloquinone is the preferred therapeutic agent to reverse the effect of anticoagulant drugs, to treat hemorrhagic disease of the newborn, to treat patients with liver disease, and whenever a prompt response is desired. Menadione also may be used to treat vitamin K deficiency, but it does not act as rapidly as phylloquinone and it can function as an oxidant drug, causing hemolytic anemia in susceptible individuals, particularly newborn infants.

REFERENCES

1 Evans HM: The pioneer history of vitamin E. Vitam Horm 20:379–387, 1962
2 Mason KE, Horwitt MK: Tocopherol. X. Effects of deficiency in animals, in Sebrell Jr WH, Harris RS (eds): *The Vitamins,* 2d ed. New York, Academic, 1972, vol 5, pp 272–292
3 Nelson JS, Fitch CD, Fischer VW, et al: Progressive neuropathologic lesions in vitamin E–deficient rhesus monkeys. J Neuropathol Exp Neurol 40:166–186, 1981
4 Drake JR, Fitch CD: Status of vitamin E as an erythropoietic factor. Am J Clin Nutr 33:2386–2393, 1980
5 Dam H: Vitamin K. Vitam Horm 6:27–53, 1948
6 Horwitt MK: Vitamin E, in Goodhard RS, Shils ME (eds): *Modern Nutrition in Health and Disease,* 6th ed. Philadelphia, Lea & Febiger, 1980, pp 181–191
7 Horwitt MK: Relative biological values of D-α-tocopheryl acetate and *all-rac*-α-tocopheryl acetate in man. Am J Clin Nutr 33: 1856–1860, 1980
8 *Recommended Dietary Allowances,* 9th ed. Food and Nutrition Board, National Research Council. Washington, D.C., National Academy of Science, 1980, pp 63–69
9 Fitch CD: Experimental anemia in primates due to vitamin E deficiency. Vitam Horm 26:501–514, 1968
10 Horwitt MK, Century B, Zeman AA: Erythrocyte survival time and reticulocyte levels after tocopherol depletion in man. Am J Clin Nutr 12:99–106, 1963
11 Gallo-Torres HE: Absorption, in Machlin LJ (ed): *Vitamin E. A Comprehensive Treatise.* New York, Marcel Dekker, 1980, pp 170–192
12 Farrell PM: Deficiency states, pharmacological effects, and nutrient requirements, in Machlin LJ (ed): *Vitamin E. A Comprehensive Treatise.* New York, Marcel Dekker, 1980, pp 520–620
13 Nitowsky HM, Tildon JT, Levin S, Gordon HH: Studies of tocopherol deficiency in infants and children. VII. The effect of tocopherol on urinary, plasma and muscle creatine. Am J Clin Nutr 10:368–378, 1962
14 Sung JH, Park SH, Mastri AR, Warwick WJ: Axonal dystrophy in the gracile nucleus in congenital biliary atresia and cystic fibrosis (mucoviscidosis): Beneficial effect of vitamin E therapy. J Neuropathol Exp Neurol 39:584–597, 1980
15 Rosenblum JL, Keating JP, Prensky AP, Nelson JS: A progressive neurologic syndrome in children with chronic liver disease. N Engl J Med 304:503–508, 1981
16 Kayden HJ: Abetalipoproteinemia. Annu Rev Med 23:285–296, 1972
17 Muller DPR, Lloyd JK, Bird AC: Long-term management of abetalipoproteinemia: Possible role for vitamin E. Arch Dis Child 52: 209–214, 1977
18 Williams ML, Shott RJ, O'Neal PL, et al: Role of dietary iron and fat on vitamin E deficiency anemia of infancy. N Engl J Med 292:887–890, 1975
19 Hittner HM, Godio LB, Rudolph AJ, et al: Retrolental fibroplasia: Efficacy of vitamin E in a double-blind clinical study of preterm infants. N Engl J Med 305:1365–1371, 1981
20 Horwitt MK: Therapeutic uses of vitamin E in medicine. Nutr Rev 38:105–113, 1980
21 Roberts HJ: Perspective on vitamin E as therapy. JAMA 246: 129–131, 1981
22 Binkley SB, Chaney LC, Holcomb WF, et al: The constitution and synthesis of vitamin K_1. J Am Chem Soc 51:2558–2559, 1939
23 Martius C, Esser HO: Uber die konstitution des im tierkörper aus methylnaphthochinon gebildeten K-vitamines. Biochem Z 331: 1–9, 1959
24 Olson RE: Vitamin K in Shils ME, Young VR (eds): *Modern Nutrition in Health and Disease*, 7th ed. Philadelphia, Lea & Febiger, 1988, pp 328–339
25 Suttie JW: Vitamin K–dependent carboxylase. Annu Rev Biochem 54:459–477, 1985
26 Vitamin K supplementation for infants receiving milk substitute infant formulas and for those with fat malabsorption. Committee on Nutrition, American Academy of Pediatrics. Pediatrics 48:483–487, 1971

Iron · Selwyn J. Baker · Elizabeth Jacob

Iron is essential for most forms of life; humans are no exception, needing iron for the formation of hemoglobin, myoglobin, and a variety of enzymes. For several reasons, in many tropical countries the iron balance is particularly precarious, with the result that iron deficiency is one of the commonest nutritional disorders. This chapter deals with some of the basic concepts of iron metabolism, the diagnosis and management of iron deficiency in the individual, and the public health approach to the prevention of iron deficiency. The subject of iron overload is not addressed, as this is seldom a problem in tropical medicine and is adequately covered in standard medical texts.

NUTRIENT

SOURCES

In early postnatal life the supply of iron is usually derived from maternal breast milk which has about 0.3 to 0.5 mg of iron per liter, irrespective of the maternal iron status [1]. In cows' milk, iron is present in similar amounts but is much less readily absorbed (about 12 percent as compared with 49 percent) so that infants fed unfortified cows' milk are very prone to develop iron deficiency [1].

In older individuals iron is obtained from many foods. However, isotopic studies have shown that there is a wide variation in the extent to which the iron in different foods can be absorbed, ranging from less than 1 percent for that in rice to 20 percent for that in meat [2,3].

PHYSIOLOGY

Absorption

Intraluminal Events. Iron absorption from the intestine can be considered as occurring from two intraluminal pools—a *heme-iron* and *non-heme-iron,* or *ionic-iron,* pool [4] (Fig. 124-1). Hemoglobin and myoglobin in the diet undergo peptic digestion, and the heme is split off and forms the heme-iron pool. The chemistry of digestion of non-heme-iron-containing foods is complex and poorly understood. To be available for absorption this iron must be in solution. Hydrochloric acid and pepsin assist in the solubilization process. Also, because of its greater solubility at the pH of the duodenum, iron(II) is better absorbed than iron(III). Other factors also play an important role. For example, phytates, oxalates, phosphates, and tannins form insoluble iron complexes and vegetable fibers bind nonheme iron thus inhibiting absorption. On the other hand, meat, fish, some amino acids, and ascorbic acid promote the absorption of nonheme iron probably by forming small-molecular-weight soluble iron complexes [5]. The intraluminal pool concept has important practical consequences since it has been shown that the iron absorption from a given meal can be quantitated by labeling the heme-iron pool with hemoglobin containing one isotope of iron and the non-heme-iron pool labeled with an iron salt containing another isotope of iron [4].

Cellular Uptake and Transport. Both heme- and non-heme-iron absorption occur maximally in the duodenum and upper jejunum [6]. The enterocyte brush borders have two different receptors, one for heme iron and the other for nonheme iron [7,8] (Fig. 124-1). The heme iron enters the cell as such and within the cell the iron is liberated from the porphyrin by the action of heme oxygenase [9]. The iron then enters the intracellular iron pool. Nonheme iron crosses the cell membrane via a separate carrier-mediated active transport mechanism and also enters the intracellular iron pool [10]. Within the cell some iron is bound to mitochondria and other organelles and the remainder is present either as ferritin or bound to a transferrinlike protein [4]. The iron–transferrinlike protein complex then exits from the enterocyte; the iron enters the plasma and becomes attached to circulating transferrin. The ferritin iron is not absorbed and is shed into the lumen with the mucosal cell.

Control. The amount of iron absorbed by the enterocyte is influenced by several factors. The more iron presented to the cell the more is absorbed, although as the amount presented increases the percentage absorption decreases. The iron status of the individual also plays a crucial role; absorption is increased in iron deficiency and decreased in iron repletion. The way in which this control is effected is not fully understood, but there is evidence to suggest that it may be both by increasing the rate of uptake of iron by the brush border and decreasing the rate at which absorbed iron is bound to apoferritin within the mucosal cell [11]. Iron absorption is also affected in some poorly understood manner by marrow activity, and by the presence of infections and chronic disease [5,6].

Body content

The total iron content of the fetus at term is of the order of 75 mg per kilogram of body weight [1]. This iron is derived from the mother by a process of active transport across the placenta which occurs even if the mother is iron-deficient. In well-nourished adult males the total iron content is about 50 mg per kilogram of body weight. Adult females have somewhat less (about 40 mg/kg), owing to their increased losses and their relatively smaller muscle mass. The major portion of body iron is present in hemoglobin, some is in myoglobin and iron-containing enzymes, and most of the remainder is in storage form, either as ferritin or hemosiderin [5].

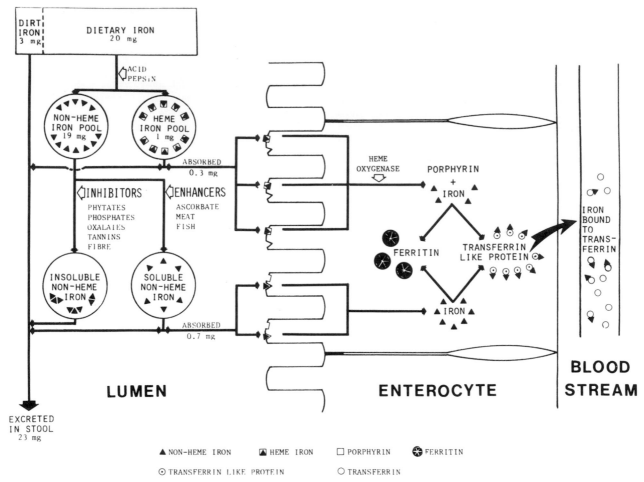

Figure 124-1. Diagrammatic representation of the digestion and absorption of food iron. The indicated quantities of iron are only illustrative and may vary widely with different diets. Each molecule of transferrin can bind up to two atoms of iron.

Requirements

Basal Requirements. Since iron is recycled in the body, the two factors affecting iron requirements are the amounts lost from the body and the amounts necessary for growth and development. Iron is regularly lost from the body via the gastrointestinal tract, urine, and skin; these have been termed the *basal* losses. In the well-nourished adult these amount to 14 μg of iron per kilogram of body weight per day [*12*]. Since normal adult males have no other requirements this is the amount that they must absorb each day to maintain iron balance (Fig. 124-2).

Women of Childbearing Age. Menstruation considerably increases body iron losses. These losses are of similar magnitude in women living in temperate and tropical countries. The frequency distribution curve of menstrual losses is skewed with

about 95 percent of women having losses which, averaged over the month, amount to 2.0 mg of iron per day or less and 5 percent of women having losses greater than this [*13*]. This means that an absorption of 2.8 mg of iron per day (2.0 mg menstrual loss and 0.8 mg basal loss) will keep 95 percent of women in iron balance (Fig. 124-2).

Pregnancy. Although menstrual losses cease, there is need for over 1000 mg of iron during the course of pregnancy. This is made up of basal losses (about 220 mg), iron needed for the increase in maternal red cell mass (about 500 mg), requirements of the fetus (about 290 mg), the iron content of the placenta and umbilical cord (about 90 mg), and the blood loss associated with delivery (about 150 mg). Iron requirements are maximal in the second half of pregnancy when they may reach 5 to 6 mg/day [*14*]. This is considerably in excess of the amount that can be absorbed from the diet. Women with iron

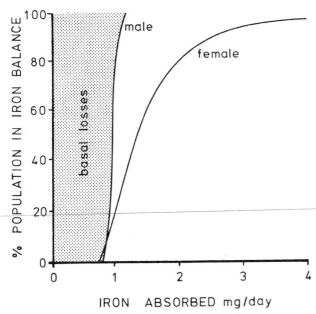

Figure 124-2. Percentage of normal adult males and normal nonpregnant females of childbearing age that will be in iron balance with a given amount of iron absorbed from the diet. The shaded area represents the amount required to make up the daily "basal" losses from the intestine, skin, and urinary tract.

stores will compensate by "borrowing" from the stores to meet these needs. However, if there are no iron stores and no iron supplements are provided, iron deficiency will develop.

Lactation. Iron is excreted in breast milk so that the nursing mother loses about 0.3 mg of iron per day by this route. Usually menstruation is in abeyance so that absorption of an amount somewhat less than that required by menstruating women should maintain iron balance [14].

Infants and Children. Basal losses in infants and children are presumably of a similar order per kilogram of body weight to those in adults. However, they also need iron for growth and development, which is most rapid in the first year or two of life and during adolescence. These are, therefore, the times when the child is most prone to develop iron deficiency [1].

Recommended Intakes. The iron requirements (i.e., the amount that needs to be absorbed) and the recommended dietary intakes to achieve this are shown in Table 124-1. Where the dietary iron has a very poor bioavailability even greater amounts may be needed.

PATIENT

PATHOPHYSIOLOGY

When iron requirements exceed the quantity of iron absorbed, the individual will be in a state of negative iron balance. In the initial stages storage iron is progressively reduced to meet the ongoing needs of the body (Fig. 124-3). When storage iron is exhausted, iron bound to circulating transferrin is utilized. This results in a fall in plasma iron concentration, an increase in the total circulating transferrin level, and a reduction in the percent saturation of transferrin. When there is insufficient iron available for heme production, there is a relative excess of protoporphyrin. As a consequence, the amount of free red cell protoporphyrin increases and the protoporphyrin-heme ratio rises. Finally, when the iron supply to the marrow is further impaired, the circulating hemoglobin concentration falls, clinically detectable anemia develops, and the red cells become hypochromic and microcytic.

PATHOGENESIS

Physiological iron requirements

Physiological iron requirements are greatest in the first 2 years of life, during adolescence, in women of childbearing age, and

Table 124-1. Iron requirements and WHO recommended daily dietary intake [11]*

	Absorbed iron required, mg	Dietary iron		
		Poor bioavailability, mg	Medium bioavailability, mg	Good bioavailability, mg
Infants 0–4 months	0.5	†	†	†
5–12 months	1.0	10	7	5
Children 1–12 years	1.0	10	7	5
Boys 13–16 years	1.8	18	12	9
Girls 13–16 years	2.4	24	18	12
Women of reproductive age	2.8	28	21	14
Postmenopausal women	0.9	9	6	5
Men	0.9	9	6	5

*WHO/FAO are revising these figures to more accurately reflect current knowledge regarding iron bioavailability and also to reflect the fact that "recommended dietary iron intakes" should meet the needs of 95 percent of the population. This will result in higher amounts especially in the "medium" and "poor" bioavailability categories.
†It is assumed that intake in breast milk is adequate.

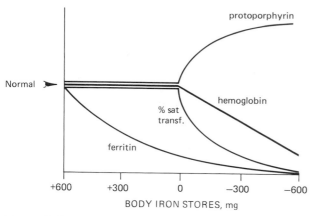

Figure 124-3. Diagrammatic representation of the changes that occur in the various parameters of iron nutrition with increasing depletion of body iron. The zero point on the X axis represents the point when all storage iron is exhausted and further movement to the right on the X axis indicates increasing deficit of body iron.

especially during pregnancy. Individuals in these categories are therefore the most vulnerable. In many developing tropical countries women tend to have more pregnancies than their western counterparts, considerably increasing their physiological iron requirements and their risk of developing iron deficiency.

Pathological iron requirements

Sweat. It used to be thought that the iron losses in sweat were a significant cause of iron deficiency in people living in hot humid environments. However, isotopic studies have shown that this is not so [15].

Intestinal Losses. Individuals living in the tropics are at risk of developing any of the lesions which may produce abnormal gastrointestinal blood loss in people in temperate climates such as ulceration, inflammation, tumors, and vascular malformations. In addition they are at risk of developing parasitic infestations which can produce significant blood loss. By far the commonest parasite is the hookworm, which affects hundreds of millions of people. The worms live mainly in the upper small intestine. Each adult *Necator americanus* worm sucks about 0.03 mL blood and each *Ancylostoma duodenale* about 0.15 mL/day [16]. The worms feed on the plasma and discharge the red cells into the lumen of the host's intestine. Some of these red cells are digested and a portion of the iron in the hemoglobin is reabsorbed and reutilized but the remainder is lost from the body. Other parasites which may cause abnormal blood loss are *Trichuris trichiuria* and schistosomiasis involving the intestine or urinary tract.

Decreased iron absorption

Low Bioavailability of Dietary Iron. Although the diet of many people living in the tropics appears to contain reasonable

amounts of iron when measured by chemical analysis, this is often misleading. Some is contaminating dirt iron which is unabsorbable. Further, in many cases the diet contains little or no heme iron; is often deficient in promoters of iron absorption such as meat, fish, and ascorbic acid; and usually contains a plentiful supply of inhibitors of absorption such as fiber, phytates, phosphates, etc. The result is that the bioavailability of the dietary iron is often of a low order [15].

Intestinal Disease. Gastric resection and other conditions producing achlorhydria reduce the absorption of both heme and nonheme iron from food. Patients with small-bowel disease such as tropical sprue and other tropical enteropathies may also have defective absorption of food iron [5].

Defective utilization

In diseases associated with chronic inflammation there is a block in release of iron from body stores and defective reutilization of iron from destroyed red cells. This may lead to a reduction in plasma iron concentration and a picture superficially resembling that of mild iron-deficiency anemia even in the presence of normal iron stores.

CLINICAL MANIFESTATIONS

Iron deficiency

Although the literature is conflicting, a variety of abnormalities are thought to be associated with iron deficiency even in the absence of anemia [14,17]. Koilonychia, angular stomatitis, glossitis, dysphagia with a postcricoid web, and achlorhydria have long been ascribed to iron deficiency, but their prevalence in different groups of iron-deficient subjects suggests that other associated deficiencies may also play a role. Children with iron deficiency have been reported to have abnormalities of the jejunal mucosa but the evidence for this is not good [18]. In pregnancy, maternal iron deficiency may be associated with a low fetal birth weight, an increased risk of premature delivery [15], and reduced serum ferritin concentration in the fetus [19]. In infants, iron defecency may lead to behavioral changes such as irritability, lack of interest in surroundings, and impaired learning ability [14,20]. In adults, fatigue and irritability have also been thought to be produced by iron deficiency but this has not been confirmed. Near-maximal work performance, as measured on a bicycle ergometer, is reduced in iron-deficient men [15] and the performance of cross-country runners with low iron stores, but no anemia, can be improved by iron therapy [21]. Whether less strenuous activity is also affected by iron deficiency is not known. This impairment in work capacity may be related to a deficiency of α-glycerophosphate oxidase activity in the muscles [22].

Iron-deficiency anemia

Mild anemia is often symptomless, but more severe degrees of anemia may be associated with nonspecific symptoms such as asthenia, weakness, dizziness, dyspnea, and dependent edema. On the other hand, because the onset of the anemia is often gradual, completely symptomless individuals may be found to have surprisingly low levels of hemoglobin. In pregnancy, mild maternal anemia may increase the risk of premature delivery and low fetal birth weight [15]. More marked degrees of anemia are associated with increased rates of maternal and fetal morbidity and mortality [14,15]. In infants, iron deficiency anemia adversely affects mental and motor development [23] and in young children there is evidence that growth may be retarded [15,17,24]. Severe anemia reduces maximum oxygen transport and limits near-maximal work performance [25]. Even mild anemia can decrease worker productivity [26,27] and this may have profound socioeconomic consequences for developing countries.

DIAGNOSIS

Iron stores

Although iron stores can be estimated by visually quantitating the stainable iron in bone marrow smears or liver biopsy sections, the best indicator of iron stores is the plasma ferritin concentration [5]. In the absence of infections or chronic diseases each microgram of ferritin (per liter of plasma) corresponds to about 8 milligrams of body storage iron. A concentration of 12 µg/L or less is diagnostic of depleted iron stores. Concentrations greater than 600 µg/L, in the absence of the above conditions, are suggestive of iron overload.

Iron-deficient erythropoiesis

The diagnosis of iron-deficient erythropoiesis is best made by the estimation of erythrocyte protoporphyrin and the saturation of transferrin. Values of erythrocyte protoporphyrin of greater than 12.5 µmol/L of red cells, and a transferrin saturation less than 16% are indicative of iron-deficient erythropoiesis.

Iron-deficiency anemia

The definition of anemia is a hemoglobin concentration below normal for the individual. The normal hemoglobin concentration differs with age, sex, and altitude of residence and can be defined as that concentration which exists in the healthy individual adequately supplied with all hemopoietic nutrients [28]. In any given demographic group, living at a given altitude, the frequency distribution of normal hemoglobin concentrations forms a gaussian curve. The frequency distribution of hemoglobin concentrations of anemic individuals is skewed to the left (Fig. 124-4). It is important to note that there is some overlap between the two populations. An otherwise healthy individual whose hemoglobin falls within the region of overlap may or may not be anemic, but the lower an individual's hemoglobin concentration the greater the chance that the individual is anemic. Although it is customary in clinical practice to use an arbitrary figure to divide anemic from nonanemic individuals, this approach is clearly a gross oversimplification [15].

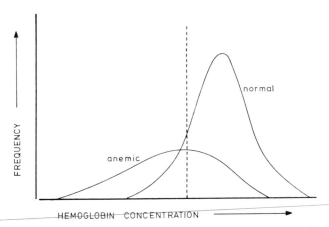

Figure 124-4. Frequency distribution of hemoglobin concentration in a "normal" and an anemic population. The dotted vertical line represents an arbitrary cutoff point defining anemia. When this is employed it will be seen that a portion of normal individuals will be classified as anemic and some anemic individuals will be classified as normal.

Evidence that a given hemoglobin concentration may in fact represent anemia for the individual may be obtained by measuring indices of iron nutrition and studying red cell morphology. However, the final proof of the presence of anemia is the demonstration of an increase in the individual's hemoglobin concentration following appropriate therapy.

MANAGEMENT

Diagnosis

Often the cause of the iron deficiency can be deduced from the history and physical examination. At other times investigations may be necessary to determine the cause. Initially, simple and cheap tests such as stool examination for parasites and occult blood may suffice. If these are negative, a therapeutic trial of iron with clinical follow-up to ensure that the iron deficiency does not recur, and/or that evidence of more serious disease does not develop, may be the most appropriate approach. If abnormal blood loss is documented, more extensive investigation may be necessary to determine its cause. At all times the physician must weigh the likelihood of an investigation showing a treatable cause against the cost of the investigation (to the patient or the health provider) and the risks (if any) associated with the procedure.

Treatment

The aim of treatment is to restore the hemoglobin concentration to normal, to rebuild the iron stores, and to treat any underlying cause.

Oral Iron. All readily soluble iron(II) (ferrous) salts are equally well absorbed [29]. Since absorption may be reduced by as much as one-fifth in the presence of food, the dose should be administered when the stomach is empty. In adults, iron tablets[1] given in divided doses to provide a total of 150 to 300 mg of elemental iron per day will usually produce a good hematological response. Infants and children may be given iron either as tablets or as an elixir in divided doses to provide 5 mg of iron per kilogram of body weight per day. In some individuals oral iron produces side effects such as epigastric pain, nausea, vomiting, and constipation or diarrhea. The prevalence of nausea and vomiting is dose-related and, for the same amount of available iron, all iron salts produce a similar prevalence of side effects [30]. The cheapest compound is therefore recommended. It is important to note, however, that the way tablets are made has a considerable influence on the availability of iron in them [31]. Some iron tablets may even be totally ineffective because they fail to disintegrate in the intestine. The bioavailability of iron in tablets may be checked by measuring the rise in plasma iron concentration 3 h after giving the tablets and comparing it with the rise produced by a subsequently administered equivalent dose of freshly prepared iron(II) sulfate in the same individual [31]. Some "slow-release" preparations are available which produce fewer side effects, but these are up to eight times more expensive so that where resources are limited their use is not justified.

Parenteral Iron. There are two forms of parenteral iron currently available, namely iron-dextran complex which may be given intramuscularly or intravenously and iron-sorbitol complex which can only be used intramuscularly. Parenteral iron is of value when iron cannot be given by mouth, where patient compliance in taking tablets is in doubt, or where the patient may only be seen on a single occasion (e.g., in dealing with nomadic people). It should be emphasized that the rate of hematological response is not greater in subjects given parenteral iron than in those given oral iron, so that severity of anemia or the desire to get a rapid response is not an indication for the use of parenteral iron. Moreover, the administration of either form of iron is not infrequently associated with reactions such as local pain, staining of the skin, headache, malaise, urticaria, and arthralgia. Rarely severe and even fatal anaphylactic reactions have occurred [15]. In massive doses in experimental animals, iron-dextran has induced sarcomas; however, although there are anecdotal reports of tumors following its use in humans, none of these are proven [32]. Another preparation, iron-poly(sorbitol gluconic acid), referred to in the first edition of this book, is no longer available.

Hematological Response. In an anemic individual, the first sign of response to iron therapy is a rise in the reticulocyte count, followed by an increase in hemoglobin concentration and hematocrit. With optimal therapy, the reticulocyte count will reach a peak on the fifth to tenth day and thereafter decline.

The rate of increase in hemoglobin is inversely related to the initial hemoglobin concentration, and whatever the initial value, it takes about 2 months for normal levels to be attained [33]. With suboptimal therapy the reticulocyte response may be lower and more delayed and the rise in hemoglobin concentration slower. Once the hemoglobin concentration has been restored to normal, iron therapy should be continued for another 3 months or so to rebuild the body iron stores.

Transfusion. In regions where there is a high prevalence of iron deficiency it is not uncommon for individuals to present with hemoglobin concentrations between 20 and 30 g/L without cardiorespiratory embarrassment. Wherever possible, the temptation to treat such individuals by blood transfusion should be avoided because of the danger of producing circulatory overload and because of the other hazards associated with blood transfusion. In the majority of such cases prompt and adequate response can be obtained by iron administration. Occasionally there may not be time to wait for a response to iron therapy, for example, in a pregnant woman at term, in someone needing emergency surgery, or in someone with associated congestive heart failure. In such cases it is advisable to give a potent diuretic such as intravenous furosemide, administer the blood as packed red cells, and, in some cases, perform a simultaneous venesection to prevent any volume overload from occurring.

POPULATION

EPIDEMIOLOGY

Since pregnant women are at great risk of developing iron deficiency, a study of their iron status provides a sensitive index of the iron status of the population [34]. Many such studies have been carried out in different parts of the tropics. The majority of these indicate a very high prevalence of iron deficiency and iron-deficiency anemia in pregnant women not receiving an iron supplement [15]. Although many of the studies have been based on hospital or clinic populations and are therefore not necessarily representative of the population as a whole, they provide evidence that iron deficiency is a very important problem in many tropical populations [35]. With the availability of simplified methods of serum ferritin estimation [36] it is possible to quantitate the iron stores of representative population samples and obtain a much more sensitive and accurate picture of their iron nutritional status.

The major factor responsible for the high prevalence of iron deficiency in tropical countries appears to be the low bioavailability of dietary iron, especially where meat and fish are not included in the diet [15,37]. The situation is made worse in areas where there are intestinal parasites. In a person with a marginal iron intake even a relatively small hookworm load may make a crucial difference, tipping them into negative iron balance. For this reason there is often a higher prevalence of anemia among rural dwellers than city dwellers, and among

---

[1] Since the rapid ingestion of large amounts of iron may produce fatal iron toxicity, all iron tablets must be kept out of the reach of young children.

those who live and work in wet areas (e.g., rice-growing lands) than in those who live in drier areas. Nevertheless, even in areas where hookworm is prevalent, people without hookworm infestation also suffer from iron deficiency, indicating that although hookworm aggravates the situation it is not the sole cause of the deficiency [37].

INTERACTION WITH INFECTION

Iron deficiency in humans produces a variety of alterations in immunological function such as impairment of lymphocyte transformation, decreased production of leukocyte migration inhibition factor, impaired delayed cutaneous hypersensitivity, and decreased bactericidal capacity of polymorphonuclear leukocytes [38]. It is, however, difficult to relate these observations to clinical susceptibility to infection. Several studies have shown that children with iron-deficiency anemia may be more prone to respiratory infections than nonanemic children [15]. It has also been shown that anemic laborers had more infections than their nonanemic iron-supplemented counterparts [26]. On the contrary, other studies have failed to confirm this relationship and it has even been suggested that in some instances iron deficiency may have a protective effect against certain infections [39,40]. More well-controlled studies are needed in this area before final conclusions can be drawn [41].

PREVENTION

The extent of the problem

If the information is not already available, an estimate of the severity of iron deficiency in the community will need to be obtained. This can be done by examining a statistically valid cross section of the population, or alternatively, by studying a representative sample of those most at risk, namely infants and young children or pregnant women [34]. In the latter case the estimation of hemoglobin concentration alone will provide considerable information. If a cross section of the population is involved, it is preferable to also include measurements of serum ferritin concentration, and, where possible, red cell protoporphyrin level and the saturation of transferrin. This will supply valuable baseline data not only about the prevalence of anemia but also the prevalence of low iron stores and of iron-deficient erythropoiesis. Once the magnitude of the problem is known, appropriate steps can be taken to deal with it, within the constraints of locally available resources [31].

Iron supplementation

Iron supplementation is employed when it is desired to improve the iron status of a segment of the population in a relatively short period of time. The greatest need for this is likely to be in pregnancy, where iron requirements are high and where it is necessary to ensure that the mother goes into labor without anemia and with reasonable iron stores. Initially, trials should

be carried out to determine the best dose of iron; whether iron alone is adequate or whether folate is also required (since in many parts of the world there is also a high prevalence of folate deficiency in pregnancy); the best methods of distributing the iron (e.g., through antenatal clinics, public health workers, etc.); and the best ways of motivating the target population to take it [31,42–44]. Once these have been determined a regional or national supplementation program can be undertaken. In some countries supplementation may also be considered for other segments of the population where there is a high prevalence of iron-deficiency anemia—for example, infants and preschool children, school children, and groups of workers covered by health care systems (e.g., plantation laborers).

Iron fortification

Fortification involves the addition of iron to some commonly consumed food or foods to increase the iron intake of the population as a whole. This has the major advantage that it is not dependent on individual compliance and needs no special distribution system. However, the amounts of extra iron that can be provided by fortification are comparatively small, so that although supplementation will produce a measurable effect in weeks or months, the results of fortification can only be seen in a period of 1 to 3 years.

In planning a food-fortification strategy for a given country or region it is necessary to first determine the most suitable vehicle or vehicles to be fortified. These must be foods which are widely consumed by the target population and are processed at relatively few points so that supervision and quality control can be carried out. The fortificant must be a source of iron which is biologically available when added to the vehicle; is stable; does not affect the taste, color, or storage properties of the vehicle or foods with which the vehicle may be mixed; and is relatively cheap [31,34]. Once a vehicle and fortificant have been chosen, a field trial should be carried out in a selected population with appropriate controls [31,43]. For a number of years many western countries have fortified bread with various iron preparations, but the efficacy of these measures has seldom been evaluated. In tropical countries bread is less widely consumed and is therefore not a suitable vehicle. Several field fortification trials have been undertaken, including fortification of fish sauce with iron(III) FeNaEDTA in Thailand, fortification of sugar with iron(III) FeNaEDTA in Guatemala, fortification of salt with iron(III) orthophosphate together with sodium hydrogen sulfate in India, and fortification of rice with iron(II) sulfate in the Philippines. To date, although some of these studies show considerable promise, none has yet reached the stage where the measure under study can be recommended for implementation on a national scale.

Fortification programs may also be aimed at specific segments of the population. The best example of this is the fortification of commercially prepared infant foods. A highly successful study using dried milk powder fortified with 15 mg of iron(II) sulfate and 100 mg of ascorbic acid per 100 g of milk powder has been carried out in Chile. This greatly reduced the prevalence of anemia and iron deficiency [45].

Reduction of nutrient losses

The single most important factor in determining the iron stores of the newborn is the time and manner in which the umbilical cord is cut. By allowing as much placental blood as possible to be returned to the baby iron stores will be maximized.

In populations where there is a high prevalence of heavy hookworm infestation, public health measures to combat this should be undertaken. It is, however, unlikely that hookworm eradication programs alone will solve the problem since hookworm infestation is not the only cause of the high prevalence of anemia in these populations [37].

Family planning programs also have an impact on iron nutrition. Reduction in the number of pregnancies decreases the total iron requirements of the women concerned. Use of the contraceptive pill reduces menstrual flow and therefore decreases iron requirements, but, on the other hand, intrauterine contraceptive devices tend to increase menstrual losses [14].

Alteration of dietary habits

Theoretically it should be possible to improve iron nutritional status by altering dietary patterns to include more sources of readily absorbable iron, especially heme iron, and to increase the consumption of promotors of iron absorption such as ascorbic acid. However, in practice this proves to be very difficult, involving the changing of long-established practices and having profound financial and, in some countries, religious implications.

An integrated approach

In most countries a multifaceted approach will be needed to solve the problem of iron deficiency. This may need to include education of the public and all members of the health care team, supplementation for those specially at risk (e.g., pregnant women), fortification of one or more foods, and control of hookworm and other parasitic infestations which increase iron losses. One example of such an approach in a temperate country can be seen in Sweden. In 1965, the prevalence of iron-deficiency anemia in women of childbearing age in Sweden was 30 percent. By 1975 this was reduced to 7 percent through a combination of factors including increased public awareness, supplementation with iron tablets, increased iron fortification, use of the contraceptive pill, and increased consumption of ascorbic acid [14]. Clearly, experience from one country cannot necessarily be transferred to another. Therefore, before large-scale programs are introduced it will usually be desirable to carry out appropriate field trials [34]. Furthermore, once programs are introduced careful ongoing monitoring will be necessary to ensure their continuing success.

REFERENCES

1 Dallman PR, Siimes MA: Iron deficiency in infancy and childhood. A report of the International Nutritional Anemia Consultative Group. New York, D.C., The Nutrition Foundation, 1980
2 Layrisse M, Cook JD, Martinez C, et al: Food iron absorption: A comparison of vegetable and animal foods. Blood 23:430–443, 1969
3 Layrisse J: Dietary iron absorption, in Kief H (ed): *Iron Metabolism and Its Disorders*. Amsterdam, Excerpta Medica, 1975, pp 25–33
4 Hallberg L, Björn-Rasmussen E: Determination of iron absorption from whole diet. A new two pool model using two radio-iron isotopes given as haem and non-haem. Scand J Haematol 9:193–197, 1972
5 Bothwell TH, Charlton RW, Cook JD, et al: *Iron Metabolism in Man*. Oxford, Blackwell, 1979
6 Forth W, Rummel W: Iron absorption. Physiol Rev 53:724, 1973
7 Hübers H, Hübers E, Forth W, et al: Binding of iron and other metals in brush borders of jejunum and ileum of the rat in vitro. Acta Pharmacol Toxicol 29(suppl 4):22–27, 1971
8 Gräsbeck R, Majuri R, Kouvonen I, Tenhunen R: Spectral and other studies on the intestinal haem receptor of the pig. Biochim Biophys Acta 700:137–142, 1982
9 Raffin SB, Woo CH, Roost KT, et al: Intestinal absorption of hemoglobin: Iron-heme cleavage by mucosal heme oxygenase. J Clin Invest 54:1344–1352, 1974
10 Cox TM, Peters TJ: The kinetics of iron uptake in vitro by human duodenal mucosa: Studies in normal subjects. J Physiol 289:469–478, 1979
11 Nathanson MH, Muir A, McLaren GD: Iron absorption in normal and iron-deficient beagle dogs: Mucosal iron kinetics. Am J Physiol 249:G439–G448, 1985
12 Requirements of Ascorbic Acid, Vitamin D, Vitamin B12, Folate and Iron. WHO Tech Rep Ser 452, Geneva, World Health Organization, 1970
13 Hallberg L, Högdahl AM, Nilsson L, et al: Menstrual blood loss— a population study. Acta Obstet Gynecol Scand 45:320–351, 1966
14 Bothwell TH, Charlton RW: Iron deficiency in women. A report of the International Nutritional Anemia Consultative Group. New York and Washington, D.C., The Nutrition Foundation, 1981
15 Baker SJ, DeMaeyer EM: Nutritional anemia: Its understanding and control with special reference to the work of the World Health Organization. Am J Clin Nutr 32:368–417, 1979
16 Roche M, Layrisse M: The nature and causes of "hookworm anemia." Am J Trop Med Hyg 15:1029–1102, 1966
17 Oski F: The nonhematologic manifestations of iron deficiency. Am J Dis Child 133:315–322, 1979
18 Baker SJ: Malnutrition and gastrointestinal disease, in Glass GBJ (ed): *Progress in Gastroenterology*. New York, Academic, 1977, vol III, pp 563–592
19 Kaneshige E: Serum ferritin as an assessment of iron stores and other hematologic parameters during pregnancy. Obstet Gynecol 57:238–242, 1981
20 Greenfield DB: Iron and behavior, in Oski FA, Pearson HA (eds): *Iron Nutrition Revisited—Infancy, Childhood, Adolescence*. Report of 82d Ross Conference on Pediatric Research. Columbus, Ohio, Ross Laboratories, 1981, pp 60–64

21 Rowland TW, Deisroth MB, Green GM et al: The effect of iron therapy on the exercise capacity of nonanemic iron-deficient adolescent runners. Am J Dis Child 142:165–169, 1988

22 Finch CA, Miller LR, Inamdar AR, et al: Iron deficiency in the rat. Physiological and biochemical studies of muscle dysfunction. J Clin Invest 58:447–453, 1976

23 Lozoff B, Brittenham GM, Wolf AW, et al: Iron deficiency anemia and iron therapy. Effects on infant developmental test performance. Pediatrics 79:981–995, 1987

24 Chwang L, Soemantri AG, Pollitt E: Iron supplementation and physical growth of rural Indonesian children. Am J Clin Nutr 47: 496–501, 1988

25 Viteri FE, Torun B: Anaemia and physical work capacity. Clin Haematol 3:609–626, 1974

26 Basta SS, Soekirman MS, Karyadi D, et al: Iron deficiency anemia and the productivity of adult males in Indonesia. Am J Clin Nutr 32:916–925,1979

27 Edgerton VR, Gardner GW, Ohira Y, et al: Iron-deficiency anaemia and its effect on worker productivity and activity patterns. Br Med J 2:1546–1549, 1979

28 Nutritional Anaemias. WHO Tech Rep Ser 503, Geneva, World Health Organization, 1972

29 Brise H, Hallberg L: Iron absorption studies II. Acta Med Scand 171(suppl 376):23–38, 1962

30 Sölvell L: Oral iron therapy—side effects, in Hallberg L, Harwerth H-G, Vanotti A (eds): *Iron Deficiency. Pathogenesis. Clinical Aspects. Therapy.* London, New York, Academic, 1970, pp 573–583

31 Guidelines for the eradication of iron deficiency anemia. A report of the International Nutritional Anemia Consultative Group. New York and Washington, D.C., The Nutrition Foundation, 1977

32 Weinbren K, Salm R, Greenber G: Intramuscular injections of iron compounds and oncogenesis in man. Br Med J 1:683–685, 1987

33 Swan HT, Jowett GH: Treatment of iron deficiency with ferrous fumarate: Assessment by a statistically accurate method. Br Med J 2:782–787, 1959

34 Control of Nutritional Anaemia with Special Reference to Iron Deficiency. Report of an IAEA/USAID/WHO Joint Meeting. WHO Tech Rep Ser 580, Geneva, World Health Organization, 1975

35 Baker SJ: Nutritional Anaemias, Part 2, Tropical Asia, in Luzzatto L (ed): *Clinics in Haematology.* London, Saunders, 1981, vol 10, pp 843–871

36 Flowers CA, Kuizon M, Beard JL, et al: A serum ferritin assay for prevalence studies of iron deficiency. Am J Hematol 23:141–151, 1986

37 Baker SJ, Mathan VI: Prevalence, pathogenesis and prophylaxis of iron deficiency in the tropics, in Kief H (ed): *Iron Metabolism and Its Disorders.* Amsterdam, Oxford, Excerpta Medica, 1975, pp 147–158

38 Weinberg ED: Iron and infection. Microbiol Rev 42:45–66, 1978

39 Masawe AEJ, Muindi JM, Swai GBR: Infections in iron deficiency and other types of anaemia in the tropics. Lancet 2:314–317, 1974

40 Murray MJ, Murray AB, Murray MB, et al: The adverse effects of iron repletion on the course of certain infections. Br Med J 2:1113–1115, 1978

41 Hershko C, Peto TEA, Weatherall DJ: Iron and infection. Br Med J 269:660–664, 1988

42 Sood SK, Ramachandran K, Mathur M, et al: WHO sponsored collaborative studies on nutritional anemia in India. Q J Med 44: 241–258, 1975

43 Baker SJ, Ramachandran K: The design and analysis of iron supplementation trials. A report of the International Nutritional Anemia Consultative Group. The Nutrition Foundation, New York and Washington, D.C., 1984

44 Charoenlarp P, Dhanamitta S, Kaewvichit R, et al: A WHO collaborative study on iron supplementation in Burma and in Thailand. Am J Clin Nutr 47:280–297, 1988

45 Stekel A, Olivares M, Cayazzo M, et al: Prevention of iron deficiency by milk fortification. II. A field trial with a full-fat acidified milk. Am J Clin Nutr 47:265–269, 1988

CHAPTER **125** / *Zinc and Other Trace Metals*

· *Noel W. Solomons* · *Manuel Ruz*

The trace elements are those elements that make up 0.01 percent of the total body mass. They include several elements of nutritional importance to mammalian species—and therefore, presumably to humans—such as iron, zinc, copper, manganese, chromium, selenium, molybdenum, cobalt, iodine, fluorine, nickel, vanadium, and lithium. The limited available knowledge about their relevance to nutrition in tropical and geographical medicine is presented in this chapter.

ZINC

NUTRIENT

Sources of zinc in the diet

Zinc is an essential trace element in human nutrition. Recommended Dietary Allowances (RDAs) for daily zinc intake by healthy individuals in the United States have been established according to age and sex: 0 to 6 months, 3 mg; 6 to 12 months, 5 mg; 1 to 10 years, 10 mg; adolescents, adult men, and nonpregnant women, 15 mg; pregnant women, 20 mg; and lactating mothers, 25 mg [1]. To meet these requirements at the usual level of daily caloric intake, a zinc density of 6 mg per 1000 kcal is needed. The zinc density of various foods and food groups is shown in Table 125-1 [2]. Clearly, inclusion of foods in the "rich" or "very rich" categories of zinc density is necessary for meeting the recommended intake levels.

The biological availability of zinc is another factor in dietary adequacy. An expert committee of WHO [3] created intake recommendations of presumably worldwide applicability based on (1) a factorial estimate of daily requirements for zinc uptake into the body and (2) a range of assumptions of intrinsic efficiency of zinc absorbability from the diet of high (40 percent), medium (20 percent) and low (10 percent) bioavailability. From these estimates, an adult needing to absorb 2.54 mg of zinc per day would require 6.3 mg of zinc in a diet of high zinc bioavailability, but 13 mg from a diet with medium availability. Fiber and phytic acid, components of unrefined cereal grains and legumes, are inhibitors of zinc absorption. The whole-wheat flatbread of rural Iran, *tanok,* and the traditional corn *tortilla* of Mexico and Central America are foods rich in these inhibitors.

Breast milk is the exclusive source of nutrients for the newborn infant. A WHO and International Atomic Energy Agency collaborative study analyzed trace element concentrations in milk samples from two developed countries (Hungary, Sweden) and four tropical nations (Zaire, Nigeria, Guatemala, and the Philippines) [4]. Extensive variability in concentrations and daily intakes was found among populations, and among subpopulations within countries. For a typical third world infant, daily median intakes would range from 0.9 mg in Zaire to 1.9 mg in Guatemala. These are well below the 3 to 5 mg recommended for infants by the RDA [1], but they were higher than the deliveries from maternal milk in Sweden (0.6 mg) and Hungary (0.8 mg). However, the biological availability of

zinc from breast milk is exceptionally high [5], and lesser quantities of zinc from human milk are likely to meet the requirements for the rapidly growing infant.

Zinc metabolism

The primary role of zinc in mammalian metabolism is as a component of metalloenzymes such as alkaline phosphatase, carbonic anhydrase, carboxypeptidase, and Zn-Cu superoxide dismutase [6]. A host of zinc-containing or zinc-activated enzymes are involved in nuclear regulation and cell proliferation. In cellular protein synthesis, zinc plays a role as a stabilizer of polyribosomes and as a component of RNA polymerases. Ionic zinc also plays a role in stabilizing membranes of circulating cellular elements such as red cells, macrophages, and platelets. Zinc is a component of thymulin and thymosin, circulating thymus-derived hormones with important regulatory roles in immune function.

Biochemistry and physiology of zinc

The adult human body contains from 2 to 3 g of zinc. It is estimated that 60 percent of total body zinc is in striated muscle, 20 percent in bone, 3.4 percent in liver, 2.1 percent in blood, 1.7 percent in the gastrointestinal tract, and 1.6 percent in skin. Homeostatic control of circulating zinc levels is not tight. About 60 percent of serum zinc is loosely bound to albumin and free amino acids while 40 percent is firmly bound to α-2-globulins. The former apparently represents the nutritionally important circulating transport pool.

Zinc absorption is only moderately efficient, but the element can be absorbed at all levels of the intestinal tract, including the colon. The majority of the absorption probably takes place in the jejunum. Because pancreatic juice is rich in zinc, a portion of the zinc that is absorbed after a meal is of endogenous origin, and *enteropancreatic* recycling of zinc is indispensable to conservation of the body reserves. The absorption of zinc is an energy-dependent, active process, and the transfer of zinc from the intestinal mucosal cell to the body is homeostatically regulated by the zinc nutriture of the host [7]. Zinc is transported from the serosal-basolateral surface of the enterocyte on serum albumin, and two-thirds of the portal zinc is cleared by the liver on the first circulatory pass.

The major route of excretion of zinc is via the feces, resulting in the loss of 1 to 2 mg of endogenous zinc daily; an additional 500 μg/day are lost through the urine. The remainder of zinc excretion proceeds by way of integumentary routes such as hair, apocrine secretions, and exfoliated skin. A liter of sweat can contain up to 1 mg of the metal.

Interaction of zinc with other nutrients

Zinc interacts with a number of nutrients. Vitamin A and zinc interact both in the transport of vitamin A from the liver on retinol-binding protein and in the conversion of retinol to its

Table 125-1. Classification of dietary zinc sources based on nutrient-energy density*

Zinc category, mg/1000 kcal	Foods
Very poor (0–2)	Fats, oils, butter, cream cheese, sweets, chocolate, soft drinks, alcoholic drinks, sugars, jams, and preserves
Poor (1–5)	Fish, fruits, refined cereal products, pastries, biscuits, cakes, puddings, tubers, plantains, sausages, chips
Rich (4–12)	Whole grains, pork, poultry, milk, low-fat cheese, yogurt, eggs, nuts
Very rich (12–882)	Lamb, leafy and root vegetables, crustacea, beef, kidney, liver, heart, mollusks

*Calculated from data in [2].

aldehyde form for the synthesis of the rhodopsin pigment ("visual purple") for night vision. High levels of dietary zinc reduce copper absorption in humans. Combined deficiencies of zinc and essential fatty acids have synergistic effects on cutaneous manifestations in rodents, but are antagonistic in fowl. The nature of the interaction of essential fatty acids and zinc deficiencies in humans has not been defined.

PATIENT

Pathogenesis of zinc deficiency

Zinc deficiency can develop by any one (or combination) of various mechanisms including insufficient dietary intake, malabsorption, excessive excretion, or increased requirements. Zinc absorption can be reduced due to inhibitory substances in the diet, as discussed above, or by pathological states such as intestinal fistulas, short-bowel syndrome, mucosal disease, pancreatic disease, diarrhea, and intestinal parasites [8]. Pathological losses of blood and sweat can contribute to zinc depletion, as can its excessive urinary excretion in renal disease, chronic inflammatory conditions, hypocaloric diets, and hormonal imbalances. Rapidly proliferating malignancies will greatly increase demand for zinc. Pregnancy and lactation also increase zinc requirements beyond the basal demands for women. An important recent observation has been a prevalence of zinc deficiency in AIDS patients [9,10].

Clinical manifestations of zinc deficiency

The clinical manifestations of human zinc deficiency are shown in Table 125-2. These represent signs and symptoms which have been shown to respond uniquely to the therapeutic administration of zinc. Some, but not all, of the manifestations are found in patients with clinical zinc deficiency. In chronically evolving zinc deficiency, growth retardation, sexual maturation delays, and nonspecific roughness predominate [11]. Zinc deficiency of acute onset is characterized by the acrodermatitis lesion, with a characteristic rash in the circumoral

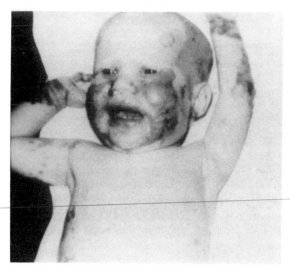

Figure 125-1. A child with acute zinc deficiency secondary to acrodermatitis enteropathica. Hyperpigmented zones are seen in the circumoral region and over flexion points at the elbow and wrists. (*Courtesy of Dr. Kenneth Nelder. From* [6]. *Reproduced with permission.*)

and pressure areas of knees, behavioral disturbances, diarrhea, and immune deficiencies. Figure 125-1 shows a child with the acute-onset form of zinc deficiency. In children with protein-energy malnutrition (PEM) and zinc deficiency, mobilization of vitamin A from the liver is stimulated uniquely by the administration of zinc; its role in retinol-binding protein synthesis appears to explain this phenomenon [12].

Assessment of nutritional status with respect to zinc

A number of body fluids and tissues have been analyzed for their content of zinc as indexes of human zinc status. They are listed in Table 125-3 along with reported ranges of normal values. The degree of correlation of many of these indexes with actual total body zinc content has never been established.

Table 125-2. Clinical manifestations of zinc deficiency

Growth retardation
Delayed sexual maturation
Hypospermia and hopogonadism
Alopecia
Skin lesions
Diarrhea
Glucose intolerance
Mental depression/apathy
Impaired wound healing
Impaired dark adaptation (night blindness)
Impaired taste acuity (hypogeusia)
Impaired phagocytic chemotaxis
Impaired T-lymphocytic function
Cutaneous allergy (anergy)

Table 125-3. Evaluation of zinc nutritional status

	Zinc content, reported ranges of normal
Serum*	140–65 μg/dL
Red cell	44–40 μg per gram of hemoglobin
White cell*	130–80 μg per 10^{10} cells
Salivary (pure parotid)	79–23 ng/g
Sweat	1.75–0.55 mg/L
Skin	80–10 μg/g
Nail*	400–100 μg/g
Hair*	230–100 μg/g
24-h urine	600–230 μg/day

*Suggested for inclusion in the battery of measures of diagnosis, including taste acuity and/or dark adaptation.

The most commonly used index—circulating zinc levels—is subject to a variety of pitfalls and caveats [*12*]. When zinc determinations are used, a *battery* of indexes should be applied. Certain *functional* indexes of zinc status are available to complement laboratory determinations of the metal [*13*]. Among these are in vitro tests (platelet aggregation, red cell uptake of ^{65}Zn), and in vivo tests (dark adaptation, taste acuity, isotopic turnover) [*6*]. Since they are not specific for zinc deficiency, caution must be exercised in their diagnostic interpretation.

Management of zinc deficiency

Oral supplements of zinc salts, in doses up to 150 mg of elemental zinc, can be used to restore zinc nutriture in zinc-deficient individuals. The sulfate, acetate, and gluconate salts of zinc are equally effective. Occasionally, zinc salts cause dyspepsia, nausea, and gastric irritation when taken on an empty stomach. Taking zinc with meals will reduce the symptoms, but will interfere with the efficiency of its absorption as well. For *chronic* administration of oral zinc, the dosage should be restricted to 45 mg daily [*15*], as higher doses consumed over periods of years have produced copper deficiency.

POPULATION

Ecological factors affecting zinc nutrition

A number of ecological factors can be postulated as having adverse effects on zinc nutrition of populations (Table 125-4). It is probable that the vegetation from zinc-poor soils will also be low in zinc. Parasitic infection and diarrhea, both common in populations of developing countries, increase wastage of endogenous zinc by the fecal route, while the hot, humid climates of the tropics increase sweat losses. Rapid succession of pregnancies and prolonged lactation periods increase maternal zinc needs. Cultural taboos often limit the offering of zinc-rich flesh foods to young children, the sick, and pregnant

Table 125-4. Ecological factors potentially reducing zinc nutriture in preindustrialized tropical countries

Geophysical factors	Low zinc content of soil
Dietary factors	High consumption of fiber, phytate
	Low consumption of meat, fermented whole-grain cereals or pulses, crustacea, and mollusks
	High consumption of fishes, tubers, refined carbohydrates, fats, and oils
Cultural factors	Geophagia
	Prolonged lactation and/or rapid succession of pregnancies
	Food taboos and food-processing methods
Climatic factors	Hot, humid climate
Zoological factors	Parasitoses
	Frequent episodes of infectious diarrhea

and lactating women. Geophagy is common in people with hookworm, in pregnancy, and in young children in the tropics, but it is not clear whether it is a cause of zinc deficiency or a response thereto. Traditional fermentation processes used in making wheat and soybean dishes may increase the biological availability of zinc by hydrolyzing the phytic acids in these foods. Milling of cereals, on the other hand, reduces the total zinc content of foods.

Zinc restriction studies in laboratory animals have demonstrated thymic atrophy, reduced thymulin, diminished T-cell blastogenesis, decreased lymphokine production, and impaired antibody production to thymus-dependent antigens: Neutrophil chemotaxis and phagocytic function are moderately impaired, whereas B-cell function is largely spared [*16*]. The hereditary disorder of zinc absorption, *acrodermatitis enteropathica,* is characterized by recurrent infections and thymic atrophy. Zinc-deficient animals develop more severe experimental parasitic infections [*17*], while in humans lepromatous leprosy, but not the tuberculoid form, is associated with depressed circulating levels of zinc. Oral administration of zinc has been reported to be adjunctive in the treatment of leprosy with dapsone [*18*]. In the West Indies [*19*] plasma zinc levels are lower in *T. trichuria*–infected persons, and an inverse association between worm burden and zinc levels has been observed.

A class of small polypeptides released by activated macrophages mediates the acute-phase response (APR) to injury and inflammation [*20*]. One of the consequences of the APR is the redistribution of zinc from the circulation to the liver. Presumably this is a "filtering" process in which the polypeptide mediators stimulate de novo hepatic synthesis of thionien, a sulfur-rich storage protein which captures and holds divalent cations such as zinc. During the prodromal phase of infection, circulating zinc levels fall precipitously. Whether or not this has survival values is uncertain, but this redistribution could prime the proliferative response of lymphocytes being activated by pathogen antigens.

Epidemiology of zinc deficiency

A syndrome of dwarfism and hypogonadism in children and adolescents in rural Egypt and Iran was attributed to zinc deficiency in the 1960s; the cause was presumed to be inhibition of zinc absorption by the fiber- and phytate-rich diet of flatbreads, as this diet provided 11 to 12 mg of zinc daily. Whether true *primary* zinc deficiency exists as a public health problem has been debated. The strongest evidence comes from the Amazon Basin of Brazil in which the diet of river fish, cassava, and refined carbohydrates had a low zinc-to-energy ratio, meeting only 40 to 50 percent of the RDA for zinc. A quarter of the population has low serum zinc levels, which show a correlation with dietary intake of the nutrient. Shrimpton [*21*] has concluded that zinc is the first limiting nutrient in this region. In the same population, serum zinc was significantly correlated with zinc content of hair in the absence—but not in the presence—of intestinal parasite infections.

Abnormally low serum zinc levels have been reported in pregnant women in Turkey and in aborigines of northwest Australia, and low hair zinc levels have been documented in natives of Papua New Guinea and in Panama. Given the unreliability of these indexes, the true state of zinc nutriture in these populations is not clear. Assuming zinc deficiency is prevalent in one or all of them, the contribution of poor intakes and impaired bioavailability has yet to be defined. Secondary (conditioned) deficiency is seen commonly in children with severe PEM. Malnourished children supplemented with zinc show faster growth, a greater restoration of lean tissue, and superior immune function [22,23]. Hair zinc levels are lower in children with a history of persistent diarrhea [24].

Prevention and control of zinc deficiency

Prevention of diarrhea, PEM, and intestinal parasitic infection will eliminate situations commonly associated with secondary zinc deficiency. Where the staple foods in the diet inhibit zinc absorption, fortification of some common food vehicle, such as sugar or salt, with an inorganic zinc compound—e.g., zinc carbonate—may be feasible. No experience with population-level zinc fortification, or its evaluation, has yet been reported, however.

COPPER

NUTRIENT

Sources of copper in the diet

The Food and Nutrition Board of the United States has established Safe and Adequate Daily Dietary Intake (SADDI) levels for trace elements for which formal RDAs cannot yet be defined [1]. For adults, the SADDI for copper is 2 to 3 mg. For infants, it ranges from 0.5 to 1.0 mg. The richest sources of copper are oysters, other shellfish, certain fish such as tuna, legumes, and whole-grain products. Milk and rice, two foods often used as weaning foods, are notably low in this element. The use of copper pipes or copper-alloy-plated utensils increases the intake of this nutrient as a contaminant of the water, beverages, and foods that come in contact with the copper-laden surfaces. The collaborative study on trace elements in breast milks [4] estimated median daily intakes of copper from maternal milk in developing countries. In micrograms per day, these were: Philippines, 198; Nigeria, 178; Guatemala, 167; and Zaire, 94. For Sweden and Hungary, the respective median daily copper intakes were 149 and 136 µg/day. The SADDI for copper for a 0- to 6-month-old infant is 500 to 700 µg/day [1]; thus, copper intakes for breast-fed infants around the world are lower than the estimated nutritional requirements.

Metabolism of copper

The adult human has between 80 and 120 mg of copper in the body. Copper is absorbed from the diet with a high efficiency, and is transported in the portal blood to the liver on albumin. The liver plays a central role in copper metabolism; the absorbed copper can be stored in reserves, distributed to other tissues as part of the hepatic protein ceruloplasmin, or returned to the gut by way of biliary secretion. The major excretion route for the metal is in the bile, with this copper having a poor chance for reabsorption. Normal pancreatic secretion tends to reduce dietary copper absorption [25]; this could be a regulatory mechanism. The urine is a minor pathway for copper elimination.

Biochemistry and physiology of copper

Copper forms part of a number of cuproenzymes, all having in common the use of molecular oxygen or a related species in biological oxidation-reduction reactions. Among the important cuproenzymes are lysyl oxidase, cytochrome c oxidase, tyrosinase, and Zn-Cu superoxide dismutase. Ceruloplasmin, the transport protein of copper, also has enzymatic activity as ferroxidase I. The physiological functions of copper in mammals include erythropoiesis, leukopoiesis, skeletal mineralization, connective tissue synthesis, myelin formation, melanin pigment synthesis, catecholamine metabolism, oxidative phosphorylation, thermal regulation, antioxidant protection, immune function, cardiac function, and glucose regulation [5].

Interactions of copper with other nutrients

The interaction of copper with zinc has been discussed above. Iron and copper exert a mutual competitive interaction at the level of hepatic storage in experimental animals. Excessive intakes of ascorbic acid can reduce the absorption of copper.

PATIENT

Pathogenesis of copper deficiency

Copper deficiency is most often the result of reduced dietary intake of the element. Overt, clinical copper deficiency has never been reported on a strictly dietary basis in an adult; in mature individuals it occurs in prolonged total parenteral nutrition or as a complication of another pathological process. In young children, especially in premature infants, copper deficiency can result from a low-copper diet. In the preterm neonate, this is aggravated by a reduction in hepatic copper stores. Chronic diarrhea reduces copper status [24], presumably due to some combination of withholding copper-rich foods, anorexia, and malabsorption of the element. PEM, specifically of the marasmic type, is associated with copper depletion [26,27].

Clinical manifestations of copper deficiency

The clinical manifestations of copper deficiency are shown in Table 125-5. Figure 125-2 shows the appearance of hand and wrist bones in two of the original patients observed in Peru [28]; bony erosion of the distal ulna is seen in both instances

Table 125-5. Manifestations of copper deficiency

Hypochromic, microcytic anemia
Neutropenia
Depigmentation of hair and skin
Defective elastin formation with arterial aneurysms
Central nervous system abnormalities
Hypotonia
Hypothermia
Skeletal demineralization
Subperiosteal hemorrhages
Epiphyseal separation

as is a "ground-glass" appearance of the metacarpal bones. The anemia of copper deficiency is a hypochromic, microcytic variety, with characteristics of iron deficiency; it does not, however, respond to the administration of iron supplements. The mechanism of bone changes appears to be analogous to scurvy, and occurs only in *growing* bone, leading to fractures and subperiosteal hemorrhages [29].

Pathogenesis of copper excess

Abnormal accumulation of copper occurs in liver, brain, cornea, and kidney in the genetic disorder Wilson's disease (hepatolenticular degeneration); and in the liver in Indian childhood cirrhosis (ICC), a familial disease of idiopathic etiology found in Pakistan, Burma, India, and Sri Lanka [30]. With onset between infancy and 10 years, ICC is characterized by the highest pathological concentrations of intrahepatic copper

of any disease, over 1 mg per gram of dry tissue. A common mode of suicide in India is intentional ingestion of cupric sulfate [31]. The lethal dose of a copper salt is thought to range from 3.5 to 35 g.

Clinical manifestations of copper excess

Hepatic cirrhosis is the common feature of copper overload states such as Wilson's disease and ICC. The inexorable course of ICC progresses from cirrhosis to cholestasis and finally to death due to portal hypertension. In acute copper intoxication, jaundice due to fulminant intravascular hemolysis and massive hepatic necrosis is seen.

Assessment of nutritional status with respect to copper

The strategies to evaluate copper status involve (1) estimates of body stores through direct measurement of copper in tissues and fluids, (2) determination of the integrity of copper-dependent functions, and (3) diagnosis of subclinical manifestations of deficiency. Table 125-6 lists the indexes that have been applied to the assessment of copper status. In copper deficiency states, circulating copper levels are usually, but not always, below 50 μg/dL. In lethal acute copper intoxication, circulating copper levels rise to 265 μg/dL or higher. However a series of nontoxic states—including pregnancy, infections and inflammations, and use of estrogens—can produce increases in ceruloplasmin concentrations that raise copper levels to 250 μg/dL or more. Activity levels of cuproenzymes in one or another tissue or fluid represent functional indexes of copper

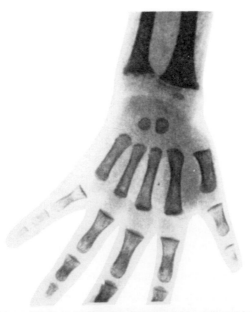

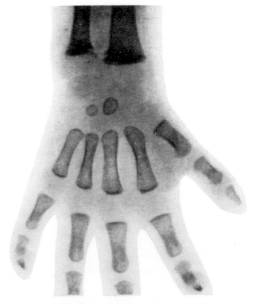

Figure 125-2. *A.* Radiograph of the hand of a malnourished Peruvian infant with copper deficiency. Note the erosion of the distal ulna and the "ground-glass" appearance of the hand bones. *B.* Shows the x-ray of another copper-deficient child with essentially similar findings. (*From* [32]. *Reproduced with permission.*)

Table 125-6. Evaluation of copper nutritional status

Hemoglobin or hematocrit
Reticulocyte count
White count and differential
Plasma or serum copper concentration
Serum ceruloplasmin
White cell copper content
Erythrocyte copper content
Copper metalloenzyme activity:
  Superoxide dismutase (red cell)
  Amine oxidase (serum)
  Cytochrome c oxidase (leukocyte)
  Lysyl oxidase (fibroblast)

status. Currently, superoxide dismutase activity shows increasing promise as a measure of copper nutriture.

Management of clinical copper deficiency

Oral doses of copper as copper salts, conventionally cupric sulfate, can be administered to treat copper deficiency states. Since ionic copper is an emetic, the amount of elemental copper per oral dose is limited to 2 mg. Higher single dosages can produce nausea and vomiting. A 2-mg dose can be repeated several times daily, however, and continued until normal copper nutriture is restored.

POPULATION

Ecological factors

A number of ecological factors can influence the predisposition to copper deficiency or marginal copper status. The use of copper tubing and copper-alloy utensils increases the level of contaminant copper leached into the diet. Cultural factors determining the offering of foods, particularly weaning foods to preschool children, will determine the susceptibility of young children to copper deficiency. Rates of twin births and preterm deliveries will also exert an effect. The state of sanitation and hygiene, determining the frequency and duration of diarrheal episodes, is yet another ecological issue in copper status at the population level.

Epidemiology of copper deficiency

Overall, there have been few reported cases of clinical copper deficiency in the two and one-half decades since its original description in malnourished Peruvian children. Among the predisposing factors are twinning and preterm births. The combination of PEM and/or persistent diarrhea in children fed low-copper formulas accounted for the occurrence of copper deficiency in the initial cases reported from Peru [33,34], and these conditions are factors in the subsequent sporadic cases in *preschool* children reported in India, Chile, and elsewhere.

Prevention and control

Special attention to copper supplementation is needed in preterm infants. Postweaning diets based on milk and/or rice should be supplemented with locally available copper-rich foods. Control of persistent diarrhea would counteract one presumed aggravating condition, and efforts to reduce protein malnutrition will also diminish the associated copper deficiency.

SELENIUM

NUTRIENT

Sources of selenium in the diet

The SADDI for selenium in adults has been established at 50 to 200 µg [1]. Selenium balance can be maintained on intakes of as little as 20 µg/day. Leading sources of selenium in the diet are fish, such as tuna and haddock; marine mollusks; organ and muscle meats; and cereal grains from high seleniferous areas. Natural yeasts are low in selenium, but when grown specially on selenium-rich nutrient broths (selenized yeast), they become a rich source of the element.

Bovine milk is a poor source of selenium. The median concentrations of selenium in breast milk from the cooperative study were consistently lower in the industrialized countries (Sweden, 13.1 µg/L; Hungary, 13.9 µg/L) than in the developing nations; the latter ranged from about 19 µg/L in Zaire and Guatemala, to 24.2 µg/L in Nigeria, to 33.2 µg/L in the Philippines [4].

Human selenium metabolism

Humans can remain in nutritional balance with from 6 to 15 mg of total body selenium reserves [35]. Selenium as selenomethionine is absorbed with over 90 percent efficiency; selenium incorporated into pork was absorbed with 87 percent efficiency [36]. The major route of excretion of endogenous selenium is in the urine, as trimethylselenomium [35].

Biochemistry and physiology of selenium

The major role of selenium is as a component of glutathione peroxidase, which contains 4 gram-atoms of the element [37]. Selenium thus functions in the antioxidant protection of the cytosolic milieu of the cell provided by this enzyme. Selenium also appears to have a role in hepatic detoxification of drugs by the cytochrome P-450 system [38].

Interactions of selenium with other nutrients

Well documented in experimental animals, livestock and poultry is an interaction between vitamin E (tocopherol) and selenium, in which excess amounts of one or the other can partially protect against the deficiency of the other in the prevention of liver necrosis and muscle disease. The extent to which this overlapping protection occurs in humans has not been determined. In animals, vitamin C favors the absorption of selenium [*36*].

Selenium appears to play a role in toxicology, protecting mammalian predators, including humans, from the toxicity of organic mercury compounds, such as methylmercury, in fish and shellfish [*39,40*]. This probably operates to the benefit of coastal populations of Japan and other Pacific Island nations.

PATIENT

Pathogenesis of selenium deficiency

The principal mechanism for human selenium deficiency is a relative or absolute lack of the element in the diet, most commonly due to total parenteral nutrition. Conditioned (secondary) selenium deficiency can occur in various types of cancer, while pancreatic insufficiency reduces the efficiency of selenium absorption. Impaired selenium nutriture has been documented in children with PEM; whether this is a primary deficiency or a consequence of abnormal wastage of the element has not been determined.

Manifestations of human selenium deficiency

The clinical manifestations of selenium deficiency are listed in Table 125-7. Both impaired granulocyte function and impaired lymphocyte function have been reported in selenium deficiency, raising the possibility of enhanced susceptibility to infection. Golden and Ramdath [*41*] have advanced the novel hypothesis that the manifestations of edematous PEM are the product of unopposed oxidant damage to cells and tissues. A relative deficit of glutathione peroxidase activity would contribute to this process.

Pathogenesis of selenium excess

A total body excess of selenium can occur with continuous ingestion of elevated amounts of the element in food and water. Self-supplementation with inorganic or organic forms of selenium (i.e., selenized yeast) can also produce total body overload.

In livestock and animals with alkali disease (chronic selenosis), the prominent features are hair loss, malformation, and hepatic cirrhosis. In humans, however, Jaffe et al. [*42*] were unable to establish any differences in clinical or biochemical features, or in frequency of congenital malformation, in a hyperseleniferous area in Venezuela. In rural China, Yang et al. [*43*] described an acute outbreak of selenium toxicity characterized by loss of hair and nails, eruptive skin lesions, peripheral neuropathy, dental mottling, and increased dental caries. The concentrations of selenium in foods and in body fluids and tissues were 1000-fold higher than those found in the hyposeleniferous areas in which Keshan disease is prevalent. The enrichment of the soil with excessive amounts of selenium was traced to leaching from coal in the subsoil by the use of lime fertilizers.

Assessment of nutritional status with respect to selenium

The laboratory indexes for assessment of selenium status are shown in Table 125-8. Circulating levels of selenium may reflect recent dietary intake. Levels of glutathione peroxidase activity in red cells or platelets have been found to be more reliable indexes of selenium status. The leakage of the muscle enzymes into the serum signifies a state of selenium-deficiency-induced myositis. Vinton et al. [*44*] have identified two additional signs of human selenium depletion, macrocytosis and pseudoalbinism.

Management of human selenium deficiency

Selenium deficiency can be treated by oral preparations of sodium selenite (Na_3SeO_2) salt or Torula yeast tablets. Treatment regimens for depleted patients have included daily amounts of 100 to 400 μg.

POPULATION

Ecological factors

The primary determinant of selenium status in populations of wildlife, livestock, or humans is the content of selenium in the soil. Belts of *hypo*seleniferous areas exist, as in New Zealand, Australia, Finland, parts of the United States, and notably China. *Hyper*seleniferous areas are also seen in the United States, China, Venezuela, and elsewhere. Concentrations of selenium in the staple grains of the former areas are as low as 0.005 to 0.01 ppm, and in the latter areas, they rise as high as 4 to 12 ppm.

Table 125-7. Clinical manifestations of selenium deficiency

Myalgias and myositis
Cardiomyopathy
Hemolytic anemias
Decreased leukocyte bactericidal activity
Depressed cellular immunity

Table 125-8. Evaluation of selenium nutritional status

Plasma or serum selenium concentration
Whole blood selenium concentration
Erythrocyte selenium concentration
Erythrocyte glutathione peroxidase activity
Platelet glutathione peroxidase activity
Serum creatine kinase activity
Serum creatinine phosphokinase activity

Epidemiology of selenium deficiency

Low circulating levels of selenium have been documented in children with PEM in Thailand, Guatemala, and Zaire. Two endemic diseases in rural China have been linked to low dietary intakes of selenium in hyposeleniferous areas. Keshan's disease is a progressive myocardiopathy of childhood and adolescence, occurring in China (Fig. 125-3) [45]. The selenium content of soil and crops, and the selenium concentration of blood and hair, are universally low in the areas endemic for Keshan's disease. In regions of China in which habitual daily intakes of selenium are greater than 30 μg, this disorder is unknown. Kashin-Beck disease is an endemic, deforming osteoarthropathy confined to distinct regions of rural China, Korea, and Siberia. Studies of the role of selenium in Kashin-Beck disease are underway [46], and a similar association with hyposeleniferous areas with the occurrence of the disease is suggested. Since low-selenium diets are universal in hypose-

leniferous areas, but the occurrence of Keshan's disease and Kashin-Beck disease are sporadic in the endemic areas, additional environmental, genetic, and/or infective factors have been implicated as cocausal influences in the development of the respective disorders.

Control and prevention

Control of primary selenium deficiency or marginal nutritional states that predispose to Keshan, and possibly Kashin-Beck, disease can be accomplished, in theory, with a variety of strategies. Treatment of agricultural soils with sodium selenite is one approach. Supplementation of animal feeds with this salt is another. Direct supplementation of at-risk segments of the population with sodium selenite is yet another. In China, supplementation with tablets containing 0.5 to 1 mg of sodium selenite weekly over a year to 4510 children produced a rate of Keshan's disease of 2.2 per 1000, as compared to the 3985

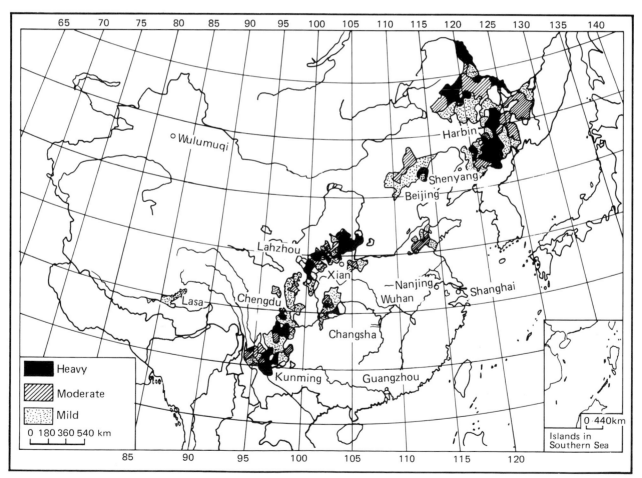

Figure 125-3. The geographical distribution of Keshan's disease incidence in distinct regions of China. (*From [45]. Reproduced with permission.*)

untreated controls, who showed a 2-year incidence of 13.5 per 1000. Prevention of PEM through dietary and hygienic measures (see Chap. 118) would eliminate the secondary selenium deficiency seen in children with kwashiorkor.

CHROMIUM

Nutrient

Sources of chromium in the diet

The SADDI for chromium for adults and adolescents is 50 to 200 μg [1]. Foods rich in chromium are brewer's yeast, mushrooms, prunes, nuts, and asparagus [47,48]. Beverages such as wine and beer also have appreciable contents of the element. Cereal products have lower amounts of chromium. Negligible amounts are found in drinking water, fish, and shellfish. Chromium introduced into foods and beverages from the chrome steel utensils and implements used to prepare them can make a substantial contribution to net intake [48]. Median breast milk chromium levels have been found to vary widely with geography [4]. The concentrations in Nigerian women's milk, 4.35 μg/L, and Filipino milk, 3.46 μg/L, are threefold higher than those found in Guatemalan milk, 1.17 μg/L, and Zairian milk, 1.07 μg/L.

Chromium metabolism

The total body content of chromium in a normal, healthy adult is estimated to be 6 to 10 mg. Inorganic chromium, as from metallic contamination of foods and beverages, is absorbed with less than 1 percent efficiency [49]. Organic complexes of chromium in food are presumably absorbed with greater efficiency. The major route of excretion of endogenous chromium is in the urine. The transport form of chromium in the circulation is on transferrin on a binding site not occupied by iron [50].

Biochemistry and physiology of chromium

The active form of chromium is an organic complex of the chromic [Cr(III)] ion with nicotinic acid and glutathione, or its constituent amino acids [51]. This has been referred to as *glucose tolerance factor*. Its exact molecular participation is not clearly understood. It interacts with insulin potentiating its hormonal interaction with target cells. Chromium also appears to play a role in nucleic acid metabolism, leading to the speculation that it has some role in gene regulation [49].

PATIENT

Pathogenesis of chromium deficiency

Given the usual clinical context of chromium deficiency in developing countries (see below), the pathogenesis of chromium deficiency is presumably a combination of decreased dietary intake and enhanced wastage of endogenous resources.

Fever and infection, physical injury and exhausting exercise, not uncommon in developing countries, are each associated with elevated excretion of chromium in urine. No amount of these factors, per se, however, seems to be able to precipitate overt deficiency in adults. The total body content of chromium, and its concentration in most tissues, decreases with aging [52]; whether this represents depletion, however, is not known.

A *theoretical* possibility that relative chromium depletion can develop due to *nutritional hemosiderosis* must be entertained. By more effective competition for binding sites on transferrin by iron, hemochromatosis has been shown to increase chromium turnover [50]. A similar state of saturation of circulating transferrin occurs in hemosiderosis, a condition common among the Bantu of South Africa [53]. One could postulate a reduced body pool of chromium in persons with nutritional overloads of iron, but this has not been documented.

Manifestations of human chromium deficiency

The clinical manifestations of chromium deficiency are listed in Table 125-9. They are consistent with an effect on insulin action, as both glucose and lipid metabolism are disordered.

Assessment of nutritional status with respect to chromium

The inaccuracy and imprecision in the determination of chromium concentration in tissues and biological fluids have hampered development of laboratory methods for assessing chromium status. Listed in Table 125-10 are potential laboratory indexes of chromium status. Anderson [49] has commented wisely that "relative chromium status can be evaluated retrospectively following daily Cr supplementation . . . for one to three months." Changes in glucose tolerance or blood lipid levels are the indexes to follow.

Management of human chromium deficiency

Given the low bioavailability of inorganic chromic salts, oral chromium supplementation usually takes the form of brewer's yeast which contains 1.1 μg of the element per gram of yeast [47]. Doses used in supplementation studies have ranged from 100 to 200 μg of yeast chromium daily. The low toxicity would suggest that these intakes would be safe over a prolonged period of time.

Table 125-9. Clinical manifestations of chromium deficiency

Hyperglycemia
Glucose intolerance
Increased insulin levels
Hyperlipidemia
Peripheral neuropathy
Encephalopathy

Table 125-10. Evaluation of chromium nutritional status

Plasma chromium concentration
Serum chromium concentration
Red cell chromium content
Whole blood chromium content
Hair chromium content
24-h urinary chromium excretion
Urinary chromium-to-creatinine ratio

POPULATION

Epidemiology of chromium deficiency

Expressed chromium deficiency in the third world is seen only in the context of children with PEM. It has been described in malnourished Turkish, Jordanian, and Nigerian infants [54]. The significance of the alterations in body chromium content with aging is not understood; however, the aging population of preindustrialized countries is expanding, and gerontological concerns are increasingly appropriate for consideration in the context of the public health of developing countries [55].

Control and prevention

Measures to prevent protein-energy depletion through maternal education, appropriate weaning foods, immunization, hygiene, and long-range economic development will reduce the incidence of PEM; this, in turn, should reduce associated chromium metabolism abnormalities.

REFERENCES

1 National Academy of Sciences: Recommended Dietary Allowances, 9th ed. Washington, DC, 1980
2 Paul AA, Southgate DAT: *McCance and Widdowson's The Composition of Foods*. London, Her Majesty's Stationery Office, 1978, p 417
3 World Health Organization: Trace Elements in Human Nutrition. WHO Tech Rep Ser 532, Geneva, 1973
4 The Composition of Breast Milk in Minor and Trace Elements. Report of a Joint World Health Organization/International Atomic Energy Agency Collaborative Study. Geneva (in press)
5 Lonnerdal B: Dietary factors affecting trace element bioavailability from human milk, cow's milk and infant formulas. Prog Food Nutr Sci 9:35–62, 1985
6 Solomons NW: Zinc and copper, in Shils ME, Young VR (eds): *Modern Nutrition in Health and Disease,* 7th ed. Philadelphia, Lea & Febiger, 1988, pp 238–262
7 Cousins RJ: Zinc metabolism—Coordinate regulation as related to cellular function, in Taylor TG, Jenking NK (eds) *Proceedings of the XIIIth International Congress on Nutrition.* London, John Libbey, pp 500–504
8 McClain CJ: Zinc metabolism in malabsorption syndromes. J Am Coll Nutr 4:49–44, 1985
9 Marilus R, Spirer Z, Michaeli D, et al: First case of AIDS in a homosexual in Israel. Results of different therapeutic regimens. Isr J Med Sci 20:249–251, 1984
10 Tong TK, Andrew LR, Albert A, et al: Childhood acquired immune deficiency syndrome manifesting as acrodermatitis enteropathica. J Pediatr 108:426–428, 1986
11 Prasad AS: Clinical manifestations of zinc deficiency. Ann Rev Nutr 5:341–363, 1985
12 Shingwekar AG, Mohonram M, Reddy V: Effect of zinc supplementation on plasma levels of vitamin A and retinol-binding protein in malnourished children. Clin Chim Acta 193:97–100, 1979
13 Solomons NW: On the assessment of zinc and copper nutriture in man. Am J Clin Nutr 32:856–871, 1979
14 Solomons NW: Assessment of nutritional status: Functional indicators of pediatric nutrition. Ped Clin N Am 32:319–334, 1985
15 Sandstead HH: Zinc interference with copper metabolism. JAMA 240:2188–2189, 1978
16 Fraker PJ, Gershwin ME, Good RA, et al: Interrelationships between zinc and immune function. Fed Proc 45:1474–1479, 1986
17 Fraker PJ, Caruso R, Kierszenbaum F: Alteration of immune and nutritional status of mice by synergy between zinc deficiency and infection with *Trypanosoma cruzi.* J Nutr 112:1224–1229, 1982
18 Mathur NK, Bumb RA, Mangal HN, et al: Oral zinc as an adjunct to Dapsone in lepromatous leprosy. Int J Leprosy 52:331–338, 1984
19 Bundy DAP: Epidemiological aspects of *Trichuris* and trichuriasis in Caribbean communities. Trans R Soc Trop Med Hyg 80: 702–718, 1986
20 Keusch GT, Farthing MJ: Nutrition and infection. Ann Rev Nutr 6:131–154, 1986
21 Shrimpton R: Studies on Zinc Nutrition in the Amazon Valley. Ph.D. thesis, University of London, 1980
22 Golden BE, Golden MHN: Effect of zinc supplementation on the dietary intake, rate of weight gain, and energy cost of tissue deposition in children recovering from severe malnutrition. Am J Clin Nutr 34:900–908, 1981
23 Castillo-Duran C, Heresi G, Fisberg M, et al: Controlled trial of zinc supplementation during recovery from malnutrition: Effects on growth and immune function. Am J Clin Nutr 45:602–608, 1987
24 Rodriguez A, Soto G, Torres S, et al: Zinc and copper in hair and plasma of children with chronic diarrhea. Acta Pediatr Scand 74: 770–774, 1985
25 Braganza JM, Klass HJ, Bell M, et al: Evidence of altered copper metabolism in patients with chronic pancreatitis. Clin Sci 60:303–310, 1981
26 Fisberg M, Castillo C, Uauy R: Factores condicionantes de hipocupremia en lactantes marasmicos. Rev Chil Pediatr 52:410–414, 1981
27 Castillo-Duran C, Fisberg M, Valenzuela A, et al: Controlled trial of copper supplementation during the recovery from marasmus. Am J Clin Nutr 37:898–903, 1983
28 Graham GG, Cordano A: Copper deficiency in human subjects, in Prasad AS (ed): *Trace Elements in Human Health and Disease,* vol 1. *Zinc and Copper.* New York, Academic, 1976, pp 363–372
29 McGill LC, Boas RN, Zerella JT: Extremity swelling in an infant with copper and zinc deficiency. J Pediatr Surg 15:746–747, 1980
30 Chopra K: Indian childhood cirrhosis. Indian Pediatr 16:533–538, 1979
31 Chuttani HK, Gupta PS, Gulati S, et al: Acute copper sulfate poisoning. Am J Med 39:849–854, 1965
32 Cordano A, Baertl JM, Graham GG: Copper deficiency in infancy. Pediatrics 34:324–326, 1964

33 Graham GG, Cordano A: Copper depletion and deficiency in the malnourished infant. J Hopkins Med J 124:139–150, 1969

34 Cordano A, Graham GG: Copper deficiency complicating severe chronic intestinal malabsorption. Pediatrics 38:596–604, 1966

35 Levander OA: Selenium, chromium, and manganese, (A) Selenium, in Shils ME, Young VR (eds): *Modern Nutrition in Health and Disease,* 7th ed. Philadelphia, Lea & Febiger, 1988, pp 263–267

36 Barbezat GO, Casey CE, Reasbeck PG, et al: Selenium, in Solomons NW, Rosenberg IH (eds): *Absorption and Malabsorption in Mineral Nutrients.* New York, Alan R. Liss, pp 231–258, 1984

37 Awasthi YC, Beutler E, Srivastaca SK: Purification and properties of human erythrocyte glutathione peroxidase. J Biol Chem 250:5144–5149, 1975

38 Burk RF: Biological activity of selenium. Ann Rev Nutr 3:53–70, 1983

39 Ganther HE, Goudie C, Sunde ML, et al: Selenium: Relation to decreased toxicity of methylmercury added to diets containing tuna. Science 175:1122–1124, 1972

40 Stillings BR, Lagally H, Bauersfield P, et al: Effect of cystine, selenium, and fish protein on the toxicity and metabolism of methylmercury in rats. Toxicol Appl Pharmacol 30:243–254, 1974

41 Golden MNH, Ramdath D: Free radicals in the pathogenesis of kwashiorkor, in Taylor TG, Jenkins NK (eds): *Proceedings of the XIIIth International Congress on Nutrition.* London, John Libbey, 1987, pp 597–598

42 Jaffe WG, Ruphael M, Mondragon MC, et al: Estudio clinico y bioquimico en ninos escolares de una zona selenifera. Arch Latinoamer Nutr 22:595–611, 1972

43 Yang GQ, Wang S, Zhou R, et al: Endemic selenium intoxication of humans in China. Am J Clin Nutr 37:872–881, 1983

44 Vinton NE, Anders Dahlstrom K, Strobel CT, et al: Macrocytosis and pseudoalbinism: Manifestations of selenium deficiency. J Pediatr 111:711–717, 1987

45 Yang GQ, Chen J, Wen Z, et al: The role of selenium in Keshan disease, in Draper H (ed): *Advances in Nutritional Research,* vol 6. New York, Plenum, 1986, pp 203–237

46 Levander OA: Etiological hypotheses concerning Kashin-Beck disease, in Levander OA (ed): *Nutrition '87,* AIN Symposium Proceedings. Washington, DC, the American Institute of Nutrition, 1987, pp 67–71

47 Toepfer EW, Mertz W, Roginski EE, et al: Chromium in foods in relation to biological activity. J Agr Food Chem 21:69–71, 1973

48 Anderson RA: Selenium, chromium, and manganese, (B) Chromium, in Shils ME, Young VR (eds): *Modern Nutrition in Health and Disease,* 7th ed. Philadelphia, Lea & Febiger, 1988, pp 268–273

49 Offenbacher EC, Pi-Sunyer X: Temperature and pH effects on the release of chromium from stainless steel into water and fruit juices. J Agr Food Chem 31:88–92, 1983

50 Sargent T III, Lim TH, Jenson RL: Reduced chromium retention in patients with hemochromatosis, a possible basis of hemochromatosis diabetes. Metabolism 28:70–79, 1979

51 Mertz W: Chromium occurrence and function in biological systems. Phys Rev 49:163–239, 1969

52 Schroeder HA, Balassa JJ, Tipton IH: Abnormal trace metals in man: Chromium. J Chron Dis 15:941–964, 1962

53 Fairbanks VF, Beutler E: Iron, in Shils ME, Young VR (eds): *Modern Nutrition in Health and Disease,* 7th ed. Philadelphia, Lea & Febiger, 1988, pp 193–226

54 Saner G: Chromium and glucose metabolism in children, in Shapcott D, Hubert J (eds): *Chromium in Nutrition and Metabolism.* Amsterdam, Elsevier/North Holland, 1979, pp 129–144

55 Solomons NW, Siu M-L, Mazariegos M: Gerontological research expanding in Guatemala. Ageing International 14:17–21, 1987

CHAPTER	*Iodine, Endemic Goiter, and Endemic*
126	*Cretinism* · John B. Stanbury · Josip Matovinovic

Endemic goiter may be said to exist when more than 10 percent of the children and adolescents in a population group have palpably enlarged thyroid glands. This definition is an epidemiological one and is arbitrary; the limits could be set higher or lower, but it should be kept in mind that 5 to 8 percent of children and adolescents and a somewhat smaller percentage of adults of any "normal" population will have enlarged thyroids for a variety of causes, including subacute or chronic thyroiditis, Graves' disease, and benign and malignant tumors [1,2].

The term *endemic cretin* is applied to persons in an endemic goiter region who are mentally deficient, with a more or less characteristic form of retarded or abnormal development. Endemic cretinism is thus defined by its association with endemic goiter and severe iodine deficiency. Correction of iodine deficiency prevents the disorder [2].

NUTRIENT

Any consideration of endemic goiter and of endemic cretinism inevitably involves iodine. A link between the disorders and lack of iodine was perceived at least a century and a half ago, and prevention by iodide supplements has been documented repeatedly.

GEOCHEMISTRY

Iodine is widely distributed over the surface of the earth, although not as a highly enriched mineral deposit. It is found in all rocks and plants, in the oceans, in soils and in salt deposits, and in association with fossil fuels. The concentration in seawater averages about 50 mg/L.

The iodine of different soils is variable. Soils accumulate iodine, in part because of recycling between successive generations of plants and accretion of iodine from fallout of atmospheric iodine derived from sea mists and evaporation from the sea. Sandy soils contain less iodine than loamy or clay soils; acid soils favor release of iodine. However, extensive cropping can remove several grams of iodine per acre per year, and it is unlikely that this amount of iodine is replaced by atmospheric fallout.

SOURCES OF IODINE

The principal commercial source of iodine is through distallation from marine algae (kelp) that concentrate iodine from seawater, forming it into diiodotyrosine (gorgonic acid) and perhaps other substances. Another commercial source of iodine is the pretroleum industry since iodine is recovered as a by-product of drilling. In spite of its relative rarity in the earth's crust, iodine from commercial sources for nutritional supplementation is exceedingly cheap; thus cost cannot be a realistic deterrent to the implementation of prophylactic programs.

IODINE IN FOOD AND WATER

The amount of iodine in plants depends largely on the iodine content of the soils on which they grow [3]. Certain plants, such as spinach, remove an unusually large amount of iodine from the soil, and may contain as much as 500 μg/kg when fresh. Kelp and related substances from the sea may contain several hundred milligrams of iodine per kilogram.

The iodine content of foods of animal origin is also variable. The iodine in milk is dependent on the concentration in the graze, but iodophors used in cleaning the udders and collecting vessels may contribute large amounts of iodine to the delivered milk. Eggs, especially the yolks, are good sources, except in iodine-deficient regions. The average amount of iodine for marine fish, 832 μg/kg, is 40-fold greater than for freshwater fish. Cereals and their products average about 50 μg/kg; fruits are poor sources of iodine. Because of the wide variability in geographical and other factors, the iodine content of diets from food tables is impossible to estimate; individual assays are required.

MINIMUM DAILY REQUIREMENTS

The minimal daily requirement for iodine may be defined as that quantity which prevents the appearance of clinical or biochemical indications of iodine deficiency. The normal thyroid is, at most, barely palpable. In persons who have long, thin necks, the gland may be both seen on swallowing and felt. A detectable increase in size occurs when the average intake of iodine falls below 40 to 50 mg/day. If intake falls below 20 mg/day, the majority of school-age children and adolescents will have distinct goiter, some with nodules; many adults will have large, multinodular goiters; and cretins will be found. When iodine intake is borderline (60 to 70 mg/day), there is evidence of compensatory increased activity of the thyroid without clinically evident thyroid enlargement.

HOST

ENDEMIC GOITER

Geographical distribution

Endemic goiter may affect as many as 200 million persons. It is chiefly a disease of the poor, isolated, and undeveloped regions of the world. It is not a tropical disorder although some of the most severe focuses, such as central Africa, Indonesia, and New Guinea, are tropical, nor is it confined to mountainous areas or to regions distant from the sea.

Pathology

The primary lesion of endemic goiter is diffuse thyroid hyperplasia [4]. Over time and with occasional access to iodine, hyperplasia evolves into diffuse goiter with colloid-filled follicles, accompanied by the development of small, nonencapsulated parenchymatous nodules. Later these areas become encapsulated, and focuses of hyperplasia may be found within and outside these nodules. This is the familiar ''puddingstone'' goiter, and its function is reflected in the irregular uptake of radioiodine as visualized in thyroid scans. Degenerative changes, cyst formation, hemorrhage into nodules, and fibrosis characterize advanced endemic goiter.

While there appears to be an increased risk of thyroid cancer associated with endemic goiter, the risk is probably small [5]. Anaplastic carcinoma is said to be excessive in populations with a long history of goiter, whereas follicular carcinoma is more often found in goiter of more recent origin. Papillary carcinoma is not associated with endemic goiter.

Pathophysiology

The altered thyroid function in endemic goiter mirrors the deficiency of iodine, which is its central cause. The avidity of the gland for iodine is increased, and the uptake is inversely proportional to the daily intake of iodine (measured as urinary excretion of iodine) [6]. Turnover of iodine may be normal or increased, and storage of iodine in the gland may be low, normal, or high, but the concentration of iodine per gram of thyroid or of thyroglobulin is reduced. There is a shift in the pattern of iodoamino acids in the gland; the ratio of mono- to diiodotyrosine rises, as does the ratio of iodotyrosines to iodothyronines and of triiodothyronine to thyroxine [7].

Plasma concentrations of thyroid hormones are unchanged in mild endemisms, but with increasing severity plasma concentrations of T_3 may remain normal or rise and those of T_4 may fall [8]. TSH may or may not rise, depending on severity of disease, and the magnitude of the TSH response to TRH administration may be increased.

Etiology

Iodine deficiency is both a necessary and a sufficient cause of endemic goiter. It and its accompanying disorders, cretinism and endemic deaf-mutism, vanish when prophylactic programs are implemented which provide the population with iodine. This etiological concept does not exclude the possibility of genetic or other nutritional factors which may accentuate the effects of a lack of iodine. For example, sulfur-containing, low-molecular-weight organic substances in drinking water in the Cauca Valley of Colombia may be responsible for persistent mild goiter in that region [9], and a cyanogenic glycoside in cassava may contribute in the endemic regions of central Africa [10].

Clinical aspects

Except when severe, endemic goiter is usually little more than an inconvenience (Fig. 126-1). In a few patients, the enlarging gland may impinge on a recurrent laryngeal nerve or the larynx to cause hoarseness, or on the esophagus to cause dysphagia. A sudden hemorrhage into a cyst will provoke pain or acute obstructive symptoms. Chronic pressure on tracheal rings can cause erosion, leading to tracheomalacia at the time of thyroidectomy. Instead of presenting as a mass in the neck, the goiter may slip behind the sternum and appear as a mediastinal mass, where it may provoke local symptoms, or, with compression of the superior vena cava, give rise to a superior mediastinal syndrome.

Since compensation for iodine deficiency in endemic goiter is usually sufficient through glandular hyperplasia to ensure normal plasma hormone concentrations, usually there are no constitutional consequences. When endemic goiter is severe, however, hypothyroidism and its effects may occur.

Treatment

Administration of iodine in any form such as tablets or drops, or as injections of iodized oil, may reduce the size of the goiter if it is due primarily to hyperplasia. Some may melt away within a few days or weeks, especially in children, but old glands with nodules, cysts, and fibrosis change little. Indeed, reduction of hyperplastic elements under iodine therapy may make preexisting nodules more apparent.

A possible complication of iodine treatment is thyrotoxicosis, also known as Jod-Basedow. It arises as areas of nodular or paranodular hyperplasia become autonomous in function and produce an excess of hormone when an abundance of iodine becomes available. An epidemic of thyrotoxicosis was observed in Tasmania, a region of mild endemic goiter, when iodide was added to bread as a dough conditioner [11].

Thyroxine may also be used in treatment of endemic goiter, with the same indications, effects, and complications as treatment with iodine. The thyroxine may be an addition to hormones already being produced by autonomous hyperplastic elements, which do not shut off as TSH is suppressed by the treatment. Thyroxine should always be given after subtotal thyroidectomy for endemic goiter, since the source of hormone has been removed, and hypothyroidism otherwise would almost surely ensue.

ENDEMIC CRETINISM

Geographical distribution

Endemic cretinism is found in association with severe endemic goiter, but only when the mean iodine intake is below 20 mg/day. The incidence is unknown because no large-scale neonatal screening program has been undertaken. Communities with prevalence rates of up to 8 percent and more of the population have been reported.

Endemic cretinism may be found today in innumerable communities and rural areas of the highland Andes, particularly in Ecuador and Bolivia, in the Himalayas, the Ubangi and Uele regions of Zaire, the Central African Republic, Indonesia, especially central Java, highland New Guinea, and in remote villages in the People's Republic of China. Older cretins may be found elsewhere, but they may have been born when iodine

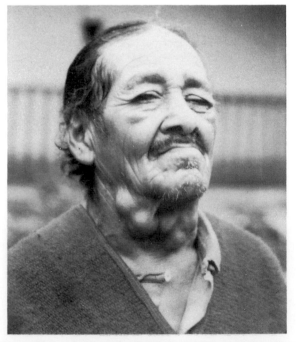

Figure 126-1. A patient with enlarged thyroid due to endemic goiter.

supplies were more limited. It appears that at extremely low levels of iodine intake, a small increase may make a large and critical difference to the fetus and newborn. Endemic cretinism is a disease of poverty, isolation, and, in contemporary terms, of official neglect.

Etiopathogenesis

Endemic cretinism is primarily a result of severe iodine deficiency during fetal and early postnatal life. The disease disappears from the community when prophylaxis is introduced. Animal models based purely on iodine deficiency mimic the human disease. Other factors, for example, consumption of thyroid antagonists such as cassava, may influence the appearance of human cretinism.

Clinical aspects

The term *endemic cretin* has been used to describe patients showing a spectrum of clinical signs. Mental deficiency must be included in the diagnosis, but other manifestations vary widely. Two major clinical forms have been described—''nervous'' cretinism and a ''myxedematous'' type—but most cretins of one type demonstrate some characteristics of the other.

The nervous cretin presents a distinctive and unique neurological picture. Frequent perceptive deafness is accompanied by proximal spasticity, with relatively good preservation of appendicular function; cerebellar signs are uncommon [12].

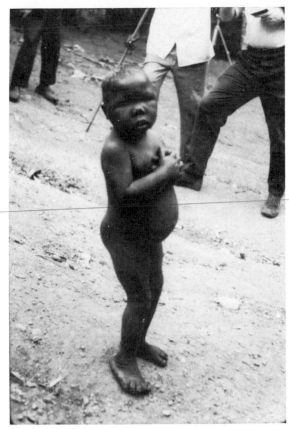

Figure 126-2. A cretin child from central Africa.

Table 126-1. The principal findings in myxedematous and nervous cretinism*

Finding	Myxedematous	Nervous
Mental deficiency	Profound	Profound
Deaf-mutism	Infrequent	Frequent
Squint	Rare	Occasional
Growth retardation	Severe	Moderate
Malformation of teeth	Frequent	Occasional
Thyroid size	Usually normal	Absent to goitrous
Proximal spasticity	Absent	Frequent
Clinical hypothyroidism	Present	Occasional
Delayed epiphyseal closure	Usual	Occasional
EKG changes	Usual	?
Delayed reflex relaxation	Present	Occasional
PBI	Low	Normal or low
T_4	Low	Normal or low
T_3	Low	Normal or low
TSH	Very high	Normal or high
TRF-TSH response	?	Exaggerated
^{131}I uptake	Normal or elevated	Elevated
^{131}I conversion ratio	Elevated	Elevated

*Endemic cretinism is considered to be a continuum; a variety of external factors influence the geographical differences which have been reported in the clinical and laboratory manifestations.

Though intellectually retarded, the patient may maintain the capacity to relate to others and to work in the household, providing there are no immobilizing deformities of the hip and knee. The clinical findings of endemic cretinism appear in Table 126-1. The cretin of central Africa belongs almost entirely in the myxedematous group. These subjects exhibit short stature and much delayed bony maturation, are without goiter, have ^{131}I uptake values lower than their normal peers, have all the clinical evidence of hypothyroidism, and are not deaf-mute (Fig. 126-2). A similar type of cretinism has been described in the People's Republic of China [13]. The nervous cretin is the dominant form in the Andes and Himalayas. In some severe endemisms, as in New Guinea and Java, both neurological and myxedematous manifestations are found.

Treatment

Treatment of the endemic cretin after the first few postnatal weeks is unavailing. Some physical growth may be achieved but there is no useful improvement in intellectual function. The benefits which might be achieved by treating with iodine or thyroxine right after birth remain unknown, and will only be learned when screening programs are established in suitable areas.

POPULATION

Grading of endemic goiter

In order that epidemiological studies and the results of preventive programs be comparable it is essential that a uniform system of grading be adopted. A recommended approach is the Pan American Health Organization (PAHO) classification system (Table 126-2).

Surveys. If endemic goiter is present, it is necessary to determine the extent of the problem in a sample of the population or in a group at special risk, such as women in the reproductive ages. Many surveys in the past have included huge numbers. It might be advantageous to examine smaller numbers but to obtain more data on each subject, depending on circumstances, logistics, and resources. The importance of employing uniform criteria in categorizing goiter should be emphasized. Minimizing the number of different observers, along with presurvey training and standardization, improves reliability of a survey.

Ideally, in addition to thyroid size and configuration, diet and daily iodine excretion are important measures to be determined. Although the latter may be based on 24-h collections, this usually imposes logistical problems and is subject to large error, so it may be better to calculate the iodine per unit volume in a sample of urine or to relate the excretion of iodine in a sample to the excretion of creatinine measured in the same sample. Radioiodine uptake studies, measurements of thyroid hormone concentrations, TSH assays, TRH responses, and so on may be done under research conditions but are not necessary for establishing the presence of an endemic or the need for a prophylactic program.

Prevention

A prevalence of 0.5 percent of endemic cretins is sufficient for implementing preventive programs, providing conditions have not changed since the birth of the youngest cretin in the community [14]. If surveys disclose grade Ia goiter in more than 15 percent of schoolchildren, then a program should be beneficial. If iodine excretion is measured, a mean value below 60 μg/day or per gram creatinine would make a program advisable, and below 40 μg/day, urgent.

Once need is established, other issues are critical to success [15]. Compliance of the health authorities must be secured, the public educated, and logistical problems anticipated and solved, such as surveillance and monitoring. This may require a national or regional laboratory. If salt is to be the vehicle for delivery of iodine, the initial survey must determine the system of salt processing and distribution, and the cooperation of the salt industry must be obtained. Projects have failed because of inattention to such details.

Certain myths must also be dispelled. Many believe that Jod-Basedow disease is a deterrent to programs. However, its occurrence is uncommon and it is easily treated; the occasional case is a small price to pay for the multiple benefits of goiter prevention. The high cost of programs is often cited as an important impediment. In fact the human requirement for iodine is so small that the cost of adding iodine to salt is minimal.

Table 126-2. Definition of goiter; classification by stages

Stages	Clinical findings
Grade 0 Persons without goiter. If the thyroid is felt, it is smaller than the distal phalanx of the subject's thumb.	Thyroid not palpable or if palpable, not larger than normal.
Grade Ia Persons with palpable goiters. The thyroid is not visible with the head in normal position. Most of these will not be readily visible with the head thrown back and the neck fully extended.	Thyroid distinctly palpable but usually not visible with the head in a normal or raised position; considered to be definitely larger than normal, at least as large as the distal phalanx of the subject's thumb.
Grade Ib Goiter easily palpable and visible only with the head thrown back.	Thyroid easily visible with the head in a normal position.
Grade II Persons with goiters visible with neck in normal position. The thyroid is smaller than those in grade III.	Thyroid easily visible with the head in a normal position.
Grade III Persons with very large goiters. Goiters can be recognized at a considerable distance, are grossly disfiguring, and may be of such size as to cause mechanical difficulties with respiration and in wearing clothes.	Goiter visible at distance.
Grade IV	Monstrous goiter.

Salt Iodization. This is the method of choice for distributing iodide to a population at risk in countries which have a well-developed salt industry and in which commercially packaged salt is the usual source for home consumption. Methods are standardized and simple, and the engineering is inexpensive [*16*]. A level of 1 in 10,000 is used in the United States but is probably higher than necessary. In general, a concentration of 1 in 20,000 to 40,000 should be adequate.

Iodized Oil. The technique of intramuscular injection of iodinated oil was introduced in the late 1950s and has been widely used [*17*]. Its effectiveness has been amply demonstrated and it is virtually free of complication. Each injection ensures an adequate supply of iodine to the recipient for 2 to 4 years. The method has lent itself admirably to use in remote regions where there is little medical infrastructure and where iodization of salt is not practicable.

Iodized Bread and Water. Programs using bread as the carrier for iodide have been tried [*11*]. Wide variability in quantity of bread consumed or the difficulty of control suggests that this is not an optimal technique for goiter prevention. A successful program of water fortification has been implemented in a community in Sicily, where the low level of water consumption makes the program economically viable [*18*].

Endemic Noncretinous Retardation in Association with Endemic Goiter. Is cretinism an all-or-none phenomenon, or are there lesser handicaps associated with endemic goiter that might be important for social and economic development of the community? Studies in different at-risk populations support the concept that associated with cretinism there are persons in the "normal" population with some deficits in motor function and perception. This becomes evident when one compares an iodine-deficient group in which there are obvious cretins with a similar group to which iodine was administered prior to conception of the study subjects. "Intelligence" is much more difficult to define and to measure, but the available information at this time supports a deleterious effect of iodine deficiency on the population, apart from cretinism as currently defined. Indeed, it may be mild retardation that is the most important effect of iodine deficiency on socioeconomic development, and its prevention the most important justification for prophylactic programs.

REFERENCES

1 Trowbridge FL, Hand KA, Nicham MZ: Findings relating to goiter and iodine in the Ten-State Nutrition Survey. Am J Clin Nutr 28:712, 1975
2 Matovinovic J: Endemic goiter and cretinism at the dawn of the third millennium. Ann Rev Nutr 13:253, 1983
3 Chilean Iodine Educational Bureau: *Iodine Content of Foods.* Bibliography, 1825–1951, London, 1956
4 Stanbury JB, Hetzel BS (eds): *Endemic Goiter and Endemic Cretinism.* New York, 1980, Wiley
5 Riccabona G: *Thyroid Cancer.* New York, Springer-Verlag, 1987
6 Stanbury JB, Brownell GL, Riggs DS, et al: *Endemic Goiter.* Cambridge, Harvard University Press, 1954
7 Ermans AM, Kinthaert J, Camus M: Defective intrathyroidal iodine metabolism in nontoxic goiter: Inadequate iodination of thyroglobulin. J Clin Endocrinol 28:1307, 1968
8 Silva JE, Sergio S: Interrelationships among serum thyroxine, triiodothyronine, reverse triiodothyronine, and thyroid-stimulating hormone in iodine-deficient pregnant women and their offspring: Effects of iodine supplementation. J Clin Endocrionol 52:4, 1981
9 Meyer JD, Gaitan E, Merino H, DeRouen TA: Geologic implications in the distribution of endemic goiter in Colombia, South America. Int J Epidemiol 7:25, 1978
10 Bourdoux P, Delange F, Gerard M, et al: Evidence that cassava ingestion increases thiocyanate formation: A possible etiologic factor in endemic goiter. J Clin Endocrinol 46:613, 1977
11 Steward JC, Vidor GI, Buttfield IH, et al: Epidemic thyrotoxicosis in northern Tasmania. Aust NZ J Med 3:203, 1971
12 Delong GR, Stanbury JB, Fierro-Benitez R: Neurological signs in congenital iodine-deficiency disorder (endemic cretinism). Dev Med Child Neurol 27:317, 1985
13 Ma T, Lu T, Tan Y, Chen B, et al: The present status of endemic goiter in China. Food Nutr Bull 4:13, 1982
14 Hetzel B, Dunn JT, Stanbury JT: *The Prevention and Control of Iodine Deficiency Disorders.* New York, Elsevier, 1987
15 Thilly CH, Delange F, Ramioul L, et al: Strategy of goiter and cretinism control in Central Africa. Int J Epidemiol 6:43, 1977
16 Hunnikin C, Wood Frank O: Iodization of salt, in Stanbury JB, Hetzel BS (eds): *Endemic Goiter and Endemic Cretinism.* New York, 1980, Wiley, p 497
17 Hennessy WB: Goiter prophylaxis in New Guinea with intramuscular injection of iodized oil. Med J Aust 1:505, 1964
18 Vigneri R, Squatrito S, Polley R, et al: Iodine prohylaxis in an endemic area in Sicily: A new method for iodine supplementation, in Reinwein D, Klein E (eds): *Diminished Thyroid Hormone Formation.* New York, F.K. Schattauer Verlag, 1982, p 187
19 Fierro-Benitez R, Cazar R, Stanbury JB, et al: Effects on school children of prophylaxis of mothers with iodized oil in an area of iodine deficiency. J Endocrinol Inv 10: August, 1987

APPENDIXES

1 *Synopsis of Etiology and Therapy*

2 *Signs and Symptoms with Possible Causes*

3 *Considerations for Travelers and Immigrants*

4 *Exotic Communicable Diseases: A Review by Region*

Synopsis of Etiology and Therapy

While it is hoped that the following pages may be used as a quick review, the complete discussion in this text should be consulted before making a commitment to diagnosis and therapy.

The Editors

Protozoan diseases

Symptoms	Distribution	Transmission	Diagnosis	Treatment
Amebiasis (dysentery)				
Diarrhea, dysentery	India, Mexico, S. Africa	Food, water	Fecal smear	Metronidazole
Amebiasis (liver abscess)				
Fever, hepatomegaly, tenderness	India, Mexico, S. Africa	Food, water	Serology	Metronidazole
Amebic meningoencephalitis (primary)				
Headache, fever, nausea	Worldwide	Fresh water contact	CSF, serology	Amphotericin B
Babesiosis				
Fever, chills, myalgias, fatigue	Worldwide zoonosis	Tick bites	Blood smears	Quinine, clindamycin
Balantidiasis				
Chronic diarrhea	Worldwide	Water	Fecal smear	Tetracycline
Cryptosporidiosis				
Chronic diarrhea	Worldwide	Water, food	Fecal smear	Experimental
Giardiasis				
Chronic diarrhea, weight loss	Worldwide	Water	Fecal smear	Metronidazole
Leishmaniasis (cutaneous)				
Skin ulcer, mucocutaneous ulceration	USSR, Middle East, Panama, Brazil	Sandfly bites	Skin biopsy	Pentostam
Leishmaniasis (visceral)				
Fever, splenomegaly, hepatomegaly, anemia	Brazil, India, east Africa, China	Sandfly bites	Bone marrow	Pentostam
Malaria				
Fever, chills, splenomegaly, anemia	Africa, Latin America, Asia	Mosquito bites	Blood smears	Chloroquinine, Fansidar, quinine/ tetracycline
Toxoplasmosis				
Fever, lymphodenopathy, retinochoroiditis, encephalopathy	Worldwide	Cat feces, raw meat	Serology, lymph node histology	Sulfadiazine, pyrimethamine
Trichomoniasis				
Vaginitis	Worldwide	Venereal	Vaginal smear	Metronidazole
Trypanosomiasis, African				
Skin nodule, fever, lymphadenopathy, mental changes	East, west Africa	Tsetse fly bites	Blood, CSF	Suramin, melarsoprol
Trypanosomiasis, American				
Fever, lymphadenopathy, heart failure, megacolon, megaesophagus	Latin America	Bug bites	Blood, serology, xenodiagnosis	Nifurtimox

Bacterial diseases

Symptoms	Distribution	Transmission	Diagnosis	Treatment
Anthrax				
Cutaneous papules, ulcers, fever, dyspnea, cyanosis	Worldwide	Contact	Skin, blood cultures	Penicillin
Brucellosis				
Fever, chills, myalgia, splenomegaly, fatigue	Worldwide	Contact, milk	Blood	Tetracycline
Campylobacter				
Diarrhea, abdominal pain, fever, dysentery	Tropics	Fecal-oral	Stool	Erythromycin
Cholera				
Watery diarrhea, hypotension	Tropics	Fecal-oral	Stool exam	Water and electrolyte replacement, tetracycline
Diphtheria				
Fever, malaise, pharyngitis, myocarditis (also cutaneous diphtheria)	Worldwide	Contact	Nasopharyngeal swabs	Antitoxin, penicillin
E. coli (enterotoxigenic)				
Watery diarrhea, abdominal cramps, malaise	Worldwide	Fecal-oral	Stool	Rehydration
Leprosy				
Skin lesions, skin anesthesia, thickened nerves, muscle weakness	Tropics	Contact	Skin smears, skin biopsies	Dapsone, rifampin
Leptospirosis				
Fever, chills, headache, malaise	Worldwide	Contact, urine	Blood serology	Penicillin
Meningococcus				
Fever, neck stiffness, headache	Worldwide	Respiratory route	CSF	Penicillin
Pertussis				
Coryza, cough	Worldwide	Aerosol, contact	Nasopharyngeal	Erythromycin
Plague				
Fever, bubo, cough, meningitis	Worldwide	Fleas, aerosols	Serology	Streptomycin
Pneumococcus				
Fever, chills, chest pains, sputum (also meningitis, otitis media)	Worldwide	Respiratory route	Blood	Penicillin
Relapsing fever				
Chills, fever, headache, fatigue	Worldwide	Tick and louse bites	Blood	Tetracycline
Rickettsial diseases				
Chills, headaches, myalgia, fever, rash, arthralgia	Worldwide	Insect bites	Serology	Chloramphenicol
Sexually transmitted diseases				
Vaginitis, urethritis, proctitis, hepatitis, genital ulcers, lymphadenopathy	Worldwide	Venereal	Blood, lesion smears	Antibiotics
Shigellosis				
Diarrhea, dysentery, fever	Worldwide	Fecal-oral	Stool	Ampicillin

Bacterial diseases (continued)

Symptoms	Distribution	Transmission	Diagnosis	Treatment
Streptococcus				
Pharyngitis, fever (also rheumatic fever, glomerulonephritis, skin infections)	Worldwide	Respiratory route	Throat swab	Penicillin
Tetanus				
Muscle spasms, stiff neck	Worldwide	Wounds	Clinical syndrome wounds	Tetanus immune globulin, penicillin, wound excision, supportive care
Tuberculosis, pulmonary				
Cough, fever, weight loss, fatigue, night sweats	Worldwide	Respiratory route	X-ray, sputum	Isoniazid, Rifampin
Typhoid				
Abdominal pain, rose spots, splenomegaly, hepatomegaly	Worldwide	Fecal-oral	Stool, serology	Chloramphenicol
Yaws				
Disseminated papillomata	Tropics	Contact	Skin smears	Penicillin

Viral diseases

Symptoms	Distribution	Transmission	Diagnosis	Treatment
Dengue				
Fever, headache, rash, myalgias, hemorrhage, shock	Tropics	Mosquito bites	Serology	Supportive care
Viral encephalitis				
Fever, headache, stiff neck, mental confusion, convulsions	Worldwide	Mosquito bites	Serology	Supportive care
Hemorrhagic fever				
Fever, headache, hemorrhage, conjunctivitis	Africa, South America	Aerosol, rodent urine	Serology	Supportive care, ribavirin
Hepatitis A				
Fever, jaundice, dark urine, anorexia	Worldwide	Fecal-oral	Serology	Supportive care
Hepatitis B				
Fever, jaundice, dark urine, anorexia, arthralgias	Worldwide	Venereal, blood	Serology	Supportive care
Measles				
Coryza, fever, cough, rash, conjunctivitis, diarrhea	Worldwide	Aerosol	Serology	Supportive care
Poliomyelitis				
Fever, headache, nausea, stiff neck, flaccid paralysis	Worldwide	Fecal-oral	CSF, serology	Supportive care

Viral diseases (continued)

Symptoms	Distribution	Transmission	Diagnosis	Treatment
Rabies				
Fever, headache, encephalitis	Worldwide	Animal bite	Corneal impression smear, skin biopsy	Supportive care
Rotavirus				
Vomiting, diarrhea, fever, respiratory symptoms	Worldwide	Fecal-oral	Fecal exam	Rehydration, supportive care
Trachoma				
Keratoconjunctivitis	Tropics and subtropics	Contact	Clinical	Tetracycline or erythromycin
Yellow fever				
Fever, headache, myalgia, jaundice, bleeding diathesis	Africa, Latin America	Mosquito bites	Serology	Supportive care

Helminthic diseases

Symptoms	Distribution	Transmission	Diagnosis	Treatment
Angiostrongyliasis				
Headache, nausea, vomiting, stiff neck	Asia, Pacific islands	Ingestion of slugs, land snails	CSF	Symptomatic
Ascariasis				
Passage of worm, abdominal pain	Tropics	Food	Fecal smear	Mebendazole
Dracunculiasis				
Worm blister on leg	India, S.W. Asia; west and central Africa	Water	Leg examination	Niridazole
Echinococcosis				
Liver enlargement, or hemoptysis, or fracture	Rural livestock areas worldwide	Dog feces	X-ray, serology	Albendazole
Enterobiasis				
Perianal pruritus	Worldwide	Fecal-oral	Anal swabs	Mebendazole
Fasciolopsiasis				
Abdominal pain, diarrhea, facial edema	Far East, S.E. Asia	Water chestnuts	Fecal smear	Praziquantel
Filariasis				
Lymphangitis, lymphadenopathy, epididymitis, hydrocoele, chyluria, elephantiasis	Tropics	Mosquito bites	Blood smears	Diethylcarbamazine
Hookworm infection				
Fatigue, pallor, shortness of breath, anemia	Tropics	Skin contact with soil	Fecal smear	Albendazole
Liver fluke infection (Clonorchis, Opisthorchis)				
Fever, abdominal pain, jaundice	USSR, Far East, S.E. Asia	Raw fish	Fecal smear	Praziquantel

Helminthic diseases (continued)

Symptoms	Distribution	Transmission	Diagnosis	Treatment
Liver fluke infection (Fasciola)				
Fever, abdominal pain, hepatomegaly eosinophilia	Worldwide	Watercress	Fecal smear	Praziquantel
Onchocerciasis				
Pruritus, subcutaneous nodules, keratitis, eosinophilia	East, west Africa	Blackfly bites	Skin snips	Ivermectin
Paragonimiasis				
Cough, chest pain, hemoptysis, epilepsy	China, Korea, Africa, Latin America	Raw crabs, crayfish	Sputum, fecal smear	Praziquantel
Schistosomiasis				
Eosinophilia, hepatomegaly, splenomegaly, hematemesis, hematuria	Asia, Africa, Caribbean, S. America	Fresh water contact	Fecal, urine exam	Praziquantel
Strongyloidiasis				
Urticaria, abdominal pain, diarrhea, eosinophilia	Worldwide	Skin contact	Fecal smear	Thiabendazole
Tapeworm infection				
Taeniasis				
Passage of segments	Worldwide	Raw pork, beef	Fecal exam	Praziquantel
Diphyllobothriasis				
Eggs, passage of segments, pernicious anemia	Worldwide	Raw freshwater fish	Fecal smear	Praziquantel
Cysticercosis				
Epilepsy	Worldwide	Raw pork	Fecal smear, x-ray, serology	Praziquantel, glucocorticoids
Toxocariasis				
Eosinophilia, fever, hepatomegaly, pneumonitis	Worldwide	Exposure to dog, cat feces	Serology, liver biopsy	Thiabendazole
Trichinosis				
Periorbital edema, myalgia, fever, diarrhea, eosinophilia	Worldwide	Undercooked pork	Serology	Thiabendazole
Trichuriasis				
Rectal prolapse	Tropics	Fecal-oral	Fecal smear	Mebendazole

Fungal diseases

Symptoms	Distribution	Transmission	Diagnosis	Treatment
Pulmonary coccidioidomycosis Fever, night sweats, cough, chest pains, fatigue	Western hemisphere	Respiratory route	Sputum, serology	Amphotericin B
Histoplasmosis Fever, headache, cough, myalgia	Worldwide	Respiratory route	Serology	Amphotericin B
Cryptococcal meningitis Headache, personality changes, cranial nerve involvement	Worldwide	Respiratory route	CSF	Amphotericin B, Flucytosine
Pneumocystosis Dyspnea, fever, cough	Worldwide	?	Pulmonary aspirates	Trimethoprim-sulfa-methoxazole
Rhinosporidiosis Intranasal growth, conjunctivitis	Worldwide	Contact	Biopsy	Surgery

Nutritional diseases

Symptoms	Distribution	Transmission	Diagnosis	Treatment
Beriberi Neurological deficiency or cardiomyopathy	Worldwide	Thiamine deficiency	Blood chemistry	Thiamine
Folate/B_{12} Numbness, tingling, ataxia, megaloblastic anemia	Worldwide	Folate/cobalamin deficiency	Blood chemistry	Folic acid, cyanocobalamin
Iodine Goiter, cretinism	Worldwide	Iodine deficiency	Clinical status	Iodine
Iron Anemia	Worldwide	Iron deficiency	Blood	Iron
Protein-energy malnutrition Growth retardation	Worldwide	Protein/calorie deficiency	Anthropometric measurements	Adequate dietary regimen
Pellagra Dermatitis, stomatitis, glossitis, diarrhea, dementia	Worldwide	Nicotinic acid deficiency	Test of cure	Nicotinamide
Scurvy Petechiae, ecchymoses, gingival hemorrhage, anemia	Worldwide	Ascorbic acid deficiency	Blood chemistry	Ascorbate
Vitamin A Xerophthalmia	Worldwide	Vitamin A deficiency	Blood chemistry	Retinyl palmitate
Vitamin D Rickets, osteomalacia	Worldwide	Vitamin D deficiency	Blood chemistry	Vitamin D

Signs and Symptoms with Possible Causes

Systemic signs and symptoms

Signs/symptoms	Possible causes
Acute fever	Dengue
	Ebola-Marburg hemorrhagic fever
	Malaria
	Plague
	Shigellosis
	Toxoplasmosis
	Trichinosis
	Trypanosomiasis, American
	Yellow fever
Chronic fever	Actinomycosis
	AIDS
	Brucellosis
	Fascioliasis
	Histoplasmosis
	Leishmaniasis (visceral)
	Relapsing fever
	Toxocariasis
	Trypanosomiasis, African
	Tuberculosis
	Typhoid fever
Recurring fever	Malaria
Exanthem with fever	Chikungunya
	Childhood exanthem
	Dengue
	Enterovirus exanthems
	Rickettsioses
Fever accompanying hemorrhage or shock	Congo-Crimean hemorrhagic fever
	Dengue hemorrhagic fever
	Dengue shock syndrome
	Ebola-Marburg hemorrhagic fever
	Hemorrhagic fever with renal syndrome
	Lassa fever
	Leptospirosis
	Plague
	Toxoplasmosis
	Trypanosomiasis, African
	Trypanosomiasis, American

Systemic signs and symptoms (continued)

Signs/symptoms	Possible causes
Life-threatening signs (eg: coma, septicemia)	Anthrax
	Congo-Crimean hemorrhagic fever
	Dengue hemorrhagic fever
	Dengue shock syndrome
	Ebola-Marburg hemorrhagic fever
	Hemorrhagic fever with renal syndrome
	Impending sudden unexplained death of adults
	Malaria
Anemia	Diphyllobothriasis
	Histoplasmosis
	Hookworm infection
	Iron deficiency
	Malaria
	Tropical sprue
	Visceral leishmaniasis
	Vitamin B_{12} deficiency
Eosinophilia	Filariasis
	Fascioliasis
	Schistosomiasis
	Strongyloidiasis
	Toxocariasis
	Trichinosis
Lymphadenopathy	Dengue
	Filariasis
	HIV infection
	Plague
	Syphilis
	Toxoplasmosis
	Trypanosomiasis, African
	Trypanosomiasis, American

Cardiovascular signs and symptoms

Heart murmur	Chagas' disease
	Enteroviral carditis
	Rheumatic heart disease
Myocarditis	Chagas' disease
	Rheumatic heart disease
	Trichinosis
	Trypanosomiasis, Rhodesian

Central nervous system signs and symptoms

Signs/symptoms	Possible causes
Altered mentation	Acute psychosis
	Trypanosomiasis, African
Coma	Cerebral malaria
	Impending sudden unexplained death of adults
	Japanese encephalitis
	Meningococcal meningitis
	Rabies
	Tick-borne encephalitis
	Trypanosomiasis, African
Localizing signs of a neurologic lesion	Angiostrongyliasis
	Botulism
	Cryptococcosis
	Cysticercosis
	Diphtheria
	Echinococcosis
	Gnathostomiasis
	Lyme disease
	Meningococcal meningitis
	Naegleria infection
	Poliomyelitis
	Schistosomiasis
	Tetanus

Dermatologic signs and symptoms

Signs/symptoms	Possible causes
Analgesia	Leprosy
Anal pruritus	Enterobiasis
Pruritus	Onchocerciasis
	Toxocariasis
Rash	Chikungunya fever
	Childhood exanthems
	Dengue
	Enteroviral exanthems
	Rickettsial diseases
Swelling or erythematous lesions	Gnathostomiasis
	Loiasis
	Lyme disease
	Pinta
Ulcer, eschar, or abscess	Anthrax
	Buruli ulcer
	Chagas' disease

Dermatologic signs and symptoms (continued)

Signs/symptoms	Possible causes
Ulcer, eschar, or abscess	Coccidioidomycosis
	Cutaneous leishmaniasis
	Lymphogranuloma venereum
	Syphilis
	Scrub typhus
	Trypanosomiasis, African
	Yaws

Gastrointestinal signs and symptoms

Signs/symptoms	Possible causes
Abdominal pain	Amebiasis
	Anisakiasis
	Fascioliasis
	Giardiasis
	Hymenolepiasis
	Salmonellosis
	Shigellosis
	Strongyloidiasis
	Taeniasis
	Typhoid fever
Diarrhea, acute	*Bacillus cereus*
	Campylobacter
	Cholera
	Clostridium perfringens
	Escherichia coli
	Rotavirus
	Salmonellosis
	Trichinosis
	Vibrio parahaemolyticus
Diarrhea, bloody	Amebic dysentery
	Balantidium coli
	Campylobacter
	Enteroinvasive *E. coli*
	Shigellosis
Diarrhea, chronic	AIDS
	Clonorchiasis
	Cryptosporidiosis
	Giardiasis
	Strongyloidiasis

Gastrointestinal signs and symptoms (continued)

Signs/symptoms	Possible causes
Hepatomegaly	Amebic liver abscess
	Chagas' disease
	Clonorchiasis
	Echinococcosis
	Fascioliasis
	Histoplasmosis
	Malaria
	Opisthorchiasis
	Schistosomiasis
	Toxocariasis
	Typhoid fever
	Visceral leishmaniasis
Jaundice	Hepatitis A, B, delta, non-A non-B (epidemic and transfusion-related)
	Leptospirosis
	Malaria (*P. falciparum*)
Splenomegaly	Chagas' disease
	Malaria
	Schistosomiasis
	Typhoid fever
	Visceral leishmaniasis
Worms	Ascariasis
	Enterobiasis
	Taeniasis

Genitourinary signs and symptoms

Signs/symptoms	Possible causes
Cervicitis	Chlamydial infection
	Moniliasis
	Trichomoniasis
Genital lesions	Chancroid
	Granuloma inguinale
	Herpes
	Lymphogranuloma venereum
	Syphilis
Hematuria	Schistosomiasis (*S. haematobium*)
Urethritis	Chlamydial and gonococcal infections

Ophthalmologic signs and symptoms

Signs/symptoms	Possible causes
Eye pain, swelling, or reddening	Chagas' disease (Romaña's sign)
	Hemorrhagic conjunctivitis
	Loiasis
	Onchocerciasis
	Trachoma
	Trichinosis

Respiratory signs and symptoms

Signs/symptoms	Possible causes
Cough	Ascariasis
	Bacterial and chlamydial respiratory infections
	Lassa fever
	Paragonimiasis
	Pertussis
	Plague
	Psittacosis
	Tuberculosis
	Upper respiratory infections
Lesions visible on chest x-ray	Blastomycosis
	Coccidioidomycosis
	Echinococcosis
	Histoplasmosis
	Melioidosis
	Pneumocystosis
	Psittacosis
	Tuberculosis
Pharyngitis	Diphtheria
	Streptococcal infections
	Viral infections
Pneumonia	AIDS
	Anthrax
	Ascariasis
	Blastomycosis
	Coccidioidomycosis
	Histoplasmosis
	Legionellosis
	Paragonimiasis
	Plague
	Pneumococcosis
	Pneumocystosis
	Psittacosis
	Q fever
	Scrub typhus
	Strongyloidiasis
	Tuberculosis

Considerations for Travelers and Immigrants: Relative Risk and Incubation Periods

Travelers relative risk in developing countries

High: More than one case in ten travelers	**Moderate:** More than one case in 200 travelers but less than one case in ten travelers	**Low:** More than one case in 1,000 travelers but less than one case in 200 travelers	**Very low:** Less than one case in 1,000 travelers
Diarrhea	Dengue	Acute hemorrhagic	Actinomycosis
Upper respiratory infection	Enteroviral infection	conjunctivitis	AIDS
	Food poisoning	Amebiasis	Angiostrongyliasis
	Gastroenteritis	Ascariasis	Anisakiasis
	Giardiasis	Childhood viral infections	Anthrax
	Hepatitis A	Chickenpox	Blastomycosis
	Malaria without prophylaxis	Measles	Boutonneuse fever
	Salmonellosis	Mumps	Chagas' disease
	Sexually transmitted diseases	Poliomyelitis	Chikungunya
	Chlamydial infection	Enterobiasis	Clonorchiasis
	Gonorrhea	Hepatitis B	Coccidioidomycosis
	Herpes simplex	Hepatitis, non-A non-B	Congo-Crimean hem. fever
	Nonspecific urethritis	(epidemic)	Cryptosporidiosis
	Shigellosis	Leptospirosis	Diphtheria
		Scabies	Ebola-Marburg hem. fever
		Sexually transmitted diseases	Echinococcosis
		Chancroid	Filariasis
		Syphilis	Gnathostomiasis
		Strongyloidiasis	Histoplasmosis
		Trichuriasis	Hookworm
		Tropical sprue	Legionellosis
		Tuberculosis	Lymphogranuloma venereum
		Typhoid fever	Malaria with prophylaxis
			Melioidosis
			Paragonimiasis
			Pertussis
			Pinta
			Plague
			Psittacosis
			Q fever
			Rabies
			Relapsing fever
			Schistosomiasis
			Toxocariasis
			Trachoma
			Trichinosis
			Trypanosomiasis
			Typhus
			Yaws
			Yellow fever

Usual incubation periods

Short (about 1 week or less)	Intermediate (1 to 4 weeks)	Long (1 to 6 months)	Very long (2 months to years)
Anthrax	Amebiasis	Ascariasis	AIDS
Boutonneuse fever	Brucellosis	Blastomycosis	Cysticercosis
Chancroid	Chagas' disease	Hepatitis B	Echinococcosis
Chikungunya	Giardiasis	Hepatitis delta	Filariasis
Chlamydial infections	Hemorrhagic fever with	Hepatitis, non-A non-B	Fluke infections
Congo-Crimean hemorrhagic	renal syndrome	(posttransfusion)	Leishmaniasis, visceral
fever	Hepatitis A	Leishmaniasis, cutaneous	Leprosy
Dengue	Hepatitis, non-A non-B	Loiasis	Schistosomiasis
Diarrhea, acute	(epidemic)	Malaria	Trypanosomiasis, African
Ebola-Marburg hemorrhagic	Katayama fever	Melioidosis	(Gambian)
fever	Lassa fever	Pinta	
Food poisoning	Leptospirosis	Rabies	
Gonorrhea	Lyme disease	Taeniasis	
Herpes genitalis	Lymphogranuloma venereum	Trachoma (scarring)	
Histoplasmosis	Malaria	Trichuriasis	
Legionellosis	Pertussis	Tropical sprue	
Plague	Q fever	Yaws	
Psittacosis	Strongyloidiasis		
Relapsing fever	Syphilis		
Salmonellosis	Trypanosomiasis African		
Tetanus	(Rhodesian)		
Trypanosomal chancre	Typhoid fever		
Viral gastroenteritis	Typhus, louse-borne		
Yellow fever	Typhus, murine		
	Typhus, scrub		

APPENDIX 4 / *Exotic Communicable Diseases: A Review by Region*

Caribbean, Mexico, Central and Tropical South America, Temperate South America, Andes Mountains

Caribbean Islands	Mexico	Central America and Tropical South America	Temperate South America	Andes Mountains
Ascariasis	Amebiasis	Amebiasis	Arenavirus infection:	Bartonellosis
Dengue	Anisakiasis	Anisakiasis	Argentine hemorrhagic	Brucellosis
Hookworm	Ascariasis	Ascariasis	fever, Bolivian	Plague
Schistosomiasis	Chagas' disease	Chagas' disease	hemorrhagic fever	Rabies
Sprue	Campylobacter	Campylobacter	Chagas' disease	Tapeworm
Trichuriasis	infection	infection	Echinococcosis	Tuberculosis
Yaws	Cysticercosis	Cysticercosis	Hepatitis	Typhus
	Dengue	Dengue	Rabies	
	E. coli enteritis	*E. coli* enteritis	Typhus	
	Echinococcosis	Filariasis		
	Hepatitis	Hepatitis		
	Hookworm infection	Hymenolepiasis		
	Leishmaniasis, cutaneous	Onchocerciasis		
	Leishmaniasis, visceral	Paracoccidioidomycosis		
	Leprosy	Paragonimiasis		
	Malaria	Pinta		
	Pinta	Rabies		
	Rabies	Relapsing fever		
	Relapsing fever	Sand fly fever		
	Trichuriasis	Schistosomiasis		
	Tuberculosis	Taeniasis		
	Typhus	Trachoma		
		Trichuriasis	Yaws	
		Tuberculosis	Yellow fever	

Africa and the Middle East

Middle East	North Africa	East, West and Central Africa	South Africa
Anthrax	Anthrax	AIDS	Amebiasis
Ascariasis	Ascariasis	Anthrax	Anthrax
Boutonneuse fever	Boutonneuse fever	Ascariasis	Ascariasis
Brucellosis	Brucellosis	Boutonneuse fever	Hepatitis
Congo-Crimean hemorrhagic fever	Congo-Crimean hemorrhagic fever	Cholera	Ebola-Marburg hem. fever
Dracunculiasis	Dracunculiasis	Congo-Crimean hemorrhagic fever	Hookworm infection
E. coli enteritis	*E. coli* enteritis	Dracunculiasis	Rift Valley fever
Giardiasis	Hepatitis	*E. coli* enteritis	Schistosomiasis
Hepatitis	Hookworm	Hepatitis	Trichuriasis
Hookworm infection	Hydatid disease	Hookworm infection	Tuberculosis
Hydatid disease	Hymenolepiasis	Lassa fever	
Hymenolepiasis	Leishmaniasis	Leishmaniasis	

Africa and the Middle East (continued)

Middle East	North Africa	East, West and Central Africa	South Africa
Leishmaniasis	Malaria	Leprosy	
Malaria	Plague	Loiasis	
Plague	Relapsing fever	Malaria	
Relapsing fever	Schistosomiasis	Onchocerciasis	
Schistosomiasis	Taeniasis	Paragonimiasis	
Taeniasis	Trachoma	Plague	
Trachoma	Tuberculosis	Rabies	
Tuberculosis		Relapsing fever	
		Rift Valley fever	
		Schistosomiasis	
		Strongyloidiasis	
		Taeniasis	
		Trachoma	
		Trichinosis	
		Trichuriasis	
		Trypanosomiasis	
		Tuberculosis	
		Typhus	
		Yaws	

Indian subcontinent and Sri Lanka; Southeast Asia; China and Korea; and the Pacific Islands

Indian Subcontinent Sri Lanka	Southeast Asia	China and Korea	Pacific Islands
Amebiasis	Angiostrongyliasis	Ascariasis	Angiostrongyliasis
Ascariasis	Anthrax	Clonorchiasis	Ascariasis
Boutonneuse Fever	Ascariasis	Dengue	Ciguatera poisoning
Cholera	Capillariasis	E. coli enteritis	Dengue
Dengue	Cholera	Fasciolopsiasis	Filariasis
E. coli	Clonorchiasis	Filariasis	Hookworm infection
Filariasis	Dengue	Hemorrhagic fever with	Leprosy
Giardiasis	E. coli enteritis	renal failure	Ross River Fever
Hepatitis	Fasciolopsiasis	Hepatitis	Scombroid poisoning
Hookworm infection	Giardiasis	Hookworm infection	Strongyloidiasis
Hymenolepiasis	Gnathostomiasis	Japanese encephalitis	Trichinosis
Japanese encephalitis	Hookworm infection	Leishmaniasis, visceral	Trichuriasis
Leishmaniasis, cutaneous	Japanese encephalitis	Leprosy	Tuberculosis
Leishmaniasis, visceral	Leprosy	Malaria	Yaws
Leprosy	Malaria	Paragonimiasis	
Malaria	Melioidosis	Rabies	
Rabies	Opisthorchiasis	Schistosomiasis	
Scrub typhus	Paragonimiasis	Shigellosis	
Shigellosis	Rabies	Strongyloidiasis	
Strongyloidiasis	Schistosomiasis	Trachoma	
Trachoma	Scrub typhus	Trichinosis	
Trichinosis	Shigellosis	Trichuriasis	
Trichuriasis	Strongyloidiasis	Tuberculosis	
Tuberculosis	Taeniasis		
	Trichinosis		
	Trichuriasis		
	Tuberculosis		

Index

Index